Brief Contents

Learn to

THINK LIKE A NURSE
FROM THE VERY FIRST DAY.

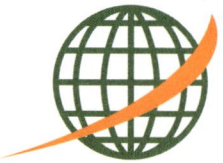

Your nursing education goes well beyond the textbook.

Davis*Plus*.com is your online home for a wealth of learning activities, study tools, and resources that make learning easier. Build your confidence as you prepare for class and clinical.

Your Davis*Plus* Resources are waiting for you.

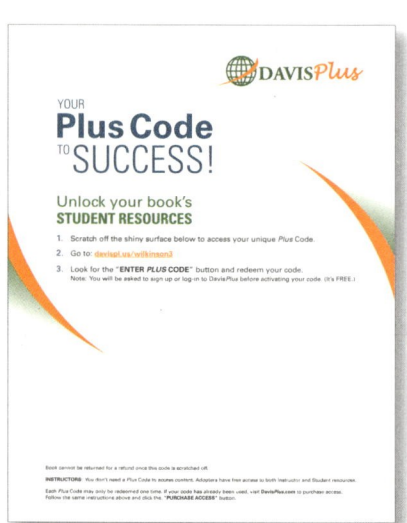

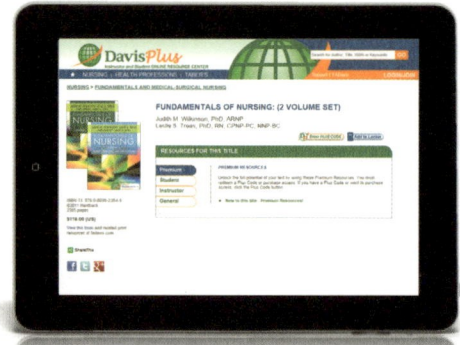

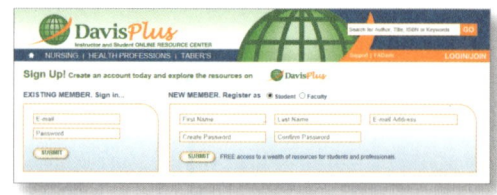

1

Scratch off the shiny surface to reveal your *Plus* Code.*

2

Go to **davispl.us/wilkinson3.** Log in or create your Davis*Plus* account. It's easy and it's FREE.

3

Look for the "Enter *Plus* Code" button to redeem your code and access your resources.

The next time you visit, look for the locker icon. You'll find all of your resources in your locker, making it easy to access the materials you need to study for class, lab, and clinical.

*Each *Plus* Code may only be redeemed one time. If your code has already been used, visit Davis*Plus*.com to purchase access.
Follow the same instructions above and click the, "Purchase Access" button.

Everything you need to prepare for class, lab, and clinical.

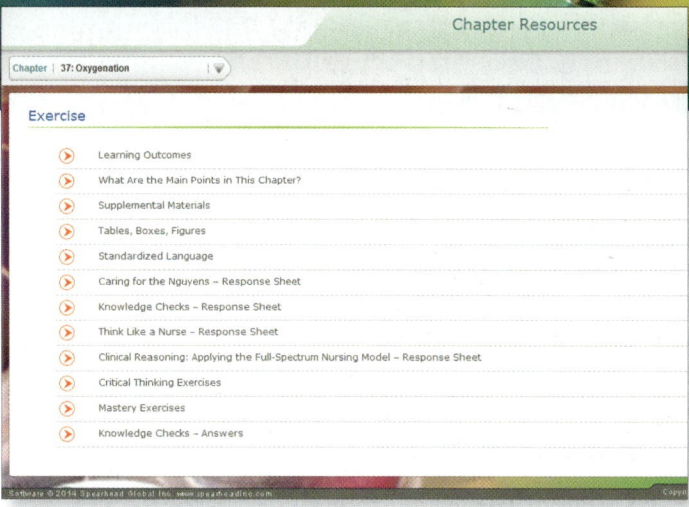

The Electronic Study Guide Chapter Resources help you master the textbook material chapter by chapter. For each chapter in the book you'll find…

- NCLEX-Style Chapter Review Questions
- Learning Outcomes
- Responses to all Critical-Thinking Questions and Exercises in the text
- Care Plans
- Care Maps
- Knowledge Maps
- Documentation Exercises
- Supplemental Materials such as tables, boxes, figures
- Resources for Caregivers & Health Professionals

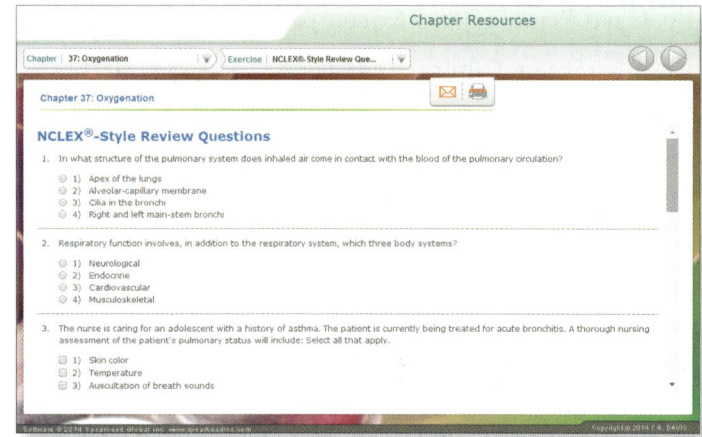

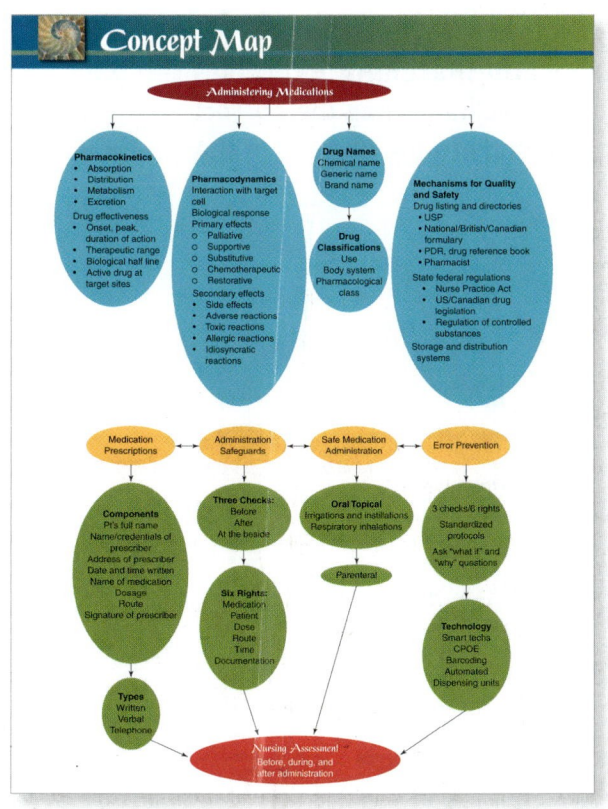

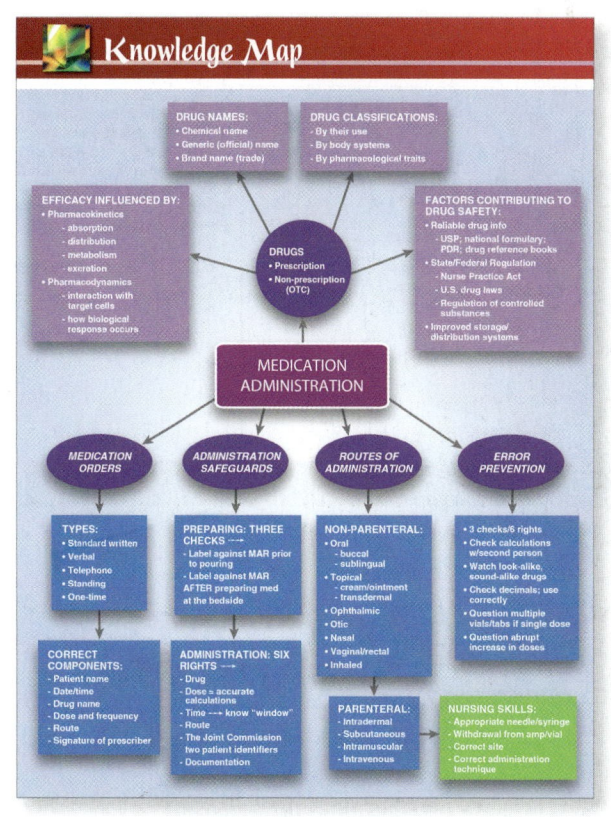

Learning Activities, Clinical Resources, and NCLEX-style quizzes prepare you for class and clinical.

- Davis Digital Version
- Student Question Bank
- Animations
- Concept Care Map Generator
- Care Planning and Care Mapping Exercises
- Interactive Clinical Scenarios
- Paragraph Matching Exercises
- Bonus Microbiology Chapter: *The Human Biome*
- Alphabetical List of NANDA Diagnoses
- Procedure Checklists
- Dosage Calculator
- Expanded Bibliography

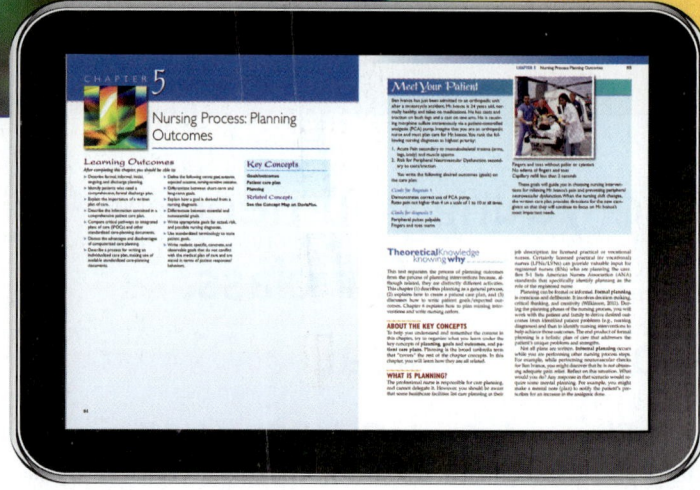

Davis Digital Version is your complete text online. Quickly search for the content you need. Add notes, highlights, and bookmarks.

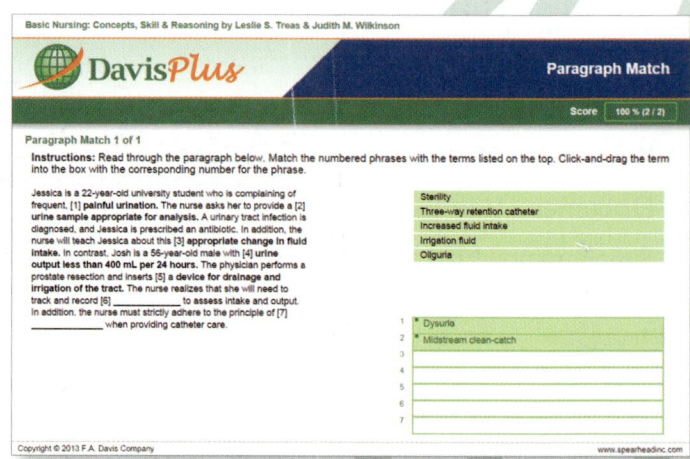

Paragraph Matching Exercises test your recall of facts. Click and drag the correct terms from the list to complete the phrases in the paragraph.

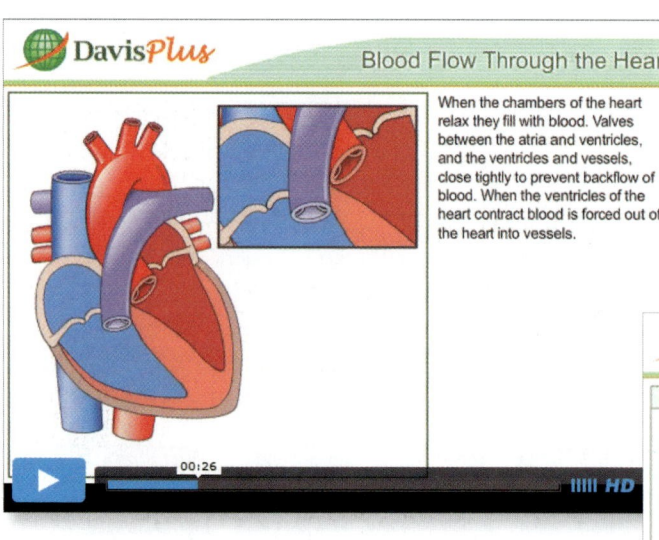

Full-Color Animations make often complex physiological processes easy to understand.

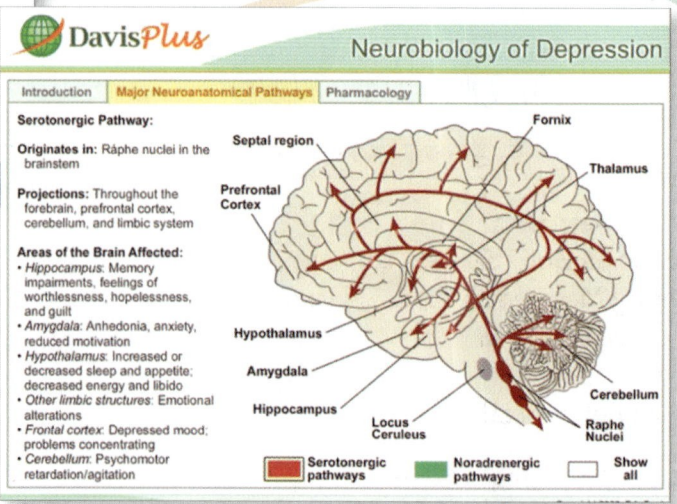

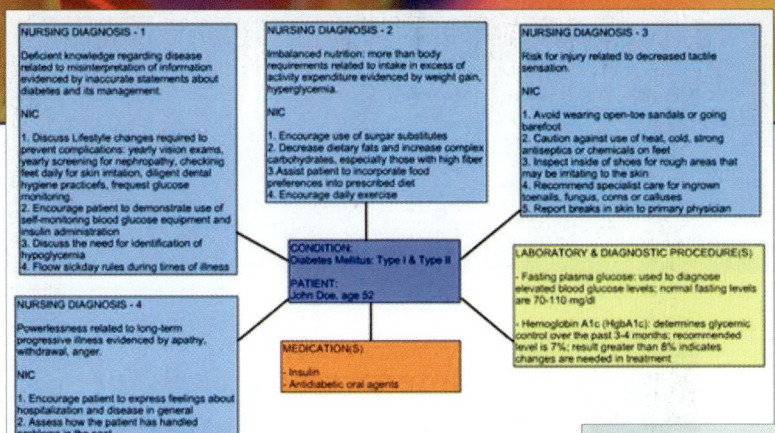

Concept Care Map Generator makes care planning easier. Use it to organize your assessment data, identify patient problems, determine the appropriate nursing diagnoses and interventions, and assess outcomes.

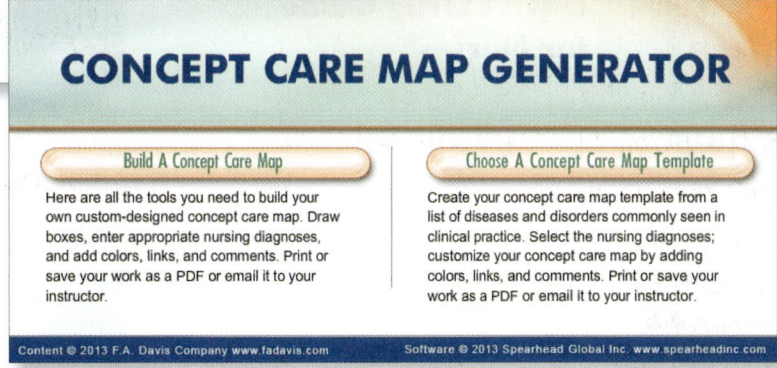

Interactive Clinical Scenarios let you apply your knowledge to virtual patient scenarios to help develop your critical-thinking skills and prepare for common clinical challenges.

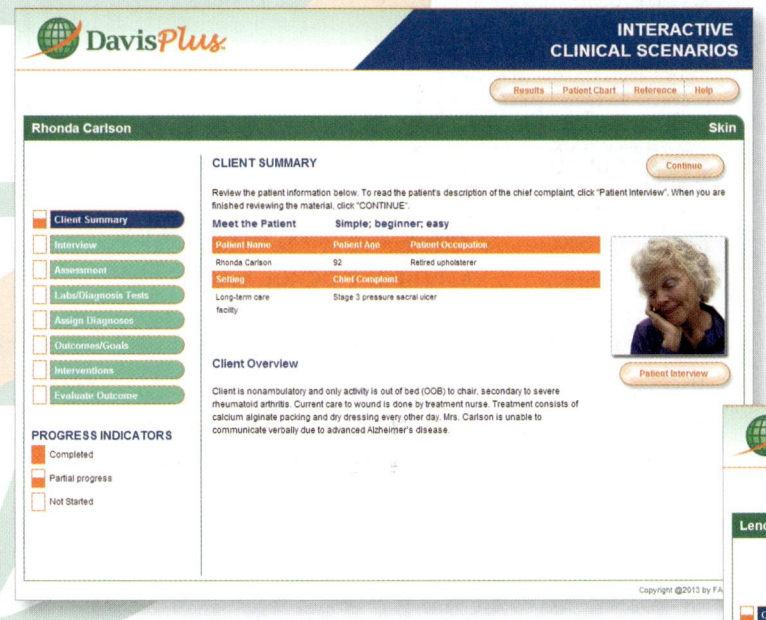

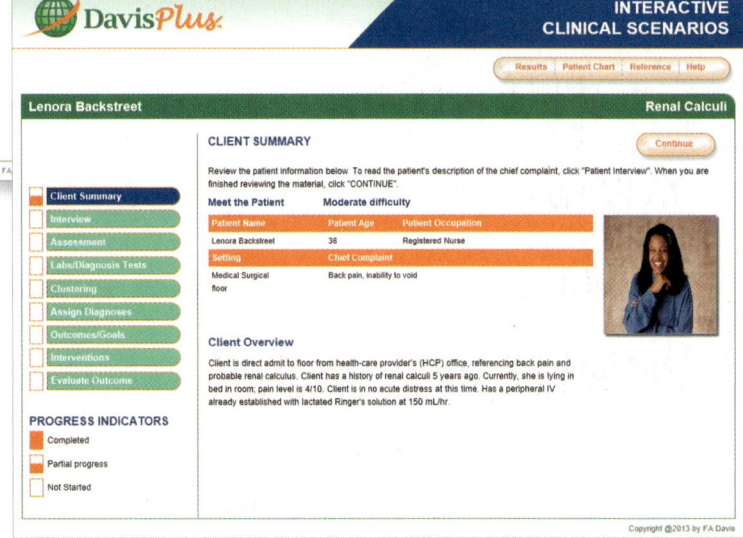

Don't miss these DavisPlus Resources

- Chapter Overviews
- Podcasts and Body Sounds Library
- Preventing Medication Errors Tutorial
- Wound Care Tutorial
- Audio Glossary
- And so much more!

Visit **www.DavisPlus.com** today!

ESSENTIAL NURSING REFERENCES

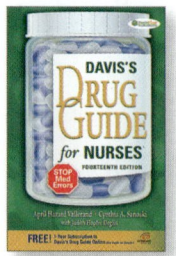

Davis's Drug Guide for Nurses®

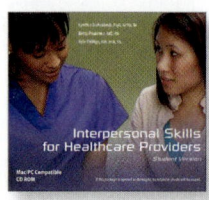

Interpersonal Skills for Healthcare Providers
Student Version

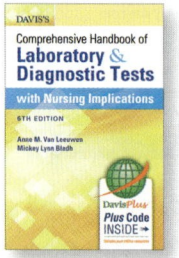

Davis's Comprehensive Handbook of Laboratory and Diagnostic Tests With Nursing Implications

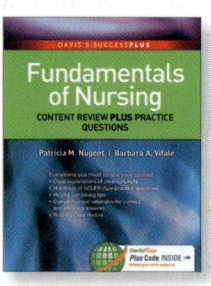

Fundamentals of Nursing
Content Review *Plus* Practice Questions

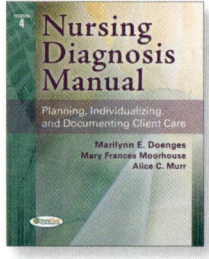

Nursing Diagnosis Manual
Planning, Individualizing, and Documenting Client Care

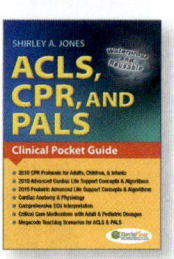

ACLS, CPR, and PALS
Clinical Pocket Guide

The road to nursing school success begins with
DAVIS'S SUCCESS SERIES

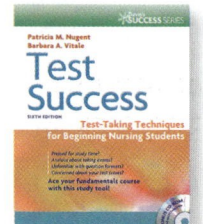
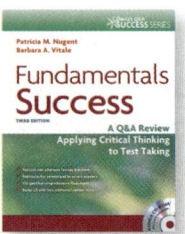
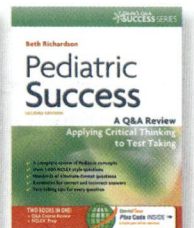
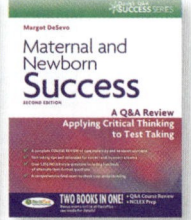
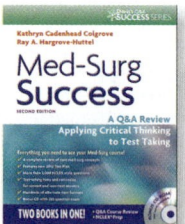
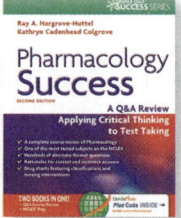
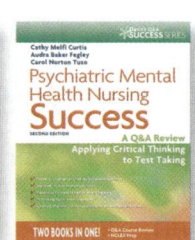

Buy today!

www.FADavis.com

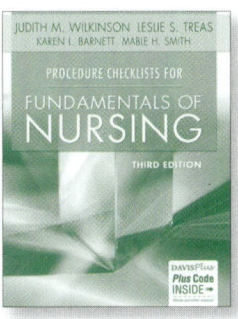
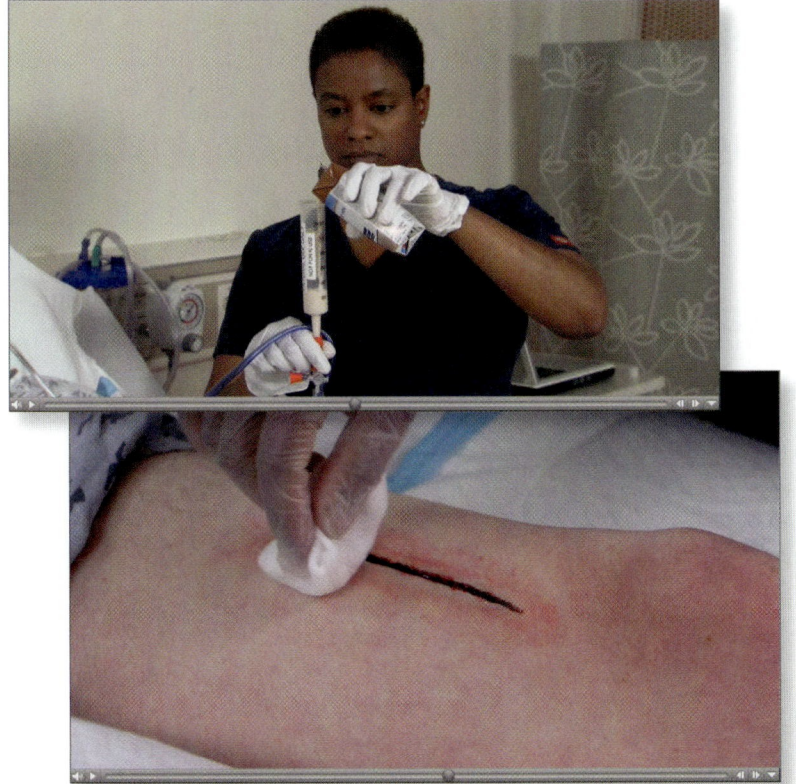
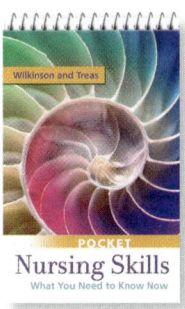

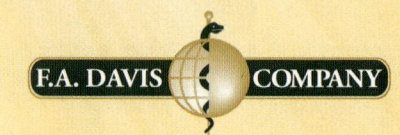

THIRD EDITION

FUNDAMENTALS OF NURSING

VOLUME 1

THEORY, CONCEPTS, AND APPLICATIONS

Judith M. Wilkinson, PhD, CNS, APRN

Leslie S. Treas, PhD, RN, CPNP-PC, NNP-BC

Karen L. Barnett, DNP, RN

Mable H. Smith, BSN, MN, JD, PhD

F.A. Davis Company • Philadelphia

F. A. Davis Company
1915 Arch Street
Philadelphia, PA 19103
www.fadavis.com

Copyright © 2016 by F. A. Davis Company

Printed in the United States of America

Last digit indicates print number: 10 9 8 7 6 5 4 3 2 1

Publisher, Nursing: Lisa B. Houck
Director of Content Development: Darlene D. Pedersen
Senior Content Project Manager: Adrienne D. Simon
Content Project Manager: Christina L. Snyder
Special Projects Editor: Shirley A. Kuhn
Electronic Project Manager: Katherine E. Crowley
Design and Illustrations Manager: Carolyn O'Brien

As new scientific information becomes available through basic and clinical research, recommended treatments and drug therapies undergo changes. The author(s) and publisher have done everything possible to make this book accurate, up to date, and in accord with accepted standards at the time of publication. The author(s), editors, and publisher are not responsible for errors or omissions or for consequences from application of the book, and make no warranty, expressed or implied, in regard to the contents of the book. Any practice described in this book should be applied by the reader in accordance with professional standards of care used in regard to the unique circumstances that may apply in each situation. The reader is advised always to check product information (package inserts) for changes and new information regarding dose and contraindications before administering any drug. Caution is especially urged when using new or infrequently ordered drugs.

Library of Congress Cataloging-in-Publication Data

Wilkinson, Judith M., 1946- , author.
  Fundamentals of nursing / Judith M. Wilkinson, Leslie S. Treas, Karen L. Barnett, Mable H. Smith.
  — Third edition.
    p. ; cm.
Includes bibliographical references and index.
ISBN 978-0-8036-4075-7 — ISBN 0-8036-4075-7
I. Treas, Leslie S., author. II. Barnett, Karen L., author. III. Smith, Mable H., author. IV. Title.
[DNLM: 1. Nursing Process. 2. Nursing Care. 3. Nursing Theory. WY 100]

RT41
610.73—dc23

                    2014025775

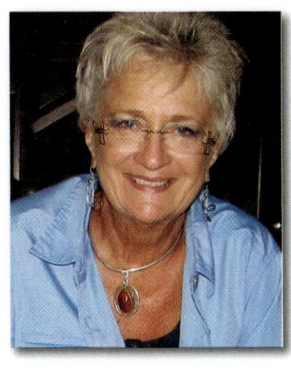

Judith M. Wilkinson, PhD, CNS, APRN, Author

Judith Wilkinson taught fundamentals of nursing for 22 years, and more recently, has taught graduate-level courses in theory, research, and health policy. She also developed, and taught for many years, an LPN-to-RN transition course. She has given numerous presentations and provided consultation and faculty development workshops for nursing and other schools—primarily in the areas of critical thinking and nursing ethics, but also in standardized nursing languages, teaching strategies, testing, evaluation, and curriculum.

She obtained her PhD in Nursing from the University of Kansas School of Nursing, and master's degrees in Nursing and Education from the University of Missouri–Kansas City. Her basic nursing degree was an ADN from Johnson County Community College, followed by a BSN from Graceland College. She was granted a National Endowment for the Humanities fellowship to study nursing ethics, and a Nurses' Educational Fund (Isabel Hampton Robb) scholarship for her nursing doctoral study. Her master's thesis was a seminal work in moral distress; her doctoral dissertation also studied nursing ethics.

Dr. Wilkinson's clinical background is broad, and includes emergency, critical care, med-surg (float), and obstetric nursing. While engaged in full-time teaching, she maintained certification in inpatient obstetric nursing; her advanced practice license is in nursing care of women.

She is co-author of another fundamentals textbook, Treas and Wilkinson, *Basic Nursing: Concepts, Skills, and Reasoning.* Her other publications include a nursing process text, a nursing diagnosis handbook (each going into multiple editions and international publication), a maternal-newborn care planning book (as a co-author), and journal articles on the topics of curriculum, critical thinking, and nursing ethics. Over the years, she has contributed chapters to several textbooks and authored many ancillary materials, including test banks, learning modules, and review modules.

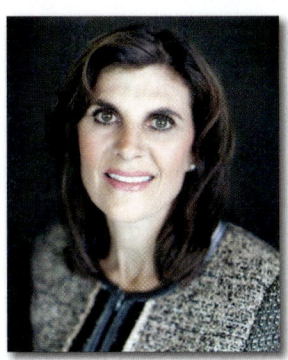

Leslie S. Treas, PhD, RN, CPNP-PC, NNP-BC, Author

Dr. Leslie Treas, one of the founders and former vice-president, Research and Development of *Assessment Technologies Institute™, LLC* (ATI) demonstrated leadership and expertise forecasting and directing the design and development of ATI product testing and educational product line since the formation of the company. In this role, Dr. Treas planned and implemented norming, test validation, and standard-setting studies to support data-driven product development, constructing tests with sound psychometric properties. Under her management, she produced a series of NCLEX-review books and nursing skills DVD set. She has conducted clinical and educational research, publishing in peer-reviewed journals of health and education.

Dr. Treas was involved in the start-up of a continuing education company for nurses, physicians, and allied health professionals, serving as Director of Education and Accreditation, *AcaMedic Institute™, LLC.*

Dr. Treas earned a BSN from Pennsylvania State University and an MSN degree with emphasis in maternal-child health at the University of Kansas. She obtained a PhD from the University of Kansas in the Educational Psychology and Research Department with dual areas of study of testing and measurement and nursing education. Her primary area of clinical expertise is the care of sick newborns in the NICU and labor and delivery settings in the clinical role of a neonatal nurse practitioner for 13 years. Dr. Treas obtained dual pediatric and neonatal nurse practitioner certifications at the Cleveland Metropolitan General Hospital, affiliate of Case Western University.

Her journal and textbook publications have featured various clinical topics ranging from fundamentals of nursing to care of neonatal patients. Other publications are education-based areas related to nursing licensure preparation and prediction, critical thinking, and others. She has also written articles geared to new graduate readers, addressing contemporary issues involving role change, employment, and communication.

Dr. Treas has presented for annual conferences for Sigma Theta Tau, National Association of Associate Degree Nurses, National Association of Neonatal Nurses, American Association of Colleges of Nursing, National Conference on Professional Nursing Education and Development, Association for the Advancement of Educational Research, to name a few.

She has test-writing expertise as a former item writer for the National Certification Examination for Pediatric Nurse Practitioners and Nurses, and also the National Certification Corporation for Neonatal Nurse Practitioner Exam.

Karen L. Barnett, DNP, RN, Co-author

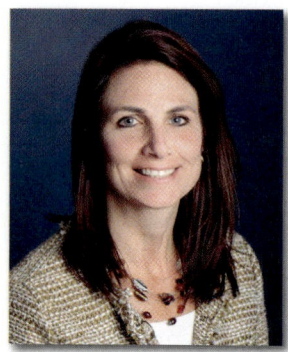

Karen Barnett has been a nurse for more than 25 years and has held various positions in nursing, including patient care, administration, and education. Most recently, Dr. Barnett serves as Dean of Nursing for St. Vincent's College in Bridgeport, Connecticut, where she oversees more than 800 pre-nursing and nursing students in AD and RN to BSN programs. Prior to that, she taught medical-surgical nursing, professional nursing theory, and clinical education to undergraduate students and has taught advanced pathophysiology to graduate nursing students. Dr. Barnett's clinical background includes critical care, medical-surgical, and cardiac-telemetry nursing. While engaged in full-time teaching, she continues to maintain clinical competence in her role as nursing supervisor at an acute care community hospital.

Dr. Barnett earned a BSN from Southern Connecticut State University and an MSN degree with a focus in nursing administration from Sacred Heart University. She earned a DNP from the Francis Payne Bolton School of Nursing at Case Western Reserve University in 2010 with a focus in nursing education. Dr. Barnett is a member of the American Nurses Association, Connecticut Nurse Association, the National League for Nursing, and Sigma Theta Tau International Nursing Honor Society. She was honored with a Nightingale Award for Excellence in Nursing in 2013. Research interests include student learning outcomes, simulation as a learning tool, and critical thinking/clinical judgment. Dr. Barnett has contributed to chapters in several textbooks and authored other ancillary material including test banks and concept maps.

Mable H. Smith, BSN, MN, JD, PhD, Co-author

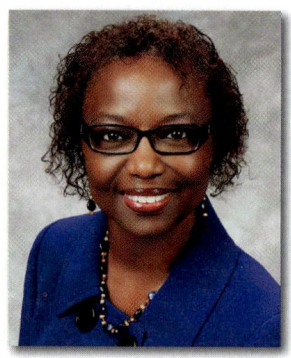

Dr. Mable Smith is the founding Dean of Nursing of the Colleges of Nursing at Roseman University of Health Sciences (formerly the University of Southern Nevada), Nevada and Utah. She has extensive experience in nursing education and has taught at all academic levels, including undergraduate courses in professional nursing, leadership and management, role transition, legal and ethical aspects of practice, and adult health nursing. Dr. Smith has published and presented in numerous arenas on legal and ethical issues in nursing education and in nursing/healthcare. Her publications have appeared in leading referred journals, and she authored the book *The Legal, Ethical and Professional Dimensions of Nursing Education,* currently in its second edition.

Dr. Smith earned a BSN from Florida State University (FSU) and an MN from Emory University, with an emphasis in education. She obtained a PhD in Higher Education Administration and JD from FSU. Dr. Smith has served on the faculties of Florida A&M

University, Old Dominion University, and the University of Southern Mississippi. Her primary area of clinical expertise is adult health nursing. Dr. Smith is a member of the American Nurses Association, Nevada Nurse Association, National League for Nursing, and the American Association of Nurse Attorneys. She was honored by the National Association of Women Business Owners as a *Woman of Distinction* for her contributions to the education field in southern Nevada and was named a Healthcare Headliner by *In Business Las Vegas*, one of southern Nevada's premier business publications. She is also a Robert Wood Johnson Executive Nurse Fellow alumna.

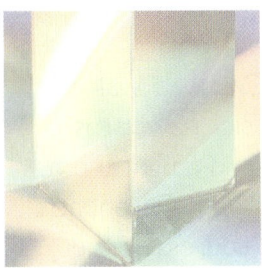

We dedicate this book to:

The people at F. A. Davis Company, who have supported us for many years and in many ways. To point out a few: the sales team, the marketing team, and especially the editorial team, with whom we have the closest relationships. They have allowed—even encouraged—us to think outside the box and to explore new paths without knowing for certain where they would lead.

My husband, Franklin Hiam, who relieves me of many (most) activities of daily living, and who I am sure expected me to have more free time during our "golden years."

My sons, Todd, Bryan, and Chris—for being kind, responsible men, who each in his own way makes the world a little better. They internalized my message that it's okay to march to the beat of a different drummer. They do that, and they accept people who step to a different beat from theirs.

My father, who when I was a small (literally) child, called me "Dynamite" when everyone else was calling me "JudyBug"; and said over and over, "You can do anything you think you're big enough to do." Almost, Daddy; almost.

—Judith M. Wilkinson

Judith Wilkinson

No work, however seemingly solitary, is ever produced in isolation. I'd like to heartily express my deep gratitude to the many people in my life who made it possible for me to pursue this textbook and arduously see it through to completion. Foremost to my loving husband, Randy, and our children, Megan, Bridget, and Jack, who have supported me with unwavering support in this journey from nurse practitioner to nurse entrepreneur to scholar and writer. Randy tirelessly carried the load and picked up the pieces all along the way. To my mother, who always urged me to tackle extraordinary tasks with persistence and diligence. She once said, "How do you eat an elephant? . . . One bite at a time." This book certainly was just that—one small bite after another, one step at a time, followed by a leap of faith that this important work could be, and would be done. My mother-in-law, Sandy Treas, has been an encourager and supporter, not only providing many meals for my family during these demanding times but her kindred spirit as a strong woman who has kept her eyes on the horizon, not succumbing to the challenges that pressed upon her.

To Diana Rieser, Nurse Manager of the NICU at Saint Luke's, Kansas City, who walked the walk of what it means to be a thinking, doing, and caring nurse to sick newborns and their families. She mentored "new nurses" with wisdom and care and taught them what it means to be the hands of compassion and competence. To Dr. John Callenbach, neonatologist, who was "all in" no matter what it took, day or night in addressing the needs of critically ill and convalescing infants; and who respected and relied on the nurses as the eyes and ears and the heart of quality care.

But mostly to my dear friend and respected colleague, Judith Wilkinson, who from the creation of this work has never once settled for good enough. Intent on perfection, committed to excellence, Judith's tenacity and wisdom raise the bar for teaching and learning. From the very design of this work, Judith passionately strives to draw students into the experience of learning throughout their journey from student to nurse. "Tell me and I forget, teach me and I may remember, involve me and I learn." — Benjamin Franklin

—Leslie S. Treas

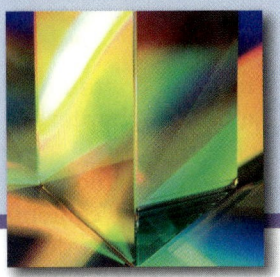

Preface

We chose our book title carefully. We have used the words *theory, concepts, application, thinking, doing,* and *caring* because we believe that excellent nursing requires an equal mix of knowledge, thought, action, and caring. It is knowledge and its application—not just the tasks nurses do—that delineate the various levels of nursing. Even so, skillful performance of tasks is essential to full attainment of the nursing role.

We chose the word *fundamentals* because this text, and its concomitant course, is truly that: the foundation for all that follows. This basic content teaches essential functions that nurses will use throughout their careers, and in that sense, we believe it is of central importance. It is—or should be—the most important course students take. We want them to say, "Everything I need to know, I learned in fundamentals—all I needed to know about how to think, what to do, and how to be" (at least at a basic level). You will see those themes integrated throughout each chapter.

The thoroughly revised and updated third edition, kept fresh by the acquisition of two new co-authors, preserves the same open, user-friendly, easy-to-read style that students have been telling us they love.

ORGANIZATION

We have organized the learning package into two volumes to make it easier for on-the-go students to have at hand the material they need in either the classroom or the clinical setting. The content of Volumes 1 and 2 is comprehensive. Our chapters are self-contained and rich in cross-references so that teachers and students can use them in any order that fits their needs. The cross-references assist them to see the relationships between Volumes 1 and 2 and among the chapters, as well as to navigate easily between the two volumes.

Content within each chapter is generally organized into two major sections: Theoretical Knowledge (Knowing Why) and Practical Knowledge (Knowing How). There is some overlap in these concepts because the two types of knowledge are interdependent. We have made this general distinction because many nursing programs begin with content learned in supporting prerequisite classes and then layer on additional Theoretical Knowledge to explain the rationale for nursing actions and activities (Practical Knowledge). The distinction also affords more flexibility in teaching fundamentals. For example, it is useful to teachers who believe students are more motivated when they present first the concrete (Practical Knowledge), and then the abstract (Theoretical Knowledge); it is equally useful for those who teach from the theoretical to the practical.

Enrichment (Supplemental Material)—We have tried to write a text that meets the needs of most students and instructors and that can be used as a reference throughout the student's career—one that is comprehensive but not overwhelming. To minimize weight and bulk, and to keep the content manageable for students, we have put some enrichment material in the Electronic Study Guide on Davis*Plus* for students who need it or who wish to pursue a subject in more depth. It is all clearly cross-referenced. Instructors who believe that content to be essential can make it a reading requirement.

PEDAGOGICAL FEATURES

The book has numerous pedagogical features to facilitate student learning.

New for Third Edition

NEW!! Key Concepts and Example Problems—In the chapter opener, we have listed the key concepts. An explanation of their use (About the Key Concepts) is found at the beginning of the Theoretical Knowledge section. A Concept Map on Davis*Plus* illustrates the relationships among the key concepts and subconcepts in each chapter. Example Problem sections (e.g., Urinary Retention in Chapter 30) help students begin to think conceptually about patient care instead of trying to organize their thinking according to medical diagnoses.

NEW!! End-of-chapter box—This is another navigation tool: a list of features to remind students and help them use Davis*Plus* to their advantage. In Volume 2, the box is in the chapter opener.

NEW!! More Key Points—We know students skim the content, so we have made visible many points we want to be certain they see and remember.

Reorganized chapters—To better address the needs of many educators, we have reorganized some chapters for this edition:

- *Life Span: Infancy Through Middle Adulthood*—To replace the summarized content contained in the second edition, we have moved and rewritten the expanded content into Chapter 9 in the book. Each stage is discussed in depth, but now more easily accessible in the book, at the request of users.

- *Life Span: Older Adults*—Because of the recent emphasis in nursing care of the growing older adult population, we now have a separate chapter on older adults (Chapter 10). The content has been expanded in this edition.
- *Oxygenation*—To allow students to focus better on one concept, we have divided the old Oxygenation chapter. The complex oxygenation content is now presented in Chapter 36, separate from the circulation content.
- *Circulation*—For the same reasons, the circulation content is now presented separately, and expanded, in Chapter 37.
- *Community & Home Health*—Because these two concepts are so interrelated, we now combine the content from the two second edition chapters (Community Nursing and Nursing in Home Care), presenting them in Chapter 43. We have not decreased the coverage of either topic – simply trimmed down redundant coverage.

Features Continued from Previous Editions

- *Learning Outcomes (Volume 1) and What Are the Main Points in This Chapter? (Volume 2)*—These focus the student's study and provide repetition to facilitate retention of material. In addition, a cross-reference is provided to a Chapter Overview podcast on the Davis*Plus* Web site.
- *Interactive Approach*—The text is written in an engaging style that speaks directly to the student. Recall and critical-thinking questions occur frequently in Volume 1 to break the reading up into small, manageable segments and maintain interest.
  - *Knowledge Checks*—These questions allow students to test their recall of the material presented in the text. Answer sheets and answers are provided on the Electronic Study Guide (ESG).
  - *Think Like a Nurse Exercises*—Thought-provoking questions in both volumes facilitate critical thinking and clinical reasoning and allow the student to synthesize content and explore personal beliefs. Response sheets are provided on the Electronic Study Guide; suggested responses are found on the Instructors' Guide on Davis*Plus*.
- *Meet Your Patient*—This chapter-opening feature in Volume 1 introduces one or more patients. The scenario is used throughout the chapter to illustrate theoretical points and make the content come alive. These patients are often followed in the clinical reasoning activities in Volume 2. This facilitates contextualizing information rather than learning facts in isolation.
- *Safety Features*—To emphasize and help students remember important aspects of safe care, we have specially marked the most important points about safety to make them visible and memorable. They are color-shaded, with an icon to draw attention to them. We do, of course, have an entire chapter on promoting safety.
- *Knowledge Maps*—In Volume 2 every chapter now has a Knowledge Map of the Volume 1 theoretical content. This serves as a content review and helps students learn visually how chapter concepts relate.
- *Care Plans*—Seventeen care plans integrating NANDA-I, NIC, and NOC are found in Volume 1 and on Davis*Plus*. They are based on case studies that allow students to see the nursing process in action. Evidence-based rationales support interventions.
- *Care Maps*—For each care plan, a Care Map allows visual learners to grasp the connection between the phases of the nursing process and illustrates an alternative method of care planning.
- *Care Planning and Care Mapping Exercises*—Several Volume 1 chapters link students to the Student Resources on the Davis*Plus* Web site for practice in constructing care plans, both in columnar format and as concept maps, using the Concept Map Generator on the Web site.
- *Practice Documentation*—Several Volume 2 chapters link students to Practice Documentation exercises on Davis*Plus*.
- *Highlights of Procedures Boxes*—This Volume 1 box contains the highlights of all chapter procedures presented in Volume 2. These boxes serve as a reference when studying the Practical Knowledge content in Volume 1, or as a quick review just before performing a procedure in the clinical area.
- *Caring for the Nguyens*—This is an ongoing case study that begins every chapter of Volume 2. It allows students to become familiar with a single family and to experience vicariously the continuity of care they may encounter in outpatient settings. As with all exercises in the two volumes, response sheets are provided on the Davis*Plus* Web site.
- *Applying the Full-Spectrum Nursing Model*—In Volume 2, these clinically based exercises guide students to safely apply their thinking skills to chapter content. At the same time, they reinforce the full-spectrum model concepts of thinking, doing, and caring introduced in Volume 1.
- *Critical Thinking and Clinical Reasoning*—This set of clinically based exercises (in Volume 2) guides students to safely practice critical thinking in preparation for doing so in the clinical area. Frequently, these clinical exercises make use of material related to the Meet Your Patient scenario in Volume 1.
- *Thinking About the Procedure*—Procedures in Volume 2 include a cross reference to Davis*Plus* for exercises that require students to watch the associated Davis's Nursing Skills Videos to answer the questions. Answers are provided on Davis*Plus*.
- *What If...*—Volume 2 procedures include a section to aid students in knowing what to do in special situations that require decisions during a procedure. For

example, what if you perform a fingerstick to monitor blood glucose, and the monitor shows a very unusual result or an error message? What should you do? We provide the answer. What If's are placed after the procedure steps so they will not distract from the steps while the student learns the procedure.

- *Diagnostic Testing Boxes*—These are found in Volume 2, and on Davis*Plus* in applicable chapters. We believe it is more meaningful to place the diagnostic test information near the related content rather than in an isolated chapter containing all the diagnostic testing content. If students need a more comprehensive reference, we recommend a diagnostic testing book.

THEMES

At least 20 themes are important in professional nursing. Our book weaves these almost seamlessly through the content of both volumes of the book. The following themes that are stressed throughout—some of them in every chapter:

- *Safety.* Safety is a central focus in nursing and healthcare. To emphasize and help students remember important aspects of safe care, we have key safety points marked for high visibility. We also have an entire chapter on Promoting Safety.
- **New for Third Edition.** *PICOT Boxes.* We have added this feature to most chapters to facilitate the skill of inquiry, especially as it relates to evidence-based practice.
- **New for Third Edition.** *More QSEN Boxes.* To promote competency-focused learning, we have introduced the Quality and Safety Education for Nurses (QSEN) competencies in the early chapters of Volume 1, and reinforced them where relevant throughout the text. To remind students that these competencies have practical implications, approximately 30 of the chapters have a QSEN box, providing an example of how a particular competency is related to a chapter concept and expressed in practice.
- **New for Third Edition.** *Gerontology.* To allow for an in-depth discussion of aging and gerontology, provided by an expert on this topic, Chapter 10 is entirely devoted to the older adult developmental stage. Assessments and interventions specifically for the young-old, middle-old, oldest-old, and frail elderly are provided. We have also included interventions specific to older adults in clinical chapters where they apply (e.g., assessing for pain, in Chapter 31; variations for older adults in the health assessment procedures in Chapter 22). Content specific to older adults is marked with a distinctive icon, and the beginning and end of the section are indicated by a colored bar. You will also find that many features and exercises use an older adult as the patient.
- **New for Third Edition.** *Developmental Stages.* The Theoretical Knowledge in most chapters devotes a

section to discussing the effects of life span on the chapter topic. In Volume 2, procedures include variations for children and older adults. The thorough discussion of life span considerations for all age groups, formerly on Davis*Plus*, has been moved to Chapters 9 and 10 by request of users.

- *Critical Thinking.* We emphasize critical thinking and clinical reasoning in various ways. The following are two examples.
  - In addition to the critical-thinking questions and exercises in Volumes 1 and 2, concepts in Volume 1 are often presented in an inductive manner, or pose a question to the student (e.g., "What would happen if . . . ?").
  - **The full-spectrum model of nursing** (presented in Chapter 2) is a comprehensive approach to care that uses critical thinking in all aspects of care. It is not rigidly used to structure the chapters. Instead, the full-spectrum model is reinforced in every chapter of Volume 2 with a set of exercises (Applying the Full-Spectrum Nursing Model) that require students to use the model concepts of thinking, doing, and caring to structure their thinking. Because students cannot focus on everything at once, different model parts are stressed at different times. Sometimes they ask, "What theoretical knowledge do you need to . . . ?" In other instances they might ask, "What biases do you have that might interfere with . . . ?"
- *Toward Evidence-Based Practice Boxes.* In every chapter, we describe research related to the chapter topic and pose critical-thinking questions for students to examine these findings. The concept of evidence-based practice is introduced in Chapter 6 (Nursing Process: Planning Interventions), further explained in Chapter 8 (Evidence-Based Practice: Nursing Theory & Research), and mentioned frequently in other chapters as well.
- *Nursing Process.* Nursing process is a common framework for nursing thinking. Chapter 2 relates nursing process and critical thinking. Chapters 3 through 7 are a comprehensive presentation of the nursing process, which is presented as reflexive rather than linear. The Practical Knowledge sections of Volume 1 are organized according to the nursing process phases; the procedures in Volume 2 have assessment and evaluation components. In addition, many of the questions and exercises provide opportunity for students to apply the nursing process.
- *Standardized Languages: NANDA-I, NIC, and NOC.* Because these are important for electronic health records, the book includes a thorough discussion of these taxonomies in the nursing process and other chapters. NOC outcomes and NIC interventions are included in every chapter of Volume 1; many are presented in tables in Volume 2 or on Davis*Plus*. The Omaha System and the Clinical Care Classification are also used in the community and home health chapters.

- *Caring.* Caring is integrated throughout many chapters and is a part of the Volume 2 book title. Chapter 1 provides historical examples of nursing as a caring profession. Chapter 8 describes the important caring theories. Watson's theory is used throughout the chapter to illustrate how theory is applied in nursing. As well, the Applying the Full-Spectrum Nursing Model exercises in Volume 2 all have questions involving caring (one of the model concepts).

- *Wellness.* Many examples and scenarios in this text refer to people who are not ill. Chapter 11 emphasizes health; Chapter 42 talks about the nurse's role in health promotion.

- *Culture.* Cultural diversity is highlighted throughout the text in clinical scenarios, illustrations, and theoretical discussion. Chapter 15 focuses on culturally sensitive nursing care. The *Caring for the Nguyens*, an ongoing case study throughout Volume 2, features an extended family; ethnic variations are described in procedures, as applicable.

- *Spirituality.* Chapter 16 is probably the most extensive presentation of spiritual care available in a fundamentals text. Spirituality is integrated within various chapters in scenarios, examples, and exercises.

- *Documentation.* All chapters include reference to documentation, where relevant. The procedures in Volume 2 all have guidelines for and examples of how to document the procedure. In addition, we have included some Practice Documentation exercises on DavisPlus. Chapter 18 contains a thorough presentation of documentation and reporting.

- *Delegation*. Delegation is introduced early, in the nursing process chapters, and is a thread in most Volume 1 chapters. Chapter 40, Leading & Managing, also discusses delegation. In Volume 2, all procedures have guidelines for delegating.

- *ANA Standards*. Nursing and other healthcare standards (e.g., The Joint Commission, Medicare) are frequently referenced. Links to pertinent Web sites are given so students can keep up with changes to standards.

- *Ethics.* In addition to the extensive treatment in Chapter 44, ethical knowledge is an aspect of our full-spectrum model. As such, many of the critical-thinking exercises ask students to grapple with ethical issues. Good examples are found in Chapter 6, Volume 2, and in the Applying the Full-Spectrum Nursing Model in every chapter.

- *Legal Issues.* Chapter 45 is devoted to legal issues that nurses face in their practice. Legal issues are integrated in many other chapters as well (e.g., licensing in Chapter 1; end-of-life legal considerations in Chapter 16).

- *Community and Home Healthcare.* Chapter 43 is devoted exclusively to these topics. In other chapters, clinical scenarios and examples involve nurses in these settings. Procedures in Volume 2 have sections for adapting skills to home care; Volume 1 has special feature boxes:

- *Home Care Boxes*—These provide guidelines for safely modifying care for delivery in the home.

- *Teaching: Self-Care Boxes*—Self-Care boxes appear throughout Volume 1. They are similar to the traditional "teaching boxes," but focus on equipping patients to perform self-care.

- *Complementary Therapies.* The book conceptualizes nursing as holistic. Chapter 46 (on DavisPlus) is devoted exclusively to complementary and alternative therapies. Several chapters in Volume 1 (e.g., Chapter 15, Culture & Ethnicity) contain material related to this topic. For example, you will find Complementary & Alternative Modalities (CAM) boxes in several chapters. Some describe a complementary therapy related to the chapter topic. Others present research concerning a particular complementary therapy (e.g., intercessory prayer in Chapter 16).

- *Contemporary Issues.* In Chapter 23, we include extensive information about bioterrorism, multidrug-resistant organisms, and emerging infectious diseases, and healthcare-related infections. Those topics are also included in Chapter 43 as relevant to Community Nursing. The safety chapter includes ways to assess for and cope with violence in the healthcare setting.

- *Nursing Informatics.* Chapter 41 is an excellent introduction to nursing informatics. Standardized languages and electronic care planning and documentation are interspersed throughout the book (for example, in the nursing process and medications chapters), and especially in standardized language tables in Volume 2 and on DavisPlus. We also emphasize electronic documentation in Chapter 18 and in our illustrations for documenting some procedures in Volume 2. We further encourage use of technology by providing students with links to material on DavisPlus and other Web sites related to the chapter topic.

THE TEXT AS A RESPONSE TO CHANGE

This book was developed to address the needs of today's nursing students and in response to the following changes in nursing education and practice.

Changes in Students

- **Nontraditional Students.** Students range from younger students just out of high school to older, second-career students. Many have work or family responsibilities that compete with school for attention. To address this change, we have followed two principles of adult learning: that learning must be relevant, efficient, and meaningful to the person. *Efficiency:* Volume 1 is intended for classroom use, while Volume 2 is for clinical use.

- *Technology:* The Electronic Study Guide on Davis*Plus* delivers enhancements to the printed text, developed with the knowledge that highly motivated students will welcome the chance to use technologies to maximize their learning.
- *Meaningfulness/Relevance:* To make the content more meaningful, each chapter opens with a patient scenario or story of a practicing nurse. This story is woven throughout the chapter to provide context for factual information and to show how concepts are applied and how nurses think.
- *Practical Application:* We stress practical application throughout the text because adults want to apply knowledge in real-life circumstances. The Nguyen family case, in all chapters of Volume 2, is a prime example of this.

- **Variety in Learning Styles.** Students learn in different ways. To address this, we have used more than 1,400 photos and many diagrams and concept maps to assist visual learners. Podcasts, animations, and sound files of body sounds and other clinical assessment findings are included on Davis*Plus* for auditory learners. To teach psychomotor skills, we have, in addition to step-by-step procedures, included skills videos and checklists that students can print out for practicing procedures or for teachers to use in evaluations.
- **Reading Comprehension.** Whether because of changes in admission requirements, or because English is a second language, or for other reasons, some schools are finding students' reading abilities to be lower than in the past. We addressed this change by writing in an informal style, addressing the student directly ("you will . . ."). We have not made the content more superficial, but have made reading about it more inviting and user-friendly. We define new terms at their first use in each chapter, and include a glossary on Davis*Plus* for additional unfamiliar terms.
- **The Technology Generation.** The newer generations of students are accustomed to using technology and multitasking. To hold their attention, in addition to our easy-to-read style, we present information in an interactive manner, and in relatively short segments interspersed with review questions and critical-thinking questions. For this same reason, the text frequently directs students to find related information on Davis*Plus* and on the Internet, often in the form of podcasts or sound files. eBooks offer the convenience of accessing the book from wherever the student has Internet access without having to lug around heavy books.

Changes in Curricula

- **Teachers say they do not have enough time to "cover the content."** One way to address this problem is not to re-teach material students have had in other classes. We provide, for example, just enough anatomy and physiology in each chapter to aid students who need to review A&P, or who are taking A&P concurrently

with nursing courses. You should not need to "cover" it in class.

- **Understanding and retention continue to be a problem.** To aid in retention, we have interspersed knowledge checks and critical-thinking questions throughout Volume 1 to allow students to check their recall and understanding of the content as they progress through the chapters. Recognizing that repetition aids retention, we provide Learning Outcomes at the beginning of each chapter in Volume 1. In addition, chapters in Volume 2 include a list titled *What Are the Main Points in This Chapter?* and a full-page Knowledge Map of the chapter content. To accompany each chapter, there is also a podcast on the Davis*Plus* Web site that overviews chapter content. And finally, the Student Resources contain an Audio Glossary.
- **Some curricula have de-emphasized mental health.** Mental health may be taught in other (e.g., medical-surgical) clinical areas, with no separate mental health course in the curriculum. In response to pleas from educators, we include expanded mental health content and tools for psychosocial assessment. In addition to the usual concepts of self-concept and self-esteem, Chapter 13 includes basic assessments and interventions for the Example Problems of anxiety and depression, which students will encounter commonly in all areas, not just on mental health units. In Chapter 21, the communication chapter, we have excellent content on the nurse-patient relationship and communication techniques that mental health teachers find so essential. Chapter 12, Stress & Adaptation, includes information about defense mechanisms.
- **The curriculum does not include separate pharmacology, nutrition, ethics, or nursing process courses.** Because all nurses need grounding in these topics, we have provided extensive coverage of these topics, both in Volume 1 and on Davis*Plus*. The medications chapter provides in-depth pharmacology information. Chapter 27, Nutrition, provides a foundational understanding of patients' nutritional needs. Chapter 44 is a comprehensive look at nursing ethics. We have, arguably, the most useful and thorough presentation of nursing process available in a fundamentals text. These chapters, as well as most others, will be a valuable reference for students when they take other clinical nursing courses.

Changes in Nursing and Healthcare

- **The nursing role is increasingly complex, requiring management, decision-making, delegation, and supervision skills early in the career.**
  To address this change, we have included a comprehensive discussion of leadership and management in Chapter 38. The critical-thinking exercises, especially in Volume 2, and the Nguyens feature help students to develop clinical decision-making skills. Delegation is presented early, in the nursing process chapters, and

stressed in the rest of the chapters in Volume 1, as applicable. Each clinical procedure in Volume 2 contains a Delegation section.

- **Healthcare has moved increasingly from the hospital to the home and community.**

  To address this change we have included a provocative discussion about the evolving healthcare system in Chapter 1. In addition, Chapter 43 discusses Community and Home Care. Those concepts are also integrated throughout Volume 1 (e.g., *Healthy People 2020* goals are cited where they are relevant to content); and the procedures in Volume 2 include home-care adaptations, as well as patient-teaching points that enable patients and caregivers to assume more responsibility for care.

- **Nurses need to be critical thinkers and life-long learners.**

  To address this change, we have organized the text around a model of Full-Spectrum Nursing, a comprehensive approach to care that uses critical thinking in all aspects of care. The model is reinforced in each chapter of Volume 2 in the feature Applying the Full-Spectrum Nursing Model. Critical thinking is integrated throughout both volumes of the text, both in discussion and in critical-thinking exercises. Discussion of this model follows.

THE FULL-SPECTRUM MODEL OF NURSING

We believe that nursing knowledge is a fusion of theoretical knowledge, practical knowledge, self-knowledge, and ethical knowledge. To function at the highest level, nurses use critical thinking and the nursing process to blend thinking and doing to put caring into action. We refer to this blend as *Full-Spectrum Nursing*. We have organized our learning package to reflect this philosophy. This model is presented in Chapter 2 and referred to and used throughout the text.

THE LEARNING PACKAGE

This is a well-integrated and cross-referenced package containing a two-volume text; an Electronic Study Guide on Davis*Plus* (Chapter Resources); and instructors' materials provided on Davis*Plus*. Although any item can be used either in classroom or clinical settings, Volume 1 will usually be used in the classroom setting, whereas Volume 2 will usually be used in the clinical setting or learning laboratory. You can also purchase a set of skills videos, a book of procedure checklists, and a *Fundamentals Skills Notes* pocket guide.

Volume 1

Volume 1 contains all the theoretical and conceptual material typically present in a fundamentals text, presented in a clinically focused, user-friendly manner,

and incorporating many examples. This presentation allows students to see how the content will be useful to them. In Chapters 8 through 46, the nursing process is used as the model to organize the Practical Knowledge section.

Unit 1—focuses on how nurses think. It begins by showing how nursing history relates to our present healthcare system. Chapter 2 focuses on critical thinking, and Chapters 3 through 7 provide an extensive treatment of the nursing process. This unit prepares students to follow the organization of subsequent chapters and provides the thinking tools and processes they need to apply the content of the other chapters. Chapter 8 contains an overview of the processes of theory building, nursing research, and evidence-based practice as they relate to the nurse in practice.

Unit 2—is about the internal and external factors that affect an individual's health (e.g., family, culture, spirituality, and life stage). Internal factors are personal beliefs or attributes that influence how the client views health, healthcare, and nursing. A groundbreaking feature is Chapter 11, which describes the health-illness-wellness continuum in an experiential way, encouraging self-knowledge, personal growth, and affective learning of that content.

Unit 3—examines essential nursing interventions. We consider these skills "essential" because nurses use some or all of these skills in *all* areas of nursing, regardless of setting or patient diagnosis. The unit begins with documentation and includes communication, teaching, taking vital signs, physical assessment, asepsis, safety, hygiene, and medication administration.

Unit 4—concentrates on nursing care that supports physiological function. We examine broad categories of physiological function (e.g., nutrition, elimination, oxygenation) and discuss related nursing care.

Unit 5—explores diverse nursing functions. For example, we look at leadership and management, the use of technology and informatics, and health-promotion activities. Chapter 41 is a more thorough introduction to informatics than you will usually find in a fundamentals text.

Unit 6—looks at the context for nurses' work. This includes chapters on community and home care, as well as the ethical and legal contexts for nursing work. And we are especially proud of Chapter 46 (on the Davis*Plus* Web site), which provides a deeper treatment of holistic healing than you will typically find. We believe that a fundamentals book, overall, provides all concepts needed for a holistic view of the patient—just scan our chapter titles to see what we mean by that. We went one step further with Chapter 46.

Volume 2

Volume 2 is designed primarily, but not exclusively, for use in the skills lab and clinical setting. As does Volume 1, it includes thinking, doing, and caring. The critical-thinking exercises require students to use their thinking skills and the nursing process to apply theoretical knowledge to specific patient situations. The clinical procedures, assessment tools, clinical forms, diagnostic testing information, and standardized language tables make up the practical knowledge sections. Throughout Volume 2, students have access to a simulated experience known as *Caring for the Nguyens*, an ongoing case study through which they learn about the nursing role, the healthcare system, and the real-world application of the content in Volume 1.

Student Resources on DavisPlus

Sometimes referred to as an Electronic Study Guide (or ESG), the Student Resources on the Davis*Plus* Web site at **DavisPl.us/Wilkinson3** contains expanded discussions of some of the Volume 1 material, mastery questions, answers to the Volume 1 Knowledge Checks, a panel of NCLEX-style and chapter review test questions for practice, a glossary, additional care plans and care maps, and procedure checklists. Also included are forms that students can print out to write their answers to Knowledge Checks, Critical Thinking questions, and Mastery questions as well as the Volume 2 critical-thinking exercises. It also provides other types of forms that students can print out and use in clinical settings, for example, some assessment tools. The questions themselves have expandable space so that answers can be typed in on the electronic form and then printed out. The large glossary provides definitions of all bolded terms used in the text as well as supplementary terms that may be helpful to students.

Procedure checklists can be used to study for skills lab or clinical, or as a means to assess skill mastery. Checklists are provided in two formats: One is a detailed list of steps for each procedure; another is a generic, principles-based list that instructors can use to evaluate all procedures.

Other Resources on DavisPl.us/ Wilkinson3

- *Podcasts*—For audio learners, podcasts for each chapter summarize the main ideas for convenient prep for class or review for quizzes or exams. There are 12 "stress buster" podcasts: one for each month. You will also find 24 clever and revealing test-taking tips to give you the "one-up" on getting a better test result.
- *NCLEX-style and chapter review questions for students*—We have added more questions to help students right from the beginning of their nursing studies to become comfortable answering NCLEX-style questions while reviewing chapter content.
- *eBook*—Tired of lugging around heavy books? Now you can access this two-volume textbook electronically. Log on to the Davis*Plus* site for on-screen reading—just as though you were turning pages in your own book.

INSTRUCTOR'S GUIDE

The Instructor's Guide contains everything in the Student Resources plus additional features to assist faculty. These include an image bank of illustrations from the book, PowerPoint lecture outlines with illustrations, "clicker" questions, and a critical-thinking question.

New for Third Edition. The PowerPoint lecture outlines now include notes you can refer to when lecturing from the slides.

New for Third Edition. The Lesson Plans have been replaced by a new feature called Flipping the Classroom. These are presented as Word files so teachers can add to or delete from them to meet their unique needs.

Also included are teaching strategies to accompany each chapter, suggested responses for the critical-thinking exercises in Volumes 1 and 2, instructions for using concept mapping, and a test bank of more than 2,300 NCLEX-style and chapter review questions, including the newer NCLEX formats. The number of learning strategies has been significantly increased.

HOW TO USE THIS LEARNING PACKAGE (FOR TEACHERS)

You are fortunate to be working with students at perhaps the most formative point in their nursing education: the fundamentals course. We are certain that each of you will bring your own special style to the teaching of this most-important-of-all nursing courses, and that you will find new and creative ways to use the many teaching and learning features we have provided. We hope your enjoyment of this new and improved learning package is equal to our pride in it.

For suggestions about how to use this integrated learning package (in both text and podcast format),

 Go to How to Use This Learning Package in the Instructor's Resources on the Davis*Plus* Web site, at **DavisPl.us/Wilkinson3.**

 Go to Getting the Most Out of This Learning Package podcast on the Davis*Plus* Web site.

Schools that adopt our textbook also have access to a PowerPoint slide presentation and a podcast explaining how to use the learning package. You can use this and/or the podcast to orient new teachers and students so they can easily navigate and make best use of the entire learning package.

GETTING THE MOST OUT OF THIS LEARNING PACKAGE (FOR STUDENTS)

For ideas about how to use your textbooks and the Electronic Study Guide (Student and Chapter Resources) to get the best results from your studying,

Go to Getting the Most Out of This Learning Package on the DavisPlus Web site.

For those times when you'd rather listen than read, we offer podcasts that describe ways for you to use the different components of your learning package—that is, your two-volume book set, nursing skills DVD set, your online Chapter Resources, NCLEX-style practice and chapter review questions, animations, documentation exercises, care mapping exercises, concept map generator, and many more, worthwhile learning tools.

 Go to Getting the Most Out of This Learning Package podcast on the DavisPlus Web site.

We also know that being a student in a nursing program is hard work and can be overwhelming. Log on to the DavisPlus Web site for 12 useful strategies to reduce your stress while you are on your journey to becoming a nurse.

 Go to Stress Busters podcast on the DavisPlus Web site.

Your goal is to do well in your courses. Knowing testing is an important part of your experience while in school, we now offer clever, test-taking tips to help you to take tests with excellence and show what you know!

 Go to Test-Taking Tips podcast on the DavisPlus Web site.

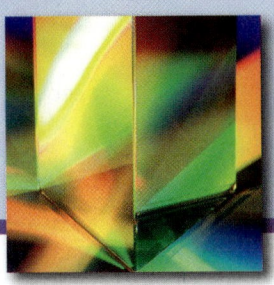

Contributors to Third Edition

The following people contributed material that was used in creating this learning package.
We are grateful for their assistance.

Pennie Sessler Branden, PhD, CNM, RN
Assistant Professor
Sacred Heart University, School of Nursing
Fairfield, Connecticut
Item Writer, Teacher Testbank

Stephanie Scovill Bronsky, RN, MSN Ed
Clinical Educator
Grand Canyon University
Chapter Contributor, Nutrition
PICOT feature

Patricia-Ann Calarco, RN, MSN
Assistant Professor
College of Nursing
Roseman University
Henderson, Nevada
Item Writer, Teacher Testbank

Lu Ann Connor, RN, BSN, MBA
Team Leader of Inpatient Adult Behavioral Health
SSM DePaul Health Care at St. Vincent's Hospital
Saint Louis, Missouri
Area Clinical Director/Home Care Director of Clinical
    Operations
Alere Health, Inc.
Saint Louis, Missouri
Chapter Contributor, Community & Home Health Nursing

Susan Johnson Garbutt, DNP, CIC, CNE
Simulation Coordinator in Nursing
University of Tampa
Tampa, Florida
Chapter Contributor, Promoting Asepsis & Preventing Infection

Kathleen C. Jones, RN, MSN, CNS
Associate Professor of Nursing
Walters State Community College
Morristown, Tennessee
Chapter Contributor, Wounds & Skin Integrity

Patricia A. Koral, RN, MSN, CNE
Associate Professor
Good Samaritan College of Nursing and Health Science
Cincinnati, Ohio
QSEN feature

Karen LoCascio, MS, RN-BC
Nursing Lab Coordinator
Southern Maine Community College
South Portland, Maine
Chapter Contributor, Urinary Elimination

Jacqueline Patton Mayer, RN, MSN
Associate Professor
Good Samaritan College of Nursing and Health Sciences
Cincinnati, Ohio
QSEN feature

Debra S. McKinney, RN, MSN/MBA/HCA
Nursing Faculty
Grand Canyon University, Ottawa University, and University
    of Phoenix
Item Writer, Teacher Testbank

Phyllis Puckett, RN, MS
Assistant Director of Nursing Program
Northern Wyoming Community College District
Sheridan, Wyoming
Contributor, Instructor Lectures

L. Jane Rosati, EdD, MSN, RN
Professor, School of Nursing
Daytona State College
Daytona Beach, Florida
Instructor's Guide Contributor, Classroom enrichment strategies

Melanie H. Simpson, PhD, RN-BC, OCN, CHPN
Pain Management Resource Team
The University of Kansas Hospital
Kansas City, Kansas
Chapter Contributor, Pain

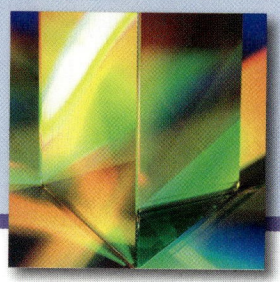

Contributors to Previous Wilkinson and Treas Textbooks

Julia Aucoin, RN, DNS, BC, CNE
Clinical consultant and literature reviews

Karen Barnett, DNP, RN
Concept maps

Linda Blazovich, RN, MSN
Procedure checklists

Diane Bligh, RN, MS, CNS
Knowledge maps, instructor's guide, lecture outlines, care planning exercises

Diane Breckenridge, RN, PhD, MSN
Assessment and diagnosis content

Leanne Cowin, RN, PhD
Literature searches

Lisa Culliton, MSN, CPN
Literature searches

Debbie Ellison, RN, MSN
Nursing care plans; oxygenation procedures

Garrett Fardon
Clerical assistance

Mary Gant, APN, ACNS-BC, RRT
Oxygenation procedures

Kathie Hayes, DNSc
Test bank items

Tracey Hopkins, RN, BSN
QSEN boxes

Lisa Lyons, RN, BSN
Procedures for sensory-perception, pain management, activity and exercise, and skin integrity chapters

Lisa LaMothe Melo, RN, BSN
Procedures for sensory-perception, pain management, activity and exercise, and skin integrity chapters

Mary N. Meyer, MSN, ARNP-BC
Procedures for safety and bowel elimination chapters

Lori Ormsby, MSN, GCNS-BC, APRN, CWOCN
Skin integrity and wound care content

Pamela Owen, BSN
Healthcare in Canada

Jessica Pedersen, ARNP, FNP-C
Nutrition procedures

Cynthia Pivec, BS
Procedure checklists

Linda Puetz, RN, BA, BSN, MEd
Documentation chapter content

Veronica Rempusheski, RN, FAAN, PhD
Older adults, expanded discussion (DavisPlus)

Elizabeth Richmond, BSN, MEd
Hygiene procedures

Sarah Kennedy Roland, RN, MSN
Documentation exercises, sample nurses notes, test bank items

Susan Simmons, ARNP-BC, PhD
Clinical consultant, literature reviews

Mable H. Smith, BSN, MN, JD, PhD
Legal issues chapter content

Lynne Sullivan, RN, MS
Procedures for sensory-perception, pain management, activity and exercise, and skin integrity chapters

Mary Pat Szutenbach, RN, CNS, PhD
Nutrition chapter content

Janet Terra, RN, MSN
Hygiene procedures

Cynthia Thompson, RN, BSN
Hygiene procedures

Diana Tilton, RN, MSN
Asepsis procedures

Lisa Watkins, RN, MS
Urinary elimination procedures

Janis Watts, RN, MSN
Nursing informatics content

Michelle Williams, RN, MSN
Nursing care plans

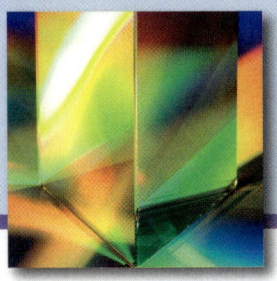

Reviewers

Special thanks to the following content reviewers:

Stephanie Adair, MSN, RN
Nursing Faculty
Bevill State Community College
Jasper, Alabama

Mary Al-Saleh, PhD, RN, CNE
Faculty, Emeritus
Mesa Community College
Mesa, Arizona

Heather Anderson, MSN, RN, FNP-BC
Lecturer
University of North Carolina at Charlotte
Charlotte, North Carolina

Ramona Anest, MSN, RNC-TNP, CNE
Associate Professor
Bob Jones University
Greenville, South Carolina

Kerri Austin, RN, MSN, CNE
Faculty Instructor
Aria Health School of Nursing
Trevose, Pennsylvania

Susan Bacher, RN, MSN, CNOR
Professor, Nursing and Surgical Technology
Cincinnati State Technical & Community College
Cincinnati, Ohio

Jenna Boothe, RN, MSN
Associate Professor
Hazard Community and Technical College
Hazard, Kentucky

Carole Boutin, MS, RN, CNE
Professor of Nursing
Nashua Community College
Bedford, New Hampshire

Nell Britton, MSN, RN, CNE, NHA
Nursing Instructor, New Student Coordinator
Trident Technical College, Nursing Division
Charleston, South Carolina

Teresa Carnevale, PhD, MSN, RN
Assistant Professor of Nursing
Appalachian State University
Boone, North Carolina

Sandra Wolf Citty, PhD, ARNP-BC (FNP)
Clinical Assistant Professor
University of Florida, College of Nursing
Gainesville, Florida

Diane Cozzi, MSN, RN
Nursing Instructor
Gateway Technical College
Burlington, Wisconsin

Ann Curtis, RN, MSN
Faculty
Central Maine Medical Center College of Nursing & Health
    Professions
Lewiston, Maine

Tammy S. Czyzewski, MS, RN-BC, NEA-BC
Associate Professor of Nursing
Sinclair Community College
Dayton, Ohio

Doreen DeAngelis, RN, MSN
Nursing Instructor
Penn State University, Fayette Campus
Lemont Furnace, Pennsylvania

Pamela K. DeMoss, MSN, RN
Assistant Professor
University of Dubuque
Dubuque, Iowa

Allison Divine, MSN, RN
Nursing Fundamentals Course Coordinator
National Park Community College
Hot Springs, Arkansas

Colleen Duncan, RN, BSN, MS, MPHA
Nursing Faculty
Portland Community College
Portland, Oregon

Kristen Fenlason, RN
Nursing Instructor
Lake Superior College
Duluth, MN

Cheryl S. Fieldhouse, MS, RN, CNE
Assistant Professor of Nursing
Greenville Technical College
Greenville, South Carolina

Kathleen Fraley, AND, BSN, MSN, RN
Lead Faculty for Principles of Nursing
St. Clair County Community College
Port Huron, Michigan

Kathleen Walsh Free, MSN, RN-C, APRN-BC
Clinical Professor
Indiana University Southeast
New Albany, Indiana

Anna E. Gryczman, DNP, RN, AHN-BC, CNE
Nursing Faculty
Century College
White Bear Lake, Minnesota

Diane Hammond, MSN, RN
Assistant Professor
Daytona State College
Daytona Beach, Florida

Anne Harner, EdS, MSN, RN
Nursing Faculty
Florida Gulf Coast University
Fort Myers, Florida

Betty Hennington, MSN, CNE
Nursing Instructor
Meridian Community College
Meridian, Mississippi

Corinne Hunter, RN, MS, FNP
Professor
Northshore Community College
Danvers, Massachusetts

Sherry Buie James, RN, MSN/Ed
Professor of Nursing
Horry-Georgetown Technical College
Myrtle Beach, South Carolina

Elizabeth Keene, MSN/Ed, RN, CNE
Assistant Professor, Nursing
Montgomery County Community College
Blue Bell, Pennsylvania

Trudy Klein, MS, RN
Associate Dean of the School of Nursing, Assistant Professor
Walla Walla University
College Place, Washington

Denise Lakous, MN, APRN, ACNP
Faculty
Butler Community College
El Dorado, Kansas

John Lazar, PhD(c), RN, MSN, FNP-BC
Associate Professor of Nursing
Shepherd University
Los Angeles, California

Sondra L. Leatherman, MSN, RN, CNE
Nursing Faculty
Hesston College
Hesston, Kansas

Karen LoCascio, MS, RN
Assistant Professor of Nursing
Southern Maine Community College
South Portland, Maine

Jocelyn Ludlow, MN, RN
Skills Lab Instructor
Bellevue College
Bellevue, Washington

Melissa Peterson Lund, MSN, RN, FNP-BC
Assistant Professor of Nursing
Gannon University, Villa Maria School of Nursing
Erie, Pennsylvania

Jeanette H. Lupinacci, EdD, MS, CRRN
Associate Professor of Nursing, Undergraduate Coordinator
Western Connecticut State University
Danbury, Connecticut

Rhonda Martin, MS, RN
Clinical Associate Professor
The University of Tulsa
Tulsa, Oklahoma

Madeline Mattern, MS, NP-C, CNE
Coordinator, Outreach Programs; Faculty
Penn State College of Nursing
University Park, Pennsylvania

Patricia McJilton, MSN, RN
Nursing Instructor
Gillette College
Gillette, Wyoming

Kathy Moore, MSN/Ed, RN
Assistant Professor, Nursing
Greenville Technical College
Greenville, South Carolina

Susan Moyer, MSN, RN
Assistant Professor
Reading Area Community College
Reading, PA

Nola Ormrod, MSN, RN
Nursing Director, Associate Professor
Centralia College, Nursing Department
Centralia, Washington

Kimberly Porter, MSNc, RN, BA
Assistant Professor
University of Arkansas at Little Rock
Little Rock, Arkansas

Joy A. Price, MSN, RN, CNE, FNP-BC
Instructor, Associate Degree Nursing
Northeast Mississippi Community College
Booneville, Mississippi

Barbara Puryear, RN, MS, CCM, CLCP
Instructor
Holmes Community College
Ridgeland, Mississippi

Cheryl Rodgers, MSN, RN, CHPN
Nursing Instructor
South University
Richmond, Virginia

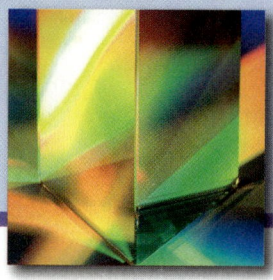

Acknowledgments

We wish to extend sincere thanks to the exceptional team that helped us create this learning package, and especially to the following people:

- **Lisa Deitch**, Acquisitions Editor and friend, for her vision and forward thinking for the first edition, and for her continued support throughout its revisions.
- **Adrienne Simon**, Senior Content Project Manager, deserves extraordinary thanks. She joined the team midway through this edition. With almost no learning curve time, she quickly grasped and managed the many interlocking details of this complex project and worked incessantly to keep this project on track. Her untiring efforts and attention to detail enabled us to better focus on content and didactic issues.

- **Shirley Kuhn**, Developmental Editor, for tirelessly facilitating communication between the authors and all elements of the production team. We dearly appreciate her integrity, work ethic, and sense of humor.
- **Jamie Elfrank**, Project Editor, for her amazing ability to organize and retrieve information and files, all the while churning out a mountain of work during the time she was with us. She kept chaos at bay, made our lives easier, and never let us down.
- **Darlene Pedersen**, Director of Content Development, for working her magic behind the scenes to support our project. We heartily thank her for throwing us a lifeline, when needed, to make things just a little bit easier.

Contents

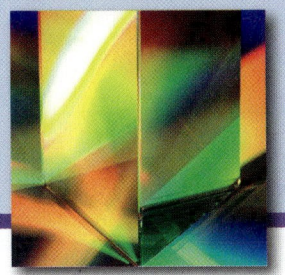

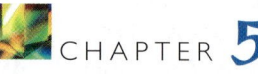
CHAPTER **4**

Nursing Process: Diagnosis 59

CHAPTER **5**

Nursing Process: Planning Outcomes 84

CHAPTER **6**

Nursing Process: Planning Interventions 105

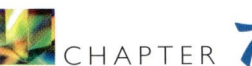
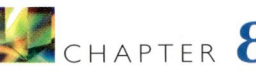
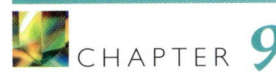

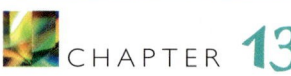
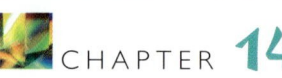

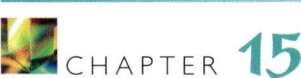
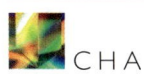

Unit 3

Essential Nursing Interventions   369

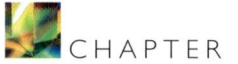

CHAPTER 18

Documenting & Reporting   371

CHAPTER 19

Teaching & Learning   396

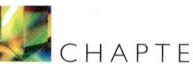

CHAPTER 20

Measuring Vital Signs   420

CHAPTER **21**

Communication & Therapeutic Relationships   458

CHAPTER **22**

Health Assessment   479

CHAPTER 23

Promoting Asepsis & Preventing Infection 516

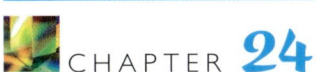

CHAPTER **24**

Promoting Safety 545

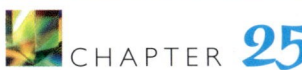

CHAPTER **25**

Facilitating Hygiene 574

CHAPTER 26

Administering Medications   604

Unit 4
Supporting Physiological Functioning   661

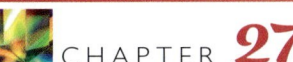

CHAPTER **27**

Nutrition   663

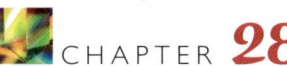

CHAPTER **28**

Urinary Elimination   714

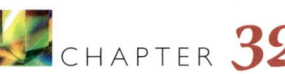

CHAPTER **31**

Pain   790

CHAPTER **32**

Physical Activity & Mobility   816

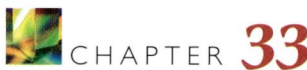

CHAPTER **33**

Sexual Health   847

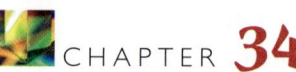

CHAPTER **34**

Sleep & Rest   878

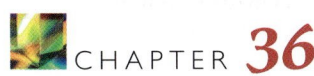

CHAPTER 35

Skin Integrity & Wound Healing   897

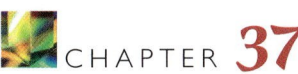

CHAPTER 36

Oxygenation   934

CHAPTER 37

Circulation   967

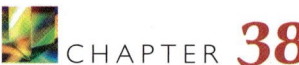

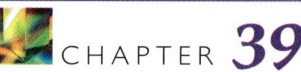

Unit 5

Nursing Functions   1023

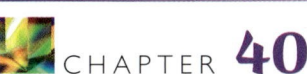

CHAPTER **40**

Leading & Managing   1056

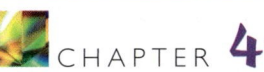

CHAPTER **41**

Nursing Informatics   1077

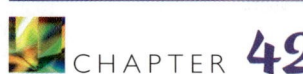

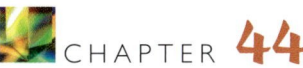

CHAPTER 44

Ethics & Values   1137

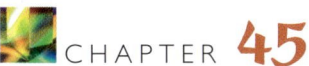

CHAPTER 45

Legal Accountability   1162

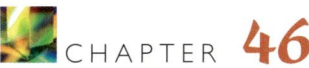

CHAPTER 46

Holistic Healing (on DavisPlus)

How Nurses Think

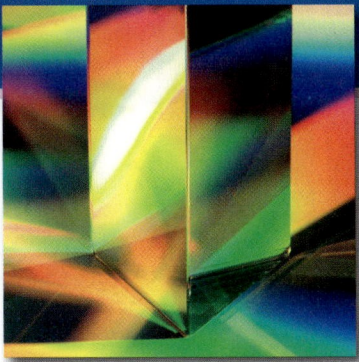

Evolution of Nursing Thought & Action

Learning Outcomes

After completing this chapter, you should be able to:

➤ Define *nursing* in your own words.

➤ Discuss the transitions nursing education has undergone in the last century.

➤ Differentiate among the various forms of nursing education.

➤ Explain how nursing practice is regulated.

➤ Give four examples of influential nursing organizations.

➤ Name and recognize the four purposes of nursing care.

➤ Describe the healthcare delivery system in the United States, including sites for care, types of workers, regulation, and financing of healthcare.

➤ Name nine expanded roles for nursing.

➤ Discuss issues related to healthcare reform.

➤ Delineate the forces and trends affecting contemporary nursing practice.

If you were assigned the Expanded Discussion on the DavisPlus, you should also be able to demonstrate the following outcomes:

➤ Identify the factors that led to the change of nursing from a vocation of men and women to a predominantly female profession.

➤ Describe the various images of nurses through history.

➤ Describe the role of religion in the development of nursing.

➤ Explain the role of the military in the development of the nursing profession.

Key Concepts

Nursing
Nursing history
Contemporary nursing education
Contemporary nursing practice
Healthcare delivery system

Related Concepts

See the Concept Map on Davis*Plus*.

This volume contains only a brief introduction to nursing history. For more detailed information,

Go to Student Resources, Chapter 1, **Evolution of Nursing Thought and Action—Expanded Discussion,** on Davis*Plus*.

Nurses Make a Difference . . .

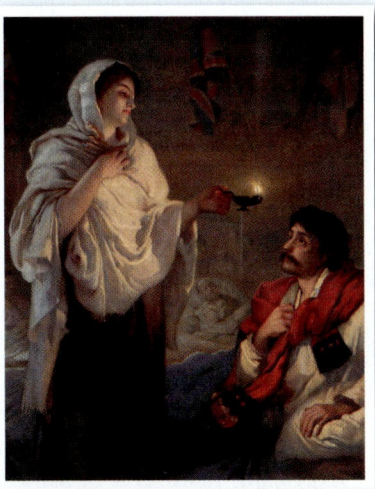

Then & Now

Time: 1854, Üsküdar (now part of Istanbul, Turkey) in the Crimea

The hospital tent is set up away from the battlefield. The injured and dying soldiers are lying upon the bare earth, soiled and covered with crusted blood. Outside the air is cool, yet the tent is stifling with the rank odor of disease and death. Scanning the scene, Florence Nightingale gathers her staff of 38 nurses. They review the environmental condition of the hospital tent, the health problems of the soldiers, and the supplies and equipment they have to work with. First, they open the tent to allow in fresh air. Then they clean the tent, bathe the wounded, and provide clean bedding. They assess and dress the wounds, feed the soldiers a nutritious meal, and comfort those dying or in pain. They offer encouragement and emotional care to the healthier soldiers and help

(Continued)

Nurses Make a Difference . . . (continued)

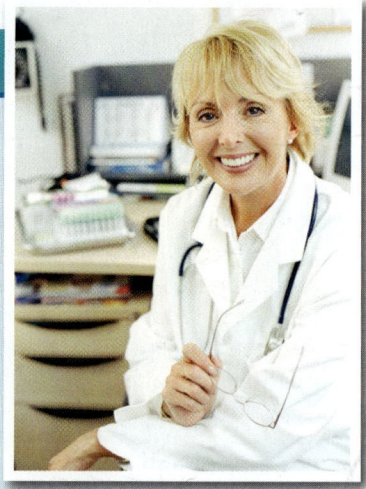

them to write letters home. Within a brief period of time the mortality rate drops from 47% to 2% and morale improves immeasurably.

Time: 2012, Your Local Hospital

While standing at the bedside mixing an antibiotic solution, Susan listens to the ventilator cycle. She notes that her patient has begun to trigger breaths on his own. In the background she hears the cardiac monitor sounds, which have become more irregular over the past hour. She mentally runs through her patient assessment. "Why is his heart so irritable?" she wonders. She calls the lab for the morning blood work results. When the lab technician e-mails the results to the unit, Susan notes that the potassium level is low (2.9 mEq/L). She notifies the physician of the lab results and the cardiac irritability. Susan tells the physician, "The patient's potassium is low from the diarrhea he's had since we began the antibiotics." Together they develop a plan to administer intravenous (IV) potassium chloride to raise the serum potassium level and to check it every 8 hours. Several hours later Susan documents that the *ectopy* (irregular heartbeat) has decreased to less than 2 beats/min.

Time: 2030, A Local Home

Yesterday, Mr. Samuels underwent cardiac surgery. He was discharged home this morning and is now under your care. As a home health nurse, your role is to assess his condition; provide skilled care; teach Mr. Samuels how to care for himself; instruct his family about his care; and coordinate any required additional services. You have been monitoring his condition remotely (telehealth) since discharge before the visit. Mrs. Samuels greets you at the front door. She tells you that her husband is in a lot of pain and that the chest drainage system appears full. She looks frightened as she says, "When my father had cardiac surgery 25 years ago, he spent 4 days in the hospital. I don't understand why my husband got sent home so quickly." You explain that changes in technology and the healthcare system allow you to take care of clients in the home who would previously have been in the hospital. As you begin your assessments, you tell Mrs. Samuels, "After I've gathered more information, we'll make a plan that will make all of us more comfortable."

In each of these scenarios, the nurses engaged in *full-spectrum nursing*; that is, they used their minds and their hands to improve the client's comfort and condition. As the scenarios illustrate, nursing roles have changed over time. Yet nursing remains a profession dedicated to client care.

 Think**Like a Nurse** I-I

The Quality and Safety Education for Nurses (QSEN) project and the Institute of Medicine (IOM) have identified quality and safety competencies for nurses: (1) patient-centered care, (2) teamwork and collaboration, (3) evidence-based practice, (4) quality improvement, (5) safety, and (6) informatics (Cronenwett, Sherwood, Barnsteiner, et al., 2007). Which of these did Florence Nightingale demonstrate? Explain your thinking.

ABOUT THE KEY CONCEPTS

The overarching concept for this chapter is **nursing**. As you come to understand key concepts (i.e., nursing history, contemporary nursing education, contemporary nursing practice, healthcare delivery system) you will grasp how nursing has emerged from historical influences to become today's contemporary nursing practice.

HISTORICAL CONTEXT OF NURSING

Key Point: *An understanding of the past can lend insight into the customs, values, and future of nursing.* When exploring history, it becomes apparent that societal beliefs, Christianity, and the military had strong influences on the evolution and images of professional nursing.

Early civilizations had numerous health practices, including massages, hydrotherapy, acupuncture, Roman baths, quarantines, prayer, and dances, to name a few. Their practices were related to societal beliefs about health and illness, as are today's practices. The following are examples:

- In the prehistoric period, illness was thought to be caused by evils spirits that had invaded the body. Care was aimed at removing the evil spirits through ceremonial rituals.
- Early Egyptians prayed to various gods and goddesses to remove illness and maintain health. Women assumed the role of nursing, providing comfort and supportive care to the sick.

Images of Nursing

As you think of each of the three scenarios at the opening of this chapter, what images of the scene and of the nurse do you see? Does each of these images reinforce nursing's legacy of caring? What is your image of yourself as a nurse?

The following are images of the nurse that have developed throughout history—and which persist to a greater or lesser extent even now.

Angel of Mercy This image grew out of the influence of religion and the risks inherent to the practice of nursing. Images of the angel-nurse are usually serene and content, with a halo or other religious symbol.

Battle-Ax The image of the nurse as a battle-ax emerged, as science and philosophy grew popular during the 17th century, when religious orders became less common. A more recent historical example is found in the 1975 film *One Flew Over the Cuckoo's Nest,* in which Nurse Ratched personifies the nurse as the battle-ax or torturer, treating her patients with cruelty and disdain.

Nurse as Professional The battle-ax image of an unprofessional nurse remained until transformed by Florence Nightingale (Fig. 1-1). Florence Nightingale kept meticulous notes and statistics that were used for advocating and obtaining changes in healthcare. She used her political connections and social standing to return nursing to a respectable profession. The Nightingale School for Nurses was opened in 1860 and is considered the first official nursing program.

Naughty Nurse The image of the sexy, risqué nurse arose in the early part of the 20th century with burlesque shows and still persists. For example, in many television programs such as *M*A*S*H* and *Grey's Anatomy*, nurses are portrayed as sexy, mindless, irrelevant, or simply potential dates for bright and talented surgeons.

Military Image Throughout the last century (the 1900s), nurses were frequently portrayed in uniform providing support at the battlefield, and nurses are still often characterized as warriors fighting disease. The impact of wars has had positive influences on the development of nursing as a profession. Nurses took the lead in providing care to the sick, wounded, and dying soldiers in each of the following wars, which highlighted the need for nurses to be trained: American Civil War, Spanish American War, World Wars I and II; and the Korean, Vietnam, Iraq, and Afghanistan conflicts.

Handmaiden Image This stereotype portrays the male physician in the dominant role, with the female nurse merely assisting the doctor, or perhaps supporting the patient at the bedside. This image grew out of the nurse's early limited role in healing, from the legal and financial authority of physicians, and from the nurse's work position as an employee.

Nursing Today: Full-Spectrum Nursing

Nurses today are highly trained, well educated, caring, and competent professionals. They are essential members of the healthcare team. The complexity of the healthcare delivery requires that nurses use their critical thinking, communication, organizational, leadership, advocacy, and technical skills to ensure that patients receive safe and effective care.

Key Point: *Nurses apply knowledge from the arts and sciences in their various roles to provide patient-centered care (Table 1-1).*

Nurses use clinical judgment, critical thinking, and problem-solving as they care for patients. (You will learn more about full-spectrum nursing in the section in Chapter 2, What Is Full-Spectrum Nursing?)

To provide safe care, nurses must carefully consider their actions and think carefully about the patient, the treatment plan, the healthcare environment, the patient's support system, the nurse's support system and resources, and safety.

Clinical judgment involves observing, comparing, contrasting, and evaluating the client's condition to determine whether change has occurred. It also involves careful consideration of the client's health status in light of what is expected based on the client's condition, medications, and treatment. These actions, collectively known as nursing process, are discussed in Chapters 3 through 7 and in each of the clinically focused chapters.

Critical thinking is a reflective thinking process that involves collecting information, analyzing the adequacy and accuracy of the information, and carefully considering options for action. Nurses use critical thinking in every aspect of nursing care. Critical thinking is discussed at length in Chapter 2 and applied in every chapter in this text.

Problem-solving is a process by which nurses consider an issue and attempt to find a satisfactory solution to achieve the best outcomes. You will often use problem-solving in your professional life. The nursing process (see Chapters 2–7) is one type of problem-solving process.

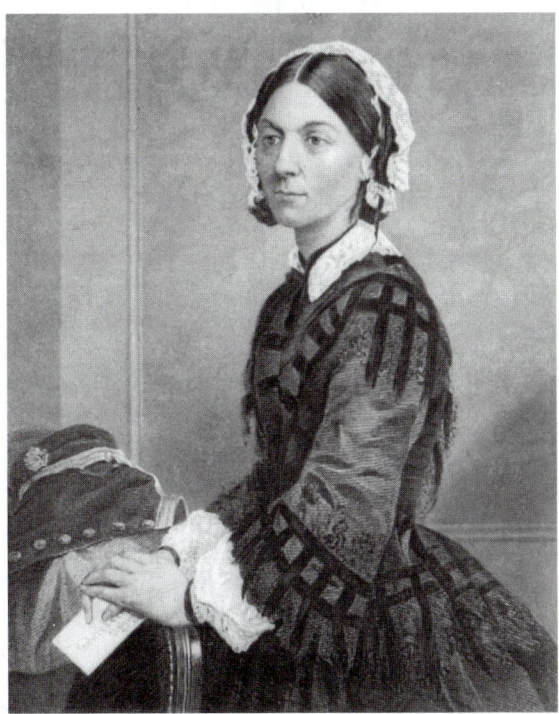

FIGURE 1-1 Florence Nightingale (1820–1910).

Table 1-1 ➤ Roles and Functions of the Nurse

ROLE	FUNCTION	EXAMPLES
Direct care provider	Addressing the physical, emotional, social, and spiritual needs of the client	Listening to lung sounds Giving medications Patient teaching
Communicator	Using interpersonal and therapeutic communication skills to address the needs of the client, to facilitate communication in the healthcare team, and to advise the community about health promotion and disease prevention	Counseling a client Discussing staffing needs at a unit meeting Providing HIV education at a local school
Client/family educator	Assessing and diagnosing the teaching needs of the client, group, family, or community. Once the diagnosis is made, nurses plan how to meet these needs, implement the teaching plan, and evaluate its effectiveness.	Preoperative teaching Prenatal education for siblings Community classes on nutrition
Client advocate	Supporting clients' right to make healthcare decisions when they are able to voice their opinions and protecting clients from harm when they are unable to make decisions	Helping a client explain to his family that he does not want to have further chemotherapy
Counselor	Using therapeutic communication skills to advise clients about health-related issues	Counseling a client on weight-loss strategies
Change agent	Advocating for change on an individual, family, group, community, or societal level that enhances health. The nurse may use counseling, communication, and educator skills to accomplish this change.	Working to improve the nutritional quality of the lunch program at a preschool
Leader	Inspiring others by setting an example of positive health, assertive communication, and willingness to improve	Florence Nightingale Walt Whitman Harriet Tubman
Manager	Coordinating and managing the activities of all members of the team	Charge nurse on a hospital unit (e.g., assigns patients and work to staff nurses)
Case manager	Coordinating the care delivered to a client	Coordinator of services for clients with tuberculosis
Research consumer	Applying evidence-based practice to provide the most appropriate care, to identify clinical problems that warrant research, and to protect the rights of research subjects	Reading journal articles Attending continuing education; seeking additional education

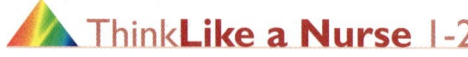 **ThinkLike a Nurse 1-2**

In the three scenarios in Nurses Make a Difference . . . Then & Now, what image of nursing predominates: thinking or doing?

CONTEMPORARY NURSING: EDUCATION, REGULATION, AND PRACTICE

As a student about to enter your new professional life, you need to realistically grasp the nature and demands of your chosen career. To help better acquaint you with nursing today, the remainder of this chapter discusses the current state of nursing, nursing education, and the trends affecting nursing. You will also be introduced to the healthcare delivery system.

How Is Nursing Defined?

As you have seen, there are many images of nursing. These images are only loosely based on fact and sometimes conflict. They make it difficult for the public to know the reality of nursing—and they are confusing to nurses and other members of the healthcare team as

What Are QSEN Competencies?

Competencies: *Patient-Centered Care, Teamwork and Collaboration, Evidence-Based Practice, Quality Improvement, Safety, Informatics**

The QSEN (pronounced cue-zen) competencies are six areas of expertise that nursing students are expected to acquire before graduation. Each competency includes a list of associated knowledge, skills, and attitudes (KSAs) that operationalize the concepts. The six competencies and their definitions are:

- **Patient-centered Care:** Recognize the patient or designee as the source of control and [a] full partner [when] providing compassionate and coordinated care based on respect for patient's preferences, values, and needs.

- **Teamwork and Collaboration:** Function effectively within nursing and interprofessional teams, fostering open communication, mutual respect, and shared decision making to achieve quality patient care.

- **Evidence-based Practice:** Integrate best current evidence with clinical expertise and patient/family preferences and values for delivery of optimal healthcare.

- **Quality Improvement (QI):** Use data to monitor the outcomes of care processes and use improvement methods to design and test changes to continuously improve the quality and safe of HC systems.

- **Safety:** Minimizes risk of harm to patients and providers through both system effectiveness and individual performance.

- **Informatics:** Use information and technology to communicate, manage knowledge, mitigate error, and support decision making.

*To see the KSAs for the QSEN competencies,

 Go to the QSEN Web site, at **http://www.qsen.org/ksas_prelicensure.php**

Source: Cronenwett, Sherwood, Barnsteiner, J., et al. (2007).

well. In addition, the constantly changing nature of nursing, healthcare, and society further complicates the definition of nursing. **Key Point: *Therefore, it is important for nurses to articulate clearly, for themselves and for the public, what nursing is and what nurses do.*** The following sections articulate the views of two important nursing organizations in answer to the question, "What is nursing?"

International Council of Nurses Definition
In 1973 the International Council of Nurses (ICN), an organization representing nurses throughout the world,

defined nursing according to the beliefs of respected theorist Virginia Henderson:

> The unique function of the nurse is to assist the individual, sick or well, in the performance of those activities contributing to health or its recovery (or to peaceful death) that he would perform unaided if he had the necessary strength, will or knowledge. (Henderson, 1966, p. 15)

In the decades since the adoption of this definition, nursing throughout the world has changed. Advances in healthcare have altered the type of care required by clients. Nurses have taken on expanded roles, and once again there is interest in providing care outside the hospital. To reflect these changes, the ICN has revised its definition of nursing, as follows:

> Nursing encompasses autonomous and collaborative care of individuals of all ages, families, groups and communities, sick or well and in all settings. Nursing includes the promotion of health, prevention of illness, and the care of ill, disabled and dying people. Advocacy, promotion of a safe environment, research, participation in shaping health policy and in patient and health systems management, and education are also key nursing roles. (ICN, 2010)

 Think Like a Nurse 1-3

Look at the three scenarios of Nurses Make a Difference ... Then & Now. What nursing actions did the nurses perform that are represented in the ICN definition of nursing?

American Nurses Association Definitions
You can see similar changes in the approach of the American Nurses Association (ANA). In 1980, the ANA defined nursing as "the diagnosis and treatment of human responses to actual and potential health problems" (p. 2). Attempts to refine this definition have been difficult. Nurses are a widely varied group of people with varying skills. They perform activities designed to provide care ranging from basic to complex in a growing number of settings. Therefore, it is not easy to describe the boundaries of the profession.

In 2010, the ANA acknowledged five characteristics of registered nursing:

- Nursing practice is individualized.
- Nurses coordinate care by establishing partnerships (with persons, families, support systems, and other providers).
- Caring is central to the practice of the registered nurse.
- Registered nurses use the nursing process to plan and provide individualized care to their healthcare consumers.
- A strong link exists between the professional work environment and the registered nurse's ability to provide quality healthcare and achieve optimal outcomes. (ANA, 2010, pp. 4–5)

As a result, the ANA redefined professional nursing as:

The protection, promotion, and optimization of health and abilities, prevention of illness and injury, alleviation of suffering through the diagnosis and treatment of human response, and advocacy in the care of individuals, families, communities, and populations. (ANA, 2010, p. 1)

Why Is a Definition Important?

Nursing organizations and leaders have pushed for accurate definitions to (1) help the public understand the value of nursing, (2) describe what activities and roles belong to nursing versus other health professions, and (3) help students and practicing nurses understand what is expected of them within their role as nurses.

From a brief review of nursing history, you can see that nursing has undergone tremendous change, from a role limited to providing kindness and support to full-spectrum work that is based in science but still focuses on care and nurturing. Undoubtedly, nursing will continue to change as nursing knowledge increases and society changes. Box 1-1 lists several additional definitions of nursing for you to consider.

BOX 1-1 ■ What Is Nursing?

- I use the word nursing, for want of a better word. It has been limited to signify little more than the administration of medicines and the application of poultices. It ought to signify the proper use of fresh air, light, warmth, cleanliness, quiet, and the proper choosing and giving of diet—all at the least expense of vital power to the patient. (Nightingale, 1876, p. 5)
- Events that give rise to higher degrees of consideration for those who are helpless or oppressed, kindliness and sympathy for the unfortunate and for those who suffer, tolerance for those of differing religion, race, color, etc.—all tend to promote activities like nursing which are primarily humanitarian. (Dock & Stewart, 1938, p. 3)
- Nursing has been called the oldest of the arts and the youngest of the professions. As such, it has gone through many stages and has been an integral part of societal movements. Nursing has been involved in the existing culture—shaped by it and yet helping to develop it. (Donahue, 1985, p. 3)
- Nurses provide care for people in the midst of health, pain, loss, fear, disfigurement, death, grieving, challenge, growth, birth, and transition on an intimate front-line basis. Expert nurses call this the privileged place of nursing. (Benner & Wrubel, 1989, p. xi)
- Nursing: The care and nurturing of healthy and ill people, individually or in groups and communities. [*Taber's* also includes as a part of the definition the ANA "essential features" involving holism, use of subjective and objective data, application of scientific knowledge, and provision of a caring relationship.] (Venes, D. *Taber's Cyclopedic Medical Dictionary*, 2013)
- Nurses provide and coordinate patient care, educate patients and the public about various health conditions, and provide advice and emotional support to patients and their family members. (Bureau of Labor Statistics, 2012c)

As a student entering nursing, you can use definitions and descriptions to understand what is expected of you. To aid you in this task, refer to Table 1-1 and review the essential components of the nursing role. While in the clinical setting, you will observe nurses functioning in each of these capacities. Nursing is a flexible career that requires you to move effortlessly among these areas to meet the needs of the patient. Nursing requires certain skills and competencies, which you will learn throughout this book. Box 1-2 identifies several qualities that are essential for safe nursing practice.

KnowledgeCheck 1-1

- What factors make it difficult to define nursing?
- Based on the ICN definition of nursing, what does a nurse do?

Is Nursing a Profession, Discipline, or Occupation?

One strategy used to describe a field of work is to categorize it as a profession, discipline, or occupation.

Profession Although the term *profession* is freely used, a group must meet certain criteria to be considered a **profession** (see Table 1-2). Nursing appears to meet all criteria of a profession as defined by Starr (1982) and Miller, Adams, & Beck (1993).

Discipline To be considered a **discipline**, a profession must have a domain of knowledge that has both theoretical and practical boundaries. The **theoretical boundaries** of a profession are the questions that arise from clinical practice and are then investigated through research. The **practical boundaries** are the current state of knowledge and research in the field—the facts that dictate safe practice (Meleis, 1991). A case can be made that nursing is both a profession and a discipline:

- It is a scientifically based and self-governed *profession* that focuses on the ethical care of others.
- It is a *discipline*, driven by aspects of theory and practice. It demands mastery of both theoretical knowledge and clinical skills.

Occupation In spite of meeting criteria for both designations (profession and discipline), nursing is often described as an **occupation**, or job. Unlike physicians, most of whom are in control of their practice environment, working conditions, and schedule, most nurses are hourly wage earners. The employer, not the nurse, decides the conditions of practice and the nature of the work. Nurse practice acts do not prevent nurses from functioning more autonomously, however.

Rather than continuing to develop arguments to "prove" that nursing is a profession, the following actions might do more to improve the status of nursing:

- Standardizing the educational requirements for entry into practice
- Enacting uniform continuing education requirements

BOX 1-2 ■ Important Qualities for Nurses

Critical-Thinking Skills

Required Action: Monitor the patient, note changes, and take actions to ensure safe and effective care.

Example: Call the physician to get a stronger pain medication for a patient who, 2 hrs after receiving pain medication, rates his pain 7 out of 10.

Caring and Compassion

Required Action: Show kindness, concern, and warmth that shows patients that you care and are concern about their well-being.

Example: Sit with and hold the hand of a patient who has just been told that he has a terminal illness.

Detail Oriented

Required Action: Pay attention to details to prevent and identify errors in care that may be harmful to the patient.

Example: Seek clarification and correct a dosage that is written as 7 mg that should be 0.7 mg.

Organizational Skills

Required Action: Prioritize the needs of your patient and meet the needs of the most critical patients first.

Example: Care for the patient with difficulty breathing prior to performing a dressing change on a postoperative patient.

Speaking Skills

Required Action: Communicate correct and pertinent information to patients and members of the healthcare team.

Example: Teach the patient how to perform a dressing change at home after discharge from the hospital.

Listening Skills

Required Action: Listen to patients' concerns and take verbal or telephone orders from providers.

Example: The provider telephones you and gives you orders to implement for your patient.

Patience

Required Action: In stressful situations in the work environment, think clearly and take the correct actions.

Example: Remains calm when a patient's condition deteriorates, provides the needed care, and transfers the patient to the ICU.

Competence

Required Action: Knowledge and skills to ensure safe, quality patient outcomes.

Example: Recognize that the correct dose for the drug is 0.10 mg rather than 10 mg.

_____

Adapted from Bureau of Labor Statistics (2012c). How to become a registered nurse. http://www.bls.gov/ooh/healthcare/registered-nurses.htm#tab-4

Table 1-2 ➤ Nursing: Is It a Profession?	
STARR CRITERION	**EXAMPLES IN NURSING**
The knowledge of the group must be based on technical and scientific knowledge.	■ Entry-level nursing education requires coursework in basic and social sciences as well as humanities, arts, and general education. ■ Nursing education and practice are increasingly based on research from nursing and related fields.
The knowledge and competence of members of the group must be evaluated by a community of peers.	■ State or provincial regulatory bodies have defined the criteria that nurses must meet to practice, and they monitor members for adherence to standards.
The group must have a service orientation and a code of ethics.	■ Nursing is clearly focused on providing service to others. ■ The major professional organizations have developed ethical guidelines to guide the practice of nursing.

- Encouraging the participation of more nurses in professional organizations
- Educating the public about the true nature of nursing practice

 ThinkLike **a Nurse** 1-4

Evaluate the status of nursing. Is nursing a respected profession? Give examples to support your opinion.

How Do Nurses' Educational Paths Differ?

The transition into the nursing profession involves formal and informal processes. **Formal education** consists of completing the initial and continuing education required for licensure. **Informal education** involves a gradual progression in skill and clinical judgment that allows the nurse to advance in the profession.

Formal Education

When the patient calls out "Nurse!" who can respond? To legally use the title *nurse,* a person must be a graduate of an accredited nursing education program and have successfully passed the National Council Licensure Examination (NCLEX). Students may enter nursing through two paths: as a practical nurse or a registered nurse. Other personnel may respond to the patient's call, but they cannot legally be considered nurses.

Practical and Vocational Nursing Education

Practical nursing education prepares nurses to provide bedside care to clients. Practical nurses are known as licensed practical nurses (LPNs) or licensed vocational nurses (LVNs) in a few states. In the United States a student who wishes to become an LPN/LVN may attend one of approximately 1,200 approved programs given at technical schools and community colleges. Educational programs for LPN/LVNs offer both classroom and clinical teaching and usually last 1 year. After completing the practical nursing education program, the student must pass the NCLEX-PN exam. Practical nurses provide basic care and work under the direction of the registered nurse (RN) or the primary care provider. The majority of LVN/LPNs work in nursing care facilities. Their job growth is expected to grow 21% between 2008 and 2018 based on the increased growth of the aging population (Bureau of Labor Statistics, 2012a).

Registered Nursing Entry Education

Currently, five educational pathways lead to licensure as a registered nurse (RN). Graduates of all these programs must successfully complete the NCLEX-RN exam to practice as RNs.

- **Diploma programs**. These hospital-based programs are the oldest type of nursing education. They were modeled after the Nightingale Schools of Nursing apprenticeship style of learning. This method of preparing nurses was the mainstay of nursing education from the mid-1800s to the 1960s. The typical program lasts 3 years and focuses on clinical experience in direct patient care. Since the 1960s the number of diploma programs has steadily decreased. In 2011, only about 4% of nursing schools were diploma programs (Kaufman, 2012). About 20% of RNs in the United States reported receiving their initial education in a diploma program in 2008 compared with 63% in 1980 (Health Resources and Services Administration, 2010). The number of diploma programs decreased from 75 in 2007 to 69 in 2008 (National League for Nursing, 2010).
- **Associate degree programs.** This type of program, conceptualized by Mildred Montag, emerged during the nursing shortage following World War II. Most associate degree (AD) programs are offered in community colleges. Although the nursing component typically lasts 2 years, students are required to take many other courses in the liberal arts and sciences. In 2008, 45% of RNs in the United States reported receiving their initial education in an AD program (Health Resources and Services Administration, 2010). The student is prepared to provide direct patient care. The number of AD programs increased from 1,023 in 2008 to 1,031 in 2009 (NLN, 2010).
- **Baccalaureate degree programs.** Students in baccalaureate (BSN) programs pursue a course of study like

that of other undergraduate students. The course of study lasts for at least eight semesters. Students are prepared to address complex clinical situations, provide direct patient care, work in community care, use research, and enter graduate education (Bureau of Labor Statistics, 2012c). In 2008, BSN graduates accounted for 34% of RNs in the United States (Health Resources and Services Administration, 2010). The number of BSN programs increased by two in 2008 to 683. Many AD graduates enter RN-to-BSN (or RN "completion") programs to obtain a baccalaureate degree in nursing. The length of time required to complete the BSN varies according to the program and the number of credits each student can transfer. The goal is to increase the proportion of baccalaureate-prepared nurses to 80% by the year 2020 (Institute of Medicine, 2011).

- **Master's entry programs.** The typical student in these programs has a baccalaureate degree in another field and has entered nursing as a second career. Programs usually are completed in 3 years of full-time study, with the first year devoted to basic nursing content. At the completion, the student is eligible to take the licensing exam and is awarded a master's degree in nursing.
- **Doctoral entry.** This is the most unusual entry pathway into nursing. The nursing doctorate (ND) path parallels the pathway through which physicians enter the healthcare field. This entry path has very limited enrollment.

For several decades, nursing leaders have debated about the most appropriate educational pathway for entry into the profession. For an overview of this debate,

 Go to Chapter 1, **Expanded Discussion: Nursing History, Entry Into Practice Debate,** on *DavisPlus*.

Graduate Nursing Education

Graduate nursing education prepares the RN for advanced practice, expanded roles, or research. **Master's degree programs** prepare RNs to function in a more independent and autonomous role, such as nurse practitioner, clinical specialist, nurse educator, or nursing administration. It typically takes 2 years or longer to complete the master's degree. **Doctoral programs** in nursing offer professional degrees. Typically the student has completed a baccalaureate and master's degree before entry into a doctoral program. Doctoral degree programs in nursing offer the Doctor of Nursing Practice (DNP) or the Doctor of Nursing Science (DSN/DNSc). The DNS/DNSc focuses on nursing research and the DNP is a practice doctorate. The popularity of the DNP has created concerns that the growth of nursing research will decline. Some nurses obtain a Doctor of Philosophy (PhD), another research degree. For additional discussion on expanded nurse roles, see the section on Expanded Career Roles later in this chapter.

Other Forms of Formal Education

Advances in healthcare have a strong influence on nursing practice. Since nurses must keep current in their practice, you will be socialized to the concept of "nurses as lifelong learners." This means that you must engage in continuing education to enhance your intellectual and practical knowledge throughout your nursing career.

- **Continuing education** is a professional strategy to help you stay current in your clinical knowledge. Continuing education programs are available at work sites, at local colleges and universities, through privately operated educational groups, on the Internet, and in professional journals. In many states, renewal of the nursing license requires successful completion of a specified number of continuing education courses. Some states allow nurses to take any approved coursework, while others have specific requirements in special areas, such as HIV/AIDS, bioterrorism, and domestic violence. The regulations for continuing education change frequently. Your state board of nursing (SBN) will notify you of continuing education requirements, if any, when you receive your initial nursing license. Thereafter, the SBN will notify you by e-mail or postal mail of any changes in the requirements. For an overview of the continuing education requirements for license renewal in the United States,

> Go to Chapter I, **ESG Table I-1, Continuing Education Requirements for Nurses,** on Davis*Plus*.

- **In-service education** is another form of ongoing education. It is offered at the work place, and usually does not count toward meeting the continuing education requirement for license renewal. In-service education is typically institution specific and product specific, and provides information on pertinent changes in nursing. For instance, in-service education might focus on the use of new equipment, the introduction of new policies, or it may resemble traditional continuing education programs. It is designed to enhance your continued competence in knowledge, skills, and attitude.

Informal Education

In addition to formal programs of study, education also requires socialization into the profession. **Socialization** is the informal education that occurs as you move into your new profession. It is the knowledge gained from direct experience, observation in the real world, and informal discussion with peers and colleagues. **Key Point:** *Professional socialization begins when you enter the educational program and continues as you gain expertise throughout your career.* Informal education complements formal education to create clinical competence.

Benner's Model

Patricia Benner (1984) described the process by which a nurse acquires clinical skills and judgment. As this process shows, expertise is not merely a demonstration of skilled application of knowledge, but rather a personal integration of knowledge that requires technical skill, thoughtful application, and insight. This is what we mean in this text when we use the term *full-spectrum nursing*. Expertise requires both thinking and doing skills.

- *Stage 1: Novice.* This phase begins with the onset of your education. The novice nurse has little nursing experience and is at the first stage of acquiring clinical knowledge. At this stage, you are task oriented and focus narrowly on "learning the rules." For example, when performing a sterile dressing change, you may be so concerned with following the steps in the skills checklist that you forget to assess the patient's reaction to the procedure.

- *Stage 2: Advanced beginner.* A new graduate usually functions at this level. An advanced beginner begins to focus on more aspects of a clinical situation, use more facts, make more sophisticated use of the rules, and recognize similarities in situations. The nurse can distinguish abnormal findings, but cannot readily understand their significance. For example, a new graduate assesses that her postoperative abdominal surgical patient's blood pressure has decreased and his pulse rate has increased, and he has become more restless during the last 2 hours. An advanced beginner will report these as changes, but does not recognize that these signs/symptoms may indicate early blood loss. After considerable exposure to clinical situations, nurses improve in performance and, through repeated experiences or mentoring, begin to recognize the elements of a situation.

- *Stage 3: Competence.* Nurses achieve competence after 2 to 3 years of nursing practice in the same area. Competent performers have gained additional experience and wrestle with more complex concerns. They are able to handle their patient load and prioritize situations. They are also more involved in their caregiving role and may be emotionally involved in the clinical choices made. Although competent nurses manage clinical care with mastery, they often do not fully grasp the overall scope and most important aspects. The competent nurse would immediately connect the changes in the vital signs with the surgical procedure, recognize possible early signs of shock, and conduct a more in-depth assessment.

- *Stage 4: Proficient.* The proficient nurse is able to quickly take in all aspects of a situation and immediately give meaning to the cluster of assessment data, and serves as a resource for less experienced nurses. Proficient nurses are able to see the "big picture" and can coordinate services and forecast needs. For example, they would immediately recognize a patient's symptoms as a possible heart attack, pulmonary embolus, or brain attack (stroke) and immediately gather the resources to initiate treatment. They are much more flexible and fluent with their role and able to adapt to nuances of various patient situations. Proficient nurses plan intuitively as well as consciously.

- *Stage 5: Expert.* Expert nurses are able to see what needs to be achieved and how to do it. They trust in and use their intuition while operating with a deep understanding of a situation, often recognizing a problem in the absence of the classic signs and symptoms. They have expert skills and are often consulted when others need advice or assistance.

Benner's model deals with the development of clinical wisdom and competence. Keep in mind that this progression is not automatic. Nurses do not simply move through the stages as they gain experience. Instead, this model assumes that to improve in skill and judgment, nurses must also be attuned to each clinical situation. This requires an ability to take in information from a variety of sources and to notice subtle variations. Although expertise (Stage 5) is a goal, not everyone can achieve this level.

Nursing Organization Guidelines

The ANA and other organizations are also involved in helping nurses to continue to improve their practice (e.g., by setting standards and articulating nursing values). For example, in the Code for Nurses, the ANA provides guidelines for nurses to conduct themselves in their day-to-day practice. These guidelines describe acceptable and unacceptable professional behaviors and identify values to help improve your practice and participation in the profession. Box 1-3 presents some values and behaviors associated with nursing. See Chapter 44 for further discussion of nursing values and the ANA Code for Nurses.

KnowledgeCheck 1-2

- Compare and contrast formal and informal education.
- Name and describe five educational pathways leading to licensure as an RN.

How Is Nursing Practice Regulated?

Nursing practice in the United States is regulated by laws and professional organizations' standards of practice.

Nurse Practice Acts In the United States, each state enacts its own **nurse practice act**—laws that regulate nursing practice. The state board of nursing is the agency responsible for regulating nursing practice. The board is charged with protecting the health, safety, and welfare of the general public. Although there are minor variations, each board of nursing is responsible for:

- Approving nursing education programs
- Defining the practice of professional nursing

- Establishing criteria that allow a person to be licensed as a registered nurse (RN) or licensed practical or vocational nurse (LPN/LVN)
- Defining professional practice, which determines the nurse's scope of practice or those activities that nurses are expected to perform (and by implications, those they may not)
- Developing rules and regulations for guidance to nurses
- Enforcing the rules that govern nursing

Key Point: *To practice nursing, you must be licensed as a nurse. Licenses are issued by the state.* All states require graduation from an approved nursing program and successful completion of the National Council Licensure Exam (NCLEX). To receive licensure in another state, the nurse simply applies for licensure by endorsement (reciprocity) or follows the guidance of the mutual recognition model. For further details about licensing and the regulation of nursing practice, see Chapter 45.

Standards of Practice Nursing is also guided by standards of practice, which "describe a competent level of nursing practice and professional performance common to all registered nurses. . . . They are authoritative statements of the duties that all registered nurses, regardless of role, population, or specialty, are expected to perform competently" (ANA, 2010, p. 2). Standards provide a guide to the knowledge, skills, and attitudes (KSAs) that nurses must incorporate into their practice to provide safe, quality care. Standards are used by individual nurses, employers of nurses, professional organizations, and other professions.

As a student of nursing, you may use the ANA standards of nursing practice to get a better understanding of nursing (Table 1-3). Practicing nurses use the standards to judge their own performance, develop an improvement plan, and understand what employers expect of them. Employers incorporate the standards into annual evaluation tools at hospitals and health facilities. Professional organizations use the standards to educate the public about nursing, to plan for continuing education programs for nurses, and to guide their efforts at lobbying and other activities that advocate for nurses. Finally, other professions read the standards of practice to examine the boundaries between nursing and other health professions.

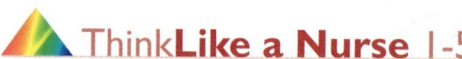 ThinkLike a Nurse 1-5

What additional information have you learned about nursing from your review of the ANA standards of practice?

What Are Some Important Nursing Organizations?

Numerous organizations are involved in the profession of nursing. Some of the most influential are discussed here.

BOX 1-3 ■ Nursing Values and Behaviors

- The nurse's primary concern is the good of the patient.
- Nurses ought to be competent.
- Nurses demonstrate a strong commitment to service.
- Nurses believe in the dignity and worth of each person.
- Nurses constantly strive to improve their profession.
- Nurses work collaboratively within the profession.

Table 1-3 ➤ American Nurses Association: Scope and Standards of Clinical Nursing Practice

STANDARDS OF CARE

Standard 1	Assessment	The registered nurse collects comprehensive data pertinent to the healthcare consumer's health and/or the situation.
Standard 2	Diagnosis	The registered nurse analyzes the assessment data to determine the diagnoses or issues.
Standard 3	Outcome Identification	The registered nurse identifies expected outcomes for a plan individualized to the healthcare consumer or situation.
Standard 4	Planning	The registered nurse develops a plan that prescribes strategies and alternatives to attain expected outcomes.
Standard 5	Implementation	The registered nurse implements the identified plan.
Standard 5A	Coordination of Care	The registered nurse coordinates care delivery.
Standard 5B	Health Teaching and Health Promotion	The registered nurse employs strategies to promote health and a safe environment.
Standard 5C	Consultation	The graduate-level prepared specialty nurse or advanced practice registered nurse provides consultation to influence the identified plan, enhance the abilities of others, and effect change.
Standard 5D	Prescriptive Authority and Treatment	The advanced practice registered nurse uses prescriptive authority, procedures, referrals, treatments, and therapies in accordance with state and federal laws and regulations.
Standard 6	Evaluation	The registered nurse evaluates progress toward attainment of outcomes.

STANDARDS OF PROFESSIONAL PERFORMANCE

Standard 7	Ethics	The registered nurse practices ethically.
Standard 8	Education	The registered nurse attains knowledge and competency that reflects current nursing practice.
Standard 9	Evidence-Based Practice and Research	The registered nurse integrates evidence and research findings into practice.
Standard 10	Quality of Practice	The registered nurse contributes to quality nursing practice.
Standard 11	Communication	The registered nurse communicates effectively in all areas of practice.
Standard 12	Leadership	The registered nurse demonstrates leadership in the professional practice setting and the profession.
Standard 13	Collaboration	The registered nurse collaborates with healthcare consumer, family, and others in the conduct of nursing practice.
Standard 14	Professional Practice Evaluation	The registered nurse evaluates his or her own nursing practice in relation to professional practice standards and guidelines, relevant statutes, rules, and regulations.
Standard 15	Resource Utilization	The registered nurse utilizes appropriate resources to plan and provide nursing services that are safe, effective, and financially responsible.
Standard 16	Environmental Health	The registered nurse practices in an environmentally safe and healthy manner.

American Nurses Association (2010). *Nursing: Scope and Standards of Practice* (2nd ed). Silver Spring, MD: Nursebooks.org.

American Nurses Association

The American Nurses Association (ANA) is the official professional organization for nurses in the United States. The ANA was formed in 1911 from an organization previously known as the Nurses' Associated Alumnae of the United States and Canada. Originally, the ANA focused on establishing standards of nursing to promote high-quality care and work toward licensure as a means of ensuring adherence to the standards.

The ANA continues to update its standards. Representatives are elected from the local branches of the state organizations to bring their concerns to the national level. As such, they track healthcare legislation, serve as liaisons with national government representatives to inform them of how current and proposed legislation will affect nursing, and develop and sponsor legislation that will have a positive effect on nursing and on patient care. The ANA publishes educational materials on nursing news, issues, and standards. The official publication of the ANA is *The American Nurse*.

National League for Nursing

Originally founded as the American Society of Superintendents of Training Schools for Nurses in 1893, the National League for Nursing (NLN) was the first nursing organization with a goal to establish and maintain a universal standard of education. The NLN sets standards for all types of nursing education programs, studies the nursing workforce, lobbies and participates with other major healthcare organizations to set policy for the nursing workforce, aids faculty development, funds research on nursing education, and publishes the journal *Nursing Education Perspectives*.

International Council of Nursing

The International Council of Nursing (ICN) represents more than 13 million nurses on a global level. It is composed of a federation of national nursing organizations from more than 130 nations. The ICN aims to ensure quality nursing care for all, supports global health policies that advance nursing and improve worldwide health, and strives to improve working conditions for nurses throughout the world.

National Student Nurses Association

The National Student Nurses Association (NSNA) represents nursing students in the United States. It is the student counterpart of the ANA. Like the ANA, this association comprises elected volunteers who advocate on behalf of student nurses. The NSNA sponsors yearly conventions to address the concerns of nursing students. Local chapters are usually organized at individual schools. The NSNA also publishes *Image*, a journal dedicated to nursing student issues.

Sigma Theta Tau International

Sigma Theta Tau International (STTI) is the international honor society for nursing. Membership includes the clinical, education, and nursing research communities and senior level baccalaureate and graduate programs. The goal of this organization is to foster nursing scholarship, leadership, service, and research to improve health worldwide. The official publication of STTI is the *Journal of Nursing Scholarship*.

Specialty Organizations

Numerous specialty organizations have developed around clinical specialties, group identification, or similarly held values. Here are some examples:

- *Clinical specialty.* Association of Operating Room Nurses (AORN), Association of Nurses in AIDS Care (ANAC), Emergency Nurses Association (ENA)
- *Group identification.* National Organization for Associate Degree Nursing (NOADN), National Association of Hispanic Nurses (NAHN), American Assembly for Men in Nursing (AMN)
- *Similar values.* Nurses Christian Fellowship (NCF), Nursing Ethics Network (NEN)

To explore Web sites of a variety of nursing organizations,

 Go to Chapter 1, **Resources for Caregivers and Health Professionals,** on Davis*Plus*.

Nursing Practice: Caring for Clients

Look again at the definitions of nursing you have read in this chapter (e.g., see Box 1-1). Notice that they all agree that nursing is about caring for clients. Recent studies show that when the proportion of RNs increases in an agency, quality of care rises, death and infection rates drop (Potera, 2007), and length of stay is shorter by at least 30% (Kane, Shamliyan, Mueller, et al., 2007). Studies also show that smaller nurse-to-patient ratios (i.e., when each nurse cared for fewer patients) were related to positive patient outcomes, lower patient mortality, improved detection of pre-discharge infections, less nurse burnout, and higher job satisfaction for nurses (Aiken, Sloane, Cimiotti, et al., 2010; Penoyer, 2010; Unruh & Zhang, 2012).

Who Are the Recipients of Nursing Care?

The recipients of nursing care may be individuals, groups, families, communities, or societies. They can be referred to as patients, clients, or persons. **Direct care** involves personal interaction between the nurse and clients (e.g., giving medications, dressing a wound, or teaching a client about medicines or care). Nurses engage in **indirect care** when they work on behalf of an individual, group, family, or community to improve their health status (e.g., restocking the code blue cart [an emergency cart], ordering unit supplies, arranging unit staffing, or serving on an ethics committee). A nurse may use independent judgment to determine the care needed or may work under the direct order of a primary care provider.

As a nurse, however, you should not view patients as passive recipients of care. Nurses should respect and actively support patients' right to make decisions about their healthcare, and facilitate their participation as collaborative members of the healthcare team.

What Are the Purposes of Nursing Care?

Nurses provide care to achieve the goals of health promotion, illness prevention, health restoration, and end-of-life care. Together these aspects of care represent a range of services that cover the spectrum from complete well-being to death. Nurses plan patient care to ensure consistency of care over time, individualize care according to patient needs, ensure that holistic care is provided, and collaborate with the interdisciplinary health team for optimal patient outcomes.

Where Do Nurses Work?

As a nurse you will have the opportunity to work in a variety of settings. During your education you will have assignments in many clinical units and environments that will allow you to see some of the options available to you upon graduation. Approximately 62% of nurses work in hospitals. The remaining 38% work in extended care facilities, ambulatory care, home health settings, public health, or nursing education (Health Resources and Services Administration, 2010).

What Models of Care Are Used to Provide Nursing Care?

Nursing care is structured in a variety of ways. The organization of the nursing team reflects the philosophy and beliefs of the institution, as well as the prevailing views on nursing. The structure of the team is often referred to as the *model of care*. The most common models include the following:

Case Method The **case method**, also called *total care*, is one-to-one care; one nurse provides all aspects of care for one patient during a single shift. An inpatient may have a different nurse on each shift. Although this method may be satisfying for patients and nurses, high costs limit its use. The case method is used in intensive care, labor and delivery, and private duty care. In this method, the patient's needs are quickly met, the nurse and patient work more closely together, and the nurse has a greater degree of autonomy.

Functional Nursing In **functional nursing**, care is compartmentalized, with each task assigned to a staff member with the appropriate knowledge and skills. For example, the nursing assistant may give bed baths and make beds, the LPN/LVN may distribute medications, and the RN may be in charge and perform ordered treatments. This approach requires a clear understanding of what tasks are required to deliver care in each unit. Although this approach is economical and efficient when the unit is short staffed, it can easily lead to fragmentation

of care—meaning that it is difficult for the nurse to fully grasp the patient's "whole picture."

Team Nursing The **team approach** is an efficient arrangement for delivering nursing care and maintains the cost saving of functional nursing while attempting to limit fragmentation. In team nursing, a licensed nurse (RN or LPN/ LVN) is paired with a nursing assistant or nursing assistive personnel. The team is then assigned to a group of patients. Teams led by RNs are assigned to high-acuity patients. Team nursing is popular during times of nursing shortages (Holt, 2011; Wood, 2007).

Primary Nursing In **primary nursing**, one nurse manages care for a group of patients. The primary nurse assesses the patient and develops a plan of care. When she is at work, she provides care for the patients for whom she is responsible. In her absence, associate nurses deliver care and implements the plan developed by the primary nurse.

Differentiated Practice **Differentiated practice** is a variation of primary nursing. It recognizes that education and experience lead to differences in the care delivered by nurses. For this system to work, each nursing unit must identify the types of expertise needed by its patients, and the nursing competencies required to deliver that care. Once this has been developed, individual nurses put together a portfolio to demonstrate their competencies. Nurses who have the necessary competencies care for patients.

HEALTHCARE DELIVERY SYSTEM

The healthcare delivery system in the United States is a unique and complex collection of patients, providers, facilities, vendors, and rules. The rest of this chapter is designed to help you gain a beginner's understanding of the U.S. healthcare system. You will need to know the various components of the system to understand the continuum of healthcare patients receive, providers involved in that care, and factors that influence the type and amount of care patients receive.

Where Is Healthcare Provided?

Patients can receive treatment in a variety of environments based on their needs. Hospitals, extended care facilities, ambulatory care centers, and home healthcare agencies are the most visible sites for delivery of healthcare. A patient who has been admitted to a healthcare facility is an **inpatient**. An **outpatient** is a person who receives treatment at a facility, but does not stay overnight. Inpatient services occur in various hospital settings.

Hospitals

Hospitals are the most expensive and the most frequently used site for care. They provide a broad range of services to treat various injuries and disease processes (Fig. 1-2). Hospitals vary in size, ownership, and the

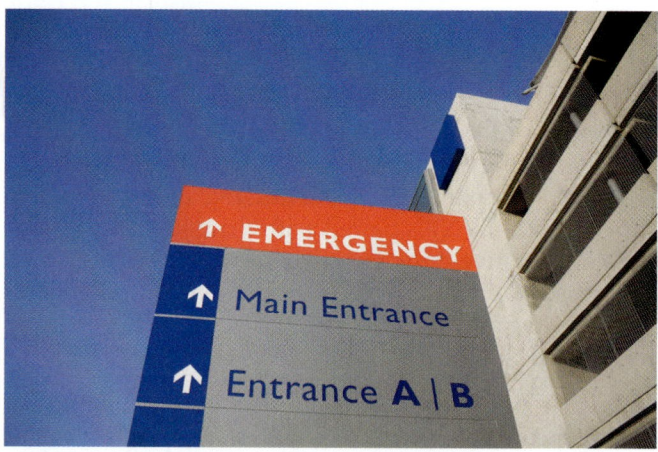

FIGURE 1-2 Emergency rooms have become the primary source of healthcare for the uninsured.

services provided. Small rural facilities may have only 8 to 12 beds. In contrast, large metropolitan medical centers might exceed a 1,200-bed capacity. Small hospitals offer basic services, whereas larger medical centers usually offer additional and specialty services. Basic services include inpatient beds, radiology, and laboratory services. Hospitals usually have an emergency department, diagnostic centers, and various units such as intensive care, medical, surgical, pediatrics, and maternal newborn.

A large percentage (62%) of RNs are employed in hospitals (Health Resources and Services Administration, 2010). Hospitals are distinguished from other healthcare facilities because they employ nurses, allied health therapists, physicians, case managers, pharmacists, and many other persons to ensure the acute care needs of the patient are met around the clock. The length of stay is limited to the amount of time that the patient requires 24-hour observation.

As a result of research and technology, many hospitals have sophisticated equipment to deliver the highest quality healthcare available. This progress has lengthened life spans in many cases but has at the same time increased the costs of care. Technological advances and efforts to control costs have had the following effects:

- *Larger Hospitals.* The number of community hospitals and hospital beds has declined, and larger regional facilities have emerged in their place.
- *Specialty Hospitals.* Hospitals may specialize in order to reduce redundancies in healthcare within a local community. For example, one hospital might be the regional tertiary cardiac care center, while another provides oncology (cancer) services. Specialization minimizes expense from duplicating costly specialized equipment and specially trained personnel for each individual site.
- *Shorter Length of Stay.* Patients' length of stay has decreased overall. For example, in the 1950s a patient having surgery for gallbladder removal would remain in the hospital for at least 10 days. Now, this surgery is

usually performed on an outpatient basis. Only those patients who require 24-hour care are hospitalized. Even after cardiac surgery, a typical patient remains hospitalized for only 4 days. As soon as the patient is stabilized, she is relocated to home or less expensive sites of care, such as extended care facilities or rehabilitation centers.

Extended Care Facilities

Extended care facilities provide care for clients for an extended period of time—usually longer than 1 month. As the length of stay in hospitals has declined, extended care facilities have begun to deliver services that were previously provided in the hospital. These facilities include nursing homes, skilled nursing facilities (also known as convalescent hospitals), and rehabilitation facilities. The distinction among them is based primarily on whether they provide skilled or custodial care.

Skilled care includes services of trained professionals that are needed for a limited period of time after an injury or illness. These "skilled" services include wound care, infusions, teaching, and ongoing monitoring of patient status. Skilled care patients are those who can be expected to improve with treatment. For example, a patient who no longer needs hospitalization may transfer to a skilled nursing facility until she is able to return home. Many extended care facilities have designated units, often called subacute units that provide post-hospitalization skilled care.

Custodial care consists of help with activities of daily living: bathing, dressing, eating, grooming, ambulation, toileting, and other care that people typically do for themselves (e.g., taking medications, monitoring blood glucose levels).

Residents in extended care facilities are most commonly older adults, but clients of any age who require assistance with self-care activities, such as hygiene, toileting, and dressing, may live in these facilities. Because of the aging population and increased longevity of patients with traumatic injuries and chronic diseases, the number of patients requiring long-term care, as well as the number of facilities providing these services, is expected to increase.

Nursing Homes A **nursing home** provides custodial care for people who cannot live on their own but are not sick enough to require hospitalization. It provides a room, custodial care, and recreation and may be a permanent residence for people who require continual supervision to ensure their safety. A physician for each patient supervises care. In the United States approximately 15,690 nursing homes provide care for approximately 1.7 million residents (Centers for Medicare & Medicaid Services, 2010).

Rehabilitation Centers Rehabilitation centers provide extended care and treatment for patients with physical and mental illness. Types of services include alcohol and drug rehabilitation, physical rehabilitation services for patients who have experienced traumatic injuries, and rehabilitation of patients after stroke or heart attack. Rehabilitation services may be inpatient, outpatient, or a combination. Nurses work in direct patient care, counseling, and coordination of care. Because of the lengthy time frame for this care, nurses at rehabilitation centers have an ongoing relationship with their patients. Rehabilitation often involves a multidisciplinary, collaborative approach with weekly team and family conferences to discuss the treatment plan. A variety of providers and therapists are involved in the patients care to help them reach their optimal level of functioning. These are discussed later in the chapter.

Assisted Living Facilities Assisted living facilities were designed to bridge the gap between independence and institutionalization for older adults who have a decline in health status and cannot live alone independently. Residents of these facilities are able to perform self-care activities, but require assistance with meals, housekeeping, or medications. Nurses have a limited presence at assisted living sites because residents typically travel from their homes to the physician and other service providers.

Ambulatory Care Centers

Ambulatory care centers are used by people to get same-day cost-effective healthcare. Ambulatory care is synonymous with *outpatient care* and provides services for clients who are able to come and go from the facility. Clients live at home or in nonhospital settings and come to the site for care. Ambulatory care sites include private health and medical offices, clinics, and outpatient therapy centers. Low-cost, walk-in, retail clinics have expanded rapidly—in shopping centers, pharmacies, and other retail sites. Typically they treat only common ailments and refer complex or serious illnesses to specialized physicians or emergency rooms (Darcé, 2007). To keep the cost of healthcare down, more and more services are being provided in ambulatory facilities, such as chemotherapy or outpatient surgeries. Ambulatory centers may be connected to hospitals (Fig. 1-3).

Home Healthcare Agencies

Home healthcare agencies provide continuing care to patients after hospitalization. Home care is provided (a) when clients are homebound or unable to get to ambulatory care centers for services; (b) when the client or family prefers to receive care in the home—particularly when the client is terminally ill; and (c) when a client still requires skilled care but is discharged from the hospital because his reimbursable length-of-stay has expired. Services are usually coordinated by a home health or visiting nurse service and include nursing care as well as various therapies and home assistance programs. Chapter 43 provides further discussion on home health nursing.

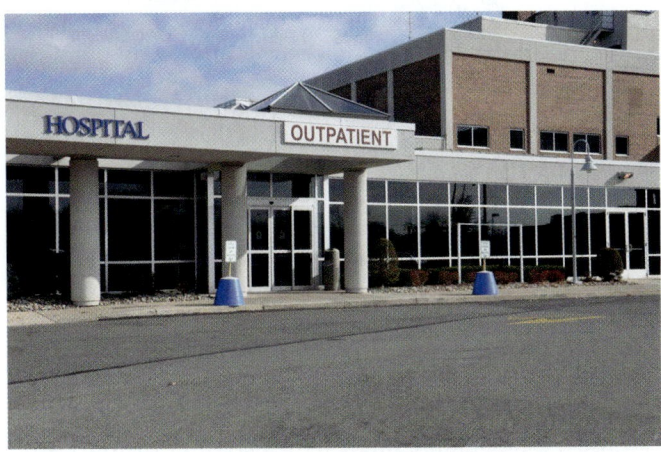

FIGURE 1-3 The shift to outpatient care is a cost-saving strategy.

Community/Public Health Centers

Community or public health centers are community-based centers that provide care for the community at large. Community health nurses provide services to at-risk populations and devise strategies to improve the health status of the surrounding community. Examples of community health programs include healthcare for the homeless and school-based programs designed to decrease the incidence of teen pregnancies.

Community care is a comprehensive term that describes the care provided to client groups at various sites, such as church, schools, shelters, the workplace, and public clinics. Care focuses on populations (e.g., older adults, pregnant women, employees at a manufacturing plant), neighborhoods, and at-risk groups (e.g., pregnant teens, victims of domestic violence, substance abusers). Chapter 43 provides further discussion of community healthcare.

Independent Living Facilities

Also known as retirement homes, **independent living facilities** are designed for seniors 55 years or older who (a) are independent in all aspects and (b) want to live in a community with other senior citizens. They may not want the responsibilities associated with owning a home, such as maintenance and yard work. Other benefits to this style of community living include a peer support network that provides socialization opportunities, structured recreational activities, transportation arrangements, fitness centers, pools, and quiet environments. Living facilities range from apartment-style homes to smaller separate residential homes. Nurses may provide periodic health screening and health information.

How Is Healthcare Categorized?

Because the boundaries of care have become fluid, it is useful to look at the system in a different light. The complexity of care no longer is a predictor of where care will be delivered. Instead, regulators, finances, and the patient's support system dictate where a patient will be located in the system. On a basic level, healthcare is categorized by degree of complexity into primary, secondary, and tertiary services.

Primary Care

Primary care services focus on health promotion, preventive services, health education, and screening for the early detection of healthcare problems. Services are directed toward keeping the patient well by preventing illness and by treating acute episodic problems. General or primary care providers provide most of the care at this level. Most of these services are offered in the community at physicians' offices, clinics, and diagnostic centers. However, hospitals may also offer primary care services. Health promotion and illness prevention by nurses are examples of primary care.

Nursing and Health Promotion In 1948, the World Health Organization (WHO) defined health as "a state of complete physical, mental, and social well-being and not merely the absence of disease or infirmity." The definition has not been amended since that time (WHO, 2007). Health promotion activities foster the highest state of well-being of the recipient of the activities. This inclusive definition can be applied to individuals, groups, families, communities, or societies. The following are examples:

- *Individual level*—Counseling a pregnant client about the importance of adequate prenatal nutrition to promote health for the client and baby.
- *Group and family level*—Teaching about nutrition during pregnancy in family education programs.
- *Community level*—Activities that focus on reaching a larger number of people, for example, advocating for prominent billboards highlighting the importance of prenatal care and nutrition, posting signs in grocery stores recommending food sources for pregnant women, and lobbying for labeling of substances that should be avoided in pregnancy.
- *Societal level*—Working with international partners to establish worldwide prenatal nutrition standards.

Nursing and Illness Prevention *Illness prevention* focuses on avoidance of disease, infection, and other co-morbidities. Activities are targeted to decrease the risk of developing an illness or to minimize the risk of exposure to disease. For example, pneumonia causes many deaths every year. It affects society's most vulnerable: the very young, the very old, and the very ill. Some nursing activities to decrease the risk of pneumonia include:

- Teaching the importance of hand hygiene to decrease the transmission of infection
- Advocating for and administering pneumonia immunizations to those at high risk
- Promoting smoking cessation
- Promoting adequate nutrition to include a diet high in vitamin C

Secondary Care

Secondary care consists of services to diagnose and treat illness, disease, and injury. Historically, we have thought of this as hospital-based care, but increasingly these services are being performed in surgery centers, offices, and outpatient centers. The trend away from the hospital is related to containing costs, increasing specialization of hospitals, and growing evidence that hospitals often harbor medication-resistant infections.

Nursing and Health Restoration Health restoration activities foster a return to health for those already ill. To restore health, the nurse provides direct care to ill individuals, groups, families, or communities. Direct care is what most people think of when they envision the nursing role. Recall that health has physical, mental, spiritual, and social dimensions. When you engage in health-restoration activities, your care should address each of those dimensions, for example:

- Providing hygiene and nutrition for someone unable to do so independently
- Counseling individuals or groups
- Lobbying for policy changes to improve access to care for an underserved group
- Identifying the significance of cultural and/or spiritual influences

Tertiary Care

Tertiary care refers to long-term rehabilitation services and care for the dying. Historically, these services were provided in extended care facilities. Now, however, many tertiary care services are provided in the home or in outpatient settings. One nursing focus in tertiary care is to provide end-of-life care.

Nursing and End-of-Life Care Death is an inevitable destination on the journey of life. Nurses have been active in promoting the respectful care of those who are terminally ill or dying. Nursing activities for the dying are designed to promote comfort, maintain quality of life, provide culturally relevant spiritual care, maintain dignity, and ease the emotional burden of death. Nurses work with dying individuals, their family members and support persons, and organizations (hospice) that focus on the needs of the terminally ill (see Chapter 17).

KnowledgeCheck 1-3

Recall the last time that you had a cold. Identify health-promotion, illness-prevention, and health-restoration activities for individuals, families, groups, and communities in relation to the common cold.

What Healthcare Providers Will You Work With?

As a nurse, you will be part of an interdisciplinary healthcare team consisting of numerous professionals whose primary role is to ensure quality patient outcomes (Fig. 1-4). The composition of the team varies depending on the healthcare needs of the patient. Typically, for an inpatient,

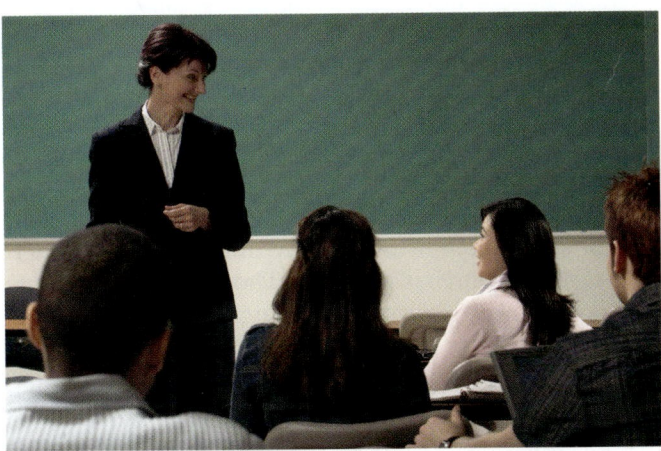

FIGURE 1-4 Quality patient outcomes require the collaboration of the entire healthcare team.

the team leader is the physician, whose primary role is to make a medical diagnosis and outline the treatment plan. The registered nurse uses this plan to develop holistic, continuous, and comprehensive nursing care to the patient, which involves the licensed practical nurse and/or nursing assistive personnel in implementing the plan. The RN administers treatments and medications, provides education, and modifies the nursing care plan based on the patient responses to treatment. The role of each provider in the interdisciplinary health team is discussed below.

Physicians   Physicians are licensed as medical doctors (MD) or doctors of osteopathy (DO). Their role is to diagnose and treat disease and illness through medical and surgical services. A physician may work independently, as part of a medical group, or as an employee of a health facility. Physicians may provide care in an office setting, in the hospital, or in a variety of clinics or ambulatory sites. Physicians who provide only hospital care are known as *hospitalists.* This is a growing specialty, as hospitals endeavor to reduce costs. More physicians are choosing employment in a hospital, rather than private practice because of guaranteed salary, attractive benefit packages, and limited practice hours. Other physicians are concerned this employment arrangement can lead to reduced autonomy and restrictions on their medical practice.

Physician's Assistants (PAs)   PAs diagnose and treat certain diseases and injuries. Although many function in a fashion similar to nurse practitioners, they are not independently licensed. Therefore, they must practice under the supervision of a physician, in contrast to NPs, who practice independently or in collaboration with a physician, and who can provide a broader range of services. Each state varies regarding the scope of practice for nurses and PAs. Check with your state nurse practice act as well as agency policies and procedures to be certain that nurses are permitted to follow a PA's orders.

Nursing Assistive Personnel (NAP)   NAP is a broad term that describes nursing assistants, aides, and technicians. NAPs provide custodial care under the direction

of nurses and physicians in a variety of settings. Some NAPs introduce themselves to patients by stating, "I'm your nurse." Because they are not licensed nurses, they are making a false claim. Be sure to clarify your role and the NAP's role with all of your patients.

Therapists   Allied healthcare providers are various therapists who focus on the rehabilitative needs of the patient. The goal of the rehabilitative team is to treat, maximize functioning, and/or assist the patient to adapt to limitations and achieve optimal outcomes. Types of therapists include the following:

- *Physiatrists*—as the rehabilitative team leader, collaborates with the team to manage the patient's rehabilitation outcomes.
- *Physical therapists* (PT)—focus on the rehabilitation of muscles and bones. They use heat, massage, ultrasound, electrical stimulation, and therapeutic exercise to treat clients with musculoskeletal problems. Their goal is to improve mobility and strength and teach motor skills, such as relearning how to walk after a stroke, exercising to promote flexibility after a knee replacement, or developing wheelchair skills.
- *Occupational therapists* (OT)—work closely with the PT to help patients regain function and independence. They concentrate on helping patients gain optimal functioning in self-care skills for activities of daily living and to learn how to use assistive devices. They also assist patients with disease or injury that limits their abilities to pursue diversional activities.
- *Respiratory therapists* (RT)—provide care for clients with respiratory problems. They provide oxygen therapy, set up and maintain mechanical ventilators, administer pulmonary tests, and provide respiratory treatments that have been prescribed by physicians or advance practice nurses.
- *Speech and language therapists* (SLT)—provide assistance to patients experiencing swallowing and speech disturbances. They evaluate the risk of aspiration, recommend food consistencies to reduce the risk of aspiration, work with patients to restore swallowing abilities, and assist patients in developing speech and language skills after neurological impairment.
- *Recreational therapists*—promote patients' physical, social, and emotional well-being through the use of leisure activities.
- *Marriage and family therapists*—provide counseling services to individuals, families, and groups.

Technologists   Technologists perform a variety of activities in hospitals, diagnostic centers, and emergency care facilities. For example, laboratory technologists examine blood, urine, tissue, and other bodily fluids to aid in the diagnosis and treatment of patients. Radiology technologists administer x-ray and specialty radiographic-type tests. Emergency medical technologists (EMTs) work for ambulance and transport services to stabilize and transport injured and ill clients.

Nutritionists Nutritionists apply specialized knowledge about nutrition and food to promote optimal health to patients with various healthcare needs. A registered dietitian (RD) is a type of nutritionist who works with inpatients to ensure they receive the prescribed diet and learn about ways to continue to follow that diet after discharge.

Pharmacists Pharmacists prepare and dispense medications and therapeutic solutions in hospitals, community pharmacies, and various health settings. They also collaborate with nurses, physicians, and other health-team members to ensure the selection of safe and effective medications to be included in the treatment plan. They provide information about medication contraindications, side effects and adverse reactions, dosage, and administration tips. Pharmacy assistants serve as support personnel for pharmacists.

Dentists Dentists diagnose and treat disorders of the mouth, gums, and teeth. They promote dental health through therapeutic cleaning services, repair of teeth, treatment of gum disorders, inspection for oral carcinomas or infection, and correct tooth alignment disorders. Although most dentists work in community settings, some visit patients hospitalized in acute care and long-term care facilities.

Social Workers Social workers provide psychosocial support and patient services throughout the healthcare system to coordinate continuity of care. They identify the patient's need for community-based support, and help arrange for services after patient discharge. Social workers also counsel clients on financial, housing, marital, and family issues affecting healthcare. Owing to rising healthcare costs, social workers are increasingly used to help move clients through the health system.

Spiritual Care Providers In the United States, chaplains and religious clergy usually provide spiritual care. However, other leaders within various faith-based groups may also do so. Many work at healthcare facilities, but most are on call from local religious facilities. As a nurse, you will likely work with chaplains to provide spiritual services in the form of organized religious services, client visits, and family and staff support, particularly at the end of life or with serious illness.

Alternative Care Providers Alternative care providers such as chiropractors, naturopaths, and herbalists offer health services outside the traditional healthcare system. To read more about alternative healthcare practices,

 Go to Student Resources, **Bonus Chapter, Chapter 46,** on Davis*Plus*.

How Is Healthcare Financed?

Payors for healthcare in the United States include individuals, individual private insurance, employment-based group private insurance, government, and charitable sources, discussed in the following sections.

Individuals

Until the latter half of the 20th century, physicians made house calls and patients paid either with cash or by bartering goods and services. Today, we refer to payments made directly by individuals as *direct payment of services* and *out-of-pocket expenses.* Many of those who do not have insurance and do not qualify for government services cannot afford healthcare if individual payment is their only means to purchase services. Those who have private insurance and government financing also bear some of these expenses through cost-sharing. **Cost-sharing** occurs in the form of insurance premiums, insurance deductibles, co-payments, costs above fixed payments, and non-covered services. **Key Point:** *Although healthcare insurance does pay for a share of the costs, even consumers with insurance sometimes avoid or delay services because of high out-of-pocket expenses.*

Individual Private Insurance

Healthcare insurance is purchased to protect individuals from having to pay the costs associated with illness and hospitalization. The average cost of an emergency room visit was $1,319 in 2009 compared with $922 in 2008. The average annual cost of medical insurance premiums in 2012 was $5,615 for single coverage and $15,745 for family coverage. Insurance is intended to protect persons from "medical bankruptcy" associated with the costs incurred by a major medical event (Fig. 1-5).

A person with private insurance pays premiums to an insurance company. The insurance company then contracts with healthcare providers to deliver care to insured members at prearranged rates. Patients share in the cost of care through out-of-pocket expenses.

Individual private insurance began in 19th-century Europe with the establishment of voluntary benefit programs through guilds and trade associations. Monthly payments were stockpiled to provide assistance in the event of illness or death. European immigrants brought this tradition to the United States. Commercial insurance programs extended this service to individuals

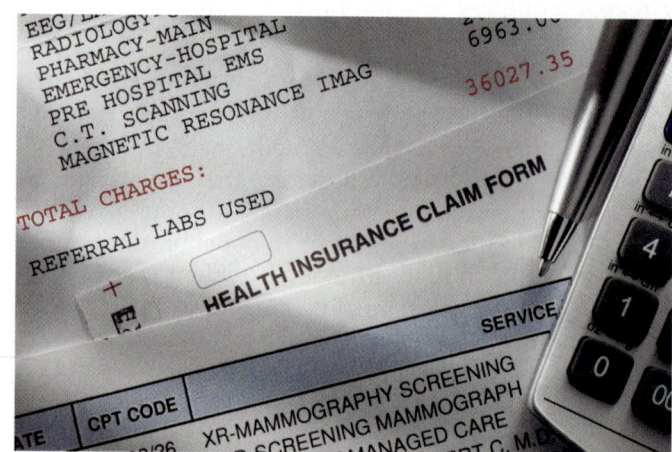

FIGURE 1-5 The high cost of healthcare is a barrier to early screening and prevention.

outside of the trades. Less than 10% of healthcare in the United States is financed through this means.

Employment-Based Private Insurance

Most private insurance in the United States is employment based. Employment-based private insurance is modeled after the individual trade plans. It developed in the United States during World War II, when a labor shortage existed and wage and price controls limited salary increases. Employers financed fringe benefits, such as health insurance, to attract and reward employees as well as to improve the health of employees. Healthy employees benefit the employers with reduced sick time and a full workforce.

With employment-based insurance, the employer pays all or a portion of the costs (e.g., premiums) of providing health insurance to its employees. Increasingly, health insurance has become a source of modern labor disputes, with employers attempting to limit their cost of doing business by reducing the amount of coverage they provide. In effect, the federal government subsidizes employer-based health insurance by not taxing health insurance and allowing employers to deduct these benefits as a business expense (Bodenheimer & Grumbach, 2005).

Government (Public) Financing

Key Point: *Government-funded programs are paid for with revenue from taxes on the citizenry. Programs include Medicare, Medicaid, children's, specialty, and categorical programs. They include federal, state, local, and jointly funded programs.*

Medicare Medicare is a federal insurance program created by Title XVIII of the Social Security Act of 1965. This Act was designed for persons aged 65 years and older. In 1972, the program was expanded to include younger people with permanent disabilities, such as end-stage renal disease. Medicare financing comes from a payroll tax levied on employers and employees and from premiums paid by Medicare subscribers (patients). The focus of Medicare reimbursement is hospital, office, and other outpatient services. Recipients can also purchase partial coverage for their outpatient medications.

Long-term care coverage is limited under Medicare. Unfortunately, as people age, the need for non-skilled care (e.g., help with bathing, dressing, and toileting) increases, yet it is not a covered benefit of Medicare, which is a program designed to care for older adults. This is a premium-based option that is available to people who are enrolled in Medicare Part A or to other eligible individuals for a monthly fee.

Medicaid Medicaid was developed under Title XIX of the Social Security Act of 1965 to provide access to healthcare services for people with low income and minimal resources. Medicaid is a joint federal and state endeavor: (1) The federal government provides the framework and

guidelines for states to use in developing and administering their Medicaid program and (2) reimburses states for their Medicaid associated expenditures. The eligibility criteria for Medicaid and the range of medical services offered vary from state to state. Medicaid offers a fairly comprehensive set of benefits, including prescription drugs.

Medicaid is funded through state and federal taxes. Most states use managed care organizations, such as HMOs, which contract with providers for healthcare services at a predetermined amount. Under the Patient Protection and Affordable Care Act, beginning in 2014, more people under age 65 years whose income falls below certain percentages of the poverty level will qualify for Medicaid coverage (Natoli, Cheh, & Verghese, 2011). The Patient Protection and Affordable Care Act is frequently referred to as the Affordable Care Act.

Children's Health Insurance Program (CHIP) CHIP is a joint venture between the federal government and states to provide health insurance to millions of children whose family income exceeds Medicaid eligibility criteria, but who cannot afford private insurance and are not covered under a parent's policy. CHIP's goal is to ensure that children have health insurance and can access healthcare, either through an expansion of Medicaid or the development of a separate program. The Patient Protection and Affordable Care Act extends CHIP's funding until October 1, 2015.

Specialty and Categorical Programs Certain programs provide distinct services. For example, the federal government supports public health service hospitals, Veterans Affairs hospitals and clinics, healthcare for military personnel and dependents, and Indian Health Services. *Categorical programs* are designated by federal laws to benefit a certain category of people, such as access to healthcare for immigrants or health screening in Head Start programs. Funded programs vary based on current laws and prevailing views.

KnowledgeCheck 1-4

- Compare and contrast privately funded and government-funded health insurance.
- How does being uninsured affect a person's health status?

Charitable Organizations

Charitable organizations are an increasingly important funding source for healthcare. Community agencies that are funded through networks like the United Way, Salvation Army, and Red Cross provide important resources to children, poor families, the aged, and vulnerable populations, such as the homeless, mentally ill, and victims of violence. Charitable organizations provide direct services and cover the costs for some traditional health services. For example, the Salvation Army provides inpatient alcohol and drug rehabilitation services, food and clothing for the needy, and social and nutritional programs for older adults in many major cities. Most participants do not pay for the cost of these services. Instead, able-bodied participants work for the Salvation Army while in the program, and donations to this charity fund the cost of these services. Charitable organizations also donate to healthcare research and healthcare organizations.

How Are Supplies and Equipment Provided?

Suppliers are the companies and corporations that bring goods to the healthcare industry. Pharmaceutical companies and medical equipment suppliers are the largest suppliers. The costs of medications, equipment, and technology have played a major role in the rising costs of care. Suppliers argue that their costs are justified because of the enormous investment required to bring a product to the market. Research, development, and testing of pharmaceuticals and medical equipment take years. Often, numerous products are tested before a successful drug or device is available for use. The cost of insurance to protect against lawsuits, in the event the product causes unforeseen harm, is tremendous. As a result, the cost of these goods is high. On the other hand, suppliers are also launching expensive direct-to-consumer marketing campaigns that urge consumers to seek new products. All of these costs are passed on to consumers in the form of higher prices, rising insurance premiums, and increased out-of-pocket expenses.

How Is Healthcare Regulated?

Regulators are governing bodies that exert influence or control over the healthcare system. They include accrediting and licensing agencies and legislators. All health professions have accrediting bodies to ensure that entry-level programs prepare personnel to deliver safe care. The Accreditation Commission on Education in Nursing (ACEN) and the Commission on Collegiate Nursing Education (CCNE) are the accrediting bodies for nursing education. The state boards of nursing are the regulatory bodies that enforce minimum standards for licensed nurses. Other healthcare providers also have regulatory agencies that govern their practice.

The most prominent regulating body in the healthcare system is The Joint Commission. Reimbursement from government and insurance sources is dependent upon accreditation by The Joint Commission. Healthcare facilities (e.g., hospitals, rehabilitation centers) must meet and maintain standards designed to promote "best practices" for patient safety.

Legislators also affect the healthcare system. For example, legislators can redefine eligibility criteria for government-funded health plans. Most recently, some states have mandated minimum nursing staffing ratios in acute-care hospitals and several others states are considering similar actions. The most notable legislation that impacts healthcare is the Patient Protection and Affordable Care Act that was signed into law by President Obama in 2010. A major provision of the Affordable Care Act is coverage options to ensure that all U.S. citizens have health insurance.

Although accreditors, licensing bodies, and legislators are the only true regulators of healthcare, several other agencies exert enormous influence on the system. Independent watchdog groups, advisory boards, and peer review groups all have the ability to effect change.

How Do Healthcare Policy and Reform Efforts Affect Care?

The U.S. healthcare system is a paradox of excess and deprivation (Bodenheimer & Grumbach, 2005). Some individuals receive too little care because they are uninsured, unable to afford out-of-pocket expenses, or have restrictive healthcare plans that deny them access to competent providers or that are not accepted by certain providers. Others receive expensive top-of-the-line care that produces results that could have been achieved through cheaper means or that result in prolonged life of questionable quality.

Sultz and Young (1997) described the U.S. healthcare system as "focused on providing excellent care for the individuals within it, while virtually ignoring the more basic health service needs of the larger populations outside of it" (p. 46). Even though our healthcare system is the model of care for the industrialized world, access to care is not available to all. Very few can afford to pay for the tremendous costs of an illness or for the ongoing expenses of a chronic illness and long-term care when supplementary resources are limited or unavailable.

During the first quarter of 2012, 47 million persons were without health insurance (Cohen & Martinez, 2012). Without some form of coverage, people forgo needed care. The indigent and working poor have access to emergency or urgent treatment, but this can require long waits for services unless the person is very ill. But primary care—such as checkups, screenings, chronic illness follow-ups, and prenatal care—can be lacking, particularly for those above the poverty level but without government support or private insurance, thus leaving many untreated and ultimately needing more costly care.

Several variables collectively account for the current situation. These include the following:

- Increased government funding of services, creating a feeling that care is without cost to the individual
- Increased use of employer-based insurance, preventing the individual from seeing the actual cost of coverage
- Inflation, escalating the costs of all goods and services
- Rising costs of pharmaceuticals and medical devices
- Direct-to-consumer advertising of medical products, increasing the demand for and use of expensive products
- Increased use of technology, which can be costly to purchase and maintain
- Defensive medicine (practices for the purpose of preventing lawsuits and malpractice claims), resulting in excessive testing, treatments, and diagnostic studies

- Increased wages of healthcare personnel
- Population changes, particularly an increasing older population and increased longevity for those with acute and chronic illness
- Increased administrative costs due to the increased complexity of care and network institutions

Medicare and Public Policy

When Medicare was initially created, health services were reimbursed using a **retrospective system**. This means that Medicare paid hospitals based on the actual cost of providing services to individuals. With no cap on expenses, Medicare payments made to hospitals increased from $3 billion in 1967 to $37 billion in 1983. In an attempt to decrease the escalating costs of healthcare, a **prospective reimbursement system** was created under the Social Security Amendment of 1983. Hospitals were then reimbursed on a per case, flat rate basis determined by patient groups having similar needs. These groups were called **diagnostic related groups (DRGs).** If the patient's hospital costs were greater than the reimbursed ("set") amounts, the hospital lost money. If the costs were less than the rate set by Medicare, the hospital made a profit. Private insurance companies, following the lead of Medicare, reimbursed in the same manner.

The introduction of DRGs forced hospitals to consider new ways of delivering care and created a number of changes in patient care, such as the following:

- *The length of stay in hospitals decreased dramatically* as care moved away from hospitals out into the community and home. For example, formerly a patient who had a hip replacement would stay in the hospital for 10 days. Under a prospective payment system, this person is discharged after 4 days.
- *The cost of delivering nursing care became an expenditure.* As a result, team nursing with NAPs replaced the comprehensive care provided by RNs at the bedside. This transition occurred in spite of research documenting that a higher proportion of RNs on staff results in fewer adverse patient outcomes (e.g., as reported by Yang, Hung, Chen, et al., 2012).
- *Fewer choices for care resulted from corporate mergers and acquisitions* in large regional facilities. In many areas, residents have only one choice for hospital care. With less choice, there are also fewer nursing positions.
- *The cost of managing these large facilities skyrocketed.* In 2000, the Healthcare Financing Administration stated that administrative costs consumed at least 25% of all health expenditures. In 2010, administrative costs had decreased to "less than 2% of program expenditures" (Potetz, Cubanski, & Neuman, 2011).
- *Reduced staffing and higher patient acuity produced a more stressful work environment for nurses.* This fact, in combination with the growing number of career choices, has contributed to a severe nursing shortage.
- *Insurance premiums and cost-sharing increased, while availability of services decreased.* This led to a growing number of people who could not afford the care they

need. As a result, most reform efforts are directed at controlling costs, improving access, and promoting appropriate distribution of resources.

Economists and policy makers agree that no matter how affluent a society is, it has limited healthcare resources—and with limited resources, rationing occurs. **Rationing** is "the limitation of access to or the equitable distribution of medical services, through various gatekeeper controls" (Farlex, 2002). Within our current system, if an individual has sufficient resources (i.e., money or insurance), then healthcare services are available. Conversely, if a person does not have the means to pay, then many services are denied. This model results in a tiered system: Those who can pay have better access to services than those who cannot pay do. The U.S. model also subsidizes healthcare via government-funded programs for some individuals who are unable to compete economically for the same services. With the passage of the Patient Protection and Affordable Care Act in 2010, the U.S. government will become more involved with funding and regulating healthcare (U.S. Department of Health & Human Services, 2010), moving toward a more European model.

In contrast, Canada, Australia, and most European countries have *socialized healthcare*, in which the government assumes responsibility for providing *necessary* services to all individuals. In a socialized model, basic services, such as office visits, prenatal care, and required surgery, are available to all. But services above the basic level, that is *desired* services, are available only to those who can afford them. In the U.S. model, rationing is implicit (hidden), whereas in the socialized model rationing is explicit (plainly visible).

Managed Care

Managed care, designed to control healthcare costs, is a competitive approach to healthcare pricing. Managed care organizations (MCOs) contract with medical providers to provide services (a) at discounted rates, or (b) based on predetermined fixed payment per individual covered under the plan (capitation). Providers treat more patients to offset their discounted rates. Employers contract with the managed care organization and select a type of health plan for its employees. There are four basic types of managed care plans:

Health Maintenance Organizations (HMOs) HMOs are a model of care based on **capitated** (per head) costs. Each HMO primary care provider receives a predetermined, fixed amount each month regardless of whether the patient receives healthcare services or not. The primary care provider coordinates all care, including referrals to specialists. Providers often choose to be a part of an HMO because of the steady income it offers. However, to compensate for the low reimbursement, they must see more patients per day, limit the number of HMO patients they are willing to provide care for, limit the number of office visits allowed, or refuse to provide care for patients with complex conditions. Patients often choose HMO coverage because they are among the most affordable insurance plans available. However, the patient sacrifices choice for affordability. The HMO will pay only for specified services, and only if the patient uses a provider on the HMO list ("in the network").

Preferred Provider Organizations (PPOs) PPOs allow patients to have greater choice among providers, medications, and devices, The PPO has many of the features of an HMO, such as a network of providers who will provide healthcare at the established contracted rate. The PPO offers patients more flexibility than an HMO, such as (a) seeing specialists within the network without having to get a referral from the primary care physician; and (b) seeing out-of-network providers, albeit at a higher cost than an in-network provider. The flexibility of a PPO comes at a financial cost, for example, the patient pays more in the form of higher premiums, deductibles, and co-insurance.

Point of Service (POS) The POS combines features from the HMO and PPO. The patient selects a physician from a list of network physicians, who will become the point of service (POS) for treatment and referrals to in-network specialists. The patient needs to see in-network providers in order to get the lower co-pays and minimal to no deductibles. There is limited out-of-network coverage, resulting in higher co-insurance and co-pay.

Integrated Delivery Networks (IDNs) Healthcare systems are moving toward a model of **integrated delivery networks**, also known as integrated delivery systems. IDNs combine providers, health facilities, pharmaceuticals, and services into one care system. Providers are employees of the facilities. They see only IDN patients, in IDN facilities, using IDN services and IDN-approved pharmaceuticals. Because all services and providers are linked, patients can be readily moved among IDN services and providers. The system is designed to promote a culture of collaboration, safety, and teamwork among the providers (Enthoven, 2009). The ability to obtain services from providers throughout the healthcare system is the chief advantage of this approach. The primary disadvantage is that care may be fragmented, as patients are rapidly moved through the system in an effort to minimize costs.

What Are the Issues Related to Healthcare Reform?

The profound changes created by the transition of the healthcare system from a retrospective open-checkbook to prospective fixed-rate payment system have created unprecedented leadership opportunities for nurse executives.

ANA Recommendations for Reform

In 1991, the ANA published *Nursing's Agenda for Healthcare Reform*, a set of recommendations to redesign the healthcare system. Although small changes were made, fragmentation of the healthcare systems, access to care barriers, and healthcare costs remained issues (ANA, 2008). The ANA

recommendations were updated in the ANA document *ANA's Health System Reform Agenda* (2008), which includes the following recommendations for change:

- Provide universal access to essential healthcare services for all citizens and residents.
- Establish health policies that support safe, effective, patient-centered, timely, efficient, and fair care based on outcomes research.
- Shift the priority from illness care to health promotion, and balance between high-tech treatment and community-based and preventive services.
- Establish a single-payer system for financing healthcare.

Work Redesign

Work redesign involves looking at the level of care required and the mix of personnel necessary to achieve the best patient outcomes. Out of this redesign, a concept known as the critical pathway emerged. A **critical pathway** is a multidisciplinary approach to care that sequences interventions over a length of stay for a given case type. Using the critical pathways model, the interdisciplinary team delivers care that yields the desired outcomes in the quickest manner, hopefully to reduce the patient's length of stay. For example, using this model, a patient who has had cardiac surgery may be assisted out of bed as soon as his vital signs are stable. In the traditional model, the patient must wait to be seen by the surgeon before an order is written to get out of bed. Advocates of critical pathways state that this model allows patients to progress at their own pace. Foes of this plan state that it is a cookie-cutter approach to healthcare. (See Fig. 5-5 and Chapter 5 for more information about critical pathways.)

Another work redesign that has emerged is case management. **Case management** is the coordination of care across the healthcare system. Many hospitals, home health agencies, and insurance companies employ nurse case managers to ensure that care is efficient, cost-effective, and of high quality. Typically, nurses case manage patients with specific diagnoses. For example, a patient with diabetes may be assigned a nurse case manager in the outpatient clinic. If the patient develops complications requiring hospitalization, the case manager coordinates care so that all providers are aware of the patient's unique needs. Later, when the patient is discharged, the case manager visits the patient at home. The case manager sets goals with the patient, monitors the cost of the care, and works with all providers to eliminate duplication of service and evaluate outcomes of care.

Is Healthcare a Right or a Privilege?

A fundamental question underlying all healthcare reform is the question of whether healthcare is a right or a privilege. This question raises more questions. For example, if healthcare is a right of all citizens, should noncitizens be offered coverage? Moreover, what responsibility does an individual have to preserve her own health? Does someone who smokes or drinks excessively have a right to receive care for illnesses brought on by these lifestyle choices—especially if the care is paid for with public funds? Even if an individual leads a healthy lifestyle, should extensive and/or expensive therapies be offered if they have little likelihood of success? Finally, if you believe that healthcare should be affordable for all, are you willing to limit the salary and benefits you receive from your own employer to help control the costs of care? Are you willing to pay higher taxes? Because of the complexity of these and countless other questions, our system remains a work in progress. These fundamental questions were discussed during the debate on the Affordable Care Act. Yet, you will continue to hear these questions and others as universal healthcare continues to evolve.

KnowledgeCheck 1-5

- Do you view healthcare as a right or a privilege?
- What are factors that impact your view (draw on your self-knowledge to answer this question)?

How Do Providers and Facilities Ensure Quality Care?

As you learned previously, a number of accrediting bodies inspect healthcare organizations. These inspections are designed to ensure that patients receive safe, quality care. To promote safety, regulators establish a minimum competency level that must be met for accreditation to be granted. However, most healthcare organizations and professionals declare that their goal is to deliver *excellent* care rather than merely meeting minimum standards.

Continuous Quality Improvement Programs

Continuous quality improvement (CQI) programs (also *total quality management* [TQM]) focus on quality (excellent) care as an ongoing goal rather than something that is periodically verified by audit or when a problem is identified.

Traditionally, quality assurance programs have consisted of **retrospective audit programs**, that is, material from the past (e.g., patient records) is reviewed for evidence of compliance with preselected criteria. For example, a nursing unit may set a goal of 100% compliance that nurses' notes will state the reason when any medication is held (not given). To conduct the audit, all charts within a selected time frame are then reviewed to identify times when medication had been held. The auditor then reviews the nursing notes to determine whether the nurse explained why it was held. The percentage of compliance is calculated based on the review. If it were determined, for example, that there were 50 occasions in which a medication was held during the past 3 months, and on 40 of those occasions the rationale is charted in the nursing notes, the compliance rate is 40/50, or 80%.

If the QA auditors determine that the goal for compliance has not been met, they will often launch a program to improve compliance. For the example above, mandatory in-service education may be provided. In addition, labels might be placed in the medication administration records and a computer-based medication system used to prompt staff to document the reason for holding a medication. At a later date, a second audit is conducted to determine whether compliance has improved.

Another form of retrospective quality improvement is **peer review**. Colleagues review medical records or patient satisfaction data that reflect the care given by their peers. Peer review requires open, honest dialogue and a willingness to improve. Objective criteria must be set to avoid complaints of favoritism and some benefit to promote participation.

ANA Model for Quality Assurance

In 1975, the ANA developed a model for QA consisting of seven steps. This model is useful to understanding the CQI process. For the steps in the QA process and an example of how each step is applied in a clinical scenario,

 Go to Student Resources, Chapter 1, **Supplemental Materials, Example of ANA Model for Quality Assurance,** on DavisPlus.

Quality and Safety Education for Nurses

Quality Improvement Competency

Chapter Key Concept: Healthcare Delivery System

Competency: Quality Improvement*

Question: The commission on Quality and Safety Education for Nurses (QSEN) identifies quality improvement (QI) as a competency you should achieve during your nursing education. QSEN defines QI as the ability to "use data to monitor the outcomes of care processes and use improvement methods to design and test changes to continuously improve the quality and safety of healthcare systems." How do you think the staffing mix in a hospital might affect care quality?

Research: Recent research shows that when the proportion of RNs increases in an agency, quality of care rises and death and infection rates drop. Consider the following examples from *Critical Care* (2007), Landon et al. (2006), Tourangeau et al. (2007), and Yang et al (2012):

➤ Hospitals with higher proportions of RNs and baccalaureate-prepared RNs have lower patient death rates.

➤ Increasing the proportion of RNS on staff by 10% resulted in 6 fewer deaths per 1,000.

➤ Hospitals with adequate staffing had lower death rates.

➤ Hospitals with a higher proportion of RNs on staff performed better on a variety of performance measures.

➤ When the ratio of nurses to patients falls (e.g., from 1:6 patients to 1:4), risk for infection falls.

Think about it: How does the QSEN competency quality improvement relate to the chapter key concept, healthcare delivery system?

*To see the KSAs for the QSEN competencies,

 Go to the QSEN Web site, at **http://www.qsen.org/ ksas_prelicensure.php**

Source: Cronenwett, Sherwood, Barnsteiner, et al. (2007).

FACTORS THAT INFLUENCE CONTEMPORARY NURSING PRACTICE

Factors that influence contemporary nursing practice include (a) those outside the profession in society at large, and (b) those within nursing and healthcare.

What Are Some Trends in Society?

As you have seen, our historical roots have influenced current nursing practice and will undoubtedly continue to do so. In addition, nursing is influenced by trends in the economy—the growing number of older adults, increased consumer knowledge, legislation, the women's movement, and collective bargaining.

The National Economy

The national economy has a tremendous impact on nursing. Consider the following examples:

- *In the United States, health insurance coverage is linked to full-time employment with health insurance benefits* (although that may be changing with recent federal legislation). Thus, when unemployment figures rise, so does the number of people without insurance. Many uninsured people delay seeking treatment, and that leads to sicker patients entering the healthcare system. This taxes the system's resources and raises the level of nursing care required.
- *The healthcare industry is very expensive to operate, even in a strong economy.* Downturns in the economy affect institutional investments and profits, as well as the amount of taxes the government can collect. These in turn limit the medications and services that are available.
- *The healthcare system employs an enormous number and variety of individuals.* If you just consider that there are 2.6 million employed RNs (Health Resources and Services Administration, 2010), 798,000 active physicians (Association of American Medical Colleges, 2011), and more than 268,000 employed pharmacists (Bureau of Labor Statistics, 2012b), you begin to understand how large the healthcare system is when all other providers are added to the count. Similarly, the salaries of healthcare providers are influenced by national economic trends.

The Growing Proportion of Older Adults in the United States

A larger older adult population creates a need for more medical and nursing care. At the same time, there are fewer younger people to provide care. The growth rate for adults 65 years and older has greatly outpaced the growth of the population at 15% (40.3 million) compared with the country as a whole (9.7%). This number is expected to grow to 20% by the year 2050. The oldest old (those 85 years and older) will continue to be the fastest growing part of the population into the next century (U.S. Census Bureau, 2010). As people age, they tend to need more assistance with activities of daily living, and they experience more acute and chronic illnesses.

Changes in Healthcare Consumers

Historically, patients relied on the knowledge and decision making of the healthcare team. Now, however, consumers are demanding greater choice in the decisions that affect their health.

- *Patients have access to vast amounts of health and medical information, particularly through the Internet* (e.g., Web sites such as WebMD and PubMed). Informed consumers tend to be active participants in discussions about their health problems and therapy options. Patients need to be taught which sites are valid for information.
- *Direct-to-consumer marketing* is another form of health information, in which corporations advertise medications and therapies directed at the potential user (e.g., on the Internet and in magazines). Such advertising generates consumer interest in new products. Clients may then request their healthcare providers to prescribe specific trade name therapies they have heard about in the media. You need to be prepared to address the truthfulness of the advertisements and to present balanced information to clients, particularly as they are appropriate for individual clients' conditions. You must also be comfortable with your knowledge and not be unduly persuaded by consumers who are relying on the latest advertisement fads. Your knowledge, standards of nursing practice, and communications with the healthcare team should be the foundation for making patient-related decisions.

Legislation

Consumer interest has also generated legislation that affects nursing care. Legislation directed at the confidentiality of patient records, treating patients who need emergency care, the patient's right to know (informed consent), and the patient's right to a dignified death (living will/advance directives) all govern the care that nurses render to patients. These acts are discussed further in Chapters 44 and 45.

The Women's Movement

Historically, only unmarried women were allowed to practice nursing. As the women's movement gained momentum, women were no longer forced out of nursing if they chose to have a family. Whereas women's careers were traditionally limited to teaching, clerical work, and nursing, the women's movement opened up more choices. As a result, nursing has become just one of many options for a career, and is no longer the only career pathway. Also, societal views of nursing as a women's profession influenced the decisions of men to enter (or not enter) nursing.

Collective Bargaining

Collective bargaining is a form of negotiating that allows nurses to seek better wages and working conditions as a group rather than individually. Not all states have collective bargaining groups for nurses. A union or organization that represents the nurses usually conducts collective bargaining. Collective bargaining has resulted in significant improvements in wages, benefits, and working conditions for nurses, as well as safer conditions for patients. These improvements have made nursing more attractive as a career choice.

ThinkLike a Nurse 1-6

What effect do you think the women's movement has had on the number of women in the nursing work force? Speculate also on the ways in which women entering nursing might have been different before and after the women's movement.

What Are Some Trends in Nursing and Healthcare?

In addition to societal factors, trends in nursing and healthcare also affect contemporary practice. We discuss the most significant trends here.

Increased Use of Complementary and Alternative Medicine

The National Institutes of Health define healthcare treatments or services outside the traditional healthcare system as **complementary and alternative medicine (CAM)**. They include medical systems, such as homeopathy, naturopathy, chiropractic, and traditional Chinese medicine, as well as specific treatments, such as herbal medications, dietary changes, massage therapy, yoga, aromatherapy, prayer, and hypnotism. There is growing interest in CAM for various reasons, including costs of traditional care and increasing cultural diversity in the population. For a more extensive discussion,

 Go to Student Resources, **Bonus Chapter 46, Holistic Healing,** under the heading Why Do People Use CAM, on Davis*Plus.*

Expanded Variety of Settings for Care

Nearly 40% of registered nurses now work outside the hospital setting, as compared with 20% in 1980 (ANA, 2010; Health Resources and Services Administration, 2010; Jonas & Kovner, 2008). As this trend continues, nurses must be prepared to function in alternative settings. This change requires entry-level education programs to prepare nurses for these types of work (Wilkinson, 1996). In the hospital, you have access to support personnel, consultation with other nurses and healthcare providers, ready access to equipment and diagnostic testing services, and increased access to the patient. As more care is delivered in

Toward Evidence-Based Practice

Numerous studies have found that a single approach, such as siderails, is not effective in preventing patient falls. These researchers have concluded that a multifactorial approach is needed.

Spoelstra, S. L., Given, B. A., & Given, C. W. (2012). Fall prevention in hospitals: An integrative review. *Clinical Nursing Research, 21*(1), 92–112.

This study found that intervention programs that included a multiple approach to preventing patient falls were more effective than relying on a single intervention. Fall prevention programs should include staff education, fall-risk assessments, environmental assessments and modifications, alarm systems, and patient assistance with transferring and toileting.

Capezuti, E. E., Wagner, L., Brush, B., et al. (2007). Consequences of an intervention to reduce restrictive siderail use in nursing homes. *Journal of the American Geriatrics Society, 55*(3), 334–341.

This study of more than 700 nursing home residents at four sites found that routine use of siderails does not reduce the risk of bed-related falls.

Brush, B. L., & Capezuti, E. (2001). Historical analysis of siderail use in American hospitals. *Journal of Nursing Scholarship, 33*(4), 381–385.

This study used social historical research methods to examine the pattern of siderail use, the value attached to siderails, and attitudes about raising siderails over time. Siderails on adult beds were rare until the 1930s; nurses used continual watchfulness to ensure patient safety. Initially siderails were used for temporary protection of confused patients. They were not a part of the bed, but had to be attached to it when they were needed. During the 1930s, litigation against hospitals and nurses for fall-related injuries, recurrent nurse shortages, and the move away from ward structure toward semiprivate and private rooms all promoted the use of siderails instead of nursing observation. They now have become a permanent fixture of the hospital bed. However, recent research has demonstrated that siderail-induced injuries may occur, and that sustained bedrest has negative physical and emotional consequences. In spite of these recent research-based findings, siderail use remains the norm in promoting patient safety.

1. What trends and factors currently affecting nursing might influence whether siderail use will change in the near future?

2. What additional information would you like to know before advocating for a change in siderail use?

 Go to Student Resources: Chapter 1, **Toward Evidence-Based Practice Suggested Responses,** on Davis*Plus.*

outpatient, community, or home settings, you must be prepared to function more autonomously and creatively.

Telehealth nursing is practiced in a variety of settings, including rural clinics, home healthcare, corrective facilities, and physicians' offices, using communication devices such as the telephone or two-way video technology. As telehealth nursing continues to evolve, you will need to combine the use of technology with your nursing knowledge to safely care for patients remotely.

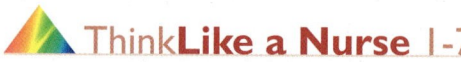

ThinkLike a Nurse I-7

What is your nursing program doing to prepare you to work outside the hospital setting?

Interest in Interprofessional Collaboration

Nursing is changing from a largely supportive role to one of increasing responsibility. This is, in part, due to the growing role of nursing in outpatient settings, the increasing complexity of care, the limited supply of nurses, and the increased use of technology. More and more, healthcare leaders are finding interprofessional teamwork to be essential to providing safe, high-quality patient outcomes.

Collaboration is the process of joint decision making among independent parties, involving joint ownership of decisions and collective responsibility for outcomes (Disch, Bellman, & Ingbar, as cited in Sterchi, 2007). However, in a relationship in which there is a power imbalance, true collaboration can occur only if the more powerful parties are willing. Physicians and nurses tend to have different values and to place different emphases on patient care. This may contribute to strained relationships and disagreements about a patient's plan of care, which may lead to undesired outcomes for patients. True collaboration occurs when institutions enforce the goal and give recognition to those who practice it.

On a typical day, a hospitalized patient may interact with six or more individuals who are involved in his plan of care. It is essential that these care providers are talking with the patient and collaborating with each other. A primary cause of serious medical errors in healthcare facilities is communication failure, which often stems from lack of collaboration. To minimize these occurrences, healthcare providers are encouraged to use a standardized system of communication known as SBAR-R (Situation, Background, Assessment, Recommendation-Readback) (see Chapter 21).

Expanded Career Roles for Nurses

Numerous **expanded roles** extend the traditional practice of the nurse. The roles may or may not be clinical.

Advanced Practice Nurses (APNs) Registered nurses, usually with a master's degree, who work in expanded roles with a clinical focus are collectively termed *advanced practice nurses (APNs)*.

- **Clinical Nurse Specialist (CNS)**—A nurse with advanced education and expertise in an area of clinical specialization (e.g., cardiovascular, pulmonary, orthopedics). The CNS may provide direct patient care; consult on client care; engage in client, family, community, or staff teaching; and/or conduct research.
- **Nurse Practitioner (NP)**—A nurse with advanced education focused on providing primary care (comprehensive healthcare) to an age group or within a specialty area. NPs may work independently or in practice with physicians. They assess, diagnose, and treat diseases and illnesses and prescribe medications and treatments. An NP can provide approximately 80% of the care offered by a physician.
- **Certified Registered Nurse Anesthetist (CRNA)**—A nurse with advanced education focused on providing anesthesia. Nurse anesthetists conduct preoperative screening and evaluation of patients, administer anesthesia during surgery, and evaluate patients' responses to anesthesia in the postoperative period.
- **Certified Nurse Midwife (CNM)**—A nurse with advanced education focused on women's health, pregnancy, and delivery. A CNM provides prenatal care, performs uncomplicated deliveries, and provides postpartum care.

Professional and public reports (e.g., Tourangeau, Doran, Hall, et al., 2007) demonstrate high patient satisfaction with APNs; comparable, and at times superior, patient outcomes over physician-provided care; better understanding of and compliance with treatment regimen; fewer hospitalizations; and greater cost effectiveness when compared with physician providers. This positive reaction to APNs has resulted in increased acceptance and support for all nurses.

Non-Clinical Expanded Roles Expanded roles with other than a clinical focus include the following:

- **Nurse Researcher**—A nurse with advanced education at the master's or doctoral level who engages in research related to clinical practice, the discipline, or nursing education.
- **Nurse Administrator**—A nurse whose practice focuses on the management and administration of nursing care, health facilities, or health resources.
- **Nurse Educator**—A nurse with advanced education and expertise who teaches in the clinical or academic setting.
- **Nurse Informaticist**—A nurse with specialized education focused on the use of technology in healthcare and the incorporation of standardized languages and classifications into nursing practice.
- **Nurse Entrepreneur**—A nurse who has creatively created an independent or innovative business. Entrepreneurs may serve as consultants, administer a health-related business, or provide educational services.

KnowledgeCheck I-6

Compare and contrast advanced practice clinical roles for nurses.

Increased Use of Nursing Assistive Personnel

Nursing assistive personnel (NAP) are healthcare providers who help nurses and physicians provide patient care. Common NAP roles include nurse aide, assistant, orderly, and technician. NAPs may perform simple nursing tasks (e.g., bathing, taking vital signs) under the direction of the licensed nurse. Some institutions even train NAPs for more complex tasks traditionally reserved for licensed nurses (e.g., inserting urinary catheters, giving certain medications). This redistribution of workload has prompted controversy about safety and quality of care.

Although it may be appropriate to allow the NAP to assume the simple tasks, this distances the licensed nurse from many aspects of direct patient care. The nurse retains ultimate responsibility for the patient, yet must base important patient care decisions on information obtained by the NAP. The nurse is able to use a higher level of critical thinking and a greater depth of knowledge, and is therefore likely to gather more in-depth patient data.

As you progress through your program, you will notice that nurses often gather different information from a client than does someone without nursing experience. For example, after bathing an older adult, a NAP will be able to tell the nurse that there are no open areas on the skin. However, a nurse performing the same task would be able to do an extensive client assessment while giving the bath. The nurse would be able to comment on the client's level of cognition (orientation to surroundings and self), tolerance for activity, breath sounds, heart sounds, bowel sounds, and the condition of the skin. The nurse might also use the time during the bath to teach the client about his condition or to gather information about the client's home and support system that can be used for discharge planning.

Influence of Nurses on Health Policy

Professional nursing organizations are actively involved in local, state, and national politics.

- The major professional organizations actively lobby and educate government officials about the role of nursing in healthcare.
- Nursing organizations sponsor legislation that promotes the interest of the profession and supports changes that positively influence health outcomes. Nurse-sponsored legislation has addressed safe staffing in hospitals, needle-exchange programs to decrease the transmission of HIV and other infectious diseases, and funding to increase nursing enrollment during times of nursing shortages.

As individuals, nurses should vote, lobby their elected representatives, and run for political office. Together, nurses represent the largest health professional group (more than 3.8 million); thus, when united as a voting block, they have strong political power. Many nurses organize local nursing groups to support candidates or legislation, or speak out in the community on health and nursing issues. Nurses are typically trusted and respected political candidates, running successful campaigns at the local, state, and national level. Another way to influence politics and policy is to serve on federal or state advisory panels. For example, nurse leaders serve on the National Advisory Committee for the Healthcare Research and Quality. They provide a voice from nursing on issues related to healthcare quality, safety, and evidence-based practice. You should consider all of these political activities as you move into the profession.

Divergence Between High-Tech and High-Touch

Advances in clinical knowledge and technology have contributed to improved care and a longer life for many patients who are critically ill (e.g., premature newborns and patients with advanced cardiovascular, pulmonary, or renal disease). This trend is in contrast to the concurrent trend toward holism and high-touch therapies, which often avoid technology. One of the challenges in healthcare is integrating these two divergent trends. For an excellent discussion on these colliding values, read *Holistic Health and Healing* by Mary Anne Bright (2002).

 To explore learning resources for this chapter,

 Go to DavisPlus at DavisPl.us/Wilkinson3.

Chapter Resources for Chapter 1:
Response sheets for all learning activities
Resources for Caregivers and Health Professionals
Reading More About Evolution of Nursing Thought & Action (suggested reading)
Concept Map of chapter content
Interactive Case Studies
NCLEX-Style and Chapter Review Questions
Chapter Overview Podcasts

For references cited in this chapter,

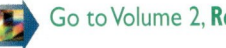 Go to Volume 2, **References Cited.**

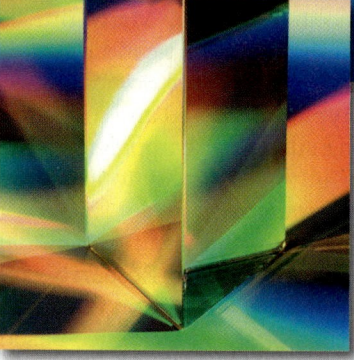
Critical Thinking & Nursing Process

Learning Outcomes

After completing this chapter, you should be able to:

➤ Give one definition and one example of critical thinking.

➤ List at least six critical-thinking skills and attitudes.

➤ Review seven attitudes of the critical thinker.

➤ Explain ways in which nurses use critical thinking.

➤ List the six overlapping and inter-dependent phases of the nursing process.

➤ Describe what the nurse is doing in each phase of the nursing process.

➤ Explain how critical thinking is used in the nursing process.

➤ Explain what is meant in nursing by the concept *caring*.

➤ Discuss, and give examples of, the differences between practical/procedural knowledge and theoretical knowledge.

➤ Name the main concepts of the full-spectrum nursing model.

➤ Explain how nursing knowledge, nursing process, and critical thinking work together in full-spectrum nursing.

Key Concepts

Critical thinking

Full-spectrum nursing

Nursing knowledge

Nursing process

Related Concepts

See the Concept Map on Davis*Plus*.

Explore Your Nursing Role

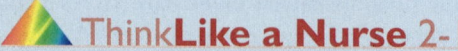

It's a pleasant Saturday afternoon, and you're meeting with an old friend whom you haven't seen in 2 years. She asks, "I hear you've decided to become a nurse. What made you choose that? I don't think I could be around people who are sick and in pain. Hospitals are such sad places."

She listens to your answer with interest. To respond to this statement, you will need to consider your motivation for entering nursing and your beliefs about the profession.

ThinkLike a Nurse 2-1

How would you reply to her question?

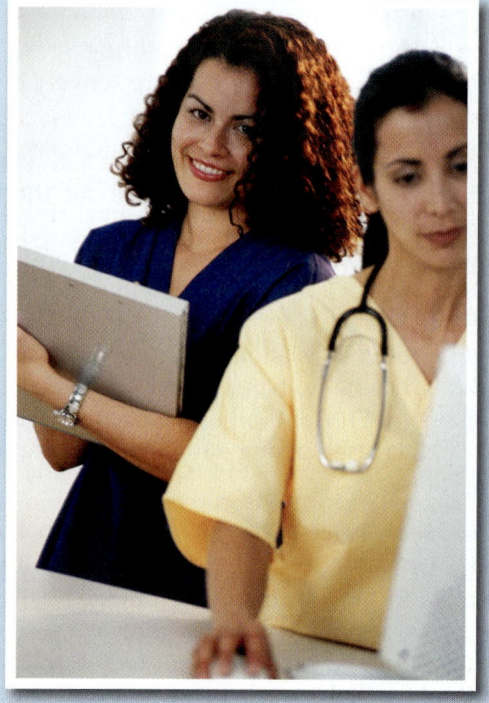

Explore Your Nursing Role (continued)

ThinkLike a Nurse 2-2

- What factors or persons influenced your decision to be a nurse?
- Have others asked you why you chose to become a nurse? How have the reactions you received before colored your explanation of your career choice?
- What makes this situation similar to or different from your prior experiences?
- What's important in this situation?

- Of the possible answers you are considering, which answer best reflects your true feelings about your career choice? Why are the other answers not appropriate?
- What beliefs and assumptions are coloring your response?

If you are able to answer these questions, then you have used critical thinking to guide your decision making. Critical thinking involves careful consideration of a situation to arrive at a solution, based on analysis of the data. Critical thinking is vital when considering important decisions. It is the kind of thinking you will use as a nurse.

ABOUT THE KEY CONCEPTS

Keep the key concepts in mind as you read this chapter. They will give you the "hooks" on which you can "hang" the other details in the chapter. As you gain understanding of **critical thinking, nursing knowledge**, and **nursing process**, you will begin to see how they all work together in **full-spectrum nursing**.

WHAT DOES NURSING INVOLVE?

Chapter 1 introduced you to nursing roles, responsibilities, and activities, and to the career of nursing. Throughout this text, you will learn much more. Thus, your view of nursing may change as you progress in your studies. To track your progress, establish a baseline by examining your current view of nursing.

ThinkLike a Nurse 2-3

What is your image of nursing? List at least five attributes a nurse should have, and at least five responsibilities that you consider to be a part of nursing.

In the preceding exercise, when you listed some nursing responsibilities, you may have mentioned activities such as "gives medications" or "performs tests and treatments." And you were correct—partially. Much of nursing is about *doing*, and nursing is activity oriented. But don't forget the importance of *caring*. And now more than ever the emphasis is on *thinking*. So, another way to describe nursing is to say that *nursing involves thinking, doing,* and *caring*.

The scientific basis for patient care changes constantly. Research continually uncovers new information that alters the practice of all healthcare providers. Therefore, you should know up front that you cannot possibly learn everything about healthcare and nursing in nursing school. In fact, to be a safe and competent nurse you must constantly update your knowledge and skills throughout your career. As a lifelong learner, you will need to develop and refine your critical-thinking skills. Critical thinking helps you to know what is important about each patient's situation, when you need more information, and when you need help to make the best decision.

Theoretical Knowledge knowing why

WHAT IS CRITICAL THINKING?

If critical thinking is so important, then you might be wondering, what exactly is it? One simple definition is that critical thinking is "the art of thinking about your thinking while you are thinking in order to make your thinking better: more clear, more accurate, or more defensible" (Paul, 1990). On closer study, this definition makes an important point. It tells us that we should reflect on the thinking process we are using to figure something out: "Why did I ask those particular questions? Do I have enough information to decide, or have I jumped to a conclusion? Have I considered all the possibilities?"

Box 2-1 provides several definitions of critical thinking, or you may want to use the following more formal definition:

Critical thinking is a combination of reasoned thinking, openness to alternatives, an ability to reflect, and a desire to seek truth.

There are many definitions of critical thinking because it is a complex concept and people think about it in different ways—none of them are "wrong." In fact, any situation that requires critical thinking is likely to have more than one "right" answer. You do not need critical thinking to add 2 + 2 and come up with the answer. However, you do need critical thinking to problem-solve important decisions.

Critical thinking is linked to evidence-based practice, which you will learn more about later in this book. Evidence-based practice is a research-based method for judging nursing interventions. An important aspect of critical thinking is the process of identifying and checking your assumptions—and this is also an important part of the research process.

- Critical thinking is the disciplined, intellectual process of applying skillful reasoning as a guide to belief or action. (Paul, Ennis, & Norris, 1996)

- Critical thinking is careful and deliberate determination of whether to accept, reject, or suspend judgment. (Moore & Parker, 2009)

- Critical thinking, as the term is generally used these days, roughly means reasonable and reflective thinking focused on deciding what to believe or do. (Ennis, 2011)

- In nursing, critical thinking for clinical decision-making is the ability to think in a systematic and logical manner with openness to questions and to reflect on the reasoning process used to ensure safe nursing practice and quality care. (Heaslip, 1992)

- Critical thinking is a purposeful, dynamic, analytic process that contributes to reasoned decisions and sound contextual judgments. (Assessment Technologies Institute, 2003)

- Critical thinking is disciplined, self-directed, rational thinking that supports what we know and makes clear what we don't know. (Wilkinson, 2011, p. 33)

- The ideal critical thinker is inquisitive, open-minded, flexible, fair-minded, well-informed, persistent in seeking the truth, wise in judgments and decision-making, logical, and honest with facing personal biases. The critical thinker uses sound reasoning and is willing to consider valid alternatives. (American Philosophical Association, 1990)

Critical thinkers are flexible, nonjudgmental, inquisitive, honest, and interested in seeking the truth. They possess intellectual skills that allow them to use their curiosity to their advantage, and they have critical attitudes that motivate them to use those skills responsibly.

What Are Critical-Thinking Skills?

Skills in critical thinking refer to the cognitive (intellectual) processes used in complex thinking operations such as problem-solving and decision making. In this example, the skills are italicized, and the complex thinking processes are in bold type:

> *When planning nursing care, nurses* gather information *about the client and then* **draw tentative conclusions** **about the meaning of the information** *to* identify the *client's problems.* *Then they* think of several different actions *they might take to help* **solve or relieve the problem**.

The following are a few examples of critical-thinking skills:

- Objectively gathering information on a problem or issue
- Recognizing the need for more information
- Evaluating the credibility and usefulness of sources of information
- Recognizing gaps in one's own knowledge

- Listening carefully; reading thoughtfully
- Separating relevant from irrelevant data and important from unimportant data
- Organizing or grouping information in meaningful ways
- Making inferences (tentative conclusions) about the meaning of the information
- Visualizing potential solutions to a problem
- Exploring the advantages, disadvantages, and consequences of each potential action

What Are Critical-Thinking Attitudes?

Attitudes are not the same as intellectual skills. They are more like feelings and traits of mind. Your attitudes and character determine whether you will use your thinking skills fairly and with an open mind. Without a critical attitude, people tend to use thinking skills to justify narrow-mindedness and prejudice, and to benefit themselves rather than others. The following are some critical-thinking attitudes (Paul, 1990):

- **Independent thinking.** Critical thinkers do not believe everything they are told; they do not just go along with the crowd. They listen to what others think and they learn from new ideas. They do not accept or reject an idea before they understand it. Nurses should challenge actions and policies with little logical support.

- **Intellectual curiosity.** Critical thinkers love to learn new things. They show an attitude of curiosity and inquiry, and frequently think or ask, "What if . . . ?" "How could we do this differently?" "How does this work?" or "Why did that happen?"

- **Intellectual humility.** Critical thinkers are aware that they do not know everything, and they are not embarrassed to ask for help when they don't know. They are not too proud to seek the wisdom of mentors with knowledge, skill, and ability. They reevaluate their conclusions or actions in light of new information and are willing to admit when they are wrong.

- **Intellectual empathy.** Critical thinkers try to understand the feelings and perceptions of others. They try to see a situation as the other person sees it.

- **Intellectual courage.** Critical thinkers consider and examine fairly their own values and beliefs, as well as beliefs of others, even when this is uncomfortable. They are willing to rethink, and even reject, previously held beliefs that are not well justified. Without intellectual courage, people become resistant to change.

- **Intellectual perseverance.** Critical thinkers don't jump to conclusions or settle for the quick, obvious answer. Important questions are usually complex, and critical thinkers give them serious thought and research, even when this takes a great deal of effort and time.

- **Fair-mindedness.** Critical thinkers try to make impartial judgments. They treat all viewpoints fairly, realizing that personal biases, customs, and social pressures can influence their thinking. They examine their own biases each time they make a decision.

Critical thinking can be used in all aspects of your life. Whenever you are trying to reach an important decision, reasoned action (critical thinking) is called for. Everyday uses of critical thinking might include deciding where you should live, choosing which nursing programs you should apply to, and deciding among several job offers. The rest of this chapter shows you why critical thinking is important to you in your chosen career, nursing.

KnowledgeCheck 2-1

- Define *critical thinking* in your own words.
- List five skills or attitudes that reflect critical thinking.

WHY IS CRITICAL THINKING IMPORTANT FOR NURSES?

Nurses use complex critical-thinking processes (e.g., problem-solving, decision making, and clinical reasoning) in every aspect of their work (Box 2-2). Because nurses care for a variety of patients with a multitude of concerns, a patient's response to therapy may not always be apparent. Nurses constantly assess their patients and determine how they are responding to nursing interventions and medical treatments. Reasoning and reflection are required for the nurse to decide what interventions to use, determine whether they worked, and, if not, figure out why.

BOX 2-2 ■ Complex Thinking Processes

Problem-Solving

Identifying a problem and finding reasonable solutions to it. Requires critical-thinking skills such as organizing data, identifying relevant and important data, making inferences, making decisions, projecting consequences of actions, and applying theoretical knowledge to a specific patient context. The nursing process is a problem-solving process.

Decision Making

Choosing the best action to take. In nursing, this is usually the action likely to produce the desired patient outcome. Requires thinking skills such as making judgments (e.g., about what is important) and making choices. Important in problem-solving; however, many decisions are made that are not related to problem-solving.

Clinical Reasoning

Reflective, concurrent, creative thinking about patients and patient care. Clinical reasoning is used in the nursing process. Reasoning is logical thinking that links thoughts together to create meaning.

Nurses Deal With Complex Situations

Critical thinking is important for nurses because they deal with complex situations daily. One such situation is that of caring for clients with **comorbidities** (more than one health problems occurring at the same time). For example, if a healthy 9-year-old fell and broke his right arm, he would experience pain and discomfort. However, with proper casting of the arm and time to heal, the child would recover. While recovering, he may have to eat using his left hand or limit the use of his injured arm. The child would likely be discharged home from the emergency department or clinic in the care of his parent(s) or guardian(s). The nurse's primary interventions would be to teach the home caregivers the care needed by the child.

 The adjustments would be quite different for an older adult who has had a stroke (a comorbidity) that limits the use of his left arm. With decreased function in the left arm, a right-arm fracture would severely affect the older person's ability to care for himself. The nurse would need to evaluate whether the adult requires care in the hospital or in a skilled-care facility and what support services he will need as he convalesces. In the inpatient setting, nursing interventions might initially include assisting the client with eating, bathing, and toileting.

Clients Are Unique

Critical thinking is important because each client is unique. Their differences (e.g., type of illness, culture, and age) make it impossible to provide strict rules for all client care.

Individual Differences Research-based care plans and protocols identify guidelines for providing care; however, nurses must evaluate and modify these guidelines to be sure they are appropriate for each client.

Consider the following example: You have undoubtedly been told to drink plenty of fluid when you have a cough, to keep the secretions moist. Now imagine you are caring for a client in renal failure. Your client no longer urinates and is being considered for dialysis. You notice that this client has a persistent cough. Should you encourage the client to drink as much fluid as possible? Do you see how you could cause harm to a client by unthinkingly doing as you have been told? Nurses must always think, "How will that work in *this* instance?" "How is this like or different from similar situations?"

Client's Culture Ethnic and cultural differences affect a person's view of health and the healthcare system, as well as his responses to health problems. Cultural beliefs influence how people define sickness, at what point they seek healthcare, what type of healthcare provider they see, and the type of treatment they consider acceptable. Critical thinking enables the nurse to assess the client's and family's cultural beliefs and adapt care so that it is culturally sensitive and responsive to their needs.

Client's Roles A person's roles also influence when, how, and why she seeks healthcare. A single mother with young children may ask to be discharged from the hospital early to meet the needs of her family. Clients with extensive support from family or friends may be willing to take more time to convalesce when they are ill. Nurses take these things into consideration, for example, when determining why a nursing intervention was (or was not) successful.

Other Factors In addition, the following factors may influence how a person responds to illness or to healthcare intervention:

- *Age*. Each of us was raised with a set of beliefs, values, and knowledge that was strongly influenced by the prevailing views of our times.
- *Personal bias*. Clients may have fixed beliefs about health and illness.
- *Personality*. Individuals have unique personalities. This means every person is different; all have individual ways of responding to stress, fear, illness, and pain. Some are hardy and show an attitude of strength, endurance, and high threshold to pain. Others are less tolerant and may outwardly express pain or other conditions associated with illness, hospitalization, and death.
- *Previous experience* with healthcare problems. For example, a boy who has experienced a painful injection in the past may be terrified when he sees the nurse approach with a syringe.

Nurses Apply Knowledge to Provide Holistic Care

In addition to the need to individualize care for each patient, there are some aspects of nursing itself that require the nurse to be a critical thinker.

- *Nursing is an applied discipline*. Nurses deal with complex, ill-defined, and sometimes confusing problems—not well-defined, straightforward problems such as you find in a math book. This means that nurses must *apply* their knowledge, not just memorize and regurgitate facts.
- *Nursing uses knowledge from other fields*. Nurses use information from chemistry, physiology, psychology, social sciences, and other disciplines to identify and plan interventions for patient problems. Nursing plays an important role within a multidisciplinary approach to patient care.
- *Nursing is fast-paced*. Nurses often deal with demanding situations. A patient's condition may change hour to hour or even minute to minute, so knowing the routine

may not be adequate. You will need critical thinking in order to respond appropriately under stress.

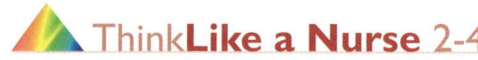

ThinkLike a Nurse 2-4

Write a short scenario (story) about a nurse that illustrates one of the reasons why nurses need to be critical thinkers.

A MODEL FOR CRITICAL THINKING

A **model** is a set of interrelated concepts that represents a particular way of thinking about something—much in the same way that the shape of a lens affects what you see. For example, you would look through a telescope to view a distant star. Looking at the star through reading glasses or a magnifying glass would give a different view. You will learn more about models in Chapter 8.

The critical-thinking model used throughout this book provides one way of making sense of critical thinking. This model organizes critical thinking into five major categories. Table 2-1 defines each category and provides questions to help you focus your thinking in patient care situations. You can use some of the questions when deciding what to think about and do; you can use others when analyzing a situation after it happens (reflecting). Figure 2-1 is a simpler representation of the model, relating it to the nursing process, which is introduced later in this chapter.

This model is not meant to be all-inclusive; there is much more to critical thinking than just the questions listed in Table 2-1. Use it as a guide when you are faced with clinical decisions or unfamiliar situations. The questions can help you to "think about your thinking" as you apply principles and knowledge from various sources to a current problem. This should help you to achieve good outcomes for your patients. You do not need to ask yourself every question in every situation—just those that are relevant. And you should not proceed from top to bottom in the table. The processes do not occur "sequentially," so you may jump back and forth among them.

Let's apply the model to a situation faced by all nursing students. Soon you will begin your clinical rotations, if you have not already done so. Many students find clinical experiences exciting, yet somewhat intimidating. ✚ How could you use the five points of the critical-thinking star to approach your first clinical day so that you will be well prepared and able to function safely?

Contextual Awareness One of the first things you need to consider is your usual response to new experiences. How do you react to change? What other tasks or assignments do you have that will dictate the timing of your preparation? Have you had any previous experiences that will aid or hamper you in your preparation? As you consider these questions, you are addressing the star point of contextual awareness.

Table 2-1 ➤ Critical-Thinking Model

THINKING PROCESS	DESCRIPTION	QUESTIONS FOR FOCUSING THINKING
Contextual awareness (deciding what to observe and consider)	An awareness of what's happening in the total situation, including values, cultural issues, interpersonal relationships, and environmental influences	■ What is going on in the situation that may influence the outcome? ■ What factors may influence my behavior and that of others in this situation (e.g., culture, roles, relationships, economic status)? ■ What about this situation have I seen before? What is different? ■ Who should be involved in order to improve the outcome? ■ What else was happening at the same time that affected me in this situation? ■ What happened just before this incident that made a difference? ■ What emotional responses influenced how I reacted in this situation? ■ What changes in behavior alerted me that something was wrong?
Inquiry (based on credible sources)	Applying standards of good reasoning to your thinking when analyzing a situation and evaluating your actions	■ How do I go about getting the information I need? ■ What framework should I use to organize my information? ■ Do I have enough knowledge to decide? If not, what do I need to know? ■ Have I used a valid, reliable source of information (e.g., patient, other professionals, references)? ■ Did I (do I need to) validate the data (e.g., with the client)? ■ What else do I need to know? What information is missing? ■ Are the data accurate? Precise? ■ What's important and what's not important in this situation? ■ Did I consider professional, ethical, and legal standards? ■ Have I jumped to conclusions?
Considering alternatives	Exploring and imagining as many alternatives as you can think of for the situation	■ What is one possible explanation for what is happening or what happened? ■ What are other explanations for what is happening? What is one thing I could do in this situation? ■ What are two more possibilities/alternatives? ■ Are there others who might help me develop more alternatives? ■ Of the possible actions I am considering, which one is most reasonable? Why are the others not as reasonable? ■ Of the possible actions I am considering, which one is most likely to achieve the desired outcomes?
Analyzing assumptions	Recognizing and analyzing assumptions you are making about the situation and examining the beliefs that underlie your choices	■ What have I (or others) taken for granted in this situation? ■ Which beliefs/values are shaping my assumptions? ■ What assumptions contributed to the problem in this situation? ■ What rationale supports my assumptions? ■ How will I know my assumption is correct? ■ What biases do I have that may affect my thinking and my decisions in this situation?

continued

Table 2-1 ➤ Critical-Thinking Model—cont'd		
THINKING PROCESS	**DESCRIPTION**	**QUESTIONS FOR FOCUSING THINKING**
Reflecting skeptically and deciding what to do	Questioning, analyzing, and reflecting on the rationale for your decisions	▪ What aspects of this situation require the most careful attention? ▪ What else might work in this situation? ▪ Am I sure of my interpretation of this situation? ▪ Why is (was) it important to intervene? ▪ What rationale do I have for my decisions? ▪ In priority order, what should I do in this situation and why? ▪ Having decided what was wrong/happening, what is the best response? ▪ What might I delegate in this situation? ▪ What got me started taking some action? ▪ What priorities were missed? ▪ What was done? Why was it done? ▪ What would I do differently after reflecting on this situation?

Sources: Model based on Brookfield, S. D. (1991). *Developing critical thinkers.* San Francisco: Jossey-Bass; McDonald, M. E. (2002). *Systematic assessment of learning outcomes: Developing multiple-choice exams.* Boston: Jones & Bartlett Publishers; Paul, R. W. (1993). *Critical thinking: What every person needs to survive in a rapidly changing world* (3rd ed.). Santa Rosa, CA: Foundation for Critical Thinking; Raingruber, B., & Haffer, A. (2001). *Using your head to land on your feet.* Philadelphia: F. A. Davis; and Wilkinson, J. M. (2011). *Nursing process and critical thinking* (5th ed.). Upper Saddle River, NJ: Prentice Hall.

Using Credible Sources You need to gather information about the clinical experience. It is important to use inquiry based on credible sources as you gather data. For example, you may ask your instructor for guidance on how to best prepare. Or you might consult a student who has successfully completed the same course. You will need to obtain accurate information about clients who have been assigned to you for care. You could use the client's chart and your textbooks to prepare. Use only knowledgeable, reliable sources of information—for example, nursing texts and nursing journals, not popular (nonscholarly) magazines (such as *Parents* magazine) or certain Internet sites. After you have more information, you should go back and analyze your response to the situation. You may find that you are feeling less anxious already! All of this is a part of inquiry.

Exploring Alternatives and Analyzing Assumptions Now that you know something about the clinical experience, you can plan your day. You need to consider alternatives and analyze your assumptions about the experience. What is expected of you? What do you expect from the experience? How should you approach your client? How will you introduce yourself? What skills do you have? How will you apply them to caring for your client?

Reflecting and Deciding After you feel that you have addressed these concerns, you need to quickly review your preparation (reflective skepticism). Have you gathered enough information to feel comfortable in the situation? Have you left anything out? Do you need more information?

This was a demonstration of how you might apply the critical-thinking model to a real experience. In this example, you also used theoretical, practical, personal, and ethical knowledge, which are explained in the next section.

Knowledge Check 2-2

In the preceding example, identify the actions that demonstrate use of each of the four types of knowledge.

WHAT ARE THE DIFFERENT KINDS OF NURSING KNOWLEDGE?

Critical thinking does not occur in a vacuum—you must have something to think about: your knowledge base. Nurses use various kinds of knowledge: theoretical, practical, personal, and ethical. Every chapter of this text is designed to help you gain practical knowledge and theoretical knowledge. Put very simply, that is *knowing what* (to do) and *knowing how* (to do it). In fact, the chapters are organized according to those two types of knowledge.

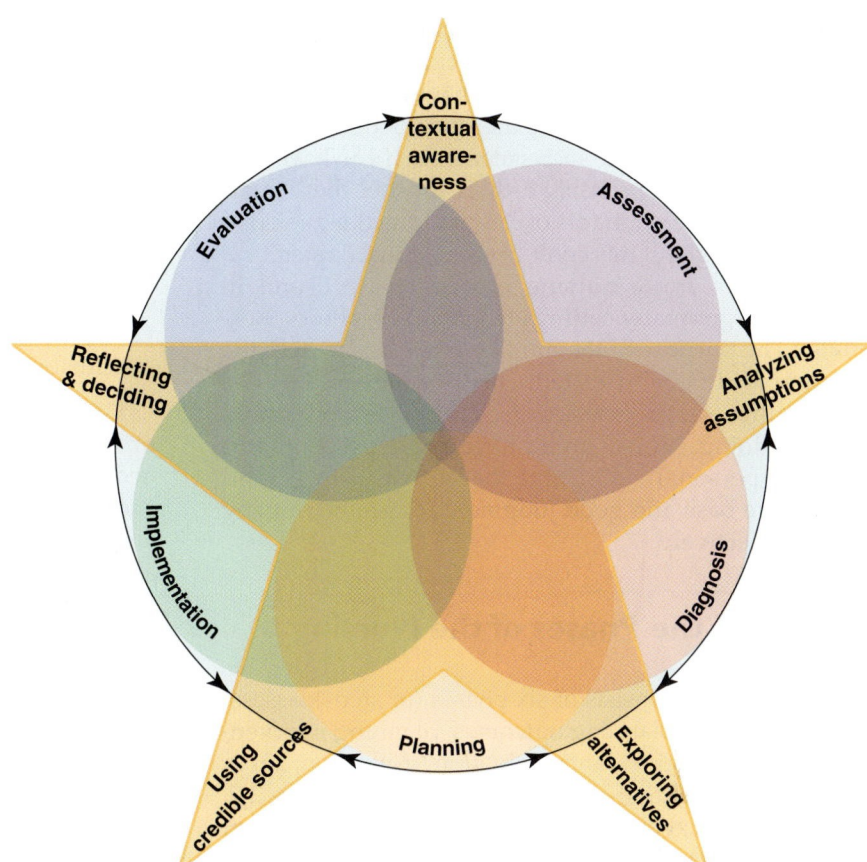

FIGURE 2-1 Model of critical thinking and nursing process.

Theoretical Knowledge Each chapter begins by presenting theoretical knowledge. Theoretical knowledge consists of information, facts, principles, and evidence-based theories in nursing and related disciplines (e.g., physiology and psychology). It includes research findings and rationally constructed explanations of phenomena. You will use it to describe your patients, understand their health status, explain your reasoning for choosing interventions, and predict patient responses to interventions and treatments.

Practical Knowledge Each chapter then provides the practical knowledge that enables you to apply your theoretical knowledge to caring for patients. Practical knowledge—knowing what to do and how to do it—consists of processes (e.g., the decision process and the nursing process) and procedures (e.g., how to give an injection), and is an aspect of nursing expertise.

Self-Knowledge In addition to theoretical and practical knowledge, nurses use self-knowledge—that is, self-understanding. To think critically, you must be aware of your beliefs, values, and cultural and religious biases. This kind of knowledge helps you to find errors in your thinking and enables you to tune in to your patients. You can gain self-knowledge by developing personal awareness—by reflecting (asking yourself), "Why did I do that?" or "How did I come to think that?"

Ethical Knowledge Finally, nurses use ethical knowledge, that is, knowledge of obligation, or right and wrong. Ethical knowledge consists of information about moral principles and processes for making moral decisions. Ethical knowledge helps you to fulfill your ethical obligations to patients and colleagues. Chapter 44 will help expand your ethical knowledge.

PracticalKnowledge
knowing **how**

WHAT IS NURSING PROCESS?

Nursing process is a systematic problem-solving process that guides all nursing actions. It is the type of thinking and doing nurses use in their practice. In fact, the American Nurses Association (ANA) organizes its standards of care around the nursing process (ANA, 2010).

ThinkLike a Nurse 2-5

Practice your critical thinking. What questions should you ask about the last paragraph you have just read? For hints, look at Figure 2-1 and Table 2-1.

When evaluating the preceding paragraph, you should ask about the credibility of the sources cited, and you should ask yourself whether you have enough information about them to judge their credibility. Do you know what the ANA is? What they do? Who are their members? What are standards of practice, and who decides what will be included in them? What effect do they have on what you will be doing as a nurse? Those are the kinds of questions you should ask when you see such statements. If you have read Chapter 1, you can probably answer most of these questions. You will see standards of care and practice quoted in chapters throughout this book, beginning in Chapter 3.

All nurses apply nursing process, to well and ill clients alike, in many settings (e.g., homes, clinics, hospitals). The purpose of the nursing process is to help the nurse provide goal-directed, client-centered care. The nursing process, like nursing itself, involves both thinking and doing. Nurses must have good psychomotor and interpersonal skills, and they must use a sound knowledge base and good judgment to use the nursing process effectively.

What Are the Phases of the Nursing Process?

Nursing process consists of six phases (or steps): assessment, diagnosis, planning outcomes, planning interventions, implementation, and evaluation (Wilkinson, 2011). A model illustrating these phases is shown in Figure 2-2. Note, though, that experts organize the phases in different ways. Many have a five-step process, combining outcomes and interventions into one planning phase. Some even have a four-step process; they combine assessment and diagnosis into one phase that they call "assessment." There is no "right" way to do it, and experienced nurses

do not use the steps separately anyway. Your text presents them as distinct and separate only to make it easier for you to learn how the process works.

Assessment The first phase of the nursing process—the data-gathering stage—is assessment. You will obtain information from many sources: the client via history or physical exam, the client record, lab or test results, other health professionals, the client's family or support system, and the professional literature. In this phase, your purpose is to gather data that you will use to draw conclusions about the client's health status.

Diagnosis This is the second phase of the nursing process. In this step you will identify the client's health needs (usually stated in the form of a problem) based on careful review of your assessment data. You need to analyze all your data, synthesize and cluster information, and hypothesize about your client's health status. The term *diagnosis* has been thought of as being medical, such as a diagnosis of cancer or diabetes. However, nursing diagnoses reflect the client's responses to actual or potential health problems and are different from medical diagnoses, as you will discover in Chapter 4.

Planning The third and fourth steps of the nursing process both involve planning. Planning can be divided into two phases: planning (predicting) outcomes and planning interventions. The finished product of the planning phases is a holistic nursing care plan, individualized to reflect the client's problems and strengths. A care plan is a written or electronic document containing detailed instructions for a client's nursing care (see Fig. 5-2).

- In the **planning outcomes** step you work with the client to decide goals for your care—that is, the client outcomes you want to achieve through your nursing activities. These outcomes will drive your choice of interventions. The following is an example of an outcome statement you might find in a care plan:

  Nutritional status will improve as evidenced by a weight gain of 3 lb (1.4 kg) by July 1.

  See Chapter 5 for more about goals and outcomes.

- In the **planning interventions** phase you develop a list of possible interventions based on your nursing knowledge and then choose those most likely to help the client to achieve the stated goals. The best interventions are evidence based; that is, supported by sound research. See Chapter 6 for more about interventions.

Implementation This is the action phase. During implementation you will you carry out or delegate the actions that you previously planned. You may delegate an action to another member of the healthcare team only if it is an action that may safely and legally be carried out by that team member. Delegation is discussed further in Chapters 7 and 40. In the implementation phase, you also document your actions and the client's responses to them.

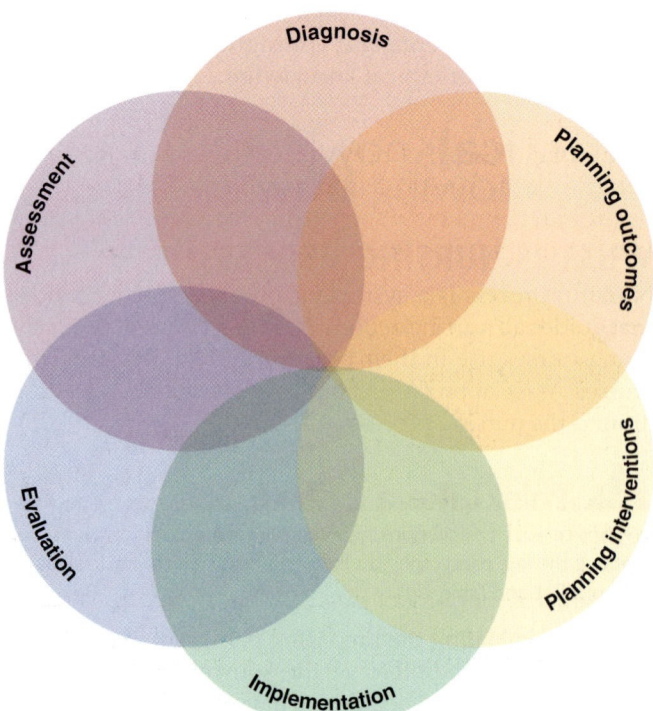

FIGURE 2-2 The phases of the nursing process.

Evaluation The final phase of nursing process is evaluation. In this phase, you determine whether the desired outcomes have been achieved, and judge whether your actions have successfully treated or prevented the client's health problems. You then modify the care plan as needed. For example, if a problem has been resolved, you delete it from the care plan; if outcomes have not been achieved, you determine why. It may be that a new intervention is needed. If so, you add it.

Key Point: *Notice that the nursing process is not intended to be linear (one step rigidly following another). Instead it is a cyclical process that follows a logical progression.* You can see that the evaluation step requires you to begin again using all the other steps. You will find that you go back and forth between the steps, especially as you gain nursing experience. In addition to being cyclical, the steps may be *concurrent*. That means that some of the steps may occur at the same time. For example, while inserting a urinary catheter (implementation step), the nurse also observes the urine that returns through the tube (assessment step). You will learn about each nursing process phase in depth in Chapters 3 through 7.

KnowledgeCheck 2-3
- List the six phases of the nursing process.
- In which stage does the nurse collect data?
- Which stage involves problem identification?
- What does the nurse do in the evaluation step?

How Is Nursing Process Related to Critical Thinking?
Key Point: *Critical thinking and nursing process are interrelated, but not identical.*

- Nurses use critical thinking for decisions unrelated to the nursing process (e.g., to decide how many nurses are needed to staff the unit).
- Some nursing activities (e.g., applying a cardiac monitor, inserting a urinary catheter), although they must be done skillfully, do not require reflective critical thinking.

Nursing process is essentially a problem-solving process. As such, it is one of the *complex critical-thinking skills* (see Box 2-2). Complex thinking skills, such as the nursing process, make use of many different critical-thinking skills (see Table 2-1 and Fig. 2-1). The following sections illustrate how nurses use critical thinking, as well as nursing knowledge, in each phase of the nursing process.

WHAT IS CARING?
Caring involves personal concern for people, events, projects, and things. It allows you to connect with others and to give help as well as receive it. One aspect of self-knowledge is to be aware of what and whom you care about. Knowing what the patient cares about reveals what is stressful for the patient, because only things that matter can create stress. Caring also enables the nurse to notice which interventions are effective.

A caring perspective highlights each person as unique and valued, so caring is always specific and relational for each nurse–person encounter. It is not an abstraction. That is, you don't just care for "suffering humankind," but you respond compassionately to *this* patient's needs right now, in the moment, even if you are busy and tired. Caring involves thinking and acting in ways that preserve human dignity and humanity, and does not treat people as objects. For example, a caring nurse drapes a patient for privacy when inserting a urinary catheter. A caring nurse's actions are never routine or impersonal.

Caring has at least five components:

- *Knowing.* Striving to understand what an event (e.g., an illness) means in the life of the patient
- *Being with.* Being emotionally present for the patient (e.g., making eye contact, actively listening)
- *Doing for.* Doing what the patient would do for himself if he could (e.g., bathing)
- *Enabling.* Supporting the patient through coping with life changes and unfamiliar events, such as hospitalization
- *Maintaining belief.* Having faith in the patient's ability to get through the change or event and to find fulfillment and meaning (Swanson, 1990)

Caring is the central concept in several nursing theories. You will learn more about them in Chapter 8.

KnowledgeCheck 2-4
List all the characteristics of caring that you can remember.

WHAT IS FULL-SPECTRUM NURSING?
Key Point: Full-spectrum *nursing is a unique blend of thinking, doing, and caring.* It is performed by nurses who fully develop and apply nursing knowledge, critical thinking, and the nursing process to patient situations for the purpose of effecting good outcomes.

What Concepts Are Used in Full-Spectrum Nursing?
When we put concepts (ideas) together to explain something, it is called a **model**. You'll learn more about concepts in Chapter 8; for now, think of them as ideas. The four main concepts that describe full-spectrum nursing are *thinking, doing, caring,* and *patient situation* (or *context*) (Table 2-2).

In order to think, you must have something to think about. When nurses think, they use the nursing knowledge that they have stored in their memory. In addition, they think about the patient situation, which they acquire through use of the nursing process. Situation, or context, refers to the context for care, the patient's

Table 2-2 ➤ Full-Spectrum Nursing Concepts			
THINKING	**DOING**	**CARING**	**PATIENT SITUATION**
Critical Thinking Enables you to fully use your knowledge and skills	**Practical Knowledge** Skills, procedures, and processes (including the nursing process)	**Self-Knowledge** Awareness of your values, beliefs, and biases	**Patient Data** Physical, psychosocial, spiritual
Theoretical Knowledge Principles, facts, theories; what you have to think *with*	**Nursing Process** *Assessment and Evaluation:* Everything you know about the patient including context *Planning and Implementation:* What you do for the patient	**Ethical Knowledge** Understanding your obligations; sense of right and wrong	**Patient Preferences and Context** Context for care, environment, relationships, culture, resources, supports

environment outside the care setting, relationships, resources available for patient care, and so on. Figure 2-3 is a simple, visual model of full-spectrum nursing. You can see that the concept's full model involves everything you have learned in this chapter—critical thinking, nursing knowledge, and nursing process—but organized under the simple concepts of thinking, doing, caring, and patient situation.

Let's see how the model concepts work together for a full-spectrum nurse. They are all interrelated and overlapping, but we divide them into simple categories to help you understand and remember them. You can see that a full-spectrum nurse needs excellent thinking skills because there is so much to think *about* and so much to *do*.

KnowledgeCheck 2-5
- What are the four main concepts of the full-spectrum model of nursing?
- Where do the four types of nursing knowledge fit into the full-spectrum model?
- What is the ultimate purpose of full-spectrum nursing?

How Does the Model Work?
The full-spectrum nursing model is used throughout this text, so it is important that you understand how it works. Nurses use critical *thinking* in all steps of the nursing process. They also apply critical thinking to the four kinds of nursing knowledge, and when they are *doing* for the patient. *Caring* motivates and facilitates

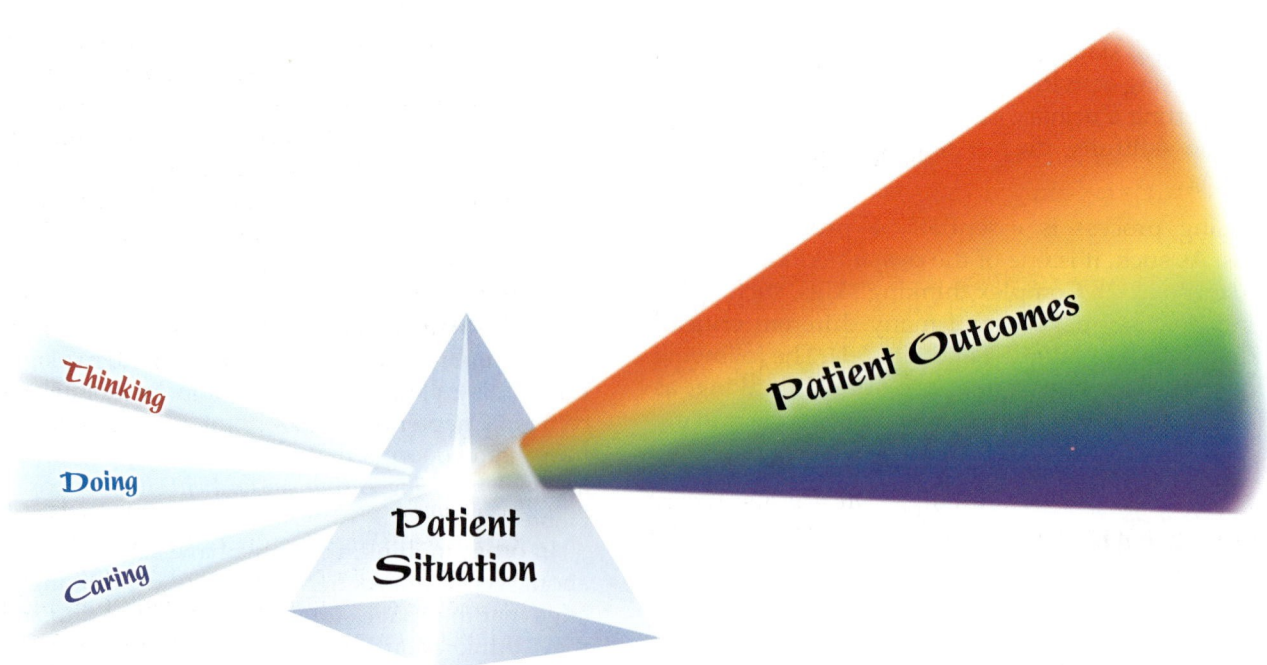

FIGURE 2-3 Model of full-spectrum nursing.

the thinking and doing. The goal of all this is to have a positive effect on a patient's health outcomes.

The following patient situations illustrate how the three main dimensions of full-spectrum nursing work together. As you read, notice the overlapping of concepts. For example, recall that nursing process and problem-solving are themselves complex critical-thinking skills. Also notice how the nurse uses critical thinking with nursing knowledge and nursing process.

Patient Situation 1

When taking a patient's oral temperature, a nurse sees a glass of ice water on the overbed table. Realizing that a cold drink can reduce the accuracy of the temperature reading, she questions the patient, "How long since you've taken a drink of water?" The nurse is busy and tired, but she returns to take the patient's temperature again at a later time.

Thinking

Theoretical knowledge. The nurse realized that a cold drink can lower the temperature reading. The nurse used interviewing principles to get more information from the patient.

Critical thinking. The nurse recognized relevant information and identified the need for more information. She used the patient's answer to decide what to do. Being aware of context is also critical thinking. The context in this scenario includes ice water within the patient's reach and that the patient was physically capable of reaching it.

Doing

Practical knowledge. The nurse used a psychomotor skill when she measured the patient's temperature to acquire more patient vital sign data and a communication process to question the patient.

Nursing process (Assessment). The nurse observed the glass of ice water on the table. The nurse asked, "How long since you've taken a drink of water?" The nurse also observed the environmental data (e.g., ice water at the bedside). *(Implementation)* The nurse took the patient's temperature.

Caring

The scenario does not say this, but a caring nurse, even a very busy one, would not be annoyed with the patient for the inconvenience of having to come back again to take the temperature. Self-knowledge might include the nurse's awareness that she is tired and feeling irritable. Ethical knowledge would tell her that she has an obligation to get an accurate temperature from the patient rather than thinking, "Oh, I'll just record the reading a degree or two higher, as it doesn't matter that much."

Patient Situation 2

Thirty minutes after giving a pain medication, a nurse checks with the patient to see whether the pain has been relieved. The nurse is using the desired outcome ("States pain relief is adequate . . .") as a criterion for evaluating the effectiveness of the nursing activity. The patient says, "I don't think that medicine is helping a bit." On a scale of 1 to 10, the patient reports her pain as 9. The nurse notifies the primary care provider to request an increase in the dosage of pain medication. She then gives the new medication to the patient and, even though it is the end of her shift, she sits with the patient to help him use guided imagery and deep-breathing strategies to reduce his pain until the medication takes effect.

Thinking

Theoretical knowledge. The nurse had theoretical knowledge of the interval needed for the medication to take effect. She also knew facts and principles about pain rating scales and strategies to relieve pain without medication.

Critical thinking. Criterion-based evaluation is a critical-thinking skill. The nurse applied knowledge of the medication's action to know when to evaluate the patient's response to it. She realized she needed more data about the patient's pain scale. She was also able to generate more interventions, such as requesting an adjustment in the dosage of medication and using guided imagery and deep breathing.

Doing

Practical knowledge. The nurse undoubtedly used practical knowledge when administering the medication (e.g., knowledge of how to administer the medication) and helping the patient with guided imagery and deep breathing to distract him from his pain.

Nursing process. The nurse had apparently previously assessed the patient, identified a nursing diagnosis of Acute Pain, set a desired outcome, implemented an intervention, and then evaluated its effect based on new patient data. She also implemented care when she called the primary provider, administered the medications, and used guided imagery and deep breathing. In addition to data about the pain, you might assume that the nurse knew the following about the context: From the way the goal is stated, we can assume that the patient can speak. The patient is most likely hospitalized because he is not administering his own medication, and the nurse plans to check on him in 30 minutes. Certainly the nurse had all that contextual information.

Caring

Ethical knowledge. The nurse served as a patient advocate when she telephoned the care provider for a new prescription. She cared enough about the patient to stay with him and help him reduce the intensity of his pain using nonpharmacological methods until the new medication took effect, even though this meant working late.

Self-knowledge. Perhaps this nurse values a stoic, "tough it out," response to pain. Knowing this about herself, she could put this aside and see the reality of suffering for the patient and how the experience of pain is individual and personal.

As a full-spectrum nurse, you will apply thinking, doing, and caring to patient situations to help benefit patients and bring about good outcomes.

Toward Evidence-Based Practice

Catlett, S., & Lovan, S. (2011). **Being a good nurse and doing the right thing: A replication study.** *Nursing Ethics, 18*(1), 54–63.

The purpose of this qualitative study was to examine nurses' perceptions of what it means to be a good nurse and to do the right thing. Researchers used open-ended questions to interview nurse subjects. They identified four categories that related to being a good nurse and doing the right thing: (1) personal traits and attributes; (2) technical skills and management of care; (3) work environment and coworkers; and (4) caring and caring behaviors.

1. What examples of full-spectrum nursing can you see in the four categories identified?

2. Based on this abstract, which of the following questions might this study answer satisfactorily for you? Explain your reasoning.
   a. What is a good nurse?
   b. Did the nurse-subjects demonstrate critical thinking?
   c. How did the nurse-subjects describe a good nurse?

 Go to Chapter 2, **Toward Evidence-Based Practice Suggested Responses** on Davis*Plus.*

 To explore learning resources for this chapter,

 Go to Davis*Plus* at DavisPl.us/Wilkinson3.

Chapter Resources for Chapter 2:
   Response sheets for all learning activities
   Resources for Caregivers and Health Professionals
   Reading More About Critical Thinking & Nursing Process (suggested readings)
   Concept Map of chapter content
Interactive Case Studies
NCLEX-Style and Chapter Review Questions
Chapter Overview Podcasts

For references cited in this chapter,

 Go to Volume 2, **References Cited.**

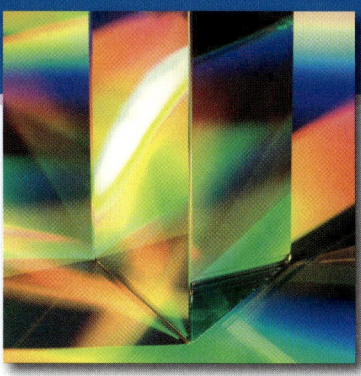

CHAPTER 3

Nursing Process: Assessment

Learning Outcomes

After completing this chapter, you should be able to:

➤ Define *nursing assessment*, including the four features common to all its definitions.

➤ Explain how assessment is related to each of the other steps of the nursing process.

➤ State the ANA position on delegating assessment.

➤ Name three requirements of The Joint Commission regarding patient assessment.

➤ Use assessment skills to gather data during a nursing assessment.

➤ Define initial, ongoing, comprehensive, and focused assessment.

➤ Explain the importance of discharge planning assessment.

➤ List five special needs assessments and state when or why you would use them.

➤ Identify the following types of data: subjective, objective, primary source, secondary source.

➤ Identify at least four components of a nursing health history and state the purpose of each.

➤ Describe the differences between directive and nondirective interviewing.

➤ Compare and contrast open-ended and closed questions, including definitions, uses, advantages, and disadvantages.

➤ Discuss how to prepare for and conduct an interview.

➤ Describe three circumstances in which you should validate data.

➤ Use nursing frameworks to organize data.

➤ State four guidelines for documenting data.

➤ Compose three questions to ask yourself when you are evaluating the quality of your assessments.

Key Concepts

Assessment
Data

Related Concepts

See the Concept Map on Davis*Plus*.

Meet Your Patient

As the intake nurse in a community-based clinic in Miami, Florida, your role is to complete a comprehensive nursing assessment and initiate a plan of care for the clients. Your first client is a 24-year-old single woman, Sami, who is requesting clinic services for her general healthcare needs. Sami is Cuban American and lives alone in a one-bedroom apartment. She works as a fitness trainer at the local fitness club while attending college part-time. Her family lives in Tampa, Florida. Sami's earnings place her below the poverty level. She realizes that she must have healthcare to prevent health problems and to detect and receive treatment of illnesses should they arise. You will be asked to apply full-spectrum thinking to Sami's case throughout the chapter as you learn the concepts of assessment.

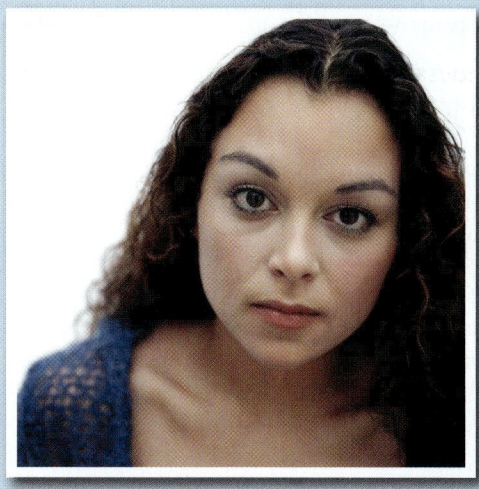

TheoreticalKnowledge
knowing**why**

In this section, you will learn about the role of assessment in the nursing process and collaborative care; about sources of data; and about various types of assessment.

ABOUT THE KEY CONCEPTS

Assessment is a key concept because it is so integral to the nursing role. It is closely tied to another key concept: *data*. The related concepts in this chapter will enable you to fully understand the notion of assessment and to see how they all fit together.

ASSESSMENT: THE FIRST STEP OF THE NURSING PROCESS

Assessment is the systematic gathering of information related to the physical, mental, spiritual, socioeconomic, and cultural status of an individual, group, or community. Although various definitions exist, all definitions of assessment include the following features: collecting data, categorizing data, recording data, and using a systematic and ongoing process.

The purpose of assessment is to obtain enough data to allow you to help the patient. The nursing interview and the physical assessment findings become a part of the **patient database** (all the pertinent patient data obtained by nurses and other health professionals). You will use the facts, impressions, and contextual information obtained in your assessment to develop a plan of care.

How Is Assessment Related to Other Steps of the Nursing Process?

Assessment is the first phase of the nursing process. Data must be accurate and complete, because the remainder of the nursing process rests on this foundation of data. Assessment is related to other nursing process steps as follows (Fig. 3-1):

- *Diagnosis*—Assessment provides the data necessary for identifying the client's health problems and strengths.
- *Planning outcomes*—Data about the patient's motivation, family, and available resources help you formulate realistic goals.
- *Planning interventions*—Assessment data help you to choose the interventions most likely to be acceptable to and effective for the client.
- *Implementation*—As you perform nursing actions, you will also gather data by observing the client's responses. For example, while helping a client ambulate, you might observe that she becomes short of breath. If this is new information, you might then identify a new diagnosis of Activity Intolerance.

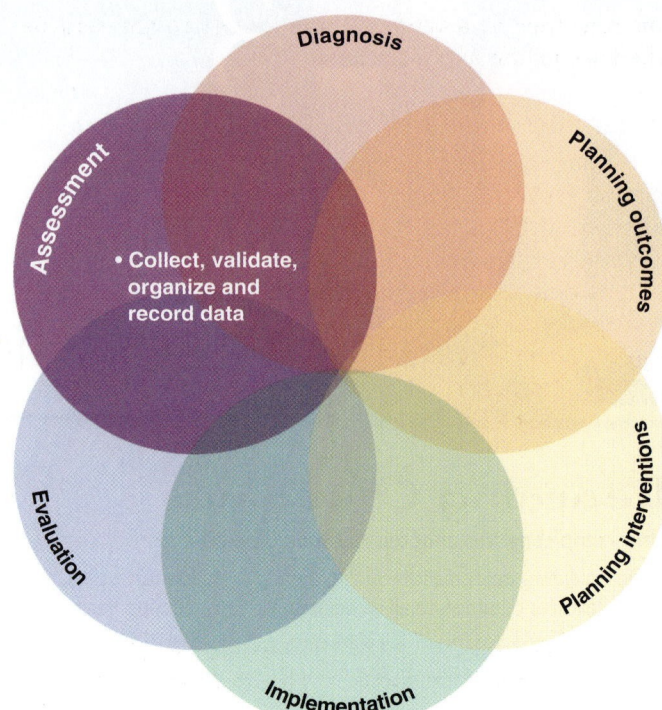

FIGURE 3-1 Nursing process: Assessment phase.

- *Evaluation*—After performing interventions for existing diagnoses, you assess the client's responses. This *reassessment* provides the basis for changes in the care plan.

How Does Nursing Assessment Fit Into Collaborative Care?

As a nurse, you will focus on your clients' *responses* to illness, which include their physical responses; their understanding of the illness and how it affects their lives and ability to care for themselves; and their emotional responses and concerns. You will also use assessment with healthy clients to help identify ways they can maintain their current level of wellness and prevent disease. This is different from traditional medical assessments, which focus on identifying disease.

Other healthcare professionals can access the database created from the nursing assessment findings. In some settings, the nurse looks at the database and delegates or makes referrals to other professionals with expertise in a particular area of healthcare. This helps ensure that clients receive the proper care by qualified individuals at the time it is needed.

Sami's case illustrates this. Sami has not had a gynecological (female) examination for 5 years. In the interview, she tells you that her mother has had breast cancer and that her sister is being treated for endometriosis. You first ask whether, because of any religious or other beliefs, Sami would be offended by an open discussion. Then you ask about her sexual activity, assuring her that you will keep all information confidential. As a result of this interview, you encourage Sami to get a women's health examination as soon as possible. She agrees, and you refer her to a women's clinic, where she will be billed according to her ability to pay.

What Do Professional Standards Say About Assessment?

Complete, skillful, and timely assessment of all clients is an important skill for nurses in all healthcare settings. Standards of governmental agencies, professional organizations, and accrediting bodies, such as the following, all address assessment.

The American Nurses Association (ANA) standards for clinical practice, which apply to all nurses, identify assessment as a professional responsibility (Box 3-1).

BOX 3-1 ■ Professional Standards for Assessment

American Nurses Association Standards of Nursing Practice[1]

Standard 1. Assessment
The registered nurse collects comprehensive data pertinent to the healthcare consumer's health and/or situation.

Competencies

The registered nurse:

- Collects comprehensive data including but not limited to physical, functional, psychosocial, emotional, cognitive, sexual, cultural, age-related, environmental, spiritual/transpersonal, and economic assessments in a systematic and ongoing process while honoring the uniqueness of the person.
- Elicits the healthcare consumer's values, preferences, expressed needs, and their knowledge of the healthcare situation.
- Involves the healthcare consumer, family, and other healthcare providers, as appropriate, in holistic data collection.
- Identifies barriers (e.g., psychosocial, literacy, financial, cultural) to effective communication and makes appropriate adaptations.
- Recognizes the impact of personal attitudes, values, and beliefs.
- Assesses family dynamics and impact on healthcare consumer health and wellness.
- Prioritizes data collection based on the healthcare consumer's immediate condition, or the anticipated needs of the healthcare consumer or situation.
- Uses appropriate evidence-based assessment techniques, instruments, and tools.
- Synthesizes available data, information, and knowledge relevant to the situation to identify patterns and variances.
- Applies ethical, legal, and privacy guidelines and policies to the collection, maintenance, use, and dissemination of data and information.
- Recognizes the healthcare consumer as the authority on her or his own health by honoring their care preferences.
- Documents relevant data in a retrievable format.

Source: American Nurses Association. (2010). *Nursing: Scope and standards of practice* (2nd ed.). Silver Spring, MD: Nursebooks.org.

Nurse practice acts regulate the practice of nurses in individual states. The National Council of State Boards of Nursing (2006, Article II, Section 2) *Model Nursing Practice Act* also asserts that the scope of nursing includes surveillance and comprehensive assessment of the health status of individuals, families, groups, and communities.

The Joint Commission (2012, pp. PC-1–PC-20), in its standards for "Provision of Care, Treatment, and Services," identifies assessment as an essential element of patient care. In agencies with an RN on staff, an RN must assess patients' needs for nursing care within 24 hours of inpatient admission (p. PC-7). The Joint Commission includes standards that require agencies to provide evidence that:

- Assessments are written, comprehensive (physical, psychological, and social status), and used to identify and assign priorities for care.
- Agency policy designates (1) when each patient is to be reassessed and (2) which disciplines can make which assessments.
- All patients are assessed for pain.

KnowledgeCheck 3-1

- What are the four features common to all definitions of assessment?
- How is a nursing assessment similar to a medical assessment?
- How is it different?

Can I Delegate Assessments?

For data to be reliable, someone with education and experience must perform the assessment. **Key Point:** *Nurse aides or other nursing assistive personnel (NAP) may collect information such as temperature, height, and weight. However, as a nurse, it is your responsibility to assign those tasks, validate the data collected, conduct the interview, and complete the physical assessment.* The ANA's *Code of Ethics for Nurses*, Provision 4 (2001) states: "The nurse . . . determines the appropriate delegation of tasks consistent with the nurse's obligation to provide optimum patient care." Also see Chapters 7 and 40 for a thorough discussion of delegation of tasks to NAPs. The following resources can guide you in deciding which caregivers are qualified to perform parts or all of an assessment.

- *State nurse practice acts.* Each state nurse practice act specifies which portions of the assessment can legally be completed by individuals with different credentials. Look for statements related to delegation. For example, the definitions in the National Council of State Boards of Nursing's (NCSBN) *Model Nursing Practice Act* (2011) differentiate between assessments by RNs and LPNs/LVNs (Box 3-2).
- *Agency policies/procedures,* such as those stating which caregivers can collect and document specified data, can provide guidelines.
- *Accrediting agencies,* such as The Joint Commission, also provide guidelines on who can perform and document assessments.

BOX 3-2 ■ NCSBN Model Nursing Practice Act (2011), Selected Definitions Related to Nursing Assessment

Comprehensive Assessment by the RN

An extensive data collection (initial and ongoing) for individuals, families, groups, and communities:

Addressing anticipated changes in client conditions as well as emerging changes in a client's health status

Recognizing alterations to previous client conditions

Synthesizing the biological, psychological, and social aspects of the client's condition

Evaluating the impact of nursing care

Using this broad and complete analysis to make independent decisions and nursing diagnoses

Planning nursing interventions

Evaluating need for different interventions

Communicating the need to communicate and consult with other health team members.

Focused Assessment by the LPN/LVN

An appraisal of an individual's status and situation at hand, contributing to comprehensive assessment by the registered nurse, supporting ongoing data collection, and deciding who needs to be informed of the information and when to inform.

Source: Reproduced from the NCSBN Web site (*www.ncsbn.org*) and used by permission from the National Council of State Boards of Nursing (NCSBN), Chicago, IL © 2011.

■ *The American Nurses Association (ANA)* definitions of nursing and *Scope and Standards of Practice* (2010) guide decisions on who is ultimately responsible and qualified to collect assessment data. To access the ANA Web site,

Go to Chapter 3, **Resources for Caregivers & Health Professionals,** on Davis*Plus.*

ThinkLike a Nurse 3-1

Think about the following situations, then answer the questions. More than one answer may be acceptable. Compare your ideas with those of other students or nurses, or consult your instructor.

■ Suppose you are a nurse in a healthcare setting in which the policy states that nursing assistive personnel (NAPs) can take vital signs (blood pressure, pulse, temperature, and respirations). You have a patient who is critically ill and whose condition is changing rapidly. Would you measure the vital signs or delegate the task to the NAP? Why?

■ Imagine that you are a nurse in the same hospital on a different day. All but one NAP have called in sick today because of an influenza outbreak. This NAP is inexperienced and overwhelmed by her tasks. Would you bathe the patients in your caseload (even though that is usually done by a NAP), or would you ask the NAP to do it? Why?

It is obvious from the previous examples that you must use good judgment when applying standards and policies and deciding when to delegate assessments.

Sources of Data

Subjective data (*covert data, symptoms*) are the information communicated to the nurse by the client, family, or community. Subjective data reveal the perspective, thoughts, feelings, beliefs, and sensations of the person giving the data. Thus, subjective data from two different people can vary. For example, people with insomnia often report getting much less sleep than their sleep partner says they do. You can use subjective data to clarify objective data (e.g., "How did you get this scar?"). Some people (e.g., infants, adults with mental illness) are unable to provide subjective data. Others can give subjective data, but you might question its accuracy. For example, how credible is a diabetic patient's response that she complies with a diabetic diet and medication regimen when the blood sugar level is markedly elevated? What could you do to double-check the subjective data?

Objective data (*overt data, signs*) are gathered through a physical assessment or from laboratory or diagnostic tests. They can be measured or observed by the nurse or other healthcare providers. Examples are vital signs, x-ray results, skin color, and urine output. You sometimes need to use objective data to validate subjective data. In the preceding example, if you thought the report of dietary intake and insulin use was inaccurate, you would measure the blood sugar and ask for a dietary journal.

You may also use objective data to verify subjective information that seems accurate. For example, when Sami told you her family and sexual history, you learned that she has significant risk factors for breast and cervical cancer and referred her for a gynecological exam. The results of the breast exam and Pap smear (Papanicolaou test, a smear of cervical cells) provide objective data related to these risk factors.

Primary data are the subjective and objective data obtained from the client: what the client says or what you observe. **Secondary data** are obtained "second-hand," for example, from the medical record or from another caregiver. A client's husband may say, "She seems more confused than usual." Or the NAP may report, "Mr. Atlas's heart rate was 100 beats per minute this morning." If you count the heart rate yourself, though, it would be primary data. Table 3-1 provides further examples of types and sources of data.

KnowledgeCheck 3-2

During Sami's appointment at the women's clinic, she has a Pap smear, breast exam, and blood work. She also informs the nurse that her menstrual flow is heavy and that she experiences severe abdominal cramping. These data are added to the database as references for future visits. Sami's Pap smear results and breast exam are normal, but she is moderately anemic. When the lab results indicate a low hemoglobin level, the nurse practitioner suspects that Sami's heavy flow may be causing her anemia. According to clinic protocol, she prescribes birth control pills for Sami to control her menstrual symptoms and provide contraception. Ongoing assessment will include visits every 6 months to manage her birth control pills and monitor the

Table 3-1 ► Examples of Data Types

DATA TYPES

Subjective Data	Objective Data
"I have been having a lot of pain in my abdomen."	Suprapubic area firm to light palpation. Lower abdomen semisoft
"My throat hurts when I swallow."	White patches noted at the back of the throat and tonsillar area reddened and swollen
"Our children have no place to go after football games. That is why they get into so much trouble."	In a windshield survey, no public facility was open after football games to allow young people to socialize under supervision.

DATA SOURCES

Primary Source (Client)	Secondary Sources (Everything Else)
Pulse rate 100 beats/min	From chart: WBC count 14,000/mm³.
States feeling short of breath	In transfer report, nurse states that the surgical dressing is dry.
Abdomen tender on palpation	Client's wife states that he has been tired a lot lately.

anemia. State whether the following data are primary or secondary, subjective or objective:

- You see in Sami's health record that her breast exam was normal.
- Sami tells the nurse practitioner that she experiences cramping with her menstrual cycle. *For the nurse practitioner*, would this be primary or secondary, subjective or objective data?
- The nurse practitioner tells you that Sami is anemic.
- You check the result of the Pap smear on the computer and see that it is normal.

Types of Assessment

Key Point: *Assessment can be broad and general or very specific. The type of assessment you do depends on the client's status.* In acute care settings, such as the emergency department, the assessments are rapid and focused on the presenting problem. In inpatient settings, you may perform an initial comprehensive assessment at admission and other, more focused assessments over time, according to the client's needs.

Initial and Ongoing Assessments

An **initial (admission) assessment** is completed when the client first comes to the healthcare agency. First obtain data related to the person's reason for seeking nursing or medical assistance. Then complete a comprehensive assessment if the client's condition permits. Data gathered from the initial assessment provide guidance for care and determine the need for further assessment. Initial assessment data tend to be static; for example, demographic data (marital status, occupation) are not likely to change often.

Ongoing assessment is performed as needed, at any time after the initial database is completed. Ideally, you will make at least some observations at every contact with a client. You use data from ongoing assessments to identify new problems or to follow up on previously identified problems. In comparison with the initial assessment, ongoing assessment reflects the dynamic state of the client. For example, vital signs may change rapidly and serve as important indicators of developing or resolving health problems.

Comprehensive Assessments

A **comprehensive assessment** (also called a *global assessment, patient database,* or *nursing database*) provides holistic information about the client's overall health status. It includes subjective and objective data about the client's body systems and functional abilities, emotional status, spiritual health, and psychosocial situation, including information about the family and community. It enables you to identify client problems and strengths. You need comprehensive data to enhance your sensitivity to a patient's culture, values, beliefs, and economic situation. Figure 3-2 shows what information is gathered in an initial comprehensive assessment (database) and how it fits into the broad concept of assessment in the nursing process. To see an example of a form for recording a comprehensive assessment,

 Go to Chapter 3, Assessment Guidelines and Tools, **Nursing Admission Data Form,** in Volume 2.

Nurses collect data through the use of all their senses. Whether assessment is initial or ongoing, comprehensive, or focused, you will use the skills of observation, physical examination, and interviewing.

Observation

Observation refers to the deliberate use of all of your senses to gather and interpret patient and environmental data. All that you see, hear, feel, or smell becomes data in the context of assessment. You should try to use the same sequence of observation at each patient contact. By making systematic observations each time you are with a patient, you are less likely to miss an assessment area. The mnemonic (memory aid) in Box 3-3 may help you.

Physical Assessment

Physical assessment (or *physical examination*) produces primarily objective data and makes use of the following techniques, which are described in detail in Chapter 22.

- **Inspection.** Observation and visual examination of the client, as well as use of equipment such as an otoscope or ophthalmoscope
- **Palpation.** Light touch, progressing to deeper touch, using the pads of the fingers
- **Percussion.** Striking a body surface with the tip of a finger, which produces different vibrations and sounds

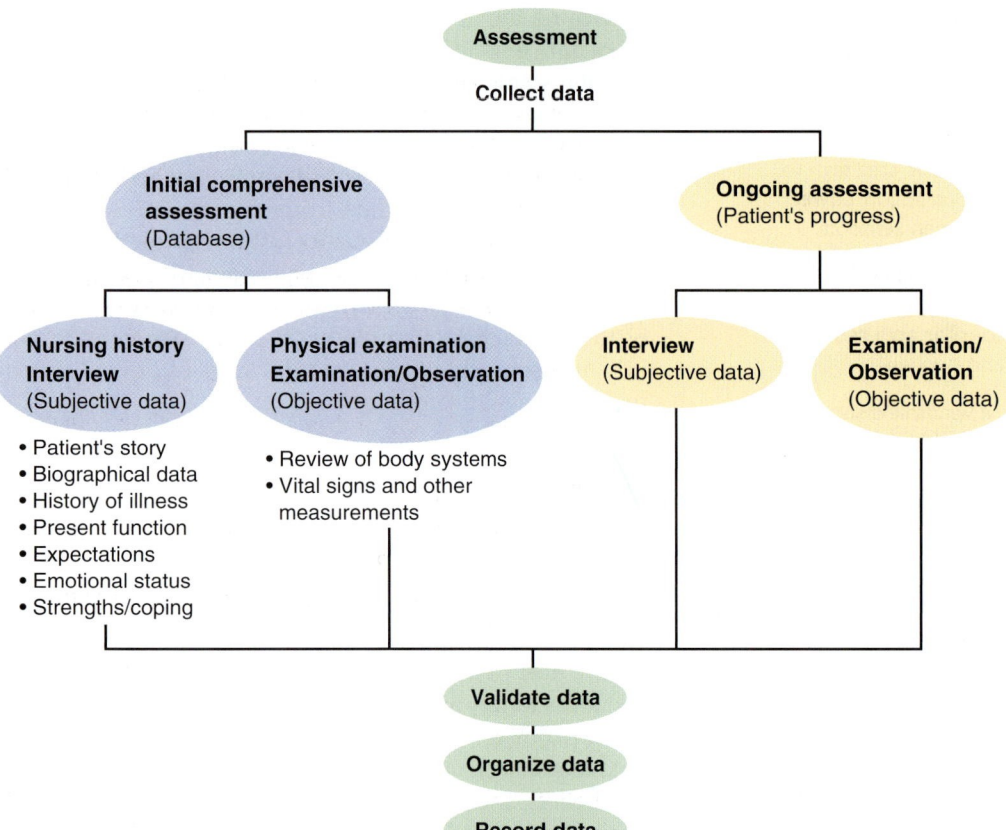

FIGURE 3-2 Overview of assessment content and methods. (*Source:* Wilkinson, J. M. (2012). *Nursing process and critical thinking* (5th ed.), p. 78. Reprinted by permission of Pearson Education, Inc., Upper Saddle River, NJ.)

depending on what is under the area that is tapped (air, fluid, or solid)

- **Auscultation.** Listening with the unaided ear for sounds made by the client (*direct auscultation*) and listening with the use of a stethoscope (*indirect auscultation*) for normal and abnormal sounds within the body

The Nursing Interview

A **nursing interview** is purposeful, structured communication in which you question the patient to gather

---

BOX 3-3 ■ Mnemonic for Systematic Observing

Use the first letter of each word to help you observe systematically as you enter a patient's room.

HELP!!

Help. Observe first signs the patient may need help. Look for signs of distress (e.g., pain, pallor, labored breathing)

Environment and equipment. Next look for safety hazards (spills, equipment cords, sharps). Check to see that all equipment is working: IV line running? Catheter draining? Oxygen working?

Look more closely. Examine the patient thoroughly for appearance, breathing, condition of dressings, correct positioning, skin color and condition, odors, condition of linens, and any other clues that might indicate a need for care.

People. Who are the people in the room? Family? Other caregivers? What are they doing?

---

subjective data for the nursing database (Fig. 3-3). The admission interview is planned, but during ongoing assessment, the interview may be informal, brief, and narrowly focused.

KnowledgeCheck 3-3

Give at least two more examples of data you might obtain with each of the following senses. One example is provided for each.

- Touch (e.g., bladder distention)
- Vision (e.g., facial expression of pain)
- Smell (e.g., fecal odor)
- Hearing (e.g., bowel sounds)

Focused Assessments

A **focused assessment** is performed to obtain data about an actual, potential, or possible problem that has been identified or is suspected. It focuses on a particular topic, body part, or functional ability rather than on overall health status. For example, focused assessments can center on pain, nutrition, spiritual health, social support, lifestyle, and family assessment. These specialized assessments add to the database created by the comprehensive initial assessment.

- An *initial focused assessment* is used to follow up on client-reported symptoms or unusual findings during the first exam (e.g., on admission to a hospital). For example, when the nurse asks Mr. Jacobs why he has come to the clinic today, he replies, "I can't get rid of this pain in my foot." The nurse asks questions to get

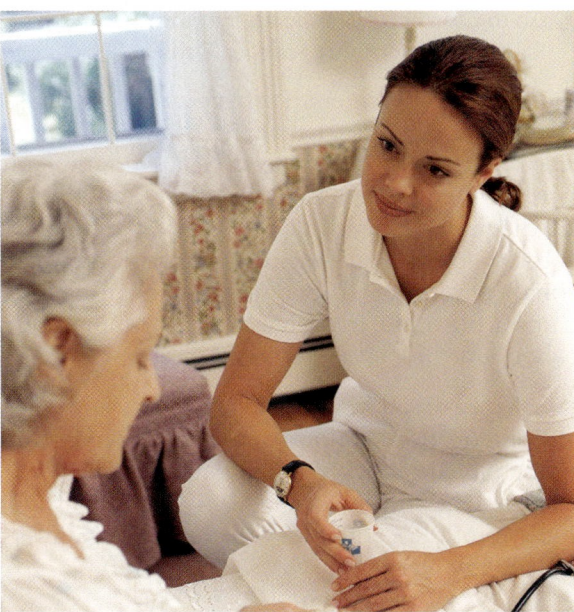

FIGURE 3-3 The nurse conducts an informal interview.

Teaching Self-Assessment

As you learned in Chapters 1 and 2, it is essential for nurses to provide information that will help clients to care for themselves. One important aspect of self-care is performing regular self-assessments to detect symptoms of disease.

Important assessments every person needs to know:

➤ Breast self-exam or testicular self-exam—monthly (Note that this is not at present recommended by all care providers or all best practice guidelines.)

➤ Skin assessment—daily but at least weekly

➤ Feet assessment—daily if diabetic or elderly, otherwise weekly

Before you begin teaching:

➤ Assess the readiness and willingness of your client to learn some type of assessment.

➤ Assess current knowledge or understanding of the topic to be discussed.

See Chapter 22 for details of these assessments.

---

in-depth information about this symptom: When did it begin? On a scale of 1 to 10, how severe is it? What makes it worse? What do you do to make it feel better? She also examines the foot for joint mobility, redness, edema, and tenderness to touch.

■ *An ongoing focused assessment* is used to evaluate the status of existing problems and goals. For examples, after surgery, Ms. King has a nursing diagnosis of Acute Pain secondary to abdominal incision. The nurse assesses her pain level at least every 2 hours and before and after administering pain medication.

▲▲ ThinkLike a Nurse 3-2

■ Give examples of each type of assessment (initial, ongoing, comprehensive, focused) using patients you have observed or cared for or your own personal experiences as a patient.

■ How might age and developmental stage make a difference in your assessment of a patient?

■ Suppose you are the triage nurse at the community clinic in the Meet Your Patient scenario. What kind of assessment do you perform at Sami's first visit (initial, ongoing, comprehensive, focused)? What type will the care provider at the women's clinic perform?

Special Needs Assessments

A **special needs assessment** is a type of focused assessment. It provides in-depth information about a particular area of client functioning and often involves using a specially designed form. The Joint Commission requires certain special needs assessments (e.g., of nutrition status and pain) for all clients. In some settings, such as hospice, home health, and rehabilitation settings, other special needs assessments (e.g., of functional abilities) are also required. You should perform a special needs assessment any time assessment cues suggest risk factors or problems in an area of client functioning.

Special needs assessments can be quite lengthy; therefore, you need to think carefully about when and how to use them. You need enough data to provide holistic care, but you must balance this need against the need not to intrude on the client's privacy. Obtain only the data you need to enhance the care provided to the client and add to the comprehensive assessment. The following are some special needs assessments:

Functional Ability Assessment Health problems and normal aging changes often bring a decline in functional status. Functional ability is especially important in discharge planning and home care. Future rehabilitation needs are derived from initial and ongoing functional ability assessments. The Joint Commission (2012, p. PC-6) requires an initial functional ability assessment "based on the patient's condition." These three functional assessment tools are commonly used:

■ **The Katz Index of ADL scale (1963).** This instrument is one of the best for assessing independent performance in very basic areas. It assigns one point for independence in each of the following areas: bathing, dressing, toileting, transfer, continence, and feeding (Shelkey & Wallace, revised 2012). Nurses often use the data to plan staffing and appropriate placement of clients. See Box 3-4 for questions to use when assessing activities of daily living (ADLs). For a link to the Katz scale,

 Go to Chapter 3, **Resources for Caregivers and Health Professionals,** on DavisPlus.

■ **Lawton Instrumental Activities of Daily Living (IADL) scale (1969).** This easy-to-use tool is particularly helpful in assessing a person's ability to independently

BOX 3-4 ■ Questions for Assessing Independence in Activities of Daily Living

Mobility

Does the client require devices (e.g., cane, crutches, walker, wheelchair) for support?

Transfer

Can the client get in and out of bed and in and out of a chair without assistance?

If not, how much help does the client need?

Is the client completely confined to bed?

Bathing

Can the client perform a sponge bath, tub bath, or shower bath with no help?

If not, specifically what assistance does the client need?

Dressing

Can the client get all necessary clothing from drawers and closets and get completely dressed without help?

If not, specifically what assistance does the client need?

Feeding

Can the client feed self without assistance?

If not, specifically what assistance does the client need (e.g., help with cutting meat, tube feeding)?

Toileting

Can the client go to the bathroom, use the toilet, clean self, and rearrange clothing without help?

If a night bedpan or commode is used, can the client empty and clean it independently?

If the client needs help with these activities, specifically what does it include?

Continence

Does the client independently control urination and bowel movements?

If not, how often is the client incontinent of bladder or bowel?

Does the client require an indwelling urinary catheter?

---

perform the more sophisticated tasks of everyday life, such as shopping. Identifying early functional decline is important for discharge planning.

 The Lawton scale is especially useful for older adults, who may begin to experience functional decline within 48 hours of hospital admission (Graf, 2008; Lawton & Brody, 1969).

■ To see the Lawton scale,

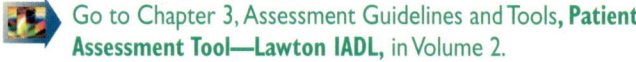
Go to Chapter 3, Assessment Guidelines and Tools, **Patient Assessment Tool—Lawton IADL,** in Volume 2.

■ **The Karnofsky Performance scale (Karnofsky & Burchenal, 1949).** This tool is used primarily in palliative care settings to assess functional abilities at the end of life. To see this tool,

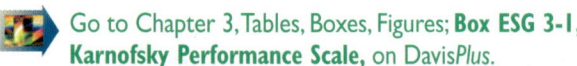
Go to Chapter 3, Tables, Boxes, Figures; **Box ESG 3-1, Karnofsky Performance Scale,** on DavisPlus.

Nutritional Assessment Perform a nutritional assessment when data suggest that the client is undernourished, is at risk for Imbalanced Nutrition, or requires nutritional therapy as an intervention (as for a person newly diagnosed with diabetes). In addition to information about food intake, it includes information related to personal, psychosocial, and economic problems that may affect nutrition. See Chapter 27 for more information about nutritional assessment.

Pain Assessment In addition, good nursing care and accrediting agency standards require you to perform a thorough pain assessment on all patients during the initial assessment and in ongoing assessments (The Joint Commission, 2012). For more information on pain assessments, see Chapter 31.

Cultural Assessment Awareness of cultural influences should guide your assessment and nursing care, but be careful not to stereotype clients based on culture. To be culturally competent, you must be able to assess and honor the diversity among all clients. For content included in a cultural assessment, see Chapter 15.

Spiritual Health Assessment For ill persons, spirituality can be a problem or a source of support. To gather useful information, you must do more than ask the client's religious preference. Spiritual health assessment provides insight into how a client interprets life events and health. See Chapter 16 for more detailed information.

Psychosocial Assessment A psychosocial assessment includes data about lifestyle, usual coping patterns, understanding of the current illness, personality style, previous psychiatric disorders, recent stressors, major issues related to the illness, and mental status (Gorman & Sultan, 2008). Perform a focused psychosocial assessment if initial assessment data indicate that social and emotional needs are not being met (e.g., if the client is very anxious or exhibiting symptoms of stress), or if sociocultural factors (e.g., unemployment) present a risk to health (see Chapter 13).

Wellness Assessment Health promotion focuses on activities of a well person to achieve a higher level of health. Well people can usually identify their own health needs, so most assessment tools are self-administered. A wellness assessment includes data about spiritual health, social support, nutrition, physical fitness, health beliefs, and lifestyle, as well as a life-stress review. See Chapter 42 for a more detailed discussion of assessing wellness.

Family Assessment Health behaviors and beliefs generally have their beginnings in family interactions. Therefore, a family assessment provides a better understanding of the client's health-related values, beliefs, and behaviors (see Chapter 14).

Community Assessment Community assessment provides information about community demographics, resources, health concerns, points of referral, environmental risks, and community norms and values (see Chapter 43).

ThinkLike a Nurse 3-3

Based on the data you have so far about Sami, consider the need to perform any of the special-purpose assessments. What is your rationale for using or not using a special needs assessment?

PracticalKnowledge
knowing **how**

In this chapter, practical knowledge involves your skill in using structured and unstructured methods of data collection, as well as validating, organizing, and documenting your assessment findings.

Interviewing to Obtain a Nursing Health History

Suppose that an elderly man has a fractured hip. The physician is interested in the cause of the fracture, the extent of the injury, and any preexisting health problems that suggest the client is a poor surgical risk. As the nurse, you too would ask about the cause of the injury. However, you would also want to (1) know what effect the injury has on the man's ability to perform everyday activities, and (2) identify supports and strengths to begin planning for his eventual discharge and self-care. **Key Point: *So you see, the nursing health history covers some of the same topics as the medical history, but the reason for the questions is different.***

Health history forms vary among agencies and according to purpose (e.g., inpatient, clinic, surgery, medical, emergency department, or newborn care), but most include the subjective information found in Table 3-2.

ThinkLike a Nurse 3-4

The Quality and Safety Education for Nurses (QSEN) competency definitions identify assessment as a necessary skill for competency in patient-centered care: Elicit patient values, preferences, and expressed needs as part of a clinical interview (Cronenwett, Sherwood, Barnsteiner, et al., 2007). Where do you think this type of patient information fits into the preceding components of a nursing health history? Why?

Types of Interviews

Interviews may be directive or nondirective. Use **directive interviewing** to obtain factual, easily categorized information (e.g., age, sex), or in an emergency situation. In this type of interview, you control the topics and ask mostly closed questions to obtain specific information. **Closed questions** are those that can be answered with a "yes," "no," or other short, factual answer. They usually begin with *who, when, where, what, do (did, does),* and *is (are, were)*. Closed questions are useful for patients who are very anxious or who have communication difficulties.

When you want to promote communication, build rapport, or help the patient to express feelings, use **nondirective interviewing.** This means that you allow the patient to control the subject matter. Your role is to clarify, summarize, and ask mostly open-ended questions that facilitate thought and communication. **Open-ended questions** specify a topic to be explored, but phrase it broadly to encourage the patient to elaborate. Ask open-ended questions when you want to obtain subjective data.

Directive interviewing is efficient but may cause you to miss topics important to the patient. Nondirective interviewing allows you to find out what is important to the patient, but it is time consuming and can produce much irrelevant data. A successful interview includes both closed and open-ended questions. Use broad, open-ended questions to guide the patient to talk about certain topics. From the answers to the broad questions, you can decide which topics to clarify or follow up with specific and closed questions. Part of the interview with Sami might have gone like this:

NURSE	When was your last physical examination? *(closed question)*
SAMI	I had a female exam about 5 years ago.
NURSE	What problems have you had in that area? *(open-ended question)*
SAMI	None, really.
NURSE	What about other women in your family? *(open-ended question)*
SAMI	Well, my mother had breast cancer about the same time that I went for my checkup. She's OK now though.
NURSE	Go on . . . *(open-ended question)*
SAMI	And my sister has been taking some pills for endometriosis. She hasn't been able to get pregnant because of that.
NURSE	Are you sexually active? *(closed question)*
SAMI	Yes.
NURSE	Tell me about that. *(open-ended question)*

See Table 3-3 for other examples of closed and open-ended questions.

Preparing for an Interview

While you are learning, you may feel uncomfortable interviewing patients. You may have one of the following concerns:

- **You are imposing on the patient, who clearly needs rest more than you need information.** This may be because you believe a "real nurse" has already obtained the information, or because you don't have a clear idea of how the information will be used to help the patient.
- **The patient won't be receptive to answering personal questions from a stranger (you).** To help set the tone for the interview, be sure to tell your patients that the information given will be kept confidential and that they can refuse to answer any question.

Table 3-2 ➤ Components of a Nursing Health History

COMPONENT	DESCRIPTION
Biographical Data	Relatively unchanging information, such as name, address, age, gender, race, religion, marital status, and occupation. Responses to these questions reflect mental status and ability to communicate.
Chief Complaint (Reason for Seeking Healthcare)	The client's perception of or reason for seeking medical or nursing advice. From this, you will be able to target your assessment to gather the most relevant and important data. Ask, for example, "Tell me why you have come to the hospital today." The client might respond, "I just don't feel right," or "I'm having chest pain." Follow up by asking him specifically what caused him to seek help (e.g., chest pain, a checkup). Be sure to document the answer in the client's words.
History of Present Illness	An in-depth exploration of the client's chief complaint. Find out when the illness or problem began, whether the onset was sudden or gradual, how often it occurs, what makes it worse, what the person does to relieve it, how the client's health has changed from his usual status, and what effect the illness has had on his daily life.
Client's Perception of Health Status and Expectations for Care	Includes the client's knowledge about his illness and its potential effects on his life. For example, does a client with arterial insufficiency believe his foot will be "normal" again? Also, ask the client what he expects will be done for him (e.g., does he understand that his foot will be amputated)? And what does he want the nurses to do to help (e.g., leave a light on at night, bring his medication)?
Past Health History (sometimes called *medical history*)	Includes childhood diseases and immunizations, previous hospitalizations, and previous surgeries. The past health history helps guide your assessment and helps you to understand some of the data you obtain. For example, if Sami tells you she had her appendix out when she was 5 years old, you would expect to find a scar on her abdomen.
Family Health History	Includes data on first-degree blood relatives such as mother, father, siblings, and maternal and paternal grandparents. It includes data about diseases they have had, their current state of health and chronic disease, whether or not they are alive, and cause of death if they are not. Risk factors for various illnesses and disorders (e.g., hypertension, allergies) are often tied to multigenerational health problems. Refer to the genogram in Chapter 14.
Social History	Includes information about family and other relationships, economic status, occupations, exposure to toxic materials, home and neighborhood conditions, and ethnicity. Also includes data about tobacco, alcohol, and drug use; and exercise habits.
Medication History and Device Use	Past and current medication usage may uncover some medical history the client has forgotten to disclose. Also ask about nutritional supplements, herbs, and other alternative medicines. As you continue with the assessment, you can direct questions toward previous episodes of medical treatment and use of medical devices, such as braces, inhalers, and home oxygen therapy. ✚ Data about current medications are essential because (1) they may interact with newly prescribed medications and (2) some may affect certain body symptoms, causing abnormalities in your assessment findings (e.g., skin color, laboratory values).
Complementary/Alternative Modalities (CAM)	Therapies used instead of or in addition to the allopathic therapies recommended by physicians—for example, chiropractics, homeopathy, aromatherapy, music therapy, massage therapy, energy work (therapeutic touch, Reiki), and acupressure or acupuncture. Such therapies can complement or interfere with conventional therapies, so this is important information.
Review of Body Systems and Associated Functional Abilities	Subjective data regarding body systems (e.g., Do you have a productive cough?). It includes functional abilities (e.g., difficulties with dressing, bathing, eating, and elimination). You can obtain these data during the physical assessment as well as in the interview.

Remember the patient is free to choose what to tell and what to withhold from you. Also, be aware that the patient may have been feeling the need to talk about something, has not known how to bring it up, and is actually relieved you have introduced the topic.

■ **Some of your questions will upset the patient—the person might cry or become angry.** Remember that patients usually feel better after releasing their emotions. Expressions of strong emotion may cause you discomfort, but you must learn to accept them. You will have large gaps in your data if you avoid difficult topics, and your patients will not get the help they need.

Your interviews will go more smoothly if you take time to prepare yourself, your patient, and the interview space before you begin asking questions. To learn how

Table 3-3 ➤ Examples of Closed and Open-Ended Questions	
CLOSED QUESTIONS	**OPEN-ENDED QUESTIONS**
Are you having any pain?	Tell me about your pain.
Do you ever drink excessively?	Tell me about your use of alcohol.
Why did you come to this clinic?	I am glad to see you here today. Could you tell me a little bit about why you decided to come see us?
Do you have any family history of heart disease?	Tell me about your family members and what kind of experiences they may have had with heart disease or problems with circulation.
Are there any parks where you can walk safely?	Tell me about safe places here in your community where you might go to take a walk.

to do that, and for tips on conducting and closing an interview,

 Go to Chapter 3, **Clinical Insights 3-1, 3-2, and 3-3,** in Volume 2.

KnowledgeCheck 3-4

- What are the 10 components of a nursing history and why are they important?
- What are two things you should do to prepare yourself before an interview?
- List several things you could do to be sure the client is comfortable before the interview. To review this information,

 Go to Chapter 3, **Clinical Insight 3-2,** in Volume 2.

- State four guidelines that will help you to obtain complete and accurate data when conducting an interview (these are also in Chapter 3, Volume 2).

HOW AND WHEN SHOULD I VALIDATE DATA?

Suppose a patient has told you that he has never had high blood pressure (BP), but you obtain an abnormal BP reading of 180/98 mm Hg. What would you do? Would you record the 180/98 mm Hg reading, or would you:

- Ask the patient some more questions, such as, "What do you mean when you say you have never had high blood pressure?" or "What have you been doing in the last 15 minutes?"
- Ask another nurse to double-check your findings?
- Check when the sphygmomanometer was last calibrated?

- Retake the BP using a different sphygmomanometer?
- Compare the reading with previous entries in the chart?
- Check the BP in the patient's other arm?
- Wait a few minutes and take the reading again in the same arm?

All of those are ways to **validate** your data—to verify it or double-check it. Validating data helps to ensure that they are accurate, complete, and factual and that you have not jumped to conclusions. If the patient tells you that he was running late and has just jogged the two blocks from the parking lot, you would know that 180/98 mm Hg does not reflect his usual BP and that you need to check it again.

Not all data must be validated. You can usually assume, for example, that laboratory results are correct and that the patient has given you correct information about data such as height, weight, and birth date. You should validate data under the following circumstances (Wilkinson, 2012):

- Subjective and objective data do not agree, or do not make sense together.
  Example: In the preceding situation, the subjective data was "never had high BP," but the objective data, BP 180/98 mm Hg, is a high reading.
- The patient's statements differ at different times in the interview.
  Example: A patient tells you he follows a low-cholesterol diet. However, later when describing his usual daily food pattern, he includes eggs for breakfast, a cheese sandwich for lunch, and a hamburger for dinner.
- The data fall far outside normal range.
  Example: A patient has no symptoms of infection or high fever, but you obtain an elevated oral temperature reading of 106°F (41.1°C). (Hint: Ask him whether he has just had something warm to drink.)
- Factors are present that interfere with accurate measurement.
  Example: The patient has very thin arms, and there are no appropriately sized BP cuffs available. Therefore, because the BP will probably not be accurate, you should measure it again after you can obtain appropriate equipment.

HOW CAN I ORGANIZE DATA?

Professional standards require systematic data collection (see Box 3-1). This means you collect and record data in predetermined categories, not just at random. Data in most initial (e.g., admissions) assessments are categorized by the agency's data-collection form. For ongoing assessments, you may need to provide your own organizing structure (framework). Because a **framework** represents a particular way of thinking about clients and health, it indicates which information is significant and guides you in deciding which patient data to observe. The major concepts of a

Toward Evidence-Based Practice

Moore, K., & Fortner, B. (2010). Utility of routine nurse assessment of the risk of chemotherapy-induced febrile neutropenia. *Canadian Oncology Nursing Journal, 20*(2), 75–79.

This study assessed the usefulness of having nurses routinely assess for the risk of febrile neutropenia (FN) in cancer patients prior to beginning chemotherapy. Using a standardized assessment tool, 15 nurses assessed 150 patients. In 94% of the patients studied, nurses detected risk factors, and interventions were provided to reduce the incidence of FN. When interviewed, 67% of the nurses said the use of a standardized tool helped them to identify patients at risk for FN.

Which of the following inferences can you make (based on this summary alone)? State whether the study summary provides *extensive, limited,* or *no evidence* to support each inference.

1. These positive results occurred because the nurses used a standardized assessment form.

2. Most of the patients in the study did not experience FN.

3. Ten of the 15 nurses in the study said the standardized tool was helpful.

4. A unit policy should require all cancer patients to be assessed with this standardized tool.

5. Assessment is faster and more efficient using a standardized assessment tool.

 Go to Chapter 3, **Toward Evidence-Based Practice Suggested Responses,** on Davis*Plus.*

---

model/framework help you to cluster data and find patterns. If you don't understand what a framework is, refer to Chapter 8.

Nonnursing Models

ANA professional standards state that nursing data collection should be holistic. Many agencies use a **body systems (medical) framework** for at least a section of the assessment form. This model is useful for identifying medical problems, but it needs to be combined with other models (e.g., a nursing model or Maslow's Hierarchy of Needs) to provide the holistic data you need to identify both nursing and medical problems.

Maslow's Hierarchy of Needs (Maslow, 1970; Maslow & Lowery, 1998) groups data according to human needs. It states that the basic needs must be met before higher needs can be addressed. Maslow's categories of needs, from most basic to highest, are:

Physiological. Basic survival needs (e.g., oxygen, water, food, and shelter)
Safety and security. The need to be safe and comfortable (e.g., safe from falls and treatment side effects as well as the need for psychological security)
Love and belonging. The need for love and affection (e.g., family, social supports)
Esteem and self-esteem. The need to feel good about oneself (e.g., body image, pride in achievements, admiration from others)
Cognitive. The need for knowledge, understanding, and exploration
Aesthetic. The need for symmetry, order, and beauty
Self-actualization. The need to achieve one's potential; the need for growth and change (e.g., extent to which goals are achieved, role performance)

See Chapter 8 for a more complete discussion of Maslow's model.

Nursing Models

Nurse theorists have developed many different theories and models for thinking about nursing, clients, health, and the environment. Nursing models produce a holistic database that is useful in identifying nursing rather than medical diagnoses. Several nursing theories are described in Chapter 8. Table 3-4 identifies the major concepts of five models frequently used to structure nursing assessments. The concepts are the categories that you would use to gather and cluster data.

HOW SHOULD I DOCUMENT DATA?

The ANA *Nursing: Scope and Standards of Practice* (2010) and The Joint Commission standards (2012) stress the importance of documenting patient information, including assessment data, in a retrievable format. Accurate, timely, and clear documentation of all assessment findings benefits patients by providing the basis for planning effective nursing care. Furthermore, since the nursing database is a permanent part of the client's record, documentation protects you, the nurse, by establishing that you actually performed the needed assessments. Malpractice suits are not unusual in our society, and court cases may be presented years after you provide care for a patient. Your documentation is the only evidence supporting the care you gave. The assumption in malpractice cases is, "If it isn't documented, it wasn't done."

Guidelines for Recording Assessment Data

Follow these guidelines when recording assessment data:

- *Document as soon as possible* after you perform the assessment.
- *Write neatly, legibly, and in black ink* or record electronically.

Table 3-4 ➤ Assessment Models: Major Concepts

MODEL	MAJOR MODEL CONCEPTS
Gordon's Functional Health Patterns	Describe common patterns of behavior that can be functional or dysfunctional. Gordon intended the model for nursing assessment. The functional health patterns are major model concepts:

Health perception/health	Self-perception/self-concept
Management	Sleep/rest
Nutritional/metabolic	Role/relationship
Elimination	Coping/stress tolerance
Activity/exercise	Value/belief
Cognitive/perceptual	

Source: Adapted from Gordon, M. (1994). *Nursing diagnosis: Process and application* (3rd ed.). St. Louis, MO: Mosby, p. 70.

MODEL	MAJOR MODEL CONCEPTS
The NANDA-International Nursing Diagnosis Taxonomy II	Consists of functional patterns and is a modified version of the Gordon model. It is intended as a model for categorizing nursing diagnoses, not as a fully developed theory of nursing. The following are the NANDA-I domains (categories):

Health Promotion	Sexuality
Nutrition	Coping/Stress Tolerance
Elimination and Exchange	Life Principles
Activity/Rest	Safety/Protection
Perception/Cognition	Comfort
Self-Perception	Growth/Development
Role Relationships	

Source: Adapted from NANDA International. (2012). *Nursing diagnoses definitions & classification 2012–2014.* Ames, IA: Wiley-Blackwell.

MODEL	MAJOR MODEL CONCEPTS
The Taxonomy of Nursing Practice (NANDA-I/NOC/NIC)	Intended as a model for categorizing nursing diagnoses, client outcomes, and nursing interventions. It consists of four domains and 28 classes.
	Functional Domain Activity exercise, comfort, growth and development, nutrition, self-care, sexuality, sleep/rest, values/beliefs
	Physiological Domain Cardiac function, elimination, fluids and electrolytes, neurocognition, pharmacological function, physical regulation, reproduction, respiratory function, sensation/perception, tissue integrity
	Psychosocial Domain Behavior, communication, coping, emotional, knowledge, roles/relationships, self-perception
	Environmental Domain Healthcare system, populations, risk management

Source: Dochterman, J. M., & Jones, D. A. (Eds.). (2003). *Unifying nursing languages: The harmonization of NANDA, NIC, and NOC.* Washington, DC: American Nurses Association, NursesBooks.org.

MODEL	MAJOR MODEL CONCEPTS
The Roy Adaptation Model	Conceptualizes patients as adapting constantly to internal and external demands within a biological and psychosocial context. Using this model, you would look at the person's ability to achieve balance in the following "adaptive modes":

Activity and rest	Temperature regulation
Nutrition	Regulation of the senses
Elimination	Physical self-concept
Fluid and electrolytes	Personal self-concept
Oxygenation	Role function
Protection	Interdependence

Source: Adapted from Roy, C., & Andrews, H. (1991). *The Roy adaptation model: The definitive statement.* Norwalk, CT: Appleton & Lange, pp. 15–17; and Roy, C., & Andrews, HA (1999). *The Roy adaptation model* (2nd ed.). Norwalk, CT: Appleton & Lange.

continued

Table 3-4 ➤ Assessment Models: Major Concepts—cont'd

MODEL	MAJOR MODEL CONCEPTS
Orem's Self-Care Model	Conceptualizes health as the ability to perform self-care. Using this model, you would gather data to identify the following universal self-care deficits that require nursing assistance:
	Maintenance of a sufficient intake of air, water, and food
	Maintenance of a balance between activity and rest
	Maintenance of a balance between time alone and time with others
	Provision of care associated with elimination processes and excrements
	Prevention of hazards to human life, functioning, and well-being
	Promotion of human functioning and development within social groups in accord with human potential, limitations, and desire to be normal (as determined by science, culture, and social values)

Source: Adapted from Orem, D. (1991). *Nursing: Concepts of practice* (4th ed.). St. Louis, MO: Mosby-Year Book, p. 126.

- *Use acronyms sparingly,* using only agency-approved abbreviations.
- *Write the patient's own words, when possible,* in quotation marks. If the comments are too long, summarize what the patient says (e.g., Patient states that he is sleepy).
- *Record only the most important patient words.* If you record everything the patient says, the narrative will probably be too long and contain irrelevant data. For example, write "Patient states, 'I hardly slept at all last night,'" even though what the patient actually said was, "I hardly slept at all last night. I tossed and turned and people kept waking me up. Then the thunder and lightning came, and then I had to get up to go to the bathroom, and my wife called early this morning."
- *Use concrete, specific information* rather than vague generalities such as *normal, adequate, good,* and *tolerated well.* For example, what does it mean to say, "Patient slept well"? Did she fall asleep easily and sleep for 6 hours? Did she fall asleep with difficulty, but sleep for 8 hours? Did she sleep only 4 hours, but state that she feels well rested? It is much better to write, "Patient fell asleep before 2100 hr and slept until 0600 hr. She states that she woke up only once during the night and feels rested now. Observed sleeping three times during the night."
- *Record cues, not inferences.* **Cues** are what the client says and what you observe. **Inferences** are judgments and interpretations about what the cues mean. In other words, "just the facts, Jack (or Jill)." When recording cues, you do not need to "waffle" with the words *appears* and *seems.* Don't write "Incision seems red" or "edges appear separated." For example:

Cues	Inferences
Incision red, draining pus, edges separated.	Incision is infected.
Tearful. States that father died of a heart attack. Trembling.	Anxious about scheduled cardiac catheterization.
States, "I hate my mother. I wish I was dead."	Patient is angry and suicidal.

Tools for Recording Assessment Data

Each organization has its own forms and formats for documenting initial and ongoing assessments. You will record data on a variety of documents, including nurses' notes and the following:

- *Graphic flow sheet.* Includes vital signs such as blood pressure, pulse, respirations, and temperature so trends over time can be seen clearly (Fig. 3-4).
- *Intake and output (I&O) sheet.* May be on the graphic sheet, as in Figure 3-4, or separate document. This form has spaces for all intake: oral, intravenous, and tube feedings. There is also space to record all output: urine, fluid from drainage tubes, wound drainage, and bowel movements.
- *Nursing admission assessment.* Although agency forms differ in organization, all collect similar data as specified by The Joint Commission for standards for initial assessment. For an example of an admission assessment form,

Go to Chapter 3, **Assessment Forms: Nursing Admission Data Form,** in Volume 2.

- *Nursing discharge summary.* This may be a part of the initial assessment form because data obtained at admission are used for discharge planning.
- *Special-purpose forms.* Examples are diabetic flow sheets and medication administration forms.
- *Electronic documentation.* In some facilities, initial data and ongoing assessment data are entered into a computer program for organization, shared communication, and easy retrieval (Fig. 3-5).

REFLECTING CRITICALLY ABOUT ASSESSMENT

After gathering and recording patient data, use critical thinking to help you evaluate the quality of your assessment. See Chapter 2 for a review of critical thinking, as

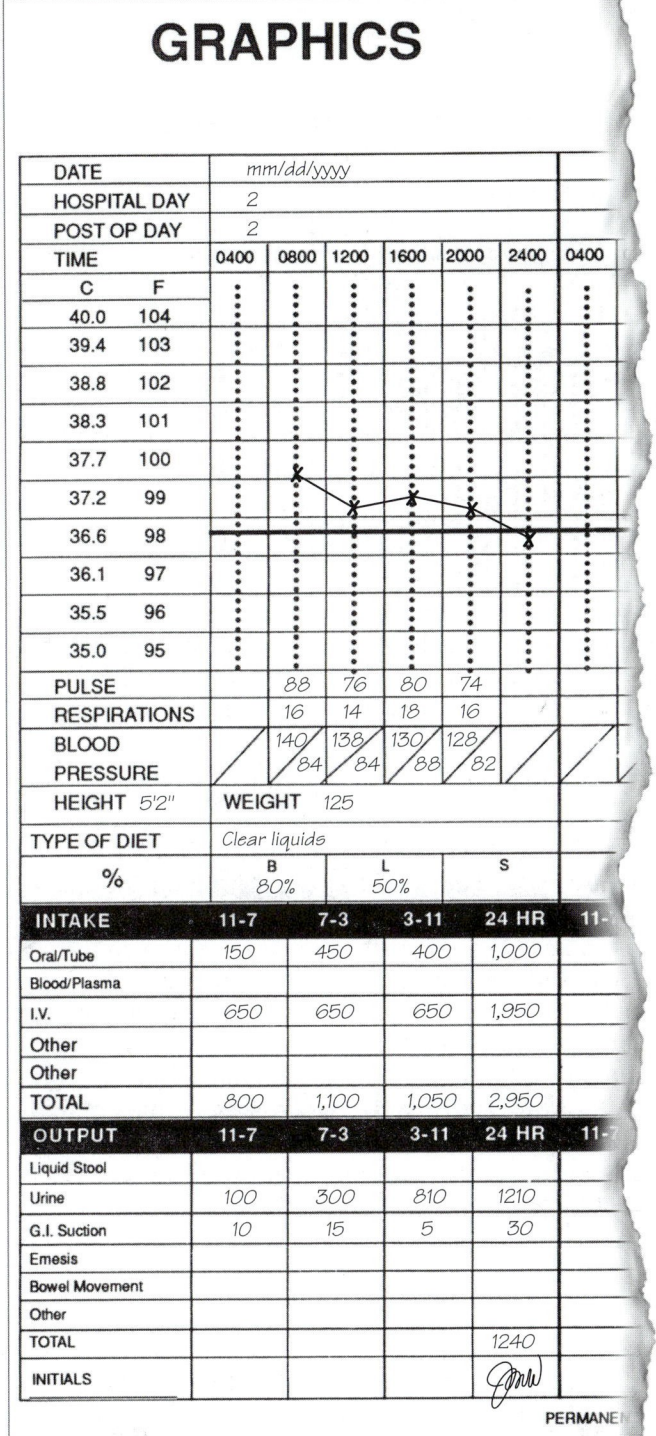

FIGURE 3-4 Graphic flow sheet. (Courtesy of Smith Northview Hospital, Valdosta, GA.)

needed. The following are questions to guide your final judgments about your data.

1. Are my data complete?
   - Have I completed all areas of the assessment form?
   - Is there anything else I need to know to identify or rule out a nursing diagnosis?
   - Have I collected holistic data: physical, emotional, interpersonal, spiritual, and cultural?
2. How do I know the data are accurate?
3. Have I recorded data rather than conclusions (cues, not inferences)?
4. Did I validate any data that do not make sense? Do any of the data conflict with other data?
5. Did I record the data in clear, specific terms, using the patient's own words, when possible, for subjective data? Did I avoid vague terms such as "normal," "good," and "slept well"?
6. Have I followed up with in-depth special needs assessments when appropriate?
7. Have I included only relevant data, taking care to protect the client's privacy?
8. The assessment interview:
   - Did I use therapeutic communication during the assessment?
   - Did I avoid asking too many questions and using too many closed questions?
   - How comfortable was I during the interview?
   - What signals did I get from the client in response to my questions? Did I follow up?
9. Physical assessment, observation, and examination:
   - Did I miss something in the environment?
   - How did the client and significant others respond to me verbally and nonverbally?
   - Did I pay attention to detail?
   - Were my assessment techniques performed skillfully (palpation, percussion, auscultation, inspection)?
10. Memory:
    - Did I have to ask questions in the sequence found on the forms?
    - Did I have to depend on the forms for all aspects of the assessment?
    - Did I have to repeat any area of assessment because I could not remember what I saw, heard, smelled, or felt?

If you have followed the recommended processes and reflected critically on your assessment, you should have the data necessary to create a holistic plan of care individualized to meet the client's needs.

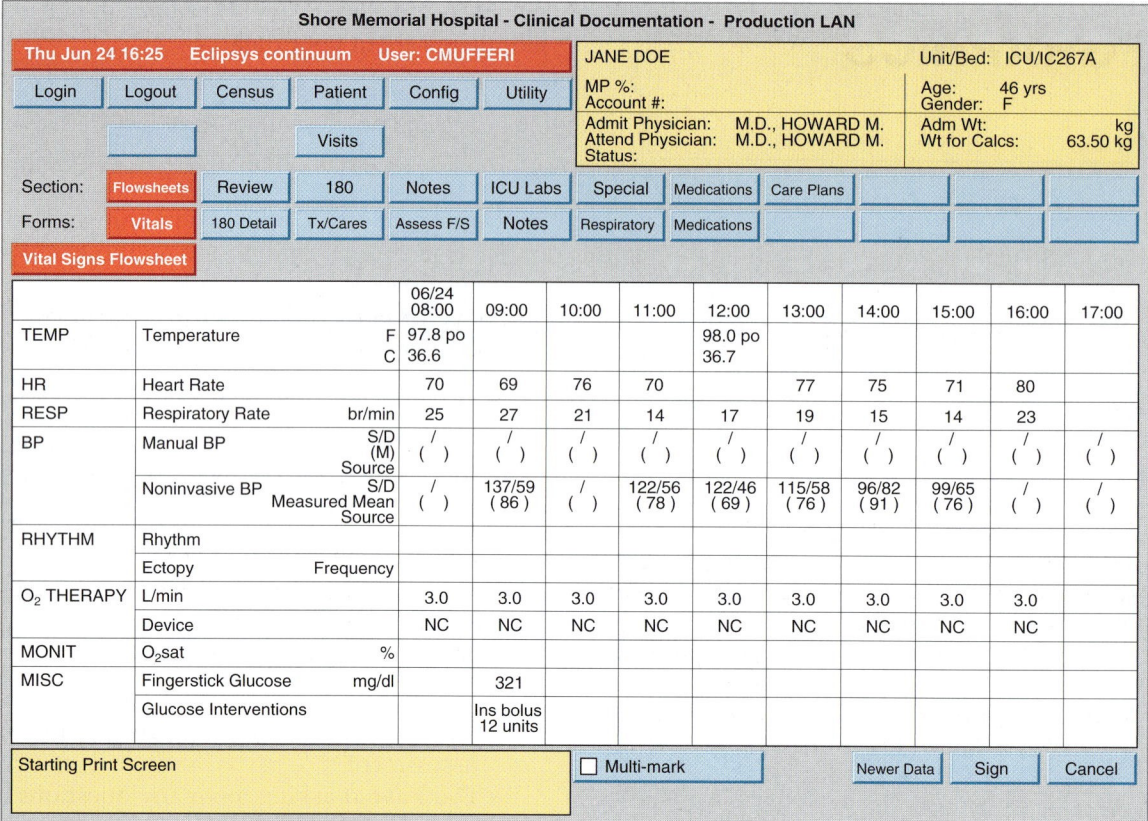

Shore Memorial Hospital - Clinical Documentation - Production LAN

Thu Jun 24 16:25	Eclipsys continuum	User: CMUFFERI			JANE DOE		Unit/Bed: ICU/IC267A

Login	Logout	Census	Patient	Config	Utility
			Visits		

MP %:
Account #:

Admit Physician: M.D., HOWARD M.
Attend Physician: M.D., HOWARD M.
Status:

Age: 46 yrs
Gender: F

Adm Wt: kg
Wt for Calcs: 63.50 kg

Section: Flowsheets | Review | 180 | Notes | ICU Labs | Special | Medications | Care Plans

Forms: Vitals | 180 Detail | Tx/Cares | Assess F/S | Notes | Respiratory | Medications

Vital Signs Flowsheet

			06/24 08:00	09:00	10:00	11:00	12:00	13:00	14:00	15:00	16:00	17:00
TEMP	Temperature	F	97.8 po				98.0 po					
		C	36.6				36.7					
HR	Heart Rate		70	69	76	70		77	75	71	80	
RESP	Respiratory Rate	br/min	25	27	21	14	17	19	15	14	23	
BP	Manual BP	S/D (M) Source	/ ( )	/ ( )	/ ( )	/ ( )	/ ( )	/ ( )	/ ( )	/ ( )	/ ( )	/ ( )
	Noninvasive BP	S/D Measured Mean Source	/ ( )	137/59 (86)	/ ( )	122/56 (78)	122/46 (69)	115/58 (76)	96/82 (91)	99/65 (76)	/ ( )	/ ( )
RHYTHM	Rhythm											
	Ectopy	Frequency										
O₂ THERAPY	L/min			3.0	3.0	3.0	3.0	3.0	3.0	3.0	3.0	
	Device			NC	NC	NC	NC	NC	NC	NC	NC	
MONIT	O₂sat	%										
MISC	Fingerstick Glucose	mg/dl		321								
	Glucose Interventions			Ins bolus 12 units								

Starting Print Screen

☐ Multi-mark | Newer Data | Sign | Cancel

FIGURE 3-5 Computer screen capture: assessment data. (Courtesy of Shore Memorial Hospital, Somers Point, NJ.)

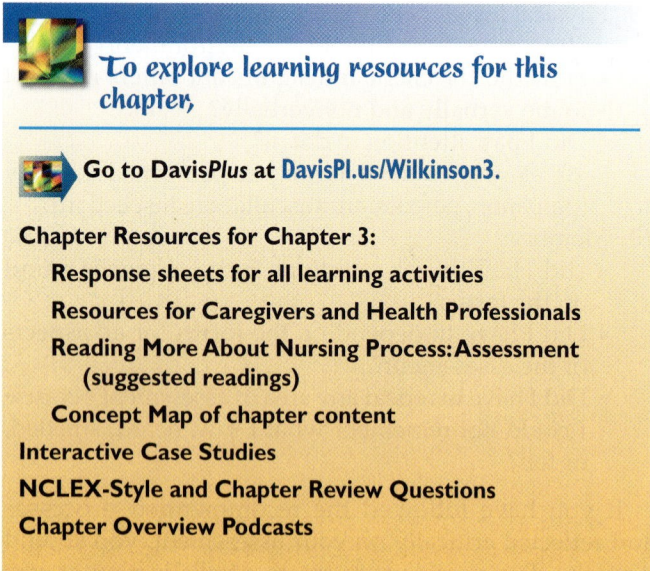

To explore learning resources for this chapter,

Go to DavisPlus at **DavisPl.us/Wilkinson3.**

Chapter Resources for Chapter 3:

Response sheets for all learning activities

Resources for Caregivers and Health Professionals

Reading More About Nursing Process: Assessment (suggested readings)

Concept Map of chapter content

Interactive Case Studies

NCLEX-Style and Chapter Review Questions

Chapter Overview Podcasts

For references cited in this chapter,

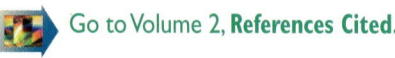

Go to Volume 2, **References Cited.**

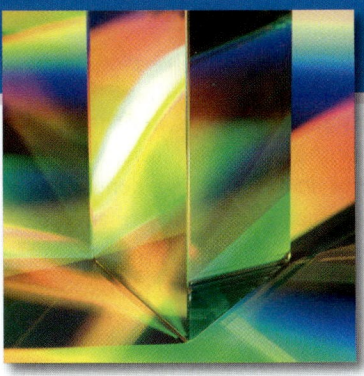

CHAPTER 4

Nursing Process: Diagnosis

Learning Outcomes

After completing this chapter, you should be able to:

➤ Define the following terms: diagnosis, nursing diagnosis, diagnostic reasoning, diagnostic label, defining characteristics, related factors, risk factors, health problem.

➤ Explain how nursing diagnosis is related to other phases of the nursing process.

➤ Differentiate between nursing diagnoses, medical diagnoses, and collaborative problems.

➤ Explain the differences between actual, risk, possible, syndrome, and wellness nursing diagnoses.

➤ Describe the diagnostic process.

➤ Explain why an etiology is always an inference.

➤ Describe at least two frameworks for prioritizing nursing diagnoses.

➤ Describe errors of theoretical and self-knowledge that may occur in diagnostic reasoning.

➤ Use standardized nursing language to write nursing diagnoses.

➤ Use collaborative problem statements appropriately.

➤ Explain the relationship between nursing diagnoses and goals/interventions.

➤ State at least five criteria for judging the quality of a diagnostic statement.

➤ Discuss issues associated with the NANDA-I diagnostic labels and with standardized language.

Key Concepts

Nursing diagnosis

Diagnostic process (diagnostic reasoning)

Diagnostic format

Related Concepts

See the Concept Map on Davis*Plus*.

Meet Your Patient

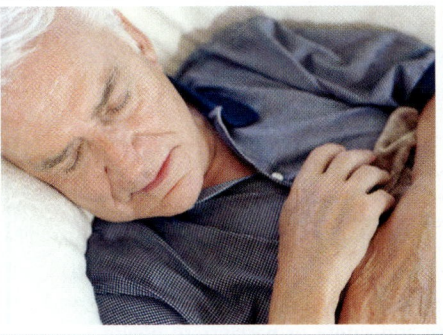

On your unit at an acute care facility, you will be admitting a client, Todd, from the emergency department (ED). Todd's ED nurse telephones you to give a report on his status. Todd's admitting medical diagnosis is chronic renal failure. He is married, 58 years old, employed, and has a longstanding history of type 2 diabetes mellitus (DM). In the past 3 days, he has developed decreased sensation in his bilateral lower extremities with slight mobility impairment.

You still have many questions concerning Todd's immediate and long-term needs. You will need to ask Todd about his medication regimen, his compliance with his diabetes treatment plan, and the extent to which his family is involved. You will also need to find out what laboratory tests have been completed and how severe his renal dysfunction has become. After you obtain necessary data, you need to organize and analyze it to form some initial impressions about what it means. For example:

■ Admitting diagnosis is chronic renal failure; anticipate a problem with fluid balance.

■ Admitted to the hospital and is acutely ill; therefore, he may be anxious and fearful.

■ Decreased sensation in lower extremities; patient may have a mobility and a safety problem.

(continued)

Meet Your Patient (continued)

- Diabetes; patient is at risk for impaired skin and tissue integrity.
- Diabetes and renal failure require complex regimens and patient self-care; therefore, it is possible that Todd may not be managing his therapy effectively, because he either is not motivated to do so or he lacks the knowledge he needs to comply with treatment.

When Todd and his family arrive on your unit, you begin gathering additional data. Using your comprehensive data, you then make a list of Todd's health problems, in order of priority. These actions illustrate the diagnosis phase of the nursing process. The purpose of diagnosing is to identify the client's health status, from which you will create an individualized plan of care.

Theoretical Knowledge
knowing why

Professional standards of nursing practice, as well as many state nurse practice acts, identify diagnosing as the unique obligation of the professional nurse (Box 4-1). Although many nursing activities may be delegated, diagnosis cannot. To meet practice expectations and professional obligations as a registered nurse, you will assume the role of diagnostician and make clinical judgments. Most state nurse practice acts limit the role of the licensed practical nurse (LPN/LVN) to gathering data that will be analyzed by the RN. However, LPN roles vary among states and agencies, and they are subject to change.

BOX 4-1 ■ Professional Standards for Diagnosing

American Nurses Association Standards of Nursing Practice
Standard 2. Diagnosis

The registered nurse analyzes the assessment data to determine the diagnoses or issues.

Competencies

The registered nurse:

- Derives the diagnoses or issues from assessment data.
- Validates the diagnoses or issues with the healthcare consumer, family, and other healthcare providers when possible and appropriate.
- Identifies actual or potential risks to the healthcare consumer's health and safety or barriers to health, which may include but are not limited to interpersonal, systematic, or environmental circumstances.
- Uses standardized classification systems and clinical decision support tools, when available, in identifying diagnoses.
- Documents diagnoses or issues in a manner that facilitates the determination of the expected outcomes and plan.

Note: There are additional measurement criteria for advanced practice registered nurses.

Source: American Nurses Association. (2010). *Nursing: Scope and standards of practice* (2nd ed.). Silver Spring, MD: Nursebooks.org.

Furthermore, LPN and RN roles are becoming more closely linked through statewide career ladder programs. Therefore, all clinicians need to stay current with updates in practice acts and standards.

ABOUT THE KEY CONCEPTS

Nursing diagnosis is the single concept in this chapter that ties all the other concepts together.

The *diagnostic process* (also called *diagnostic reasoning*) represents the thinking aspect of nursing diagnosis, and the *diagnostic format* is the concrete product. Other, related, concepts will clarify what is *not* a nursing diagnosis, explain various types of nursing diagnoses, and expand on the concept of diagnostic format.

DIAGNOSIS: THE SECOND STEP OF THE NURSING PROCESS

After gathering the data you will use your critical-thinking skills to analyze the data—that is, identify patterns in the data and draw conclusions about the client's health status. This describes **nursing diagnosis,** the second step of the nursing process. As in all phases of the nursing process, involve the patient and family as much as possible.

Overlapping As you can see in Figure 4-1, diagnosis overlaps with the other nursing process steps. Most nurses actually begin diagnostic reasoning during the assessment phase. For example, you probably formed your initial impressions about Todd while you were still gathering data. On learning the medical diagnosis, chronic renal failure, you would have immediately considered the diagnosis Risk for Imbalanced Fluid Volume, but you would have obtained more data before actually recording that as a nursing diagnosis. So your tentative diagnostic conclusion would actually lead you to collect more data: *Is he still producing urine? What is his oral intake? Does he have edema?* Do you see how you would move back and forth between assessment and diagnosis? The two stages are not separate at all, but we present them that way to make it easier for you to learn.

Diagnosis is critical because it links the assessment step, which precedes it, to all the steps that follow it (Fig. 4-2). Assessment data must be complete and

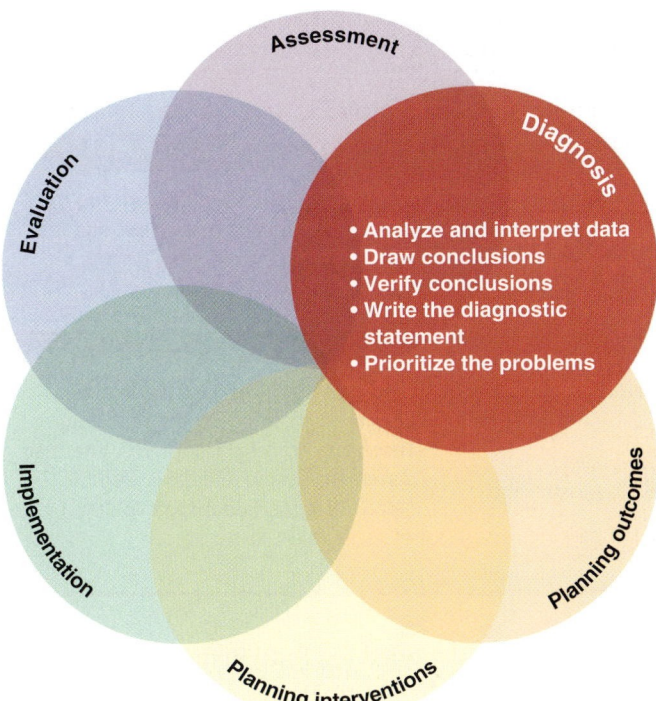

FIGURE 4-1 Nursing diagnosis: Second phase of the nursing process.

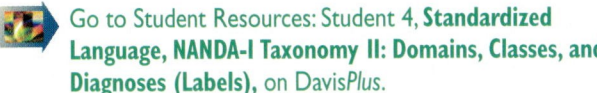

Go to Student Resources: Student 4, **Standardized Language, NANDA-I Taxonomy II: Domains, Classes, and Diagnoses (Labels),** on Davis*Plus*.

Table 4-1 summarizes and provides examples of how we use nursing diagnosis terminology in this text.

What Are the Origins of Nursing Diagnosis?

Before the 1950s, nurses assisted physicians by collecting data to help them diagnose and treat disease. Nursing care was thought of as a set of tasks and organized as a list of things to do. The term *nursing diagnosis* was first used in 1953 to differentiate nursing from medicine, when Fry (1953) stated that a nursing diagnosis identifies the client's needs for nursing rather than for medical care. Until the early 1970s, nursing diagnosis was not widely used in nursing practice, but two major events in 1973 spurred change:

- The First Conference on Nursing Diagnosis was held (Gebbie, 1976). A national task force was formed to begin developing a language to describe the health problems treated by nurses.
- The American Nurses Association (ANA) *Standards of Nursing Practice* included nursing diagnosis as an expectation of professional nurses.

In 1980, the ANA published *ANA Social Policy Statement,* which characterized nursing as "the diagnosis and treatment of human response to actual or potential health problems" (ANA, 1980, p. 2). As a result of this definition and the work of the nursing diagnosis task force, most state nurse practice acts began to designate nursing diagnosis as an exclusive responsibility of registered nurses. Nursing diagnosis is now widely used in nursing education and practice. **Key Point:** *The formal list of nursing diagnostic labels describes health problems that can be addressed by independent nursing actions and, in that sense, forms the body of knowledge that is unique to nursing.*

Since the first conference, the nursing diagnosis group has continued to meet every 2 years. In 1982 it adopted the name North American Nursing Diagnosis Association (NANDA). In 2002 the organization changed its name to NANDA International (NANDA-I), to reflect its large number of members from countries outside the

accurate for you to make an accurate nursing diagnosis. **Key Point:** *Nursing diagnosis is the basis for planning client-centered goals and interventions, so accuracy is essential.*

Terminology The term **diagnosis** is used in the nursing literature to refer to:

- The second phase of the nursing process
- The reasoning process used in interpreting assessment data
- A formal diagnostic statement of the client's health status, containing both the problem and etiology (factors contributing to the problem)
- The list of standardized terms (labels) used to write diagnostic statements. Those terms are actually problem labels; you must add a second part (etiology) in order to create a complete diagnostic statement. To see the entire list of NANDA-I diagnostic labels,

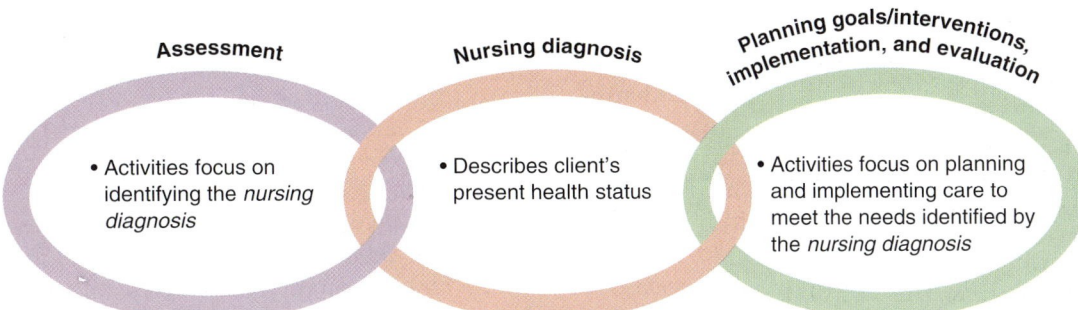

FIGURE 4-2 Diagnosis links the assessment phase to the rest of the nursing process.

Table 4-1 ➤ Nursing Diagnosis Terminology

TERM AND EXISTING MEANINGS	TERMINOLOGY USED IN THIS BOOK	EXAMPLE
Diagnosis		
1. The second phase of the nursing process 2. The reasoning process used in identifying patient problems and strengths	1. Diagnosis 2. Diagnostic process, diagnostic reasoning, or diagnosing	With Todd (Meet Your Patient), you used *diagnostic reasoning* to *diagnose* and list his problems. This was the *diagnosis phase* of the nursing process.
Nursing Diagnosis		
1. The end product of the diagnostic reasoning process: a full diagnostic statement describing client health status. It contains both problem and etiology. 2. A standardized problem label from the NANDA-I taxonomy (e.g., Anxiety)	1. Nursing diagnosis, diagnostic statement 2. Label, NANDA-I label, problem label, diagnostic label	For Todd, you might have made a *nursing diagnosis* of Excess Fluid Volume secondary to renal failure. To write that statement, you would have used the *NANDA-I label* Fluid Excess Volume.

United States and Canada. NANDA-I continues to review and refine the diagnostic labels and to discuss new and revised labels at each biannual conference. The diagnoses on the official list are approved for clinical use and further study; the list is not intended to represent a finished product, because many of the diagnoses are only partially substantiated by research. NANDA-I encourages individual nurses and nursing organizations to submit new and revised diagnoses.

KnowledgeCheck 4-1

- Why is the diagnosis step so critical to the other phases of the nursing process?
- Which two nursing organizations have been responsible for making diagnosis a part of the professional nursing role?

What Are Health Problems?

A **health problem** is any condition that requires intervention to promote wellness or to prevent or treat disease or illness. After you identify a health problem, you must decide how to treat it: independently or in collaboration with other health professionals. The answer determines whether it is a nursing diagnosis, a medical diagnosis, or a collaborative problem. See Table 4-2 for a comparison of these problem types.

Recognizing Nursing Diagnoses

A **nursing diagnosis** is a statement of client health status that nurses can identify, prevent, or treat independently. It is stated in terms of **human responses** (reactions) to disease, injury, or other stressors, and it can be either a problem or a strength. Human responses can be biological, emotional, interpersonal, social, or spiritual. For example, in the Meet Your Patient scenario, Todd's medical diagnosis is chronic renal failure. A *physical response* to renal failure might be Excess Fluid Volume. Admission to the ED is also a stressor, to which his *emotional response* might be Anxiety or Fear. What other actual or possible

responses were identified for Todd in the situation? Take a moment to write them down.

Recall that Todd has decreased sensation in his lower extremities. This is a stressor, to which he has responded with slightly impaired mobility. Perhaps you identified that because of diminished feeling in his feet, Todd might be at risk for falling (safety), impaired skin or tissue integrity, and ineffective management of his therapy. All of those are responses to disease, illness, or stressors. Also note that in addition to being a stressor, the decreased sensation in Todd's lower extremities can be considered a physical response to type 2 DM. Was this response on the list you just made?

ThinkLike a Nurse 4-1

Imagine that you have been in an automobile accident. You have internal injuries and broken bones and will be hospitalized for at least 2 weeks, right before your final exams. What human responses (physical, emotional, interpersonal, social, spiritual) would you have?

NANDA-I officially defines *nursing diagnosis* as "a clinical judgment about individual, family, or community experiences/responses to actual or potential health problems/life processes. A nursing diagnosis provides the basis for selection of nursing interventions to achieve outcomes for which the nurse has accountability" (approved at the ninth NANDA conference; amended in 2009) (NANDA-I, 2012, p. 514). This definition emphasizes the clinical judgment aspect of diagnosing.

Recognizing Medical Diagnoses

Todd has two medical diagnoses: chronic renal failure and type 2 DM. A **medical diagnosis** describes a disease, illness, or injury. Its purpose is to identify a pathology so that appropriate medical treatment can be given. A medical diagnosis is more narrowly focused than is a nursing diagnosis.

Table 4-2 ➤ Comparison of Nursing Diagnoses, Medical Diagnoses, and Collaborative Problems

	NURSING DIAGNOSIS	MEDICAL DIAGNOSIS	COLLABORATIVE PROBLEM
Definition	A clinical judgment about individual, family, or community responses to a health problem	Disease, illness, injury, or condition validated by signs and symptoms and medical diagnostic studies	Certain potential physiological complications that are always associated with a disease, test, or treatment
Focus	The individual/person	Disease, pathology, and medical treatments/procedures	Pathophysiology (complications caused by the disease process)
Characteristics	Holistic; describes physiological, psychological, social, interpersonal, and spiritual responses	Describes disease or pathology; does not consider the broader range of human responses	Describes potential physiological complications only; not holistic
Who Diagnoses?	Professional nurse	Physicians, advanced practice nurses, physician's assistants	Nurses
Who Orders Treatment?	Professional nurse, primarily	Physician, advanced practice nurse, physicians' assistants	Physician prescribes primary interventions; however, the nurse can order some as well.
Problem Status	Can be actual, potential, or possible	Actual or possible (rule out)	Always potential; if the problem actually develops, it is then a medical diagnosis.
Purpose of Nursing Interventions	Treat or prevent the problem; relieve the symptoms	Carry out medical prescriptions for treatment; monitor for improvement or worsening of the condition.	Monitor for development of the complication; institute some, but not all, preventive interventions.
Example of Diagnostic Statement	Ineffective Denial related to difficulty coping with new diagnosis of "heart attack"	Myocardial infarction	Potential Complication of myocardial infarction: congestive heart failure
Example of Data to Support the Diagnosis	Waited more than 6 hours before coming to hospital. Minimizes symptoms, refuses pain medications. States, "I've got to get back to work. I can't stay in the hospital." Laughing, joking, saying, "It's nothing."	Cardiac enzyme levels elevated; has had severe chest pain; elevated white blood cell count; electrocardiogram (ECG) and echocardiogram diagnostic of cardiac muscle ischemia	58-year-old man with diagnosis of myocardial infarction (MI); acknowledges chest pain; ECG and lab work diagnostic of MI

Key Point: *Except for advanced practice nurses, nurses cannot legally diagnose or treat medical problems.* Your assessment data will help the medical team to identify disease states and evaluate the effects of medical therapies. For example, if your assessment indicates that a medication does not adequately relieve a patient's pain, you would inform the primary care provider, who would prescribe a different medication or dosage. You need to know the pathophysiology of the patient's illness to understand and evaluate the effects of medical treatments and to know how to focus your assessments. The following are differences between medical and nursing diagnoses:

- **You cannot predict a patient's nursing diagnoses just by knowing his medical diagnosis or pathology.** Nursing diagnoses are human responses, which are complex and unique to each person. A medical diagnosis, in contrast, remains the same as long as a particular injury or pathology is present. In the Meet Your Patient scenario, Todd's medical diagnosis of type 2 DM will not change, because the fact that his body cannot use glucose normally will not change. This is not true for nursing diagnoses. Suppose Todd has a nursing diagnosis of Noncompliance with diabetic diet r/t (related to) lack of knowledge about food groups. If he learned about the foods and began following his diet, he would no longer have this nursing diagnosis. But he would still have the medical diagnosis of type 2 DM.

- **A medical diagnosis, disease, or pathological condition can have any number of nursing diagnoses associated with it.** For example, in response to his type 2 DM, Todd might have nursing diagnoses of Noncompliance and Risk for Impaired Skin Integrity.

- **Clients with the same medical diagnosis may have different nursing diagnoses.** Another client with type 2 DM may not have a diagnosis of Noncompliance, but instead may have a diagnosis of Ineffective Denial because he simply cannot accept that he truly has diabetes. Other patients with type 2 DM might have diagnoses of Anxiety, Deficient Knowledge, Disturbed Body Image, and perhaps others, depending on their unique responses to the stressor, type 2 DM.

Recognizing Collaborative Problems

Collaborative problems are "certain physiologic complications [of diseases, medical treatments, or diagnostic studies] that nurses monitor to detect onset or changes in status" (Carpenito, 2006, p. 19). They have the following characteristics:

- **All patients who have a certain disease or medical treatment are at risk for developing the same complications.** That is, the collaborative problems (complications) are determined by the medical diagnosis or pathology. Consider these examples:

    Todd, because he has type 2 DM, has the collaborative problem Potential Complication of type 2 DM: hyperglycemia and/or hypoglycemia. All other patients with type 2 DM also have those potential complications.

    All patients having surgery have the collaborative problem Potential Complication of surgery: infection.

    Use your theoretical knowledge of anatomy, physiology, microbiology, pathophysiology, and so on as the basis for identifying the complications associated with a particular disease or treatment.

- **A collaborative problem is always a potential problem.** If it becomes *actual*, then it is no longer a collaborative problem, but a medical diagnosis requiring physician interventions. Consider what would be needed if the preceding potential complications became actual problems:

    Actual hyperglycemia (high blood glucose) or actual hypoglycemia (low blood glucose)

    Actual infection of a surgical incision

    Either condition would require medical intervention to prevent serious harm to the patient.

- **If you can prevent the complication with independent nursing interventions alone, it is not a collaborative problem.** Collaborative problems require both medical and independent nursing interventions to prevent them or minimize the complications. The purpose of independent nursing interventions is primarily to monitor for onset of the complication, although nurses can provide some independent preventive measures.

See Figure 4-3 for an algorithm to help you differentiate nursing diagnoses from medical diagnoses and collaborative problems.

KnowledgeCheck 4-2

State whether each of the following represents a nursing diagnosis, medical diagnosis, or collaborative problem:

- After giving birth, all women are at risk for developing postpartum hemorrhage.

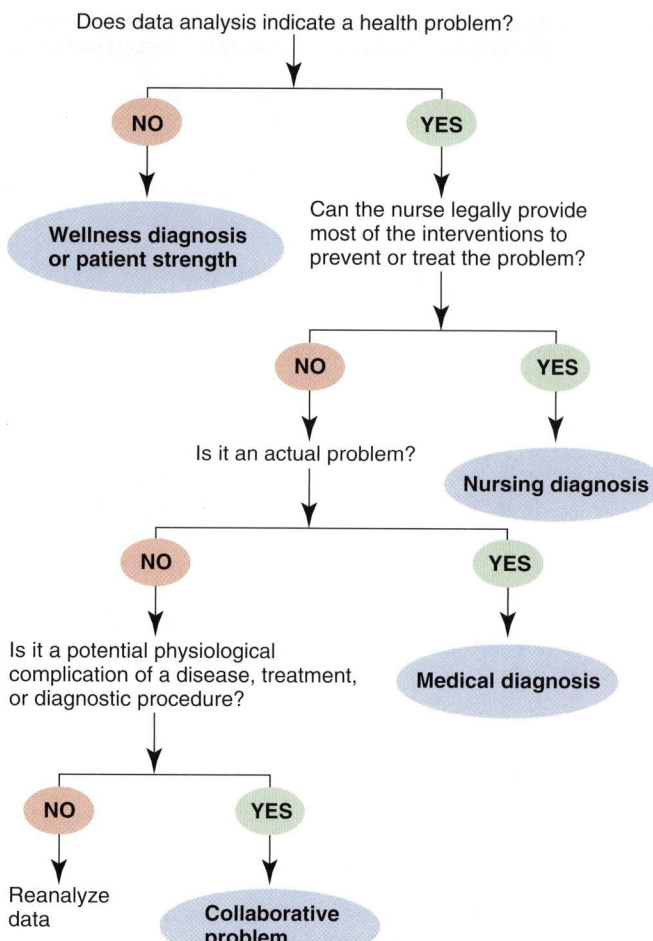

FIGURE 4-3 Algorithm for distinguishing among nursing, medical, and collaborative problems.

- A patient has signs and symptoms of appendicitis, which must be treated with surgery and antibiotics.
- A client is at risk for constipation because he postpones defecation and also does not consume enough dietary fiber and fluids. The problem can be prevented by patient teaching, which the nurse is licensed to do.

Types of Nursing Diagnoses

You must determine the status, or type, of each nursing diagnosis: Is it an actual, risk (potential), possible, syndrome, or wellness nursing diagnosis? Figure 4-4 provides an algorithm for determining the type of diagnosis, and Table 4-3 compares the diagnosis types. Identifying the type is important because each status requires (1) different wording in the diagnostic statement and (2) different nursing interventions.

KnowledgeCheck 4-3

- What are the five types (statuses) of nursing diagnoses?
- What type of nursing diagnosis is each of the following?
    a. Jane Thomas regularly engages in exercise but tells you she would like to increase her endurance.
    b. Mrs. King has several of the signs and symptoms (defining characteristics) of the nursing diagnosis Ineffective Coping.

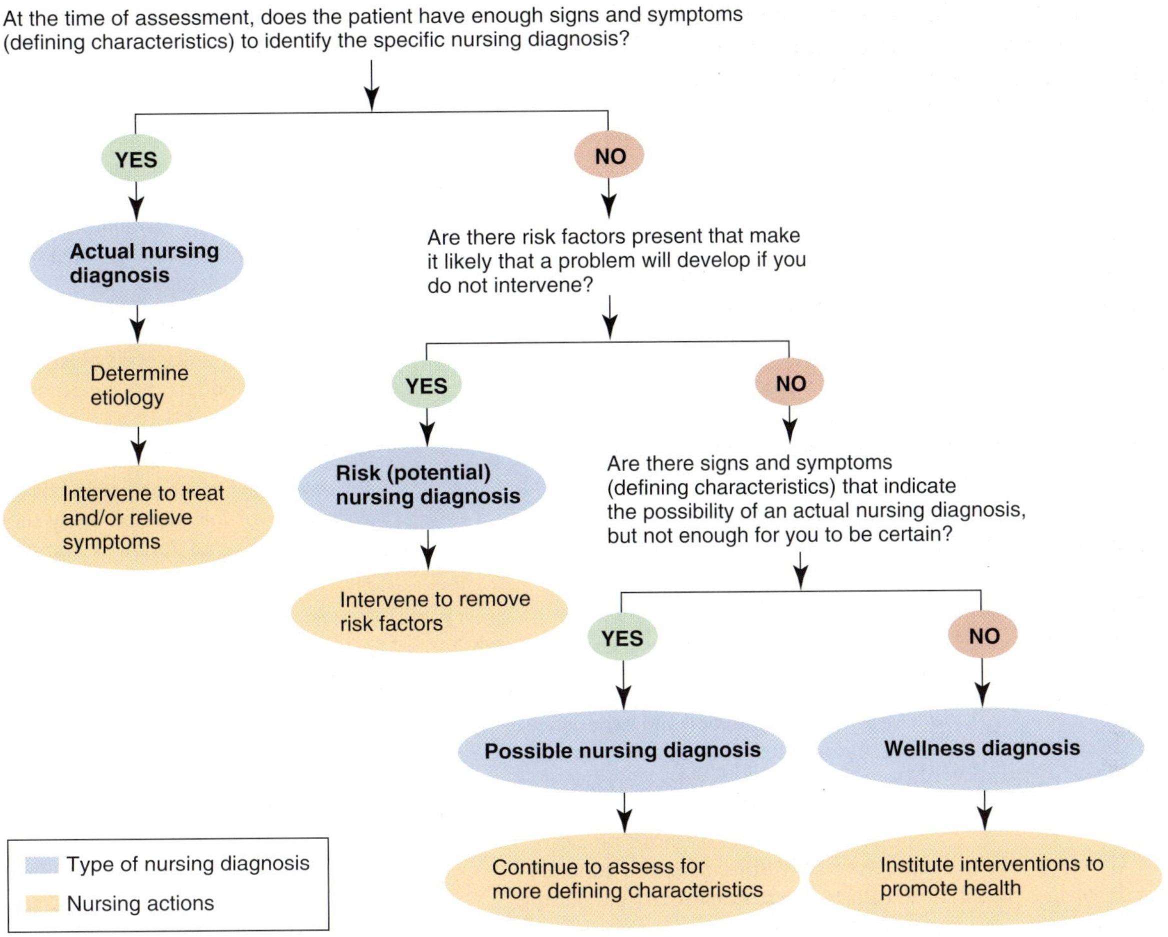

At the time of assessment, does the patient have enough signs and symptoms (defining characteristics) to identify the specific nursing diagnosis?

FIGURE 4-4 Algorithm for determining whether a nursing diagnosis is an actual diagnosis, a risk (potential) diagnosis, a possible diagnosis, or a wellness diagnosis.

c. Alicia Hernandez seems anxious, but you are not sure whether she actually is. You would like to have more data in order to diagnose or rule out a diagnosis of Anxiety.

d. Charles Oberfeldt has no symptoms of constipation. However, he reports that he does not include many fiber-rich foods in his diet and drinks few liquids. In addition, he is now fairly inactive because of a back injury. These are all risk factors for a diagnosis of Constipation.

WHAT IS DIAGNOSTIC REASONING?

A comprehensive patient assessment produces a great deal of data. **Diagnostic reasoning** is the thinking process that enables you to make sense of it. This text presents diagnostic reasoning (also referred to as **analysis**) in separate steps so that it is easier to learn, but that is not the way it really occurs (Fig. 4-5). When you first begin to use diagnostic reasoning, follow the steps in the order presented so that you will not miss anything. But just as you move back and forth between assessing and diagnosing, you will soon find yourself moving back and forth among the steps of diagnostic reasoning, skipping steps, returning to previous steps, and doing some steps simultaneously.

In diagnostic reasoning, you will use your critical thinking to analyze and interpret data, draw conclusions about the patient's health status, verify problems with the patient, prioritize the problems, and record the diagnostic statements.

Analyze and Interpret Data

As you analyze and interpret the data, you will gradually narrow the quantity of data you must deal with. But even as you narrow the field of data to the significant points and patterns, you will note the need for new information and further assessments. To analyze and interpret data, follow three steps: (1) Identify significant data, (2) cluster cues, and (3) identify data gaps and inconsistencies.

Step 1. Identify Significant Data

Significant data (also called **cues**) are data that influence your conclusions about the client's health status. A cue should alert you to look for other cues that might be related to it (form a pattern). You may be thinking, "How will I recognize a cue?"

Table 4-3 ➤ Types of Nursing Diagnoses: Actual, Risk, Possible, Syndrome, and Wellness

DIAGNOSIS TYPE	DEFINITION AND CHARACTERISTICS	MEET YOUR PATIENT OR OTHER EXAMPLE
Actual Nursing Diagnosis: Problem Is Present	▪ A problem response that exists at the time of the assessment ▪ Signs and symptoms (cues) that are present	Todd (Meet Your Patient) may have at least one actual nursing diagnosis (Impaired Walking or perhaps Impaired Physical Mobility), related to his lack of peripheral sensation; however, no signs and symptoms were given in the scenario to support that diagnosis.
Risk (Potential) Nursing Diagnosis: Problem May Occur	▪ A problem response that is likely to develop in a vulnerable patient if the nurse and patient do not intervene to prevent it ▪ No signs/symptoms of the problem, but the risk factors are present that increase the patient's vulnerability ▪ The patient is more susceptible to the problem than others in the same or a comparable setting (e.g., one who is undernourished or who has a compromised immune system).	1. Todd's (MYP) loss of lower limb sensation is a risk factor for a diagnosis of Risk for Falls even though Todd has no symptoms or history of falling. 2. All surgical patients have at least some risk for developing infection, so do not routinely write Risk for Infection on every surgical care plan. Instead, write Potential Complication of surgery: infection (incision and systemic).
Possible Nursing Diagnosis: Problem May Be Present	▪ Use when your intuition and experience direct you to suspect that a diagnosis is present, but you do not have enough data to support the diagnosis. The main reason for including this type of diagnosis on a care plan is to alert other nurses to continue to collect data to confirm or rule out the problem.	Todd (MYP) has a symptom, mildly impaired mobility. This could indicate the diagnoses Impaired Physical Mobility, Impaired Walking, or Risk for Falls. You need more data to decide which nursing diagnosis is appropriate, so you might write a nursing diagnosis of Possible Risk for Falls related to decreased sensation in both legs.
Syndrome Nursing Diagnosis: Several Related Problems Are Present	▪ Represents a collection of nursing diagnoses that usually occur together. ▪ Use when you notice that the patient has more than one nursing diagnosis with the same etiology (cause, contributing factors).	The NANDA-I label Risk for Disuse Syndrome is used to represent all the complications that can occur as a result of immobility (e.g., pressure ulcer, constipation, stasis of pulmonary secretions, thrombosis, body image disturbance).

Wellness Nursing Diagnosis: No Problem Is Present	▪ Describes health status, but does not describe a problem; can apply to an individual, family, group, or community
	▪ Use when the client is in transition from one level of wellness to a higher level
	▪ Two conditions must be present:
	  1. The client's present level of wellness is effective.
	  2. The client wants to move to a higher level of wellness.
		Suppose that Todd (MYP) tells you that he prays, participates in religious activities, and trusts in God, but he would like to feel even closer to God. He asks to meet with the minister from his church. You might make a diagnosis of Readiness for Enhanced Spiritual Well-Being.

A cue is usually an unhealthy response. One way to recognize cues is to draw on your theoretical knowledge (e.g., of anatomy, physiology, psychology) and compare each piece of data with standards and norms. For example, suppose you have noted that a woman's pulse rate is 110 beats/min. Is this an unhealthy response—a cue? You would of course use as one standard the average rate (80 beats/min) and normal range (60–100 beats/min) for an adult pulse. But this woman is a long-time cigarette smoker who also drinks coffee and caffeinated energy

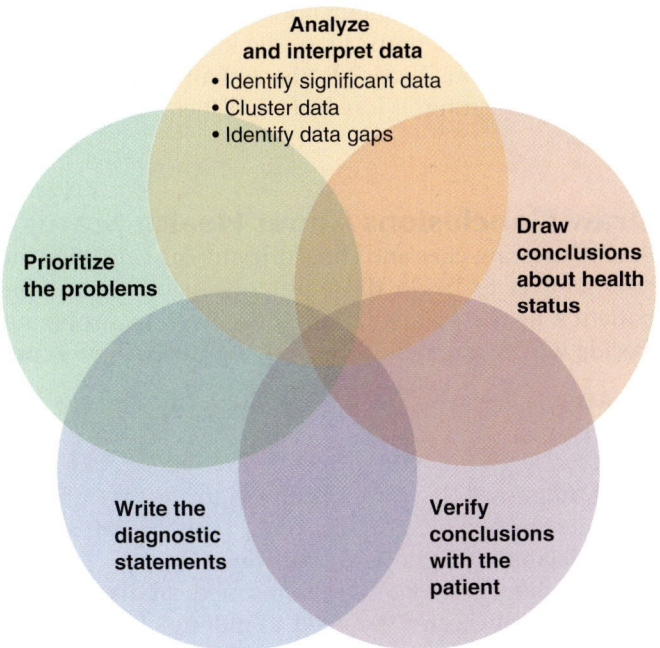

FIGURE 4-5 The process of diagnostic reasoning.

drinks. These habits increase pulse rate, so 110 beats/min may be a normal finding for this client. See Box 4-2 for other indications of cues.

KnowledgeCheck 4-4

- What is a cue?
- What are five ways you can recognize a cue?

Step 2. Cluster Cues

A **cluster** is a group of cues that are related to each other in some way. The cluster may suggest a health problem. To help ensure accuracy, you should always derive a nursing diagnosis from data clusters rather than from a single cue.

Consider this example: Alma was transferred to the hospital from a long-term care facility. Because of a CVA (cerebrovascular accident, or stroke), Alma can make sounds but cannot speak; and because of joint contractures, she cannot use her hands and arms. Alma is frequently incontinent of urine, so the nurses have diagnosed Overflow Urinary Incontinence and are re-signed to the idea that Alma will not be able to control her urine. Because Alma makes loud vocal noises, they have placed her in a room near the nurses' station. When a nursing student is assigned to the care for Alma, the student looks for cues in addition to urinary inconti-nence. The student notices that Alma is often inconti-nent after loud vocalizing. She sees a pattern in these cues: urinary incontinence, cannot use hands and arms, and cannot communicate verbally. The student changes the nursing diagnosis to Self-Care Deficit: Toileting related to immobility and inability to communicate the

---

---

need to void. After the student provides a call device that fits under Alma's arm, Alma is able to press the device and call the nurse when she needs to void. She is no longer incontinent of urine.

 ThinkLike a Nurse 4-2

For each of the following cue clusters, decide whether the cues represent a pattern; that is, are all the cues related in some way? If so, explain how they are related. If not, state which cue does not fit. If you do not have enough theoretical knowledge to know for sure, draw on your past experiences and discuss the clusters with other students.

a. Dry skin, abnormal skin turgor (more than 4 seconds), thirst, and scanty, dark yellow urine
b. Pain and limited range of motion in knees, uses walker, medical diagnosis of osteoarthritis
c. Hard, painful bowel movement about every 3 days; does not exercise regularly; eats very little dietary fiber; skin is dry.

Clustering data forces you to think about the relation-ships between the cues. For item (c) in the preceding example, you would think, "What might cause hard, painful bowel movements? I know that dietary fiber promotes peristalsis, so lack of fiber might contribute to constipation. And I remember that lack of exercise is associated with constipation. I don't see how dry skin would be related to constipation."

Step 3. Identify Data Gaps and Inconsistencies

As you cluster and think about relationships among the cues, you will identify the need for data that was not apparent before. In Think Like a Nurse item (c), you have enough data to support a diagnosis of Constipation. However, you still need to identify factors contributing to the problem. You have two: lack of dietary fiber and lack of exercise. But you should also ask about other causes of Constipation. Does the patient postpone defecation? Does he have a history of relying on laxatives? How much fluid does the client drink? (For example, Todd's skin is dry [Meet Your Patient]. Could that be because he is fluid deficient?)

Data Gaps As another example, look again at Todd's data. Except for medical diagnoses, there are very few data. The following data gaps exist:

- His admitting diagnosis, chronic renal failure, suggests the possibility of fluid imbalance; however, there are no other data to support that. What is his intake? His output? His skin turgor? The appearance of his urine? Does he have edema? Does he complain of thirst? What are his hemoglobin and hematocrit levels?
- Admission to the ED could cause Anxiety. To pursue that line of thinking, observe for physical and verbal symptoms of Anxiety.
- Decreased sensation in his lower extremities might create mobility or safety problems. You would need to know the degree of sensation loss and the exact meaning of "slight loss of mobility" to determine whether to focus on the mobility or the safety issue.
- The effect of diabetes on circulation and skin certainly places Todd at risk for skin problems. However, you need more data to determine whether he has any actual skin problems (e.g., presence or history of sores on his feet).

Inconsistencies In addition to missing data, look for inconsistencies in the data. Suppose a client tells you, "I really don't eat much. Three meals a day, and I don't snack between meals." However, she is 5 ft tall and weighs 190 lb. This seems inconsistent because your theoretical knowledge tells you that obesity is often caused by excessive intake of calories. Even though there are many causes for overweight, you wonder if someone could be so much overweight without "eating much." You would need more specific data about what this client actually eats, so consider having her keep a food diary of everything she eats for a week or two. What else would you want to know? For example, does she have any medical problems that might cause obesity (e.g., hypothyroidism)?

Is there any reason she might not want to tell you the truth about her eating pattern? Does she know the number of calories in various foods? Is she actually aware of how much she is eating? More data will help answer your questions.

Draw Conclusions About Health Status

After clustering cues and collecting any missing data, the next step is to begin drawing conclusions about the patient's health status—strengths as well as problems. Decide which one of the following the cluster represents:

- *Nursing Diagnosis: Possible, actual, risk, or wellness* (see Table 4-3)
- *Medical diagnosis.* Nurses are not licensed to make medical diagnoses. If you recognize signs and symptoms suggestive of a medical diagnosis, refer the patient to a physician for diagnosis and treatment.
- *Collaborative problem.* The client's medical diagnosis or treatment indicates the need to monitor for development of complications and to take some measures to prevent the complication, but you cannot prevent or treat the problem independently.
- *Patient strength.* If data seem to meet standards and norms, you can conclude the patient has a strength in that area. For example, Todd's strengths might be his marital status, family involvement, and employment status.
- *No problem.* If data seem to meet standards for normal and no nursing interventions are needed, you can conclude no problem exists in that area. If, in addition, the patient expresses the wish to achieve a higher level of wellness, you would make a wellness diagnosis.

Step 1. Make Inferences

Making inferences is a critical-thinking skill. Recall that cues are facts (or data), whereas inferences are conclusions (judgments, interpretations) that are based on the data. An inference is not a fact, because you cannot directly check its truth or accuracy. For example:

Fact: Patient is crying. (You can observe that directly.)
         Patient is trembling. (You can observe that directly.)
Inference: Patient is anxious. (You cannot observe anxiety, but you know that crying and trembling may be signs of anxiety.)

Even though you can never be completely sure that an inference is accurate, clearly some inferences are supported by more complete and reliable data than others. In the preceding example, suppose you said to the patient, "You seem upset. Can you tell me what's going on?" And the patient replied, "I've never been in the hospital before. So much has been happening, I guess I'm just anxious about everything." Now you have enough data to support your inference, and you can be reasonably sure that it is accurate (valid). But remember, you can't be absolutely certain. For example, although it is unlikely, the patient might be exaggerating or not telling you the truth. Perhaps she is crying because her husband said hurtful things to her, and she is too embarrassed to share that with you. Or perhaps she is a spy and is trying to divert your attention while an accomplice finds the hospital's hidden secrets. Yes, that is far-fetched, but that exaggerated example should convince you that an inference—even one that appears to be more valid than this one—is not a *fact*.

Key Point: *Nursing diagnoses, because they are inferences, are only your reasoned judgment about a patient's health status. So try not to think of a diagnosis as being right or wrong, but instead as more accurate or less accurate. Realize that you can never construct a perfect diagnosis, but strive to make your diagnostic statements as accurate as possible. Incorrect diagnoses result in ineffective care.*

KnowledgeCheck 4-5

- What are the possible conclusions you can draw about a client's health status (e.g., that no problem exists)?
- What is the difference between a cue and an inference?
- How can you be satisfied that you have made a valid inference?

Step 2. Identify Problem Etiologies

An **etiology** consists of the factors that are causing or contributing to the problem. Etiologies may be pathophysiological, treatment related, situational, social, spiritual, maturational, or environmental. It is important to correctly identify the etiology because it directs the nursing interventions. Consider this nursing diagnosis:

Constipation related to inadequate intake of dietary fiber

The etiology suggests that you encourage the client to eat more high-fiber foods. You might also teach the client about foods that are high in fiber. But what if that etiology is incomplete? What if you overlooked the fact that the client does not drink enough fluids? Or that he gets very little exercise? And what if you didn't realize that he often postpones defecation because he is a kindergarten teacher in a crowded, bustling classroom, and he simply cannot leave the children unattended except at scheduled times? In that case, your efforts to increase intake of high-fiber foods would probably not help relieve the client's constipation.

To identify the etiology of a health problem, use your theoretical knowledge (e.g., of psychology, physiology, disease processes) and the patient data to answer questions such as the following:

- What factors are known to cause this problem?
- What patient cues are present that may be contributing to this problem?
- How likely is it that these factors are contributing to the problem?
- What past experiences do I have that support my judgment that these factors are linked to the problem?

- Are these cues *causing* the problem, or are they merely *symptoms* of the problem?

Key Point: *An etiology is always an inference because you can never actually observe the "link" between etiology and problem.* For example, in the preceding Constipation diagnosis, you could measure (observe) the person's fiber intake. You could also observe infrequent, hard stools (Constipation). But you cannot observe that the lack of fiber is the cause of the Constipation. You have to infer that link based on your knowledge of normal elimination and your experiences with other patients.

ThinkLike a Nurse 4-3

- How would your nursing interventions be different for the following diagnoses?
  a. Constipation related to lack of knowledge about laxative use
  b. Constipation related to weak abdominal muscles secondary to long-term immobility
- How would your nursing interventions be different for the following diagnoses?
  a. Ineffective Breastfeeding related to lack of knowledge about breastfeeding techniques
  b. Ineffective Breastfeeding related to inability of infant to latch on to the breast and to coordinate sucking and swallowing, secondary to prematurity

Verify Problems With the Patient

After identifying problems and etiologies, verify them with the patient. A diagnostic statement is an interpretation of the data, and the patient's interpretations may differ from yours. For example, if you have diagnosed Ineffective Breastfeeding related to lack of knowledge about breastfeeding techniques, you might verify it by saying, "It seems to me you are having difficulty breastfeeding your baby because you are not sure how to position him and get him to latch on to your breast. Does this seem accurate to you?" The woman might confirm your diagnosis, or she might say, "No. I *do* know how to do it; I am just tired and a little nervous with you watching me." Think of nursing diagnoses as tentative, and remain open to changing them based on new data or insights from the patient.

Prioritize Problems

Up to this point, the diagnostic process has focused on identifying and validating health problems. However, clients often have more than one problem, so you must use nursing judgment to decide which ones to address first and which it is safe to address later. This is **prioritizing**. Prioritizing places the problems in order of importance, but it does not mean you must resolve one problem before attending to another.

You will usually prioritize problems when you are recording them. You can indicate the priority by designating each problem as high, medium, or low priority or by ranking all the problems in order from highest to lowest (i.e., 1, 2, 3, and so on). For example:

Labeling Each Problem	*Ranking the Problems*
Pain (high)	1—Risk for Falls
Risk for Falls (high)	2—Pain
Chronic Low Self-Esteem (low)	3—Imbalanced Nutrition
Imbalanced Nutrition (medium)	4—Chronic Low Self-Esteem

Notice that risk problems can have a higher priority than actual problems. In this example, it is more urgent to prevent falls than to treat low self-esteem.

Problem priority is largely determined by the theoretical framework you use (e.g., whether your criteria are human needs, problem urgency, future consequences, or patient preference).

Maslow's Hierarchy of Human Needs

Even though it is not a nursing framework, many nurses use Maslow's hierarchy to prioritize nursing diagnoses (Fig. 4-6). In Maslow's model, basic needs must be met

Transcendence
of self; helping others self-actualize

Self-actualization
Personal growth, reaching potential

Aesthetic
Symmetry, order, beauty

Cognitive
Knowledge, understanding, exploration

Self-esteem
Pride, sense of accomplishment, recognition by others

Love and belonging
Giving and receiving affection, meaningful relationships, belonging to group(s)

Safety and security
Protection, emotional and physical safety and security, order, law, stability, shelter

Physiological
Food, air, water, temperature regulation, elimination, rest, sex, and physical activity

FIGURE 4-6 Maslow's Hierarchy of Human Needs can be used for prioritizing problems. Most nursing diagnoses fall at the cognitive and lower levels. (*Source:* Adapted from Maslow, A. (1971). *The farther reaches of human nature.* New York: The Viking Press; and Maslow, A., & Lowery, R. (Eds.). (1998). *Toward a psychology of being* (3rd ed.). New York: John Wiley & Sons.)

before a person can focus on higher needs. Maslow (1970) ranks human needs on eight levels, beginning with the most basic needs. Table 4-4 shows examples of nursing diagnoses at various levels of Maslow's hierarchy. For further information on the Maslow theory, see Chapter 8.

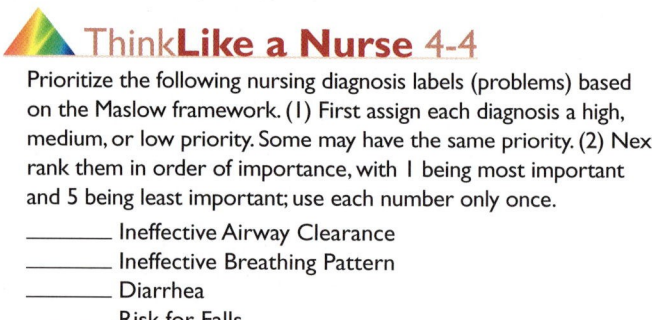

ThinkLike a Nurse 4-4

Prioritize the following nursing diagnosis labels (problems) based on the Maslow framework. (1) First assign each diagnosis a high, medium, or low priority. Some may have the same priority. (2) Next rank them in order of importance, with 1 being most important and 5 being least important; use each number only once.

_____ Ineffective Airway Clearance
_____ Ineffective Breathing Pattern
_____ Diarrhea
_____ Risk for Falls
_____ Impaired Memory

Problem Urgency

If you use problem urgency as your ranking criteria, you would rank the problems according to the degree of threat they pose to the patient's life or to the immediacy with which treatment is needed. Assign:

High priority to problems that are life threatening (e.g., Ineffective Airway Clearance) or that could have a destructive effect on the client (e.g., substance abuse)

Medium priority to problems that do not pose a direct threat to life, but that may cause destructive physical or emotional changes (e.g., Ineffective Denial, Unilateral Neglect)

Low priority to problems that require minimal supportive nursing intervention (e.g., Risk for Delayed Development, Interrupted Breastfeeding, mild Anxiety)

Future Consequences

Even though a problem is not life threatening, and even though the patient does not see the problem as a priority, it may result in harmful future consequences for the patient. For example, suppose that Todd (Meet Your Patient) is hospitalized for 5 days and undergoes inpatient dialysis. His physician prescribes a renal diet and insulin (instead of his previous oral medications) to treat the diabetes. Todd announces that he would like to go home as soon as possible. "I need to get back to my job and my family," he tells you. He resists learning about his medicines and how to administer his insulin. "Just give me a list of my medicines, and I'll take them when I get home," he says. You are aware that his renal failure is secondary to uncontrolled DM and that he often neglected to take his medication in the past. You suspect that he has not been taking his medicines because he is in denial about his health problems. Clearly his Ineffective Denial may lead to further problems with his treatment plan. You would assign high priority to this problem and address it before attempting to provide teaching for his nursing diagnosis of Deficient Knowledge (insulin).

Table 4-4 ➤ Using Maslow's Hierarchy to Prioritize Diagnoses

BASIC NEEDS (MOST BASIC TO HIGHEST)	EXAMPLES OF HUMAN NEEDS	EXAMPLES OF NURSING DIAGNOSES
Physiological	Food, air, water, shelter, sleep and rest, elimination, activity, temperature regulation	Imbalanced Nutrition: Less Than Body Requirements Impaired Gas Exchange
Safety and Security	(Includes both physical and psychological safety); law, order, shelter, stability	Risk for Falls Fear Risk for Self-Directed Violence
Love and Belonging	Roles, relationships, the need to give and receive affection, the feeling of belonging	Impaired Social Interaction Ineffective Sexuality Pattern Risk for Impaired Attachment
Self-Esteem	Feelings of confidence, capability, and independence; respect, recognition, and appreciation from others	Chronic Low Self-Esteem Social Isolation
Cognitive	Knowledge, understanding, exploration	Acute Confusion Impaired Memory Delayed Growth and Development
Aesthetic	Symmetry, order, beauty	(It is unusual for nursing diagnoses to fall into this, or the two higher, categories.)
Self-Actualization	Personal growth, reaching one's highest potential	
Transcendence	Connecting to something beyond self, helping others reach their potential	Readiness for Enhanced Spiritual Well-Being Spiritual Distress (and Risk for Spiritual Distress)

Sources: Adapted from Maslow, A. (1971). *The farther reaches of human nature.* New York: The Viking Press; and Maslow, A., & Lowery, R. (Eds.). (1998). *Toward a psychology of being* (3rd ed.). New York: John Wiley & Sons.

Patient Preference

Give high priority to problems the patient thinks are most important, provided that this does not conflict with basic/survival needs or medical treatments. Patients cooperate more fully with interventions they consider important. In addition, they may be more motivated to work on other problems after their own priorities are addressed.

Consider this example. Mr. Amani has had a major surgery within the past 24 hours. His main concern is to obtain pain relief. He refuses to turn, deep-breathe, and cough (TDBC) because it causes pain. However, as his nurse, you realize that these activities are essential for preventing Ineffective Airway Clearance, so you cannot safely support Mr. Amani's priorities. You should of course provide pain medication before helping him TDBC, but it may be impossible for him to be entirely pain free during these activities. You would explain your actions and continue to emphasize the importance of TDBC. When you explain the importance of your priorities, patients often come to agree with them.

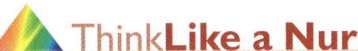 ThinkLike a Nurse 4-5

Suppose that on Todd's transfer from the ED (Meet Your Patient), you made the following nursing diagnoses for him. Using problem urgency as your criterion, assign each of these diagnoses a low, medium, or high priority. You may not have much theoretical knowledge about type 2 DM and chronic renal disease, but use the information provided in the scenario and in the etiologies to prioritize as well as you can. Discuss the case with your classmates and your instructor.

■ Risk for Imbalanced Fluid Volume secondary to renal failure
■ Risk for Falls related to decreased sensation and mobility in legs
■ Anxiety r/t unknown prognosis of renal failure and ED environment
■ Deficient Knowledge (renal disease process) r/t new diagnosis of renal involvement secondary to type 2 DM

Computer-Assisted Diagnosing

Many institutions use computers for planning and documenting patient care. Some expert (knowledge-based) systems allow you to enter assessment data, and the computer program will generate a list of possible problems. After you choose a problem label, the computer will provide a screen with the definition and defining characteristics of the problem so you can compare them to the actual patient data. After you "accept" the diagnostic label, you complete the problem statement by choosing etiologies from the next computer screen. To see examples of such computer screens,

 Go to Student Resources: Chapter 4, **Tables, Boxes, Figures: ESG Figures 4-1 and 4-2,** on DavisPlus.

KnowledgeCheck 4-6
List the steps in the diagnostic process.

REFLECTING CRITICALLY ON YOUR DIAGNOSTIC REASONING

Diagnostic reasoning is complex and vulnerable to error. Therefore, after prioritizing your list of problems, you need to evaluate the list for accuracy. With the implementation of electronic health records, there is an even greater need for accuracy of nursing diagnoses (Häyrinen, Lammintakanen, & Saranto, 2010; Lunney, 2008). When diagnosing, you apply critical thinking to your theoretical and self-knowledge and to the patient data and situation (recall the full-spectrum nursing model in Chapter 2).

Critical thinking + Knowledge + Data = Statement of health status

Think About Your Theoretical Knowledge

The better your knowledge base is, the better is your diagnostic reasoning. Ask yourself the following questions:

- Is this diagnosis based on sound knowledge (e.g., of pathophysiology, psychology, nutrition, and other related disciplines)?
- Do I have sound knowledge about the defining characteristics associated with various nursing diagnoses?
- Do I feel reasonably sure I have interpreted the data correctly?
- Have I identified the problem type correctly—that is, can this problem be treated primarily by nursing interventions?
- Am I qualified to make this diagnosis, or should I consult with a more experienced nurse or other member of the collaborative healthcare team?

To avoid diagnostic error, build a good knowledge base and learn from your clinical experiences. If you lack knowledge in an area, review the literature. Solid theoretical knowledge will help you (1) to recognize cues and patterns, (2) to associate patterns with the correct problem, (3) gain confidence in your ability to reason, and (4) keep from relying too much on authority figures (Wilkinson, 2011).

Think About Your Self-Knowledge

Realize that your beliefs, values, and experiences affect your thinking and can be misleading. For example, imagine that a nurse in a labor and delivery unit believes it is important to be strong and uncomplaining, even when experiencing severe pain. When this nurse cares for a woman in early labor who cries out and complains of pain, the nurse sees it as a problem of either Anxiety or Ineffective Coping, not as a problem of Pain. Can you see how that changes the focus of the nurse's care? Ask yourself the following questions (Wilkinson, 2011):

What biases and stereotypes may have influenced my interpretation of the data? A **bias** is the tendency to slant your judgment based on personal opinion or unfounded beliefs, as the nurse did in the preceding example. **Stereotypes** are judgments and expectations about an individual based on the personal beliefs you have about this group (e.g., men are unemotional; Asians are intelligent; teenagers are irresponsible). Referring to patients by their diagnosis or developmental group is a form of stereotyping (e.g., "the elderly man in room 110"; "the broken hip in 288"). You form stereotypes by making flawed assumptions when you have little or no actual experience with a person or group.

Did I rely too much on past experiences? This is like stereotyping in that you draw conclusions about an individual based on what you know about people in similar situations. Consider, for example, a nurse who has cared for many first-time mothers (primiparas) during labor. Most of these women experienced moderate anxiety even during early labor. Now each time the nurse cares for a primipara, she expects to see anxiety, and she tends to identify cue clusters as Anxiety, failing to check for other explanations such as Pain or Deficient Knowledge.

Did I rely too much on the client's medical diagnosis, the setting, or what others say about the client instead of on the data? Medical diagnoses and statements from others can help you to think of possible explanations for your data, but they can also bias your thinking and prevent you from gathering your own data. For example, Ms. Grayson has cancer. She returned to the unit last evening after undergoing a total colectomy and colostomy (removal of the colon and creation of an artificial opening for removal of stool). She had expected her surgery to be only an exploratory laparotomy to evaluate abdominal symptoms. This morning in report, the night shift nurse stated, "Ms. Grayson is aware that she has cancer and is coping well." While bathing Ms. Grayson, you begin to talk to her about her colostomy. She seems shocked. "I didn't know they did that! What's wrong with me?" As you answer her questions, you realize that she has been very groggy from the anesthesia and pain medication and does not recall being told about her surgery and cancer.

Think About Your Thinking

After reflecting on your knowledge, think about how you used the diagnostic process. Be sure your analysis of the data was thorough, that you have accurately identified the patient's problems, and that they are logically linked to the etiologies. Review your interactions with the patient: Do the diagnostic statements reflect his perceptions and priorities, or did he just give you the answers he thought you wanted? Use the questions in Box 4-3 to critique your thinking during the diagnostic process.

KnowledgeCheck 4-7

To help you fix them in your mind, list at least 10 questions to ask yourself when evaluating your diagnostic reasoning. Refer to Box 4-3 if you need help preparing this list.

Practicalknowledge
knowing **how**

After you have completed the diagnostic reasoning process, the final activity in the diagnosis step is to record patient strengths and problem statements. Practical knowledge regarding nursing diagnosis involves selecting the correct standardized problem labels and writing the diagnostic statements. The remainder of this chapter will help you learn to apply the concepts you learned in the Theoretical Knowledge section.

STANDARDIZED NURSING LANGUAGES

In order to communicate, people need a shared language. A **standardized language** is one in which the terms are carefully defined and mean the same thing to all who use them. One example is the periodic table for chemical elements. When a chemist in the United States writes Fe or Zn, all other chemists in the world know that she means iron or zinc. Moreover, they know exactly what is meant by iron and zinc, because each is defined by its own atomic number, atomic mass, number of protons, number of neutrons, and so on. There is no confusion. **Standardized nursing languages** are a comparatively recent attempt to bring such clarity to communication about nursing knowledge and nursing thinking. Nurses need clear, precise, consistent terminology when referring to the same clinical problems and treatments. A standardized language can do the following:

- Support electronic health records.
- Define, communicate, and expand nursing knowledge.

BOX 4-3 ■ Critiquing Your Diagnostic Reasoning Process

Data Analysis

Did you:

- Identify all the significant data (cues)?
- Omit any important cues from the cluster?
- Include unnecessary cues that may have confused your interpretation?
- Try more than one way of grouping the cues?
- Consider the patient's social, cultural, and spiritual beliefs and needs?
- Identify all the data gaps and inconsistencies?

Drawing Inferences and Interpretations of the Data

- Did you consider all the possible explanations for the cue cluster?
- Is this the best explanation for the cue cluster? Remember that a variety of explanations may be possible.
- Did you have enough data to make that inference? If not, suspend judgment until you gather more data.
- Did you look at patterns, not single cues?
- Did you look at behavior over time, not just isolated incidents?
- Did you jump to conclusions? Or did you take the time to carefully analyze and synthesize the data?

Critiquing the Diagnostic Statement (Problem + Etiology)

- Is the diagnosis relevant, and does it reflect the data?
- Does the diagnostic statement give a clear and accurate picture of the patient's problem or strength?

- When identifying the problem and etiology, did you look beyond medical diagnoses and consider human responses?
- Did you consider strengths and wellness diagnoses?
- Can you explain how the etiology relates to the problem—that is, how it would produce the problem response?
- Does the complete list of problems fully describe the patient's overall health status?

Verifying the Diagnosis

- Did the patient verify this diagnosis?
- When you verified the diagnosis are you certain the patient understood your description of his health status?
- Did you obtain feedback from the patient, or did you merely assume that the patient agreed?
- Did you keep an open mind, realizing all diagnoses are tentative and subject to change as you acquire more data?

Prioritizing

- Considering the whole situation, what are the most important problems?
- What aspects of the situation require immediate attention?
- Did you consider patient preferences when setting priorities? If not, was there a good reason?

- Increase visibility and awareness of nursing interventions.
- Facilitate research to demonstrate the contribution of nurses to healthcare and influence health policy decisions (Shever, 2011).
- Improve patient care by providing better communication among nurses and other healthcare providers and facilitating the testing of nursing interventions.

For a full discussion of the benefits of a uniform nursing language,

 Go to Student Resources, Chapter 4, **Supplemental Materials: Why Do We Need a Standardized Nursing Language?** on Davis*Plus*.

What Is a Taxonomy?

A **taxonomy** is a system for classifying ideas or objects based on characteristics they have in common. Classifications are created and used for various reasons. As mentioned earlier, the periodic table classifies elements according to their atomic mass, number of protons, and so on. Medications are classified in various ways; one way is to classify them according to their use (e.g., analgesics, antibiotics). The following classification systems are widely used in healthcare:

- The American Psychiatric Association's (APA) *Diagnostic and Statistical Manual (DSM-5)* describes mental disorders (e.g., bipolar disorder, schizoaffective disorder) (APA, 2013).
- The *Manual of the International Classification of Disease and Related Health Problems (ICD-10)* names and classifies medical conditions (World Health Organization [WHO], 1992).
- The *Current Procedural Terminology: CPT 2010*, used for reimbursement of physician services, names and defines medical services and procedures (American Medical Association [AMA], 2010).

The following are classification systems that the American Nurses Association (ANA) has recognized for describing nursing diagnoses (some describe outcomes and interventions as well):

- *NANDA International*. The first use of standardized nursing language began in the 1970s, with the NANDA classification of nursing diagnoses. This taxonomy includes more than 200 diagnostic labels with etiologies, risk factors, and defining characteristics. Most chapters of this textbook use NANDA-I terminology.
- *Clinical Care Classification (CCC)*. Similar to the NANDA-I system; includes nearly 200 labels. Contains interventions as well as nursing diagnoses. The CCC was developed for home health use, but can be used in any setting.
- *Omaha System*. Contains about 42 nursing diagnosis "concepts" (also interventions and outcomes). The Omaha system is primarily for community health use, but can be used in other settings.

- *Perioperative Nursing Data Set (PNDS)*. For use in perioperative nursing only. Consists of 64 nursing diagnoses (also includes nursing interventions and patient outcomes). This was the first nursing language developed by a nursing specialty.
- *International Classification for Nursing Practice (ICNP)*. Includes diagnoses, outcomes, and nursing actions. The ICNP intends to provide a common language for nurses in various clinical settings worldwide (International Council of Nurses, 2011).

NANDA-I Taxonomy of Diagnostic Terminology

Which of the following could you group together? In what ways are the grouped objects similar?

a five-dollar bill	a penny
weeds (still growing)	new grass
an iron skillet	a needle

You could make these groupings:

A $5 bill and a penny (because they are both money).
A penny, an iron skillet, and a needle (because they are all metal).
A $5 bill, grass, and weeds (because they are all green).

Maybe you thought of other groupings, too. Any number of principles can be used to classify things and to organize a taxonomy.

The first NANDA taxonomy was simply an alphabetical list. To see that taxonomy,

 Go to Additional Resources: **NANDA-I Nursing Diagnoses, 2012-2014 Alphabetical List,** on Davis*Plus*.

NANDA's *Taxonomy II* categorizes nursing diagnoses into 13 domains and 47 classes (NANDA-I, 2012). A **domain** is an area of activity, study, or interest (e.g., health promotion, nutrition). A **class** is a subdivision of a domain (e.g., health awareness is a class under health promotion; digestion is a class under nutrition). To see Taxonomy II,

 Go to Student Resources: Chapter 4, **Standardized Language, NANDA-I Taxonomy II: Domains, Classes, and Diagnoses (Labels),** on Davis*Plus*.

One strength of the NANDA taxonomy is that it has been developed by nurses from the areas of administration, education, practice, and research, and from all specialties (e.g., maternity, mental health, medical-surgical, community). Because they represent the thinking of a broad spectrum of nurses, the diagnostic labels can be used in any setting or specialty.

What Are the Components of a NANDA-I Nursing Diagnosis?

Each nursing diagnosis in the NANDA-I taxonomy has four parts: label, definition, defining characteristics, and related or risk factors. You must consider all four parts when formulating a nursing diagnosis.

Diagnostic Label The **diagnostic label** (**title** or **name**) is a word or phrase that represents a pattern of related cues and describes a problem or wellness response, such as Disturbed Body Image or Readiness for Enhanced Nutrition. Some labels include descriptors for time, age, and other factors (e.g., acute, deficient, delayed). For the complete list of descriptors for NANDA-I nursing diagnoses,

 Go to Chapter 4, **Descriptors for NANDA-I Nursing Diagnoses,** in Volume 2.

Definition The **definition** explains the meaning of the label and distinguishes it from similar nursing diagnoses. For example, for a patient with a sleep problem, would you label the problem Sleep Deprivation or Disturbed Sleep Pattern? The following definitions can help you to decide:

Sleep Deprivation: Prolonged periods of time without sleep

Disturbed Sleep Pattern: Time limited disruption of sleep amount and quality

Defining Characteristics The cues (signs and symptoms) that allow you to identify a problem or wellness diagnosis are called **defining characteristics**. To use a problem label appropriately, a cluster of defining characteristics must be present in the patient data. For example, you cannot decide to use the label Sleep Deprivation merely by reading the definition. You must be sure the patient actually has some of the defining characteristics for Sleep Deprivation.

Related Factors The cues, conditions, or circumstances that cause, precede, influence, contribute to, or are in some way associated with the problem (label) are called **related factors**. They can be pathophysiological, psychological, social, treatment related, situational, maturational, and so on. NANDA-I lists the related factors that are most often associated with each problem label, but keep in mind that:

- *The list is not exhaustive.* Factors other than those listed by NANDA-I could also be associated with the problem. For example, imagine the vast number of factors that might cause someone to have Chronic Low Self-Esteem.
- *The problem may have more than one related factor.* Human beings are complex, and their problems rarely have one single cause. Nursing diagnoses may have multiple factors as their etiology.
- *An individual patient's etiology will not include all the related factors* that NANDA-I lists for the diagnosis.

Risk Factors Events, circumstances, or conditions that increase the vulnerability of a person or group to a health problem are called **risk factors**. They can be environmental, physiological, psychological, genetic, or chemical. For example, ignoring the urge to defecate and being pregnant increase the risk a person will become constipated. The diagnostic statement would be: Risk for Constipation r/t pregnancy and habitually ignoring the urge to defecate.

For potential (risk) nursing diagnoses, risk factors function as the defining characteristics. They must be present to make the diagnosis, and they almost always form at least a part of the etiology of the diagnostic statement. If **related factors** are present, an actual, rather than potential, problem exists.

Key Point: *To help you remember, as a rule:*

Related factors are similar to signs and symptoms (of actual problems)

Risk factors are similar to etiologies (of potential problems)

KnowledgeCheck 4-8

- What are the four parts of a NANDA-I nursing diagnosis?
- What purpose does each part of the nursing diagnosis serve for directing the care of the client?

How Do I Know Which Label to Use?

For the following sections, you will need access to the NANDA-I labels, definitions, and so on, as well as to *Taxonomy II.* You can use either a NANDA-I handbook or a nursing diagnosis handbook; or if you wish, print out NANDA-I *Taxonomy II* and use that,

 Go to Student Resources: Chapter 4, **Standardized Language, NANDA International—Approved Nursing Diagnoses (2012–2014), Taxonomy II: Domains, Classes, and Diagnoses (Labels),** on DavisPlus.

During the diagnostic process, you will already have determined the general topic of the problem and perhaps even have some tentative problem labels in mind. Follow these steps:

1. *First, identify the broad topic (or domain) that seems to fit the cue cluster.* You can look at the NANDA-I taxonomy to see which domain the problem seems to fit. For example, suppose that after further assessment, you find that Todd (Meet Your Patient) has the following defining characteristics:

   Intake exceeds output.
   Oliguria (low volume of urine)
   Generalized edema
   Recent rapid weight gain

   Which of the following NANDA domains are suggested by those cues?

Health Promotion	Role Relationships
Nutrition	Self-Perception
Elimination	Activity/Rest

   The most logical guesses would be Nutrition and Elimination. However, you would need to read the domain definitions in the table, NANDA International—Approved Nursing Diagnoses (2012–2014), Taxonomy II: Domains, Classes, and Diagnoses Labels (on the ESG); also look at the classes to be sure.

2. *Narrow your search (to the class or most likely labels).* In the NANDA-I taxonomy, read the definitions for the Nutrition and Elimination domains. Then look at the classes in each. Under Elimination,

you will find that Class 1 is Urinary Function. Because Todd has renal failure, you may think that his nursing diagnosis will be found in this class. However, remember that renal failure is a pathology or pathological condition; you are looking for Todd's *responses* to renal failure. On examining the diagnosis labels in the Urinary Function class, you will see none of those really represents Todd's defining characteristics.

Now look at the Nutrition domain. You will see the classes Ingestion, Digestion, Absorption, Metabolism, and Hydration. Look at the diagnostic labels listed for the class Hydration. All five of those labels describe fluid balance. You can easily eliminate both risk labels because Todd has an actual problem (he has symptoms). You can eliminate Readiness for Enhanced Fluid Balance because it is a wellness diagnosis. So, you must choose between Deficient Fluid Volume and Excess Fluid Volume. From this point, you simply compare Todd's cue cluster to the defining characteristics and definitions of those two labels and choose the best match.

3. *Using a nursing diagnosis handbook, compare definitions and defining characteristics of the diagnostic labels to your cue cluster.* A brief look at a NANDA-I alphabetical list should convince you that you cannot know exactly what a diagnostic label means from the label name alone. For example, suppose you have a patient who is not sleeping well at night. As a result, she is too tired to concentrate during the day. Which label would you use to describe this problem: Activity Intolerance, Fatigue, or Acute Confusion? You can answer that question only if you know the definition and defining characteristics of those nursing diagnosis labels.

Not all of the defining characteristics need to be present, but recall that the more data you have when you make an inference, the more certain you can be that your inference is correct. For example, NANDA-I lists 14 defining characteristics for Ineffective Thermoregulation, including the following:

- Fluctuations in body temperature above and below normal range
- Cyanotic nailbeds
- Pallor
- Slow capillary refill
- Tachycardia

You could diagnose Ineffective Thermoregulation on the basis of the first defining characteristic alone, but you might be more certain of your diagnosis if the other cues were also present.

▲ ThinkLike a Nurse 4-6

- In the preceding example, what if the first defining characteristic (temperature fluctuations) were not present and you had only cyanotic nailbeds, pallor, and slow capillary refill as cues? Could you conclude that Ineffective Thermoregulation is causing those signs? What other explanations might there be for cyanotic nailbeds, pallor, and slow capillary refill?

- What if the tachycardia was present without fluctuations in body temperature above and below normal range? What could cause tachycardia? Do you see the importance of using clusters rather than individual cues?

WRITING DIAGNOSTIC STATEMENTS

A diagnostic statement consists of a problem and an etiology linked by a connecting phrase.

Problem   The **problem** describes the client's health status (or a human response to a health problem) and identifies a response that needs to be changed. Use a NANDA-I label when possible. As noted earlier, many NANDA-I labels include a descriptor such as acute, impaired, or deficient. You will see them arranged in alphabetical lists with the descriptor after the main word (e.g., Physical Mobility, Impaired). However, you should record them as you would say them; for example:

Incorrect: Physical Mobility, Impaired r/t pain in left knee
Correct: Impaired Physical Mobility r/t pain in left knee

Etiology   As discussed earlier, the **etiology** contains the factors that cause, contribute to, or create a risk for the problem. The etiology may include a NANDA-I label, defining characteristics, related factors, risk factors, or other factors. Remember that an etiology may consist of several factors.

- *The etiology will help you to individualize nursing care because etiologies are unique to the individual.* For example, suppose two patients have the following nursing diagnoses:

    John: Anxiety r/t lack of knowledge of the treatment procedure
    Janet: Anxiety r/t prior negative experiences and lack of trust in health professionals

    The problem, Anxiety, has the same definition for both patients. They probably share some of the same defining characteristics, and you would use some of the same interventions for both John and Janet. For example, for all anxious patients, regardless of etiology, a calm, reassuring approach is important. However, to prevent the anxiety from recurring, you would need to treat its cause. To relieve John's anxiety, you would teach him what to expect from the impending procedure. But teaching would do nothing to relieve Janet's anxiety. For her, you would need to spend time building a relationship that demonstrates you can be trusted. You would also encourage her to talk about her fears and feelings.

- *Because the etiology directs the nursing interventions, include only factors that are influenced by nursing interventions.* For example, do not use a medical diagnosis or treatment as an etiology, because you cannot write nursing orders to change it. As another example, there are no independent nursing actions that would change the etiologies in the following diagnosis: Deficient Fluid Volume related to medical order of NPO (nothing by mouth).

- *Most NANDA-I–related factors are listed in nonspecific terms, so you will usually need to individualize them to reflect each person's unique problem etiology.* For example, one of the related factors for Impaired Skin Integrity is "extremes in age." To plan care, you need to know whether this means very old or very young; even better, you should specify the exact age. You would write the diagnostic statement as Impaired Skin Integrity r/t very young age (2 days).

Connecting Phrase (related to) Most nurses use **related to (r/t)** to connect the problem and etiology, believing that the phrase *due to* implies a direct causal relationship. Because humans are complex, there are usually many factors that combine to "cause" a problem, so it is nearly impossible to prove an exact cause. In fact, even if you eliminate the etiological factors, the problem might remain. For example, even if Janet begins to trust health professionals, she may become anxious for another reason.

Formats for Diagnostic Statements

A diagnostic statement should describe the client's health status as specifically as possible. The format will vary depending on the type of problem you are describing (Table 4-5).

Basic Two-Part Statement

The two-part statement is used for actual, risk, and possible diagnoses. The format is:

Problem	r/t	Etiology
Or		
NANDA-I label	r/t	related factors

For actual diagnoses, the etiology consists of related factors; for risk diagnoses, it consists of risk factors. For example, for a client with excessive vomiting you might write Risk for Deficient Fluid Volume r/t excessive losses through vomiting.

Basic Three-Part Statement

The three-part statement is also called the **PES format** (problem, etiology, and symptom). Some nurses use *AEB (as evidenced by)* whereas others use *AMB (as manifested by)*. The format is:

Problem r/t etiology as manifested by (AMB) signs or symptoms

This format adds the patient signs or symptoms that led you to make the diagnosis. For example:

Constipation r/t inadequate intake of fluids and fiber-rich foods AMB painful, hard stool and bowel movement every 3 or 4 days.

This is a good method for students because it helps to ensure that you have enough data to support the problem you have identified.

Although ideally the problem and etiology should thoroughly describe the patient's health status, you can sometimes make the description more clear and useful by including the cues in the statement. However, this method can create a long, unwieldy statement. For example:

Decisional Conflict (whether to accept chemotherapy) r/t desire to protect family from financial hardship of a lingering illness AMB verbalizing uncertainty about what to do and feelings of distress; indecision about having and not having chemotherapy; exhibiting physical signs of anxiety (increased heart rate, restlessness); questioning personal values and beliefs ("I'm not sure what to do. I hate to leave them any sooner than I have to, but I don't want to ruin them financially, either").

For such situations, you can record the cues in the nurses' notes instead of in the diagnostic statement. Another alternative is to list the signs and symptoms below the nursing diagnosis on the care plan instead of including it as part of the statement, as in the following example:

Decisional Conflict (whether to accept chemotherapy) r/t desire to protect family from financial hardship of a lingering illness

Subjective cues: Verbalizes uncertainty about what to do and feelings of distress; vacillates between having and not having chemo; questions personal values and beliefs ("I'm not sure what to do. I hate to leave them any sooner than I have to, but I don't want to ruin them financially, either").

Objective cues: Exhibits physical signs of anxiety (increased heart rate, restlessness)

Obviously you cannot use the PES format for risk nursing diagnoses, because symptoms are not present with risk diagnoses.

One-Part Statement

You can omit the etiology from certain kinds of diagnostic statements:

Syndrome Diagnoses Recall that a syndrome diagnosis is a label that represents a collection of several nursing diagnoses. A syndrome diagnosis usually does not need an etiology.

Wellness Diagnoses As a rule, NANDA-I wellness diagnoses are one-part statements beginning with the phrase Readiness for Enhanced (e.g., Readiness for Enhanced Parenting). Because the wellness label does not describe a problem, no etiology ("cause") is needed.

Very Specific Labels A few NANDA-I labels are so specific that they imply the etiology, or the only possible etiology is a medical diagnosis (e.g., Death Anxiety, Latex Allergy Response). For Latex Allergy Response, it would be redundant to write Latex Allergy Response

Table 4-5 ➤ Examples of Diagnostic Statements

FORMAT	PROBLEM TYPE	PROBLEM (CLIENT RESPONSE; NANDA LABEL)	ETIOLOGY (RELATED OR RISK FACTORS)	DEFINING CHARACTERISTICS OR "SECONDARY"
Basic One-Part	Wellness diagnosis	Readiness for Enhanced Nutrition	None	
	Syndrome diagnosis	Disuse Syndrome	None	
	Very specific label	Death Anxiety	None	
Basic Two-Part	Actual problem	Impaired Social Interaction	r/t self-consciousness following amputation of bilateral lower extremities	
	Potential problem	Risk for Impaired Attachment	r/t separation from infant at birth because of mother's illness	
	Possible problem	Possible Impaired Attachment	r/t separation from infant at birth because of mother's illness	
Basic Three-Part	Actual Problem	Impaired Social Interaction	r/t self-consciousness following amputation of bilateral lower extremities	AEB avoidance of others, social isolation, blaming others for current condition
	Possible Problem	Impaired Social Interaction	r/t self-consciousness following amputation of bilateral lower extremities	AEB blaming others for current condition
Variations	(Specify)	Decisional Conflict (whether to accept chemotherapy)	r/t desire to protect family from financial hardship of a lingering illness	Secondary to diagnosis of terminal cancer
	Secondary to	Decisional Conflict (whether to accept chemotherapy)	r/t desire to protect family from financial hardship of a lingering illness	Secondary to side effects of chemotherapy
	Two-part NANDA-I label	Imbalanced Nutrition: Less Than Body Requirements	r/t loss of appetite from nausea	Secondary to residual effects of stroke
	Adding words to the label	Impaired Physical Mobility: Inability to turn self in bed	r/t generalized weakness	
	Unknown etiology	Parental Role Conflict	r/t unknown etiology or possibly r/t recent divorce	
	Complex etiology	Chronic Low Self-Esteem	r/t complex etiology	
Collaborative Problems	Potential complications of disease, test, or treatment	Potential Complication of preeclampsia: renal failure	None	

AEB = as evidenced by

r/t sensitivity to latex. The etiology adds nothing to your understanding of the problem, nor does it suggest interventions different from those suggested by the problem label. The same is true for Death Anxiety.

Format Variations

The following are some variations of the basic two- and three-part formats.

"Specify" You will see the word *specify* in some NANDA-I labels, for example, Decisional Conflict (specify). This means that the label is useful only if you describe the problem more specifically (see Table 4-5 for an example).

"Secondary to" When the defining characteristics are vague (e.g., Chronic Pain r/t chronic physical disability) you may need to add a second part to the etiology following the words *secondary to* (2°). This second part is usually a pathophysiology or disease process (e.g., Chronic Pain r/t chronic physical disability secondary to rheumatoid arthritis). As a rule, you should avoid using pathophysiology or medical diagnoses in the etiology because they cannot be addressed by independent nursing interventions. The words *secondary to* make it clear the nurse is not ultimately responsible for the pathophysiological part of the etiology. Do not use this phrase routinely. Use it only if it adds to the understanding of your diagnostic statement.

Two-Part NANDA-I Label Some NANDA-I labels have two parts. The first part describes a general response; the second part, following a colon, makes it more specific (see Table 4-5).

Adding Words to the NANDA-I Label The problem phrase must describe the client's health status precisely because general categories are not useful for planning nursing care. For example, what do you think the problem label Impaired Physical Mobility means? Does it mean that the patient cannot grasp objects with her hands, or that she cannot walk, or that she cannot move at all? For such labels, you will need to add your own words to the label to make it more descriptive (see example in Table 4-5).

Other labels that often need to be clarified include: Acute Pain, Chronic Pain, Risk for Infection, and Risk for Injury. Think carefully about whether the clarifying words belong in the problem or the etiology. For example, you may see a pain diagnosis written as: Acute Pain r/t surgical incision. However, surgical incision is a medical treatment and should not be used as the etiology. It would be better to write: Acute pain (abdominal incision) r/t turning and moving secondary to abdominal surgery.

Key Point: *The "rule" for adding words is to first try to make the statement specific or descriptive by writing a good etiology, using the PES format, or adding secondary to. If that does not fully describe the health status, add descriptive words to the problem label.*

Unknown Etiology Sometimes you will be able to identify the patient's problem but not know the etiology. For example, your patient might have defining characteristics for Parental Role Conflict, but you may need more information to determine the cause. Perhaps there is an impending divorce; perhaps she has just had to take on the care of an elderly parent, and so on. In this case, you could write Parental Role Conflict *r/t unknown etiology*. Later, when you obtain more data, you will be able to complete the etiology. A similar situation exists when you have some, but not enough, information about the etiology. In this case you would write Parental Role Conflict *possibly r/t recent divorce*.

Complex Etiology Some problems have too many etiological factors to list, or the etiology is too complex to explain in a brief diagnostic statement. For example, imagine the number of factors that might contribute to problems such as Chronic Low Self-Esteem, Disabled Family Coping, and Adult Failure to Thrive. For such problems you can replace the etiology with the phrase *complex factors* (e.g., Disabled Family Coping r/t complex factors).

Collaborative Problems

A collaborative problem is always a potential problem (e.g., a complication of a disease, test, or medical treatment). The disease, test, or treatment is actually the etiology of the problem. Because you cannot treat the etiology with independent nursing interventions, you should not use the problem + etiology format. The focus of your interventions is monitoring for and preventing the complication. The format is:

Potential Complication of thrombophlebitis: Pulmonary embolism

Can you see that the word(s) following the colon represent the problem you are monitoring and trying to prevent?

Key Point: *In actual practice, you would not write an etiology for a collaborative problem.* However, as a student, you may wish to do so when it clarifies your diagnostic statement or when it helps to suggest nursing interventions (Wilkinson, 2011). For example, a student statement might be:

Potential Complication of magnesium sulfate therapy: Respiratory depression r/t increased blood levels of magnesium because of decreased kidney function secondary to preeclampsia (a pregnancy-related disorder with hypertension as a major pathology).

In addition to alerting you to monitor for respiratory depression, this statement might remind you to monitor the serum magnesium level, assess for other data related to kidney function, and monitor blood pressure.

KnowledgeCheck 4-9

Write an example of each of the following diagnostic statement formats, using the listed components—mix and match:

Problem labels: Anxiety, Pain (lower back)

Etiologies: Unknown outcome of surgery; muscle strain and tissue inflammation

Cues: Exhibits physical manifestations of anxiety (e.g., hands shaking); states pain is 9 on a scale of 1 to 10.

- Basic two-part statement
- Basic three-part statement
- Basic two-part statement, using "secondary to" (create your own disease/pathology)
- Statement with unknown etiology
- Possible nursing diagnosis
- Risk nursing diagnosis

How Does the Nursing Diagnosis Relate to Outcomes and Interventions?

Key Point: *As a general rule, the problem suggests goals, and the etiology suggests interventions.* Keep in mind that there are exceptions to this rule.

The Problem Suggests Goals

The problem describes a health status that needs to be changed. From the problem, you can determine the patient outcomes for measuring this change. Consider the following diagnostic statement: Risk for Impaired Skin Integrity r/t complete immobility 2° spinal cord injury.

- *The goal, or outcome, is the opposite of the unhealthy response:* Skin will remain intact and healthy.
- *The goals suggest assessments*, which are actually a type of nursing intervention. For example, the diagnosis Risk for Impaired Skin Integrity tells you to monitor the patient's skin condition.
- *If the problem is not an accurate statement of health status, then your goals and resulting assessments will be wrong.* If you incorrectly identified the previous problem as Impaired Physical Mobility 2° spinal cord injury, then the goal would suggest that you monitor the patient's mobility—which would not improve—and you might miss a developing skin problem.

The Etiology Suggests Interventions

Key Point: *The aim of the nursing interventions is to remove or alter the factors contributing to the problem.* In the preceding example, Impaired Physical Mobility 2° spinal cord injury, you could not cure the spinal cord injury or restore the patient's ability to move about. However, you could provide some mobility by turning and repositioning the patient frequently. This would help prevent Impaired Skin Integrity (which is the best diagnosis).

If the etiology is incorrect or incomplete, you might omit important nursing interventions. For the diagnosis Risk for Impaired Skin Integrity *r/t complete immobility 2° spinal cord injury*, you would focus on supporting mobility in order to prevent Impaired Skin Integrity. However, what if that etiology is incomplete, and the diagnosis should have been Risk for Impaired Skin Integrity *r/t poor nutritional status and complete immobility 2° spinal cord injury*? Now you can see that interventions that focus only on supporting mobility would not be adequate to prevent Impaired Skin Integrity.

REFLECTING CRITICALLY ABOUT DIAGNOSTIC STATEMENTS

Just as you critiqued your diagnostic reasoning process, you must reflect on the content, format, and meaning of your diagnostic statements. In this section, you will also begin to reflect on the nature of standardized language and the NANDA-I taxonomy of nursing diagnoses.

Guidelines for Judging the Quality of Diagnostic Statements

After you have written your diagnostic statements, use the following criteria to judge their quality (Wilkinson, 2011).

In choosing a NANDA-I label, do not rely on the label definition alone. Always compare patient data with the defining characteristics of the label as well as with the definition. Consider the diagnosis Parental Role Conflict:

Definition: Parental experience of role confusion and conflict in response to crisis

Defining Characteristics: Include "Reluctant to participate in usual caretaking activities"

Notice that you cannot actually observe role confusion and conflict in a patient; however, the defining characteristics for this label include more specific cues to help you make the diagnosis.

Include both problem and etiology, with cause and effect stated correctly. A quick check of this is to read your statement backward: "Etiology causes problem," and see if it makes sense.

Correct example: Ineffective Breastfeeding r/t Deficient Knowledge (positioning infant at breast)
   Read backward, this statement says deficient knowledge about positioning the infant at breast "causes" Ineffective Breastfeeding. This makes sense.

Incorrect example: Deficient Knowledge r/t Ineffective Breastfeeding (incorrect positioning infant at breast)
   Read backward, this statement says Ineffective Breastfeeding causes deficient knowledge. This does not make sense.

Be sure that the etiology does not merely restate the problem.

Incorrect example: Impaired Physical Mobility r/t inability to walk

Correct example: Impaired Physical Mobility: Inability to walk r/t weakness and pain in legs

In the incorrect example, inability to walk is the specific impaired physical mobility. The etiology should state the factors that are causing the inability to walk.

Avoid using medical diagnoses and treatments as etiological factors. The nurse should be able to provide interventions to change or remove the etiological factors. What could the nurse do to change the following etiology?

Incorrect example: Risk for Impaired Skin Integrity (ulcers, infection) r/t diabetes mellitus

The answer, of course, is that the nurse can do nothing to change or get rid of the DM. Try the following approaches to reword the diagnosis:

- Reword the etiology in terms of something the nurse can change, as follows:
  Correct example: Risk for Impaired Skin Integrity (ulcers, infection) r/t lack of knowledge of self-care measures for inspecting feet and trimming toenails
- If you cannot reword the etiology in terms of something the nurse can change, you may have identified the problem incorrectly; perhaps it is merely the stimulus for another patient problem that you can address independently. In the following example, Risk for Impaired Skin Integrity is one possible response to the stimulus, Impaired Physical Mobility.
  Incorrect example: Impaired Physical Mobility (total) r/t paralysis secondary to high spinal injury
  Correct example: Risk for Impaired Skin Integrity (pressure ulcers) r/t Impaired Physical Mobility (total) secondary to high spinal injury
- If none of these seem to work, you can resort to using "secondary to" instead of "related to," as in the following example: Risk for Deficient Fluid Volume secondary to prescribed NPO.

Write the statement clearly. The statement should give a clear picture of the client's health status, and other health professionals should be able to understand it readily. Avoid abbreviations and jargon as much as possible. For example, do you know what the first statement below means?

Incorrect example: Imp. Phys. Mobility (inability to get OOB w/o assist.) r/t muscle weakness and pain in LL
Correct example: Impaired Physical Mobility (inability to get out of bed without assistance) r/t muscle weakness and pain in left leg

Write the statement concisely. A wordy statement is likely to be unclear. The following will help limit statement length:

- Use "complex etiology" instead of listing numerous etiological factors.
- If there are numerous signs and symptoms, either do not use PES format, or describe the signs and symptoms in the nurses' notes.
  Incorrect example: Constipation r/t habitually ignoring the urge to defecate, insufficient exercise, weak abdominal muscles, side effects of iron medications, insufficient intake of fluids and fiber, and longstanding reliance on laxatives.

Correct example: Constipation r/t complex factors (see nurses' notes)

Be sure the statement is descriptive and specific. A vaguely stated problem and/or etiology cannot provide guidance for formulating goals and nursing interventions. Follow this guideline even if it means the statement is not as concise as you'd like. You can make the NANDA-I labels more specific by doing the following:

- Include all appropriate etiological factors.
- Review the label definition. Do not write the definition, but when you know the meaning of the label, you may find that it is descriptive enough.
- Use PES format to add the patient's signs and symptoms.
- Add qualifying words (e.g., mild, severe, occasional, or constant) to the label.
  Example: Severe Neck Pain r/t muscle spasms 2° herniated intervertebral disc
- Add "secondary to" to the etiology.
  Example: Severe Neck Pain r/t muscle spasms 2° herniated intervertebral disc
- Add a colon and descriptors to the label.
  Example: Impaired Physical Mobility: Inability to walk r/t weakness and pain in legs

State the problem as a patient response.
- **A problem is not a patient need.** As a rule, avoid using the word *need* in a problem statement. A need may cause a problem, but it is not a human response.
  Incorrect example: Needs increased fluids related to . . .
  Correct example: Risk for Deficient Fluid Volume, or Deficient Fluid Volume related to . . .
- **A problem is not a medical test, treatment, diagnosis, or equipment.**

Incorrect examples	Correct examples
Starting on diabetic diet	Deficient Knowledge, Ineffective Denial
Foley catheter in place	Risk for Infection, Urinary Retention
Risk for pneumonia	Risk for Ineffective Airway Clearance
Traction to left leg	Impaired Physical Mobility

- **A problem is not a nursing goal, a nursing problem, or a nursing action.**

Incorrect examples	Correct examples
Prevent urinary tract infection (nursing goal)	Risk for Urinary Tract Infection
Combative, hits (nursing problem) caregivers	Risk for Other-Directed Violence, Ineffective Coping, Acute Confusion
Provide emotional support (nursing action)	Anxiety, Decisional Conflict, Grieving

Use nonjudgmental language. If you examined your biases during the diagnostic process, your statements will probably be neutral. Look for phrases that may imply criticism of a patient, for example:

Incorrect: Risk for Infection r/t poor hygiene and housekeeping

Better: Risk for Infection r/t lack of information about sanitation and hand washing

Avoid legally questionable language. Be alert for legal implications. Look for phrases that seem to blame caregivers or patients or that refer negatively to patient care. For example, do not write: Risk for Falls r/t lack of staff to adequately supervise ambulation.

 ThinkLike a Nurse **4-7**

Rewrite the preceding diagnostic statement so it contains no legally questionable language. Use imaginary etiological factors if you need to.

Critiquing the NANDA-I System

Despite the potential benefits, some nurses have criticized the use of standardized language and the NANDA-I taxonomy in particular. The following are some objections and responses to counter them:

1. *Criticism:* **The labels are hard to use or not useful.**
   - They are too abstract to be useful (e.g., Ineffective Coping).
   - Some labels are merely reworded medical diagnoses (e.g., Decreased Cardiac Output).
   - Few people outside nursing know what the labels mean (e.g., "Why not just say 'tooth decay' or 'missing teeth' instead of 'Impaired Dentition'?").

   Response: These are legitimate concerns, but when you know the label definition, the term is more meaningful. Also, you can make the labels more specific and useful by adding descriptors, etiological factors, and defining characteristics to the diagnostic statement. Compared with the terminology for describing medical diagnoses, the NANDA-I system is relatively new (recall that it was begun just over 30 years ago). Consider that not long before that time, AIDS was not a medical diagnosis. All classification systems evolve and change, so many of the difficulties with individual labels will be revised as the terminology is refined.

2. *Criticism:* **The NANDA-I diagnoses have not been researched.** Historically, this has been true.

Response:
- An elected diagnostic review committee evaluates each submitted diagnosis to determine whether it complies with the criteria for inclusion in the taxonomy. Also, a label can be approved for testing. It must be validated by the literature, preferably research based, to remain on the approved list.
- Research on the labels has been conducted and is continuing. In 1994, a research team at the University of Iowa (the Nursing Diagnosis Extension Classification [NDEC]) began collaborating with NANDA-I to extend and refine the NANDA-I work. They have begun to address some of the difficulties with the labels, such as specificity, clinical usefulness, and clinical testing.

3. *Criticism:* **Using a NANDA-I label to describe health status is "labeling"—it dehumanizes and stereotypes the patient.** The most serious criticisms are leveled by those who say that nurses should not use *any* standardized languages to describe nursing knowledge and nursing work.

Response:
- If this is true, then medical diagnoses would meet the same objection.
- This objection ignores the fact that we must name objects and ideas in order to communicate them to other people.
- Many of the criticisms arise out of disillusionment. It may be that nurses expect too much from nursing diagnosis. Although it is important, it is, after all, merely a process for identifying, naming, and communicating patient health status. We should not expect it to be the "magic bullet" that single-handedly cures all problems of the nursing profession and the patients.

Try not to reject the idea of standardized language just because of a few problematic labels. You do not need to use the official NANDA-I labels exclusively. If you are uncomfortable with a label, change the wording to make it more useful, or write a completely new label. **Key Point:** *Remember, the point of a standardized language is to more clearly communicate the nature of the patient problem in nursing terms.*

For a more comprehensive critique of standardized nursing language, and the NANDA-I system in particular,

 Go to Student Resources: Chapter 4, **Supplemental Materials: Critique of Standardized Nursing Language,** on Davis*Plus.*

Toward Evidence-Based Practice

Müller-Staub, M., Lavin, M.A., Needham, I., et al. (2006). **Nursing diagnoses, interventions and outcomes—application and impact on nursing practice: Systematic review.** *Journal of Advanced Nursing, 56*(5), 514–531.

Researchers analyzed the content of 36 published studies to examine the outcomes of using nursing diagnosis. Specifically, they looked at effects on quality of patient assessments, accuracy, and completeness of nursing diagnoses, and on coherence among nursing diagnoses, interventions, and outcomes documented. They found the following:

- Nursing diagnosis use improved the quality of documented patient assessments.
- The completeness of nursing diagnoses in practice is problematic; signs and symptoms or etiology were often lacking or incompletely described.
- There was some evidence for coherent use of documented nursing diagnoses, interventions, and outcomes.

- There was some evidence that nursing diagnosis improved the quality of interventions documented.
- There was no evidence that use of nursing diagnosis improved outcomes in patients.

1. What do you think "coherence among nursing diagnoses, interventions, and outcomes" means?

2. From this study, could you reasonably infer that using nursing diagnosis would improve the quality of your nursing assessments? Why or why not?

3. From this study, could you reasonably infer that using nursing diagnosis led to nurses' documenting their interventions better? Why or why not?

 Go to Student Resources: Chapter 4, **Toward Evidence-Based Practice Suggested Responses,** on *DavisPlus.*

 To explore learning resources for this chapter,

 Go to *DavisPlus* at **DavisPl.us/Wilkinson3.**

Chapter Resources for Chapter 4:
  Response sheets for all learning activities
  Resources for Caregivers and Health Professionals
  Reading More About Nursing Process: Diagnosis (suggested readings)
  Concept Map of chapter content
Interactive Case Studies
NCLEX-Style and Chapter Review Questions
Chapter Overview Podcasts

For references cited in this chapter,

 Go to Volume 2, **References Cited.**

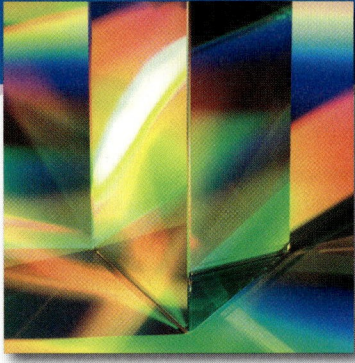

CHAPTER 5

Nursing Process: Planning Outcomes

Learning Outcomes

After completing this chapter, you should be able to:

- ➤ Describe formal, informal, initial, ongoing, and discharge planning.
- ➤ Identify patients who need a comprehensive, formal discharge plan.
- ➤ Explain the importance of a written plan of care.
- ➤ Describe the information contained in a comprehensive patient care plan.
- ➤ Compare critical pathways to integrated plans of care (IPOCs) and other standardized care-planning documents.
- ➤ Discuss the advantages and disadvantages of computerized care planning.
- ➤ Describe a process for writing an individualized care plan, making use of available standardized care-planning documents.

- ➤ Define the following terms: *goal, outcome, expected outcome, nursing-sensitive outcome.*
- ➤ Differentiate between short-term and long-term goals.
- ➤ Explain how a goal is derived from a nursing diagnosis.
- ➤ Differentiate between essential and nonessential goals.
- ➤ Write appropriate goals for actual, risk, and possible nursing diagnoses.
- ➤ Use standardized terminology to state patient goals.
- ➤ Write realistic specific, concrete, and observable goals that do not conflict with the medical plan of care and are stated in terms of patient responses/behaviors.

Key Concepts

Goals/outcomes
Patient care plan
Planning

Related Concepts
See the Concept Map on Davis*Plus*.

Meet Your Patient

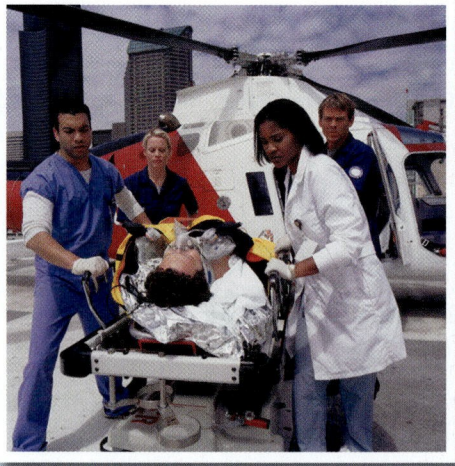

Ben Ivanos has just been admitted to an orthopedic unit after a motorcycle accident. Mr. Ivanos is 24 years old, normally healthy, and takes no medications. He has casts and traction on both legs and a cast on one arm. He is receiving morphine sulfate intravenously via a patient-controlled analgesia (PCA) pump. Imagine that you are an orthopedic nurse and must plan care for Mr. Ivanos. You rank the following nursing diagnoses as highest priority:

1. Acute Pain secondary to musculoskeletal trauma (arms, legs, body) and muscle spasms
2. Risk for Peripheral Neurovascular Dysfunction secondary to casts/traction

Meet Your Patient (continued)

You write the following desired outcomes (goals) on the care plan:

Goals for diagnosis 1

Demonstrates correct use of PCA pump.
Rates pain not higher than 4 on a scale of 1 to 10 at all times.

Goals for diagnosis 2

Peripheral pulses palpable
Fingers and toes warm

Fingers and toes without pallor or cyanosis
No edema of fingers and toes
Capillary refill less than 3 seconds

These goals will guide you in choosing nursing interventions for relieving Mr. Ivanos's pain and preventing peripheral neurovascular dysfunction. When the nursing shift changes, the written care plan provides directions for the new caregivers so that they will continue to focus on Mr. Ivanos's most important needs.

Theoretical Knowledge
knowing why

This text separates the process of planning outcomes from the process of planning interventions because, although related, they are distinctly different activities. This chapter (1) describes planning as a general process, (2) explains how to create a patient care plan, and (3) discusses how to write patient goals/expected outcomes. Chapter 6 explains how to plan nursing interventions and write nursing orders.

ABOUT THE KEY CONCEPTS

To help you understand and remember the content in this chapter, try to organize what you learn under the key concepts of **planning**, **goals** and **outcomes**, and **patient care plans**. Planning is the broad umbrella term that "covers" the rest of the chapter concepts. In this chapter, you will learn how they are all related.

WHAT IS PLANNING?

The professional nurse is responsible for care planning, and cannot delegate it. However, you should be aware that some healthcare facilities list care planning in their job description for licensed practical or vocational nurses. Certainly licensed practical (or vocational) nurses (LPNs/LVNs) can provide valuable input for registered nurses (RNs) who are planning the care. Box 5-1 lists American Nurses Association (ANA) standards that specifically identify planning as the role of the registered nurse.

Planning can be formal or informal. **Formal planning** is conscious and deliberate. It involves decision making, critical thinking, and creativity (Wilkinson, 2011). During the planning phases of the nursing process, you will work with the patient and family to derive desired outcomes from identified patient problems (e.g., nursing diagnoses) and then to identify nursing interventions to

help achieve those outcomes. The end product of formal planning is a holistic plan of care that addresses the patient's unique problems and strengths.

Not all plans are written. **Informal planning** occurs while you are performing other nursing process steps. For example, while performing neurovascular checks for Ben Ivanos, you might discover that he is not obtaining adequate pain relief. Reflect on this situation. What would you do? Any response in that scenario would require some mental planning. For example, you might make a mental note (plan) to notify the patient's prescriber for an increase in the analgesic dose.

How Is Planning Related to Other Steps of the Nursing Process?

Nursing process steps are overlapping and interdependent. To develop a plan of care with realistic goals and effective nursing orders, you must have accurate, complete *assessment* data and correctly identified and prioritized *nursing diagnoses*. The *goals/desired outcomes* flow logically from the nursing diagnoses. By stating what is to be achieved, the goals then suggest nursing interventions (which are written as nursing orders in the *planning interventions* phase). The plan of care is carried out in the *implementation* phase. In the *evaluation* step, the goals/desired outcomes serve as criteria for evaluating whether the nursing care has been effective. Figure 5-1 illustrates the relationship of planning outcomes to the other stages of the nursing process.

Initial and Ongoing Planning

Initial planning begins with the first patient contact. It refers to the development of the initial comprehensive care plan, which should be written as soon as possible after the initial assessment. The nurse who performs the admission assessment has the benefit of personal contact (rather than relying completely on the written database), has the best information about the patient, and, ideally, is the one who should initiate the care plan.

BOX 5-1 ■ American Nurses Association Standards of Nursing Practice for Outcomes and Planning

Standard 3. Outcomes Identification

The registered nurse identifies expected outcomes for a plan individualized to the patient or the situation.

Competencies

The registered nurse:

Involves the healthcare consumer, family, healthcare providers, and others in formulating expected outcomes when possible and appropriate.

Derives culturally appropriate expected outcomes from the diagnoses.

Considers associated risks, benefits, costs, current scientific evidence, expected trajectory of the condition, and clinical expertise when formulating expected outcomes.

Defines expected outcomes in terms of the healthcare consumer, healthcare consumer culture, values, and ethical considerations.

Includes a time estimate for attainment of expected outcomes.

Develops expected outcomes that facilitate continuity of care.

Modifies expected outcomes based on changes in the status of the healthcare consumer or evaluation of the situation.

Documents expected outcomes as measurable goals.

Standard 4. Planning

The registered nurse develops a plan that prescribes strategies and alternatives to attain expected outcomes.

Competencies

The registered nurse:

Develops an individualized plan in partnership with the person, family, and others considering the person's characteristics or situation, including, but not limited to, values, beliefs, spiritual and health practices, preferences, choices, developmental level, coping style, culture and environment, and available technology.

Establishes the plan priorities with the healthcare consumer, family, and others as appropriate.

Includes strategies in the plan that address each of the identified diagnoses or issues. These may include, but are not limited to, strategies for:

- Promotion and restoration of health
- Prevention of illness, injury, and disease
- The alleviation of suffering
- Supportive care for those who are dying

Includes strategies for health and wholeness across the life span.

Provides for continuity in the plan.

Considers the economic impact of the plan on the healthcare consumer, family, caregivers, or other affected parties.

Integrates current scientific evidence, trends, and research.

Utilizes the plan to provide direction to other members of the healthcare team.

Explores practice settings and safe space and time for the nurse and the healthcare consumer to explore suggested, potential, and alternative options.

Defines the plan to reflect current statutes, rules and regulations, and standards.

Modifies the plan according to the ongoing assessment of the healthcare consumer's response and other outcome indicators.

Documents the plan in a manner that uses standardized language or recognized terminology.

_____

Note: There are additional standards for advanced practice nurses.
Source: American Nurses Association. (2010). *Nursing: Scope and standards of practice* (2nd ed.). Silver Spring, MD: Author.

You may sometimes need to begin care planning even though the initial database is incomplete. For example, the patient may require emergency care before assessment is complete. Or a different patient may need your immediate attention. In such situations, make a preliminary plan with whatever information you have. You can complete and refine the plan when you are able to perform a more detailed assessment.

Ongoing planning refers to changes made in the plan (1) as you evaluate the patient's responses to care or (2) as you obtain new data and make new nursing diagnoses. For example, the nurses discovered that Ben Ivanos (Meet Your Patient) had not slept well on his first night in the hospital. They identified a new nursing diagnosis for him: Disturbed Sleep Pattern r/t unfamiliar environment and pain. They then developed a plan for addressing this problem. Ongoing planning allows you to decide which problems to focus on each day that you care for the patient.

Discharge Planning

If the recommended length of stay for patients with surgical reduction of fractures is 2 days, then Ben Ivanos will still have casts on his arm and both legs when he leaves the hospital. Obviously, he will not be able to manage his own activities of daily living (shopping, cooking, bathing, etc.). What questions come to your mind when you think about how he will manage after he leaves the hospital? Stretch your mind—take a moment now to jot down your ideas.

You may have thought of some questions: Is there anyone who can help Mr. Ivanos with his personal care? Will he need to go up and down stairs? Who will drive him home from the hospital? Can he be discharged home or will he need to go to a rehabilitation facility? How soon does he need to see his primary care provider? Can he get to the provider's office? How will he manage his pain at home; what will he use in place of the PCA narcotics?

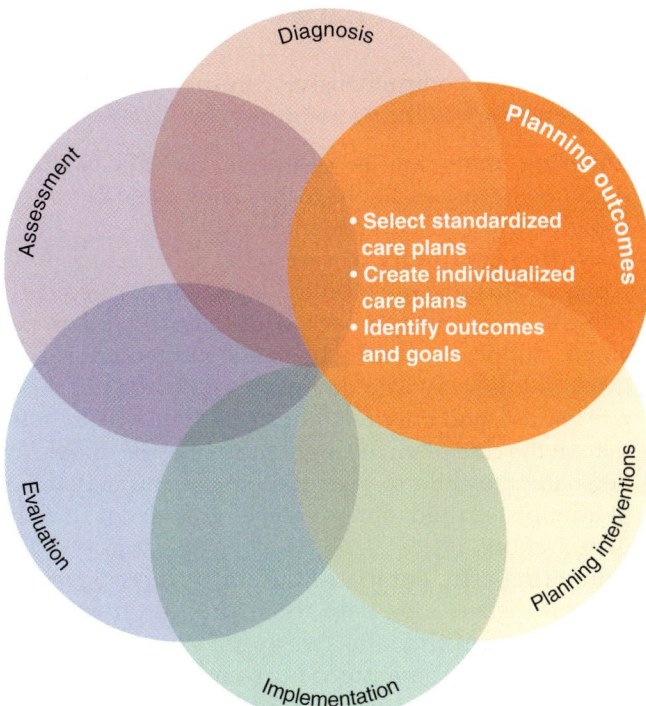

FIGURE 5-1 Nursing process phases: Planning outcomes.

Discharge planning is the process of planning for self-care and continuity of care after the patient leaves a healthcare setting. Ben Ivanos's case is not unusual. In the United States, outpatient surgeries and short hospital stays are the norm. Many patients are discharged despite ongoing need for nursing care and complex treatments. Therefore, nurses must prepare family members to perform tasks such as bathing, changing sterile dressings, and monitoring intravenously administered medications. If family members are not available or if skilled nursing care is needed, arrangements must be made for home healthcare or transfer to a skilled nursing or rehabilitation facility. Sometimes a case manager is assigned, but often staff nurses must plan and coordinate services. If appropriate services are not provided or if family members perform care incorrectly, the patient may experience delayed recovery or complications that require further treatment or hospital readmission.

To learn more about the process of discharging patients from an institution, refer to the section Maintaining Trust During Transitions in Chapter 11 and

 Go to Chapter 11, **Procedure 11-4, Discharging a Patient from the Healthcare Facility,** in Volume 2.

Discharge Planning Begins at Assessment

Because patients are in the surgery center or hospital for such a short time, discharge planning must begin at the initial assessment, which should include the following patient data:

- Physical condition and functional and self-care limitations
- Emotional stability and ability to learn
- Financial resources (e.g., personal finances, insurance, community resources such as food stamps, Medicaid)
- Family or other caregivers available
- Caregiving responsibilities the patient may have for others
- Environment, both home and community (e.g., stairs, space for supplies and equipment, availability of transportation to healthcare services)
- Use of community services before admission
- Estimated date of discharge. Some agencies require this be done at the time of admission, except for situations such as admission from the emergency department or a critical care unit. This may require collaborative effort.

Written Discharge Plans

All patients need at least some discharge planning, but you will not always need a separate, written discharge plan. For example, a middle-aged patient who has been hospitalized for deep vein thrombosis (a blood clot in a major vein, usually the lower leg) will be able to care for herself independently when she goes home. For this patient, you could simply write on the comprehensive care plan a nursing order to teach her about the side effects of the warfarin (Coumadin, an anticoagulant) she will be taking at home. In contrast, you will probably need a comprehensive, formal discharge plan if the patient is an older adult or has one or more of the following (Jweinat, 2010; NSW Department of Health, 2011; Walker, Hogstel, & Curry, 2007):

- *Personal characteristics that interfere with self-care, such as the following:*
  Difficulty learning or a memory deficit
  Emotional or mental illness
  Poor mobility
  Self-care deficits (e.g., dressing, feeding, bathing, toileting)
  Incontinence
- *Disease or treatment characteristics; coexisting illness*
  Terminal illness
  Complicated major surgery
  Complex treatment regimen or more than three medications to continue at home
  An illness with an expected long period of recovery
  A newly diagnosed or multiple chronic health problems (e.g., diabetes, chronic pain)
  Preexisting wound
  Malnutrition
- *Social or family factors*
  Inadequate services available in the community

Inadequate financial resources
No family or significant others to help provide care

For an example of a discharge planning form,

 Go to Chapter 5, **Discharge Planning Form,** in Volume 2.

Discharge Planning for Older Adults

The percentage of older adults in hospitals is quite high, and they tend to have complex needs when discharged. Therefore, when an older adult is hospitalized, it is especially important to start discharge planning at the initial admission assessment. This means that assessment of functional abilities, cognition, vision, hearing, social support, and psychological well-being must be a part of the initial assessment so that you can identify needed services at discharge. A comprehensive discharge process for older adults should help to achieve the following objectives:

- Maintain functional ability.
- Lengthen the time between rehospitalizations.
- Involve all concerned parties in decision making.
- Improve interagency communication (e.g., hospital to nursing home).
- Emphasize client and family involvement and interdisciplinary collaboration (Walker, Hogstel, & Curry, 2007).

Discharge Planning Requires Collaboration

Comprehensive discharge planning involves significant collaboration. Ideally, it is done *with,* not *for,* the patient—patient involvement is important for achieving desired outcomes. In addition, a patient's postdischarge needs often call for services from a multidisciplinary team, which may include home care service personnel; private-duty nurses; physical therapists; social service professionals; speech, occupational, and hearing therapists; physicians; and members of the patient's family.

KnowledgeCheck 5-1

- What does the nurse do in the planning phases of the nursing process?
- What is the purpose of initial planning? Ongoing planning? Discharge planning?

PATIENT CARE PLANS

The **comprehensive patient care plan** (also called *nursing care plan*) is the central source of information needed to guide holistic, goal-oriented care to address each patient's unique needs. It is a document—usually several documents—that specifies dependent, interdependent, and independent nursing actions necessary for care of a specific patient. It usually combines both standardized and individualized approaches to care.

Why Is a Written Patient Care Plan Important?

A well-written comprehensive care plan benefits the patient and the healthcare institution by:

- **Ensuring that care is complete.** Specific written directions are less likely to be overlooked by busy caregivers (e.g., "Turn patient hourly").
- **Providing continuity of care.** This helps ensure that when an effective intervention is found, all caregivers will use the same approach with the patient. For example, suppose a child who is dehydrated refuses to drink any liquids. The day nurse discovers the child will eat red, and only red, popsicles. If he fails to note that on the care plan, the night nurse may be unable to persuade the child to take oral liquids and may have to administer fluids intravenously to prevent further dehydration.
- **Promoting efficient use of nursing efforts.** Specific, written instructions help to ensure that nurses do not waste time on ineffective approaches. In the preceding example, the night nurse may waste a great deal of time trying to persuade the child to drink liquids.
- **Providing a guide for assessments and charting.** Nursing orders and goals/expected outcomes on the care plan can help you plan your activities and ensure nothing is omitted from your documentation.
- **Meeting the requirements of accrediting agencies.** The Joint Commission and professional standards review organizations (PSROs) require a patient-specific plan of care.

What Information Does a Comprehensive Patient Care Plan Contain?

Regardless of their format, comprehensive care plans include directions for four different kinds of care and include both medical and nursing interventions:

1. *Basic needs and activities of daily living (ADLs).* This includes the routine assistance that the patient needs with hygiene, nutrition, elimination, and so on, regardless of her nursing diagnoses.
2. *Medical/multidisciplinary treatment.* Nurses need to know the medical orders for each patient (e.g., prescriptions for IV fluids and medications) and the nursing activities necessary for carrying out those orders.
3. *Nursing diagnoses and collaborative problems.* This section may be referred to as the *nursing diagnosis care plan.* It contains goals and nursing orders for the patient's nursing diagnoses and collaborative problems.
4. *Special discharge needs or teaching needs.* Finally, the plan should contain instructions for formal discharge planning and special teaching if they are needed.

What Documents Make Up a Comprehensive Patient Care Plan?

You will use a variety of documents to create a care plan. Care plans vary widely in format, appearance, and use. In most healthcare organizations, caregivers use preprinted, standardized plans that can be adapted to meet individual needs. Figure 5-2 shows the documents that are most commonly included in a comprehensive patient care plan.

Form for Client Profile and Basic Needs

Some essential client data either do not change or are used or updated often. This includes the client's profile (e.g., age, providers, drug allergies, and so on), basic needs (e.g., for hygiene, nutrition, and elimination), and diagnostic tests and treatments (e.g., laboratory tests, radiology procedures, and respiratory therapy). To provide quick and easy access, such information is usually recorded on standardized forms and not organized according to medical or nursing diagnoses (see Fig. 5-2A). These are often in electronic format, but may be printed on cardstock and kept in a central location easily accessible to all care providers. For an example of a printed Kardex,

 Go to Student Resources: Chapter 5, **Tables, Boxes, Figures: ESG Figure 5-1,** on Davis*Plus*.

For clients who require more than routine attention to their basic needs, you may need to write a nursing diagnosis care plan. Examples include a client with no appetite and the nursing diagnosis Imbalanced Nutrition: Less Than Body Requirements, or an immobile client with the diagnosis Risk for Impaired Skin Integrity.

Preprinted, Standardized Plans

As shown in Figure 5-2B, a comprehensive care plan usually includes one or more preprinted, standardized documents. It would be too time consuming to handwrite a complete care plan for every patient. Standardized plans save nursing time, promote consistency of care, and help ensure that nurses do not overlook important interventions. You will find standardized instructions for patient care in a variety of documents. A document may (1) contain nursing or multidisciplinary interventions and (2) prescribe care for one or more nursing diagnoses (e.g., Anxiety) or a disease or medical condition (e.g., pneumonia). The following are examples of standardized, preprinted instructions for care.

Policies and Procedures

Policies and **procedures** are similar to rules and regulations. When a situation occurs frequently or requires a consistent response regardless of who handles it, management develops a policy to govern how it is to be handled. You should consider individual needs and use critical thinking to interpret policies in a caring manner. For example, in some critical care units a patient is allowed one visitor for 10 minutes each hour. Imagine, though, that a patient is expected to die soon, and that his daughter has come from a distant state

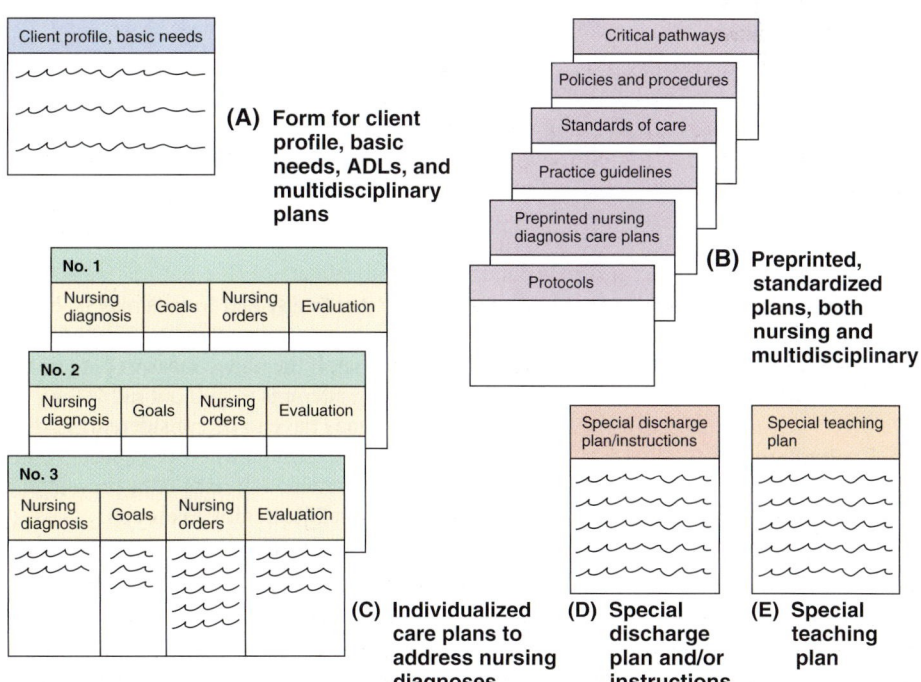

FIGURE 5-2 Components of a patient care plan. *A*, Form for client profile, basic needs, ADLs, and multidisciplinary plans. *B*, Preprinted, standardized plans, both nursing and multidisciplinary. *C*, Individualized care plans to address nursing diagnoses. *D*, Special discharge plan and/or instructions. *E*, Special teaching plan.

and brought her three children for one last visit. Would you tell the daughter to take the children in to see their grandfather? Would you insist that she follow the rule and send them in without her, one at a time over a period of 3 hours?

Protocols

Protocols cover specific actions usually required for a clinical problem unique to a subgroup of patients. For example, not every patient on a medical-surgical unit is at risk for falls, but many are. Therefore the nurse would add a falls protocol to the care plan for a patient in that subgroup, such as in Figure 5-3. Protocols may be written for a particular medical diagnosis (e.g., seizure), treatments (e.g., administration of oxytocin to induce labor), or diagnostic tests (e.g., barium enema). They contain both medical and nursing orders. Some include definitions and rationales for interventions.

Unit Standards of Care

Unit standards of care describe the care that nurses are expected to provide for all patients in defined situations (e.g., all women admitted to a labor unit or all patients admitted to the critical care unit). In this way, they are similar to protocols. Unlike protocols, however, they (1) apply to every patient in a defined situation, rather than a subgroup; (2) do not become part of the patient's care plan but are kept on file on the unit; and (3) do not usually include specific medical orders. Instead of describing ideal care, standards of care describe the minimum level of care the nurses are expected to achieve given the institution's resources and the client population. Unit standards of care usually are not organized according to nursing diagnoses and they usually resemble a list of "things to do" (e.g., complete comprehensive assessment within 2 hours of admission) rather than detailed instructions for care.

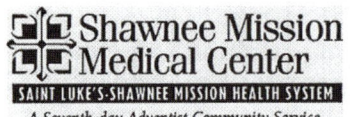

Patient Care Protocol

Title: Fall or Injury/Disruption of Care, Care of the Patient at Risk for   **Effective Date:** mm/dd/yyyy

Expected Outcome: The patient at risk for falls will be identified and preventive measures initiated.
The patient will not pull out indwelling devices.

Relevant Information: Initiate this protocol for adult patients who have a Conley Fall Scale score of ≥3.

Assessment: 1. The Conley Fall Scale will be administered on admission to adult inpatients. Further assessment will be based on patient population and identified patient need.

Interventions: Make alterations in environment, such as:
- Avoiding clutter in room.
- Moving patient closer to Nursing Station if indicated.
- Making sure call light, telephone, and other personal items are within reach

Educate patient and family about:
- The possibility that family and friends may be called upon to stay with patient with high risk for fall or injury or who attempts to pull out indwelling devices.
- The possibility that, if the above measures are not successful in reducing the patient's fall risk or preventing attempts to pull out indwelling devices, alternative measures such as the use of restraints may have to be considered.

Evaluation: 1. Evaluate frequently to determine whether expected outcome is being met. Change strategies as needed to reduce fall risks or to prevent disruption of indwelling devices.
2. **Criteria for initiation of Restraint Protocol:**
- If interventions have been implemented and patient continues to be at risk of falling or disrupting medical treatment, the protocol Care of the Patient in Restraint for Medical/Surgical Management is initiated.
- The CRN/Supervisor is notified at the time the restraint is initiated for med/surg management and reviews the need for restraint.

FIGURE 5-3 Portion of Patient Care Protocol for patient at risk for falls. (*Source:* Courtesy of Shawnee Mission Health System, Shawnee Mission, KS, 66204.)

ThinkLike a Nurse 5-1

- Think of some other "defined situations" for which unit standards of care might be useful.
- Suggest some other subgroups for which a protocol might be appropriate.

Standardized Patient Care Plans

Standardized (model) patient care plans detail the nursing care that is usually needed for a particular nursing diagnosis or for all nursing diagnoses that commonly occur with a medical condition. Figure 5-4 is a standardized care plan for a single nursing diagnosis. Although similar to unit standards of care, model care plans are different in that they usually:

- Provide more detailed interventions. They may add to or delete from unit standards of care.
- Are organized by nursing diagnosis and include specific patient goals and nursing orders.
- Are a part of the patient's comprehensive care plan and become a part of the permanent record.
- Describe ideal rather than minimum nursing care.
- Allow you to incorporate addendum care plans.
- Include checklists, blank lines, or empty spaces so that you can individualize goals and interventions.

Students sometimes purchase model care plan books. You can use them as guides, but be aware that they do not address a client's individual, specific needs. For this reason, they may lead you to focus on the common, predictable problems and overlook an unusual—and perhaps more important—problem the person is experiencing. Beginning with the standardized plan may stifle your creativity. It is best to first use the process for writing a patient care plan (see What Is the Process for Writing an Individualized Patient Care Plan? later in this chapter) and then consult the model plan to see whether you have missed anything.

Critical Pathways

Critical pathways are often used in managed care systems. They are outcomes-based, interdisciplinary plans that sequence patient care according to case type. They specify predicted patient outcomes and broad interventions for each day, or in some situations, for each hour (Fig. 5-5). They describe the minimal standard of care required to meet the recommended length of stay for patients with a particular condition or *diagnosis-related group* (*DRG*; e.g., postpartum, myocardial infarction, or total hip replacement). An agency usually develops critical pathways for its most frequent case types or for situations in which standardized care can produce predictable outcomes. Although critical pathways are developed by a multidisciplinary team, they tend to emphasize medical problems and interventions. Because critical pathways describe the expected outcomes of multidisciplinary care, they do not provide a way to judge *nursing* effectiveness—you will learn about *nursing-sensitive outcomes* later in the chapter.

Integrated Plans of Care

Integrated plans of care (IPOCs) are standardized plans that function as both care plan and documentation form. Therefore, there is a different form—or sometimes a different column—for each day of care. Many critical pathways are designed as IPOCs; however, IPOCs do not necessarily (1) organize care according to diagnosis, (2) describe minimal standards of care, or (3) specify a timeline for interventions and outcomes. For an example of an IPOC,

 Go to Chapter 5, **Tables, Boxes, Figures: ESG Figure 5-2,** on Davis*Plus.*

Individualized Patient Care Plans

Nurses use individualized patient care plans to address nursing diagnoses unique to a particular client (Fig. 5-2C). These care plans reflect the independent component of nursing practice, and therefore best demonstrate the nurse's critical thinking and clinical expertise. In addition to including goals and nursing orders that you write specifically for a patient, a complete individualized care plan may contain standardized single-problem care plans (see Fig. 5-4).

Standardized plans focus on the common problems and interventions needed by most patients. They do not address unusual problems and may not meet a patient's individual needs. You should always adapt standardized plans by adding the necessary nursing diagnoses, goals/outcomes, and nursing orders they do not include. For example, a standardized plan for a client with a myocardial infarction (heart attack) would undoubtedly prescribe care for the nursing diagnosis Pain and the potential complication of heart failure. However, it might not address the needs of a person who is not complying with treatments because he is in denial about his illness (nursing diagnosis: Ineffective Denial). An individualized plan for resolving the patient's denial would improve the likelihood that the rest of the plan will be successful.

You may sometimes include medical orders in a nursing diagnosis or collaborative problem care plan, especially in a student care plan. For example, for a client with a nursing diagnosis of Deficient Fluid Volume, you might list the medical prescription for intravenously administered fluids in the Nursing Orders column.

Nursing Diagnosis	Nursing orders
Deficient Fluid Volume related to vomiting and diarrhea	1. Check skin turgor q4hr 2. Medical order: IV normal saline, 150 mL/hr

Special Discharge or Teaching Plans

A nursing plan of care may also contain one or more discharge or teaching plans (see Fig. 5-2D). These are sometimes referred to as *special-purpose* or *addendum* care plans. You can address routine discharge planning and teaching needs by using standardized plans or by

PATIENT PLAN OF CARE - GENESIS MEDICAL CENTER - Davenport, Iowa

PAIN, ACUTE: Experience of an unpleasant sensory and emotional sensation for a duration of less than 6 months.
SIGNS & SYMPTOMS: Observed or reported (select at least 2)

☐ Change in BP   ☐ Restlessness   ☐ Grimacing   ☐ Crying
☐ Patient's self-report of pain   ☐ Diaphoresis   ☐ Increased muscle tension   ☐ Change in pulse rate
☐ Change in respiratory pattern   ☐ Whimpering   ☐ Whining

OUTCOME SCORING

RELATED FACTORS	OUTCOMES	ADM			DC	INTERVENTIONS
☐ Physical injuring agent ☐ Psychological injuring agent	4 Pain-control behavior – Recognizes causal factors – Uses non-analgesic relief measures – Uses analgesics appropriately – Reports pain controlled 3 Pain level – Oral/facial expressions of pain – Change in respiratory rate, heart rate, BP – Restlessness – Reported pain 3 Comfort level – Reported satisfaction with symptom control – Expressed satisfaction with pain control – Reported physical well-being					☐ Pain management ☐ Analgesic administration ☐ Patient-controlled analgesic (PCA) assistance ☐ Analgesic administration: Intraspinal ☐ Environmental management: comfort ☐ Anxiety reduction ☐ Transcutaneous electrical nerve stimulation (TENS) ☐ Heat/cold application ☐ Distraction ☐ Simple relaxation therapy ☐ Simple massage ☐ Developmental care ☐ Preparatory sensory information ☐ Positioning

Definition of scoring scales	1	2	3	4	5
Pain control — Personal actions to control pain	Never demonstrated	Rarely demonstrated	Sometimes demonstrated	Often demonstrated	Consistently demonstrated
Pain level — Severity of reported pain	Severe	Substantial	Moderate	Slight	None
Comfort level — Extent of physical and psychological ease	None	Limited	Moderate	Substantial	Extensive

Diagnosis _____

Date Initiated _____ RN Initials _____

Date Resolved _____

FIGURE 5-4 Computer printout of standardized care plan for a single nursing diagnosis using standardized language. (*Source:* Adapted from Genesis Medical Center, Davenport, IA, 52804. Used with permission.)

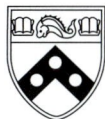

HOSPITAL OF THE UNIVERSITY OF PENNSYLVANIA

TOTAL LOWER JOINT (HIP/KNEE)
CLINICAL PATHWAY

ELIGIBILITY CRITERIA: All primary unilateral total hip or total knee
replacements

EXPECTED LOS: 3 Days   ADDRESSOGRAPH

CLINICAL KEYS:

1.	Pain managed midpoint on painscale
2.	Transfer to chair/commode with assistance POD 1; Ambulate in room, bathroom POD2
3.	DVT precautions
4.	Discharge plan completed by POD2
5.	Patient verbalizes knowledge of hip or knee precautions
6.	Knee motion 10 to 70 or better (TKA patients only)

	PACU	IMMED. POST- OP	POD 1	POD 2	POD 3-4
ASSESSMENTS	• NV checks with VS q1h × 4 • Pain • Effects of narcotics/ tolerance • I & O × 24hr • Pulse Ox q8 if on O2	• NV check / VS q 4hr → → • S/S DVT →	→ → → → • Pulse Ox × 1 on RA • Dsg/wound status q4	• NV check / VS q 8hr → → → • D/C pulse ox if O2 D/C • Dsg/wound status q8	→ → → → →
CONSULTS		• PT • PMR	→ (If not done already) → (If not done already)		
TESTS	• A/P hip X-ray (THA) • A/P knee X-ray (TKA)		• CBC	→ • INR (if on warfarin)	• A/P hip X-ray →
TREATMENTS	• O2	• D/C O2 if sat 94% • Incentive spirometry • Order walker (hip chair, elevated commode if needed) • Pneumatic compression device (ankle for knees, calf for hips)	→ → • D/C foley • Dressing change (1st dsg change by MD) →	→ → • Dressing change q day and pm	→ → →
MEDICATIONS	• PCA or epidural	→ • Anticoagulation	• IV heplock → • Consider conversion to oral pain meds	• D/C heplock → • D/C PCA/PCEA • PO pain meds	→
ACTIVITY	• Bedrest • Hip precautions if THA • CPM for total knee	→ → →	• OOB to chair BID → → • Weight bear per order • Ambulate with assistive device	• OOB TID → → → → • PT ×2	→ → → → → →
NUTRITION	• NPO	• NPO → ice → advance to full as tolerated	• Regular	→	→
EDUCATION / D/C PLANNING	• Deep breathing exercises	• Pain management • Initiate d/c plan	→ • Home vs rehab decision • Anticoagulation if indicated	→ • S/S wound infection • Medications • Activity level • D/C plan in place	→ → → • Car transfer

Transfer to rehab when:	Discharge to home when:
1. Able to participate in care 2. Tolerating 2 physical therapy sessions 3. Not requiring IV pain medicine 4. Blood values are stable 5. Motivation is commensurate with projected functional status	1. Mobility and ADL's appropriate for degree of assistance at home and home environment 2. Appropriate assistive device and necessary adaptive equipment is used 3. Independent with hip/knee precautions 4. Independent with home exercise program or ongoing PT in the home or outpatient **IF D/C TO HOME, ENSURE APPROPRIATE CONSULTS TO ARRANGE HOME CARE FOLLOW-UP AND EQUIPMENT

FIGURE 5-5 Portion of a critical pathway. (*Source:* Hospital of the University of Pennsylvania, Philadelphia, PA. Used with permission.)

including teaching as part of the nursing orders on an individualized care plan. For example, a care plan for the diagnosis Acute Pain might include the nursing order, "Teach patient to splint incision when turning in bed." Chapter 19 shows an example of a teaching plan for the diagnosis Deficient Knowledge.

Computer Plans of Care

Many healthcare organizations use electronic health records, including *computer-generated care plans*. The computer stores standardized plans (e.g., for nursing diagnoses, medical diagnoses, or diagnosis-related groups [DRGs]). When you enter a diagnosis or a desired outcome, the computer generates a list of suggested interventions. You then choose appropriate interventions from the list, individualize by choosing from checklists, or type in your own interventions and strategies.

Computer prompts help ensure that you consider a variety of actions and keep you from overlooking common and important interventions. After the initial learning curve, they also reduce the time spent on paperwork. However, computerized planning requires constant use of a step-by-step thinking process, which may cause a decrease in intuition, insight, ability to care, and nursing expertise (Harris, 1990; Kossman & Scheidenhelm, 2008). You must resist the temptation to accept "one size fits all" solutions. Always look for creative approaches that might be more effective for a particular individual. Think, "What would work for *this* person?"

ESG Figure 5-3 at Davis*Plus* shows a computer screen displaying a care plan for the nursing diagnosis Impaired Mobility. Most computer programs allow you to print the plan.

 Go to Student Resources: Chapter 5, **Tables, Boxes, Figures: ESG Figure 5-3,** on Davis*Plus*.

KnowledgeCheck 5-2

- In addition to care related to the patient's basic needs, what other types of information does a comprehensive care plan contain?
- How are critical pathways different from other standardized care plans?
- What is the main disadvantage of computerized and standardized care plans?

ThinkLike a Nurse 5-2

Suppose a nurse sees one of your student care plans and says to you, "You're wasting your time writing those things. We never use the nursing process in the real world." Take a few minutes to write how you might respond.

Student Care Plans

You may have noticed that the care plans you see in clinical settings look different from the ones you create as a part of your clinical preparation. This is because student care plans are a learning activity as well as a plan of care. They are designed to help you learn and apply concepts

from the nursing process, physiology, and psychopathology. For this reason, they may contain more detailed nursing orders as well as other information the instructor requires (e.g., information about lab tests, medications, and assessment data to support the nursing diagnoses). Some instructors may ask you to write rationales and cite references to support them. **Rationales** state the scientific principles or research that supports nursing interventions. Writing rationales helps ensure that you understand the reasons for the interventions. **Key Point:** *Understanding why you do what you do is one aspect of functioning as a professional.* For an example of a student care plan,

 Go to Student Resources: Chapter 5, **Student Care Plan Example,** on Davis*Plus*.

Mind-Mapping Student Care Plans

Mind-mapping is a technique for showing relationships among ideas and concepts in a graphical, or pictorial, way. Mind-mapping is thought to stimulate "whole-brain" and critical thinking, and to foster the development of holistic plans of care (Mueller, Johnston, Bligh, & Wilkinson, 2002). A mind-mapped care plan uses shapes and pictures to represent the parts of the nursing process (i.e., assessment data, nursing diagnoses, patient goals, interventions, and evaluation), as well as the patient's pathophysiology, medications, and other pertinent information. For complete information about mind-mapping,

 Go to Student Resources: Chapter 5, **Supplemental Materials: Mind-Mapping Student Care Plans,** on Davis*Plus*.

PracticalKnowledge
knowing **how**

The rest of this chapter will help you learn how to apply your knowledge of the key concepts, *goals, outcomes, patient care plan, and planning*, as well as the many related concepts you have learned.

WHAT IS THE PROCESS FOR WRITING AN INDIVIDUALIZED PATIENT CARE PLAN?

In this section, you will need to use your theoretical knowledge of concepts related to care planning (e.g., standardized plans, protocols, individualized patient care plans. Writing an individualized patient care plan follows in natural sequence from the assessment and diagnosis phases of the nursing process:

1. *Make a Working Problem List*. Earlier in the nursing process, you will already have developed and prioritized a list of the patient's nursing diagnoses, collaborative problems, and strengths. Suppose that after

assessment you prioritized Ben Ivanos's (Meet Your Patient) problems as follows:

A. Acute Pain secondary to musculoskeletal trauma (arms, legs, body) and muscle spasms

B. Risk for Peripheral Neurovascular Dysfunction secondary to casts/traction

C. Self-Care Deficit (Bathing, Dressing, Feeding, Toileting) r/t immobility secondary to casts, especially cast on dominant right arm

D. Potential Complication of fracture: delayed, union, malunion, or nonunion of bone

2. *Decide which problems can be managed with standardized care plans or critical pathways.* What institutional documents are available? Suppose that the hospital unit has a critical pathway for "Patients with Casts and/or Traction." This critical pathway would contain goals and interventions to guide the care for problems B and D above. It would specify regular neurovascular assessments and management of the traction apparatus, for example.

3. *Individualize the standardized plan as needed.* Cross out any instructions that do not apply to your patient, and add or adapt nursing orders as appropriate. For example, the plan might say "Perform neurovascular checks q_____." You would fill in the frequency of the assessment according to Mr. Ivanos's needs.

4. *Transcribe medical orders to appropriate documents.* For example, you might write orders for pain medications on a special medication administration record. Details about Mr. Ivanos's traction would probably go on a Kardex or special section of the critical pathway.

5. *Write ADLs and basic care needs in special sections of the Kardex, care plan, or computer screen.* For Ben Ivanos, you might note on the Kardex that he requires a complete bed bath and help with eating.

6. *Develop individualized care plans for problems not addressed by standardized documents.* For Ben Ivanos, you would need to write a plan for problems A and C above. The critical pathway probably contains some expected outcomes and basic interventions for problem A, Pain, but you might need to individualize them to make them more effective. If your unit had a Pain protocol, similar to the Falls protocol in Figure 5-3, you would add it to Mr. Ivanos's care plan. If not, you would hand-write goals and interventions for the Pain diagnosis.

Problem C, Self-Care Deficit, would be partially addressed in the basic care section of Mr. Ivanos's Kardex, but he has special needs. For example, he will need teaching and therapy to increase his ability to care for himself. So you would need to hand-write a plan for this nursing diagnosis.

KnowledgeCheck 5-3

Briefly describe a process for creating a comprehensive, individualized care plan that incorporates collaborative care and standardized planning documents.

PLANNING PATIENT GOALS/OUTCOMES

In this section you will learn about the key concepts of goals and outcomes, and also about a number of related concepts that will expand your understanding of goals and outcomes (e.g., short-term and long-term goals). Then you will learn how to apply your knowledge of goals and outcomes in creating a patient care plan.

After assessment and diagnosis, the next step in individualized care planning is to formulate goals for improving or maintaining the patient's health status. **Goals** (also called **expected outcomes, desired outcomes,** or **predicted outcomes**) describe the changes in patient health status that you hope to achieve. **Nursing-sensitive outcomes** are those that can be influenced by nursing interventions. The rest of this chapter discusses individualized care planning and nursing-sensitive outcomes.

Importance of Goals The purposes of precise, descriptive, clearly stated goals/expected outcomes are to:

- Provide a guide for selecting nursing interventions by describing what you wish to achieve.
- Motivate the client and the nurse by providing a sense of achievement when the goals are met. This is especially important when the client must make difficult lifestyle changes.
- Form the criteria you will use in the evaluation phase of the nursing process.

Nursing Responsibility Goal/expected outcome formulation is the responsibility of the professional nurse (see Box 5-1). You should involve the client as much as possible in goal setting, because goal achievement is more likely if the client believes the goals are important and realistic. Of course, the client must be alert and independent enough to participate. If physical or mental impairments prevent active participation, the nursing team acts on the client's behalf to develop client-centered goals.

How Should I Use the Terms Goal and Outcome?

Many nurses use the terms *goal* and *outcome* interchangeably. In this text, we usually use the Nursing Outcomes Classification (NOC) terminology: the word *outcome*, used alone, means *any* patient response (positive or negative) to interventions (e.g., the pain could become better or worse; both are outcomes). When referring to desired (positive) patient responses, we use *goals, expected outcomes, desired outcomes,* or *predicted outcomes.* For example:

Outcome	Decision Making
Goals/expected outcomes	Participates in decisions about own care.
	Chooses between two or more alternatives.

Some nurses use the term *goal* to mean a broad, nonspecific statement about the desired results of nursing activities. They use *outcomes* (and other outcome terms such as *expected outcomes*) to mean the more specific, observable responses you would use to judge whether the goal has been met. When goals are defined in this way, you must include both goals and expected outcomes on the care plan because a broad goal does not provide enough guidance for evaluating patient responses to care. You can combine the broad goal and specific expected outcome into a single statement by writing, "as evidenced by," as in the following example:

Broad statement (goal)	Constipation relieved
Specific expected outcome (evaluation criteria)	Will have soft, formed bowel movement within 24 hours
Combined statement (goal + outcome)	Constipation will be relieved *as evidenced by* soft, formed bowel movement within 24 hours

Key Point: *Use of broad goals on the care plan is optional; however, expected outcomes are not optional. You must include them on the care plan.*

How Do I Distinguish Between Short-Term and Long-Term Goals?

Short-term goals are those you expect the patient to achieve within a few hours or days. They are important:

- In situations in which the patient may be discharged before you can evaluate progress toward long-term goals (e.g., as in a same-day and outpatient surgery).
- For providing positive reinforcement to clients who are working toward long-term goals.

Long-term goals are changes in health status that you wish to achieve over a longer period—perhaps a week, a month, or longer. They describe the optimal level of functioning you expect the patient to achieve, given health status and available resources. Ideally, this is a return to normal functioning, but that is not always possible. See Table 5-1 for a comparison of short-term and long-term goals.

KnowledgeCheck 5-4

Refer to Meet Your Patient, at the beginning of the chapter. State whether each of Mr. Ivanos's goals was a short-term or long-term goal.

What Are the Components of a Goal Statement?

Every expected outcome/goal statement must have the following parts:

Subject The subject is understood to be the client, but it can also be a function or part of the client. For example:

[Mrs. Johnson] Will walk to the doorway with the help of one person by 12/13/15.
Lung sounds will be clear to auscultation within 2 days after receiving antibiotics.

Assume that the subject is the client unless otherwise stated. Think, "Client will . . ." to help you phrase the goal statement correctly, but do not write it. For example, in the first goal, you should not write "Mrs. Johnson."

Action Verb Use an action verb to indicate the action the client will perform: what the client will learn, do, or say (e.g., Will *walk* to the doorway). Use concrete verbs

Table 5-1 ▶ Comparison of Short-Term and Long-Term Goals

	DEFINITION	SITUATIONS FOR USE	EXAMPLES
Short-Term Goals	■ Can be achieved in a few hours or a few days.	■ Acute care ■ Day surgery ■ Clinics ■ Focus on immediate needs ■ Students ■ Evaluation of progress toward long-term goals	■ Describes pain as < 3 on a 1–10 scale within 30 min after receiving analgesic. ■ Limits food intake to 1,500 calories per day.
Long-Term Goals	■ Expected changes that occur over a week, a month, or more ■ Optimal level of functioning given health status and resources	■ Home healthcare ■ Extended-care facilities ■ Rehabilitation centers ■ Chronic illness ■ Conditions that are managed, not cured	■ Infant will double birth weight within 5 months. ■ Within 3 months after physical therapy treatments, will dress self except for buttons.

(i.e., describing actions that you can see, hear, smell, feel, or measure), such as the following:

apply	explain	report
choose	eat	select
demonstrate	list	transfer
describe	measure	turn
drink	prepare	verbalize

Performance Criteria These are the standards for evaluating the client's performance. They describe the extent to which you expect to see the action or behavior. Write them in concrete, observable terms because they indicate what you need to measure in order to evaluate outcomes. Performance criteria specify:

(a) How, what, when, or where something is to be done
(b) Amount, quality, accuracy, speed, distance, and so forth

The following example specifies the distance the client is expected to walk: [Client] Will walk *to the doorway* with the help of one person by 12/13/16.

Target Time This is the realistic date or time by which the performance/behavior should be achieved. The target time is the "when" part of the performance criterion: [Client] will walk to the doorway with the help of one person *by 12/13/16.*

Other examples of target times are *by discharge, within 24 hours, at the next visit, each hour, at all times.* For risk (potential) nursing diagnoses, the desired outcome is that the problem will never occur. You assume that the desired response should occur "at all times," but you may wish to schedule times for evaluating the outcome. For example:

Nursing diagnosis: Risk for Constipation r/t inadequate fluid intake
Expected outcome: Bowel movements will be of normal frequency and consistency.
Target time: At all times
Evaluate: Daily

Special Conditions These describe the amount of assistance or resources needed or the experiences/treatments the client should have to perform the behavior. Include special conditions when it is important for other nurses to know them. For example:

[Client] Will walk to the doorway *with the help of one person* by 12/13/16.
After two teaching sessions, [client] will be able to identify foods to avoid on a low-fat diet by 3/1/15.

KnowledgeCheck 5-5

In the following predicted outcomes, identify the subject, action verb, performance criterion, target time, and special conditions (if any). State which components are assumed, if any.

- Will walk to the doorway with the help of one person by 12/13/16.
- After two teaching sessions, [client] will be able to identify foods to avoid on a low-fat diet by 3/1/16.
- Bowel movements will be soft and formed and of his usual frequency.
- Lungs clear to auscultation at all times.

How Do Goals Relate to Nursing Diagnoses?

Expected outcomes are derived directly from the nursing diagnosis. Therefore, they will be appropriate only if you identify the nursing diagnosis correctly. The problem clause (the clause at the left) of a nursing diagnosis describes the response or health status you wish to change. A desired outcome states the *opposite* of the problem and implies this response is what the interventions are intended to achieve (Table 5-2).

 ThinkLike a Nurse 5-3

Answer the following questions for Ben Ivanos's nursing diagnosis of Acute Pain secondary to musculoskeletal trauma (arms, legs, body) and muscle spasms:

- What would be the opposite, healthy response to his problem?
- What changes should you see in appearance, body functions, symptoms, knowledge, and emotions?
- If the problem is prevented or solved, how will Mr. Ivanos look or behave? What will you be able to observe (e.g., see, hear, smell, taste, or touch)?
- What should Mr. Ivanos be able to do to demonstrate a positive change? How well, or how soon, should he be able to do it?

Table 5-2 ➤ Comparison of Nursing Diagnoses and Goals	
NURSING DIAGNOSIS (PROBLEM SIDE)	**GOAL/EXPECTED OUTCOME**
Problem response	Opposite of problem response
Present health status	Desired health status
Response that you hope to change	Response that you hope to achieve
Example:	*Examples:*
Ineffective Airway Clearance ⟶	Lungs clear to auscultation
r/t ineffective cough secondary to incision pain ⟶	Coughs productively

After thinking about those questions, you might have said that the opposite response to pain would be absence of (or relief from) pain, but you couldn't really observe that. "Absence of pain" might serve as a broad goal statement. But how about more specific, observable expected outcomes? How would you know that Mr. Ivanos's pain was relieved? Specific, observable behaviors that demonstrate absence of pain include the following: Relaxed body posture, relaxed facial expression, states that his pain is relieved, rates pain as less than 3 on a scale of 1 to 10.

Essential Versus Nonessential Goals

In general, the problem side of the nursing diagnosis suggests the goals, and the etiology suggests nursing interventions. You can also derive some goals from the etiology; however, the **essential patient goals** flow from the problem side of the nursing diagnosis (see the bold print in Table 5-3) because the problem side describes the unhealthy response you intend to change.

Notice in Table 5-3 that the goals derived from the etiology may help resolve the problem, but they could also be achieved without resolution of the problem. Suppose that for a patient with Ineffective Airway Clearance you had written only the goals in regular type. If the patient coughs forcefully and effectively, rates pain as less than 3, and splints his incision while coughing, you might discontinue the interventions for Ineffective Airway Clearance. However, the problem might still exist. Even a client who demonstrates all three of those responses might not be coughing productively enough to clear the airways and might still not have clear lung sounds. This means you should follow this rule:

Key Point: *For every nursing diagnosis, you must state one goal that if achieved would demonstrate resolution or improvement of the problem.*

Goals for Actual, Risk, and Possible Nursing Diagnoses

You will develop expected outcomes to promote, maintain, or restore health, depending on the status of the nursing diagnosis. See Table 5-4 for explanations and examples. Review Chapter 4 as needed.

Goals for Collaborative Problems

Recall that collaborative problems are physiological complications of diseases (e.g., diabetes) or medical treatments (e.g., cardiac catheterization) that nurses monitor to detect onset or changes in status. The desired outcome is always that the complication will not develop. However, unlike outcomes for nursing diagnoses, these outcomes are not nurse-sensitive; that is, they do not result primarily from nursing interventions. They occur as a result of interventions by several disciplines. Consider the following example:

Collaborative problem: Potential Complication of abdominal surgery: paralytic ileus (paralysis of the ileum of the small intestine)
Goal: Patient will not develop paralytic ileus

Suppose that 36 hours after the surgery, the patient's bowel sounds are absent, his abdomen is distended and painful, and he begins vomiting. What could the nurse have done to prevent this situation? What can the nurse do to relieve the ileus and bring about return of peristalsis? Very little, actually. The primary interventions are medical, and if there is obstruction, probably surgical. Therefore, it would not be appropriate to include a goal for this problem on a patient care plan, because that would imply that nurses are primarily accountable for the outcome.

Collaborative goals are appropriate on multidisciplinary care plans and critical pathways. However, all goals on a patient care plan should be nursing-sensitive goals. For collaborative problems, instead of a patient outcome, you might wish to write a *nursing goal* such as "Early detection of complication, should it occur." See Table 5-4.

On student care plans, to aid your learning, you can write the symptoms of the complication or the normal physiological response you hope to observe (e.g., Bowel sounds present within 24 hours; no abdominal distention; no vomiting), but these are not appropriate on an institutional care plan.

Table 5-3 ➤ Deriving Goals and Interventions From Nursing Diagnoses

NURSING DIAGNOSIS	GOALS/EXPECTED OUTCOMES	NURSING ACTIVITIES
Problem: ⟶	**Lungs clear to auscultation.** ⟶	Teach deep breathing and coughing.
Ineffective Airway	**Coughs productively.**	Auscultate lungs q4hr.
Clearance	**Respirations 12–20/min.**	Assess respiratory rate, breathing, and
r/t	**No pallor or cyanosis.**	skin color q4hr.
	No dyspnea or shortness of breath (SOB)	
Etiology: ⟶	Coughs forcefully/effectively. ⟶	Teach to splint incision while coughing.
Ineffective cough secondary to incisional pain	Rates pain as < 3 on 1–10 scale.	Turn, cough, and deep-breathe (TCDB) hourly.
	Splints incision while coughing.	Medicate for pain 30 min before TCDB.

Table 5-4 ➤ Expected Outcomes for Various Problem Types

TYPE OF PROBLEM	EXAMPLE OF DIAGNOSIS	EXPLANATION OF DIAGNOSIS	EXAMPLE OF EXPECTED PATIENT OUTCOME	FOCUS OF NURSING INTERVENTIONS
Actual Nursing Diagnosis	Constipation r/t inadequate dietary fiber and fluids	Symptoms of constipation present (e.g., no bowel movement [BM]).	Will have normal, formed BM within 24 hours after receiving stool softener.	Resolution or reduction of problem; prevention of complications
Risk (Potential) Nursing Diagnosis	Risk for Constipation r/t inadequate dietary fiber and fluids	Risk factors present (e.g., not drinking enough or eating adequate fiber).	Will have bowel function within normal limits for patient (e.g., daily bowel movement with no need for stool softener or laxative).	Prevention and early detection of problem
Possible Nursing Diagnosis	Possible Constipation r/t suspected inadequate intake of dietary fiber and fluids	Not enough data (e.g., no BM for 2 days, but no data on intake or on his usual bowel habits).	No patient goal. The nursing goal is "Confirm or rule out the problem."	Confirm or rule out problem.
Collaborative Problem	Potential Complication of abdominal surgery: ileus	Medical treatment creates risk for complication that is prevented by collaborative care.	None. Patient responses depend on collaborative care. The broad nursing goal is early identification of the problem.	Primarily detection; prevention is collaborative.
Wellness Diagnosis	Readiness for Enhanced Nutrition	Bowel habits and dietary intake within normal limits, but can be improved	Reports increased intake of dietary fiber and fluids; reports bowel functioning within normal limits.	Maintain or promote higher level of health.

How Do I Use Standardized Terminology for Outcomes?

In Chapter 4, you learned about the NANDA-I standardized terminology for nursing diagnoses. The ANA has also approved several standardized vocabularies for describing client outcomes. The one used throughout most of this book is the Nursing Outcomes Classification (NOC) (Moorhead, Johnson, Maas, et al., 2013).

The NOC is a standardized vocabulary of 385 nursing-sensitive outcomes developed by a research team at the University of Iowa. In the NOC vocabulary, an **outcome** is "an individual, family, or community state, behavior, or perception that is measured along a continuum in response to nursing interventions" (Moorhead, Johnson, Maas, et al., 2013, p. 2). Thus, the NOC is versatile because it is appropriate for use in all specialty and practice areas.

Components of an NOC Outcome

Each NOC outcome consists of an outcome label, indicators, and a measurement scale.

Outcome Label The **outcome label** (usually referred to as *the outcome*) is broadly stated (e.g., Decision Making, Mobility Level, Concentration). It is a neutral label

(a variable), to allow for positive, negative, or no change in patient health status. Because NOC outcomes are linked to NANDA-I nursing diagnoses, you can look up a nursing diagnosis to see the list of outcomes suggested for it (Box 5-2). You can find suggested outcomes for each NANDA-I diagnosis in the NANDA/NIC/NOC "linkages" book (Johnson, Moorhead, Bulechek, et al., 2012). You can find Additional Associated Outcomes for each diagnosis in Part IV of the *Nursing Outcomes Classification (NOC)* (Moorhead, Johnson, Maas, et al., 2013).

Indicators The **indicators** are the observable behaviors and states you can use to evaluate patient status. In Table 5-5 the indicators are in the first (left) column. The first one is "Identifies relevant information." This indicator helps you evaluate whether Decision Making (the broad outcome) is being achieved. For each outcome, you select the indicators that are appropriate to the patient. You can add to the list of indicators if necessary.

Measurement Scale For each outcome, NOC has a five-point **measurement scale** (the numbers in Table 5-5) for describing patient status for each indicator. As a rule, 1 is least desirable and 5 is most desirable. If you are using

---

BOX 5-2 ■ Outcomes Linked to NANDA-I Diagnosis

Nursing Diagnosis
Situational Low Self-Esteem

Definition
Development of a negative perception of self-worth in response to a current situation (specify)

Suggested Outcomes
Adaptation to Physical Disability

Grief Resolution

Personal Resiliency

Psychosocial Adjustment: Life Change

Self-Esteem

Sources: Johnson, M., Moorhead, S., Bulechek, G., et al. (2012). *NOC, and NIC linkages to NANDA-I and clinical conditions* (p. 196). St. Louis, MO: C.V. Mosby; NANDA International (2012). *Nursing diagnoses: Definitions & classification 2012–2014.* Ames, IA: Wiley-Blackwell, p. 287.

Additional Associated Outcomes
Abuse Recovery

Abuse Recovery: Emotional

Abuse Recovery: Physical

Abuse Recovery: Sexual

Anxiety Level

Body Image

Burn Recovery

Coping

Development: Late Adulthood

Development: Middle Adulthood

Development: Young Adulthood

Fear Level

Fear Level: Child

Neglect Recovery

Personal Autonomy

Role Performance

Stress Level

Source: Moorhead, S., Johnson, M., Maas, M., et al. (2013). *Nursing outcomes classification* (5th ed.). St. Louis, MO: Mosby/Elsevier.

NOC, you do not need to write traditional goal statements. You simply write the label, choose the appropriate indicators, and assign a number from the measurement scale. In your initial assessment, you assign the number that represents the patient's present health status. To form the "goal," you assign the scale number that the patient can realistically achieve after the interventions. Using Table 5-5, you might assign the following numbers:

(NOC Outcome) **Decision Making**
Goals (Indicators + measurement scale)

Identifies relevant information (4, mildly compromised)

Identifies alternatives (4, mildly compromised)

Identifies potential consequences of each alternative (5, not compromised)

For a list of the NOC measurement scales,

 Go to Chapter 5, **Standardized Language,** in Volume 2.

KnowledgeCheck 5-6
Figure 5-4, a patient plan of care for Acute Pain, uses NOC language.

■ What outcomes did the nurse choose for this patient?

■ List two indicators for each of the outcomes.

■ For which outcome does the nurse expect the highest level of functioning to occur after interventions? (Note that in this care plan the measuring scale has been applied to the outcomes rather than to the indicators.)

ThinkLike a Nurse 5-4
In Figure 5-4, what do you think the nurse expects to happen? Why do you think she ranked the outcomes this way?

Using NOC With Computer Care Plans
Standardized language (e.g., NOC) is especially useful in computerized care systems. To see computer screens for locating and choosing NOC outcomes and for choosing NOC indicators, respectively,

 Go to Student Resources: Chapter 5, **Tables, Boxes, Figures: ESG Figures 5-4 and 5-5,** on Davis*Plus.*

In those figures, the nurse chose Circulation Status as a patient outcome, and the program provided the definition and the NOC indicators for that outcome. The nurse would then check the indicators that apply to the patient.

Key Point: *The computer does not think for you. You are responsible for deciding which outcomes and indicators to use for each patient, and for identifying a target time.* Most electronic health records have a screen that allows you to type in your own goals as well.

How Do I Write Goals for Groups?
Home and community health nurses are especially likely to write goals for aggregates (groups), such as families and communities. **Community health goals (public health goals)** are those you would use to specify and evaluate the health of groups, aggregates, or populations. They tend to emphasize health promotion, health maintenance, and disease prevention outcomes. The following are examples.

The U.S. Public Health Service (USPHS) has proposed four group goals—the following broad, overarching goals for improving the health of the nation by a target date of 2020 (*Healthy People 2020*, 2010):

■ Attain high-quality, longer lives free of preventable disease, disability, injury, and premature death.

Table 5-5 ➤ Example of an NOC Outcome

Decision Making (0906)

Domain—Physiologic Health (II)

Class—Neurocognitive (J)

Scale(s)—Severely compromised to Not compromised

Definition: Ability to make judgments and choose between two or more alternatives

DECISION MAKING OVERALL RATING	SEVERELY COMPROMISED 1	SUBSTANTIALLY COMPROMISED 2	MODERATELY COMPROMISED 3	MILDLY COMPROMISED 4	NOT COMPROMISED 5
Identifies relevant information.	1	2	3	4	5
Identifies alternatives.	1	2	3	4	5
Identifies potential consequences of each alternative.	1	2	3	4	5
Identifies needed resources to support each alternative.	1	2	3	4	5
Identifies time frame necessary to support each alternative.	1	2	3	4	5
Identifies sequence necessary to support each alternative.	1	2	3	4	5
Recognizes contradiction with others' desires.	1	2	3	4	5
Acknowledges social context of the situation.	1	2	3	4	5
Acknowledges relevant legal implications.	1	2	3	4	5
Weighs alternatives.	1	2	3	4	5
Selects among alternatives.	1	2	3	4	5

Source: Moorhead, S., Johnson, M., Maas, M., et al. (2013). *Nursing outcomes classification* (5th ed.). St. Louis, MO: Mosby/Elsevier.

- Achieve health equity, eliminate disparities, and improve the health of all groups.
- Create social and physical environments that promote good health for all.
- Promote quality of life, healthy development, and healthy behaviors across all life stages.

NOC currently includes 16 outcomes targeted to Community Health, which they define as "outcomes that describe the health, well-being, and functioning of a community or population" (Moorhead, Johnson, Maas,

et al., 2013, pp. 66–67). Two examples are Community Competence and Community Risk Control: Lead Exposure. NOC also has 14 outcomes that describe the health of a family as a unit. Two examples are Family Coping and Family Health Status. NOC outcomes can be used in all settings, including home and community nursing. For further explanation, see Chapters 14 and 43. Also, search for Nursing Outcomes Classification on the Web or

 Go to the NOC Web site at http://www.nursing.uiowa.edu/ excellence/nursing_knowledge/clinical_effectiveness/index.htm

The Clinical Care Classification (CCC) was developed by Virginia Saba, a nurse-researcher, for use in home health nursing. In the CCC, you form goals by adding modifiers to the nursing diagnoses. This system has four nursing diagnoses that are clearly for family units: Family Coping Impairment, Compromised Family Coping, Disabled Family Coping, and Family Processes Alteration. The CCC includes one diagnosis specifically for communities: Community Coping Impairment. For a complete description of the CCC system,

 Go to the CCC Web site at http://www.sabacare.com

The Omaha System was developed specifically for community health nursing. In that system, you must label all nursing diagnoses as *individual, family,* or *group.* You can write aggregate outcomes by specifying a *family* or *group* diagnosis and then creating a goal from it, by using terms in a Problem Rating Scale for Outcomes, as in the following example.

> *Omaha Nursing Diagnosis:* Personal Hygiene. Family. Deficit (Actual Problem)

Present status	*Expected outcome*
Minimal knowledge of family personal hygiene	Adequate knowledge of family personal hygiene

For a complete description of the Omaha System, and to see the Problem Rating Scale for Outcomes,

 Go to the Omaha System Web site at http://www.omahasystem.org

KnowledgeCheck 5-7

- Which standardized classification system was designed specifically for community health nursing?
- Which standardized classification system was designed specifically for home healthcare?
- Which standardized classification system was designed for use in all areas and specialties of nursing?

How Do I Write Goals for Wellness Diagnoses?

Whether standardized or individualized, expected outcomes for wellness diagnoses describe behaviors or responses that demonstrate health maintenance or achievement of an even higher level of health. For example: "Over the next year, [Mr. Needham] will continue to eat a balanced diet with more emphasis on including whole grains and fiber." By using the highest number (5) on the rating scale, you can use the NOC to write wellness outcomes. For example:

> *Nursing diagnosis:* Readiness for Enhanced Nutrition
> *Expected outcome:* Nutritional Status: (5) Not compromised

In addition, many NOC outcomes can be used to measure health (e.g., Activity Tolerance, Child Development,

Growth, Nutritional Status). See Chapter 42 or go to the NOC Web site for a complete list of wellness outcomes.

Outcomes for Special Teaching Plans

As discussed earlier, some patients need a special teaching plan to address learning needs. Expected outcomes are written in the same way as any other type of care plan, but they are usually called teaching objectives. **Teaching objectives** describe what the patient is to learn and the observable behaviors that will demonstrate learning; they should state whether learning is to be cognitive, psychomotor, or affective. Consider the following examples:

> *Cognitive*: By May 1, will list four foods to avoid on a low-fat diet.
> *Affective:* By May 1, will verbalize feeling less anger about diet limitations.
> *Psychomotor:* By May 1, will demonstrate how to use grasp extender to obtain food from the top shelf.

For further information about teaching objectives, see Chapter 19.

REFLECTING CRITICALLY ABOUT EXPECTED OUTCOMES/GOALS

After writing the expected outcomes for a client, use the full-spectrum nursing model to help you evaluate their quality. Use the following questions as a guide.
For each nursing diagnosis:

1. *Is there at least one goal that, when met, would demonstrate problem resolution;* that is, does at least one goal flow from the problem clause?
2. *Do the predicted outcomes completely address the nursing diagnosis?* If you have written outcomes in very specific, measurable terms, you may need several for a single nursing diagnosis. Review Table 5-3.

For each expected outcome:

3. *Is the outcome appropriate for the nursing diagnosis?* If not, a new nursing diagnosis should be written rather than adding a not-quite-related goal to the existing plan. In Table 5-3, for example, "Obtains 8 hrs sleep at night" would not be appropriate for the nursing diagnosis Ineffective Airway Clearance, because it does not flow from either the problem or etiology clause.
4. *Is each outcome derived from only one nursing diagnosis?* That is, does it describe only one patient response? Consider the following outcomes for a diagnosis of Diarrhea.

Examples:
Incorrect: Will have no diarrhea in the next 12 hours, and skin will be intact and without redness in the perianal area. (*Explanation:* Even though diarrhea may cause excoriation of perianal skin, obtaining a good skin outcome would not tell you anything about the status of the Diarrhea diagnosis.)

Correct: Will have no diarrhea in the next 12 hours.

Correct: Then write a new diagnosis of Impaired Skin Integrity, and a goal, "Skin will remain intact and without redness in the perianal area."

5. ***Does each outcome describe only one patient response or behavior?*** Look at the "correct" example in item 4, preceding, for the new Impaired Skin Integrity diagnosis. How many patient responses does it contain? It has two responses: Skin will remain intact, and skin will not be red. So our "correct" example meets the criteria for item 4 but not for item 5.

 ThinkLike a Nurse 5-5

Why is it not a good idea to write the Skin Integrity outcome as shown in Item 4?

6. ***Is the outcome stated as a patient behavior, not a nurse activity?***
   Incorrect (nurse activity): Prevent skin irritation.
   Correct (patient response): Skin will not show signs of irritation.

7. ***Is the outcome stated in positive terms?*** When possible, state what you intend to occur, rather than what should not occur. For example, use "incision dry," rather than "no incision drainage." This is not always possible, especially for potential problems. It is better, for example, to write "No redness" (even though it is negative) than to write "Skin color normal," because "normal" is too vague. For potential problems, a negatively worded outcome is actually a list of the patient responses you are trying to prevent.

8. ***Is the outcome measurable or observable?***
   Correct: Explains the actions and side effects of Coumadin, by 8/11/16.
   Incorrect: Understands the actions and side effects of Coumadin, by 8/11/16.
   There is no way to observe someone's understanding, so you could not use the second (incorrect) goal to evaluate client progress. Use action verbs; think, "What do I want to see, hear, feel, or smell?"

9. ***Are the performance criteria specific and concrete?*** Avoid words such as *normal, sufficient, enough, more, less, adequate, increased.* Vague words can be interpreted differently by different people. Does *"adequate* sleep" mean that the patient will sleep 8 hours per night, will fall asleep within an hour of going to bed, will feel rested in the morning, or will not become sleepy during the day?

10. ***Does each goal include all the necessary parts?*** Is there a subject (implied or actual), action verb, performance criterion, target time, and special condition (when needed)?

11. ***Is the expected outcome realistic and achievable by this patient, given the available resources?*** People usually will not work toward goals unless they believe they are possible to achieve. The outcome "Will rest for an hour twice a day" may not be realistic for a single mother with several small children and no help at home. Be sure to consider the patient's support system, financial status, available community services, and physical and mental status. Also consider institutional resources. For example, there is no point in writing, "Will express anxieties freely to the nurse" if staffing is not adequate to allow the nurse to spend time with the patient to develop a relationship.

12. ***Does the outcome conflict with the medical or other collaborative treatment plan?*** For example, an outcome of "Ambulated to end of hall" would not be compatible with the medical treatment plan for a patient who is sleepy and lethargic from the side effects of medications.

13. ***Does the patient, family, or community value the outcome?*** The care plan is more likely to be effective if the goal is important to the client. You may, for example, believe that smoking cessation is an important goal for the patient. However, the patient might not be motivated to stop smoking, even when given all the related information. When your goals conflict with the patient's, explore the patient's thinking. Explain your reasoning and try to find a compromise or an alternative approach.

14. ***Does the goal conflict with any religious or cultural values?*** You may know that early ambulation (e.g., "Ambulates to bathroom within 4 hours after birth of the baby") helps to prevent thrombophlebitis. However, in some cultures, childbirth is viewed as an illness, and the mother expects to remain in bed for several days with family members taking care of her needs. When a patient is "noncompliant," the reason may be that she is complying with her cultural beliefs rather than the caregiver's plan of care.

KnowledgeCheck 5-8

List at least eight questions you could use to critically evaluate the quality of your goal/outcome statements.

Toward Evidence-Based Practice

Scherb, C. A., Stevens, M. S., & Busman, C. (2007). **Outcomes related to dehydration in the pediatric population.** *Journal of Pediatric Nursing, 22*(5), 376–382.

The purpose of this pilot study was to (1) determine whether there was a meaningful difference (in statistical terms) in nursing-sensitive patient outcome ratings from admission to discharge and (2) to describe nursing interventions used for children (younger than age 18 years) admitted with a primary diagnosis of dehydration. During the study period, researchers examined 29 patient care records that were a part of a computerized clinical documentation system in a Midwestern hospital. The documentation system used the standardized nursing languages of NANDA-I, NOC, and NIC.

Standardized care plans (also using NANDA-I, NOC, and NIC) were initiated upon a child's admission, and

individualized as needed. NOC outcomes were rated upon admission and at discharge. Examples of outcomes on the care plan include Nutritional Status, Fluid Balance, and Urinary Elimination. Of the eight outcomes on the care plan, seven had statistically significant changes (showing the child's improvement).

1. If you had to decide on the basis of this study alone, would you be for or against using standardized nursing languages for documentation and patient care plans in your organization? Explain your reasoning.

 Go to Student Resources: Chapter 5, **Toward Evidence-Based Practice Suggested Responses,** on *DavisPlus*.

 To explore learning resources for this chapter,

 Go to *DavisPlus* at **DavisPl.us/Wilkinson3.**

Chapter Resources for Chapter 5:
   Response sheets for all learning activities
   Knowledge Check Answers
   Resources for Caregivers and Health Professionals
   Reading More About Nursing Process: Planning Outcomes (suggested readings)
   Concept Map of chapter content
Interactive Case Studies
NCLEX-Style and Chapter Review Questions
Chapter Overview Podcasts

For references cited in this chapter,

 Go to Volume 2, **References Cited.**

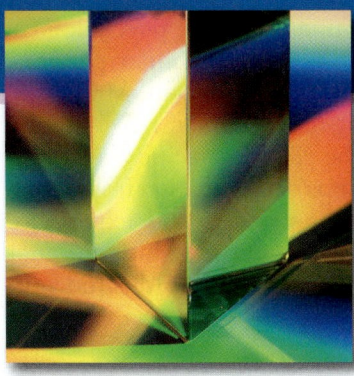

CHAPTER 6

Nursing Process: Planning Interventions

Learning Outcomes

After completing this chapter, you should be able to:

➤ Define the term *nursing intervention*.

➤ Compare and contrast independent, dependent, and interdependent (collaborative) nursing interventions.

➤ Explain how theories, research, and evidence-based practice influence the choice of nursing interventions.

➤ Explain how nursing interventions are determined by problem status (i.e., actual or potential problem).

➤ Describe a process for generating nursing interventions for a client.

➤ Explain how to use a standardized vocabulary for nursing interventions and activities.

➤ Give one example of a standardized wellness (health promotion) intervention and one individualized nursing order for performing that intervention.

➤ Give one example of a standardized spirituality intervention and one individualized nursing order for performing that intervention.

➤ Write complete, detailed nursing orders, in correct format, for patients.

➤ Give examples of some questions for reflecting critically about nursing orders you have written.

Key Concepts

Evidence-based practice
Nursing interventions

Related Concepts
See the Concept Map on Davis*Plus*.

Meet Your Patient

Ben Ivanos, whom you met in Chapter 5, is confined to bed after a motorcycle accident. He has casts and traction for both legs and a cast on one arm. Since admission to the hospital 3 days ago, he has been receiving narcotic analgesics for severe pain. He has a new nursing diagnosis today: Constipation related to immobility and decreased gastrointestinal (GI) motility secondary to narcotic analgesics. The nurse enters the diagnosis into a care-planning program. In addition to a list of suggested assessments, the computer database generates the following list of suggested treatment interventions:

1. Institute a program to establish a regular pattern of bowel movements.
2. Administer laxative or stool softener, as prescribed.
3. Administer enema.
4. Remove stool manually.
5. Encourage increased fluid intake, including warm liquids.
6. Instruct about and encourage a high-fiber diet.
7. Encourage a regular program of activity and exercise.
8. Perform manual reduction of rectal prolapse.

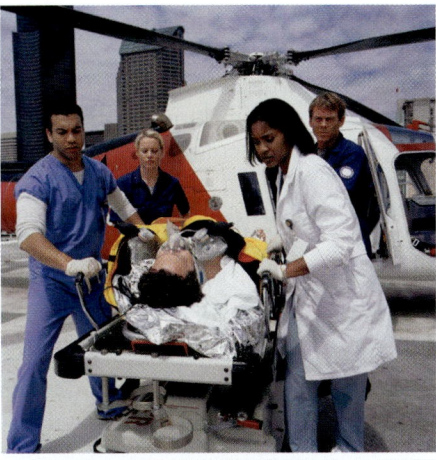

Which interventions should the nurse choose? Which can he eliminate, based on the information provided? You may not yet have enough nursing knowledge to be sure about your answers to these questions, but before reading on, try to think it through with the information and life experience available to you.

The nurse eliminated interventions 1, 3, 4, 7, and 8. Take a few moments to see if you can explain the nurse's reasons for deleting these interventions.

Theoretical Knowledge
knowing **why**

Compare your explanations to the following reasons given by the nurse in the Meet Your Patient scenario. The nurse eliminated the following interventions:

- **1**—because it is useful for patients who are constipated as a result of irregular bowel habits, whereas Mr. Ivanos's problem is caused by immobility and narcotic side effects.
- **3 and 4**—because Mr. Ivanos's symptoms did not seem severe enough to warrant an enema or manual removal of stool.
- **7**—because it is not practical: Mr. Ivanos cannot exercise in his present condition.
- **8**—because it is not relevant: Mr. Ivanos does not have rectal prolapse.

The nurse chose the following interventions to include in the care plan:

- **2**—because it directly addresses the problem, Constipation.
- **5 and 6**—because they address the etiology of the problem. Fluid and fiber soften the stool and help to stimulate bowel activity.

The nurse also reasoned that because narcotics cause constipation, it would be good to administer them less frequently to Mr. Ivanos if other satisfactory pain-relief measures could be found. So he added the following nursing orders to the care plan:

Assist to change position every 1–2 hours.
Encourage distraction (e.g., watching TV, reading, listening to music).
Assist with relaxation and visualization techniques.
Obtain medical prescription for nonnarcotic analgesics to enhance nonpharmacological pain-relief measures.
Assess effectiveness of nonpharmacological interventions for pain.
Give prescribed narcotic analgesics if other measures are ineffective.

The nurse knows people are often self-conscious or embarrassed about using a bedpan, especially in the presence of others. So he also added the following to the care plan:

Encourage Mr. Ivanos to summon the nurse when he feels the urge to defecate (place call light within reach). If he does not, then ask at least every 4 hr whether he needs the bedpan.
Warm the bedpan and provide privacy. Pull the bed curtain; turn on the TV or radio if he has a roommate; explain that you will leave the room and that he should call when he is ready for you to return; and shut the door.

As you can see, to develop interventions to meet Mr. Ivanos's needs, the nurse needed to do more than just look at a list and follow physician orders. He thought critically about (1) his theoretical knowledge (of narcotics, bowel elimination, and psychological needs), (2) his past experiences with similar patients, and (3) the patient situation (the data about Mr. Ivanos and the factors contributing to his problem). By thinking of interventions to meet the client's specific needs, this nurse may prevent Mr. Ivanos's constipation from worsening. A nurse with less knowledge and experience might have used only the interventions in the computer database, failing to effectively meet the desired outcomes (goals) for Mr. Ivanos.

ABOUT THE KEY CONCEPTS

As you study this chapter, try to think about how related concepts (such as theories, standardized language, nursing orders, and so on) are linked to the key concepts of **evidence-based practice** and **nursing interventions**. This should help you to understand and remember chapter content. The deeper your understanding, the better you will be able to apply your knowledge in caring for patients.

WHAT ARE NURSING INTERVENTIONS?

Nursing interventions are actions, based on clinical judgment and nursing knowledge, that nurses perform to achieve client outcomes. Interventions are also referred to as *nursing actions, measures, strategies,* and *activities*. This chapter uses those terms interchangeably except when referring to the Nursing Interventions Classification (NIC) standardized labels (discussed later in the chapter), which are always called *interventions*. Figure 6-1 shows how planning interventions relates to the other phases of the nursing process.

No matter what term is used, nursing interventions include a broad range of activities.

- **Direct-care interventions** are performed through interaction with the client(s). Examples are physical care, emotional support, and patient teaching.
- **Indirect-care intervention**s are performed away from the client but on behalf of a client or group of clients. They include advocacy, managing the environment, consulting with other members of the healthcare team, and making referrals.

Think Like a Nurse 6-1

- Give one example of a direct-care intervention.
- Give one example of an indirect-care intervention.

Nurses work collaboratively with other healthcare providers. Some things you do for patients will require a physician's order; many will not. Sometimes the activities of care providers overlap. For example, physicians, nurses, and respiratory therapists may all measure a client's blood pressure; and a nurse and a dietitian may both teach the client about a diet to help manage hypertension. Nursing

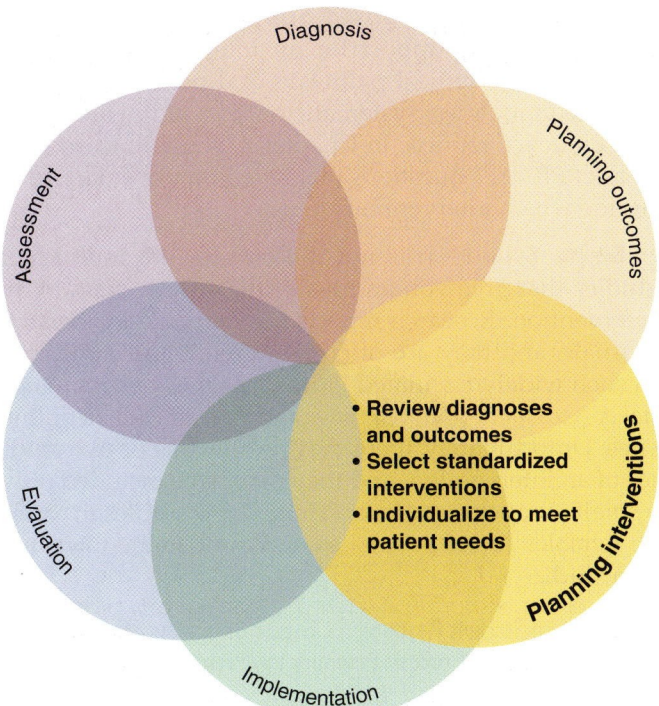

FIGURE 6-1 Nursing process: Planning interventions.

interventions may be independent, dependent, or collaborative (interdependent).

Independent Interventions *Nurse A makes a nursing diagnosis of Anxiety related to deficient knowledge about barium enema; she writes a nursing order to teach the patient what to expect from the upcoming diagnostic test.* This is an **independent intervention**—one that registered nurses are licensed to prescribe, perform, or delegate based on their knowledge and skills. It does not require a provider's order. Knowing how, when, and why to perform an activity makes the action **autonomous** (independent). As a rule, nurses prescribe and perform independent interventions in response to a nursing diagnosis. Understand you are **accountable** (answerable) for your decisions and actions with regard to nursing diagnoses and independent interventions. If patient teaching did not relieve the patient's anxiety in this example, it might be that the nurse misdiagnosed or chose an ineffective intervention.

Dependent Interventions *Nurse B reads a physician's prescription in a patient's chart: Give cephalothin sodium (Keflin) 1 g IV [through the intravenous line] before surgery, and then every 6 hr for 24 hr. She prepares and administers the medication.* This is a **dependent intervention**—one that is prescribed by a physician or advanced practice nurse but carried out by the bedside nurse. Dependent interventions are usually orders for diagnostic tests, medications, treatments, IV therapy, diet, and activity. In addition to carrying out medical prescriptions, you will be responsible for assessing the need for the prescription, explaining the activities to the patient, and evaluating the effectiveness of the order. For example, after giving the Keflin (an antibiotic), Nurse B observes

that the patient has developed a severe rash. Suspecting an allergic reaction, she contacts the prescriber so that the prescription can be changed and antibiotic prophylaxis can be continued after surgery without danger to the patient.

You may write nursing orders to individualize a medical order, based on the patient's condition. For example, the provider may prescribe, "Give oral fluids up to 3,000 mL every 24 hours." You might individualize the order to give 1,500 mL on the day shift, 1,000 mL on the evening shift, and 500 mL during the night, so that the patient will not have to be awakened frequently during the night.

Collaborative (Interdependent) Interventions *Nurse C notes that a client newly diagnosed with diabetes has been seen by a dietitian, who taught and provided materials about a diabetic diet. The nurse observes the client's menu choices. She notes that the client is eating candy brought by visitors. She explains to the client how concentrated sugar affects his diabetes; she also communicates her assessments and teaching to the dietitian.* This is an **interdependent (collaborative) intervention**—one that is carried out in collaboration with other healthcare team members (e.g., physical therapists, dietitians, and physicians). Because nurses care for the whole person, their responsibilities often overlap with those of other team members.

 Think**Like a Nurse** 6-2

- What are some other examples of independent interventions?
- What are some other examples of dependent interventions?
- What are some other examples of collaborative interventions?

HOW DO I DECIDE WHICH INTERVENTIONS TO USE?

To review American Nurses Association (ANA) (2010) standards of care related to care planning and interventions, refer to Box 5-1, Standard 4, in Chapter 5. Use the ANA standards to guide you in selecting interventions appropriate for the client's nursing diagnoses (or collaborative problems) and the desired outcomes. In addition to these standards, a variety of theories, nursing research, and the client's problem status will all influence your choice of interventions.

Key Point: *As a nurse, you will be responsible for choosing nursing interventions. You cannot delegate this responsibility to nursing assistive personnel.*

As a rule, licensed practical/vocational nurses (LPN/LVNs) give care according to a plan created by the RN. In many situations, the LPN/LVN contributes to the plan by providing data or by giving feedback about the effectiveness of the interventions. For more information about delegation, see Chapter 7.

How Do Theories Influence My Choice of Interventions?

A **theory** is a set of interrelated concepts (ideas) that describes or explains something—nursing, for example.

A theory, like a lens, influences your perspective: What you notice, what you consider to be a problem—and how you define a problem—more or less determine what you choose to do about it. For example, suppose a patient is pale and fidgeting and has sweaty palms and a rapid pulse. If you looked at this person through the lens of psychological theory, your first thought might be that the patient is anxious. Your first intervention, then, would probably be to assess for the cause of his anxiety. If you were using a physiological lens, you might suspect pain. Your first intervention, then, might be to ask the patient whether he is having pain. For more information about nursing theories, see Chapter 8.

How Does Nursing Research Influence My Choice of Interventions?

Although much nursing and medical practice is still based on tradition, experience, and professional opinion, this is not an ideal basis for choosing an intervention. Ideally, a nurse should choose an intervention because of firm evidence that it is the best possible approach for the patient. You would expect that such interventions should be those that were developed from a sound body of scientific research.

American Nurses Association (ANA) Standards Standard 9 of the ANA Scope and Standards of Practice, Nursing (ANA, 2010, p. 51), states that the registered nurse:

- Utilizes current evidence-based nursing knowledge, including research findings, to guide practice decisions.
- Incorporates evidence when initiating changes in nursing practice.
- Participates, as appropriate to education level and position, in the formulation of evidence-based practice through research.
- Shares personal or third-party research findings with colleagues and peers.

To see if you have the most current ANA standards,

 Go to http://www.nursingworld.org/, or more directly, go to http://www.nursingworld.org/MainMenuCategories/ThePracticeofProfessionalNursing/NursingStandards.aspx

QSEN Competencies According to the Quality and Safety Education for Nurses (QSEN) group, one competency you should achieve in nursing school is to differentiate clinical opinion from research and evidence summaries. To see an expanded discussion of this competency,

 Go to **the Cronenwett, et al. (2007) reference, in** Student Resources: Chapter 6, **Reading More About Nursing Process: Interventions,** on DavisPlus
or

 Go to http://qsen.org/competencies/pre-licensure-ksas/

Types of Research-Based Support

Research-based support for an intervention includes single studies, critical pathways and protocols, clinical practice guidelines, systematic reviews of the literature, and evidence reports. In Chapter 8, you will learn how to ask "PICOT" questions that help you use evidence to decide which interventions to use.

Single Studies It is not difficult to find individual studies that give you an idea of the effectiveness of an intervention. Research reports are available in research journals, and they are often interpreted and published in such widely circulated journals as the *American Journal of Nursing (AJN), Nursing,* and *RN,* as well as online sites. Unfortunately, there may be only one or two studies of an intervention, and they may have included only a small number of patients. Thus, single studies may not be reliable. To see several examples of single intervention studies,

 Go to Student Resources: Chapter 6, **Reading More About the Nursing Process: Planning Interventions,** on DavisPlus.

Critical Pathways and Protocols Critical pathways (also called *clinical pathways* and *collaborative care plans*) are standardized plans of care for frequently occurring conditions (e.g., total hip replacement) for which similar outcomes and interventions are appropriate for all patients who have the condition. They are tools developed by an organization for its own use and are intended to guide best practice at the local level. However, they may not be based on research if the practitioners who develop them are reluctant to change traditional practices they believe to be effective. Furthermore, issues of cost to the organization influence the decision to include an intervention in the plan of care. Nevertheless, critical pathways have, at the very least, been developed on the basis of expert opinion. So they do provide some guidance for nursing interventions. See Chapter 5 for discussion and examples of critical pathways and protocols.

What Is Evidence-Based Practice?

You can feel more confident about an intervention if several studies have supported it. **Evidence-based practice (EBP)** is an approach that uses firm scientific data rather than anecdote, tradition, intuition, or folklore in making decisions about medical and nursing practice. In nursing it includes blending clinical judgment and expertise with the best available research evidence and patient characteristics and preferences. The goal of evidence-based practice is to identify the most effective and cost-efficient treatments for a particular disease, condition, or problem. Steps in the EBP process include the following:

1. Formulating an answerable question about prevention, diagnosis, prognosis (likely outcome), and interventions
2. Conducting a systematic review of published evidence (research) to find studies that shed light on the desired topic

3. Evaluating or grading the quality of the evidence obtained. Quality involves *validity* (closeness to the truth), *applicability* (usefulness), and *impact* (extent of the effect). Figure 6-2 lists evidence from strongest to weakest. For more information about "levels of evidence," or how evidence is evaluated,

 Go to Student Resources: Chapter 6, **Supplemental Materials, Levels of Evidence,** on Davis*Plus*.

4. Compiling and analyzing the data to prepare a structured report of the review
5. "Translating" the evidence into guidelines for practice
6. Integrating the guidelines and evidence with clinical expertise and the patient's preferences and characteristics

A number of healthcare organizations and groups are devoted to compiling study results that provide evidence to use in formulating guidelines for medical and nursing practice. Online examples include The Joanna Briggs Institute and the Cochrane Database of Systematic Reviews. You will find such compiled information in clinical practice guidelines, evidence reports, and sometimes in local healthcare agency tools (e.g., clinical pathways and protocols). For full discussion on the importance of research and evidence-based nursing practice, see Chapter 8.

Evidence Reports

Evidence reports are state-of-the-art, systematic reviews of clinical topics for the purpose of providing evidence for practice guidelines, quality improvement, quality measures, and insurance coverage decisions (Cronenwett, 2002). Evidence reports are usually developed by scientists rather than by clinicians, patients, and advocacy groups. One source of such reports is the Evidence-Based Practice Center (EPC) Program of the federal Agency for Healthcare Research and Quality (AHRQ). The EPC uses explicit grading systems to review studies and rank the strength of their evidence. For free access to online reviews,

 Go to the AHRQ Web site at http://www.ahrq.gov/clinic/ epcindex.htm

- Meta-analysis of randomized clinical trials
- Individual randomized clinical trials
- Individual cohort study
- Outcomes research
- Individual case-control study
- Case studies
- Expert opinion

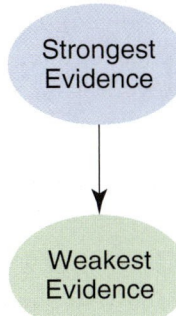

FIGURE 6-2 Hierarchy of research evidence. (*Source:* Courtesy of Fain, J. A. (2008). *Reading, understanding, and applying nursing research: A text and workbook* (3rd ed., p. 279). Philadelphia: F. A. Davis.)

Clinical Practice Guidelines

Evidence reports often form the basis for developing clinical practice guidelines. **Clinical practice guidelines** are statements developed by a systematic review of evidence and an assessment of the benefits and harms of care options. They include recommendations made to assist practitioners and patients in making decisions about appropriate healthcare for a particular disease or procedure (Field & Lohr, 1992; Institute of Medicine, 2011). Clinical practice guidelines are usually developed by clinicians, patients, and advocacy groups and are published by specialty organizations, universities, and government agencies. The following are examples:

- The Joanna Briggs Institute *Best Practice* information sheet on Topical Skin Care in Aged Care Facilities (JBI, 2007)
- University of Iowa research-based guidelines for care of the elderly (Titler, Mentes, Rakel, et al., 1999)
- National Guideline Clearinghouse, initiative of the Agency for Healthcare Research and Quality (AHRQ), U.S. Department of Health and Human Services, is a comprehensive database of guidelines for health professionals (http://www.guideline.gov/)

Clinical practice guidelines form the basis for nursing interventions. One example of clinical practice guidelines is found in Box 6-1. For years, relying on conventional

---

BOX 6-1 ■ Portion of a Clinical Practice Guideline on Pressure Ulcer Formation

Note: This is not the complete practice guideline.

Assessment*

- Use a reliable and standardized tool for doing a risk assessment, such as the Braden Scale.
- Risk assessment documentation on admission to a facility and whenever the client's condition changes and based on patient care setting (e.g., acute care, every 48 hr)

Nursing Care Strategies and Interventions

 Do not massage bony prominences.

- Use pressure-reducing devices (static air, alternating air, gel, water mattresses). (Evidence Level II)
- Raise heels of bedbound clients off the bed; do not use donut-type devices. (Evidence Level III)
- Avoid hot water and soaps that are drying when bathing elderly. Use body wash and skin protectant. (Evidence Level III)

---

*"Strength of evidence" is an AHRQ ranking (I to VI) of the amount and quality of research supporting the guideline. The best ranking is I.
Source: Agency for Healthcare Research and Quality (AHRQ). (2003; updated June 2008). Guideline summary. Preventing pressure ulcers and skin tears. In: *Evidence-based geriatric nursing protocols for best practice.* Retrieved July 13, 2012, from http://www.guideline.gov/content.aspx?id=12262&search=pressure+ulcer#Section442

wisdom and word of mouth, nurses tried to prevent pressure ulcers by writing the nursing order, "Massage skin over bony prominences." They reasoned that because poor circulation can contribute to the formation of pressure ulcers, improving circulation to the area would prevent them. But as you can see in Box 6-1, research-based practice guidelines show that massage may actually be harmful. This report would certainly motivate you, as a full-spectrum nurse, to remove this "standard" intervention from your practice.

KnowledgeCheck 6-1

- Explain how theory influences your choice of nursing interventions.
- Why does a clinical practice guideline provide better support for an intervention than does a single study?
- Why does a clinical practice guideline provide better support for an intervention than does an agency's critical pathway?

How Does Problem Status Influence Nursing Interventions?

Nursing interventions include activities for observation/assessment, prevention, treatment, and health promotion. As you can see in Table 6-1, the status of the problem (i.e., whether it is a collaborative problem or an actual, potential, possible, or wellness nursing diagnosis)

determines which types of activities are required (to review problem status, see Chapter 4).

A nursing strategy can be a preventive measure in one situation and a treatment in another. For example, you might write the nursing order, "Teach the importance of adequate fluids," to treat a patient with an actual diagnosis of Constipation or to help prevent the problem for a woman with a diagnosis of Risk for Constipation.

KnowledgeCheck 6-2

Review problem status (actual, potential, or possible nursing diagnosis; collaborative problem; or wellness diagnosis) in Chapter 4. For which type(s) of problem(s) would you write the following:

- Nursing orders for observation/assessments?
- Nursing orders for treatments?
- Nursing orders for health promotion interventions?
- Preventive nursing orders?

What Process Can I Use for Generating and Selecting Interventions?

As you can see from the case of Ben Ivanos (Meet Your Patient), there are usually several nursing measures that might be effective for any one problem. The idea, of course, is to select those most likely to achieve the

Table 6-1 ➤ Relationship of Problem Status to Intervention Type

PROBLEM STATUS	INTERVENTION TYPE			
	Observation	Prevention	Treatment	Health Promotion
Actual nursing diagnosis	To detect change in status (improvement, exacerbation of problem).	To help keep the problem from becoming worse.	To relieve symptoms and resolve etiologies (contributing factors).	
Potential (risk) nursing diagnosis	To detect (1) progression to an actual problem or (2) an increase or decrease in risk factors.	To remove or reduce risk factors in an effort to keep the problem from developing.		
Possible nursing diagnosis	To obtain more data to confirm or rule out a suspected nursing diagnosis.			
Collaborative problem	To detect onset of a complication for early provider notification.	To implement nursing and medical orders to help prevent development of a complication.	To implement nursing and medical orders for relieving or eliminating the underlying condition for which complications may develop.	
Wellness diagnosis	To assess a client's wellness practices.	To prevent specific diseases (e.g., giving immunization).	Clients usually manage their own wellness treatment.	To support a client's health promotion efforts and achieve a higher level of wellness.

desired goals. In doing that, you must consider the patient's abilities and preferences; the education, experience, and capabilities of the nursing staff; the resources available (e.g., time, equipment); medical orders; and institutional policies and procedures. When generating interventions, you will use critical thinking skills.

For example, imagine you are caring for a hospice patient who has cancer and is dying. She has told you that she is experiencing significant pain, but also that she wants to spend her last hours with her husband and two daughters, who are staying with her. Critical thinking skills you might use include the following:

- *Making interdisciplinary connections* (e.g., "What did I learn in psychology class that might help me here?")
- *Predicting* (e.g., "If I give morphine to the patient, it should relieve her pain, but she will probably become drowsy.")
- *Generalizing* (e.g., "I have used touch to relieve anxiety many times in similar situations; perhaps it will also help for this patient.")
- *Explaining* (e.g., "The morphine causes drowsiness by depressing the central nervous system.")
- *Therapeutic judgment* (e.g., "The patient wants to spend quality time with her family before she dies. Because the morphine will make her drowsy, I should find out if she wants me to give a smaller dose, even though it will not provide good pain relief, along with some nonpharmacological measures.")

You must always rethink an intervention for each patient. You cannot assume a strategy that was useful in the past will be effective in every situation. Mr. Ivanos's nurse may have used distraction successfully to relieve the pain of other patients in the past. However, if Mr. Ivanos has severe pain, or if he has difficulty concentrating, then distraction may not be effective. A full-spectrum nurse takes such details into account before choosing an intervention. The following five-step process will help you to select the best interventions (Wilkinson, 2011):

1. Review the Nursing Diagnosis

The etiology of a nursing diagnosis describes the factors that contribute to the unhealthy response. Choose strategies you expect will reduce or remove the etiological factors of actual problems, or that will reduce or remove risk factors for potential problems.

- ***When it is not possible to change the etiology***, choose strategies to treat the patient's symptoms (the AMB part of a diagnosis referred to in Chapter 4). For example, if the cause of pain is a surgical incision, you cannot suddenly "cure" the incision. Your nursing actions should focus on measures to relieve the pain.
- ***You may not always know the etiology of the problem***. However, some interventions may relieve a problem regardless of its cause. For example, when you have a client with Anxiety, regardless of its cause, it is helpful to approach the patient calmly; and when you

have a client with Constipation, regardless of its cause, it is always appropriate to assess the characteristics of the stool. Consider the nursing diagnosis and interventions for Mr. Ivanos in Figure 6-3.

Obviously, some people with constipation do not have pain. The pain-relief nursing order, which flows from the etiology of the problem, is specific to Mr. Ivanos's needs. Administering a stool softener and laxative, however, is a common strategy for constipation, whatever its cause.

Key Point: *As a rule, standardized interventions (care common to all patients with a particular condition) flow from the problem side of a nursing diagnosis; individualized interventions, from the etiology.*

ThinkLike a Nurse 6-3

For the following nursing diagnoses, write one intervention to address the problem and one for the etiology of the problem.

- Ineffective Airway Clearance r/t thick secretions and decreased chest expansion secondary to dehydration and pain
- Self-Care Deficit: Bathing and Dressing r/t fatigue secondary to disturbed sleep pattern

2. Review the Desired Patient Outcomes

Desired outcomes (goals) suggest nursing strategies that are specific to the individual patient. For example, Table 6-2 shows some goals and outcomes for Mr. Ivanos's Constipation diagnosis. For each goal on the care plan, ask, "What intervention(s) will help to produce this patient response?" As you can see in the table, there may be one or more interventions for each goal. There is no

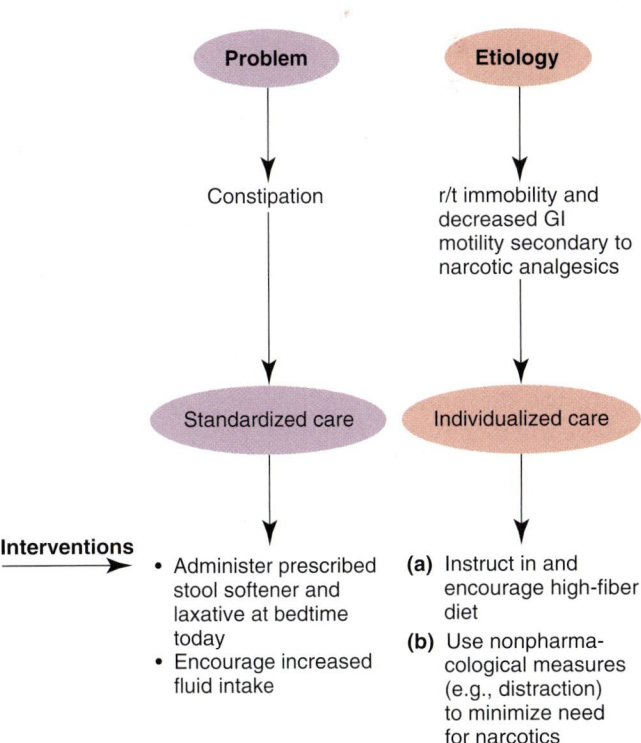

FIGURE 6-3 Nursing interventions flow from the nursing diagnosis.

Table 6-2 ➤ Interventions Flow from Desired Outcomes

GOALS/OUTCOMES	STRATEGIES SUGGESTED BY GOALS
1. **Will have bowel movement within 12 hours after receiving stool softener and laxative.**	A. **Administer prescribed stool softener and laxative at bedtime today.**
2. Will have daily soft, formed bowel movement during rest of hospital stay.	B. Instruct in and encourage high-fiber diet.
	C. Encourage increased fluid intake.
3. <u>Within 24 hours, will need narcotics to manage pain < 2x/day.</u>	D. <u>Use nonpharmacological measures (e.g., distraction) to minimize need for narcotics.</u>
4. *Calls nurse when urge to defecate is felt; does not delay defecation.*	E. *Encourage Mr. Ivanos to summon the nurse when he feels the urge to defecate.*
	F. *Provide privacy (e.g., pull the bed curtain, turn on the TV, leave room).*

Discussion:

Strategy A would help to achieve goal 1; but because the effects of these medications are short lived, it would do nothing to achieve goals 2 through 4.

Strategies B and C both help to achieve goal 2.

Strategy D (minimize narcotics), in contrast, directly addresses goal 3 and indirectly helps to achieve goal 2.

Strategies E and F both directly address goal 4 and indirectly address goal 2.

Note: Dotted lines indicate indirect contribution to goal.

strict one-to-one correspondence between goals and interventions.

3. Identify Several Interventions or Actions

The next step in choosing interventions is to think of several nursing activities that might achieve the desired outcomes. Don't try to narrow your list at this point; include unusual and creative ideas. You can refer to a standardized list of interventions (e.g., the Nursing Interventions Classification list on Davis*Plus*) or choose interventions from standardized care plans and agency protocols. Alternatively, you can generate the interventions yourself, based on your knowledge; experience; and use of nursing texts, journal articles, and professional nurses. To get started, ask yourself: For this nursing diagnosis, (1) What assessments/observations do I need to make? (2) What do I need to do for the patient? Include both dependent and independent activities as appropriate.

4. Choose the Best Interventions for the Patient

The best interventions are those you expect to be most effective in helping to achieve client goals. When possible, choose interventions based on research and scientific principles. Use the following critical-thinking questions from the full-spectrum nursing model (in Chapter 2) to help you determine the best actions.

Contextual awareness

- Is this intervention acceptable to the client (e.g., congruent with the patient's values and wishes)?

- Is this intervention culturally sensitive?
- What is going on in the patient's life (e.g., family, work situation, financial status) that may enhance or interfere with the effectiveness of the intervention?
- What is going on in the patient's health status (e.g., knowledge, abilities, resources, severity of illness) that may enhance or interfere with the effectiveness of the intervention?

Credible sources

- Have I used valid, reliable sources of information to identify this intervention (e.g., patient, other professionals, references)?
- Did I consider professional, ethical, and legal standards?
- What is the research basis for this intervention, if any?

Considering alternatives

- Is there adequate rationale for this intervention (e.g., principles, theory, facts)?
- Which action(s) is (are) most reasonable? Why are the others not as reasonable?
- Which action(s) is (are) most likely to achieve stated goals?

Analyzing assumptions

- What beliefs, values, or biases do I have that may affect my thinking and my choice of interventions?
- Do I feel any discomfort with this intervention?

Reflecting skeptically

- Are there other interventions I have overlooked?
- What might be the consequences of this intervention?
  - "What will happen if . . .?"

- Does it have any potential ill effects? If so, how will we manage them?
- Is this intervention feasible? For example, is it cost effective, are the time and personnel available for it? Can the patient or family manage it at home?
- How will the intervention interact with medical orders? For example, you cannot order "elevate head of bed" to facilitate breathing if there is a medical order to keep the patient flat to improve circulation to the neck and head.
- In priority order, what should I do in this situation and why?
- Do I have the knowledge and skills needed for the intervention, or do I need to consult with someone more qualified in this area?
- What might I delegate in this situation?

5. Individualize Standardized Interventions

Practice guidelines, systematic reviews of the literature, protocols, critical pathways, and even textbooks describe interventions that are appropriate for most people or the average person. However, they cannot take into account all the individual factors that contribute to a problem or that might affect the effectiveness of an intervention. You must always consider how an intervention can be used with a particular person. For example, after Ben Ivanos's nurse decided which of the computer-generated list of interventions to use, he adapted them to fit Ben's unique needs and preferences. Table 6-3 provides examples of standardized and individualized interventions for Mr. Ivanos.

KnowledgeCheck 6-3

Describe a five-step process for generating and choosing nursing interventions.

Computer-Generated Interventions

Most electronic care planning programs will generate a list of suggested interventions when you enter either a problem (nursing diagnosis, medical, collaborative) or an outcome (Fig. 6-4). You then choose the interventions appropriate for the patient (as in the case of Ben Ivanos) or type in nursing actions of your own. Computer prompts provide a wide range of interventions for your consideration. However, you must resist the temptation to settle for the ready-made solutions. Always look for other, perhaps more effective, strategies based on the patient data. Always think, "Are there other interventions I have overlooked? How should I adapt this for *this* patient?"

To see a computer screen showing how an intervention (Pain Control Techniques Education) is converted to nursing orders,

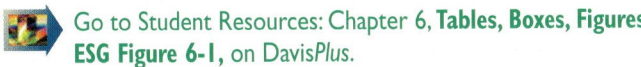 Go to Student Resources: Chapter 6, **Tables, Boxes, Figures: ESG Figure 6-1,** on Davis*Plus.*

Table 6-3 ➤ Individualizing Nursing Actions for Ben Ivanos	
STANDARDIZED INTERVENTIONS	**INDIVIDUALIZED NURSING ORDERS**
1. Encourage increased fluid intake.	1. Remind patient to drink a glass of water every hour; also keep ice and tea available at the bedside.
2. Instruct on and encourage a high-fiber diet.	2. Assist with menu choices to obtain more fiber; encourage family to bring salads and fruits from home for snacks.
3. Encourage distraction (e.g., watching TV, reading, listening to music).	3. Provide books from hospital library (he does not enjoy TV); have family bring radio, iPad, or tablet and headphones from home.
4. Give prescribed narcotic analgesics if other measures are ineffective.	4. Give Tylenol #3 every 4 hr if relaxation, visualization, and distraction are not effective. If orally administered Tylenol #3 is not effective, advise patient to administer IV morphine via patient-controlled analgesia pump.

HOW CAN I USE STANDARDIZED LANGUAGE TO PLAN INTERVENTIONS?

As a review before reading this section, you may wish to read the discussion of standardized language in Chapter 4 (NANDA-I for nursing diagnoses), and in Chapter 5 (NOC for patient outcomes).

Recall that standardized nursing terminologies are important for electronic health records (EHR), for research, and for clear, precise, consistent communication among nurses and with other disciplines. The American Nurses Association (ANA, 2006) has recognized 12 standardized vocabularies for recording and tracking the clinical care process. Those most commonly used for describing nursing interventions are the Nursing Interventions Classification (NIC), the Clinical Care Classification (CCC), and the Omaha System. NIC classifies only interventions. The CCC and the Omaha System also include nursing diagnoses and outcomes.

What Is the Nursing Interventions Classification?

Developed by a research team at the University of Iowa, the *Nursing Interventions Classification (NIC)* was the first comprehensive standardized classification of nursing interventions (McCloskey & Bulechek, 1992). The fifth edition NIC (Bulechek, Butcher, & Dochterman, et al.

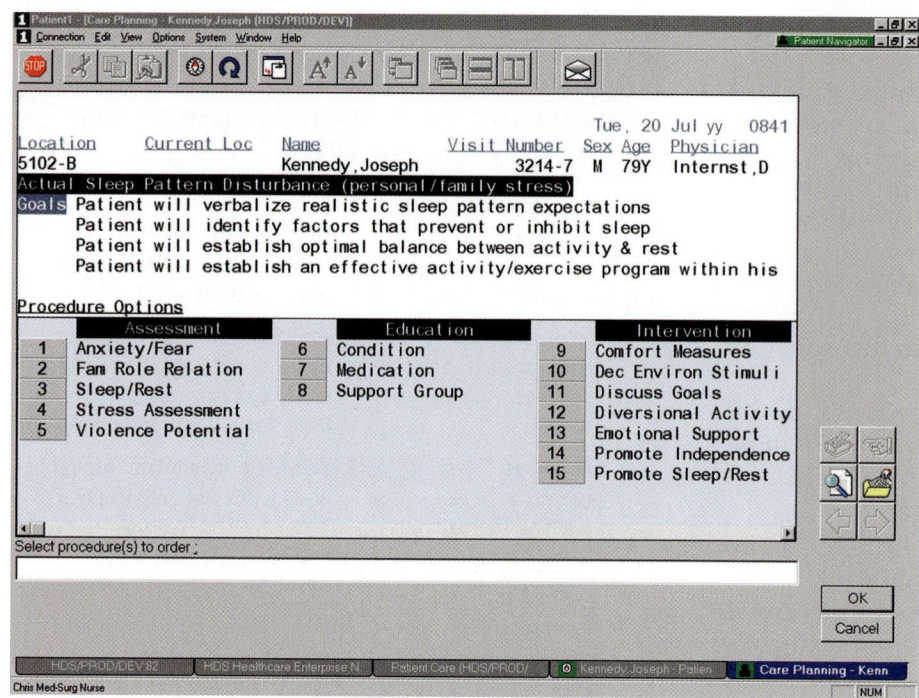

FIGURE 6-4 Computer care planning: When the nurse selects a nursing diagnosis of Sleep Pattern Disturbance, the computer database generates a list of suggested goals and "procedure options" (interventions); the nurse then chooses those best suited for the patient. (*Source:* Copyright© Ergo Partners, L.C. All rights reserved. Used with permission.)

2013) describes 554 direct and indirect-care activities performed by nurses. The NIC (pronounced "nick") is versatile—appropriate for use in all specialty and practice areas, including home health and community nursing.

Each NIC intervention consists of a label, a definition, and a list of the specific **activities** nurses perform in carrying out the intervention (Box 6-2). The **label**, usually consisting of two or three words, is the standardized terminology. The **definition** explains the meaning of the label. You are free to word the activities any way you choose in a care plan or client record. For a complete list of NIC intervention labels and definitions,

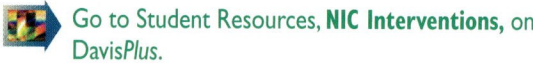 Go to Student Resources, **NIC Interventions,** on Davis*Plus*.

Locating Appropriate NIC Interventions and Activities

NIC interventions are linked to NANDA-I nursing diagnoses and NOC outcome labels in a "linkages" book, *NOC and NIC Linkages to NANDA-I and Clinical Conditions,* referred to by most nurses as the NNN linkages book (Johnson, Moorhead, Bulechek, et al., 2012). In this book, you can look up a nursing diagnosis to see the list of outcomes suggested for it and the interventions for achieving each outcome. Refer to Table 6-4 for an example of interventions linked to the nursing diagnosis Risk for Aspiration. Notice there are 5 "major" interventions and 17 "suggested" interventions from which to choose.

Once you have chosen the interventions (based on your knowledge and judgment), you then choose the

---

BOX 6-2 ■ NIC Intervention: Bathing

Definition

Cleaning of the body for the purposes of relaxation, cleanliness, and healing

Activities

Assist with chair shower, tub bath, bedside bath, standing shower, or sitz bath, as appropriate or desired.

Wash hair, as needed and desired.

Bathe in water of a comfortable temperature.

Use playful bathing techniques with children (e.g., wash dolls or toys; pretend a boat is a submarine; punch holes in bottom of plastic cup, fill with water, and let it "rain" on child).

Assist with perineal care, as needed.

Assist with hygiene measures (e.g., use of deodorant or perfume).

Administer foot soaks, as needed.

Shave patient, as indicated.

Apply lubricating ointment and cream to dry skin areas.

Offer handwashing after toileting and before meals.

Apply drying powders to deep skinfolds.

Monitor skin condition while bathing.

Monitor functional ability while bathing.

Source: Bulechek, B. M., Butcher, H. K., & Dochterman, J. M. (Eds.). (2013). *Nursing interventions classification (NIC)* (6th ed). St. Louis, MO: C.V. Mosby, p. 81. Used with permission from Elsevier Science.

Table 6-4 ➤ NIC Interventions Linked to NANDA-I Diagnosis, Risk for Aspiration	
Aspiration, Risk for:	
The state in which an individual is at risk for entry of gastrointestinal secretions, oropharyngeal secretions, or solids or fluids into tracheobronchial passages.	
NICS Associated With Prevention of Aspiration	
Airway Management	Neurologic Monitoring
Airway Suctioning	Positioning
Artificial Airway Management	Postanesthesia Care
Aspiration Precautions	Respiratory Monitoring
Chest Physiotherapy	Resuscitation: Neonate
Cough Enhancement	Risk Identification
Dementia Management	Sedation Management
Enteral Tube Feeding	Seizure Management
Feeding	Self-Care Assistance: Feeding
Gastrointestinal Intubation	Surveillance
Mechanical Ventilation Management: Invasive	Swallowing Therapy
Mechanical Ventilatory Weaning	Tube Care: Gastrointestinal
Medication Administration: Oral	Vomiting Management

Johnson, M., Moorhead, S., Bulechek, G., et al. (2012). *NOC and NIC linkages to NANDA-I and clinical conditions* (3rd ed.). St. Louis, MO: C.V. Mosby.

appropriate activities to carry out the intervention. As you might guess from looking at Box 6-2, you will probably never need to perform all the activities for a client. Choose the best ones for the situation and individualize them to fit the client and the resources (e.g., supplies, equipment) available.

Using NIC in Electronic Care Plans

Standardized language is especially useful in electronic care systems. For a computer screen with suggested NIC interventions for a NANDA-I nursing diagnosis,

 Go to Student Resources: Chapter 6, **Tables, Boxes, Figures: ESG Figure 6-2,** on Davis*Plus.*

For any NIC intervention, the program will also list the more specific nursing activities, which you can individualize as nursing orders.

 Go to Student Resources: Chapter 6, **Tables, Boxes, Figures: ESG Figure 6-3,** on Davis*Plus.*

Remember that you, not the computer, are responsible for choosing which interventions to use for each patient, when to use them, and which activities to write as specific nursing orders. You can reject *all* of the suggested interventions if they do not fit the patient's

unique needs. Most computer programs have a field that allows you to type in your own interventions and activities.

Standardized Languages for Home Health and Community Care

The NIC includes interventions applicable in all settings, including home health and community nursing. However, the following taxonomies were created specifically for those uses:

- **The Clinical Care Classification (CCC).** Previously called the *Home Healthcare Classification,* the CCC was developed for use in home healthcare (Saba, 1995, 2006). In addition to terminology for nursing diagnoses and outcomes, the CCC has 198 interventions. For a complete description of the CCC system, see the nursing process section of Chapter 43 and

 Go to the CCC Web site at http://www.sabacare.com

- **The Omaha system.** The Omaha system was developed for community health nurses to use in caring for individuals, families, and **aggregates** (community groups or entire communities) (Martin, 2005). It includes terminology for diagnoses, outcomes, and interventions. For a complete description of the Omaha system, and for NIC community interventions, see the nursing process section of Chapter 43 and

 Go to the Omaha system Web site at http://www. omahasystem.org

KnowledgeCheck 6-4

- Name and describe three standardized intervention vocabularies recognized by the ANA.
- In the NIC system, what is the difference between interventions and activities?

Does Standardized Language Interfere With Holistic Care?

Some nurses have criticized standardized terminologies for focusing on illness and physical interventions. However, NIC, Omaha, and CCC do include interventions to address health promotion and cultural and spiritual needs. If you have a holistic attitude, you will give holistic care. Using a common language should help rather than hinder your choice of interventions. CAM performed and documented according to one of the standard taxonomies makes clear that the techniques are appropriate as nursing interventions (Frisch, 2001). For further discussion of holistic nursing care,

 Go to Student Resources: Chapter 46, on Davis*Plus.*

The following sections discuss interventions focused on wellness, spiritual needs, and culturally sensitive care.

Wellness Interventions When you are caring for a healthy client, the client is the primary decision maker. You will function mainly as a teacher and health counselor. Frequently, the nursing orders outline lifestyle modification or behavior changes the client wants to make, along with self-rewards to reinforce the behaviors. For example:

Specific behavior change: I will consume fewer than 1,400 calories per day for the next week.
Self-reward: I will reward myself with an evening out to hear my favorite band.

The NIC contains most of the wellness interventions you will need. However, they are not all grouped together in one class. Some examples are Decision-Making Support, Exercise Promotion, and Health Screening. For more information on using standardized languages to describe wellness interventions, see Chapter 42.

Spiritual Care Interventions NIC, CCC, and the Omaha system all include terminology to describe spiritual interventions. The following are just a few examples:

NIC: Spiritual Growth Facilitation, Religious Ritual Enhancement
CCC: Spiritual Care, Coping Skills
Omaha: Spiritual Support, Bereavement Support

Chapter 16 provides full discussion of standardized nursing interventions to address spiritual needs. As you will see, you could also use most of those interventions (e.g., Coping Skills) for other than spiritual problems.

Culturally Sensitive Care Except for the NIC Culture Brokerage intervention, there are no standardized interventions that are unique to culturally based needs. All standardized interventions will result in culturally sensitive care if they are delivered by a culturally competent nurse.

PracticalKnowledge
knowing **how**

WHAT ARE NURSING ORDERS, AND HOW DO I WRITE THEM?

Nursing orders are instructions that describe how and when nursing interventions are to be implemented. They are usually written on a patient care plan. Other nurses and nursing assistive personnel (NAP) are responsible and accountable for implementing nursing orders.

 Think**Like a Nurse** 6-4

Suppose you are caring for a patient 24 hours after a major surgery. You see the following order on the nursing care plan: Ambulate 24 hours postoperatively.

- When you care for the patient, how will you go about implementing this nursing order?
- What else do you need to know to effectively carry out this order?

Components of a Nursing Order

Did you have trouble answering the preceding questions? Even experienced nurses would, because this nursing order is incomplete. As you see from this example, nursing orders must be specific and detailed because many caregivers will use the care plan, and they need to be able to interpret the orders correctly. A well-written nursing order, whether on paper or as an electronic care plan, contains the following components:

- **Date.** Indicate the date the order was written. Change the date each time you review or revise the order. Why do you think it is important to have the date?
- **Subject.** Nursing orders are instructions to nurses, so they are written in terms of *nurse* behaviors. Therefore, the subject of the order is "the nurse." Because anyone reading the care plan should understand this, you do not actually need to write "the nurse" in your orders. For each order, think, but do not write, "The nurse will . . ." or "The nurse should . . ." This will help you to state the order properly so that it doesn't sound like a goal statement. Goals state patient behaviors; nursing orders state nurse behaviors. For example:

Goal/expected outcome	Nursing order
(Patient) Drinks 100 mL fluids per hour	(Nurse will) Offer 100 mL water or juice per hour on day shift

- **Action verb.** This tells the nurse what action to take— what to do. Examples of action verbs are *assist, assess, auscultate, bathe, change, demonstrate, explain, give, teach,* and *turn.* The following nursing orders show the action verbs in italics:

Teach the components of a healthy diet, 9/15, day shift
Offer 100 mL water every hour
Administer acetaminophen 500 mg orally at least 30 min before dressing change

- **Times and limits.** State when (e.g., which shift, what day), how often, and how long the activity is to be done. Consider the unit routines (e.g., visiting hours, mealtimes), the patient's usual rest times, scheduled tests and procedures (e.g., chest x-ray), and treatments (e.g., physical therapy). The following nursing orders show times and limits

Teach the components of a healthy diet *on 9/15, day shift.*
Offer 100 mL water *every hour between 0700 and 1900.*
Administer acetaminophen 500 mg orally *at least 30 min before dressing change.*

If you omit specific times, such as "day shift," the order may not be followed. It is easy for a nurse to think, "Perhaps someone else will do it (or has done it)."

- **Signature.** The nurse writing the order should sign it. A signature indicates that you accept legal and ethical accountability for your orders and allows others to know whom to contact if they have questions or comments about the order. If interventions are chosen on an electronic care plan, there may not be an actual signature. However, the name of the nurse who chose the intervention should be indicated in some manner.

KnowledgeCheck 6-5

List the five components of a nursing order.

Reflecting Critically About Nursing Orders

After writing the nursing orders, reflect on the interventions you have chosen. If you followed the process in the section What Process Can I Use for Generating and Selecting Interventions? you will already have thought critically and made some considered decisions as you were choosing the interventions and activities. The following are questions to guide your final judgments about the plan of care.

1. *Is the set of orders complete?* That is, do they address all aspects of the problem?
   — Do they address the etiology of the problem?
   — If the etiology cannot be changed, do the orders focus on the symptoms of the problem?
   — Have I considered physical, emotional, interpersonal, spiritual, and cultural needs?
2. *Is each order technically complete?* That is, does it contain all the required components?
3. *Are the orders clear, specific, and precise?* If you have included all the required components, the orders will usually provide specific enough directions (e.g., when, how often, and so on) to be useful to other nurses. Avoid vague language. For example, "Offer emotional support" is too general to provide direction for care. One nurse might think this means to ask the client about his family, another might sit quietly with the patient, and still another might use a therapeutic statement such as, "This must be difficult for you." Ask yourself, "Would all nurses interpret this order in the same way? Would they all do the same thing after reading it?"
4. *Is the order individualized for this particular patient?* For example, even if you have written an order to "Offer 100 mL fluids every hr," it is even better if you make a note of the kinds of fluids the patient likes or can tolerate.

Toward Evidence-Based Practice

Paradis, V., Cossette, S., Frasure-Smith, N., Heppell, S., & Guertin, M-C. (2010). The efficacy of a motivational nursing intervention based on the stages of change on self-care in heart failure patients. *Journal of Cardiovascular Nursing*, 25(2), 130–141.

It is known that adherence to self-care recommendations is not optimal in heart failure patients. This study evaluated the effect of a specific type of motivational interviewing based on the stages of change (MISC). Thirty patients were randomly assigned to an experimental (EG) or control group. The EG patients each received one in-person intervention and two phone interventions. The effect of the interventions was evaluated on five self-care outcomes specific to heart failure. In the group receiving the interventions, significant results were obtained regarding patients' confidence in performing self-care specific to heart failure. Researchers concluded that an MISC intervention is useful in increasing patients' confidence in self-care and has the potential to improve self-care.

1. Based on this brief report, what facts do you know about the 30 patients who took part in the study?

2. Which of the following statements is most accurate based on the information in this report?
   a. The MISC intervention increased patient confidence in self-care.
   b. The MISC intervention increased patient confidence in self-care related to heart failure

3. If you wanted to begin using the MISC intervention to increase confidence in self-care for all heart failure patients on your unit, which of the following additional information would be most important to know?
   a. Did the same nurse provide the interventions to all the EG patients?
   b. How many patients were men and how many were women?
   c. Does increased confidence in self-care actually result in better performance of self-care?

4. Which of the following questions would be the best to use as the basis for a future related study? Why?
   a. Did the same nurse provide the interventions to all the EG patients?
   b. How many patients were men and how many were women?
   c. Do increased confidence in self-care actually result in better performance of self-care?

 Go to Student Resources: Chapter 6, **Toward Evidence-Based Practice Suggested Responses,** on DavisPlus.

5. *Are the orders concise?* Long, complex statements may be unclear. Keep the orders as brief as possible without sacrificing clarity and specificity. If the patient requires complex procedures (e.g., insertion of a urinary catheter), don't write the details of the procedure on the care plan. Simply refer to the source of instructions for the procedure: perhaps an agency procedure manual, or a list of instructions to be found at the bedside. You will, however, need to write in the care plan any modifications to a procedure (e.g., "Do not use alcohol; client's skin is very dry").

6. *Which orders have priority?* Which nursing orders must be implemented immediately? Which must be done on this shift? Which must be done today? If possible, write them in priority order. In Chapter 4 you learned about frameworks for prioritizing nursing diagnoses (e.g., Maslow's hierarchy, problem urgency, future consequences, and patient preference). You can use these same frameworks to help you prioritize nursing orders.

If you have followed the recommended processes and reflected critically on your interventions, you should have a holistic plan of care individualized to meet the client's needs.

To explore learning resources for this chapter,

 Go to Davis*Plus* at DavisPl.us/Wilkinson3.

Chapter Resources for Chapter 6:

> **Response sheets for all learning activities**
> **Resources for Caregivers and Health Professionals**
> **Reading More About Nursing Process: Planning Interventions (suggested readings)**
> **Concept Map of chapter content**

Interactive Case Studies

NCLEX-Style and Chapter Review Questions

Chapter Overview Podcasts

For references cited in this chapter,

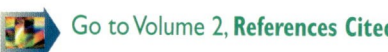 Go to Volume 2, **References Cited.**

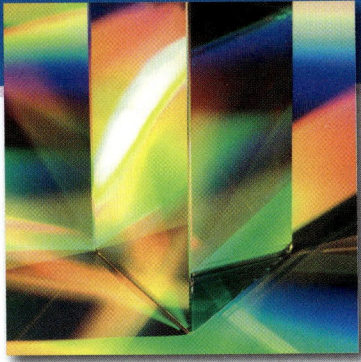
Nursing Process: Implementation & Evaluation

Learning Outcomes

After completing this chapter, you should be able to:

➤ Define implementation.

➤ State the three broad phases of the implementation process (doing, delegating, recording).

➤ Describe what nurses do in the implementation phase of the nursing process.

➤ Define the terms *delegation* and *supervision*.

➤ Identify and describe the "five rights" of delegation.

➤ Explain how standards and criteria are used in evaluation.

➤ Explain how structure, process, and outcomes evaluation are related.

➤ Distinguish between ongoing, intermittent, and terminal evaluation.

➤ Describe a process for evaluating client health status (outcomes) after interventions.

➤ Describe a process for evaluating the effectiveness of the nursing care plan.

➤ List variables that may influence the effectiveness of a nursing intervention; state which ones the nurse can and cannot control.

➤ Discuss the importance of nurses' involvement in evaluating the quality of care in an organization.

Key Concepts

Evaluation

Implementation

Quality improvement

Related Concepts

See the Concept Map, on Davis*Plus*.

Meet Your Patients

Patient 1. Jeannette Wu is a frail 80-year-old woman who is in the hospital after surgical repair of a fractured hip 4 days ago. Because of her overall fragile health and some postsurgery confusion, her recovery is slower than usual. One of her nursing diagnoses is Self-Care Deficit (Bathing, Dressing, and Toileting) related to weakness, pain, confusion, and decreased mobility. Her nursing orders (NIC) include Bathing and Self-Care: Activities of Daily Living (ADLs). As the nurse is helping a nursing assistive personnel (NAP) with Mrs. Wu's bath, she notices a reddened area on Mrs. Wu's sacrum. Realizing that this may be the beginning of a pressure ulcer, the nurse observes closely and notes a small skin excoriation (abrasion) in the reddened area. She repositions Mrs. Wu to prevent further pressure on her sacrum. After finishing the bath, the nurse records her findings and enters on Mrs. Wu's care plan a nursing diagnosis of Impaired Skin Integrity related to impaired bed mobility and minimal

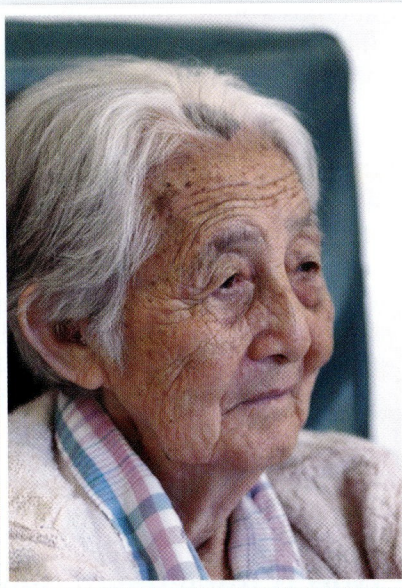

subcutaneous tissue. She writes nursing orders, including an order to observe skin over bony prominences every 4 hours, and then delegates to the NAP the task of turning and repositioning Mrs. Wu every 2 hours. The nurse also sends a consultation request to a wound care nurse specialist.

Patient 2. Patsy Jimenez is a healthy 25-year-old woman with no medical problems. She eats a balanced diet but does not exercise much. She and the nurse have created a plan to help her increase her physical activity. Ms. Jimenez will try

(continued)

to walk for 30 minutes at least 5 days a week. Each week she is successful, she plans to reward herself with a movie or a milkshake, which she usually avoids because of the fat content. The nurse would prefer that Ms. Jimenez not reward herself with food, but respects her decision and realizes that if it is to serve as motivation, the reward must be something that Ms. Jimenez values.

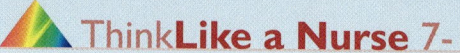

ThinkLike a Nurse 7-1

- For Jeannette Wu, which parts of the scenario illustrate *doing* by the nurse?
- For Jeannette Wu, which parts of the scenario illustrate *thinking* by the nurse?
- For Patsy Jimenez, who will be implementing (carrying out) the plan of care?

ABOUT THE KEY CONCEPTS

As you study this chapter, keep the key concepts of **implementation, evaluation**, and **quality improvement** in mind. Everything in the chapter relates to those concepts in some way and as you read, you will begin to understand how they are related to each other and to your role as a nurse.

IMPLEMENTATION: THE ACTION PHASE OF THE NURSING PROCESS

Implementation is the action phase of the nursing process. Of course, it involves thinking, but the emphasis is on doing. During **implementation**, you will perform or delegate planned interventions—that is, carry out the care plan. The implementation phase ends when you document the nursing actions; it evolves into evaluation as you document the resulting client responses (Fig. 7-1). In short, implementation is doing, delegating, and documenting. For professional standards relating to implementation see Box 7-1.

As in all phases of the nursing process, think of the client as a collaborative partner. Encourage the client and family to participate as much as possible in the client's care. When Mrs. Wu is less confused and better able to move about, for example, the nurse will encourage her to help with her own bath. Keep in mind that clients vary in their ability and desire to participate. In the opening scenarios, Mrs. Wu was able to participate very little, but Patsy Jimenez participated fully. Typically, the client implements health-promotion interventions, with little or no involvement by the nurse.

How Is Implementation Related to Other Steps of the Nursing Process?

Nursing process phases are interdependent (see Fig. 7-1). Each phase affects and is affected by other phases. Without the assessment, diagnosis, and planning steps, implementation would reflect only dependent functions, such as carrying out policies, protocols, and medical orders. The autonomous nursing activities

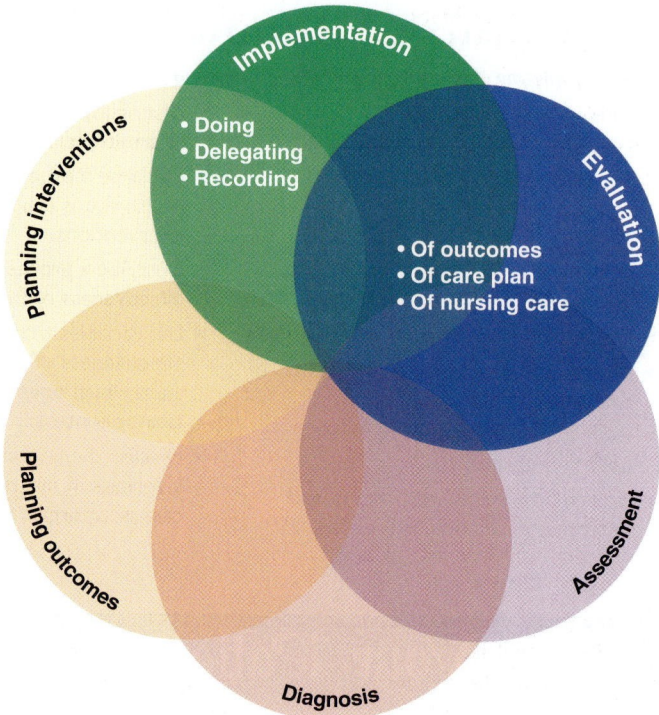

FIGURE 7-1   Nursing process phase: Implementation and evaluation.

performed during implementation are built on the nurse's reasoning in the previous three steps. Implementation overlaps in some way with every other phase of the nursing process.

Implementation Overlaps With Assessment Nurses use assessment data to individualize interventions for a specific person rather than just giving "routine care." For example, a nursing order may read, "Offer clear liquids hourly; patient likes tea." When taking the tea to the patient, you may discover that she prefers it without ice. This information allows you to individualize the nursing order further. Implementation also provides the opportunity to assess your patients at every contact. In Meet Your Patients, what data did the nurse obtain while bathing Mrs. Wu? When performing an ordered ongoing assessment, you are both

BOX 7-1 ■ American Nurses Association Standards of Practice for Implementation

Standard 5. Implementation

The registered nurse implements the identified plan.

Competencies

The registered nurse:

Partners with the person, family, significant others, and caregivers to implement the plan in a safe, realistic, and timely manner.

Demonstrates caring behaviors towards healthcare consumers, significant others, and groups of people receiving care.

Utilizes technology to measure, record, and retrieve healthcare consumer data; implement the nursing process; and enhance nursing practice.

Utilizes evidence-based interventions and treatments specific to the diagnosis or problem.

Provides holistic care that addresses the needs of diverse populations across the life span.

Advocates for healthcare that is sensitive to the needs of healthcare consumers, with particular emphasis on the needs of diverse populations.

Applies appropriate knowledge of major health problems and cultural diversity in implementing the plan of care.

Applies available healthcare technologies to maximize access and optimize outcomes for healthcare consumers.

Utilizes community resources and systems to implement the plan.

Collaborates with healthcare providers from diverse backgrounds to implement and integrate the plan.

Accommodates for different styles of communication used by healthcare consumers, families, and healthcare providers.

Integrates traditional and complementary healthcare practices as appropriate.

Implements the plan in a timely manner in accordance with patient safety goals.

Promotes the healthcare consumer's capacity for the optimal level of participation and problem solving.

Documents implementation and any modifications, including changes or omissions, of the identified plan.

Standard 5A: Coordination of Care

The registered nurse coordinates care delivery.

Competencies

The registered nurse:

Organizes the components of the plan.

Manages a healthcare consumer's care in order to maximize independence and quality of life.

Assists the healthcare consumer in identifying options for alternative care.

Communicates with the healthcare consumer, family, and system during transitions in care.

Advocates for the delivery of dignified and humane care by the interprofessional team.

Documents the coordination of the care.

Standard 5B: Health Teaching and Health Promotion

The registered nurse employs strategies to promote health and a safe environment.

Competencies

The registered nurse:

Provides health teaching that addresses such topics as healthy lifestyles, risk-reducing behaviors, developmental needs, activities of daily living, and preventive self-care.

Uses health promotion and health teaching methods appropriate to the situation and the healthcare consumer's values, beliefs, health practices, developmental level, learning needs, readiness and ability to learn, language preference, spirituality, culture, and socioeconomic status.

Seeks opportunities for feedback and evaluation of the effectiveness of the strategies used.

Uses information technologies to communicate health promotion and disease prevention information to the healthcare consumer in a variety of settings.

Provides healthcare consumers with information about intended effects and potential adverse effects of proposed therapies.

Standard 15. Resource Utilization

The registered nurse utilizes appropriate resources to plan and provide nursing services that are safe, effective, and financially responsible.

Competencies

The registered nurse:

Delegates elements of care to appropriate healthcare workers in accordance with any applicable legal or policy parameters or principles.

Modifies practice when necessary to promote positive interaction between healthcare consumers, care providers, and technology.

Assists the healthcare consumer and family in identifying and securing appropriate services to address needs across the healthcare continuum.

Source: American Nurses Association. (2010). *Nursing: Scope and standards of practice* (2nd ed.). Silver Spring, MD: Author.

implementing and assessing. What ongoing assessment was ordered for Mrs. Wu?

Implementation Overlaps With Diagnosis Nurses use data discovered during implementation to identify new diagnoses or to revise existing ones. What new nursing diagnosis did the nurse make for Mrs. Wu after bathing her?

Implementation Overlaps With Planning Outcomes and Interventions Patient responses to interventions provide the data you need for revising the original goals and nursing orders. As you care for a client, you begin to know her better, and her unique needs become more apparent.

Implementation Overlaps With Evaluation When evaluating patient health status and progress toward goals, you will compare the responses you observe during implementation to the existing goals (which were written in the planning outcomes phase).

Preparing for Implementation?

Implementation involves some preparation. Although the care plan will already have been developed in the planning stages of the nursing process, you should do some more planning just before implementing the plan—as explained in the following sections. Notice how important critical thinking and nursing knowledge are to this "doing" phase of the nursing process. To see how the concept *preparation* is related to the key concept *implementation*,

 Go to the **Knowledge Map**, at the end of Chapter 7, in Volume 2.

Check Your Knowledge and Abilities

Before beginning a nursing activity, review the care plan and reflect critically on the nursing and medical prescriptions. As a nurse, you are obligated ethically and legally to clarify or question orders that you believe to be unclear, incorrect, or inappropriate. At the same time, you must decide whether you are qualified to carry out the orders.

✚ You should ask for help when:

- You do not have the knowledge or skill needed to implement an order (e.g., when administering an unfamiliar medication, or when you have never performed an ordered procedure).
- You cannot perform the activity safely alone (e.g., helping an obese, weak patient to ambulate).
- Performing the activity alone would cause undue stress for the patient (e.g., giving back care to a patient with multiple fractures).

For a decision tree to help you check whether you are ready to implement care,

 Go to Student Resources: Chapter 7, **Resources for Caregivers and Health Professionals**, and follow the link for **"Decision Tree,"** on DavisPlus.

Organize Your Work

Because you will be providing care for more than one patient on each shift, you will need to make a time-sequenced work plan (worksheet) to prioritize your patient care for the day. Because of the need to control healthcare costs, you must work efficiently. To make the most of every patient contact, think ahead which interventions you can perform at the same time. Mrs. Wu's nurse performed a skin assessment while she was giving a bed bath. As another example, you might conduct patient teaching while assisting with breathing exercises. While changing a dressing, you might also use that time to show interest and concern for an anxious patient.

Many institutions have forms for this type of scheduling, or you may need to write your own list of "things to do" in the order you need to do them. For a worksheet you can print and use in clinical,

 Go to Student Resources: Chapter 7, Tables, Boxes, Figures: **ESG Figure 7-1, Worksheet for Organizing Nursing Care,** on DavisPlus.

At first, you may also need to make a time-sequenced list, the size of a 3 × 5 card, to help you organize your day. For example, it might read in part:

0700—Assessments, all patients, begin with Room 310.
0730—Ambulation: 315, 318
0800—Change IV, meds 310; check intake
0815—Meds 315, 318, 319; check intake
0845—Toilet and bath, 310

Key Point: *Room numbers take up less space than names on the form, but do not fall into the habit of thinking of your patients by room number or diagnosis. They are people, with names.*

Establish Feedback Points

You cannot assume you will be able to carry out a nursing order in exactly the way it was written. For example, suppose the nursing order states, "Help to ambulate in the hall bid." When you help the patient to stand, he becomes pale, dizzy, diaphoretic, and short of breath. Would you still carry out the order? Of course you would not. You must always be ready to alter the activity on the spot as the patient's responses demand. This means that you must look for **feedback** (how the patient is responding to the activity) as you perform care. In a sense, this is evaluating. However, because it is done before the intervention is complete, we call it *feedback*.

When organizing your work, identify points in each intervention where you want to pause for feedback. For example, if you are assisting with range-of-motion exercises, you might plan to assess for pain during movement of each joint and to assess for activity intolerance after exercising both arms and again after exercising the legs. Feedback is not always verbal; it could be a change in vital signs, skin color, or level of consciousness.

Key Point: *Notice how the concept of feedback relates to the concept organization, and how they both relate to the key concept, implementation.*

Prepare Supplies and Equipment

Gather all the supplies and equipment you need before you go to the patient's room. This allows you to work efficiently by eliminating the need to go to the supply room for items you have overlooked. Also, it prevents the stress to your patient that occurs when you interrupt a procedure to go get a needed item.

Suppose that when you insert an intravenous (IV) catheter, you "blow" the vein. You discover that you do not have another IV catheter; you have used the last one. What are your options at this point? Are there any *good* options?

The answer is that there are no good options. You might call another busy caregiver (provided that one is available) to bring you a sterile IV catheter. Or you could interrupt the procedure and get it yourself, making it necessary to leave the patient, and don another pair of gloves to prep another site. Either way, time and money would be lost, as might your patient's confidence in you. You may not be able to prevent "blowing" an IV; but by preparing ahead, you can prevent inefficiency and waste. In this case, that would mean being sure your IV tray is fully stocked before beginning the procedure.

Prepare the Patient

Before performing a nursing activity, identify the patient and reassess him to make sure the activity is still necessary and the patient is physically and psychologically ready for the intervention.

Check Your Assumptions This is just good critical thinking. Don't assume that an intervention is still needed simply because it is written on the care plan. For example, on postoperative day 6 after Jeannette Wu's surgery, the NAP is preparing to give her a bed bath, as instructed on the care plan (Table 7-1, section of plan dated December 18). However, Mrs. Wu has regained some of

her strength and is able to sit in a chair. So the nurse and the assistant agree that, with help, Mrs. Wu can bathe at the sink instead of requiring a complete bed bath.

Assess the Patient's Readiness To obtain the most benefit from an intervention, a client must be physically and psychologically ready. The hospital's critical pathway for hip fractures recommended a "help bath" on postoperative day three. The nurse did not assume Mrs. Wu was ready to progress just because the critical pathway dictated it, and a complete bed bath was given, as indicated by Mrs. Wu's physical condition. The following are more examples of ensuring readiness:

- Because her patient was anxious about his test results, a nurse postponed a teaching session until he was feeling calmer.
- While preparing to perform a painful dressing change, a nurse discovered the patient had visitors. The nurse waited until the visitors had gone to do the procedure.

Explain What You Will Do and What the Patient Will Feel Clients are not merely passive recipients of your care. Many interventions require their participation or cooperation. Caring nurses take time to explain because

Table 7-1 ▸ Portions of the Care Plan for Jeannette Wu

Date: 12/16/15 Care Plan Before Implementation on Post-Op Day 4

NURSING DIAGNOSIS	DESIRED OUTCOMES	NURSING ORDERS	EVALUATION
12/16/15 Self-Care Deficit (Bathing/Hygiene, Dressing/Grooming, and Toileting) related to weakness, pain, confusion, and decreased mobility	By post-op day 6 (12/18/15) will assist with bath and oral hygiene.	■ Complete bed bath daily in a.m. ■ Give prescribed analgesic ½ hr before bath. ■ Assist with range-of-motion exercises.	

Date: 12/16/15 Care Plan After Implementation on Post-Op Day 4

NURSING DIAGNOSIS	DESIRED OUTCOMES	NURSING ORDERS	EVALUATION
12/16/15 Self-Care Deficit (Bathing/Hygiene, Dressing/Grooming, and Toileting) related to weakness, pain, confusion, and decreased mobility	By post-op day 6 (12/18/15) will assist with bath and oral hygiene.	■ Complete bed bath daily in A.M. (NAP) ■ Give Tylenol #3, tabs i by mouth, ½ hr before bath ■ Assist with range-of-motion exercises tid. (RN).	12/16/15 Too soon to evaluate
12/16/15 Impaired skin integrity (sacrum) r/t pressure 2° immobility	*By 12/23/15, skin healed over sacrum; skin intact and normal color over all bony prominences*	■ *Turn and reposition q2hr; do not place supine (NAP).* ■ *Observe skin over bony prominences q4hr (RN).*	

continued

Table 7-1 ➤ Portions of the Care Plan for Jeannette Wu—cont'd

Date: 12/18/15 Care Plan After Implementation on Post-Op Day 6

NURSING DIAGNOSIS	DESIRED OUTCOMES	NURSING ORDERS	EVALUATION
12/16/15 Self-Care Deficit (Bathing, Dressing, and Toileting) related to weakness, pain, confusion, and decreased mobility	By post-op day 6 (12/18/15) will assist with bath and oral hygiene.	▪ ~~Complete bed bath daily in A.M.~~ 12/18/15 NAP help with bath at sink daily in A.M. Patient can wash hands and face and perform oral hygiene. ▪ Give prescribed analgesic ½ hr before bath. ▪ Assist with range-of-motion exercises tid (RN).	12/18/15 Goal met. Sat in chair for help with bath. Performed oral hygiene and washed hands and face.
12/16/15 Impaired skin integrity (sacrum) r/t pressure 2° immobility	By 12/23/15, skin healed over sacrum; skin intact and normal color over all bony prominences	▪ Turn and reposition q2hr; do not place supine (NAP). ▪ Observe skin over bony prominences q4hr (RN). ▪ 12/18/15 Requested foam and fatty mattress pad. ▪ 12/18/15 Refer to nutritionist for evaluation.	12/18/15 Skin excoriation over sacrum is larger: now 2 cm × 2 cm, and about ½ cm deep

it helps to motivate the person and gives him the information he needs to participate. Knowing what to expect helps to relieve anxiety, enables the person to cope with unpleasant or painful sensations, and promotes a trusting relationship.

KnowledgeCheck 7-1

▪ Why is it important to organize your work before implementing care?
▪ In addition to organizing your work, what other preparations should you make before implementing care?

 ThinkLike a Nurse 7-2

Suppose your patient, Jeannette Wu, has become incontinent of bowel and bladder. Because she already has Impaired Skin Integrity, the physician writes a new prescription to insert an indwelling urinary catheter (a drainage tube inserted through her urinary meatus into her bladder). Urinary catheterization is a sterile technique. You have practiced this procedure in the skills lab, but you have never actually performed it on a patient.

▪ As a student, what should you do?
▪ If you were a licensed nurse, what are some things you could do to ensure that both you and the patient are prepared for the procedure?

Implementing the Plan: Doing or Delegating

After both you and the patient are prepared, it is time to act. Nursing actions include both those you do yourself and those you delegate to others; and they may be collaborative, independent, or dependent (see Chapter 6 if you do not recall the meaning of these terms). During implementation, you will coordinate and carry out both the nursing orders on the nursing care plan and the medical orders that relate to the patient's medical treatment.

What Knowledge and Skills Do I Need?

There is almost no limit to the number and kinds of nursing interventions you might perform. The *Nursing Interventions Classification* (Bulecheck, Butcher, & Dochterman, et al., 2013), for example, lists 554 broad interventions (e.g., Hypothermia Treatment), each of which includes approximately 15 to 20 specific activities. For example, one activity for Hypothermia Treatment is to "remove patient's cold, wet clothing" (p. 224). During implementation, then, you can expect to use all the types of knowledge presented in Chapter 2: theoretical, practical, personal, and ethical knowledge, as well as knowledge about the patient situation.

You will also use various combinations of cognitive, interpersonal, and psychomotor skills to perform nursing activities (thinking, doing, caring). For example, when you are inserting an IV catheter, you need cognitive knowledge of sterile procedure, interpersonal skills to reassure the patient, and psychomotor skills to apply the tourniquet and insert the IV catheter.

 ## Think**Like a Nurse** 7-3

Use the examples provided in the preceding paragraph to help you write a definition for each of the following terms:

- Cognitive skills
- Interpersonal skills
- Psychomotor skills

How Can I Promote Client Participation and Adherence?

Different interventions require differing levels of participation. However, even a nurse-initiated intervention, such as inserting a urinary catheter, goes more smoothly if the patient participates at least to the extent of holding still while you perform the procedure. Many interventions (e.g., instituting a low-calorie diet) depend almost entirely on the patient's adhering to the therapy. In the case of Ms. Jimenez (Meet Your Patient), implementation of the intervention, walking for 30 minutes five times a week, depends entirely on the client.

People fail to follow therapeutic regimens for various reasons: pain, lack of understanding of the routines or their rationale, cultural objections, lifestyle difficulties (e.g., no time to exercise), fear of failure, embarrassment, or hesitation to ask questions of a "busy" nurse or physician. You can promote cooperation with treatments and therapies by following these guidelines:

- **Assess the client's knowledge.** Assess the client's understanding of his illness and the treatments and provide the necessary information.
- **Provide teaching.** Be as specific as possible with your instructions. Keep instructions simple and clear, and provide a written copy.
- **Assess the client's supports and resources.** You cannot assume that every patient has transportation to the healthcare facility. Even if they wish to follow the therapy, some people do not have enough money for food or medicine; some people cannot read printed instructions; some do not have family or friends to help with their care at home, and so on.
- **Be sensitive to the client's cultural, spiritual, and other needs and viewpoints.** For example, regardless of the need for dietary protein, some people do not like the taste of meat, poultry, or fish. Others might have religious or cultural objections to eating these foods. You will need to modify your recommendations to reflect client preferences and beliefs.
- **Realize and accept that some attitudes cannot be changed.** For example, regardless of the effects of obesity on blood pressure, a client will not lose weight simply because you tell him it is important. The client must *want* to lose weight.
- **Key Point:** *Information alone will not change a person's behavior.*
- **Determine the client's main concerns.** For example, you may be concerned that lack of exercise makes it difficult to regulate a client's blood sugar; the client's main concern may be that exercise makes her joints hurt.
- **Help the client to set realistic goals.** Clients usually more readily accept small, rather than drastic, behavioral or lifestyle changes. Perhaps a client with a child who has asthma cannot even imagine that she could stop smoking. But you may be able to convince her it would be better for her child if she would smoke outdoors rather than in the house or in the car (U.S. Environmental Protection Agency [EPA], 2009).
- **Talk openly and regularly about adherence.** Let the client know you understand how difficult treatment can be and that others struggle with adherence as well.

After reading this section, can you define the concept of *adherence*? Can you explain how this concept relates to the key concept, implementation?

What Should I Know About Collaborating and Coordinating Care?

For successful implementation, you need the skills of collaboration and coordination.

Collaboration As discussed in Chapter 6, **collaboration** simply means working with patients and other caregivers (e.g., physicians, respiratory therapists) to plan, make decisions, or perform interventions. Unlike delegated activities (discussed in the following section) true collaboration requires shared decision making.

According to the Quality and Safety Education for Nurses (QSEN) project, one of the competencies you should acquire in nursing school is the ability to function and collaborate on an interdisciplinary team, as well as with other nurses. This means, in part, that you will learn to be assertive in discussions about patient care. At the same time, you should recognize the differences in authority and power that exist on interdisciplinary teams and choose your communication style carefully, taking that into account (Cronenwett, Sherwood, Barnsteiner, et al., 2007).

Coordination Coordinating care includes scheduling treatments and activities with other departments (e.g., laboratory, physical therapy, radiology), but it is more than that. In the hospital, nurses are the professionals who have the most frequent and continuous contact with the patient, so they have the most complete picture of the person. Most other caregivers focus on only a very specific aspect of the patient (e.g., breathing, eating, surgical incision). You will be expected to put together the bits and pieces of information (e.g., the patient's response to physical therapy, dietary intake, emotional status, and vital signs) to provide a holistic view of the person. You will need to read the reports of other professionals; help interpret the results for the patient and family; and make rounds with other professionals to be sure that everyone sees the whole picture.

Outside the hospital, the health professional who has the most contact with the client usually assumes the coordination role. For example, if a client is receiving episodic care for ongoing health problems, the primary care provider (e.g., physician or advanced practice nurse) may coordinate care. For a client discharged home after a hip fracture, the physical therapist may coordinate care.

KnowledgeCheck 7-2

- What are some reasons that a client may not follow a recommended treatment regimen?
- List at least four things you can do to promote client participation in care or adherence to recommendations for treatment.

What Should I Know About Delegation and Supervision?

Delegation is the process of directing another person to perform a task or activity; it is a transfer of authority or responsibility. The person delegating retains accountability for the outcome of the activity (American Nurses Association [ANA] & the National Council of State Boards of Nursing [NCSBN], 2006). As a registered nurse, you will frequently delegate patient care activities to licensed vocational (or practical) nurses (LVN/LPNs) and NAPs, although in some states LVN/LPNs are considered accountable for their actions because they are licensed.

Delegating Is Not the Same as Assigning You may also *assign* tasks to other registered nurses (RNs) (e.g., as a nurse in charge tasks making unit assignments for the day). However, this is not delegation because those RNs are accountable for the outcome of their activities. **Key Point:** *Remember, you can only delegate down in the chain of command.*

Understand That You Cannot Delegate Nursing Care Decisions You can delegate only the responsibility for performing a defined activity in a particular situation. So, even though the nurse has delegated to the NAP the task of turning Mrs. Wu (Meet Your Patients) every 2 hours, it is *the nurse* who must assess her skin condition and take action if it does not improve.

Use NAPs Appropriately In some healthcare settings, NAPs are used inappropriately to perform functions that are legally nursing functions (e.g., administering medications) (Dickens, Stubbs, & Haw, 2008). Many nurses are concerned that inappropriate delegation is a threat to patient safety. Nurses may find themselves in a difficult position of caring for sicker patients, using new technologies, administering medications, and juggling

these activities with overseeing delegated work. According to the ANA, any nursing intervention that requires critical thinking or professional judgment cannot be delegated. However, the ANA takes the position that RN delegation and direction of specific tasks to NAPs in accordance with state nurse practice acts is appropriate, safe, and resource-efficient (ANA, 2007). Standard 15 of *Nursing: Scope and Standards of Practice* (2nd ed.) (ANA, 2010) states that the registered nurse "delegates elements of care to appropriate healthcare workers in accordance with any applicable legal or policy parameters or principles."

The Five Rights of Delegation

When deciding whether to delegate tasks, think critically about the task, the circumstance, the person, the direction or communication, and the supervision and evaluation. For a checklist to help you consider these five critical elements, or "five rights" of delegating,

 Go to Chapter 7, **Implementation and Evaluation Tools, The Five Rights of Delegation—Checklist,** in Volume 2.

Right Task

The first question to ask is, "Can I delegate this task?" As a rule, you should delegate an activity only if it meets *all* of the following criteria (ANA, 1996; ANA/NCSBN, 2006). The activity:

- Is within your scope of practice to perform and delegate, as defined by your state nurse practice act.
- Is within the LVN/LPN's or NAP's scope of practice.
- Is in accordance with agency policies, if they exist.
- Is performed according to an established sequence of steps and requires little or no modification from one situation to another.
- Does not require ongoing nursing assessments, interpretation, or decision making.
- Occurs frequently in the daily care of patients on the unit.
- Has reasonably predictable results.
- Does *not* require independent or specialized nursing knowledge, skills, or judgment.
- Is *not* health teaching or counseling.
- Does not endanger a client's life or well-being.

Examples of tasks you might assign to a NAP are bathing a stable patient, ambulating steady patients, obtaining routine vital signs, changing linens, assisting patients with meals, clerical duties, and transporting non-acute patients and specimens.

LPNs can usually provide care to medically stable patients according to an established plan of care; they can give you feedback about patient responses for patients who are expected to respond predictably. Tasks you can usually assign to an LPN include administering some medications (except for IV medications and some controlled substances), starting an IV infusion and administering plain IV solutions, and assisting with identification of blood units for transfusion. You would not assign an

LPN to start a blood transfusion, administer chemotherapy, administer or monitor parenteral nutrition, give IV push medications, or create and modify nursing care plans (Ayers & Montgomery, 2008).

Key Point: *Remember that you are assigning staff members to a task, not to a patient. You cannot delegate the responsibility for total patient care; and you cannot allow a NAP to delegate care to other NAPs.*

Right Circumstance

NAPs are being used in settings in which acuity and technology have increased while length of stay has decreased. This means they are caring for sicker patients. Even tasks such as bathing, feeding, and turning patients may not be appropriate if the patient is seriously ill. Before deciding to delegate, assess your patient to be certain that her needs match the abilities of the NAP or LPN. It is best if the patient is relatively stable (e.g., with a chronic rather than an acute condition) and does not need extensive help with self-care activities. If the client is very ill or if the results of the task are unpredictable, the task should probably not be delegated. For a tool to help you make appropriate delegation decisions,

 Go to Chapter 7, Implementation and Evaluation tools, **NCSBN Delegation Grid**, in Volume 2.

Right Person

You must also be sure that the LPN or NAP is competent to perform the task and that his workload allows time to do the task properly. Consider the person's experience, training, and cultural competence. The following are evidence of competence:

- The facility has documented proof that the person has demonstrated competence.
- The NAP has performed the task often or has worked with patients with similar diagnoses.

If evidence is lacking, you need to establish the NAP's competence. For example, you might observe and evaluate his performance, or you might ask the NAP, "How many times have you done this procedure?" or "Will you need help with this procedure?" Only a professional nurse can evaluate an LPN's or NAP's ability to perform a nursing task.

Right Communication

Right communication means that when you delegate, you should communicate clearly and specifically about each task. You can communicate orally or in writing, but leave no room for misinterpretation.

- **Explain exactly what the task is.** Include what to do and what not to do. For example, "Empty the catheter bag, and measure the amount of urine using the clear, marked plastic container"—not just, "Measure the urine."
- **Include specific times and methods for reporting.** For example, "Come tell me the patient's temperature every hour."

- **Explain the purpose or objective of the task.** For example, "Change Mrs. Wu's position every 2 hours to prevent bedsores; she is not able to turn by herself."
- **Describe the expected results or potential complications to expect.** For example, "She will probably cry out when you turn her, but that is more from fear than from pain," or "I have given her medications, so her temperature should be below 100°F by 0900. If not, let me know immediately."
- **Be specific in your instructions.** For example, "Let me know whether Mrs. Wu has any red spots or broken skin areas when you turn her"—not "Tell me what her skin looks like."

Right Supervision

Supervision is the process of directing, guiding, and influencing the performance of the delegated task. When you delegate tasks to a NAP or LVN/LPN, you or another RN must be available to answer questions and provide help, if necessary. You are responsible for providing supervision and evaluating the outcomes. This includes the following:

- **Monitor the NAP/LVN/LPN's work.** This is important to be sure it complies with agency policies and procedures and standards of practice. For example, after the NAP bathes a patient, you could check to see whether the patient is clean; or you might choose to observe for a few minutes while the NAP is working. Make frequent patient rounds and get regular reports from those you have assigned to do tasks.
- **Intervene, if necessary.** Many NAPs receive little training, so you may need to demonstrate some caregiving activities.
- **Obtain and provide feedback from the worker.** Give positive, as well as negative, feedback often. If performance is not acceptable, speak privately with the NAP to explain the specific mistakes that were made. Listen to the NAP's view of the situation. For example, there may have been too many tasks to complete in the time allowed.
- **Evaluate client outcomes.** Evaluate both the physical response and the relationship with the NAP. Ask the client for input after the care is given.
- **Ensure proper documentation.** Some agencies permit NAPs to record vital signs and other patient data. You are responsible for seeing that all necessary data are recorded and that they are accurate.

KnowledgeCheck 7-3

- List the five rights of delegation.
- List at least four characteristics of a "right task"—that is, a task that would be acceptable to delegate.
- As an RN, how could you establish that a NAP is competent to perform a task?
- List at least three ways to help ensure that the NAP will understand clearly what she needs to do when you delegate a task.
- List at least three things you should do when providing supervision to an unlicensed caregiver.

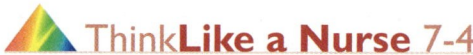

ThinkLike a Nurse 7-4

For your patient, Jeannette Wu:

- Which activity did the nurse delegate to someone else?
- What collaborative activities should the nurse consider?

Documenting: The Final Step of Implementation

After giving care, you will record the nursing activities and the patient's responses. Documentation is a mode of communication among the members of the health team, and it provides the information you need to evaluate the patient's health status and the nursing care plan. For a thorough discussion of documenting, refer to Chapter 18.

Reflecting Critically About Implementation

During the implementation phase, perhaps more than at any other time, nurses combine thinking and doing. You should always be prepared to modify the activity based on the patient's responses. Afterward, when you have some time to reflect, you can think critically about what happened (good or bad) and why. Use the following questions, or refer to the critical thinking model. (See Chapter 2, Table 2-1 if you would like other ideas.)

- What was done? Why was it done? What were the patient's responses?
- Did I forget to do anything?
- What was going on in the situation that may have influenced the outcome?
- What factors influenced my behavior (or others' behavior) in this situation?
- Would the activity have been more successful if I had had more knowledge or skill? If so, why did I not realize that ahead of time, and how can I avoid such lack of insight in the future?
- What assumptions or biases (mine or the patient's) contributed to the problem in this situation?
- Did I communicate clearly to the patient?
- Did I convey respect and caring?
- What could I have delegated? What did I delegate that I should *not* have? Why?
- After reflecting on it, what would I do differently in this situation?

Refer to Table 7-2 for examples that demonstrate how the reflection questions might be used in a clinical situation.

Toward Evidence-Based Practice

Read about the following studies, and then answer the questions at the end of the box.

> Potter, P., Deshields, T., & Kuhrik, M. (2010). **Delegation practices between registered nurses and nursing assistive personnel.** *Journal of Nursing Management, 18*(2), 157–165.

The authors of this qualitative study conducted a series of small-group, semi-structured interviews with ten RNs and six NAPs. They asked participants to describe their experiences of delegation practices on their units, and then analyzed transcripts of the interviews. Participants described conflict as a central theme. Researchers concluded that successful delegation depends on the quality of RN and NAP working relationships, timely ongoing communication, initiative, and a willingness to collaborate.

> Standing, T., & Anthony, M. K. (2008). **Delegation: What it means to acute care nurses.** *Applied Nursing Research, 21*(1), 8–14.

The authors of this qualitative study conducted 17 in-depth interviews with acute care nurses, both novice and experienced, to examine the nature of delegation. Nurses expressed frustration that they were being held accountable for the NAPs' tasks, while the NAPs themselves were not. Several nurses described NAPs' resentment of RNs. They indicated that the RN-NAP relationship and good communication are at the heart of delegation. The RNs recognized the importance of acknowledging the contribution of the NAP. The RNs pointed out that one negative aspect of delegation is that the NAP sometimes did not perform tasks well, or at all, and sometimes communicated improperly with patients. A positive aspect is that delegation allows the RN time to monitor patient changes, review charts, and focus on "more important things." They concluded nursing education should provide more content on communication and interpersonal relationships.

1. What similarities do you see between the methods used in the two studies?

2. What differences do you see in the participants in the two studies?

3. What similarities in results are reported?

4. With your answer to question 3 in mind, what skill(s) do you think you need to learn and practice to prepare for working with and delegating to NAPs?

 Go to Student Resources: Chapter 7, **Toward Evidence-Based Practice Suggested Responses,** on Davis*Plus.*

Table 7-2 ➤ Examples of Reflecting Critically About Implementation

SITUATION	QUESTION FOR REFLECTION	WHAT MIGHT HAVE HAPPENED?
The nursing order read, "Assist to ambulate to the end of the hall. . . ." However, the patient was able to walk only about half that distance before becoming too weak to stand.	What was going on in the situation that may have influenced the outcome?	Perhaps the patient was weak because he had not slept well the night before; or perhaps he had just had a long, tiring session of physical therapy.
When the patient became too weak to walk, the nurse called for help. Why did she do that instead of helping the patient to sit where he was, or instead of helping him back to the room by herself?	What factors influenced the nurse's behavior in this situation?	Perhaps the patient was very large and the nurse realized she was not strong enough to provide support. Can you think of other reasons that the nurse might have chosen that action?

EVALUATION: THE FINAL STEP OF THE NURSING PROCESS

Evaluation, the final step of the nursing process, is a planned, ongoing, systematic activity in which you will make judgments about:

- The client's progress toward desired health outcomes.
- The effectiveness of the nursing care plan.
- The quality of nursing care in the healthcare setting.

How Is Evaluation Related to Other Steps of the Nursing Process?

The patient outcomes stated in the *planning outcomes* stage must be concrete, observable, and appropriate for the patient in order to be useful as evaluation criteria. Appropriate outcomes, in turn, depend on complete and accurate *assessment* data and *nursing diagnoses*. You will observe and evaluate client responses during *implementation* in order to make on-the-spot changes in activity. And, of course, *interventions* must be *planned* and *implemented* to produce the patient behaviors that you evaluate. Evaluation overlaps greatly with the assessment step—both involve data collection.

   Key Point: *The difference is in when you collect and how you use the data.*

- *Assessment data* are collected before interventions are performed to determine initial or baseline health status and to make nursing diagnoses.
- *Evaluation data* are collected after interventions are performed to determine whether client goals were achieved.

Why Is Evaluation Essential to Full-Spectrum Nursing?

Evaluation is a key concept in this chapter, and it is an essential part of the full-spectrum nursing role for the following reasons:

- **The patient is the nurse's first priority.** The aim of all nursing activity is to achieve positive outcomes for patients. Evaluation lets you know whether your interventions are helping the patient as intended, and guides your next actions. No matter how carefully and conscientiously you implement, if the intervention does not help the patient achieve desired outcomes, you may need to revise the plan of care.

- **Evaluation helps nurses to conserve scarce resources.** Healthcare resources are limited and fewer nurses are hired to care for more and sicker patients. Workloads are heavy. Therefore, nursing time must be used wisely. Evaluation allows you to discard interventions that are not working well and focus on more effective, and perhaps more cost-effective, ones.

- **Professional standards of practice require evaluation.** For an example, see the ANA practice standards in Box 7-2.

- **The ANA Code of Ethics requires evaluation.** "The nurse's primary commitment is to the recipient of nursing and healthcare services—the patient—whether the recipient is an individual, a family, a group, or a community. . . . The nurse has a responsibility to implement and maintain standards of professional nursing practice. The nurse should participate in planning, establishing, implementing, and evaluating review mechanisms designed to safeguard patients and nurses, such as peer review processes or committees, credentialing processes, quality improvement initiatives, and ethics committees" (ANA, 2001, Section 2.1 and Standard 3.4).

- **The Joint Commission and professional standards review organizations (PSROs) require evaluation.** These organizations use outcomes and performance measures to evaluate the quality of care in healthcare institutions. They conceptualize quality of care as the degree to which health services increase the likelihood of desired health outcomes.

- **Evaluation helps demonstrate the value of nursing.** Linking nursing interventions to achievement of client outcomes demonstrates the value of nursing. In today's competitive healthcare market, that is essential for ensuring continued funding for nursing services, education, and research.

BOX 7-2 ■ ANA Standards of Practice for Evaluation

Standard 6. Evaluation

The registered nurse evaluates progress toward attainment of outcomes.

Competencies

The registered nurse:

Conducts a systematic, ongoing, and criterion-based evaluation of the outcomes in relation to the structures and processes prescribed by the plan of care and the indicated timeline.

Collaborates with the healthcare consumer and others involved in the care or situation in the evaluation process.

Evaluates, in partnership with the healthcare consumer, the effectiveness of the planned strategies in relation to the healthcare consumer's responses and attainment of the expected outcomes.

Uses ongoing assessment data to revise the diagnoses, outcomes, the plan, and the implementation, as needed.

Disseminates the results to the healthcare consumer, family, and others involved, in accordance with federal and state regulations.

Participates in assessing and assuring the responsible and appropriate use of interventions in order to minimize unwarranted or unwanted treatment and healthcare consumer suffering.

Documents the results of the evaluation.

Source: American Nurses Association. (2010). *Nursing: Scope and standards of practice* (2nd ed.). Silver Spring, MD: Author.

- **Evaluation demonstrates caring and responsibility.** Without evaluation, you would not know whether your care was effective. Examining outcomes implies that you care about how your activities affect your clients.
- **Quality and Safety Education for Nurses (QSEN).** This task force includes quality improvement, which involves evaluation, as one of the competencies to be achieved during your education in nursing.

How Are Standards and Criteria Used in Evaluation?

In a broad sense, evaluation is the systematic process of judging the quality or value of something by comparing it with one or more standards or criteria. In our daily lives, we evaluate many things: for example, a meal, a TV program, an insurance policy we are thinking of buying. **Key Point:** *However, for formal evaluation, you must decide* in advance *which standards and criteria you will use.*

As you learned in Chapter 1, **standards** represent expected or accepted levels of performance; they provide a model of what ought to be done. In nursing, standards

are used to describe quality nursing care. The ANA's standards of practice are a good example of broadly written standards (see Boxes 7-1 and 7-2).

Notice that each of the ANA standards includes a set of measurement criteria, called competencies, to help describe the standard. **Criteria** are measurable or observable characteristics, properties, attributes, or qualities. They describe the specific skills, knowledge, behaviors, and attitudes that are desired or expected. Judges at a diving competition, for example, might evaluate a dive by using criteria for difficulty, technique, and style.

The patient goals and outcomes discussed in Chapter 5 are also examples of criteria. As you learned there, these criteria should be concrete and specific enough to serve as guides for collecting evaluation data. In addition, they should be reliable and valid. A criterion is **reliable** if it yields consistent results—that is, the same results every time, regardless of who uses it. For example, suppose you and another nurse measure a patient's temperature by (1) using an oral thermometer and (2) placing the back of your hand on the patient's forehead. Which method would probably give the same (or nearly same) results every time? As you probably concluded, the oral thermometer is more reliable.

A criterion is **valid** if it is really measuring what it was intended to measure. For example, fever is often used as a criterion for concluding that a person has an infection. However, if used alone, it is not a valid indicator because (1) other conditions, such as dehydration, can cause a fever and (2) elevated temperature is not present in all infections. However, validity of that criterion is increased when you use additional criteria (e.g., elevated white blood cell count, presence of signs of infection, such as redness and pus).

🔺 ThinkLike a Nurse 7-5

- The outcome "Patient will not complain of pain" by itself is not a valid criterion for measuring pain. Why? What would be a more valid criterion for pain?
- A criterion reads, "Measures client vital signs once per shift, or as prescribed." For which of the following standards would it be valid (that is, which conclusion could you draw if you knew that a nurse measured the vital signs once per shift, or as prescribed)?
  Follows unit policies.
  Performs skills accurately.

What Are the Types of Evaluation

Evaluation is categorized according to (1) what is being evaluated (structures, processes, or outcomes) and (2) frequency and time of evaluation.

Evaluation of Structures, Processes, and Outcomes

Structures, processes and outcomes all work together to affect care; however, each requires different criteria and methods of evaluation.

Structure evaluation focuses on the setting in which care is provided. It explores the effect of organizational characteristics on the quality of care. It requires standards and data about policies, procedures, fiscal resources, physical facilities and equipment, and number and qualifications of personnel. Examples of criteria for structure evaluation include the following:

At least one registered nurse is present on each unit at all times.
A resuscitation cart is available on each floor.

Process evaluation focuses on the manner in which care is given—the activities performed by nurses (and other personnel). It explores whether the care was relevant to patient needs, appropriate, complete, and timely. Your instructor uses process evaluation to evaluate your clinical performance. Your clinical evaluation describes what you did and how well you did it. As a rule, it does not describe the *results* of your activities. Examples of criteria for process evaluation include the following:

Protects patient's privacy when performing procedures.
Washes hands before each patient contact.

Outcomes evaluation focuses on observable or measurable changes in the patient's health status that result from the care given. Although structure and process are important to quality, the most important aspect is improvement in patient health status. The evaluation step of the nursing process uses outcomes evaluation. Examples of outcomes criteria include the following:

Patient will walk, assisted, to end of hall by postoperative day 5.
Patient reports pain less than 4 on a scale of 1 to 10 within 1 hour after analgesic administration.

Outcomes evaluation is also used when evaluating quality of care in an organization. When used for that purpose, the criteria also state the percentage of clients expected to have the outcome when care is satisfactory—as in the following example:

Post-catheterization urinary tract infection does not occur.
Expected compliance: 100%

This means that the criterion would be met only if no patients developed a urinary tract infection after being catheterized.

Ongoing, Intermittent, and Terminal Evaluation

Evaluation begins as soon as you have completed the first nursing activity and continues during each client contact until all goals are achieved or the client is discharged from nursing care. The client's status determines how often you evaluate. A critically ill patient may need a nurse constantly at the bedside; after a patient undergoes surgery, you may measure vital signs every 15 minutes; as the patient nears discharge, you may evaluate once a day. In long-term care settings, in contrast, residents often have chronic health problems that require evaluation over an extended period of time.

Most care is provided by LVN/LPNs and NAPs, and the RN may participate in weekly care conferences to evaluate the resident's response to the current plan of care.

You will perform **ongoing evaluation** while implementing, immediately after an intervention, and at each patient contact. In contrast, **intermittent evaluation** is performed at specified times. Both kinds of evaluation enable you to judge the progress toward goal achievement and to modify the care plan as needed. Goals and expected outcomes should designate times for collecting evaluation data. For example:

Will rate pain as < 3 on a scale of 1 to 10 *within 1 hr after medication.*
Will lose 1 lb *per week* until weight of 125 lb is achieved.
By the second home visit, mother will demonstrate proper techniques for breastfeeding.

Terminal evaluation describes the client's health status and progress toward goals at the time of discharge. Most institutions have special discharge forms for terminal evaluation that also include instructions about medications, treatments, and follow-up care.

As in all phases of the nursing process, collaborate with the patient and family in the evaluation to the extent they are able. As the nurse, you are responsible for drawing evaluative conclusions; however, you should use input from the patient, the family, NAPs and other caregivers (see Box 7-2).

 Think**Like a Nurse** 7-6

For each of the following goals, when or how often should the nurse collect evaluation data?

- Will rate pain as < 3 on scale of 1 to 10 within 1 hr after medication.
- Will lose 1 lb per week until weight of 125 lb is achieved.
- By the second home visit, mother will demonstrate proper techniques for breastfeeding.

Knowledge Check 7-4

- Explain what is evaluated in each of the following types of evaluation (i.e., the focus of each type of evaluation): structure, process, and outcomes.
- Identify what is evaluated using the following criteria: structure, process, or outcomes.
    In the Emergency Department the time from patient sign-in to assessment by a healthcare worker will be less than 15 minutes.
    A fire extinguisher is located in an accessible spot on each unit.
    No patients with indwelling urinary catheters will develop urinary tract infection.
- Define the following: ongoing evaluation, intermittent evaluation, terminal evaluation.

How Do I Evaluate Patient Progress?

Evaluation does not "end" the nursing process. It merely provides the information you need to begin another cycle. After giving care, you compare patient responses to the desired outcomes (goals) and use that information to reflect critically on (1) the care plan and (2) each step of the nursing process as it applies to that patient. When evaluating patient progress, you review the desired outcomes, collect reassessment data, judge whether goals have been met, and record the evaluative statement (Wilkinson, 2011). Figure 7-1 illustrates the relationship of the evaluation phase to the rest of the nursing process.

Review Outcomes

First, review the goals/outcomes on the patient's care plan. The goals and indicators you identified in the planning outcomes phase suggest the kind of assessments you need to make and provide criteria by which to judge the data.

Collect Reassessment Data

Next, assess client responses to the interventions. To minimize confusion, assessments made for the purpose of evaluation may be called **reassessment**. Reassessments are always focused assessments (see Chapter 3). As already mentioned, the care plan goals determine their focus.

- Suppose, for example, that the nursing care plan lists the following goal: "By 8/24/16, will walk, unassisted, to the end of the hall without pallor or shortness of breath." What kind of assessments would you make to know whether this goal has been met?
- Suppose the care plan includes the following goal: "By 8/24/16, will notify nurse as soon as pain begins." How would you obtain the data you need to evaluate this goal?

For the first example, you would observe the patient's skin color as he walked, observe and count his respirations, and ask him whether he felt short of breath at any time. The second example is a little less obvious. If the patient doesn't call you, you cannot assume this means there is no pain. You would need to ask him whether he has had pain (e.g., "I notice that you have not put your call light on. Have you had any pain at all today?"). If the patient does call you, you still cannot assume it is because of pain, or that he called as soon as the pain began. You must question to clarify, for example, "How can I help you?" "Are you in pain?" "When did it start?"

 ThinkLike a Nurse 7-7

In the examples in the preceding paragraph, which aspects of critical thinking (in the full-spectrum nursing model in Chapter 2) did you use in order to decide what data you needed?

Goals can be cognitive, psychomotor, or affective, or they may refer to body appearance and function. The nature of the goal determines the kind of data you need to collect. See Table 7-3 for examples of goal types and the kind of reassessment data they require. As in the assessment phase, you will collect data from the client,

family, friends, and health team members, as well as from the client's chart (e.g., laboratory results). The RN is responsible for evaluating goal achievement, even though someone else may have supplied the data.

Judge Goal Achievement

Next, compare the reassessment data with the patient's goals. Are the responses (actual outcomes) the same as the expected or desired outcomes? If so, the goal has been met. As always, get the patient's input. Ask her whether she thinks the goals have been achieved. You can draw the following conclusions about a goal or outcome:

- *Achieved.* The actual responses are the same as the desired outcome.
- *Partially achieved.* Some, but not all, of the desired behaviors were observed, or the desired response occurs only some of the time (e.g., the desired heart rate is < 100 beats/min, a goal that is achieved except for one or two episodes a day, when it is 110 beats/min).
- *Not achieved.* The desired response did not occur (actual outcome does not match desired outcome or goal).

Record the Evaluative Statement

Professional standards require that you record your evaluations. You may write an evaluative summary in the nursing notes or on the care plan, depending on the procedure specified by the institution. An evaluative statement should include:

- The conclusion about whether the goal was achieved
- Reassessment data to support the judgment

An evaluative statement for the pain goal "By 8/24, will notify nurse as soon as pain begins" might be:

> 8/25/16, 0100. Goal not met. Has not used call light at all this a.m. Restless and grimacing with movement during a.m. care. When asked, described pain as 8 on a scale of 1 to 10. ———— J. Hiam, RN

When using standardized outcomes (e.g., Nursing Outcomes Classification [NOC]) or electronic care plans, your evaluative statements may be different. In the NOC system, each outcome (label) has a scale and indicators (specific patient responses), numbered 1 through 5, which you can use to write goals (see Chapter 5). For example, a patient with a problem of decreased peripheral circulation might have this goal: "Circulation status not compromised." Using standardized language from NOC, you might write a goal (*desired* status) of:

> *Goal:* Circulation Status: 5 (5 means "no deviation from normal range" in the NOC scale).

Each of the indicators could also be made into a goal by adding the desired scale numbers, as follows:

> Systolic BP in expected range: 5
> Diastolic BP in expected range: 5
> Mean BP in expected range: 5

Table 7-3 ➤ Reassessments for Different Types of Goals

TYPE OF GOAL	INVOLVES	EXAMPLE OF GOALS	REASSESSMENT TECHNIQUES
Cognitive	Increases in patient knowledge	■ By 8/24/16 accurately describes schedule for taking medications. ■ By 8/25/16 correctly describes the procedure for pouring liquid medications.	Ask the person to repeat information or to apply new knowledge (e.g., to describe to you the schedule for taking her medications).
Affective	Changes in feelings, values, beliefs, and attitudes	■ By 8/24/16 expresses positive feelings for the newborn. ■ By 8/24/16 states he is only mildly anxious about changing his own dressing.	Observe client behavior reflecting values and beliefs; talk to the client about feelings and beliefs; observe nonverbal expression of feelings (e.g., laughing, crying).
Psychomotor	Patient's ability to perform skills	■ By 8/24/16, performs own dressing change, using proper aseptic technique. ■ By 8/24/16, measures liquid medication accurately.	Ask the person to demonstrate the new skill (e.g., change a dressing, measure a liquid medication).
Body appearance and function	Changes in body systems and functions	■ Heart rate will be 100 beats/min after ambulation to end of hall. ■ By 8/24/16 can dress self and fasten own zipper.	Observe functioning, examine the body, perform measurements, read laboratory reports (e.g., measure vital signs, observe skin color, assess for pain).

Evaluation statements are written exactly the same as goals, but the scale number describes the patient's *actual* status. So, if on reassessment the patient's blood pressure is quite low and he has orthostatic hypotension, the evaluative statement might be:

Evaluative Statement: Circulation Status: 3 (3 means "moderately compromised" on this NOC scale)

Figure 7-2 is a computer screen showing the NOC outcome of Acceptance: Health Status. The Initial Scale shows the initial assessment; the Expected Scale is the goal; and the Outcome Scale is the evaluative statement after intervention and reassessment. Did the interventions achieve the desired effect, or not? If you want to see a computer screen showing a single NOC outcome with a definition and indicators,

 Go to Student Resources: Chapter 7, **Tables, Boxes, Figures: ESG Figure 7-2,** on DavisPlus.

KnowledgeCheck 7-5

Using the following outcomes and reassessment data, determine whether each goal has been met, partially met, or not met.

Goal: By 8/24/16, will walk, unassisted, to the end of the hall without pallor or shortness of breath.
Reassessment data: 8/24/16. Walked, unassisted, to end of hall; states no shortness of breath, but skin color was noticeably pale.

Goal: By 8/24/16, will walk, unassisted, to the end of the hall without pallor or shortness of breath.

Reassessment data: 8/23/16. Walked, unassisted, to end of hall. Skin color pink; respirations 14/min; no dyspnea observed; states no shortness of breath.

Goal: By 8/24/16, will walk, unassisted, to the end of the hall without pallor or shortness of breath.
Reassessment data: 8/25/16. Walked halfway to end of hall before becoming pale and short of breath.

How Do I Evaluate Collaborative Problems?

If a patient's collaborative problem is Potential Complication of myocardial infarction: congestive heart failure (CHF), the logical goal is that CHF will not occur. Clearly, nursing actions alone cannot prevent CHF. Collaborative efforts are required.

Because collaborative problems are the responsibility of the entire healthcare team, goals for collaborative problems are not included on the nursing care plan, and the evaluation process is slightly different. The desired outcome for all collaborative problems is that no complication will occur. To evaluate, you will compare the reassessment data with established norms (e.g., normal temperature, normal electrocardiogram patter) and determine whether data are within an acceptable range. If the data indicate the client's condition is worsening, notify the medical provider.

Example: If a patient with the collaborative problem, Potential Complication of myocardial infarction: CHF, develops fatigue, dyspnea, a productive cough, or abnormal lab results (e.g., elevated blood urea nitrogen [BUN] and creatinine levels), you would suspect CHF and notify the provider.

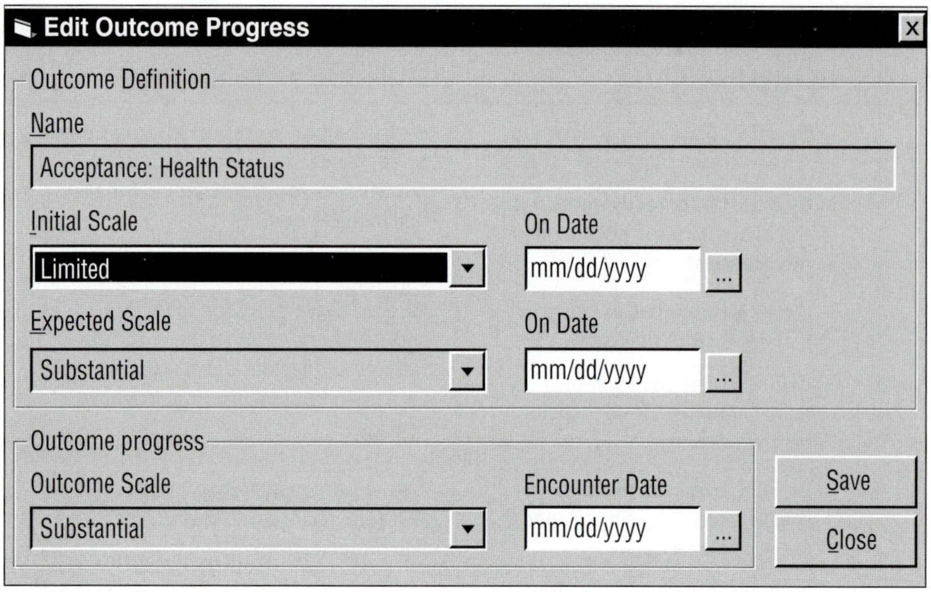

Edit Outcome Progress   ☒

Outcome Definition

Name

| Acceptance: Health Status |

Initial Scale   On Date

| Limited   ▼ | | mm/dd/yyyy | ... |

Expected Scale   On Date

| Substantial   ▼ | | mm/dd/yyyy | ... |

Outcome progress

Outcome Scale   Encounter Date   Save

| Substantial   ▼ | | mm/dd/yyyy | ...   Close

Explanation of Figure

Computer field	Nursing process terminology	Represents	Status recorded on computer
Initial scale	Initial assessment	*Actual* status *before* intervention	Limited acceptance of health status
Expected scale	Goal	*Desired* status *after* intervention	Substantial acceptance of health status
Outcome scale	Evaluative statement	*Actual* status *after* intervention	Substantial acceptance of health status

FIGURE 7-2 Computer screen showing outcome progress, using NOC. (*Source:* Courtesy of Ergo Partners, L.C., Boulder, CO. Used with permission.)

If the reassessment data are within normal limits, this does not mean that the collaborative problem is resolved—only that the complication has not occurred. As long as the patient has the medical condition (e.g., myocardial infarction), the collaborative problem (e.g., CHF) still exists. See Chapter 4 if you need to review collaborative problems.

Evaluating and Revising the Care Plan

After evaluating patient progress, you will use your conclusions about goal achievement to decide whether to continue, modify, or discontinue the care plan.

Relate Outcomes to Interventions

Even when goals have been met, you cannot assume that the nursing interventions caused the patient outcomes. You need to use critical reflection to identify factors that might have supported or interfered with the effectiveness of an intervention. Recall that organizational structures and processes can also affect patient care. The following are variables that can affect the ability of an intervention to produce the desired outcome:

- The client's ability and motivation to follow directions for treatment
- Availability and support from family and significant others
- Treatments and therapies performed by other healthcare team members

- Client failure to provide complete information during assessment
- Client's lack of experience, knowledge, or ability
- Staffing in the institution (ratio of licensed to unlicensed caregivers; number of patients for whom a nurse is responsible)
- Nurse's physical and mental well-being

Identifying these factors allows you to reinforce or change them. For example, if Jeannette Wu does not achieve a goal of "Intact skin over sacrum" even after being turned every 2 hours by the NAP, you may discover Ms. Wu's skin is more fragile than expected because her hydration and nutrition are not adequate. You could then take measures to support her intake of food and fluids, increasing the effectiveness of the turning intervention. Notice, though, that you cannot control all the variables that might affect the success of an intervention (e.g., the client's lack of experience, staffing in your institution).

Draw Conclusions About Problem Status

Whether you retain or remove a nursing diagnosis from the care plan depends on whether or not goals were met, as follows:

Goals met: If all goals for a nursing diagnosis have been met, you can discontinue the care plan for that diagnosis.

Goals partially met: If some outcomes are met and others not, you may revise the care plan for that problem;

or you may continue with the same plan but allow more time for goal achievement.

Goals not met: If goals are not met, you should examine the entire plan and review all steps of the nursing process to decide whether to revise the care plan.

For an example of electronic evaluation of problem status for a client with multiple nursing care needs,

 Go to Student Resources: Chapter 7, **Tables, Boxes, Figures: ESG Figure 7-3,** on Davis*Plus*.

Revise the Care Plan

To decide how to revise the care plan, you must review each step of the nursing process. You cannot merely discontinue the ineffective interventions and try new ones. The interventions may not need to be changed at all. When goals have not been met, errors in other steps of the nursing process may be the reason. To find a checklist you can use to evaluate the care plan and the process by which it was developed (Wilkinson, 2011),

 Go to Chapter 7, Implementation and Evaluation Tools, **Evaluation Checklist,** in Volume 2.

1. *Review of assessment.* Review all initial and ongoing assessment data. All steps of the nursing process depend on complete and accurate data. So if there are errors or omissions, you may need to revise any or all sections of the care plan (i.e., nursing diagnosis, outcomes, nursing orders). Also, the data may have changed since the care plan was written: The client's condition may have changed, or new data may have been identified.

2. *Review of diagnosis.* Even if there were no assessment errors, you may need to revise or add new nursing diagnoses. Perhaps the nurse who wrote the diagnostic statement did not communicate the patient's condition clearly, or perhaps it was not validated with the patient. This might have caused an incorrect focus for outcomes and interventions.

3. *Review of planning outcomes.* You will probably need to revise the outcomes if you have added data or revised the nursing diagnosis. If assessment and diagnosis are satisfactory, perhaps the outcomes were unrealistic, written too broadly, or had unrealistic target times. Or perhaps the client's priorities have changed, or the outcomes did not address all aspects of the patient's problem.

4. *Review of planning interventions.* You will probably need to modify nursing orders (a) if you determine that interventions were not effective or (b) if you have revised nursing diagnoses or outcomes.

5. *Review of implementation.* It could be that goals were not met because of a failure to implement the nursing orders or because of the manner in which they were implemented. Get input from the client, significant others, other caregivers, and the client records to find out what went wrong. For example, the person implementing care may have been tired, in a hurry, or menting care may have been tired, in a hurry, or abrupt with the client; or maybe he did not have the necessary skills. See Delegating and Supervising Care, earlier in this chapter, if you need a review.

Reflecting Critically About Evaluation

After evaluating the patient's health status and the nursing care plan, you should think critically about your thinking during the evaluation process. That's right: Think about your thinking, not just about your actions. The critical thinking model from Chapter 2, Table 2-1, suggests some questions you might use for reflection.

Inquiring

Is my evaluation statement clearly stated (goal met or not met, plus supporting data)?

Were my information sources reliable (e.g., was the patient being honest or merely trying to please me)?

Did I jump to conclusions about goal achievement? Do I need any other data to validate my conclusion?

Noticing context

What was going on either before or during evaluation that might have influenced my ability to gather data or draw conclusions (e.g., Was I in a hurry? Did the patient have visitors?)

What emotional responses influenced my conclusions about goal achievement (e.g., Would I feel as though I had failed if the goal was not met?)

Analyzing assumptions

What biases do I have that may have affected my ability to reassess or evaluate goal achievement?

Reflecting skeptically

Did I make evaluating a priority? Did I schedule time for it, the same as I do for interventions?

Could I have done it better?

What would I do differently next time?

The most common errors of evaluation are failing to:

- Evaluate systematically.
- Record the results.
- Use the reassessment data to examine and modify the care plan.

Because nurses are action oriented, it is easy for most to make a plan and take action. And most nurses regularly observe the patient's responses to the actions. But you will need determined effort to make time to *observe regularly and systematically* and *document the patient's responses* to your actions. Only in that way can you be sure the care has met the client's needs.

Evaluating the Quality of Care in a Healthcare Setting

As a nurse, you may be involved in evaluating and improving the overall quality of nursing care in an organization or a geographical area. At a minimum, your documentation will provide data that regulatory agencies (e.g., The Joint Commission, state boards of

Quality and Safety Education for Nurses

Learning About the Outcomes of Care

Chapter Key Concept: *Quality Improvement*

Competency: *Quality Improvement (Knowledge, Skill, Attitudes)**

Situation. Quality improvement (CQI) is an essential element of everyday nursing practice. You are in a unique position to identify problems in the patient populations for which you provide care, but first you must be able to quantify (measure) the outcomes and determine the cause (or root) of the outcome. For example, suppose you suspect that the number of central line infections has increased on your pediatric unit. You have noticed a lot of variation in how different nurses provide central line care. Knowing that variation in treatment often leads to variations in outcomes, what data do you need to support your suspicions? What outcome must you measure? What root cause should be assessed (i.e., what nursing practice may be causing the infections)?

Actions. If you identified the *outcome* as rate of central line infection, and the *nursing practice* as how central line dressing changes are performed, you are correct. Now, how can you obtain data about those two factors? Sources might include databases kept by QI, safety, and/or infection control departments. Some patient care units also track quality measures. The medical records department can develop electronic reports or you can review charts, or collect data prospectively.

Improving the quality of care is possible only with clear measurements. They provide insight into the problem and a baseline against which practice changes can be judged.

Think about it. Do you see how this box relates to the QSEN competency of QI? Notice that this QSEN competency is one of the key concepts of this chapter.

Source: Draper, D., Felland, L., Liebhaber, A., & Melichar, L. (2008). *The role of nurses in hospital quality improvement* (HSC Research Brief No. 3). Retrieved January 10, 2014, from http://hschange.org/CONTENT/972/ *For specific Knowledge, Skills, and Attitudes,

 Go to the QSEN Web site at http://www.qsen.org/ksas_prelicensure.php

---

nursing) use to determine whether nursing care meets nursing standards.

QSEN Competency Quality improvement is one of the QSEN competencies. That means that by the time you graduate, you should be able to "use data to monitor the outcomes of care processes and use improvement methods to design and test changes to continuously improve the quality and safety of healthcare systems (Cronenwett, Sherwood, Barnsteiner, et al., 2007).

Quality Assurance (QA) Programs QA programs are specially designed programs to promote excellence in nursing. Variations of quality assurance are quality improvement (QI), continuous quality improvement (CQI), total quality management (TQM), and persistent quality improvement (PQI). Whatever the approach, the goal is to evaluate and improve the care provided in an agency or for a group of patients. One hospital reports reduction in patient falls and medication errors, as well as improvement in nursing documentation after implementation of a QI program chaired by a staff nurse (Johnson, Hallsey, Meredith, et al., 2006). For more information about quality assurance, refer to Chapter 1.

Summary

This chapter has described (1) outcomes evaluation of *client progress* and (2) process evaluation of the *effectiveness of the nursing care plan*. Quality improvement involves evaluation of structures, as well as outcomes and processes. All are important because structures and processes affect patient outcomes. Adequate structures (e.g., staffing, money) and processes (e.g., policies and procedures) do not guarantee desired patient outcomes;

however, without them, it is very difficult to obtain good outcomes. For example, a unit could be well staffed (structure) and follow infection-control procedures carefully (process), yet have a higher-than-average rate of urinary tract infections (outcome). The reason may be that most of the patients treated on that unit have compromised immune systems, making them especially susceptible to infection. For more discussion of QSEN QA/QI evaluation, see Chapter 1.

 To explore learning resources for this chapter,

 Go to DavisPlus at DavisPl.us/Wilkinson3.

Chapter Resources for Chapter 7:
   Response sheets for all learning activities
   Resources for Caregivers and Health Professionals
   Reading More About Nursing Process: Implementation & Evaluation (suggested readings)
   Concept Map of chapter content
Interactive Case Studies
NCLEX-Style and Chapter Review Questions
Chapter Overview Podcasts

For references cited in this chapter,

 Go to Volume 2, **References Cited.**

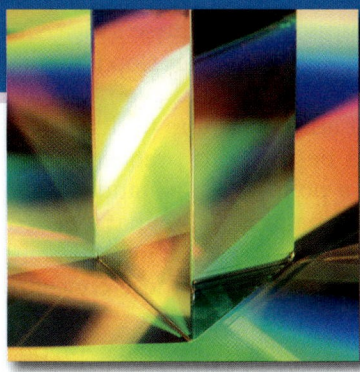

CHAPTER 8

Evidence-Based Practice: Theory & Research

Learning Outcomes

After completing this chapter, you should be able to:

➤ Define *nursing theory.*

➤ List four components of a theory.

➤ Describe how a nursing theory is developed.

➤ List the four essential concepts in a nursing theory.

➤ List three ways nurses can use nursing theory.

➤ Name three predominant thinkers who proposed theories of caring.

➤ Describe three nonnursing theories and their contributions to nursing.

➤ Define *nursing research.*

➤ Describe the significance of evidence-based nursing practice.

➤ Compare and contrast quantitative and qualitative nursing research.

➤ List three components of the research process, and explain their importance.

➤ Name three priorities in the process of protecting research participants, and explain the significance of these to the nursing research process.

➤ Describe the PICOT method of formulating a question to guide a literature search.

➤ Discuss the process of analytical reading of research reports, and explain its significance to the appraisal of research.

➤ Describe how to use nursing research in nursing practice.

Key Concepts

Evidence-based practice

Nursing research

Nursing theory

Theory

Related Concepts

See the Concept Map on Davis*Plus*.

Meet Your Patient

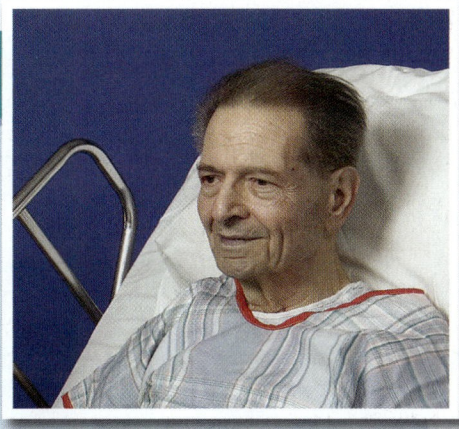

Imagine you are the charge nurse on the night shift at a long-term care facility. You hear the certified nursing assistant (CNA) and another person speaking loudly down the hall. You immediately go to see what has happened. You are startled by what you see. An older patient, Mr. Wilkey, is sitting on the bed of another patient, Mrs. Fredrickson, who is crying and shouting, "Get out! Get out!" Mr. Wilkey is tearful and looks frightened. He keeps repeating, "Where is Momma? Where is Momma?" The CNA is visibly upset and is grabbing at Mr. Wilkey in an effort to get him off the bed.

What are you going to do, and why do you think it will help? Don't be concerned if you don't think you know enough to answer this question. Before you read on, try to answer it based on the knowledge and experience that you *do* have.

There are two general ways to approach this problem. One way is to be upset with Mr. Wilkey and take him from the room immediately, explaining sternly that his behavior

is not acceptable and he must stay in his room. Another possibility is to ask the CNA to calm Mrs. Fredrickson while you talk quietly to Mr. Wilkey and gently guide him out of the room, not rushing him. While you are talking to him, you might ask, "Who is Momma? What does she look like? Do you miss her?" By the time you lead him to his room, you might realize he is exhibiting stage II dementia. You infer that he probably woke up scared and confused and began looking for his long-dead mother. Seeing Mrs. Fredrickson, Mr. Wilkey thought he had found his mother and crawled into her bed.

If you chose the first approach in the scenario, you were demonstrating **mechanistic nursing**, which is based on getting the tasks done. If you chose the second solution, you based your behavior on **holistic nursing**, which requires meeting the needs of the whole person. This scenario demonstrates the powerful impact of nursing theory and research on your daily practice as a nurse.

ABOUT THE KEY CONCEPTS

The overall goal of this chapter is for you to understand the concepts of **nursing theory, nursing research, and evidence-based practice** well enough to see how they are related and how they form the foundations for patient care.

Think of full-spectrum nursing as a jigsaw puzzle of concepts (Fig. 8-1). Initially, a nurse has an idea, which usually comes out of experiences in practice (the first puzzle piece). Perhaps the idea is something simple like: "Why don't I slow down and spend more time with the patients' families? It would really help them if I took more time." After seriously considering the new idea, the nurse may decide the idea is worth investigating with *research* (the second puzzle piece). The research

question might be: "How does spending more time with family members affect the quality of care the patient receives?" If the research supported the nurse's idea, she could then use the research findings to develop a **theory** (the third puzzle piece). The nurse could even take the research results to nursing administrators to determine whether the theory could be put into practice in the organization—perhaps as a policy or in a standardized care plan. That would be the beginning of what is called a **clinical practice theory**, a theory that is immediately applicable in the clinical setting. All of these concepts are essential to **evidence-based practice**.

You will also need a grasp of the related concept, *caring*. This chapter uses theories of caring to illustrate key points because we believe caring is central to nursing and influences all the actions that nurses take. You may recall that it is an important concept in the full-spectrum model introduced in Chapter 2.

TheoreticalKnowledge
knowing **why**

This chapter introduces you to nursing theory and research and how they form the foundations for patient care. It draws heavily on caring theory for examples. However, you will find other theories that pertain to specific aspects of practice in later chapters. For example, developmental theories are discussed in Chapter 9, theories of self-concept in Chapter 12, and family theories in Chapter 14.

 Go to Student Resources: Chapter 8, **Resources for Caregivers and Health Professionals,** on Davis*Plus.*

THE IMPORTANCE OF NURSING THEORY AND RESEARCH

Following are three examples that demonstrate how important theory and research are to the foundations for patient care.

The Framingham Heart Study The Framingham Heart Study is a longitudinal, multidisciplinary research project (*longitudinal* means done over a long period of time). It consisted of several studies carried out over 50 years (from 1948 to 1998) to identify the health and healthcare practices of one specific community: Framingham, Massachusetts. The results of the various Framingham studies influenced healthcare practices for diabetes mellitus, breast cancer, heart disease, osteoarthritis in older adults, and other disease entities. For example, one commonly accepted practice that came out of the Framingham study is the use of mammography to screen for breast cancer. There was a time when mammography was considered unreliable and unimportant. The Framingham project changed that attitude and, as a result, improved the healthcare of women.

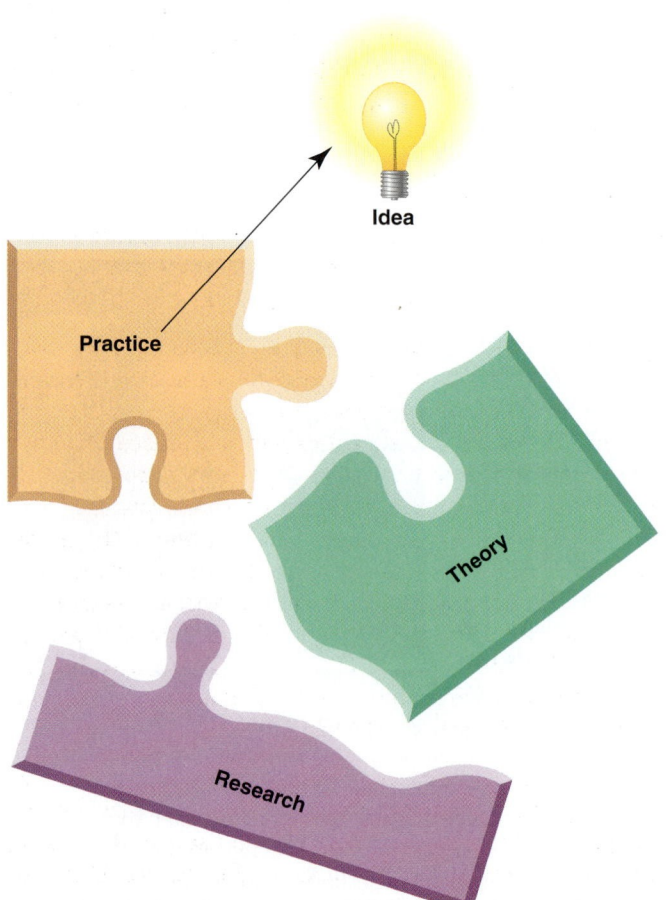

FIGURE 8-1 Practice, theory, and research are interrelated: A nurse has an idea, conducts research to test the idea, and finally develops a theory.

Watson's Science of Human Caring Dr. Jean Watson (Fig. 8-2) developed a nursing theory called the **Science of Human Caring** (Watson, 1988). This theory describes what *caring* means from a nursing perspective. It may not seem that nurses need to be taught how to care, but Dr. Watson and other nursing theorists found they did. Before the "caring theorists," nurses were somewhat mechanistic in the work they did, much like the first alternative for dealing with Mr. Wilkey (Meet Your Patient). A mechanistic nurse has a list of things to do, completes the list, and does nothing more. The "something more" behaviors often are the caring behaviors, such as singing to a frightened child or taking the time to teach a new mother for the second time how to bathe her baby.

This is not to say that nurses didn't care about their patients before Watson. The point is that a theory of caring (such as Watson's) changes the *focus* of nursing. Certainly Nightingale must have cared about the soldiers who were her patients. But what she wrote about and what she taught the nurses was a set of "things to do." Nurses were valued for the tasks they performed in patient care. Caring theories demonstrate the value of the non–task-oriented aspects of nursing.

Benner's "Novice to Expert" Dr. Patricia Benner, in the book *From Novice to Expert* (1984), proposed a theory that should be of special interest to you. This theory, which was explained in Chapter 1, describes the progression of a beginning nurse to increasing levels of expertise. You are a **novice**, or a beginning nurse, simply because you are new to the nursing profession. Benner's theory provides the information necessary to understand how you learn and perform your nursing

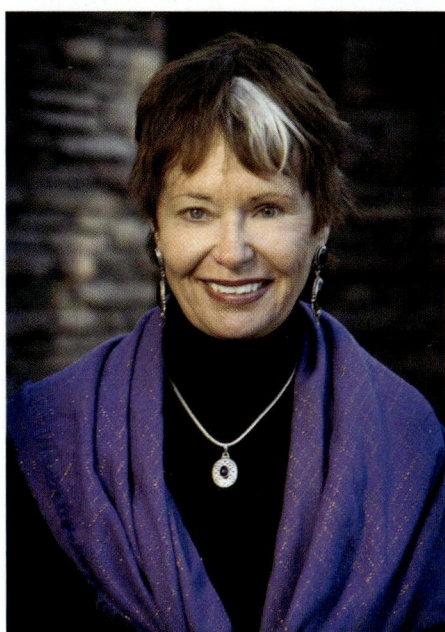

FIGURE 8-2 Dr. Jean Watson, distinguished professor and nursing theorist.

responsibilities. Benner's theory of caring is discussed later in this chapter.

KnowledgeCheck 8-1

- Compare mechanistic and holistic nursing. Select one of these concepts and describe a scenario in which it is used.
- Briefly describe the Framingham Heart Study, and list three diseases for which this study influenced care.

NURSING THEORIES

Florence Nightingale (1859/1992) stated that nursing theories describe and explain what is and what is not nursing. Therefore, it is helpful to learn them in the beginning of your nursing education. Before focusing on nursing theory, though, you need to learn a little more about theory in general. Exactly what *is* a theory? And how is a theory created?

A **theory** is an organized set of related ideas and concepts that helps us:

- Find meaning in our experiences (such as nursing)
- Organize our thinking around an idea (such as caring)
- Develop new ideas and insights into the work we do

Put simply, a theory answers the questions: *What is this? And how does it work?* Although a theory is based on observations of facts, the theory itself is *not* a fact. A theory is merely a way of viewing phenomena (reality); it defines and illustrates concepts and explains how they are related or linked. Theories can be, and are, changed.

What Are the Components of a Theory?

Theories are made up of assumptions, phenomena, concepts, definitions, and statements (or propositions). You can think of these as the building blocks of a theory.

Assumptions **Assumptions** are ideas that we take for granted. In a theory, they are the ideas that the theorist or researcher presumes, or takes for granted, to be true and does not intend to test with research. They are statements about concepts or relationships between concepts. For example, Watson assumed nursing had its own professional concepts and that one of them was caring. Assumptions may or may not be stated in a theory. For example, most nursing theorists assume but do not state that human beings are complex. One exception is Martha Rogers (1970), who states outright that human beings are unified wholes that are more than and different from the sum of their parts.

Phenomena Aspects of reality that you can observe and experience are called **phenomena**. They are the subject matter of a discipline (when used in this sense, they are often called *phenomena of concern*). Think of phenomena as marking the boundaries (*domain*) of a discipline—making one discipline unique from another. For example, for pharmacists, the phenomena of concern are medications: their chemical composition and their effects on the body. For nurses, the phenomena of concern are human beings and, more specifically, their body-mind-spirit responses to illness and injuries. It may seem a subtle difference, but Watson's theory of caring gave us the words and ideas for describing the nursing phenomena of concern in terms of *human beings in their environments.*

Concepts A **concept** is a mental image of a phenomenon. It is formed by generalizing an abstract idea from your experiences and observations of events, objects, and properties, and it exists as a symbol (e.g., a word or picture) in your mind. For example, what does the word *fever* bring to mind? From your own experience with fever, you know the subjective feeling that fever produces. You have the theoretical knowledge that it is an elevated body temperature; you know the physiology of temperature regulation, so you know what is going on in the body. You may have the visual image of a thermometer or someone who is warm to the touch and possibly perspiring. The word *fever* is a symbol for all of those ideas and images. It is a concept.

Concepts range from simple to complex and from fairly concrete to very abstract. Simple, concrete concepts are those you can observe directly (e.g., height, weight, gender, body type). More abstract and complex concepts are those you observe indirectly (e.g., hematocrit, brain activity, nutritional status). Abstract concepts are those you must infer from many direct and indirect observations (e.g., self-esteem, wellness).

A theory usually contains several concepts. For example, Watson includes ten "caring processes" in her original theory (Box 8-1). Each of those is a complex concept. To see how those caring factors have evolved in her theory,

 Go to Student Resources: Chapter 8, **Tables, Boxes, Figures: ESG Table 8-1, Watson's Caritas Processes,** on Davis*Plus.*

Definitions A **definition** is a statement of the meaning of a term or concept that sets forth the concept's characteristics or indicators—that is, the things that allow you to identify the concept. A definition may be general or specific. A **theoretical definition** refers to the conceptual meaning of a term, whereas an **operational definition** specifies how you would observe or measure the concept (e.g., when doing research). For example, for pain:

> *Theoretical definition:* Pain is an unpleasant sensory and emotional experience associated with actual or potential tissue damage.
> *Operational definition:* Pain is the patient's verbal statement that he is in pain.

Statements (Propositions) **Statements**, or propositions, systematically describe the linkages and interactions among the concepts of a theory. The statements, taken as a whole, make up the theory. In Maslow's theory, for example, two concepts are *physiological needs* and *self-esteem needs.* An example of a statement in that theory would be: "*Physiological needs* must be met to an acceptable degree before a person can attempt to meet his *self-esteem needs.*"

Theory, Framework, Model, or Paradigm?

In any discussion of nursing knowledge, you may hear the terms *theory, framework, model,* or *paradigm.* It may be difficult for you to differentiate among these terms because (1) they are so abstract, (2) they are defined differently by theorists, and (3) you may hear them used interchangeably in general conversation among nurses. As you progress in your career and education, you will need to pay more careful attention to the similarities and differences among these terms. For now, you can use the following basic definitions (*theory* was defined earlier):

A **paradigm** is the worldview or ideology of a discipline. It is the broadest, most global conceptual framework of a discipline. It includes and guides the values, philosophy, knowledge, theories, and research processes of the discipline. It is a way of thinking that is shared by a community of scholars who are studying and working on the same phenomena. Compare the two following examples:

- *The medical paradigm* views a person through a lens that focuses on identifying and treating disease. This lens causes you to look in depth at the person's "parts" (e.g., cells, organs).
- *The nursing paradigm* views the person through a lens that focuses more broadly on the entire person and how he responds to isolated changes in his cells and organs.

Key Point: *Paradigms are not theories; they are just "how we see things."*

BOX 8-1 ■ Watson's Ten Caring Processes

1. Forming a humanistic–altruistic system of values
2. Instilling faith and hope
3. Cultivating sensitivity to self and others
4. Forming helping and trusting relationships
5. Conveying and accepting the expression of positive and negative feelings
6. Systematic use of the scientific problem-solving method that involves caring process
7. Promoting transpersonal teaching–learning
8. Providing for supportive, protective, and corrective mental, physical, sociocultural, and spiritual environment
9. Assisting with gratification of human needs
10. Sensitivity to existential–phenomenological forces

Source: Watson, J. (1988). *Nursing: Human science and human care. A theory of nursing.* Publication No. 15-2236. New York: National League for Nursing Press.

A **conceptual framework** (also referred to as a *theoretical framework*) is a set of concepts that are related to form a whole or pattern. Frameworks (and models) tend to be broader and more philosophical than theories. As a rule, frameworks are not developed using research processes and have not been tested in practice. The relationships among the concepts are described in less detail than in a theory, and assumptions are not stated. Don't be alarmed if you can't tell the difference between a theory and a theoretical framework. The experts don't always agree, either. Many theorists, for example, classify the early nursing theories (e.g., Orem's self-care deficit theory and others presented in this chapter) as conceptual frameworks; others classify them as theories.

A **model** is a symbolic representation of a framework or concepts—a diagram, graph, picture, drawing, or physical model. The plastic body parts you have seen in anatomy class are models of the real human body; Figure 8-1 is a simple model of the relationships between nursing practice, theory, and research, for example. Many models are more complex than Figure 8-1.

A **conceptual model** (sometimes referred to as a *conceptual framework*) is a model that is expressed in language—the symbols are words. Figure 2-3 is a model of full-spectrum nursing. In comparison, the *description* of the full-spectrum model in Chapter 2 is a conceptual model or framework. In one sense, all models are "conceptual" because they all represent ideas.

For now, it is enough for you to remember these three points:

1. The terms *theory, model,* and *framework* all refer to a group of related concepts.
2. The terms differ in meaning, depending on the extent to which the set of concepts has been used and tested in practice and on the level of detail and organization of the concepts.
3. A theory has a higher level of research, detail, and organization of concepts than do models and frameworks.

 ## ThinkLike a Nurse 8-1

 Go to Student Resources: Chapter 4, **Standardized Language, NANDA-International Taxonomy II: Domains, Classes, and Diagnoses (Labels),** on DavisPlus.

Do you think this is a theory, a conceptual framework, or a model?

KnowledgeCheck 8-2

- Name the five building blocks of a theory.
- How is a paradigm different from a theory?

How Are Theories Developed?

To begin developing a theory, a nurse has an idea that seems worth exploring through research. As an example, Dr. Jean Watson had an idea about caring behaviors toward patients. Once the idea was clear in her mind, she performed research to see whether her ideas made sense. She validated her ideas to develop her theory. Once she had a research-based theory, she shared it with others, and it changed nursing practice.

Theories are developed through a specific way of thinking called logical reasoning (Alligood & Marriner Tomey, 2009). Generally, you can think of **reasoning** as connecting ideas in a way that makes sense. The purpose of **logical reasoning** is to develop an argument or statement based on evidence that will result in a logical conclusion. Nursing theories cannot be based on guesswork; they must be developed on a solid foundation of logical reasoning. The most commonly used types of logical reasoning are inductive and deductive reasoning.

Inductive reasoning is often used in nursing process. If you walk into a person's room and note that the patient has a temperature of 101°F (38°C), a pulse of 104 beats/min, and respiration rate of 20 breaths/min, you could reasonably *induce* (conclude) that the person is ill, possibly with an infection. Induction moves from the specific to the general. You gathered separate pieces of information, recognized a pattern, and formed a generalization. Remember induction by thinking, "IN-duction: I have specific data 'out there,' and I bring the data 'IN' to make the generalization" (Fig. 8-3).

Deductive reasoning is the opposite of inductive reasoning. Deduction starts with a *general premise* and moves to a *specific deduction*. Suppose you receive a call from the emergency department stating they will be receiving a new patient with acute pyelonephritis (kidney infection). Because you know what is involved in the general premise (pyelonephritis), you deduce the patient will probably have an elevated temperature and back pain. You have the "big picture" about what is true in general, and from that you can figure out logically what is likely to be true for a particular individual.

Understanding logical thinking, even on this basic level, will help you understand the thinking that goes into both nursing theory and nursing research.

 ## ThinkLike a Nurse 8-2

- Your patient is grimacing, groaning, and holding his hands over his abdominal incision. You induce that the patient is having incision pain. How could you be sure your induction is factual (true)?
- In the example of deductive reasoning (above) you deduced that your emergency department patient with pyelonephritis will have a temperature and back pain. How confident are you that this is actually so? How could you be more certain your deduction is correct?

The preceding exercise should demonstrate that inductions and deductions are not "facts" or "truth," but rather that they point you in the direction to go in seeking truth (reality). They also allow you to make connections between ideas when you are developing a theory. The more

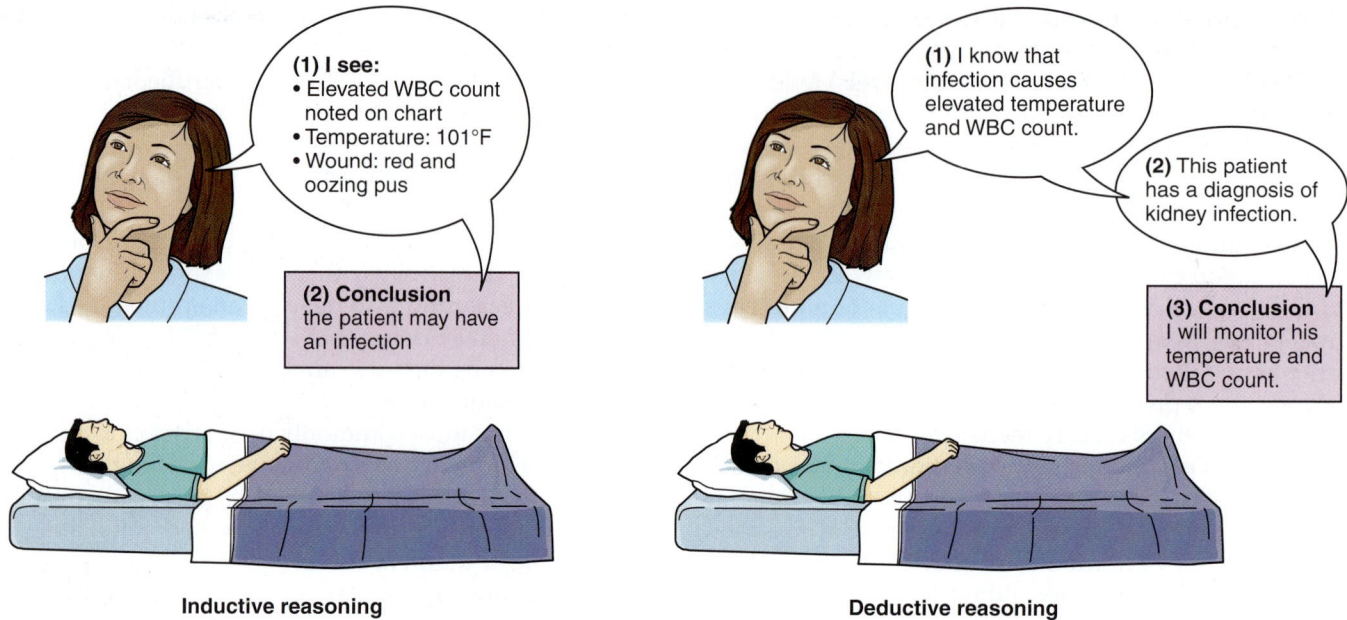

Inductive reasoning   Deductive reasoning

FIGURE 8-3 A comparison of inductive and deductive reasoning. Theorists and nurses in practice use both types of reasoning.

information you have to support your conclusions, the more confident you can be that they are correct.

What Are the Essential Concepts of a *Nursing* Theory?

Any nursing theory should address the four basic concepts that are said to be the phenomena of concern for nursing: **person, environment, health,** and **nursing** (Yura & Torres, 1975). Notice that these concepts further divide the puzzle piece for nursing theory into four more pieces (Fig. 8-4).

A meaningful nursing theory defines these four puzzle pieces and explains how they are related to each other. Consider a theory that does not include the concept of person. Such a theory would describe the needs of the *nurse* and the condition of the *environment*, as well as the *health* of the person. However, it would not deal with the *person's* reaction to her health or lack of health. As a result, the person's learning needs, fears, family concerns, or discharge arrangements would not be considered. That sounds quite mechanistic, doesn't it?

The following illustrates how Watson (1988) viewed the four basic concepts. In her science of human caring, she explored the concept of *caring* as it relates to the person, environment, health, and nursing. Watson focused heavily on the *person* and the *nurse*. She talked about the "transpersonal" caring moments that exist between the two. She presented the *environment* as another way to show caring: by keeping it clean, colorful, or quiet or including whatever promotes health for the person. All of the caring behaviors (see Box 8-1) listed in Watson's theory focus on improving the *health* of the person.

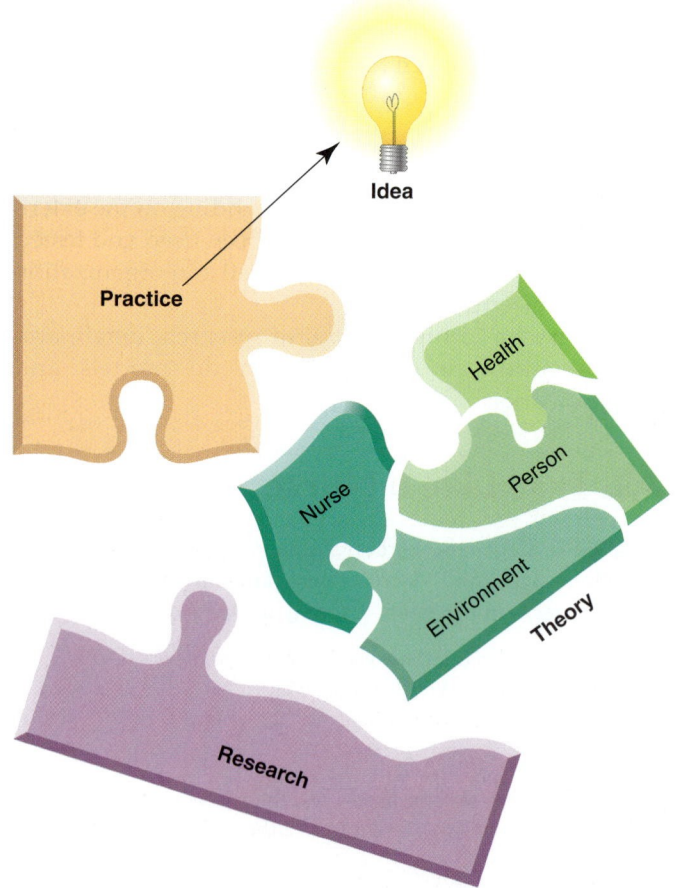

FIGURE 8-4 The four components of a nursing theory are person, nurse, health, and environment.

Observing nursing situations within the framework of the four components of nursing theory will help you understand the importance of each. This is very important because the finished puzzle reflects excellent (full-spectrum) nursing care.

ThinkLike a Nurse 8-3

Think of an experience you have had in clinical. Perhaps it was taking vital signs or bathing a confused patient. Describe how each of the four components of a nursing theory occurred in your clinical situation. Share your thinking with a classmate or coworker.

- Who was the *person(s)* involved (*person* refers to the patient or resident or the family and support persons)?
- What was the *environment*? A community center? A bathing room in a nursing home? The person's bedside in a hospital?
- What was the *health* condition of the person? For example, was the person seeking information for self-care? Critical? In pain? Ready for discharge?
- How was *nursing* involved? For example, was the nurse compassionate? Angry? Efficient? A novice or an expert?

KnowledgeCheck 8-3

- What are the four essential concepts in a nursing theory?
- What is the title of Dr. Watson's theory?
- Caring processes are critical to her theory. What is the purpose of the caring processes?

How Do Nurses Use Theories?

Nursing theories try to describe, explain, and predict human behavior. The case of Mr. Wilkey (Meet Your Patient) shows how the use of a certain theory might guide the nurse to more compassionate care. Think of a theory as a lens. You can see the stars more clearly if you look at them through a telescope than you can by using binoculars. As another metaphor, the lenses of your sunglasses remove glare, allowing you to see more clearly in bright sunlight but decreasing your ability to see in dim light. Theories offer a lens for looking at nursing, and in this way they affect your entire perspective. The theory you use influences what you look for, what you notice, what you perceive as a problem, what outcomes you hope to achieve, and what interventions you will choose.

In Nursing Practice

Nursing theories serve as a guide for assessment, problem identification, and choice of nursing interventions. They help nurses communicate to other members of the health team what it is that makes nurses unique and important to the interdisciplinary team.

Clinical practice theories very specifically guide what you do each day. They are limited in scope—that is, they do not attempt to explain all of nursing. A theory on human interaction directs nurse–client communication;

another theory provides a guide for teaching people how to be self-reliant. The following are other examples:

1. Nightingale's theory emphasized the importance of the environment in the care of patients. Her work affected the design and building of hospitals for decades.
2. Dr. Imogene Rigdon developed a theory about bereavement of older women after noticing (and having an idea!) that older women handled grief differently from men and younger women (Rigdon, Clayton, & Dimond, 1987). Hospice organizations all over the country now use this theory to work with older women who have lost a significant other.
3. Nola Pender's theory on health promotion (see Chapter 42) is the basis for most health promotion teaching done by nurses (Pender, Murdaugh, & Parsons, 2011).
4. Dr. Katharine Kolcaba (1994) developed a theory of holistic comfort in nursing, which provides a more holistic view than earlier theories of pain and anxiety.

In Nursing Education

Some schools of nursing use theories to guide curriculum planning, programs, and projects. These are frequently grand theories, such as Watson's theory of caring or Rogers's science of unitary human beings. A **grand theory** covers broad areas of concern within a discipline. A grand theory is usually abstract and does not outline specific nursing interventions. Instead, it tends to deal with the relationships among nurse, person, health, and environment.

A school using Watson's theory, for example, would include aspects of her theory in each class. A course might even be organized around the caring factors listed in Box 8-1. As another example, an inservice education director in a nursing home may choose a narrower and more specific theory (*mid-range* or *practice theory*) of comfort, using it to create policies and procedures and design educational programs.

In Nursing Research

Theories help generate new knowledge by suggesting questions for researchers to study. Researchers also use theories and models as a framework for structuring a study. Theories provide a systematic way to define the questions for study, identify the variables to measure, and interpret the findings. For example, Kolcaba tested her statement that comfort interventions, as defined in her theory, would improve the health of the whole person.

Who Are Some Important Nurse Theorists?

You will need to thoroughly understand the theories you use in practice and the one (or more) used by your school of nursing. As an educated nurse, you should also have at least a nodding acquaintance with the nurse theorists who have influenced nursing practice. The first three theorists below, along with the caring theorists that follow, are presented in detail because of their historical significance. The description of their theories is simple and applicable to what you do every day as a nurse.

Florence Nightingale

As you learned in Chapter 1, Florence Nightingale revolutionized nursing. When she went to the hospital in Scutari during the Crimean War, the soldiers slept on mats on the floor, where rats scampered and raw sewage flowed. Nightingale's "idea" was that *more men would survive if they had a clean and healthy environment and nutritious food (so that the body could heal itself).* That may not seem remarkable to you, but consider that the germ theory of infectious disease had not yet been identified.

Nightingale also was an outstanding researcher. She stayed awake late at night to keep records of what was happening at the hospital before and after she introduced her ideas (research). She used her research to develop her theory that a clean environment would improve the health of patients. Because of her theory and research, Nightingale dramatically reduced the death rate of the soldiers and changed the way the entire British Army hospital system was managed (Dossey, 1999). For links to more information about Nightingale,

 Go to Student Resources: Chapter 8, **Resources for Caregivers and Health Professionals,** on Davis*Plus*.

Virginia Henderson

Virginia Henderson began her career as a U.S. Army nurse in 1918. She also was a visiting nurse in New York City and then a teacher of nursing. Her pamphlet, *Basic Principles of Nursing Care,* published in 1960 by the International Council of Nursing, has been translated into 20 languages.

While a nursing student at Walter Reed Army Hospital, Henderson began to question the mechanistic nursing care she was taught to give, as well as the fact she was expected to be the physicians' handmaiden. As a teacher of nursing, she came to recognize there was no clear description of the purpose and function of nursing. She was the first nurse to identify that as a concern. Her "idea" was that *nurses deserve to know what it means to be a nurse.*

Henderson's 1966 book, *The Nature of Nursing,* described her theory of nursing's primary, unique function. She identified 14 basic needs that are addressed by nursing care (Box 8-2). Although the simple things on that list are commonplace today, they had not been identified as components of nursing care until Virginia Henderson did so. Henderson's (1966, p. 3) definition of nursing states: "The unique function of the nurse is to assist the individual, sick or well, in the performance of those activities contributing to health or its recovery (or to a peaceful death) that he would perform unaided

---

> ### BOX 8-2 ■ Virginia Henderson's List of Basic Needs
>
> 1. Breathe normally.
> 2. Eat and drink adequately.
> 3. Eliminate body wastes.
> 4. Move and maintain desirable posture.
> 5. Sleep and rest.
> 6. Select suitable clothes—dress and undress.
> 7. Maintain body temperature within normal range by adjusting clothing and modifying the environment.
> 8. Keep the body clean and well groomed, and protect the integument.
> 9. Avoid dangers in the environment and avoid injuring others.
> 10. Communicate with others in expressing emotions, needs, fears, or opinions.
> 11. Worship according to one's faith.
> 12. Work in such a way that there is a sense of accomplishment.
> 13. Play or participate in various forms of recreation.
> 14. Learn, discover, or satisfy the curiosity that leads to normal development and health and use of the available health facilities.
>
> *Source:* Alligood, M., & Marriner Tomey, A. (2009). *Nursing theorists and their work* (7th ed.). St. Louis, MO: C.V. Mosby.

---

if he had the necessary strength, will or knowledge. And do this in such a way as to help him gain independence as rapidly as possible." Henderson defined what nursing was in the 20th century. If you would like more information on Henderson,

 Go to Student Resources: Chapter 8, **Resources for Caregivers and Health Professionals,** on Davis*Plus*.

Hildegard Peplau

Hildegard E. Peplau was born in 1909 to immigrant parents in Pennsylvania. She was a psychiatric nurse and contributed much to nursing in general. She influenced the advancement of standards in nursing education, promoted self-regulation in nursing through credentialing, and was a strong advocate for advanced nursing practice.

Dr. Peplau's "idea" was that *health could be improved for psychiatric patients if there was a more effective way to communicate with them.* You may feel this is an unnecessary theory because nurses communicate with patients all the time. But remember that in the early 1900s actually talking to and developing a personal relationship with psychiatric patients simply was not done. Psychiatric patients did not have the benefit of psychotropic drugs currently available to manage their symptoms. They were often agitated and extremely difficult to communicate with.

Peplau's research showed that developing a relationship with psychiatric patients does make their treatment more effective. She developed the theory of interpersonal relations, which focuses on the relationship a nurse has with the patient. This is a theory you use every day without even knowing it existed. For more information on Peplau's theory,

 Go to Student Resources: Chapter 8, **Resources for Caregivers and Health Professionals,** on Davis*Plus.*

The Caring Theorists

It could be argued that the three leading caring theorists in nursing are Dr. Jean Watson, Dr. Patricia Benner, and Dr. Madeleine Leininger. We have been using Watson's ideas to illustrate principles and concepts of theory. In this section, we discuss Benner and Leininger.

Patricia Benner

Caring is the central concept in Benner and Wrubel's *primacy of caring model.* The nurse's caring helps the client cope. Moreover, it offers opportunity for the nurse to connect with others and to receive as well as give help (Benner & Wrubel, 1989). Caring involves personal concern for persons, events, projects, and things. Therefore, it reveals what is stressful for a person (because if something does not matter to a person, it will not create stress) and provides motivation. Caring also makes the nurse notice which interventions are effective. This theory stresses that each person is unique, so that caring is always specific and relational for each nurse–person encounter.

In Chapter 1, we discussed another of Benner's theories. A critical care nurse, she wanted to find out *what makes an expert nurse.* In this case, the idea took the form of a question. An example of an expert nurse, for her, was an intensive care unit (ICU) nurse who "knew" intuitively when it was time to extubate a critical patient. Benner wanted to know what makes a nurse expert enough to know that and other critical information. She therefore interviewed ICU nurses and, from her research, identified five stages of knowledge development and acquisition of nursing skills. As you may recall, the first level is that of a novice nurse (you). The others are advanced beginner, competent, proficient, and expert nurse (see Chapter 1 if you need to review).

Let's see whether this novice-to-expert theory addresses the four components of a nursing theory. *Person* and *nurse* are very clearly points of focus. Knowing the nurse's skill level (novice, advanced beginner, competent, proficient, or expert) provides for an intelligent way to match the nurse's skill with the patient's (*person*) acuity. This is the basis of the theory. The theory also indicates the nurse contributes to the person's *health* according to her skill level.

The *environment* is clearly stated as the ICU. Benner's theory does meet the criteria of the four components of a theory, although some are emphasized more than others. Differences in emphasis are typical of theories, by the way.

Madeleine Leininger

Leininger is the founder of transcultural nursing and was the first nurse in the United States to earn a doctoral degree in cultural and social anthropology. Her theory focuses on caring as **cultural competence** (using knowledge of cultures and of nursing to provide culturally congruent and responsible care). Her "idea" came from working with children from diverse cultures who were under her care in a psychiatric hospital: *Would the psychotherapy for the children be more effective if delivered within the framework of the child's culture* (Alligood & Marriner Tomey, 2006)?

Leininger performed the research to confirm her idea that culturally competent care made a difference, and then she developed her theory. She followed the pattern of the puzzle pieces referred to throughout this chapter. The *person* in Leininger's theory is an individual with cultural beliefs that are specific to herself and that may differ from the beliefs of others. Human beings can feel concern for others, but ways of caring vary across cultures. The *nurse* is the professional who values the cultural diversity of the person and is willing to make cultural accommodations for the health benefit of the person. This requires specialized cultural knowledge. The *environment* is wherever the nurse and the person are together in the healthcare system. *Health* is defined by the person and may be culturally specific in its definition. You will learn more about Leininger's theory in Chapter 15.

You may be thinking, "This is all about culture; what does that have to do with caring?" Leininger's theory brings together the cultures of the *person,* the *nurse,* and the *healthcare system* (indeed, there is a culture of healthcare, as you will discover in Chapter 15) to improve healthcare delivery and its effectiveness. For example, as a nurse, you may need to welcome the Shaman from a Native American tribe who has been asked to perform a sacred dance in the hospital room. This is one way to demonstrate caring and respect for the person who is ill.

A nurse tells a true culture-care story. It is an example of applying a theory directly to the needs of an ill person.

As a young nurse, I was caring for a monk who had just had surgery, and he would not take any pain medication. He wanted to "offer the pain up to God." That was a serious values clash for me because I believed the patient was jeopardizing his health, yet I did respect his right to live his cultural beliefs. We worked out a compromise. The monk agreed to take pain medication every 8 hours (instead of the prescribed every 3–4 hours), and I made sure to ambulation, hygiene, and his other needs during the times the medication was in effect.

Other Selected Nurse Theorists

You will find a list of selected nurse theorists and a brief description of their theories in Table 8-1. For a more complete discussion of those theories, you could see the Web sites listed there, and

 Go to Student Resources: Chapter 8, **Supplemental Materials: Other Selected Nurse Theorists,** on Davis*Plus.*

Table 8-1 ➤ Selected Nurse Theorists

THEORIST	DATE	THEORY
Peplau, Hildegard E.	1952	Interpersonal relations model: Interpersonal communication can improve mental health.
Henderson, Virginia	1955	14 basic needs addressed by nursing care; definition of nursing; do for the patient what he cannot do for himself.
Abdellah, Faye G.	1960	21 nursing problems; deliver care to the whole person.
Orlando, Ida Jean	1961	Interpersonal process; nursing process theory.
Wiedenbach, Ernestine	1964	The purpose of nursing is to support and meet patients' needs for help. Nursing is a helping art.
Levine, Myra	1967, 1973	Conservation model; designed to promote adaptation of the person while maintaining wholeness, or health.
Johnson, Dorothy	1968, 1980	The behavioral system model: Incorporates five principles of systems thinking to establish a balance or equilibrium (adaptation) in the person. The patient is a behavioral system consisting of subsystems.
Rogers, Martha	1970	The science of unitary human beings focuses on the betterment of human kind through new and innovative modalities. Maintaining an environment free of negative energy is important.
Orem, Dorothea	1971	The self-care deficit nursing theory explains what nursing care is required when people are not able to care for themselves. Goal is to help client attain total self-care.
King, Imogene	1971	First of two theories was the interacting systems framework, designed to explain the organized wholes within which nurses are expected to function, i.e., society, groups, and individuals. The first theory led to the theory of goal attainment, which focuses on mutual goal setting between a nurse and patient and the process for meeting the goals.
Neuman, Betty	1972	Neuman systems model is based on general system theory (a nonnursing theory) and reflects the nature of living organisms as open systems.
Roy, Sr. Callista	1974	Adaptation model was inspired by the strength and resiliency of children. The model relates to the choices people make as they adapt to illness and wellness.
Leininger, Madeleine M.	1978, 1984	Cultural care diversity and universality theory. Caring theory.
Newman, Margaret	1979	Theory of health as expanding consciousness describes nursing intervention as nonintervention, where the nurse's presence helps patients recognize their own pattern of interacting with the environment.
Watson, Jean	1979	Caring theory. Nursing is an interpersonal process.
Parse, Rosemarie Rizzo	1981	Theory of human becoming focuses on the human–universe–health process and knowledge related to human becoming (or reaching one's potential).
Benner, Patricia, and Wrubel, J.	1989	Primacy of caring model. Caring is central to the model and helps the client cope with stressors of illness.

For more information on these theorists,

 Go to Chapter 8, **Supplemental Materials,** on DavisPlus.

KnowledgeCheck 8-4

Define in a brief conceptual form or title the nursing theory of each theorist listed below:

- Florence Nightingale
- Virginia Henderson
- Hildegard Peplau

How Do Nurses Use Theories From Other Disciplines?

Theory development is relatively new in nursing. Except for Nightingale (1859/1992), it was not until the mid-1950s that nursing leaders began to publish their theories about nursing. The profession relied heavily on the theories of other disciplines. Nurses still use knowledge from other disciplines as a part of their scientific knowledge base. The following are a few of the many "borrowed" theories you will use in nursing.

Maslow's Hierarchy of Basic Human Needs

One of the classic theories still used in most nursing education and practice settings is Maslow's Hierarchy of Needs (1970). Maslow observed that certain human needs are common to all people, but some needs are "more basic" than others. The lower-level (e.g., physiological) needs must be met to some degree before the higher needs (e.g., self-esteem) can be achieved (Fig. 8-5). For example, if you sit down to study but the room is cold, you will likely decide to put on a sweater or turn up the heat before opening your books. Nevertheless, a person may consciously choose to ignore a lower-level need in order to achieve a higher need. For example, the rescuers at the World Trade Center on 9/11 and in Haiti after the 2010 earthquake ignored their need for safety and security to help others (transcendence of self). In daily life, most people are partially satisfied and partially unsatisfied at each level.

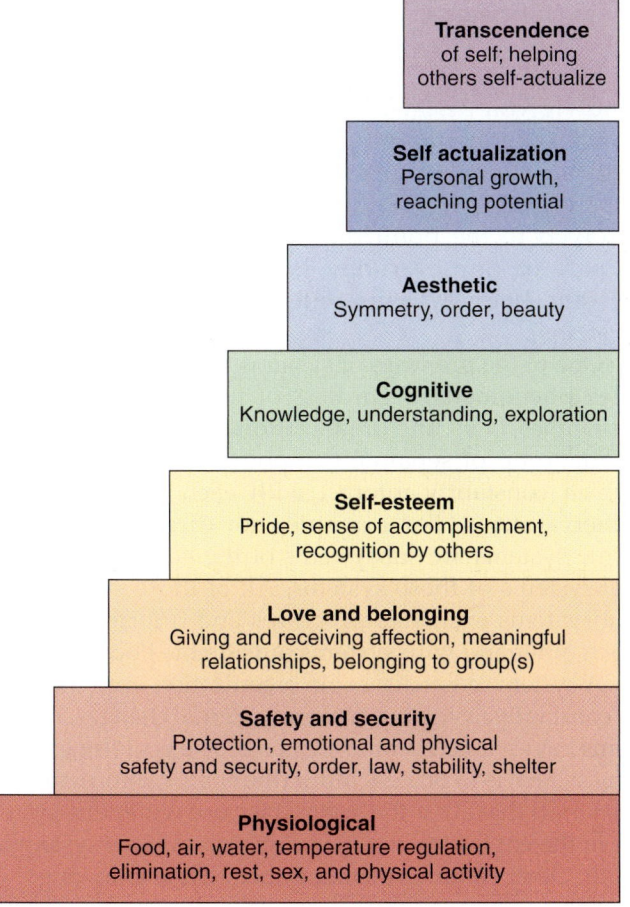

FIGURE 8-5 Maslow's Hierarchy of Human Needs is a theory nurses use every day. (*Sources:* Adapted from Maslow, A. (1971). *The farther reaches of human nature.* New York: Viking Press; and Maslow, A., & Lowery, R. (Eds.). (1998). *Toward a psychology of being* (3rd ed.). New York: John Wiley & Sons.)

Everyone has a dominant need, but it varies among individuals. For example, a teenager may have a (self-esteem) need to be accepted by a group. A heroin addict needs to satisfy her cravings for heroin and will not worry much about being accepted by others.

Physiological Needs Physiological needs, the most basic, are those that must be met to maintain life. They include the needs for food, air, water, temperature regulation, elimination, sleep and rest, sex, and physical activity. Most healthy adults meet their physiological needs through self-care. However, many of your nursing interventions are intended to support patients' physiological needs.

Safety and Security Needs The needs for safety and security are the next priority. Safety and security may refer to either physical or emotional needs. *Physical safety and security* mean protection from physical harm (e.g., falls, infection, and effects of medications) and having adequate shelter (e.g., housing with sanitation, heat, and safety). *Emotional safety and security* involve freedom from fear and anxiety—feeling safe in the physical environment as well as in relationships. We need the security of a home and family. If there is an abusive husband, for example, the wife will spend most of her time and energy trying not trigger episodes of violence or abuse. This leaves little attention for meeting self-esteem needs, for example.

Love and Belonging Needs Needs for love and belonging are sometimes called social or affiliation needs. When they dominate, the person strives for meaningful relationships with others. Everyone has a basic need to love and be loved, give and receive affection, and have a feeling of belonging, (e.g., in a family, peer group, or community). When these needs are not met, a person may feel isolated and lonely and may withdraw or become demanding and critical.

Self-Esteem Needs People who have begun to satisfy the need to belong may begin to feel the need for self-esteem. Self-esteem comes through a sense of accomplishment and recognition from others and brings confidence and independence. As we discuss in Chapter 13, illness can affect self-esteem by causing role changes (e.g., inability to perform one's job), or a change of body image (e.g., loss of a body part). When recognition cannot be obtained through positive behaviors, the person may resort to disruptive or irresponsible actions.

Self-Actualization Needs The highest level on Maslow's original hierarchy, self-actualization refers to the need to reach your full potential and to act unselfishly. At this level, a person develops wisdom and knows what to do in a variety of situations. Maslow studied self-actualized people to develop a list of their characteristics. To see this list,

 Go to Student Resources: Chapter 8, **Tables, Boxes, Figures: ESG Box 8-1,** on Davis*Plus.*

In his later work, Maslow identified two growth needs that must be met before reaching self-actualization (Maslow & Lowery, 1998):

1. *Cognitive needs* to know, understand, and explore
2. *Aesthetic needs* for symmetry, order, and beauty

Transcendence of Self   Later research led Maslow to identify another, even higher need (Maslow, 1971): the need for *transcendence of self*. This is the drive to connect to something beyond oneself and to help others realize their potential. Some people include spirituality at this level, which is also the basis for acts of self-sacrifice (for example, donating a kidney so that another person can live).

Applying Maslow's Theory

The following example illustrates how you might use Maslow's theory when teaching patients. Suppose you have been assigned to teach your patient, Mrs. Gallegos, about her colostomy before her discharge. Because she speaks little English, you put a great deal of effort into obtaining materials in her primary language, and you have arranged for an interpreter in case she has some questions you can't understand or answer. As you walk in the door to begin teaching, you immediately observe that Mrs. Gallegos seems to be in a great deal of pain. What will you do?

Maslow's Hierarchy of Needs tells you clearly that until the pain (a physiological need) is controlled, Mrs. Gallegos cannot learn. (Maslow considers pursuit of knowledge a self-actualization need.) You arrange for pain medication to be administered and reschedule the teaching session. If you went ahead with the teaching, the experience would be for the sole purpose of "crossing it off your list" (remember mechanistic nursing?) rather than actually teaching Mrs. Gallegos.

Validation Theory

Validation theory (Feil, 2003) arises from social work and provides for a way to communicate with older people with dementia. The theory asks the caregiver to *go where the demented person is in his own mind*. For example, if Mr. Wilkey (Meet Your Patient) is talking about his mother, who has been dead for many years, you would ask questions about her rather than tell him that she is dead. Learning of his mother's death would be a shocking and traumatic experience, which he would relive each time he heard the news. So instead of telling him that she is dead, you would go where Mr. Wilkey is in his own mind by asking him, for example, about the color of his mother's eyes, what songs she sings to him, or other personal questions that will likely stimulate meaningful conversation about the mother.

Stress and Adaptation Theory

Hans Selye (1993) developed the stress and adaptation theory. There are many theories about stress, but Selye's was the forerunner of them all. His theory states that a certain amount of stress is good for people; it keeps them motivated and alert. However, too much stress, called *distress*, results in physiological symptoms and eventual illness. Does that happen to you at the end of the semester when you are "distressed" over the number of papers due and the difficulty of the tests for which you are studying? Generally the human body will respond to distress with an illness, such as a cold, that will force the body to slow down or simply go to bed. Selye's theory is discussed more in Chapter 12.

Developmental Theories

Developmental theories look at stages through which individuals, groups, families, and communities progress over time. The following are some important examples:

- Erickson's psychosocial developmental theory (discussed in Chapter 9)
- Theories of family development (discussed in Chapters 13 and 14)
- Kohlberg's and Gilligan's theories of moral development (discussed in Chapters 9 and 44).

These theories are useful in nursing practice because they identify norms and expectations at various stages of development and help you identify activities and interventions that are appropriate for your client.

System Theory

Ludwig von Bertalanffy created system theory in the 1940s (von Bertalanffy, 1976). He intended it to be abstract enough to use for theory and research in any discipline. Today the understanding of systems has evolved to the point that many of the concepts are a part of our everyday language (e.g., healthcare system, body systems, information systems, family systems).

One of the premises of systems theory is that all complex phenomena, regardless of their type, have some principles, laws, and organization in common. A **system** is made up of separate components (or **subsystems**), which constantly interact with each other and with other systems. For example, the cardiovascular and renal systems are subsystems of the body; the cells are subsystems of those systems. All of those systems and subsystems exchange processes and information with each other and with systems outside the body.

A system maintains some organization even though it is constantly facing internal and external changes. All systems have some common elements. The goal (function) of any system is to process **input** (the energy, information, or materials that enter the system) for use within the system or in the **environment** (everything outside the system) or both. Other common elements include the following:

- **Throughput** consists of the processes the system uses to convert input (raw materials) into output (products to be used by the system or environment). Examples are thinking, planning, sorting, meeting in groups, sterilizing, hammering, and cutting.

- **Output** is the product or service that results from the system's throughput. Examples of output are documents, money, nursing diagnoses, and cars.
- **Feedback** is information about some aspect of the processing that is used to monitor the system and make its performance more effective (e.g., evaluation in the nursing process: how the patient responded to the interventions).
- **Open systems** exchange information and energy freely with the environment. Open systems are capable of growth, development, and adaptation. Examples of open systems include people, body systems, hospitals, and businesses.
- **Closed systems** have fixed, automatic relationships among their components and little give-and-take with the environment. One example is a rock. A nursing example is a family that is isolated from the community and resists outside influences.

Several nursing theories have been built on system theory, for example, Johnson's (1968, 1980) behavioral system model, King's (1971) interacting systems framework, and the Neuman systems model (Neuman & Young, 1972), to name a few. If you need more information about these theorists,

 Go to Student Resources: Chapter 8, **Supplemental Materials: Other Selected Nurse Theorists,** on Davis*Plus.*

KnowledgeCheck 8-5

- Name four theories nurses "borrow" from other disciplines.
- What are the five original levels of Maslow's basic human needs (not including cognitive needs, aesthetic needs, and transcendence)?

PracticalKnowledge
knowing **how**

Practical knowledge about theory means using theories to guide you in your use of the nursing process. Recall the lens metaphor: A theory's concepts and principles determine what you look for and what you notice. In the assessment step of the nursing process, your theory tells you what to assess and provides the rationale for the assessments. Its major concepts serve as categories for organizing the data. In the diagnosis step, your theory guides you in defining patient problems; in fact, it determines whether you will even recognize a cluster of cues as a problem. The theory helps you to generate appropriate, achievable client outcomes, to choose effective nursing interventions, and to provide rationales for your actions.

There is no reason to read about theory in this book unless you can apply the information. To show you how, this section applies caring theory to the planning of nursing interventions. Of course you can use *any* theory for this purpose. We use caring theory because of the powerful and positive impact it can have on

your nursing care. In reading this chapter, you should have become familiar with two well-known caring theories. Test your recall by writing the theorists' names and basic ideas. If you have difficulty, be sure to review the information about caring theorists before proceeding.

 ## Think**Like a Nurse** 8-4

Write a paragraph describing a clinical experience in which you applied or observed one or both of the caring theories. Record your thinking on a piece of paper, and be prepared to share it with your classmates. You may title it "My Experience in Caring."

Planning Theory-Based Interventions/ Implementation

The Nursing Interventions Classification, or NIC (Bulechek, Butcher, Dochterman, et al., 2013), introduced in Chapter 6, is theory development in an early stage. Each of the standardized intervention labels (e.g., Exercise Promotion, Infection Control) is a concept, and defining or describing concepts is an important step in theory development. In this section, we use nine key concepts of Watson's caring theory to describe important nursing activities and approaches.

1. **Holistic Nursing Care.** The basis of modern nursing, holistic nursing care allows nurses to examine the entire person and the person's world when making healthcare decisions. It goes beyond just giving the medication or dressing a wound. These are important tasks, but try to see nursing as giving care to the entire person and all that this entails (e.g., family, friends, fears, cultural beliefs).
2. **Honoring Personhood.** None of the three caring theorists refers to the person in the healthcare system as a patient unless they need to for clarification. They believe the "patient" is someone who deserves to be honored for individuality in behavior as well as needs. If you accept the need to honor personhood, you will learn the names of the people in your care and will refer to them by name instead of "Room 331," or "the kidney infection down the hall." Honoring personhood requires you to control the fast pace of nursing and hurried care and take time with your patients. You need to look at, talk to, and touch the person to understand what his personhood is.
3. **Transpersonal Caring Moments.** The concept of transpersonal caring is a moral ideal rather than a task-oriented behavior. Transpersonal caring moments occur when an actual caring occasion or caring relationship exists between the nurse and the person. This can be a challenge! The current healthcare environment moves people rapidly through the system. How can you find the time to develop authentic caring relationships? The first step is to make a commitment to be a caring nurse: to go to

work with the thought, "Today I will be authentic (genuine, real) with the people in my care." Or you might think, "I will focus on creating transpersonal caring moments instead of rushed and harried ones." As a student, you might think, "Today I will practice changing sterile dressings, starting intravenous solutions, or giving intramuscular injections." However, developing the ability to have transpersonal caring moments is just as important. Think about Mr. Wilkey (Meet Your Patient). Where did opportunities for transpersonal caring moments with him arise?

4. **Personal Presence.** Another phrase for being authentic and in the moment is *personal presence*. The concept of presence suggests that you, the nurse, are emotionally and physically *with* the person for the time you are there. You are not thinking about a medication you need to give or medical orders you need to get. If the person in the bed is fearful, you should be fully present, recognize the fear, and support the person experiencing it. Your support may take the form of answering simple questions or providing more in-depth education. It may simply be staying with the person for 2 or 3 minutes while quietly listening and holding the person's hand. As your psychomotor and nursing process skills become second nature to you, you will find it easier to remain in the moment.

5. **Comfort.** Some nurses think of comfort as the relief of pain, but it is much more. In Kolcaba's (1994) theory, comfort occurs in four contexts: physical, psychospiritual, social, and environmental. For example, is the person comfortable with you as the caregiver? Some women, especially from Middle Eastern or Asian cultures, are uncomfortable with male nurses. Other questions to consider are whether
   - the patient's modesty is being respected.
   - there is too much or too little environmental stimuli.
   - the room temperature is neither too cold nor too warm.
   - the patient needs more rest periods in order to heal.
   - the patient needs someone to spend a transpersonal caring moment with him so he can express fears and anxiety.

   This is the complex picture of comfort.

6. **Listening.** Listening requires you to quiet your mind and truly listen with your mind *and* heart. The caring theorists also talk about listening from within yourself. Some call that *intuition*. Benner believes it is intuition that allows nurses to advance to expert level practice.

7. **Spiritual Care.** Spiritual care is a critical aspect of holistic nursing care (see Boxes 8-1 and 8-2). You need to know what an individual's spiritual needs are and make appropriate plans to meet them. If the person does not want to talk about or deal with her spirituality, you will listen and follow her instructions. However, generally the opposite is true. People who are ill often want to talk about their spiritual needs, but they may be uncomfortable doing so. Helping someone to meet spiritual needs may be as simple as offering to call a clergy member or praying with the person who is sick. Chapter 16 provides more information about spiritual care.

8. **Caring for the Family.** All nurses who base their practice on caring theories recognize the importance of including the family of the person who is receiving care. Nontraditional family structure (e.g., a same-sex couple, a polygamist family) is not a reason to withdraw support, even if it conflicts with your values. What about an older family member with dementia? This person deserves to know what is happening to his loved one even though he most likely will forget the information. If he does forget, patiently repeat what he needs to know. You will find more information about family care in Chapter 14.

9. **Cultural Competence.** This was discussed in the explanation of Leininger's cultural care theory. Also see Chapter 15 if you want more information.

Do you see the value of each of these nine abstract concepts? From them flow very real, concrete nursing actions that make a difference in the lives of patients. Theory is not just "pie in the sky." Understanding nursing theories and applying them throughout your career are essential to full-spectrum nursing care. To perform the essential clinical tasks of nursing within the framework of caring is the highest possible performance of the profession.

KnowledgeCheck 8-6

List and explain three ways to incorporate caring theory into your nursing care.

NURSING RESEARCH

You now have a good beginning (novice) background in nursing theory. Remember the puzzle pieces (Fig. 8-2)? A nurse has an idea, does research to determine whether the idea is a valid one, and then develops a nursing theory. It is now time to study the research piece of the puzzle.

TheoreticalKnowledge knowing **why**

Many people, including some nurses, do not know that nurses do research. They see nurses as people who work in hospitals, wear scrubs, and carry a stethoscope in their pocket. Were you aware of the research done in the field of caring before reading this chapter? Most novice nurses would not be. Remember the Framingham Heart Study, which changed medical and nursing practice? Had you heard of that before? To be an effective professional nurse in the 21st century, you need to understand the basic principles of nursing research and their powerful impact on healthcare and the nursing profession. This section of the chapter is designed to show you what research is and how to incorporate it into your practice.

Although there are many definitions of nursing research, this chapter defines **nursing research** as the systematic, objective process of analyzing phenomena of importance to nursing (Nieswiadomy, 2008). Its purpose is to develop knowledge about issues that are important in nursing. Nursing research encompasses all clinical practice arenas, nursing education, and nursing administration.

Nurse researchers currently are making important contributions to the evidence-based practice necessary for professional nursing. Consider this example: When you are in the clinical setting, you will notice that when a nurse discontinues an intravenous (IV) fluid infusion, she sometimes replaces it with a lock, or plug, to maintain a route for IV medications, even though the patient no longer needs the fluids. Not many years ago, she would periodically flush the plug with heparin to keep blood from clotting and blocking the IV catheter. But heparin is a drug, and it has side effects. Nurses and other professionals performed several studies to see whether saline (which has no side effects) would work just as well. Goode and others (1996) performed a meta-analysis of those studies showing that saline was indeed just as effective; that is now the standard of care in most institutions. (A **meta-analysis** combines and analyzes the data from several different studies.)

Why Should I Learn About Research?

The best reason, of course, is that the ability to read and use nursing research enhances your ability to give quality patient care. Like theory, research affects you every day you are a nurse. Full-spectrum nurses participate in research by:

- Identifying ideas that should be examined through the research process
- Assisting in, designing, and/or performing research
- Using research as a basis for their practice

In fact, educational and practice standards require that you acquire a degree of research competence.

ANA Standards

The position of the American Nurses Association (ANA) is that all nurses share a commitment to the advancement and ethical conduct of nursing science. The following two items from The ANA Standards of Practice (2010) include the ability to use research in planning care:

Standard 4, Planning—Measurement Criterion: The registered nurse integrates current trends and research affecting care in planning.

Standard 5, Implementation—Measurement Criterion: The registered nurse utilizes evidence-based interventions and treatments specific to the diagnosis or problem.

The ANA Standards of Professional Performance include a separate research standard (Standard 9, Evidence-Based Practice and Research). Four criteria for it follow. The registered nurse:

- Utilizes current evidence-based nursing knowledge, including research findings, to guide practice decisions.
- Critically analyzes evidence-based practice and research findings for application to practice.
- Participates in the development of evidence-based practice through research activities. Participation levels occur appropriate to the nurse's education and position.
- Shares research activities and/or findings with peers and others.

Educational Competencies

The Quality and Safety Education for Nurses (QSEN) project has identified competencies for nurses. One important competency is evidence-based practice, the ability to "integrate the best available current evidence with clinical expertise and patient/family preferences and values for delivery of optimal healthcare" (Cronenwett, Sherwood, Barnsteiner, et al., 2007, pp. 122–131). To achieve this competency, you will need a basic understanding of nursing research. If you would like to see a description of the knowledge, skills, and attitudes you need for achieving this competency,

 Go to Student Resources: Chapter 8, **ESG Table 8-2** on Davis*Plus*,

or

 Go to the QSEN Web site at **http://www.qsen.org/ksas_prelicensure.php**

What Is the History of Nursing Research?

The records Florence Nightingale kept while nursing soldiers in the Crimea were the beginning of formalized nursing research. As she developed schools of nursing throughout Britain and the United States, Nightingale urged her students to do clinical research. Yet because she had passed on to them the authoritarian tradition of her time, she found they were not prepared to perform it. Authority-based education does not promote intellectual inquiry or critical thinking, two characteristics essential for research. This is one reason nursing research was slow to develop.

As baccalaureate, master's, and doctoral programs grew in number, so did the number and quality of research projects nurses performed. Nursing research is now supported by federal funds and private grants, and results are reported in a growing number of nursing (and other) research journals. Nurses present their research at national and international conferences and publish their results in national and international journals.

The preparation of doctoral-level nurses with a strong background in research has enhanced the quality and diversity of nursing research.

How Are Priorities for Nursing Research Developed?

Nursing research provides evidence on which to base nursing care. Ideally, all nursing interventions should be validated through research to show their safety and effectiveness. Professional organizations, such as the ANA and specialty organizations (e.g., the Oncology Nurses Association), have established research priorities that will assist nursing to build a strong knowledge base in areas of importance to society. In the present healthcare system, which emphasizes the need for cost-effective interventions, it is likely that nursing research will continue to be focused on clinical issues. The National Institute of Nursing Research (NINR), a federally funded agency that is a part of the National Institutes of Health (NIH), periodically identifies research themes and priorities for funding (NINR, n.d., 2006, 2010). For more information about nursing research priorities,

 Go to Student Resources: Chapter 8, **Supplemental Materials: What Are the Priorities for Research in the 21st Century?** on Davis*Plus*.

KnowledgeCheck 8-7

- Define *nursing research*.
- According to the text, why has nursing research been slow to develop?

What Educational Preparation Does a Researcher Need?

At each level of educational preparation, nurses function in different roles in the research process.

Associate Degree and Diploma Nursing At this educational level, there are three research roles you can fulfill. You can (1) be aware of the importance of research to evidence-based practice, (2) help identify problem areas in nursing, (3) help collect data with a more experienced nurse researcher, and (4) use evidence-based practice in planning nursing interventions.

Baccalaureate Degree in Nursing If you are a baccalaureate-prepared nurse, you should be able to (1) critique research for application to clinical practice, (2) identify nursing research problems and help implement research studies, and (3) apply research findings to establish sound, evidence-based clinical practice.

Master's Degree in Nursing Nurses with graduate degrees should be able to (1) analyze problems so that appropriately designed research can be used to solve the problem, (2) through clinical expertise, apply evidence-based practice to nursing care situations, (3) provide support to ongoing research projects, and (4) conduct research for the purpose of assuring quality nursing care.

Doctoral Degree in Nursing or Related Field Doctorally prepared nurses are specifically educated to be nurse researchers. They are qualified to (1) conduct nursing research, (2) serve as leaders in applying research results to the clinical arena, and (3) develop ways to monitor the quality of nursing care being administered by nurses (adapted from ANA, 1981). In addition, they should disseminate their research findings via publications and conferences.

PracticalKnowledge knowing **how**

No one expects you to have a sophisticated understanding of research at this point in your career. However, you do need some basic practical knowledge, including information about the scientific method, types of research design, the research process, how to find practice-related research articles, how to identify researchable problems, and how to critique research reports.

How Do We Gain Knowledge?

Recall that in Chapter 2 you learned the different kinds of nursing knowledge: theoretical, practical, ethical, and self-knowledge. There are also various ways to *gain* knowledge.

Trial and Error Plus Common Sense Suppose a patient has been medicated but is still in pain. You might try repositioning him. If that doesn't help, you might try distraction or visualization techniques. And so on. If visualization provides some relief, you would probably try that technique first when a similar situation occurs with another patient.

Authority and Tradition This means to rely on an expert or to do "what has always been done." For the patient with unrelieved pain, this would mean you might ask a more experienced nurse what to do. Or you could consult a procedure manual.

Intuition and Inspiration Intuition is a "feeling" about something—an inner sense. Nurses say, "I just had a feeling something was wrong with the patient, but I can't explain why." For the patient in pain, you might "have a feeling" that a complication was developing, that the pain was due to more than just ineffective pain medication. However, as a novice, you should always check with a more experienced nurse before acting on your intuition.

Logical Reasoning Using your knowledge and the facts available, you form conclusions (refer to How Are Theories Developed?). For the patient in pain, you might think, "This man weighs 300 lb, but I gave him only the standard dose of medication. Probably he needs a higher dose."

Scientific Method Research is based on the scientific method (or scientific inquiry). **Scientific inquiry** is the process in which the researcher, through use of the senses, systematically collects observable, verifiable data to describe, explain, or predict events. The goals of scientific inquiry are to find solutions to problems and to develop explanations of the world (theories). The scientific method has two unique characteristics that the other ways of gaining knowledge do not:

- *Objectivity,* or *self-correction.* This means that the researcher uses techniques to keep her personal beliefs, values, and attitudes separate from the research process.
- *The use of empirical data.* Researchers use their senses to gather empirical data through observation. They attempt to verify the information gathered through a variety of methods so that the research conclusions are based in "reality" rather than on the researcher's beliefs, biases, or hunches.

Box 8-3 summarizes the characteristics of the scientific method.

BOX 8-3 ■ Characteristics of the Scientific Method

Begins with an identified problem or need to be studied.

Uses theories, models, and conceptual themes that have been empirically tested.

Uses systematic, orderly methods to acquire empirical evidence to test theories.

Uses methods of control for ruling out other variables that might affect the relationships among the variables they are studying.

Avoids explanations that cannot be empirically tested.

Prefers to generalize the findings (knowledge) so that it can be applied in cases other than those in the study.

Uses built-in mechanisms for self-correction.

Source: Adapted from Wilson, H. S. (1993). *Introducing research in nursing* (2nd ed.). Redwood City, CA: Addison-Wesley Nursing.

What Are Two Approaches to Research?

The scientific method makes use of a variety of procedures and study designs aimed to increase the chances that the data collected will be reliable, relevant, and unbiased. You should recognize the two major categories of research design: quantitative and qualitative. Each category has within it several specific types of research methodologies; however, for now you need to understand only the basic differences (Table 8-2). For an expanded discussion,

 Go to Student Resources: Chapter 8, **Supplemental Materials: Quantitative Research and Qualitative Research,** on Davis*Plus*.

Quantitative Research

The main purpose of **quantitative research** is to gather data from enough **subjects** (people being studied) to be able to generalize the results to a similar population. **Generalizing results** means that you think, "What I found to be so for this group of people will probably be the same for all people who are similar" (e.g., "My findings for *this* group of women over age 40 in the United States will probably be useful for *all* women over age 40 in the United States"). In quantitative research, researchers carefully control data collection and are careful to maintain the objectivity of the process. Quantitative data are reported as numbers. The Framingham Study is a classic example of a quantitative study—actually of several quantitative studies. To read more about this landmark research,

 Go to the Framingham Study Web site at http://www. framinghamheartstudy.org/index.html

Another classic example of quantitative nursing research is the Conduct and Utilization of Research in Nursing (CURN) project, which was intended to increase the use of research by direct-care nurses (Horsley, Crane, Crabtree, et al., 1983). Many of the protocols (procedures)

Table 8-2 ➤ Comparison of Quantitative and Qualitative Research

	QUANTITATIVE RESEARCH	QUALITATIVE RESEARCH
Data	Numerical data, e.g., questionnaires, number of incidents, or reactions to a medication	Nonnumerical data; data may consist of words from interviews, observations, written documents, and even art or photos.
Persons Studied	Large numbers of *subjects* so it can be generalized to other similar populations	Often uses small numbers of *participants*; is not designed with the intent to generalize.
Hypothesis	Has a hypothesis	No hypothesis because it is the research of the "lived experience" of the person or persons being studied; study may be guided by research questions.
Environment	Can be in a laboratory setting; needs to be a controlled environment	Is often done in the "natural" setting (i.e., the person's home or work setting).
Analysis	Objective data, tested with statistical methods	Subjective data; identifies themes; sometimes converted to numerical data (e.g., by counting categories).

developed from these studies are used today with some modification. The following are some CURN protocol examples:

Clean intermittent catheterization
Intravenous cannula change
Distress reduction through sensory preparation
Preventing decubitus ulcers

Qualitative Research

Qualitative research focuses on the lived experience of people. The purpose is not to generalize the data, but to share the experience of the person or persons in the study. There is no need for large numbers. A case study of one person can examine the lived experience, for example, of a 19-year-old single mother of triplets or a middle-aged woman with HIV. Qualitative research uses words, quotations from persons interviewed, observations, and other nonnumeric sources of data. The Nun Study, a long-term, multidisciplinary project involving a convent of Catholic nuns in Minnesota, included some qualitative research (e.g., data obtained by interviews and reported in the nuns' own words, and samples of writing from the nuns' diaries, reports, and letters). For an example of research from the Nun Study,

 Go to the University of Minnesota Web site, **The Nun Study,** at http://www.apa.org/pubs/journals/releases/psp805804.pdf

KnowledgeCheck 8-8
- Define *quantitative research.* Name one study presented as an example in this chapter.
- Define *qualitative research.* Name one study presented as an example in this chapter.

What Are the Phases of the Research Process?

At the novice level, you will be using but not performing research. But in order to evaluate the research you read, you should have a general idea of the steps for conducting valid, reliable research. The research process is a problem-solving process, similar to but not the same as the nursing process. Different study designs require different steps, and you will find some variation in how different authors present the research process steps. However, in general, the steps include the following five phases (Fain, 2013):

1. Select and define the problem.
2. Select a research design.
3. Collect data.
4. Analyze data.
5. Use the research findings.

If you need a more detailed description of those phases,

 Go to Student Resources: Chapter 8, **Supplemental Materials, What Are the Steps of the Research Process?** on Davis*Plus.*

 ThinkLike a Nurse 8-5

Take 10 minutes to sit quietly and think about nursing research. Do you have an idea or a problem you would like to see investigated with a research project? If nothing comes to mind quickly, then ponder for a few moments more. Write the information on a sheet of paper. Take the time to do your best thinking. Then share what you have written with your instructor and other students.

- What would you like to have more information about in nursing? Explain why it is a problem or what brought about your idea.
- If you were the research assistant on a nursing research project on your topic, what one-sentence problem statement would you write regarding your research idea?
- What is the purpose of doing this research project? Why should it be done?

You may struggle with this assignment and wonder about its value to you, yet one of the most important things that nurses do is identify problems. Here is your chance to practice.

What Are the Rights of Research Participants?

Every nurse has a moral and legal responsibility to protect research participants from being harmed during the research process. Although research is crucial to the development of the profession, it should never be held in higher regard than the rights of the individuals being studied.

The current ethical standards for research, from all disciplines, are a direct result of the atrocities committed in the name of research in the German prison camps during World War II. After the trials for war crimes committed at that time, the Nuremberg Code was developed in 1949 to protect research participants from unethical behavior. The Nuremberg Code prompted many other codes and standards for performing ethical research (Code of Federal Regulations, 2009; Ghooi, 2001; The Nuremberg Code, 1949). The United States government, through the Department of Health and Human Services (DHHS), has a complex set of standards that all researchers must follow.

Informed Consent

As a rule, **informed consent** must be obtained from every participant in a study. Consent is obtained by discussing what is expected of the participant, providing written information on the project to the participant, and obtaining the participant's written consent to be a subject. The following critical concepts are part of the informed consent.

- *Right to not be harmed.* The information given to the participant outlines the safety protocols of the study. If at any time preliminary data indicate potential harm to the participant, the study must be stopped immediately.
- *Right to full disclosure.* Participants have a right to answers to such questions as: What is the purpose of this

research? What risks are there? Are there any benefits? Will I be paid? What happens if I get sick or feel worse? Whom do I contact with questions and concerns?

■ *Right to self-determination.* This refers to the right to say no. At any time in a study, the participant has the right to stop participating, for any reason. As the nurse, you are responsible to support a participant during the process of withdrawing from a study. Do not allow anyone to coerce the participant into remaining in the study.

■ *Rights of privacy and confidentiality.* All research participants have the right to have their identity protected. Generally they are given a code number rather than being identified by name. Once the study is completed and the data are analyzed, the researcher is responsibility for protecting the raw data (such as questionnaires and taped interviews).

Institutional Review Boards

The mechanism for overseeing the ethical standards established by the U.S. DHHS is the Institutional Review Board (IRB). Every hospital, university, and other healthcare facility where federal funds are involved has an IRB. It consists of healthcare professionals and people from the community who are willing to review and critique research proposals. The two main responsibilities of the IRB are to (1) protect the research participants from harm and (2) ensure that the research is of value.

KnowledgeCheck 8-9

■ List the phases of the research process.
■ List four critical concepts that make up informed consent.

How Can I Base My Practice on the Best Evidence?

Recall from Chapter 6 that research provides the data for evidence-based practice. When there is a body of research on a topic, experts and professional groups evaluate the quality of the research reports and translate them into guidelines for practice. In your own evidence-based practice, you should use research findings and practice guidelines when they are available. When they are not, you will need to rely on the research reports themselves. Similar to the phases of research, the following process should assist you in finding the best evidence for your own interventions:

■ Identify a clinical problem.
■ Formulate a searchable question.
■ Search the literature.
■ Evaluate the quality of the research you find in the literature.
■ Integrate your findings into your practice.

Identify a Clinical Nursing Problem

Even as a novice nurse, you should be prepared to identify clinical problems for research. Identifying a clinical nursing problem comes from being alert and interested in what you are doing each day in your clinical setting. How do you think the tympanic thermometer came into being? Someone became frustrated with the discomfort patients experienced when temperatures were taken rectally. At the same time, there was a great deal of concern over the inaccuracy of axillary temperatures. Someone noticed the problem and wondered: "Is there a better way to do this?"

Common sources of clinical problems are experience, social issues, theories, ideas from others, and the nursing literature (Polit & Beck, 2007). Most of these sources are relevant whether you are identifying a problem for a research study or for doing a literature search.

Experience As you go about your work, you will notice interventions that may not be working or that require a great deal of effort for the minimal good they do. You will wonder, "How could we do this better?" Or you may notice that for clients with a particular health problem, the outcomes are often not good. You will wonder, "How could we improve the care so the patient's health improves?" Other questions might be, "Why do we do this procedure this way? "What do I need to know in order to plan new interventions for patients with this health problem?" If you are curious about why things are done and about what might happen if changes were mad, you will find plenty of problems—for example, problems to staffing, equipment, nursing interventions, or coordination among health professionals.

Social Issues You may be concerned about broader social issues that affect or require nursing care, such as issues of gender equity, sexual harassment, and domestic violence. You may be concerned about patients who do not have access to healthcare or about the health problems of a particular group or subculture.

Theories Recall that theories must be tested in order to be useful in nursing practice. You might want to suggest research to test a theory you are interested in. If the theory is accurate, what behaviors would you expect to find, or what evidence would you need to support the theory?

Ideas From Others Your instructor may suggest a topic to research, or perhaps you might brainstorm with nurses or other students. Agencies and organizations that fund research often ask for proposals on certain topics (e.g., the ANA and the NINR).

Nursing Literature Read widely in your field of interest. You may identify clinical problems by reading articles and research reports in nursing journals. This may occur in one of the following ways:

■ An article may stimulate your imagination and interest in a topic.
■ You may notice a discrepancy in what staff nurses are doing and what the literature recommends.

- You may notice inconsistencies in the findings of two different studies on the same topic.
- You may read a study on a topic of interest to you (e.g., a technique for measuring blood pressure) and wonder whether the results would be the same if the study had been done in a different setting (e.g., a clinic instead of a hospital) or with a different population (e.g., healthy instead of ill people).

Formulate a Searchable Question

When you have found a topic of interest, the next step is to state it in such a way that you can find it in the vast amount of nursing literature that is published. Stated too broadly, the search may yield thousands of irrelevant results. Stated too narrowly, you may get no results. Using the acronym PICO enables you to search efficiently. The acronym stands for *P*atient or problem, *I*ntervention, *C*omparison intervention, *O*utcomes, and *T*imes. You may not always need a comparison intervention (C), and sometimes not a (T) (Box 8-4).

Search the Literature

Once you have stated your guiding question, the next step is to look for research articles related to the question (or problem statement). You may be thinking, "Where do I look for research articles?" As previously stated, evidence reports and practice guidelines may already exist for your clinical problem, so look first for those. If there are none, proceed to search for your topic in research reports in scientific journals.

Indexes and Databases

Obviously you need to go to a library or online and search a database or index for appropriate journal references. A **database** is an electronic bibliographic file that can be accessed either online or on a CD-ROM. The best database for you, as a novice nurse, is the Cumulative Index to Nursing and Allied Health Literature (CINAHL). This is a comprehensive database that includes nearly 3,000 nursing and allied health journals. Generally, you will be able to find in CINAHL whatever you are looking for in clinical nursing. Most university libraries have access to CINAHL and other indexes online. If you are an online user, it will be worth your time to get information from the library about conducting online searches. In the library, you will find the printed version of CINAHL in a set of large books in the reference section.

Once you have access to CINAHL in either format, select words that relate to your topic (e.g., dementia or nursing ethics). The index or database will list journal articles related to the key words. Sometimes, you will get a large number of articles (more than 1,000) that carry that word. A PICO question should help you narrow your search, but you may need to ask the librarian for assistance. It is beyond the scope of this chapter to provide detailed instructions for literature searches. For more information about literature databases, see Chapter 41.

BOX 8-4 ■ PICOT Questions

	Sample Questions	Example
P—Patient Population, or Problem	What is the medical diagnosis, nursing diagnosis, patient problem, symptom, situation, or need that requires an intervention?	For patients with Impaired Skin Integrity (perineum) related to urinary incontinence
	How would you describe a group of similar patients?	
I—Intervention, treatment, cause, contributing factor	Which intervention are you considering? Specifically, what might help the problem (improve the situation, etc.)?	Would applying a barrier cream help?
C—Comparison Intervention, control	What other interventions are being considered or used?	As compared with washing with soap and water, rinsing well, and air-drying?
O—Outcome	What effect could the intervention realistically have? What do you hope to achieve?	Prevent or achieve less perineal excoriation? Are there any expected undesired effects associated with the intervention?
T—Time	How often, or when, will the outcome be measured? How often or how long will the intervention or treatment be administered?	After incontinent episodes?

Sources: University of Southern California, Health Sciences, Los Angeles. (n.d.). Evidence based decision making, "asking a good question (PICO)." Retrieved December 10, 2012, from www.usc.edu/hsc/ebnet/ebframe/PICO.htm; Center for Evidence Based Medicine. (Page last edited April 7, 2009). Asking focused clinical questions. Retrieved December 3, 2012, from www.cebm.net/index.aspx?o = 1036; Sacket, D. L., Richardson, W. S., Rosenberg, W., et al. (1997). *Evidence-based medicine: How to practice and teach EBM.* New York: Churchill Livingstone; Stilwell, S., Fineout-Overholt, E., Melnyk, G., et al. (2010). Evidence-based practice, step by step: Asking the clinical question: A key step in evidence-based practice. *American Journal of Nursing, 110*(3), 58–61.

KnowledgeCheck 8-10

Where can you go to use CINAHL?

Journals

It also is easy to search in a specific journal for articles. The title of a journal provides clues to the content. The critical care journals will have, obviously, articles about critical care. Oncology, orthopedics, and other specialty journals carry information specific to their own specialty. Looking for such journals is another way to do a casual search for articles of interest.

You will find the best research articles in refereed journals. **Refereed journals** are professional journals (not lay magazines, such as *Men's Health* or *Fitness*) in which professionals with expertise in the topic review each article and then recommend whether the article should be published. The easiest way to identify a refereed journal is to see whether it has an extensive editorial board listed in the front of the journal. Refereed journals meet a higher standard for publishing, which makes the information you read more credible (and therefore more useful to your work). Two examples of refereed nursing research journals are *Advances in Nursing Science* and *Nursing Research*. For a more extensive list,

 Go to Chapter 8, **Supplemental Materials: Nursing Research Journals,** on Davis*Plus.*

How can you tell whether the article you retrieve is a research article? Simply look for the steps in the research process described earlier in this chapter. Does the article have a problem statement and a purpose? Is there a section on the sample and site of the research? And so on.

If your focus is clinical practice, you should not overlook specialty journals, such as *Geriatric Nursing* or the *Journal of Gerontological Nursing,* if you really want information on, say, older adults with dementia. They are not research journals, but they generally have one or two research articles in each issue. If you do not have a specialty interest, review the *American Journal of Nursing, Nursing,* or *RN* for articles of general interest. Again, remember that it is up to you to identify whether the article is research or another form of information sharing.

Evaluate the Quality of the Research

As mentioned previously, you may be fortunate enough to find clinical practice guidelines related to your topic. If so, the related research has already been evaluated by experts, and should have a notation about the level of evidence supporting the guideline. For a description of the different levels of evidence described by guidelines panels,

 Go to Student Resources: Chapter 6, **Supplemental Materials, Levels of Evidence,** on Davis*Plus.*

If no practice guidelines are available, you will need to critically appraise the individual research articles you find. You can do this by reading analytically and performing a careful appraisal of the research you read.

Analytical Reading

You cannot expect to do a sophisticated critique of a research report at this stage of your education, or probably even on graduation from your basic education. However, you need to know enough to help you decide which articles are worthy of using in your practice. You will make that decision after you have examined the research to determine whether it is well done and meaningful to your work. Begin this process by learning to read analytically. Wilson (1993, p. 25) says that **analytical reading** occurs when you "begin asking questions of what you are reading so that you can truly understand it." For questions to use when reading analytically, see Box 8-5.

Research Appraisal

Not all research is good research. Some published studies contain serious flaws, and you need to be able to recognize them. An effective strategy for conducting a research appraisal is to read the entire article, using the four "analytical reading" questions in Box 8-5 and making notes of questions you have. Then go back and evaluate the article section by section, thinking critically about each (Wilson, 1993).

- *Researcher qualifications* are an easy place to start. Was the researcher qualified as an expert on the study topic? Try to determine whether the author's credentials and background "fit" with the topic.
- *The title* should be concise and clear. Key words in the title should provide clues to the research topic.
- *The abstract* is a brief (perhaps 500 words) summary of the study. It should be interesting and usually describes at least the purpose, methods, sample, and findings of the study.
- *The introduction* should catch your interest and set the stage for the rest of the report. The introduction

---

BOX 8-5 ■ Reading Analytically

When reading analytically, ask yourself the following questions:

1. *What is the book, journal, or article about as a whole?* That is, what is the theme of the article, and how is it developed?

2. *What is being said in detail, and how?* What are the author's main ideas, claims, and arguments? In a research article, you will find this mainly in the abstract and the conclusions.

3. *Is the book, journal, or article "true" in whole or part?* You must decide this for yourself. The strategies in the section, Research Appraisal, may help you to determine the truth of a research report.

4. *What of it?* Is it of any significance? Is there any way to use the information to improve patient care, education, or other areas of nursing?

may contain the *review of the literature, theoretical (conceptual) framework, assumptions, and limitations.* At this stage of your expertise, you should primarily just check that these are present; however, some explanation follows.

■ *Review of the literature* should be thorough and relevant. The references should logically pertain to the study topic and methods and consist primarily of research and theory articles. The references should support the researcher's variable definitions, methodology, and choices of data-collection tools; it should also present background work on the topic being studied.

■ *Identify the study assumptions.* Recall that assumptions are beliefs that you "take for granted" as true but that have not been proved. For example, you assume that when people are in bed, they sleep; and you assume that study participants answer truthfully to the researcher's questions. Assumptions should be clearly stated to avoid confusion regarding the study.

■ *Recognize the limitations of the study.* Every study has limitations or weaknesses. Look for the author to admit the things that could not be controlled. For example, a study may test a population of people that would not generalize to other populations, (e.g., testing only Caucasian students instead of testing a variety of students who represent the ethnic diversity of the university).

■ *The purpose* should be stated clearly. It should give the reasons for doing the study. Ask these three questions to help you judge it: Will the study (1) solve a problem relevant to nursing, (2) present facts that are useful to nursing, or (3) contribute to nursing knowledge?

■ *The problem statement* should be presented early in the report, and it should be "researchable"; that is, it (1) is stated as a question, (2) involves the relationship between two or more variables, and (3) can be answered by collecting empirical data.

■ *Definition of terms* is essential in a formal research report. However, it often is not included in a published article because of the lack of space.

■ *The research design* indicates the plan for collecting data. As a novice, you probably cannot judge the adequacy of the design, but you should be sure the researcher names and describes it and discusses its strengths and weakness. The researcher should include an explanation of what was done to enhance the validity and reliability of the study. To oversimplify, **validity** means the study actually measures the concept it claims to measure. **Reliability** refers to the accuracy, consistency, and precision of a measure. That is, if someone else repeated the study using the same design, would they obtain similar results? For example, if you weighed the same item on a scale each day and obtained the same weight each time, you could say that the scale is reliable—but a scale would not give you a valid measure of body fat.

■ *Identify the setting, population, and sample.* The researcher should identify the type of setting where the data was collected, describe the population and sample, and state the criteria that were used for choosing study participants. This section may also contain information about how informed consent was obtained.

■ *Data-collection methods* answer the basic questions of what, how, who, where, and when. Data-collection instruments are the "tools" used to gather the data (e.g., questionnaires or a laboratory instrument). The researcher should provide evidence (pilot tests, literature) that the tools used were reliable and valid.

■ *Determine the data analysis used.* A quantitative report would include statistical analyses of the data. A qualitative report would include quotes from the participants. The analyses of both types of data are very specific and beyond the scope of this textbook.

■ *Discussion of findings and conclusion* are the sections of a research report that you may find most interesting. They are the "So what was learned?" sections. All findings should be presented in an objective manner, and compared with information found in the literature. The easiest errors for you to recognize with your present knowledge level are that the researcher:

1. Generalizes beyond the data or the sample. For example, the sample may have been young adult women in a clinic setting, but the researcher might have suggested that the same intervention be used for all women in the clinic, regardless of age.

2. Does not mention any limitations that might have influenced the results.

3. Does not present findings in a clear, logical manner (i.e., you have trouble figuring out what the findings actually are).

■ *Implications and recommendations* are the final pieces of the research critique. The implications are the "shoulds" of the research. In essence, the researcher says, "Now we know this fact; therefore, nurses should . . ." For example, the research "should" be replicated with another population, or the instrument "should" be revised and retested, or that nurses "should" use the study intervention in their practice.

When you read a research article, examine it for each of the preceding items. Although you have limited knowledge and experience, every time you review an article thoroughly, you will learn more about the research process. As you learn, you will be better able to determine the quality of research you will accept as a basis for changing your nursing practice.

KnowledgeCheck 8-11

■ Explain the difference between analytical reading and research appraisal.
■ What are the parts of a PICOT question?

Integrate the Research Into Your Practice

True evidence-based practice requires that after discovering and critiquing the best available evidence, nursing expertise must be applied to see how the recommended interventions fit into the practice setting and whether they are compatible with patient preferences. If the intervention is to involve more than just an individual nurse, nurse managers must consider costs, barriers to change, facilitators for change, and staff education before deciding to implement the clinical practice guideline in their unit or hospital.

Research is more than just an exercise that nurses engage in to earn master's and doctoral degrees. The ultimate reason for conducting research is to establish an evidence-based practice or to gain greater understanding of a phenomenon. This means that nurses in practice have a responsibility for finding and using the research that others do. Remember the discussion of authority-based practice during Florence Nightingale's era? Even in the 21st century, much nursing practice is still based on authority and tradition. That is not acceptable for full-spectrum professional nurses. You must have reasons for what you do. Research can provide those reasons.

Although there are barriers (see Box 8-6), you can use nursing research to enhance your practice by acting on the information in this chapter. Read and talk about research with your colleagues and instructors. Once you have a research-based idea clear in your mind, try it out in your clinical setting (with approval from the nurse manager or instructor). Then discuss it with others. You can learn to effectively read and use research, and then you can motivate others to do the same.

To explore learning resources for this chapter,

 Go to DavisPlus at DavisPl.us/Wilkinson3.

Chapter Resources for Chapter 8:
  Response sheets for all learning activities
  Resources for Caregivers and Health Professionals
  Reading More About Evidence-Based Practice: Theory & Research (suggested readings)
  Concept Map of chapter content
Interactive Case Studies
NCLEX-Style and Chapter Review Questions
Chapter Overview Podcasts

For references cited in this chapter,

 Go to Volume 2, **References Cited.**

BOX 8-6 ■ Barriers to Using Research

According to Nieswiadomy (2008), there are five reasons nurses *do not* use research as the basis for their practice:

1. Lack of knowledge of nursing research
2. Negative attitudes toward research
3. Inadequate forums for disseminating research
4. Lack of support from the employing institution
5. Study findings that are not ready for the clinical environment

Factors Affecting Health

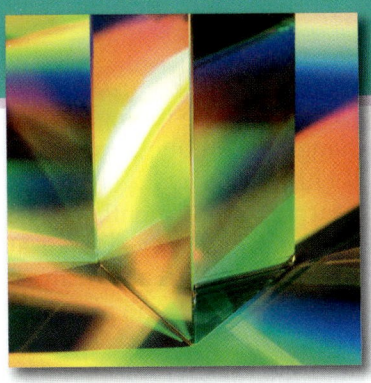

CHAPTER 9

Life Span: Infancy Through Middle Adulthood

Learning Outcomes

After completing this chapter, you should be able to:

➤ Discuss the principles of growth and development.

➤ Compare and contrast developmental task theory, psychoanalytic theory, cognitive theory, and the psychosocial theory of growth and development.

➤ Outline the major principles involved in moral and spiritual development.

➤ Identify conditions that influence growth and development at all ages.

➤ Discuss the cognitive and psychosocial challenges for each age group, infant through middle age.

➤ Identify common health problems seen in each stage of development.

➤ Describe special assessments unique to each age group.

➤ Discuss age-appropriate interventions for each age group.

➤ Incorporate developmental principles into nursing care.

Key Concepts

Growth
Development
Stages

Related Concepts

See the Concept Map on Davis*Plus*.

Example Problems

Abuse, neglect, and violence
Substance abuse

Meet Your Patients

At the end of your first clinical day on the pediatric unit, you reflect on your experiences. You provided care for three children who were diagnosed with pneumonia:

- Tamika, a 3-year-old, lives with her grandparents. Her grandmother is present only during afternoon visiting hours because she must care for her husband, who suffers from numerous health problems.
- Miguel, a 2-month-old, lives with his mother. Since his admission yesterday, Miguel's mother has stayed at his bedside and provided most of her son's care.
- Carrie, a 13-year-old, lives with her parents. Both parents are able to visit only during evening visiting hours, when they leave work.
- You think back to another clinical day when you were assigned to care for Ms. Lowenstein, a middle-aged patient with pneumonia who lives alone.

Each of these patients is unique. Although they share the same medical diagnosis, their needs and your nursing care differ dramatically. These differences stem from a

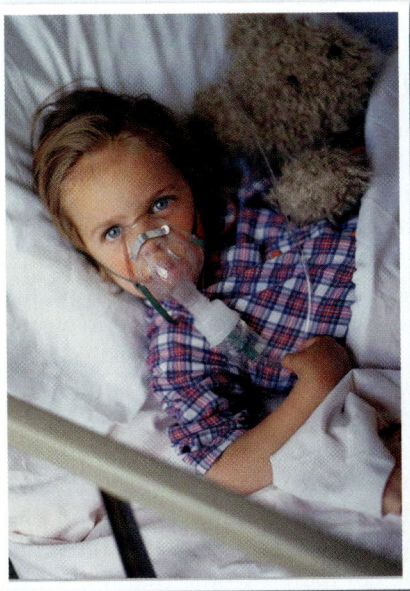

variety of factors, one of the most significant of which is each patient's developmental stage. Throughout the life span, human beings are in a constant process of physical, cognitive, and emotional change, whether or not it is visible to the eye.

Theoretical Knowledge
knowing why

In this chapter, you will learn principles and theories of growth and development that can form the foundation for planning and delivering effective patient care. You will also find a discussion of normal growth and development across the life span. A fundamentals course or textbook can provide only a basic foundation covering infant and child development. For situations in which you need more in-depth or specialized knowledge, refer to a child development or pediatric nursing textbook.

ABOUT THE KEY CONCEPTS

Development refers to the process of adapting to one's body and environment over time, which is enabled by increasing complexity of function and skill progression. A few examples of development are a child who comes to recognize right from wrong, an adolescent who decides on a vocation, and an older adult who recognizes the nearness of death. **Growth** refers to physical changes that occur over time, such as increases in height, sexual maturation, or gains in weight and muscle tone. Growth is the physical aspect of development; the rest is behavioral. As you read this chapter, you will see how the key concept of **stages** is intertwined with the concepts of growth and development.

HOW DOES DEVELOPMENT OCCUR?

The Greek philosopher Heraclitus said, "Nothing is permanent but change." We readily see this truth in the dramatic physical, cognitive, and emotional growth that children undergo from one month to another, but it is true also for adults. **Key Point:** *Change is constant throughout the life span.*

What has been the most important force in your becoming the person you are now: characteristics that you inherited from your parents, or the environment in which you were raised?

For centuries, scientists have debated the effects of nature versus nurture on growth and development. **Nature** refers to genetic endowment, whereas **nurture** is the influence of the environment on the individual. The birth of a child can be compared to the planting of a tulip. Within the bulb is nearly everything it needs to sprout; but whether it reaches its full potential—that is, grows into a flowering plant—also depends on the environment. Is the soil rich in nutrients? Is there adequate sunshine? Water? Similarly, the joining of ovum and sperm forms chromosomes that determine appearance, characteristics, and affect how the child will grow and develop. However, environmental factors, such as access to food, love, affection, and education, also affect how the child develops and thrives.

Principles of Growth and Development

Important principles of growth and development include the following.

Growth and Development Usually Follow an Orderly, Predictable Pattern However, the timing, rate of change, and response to change are unique for each individual. For example, all children learn to sit before they walk. One child may learn to sit at 6 months of age and walk at 10 months; another child may first sit at 7 months and not walk until 15 months. Each of these children is developing in the same pattern, and progressing within a normal time frame.

Growth and Development Follow a Cephalocaudal Pattern, Beginning at the Head and Progressing Down to the Chest, Trunk, and Lower Extremities To illustrate cephalocaudal *growth*, when an infant is born, the head is the largest portion of the body. In the first year, the head, chest, and trunk gain in size, yet the legs remain short. Growth of the legs is readily apparent in the second year. An example of cephalocaudal *development* is the tendency of infants to use their arms before their legs.

Growth and Development Proceed in a Proximodistal Pattern beginning at the center of the body and moving outward. Proximodistal *growth* occurs in utero, for example, when the baby's central body is formed before the limbs. As an example of proximodistal *development*, the infant first begins to focus his eyes; then lifts the head; later pushes up and rolls over. As the infant gains strength and coordination distally, he will crawl and later walk.

Simple Skills Develop Separately and Independently Later they are integrated into more complex skills. Many complex skills represent a combination of simple skills. For example:

- Feeding yourself requires the ability to find your mouth, grasp an object, control movement of that object, coordinate movement of the hand from the plate to the mouth, and swallow solid food.
- If you have ever tried to learn to play a musical instrument, you are familiar with this principle. You must master simple steps before you are able to play a tune.

Each Body System Grows at its Own Rate This principle is readily apparent in fetal development and at the onset of puberty. In the years leading up to puberty, the cardiovascular, respiratory, and nervous systems grow and develop dramatically, yet the reproductive system changes very little. Puberty is a series of changes that leads to full development of the reproductive system and also triggers growth in the musculoskeletal system.

Body System Functions Become Increasingly Differentiated Over Time Have you ever seen a newborn respond to a loud noise? The newborn's startle response involves the whole body. With maturity, the response becomes more focused, for example, covering the ears. An adult is often able to state the location of the sound and distinguish the origin of the sound.

Theories of Development

Theories of development describe and explain patterns of development common to all people. Such theories provide a basis for your nursing interventions and clinical decision making. The needs of a 6-year-old differ greatly from those of a 25-year-old or a 65-year-old, even though they all may have the same medical diagnosis (e.g., asthma) or even the same nursing diagnosis (e.g., Anxiety). Understanding the tasks associated with a person's developmental stage (1) provides a basis for assessing whether behaviors are as expected or if they need further assessment, and (2) suggests specific ways in which to support and encourage the person's progress through the developmental stage.

Each developmental theory examines how humans develop and divides the life span into stages. Each stage represents a period of time that shares common characteristics. Most theories also identify tasks that are usually accomplished in each stage. An understanding of the following key developmental theories is essential to full-spectrum nursing practice.

Developmental Task Theory

Robert Havighurst theorized that learning is a lifelong process. He believed that a person moves through six life stages, each associated with a number of tasks that must be learned. Havighurst characterizes **developmental task** as "midway between an individual need and societal demand. It assumes an active learner interacting with an active social environment" (1971, p. vi). Failure to master a task leads to imbalance within the individual, unhappiness, and difficulty mastering future tasks and interacting with others. Table 9-1 presents the tasks associated with each stage of life. It is easy to evaluate a client's completion of Havighurst's broadly written tasks, but the nonspecific time frame limits this theory's usefulness for assessing whether an individual is developing within an expected range.

 ThinkLike a Nurse 9-1

Which stage in Havighurst's developmental task theory contains the most complex tasks and would be the most difficult to master? Why?

Psychoanalytic Theory

Sigmund Freud was a pioneer in the science of human development. His psychoanalytic theory focuses on the motivation for human behavior and personality development. Freud believed human development is maintained by instinctual drives, such as libido (sexual instinct), aggression, and survival (Sadock & Sadock, 2010). Different drives predominate, depending on the age of the individual. Psychoanalytic theory became the foremost theoretical foundation of early 20th century

psychotherapy. However, Freud developed his theory in the Victorian era, when societal norms were very strict. Sexual repression and male dominance over female behavior were the cultural standard. Many of today's social scientists question whether his theory should be applied to life in the 21st century.

In Freud's theory, the personality consists of the id, ego, and superego—different "parts" that develop at different life stages. Each factor, or force, has a unique function.

- The **id** represents instinctual urges, pleasure, and gratification, such as hunger, procreation, pleasure, and aggression. We are born with our id. It is dominant in infants and young children, as well as in older children and adults who cannot control their urges.
- The **ego** begins to develop around 4 to 6 months of age and is thought to represent reality. It strives to balance what is wanted (id) and what is possible to obtain or achieve.
- The **superego** is sometimes referred to as the conscience. This force develops in early childhood (age 5 or 6) as a result of the internalization of primary caregiver responses to environmental events.
- The **unconscious mind** is composed of thoughts and memories that are not readily recalled but unconsciously influence behavior.

In the mid-1950s, Freud's daughter, the psychologist Anna Freud, identified a number of **defense mechanisms**, which she described as thought patterns or behaviors that the ego makes use of in the face of threat to biological or psychological integrity (Townsend, 2011). In other words, defense mechanisms protect us from excess anxiety. For example, after receiving a failing grade in chemistry, a student might refuse to think about it, intellectualize reasons why she failed, blame her teacher, or compensate by emphasizing her A grade in psychology. All people use defense mechanisms to varying degrees. For a comprehensive discussion of defense mechanisms, see Chapter 12 and Table 12-1.

Freud identified five stages of psychosexual development (Table 9-2). He believed that human development is perpetuated by instinctual drives, such as libido (sexual instinct), aggression, and survival (Sadock & Sadock, 2010). These drives have varying emphases, depending on the age of the individual.

KnowledgeCheck 9-1

- According to Freud, which motivator of personality is based in reality?
- Which is referred to as our conscience?
- What is the purpose of defense mechanisms?

Cognitive Development Theory

Swiss psychologist Jean Piaget studied his own children to understand how humans develop **cognitive abilities** (i.e., the ability to think, reason, and use language).

Table 9-1 ➤ Havighurst's Developmental Task Theory

STAGE	TASKS
Infants & Toddlers	**Physical Development** ■ Walking ■ Taking solid foods ■ Talking ■ Controlling bowel and bladder elimination ■ Learning sex differences and sexual modesty **Cognitive & Social Development** ■ Acquiring psychological stability ■ Forming concepts; learning language ■ Getting ready to read
Preschool & School Age	**Physical Development** ■ Learning physical skills necessary for ordinary games **Cognitive & Social Development** ■ Building wholesome attitudes toward oneself as a growing organism ■ Learning to get along with age-mates ■ Learning masculine or feminine social role ■ Acquiring fundamental skills in reading, writing, and calculating ■ Developing concepts necessary for everyday living ■ Developing a conscience, morality, and a scale of values ■ Achieving personal independence ■ Acquiring attitudes toward social groups and institutions
Adolescents	**Physical Development** ■ Accepting one's physique and using the body effectively **Cognitive & Social Development** ■ Achieving new and more mature relations with age-mates of both sexes ■ Achieving a masculine or feminine social role ■ Developing emotional independence from parents and other adults ■ Preparing for future marriage and family life ■ Preparing for a career ■ Acquiring a set of values and an ethical system to guide behavior; developing an ideology ■ Aspiring to and achieving socially responsible behavior
Young Adults	■ Choosing a mate ■ Achieving a masculine or feminine social role ■ Learning to live with a partner ■ Rearing children ■ Managing a home ■ Establishing an occupation ■ Taking on community responsibilities ■ Finding a compatible social group
Middle Adults	**Physical Development** ■ Adjusting to the physiological changes of middle age

Table 9-1 ▶ Havighurst's Developmental Task Theory—cont'd

STAGE	TASKS
	Cognitive & Social Development ■ Assisting teenage children to become responsible and happy adults ■ Achieving adult civic and social responsibility ■ Reaching and maintaining satisfactory performance in one's occupational career ■ Developing adult leisure-time activities ■ Relating oneself to one's spouse as a person
Older Adults, refer to Chapter 10.	

Source: Havighurst, R. J. (1971). *Developmental tasks and education* (3rd ed.). New York: Longman.

Table 9-2 ▶ Freud's Stages of Psychosexual Development

AGE	STAGE	DESCRIPTION
Birth–18 mo	Oral	The infant's primary needs are centered on the oral zone: lips, tongue, mouth. The need for hunger and pleasure are satisfied through the oral zone. Trust is developed through the meeting of needs. When needs are not met, aggression can manifest itself in the form of biting, spitting, or crying.
18 mo–3 yr	Anal	Neuromuscular control over the anal sphincter allows the child to have control over expulsion or retention of feces. This coincides with the child's struggle for separation and independence from caregivers. Successful completion of this stage yields a child who is self-directed, cooperative, and without shame. Conversely, the anal child will exhibit willfulness, stubbornness, and need for orderliness.
3–6 yr	Phallic	The focus is on the genital organs. This coincides with the development of gender identity. Unconscious sexual feelings toward the parent of the opposite sex are common. Children emerge from this stage with a sense of sexual curiosity and a mastery of their instinctual impulses.
6–12 yr	Latency	Ego functioning matures, and sexual urges diminish. The child focuses his energy on same-sex relationships and mastery of his world, including relationships with significant others (teachers, coaches).
13–20 yr	Genital	Puberty causes an intensification of instinctual drives, particularly sexual. The focus of this stage is the resolution of previous conflicts and the development of a mature identity and the ability to form adult relationships.

According to Piaget, cognitive development requires three core competencies: adaptation, assimilation, and accommodation. **Adaptation** is the ability to adjust to and interact with one's environment. To be able to adapt, one must assimilate and accommodate. **Assimilation** is the integration of new experiences with one's own system of knowledge. **Accommodation** is the change in one's system of knowledge that results from processing new information. For example, an infant is born with an innate ability to suck. Presented with the mother's nipple, the infant is able to assimilate the nipple to the behavior of sucking. If given a bottle, the infant can learn to accommodate the artificial nipple. However, the baby may adapt by accepting the artificial nipple only from the father, crying and fussing if the mother offers a bottle instead of her breast.

According to Piaget, cognitive development occurs from birth through adolescence in a sequence of four stages: sensorimotor, preoperational thought, concrete operations, and formal operations (Table 9-3). A child must complete each stage before moving to the next. The rate at which a child moves through the four stages is determined by the inherited intellect and the influence of the environment. Piaget does not address cognitive development after adolescence.

KnowledgeCheck 9-2

- According to Piaget, what core competencies are necessary for cognitive development?
- During which stage is the child the most egocentric?
- When does abstract thinking develop?

Table 9-3 ➤ Piaget's Stages of Cognitive Development

STAGE	AGE	CHARACTERISTICS OF DEVELOPMENT
Sensorimotor	Birth–2 yr	▪ Learns the world through the senses. ▪ Displays curiosity. ▪ Shows intentional behavior. ▪ Begins to see that objects exist apart from self. ▪ Begins to see objects as separate from self.
Preoperational	2–7 yr	▪ Uses symbols and language. ▪ Sees himself as the center of the universe: egocentric. ▪ Thought based on perception rather than logic.
Concrete operations	7–11 yr	▪ Operates and reacts to the concrete: What is perceived is actual. ▪ Egocentricity diminishes, can see from others' viewpoints. ▪ Able to use logic and reason in thinking. ▪ Able to conserve: to see that objects may change but recognizes them as the same. (e.g., water may change to ice, or a tower of blocks is the same as a long fence of blocks).
Formal operations	11–adolescence	▪ Develops the ability to think abstractly: to reason, deduce, and define concepts in a logical manner. ▪ Some individuals do not develop the ability to think abstractly.

Psychosocial Development Theory

In the 1950s Eric Erikson introduced his theory of psychosocial development. He was strongly influenced by Freud but believed that personality continues to evolve throughout the life span as the person interacts with the social world. He hypothesized that individuals must negotiate eight stages as they progress through the life span. Most people successfully move from stage to stage; however, a person can regress during times of stress to earlier stages or be forced to face tasks of later stages because of unforeseen life events, such as terminal illness. Failure to successfully move through a stage leads to maladjustment. Erikson's theory is widely used in nursing and healthcare. Below are Erikson's eight stages.

Stage 1: Trust Versus Mistrust (Birth to About 18 Months) The child develops a sense of trust in himself and the external world as a result of having his needs consistently met. This is the beginning of self-confidence. An infant who does not have his needs met develops a sense of mistrust and suspiciousness in others that will affect future interpersonal relationships.

Stage 2: Autonomy Versus Shame and Doubt (About 18 Months to 3 Years) The goal is for the child to develop self-control and independence while maintaining self-esteem. This requires an ability to cooperate and express feelings and thoughts. Failure to successfully complete this stage will lead to an adult who lacks self-confidence and feels controlled by others and who may exhibit extreme compliance (self-restraint) or defiance.

Stage 3: Initiative Versus Guilt (3 to 5 Years) The focus of this stage is to develop initiative by gradually assuming responsibility and developing self-discipline. During this stage, the superego (conscience) develops, and the child learns to manage impulses. Failure to develop initiative leads to guilt, limited creativity, lack of self-confidence, and pessimism.

Stage 4: Industry Versus Inferiority (6 to 11 Years) In this stage, the child learns that recognition comes through achievement and completion of tasks. This success occurs primarily in school. The adult who has not fulfilled the tasks of this stage will demonstrate a sense of inadequacy in all areas of life.

Stage 5: Identity Versus Role Confusion (11 to 21 Years) This stage coincides with puberty. The adolescent develops a sense of self and begins to make decisions about the future. Social groups serve as a place to test out ideas and behaviors. Healthy role models facilitate the development of identity. A person who fails to recognize his abilities and sense of self is unable to experience a solid place in the world. This is manifested by dysfunctional interpersonal relationships and occupational performance. Delinquent and rebellious behavior may be prominent when the task of identity formation is not met.

Stage 6: Intimacy Versus Isolation (21 to 40 Years) Erikson (1963) defines intimacy as "the capacity to commit himself to concrete affiliations and partnerships and to develop the ethical strength to abide by such commitments" (p. 263). Isolation is the avoidance of intimacy. The task at this stage is to develop a commitment to work and relationships. Failure to do so will result in impersonal relationships and difficulty with maintaining a job.

Stage 7: Generativity Versus Stagnation (40 to 65 Years) The goal of this stage is to be creative and productive. Often this is accomplished through work or relationships, such as raising healthy, functional children or contributing to society by developing a distinguished career, for example in nursing. The person who fails to achieve generativity (the desire and motivation to guide the next generation) may manifest stagnation in the form of superficial relationships and self-absorption.

Stage 8: Ego Integrity Versus Despair (Over 65 Years) The task of this stage is the acceptance of one's life, worth, and eventual death. Ego integrity reflects a satisfaction with life and an understanding of one's place in the life cycle. In despair, a sense of loss, discomfort with life and aging, and a fear of death are seen.

 ThinkLike a Nurse 9-2

Review the case study in the Meet Your Patients section of the chapter. Based on Erikson's psychosocial development theory, what kind of behavior would you anticipate from Carrie?

Moral Development Theory: Kohlberg

Lawrence Kohlberg (1968) developed his theory of moral development by studying the development of 84 boys over a period of 20 years. Observing their responses to moral dilemmas, Kohlberg hypothesized that a person's level of moral development can be identified by analyzing the rationale he gives for action in a moral dilemma. In this theory, moral reasoning appears to be somewhat age-related, and moral development is based on one's ability to think at progressively higher levels. Increased maturity provides some degree of higher-level thinking but does not guarantee the ability to function at the highest cognitive or moral levels. Kohlberg described the following levels; each has two stages (Kohlberg, 1968, 1981; Waugh, 1978). Not all people are able to achieve the higher levels. To see a table with expanded information about the stages,

 Go to Student Resources: Chapter 44, **ESG Table 44-1, Stages of Moral Development: Kohlberg,** on *DavisPlus.*

Level I. Preconventional The person conforms to cultural rules and labels of good and bad, but interprets them in terms of punishment and reward or in terms of the physical power of those who enforce the rules. Children ages 4 to 10 years are usually at this level; some adults are, as well.

Stage 1—punishment–obedience orientation (right action is that which avoids punishment)
Stage 2—personal interest orientation (right action is that which satisfies personal needs)

Level II. Conventional The person perceives that meeting the expectations of the family, group, or society is valuable in its own right, regardless of the consequences of the actions. More than just conforming, the person is loyal to the social order and identifies with those involved in it. Others set the standards, but motivation to follow them is internal.

Stage 3—"good boy–nice girl" orientation (right actions are those that please others)
Stage 4—law-and-order orientation (right action is following the rules)

Level III. Postconventional, Autonomous, or Principled The person makes an effort to define moral values and principles that have validity apart from society, groups, or persons in power. At this level it becomes possible for conflict to occur between two socially accepted standards, and the person attempts to decide rationally between them. Both the standards and the decision are internal.

Stage 5—legalistic, social contract orientation (right action is decided in terms of individual rights and standards agreed upon by the whole society)
Stage 6—universal ethical principles orientation (right action is determined by conscience and abstract principles such as the Golden Rule)

Moral Development Theory: Gilligan

Although all of his research subjects were male, Kohlberg claimed that his sequence of stages applies equally to everyone. The validity of his theory for women has been sharply criticized, most prominently by Carol Gilligan (1982, 1993). To address the moral development of women, Gilligan proposed an alternative theory that incorporates the concepts of caring, interpersonal relationships, and responsibility. She described a three-stage approach to moral development.

Stage 1: Caring for Oneself In this stage, the focus is providing for oneself and surviving. The individual is egocentric in thought and does not consider the needs of others. When concerns about being selfish begin to emerge, the individual is signaling a readiness to move to stage 2.

Stage 2: Caring for Others At this level, an individual recognizes the importance of relationships with others. The person is willing to make sacrifices to help others, often at the expense of her own needs. When she recognizes the conflict between caring for oneself and caring for others, the individual is ready to move to stage 3.

Stage 3: Caring for Self and Others This represents the highest stage of moral development. In this stage, care is the focus of decision making. The individual carefully balances her own needs against the needs of others to decide on a course of action.

See Chapter 44 for more discussion of moral development.

Spiritual Development Theory

James Fowler, a minister, defined faith as a universal human concern and as a process of growing in trust. He noticed that his congregants had very different approaches to faith, depending on their age. Basing his studies on the work of Piaget, Erikson, and Kohlberg, he developed a theory of faith development, which includes a pre-stage (stage 0) and six stages of faith (Fowler, 1981).

- **Stages 0, 1, and 2** are closely associated with evolving cognitive abilities. In these stages, faith depends largely on the views expressed by the parents, caregivers, and those who have significant influence in the life of the person.
- **Stage 3** coincides with the ability to use **logic** and **hypothetical thinking** to construct and evaluate ideas. At this point, faith is largely a collection of conventional, unexamined beliefs. Fowler's studies demonstrated that approximately one-fourth of all adults function at this level or lower.
- **Stages 4, 5, and 6** represent increasing levels of refinement of faith. With each increase in level there is decreasing likelihood that an individual can attain this stage of development. Fowler found that very few people achieve stage 6.

To see more details about Fowler's stages,

 Go to Student Resources: Chapter 9, **ESG Table 9-1, Fowler's Theory of Faith Development,** on Davis*Plus*.

The rest of this chapter describes the human life span as a series of developmental stages: physical, cognitive, and psychosocial. Development and common health problems are discussed for each stage. To simplify organization, you will find nursing assessments and interventions included with each stage rather than together in a single Practical Knowledge section.

THE GESTATIONAL PERIOD: CONCEPTION TO BIRTH

The time between conception and birth is called the **gestational period.** Human gestation (pregnancy) is calculated from the first day of the mother's last menstrual period and lasts approximately 40 weeks (280 days). Full discussions of pregnancy and childbirth are beyond the scope of a fundamentals text. If you need more information, refer to a maternal–child health textbook.

Fetal Development During Gestation

Pregnancy is usually divided into three trimesters, each lasting about 13 weeks.

First Trimester The first 8 weeks is known as the **embryonic phase**. It begins when an egg released from a woman's ovary unites with a sperm cell, usually in one of the woman's fallopian tubes. This is called **fertilization (or conception)**. Continual cell division leads to the development of a tiny ball of cells called the **morula**, which travels toward the woman's uterus for a period of about 7 days before implanting there as a multicelled **blastocyst**. Upon implantation, three primary germ layers begin to differentiate, and the **embryo** begins to resemble a tiny organism with a head and tail. By week 4, the brain, heart, and liver have begun to form, and tiny limb buds are present. As early as 6 to 7 weeks, you can hear the fetal heartbeat with a fetal ultrasound Doppler. By the end of week 8, all organs are formed, and the embryo is then called a **fetus**.

Second Trimester Rapid fetal growth and further development of the body systems characterize the second trimester. At about 16 to 20 weeks of pregnancy, the mother can feel her fetus move, a sensation called *quickening*. At the end of the second trimester, the fetus has all organs and body parts intact that will develop during the last trimester. The kidneys are intact and begin to produce urine, although they do not effectively concentrate it until late in the third trimester. The lungs are formed, but they do not contain enough of the substance to keep air sacs open after birth until late in the third trimester.

Third Trimester The fetus continues to grow in size and add subcutaneous fat. Body systems mature in preparation for extrauterine life. If born prematurely during this trimester, the newborn may be able to survive with intensive care. By week 37, the fetus is considered full term; after 41 weeks it is considered post-term. A normal full-term baby weighs, on average, 5 lb 8 oz to 8 lb 13 oz (2,500 to 4,000 g) and is 20 in. (50 cm) long. If you would like to see a concise timeline of fetal growth,

 Go to Chapter 9, **Tables, Boxes, Figures: ESG Table 9-2,** on Davis*Plus*.

Maternal Changes During Pregnancy

A woman's health during pregnancy is essential for healthy, sustained growth and development of the fetus. It is important for young women to develop good health practices well before conception, including exercise, a balanced diet, smoking cessation, avoidance of alcohol, and regular dental checkups. The growing fetus depends entirely on the placenta for oxygen and nutrition. Therefore, many of the physical changes that the woman experiences during pregnancy are for the purpose of increasing blood flow through the placenta to the baby. A pregnant woman's heart enlarges slightly and the chest wall expands so that respiratory rate and cardiac output increase significantly. In fact, the woman's normal blood flow increases by about 30% by the 35th week of pregnancy.

First Trimester Menses typically cease. Hormone shifts, primarily in progesterone and estrogen, may cause the pregnant women to experience morning sickness, fullness in the pelvic area, breast enlargement and tenderness, urinary frequency, and fatigue.

Second Trimester The uterus enlarges and hyper-pigmentation of the skin occurs, often creating a dark line from the umbilicus to the symphysis pubis and causing the nipples to darken. Other common changes include mottling of the cheeks and forehead, swelling and bleeding of the gums, and "stuffiness" from swelling in the mucous membranes in the nose. The woman begins to feel the fetus moving and may experience mild contractions (called Braxton Hicks).

Third Trimester Fetal movement is the predominant feature of the latter period of pregnancy. The breasts begin to produce and secrete colostrum in preparation for lactation. Pressure from the enlarged fetus may cause shortness of breath and urinary frequency.

Psychosocial Challenges As the birth of a child is a life-changing condition, it is normal for women to feel ambivalent about pregnancy at first, but these feelings usually resolve in the second trimester. The pregnant woman must adapt to changes in body image, role changes, concerns about sexuality, fears about labor and delivery, concern for the baby's health and safety, planning for care of the child after delivery, financial pressures, and stresses involving employment during pregnancy.

Common Health Problems During Gestation

Blood circulating through the placenta carries nutrients and oxygen to the fetus and toxins and metabolic wastes away from the fetus. Other substances also cross the placenta. For example, **teratogens** are substances that interfere with normal growth and development.

   Key Point: *Because the brain and other vital organs develop during the first trimester, this is the time when the fetus is most vulnerable to teratogens.*

- *Alcohol* can cause birth defects, growth retardation, developmental delay, and impaired intellectual development.
- *Nicotine* interferes with the transport of oxygen to the fetus, contributing to premature birth, low birth weight, and learning disabilities.
- *Morphine, heroin, methadone, and other narcotics,* when used during pregnancy, cause the newborn to suffer from withdrawal at birth. Symptoms include tremors, restlessness, hyperactive reflexes, poor temperature control, vomiting and diarrhea, high-pitched cries, seizures, and sometimes death.
- *Cocaine, including crack, and methamphetamines* are highly addictive and potentially harmful to the fetus. Infants born to cocaine users and crack users are more likely to suffer from growth retardation and to have sleep disturbances, hyperactive reflexes, irritability, feeding difficulties, attention and behavioral disorders, and learning disabilities at school age. These infants are also more likely to die from **sudden infant death syndrome (SIDS)**, the sudden, unexplained

death of an infant (discussed in more detail in the section about infancy).

- ✚ *Medications,* both prescribed and over the counter, can have teratogenic effects. Examples include the acne medication isotretinoin (Accutane), tetracycline (Achromycin), phenytoin (Dilantin), and lithium (Lithobid). Pregnant women should check with their primary care provider before taking any medications or herbal remedies.

Effects of Maternal Age The risk for preterm birth, low birth weight, and fetal death is higher for babies born to adolescent mothers. The risk of fetal death is also higher for mothers over age 40 (Centers for Disease Control and Prevention [CDC], n.d.d.). Furthermore, the risk of conceiving a child with Down syndrome (trisomy 21) and other congenital anomalies increases for each year over the age of 35, but dramatically after age 42.

Effects of Maternal Health Maternal diseases, such as *rubella, syphilis, and gonorrhea,* although not common, can cause fetal blindness, deafness, or fetal loss. *Cytomegalovirus (CMV)* is a common, flu-like viral infection in adults. If the mother acquires CMV during pregnancy, the fetus can suffer intrauterine growth retardation, poor brain growth, enlarged liver (hepatomegaly) with jaundice, irritation of the lung (pneumonitis), and bleeding problems. *Toxoplasmosis* can be transmitted to the unborn fetus through handling of contaminated cat litter. If the mother experiences an outbreak of genital herpes at the time of delivery, there is risk of passing the virus to the infant. *Maternal diabetes* can result in a low blood sugar after birth and also have lasting effects on the fetus. Failure to control the diabetes may lead to neural tube and heart defects, as well as **macrosomia** (large body size).

Effects of Maternal Nutrition Even before pregnancy, nutrition is vital to the fetus. Appropriate healthy weight management before conception and appropriate maternal weight gain during pregnancy contributes to appropriate fetal birth weight and reduce the risk of fetal illness and infections. The recommended average weight gain for a pregnancy is 25 to 35 pounds. The expected weight gain is higher for underweight women and lower for overweight women.

✚ Folic acid deficiency in the first weeks of pregnancy—typically before the woman even knows she is pregnant—is a risk factor for neural tube defects, such as spina bifida. Neural tube defects occur during the first weeks of fetal development.

▬ ASSESSMENT

Routine prenatal visits and screenings usually take place monthly until 28 weeks, then every 2 weeks until 36 weeks, then weekly until birth. In addition to vital signs, weight, fetal heart tones, nutritional status, and other measures of maternal–fetal well-being should be assessed at each visit (Fig. 9-1).

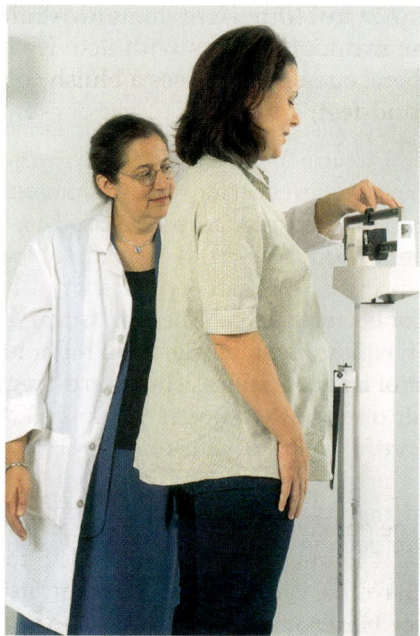

FIGURE 9-1 After establishing a baseline weight in early pregnancy, monitor for appropriate weight gain at each prenatal visit.

Assess for common discomforts associated with pregnancy, such as nausea, fatigue, and back pain. Preexisting conditions (e.g., diabetes) must be carefully monitored. Inquire about medication use, including over-the-counter drugs (OTCs), the use of alternative therapies, and other substances. Also screen for risk factors for complications of pregnancy, such as the following:

- **Birth defects.** Women who are at higher risk for a fetus with a birth defect are those with advanced maternal age (over age 40), family history of congenital anomalies, maternal diabetes with insulin use, viral infection during pregnancy, and exposure to high levels of radiation. Blood markers and ultrasound screening are done to detect neural tube defects, abdominal wall defects, trisomy 21 (Down syndrome), and trisomy 18.
- **Gestational diabetes.** Screening for gestational diabetes is most often done between 24 and 28 weeks' gestation—earlier if there is a history of gestational diabetes with a previous pregnancy.
- **Group B streptococcus.** The Centers for Disease Control and Prevention (CDC), the American Academy of Pediatrics (AAP), and the American College of Obstetricians and Gynecologists (ACOG) recommend that pregnant women be screened for group B streptococcus between 35 and 37 weeks' gestation.

▒▒ INTERVENTIONS

Key Point: *One of the most important nursing interventions for promoting maternal and fetal health is to facilitate and teach the importance of early and continuing prenatal care.* Early prenatal care can identify complications of pregnancy, prevent some of the effects of maternal diseases such as diabetes, and provide an opportunity for patient education.

Key Point: *You should stress that maternal nutrition is important for a healthy baby. The mother's food intake should be well balanced.* The recommended dietary allowances of vitamins and minerals for the pregnant woman range from 25% to 50% higher than for the nonpregnant woman. Pregnant women should increase their caloric intake by 10% to 15%. Inadequate protein affects formation of the placenta and fetal brain development. Increasing folic acid (also called folate) intake to 400 to 800 mcg daily reduces the risk of neural tube defects. Women who are of childbearing age should follow these guidelines daily rather than waiting for pregnancy to occur. This will help achieve a national goal for the year 2020 of reducing the incidence of neural tube defects (U.S. Department of Health and Human Services [USDHHS], 2010b). You can find the national goals for 2020 on the Healthy People 2020 Web site,

 http://www.healthypeople.gov/

Other teaching topics include the following:

Information regarding sexually transmitted infections (STIs) and vaginal infections
Information about urinary tract infections
Exercise patterns
Child care
Fetal growth and development
Hazardous substances to avoid
Avoiding use of OTCs medication without approval from the supervising provider
Self-care measures for common discomforts of pregnancy
Danger signs that alert the woman to call her care provider
Signs of impending labor; when to go to the birthing unit

Knowledge Check 9-3

- What are the most common health concerns to monitor for in the gestational period?
- Identify at least four important topics for health teaching with the expectant mother.
- Why is early prenatal care so important?

THE NEONATAL PERIOD: BIRTH TO 28 DAYS

During the **neonatal period** (the first month of life), the newborn's primary task is to stabilize the body's major organ systems and adapt to life outside the uterus. Behaviors are primarily reflexive.

Physical Development of the Neonate

Growth The normal full-term newborn weighs between 2,500 and 4,000 g (5 lb 8 oz to 8 lb 13 oz). Lower birth weights are seen with prematurity, whereas higher birth weights are associated with gestational diabetes. The neonate measures between 18 and 22 in. (46 and 56 cm) in length (Fig. 9-2) and the arms are slightly longer than the legs.

At birth, the head is one-fourth the total body length, with a head circumference of 33 to 35 cm (13 to 14 in.). For a few days, it may appear asymmetrical because of molding during vaginal birth. The skull consists of six soft bones separated by sutures composed of cartilage (Fig. 9-3), with anterior and posterior **fontanels** (soft spots). These spaces allow room to accommodate the rapid growth of the infant's brain during the first months of life.

Respirations   At birth, the most critical adaptation is the *establishment of respirations*. Pressure on the baby's chest during vaginal birth helps eliminate amniotic fluid from the lungs in preparation for breathing. The normal newborn's respirations are irregular, shallow, and 30 to 50 breaths/min, with brief periods of **periodic breathing** (pauses in breathing).

Cardiovascular System   The cardiovascular system must also adapt to the change from placental blood flow to independent circulation. The average heart rate of a newborn is 120 to 140 beats/min, with slightly lower rates at rest and higher rates with activity or crying. Poor peripheral circulation causes a bluish coloration of the hands and feet; this is normal and usually disappears within a few hours of birth.

Thermoregulation   Thermoregulation is another critical task at birth. The newborn can produce adequate heat but cannot protect against heat loss. Heat may be lost by exposure to cool air temperatures, by contact with cooler solid surfaces, or by evaporation of moisture from the skin. The normal newborn's temperature is close to that of an adult. To assist in thermoregulation, it is important to keep the newborn warm and dry, with a cap on his head.

Elimination   At birth, the kidneys produce 15 to 60 mL of urine per kilogram of body weight per day. During the first 24 hours, the newborn voids 5 to 25 times. Newborns have limited ability to concentrate urine. At birth, the newborn's lower intestine is filled with **meconium**, a sticky, greenish-black substance formed from amniotic fluid and intestinal secretions. Meconium is usually passed within 12 hours of birth, and the stool progressively changes in color to yellow. The full-term infant is able to swallow, digest, metabolize, and absorb proteins and simple carbohydrates. Stomach capacity varies from 30 to 90 mL, depending on the infant's weight. Normal colonic bacteria are established within a week of birth.

Epidermis and Dermis   The epidermis and dermis are very thin at birth and can be easily damaged. Infants are born with varying degrees of **vernix caseosa**, a cheese-like protective covering for the skin. **Milia**, tiny white spots, may be present on the newborn's face, and the area over the sacrum may show a darkly pigmented area called a **mongolian spot**. All such features disappear spontaneously.

Neuromuscular System   The neuromuscular system is not completely developed at birth. However, the following **reflexes** (automatic responses) are present at birth. Selected reflexes are illustrated in Figure 9-4.

- **Rooting.** Rooting is elicited by stroking the infant's cheek with the nipple or finger. In response, the newborn turns his head toward the stimulus, opens his mouth, takes hold and sucks. This reflex disappears by 3 to 4 months of age.
- **Sucking Reflex.** The sucking reflex is elicited by touching the infant's lips.
- **Swallowing Reflex.** The swallowing reflex is coordinated with sucking and usually occurs without gagging, coughing, or vomiting. This response is weak with prematurity or neurological defect.
- **Grasp Reflex.** The grasp reflex is triggered by placing a finger in the palm of the infant's hand (palmar) or at the base of the toes (plantar). The infant's fingers curl around the examiner's fingers, or the toes curl downward. The palmar reflex lessens by 3 to 4 months, and the plantar reflex lessens by 8 months.

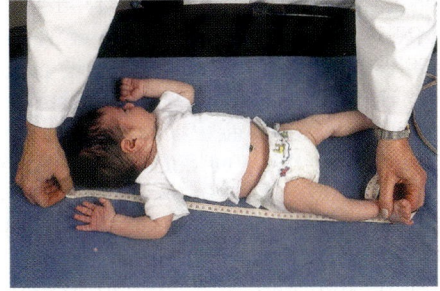

FIGURE 9-2 Measuring the length of a newborn.

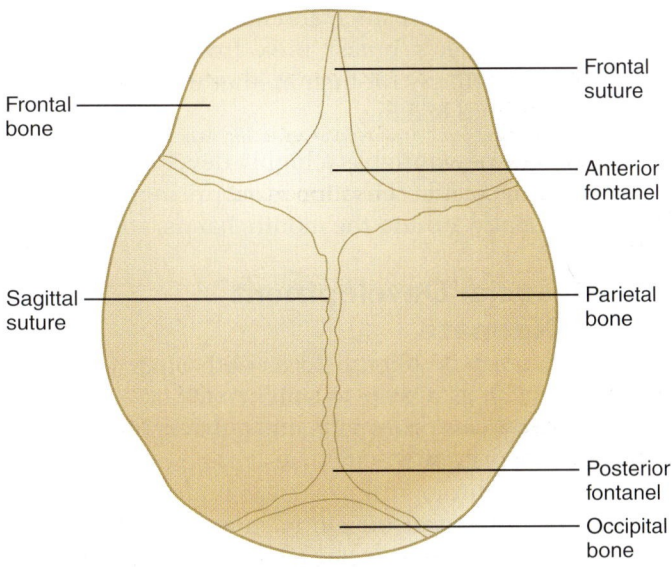

Frontal bone

Sagittal suture

Frontal suture

Anterior fontanel

Parietal bone

Posterior fontanel

Occipital bone

FIGURE 9-3 Sutures and fontanel of the newborn's skull.

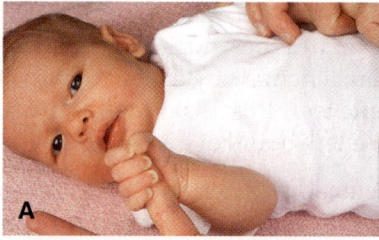

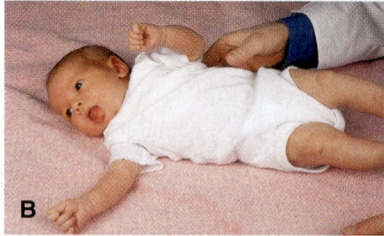

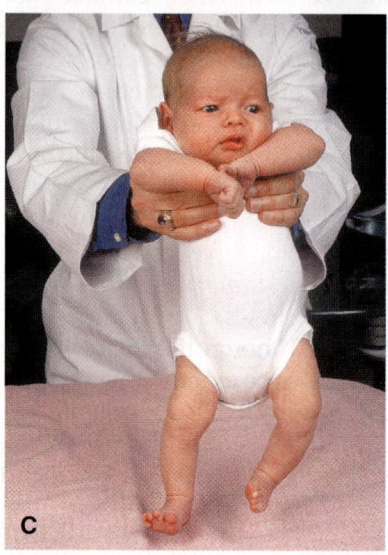

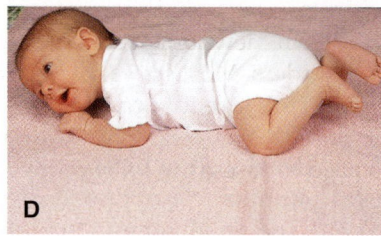

FIGURE 9-4 Several infant reflexes: *A*, the palmar grasp reflex; *B*, tonic neck reflex; *C*, stepping reflex; and *D*, crawling reflex.

- **Tonic Neck or Fencing Reflex.** The tonic neck, or fencing, reflex is elicited by rotating the infant's head to the left with the left arm and leg extended and the right arm and leg flexed. Turn the head to the right, and the extremities assume the opposite posture. The response disappears by 3 to 4 months.
- **Moro or Startle Reflex.** This reflex is elicited by placing the infant on a flat surface and striking the surface to startle the infant. Symmetrical abduction and extension of the arms are expected as an indicator of overall neurological health. The fingers fan out and form a C with the thumb and forefinger. This response is absent by 6 months.

- **Stepping Reflex.** Elicit the stepping reflex by holding the infant vertically, allowing one foot to touch a surface (e.g., tabletop). The infant will simulate walking by alternating flexion and extension of the feet during the 3 to 4 weeks of life.
- **Crawling Reflex.** The crawling reflex is noted by placing the infant on her abdomen. The newborn makes crawling movements with her arms and legs. This response should disappear by 6 weeks of age.
- **Babinski Reflex.** The Babinski reflex is elicited by stroking upward along the lateral aspect of the sole. A positive response occurs when the toes hyperextend and the great toe dorsiflexes. An infant who does not respond in this manner should undergo a neurological evaluation. This reflex disappears as the infant begins to walk or between 12 and 18 months.

Cognitive Development of the Neonate

In the first month of life, the neonate responds to stimuli in a reflexive manner. Piaget described this as the *sensorimotor phase.* Despite the newborn's limited voluntary abilities, the sensory functions are well developed.

Vision   At birth, the eyes are treated with antibiotics to prevent blindness caused by gonorrhea. After the ointment has been absorbed, the newborn begins to fixate on an object. During the first few weeks of life, the infant focuses on objects, following from side to side with his gaze. The infant has visual preferences for the human face, black-and-white contrasting patterns, and large objects. Some newborns appear cross-eyed because of undeveloped ocular muscle control; this normally resolves in 3 to 4 months. Eye color varies from dark to slate gray to pale blue. Because the lacrimal apparatus is not fully developed, the newborn does not produce tears until at least week 4 of life.

Hearing and Smell   Once the amniotic fluid drains from the ears, hearing is equivalent to that of an adult. Newborns react strongly to pungent odors by turning the head away from a smell and are able to distinguish their own mother's breast milk from that of other women. They will cry for their mother when her breasts are engorged and leaking.

Touch   The newborn has a highly developed sense of touch, and his tactile sensation is surprisingly sophisticated, especially around the mouth, hands, and feet.

Psychosocial Development of the Neonate

The neonate calms when held or with other pacifying measures, such as a warm blanket, pacifier, and swaddling. Crying is the principal method for communicating a need or displeasure. Sometimes crying occurs simply because the neurological system is immature. Erikson identified the central developmental task of the first 18 months of life as developing a sense of trust. The neonate is completely dependent on his caretakers for all needs. Prompt responses to cries of discomfort create security and trust and promote **attachment**, emotional bonding between parent and child.

Common Health Problems of the Neonate

Respiratory Distress   Respiratory distress is one of the most serious problems facing newborns. It occurs most commonly in infants born before the lungs mature, but can also be caused by aspiration of meconium during the birthing process. Newborns in respiratory distress are typically pale or mottled, with labored respirations, hypothermia, and flaccid muscle tone.

Birth Injuries   Birth injuries may occur at the time of the birthing process. The following are three examples:

- **Caput succedaneum**, edema of the scalp that crosses the suture lines, results from head compression against the cervix during labor. The fluid is reabsorbed in 1 to 3 days.
- **Fracture of the clavicle** occurs with breech presentation or as a result of difficulty delivering a large baby whose shoulder gets stuck behind the mother's pelvic bones. Often no intervention is needed except for careful handling and supporting the affected bone.
- **Birth asphyxia** is a serious and potentially permanent injury resulting from perinatal events, such as a *cord prolapse* (compression of the umbilical cord), *placental abruption* (bleeding secondary to tear of the placenta), other interruptions of the blood supply between the baby and placenta, or delay in infant respiration after birth.

Congenital Anomalies   Congenital anomalies (birth defects) may be visible at birth or may become apparent in the neonatal period. Treatment may be initiated, if appropriate. Congenital heart defects, fistulas, cleft lip and palate, and inborn metabolic problems are some common birth defects.

Infectious Microorganisms   Infectious microorganisms that do not cause illness in older babies can cause sepsis for newborns, especially those born prematurely. Pregnant women should be screened prenatally for STIs, and treatment initiated, if possible. Newborns exposed to infections during the gestational period should be tested as soon as possible after birth.

Jaundice   Jaundice is another risk for newborns. Within 48 to 72 hours after birth, the newborn's red blood cell (RBC) count normally begins to decrease. One by-product of RBC destruction is **bilirubin**, a yellowish pigment. If the newborn is not successful in eliminating the excess bilirubin, jaundice develops, giving the newborn's skin a yellowish cast. If the bilirubin level becomes too high, the newborn can suffer neurological consequences as the pigment enters the brain. Sunlight breaks down bilirubin; thus, phototherapy is a treatment of choice for jaundice.

Fetal Alcohol Syndrome   Fetal alcohol syndrome may occur in infants of pregnant women addicted to alcohol. It is characterized by irregular facial features and cognitive deficits.

Women With Substance Addiction   Newborns born to women who abuse substances during pregnancy are at risk for respiratory distress, behavioral abnormalities, and birth defects, as well as drug withdrawal.

ASSESSMENT

Physical assessment begins at birth. The initial assessment tool is the **Apgar scoring system**. The score is based on heart rate, respiratory effort, muscle tone, reflex irritability, and skin color. Each category is scored at 1 and 5 minutes after birth. The 1-minute score indicates how well the baby tolerated the birthing process; the 5-minute score indicates how well the baby is adapting to his new environment. A high score indicates fetal well-being. Prematurity, neuromuscular disease, and maternal sedation during the birthing process are all factors that can lower the Apgar scores. For a table to assist you with Apgar scoring,

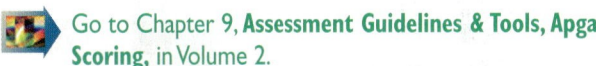 Go to Chapter 9, **Assessment Guidelines & Tools, Apgar Scoring,** in Volume 2.

During the first 24 hours after birth, the nurse assesses the infant's transition to extrauterine life. For the first 6 to 8 hours, the newborn alternately cries and appears interested in the environment. The baby then enters the sleep stage, which lasts 2 to 4 hours. The heart and respiratory rates decrease and the infant is in a state of calm. After this restful phase, the infant is alert and responsive. The heart and respiratory rates again increase.

Shortly after birth, newborns are screened for a variety of genetic disorders. Most states require screening for phenylketonuria (PKU) (an inborn error of metabolism), hypothyroidism, galactosemia, and sickle-cell disease. You will also need to assess the following parameters:

Vital signs
Elimination (first urine and meconium)
Presence of congenital anomalies
Reflexes
Ability to breastfeed or take formula from a bottle
Skin integrity
Parent–infant attachment

INTERVENTIONS

The neonatal period is a time of transition. Feeding concerns and uncertainty about appropriate care are the primary reasons parents seek healthcare advice. Nursing interventions for the neonate are designed to smooth the transition to extrauterine life and help the neonate adjust to his new environment. Activities include the following:

- Thoroughly dry the neonate at birth and after bathing to prevent heat loss via evaporation. Also, wrap the neonate in blankets, and place her in her mother's arms or in a warmed crib.

- Assist the mother with breastfeeding or formula feeding. Often assistance is needed with the first few feedings as the newborn learns to latch on to the nipple.
- Teach parents the importance of providing warmth, nutrition, and a clean environment to prevent infection.
- Teach the caregivers about expected behavior, including crying, eating, and elimination.
- Provide circumcision care. **Circumcision** is surgical removal of the foreskin of the penis. Many male infants are circumcised a day or two after birth, although there is controversy over risks and benefits. Risks include hemorrhage, infection, and meatal stenosis. Benefits are said to include prevention of penile cancer and cervical cancer in a sexual partner. The main reason most parents elect circumcision for their infant is social, so their child looks like other family members and peers. Parental consent is required for this procedure. Care of the site depends on the procedure used. Whatever the procedure, regularly observe and teach parents to observe for hemorrhage, swelling, or oozing (signs of infection).

INFANCY: 1 MONTH TO 1 YEAR OF AGE

The remainder of the first year is known as **infancy**. This is a time associated with dramatic physical changes and acquisition of numerous skills.

Physical Development of the Infant

Growth During the first year of life, growth is very rapid. The full-term newborn loses approximately 8% to 10% of birth weight in the first days of life but will regain it by 2 weeks of age. The infant gains about 1½ pounds per month for the first 3 months. Birth weight doubles by 5 months of age and triples by 1 year. Length increases approximately 1 inch per month until 6 months of age; it then slows to 1 inch over the next 6 months. Head circumference increases by about 33% in the first year.

Eruption of Primary Teeth Eruption of teeth varies among children, but there is a distinct, predictable pattern. The first tooth typically appears between 6 and 8 months of age. First to appear are lower central incisors, followed by the upper central incisors.

Feeding Infants typically consume about 30 ounces of breast milk or formula per day by 4 months of age. Breastfeeding is recommended because it is considered the most complete nutritional source for infants up to 6 months of age. **Key Point:** *Breastfeeding is accompanied by a lower incidence of food allergies, gastroenteritis, ear infections, and overweight in childhood, adolescence, and adulthood (Waldrop, 2008). In addition, breast milk supplies immunoglobulins that help the infant to resist infection.* However, if breastfeeding is not possible or acceptable to the parents, the nurse should support the parents' choice of method. Most infants are physiologically ready to take solid foods between 4 and 6 months of age, but adequate nutrition

can be maintained with breast milk or formula for a full year. The choices of when to begin introducing solid foods and what to use are often culturally determined, as is choice of when to wean.

Sleep Patterns Sleep patterns vary among infants. Generally by 3 to 4 months the infant has developed a night pattern of sleeping and can sleep approximately 10 hours. Infants vary in the number and length of naps they take, but the total numbers of hours they sleep per day is about 15.

Motor Development Motor development follows a predictable pattern. Box 9-1 lists typical milestones.

Cognitive Development of the Infant

Piaget describes the infancy phase of cognitive development as the *sensorimotor phase*. Although the neonate responds in a reflexive manner, the infant makes major strides in motor development and is able to vocally interact with caregivers. An infant's visual acuity and color discrimination allow her to see and explore the environment. Hearing becomes more discriminating, and infants please themselves by vocalizing with cooing, laughing, and repeating sounds they find pleasurable. By the 12th month, the infant is able to imitate sounds and understand simple words and may have a vocabulary of four or five simple words, such as "da-da."

BOX 9-1 ■ Milestones of Infant Development

- Infants can smile by the age of 3 months.
- By the age of 5 months, an infant can roll from abdomen to back.
- By 6 months, an infant can turn from back to abdomen.
- At 7 months, most infants can sit alone.
- Crawling on hands and knees occurs around 9 months.
- By the age of 10 months, the infant's pincer grasp is well enough developed to pick up finger foods; the child can move from a prone to sitting position.
- At 11 months, the infant can "cruise"—walk holding on to furniture.
- Many infants attempt their first independent steps by 12 months.
- By 12 months, many infants can pick up objects and let them go, put objects into a container, and take them out again. They typically can also find an object that has been hidden and are beginning to use objects, such as cups and combs, correctly, as when "combing dolly's hair."
- By 12 months, infants can typically respond to simple verbal requests and commands, such as "Stop!" or "No." They may also use simple gestures such as waving bye-bye or shaking their head no, and they may try to imitate adults' words.
- Psychosocial milestones include testing of caregivers to see what response is elicited by crying, refusals, and so on; anxiety with strangers; and strong preference for the primary caregiver (usually the mother).

At this stage, infants learn by doing. They develop a simple sense of cause and effect, delighting in the fact that squeezing a ball, for example, causes it to squeak, and repeating their experiment over and over again. By 12 months of age, the infant recognizes familiar objects and searches for them when they are out of sight.

Psychosocial Development of the Infant

In infancy the central task remains the development of trust. The response of the caregivers in the neonatal phase has set the tone for ongoing interaction between caregivers and child. Continued prompt responses to discomfort, cuddling, and stimulating interaction provide the infant with a sense of trust in the world.

Freud refers to infancy as the *oral stage.* The infant receives pleasure in sucking and learns to quiet herself by oral stimulation such as eating, sucking on a pacifier, or placing her hand in her mouth. At 2 or 3 months of age, infants begin to smile in response to others. At about 9 months they interact more with their environment and socialize with others. They enjoy simple games such as peek-a-boo and patty-cake.

Common Health Problems of the Infant

Common problems that cause distress for infants and their caregivers include the following.

Crying and Colic

Crying often alarms parents; however, it is a form of communication for the infant and a normal infant reaction to discomfort, cold, or hunger. A healthy infant will have "fussy" periods each day that may last up to 1 to 2 hours. Extended crying may be a sign of colic, a term used to describe frequent episodes of abdominal pain. The infant is often inconsolable during these episodes. The cause is unknown. Current theories include gulping of air, allergy or intolerance to formula or something that the breastfeeding mother ate, inability to digest the carbohydrates consumed, overstimulation, and parental anxiety. Colic typically disappears at about 3 months of age.

Failure to Thrive

Infants depend upon their caregivers for food, water, warmth, comfort, and love. An infant who is deprived of a comforting, responsive relationship with a mother or caregiver will not thrive even if supplied with adequate nutrition. The infant will fail to gain weight, be unable to meet age-appropriate developmental tasks, be malnourished, and may have difficulty interacting with others. This syndrome, known as failure to thrive, is exhibited, for example, in some infants in orphanages. Erikson believed the syndrome was proof of the essential nature of the trust versus mistrust stage. Notice, however, that failure to thrive can also stem from organic causes, such as disease or drug withdrawal.

Dental Caries

Dental caries (tooth decay) can develop as early as the end of the first year in infants allowed to sleep with a bottle containing anything other than water. Caries are caused by pooling in the back of the mouth of fluids containing sugar, such as breast milk, formula, or juice. If you need more information about dental problems, see Chapter 25.

Example Problem: Abuse, Neglect, and Violence

We have chosen abuse, neglect, and violence as the classic example of a problem of development because they form a problem that occurs in all developmental stages. You will read about it again and again in sections about other developmental stages, where we discuss how it manifests in those stages and suggest appropriate nursing interventions.

About 1 in 50 infants in the United States are neglected or abused, according to a national study (Brodowski, Nolan, Gaudiosi, et al., 2008). Nearly a third of the infants were 1 week old or younger when the maltreatment was reported. Child abuse may take the form of physical abuse, psychological maltreatment and neglect, or sexual abuse. Neglect is most commonly seen. Unexplained injuries, neurological defects, seizures, and respiratory difficulty are all overt signs of abuse. **Key Point:** *Abusive head trauma (AHT) (previously known as shaken-baby syndrome), caused by violent shaking of an infant, is a form of abuse that causes severe brain injury but may not produce visible evidence of trauma. It can cause blindness and spinal cord damage, as well as broken bones.*

Factors associated with child abuse and neglect include low income status, low maternal education, nonwhite race, large family size, young maternal age, single-parent household, and parental psychiatric disturbances (National Guideline Clearinghouse [NGC], 2007; Schnitzer & Ewigman, 2008). Household composition is another risk factor: Young children living with unrelated adults, step-parents, or foster parents are at increased risk of fatal injury from maltreatment. Mothers, especially mothers in single-parent households, are two times more likely than fathers to be perpetrators of abuse (Schnitzer & Ewigman, 2008; Wilcox & Dew, 2008).

Unintentional Injury

Automobile accidents are a major cause of death in infants, often because the child was not properly restrained. Falls, burns, choking, and drowning are other common causes of accidental injury and death in infants. As infants mature, they may attempt to climb from cribs onto chairs or tables, or up or down ungated stairs. Their tendency to explore things with their mouths may lead to choking on small objects, such as bottle caps, buttons, and parts of toys. If you require more information about infant safety, refer to Chapter 24.

Sudden Infant Death Syndrome (SIDS)

SIDS is the sudden death of a previously healthy infant with no explainable cause. Even postmortem examinations fail to reveal a cause of death. The peak incidence is usually around 3 to 4 months of age, although it may occur up to 12 months of age. An increased incidence is associated with prematurity, low birth weight, male gender, African American race, smoking in the household, swaddling, and putting an infant to sleep in the prone position (Fig. 9-5). Breastfeeding and offering a pacifier at naptime and bedtime are thought to be preventive measures (Adams, Good, & Defranco, 2009).

◼ ASSESSMENT

The infant typically has regular appointments with the pediatrician or primary care provider until at least 6 months of age. As a rule, visits are timed to coincide with the immunization schedule at 2, 4, 6, and 12 months. More frequent visits may be required if problems are identified. At each visit, measure the infant's growth and development and compare against standards for height, weight, head circumference, and gross and fine motor skills.

The Denver Developmental Screening Test (Denver II, 1990) is a frequently used standardized test to assess development. The Denver II evaluates four major areas: personal-social, fine motor skills, language, and gross motor skills. It requires specialized training to administer and evaluate.

✚ You should be aware of factors that increase the risk for child abuse, and assess for abuse any time there is an injury that is not well explained by the parent's account of how it occurred. For further discussion about assessing for abuse,

 Go to Chapter 9, **Procedure 9-1: Assessing for Abuse,** in Volume 2.

Also see the accompanying Highlights of Procedures box.

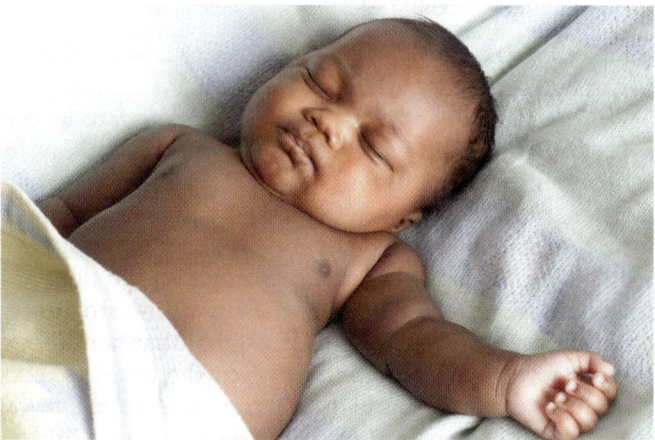

FIGURE 9-5 The "Back to Sleep" campaign teaches parents to place the infant in the supine position for sleeping.

Highlights of Procedures 9-1

 For steps to follow in all procedures, refer to the Universal Steps for All Procedures found on the inside back cover of Volume 2. Go to the full procedures in Volume 2 to practice and learn the skill. Use these Procedure Highlights later to help you review key steps.

Procedure 9-1: Assessing for Abuse

➤ Use a nonjudgmental approach. Do not make assumptions.

➤ Take a health history, assessing for physical, sexual, and psychological abuse.

➤ Perform a physical assessment; ensure the integrity of evidence that may be needed for criminal prosecution.

➤ Assess whether injuries are consistent with history.

➤ Observe for signs of neglect.

➤ If appropriate, refer for help in escaping the abusive situation.

➤ If appropriate, refer parent, caregiver, or partner involved in abuse to hotlines or agencies focused on stopping the abuse.

➤ Report abuse according to agency and state guidelines.

◼ INTERVENTIONS

Nursing interventions for the infant focus on health promotion, safety, and growth and development.

Nutrition Teach parents about adequate nutrition, adding foods to the diet, and expected elimination patterns. If breastfeeding is not possible, or is not the parents' method of choice, commercially prepared formulas

---

Quality and Safety Education for Nurses

Detecting and Preventing Abuse

Chapter-Related Concepts: *Age-Specific Assessments, Age-Specific Interventions*

Competency: *Teamwork and Collaboration: (Knowledge, Skills, Attitudes)**

Detection and prevention of abuse require collaborative efforts of the healthcare team. The goal of the collaborative approach is to reduce trauma to the victims during the investigation and assessment of the patient. The team (comprising members from Child Protective Services [DCFS], Law Enforcement, State's Attorney's Office, Medical Personnel, and Mental Health Counselors) employs a multidisciplinary approach in dealing with issues of child abuse. The team approach decreases the number of interviews and invasive procedures a child must endure, thereby reducing the trauma that children face when they have been victims of sexual or physical abuse.

Think about it: Do you see how teamwork and collaboration relate to the key concepts of development and stage?

For specific Knowledge, Skills, and Attitudes,

 Go to the QSEN Web site at http://www.qsen.org/

fortified with vitamins and minerals are acceptable. Cow's milk should not be used during the first year of life because infants have difficulty digesting the fat in it, and it is low in iron.

Colic Provide information about using warmth, motion, and security to relieve colic. For example, parents might try swaddling the baby, cuddling him close to their body, rocking him, placing him in a "kangaroo" pouch or a back pack, or placing him in a swinging chair.

 SIDS In accordance with recommendations in *Healthy People 2020*, teach parent to place infants on their backs to sleep. Research shows that this greatly decreases the risk for SIDS. Additional interventions are discussed in Chapter 24.

 Car Seats Stress the importance of car seats. Under federal law, infants must be secured in the back seat in an approved car seat every time they are in a vehicle. Because of poorly developed musculoskeletal head support, infants should be placed in a rear-facing position until 2 years of age and until they reach the height and weight recommended by the seat manufacturer (AAP, 2011). For more information about car seat restraints, refer to Chapter 24 in this book and

 Go to the American Academy of Pediatrics Web site, at http://www.aap.org/family/carseatguide.htm

Immunizations Immunizations are a major aspect of health promotion for the infant. The infant receives immunizations at 2, 4, 6, and 12 months. The CDC is no longer expressing a preference for administering the combined MMRV vaccine rather than two shots (MMR for measles, mumps and rubella, and a separate one for varicella [chicken pox] [CDC, 2011a]). To see the CDC's optimal immunization schedule for children up to 6 years of age,

 Go to Student Resources: Chapter 9, Tables, Boxes, Figures: **ESG Figure 9-1,** on *DavisPlus*.

Recommendations change frequently. You can always find the most current schedule on the CDC Web site, at

 http://www.cdc.gov/vaccines/schedules/index.html

 Unintentional Injury Stress the importance of constant supervision. As the infant gains greater mobility, potential dangers (e.g., for drowning, falls, and burns) increase. To prevent drowning, infants should never be left unattended in sinks, shallow baths, and plastic wading pools, even for a few seconds. To prevent scalding, caregivers should not drink or carry hot foods or fluids while holding the baby.

Play Encourage sensory stimulation for the infant through parental interaction and age-appropriate toys.

Interventions for Example Problem: Abuse, Neglect, and Violence

 Teach parents about the dangers of shaking a baby or picking him up by an arm or leg.

If you suspect abuse, you are legally responsible for reporting your observations. As a beginning student, it is best to discuss your concerns with your instructor or the nurse assigned to the client before you make a report. Federal funds support a variety of home visit programs directed at high-risk mothers (identified on the basis of risk factors). Further information on abuse and reporting is included in Chapter 45, under Mandatory Reporting Laws.

 Think**Like a Nurse** 9-3

Recall Miguel, a 2-month-old, in the Meet Your Patients scenario. How might a prolonged hospitalization affect his growth and development? What nursing actions would you take to offset developmental delays?

KnowledgeCheck 9-4

- Identify at least two reflexes present in the neonate.
- According to Erikson, what is the developmental stage of the infant?
- What teaching guideline is important in reducing the risk of SIDS?

TODDLERHOOD: AGES 1 TO 3 YEARS

The toddler period lasts from 12 to 36 months of age. This is a period of increased mobility, independence, and exploration. This is also the time of temper tantrums and negative behavior, stemming from a toddler's desire to gain autonomy.

Physical Development of the Toddler

Compared with that of infants, toddlers' *growth rate* is much slower. The average toddler gains 5 lb (2.3 kg) per year and increases in height by 3 in. (7.6 cm). Length is added mainly in the legs. By the second birthday the typical toddler weighs 27 lb (12.25 kg), is 34 in. (86 cm) tall, and has a head circumference equal to the chest circumference. Between 12 and 18 months, the anterior fontanel closes (see Fig. 9-3).

- *Respirations and heart rate* slow in comparison with infancy, but blood pressure increases.
- *The stomach* increases in size to accommodate larger portions. Toddlers typically eat about 6 times a day, in relatively small portions, and join the family at mealtimes. Most toddlers enjoy picking up food with their hands to feed themselves.
- *The physical ability to control the anal and urethral sphincters* develops between 18 and 24 months. However, the child is ready when she can signal that her diaper is wet or soiled, or is able to say that she would like to go to the potty. This usually occurs at about 18 to 24 months of age, but it is not uncommon for a child to be in diapers until 3 years of age (American Academy of Family Physicians [AAFP], 2006, updated 2010).

- *Gross motor skills* continue to be refined during toddlerhood. By 10 to 15 months, the toddler can walk using a wide stance. At the age of 24 months, many toddlers can walk up and down stairs one step at a time. At 30 months, the toddler can jump using both feet. Before the age of 3, he can stand on one foot and climb steps alternating feet.
- *Fine motor skills* also continue to be refined. By 1 year, infants can grasp small objects, yet are unable to release the object. However, by 15 months the toddler can release objects as well. By 18 months he can throw a ball overhand (Fig. 9-6). The toddler uses his new motor skills and all five senses to explore his environment, and safety continues to be an important concern.
- *Visual acuity* improves to 20/40 by the end of the toddler stage, and **strabismus** (crossed eyes) may still be seen transiently.
- *Hearing* should be fully developed by toddlerhood.

Developmental milestones of toddlerhood are listed in Box 9-2.

Cognitive Development of the Toddler

During toddlerhood the child completes Piaget's *sensorimotor phase* and moves into the *preconceptual phase*. This is a time of rapid language development and increasing curiosity. The toddler is able to name many things and begins to recognize that different objects (such as a ball, a block, and a puzzle) may be named the same thing (toys). This is the beginning of categorization and concept development. The child abandons trial and error and begins to solve problems by thinking. However,

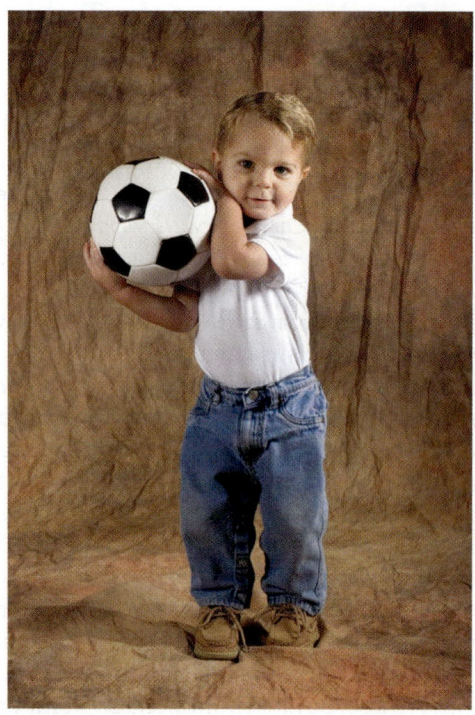

FIGURE 9-6 By 18 months, the toddler can throw a ball overhand.

reasoning and judgment lag far behind. This discrepancy places the child at risk for accidents and injuries.

Psychosocial Development of the Toddler

The most important psychosocial developmental task for the toddler is to initiate more independence, control, and autonomy. Erikson refers to this stage as *autonomy versus shame and doubt*. To successfully negotiate this stage, the child must learn to see herself as separate from mother, tolerate separation from the parents, withstand delayed gratification, learn to control anal and urinary sphincters, and begin to verbally communicate and interact with others.

Toddlers exert their independence by saying no to parental requests or actions or by "throwing a tantrum" to protest a parental decision they don't like. This behavior is best understood as a necessary attempt to define boundaries and test parental limits, rather than stubbornness or naughtiness. A firm but calm parental response to such "misbehavior" allows toddlers to feel secure while exploring their boundaries.

Freud defined this phase as the *anal stage*. To Freud, a successful toilet training experience accompanied by praise is necessary to becoming a well-functioning adult; difficulty in this phase leads to obsessive-compulsive behavior in adulthood. Contemporary theorists find this view somewhat narrow.

Common Health Problems of Toddlers

Unintentional Injury Drowning is the leading cause of accidental death in this age group (Reinberg, 2012). Most drowning accidents are due to unsupervised access to swimming pools or other water sources (bathtubs). Other common causes of injuries to toddlers are falls, motor vehicle accidents, burns and scalds, and choking. As toddlers gain increasing mobility, poisoning from household medications and toxic cleansers, as well as access to knives, guns, and other dangers become concern. For further discussion of safety concerns for toddlers, see Chapter 24.

Infections The shorter and wider eustachian tube in infants and toddlers increases their risk for multiple ear infections, which in turn increases the risk for hearing loss. Upper respiratory infections are common among toddlers. They no longer have the passive immunity acquired in utero, and because most breastfeeding ends before the first birthday, most toddlers no longer receive maternal antibodies in breast milk. Furthermore, as toddlers enter into more public and social settings, they are increasingly exposed to other children. Those in day care and those who have school-age siblings are particularly at risk. The most common infections are colds, ear infections, and tonsillitis. Other common infections include parasitic diseases, such as lice and tapeworms.

Immunizations The CDC (2011a) recommendations for immunization are designed to protect infants and children early in life, when they are most vulnerable and before they are exposed to potentially life-threatening diseases. Vaccines should be administered at the recommended age; but if not done, a vaccine can be administered at a later well child visit. Catch-up schedules and minimum intervals between doses for children whose vaccinations have been delayed are included in the recommendations. The CDC updates the immunization schedules periodically. To see the CDC's optimal immunization schedule for children up to 6 years of age,

 Go to Student Resources: Chapter 9, **Tables, Boxes, Figures: ESG Figure 9-1,** on Davis*Plus*, or the CDC Web site, at http://www.cdc.gov/vaccines/schedules/index.html

The CDC (2011a) immunization schedule for toddlers includes the following vaccines: hepatitis A, hepatitis B, *Haemophilus influenzae,* meningococcal conjugate, tetanus and diphtheria toxoids (Td) and acellular pertussis (Tdap), pneumococcal pneumonia, inactivated poliovirus, varicella, measles/mumps/rubella (MMR), and rotavirus.

Delayed Toilet Training Although not strictly speaking a "health" problem, many parents are concerned about what they perceive as delayed toilet training. Physiologically, most children develop sphincter and neurological control by age 2, but more is involved in successful toileting. Toddlers must learn to unfasten their clothing and pull down their pants, use toilet paper effectively, dress again, and wash their hands before they are completely independent. The child also must be able to sense the need to go to the bathroom, even when preoccupied with play activities, before it is "too late." Accidents are frequent and parents should expect them.

ASSESSMENT

Children of this age are generally fearful of strangers. Thus, before beginning your assessment, you will need to establish rapport. To do so, you might engage the child in play—for example, by playing catch with a soft ball or asking the child to introduce you to the stuffed animal he may have brought along. This is also a nonthreatening way to assess language skills and motor development. Encourage parents to relieve their child's stress and anxiety by holding him during the exam and speaking to him in a calm and reassuring voice.

Toddlers need regular physical examinations. At each office visit, evaluate the child's weight, height, growth, and development against standard growth charts and by comparing his skills against age-appropriate norms. Beginning at age 3, blood pressure should be checked at least once yearly and results recorded with age/gender/height percentile and reviewed with parents (National Heart, Lung and Blood Institute, 2012).

INTERVENTIONS

Health Teaching You cannot stress safety enough to parents. Teach them how to childproof the environment. Emphasize that increasing motor skills and dexterity allow the toddler to find many dangerous areas, including stairways, windows, and electrical outlets. To prevent injury or death from such hazards, parents must provide constant supervision. They should use consistent, firm limits to help the toddler remain safe. Parents should also be vigilant about their children's toys, in light of recent recalls of toys that contained lead and other toxic substances. Toys should be larger than the diameter of the trachea in order to avoid choking accidents.

Plan ahead by teaching parents basic first aid and the choking rescue maneuver (see Chapter 24). Encourage parents to enroll in a basic life support class. You will also find a detailed list of safety measures for toddlers in Chapter 24.

Health Promotion Interventions At each wellness visit, reinforce the need for handwashing, tooth brushing, regular dental exams, and a balanced diet. This is also a time for additional immunizations and boosters. Oral health teaching should include information on brushing, fluoride, non-nutritive oral habits, and dental injury prevention (AAP, 2008). Children should see a dentist at between 12 and 36 months of age—certainly by age 3, when all teeth have erupted

Methicillin-Resistant Staphylococcus aureus (MRSA) and Vancomycin-Resistant Enterococci (VRE) These organisms have put a spotlight on the threat posed by drug-resistant bacteria. **Key Point:** *Teach parents that antibiotics should not be used for simple colds and "flu." Explain the importance of taking the entire prescription when an antibiotic is prescribed, even after the child's symptoms resolve.* These actions help prevent the development of drug-resistant strains of bacteria.

 Remind parents that many cough and cold medicines marketed to children have not been approved for use in children, and that they should be certain that any OTC medicines are truly safe for children.

KnowledgeCheck 9-5

- According to Erikson, what is the developmental stage of the toddler?
- What is the leading cause of accidental death in toddlers?

ThinkLike a Nurse 9-4

Recall Tamika, a 3-year-old girl, in the Meet Your Patients scenario. Her grandmother, who is also caring for her ill husband, is raising Tamika. What concerns does that raise about the home environment?

PRESCHOOL STAGE: AGES 4 AND 5 YEARS

The preschooler is becoming increasingly verbal and independent and is refining gross and fine motor skills. He is able to maintain separation from parents, use language to communicate needs, control bodily functions, and cooperate with children as well as adults. These skills prepare the child to enter school.

Physical Development of the Preschooler

Growth By 4 years of age, the average preschooler weighs about 36 lb (16.3 kg) and is 40 in. (1 m) tall. By age 5, the preschooler has gained an additional 5 lb (2.3 kg) and grown 3 more in. (7.6 cm) in height. The proportions of head to trunk are somewhat closer, and the "pot belly" and exaggerated lumbar curve of toddlerhood gradually disappear. The average pulse rate is 90 to 100 beats/min, and respirations are 22 to 25 breaths/min.

Sensorimotor Development The preschooler has mature depth and color perception and 20/20 vision. Hearing is also mature. The preschooler continues to develop eye–hand coordination. Improvement in fine motor skills is most evident in artwork. Drawings

become much more precise and detailed. Developmental milestones for preschoolers are listed in Box 9-3.

Cognitive Development of Preschoolers

According to Piaget, the preschooler has entered the phase of *intuitive thought*. She is able to classify objects and continues to form concepts. She still uses trial and error as a way to solve problems but increasingly uses thought to reason them out. Verbal skills expand dramatically during this phase, allowing the child to interact with more people. Preschool children are very interested in books, learning to read, and counting.

Preschoolers lack the ability to reason formally and are unable to understand that two objects that appear different may in fact be the same (e.g., two balls of clay in two different shapes). They have a limited ability to tell time or understand the passage of time, and they may say "yesterday" in describing an event of several months ago. They also retain a strong belief in magic, monsters, and mythic figures, such as Santa Claus. Preschoolers often have irrational fears, for example, of tigers lurking in the basement. Their fascination with powerful figures, such as dinosaurs and superheroes, is one way of coping with their feelings of powerlessness.

BOX 9-3 ■ Milestones of Preschool Development

- By age 5, most children can stand on one foot for 10 sec, skip, jump, hop on one foot or both feet together, climb play structures with ease, repeat simple dance steps, and begin to learn to skate.

- Most preschoolers can copy a triangle, square, and stick figure; print at least some letters; and use a fork and spoon.

- Most can dress and use the bathroom without assistance.

- Language abilities continue to be variable, but most preschoolers can tell stories, recall parts of a story told to them, and speak in sentences of more than five words. Most can state their name, age, and address, and many can repeat their home phone number. A toddler who is not speaking intelligibly by age 4 requires evaluation.

- Preschoolers can count 10 or more objects, such as buttons or coins, and may be able to name several colors and shapes. They can compare big and small, long and short, and so on, and often delight in completing simple mazes and "connect the dots" games.

- Preschoolers become increasingly aware of sex organ differences and curious about sexuality.

- Preschoolers may begin to ask about God, death, how babies are born, and other questions of a philosophical or scientific nature.

- Preschoolers typically can distinguish fantasy from reality and enjoy jokes and simple riddles.

- Psychosocial milestones include assertion of independence; pride in showing off skills, new toys and clothes, and prize possessions to friends; and a strong desire to socialize with peers.

Psychosocial Development of Preschoolers

The preschooler is in Erikson's stage of *initiative versus guilt*. In this stage, the child develops a conscience and readily recognizes right from wrong. The child becomes socially aware of others and develops the ability to consider other people's viewpoints. At this age, play is often used to teach life experiences.

The preschool child begins to fully express his personality and develop a self-concept (see Chapter 13 if you need to learn more about self-concept). He readily expresses likes and dislikes. Encouraging the child to participate in his favorite activities helps foster a positive self-concept (Fig. 9-7). Preschool children enjoy playing in small groups and use their language skills to facilitate imaginative play. Often elaborate stories, improvised costumes, and role-playing become part of the play experience. Many preschoolers have a best friend.

Freud identified the preschool years as the *phallic stage* of development. The child is aware of gender differences and often imitates the same-sex parent. The child also develops an attraction to the opposite-sex parent and may feel jealousy toward the same-sex parent.

Common Health Problems of Preschoolers

The preschooler experiences health problems similar to those of the toddler.

Communicable Diseases Communicable diseases (e.g., respiratory infections, intestinal viruses, and parasitic infections such as scabies and lice) remain a major health issue as preschoolers expand their social groups and come in contact with more children in play and

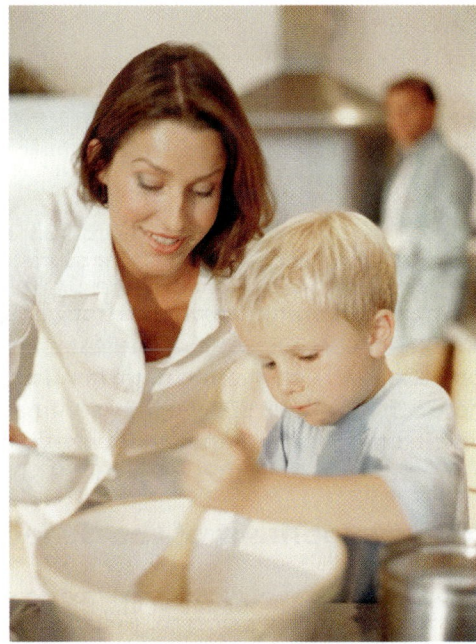

FIGURE 9-7 Preschoolers typically enjoy helping a parent in the kitchen.

structured preschool experiences. They are "hands-on," so they tend to readily transmit viruses through direct contact and airborne vectors.

✚ **Poisoning** Poisoning remains a significant risk for preschoolers, who often use imitation as a way to learn about new things. This predisposes the child to ingesting substances used by the adults in the house, such as prescription medicines and alcohol, or substances that look similar to these products

Enuresis Parents of preschoolers may report a concern about bed-wetting (**enuresis**), especially in boys. The causes of enuresis are not fully understood. However, it is known that in some children, the bladder is simply unable to hold a full night's output of urine until later in childhood, whereas others lack the neurological ability to waken in response to a full bladder. Most cases resolve spontaneously, with only very occasional episodes past age 6. In contrast, daytime wetting or soiling (**encopresis**) requires evaluation.

Example Problem: Child Abuse, Neglect, and Violence

Child abuse can occur at any age. It is often detected in the toddler and preschool period as children come in contact with more people outside the home. Abuse may be physical, emotional, or sexual or due to neglect. Of the confirmed cases of abuse and neglect reported to Child Protective Services, more than half are under the age of 7. Child abuse is not isolated to any one socioeconomic or education level group. The following are a few of the reasons why some people have difficulty meeting the demands of parenthood:

- **Parental characteristics:** Parents who were abused as a child are more likely to abuse their own children, especially when faced with high levels of stress and little support. Abuse can occur when parents or caregivers have unrealistic expectations of the child or unmet emotional needs of their own. Other factors include immaturity, lack of parenting knowledge, difficulty in relationships, depression, anxiety, mental health problems, and alcohol and drug addiction.
- **Characteristics of the child:** Statistical data indicate that children with a physical or mental disability and those who are born to unmarried parents or who are unwanted are more likely to suffer abuse.
- **Situational characteristics:** Crowded living space, financial difficulty, stresses of child care, employment pressures or unemployment, poor housing, domestic violence in the home, and frequent household moves are all environmental stressors that can contribute to child abuse. One recent study found that hospital visits for abuse were associated with the mortgage delinquency and foreclosure rates (Wood, Medina, Feudtner, et al., 2012). Obviously, most parents do not abuse their children, despite the presence of those characteristics. However, you should be aware

of the statistical risks. For further discussion of child abuse, refer to the section on Infancy, preceding, and

 Go to Chapter 9, **Procedure 9-1: Assessing for Abuse,** in Volume 2.

ASSESSMENT

Assessments for preschoolers should include the following:

Height, Weight, and Vital Signs Gather the data and compare your findings with age-appropriate norms. Calculate and plot body mass index (BMI) at every well-child visit. To obtain information about this from the CDC Web site,

 Go to "BMI—Body Mass Index," at http://www.cdc.gov/nccdphp/dnpa/bmi/index.htm

Nutrition Assess for food preferences, habits, and amount eaten. The preschool child often has strong food preferences.

Sleep Habits Assess the numbers of hours slept, bedtime rituals, and problems with night awakenings. Preschoolers are generally very active but require adequate rest. This is also the stage when children stop taking afternoon naps.

Vision Screening U.S. Preventive Services Task Force (USPSTF) (2011a) recommends vision screening for all children at least once between the ages of 3 and 5 years, to detect the presence of vision loss or its risk factors (Couser, Esmail, & Hutchinson, 2012).

Dental Hygiene During the preschool years, all deciduous teeth have erupted. Therefore, dental hygiene is very important. At each visit, ask the child about toothbrushing habits. If possible, have him demonstrate how he brushes. The child should already have made at least one visit to a dentist by age 3. *Healthy People 2020* oral health goal includes prevention and control of oral and craniofacial diseases, by providing access for all school-age children to fluoridated water, tooth sealants, and preventive oral care (USDHHS, 2010b).

✚ Safety Risks Assess for parent and child knowledge of hazards and precautions. Because the preschool child is mobile and involved in activities such as riding a tricycle, chasing a ball, and crossing streets, accidents increase.

School Readiness A physical examination is required before the child enters school. This exam should include an assessment for "readiness"—whether the child has acquired skills such as an ability to converse with adults, follow instructions, hold a pencil, and perform a variety of motor skills, such as jump, hop, and walk a straight line. At the readiness exam, you will also need to review the immunization record. Several boosters and immunizations are due at this time. Any missed immunizations must be administered before the child enters school. For other information, refer to Common

Health Problems of Toddlers earlier in this chapter. To see the CDC's Catch-Up Immunization Schedule for Persons Aged 4 Months–18 Years,

 Go to Student Resources: Chapter 9, **Tables, Boxes, Figures: ESG Figure 9-2,** on Davis*Plus*, or to the CDC Web site at http://www.cdc.gov/vaccines/schedules/index.html

INTERVENTIONS

The preschool child is interactive and curious. Speak directly to the child, and include her in your teaching sessions. Teaching topics include the following:

- *Frequent handwashing to prevent the spread of disease.* Teach the child handwashing technique, and encourage parents to model frequent handwashing.
- *Proper brushing and flossing of teeth.* At this age, most children still need supervision while brushing their teeth.
- *The essentials of a balanced diet.* Encourage parents to offer a well-balanced diet and to instill healthy eating habits. By age 5 most children are willing to try new foods and are better able to sit during an entire meal. Generally, preschoolers eat half of the food portion of an adult.
- *The importance of adequate rest.* The average preschooler requires at least 12 hours of sleep each night.

- ✚ *The hazard of "stranger danger."* Increasing independence and mobility place the preschool child at risk for abduction. Teach the child to avoid talking to strangers and to never enter a stranger's home or car. This topic is explored in depth once the child is in school.
- ✚ *The importance of seat belts and car seats.* Current recommendations are to use a booster seat for children weighing between 40 and 80 lb and to continue using the seat until the child is at least 4 ft 9 in. tall.

KnowledgeCheck 9-6

- According to Erikson, what is the developmental stage of the preschooler?
- Identify at least two important assessments to make when providing care to a preschooler.

SCHOOL-AGE: AGES 6 TO 12 YEARS

The school-age child undergoes many changes; the child becomes more independent, places more importance on relationships outside the immediate family, and becomes more confident. See Box 9-4 for a summary of the developmental milestones of the school-age period.

Physical Development of the School-Age Child

Growth During the school-age years, the child grows about 2 in. (5 cm) taller and gains 4 to 7 lb (2.3 to 3 kg) per year. The child takes on a slimmer appearance, with longer legs and a lower center of gravity. Muscle mass rapidly increases and ossification of bones continues

BOX 9-4 ■ Milestones of School-Age Development

- By age 7, most children can tie their own shoelaces, print their names, and perform self-care, such as bathing and feeding themselves. Many can even prepare simple meals.
- By age 8, improved fine motor skills allow the child to begin to write, learn to knit or crochet, and/or take up a musical instrument.
- By age 9, motor development approaches that of an adult.
- School-age children understand the concept of payment for work and the value of money.
- Fears of ghosts and monsters may continue through age 7 but give way to more realistic fears, such as of school failure or divorce of parents, by age 8 or 9.
- By age 6, the child has a vocabulary of 3,000 words and usually can read. By the end of the school-age period, the child can write complex compositions with appropriate grammar, spelling, and accurate description.
- Psychosocial development includes team play, peer friendships, and ability to look beyond family members for social support.

throughout this stage. Strength and physical abilities rapidly improve, and the child gains more poise and co-ordination. The brain and skull grow slowly, and facial characteristics mature. The gastrointestinal system matures and stomach capacity increases, although caloric demands decrease. As the immune system develops, the school-age child begins to produce antibodies and antigens. Initially boys and girls vary little in size. Toward the end of the school-age phase, marked differences become apparent. Girls grow rapidly in the latter school-age years, as puberty begins. They experience onset of puberty approximately 2 years before boys do.

Visual Acuity Visual acuity improves with age. Because children do not complain of visual difficulties, the AAP (2003) recommends visual acuity measurement (vision screening) beginning at age 3 years. AAP Vision Screening Guidelines specify that all children over age 8 should be able to achieve 20/20 visual acuity using their best eyeglass correction. Younger children should be referred to an ophthalmologist if there is a difference between the right and left eyes of two or more lines on a Snellen chart evaluation (Broderick, 1998).

Dentition School-age children begin to lose their primary teeth (baby teeth) at about age 6 or 7, and the permanent teeth appear soon after. Their large size in relation to the remaining primary teeth and the child's jaw, as well as the gaps left by teeth not yet replaced, can make even the most beautiful children look somewhat awkward at this stage.

Cognitive Development of the School-Age Child

School-age children use their thought processes to experience actions and events. Piaget describes this as *concrete operations*. The child's thinking is concrete and systematic;

magical beliefs are gradually replaced with a passion to understand how things really are. He is also able to see another person's point of view and develops an understanding of relationships. The school-age child learns to classify objects according to similarities, and enjoys learning by handling and manipulating objects. The child learns to tell time and gains an experiential understanding of the length of days, months, and years. He reads independently and does numerical calculations without representative objects such as fingers or beads. By the end of this stage, mental capacity develops to the point where the child is able to think through a task and understand it without actually performing the task.

Psychosocial Development of the School-Age Child

Erikson describes this stage as a time of *industry versus inferiority*. During this stage, the child is able to work at more complex projects independently. Through participation in school, she is recognized for achievements and accomplishments. For the child to progress through this stage, the parent must also provide praise for accomplishments. This recognition builds self-confidence. The child will develop a sense of inferiority and lack of self-worth if her accomplishments are met with a negative response.

Peers take on increasing importance, influencing the child's choices of what to eat, wear, and do. Friendships during the school-age years are usually with children of the same gender and may be intense but short-lived (Fig. 9-8). However, some children have one best friend throughout their childhood. In the later school-age years, friendships become more reciprocal with each child recognizing the unique qualities of the other.

Common Health Problems of School-Age Children

School-age children are at risk for problems similar to those of preschoolers, including upper respiratory tract infections, parasitic infections such as scabies and lice, and dental caries. Although violence, bullying, smoking, and

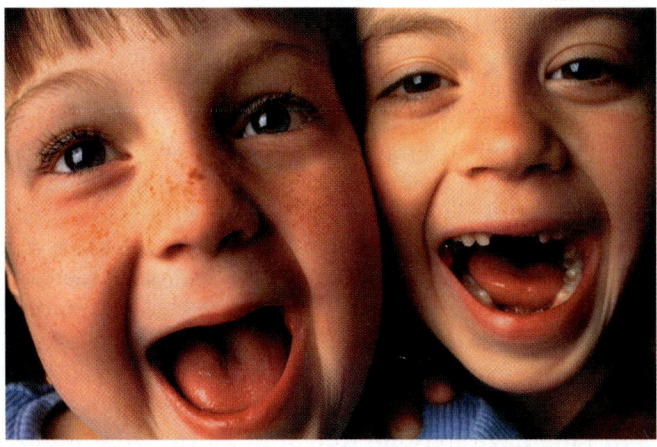

FIGURE 9-8 Same-gender friendships are important to school-age children.

experimentation with alcohol, drugs, and sex are more common among adolescents, these problems are also seen toward the end of the school-age years. The presence of a gun in the home significantly increases the risk of accidental death, even in the school-age population.

Childhood Obesity

Obesity among school-age children has become a growing health concern. In 1994, 11% of children ages 6 to 11 were obese (defined as being in the 95th percentile of body mass index); by 2006, that figure had risen to 17%, to what is viewed as epidemic proportions (American Heart Association, 2012). Nutrition and lifestyle are primarily responsible. Children spend much less time playing outside than in past generations, and more time watching television and playing on electronic devices. They consume more fast food, bigger portions, and fewer vegetables. Thirty percent of all meals are taken outside of the home and fast food contributes to 10 percent of overall calorie intake (American Heart Association, 2010). As a result of the obesity epidemic, prevalence of obesity-related diseases, such as type 2 diabetes mellitus (type 2 DM), hyperlipidemia, and hypertension, have risen in children.

Type 2 DM is an endocrine disorder characterized by insulin resistance; that is, insulin fails to effectively transfer glucose from the bloodstream into the body's cells. Treatment involves dietary changes, weight loss, and exercise. Medications are required if these lifestyle changes are not sufficient to control blood sugar.

Childhood Asthma

Asthma, a chronic inflammatory disorder of the airways, affects about 6.8 million children in the United States. From 2001 through 2009 asthma rates rose most among African American children, increasing almost 50% (CDC, 2006, 2010a). Asthma is the leading cause of school absenteeism owing to chronic illness and of childhood emergency department (ED) visits. It accounts for one-third of all pediatric ED visits. Even in children who do not require emergency care, asthma can decrease attention span in school, make participation in school activities difficult, and cause social problems. For example, children are often teased and stigmatized as being "wheezers" or "lazy." Asthma has complex causes, including a strong genetic component, but poverty appears to play at least some role. Recent research has focused on indoor air pollutants, such as dust mites, mouse urine, and the decomposing corpses of cockroaches as significant triggers.

Unintentional Injuries in School-Age Children

School-age children experience fewer injuries than do preschoolers because of their increased coordination and improved reasoning abilities. Nevertheless, they do have a high incidence of fractures, sprains, strains, cuts, and abrasions. Falls are the most common form of nonfatal injury for children ages 6 to 12 years, while the leading cause of death from unintentional injury is motor vehicle and traffic injury (54% of the deaths for this group) (CDC, 2012a).

Concussions are one of the most commonly reported injuries in children and adolescents who participate in sports and recreation activities. Most sports- and recreation-related concussions seen in EDs each year (65%) occur among youth ages 5 to 18. While many of these injuries may be considered mild, they can result in health consequences such as impaired thinking, memory problems, and emotional or behavioral changes (USDHHS, 2007–2008). Injuries also occur from riding bicycles on the street, skiing, skateboarding, sledding, and the use of trampolines. If you would like more information about unintentional injuries, see Chapter 24.

ASSESSMENT

The school-age child should have a routine health maintenance visit every 1 or 2 years. Many children participate in sports, so annual physical exams are scheduled for them. Allow time to meet with the child alone as well as time with the caregiver present. School-age children often have questions about puberty and the changes their bodies are undergoing. Private time with the child may encourage the child to be more open as you explore these concerns.

Nursing Interview The nursing interview should cover the following topics:

- **Nutrition.** Assess the child's nutrition, including intake of key nutrients such as calcium, vitamin D, and iron.
- **Allergies.** Ask the child whether he ever experiences difficulty breathing or feels too tired to play. Ask about allergy symptoms, including clear nasal discharge, frequent sneezing, or watery eyes. Listen to breath sounds, and observe for allergy symptoms.
- **Dental hygiene.** Determine the child's knowledge of dental hygiene. Inspect the mouth for secondary teeth eruption according to expected patterns, as well as for tooth decay and gum disease.
- **Sleep pattern.** Assess the child's sleep pattern. To remain healthy and function well at school, the school-age child needs 9 to 10 hours of sleep each night.
- **Safety.** Determine the child's awareness of safety. Be sure to assess risk-taking behavior. Has the child tried smoking? Does he have friends who are smoking? What is the child's experience with alcohol and drugs? Has he tried them? What does his peer group think about drinking and drugs? Has he ever been sexually active? Does he have friends who are sexually active? Has the child engaged in fistfights or fights with knives or other weapons? Is there a gun in the home? Does the child have access to it? Although these concerns are seen with greater frequency in adolescence, you should assess for them among school-age children.

BMI At each visit, assess the child's vital signs, height, weight, and developmental skills. After weighing the child, correlate your measurements with growth charts. The American Heart Association (2012) BMI classifications are as follows:

- At 85th percentile—mild to moderately overweight
- At or above the 95th percentile—obese

Because health risk increases with degree of obesity, at-risk and obese school-age children should be identified and counseled. For more information about BMI for children,

 Go to **BMI—Body Mass Index, at http://www.cdc.gov/ nccdphp/dnpa/bmi/index.htm**

Vision Screening Many school systems have regular vision screening programs that are carried out by volunteer professionals, school nurses, and/or properly trained laypersons. Screening can be done quickly, accurately, and with minimal expense by one of these individuals.

Scoliosis Screening **Scoliosis** is an abnormal spinal curvature that affects primarily females. Screening is done in the preadolescent period, usually in the 6th grade. Refer to an orthopedic surgeon for evaluation and follow-up if an abnormal curvature is discovered.

Immunizations Review the immunization record. Although immunization against hepatitis B is recommended in infancy, many parents skip these immunizations. Several states require students to complete the hepatitis B series prior to entry into 7th grade. The child must begin the series at or before 12 years of age to complete it in time for 7th grade. The CDC (2011a) recommends the following vaccines for school-age children: tetanus, diphtheria, and pertussis booster; human papillomavirus; meningococcal; pneumococcal; influenza; hepatitis A; hepatitis B; inactivated poliovirus; measles, mumps, and rubella; and varicella. To see this schedule,

 Go to the CDC, **2012 Recommended Immunizations for Children from 7 Through 18 Years Old,** at http://www.cdc. gov/vaccines/who/teens/downloads/parent-version-schedule-7-18yrs.pdf

Also refer to the section Common Health Problems of Toddlers.

INTERVENTIONS

The *Healthy People 2020* campaign focuses on preventing injury rather than on treating illness. Your efforts in patient teaching will help promote the national *Healthy People 2020* population objectives (USDHHS, 2010b). Use age-appropriate teaching materials and methods.

Teaching for Safety

To help prevent injury in the school-age child, educate the child and parents on safety and the proper use of equipment and gear. Teach them to wear seat belts at all times. Encourage parents to be firm about the use of helmets for bicycle safety, stressing that head injury is the most common cause of death

in this group. Also stress the importance of warming up before playing sports, using safety equipment that is properly fitted, and avoiding overtraining.

Teaching About Nutrition, Exercise, and Overweight

Counsel overweight and obese children about nutrition for weight loss. Encourage them to develop good eating habits by choosing nutritious foods and snacks. For example, they should avoid junk foods, and instead of sodas choose milk, calcium-fortified orange juice, or plain water. If the diet is severely restrictive, and if it has none of the child's favorite foods, it is likely to fail. Focus on making small but permanent changes. Refer for further counseling, if indicated.

Recommend 60 minutes of moderate-intensity exercise 7 days per week (American Heart Association, n.d., updated June 2012). USDHHS guidelines recommend even more exercise: 1 hour or more of vigorous aerobic physical activity every day. Explain how important exercise is to weight loss—diet alone will not achieve it for them. Exercise does not necessarily need to be structured. For example, it might consist of family walks in the community, bike riding, skateboarding, or swimming in a neighborhood pool. Even table tennis requires more activity than watching television. The AAP (2006) recommends the following:

- Limit TV viewing and video game playing to 2 hours a day.
- Boys should take at least 11,000 steps daily.
- Girls should take at least 13,000 steps daily.

You could suggest that parents buy a pedometer so the child can track the number of steps.

Teach children about self-regulation of impulse control, decision-making skills, and social competence. The most effective programs for preventing obesity focus on children, rather than their parents. However, management of obesity does involve the whole family. Parents can help by modeling healthy eating. Recommend group-based or family-based counseling. Many parents do not perceive that their child is overweight, and they must come to recognize this if they are to cooperate with needed changes.

Work with the community to involve the schools in obesity prevention. Many schools have removed soda from their campuses and are now offering healthy menus in their cafeterias. In addition, physical education in public schools has been mandated in many U.S. states.

Teaching About Asthma

Teach parents and children about indoor environmental asthma triggers, such as secondhand smoke, dust mites (in mattresses, carpets, and furniture), mold, cockroaches, pets, and nitrogen dioxide (a gas that is a byproduct of indoor fuel-burning appliances such as gas stoves, fireplaces, or wood stoves (U.S. Environmental Protection Agency [EPA], last updated October, 2010)).

Provide and help fill out, as necessary, an asthma action plan card for the child to carry when away from home. An action plan should include (1) the child's asthma triggers, (2) instructions for asthma medicines, (3) what to do if the child has an attack, (4) when to call the doctor, and (5) emergency telephone numbers. To obtain a plan form from the EPA's Asthma home page,

 Go to http://www.epa.gov/asthma/pdfs/asthma_action_plan.pdf

Intervention for Example Problem: Violence

At the community health level, school violence can be addressed through psychological counseling, weapons-screening devices, schoolwide educational programs, and policies calling for the suspension or expulsion of students who are caught intimidating other children or participating in fights on school property. The school-age period also offers many opportunities to educate children about the hazards of smoking, drinking, and using drugs, which often contribute to violence.

Helping the Hospitalized Child

Finally, help children express their fears so you can respond to specific needs. Hospitalized children may fear the unknown, the strange environment, and strange professionals. They are afraid of tests and treatments (e.g., operations, needles), pain, and dying. They miss the comforts of home: their mother's cooking, their own room, and so on. They are bothered by separation from family and friends and by loss of control over their personal needs. You can help by maximizing their contact with friends and school. Offer children choices, when possible, to restore some sense of control (e.g., whether to have a tub or shower bath or what they'd prefer to eat for meals). Encourage parents to bring familiar items from home to personalize their space. Involve parents in their care, and provide them accurate information so they can relieve children's anxieties.

KnowledgeCheck 9-7

- What important physical changes occur in the school-age group?
- According to Piaget, what is the cognitive developmental stage of the school-age child?

ADOLESCENCE: AGES 12 TO 18 YEARS

Adolescence marks the transition from child to adult. **Puberty** refers to the beginning of reproductive abilities. In this period, the child experiences progressive physical, cognitive, and psychological change.

Physical Development of Adolescents

Physical and hormonal changes are readily apparent during the adolescent years. Developmental milestones of adolescence are summarized in Box 9-5.

BOX 9-5 ■ Milestones of Adolescent Development

- The adolescent reaches adult height and about 90% of peak bone density by the end of this stage.
- Menarche occurs by age 14 in most girls, who develop adult primary and secondary sex characteristics by about age 16.
- Boys have developed adult primary and secondary sex characteristics by about ages 17 to 19.
- Motor development is equal to that of adults.
- Maturation of the central nervous system allows formal operational thought processes, logic, and abstract reasoning.
- Psychosocial development includes the teen's increasing reliance on peers, ambivalent feelings toward family, anxiety over and/or preoccupation with sex and sexuality, and determination of sexual orientation.

Growth *Females* undergo a growth spurt between 9 and 14 years of age. Height increases 2 to 8 in. (5.1 to 7.6 cm), and weight gain varies from 15 to 55 lb (6.8 to 24.9 kg). By the onset of menstruation, females have attained 90% of their adult height. *Males* undergo a growth spurt between the ages of 10 and 16 years. Height increases by 4 to 12 in. (10.2 to 30.5 cm), and weight increases by 15 to 65 lb (6.8 to 29.5 kg). Boys continue to grow until 18 to 20 years of age. Bone mass continues to accumulate until about age 20.

In both males and females, the blood pressure and the size and strength of the heart increase. The pulse rate decreases. By the end of adolescence, blood values are that of the adult. Respiratory rate, volume, and lung capacity also reach the adult rates. By the end of the adolescent period, all vital organs reach adult size.

Onset of Puberty The onset of puberty varies widely, but the sequences of these changes are standard (Tanner, 1962).

- In females, the time from the first appearance of breast tissue to full sexual maturation is 2 to 6 years. **Menarche** (first menstruation) occurs approximately 2 years after the beginning of puberty. The average age of menarche is 12 years, depending on race and body mass.
- In males, the onset of puberty occurs between 9 and 14 years of age. Throughout puberty, boys become more muscular, the voice deepens, and facial hair begins to grow and coarsen. It may take 2 to 5 years for the genitalia to reach adult size.

In both males and females, hormonal changes are accompanied by increased activity of the sweat (apocrine) glands, and heavy perspiration may occur for the first time. At the same time, the sebaceous glands become active, and the adolescent may experience acne. For more information about the changes in secondary sexual characteristics associated with puberty for males and females,

Go to **Procedures 22-17 and 22-18,** respectively, in Volume 2, and

 Go to Student Resources: Chapter 9, **Tables, Boxes, Figures: ESG Table 9-3, Tanner Staging System,** on Davis*Plus.*

Cognitive Development of Adolescents

Piaget refers to adolescence as the period of *formal operations*. The adolescent develops the ability to think abstractly and is receptive to more detailed information. She can now imagine what may occur in the future as well as the consequences of her own decisions. Despite their more refined cognitive abilities, adolescents may still lack judgment and common sense. These develop later through life experiences.

Psychosocial Development of Adolescents

The major psychosocial task of the adolescent is to develop a *personal identity*. Teenagers shift emotional attachment away from their parents and create close bonds among their peers (Fig. 9-9). This helps the teenager to further characterize the differences between himself and his parents. The adolescent often takes on a new style of dress, dance, music, or hairstyle; develops personal values; and begins to make choices about career and further education.

Group Acceptance One of the strongest needs for teens is to feel accepted within a group of their own choosing. Acceptance onto a sports team, into a club, or into a clique or gang increases the teen's sense of self-esteem. In contrast, unpopular teens feel alienated, resentful, and antagonistic and may react with violence directed at themselves or others (Polan & Taylor, 2010).

Tattoos and Piercings Adolescents may engage in the trend of body art and piercings for a number of reasons, including a desire for social bonding, desire to look like their peers, and the wish to commemorate a friend or loved one. In the 10-year period after the mid-1990s, the

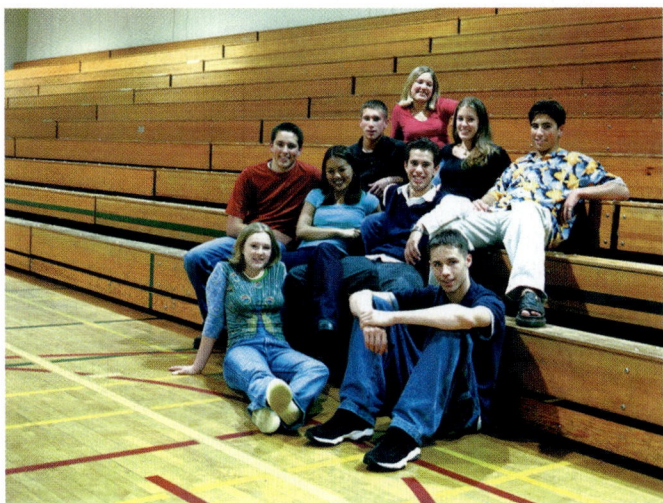

FIGURE 9-9 Teenagers create close bonds among their peers.

number of teens who had tattoos increased from 4.5% to 14%. The average age at time of tattooing is around 17 years (Scudder, 2007). Body piercings, likewise, are not unusual. Some studies have reported a significant relationship between piercing and substance abuse, leading some to speculate that body piercing may serve as a marker of an at-risk teen (Roberts, Auinger, & Ryan 2004). Both tattoos and piercings can cause skin infections and bloodborne diseases such as HIV and hepatitis.

Emerging Sexual Orientation Most adolescents have a sense of their emerging sexual orientation. Approximately 4.5% of people between 18 and 44 years of age identify themselves as homosexual or bisexual (CDC, 2011b). A higher percentage report having had same-sex intercourse at least once, but consider themselves heterosexual. Some youth are bisexual, that is, attracted somewhat equally to both males and females.

Common Health Problems of Adolescents

In the United States, 77% of all deaths among young people ages 10 to 25 result from four causes: motor vehicle crashes (30%), other unintentional injuries (15%), homicide (15%), and suicide (12%). Illnesses are responsible for less than one-fourth of deaths; cancer and heart disease are the most common. Many students engage in behaviors that increase their likelihood of death or injury including: texting while driving, drinking while driving, carrying a weapon, using alcohol, and using other drugs. In a recent year, 32.8% of high school students reported having been in a physical fight (CDC, 2012b).

Example Problem: Substance Abuse

Substance abuse is the regular use of drugs or other substances for purposes other than medical use that causes physical or psychological harm to the person. Substance abuse is a major concern because of the physical, mental, and spiritual toll it takes on teens, families, and the community. Substance abuse is associated with risk-taking behaviors resulting in injury and death (e.g., car accidents, suicide).

Alcohol and Other Substances

An adolescent may try alcohol and other drugs out of curiosity or to alter the consciousness to gain a feeling of power, excitement, or confidence. Peer pressure also exerts a powerful influence. Boys and girls are starting to drink at younger ages. In a recent survey, alcohol use among those ages 12 to 17 years was 15%; youth binge and heavy drinking rates were 9% and 2%, respectively. Three out of four students have consumed more than just a few sips of alcohol by the end of high school. An estimated 11% of those in grades 9 through 12 report having driven a motor vehicle when they had been drinking alcohol (CDC, 2012b; Substance Abuse and Mental Health Services Administration [SAMHSA], 2010).

Heroin, cocaine, crack, methamphetamine, and the "designer drugs" (ecstasy, bath salts and others) may be abused. Abuse of over-the-counter and prescription drugs used by the teen's parents, such as OxyContin, is also common.

Tobacco

It is illegal to sell tobacco to minors, yet 9.5% of middle school students and 25.6% of high school students currently use some form of tobacco (American Lung Association, 2010, updated July 2011; SAMHSA, 2010) and over 54% say they have tried a cigarette. A majority of these students report that they were not asked to show proof of age when they, themselves, bought cigarettes. Tobacco use is associated with alcohol use, and acts as a "gateway drug" to using illegal drugs. Cigarette use causes an increase in the number and severity of respiratory illness, and decreased physical fitness. Smoking during childhood often forms an addiction that persists into adulthood.

Depression

Depression affects up to 8.3% of adolescents in the United States (About Teen Depression, n.d.), compared with 11% of the adult population. A government survey found an even higher rate: During the 12 months preceding the survey, 28.5% of students nationwide had felt so sad or hopeless almost every day for more than 2 weeks in a row that they stopped doing some usual activities (CDC, 2012a). Defining features of depression are the same as for adults, but the way symptoms are expressed varies with the developmental stage. Young adolescents may have difficulty identifying and describing their emotional or mood states. Instead of saying how bad they feel, they may be irritable or act out by disobeying or misbehaving, or they may use tobacco and other substances. They may sulk, be negative or grouchy, feel misunderstood, and get into trouble at school.

Risk factors for adolescent depression include a family history of depression, cigarette smoking, stress, loss of a loved one, break up of a romantic relationship, learning disorders, attention or behavioral disorders, chronic illnesses (e.g., diabetes), abuse, neglect, or other trauma. If you would like more information about depression, see Chapter 13.

Suicide

Suicide is the third leading cause of death in teenagers. It is estimated that 7.8% of high school students have attempted suicide (CDC, 2012b). Rates are higher among females (19.3%) than among males (12.5%), but because boys tend to use more lethal methods, such as guns and hanging, they are more likely to die from the attempt. Risk factors include problems at school or in romantic or family relationships, low self-esteem, social isolation, substance abuse, and depression.

Eating Disorders

Although anorexia and bulimia create nutritional problems and manifest as eating disorders, they are psychiatric disorders that require medical and psychiatric intervention.

Anorexia Nervosa A person with **anorexia nervosa** dramatically restricts food intake and may exercise excessively in an attempt to lose weight. It is the third most common chronic illness among adolescents. It occurs predominately in, but is not limited to, high-achieving adolescent females from upper-middle-class backgrounds. Anorexia is characterized by a distorted body image; often the girl sees herself as fat in spite of being markedly thin. Physical consequences include amenorrhea, bradycardia, low white blood cell count, anemia, infertility, and bone loss. Eating disorders have the highest mortality of any mental illness: 5% to 10% of patients die within 10 years of developing anorexia nervosa (Lippert, Shea, & Seagrave, 2008).

Bulimia Bulimia is another eating disorder seen in adolescent girls, as well as in boys who participate in sports that require them to maintain a specific weight. Bulimia is characterized by binge eating followed by inappropriate mechanisms to remove the food that was consumed (usually, inducing vomiting, using laxatives, or excessive exercise). Binge eating may occur every few days or as often as several times a day. People with bulimia frequently experience electrolyte imbalances, decayed teeth from gastric acid exposure, or abdominal pain from gastric overload or laxative use.

Overweight and Obesity

Overweight and obesity continue to be a concern during adolescence. The numbers are staggering. Consider these facts:

- In 1994, 11% of adolescents (ages 12 to 19) were classified as obese; by 2008, that number had reached 18% (National Center for Health Statistics, 2011a). By 2011, about 1 in 3 American children and teens was overweight (American Heart Association, 2012).
- Causes of teen obesity are similar to those of childhood obesity: sedentary lifestyles, eating larger portions, eating fast foods, and substituting high-calorie, nutrient-poor snacks for balanced meals. Even school vending machines contain junk food such as soda, snack cakes, candy, and chips, although this is changing in some areas.
- One-third of American children ages 4 to 19 years eat fast food daily. The percentage is undoubtedly higher for adolescents, who eat fewer meals at home and have more freedom to choose their own foods. Food preferences are influenced by television and other marketing strategies; on children's television shows, most of the advertising is for foods of poor nutritional value.
- Type 2 DM, hypertension, high cholesterol, and heart disease are disorders that were previously seen mainly in adults. Now that obesity has become a major health problem among youth, these disorders are occurring with increasing frequency in adolescents. Moreover,

overweight children are more likely to become overweight adults.

Risky Sexual Behaviors

Sexual activity is common among teenagers. By age 13, 3.4% of girls and 9% of boys have had sexual intercourse. This tends to increase with age, with 34% of students in grades 9 to 12 being sexually active. About 15% of students have had sexual intercourse with four or more persons (CDC, 2011b; DeNoon, 2012).

Condom Use About two-thirds of sexually active high school students report having used a condom during their most recent sexual intercourse. Child Trends (2012) reports that males are far more likely to use condoms than are females; and black males were more likely to use condoms than Hispanic males. Through its *Healthy People 2020* initiative, the federal government has set a national goal of increasing effective condom use among sexually active adolescents ages 15 to 19 years, with the goal of preventing pregnancy and providing barrier protection against disease.

Oral Sex A fairly recent trend among youth is engaging in oral sex, in the belief that it is not "real sex." In one survey of university students, 62% of females and 56% of males believed that oral sex is not "actually sex" and does not take away their virginity (Halpern-Felsher, 2008, Lindberg, Jones, & Santelli, 2008).

Web-Based Social Networking A recent study of young men (ages 16 to 24 years) who have sex with men examined the use of the Internet or Web-based social networking sites for meeting sexual partners. Forty-eight percent of the sample had sexual relations with a partner they met online. Of these, only 53% used condoms consistently, and 47% reported having sexual partners more than 4 years older than themselves. A history of unprotected anal intercourse, multiple anal intercourse partners, and engaging in sexual activity at a sex club or a bathhouse was associated with meeting sexual partners through the Internet. Researchers concluded that young men who have sex with men and who seek partners online also engage in other behaviors that place them at risk for HIV and other STIs (Garofalo, Herrick, Mustanski, et al., 2007).

Sexually Transmitted Infections (STIs) Approximately 1 in 4 U.S. teens has an STI. STIs, including HIV/AIDS, are a major health consequence associated with sexual activity, especially with unprotected sexual activity. A majority of adolescents believe that sex without a condom is not worth the risk, but most also mistakenly believe that condoms are a foolproof method of preventing STIs and HIV/AIDS. Among adolescents, trichomonal and monilial infections and human papillomavirus are common. Chlamydial infections, syphilis, and herpes simplex type II (genital herpes) occur in both males and females, and can have serious complications.

AIDS is a major cause of death worldwide, reaching epidemic proportions in some countries. It is transmitted primarily through genital, oral, or anal sexual activities, but it can be transmitted by other ways (e.g., by sharing needles with an infected person). The annual rate of AIDS diagnoses reported among males ages 15 to 19 has nearly doubled in the past 10 years (Gavin, MacKay, Brown, et al., 2009). For more information about STIs, see Chapter 33.

Adolescent Pregnancy Except for an increase between 2005 and 2007 (Gavin, MacKay, Brown, et al., 2009), teenage birth rates have declined each year since 1991. The 2010 rate of 34.3 births per 1,000 teens (ages 15 to 19) was the lowest in 70 years (CDC, 2010b). Nevertheless, rates are still high, especially among black and Hispanic teens in the South; and the United States has substantially higher teen pregnancy and birth rates than other industrialized nations (CDC, 2010b). Although a similar percentage of teens are sexually active in the United States, consistency and effectiveness of condom use are lower.

Adolescents who become pregnant face physiological risks, such as bone density loss and iron deficiency anemia, the interruption of progress in their own developmental tasks, and loss of educational opportunities. Teen mothers are less likely to complete high school and more likely live in poverty than other teens. They are less likely to be married, to receive prenatal care, and gain appropriate weight; and more likely to smoke than older mothers. This puts them and their babies at higher risk for complications of pregnancy and low-birth-weight infants.

Example Problem: Abuse, Neglect, and Violence

There is no age limit on abuse and neglect. One study of children age 13 to adulthood reported that more than 9% of the nearly 1,000 subjects had substantiated maltreatment. Maltreatment included sexual abuse, physical abuse, emotional abuse, and neglect. Abuse may be linked to later violent crimes and illicit drug use (Leeb, Lewis, & Zolotor, 2011; Mersky, Topitzes, & Reynolds, 2011). Adults often ignore symptoms and complaints of adolescent abuse. Young children are perceived as defenseless, but people tend to stereotype adolescents as provoking their own abuse. Fewer than 40% of adolescent maltreatment cases are reported to child protection agencies, compared with 76% of cases involving younger children (McFarlane & Miller, 2005).

▉ ASSESSMENT

Adolescents should have a general health examination every 2 years. Communicating with adolescents can be challenging because they are sometimes rebellious. Try to establish rapport, and reassure the teenager that you will maintain confidentiality.

Toward Evidence-Based Practice

Perry, R., Kayekjian, K., Braun, R., et al. (2011). Adolescents' perspectives on the use of text messaging service for preventive sexual health promotion. *Journal of Adolescent Health, 51*(3), 220–225.

This study investigated the perspectives of 26 adolescents (ages 15 to 20 years) regarding a preventive sexual health text messaging service. Participants reported that they generally enjoyed receiving health-related text messages that were relevant to and directly helpful in their daily lives. They stated that receiving the text messages helped to stimulate or guide positive discussions with peers about sexual health. Findings indicated that using text messaging to relay health information to teens was convenient for the participants, did not pose financial concerns for most, and generally created a greater sense of privacy than did traditional communication tools.

Kogan, S., Yu, T., Brody, T., et al. (2012). Integrating condom skills into family-centered prevention: Efficacy of the strong African American families–teen program. *Journal of Adolescent Health, 51*(2), 164–170.

In this research study 16-year-old African American youths and their primary caregivers were randomly assigned to a group that participated in a 5-week family skills training program with a condom skills unit, or to the control group, which was not offered the condom skills unit as part of the intervention. The results of this study indicate that the intervention with its condom skills unit was effective in reducing the frequency of unprotected intercourse and increasing condom efficacy among rural African American high school students. These results suggest that integrating condom skills education into a family-centered prevention programs is effective when caregivers' input on the issue is respected.

1. What important points does the first research study make pertaining to adolescent learning needs that you could use in your preventive healthcare teaching?

2. What implications do the findings from the research studies have on how you might provide preventive services to adolescents?

Obtain a Thorough Health History Obtain information in the following areas:

- *Medications and other drugs.* Be sure to ask about use of prescription and OTC medications, tobacco, and recreational drugs. If so, find out what, how much, and for how long?
- *Psychosocial profile.* Obtain a psychosocial profile focusing on health practices and behaviors. Assess the adolescent's ability to cope with stressors. **Key Point:** *A change in academic performance or lack of interest in school may indicate a problem such as depression.*
- *Peer relationships.* Assess the quality of the adolescent's peer relationships, to assess risk for social isolation and to determine risk for school-related and/or gang-related violence.
- *Nutrition and body image.* Ask questions about body image in relation to the adolescent's nutritional status. Assess eating patterns, as well as intake of key nutrients such as protein, iron, calcium, and vitamin D.
- *Tattoos and piercings.* The tattoo or piercing may be in a concealed location, so ask about tattoos and piercings and ask to look at them during the visit. Discuss the risks of body art and modification.
- *Activity and exercise patterns.* If the adolescent engages in activities that increase the risk for injuries, ask about the use of protective *equipment,* such as helmets, mouth guards, or padding. If the adolescent reports no regular physical activity, assess his or her understanding of the benefits of exercise.

- *Sleep patterns.* Teens often get little sleep during school days and sleep late on weekends. Ask whether the teen feels refreshed after a night's sleep.
- ✚ *Safety.* Determine whether the adolescent wears a seat belt. Determine whether he is aware of the hazards of driving under the influence of drugs and alcohol and while texting or talking on the phone. Other distractions, including loud music and other teens in the car, can compete with the attention and focus needed for traffic and driving safety.
- *Sexual activity.* Determine whether the adolescent is sexually active. If so, ask about condom use.
- *Review all body systems.* While doing so, keep in mind changes or problems that are specific to the adolescent.

General Survey Complete a general survey after you have gathered the subjective data. Include vital signs, height, and weight. Follow with a head-to-toe physical exam. If you identify any problems in the course of the history and physical examination, actively involve the adolescent and the parents in a plan of care.

Calculate the BMI using a BMI calculator and BMI-for-age percentiles for children and teens. Adult calculators will not give accurate results for teens. The following are the CDC weight status categories:

Underweight	Less than 5th percentile
Healthy weight	5th to less than 85th percentile
At risk of overweight	85th to less than 95th percentile
Overweight	95th percentile or greater

To use the CDC BMI Calculator for Child and Teen,

 Go to the CDC Web site at http://nccd.cdc.gov/dnpabmi/

To see the CDC body mass index-for-age percentile charts for boys and girls ages 2 to 20,

 Go to Student Resources: Chapter 9, **Tables, Boxes, Figures: ESG Figures 9-4 and 9-5,** in the Chapter Resources on Davis*Plus.*

INTERVENTIONS

When working with adolescents, your goal is to help the adolescent make informed decisions. Avoid scare tactics, and encourage open discussion. Often a teenager will feel more comfortable asking a nurse or other health professional about sensitive topics than asking a parent. **Key Point:** *Reassure the adolescent that you will maintain confidentiality. However, if there is concern about suicide, explain to the adolescent that you are required to share this information with others. Provide mental health referrals immediately when an adolescent contemplates suicide.*

Focus your age-specific interventions on educating the teenager about common health problems and avoidance of injury and disease. Include the following topics in your discussions:

Preventing and Treating Obesity

Help the patient to make small but permanent changes in eating and exercise. These usually work better than a series of extreme short-term diets and exercise plans that cannot be sustained. Gradual weight loss is the healthiest approach. Even for teens, parental involvement is important, primarily to model healthy eating and physical activity.

Calorie Intake Reducing calorie intake is usually the easiest change to make. As a rule, avoid highly restrictive diets that forbid favorite foods. It is important to encourage strong support from parents and others involved in buying and preparing food. Teach the teen how to choose highly nutritious foods at school, to replace junk foods with healthier choices as snacks, and to limit fruit juices and sodas. Recommend eating a balanced diet, but with smaller portions.

Physical Activity Stress the importance of regular physical activity. Suggest walking to school instead of driving or taking a bus. If this is not practical, involve the family in planning regular physical activities, for example, a long walk after dinner. Even mild exercise, such as shooting hoops or swimming, provides more activity than watching television or playing computer games. You might start with the following goals:

- *Limit television and video game use* to 1 or 2 hours a day. Discourage use before school, during homework, and late at night. Keep the television off during family mealtimes.

- *Engage in 30 minutes of outdoor activity every day*, no matter how mild the activity. Then work up to an hour a day of more strenuous exercise.

Intervention for Example Problem: Substance Abuse

Discuss with the adolescent the effects of drugs, alcohol, and tobacco and the hazards associated with their use. If your assessment has identified drug or alcohol use, make appropriate referrals.

Provide information on smoking cessation programs, if appropriate. Remind teens that the earlier a person begins smoking, the harder the addiction is to break. Stress the unattractive physical effects, such as bad breath, stained teeth and fingers, and a long-term cough, not to mention the expense and inconvenience of purchasing cigarettes. More and more teens are using smokeless tobacco products, and some have the mistaken idea that these are safer than smoking.

Preventing Pregnancy and STIs

One of the *Healthy People 2020* national goals is to increase the percentage of adolescents who either abstain from sex or use condoms with hormonal or intrauterine contraception. To see the *Healthy People 2020* objectives,

 Go to the *Healthy People 2020* Web site at http://www.healthypeople.gov/2020/default.aspx

Abstinence is the only 100% effective way to prevent pregnancy and STIs. However, if the adolescent is sexually active, explain that using condoms can greatly reduce, although not eliminate, the risk of STIs and unwanted pregnancies. Be sure he understands that STIs can be transmitted orally and anally, as well as vaginally, so it is important that he uses a condom, regardless of the type of sexual activity.

A practice guideline from the AAP (2005) recommends that schools make condoms available for adolescents and, with community involvement, develop a comprehensive sequential sexuality education as a part of a K–12 health education program. Some parents may worry that sex education and condom availability encourage teenage sex but data show that making condoms available does not increase the rate of sexual activity (Agency for Healthcare Research and Quality, 2008). School and community collaboration is essential to promote sexual responsibility by increasing the use of condoms.

Breast Self-Exam

Currently there is some controversy about whether or not we should continue to encourage breast self-examination (BSE). The American Cancer Society (n.d., updated 2012) advises that monthly BSE is optional for women under age 30. BSE is recommended by certain medical groups, such as the ACOG (2009; NGC, 1998, revised March 2012), but not by the USPSTF (2009). Some studies indicate that BSE does not reduce death rates from breast cancer (National Cancer Institute, 2008); however, others found that more cancers are discovered and that the cancers detected are smaller in groups who perform BSE (Gemignani, 2011; Kösters & Gøtzsche, 2004, updated October 8, 2009; Meissner, Klabunde, Han, et al., 2011).

There is a trend away from teaching BSE and toward promoting *breast self-awareness*, defined as women's awareness of the normal appearance and feel of their breasts. Breast self-awareness can include BSE, and if patients choose to perform BSE, they should be trained in proper technique to avoid false-negative findings (ACOG, 2009; USPSTF, 2009; NGC, 1998, revised March 2012). To see how to perform a BSE,

 Go to Chapter 9, **Assessment Box: Breast Self-Exam**, in Volume 2.

Testicular Self-Exam

Males over the age of 14 should perform a testicular self-examination once a month. This is an effective way to become familiar with the body and to detect testicular cancer early, when it is most curable. However, the USPSTF (2011b) recommends against routine screening, even though they acknowledge that most testicular cancers are discovered by TSE. They concluded that screening does not reduce the deaths population-wide from testicular cancer sufficiently to merit routine TSE. If your patient chooses to perform TSE, advise him to perform the exam after a warm bath or shower (heat relaxes the scrotum, making it easier to find abnormalities). To learn how to do a testicular self-exam,

 Go to Chapter 9, **Assessment Box: Testicular Self-Exam**, in Volume 2.

To find information about testicular self-examination,

 Go to the Testicular Cancer Resource Center Web site at http://tcrc.acor.org/tcexam.html

Immunizations

For adolescents ages 13 to 17, none of the *Healthy People 2010* objectives for vaccinations were met. Fewer than half have current tetanus, diphtheria, and pertussis immunization. About double that number have been vaccinated for hepatitis B, measles, mumps, and rubella. To see the national goals for 2020,

 Go to the *Healthy People 2020* Web site at http://www.healthypeople.gov/2020/topicsobjectives2020/default

For the recommended immunization schedule for adolescents,

 Go to Student Resources: Chapter 9, **Tables, Boxes, Figures: ESG Figure 9-3,** on DavisPlus. Also go to Immunizations Recommended for Children Ages 7 to 18 years, on the CDC Web site, at http://www.cdc.gov/vaccines/schedules/Schedulers/adolescent-scheduler.html

Other Health Promotion Activities

Other nursing activities include promoting adolescent health and safety.

- *Rest.* Explain the importance of adequate rest. Teens need 8 hours of sleep a night for maximum performance in academics and sports.
- *Nutrition.* Stress the importance of adequate nutrition, including intake of 1,300 mg of calcium and 400 IU of vitamin D daily to reach maximum bone density during this critical period of rapid increase in growth and bone mass. Teach teens how to include fruits, vegetables, cereal and grains, lean meats, chicken, fish, and low-fat dairy products in their diet, and to avoid foods and drinks that are high in sugar, fat, or caffeine.
- *Dental Hygiene.* Advise parents that the adolescent should have a preventive dental care visit once a year. Teach the teen to brush twice a day with a soft toothbrush, and to floss daily.
- *Safety.* Remind teens to wear a seat belt when riding in the car, and avoid distractions while driving (e.g., talking or texting on a cell phone, changing a radio station). Ask them *never* to drive under the influence of alcohol or drugs. Remind them to wear a helmet and protective gear for activities such as bicycling, in-line skating, and skateboarding. Teach the importance of sun safety (e.g., applying a sunscreen of at least SPF 15, avoiding tanning beds, wearing sunglasses when in the sun).

KnowledgeCheck 9-8
- According to Erikson, what is the developmental stage of the adolescent?
- Name two common health problems of adolescents.

ThinkLike a Nurse 9-5
Recall Carrie, a 13-year-old, in the Meet Your Patients scenario. Carrie is hospitalized for pneumonia. What effect might this have on her behavior? As her nurse, how might you intervene?

YOUNG ADULTHOOD: AGES 19 TO 40 YEARS

Young adulthood is the time of transition to independence and responsibility. This transition involves important life events, such as high school graduation, entering college or starting a career, and leaving home and functioning independently. The 20s are spent exploring occupations, marriage, or alternative relationships.

Physical Development of Young Adults

Young adulthood is usually the healthiest stage of a person's life. Maturation of the body systems is complete. Peak bone density is achieved for both females and males by age 25. Vision and hearing are typically acute. For women, the ages between 20 and 30 years are the optimal years for childbearing. For men, male hormone levels that surged in adolescence begin to slowly decrease and stabilize around age 24.

Cognitive Development of Young Adults

According to Piaget, cognitive development terminates in adolescence around age 15. At this point, thought processes and mental abilities are well established. Learning continues throughout life but patterns of thinking do not alter.

Contemporary psychologists have proposed an additional stage of cognitive development called *post-formal operations*. In the *formal operations* phase, one is able to think rationally, predict outcomes, and hypothesize about the future. *Post-formal operations* add a dimension of complexity. In this phase, the young adult is able to accept contradictions and fine points in thinking. For example, the post-formal thinker recognizes that her opinion on a social controversy has aspects of two opposing viewpoints. She sees merit in both parts of the argument and is comfortable with the discrepancy.

Psychosocial Development of Young Adults

Young adults begin to explore options for careers and intimate relationships. They strive to become less dependent and more self-sufficient. Around age 30, most young adults experience a period of self-evaluation. This often results in job, career, or relationship changes. Erikson describes this period as the stage of *intimacy versus isolation*. Successful completion of this phase requires establishment of lasting friendships and associations. Freud described this phase of life as the *genital stage*. He believed that young adults are instinctively driven to form a sexually intimate relationship.

Common Health Problems of Young Adults

Young adults are generally active and in good physical health. Health problems may include STIs, unplanned pregnancies, traumatic injury, suicide attempts, substance abuse, domestic violence, obesity, diabetes, and hypertension.

Sexually Transmitted Infections

Sexual experimentation often continues in this stage. Among adults 15 to 44 years of age, nearly all have had vaginal intercourse and most have had oral sex with an opposite-sex partner. More than one-third of women and 44% of men have had anal sex with an opposite-sex partner. Twice as many women ages 25 to 44 (12%) reported any same-sex contact in their lifetime, compared with men (5.8%) (Chandra, Mosher, & Copen, 2011). Some common STIs include chlamydia, genital warts (condyloma acuminata), gonorrhea, and genital herpes. Also, the large majority of newly diagnosed cases (nearly 39%) of acquired immunodeficiency syndrome

(AIDS) are among young adults (CDC, 2008, 2010b, revised 2011). For more information about STIs, see Chapter 33, and

 Go to Chapter 9, **Supplemental Resources, Sexually Transmitted Infections,** on Davis*Plus*.

Example Problems: Substance Abuse and Violence

Drug abuse is commonly thought of as an adolescent problem; however, cocaine use is on the rise among young adults with families and careers. In the young adult years, there is a strong emphasis on "getting ahead," establishing a career and family, and becoming independent. These tasks are emotionally difficult. Substance abuse and mental health problems, particularly depression and suicide, may result from the tensions that arise. Substance abuse is often associated with acts of violence.

Unintentional injury is the leading cause of death in young adults (National Center for Health Statistics, 2011b). Suicide, a potential result of untreated depression, is another cause of death among young adults. Roughly 40,000 people a year die from firearm injuries; most of these are suicide and homicide rather than accidental injury. This is a rate of about 1 death per 10,000 people. The male death rate is about 7 times that for females (Heron, Hoyert, Murphy, et al., 2009).

Example Problem: Intimate Partner Abuse, Neglect, and Violence

Domestic violence is the abuse of power and control within an intimate relationship, most often between spouses or domestic partners. The CDC recognizes four categories of intimate partner violence (IPV), including physical violence, sexual violence, threat of physical or sexual violence, and psychological or emotional abuse.

Incidence Surveys typically report that 1 in 3 U.S. women is physically assaulted by a spouse or partner at some point in their lives—an estimated 1 to 5 million each year. About half of these incidents result in injury (Moracco, Runyan, Bowling, et al., 2007; Nelson, Bougatsos, & Blazina, 2012; U.S. Department of Justice, 2000). Many victims do not report the abuse, so survey results vary. Violence against women and girls is a worldwide epidemic. Globally, 1 in every 3 women has been assaulted, coerced into sex, or otherwise abused at some point in her life. More often than not, the abuser is a spouse or domestic partner, but it is sometimes another family member.

Risk Factors Abuse occurs in all ethnic and socioeconomic groups. Factors associated with intimate partner violence include young age, low income status, pregnancy, mental health problems, alcohol or substance abuse by victims or perpetrators, separated or divorced status, and history of childhood sexual or physical abuse (Nelson, Bougatsos, & Blazina, 2012). Females 16 to 24 years of age are the most vulnerable to nonfatal violence. In the United States, women are 7 to 14 times more likely to be abused than are men. About 31% of female murder victims are killed by an intimate, compared with 3% of male victims.

Health Consequences Intimate partner violence has negative consequences for physical, sexual, and psychological health. Abuse victims can suffer acute and chronic pain, disability, damage to the eyes, sleep disorders, miscarriage, STIs, poor self-esteem, depression, anxiety, and even suicidal behavior.

Obesity

Obesity rates have increased during the past 25 years. It has now become a public health crisis. In 2010, 35.7% of U.S. adults were obese, with no difference between men and women. With the increase in obesity, the incidences of type 2 DM and hypertension have grown dramatically among young adults (National Center for Health Statistics 2011a; Ogden, Carroll, Kit, et al., 2012).

■ ASSESSMENT

Young adults should have an annual physical examination, including assessment of physical health, mental health, and lifestyle. Be sure to assess diet, exercise, smoking, drinking, and drug use. For women the exam should include a pelvic examination.

Screening Screening for diabetes and hypertension is very important in the young adult years, especially for those who are overweight or who have a family history of these disorders.

The American Cancer Society recommends a clinical breast examination at least once every 3 years. The USPSTF (2011b) no longer recommends clinical testicular exams because there is not enough evidence to show that screening reduces the deaths population-wide from testicular cancer. Nor do they recommend monthly TSE.

Example Problem: Assessment — Violence Screening

Intimate partner violence (IPV) is common, but often remains undetected, so the USPSTF recommends that clinicians screen women of childbearing age for abuse or domestic violence, and provide or refer women who screen positive to intervention services (Smith & Segal, 2012; USPSTF, 2012a). If there is any reason to suspect abuse, conduct a thorough assessment.

If a patient discloses domestic violence, act immediately. Ask the patient whether she would like you to contact the agency's domestic violence advocate (if there is one). If not, provide contact information for community domestic violence programs. Patients are often fearful, isolated, and in real danger, but they may refuse help the first time it is offered. For further information on abuse assessment and reporting,

 Go to **Procedure 9-1,** in Volume 2.

Also see Mandatory Reporting Laws, in Chapter 45, Legal Issues.

■ INTERVENTIONS

Nursing interventions for the young adult are similar to those for the adolescent. As a newly independent person, the young adult is establishing health patterns, including how she will interact with healthcare providers. Reinforce the teaching that was begun in the earlier age group. Stress the importance of health promotion activities such as Papanicolaou (Pap) test (for cervical cancer) every 3 years for women between the ages of 21 and 30 (NGC, 2012a; USPSTF, 2012b).

Breast Cancer Prevention Teach BSE if the client chooses to do it for early detection of cancer (see the section Breast Self-Exam in the part of this chapter on adolescents, preceding). Self-exam does not replace screening mammograms, and women younger than 40 who have risk factors for breast cancer should ask their healthcare provider whether they need mammograms. Risk factors include personal and family history of breast cancer, having the first child late in the childbearing cycle, having the first menstrual period before age 12, and certain breast changes (e.g., cells that look abnormal under a microscope). Studies have shown no link between abortion, or miscarriage, and breast cancer (National Cancer Institute, 2009). For a BSE procedure,

Go to **Assessment Guidelines & Tools, Assessment Box: Breast Self-Examination (BSE),** in Volume 2.

Exercise Recommend that adults engage in 2½ hours a week of moderate-intensity or 75 minutes a week of vigorous-intensity aerobic physical activity. Increasing exercise to 300 minutes a week provides even more health benefits (USDHHS, 2008).

KnowledgeCheck 9-9

- According to Erikson, what is the developmental stage of the young adult?
- What is the leading cause of death for this age group?
- What gender-specific assessments should be emphasized with this age group?

MIDDLE ADULTHOOD: AGES 40 TO 64 YEARS

The middle adult years are a time when people realize the difference between their early aspirations and their actual achievements. For families with children, this is a time when the children mature and leave the home. As a result, many middle adults and their children feel a need to redefine family roles.

Physical Development of Middle Adults

Physiological changes that occur during the middle adult years include graying hair, decreases in elasticity of the blood vessels, muscle tone, skin moisture and turgor, and gastrointestinal (GI) motility. A decrease in bone mass often causes a slight loss of height.

Menopause One of the principal changes that middle-adult women experience is menopause, the cessation of menstrual periods for at least 12 months. The ovaries no longer produce eggs on a cyclical basis, and reproductive ability is lost (although some women do become pregnant after not having menses for a year). The average age of menopause is 51 years. Most women experience a transition that takes place over several years. *Perimenopausal symptoms* are related to a decline in estrogen levels and may precede menopause by as much as 5 to 7 years. These symptoms include hot flashes, a decrease in breast size, changes in the length of the menstrual cycle and menstrual flow, vaginal dryness, nighttime awakenings, and moodiness.

Hormone replacement therapy (HRT) has been used extensively in the past to treat these symptoms, but recent studies have raised questions about the safety of hormone therapy to treat a naturally occurring phenomenon. HRT can relieve symptoms such as hot flashes and vaginal dryness. It may also protect against osteoporosis and age-linked eye disease. Some studies show that it may help prevent dementia; others show that it does not. Risks of HRT include increased risk of heart disease, breast cancer, stroke, and blood clots. The National Heart, Lung, and Blood Institute (National Institutes of Health, 2008) concludes that the risks of long-term combination hormone (estrogen and progestin) therapy outweigh the benefits for postmenopausal women. Women should be advised to consult their physician about estrogen-alone therapy, bioidentical therapies, and certain natural remedies that can provide symptom relief.

Andropause Men do not experience such a clear-cut transition as do women; however, many men do experience a transitional period known as andropause. Andropause is characterized by a decline in testosterone production, a lower sperm count, and a need for more time to achieve an erection. Andropause does not result in an inability to reproduce but does limit reproductive abilities.

Cognitive Development of Middle Adults

Piaget theorizes that the middle adult moves freely between formal operations, concrete operations, and problem-solving as the task demands. The middle adult is able to reflect on the past and anticipate the future. Creativity may reach its peak during this stage. Memory is intact, but reaction time begins to diminish because of diminishing nerve impulses.

Psychosocial Development of Middle Adults

Erikson describes middle adulthood as a stage of *generativity versus stagnation. Generativity* is the process of guiding the next generation or improving the whole of society. *Stagnation* occurs when development ceases: A stagnant middle adult cannot guide the next generation or contribute to society. Erikson believes that an inability to meet the developmental tasks of the middle adult years results in lack of preparedness for the final life stage of old age.

Middle adults often complain of declining energy and competing demands as they raise children, care for aging parents, and work at the peak of their career (Fig. 9-10). These stressors in combination with visible signs of aging may produce a **midlife crisis**—a recognition that youth is over and that life is limited. Coping skills learned in earlier years are important predictors of how the middle adult reacts to these changes.

Common Health Problems of Middle Adults

In the middle adult years, chronic diseases emerge as a major health problem. The most common chronic diseases are cancer, obesity, diabetes, hypertension, and cardiovascular disease. Many interventions for younger age groups are directed at preventing the development of these disorders.

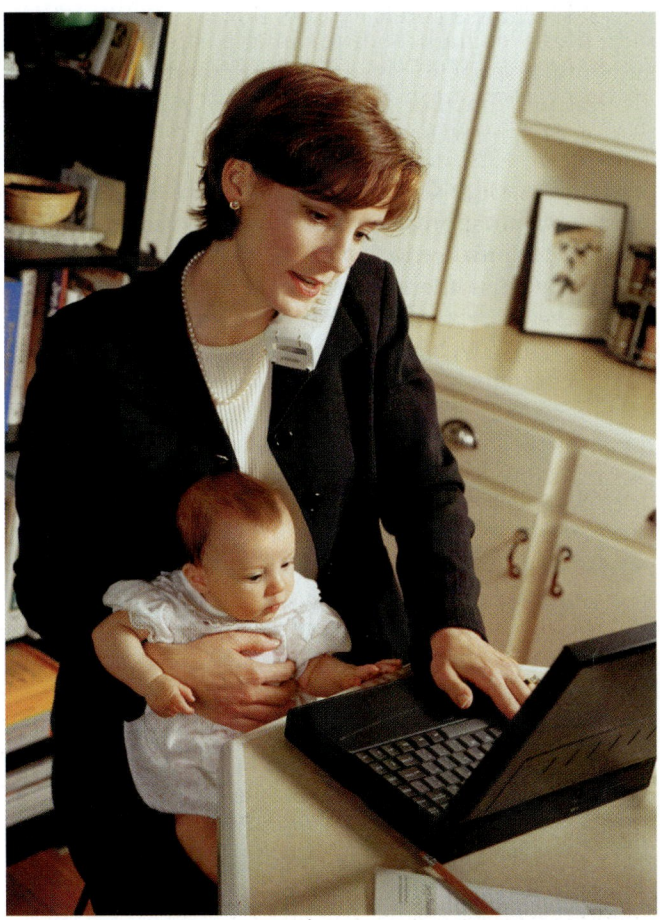

FIGURE 9-10 Middle adulthood is a time of competing demands.

Cancer Cancer is the second leading cause of death in this age group. The majority of cancer diagnoses occur in the middle and older adult years. Cancers of the lung, breast, colon, prostate, and bladder are among the most common. A man's risk of **prostate cancer** increases as he ages. Nearly 65% of prostate cancer cases occur after the age of 65. Other factors that increase the risk of developing prostate cancer are family history, race (African American men have the highest rate), and possibly diet. There is some evidence that a diet high in animal fat may increase the risk.

Obesity As we have seen, obesity is a major health problem in all age groups. It often triggers development of type 2 DM, hypertension, joint pain, and cardiovascular diseases, such as coronary artery disease, atherosclerosis, and venous insufficiency. Diet and exercise must be consistently used together to combat obesity. Ironically, obesity leads to a variety of problems that make it even harder to exercise.

Hypertension Hypertension (high blood pressure) is a complex disorder. As the elasticity of the vascular system declines with each passing year, the incidence of hypertension increases. If there is a strong family history of hypertension, the likelihood of needing treatment escalates sharply. Except for age and family history, factors that increase the risk of hypertension are under the patient's control. They include excess weight, sedentary lifestyle, high sodium intake, high fat intake, smoking, and the ingestion of more than 1.5 ounces of alcohol per day. For further discussion of hypertension, see Chapter 20.

Cardiovascular Disease Cardiovascular disease (CVD) is often the end product of poor lifestyle choices. Atherosclerotic plaque develops in the peripheral vascular system, the heart, major vessels, or any combination of these areas. CVD is the result of inadequately treated hypertension, ongoing weight gain or obesity, an aftermath of poorly controlled type 2 DM, and an outcome of sedentary lifestyle. Smoking and excess alcohol use are additional risk factors, as is long-term hormone replacement therapy for women. CVD is among the leading causes of death in the middle adult years.

Example Problem: Domestic Abuse, Neglect, and Violence.

Although younger women are more likely to experience nonfatal violence, women ages 35 to 49 are the most at risk for intimate murder (U.S. Department of Justice, n.d., last reviewed 2012). Also see Common Health Problems of Young Adults and the Example Problem: Intimate Partner Abuse, Neglect, and Violence, preceding. The assessments and interventions for middle adults are similar to those for young adults.

■■■ ASSESSMENT

Middle adults should undergo an annual physical exam. In addition to height, weight, BMI, and vital signs, the exam should include the following:

- *Lipid panel screening*; total cholesterol, triglycerides, high-density lipoprotein (HDL), low-density lipoprotein (LDL), and ratios.
- *Blood glucose screening.*
- *Clinical breast and pelvic examination* for women. There is still controversy about whether to encourage BSE (*The Guide to Clinical Preventive Services 2010–2011*; NGC, 1998, revised 2012); however, many clinicians believe it to be useful. See Breast Self-Exam, in the section on adolescents. Women older than age 30 should have a Pap test every 3 to 5 years based on health history and discussion with their primary care provider.
- *Annual or biannual mammogram* for women (American Cancer Society, n.d.b, last revised June 2012; NGC, 1998, revised March 2012).
- *Digital rectal exam for prostate evaluation* in men should be offered but not routinely done (American Cancer Society, n.d.b). An enlarged prostate can indicate either benign prostatic hypertrophy or prostate cancer. In men, serum prostatic specific antigen (PSA) level is a sensitive indicator of prostate disorders. Recommendations vary. Some caution against routine screening; however, the American Cancer Society (n.d.b, revised June 2012) says this test should be given beginning at age 45 to men who want to be screened, and at age 40 for those who are at higher risk.
- *Annual eye exam*. Visual changes are common in this age group and include the development of presbyopia (far-sightedness) and the onset of glaucoma and cataracts.
- *Colorectal cancer screening.* Regular screening, beginning at age 50, is the key to preventing colorectal cancer. The USPSTF and an NGC Guideline Summary recommend screening for colorectal cancer using stool for occult blood testing, and sigmoidoscopy or colonoscopy beginning at age 50 years (or at age 40 for high-risk patients) and continuing until age 75 years (NGC, 2012b; Qaseem, Denberg, Hopkins, et al., 2012; USPSTF, 2008). The frequency of repeat exams depends on the findings.
- *Osteoporosis screening* at or prior to menopause for at-risk women who elect it. Most guidelines recommend assessing all adults age 50 years and older for risk factors (e.g., smoking, low body weight), with bone density measurement (e.g., a DXA test) based on the risk profile (NGC, 2008, revised 2012).

■■■ INTERVENTIONS

Care for middle adults focuses on identifying risk factors and promoting a healthy lifestyle. At each annual exam and at periodic health visits, you should discuss the hazards of alcohol and tobacco use, stress-management techniques, and safety, as well as the following three topics. You will also need to add teaching interventions if any chronic problem is discovered.

Nutrition For menopausal women, encourage daily intake of 12,00 milligrams of calcium and 600 IU of vitamin D, as well as regular weight-bearing exercise, to promote optimal bone density (Institute of Medicine, Food and Nutrition Board, 2010, updated 2012; Office of Dietary Supplements, National Institutes of Health, 2011). There is growing consensus that even this amount may be too low. Many clinicians are prescribing higher doses, especially in cases of known deficiency.

Exercise Although the usual recommendation is for 60 minutes of exercise daily, and that amount brings the most health benefits, researchers now suggest that even smaller amounts of exercise can improve the quality of life for sedentary, overweight or obese postmenopausal women. Even just 10 to 30 minutes a day can improve in social functioning and decrease limitations in work and other activities due to physical or emotional problems (American Heart Association, 2011).

Immunizations Review the patient's immunization record regularly. Middle adults often require periodic boosters, for example, for tetanus. For clients who have a chronic disease, recommend an annual flu vaccination. Strongly encourage clients with respiratory problems to receive pneumonia vaccination as well.

KnowledgeCheck 9-10

- According to Erikson, what is the developmental stage associated with middle adulthood?
- Identify at least five appropriate topics for health teaching during middle adulthood.

PracticalKnowledge
knowing **how**

This section of the chapter focuses on using standardized nursing language for nursing diagnoses, patient outcomes, and interventions for patients in infancy through middle-adulthood. Specific assessments and interventions were discussed within each of the developmental stages in the Theoretical Knowledge section.

ANALYSIS/DIAGNOSIS

Although most NANDA-I diagnoses can be used for any age group, the following focus specifically on growth and development (NANDA-I, 2012):

Adult Failure to Thrive
Delayed Growth and Development
Risk for Delayed Development
Risk for Disproportionate Growth

Refer to the clients in the Meet Your Patients scenario. You would, of course, consider their growth and development needs in your assessments and care. However, they are unlikely to experience any of the four growth and development diagnoses. Short-term illness does not usually lead to delays in growth and development. Growth and development problems are more likely to be caused by family dysfunction, inadequate nutrition, or severe or long-term illness (e.g., Risk for Delayed Development r/t inadequate stimulation secondary to parental substance abuse).

Delayed growth and development is more often a part of the defining characteristics (signs and symptoms) of a problem rather than the diagnosis (e.g., Impaired Parenting r/t mother's chronic disability and absent father, as evidenced by height, weight, and verbal skills behind norms for age group).

When used to describe a client's *problem,* Delayed Growth and Development is too broad to suggest nursing actions. For example, the label is not useful for a mentally handicapped child (e.g., do not write, Delayed Growth and Development r/t Down syndrome). Instead, write a nursing diagnosis describing the specific functional task(s) the child cannot perform (e.g., Toileting Self-Care Deficit r/t inability to recognize the urge to void in time to ask for help secondary to Delayed Growth and Development). This label is also not appropriate for a child with failure to thrive. Instead, use one of the family functioning diagnoses (e.g., Impaired Parenting) or Imbalanced Nutrition: Less Than Body Requirements (Wilkinson, 2013).

Although there are only four NANDA-I diagnoses that specifically address growth and development, some other NANDA-I diagnoses do address age-specific problems. Because they provide more specific direction for nursing care than the growth and development diagnoses, use these when possible. Those diagnoses are as follows:

- Ineffective Breastfeeding
- Ineffective Infant Feeding Pattern
- Interrupted Breastfeeding
- Readiness for Enhanced Breastfeeding
- Disorganized Infant Behavior
- Risk for Disorganized Infant Behavior
- Readiness for Enhanced Organized Infant Behavior
- Risk for Impaired Attachment
- Impaired Parenting
- Readiness for Enhanced Parenting
- Risk for Impaired Parenting
- Parental Role Conflict

PLANNING OUTCOMES/EVALUATION

NOC outcomes specifically related to growth and development include the following; however, many other NOC outcomes may be appropriate depending on the

NANDA-I label you use (e.g., Imbalanced Nutrition, Self-Care Deficit).

- Child Development: (specify 2 Months, 4 Years, and so on)
- Fetal Status: Antepartum
- Fetal Status: Intrapartum Growth
- Newborn Adaptation
- Physical Aging
- Physical Maturation: Female
- Physical Maturation: Male
- Will to Live

Individualized goals/outcome statements for the other NANDA-I growth and development diagnoses might include the following examples:

- *Diagnosis*: Risk for Disproportionate Growth
  Goal: The child will continue to gain weight and length as measured at the next well-child check.
- *Diagnosis*: Risk for Delayed Growth and Development
  Goal: The child will continue to gain weight and length and meet developmental milestones as measured at the next well-child check.

▰ PLANNING INTERVENTIONS/IMPLEMENTATION

NIC *standardized interventions* associated with growth and development diagnoses include the following:

- Coping Enhancement
- Developmental Care
- Hope Inspiration
- Parent Education: Childrearing Family
- Risk Identification
- Self-Care Assistance
- Self-Responsibility Facilitation
- Teaching: Infant Nutrition, Infant Safety, Safe Sex, Sexuality, Toddler Nutrition, Toddler Safety

PUTTING IT ALL TOGETHER

Recall the case of 3-year-old Tamika, who is being raised by her grandmother and has been hospitalized with pneumonia (Meet Your Patients scenario). Imagine that Tamika has been abandoned by her mother, who is addicted to heroin. If you observe that Tamika is small for her size and has not met developmental milestones appropriate for a 3-year-old, you could write the following *diagnostic statement*:

> *Delayed Growth and Development r/t abandonment by mother, recent change in living status, and gestational heroin exposure as evidenced by underweight status, short stature, limited verbal skills, and onset of walking at 36 months of age*

To address Tamika's diagnosis you might use the following *outcomes*:

> *NOC outcome:* Child Development: 3 Years
> *Individualized goal:* Tamika will achieve growth between the 35th and 65th percentiles for her age group and be able to walk up steps, verbalize with 2- to 3-word sentences, and eat a variety of foods within 6 months.

Tamika will need care that helps her catch up developmentally and allows her to establish a strong relationship with her grandmother. Because the grandmother is also caring for an ailing spouse, you may need to refer this family to community support services for ongoing help.

> *NIC interventions* appropriate for Tamika are as follows:
> Developmental Care
> Teaching: Toddler Nutrition and Toddler Safety
> *Specific interventions* for Tamika might include therapeutic play with age-appropriate toys, reading stories, and engaging in conversation, as well as teaching the grandmother about these activities. This family may need counseling to assist with this transition.

To explore learning resources for this chapter,

 Go to DavisPlus at DavisPl.us/Wilkinson3.

Chapter Resources for Chapter 9:

Response sheets for all learning activities

Resources for Caregivers and Health Professionals

Reading More About Life Span: Infancy Through Middle Adulthood (suggested readings)

Concept Map of chapter content

Interactive Case Studies

NCLEX-Style and Chapter Review Questions

Chapter Overview Podcasts

For references cited in this chapter,

 Go to Volume 2, **References Cited.**

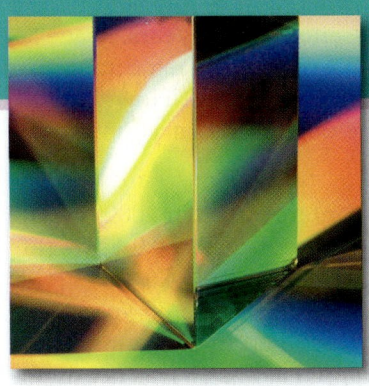

CHAPTER 10

Life Span: Older Adults

Learning Outcomes

After completing this chapter, you should be able to do the following:

➤ Discuss the relationship of life expectancy and livable communities.

➤ Discuss the developmental challenges for each older adult age group.

➤ Identify common health problems seen in each group and for all older adults.

➤ Describe any special assessments unique to each group of older adults.

➤ Discuss age-appropriate interventions for older adults and for each group.

➤ Incorporate developmental principles of aging into nursing care.

Key Concepts

Developmental changes
Functional status
Older adulthood

Related Concepts

See the Concept Map on Davis*Plus*.

Example Problems

Dementia
Elder abuse
Frail elderly

Meet Your Patient

Ethel Higginbotham, an 80-year-old woman, is in the hospital with pneumonia. She lives alone. Her son tells you that she began to lose weight rapidly, complains of no appetite, and became withdrawn after the death of her husband. At a recent visit to her home, he found his mother confused, with a productive cough, and with small open lesions on her lower legs. This led to her hospitalization. Even though she is no longer receiving oxygen, you observe that she is very thin and weak, sleeps most of the time, and refuses to eat. "I just want to die," she tells you.

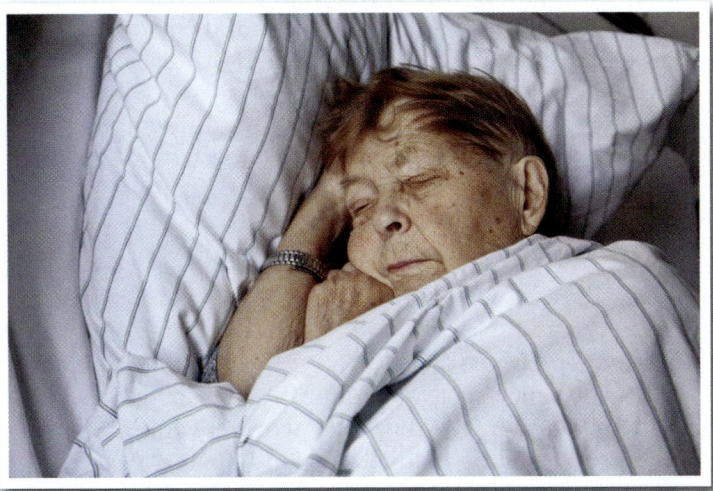

Theoretical Knowledge
knowing why

Why should you learn about older adults? One very important reason is that most of your patients are likely to be older adults. Half of all hospitalized patients are older adults, and because older adults are more likely to have disabilities and chronic health problems, they will make up a sizeable number of the patients you see in clinics, home care, and other settings, as well. This chapter presents the most important topics and issues about aging and the development of older adults.

ABOUT THE KEY CONCEPTS

You may have thought of **developmental stages** as something that applies mostly to children. However, as you learned in Chapter 9, developmental changes occur throughout life, even in **older adulthood.** Many normal changes occur in **older adulthood**. You will learn how normal changes, as well as illness, can affect **functional status**—a major focus in caring for older adults.

PERSPECTIVES ON AGING

Older adulthood is the fastest growing age group in developed nations. To understand this, you will need to look at some statistics. In 1900, a mere 4.1% of the U.S. population was 65 or older. By 2008, life expectancy had increased, and older adults made up 13% of the population. It is expected that by 2050 one-fifth of the population will be over 65.

This chapter examines aging from different angles. We will discuss the concepts of life expectancy, distribution of age groups, life-span perspective, and percentage of total population. All of these concepts require you to think about numerical descriptions of population characteristics.

Life Expectancy

Life expectancy, measured at birth and at age 65, is one way to view aging. Around the world, people in developed countries are living longer and having fewer children. Consider the following data from the National Center for Health Statistics (2012).

- **Life expectancy at birth** has risen dramatically in the United States:
  In 1900, average life expectancy was 49.2 years.
  In 2009, average life expectancy was 78.5 years.
- **Life expectancy measured at age 65** has risen as follows:
  In 1900, a 65-year-old person could expect to live 11.9 more years.
  In 2009, a 65-year-old person could expect to live 19.2 more years.

This means that a baby born in 2009 could expect to live for nearly 78.5 years, whereas a 65-year-old person in 2009 could expect to live another 19.2 years, to age 84. Those numbers reflect the average life expectancy for both sexes and all ethnic/racial groups. However, differences in life expectancy emerge when you examine sex and ethnic group data.

Gender Disparities For infants born in 2009, the average total life expectancy for females is 80.9 years (life expectancy at birth). For males it is only 76 years. This difference is especially noticeable in the 85-years-and-older population, in which women greatly outnumber men. Life expectancy measured at age 65 was nearly the same for men and women in 1900; however, women had a lead of about 5 years over men in 2009, narrowing the gap as men age. So the longer men live, the longer they *will* live.

Racial Disparities In 1900, race defined U.S. life expectancy at birth. As of 2009, the picture was less clear (as you can see in the following data from National Center for Health Statistics, 2012).

- *Life expectancy at birth:* White females continued to have the highest life expectancy at birth but following closely behind were white males and black females. In 2009, the life expectancy of black males at birth was a little over 10 years less than for white females.
- *Life expectancy at age 65*: White women led life expectancy with 20 years, followed closely by black women at 19.3 and white men at 17.7 years, whereas black men at age 65 had the lowest life expectancy (15.8). Notice, though, that the gap for ethnicity decreases as a person ages.
  A black baby boy born in 2009 can expect to live to about age 71.
  A black man at age 65 in 2009 can expect to live another 15.8 years, to age 81.

The future population of older adults will be more ethnically and racially diverse, with minority groups (everyone except non-Hispanic, single-race whites) representing 54% of the population in 2050. The non-Hispanic white population—66% of the population in 2008—is projected to decrease and to compose only 46% of the total population in 2050 (U.S. Census Bureau, 2008).

Migration and Distribution of Age Groups

In addition to life expectancy, in-migration and out-migration within countries and between countries contribute to the distribution of age groups within each country and the median age of a population. For example, between 1995 and 2000, five states had the highest in-migration of newly retired persons: Nevada, Arizona, Florida, North Carolina, and Delaware. By 2020, these five states will begin to face an accelerated growth in the

85+ population. In 2010, the median age (years) (U.S. Census Bureau, 2008):

Of the U. S. population	was	37.2
Of the state of Maine	was	42.7
Of the state of Utah	was	29.2

The median age of the population in the United States is increasing:

In 2005, the median age of the U.S. population was 37.2 years.

In 2050, the median age of the U.S. population is expected to be 39 years.

KnowledgeCheck 10-1

- About what percentage of people over age 65 live in nursing homes?
- What percentage of people over 85 years old live in nursing homes?
- Who has the longer life expectancy, women or men?

Percentage of Total Population

Yet another way to view aging is by the *percentage of total population* each age group represents. In the United States, older adults composed approximately:

4.1% of the population in 1900

13% of the population in 2010

21% of the population in 2050 (projected by the U.S. Census Bureau, 2008)

Age distribution of a population is often illustrated in a pyramid with the youngest age group (0–4) at the base and the oldest age group (85+) at the peak, men on the left of the figure and women on the right. The shape of a population pyramid changes to that of a rectangle in developed countries with fewer births and increased life expectancy. To view a population pyramid that illustrates the projected age distribution of the U.S. population in 2025 and 2050, see Figure 10-1.

Notice that also that the percentage for centenarians almost doubles from 2025 to 2050. The Census Bureau reports the following in total number of centenarians (U.S. Census Bureau, 2006, 2008, 2011):

53,000 centenarians—actual total number in 2010

600,000 centenarians—projected total number in 2050

 Think**Like a Nurse** 10-1

- What factors do you think account for the overall increase in life expectancy?
- What effect will the distribution of the population by age within your state have on your nursing practice?
- Refer to Figure 10-1 to answer the following three questions.
  In the 85 to 89 age group in the 2025 data, what percentage of the population are men? What percentage are women?
  In the 85 to 89 age group in the 2050 data, what percentage of the population are men? What percentage are women?
  In the 85 to 89 age group, which group increases the most between 2025 and 2050: women or men?

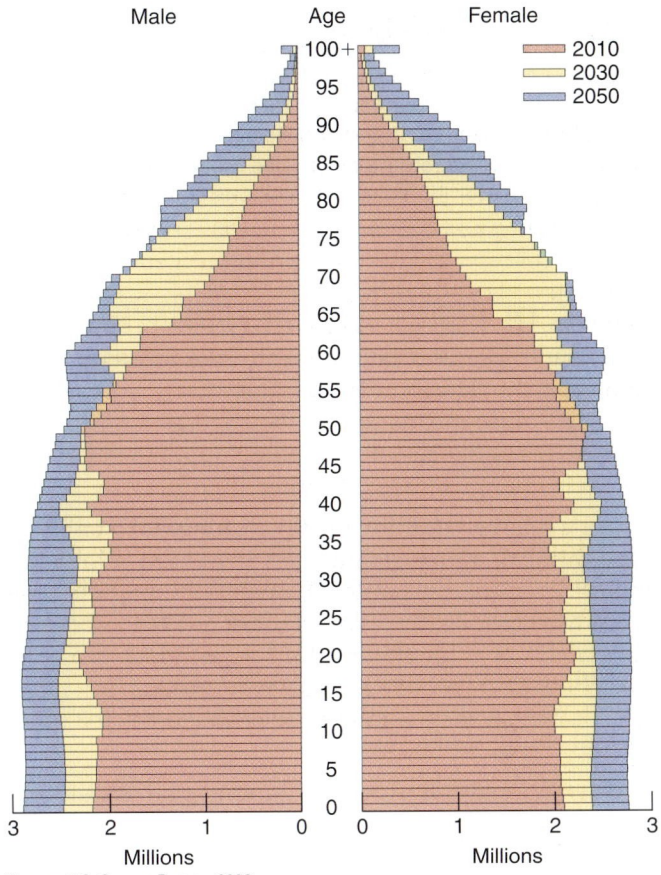

Source: U.S. Census Bureau, 2008.

FIGURE 10-1 Age and sex structure of the population for the United States: 2010, 2030, and 2050. (*Source:* Retrieved December 9, 2012, from http://www.census.gov/prod/2010pubs/p25-1138.pdf.)

Life-Span Perspective

Another way to view aging is from a *life-span perspective.* In this perspective, *genes* inherited at conception, *behaviors* expressed throughout a lifetime and *environments* within which a person lives, works, and plays interact with each other over time. The cumulative effect of these interactions is seen in older adulthood.

Think of the genetic–behavior–environment interaction as a survival mechanism of aging. Attending to healthy behaviors (e.g., daily exercise) and avoiding unhealthy behaviors (e.g., tobacco use) is a lifelong process. A lifetime of positive health behaviors interacting with a healthful environment has the potential to shift effects of a harmful genetic trait—that is, a person may have the genetic trait for a particular disease but never show signs of the disease.

Remember the Nun Study discussed in Chapter 8? Some of the nuns demonstrated no symptoms of Alzheimer's disease during their lifetime, yet upon autopsy scientists discovered the typical neurological changes associated with Alzheimer's disease (Snowdon, 2003). The Nun Study results illustrate strong evidence of the power of behaviors and the environment over genes, resulting in centenarians who are cognitively intact and asymptomatic for Alzheimer's disease.

ThinkLike a Nurse 10-2

Plot your birth year on a time line that extends in 10-year increments through your 65th and 100th year. What is the projected distribution of age and gender when you are an older adult? What genetic, environmental, and behavioral attributes will influence your life expectancy and state of health as an older adult?

AGING IN PLACE AND ALTERNATIVES

Contrary to popular belief, most older adults live independently (Houser, Fox-Grage, & Gibson, 2012). **Aging in place** means that as they age, persons live in their own residences and receive supportive services for their changing needs, rather than moving to another type of housing. Aging in place requires an elder-friendly residence and an elder-friendly or livable community that provides maximum accessibility, minimal barriers, and adequate resources and services to maintain independence for as long as possible. The goal of an elder-friendly residence is safe daily interaction with a living environment for persons with normal changes of aging.

Elder-Friendly Residences Among the considerations for an *elder-friendly residence* are the following:

- Ground-level entry or no-step entry
- One-level living area
- Wide doorways to allow for assistive devices such as walkers and wheelchairs
- Lever-style door and faucet handles for easy grasp
- Grab bars, shower seats, and elevated toilet seat in bathrooms
- Kitchen appliances, cabinets, and surfaces no higher than 48 inches above the floor
- Shelves no more than 10 inches deep, for easy accessibility
- Adequate light in all areas inside and outside the residence
- Walking areas free of clutter, including area rugs.

Elder-Friendly Communities Livable communities (also referred to as *elder friendly*) "actively involve, value, and support older adults" (Alley, Liebig, Pynoos, et al., 2007, p. 1). To illustrate the need for elder-friendly communities, consider these facts about older adults in 2007 (Houser, Fox-Grage, & Gibson, 2009):

1 in 3 persons age 75+ lived alone
A little less than half the persons age 65+ lived at or below 250% of the poverty line (about $27,000 for a single person or $36,000 for a family of two)
Nearly 1 in 5 persons age 65+ had a bachelor's degree or higher
37% have a sensory, physical, mobility, self-care, or cognitive disability

Many older adults spent at least 30% of their income on housing (Harrell, 2011). This includes the approximately 48% who owned their own homes, and the 59% of older adults who were renters.

Livable communities offer:

- Affordable and appropriate housing for all ages
- Supportive services and features
- Dependable and affordable transportation and housing
- Resources that facilitate individual independence and socialization of residents (AARP Public Policy Institute, 2011)
- Affordable and accessible healthcare
- Safe, low-crime environment
- Community engagement

Naturally Occurring Retirement Communities

When persons "age in place" within a specific apartment building or a community/street of single-family homes, that area is referred to as a **naturally occurring retirement community (NORC)**. Persons within a NORC have aged together. More often than not, they have, over the years, developed access to services needed to maintain the highest quality of life for all within the NORC. When one neighbor needs assistance, others pitch in to help or to obtain help. The U.S. Administration on Aging provides competitive funding to support the development and maintenance of services within a NORC.

Retirement Communities

Some housing developments are built specifically as **retirement communities**. They are planned to provide elder-friendly dwellings and environments for independent living and allow older adults to "downsize" into a house that has less than 2,000 square feet in single-level, livable space. Purchase of a home in a retirement community usually includes, for an annual association fee, services such as home maintenance and repair; landscaping; snow, leaf, and trash removal; some home utilities; security; home fire and theft insurance; recreational amenities, such as pool, spa, walking track, and golf and tennis facilities; and planned activities. They usually have a minimum age restriction of 55, 60, or 62 either for one of the residents in a household or for all occupants. Age restriction may be problematic if grandparents become the primary care providers for a grandchild.

Continuing Care Retirement Communities

Continuing care retirement communities (CCRC), or *life care communities*, offer a wide range of living accommodations from residential living (e.g., cottages, cluster homes, apartments), assisted living, skilled nursing care, rehabilitation, and dementia care on a large campus-like setting. CCRCs include many amenities, ranging from golf courses, pools, and indoor sport facilities to a full range of hobby and clubrooms and personal services. A CCRC is another example of aging in place, except that an older adult must first move to it. So in that sense, it is not a NORC.

Entrance requirements include physical, mental, and financial health evaluations. CCRCs are usually expensive, requiring a contract, an entrance fee, and monthly fees that may increase with annual cost-of-living estimates. Depending on the contract, monthly fees may cover a set number of meals per month, transportation, housekeeping, unit maintenance, laundry service, health monitoring, some utilities, coordinated social activities, emergency call monitoring, and round-the-clock security. A health clinic is usually on site. Healthcare providers may include a registered nurse, nurse practitioner, physician, dentist, and physical therapist.

CCRCs vary by their affiliation (e.g., ethnic or religious group, university, corporation) and whether the living space is rented or purchased. University-affiliated CCRCs incorporate all aspects of academic life into the lives of residents and provide opportunities for cross-generation interactions on the CCRC and university campuses. These interactions are especially important for students interested in careers in gerontology, because they have an opportunity to work or conduct research with CCRC residents in areas that fit their disciplinary focus.

Assisted-Living Facilities

Assisted-living facilities (ALFs) are congregate residential settings that provide or coordinate personal services, 24-hour supervision and assistance (scheduled and unscheduled), activities, and health-related services. ALFs are *not* aging in place environments. State regulations and level of services do not allow residents to stay in an ALF when their needs become greater than the resources and services provided can handle. ALFs are designed to:

- minimize the need to move
- accommodate individual residents' changing needs and preferences
- maximize residents' dignity, autonomy, privacy, independence, and safety
- encourage family and community involvement (Total Living Choices, 2000–2012)

There are multiple definitions and goals of ALFs and no common physical size, design, or model. ALFs might be self-standing or housed within a CCRC as one level of housing and service. Each ALF has its own culture, rules, norms, values, and rituals that are created by the residents (Al Omari, Kramer, Hronek, et al., 2005). An ALF may have limitations such as reduced consumer choice, little flexibility, and an illusion of certainty (Zimmerman & Sloane, 2007).

Nursing Care Facilities (Nursing Homes)

Nursing care facilities, or nursing homes, provide skilled and unskilled nursing care for older adults and adults with disabilities. To understand the scope of nursing care facilities in the overall picture of aging, consider the following facts. In 2009:

- About 1.5 million residents lived in more than 16,000 U.S. nursing facilities.
- Only 3.1% of persons age 65+ lived in nursing facilities; however, this rises to 10.4% for people over 85 years.
- Nearly half of the residents of nursing homes had dementia, and one-fifth had other psychological diagnoses (Houser, Fox-Grage, & Gibson, 2009).
- Women composed more than 70% of the nursing home population.
- Nearly 75% of residents are age 75 or older; the median age is 83.2 (U.S. Census Bureau, 2007, revised September 19, 2012).
- Medicaid is the primary source of payment for most (65%) of the residents; Medicare pays for about 13%, primarily for short stays; and individual long-term care insurance or private sources pay for 22% (Houser, Fox-Grage, & Gibson, 2009).

KnowledgeCheck 10-2

What is the difference between a retirement community and a continuing care retirement community (CCRC)?

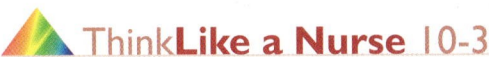 ThinkLike a Nurse 10-3

How elder-friendly is the community in which you live?

THEORIES OF AGING

There is no single explanation for how the body ages, but four groups of physiological theories predominate. Despite wide debate on these theories, most scientists consider aging to be a combination of factors, including inherited traits and the cell's response to environmental stressors.

Wear-and-Tear Theory This theory of aging proposes that repeated insults and the accumulation of metabolic wastes eventually cause cells to wear out and cease functioning.

Genetic Theories Genetic theories of aging propose that cells have a preprogrammed, finite number of cell divisions. Hence, the time of death is determined at birth. The genetic messages within the various body cells specify how many times the cell can reproduce, thus defining the life of that cell.

Cellular Malfunction These theories hypothesize that a malfunction in the cell causes changes in cellular DNA, leading to problems with cell replication. The cellular malfunction can be the result of a chemical reaction with the DNA (cross-linking theory), an abundance of free radicals that damage cells and impair their ability to function normally (free-radical theory), or a buildup of toxins over time that causes cell death (toxin theory).

Autoimmune Reaction This theory hypothesizes that cells change with age. Over time the changes result in the immune system's perceiving some cells as foreign substances and triggering an immune response to destroy the cells.

STAGES OF OLDER ADULTHOOD

Most references use 65 years as the age when older adulthood begins. The stages of older adulthood are typically referred to as the *young-old* (age 65 to 74), *middle-old* (age 75 to 84), and *oldest-old* (age 85 and older). The fastest growing segment of older adults is the oldest-old, some of whom are the frail elderly and *centenarians* (people older than 100 years). For more in-depth information about aging and older adults, refer to a life-span development or gerontology book.

Young-Old: Age 65 to 74

Physical and psychological adaptations to retirement are paramount in this age group. At retirement, a person's usual social contacts and structure for daily activities may change markedly. A newly retired older adult may be searching for new interests outside of the previous work environment. One key indicator of well-being is use of leisure time. On an average day, young-old persons spend most of their time (57%) watching television; 18% in solitary activities of reading, relaxing, and thinking; 11% socializing and communicating; 3% participating in sports, exercise, and recreation; and the remaining time in other activities, including related travel (Federal Interagency Forum on Aging Related Statistics, 2010).

By the time they reach age 65, young-old persons are already experiencing the effects of chronic illnesses that began in middle adulthood, along with the effects of lack of time to care for self because of the demands and stressors of work during that period. Retirement frees up time for the young-old to make up for these effects and focus on health-promoting behaviors to help prevent the decline of health as they age. However, young-old persons face barriers to health, such as a lack of supplemental insurance for health screening or physicals that are not covered under Medicare, self-perception of aging, changes in physical activity, and being in a deconditioned state by not participating in exercise in earlier life stages. There is some evidence that physical activity declines as early as age 63 for some, and by age 70 for most people (Wilson & Palha, 2007).

Middle-Old: Age 75 to 84

The developmental challenge of middle-old persons is an increasingly solitary, sedentary lifestyle. This age group spends one-fourth of their leisure time reading, relaxing, and thinking—more than their younger cohort. They spend only 3% of their time participating in sports, exercise, and recreation—less than their younger cohort (Federal Interagency Forum on Aging Related Statistics, 2010). Without physical activity, the risk of disability associated with chronic conditions increases during the middle-old years.

Adapted Physical Activity (APA) programs are group exercise programs designed for persons with chronic conditions, to correct sedentary lifestyle and prevent disability secondary to the disease. The focus of APA programs is on functional ability rather than disability, and they are beneficial throughout the older adult years. Even after critical incidents such as a stroke, APA can prevent further disability, maximize function, increase quality of life, and curtail the side effects of social isolation and depression (Macko, Benvenuti, Stanhope, et al., 2008).

Senior centers are beginning to offer APA programs as they update their programming for the active baby-boomer generation. Some health and fitness facilities may also offer senior health programs that include adapted strategies for lifelong walkers and marathon runners. Although physical activity declines in the middle-old group overall, there is some evidence that older adults represent the fastest-growing segment of participants in competitive sports, with a rise in the 80-plus-year-old finishers at road races such as the New York City Marathon (Futterman, 2008).

Oldest-Old: Age 85 and Older

The developmental challenges of the oldest-old are sensory impairments, oral health, inadequate nutritional intake, and functional limitations. The following incidence figures are from 2010 (Federal Interagency Forum on Aging Related Statistics, 2010):

- *Hearing.* Nearly half of older men and more than one-third of older women reported difficulty hearing. This was higher for the 85+ age group than it was for the young-old and the middle-old.
- *Vision.* 27% of the 85+ age group reported trouble seeing.
- *Edentulism.* 34% of those over 85 years old reported **edentulism** (having no natural teeth). This tends to be income related: 42% of older adults below the poverty line reported edentulism, whereas for those above the poverty line, incidence was only 23%.
- *Nutrition.* Edentulism compromises an already inadequate nutritional intake of older adults and fosters a diet of "soft" foods that may be higher in fats, carbohydrates, and calories. For the oldest-old, this occurs at a time when they need to decrease intake of these foods to combat obesity and counter decreased activity levels.
- *Functional limitations.* Ability to stoop/kneel, reach overhead, walk two or three blocks, and lift 10 pounds

are common parameters for determining functional abilities of older adults. Forty percent of men and more than half of women in the oldest-old group reported they were unable to perform at least one of these activities. There were minimal to no differences across ethnic and racial groups.

Centenarians People aged 100 years and older (**centenarians**) are a subgroup of the oldest-old. It appears that surviving to an extreme old age is the result of favorable interactions between genetic composition, environment, and lifestyle (behaviors). The most significant factor may be the presence of a loved one in the life of the older adult. One genetic variation of centenarians has been linked with longevity, but mapping the centenarian genome is essential to determine whether they do, in fact, carry a so-called longevity gene (Perls, 2006; Perls, Silver, & Lauerman, 1999). Among the characteristics of centenarians are that 12% live independently, 90% are cognitively intact into their 90s, and their commitment to community is linked to their longevity.

Example Problem: Frail Elderly

As humans age, they are gradually less able to adapt to challenges from internal (disease) and external (injury) environments. Frailty was at first used to mean the oldest-old, believing they were the least able to adapt and survive. However, as the oldest-old population increased and more is known about their survival, **frailty** has been distinguished in the following ways:

- A syndrome, or a set of characteristics, that describes a heightened state of vulnerability for developing adverse health outcomes.
- A multisystem reduction in the person's physiological capacity.
- The point at which the human organism is believed to have its least capacity for survival, and will fail in response to a minor internal or external insult. For example, a frail older adult might die merely as a result of falling ill to an upper respiratory infection (such as a cold).

KnowledgeCheck 10-3

- Name and give the age ranges for the four stages of older adulthood.
- Name and briefly describe four theories of aging.

DEVELOPMENTAL CHANGES OF OLDER ADULTS

Although not all people age at the same pace, there are predictable patterns of physical, cognitive, and psychosocial change. Older adults also have several, often chronic, health problems in common.

Physical Development of Older Adults

Although there is variation among individuals, patterns of change can be predicted in each body system. Table 10-1 presents an overview of changes seen with aging as well as corresponding areas for assessment.

Cognitive Development of Older Adults

Reaction time slows in older adults, and short-term memory declines; it takes longer to respond to a stimulus, and it takes more time to process incoming information. Thus, older adults learn new material more slowly. **Key Point:** *However, there is no loss of intelligence as a person ages.* Loss of short-term memory is more common than loss of long-term memory; thus, older adults may remember incidents from many years ago in vivid detail but may have trouble recalling what they did earlier in the day.

Physical health problems or medications may also affect memory. Research indicates that an active social life with complete engagement and participation in the community delays memory loss with aging (Ertel, Glymour, & Berkman, 2008). Regular mental exercises (e.g., crossword puzzles, conversation) appear to stimulate the brain and enhance memory. Other factors that slow memory loss are getting adequate sleep and rest, eating a nourishing diet, and avoiding drugs and alcohol.

Psychosocial Development of Older Adults

Rather than explaining how the body ages, psychosocial theories of aging attempt to explain the psychological and social adjustment associated with aging.

Disengagement Theory (1961) Cumming and Henry hypothesized that the older adult and society gradually and mutually withdraw or disengage from each other. Mandatory retirement, chronic illness, the deaths of relatives and friends, and poverty are among the factors that may contribute to this phenomenon. As the interaction between a person and his world decreases, there is (a) more time for reflection and (b) freedom from societal roles. Power transfers to younger members of society as the older adult withdraws. Disengagement is not the norm for the current generation of older adults in America, nor is it universally true for cultures that value older adults' advice as essential for family decision making.

Activity Theory (1963) Activity theory posits that the individual should stay as active and engaged as possible to enjoy the highest life satisfaction. On retirement, another activity, such as travel, sports, hobbies, or volunteering, replaces time spent at work. The more engaged the older adult is, the greater his life satisfaction will be (Fig. 10-2). Havighurst's theory is the counterpart of disengagement theory. According to Havighurst

Table 10-1 ➤ Age-Related Changes and Areas for Assessment

	NORMAL AGING CHANGE	AREAS FOR ASSESSMENT
Musculoskeletal	Decreased muscle strength, body mass, bone mass, joint mobility Increased fat deposit	■ Activity/exercise tolerance ■ Joint pain, range of motion ■ Gait, balance, posture, change in height ■ Susceptibility to falls ■ Ability to perform ADLs
Cardiovascular	Decreased cardiac output Increased peripheral resistance, systolic blood pressure	■ Activity tolerance ■ Blood pressure ■ Orthostatic hypotension ■ Susceptibility to arrhythmia
Respiratory	Decreased elasticity of chest wall, intercostals muscle strength, cough reflex Increased anteroposterior diameter of chest, rigidity of lung tissue	■ Cough reflex ■ Use of accessory muscles ■ Gas exchange ■ Mouth breathing
Gastrointestinal	Decreased saliva production, GI motility, gastric acid production	■ Ability to chew ■ Dentition ■ Pattern of elimination ■ Frequency/size of meals
Integument	Decreased skin elasticity, nail growth Increased dryness of skin, thinning of skin layers, nail thickening, hair thinning	■ Susceptibility to hypo/hyperthermia ■ Intact skin, bruising ■ Dry skin ■ Bathing pattern
Genitourinary	Decreased glomerular filtration rate, blood flow to kidneys, bladder capacity, vaginal lubrication, hardness of erection	■ Continence ■ Urgency, frequency, nocturia ■ Hydration status ■ Drug levels ■ Sexual pattern
Nervous	Decreased nerve cells, neurotransmitters, REM sleep, blood flow to CNS	■ Diminished reflexes ■ Sleep pattern ■ Depression
Endocrine	Decreased insulin release, thyroid function, estrogen and testosterone	■ Change in weight ■ Libido ■ Energy level
Sensory	Decreased visual acuity (presbyopia, or impaired near vision) and depth perception, tear production, pupil size, accommodation, acuity of smell and taste, hearing of high-frequency sound, sense of balance changes in pain sensation Increased glare sensitivity, thickening of lens of the eye, changes in pain sensation	■ Adequate lighting with a glare-free bulb ■ Cerumen buildup ■ Home safety ■ Pain sensation ■ Driving ability ■ Environmental stimulation

Table 10-1 ➤ Age-Related Changes and Areas for Assessment—cont'd		
	NORMAL AGING CHANGE	**AREAS FOR ASSESSMENT**
Cognition	Decreased short-term memory Increased reaction time, information-processing time	■ Memory changes ■ Learning barriers ■ Adaptive coping
Personality	Increased cautiousness Retirement, widowhood, grandparenthood	■ Sources of social support ■ Social network

CNS = central nervous system; REM = rapid eye movement.

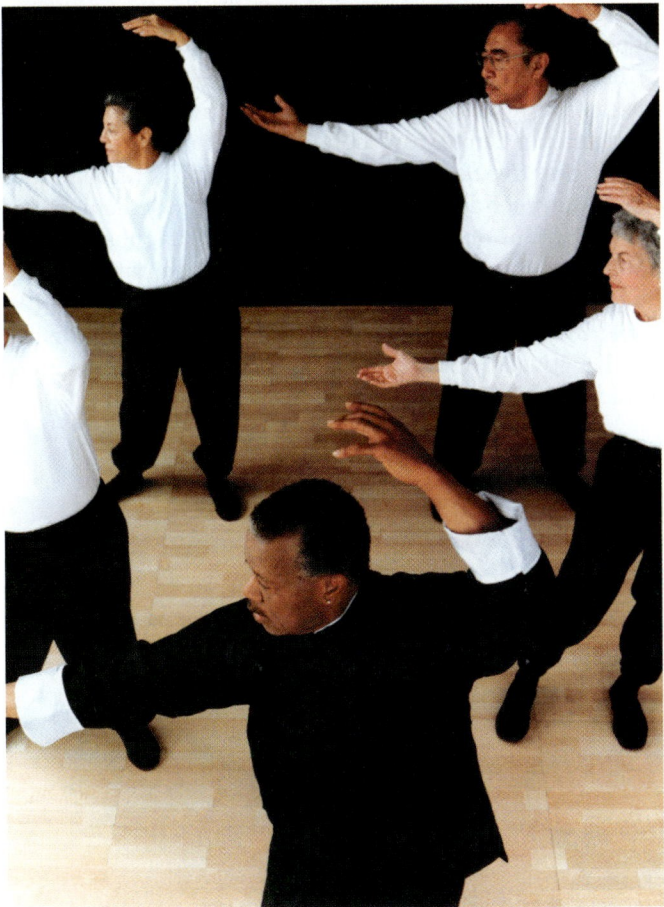

FIGURE 10-2 Many older adults are able to remain active and engaged well into their later years.

(1971), the following are physical, cognitive, and social developmental tasks of older adults:

Adjusting to decreasing physical strength and health
Adjusting to retirement
Adjusting to a lower income
Adjusting to death of a spouse
Establishing an open affiliation with one's age group
Adopting and adapting flexible social roles
Establishing satisfactory physical living arrangements

Psychosocial Development Theory (1963) Erikson's developmental theory identifies *ego integrity versus despair* as the task of the older adult. This stage of development has as its cornerstone the acceptance that one's life has had meaning and that death is a part of the continuum of life. This outlook allows a person to accept the inevitable changes in health and life circumstances. The basic virtue gained at this stage is wisdom. Recall that Erikson's theory is discussed in Chapter 9.

Psychosocial changes in this age group are many and significant. The older adult must face multiple losses, including the death of a spouse or partner, family members, and friends, as well as challenges to health, independence, and youthful vitality. Loss of independence and the ability to live without assistance often have a negative psychological affect on the older adult. Loss is discussed in detail in Chapter 17.

Common Health Problems of Older Adults

The 10 leading causes of death for older Americans are as follows (Murphy, Xu, & Kochanek, 2012):

1. Heart disease
2. Cancer
3. Chronic lower respiratory diseases
4. Stroke
5. Alzheimer's disease
6. Diabetes mellitus
7. Influenza and pneumonia
8. Nephritis, nephritic syndrome, and nephrosis
9. Accidents
10. Septicemia

Six of the seven leading causes of death among older adults are chronic diseases. Heart disease, cancer, stroke, and diabetes not only are among the most common but also are the most costly health conditions. These are long-term illnesses that are rarely cured, but many can be prevented or modified with healthy behavioral interventions. Prevalence of chronic conditions differs by race and ethnicity. For example, consider the different prevalence in diabetes in older adults in 2007–2008 (American Diabetes Association, 2011; Federal Interagency Forum on Aging Related Statistics, 2010):

Non-Hispanic blacks	30%
Hispanics	27%
Non-Hispanic whites	16%
Asian Americans	8.4%

In addition, an estimated 10 million Americans have *osteoporosis*, a loss in bone mineral density that increases the risk of fracture. In advanced cases, bones become so porous that they fracture spontaneously, merely from the stress of bearing the person's weight. The risk increases with age and is much greater for women, in part because of their normal bone density is less than that of men, but also because of hormonal changes at menopause and inadequate calcium intake. Cigarette smoking, moderate to heavy alcohol consumption, and lack of weight-bearing exercise also increase risk.

Example Problem: Dementia

Key Point: *Dementia is not a normal result of aging.* Dementia is an irreversible, progressive decline in mental abilities that affects about 1 in 5 adults older than age 70.

Dementia involves both memory impairments and a disturbance in at least one other area of cognition such as the following:

- Aphasia (loss of ability to communicate)
- Apraxia (loss of ability to carry out purposeful movements)
- Agnosia (impaired ability to recognize or identify objects). Agnosia can lead to the inability to recognize family members or even one's own reflection in the mirror.
- Disturbance in executive functioning (ability to organize, manage, and make decisions)

Dementia makes it more and more difficult for the older adult to remember things, think clearly, communicate with others, or take care of himself. In addition, dementia can cause mood swings and even change a person's personality and behavior.

Risk factors for dementia include old age, family history, cardiovascular disease, and environmental factors such as a head injury or alcohol abuse (Fletcher, 2012). The U.S. Preventive Services Task Force (USPSTF) (2003a) does not recommend for or against routine screening for dementia, but does recognize that early diagnosis allows clinicians to anticipate future problems the patients may have (Registered Nurses' Association of Ontario, 2010). Table 10-2 includes information that may help you distinguish between normal changes in older adults as compared with changes resulting from dementia.

Table 10-2 ▶ Distinguishing the Changes of Typical Aging From Dementia

TYPICAL AGING	DEMENTIA
Independence in daily activities preserved	Dependent on others for key independent-living activities
Complains of memory loss but able to provide considerable detail regarding incidents of forgetfulness	May complain of memory problems only if specifically asked; unable to recall instances in which memory loss was noticed
Patient is more concerned about alleged forgetfulness than are close family members	Close family members much more concerned about incidents of memory loss than patient
Recent memory for important events, affairs, conversations is intact	Notable decline in memory for recent events and ability to converse
Occasional word-finding difficulties	Frequent word-finding pauses and substitutions
Does not get lost in familiar territory; may have to pause momentarily to remember way	Gets lost in familiar territory while walking or driving; may take hours to eventually return home
Able to operate common appliances even if unwilling to learn how to operate new devices	Becomes unable to operate common appliances; unable to learn to operate even simple new appliances
Maintains prior level of interpersonal social skills	Exhibits loss of interest in social activities; exhibits socially inappropriate behaviors
Normal performance on mental status examinations, taking education and culture into account	Abnormal performance on mental status examination not accounted for by education or cultural factors

Source: Adapted from Agency for Healthcare Research and Quality. (1996, November). *Clinical practice guidelines.* No. 19. Publication #97-0702, Washington, DC: U.S. Department of Health and Human Services. Retrieved October 25, 2012, from http://www.dartmouth-hitchcock.org/dhmc-internet-upload/file_collection/111609_aging_vs_dementia_table.pdf

Alzheimer's disease is the primary form of dementia and is considered progressive. Increasing age is the greatest known risk factor for Alzheimer's disease. The odds of developing Alzheimer's disease double about every 5 years after age 65. About half the adults age 85 and older have Alzheimer's disease (Alzheimer's Association, 2008).

Other dementias may be treatable—for example, those resulting from medication toxicity, sensory deficits, and some physiological problems. The diagnosis of dementia is often complicated by the fact that older adults may have comorbidities. It is important to differentiate dementia from acute confusion or delirium that may be precipitated by dehydration, infection, or a medication side effect or overdose. If you need more information about differentiating dementia, delirium, and depression, see Chapter 13.

Polypharmacy

Polypharmacy, the use of multiple medications, is a risk factor for acute confusion, delirium, and depression in older adults (see Chapter 26). The mapping and continued growth in knowledge about the human genome has accelerated the field of **pharmacogenomics** (the discipline that blends pharmacology with genomic capabilities); therefore, the future of drug therapy for older adults will take into consideration DNA variants and individual responses to medical treatments to identify particular subgroups of older adults and develop drugs customized for those subgroups. This technology is expected to increase the efficiency of the drug industry and result in cheaper, more effective drug therapies for older adults.

Depression

Medical problems can cause depression in older adults either directly or as a psychological reaction to the illness. Any chronic medical condition, particularly if it is painful, disabling, or life threatening, can lead to depression or make depression symptoms worse. In 2008, 17% of older women reported depressive symptoms compared with 10% of older men, numbers that have remained fairly stable for nearly a decade and may be related to appropriate antidepressant drug treatment for older adults (Federal Interagency Forum on Aging Related Statistics, 2010).

Depression not only affects mood but also impacts energy, sleep, appetite, and physical health. Many of the symptoms of depression are similar to those of dementia (memory problems, sluggish speech and movements, and low motivation) so it may be difficult to tell the two apart. ✚ Symptoms of depression can also be the side effect of many commonly prescribed drugs, especially if the person is taking multiple medications. Older adults are more sensitive to mood-related side effects of prescription medication because, as they age, their bodies become less efficient at metabolizing and processing drugs.

Example Problem: Elder Abuse

Elder abuse takes many forms, including the following:

- Battering
- Inappropriate use of drugs and physical restraints
- Force-feeding, physical punishment
- Nonconsensual sexual contact
- Treating an older person like an infant, including infantilizing communication (also referred to as *elderspeak*)
- Giving an older person the "silent treatment"
- Enforced social isolation
- Demeaning an older adult
- Neglect
- Abandonment
- Financial or material exploitation, such as illegal or improper use of an older adult's funds, property, assets, or Social Security checks
- Risk of abuse is higher for women and those with physical and cognitive vulnerabilities (Laumann, Leitsch, & Waite, 2008; Williams, Herman, Gajewski, et al., 2008)

Like domestic violence, elder abuse is seen in all cultures and socioeconomic groups. Risk factors for elder abuse include the following: advanced age; physical, functional, or cognitive impairment; mental illness, alcoholism, or drug abuse in elder or caregiver; social isolation or poor social network; dependence on others; past history of abusive relationships; low income status; financial or other family problems (of elder or caregiver); inadequate or unsafe housing; depression; low self-esteem; poor health of patient or caregiver; caregiver stressed or frustrated with difficult caregiving tasks.

Keep in mind that if there an older adult has an injury such as maxillofacial trauma, dental trauma, subdural hematomas, periorbital and laryngeal trauma, rib fractures, or upper extremity injuries, along with a wasted and unkempt appearance, there is the possibility that it was inflicted (Lowry, 2012). **Key Point:** *If you suspect abuse, your care priority is to assure the client is safe and cared for. Next, suspicion of elder abuse must be reported to adult protection services and/or the authority designated by law in each state to investigate and prosecute elder abuse.* For some elder abuse resources,

 Go to the National Center on Elder Abuse (NCEA) **(http://www.ncea.aoa.gov)** and the Clearinghouse on Abuse and Neglect of the Elderly (CANE) **(http://www.cane.udel.edu).**

To assess for elder abuse, see the Assessment section, and

 Go to **Procedure 9–1,** in Volume 2.

Ageism

Ageism is age-based discrimination. Negative expectations for older adults can cloud nursing assessments, planning, and interventions. Box 10-1 presents a quiz to test your knowledge of aging. Take the quiz so that you can be prepared to best assist your older adult clients. For answers,

 Go to Chapter 10, **Supplemental Materials: Answers to "What's Your Aging IQ?"** on Davis*Plus*.

KnowledgeCheck 10-4
- Name two age-related changes seen in older adults.
- According to Erikson, what is the developmental stage of the older adult?
- What are the top two causes of death among older adults?

Practical Knowledge
knowing **how**

You would expect differences in functioning in older adults who are relatively healthy and those who have one or more illnesses. You will, of course, base nursing care on individual needs, not on a person's age category. And yet, in general, you would expect a patient's needs to be different at age 65 than at age 85. **Key Point:** *Remember, though, that an individual's health status and needs are affected by many more variables than just his or her age (e.g., chronic illness, stressors).*

ASSESSMENT

This section presents information to use in caring for all older adults, as well as interventions specific to the young-old, the middle-old, the oldest-old, and the frail elderly.

Assessment for All Older Adults

Recommend to older adults that they have an annual physical and dental examinations. The exam should include the same categories as in middle adulthood (see Chapter 9), as well as screening for mood, cognition, and ability to perform activities of daily living (ADLs) (e.g., bathing and dressing), and instrumental activities of daily living, or IADLs (e.g., shopping, doing laundry). A focused nutritional assessment becomes increasingly important for those in the old-old category. Table 10-1 summarizes the areas for physical assessment related to the aging process. **Key Point:** *Expect frequent changes to recommendations for screening exams (e.g., for breast, cervical, and colon cancer).*

- *Vital signs.* When assessing vital signs, keep in mind that the normal ranges for vital signs are slightly different for older adults (see Chapter 20). The average body temperature, for example, is lower.
- *Height measurement.* Compare with previous height (a screen for osteoporosis). This begins to be especially important past age 65.
- *Weight and body mass index (BMI) calculation.*

BOX 10-1 ■ What's Your Aging IQ?

The following quiz is adapted from one created by the National Institute on Aging to test your knowledge of aging.

1. Which of the following age groups is one of the fastest growing segments of the American population?
   (a) Babies and children under age 5
   (b) Children age 15 to 19
   (c) People over age 85

2. You can be too old to exercise.   True/False

3. Diet and exercise reduce the risk for osteoporosis. True/False

4. Heart disease is a much bigger problem for older men than for older women.   True/False

5. Screening older people for cancer is not beneficial because they can't be treated.   True/False

6. Everybody gets cataracts.   True/False

7. People who are older than 80 years should stop driving a car.   True/False

8. Most older people are depressed.   True/False

9. The older you get, the less you sleep.   True/False

10. Everyone becomes confused or forgetful if they live long enough.   True/False

11. If your parents had Alzheimer's disease, you will inevitably get it.   True/False

12. Older people take more medications than younger people.   True/False

13. People should control their weight as they age. True/False

14. People begin to lose interest in sex around age 55. True/False

15. Older adults are not at risk for HIV/AIDS.   True/False

16. Families do not take responsibility for care of their older relatives.   True/False

17. As your body changes with age, so does your personality. True/False

18. Older people can accept urinary accidents as a fact of life. True/False

19. Falls and injuries "just happen" to older people.   True/False

20. "You can't teach an old dog new tricks."   True/False

21. Extremes in environmental heat and cold can be especially dangerous for older people.   True/False

22. Suicide is most often a risk among teens.   True/False

Source: Adapted from U.S. Department of Health and Human Services, Public Health Service, National Institutes of Health. (2003). *What's your aging IQ* (Reprinted 2006). Retrieved September 18, 2012, from \http://www.nia.nih.gov/sites/default/files/AgingIQ_web.pdf

- *Lipid panel screening*. Total cholesterol, triglycerides, high-density lipoprotein (HDL), low-density lipoprotein (LDL), and ratios.
- *Blood glucose screening*.
- *Annual clinical breast and pelvic examination* for women (American Cancer Society, 2010).
- *Breast self-examination (BSE)*. There is still controversy about whether to encourage BSE. There is insufficient research evidence to support BSE (National Cancer Institute, 2008, last modified January, 2011; *Guide to Clinical Preventive Services, 2010–2011*, 2010), but many clinicians believe it to be useful until at least age 85 (American College of Obstetricians and Gynecologists [ACOG], 2009; Flaherty, Morley, Murphy, et al., 2002; Gemignani, 2011, updated 2009; Meissner, Klabunde, Han, et al., 2011; Smith, Cokkinides, Eyre, et al., 2003).
- *Annual or biannual mammogram or thermography* for women over age 65. A woman should have mammograms as long as she is in good health and would be a candidate for treatment. Age alone is not a reason to stop having mammograms (American Cancer Society, 2010). The USPSTF (2002, updated 2009, 2009b) does not recommend biannual mammograms after age 74. However, other guidelines recommend them even beyond age 80 or 85 if the woman is in good health (ACOG, 2011; Flaherty, Morley, Murphy, et al., 2002; Smith, Cokkinides, Eyre, et al., 2003).
- *Pap test*. Some guidelines do not recommend a routine Pap test for women past age 65 (National Guideline Clearinghouse [NGC], 2012; USPSTF, 2012, but the American Cancer Society recommends that they be continued until age 70. The ACOG (2012) recommends that women stop cervical cancer screening at age 65 if they've had three or more normal Pap results in a row and no abnormal Pap in the previous 10 years.
- *Colon cancer screening*. The USPSTF recommends screening for colorectal cancer (CRC) using fecal occult blood testing, sigmoidoscopy, or colonoscopy in adults, beginning at age 50 years and continuing until age 75 years. Intervals for recommended screening strategies include (USPSTF, 2009a):
  - Annual screening with high-sensitivity fecal occult blood testing
  - Sigmoidoscopy every 5 years, with high-sensitivity fecal occult blood testing every 3 years
  - Screening colonoscopy every 10 years
- *Screening CT colonographies*, or "virtual colonoscopies," are particularly safe for older adults as a noninvasive test that does not require sedation or anesthesia. The American Cancer Society considers CT colonography, as a first-line colon cancer screening test, to be as effective as the traditional colonoscopy.
- *Digital rectal exam* for prostate evaluation in men. An enlarged prostate can indicate either benign prostatic hypertrophy or prostate cancer. The USPSTF (2012b) recommends against routine screening for prostate cancer.
- *Serum prostatic specific antigen (PSA) level* (for men) is a more sensitive indicator of prostate disorders than

is digital rectal exam. Some guidelines encourage yearly screening for men over age 50; some caution against routine screening; others make decisions on an individual basis. The USPSTF recommends that regardless of age, men without symptoms should not routinely have the PSA blood test to screen for (USPSTF, 2012b). However, at this writing, Medicare does provide coverage for an annual PSA test for all men age 50 and older.

- *Eye exam every 2 years* if there are no problems; otherwise annually, particularly if the older adult has chronic conditions such as hypertension, cardiovascular disease, or diabetes. Macular degeneration is a problem that may occur in older adults that an eye exam can pick up.
- *Bone density scan* is recommended for all women age 65 and older as a routine screening for osteoporosis and for women at increased risk for osteoporotic fractures (postmenopausal, tobacco smoking, history of fragility fracture, low body weight) screening should begin at age 60 years (NGC, 2008, April, revised November 2012). The test is also recommended for men older than age 70.

 ThinkLike a Nurse 10-4

To determine whether Mrs. Higginbotham's pneumonia is resolving (Meet Your Patient), you are monitoring her vital signs. Her oral temperature is 98.9°F (37.2°C). What do you need to keep in mind when evaluating the meaning of this reading? Do you think this represents a fever?

Assessing Functional Status

Functional status is the ability to perform self-care and other activities of daily living (ADLs) and instrumental activities of daily living (IADLs).

- **Activities of Daily Living.** You can use the Katz Index of Independence in Activities of Daily Living to assess for ADLs. It allows you to rate a client's independence in bathing, dressing, toileting, transferring, continence, and feeding (Katz, Down, Cash, et al., 1970; "Katz Index," 2007). To use the Katz assessment tool,

 Go to http://consultgerirn.org/uploads/File/trythis/try_this_2.pdf

- **Instrumental Activities of Daily Living. IADLs** are the activities needed to maintain one's immediate environment, for example, shopping, using the telephone, housekeeping, managing money, preparing food, and managing one's medications. Loss of ability to perform IADLs frequently marks a need for assisted living, nursing home placement, or the aid of family or homemaker services to allow an older adult to age in place. For a tool to help you assess IADLs,

 Go to Chapter 3, Assessment Guidelines & Tools, **Lawton Instrumental Activities of Daily Living,** in Volume 2.

Assessing for Depression

For more information about depression in older adults, see Chapter 13, Example Problem: Depression, as well as the entire section entitled Assessment: Depression. To assess for depression, you may wish to use the Geriatric Depression Scale (GDS), a 30-item questionnaire that screens for depression. It is tailored to the concerns that older adults face. To see the Geriatric Depression Scale,

 Go to Chapter 10, **Resources for Caregivers & Health Professionals** on DavisPlus, and click the links under **Web Sites for Mental Status Exams.**

Assessing Cognitive Status (Example Problem: Dementia)

The Mini Mental State Exam (MMSE) (Folstein, Folstein, & McHugh, 1975) and other similar tools are used to obtain a baseline of cognitive function and to evaluate any interventions. The MMSE assesses various aspects of cognition, including short-term memory. A total score of 30 is possible. Typically, a score of 25 or lower indicates some degree of cognitive impairment. Further work-up is required to determine the stability and cause of the impairment.

The "Sweet 16" is a newer cognitive assessment screening tool that is useful for identifying problems in thinking, learning, and memory in older adults who might need further evaluation by a specialist (Fong, Jones, Rudolph, et al., 2010). It consists of 16 items that test orientation, registration, sustained attention, and short-term memory. It is easy to use and correlates highly with the MMSE. For a step-by-step procedure for assessing mental status, see Procedure 22-16, Assessing the Sensory-Neurological System. To see the MMSE and the Mini-Cog (a mental status assessment for older adults),

 Go to Chapter 9, **Resources for Caregivers & Health Professionals** on DavisPlus, and click the links under **Web Sites for Mental Status Exams.**

Assessing for Example Problem: Abuse

It is important to assess older adults for abuse routinely and any time there is a possibility that an injury may have been inflicted rather than accidental (USPSTF, 2012c). For a screening tool and a procedure to aid you in assessing for abuse,

 Go to Chapter 9, **Procedure 9-1,** in Volume 2.

Assessment (Young-Old)

Assessments focused on young-old patients should include the following:

- Assess daily routines, social interactions, and short- and long-term goals. This will help determine the degree to which the person has adapted to retirement.

- Determine the level of fitness and the level of effort for physical activity. This and the following point are essential before beginning a program of routine exercise.
- Gain an understanding about how a chronic condition affects the client's ability to do regular physical activities safely.
- Assess the client's barriers to exercise.
- Assess the client's self-confidence in her ability to maintain an exercise program.

Assessment (Middle-Old)

It is critical for you to assess the function, support system, social network, and mental health of the middle-old client. ✚ Observe for cues to triggers that the client is entering a *spiral of vulnerability*. For example, a decrease in an older adult's mobility and the use of an assistive device such as a cane may indicate prolonged inactivity associated with physiological changes. These may be associated with an unsteady or slow gait and slower response and reaction times—all resulting in deliberate, slow actions. Thus begins a spiral of vulnerability: The older adult may become a victim of abuse, fall, and sustain an injury; the injury may require hospitalization, giving rise to the potential complications of infection and pressure ulcers and the need for rehabilitation. The impact of this spiral of vulnerability is felt in psychological and financial costs to the client and society, as well as loss of client independence. It is easier to intervene and stop the spiral if cues are found early (Fig. 10-3).

Some research indicates that regular mammography or thermography for women over 80 years of age is associated with diagnosing cancer at an earlier disease

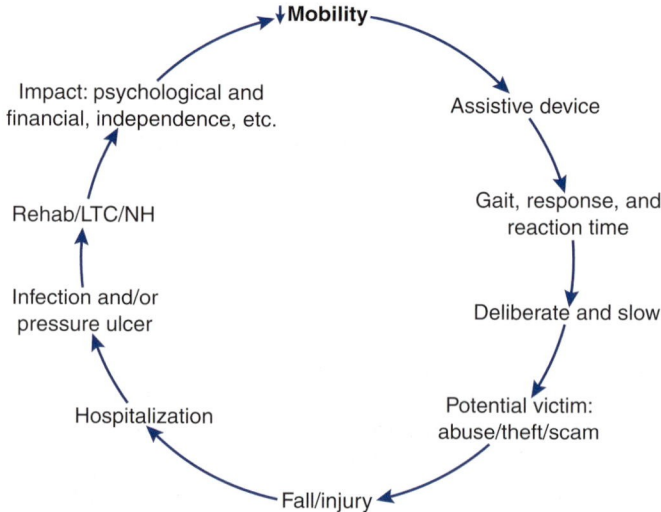

Assessment of the Middle-Old
Spiral of Vulnerability Example

FIGURE 10-3 A seemingly small event for a middle-old adult may trigger a spiral of vulnerability. (Courtesy of V. Rempusheski, PhD.)

stage, and with fewer positive lymph nodes at surgery. However, only about 1 in 5 women of this age actually have regular mammograms (Badgwell, Giordano, Duan, et al., 2008).

Assessment (Oldest-Old)

The oldest-old need similar assessments as the middle-old. Keep in mind that assessment of physical, psychosocial, and cognitive abilities and social engagement and living conditions are crucial for the oldest-old. Psychosocial and environmental factors may be the cues for frailty when subtle physiological changes are not obvious.

Assessing for Example Problem: Frail Elderly

Assess older adults for risk factors and characteristics associated with frailty. Frail older adults are weak, have little ability for independent living, and often need assistance with ADLs. They may have impaired mental abilities. Most are women, are older than 80 years, and receive care from an adult child. To be considered frail, a person must have three or more of the following characteristics:

- Low physical activity
- Muscle weakness
- Slowed performance
- Fatigue or poor endurance

Recall an earlier discussion of genetic–behavior–environment interaction as a survival mechanism of aging. Psychosocial and behavioral factors, including depression, caregiver problems, and housing conditions, are important to a person's interactions with the environment and are believed to predict vulnerability (frailty) and ability to survive (Martin & Brighton, 2008; Rockwood, 2005; Woodhouse & O'Mahony, 1997). Other risk factors include smoking and being underweight.

ANALYSIS/DIAGNOSIS (ALL OLDER ADULTS)

Although most NANDA-I diagnoses can be used for any age group, the following NANDA-I diagnoses focus specifically on growth and development:

Risk for Disproportionate Growth
Adult Failure to Thrive
Delayed Growth and Development
Risk for Delayed Development

An understanding of age-related changes can help older adults identify normal changes, adapt their routine, and report alterations in ADLs and IADLs that are outside the expected changes for their age. Many such changes signal conditions that are treatable. Consider these examples:

- Frequent falls or loss of balance is not the result of normal age-related changes but could signal a neuropathology such as Parkinson's disease or early symptoms of dementia and should be reported to a healthcare provider.
- Urinary incontinence is not the result of usual age-related changes. It may signal a urinary tract infection, a prostate problem, excessive urogenital drying, or the need for in-home assistance.

OUTCOMES/EVALUATION (ALL OLDER ADULTS)

Nursing goals for all older adults should be to maintain the person's ability to function independently for as long as possible, arrange for appropriate care, and teach clients and caregivers how and when to call for professional help.

INTERVENTIONS/IMPLEMENTATION

As you already know, interventions depend on the nursing diagnoses that you identify for each individual. This section presents interventions specific to each of the older-adult age groups, as well as interventions that apply to all older adults.

Interventions (Young-Old)

Young-old adults may need support for positive retirement, identifying and overcoming barriers to health promotion, evaluating methods for introducing health promotion for positive long-term change, and describing short- and long-term benefits of health promotion (Wilson & Palha, 2007). Providing resources for social and civic engagement will help a new retiree reestablish a satisfying and rewarding retirement.

It is also important to teach and help the client plan for physical exercise. Research indicates that a sedentary lifestyle increases the risk of aging-related diseases and premature death. DNA changes occur partly as a result of stress and oxidative damage to cells. By reducing stress, exercise may slow some of these oxidative changes and thereby the aging process (Cherkas, Hunkin, Kato, et al., 2008). More research is needed.

The Centers for Disease Control and Prevention (CDC) (2011) recommends the following activities for older adults:

- *Regular aerobic physical activity.* Encourage clients to engage in 150 minutes a week of moderate-intensity aerobic exercise. Alternatively, they can engage in 75 minutes a week of vigorous-intensity activity. Each episode of activity should last for at least 10 minutes, and the client should spread the exercise throughout the week. Advise clients that additional benefits can be obtained by gradually increasing the amount of exercise (perhaps up to 300 minutes a week).
- *Muscle-strengthening activities.* Clients should perform moderate or high-intensity muscle-strengthening activities on 2 or more days a week. The weight-bearing and toning exercises should involve all major muscle groups.

- *Balance activities.* These are especially important for older adults at risk for falls.
- *Adapted physical activities.* Encourage older adults with chronic conditions to be as physically active as abilities and conditions allow. Help them to make adaptations that allow them to do so, or refer them to an exercise therapist.

Key Point: *Some activity is better than none; and more is better.* Remind clients that doing some activity at least 3 days a week produces health benefits and helps avoid excessive fatigue. Some practical suggestions for exercising include the following:

- A brisk 15-minute walk twice a day, every day of the week would easily meet the minimum guidelines for aerobic activity.
- Muscle-strengthening activities at least 2 days a week can include use of exercise bands, handheld weights, digging, lifting and carrying as part of gardening, carrying groceries, and some yoga and tai chi exercises.
- Inactive older adults or those with a very low level of fitness should begin with 10 minutes of walking and increase minutes and intensity slowly with subsequent walks.

You can provide support for the client's exercise regimen by suggesting a range of choices and a list of community resources (e.g., parks, organizations, recreation centers). Also, teach the client how to walk, as needed, and safety considerations. Help the young-old adult institute self-monitoring methods to help her see her progress (e.g., a graph, a chart, a step counter), and reinforce personal progress, such as decreased fatigue and weight loss.

Interventions (Middle-Old)

Older adults who have maintained healthy behaviors throughout their lifetime are likely to remain vital and actively engaged. However, the occurrence of a health crisis and even a short period of restrictive activity will lead to decreased functional ability and the need for encouragement, support, and a planned program of limited activity progressing to optimal function for clients in this age group.

Interventions (Oldest-Old)

The goal of interventions for the oldest-old is to maximize function and prevent loss of function or disability, thus ensuring independence for as long as possible. Broad interventions important for the oldest-old include the following:

- Supportive environments and conditions that allow a person to function are vital.
- Modified adapted activity may include walking, flexibility exercises, yoga, tai chi, and water aerobics.
- Nutrition should include whole grains, dark green and orange vegetables and legumes, all types of fruits and vegetables, and fat-free and low-fat milk and milk products. These are among the food groups most needed in the diet of the oldest-old to combat obesity and inactivity.

Interventions/Implementation for Example Problem: Frail Elderly

Prevention of frailty and care of the frail elderly are complex and specialized. The following are examples of

---

PICOT

Physical Activity and Well-Being of Older Adults

Situation: While caring for patients in the rehab unit, the nurse notes that there is a wide range of health among the elderly patients, and that not all 75-year-old clients heal at the same rate.

PICOT Components:

P	Population/patient	=	Older adults
I	Intervention/indicator	=	Regular exercise and physical activity
C	Comparator/control	=	No regular exercise, sedentary
O	Outcome	=	Improved well-being into aging
T	Time	=	None

Seachable Question: Do _____ (P) who receive/are exposed to _____ (I) demonstrate _____ (O) as compared with _____ (C) during _____ (T)?

Example of Evidence: Advances in healthcare have increased the life span as well as the quality of life for many people. Physical fitness as a younger adult may improve the physical and emotional well-being later in life. One of the specific goals of *Healthy People 2020* is to increase physical activity, with the expectation that it will slow the decline in physical functioning associated with age. This should help to improve the quality of life in later adulthood, promote faster recovery time, and therefore help decrease the dollars spent each year on medical care.

Practice Change: The nurse emphasizes to all her patients the importance of regular exercise, and helps them think of ways they might incorporate more activity into their present routines. She also discusses with the unit manager the possibility of incorporating this nursing action into unit routines.

Reference: Tahmaseb-McConatha, J., Volkwein-Caplan, K., & DiGregorio, N. (2011). Culture, aging and well-being: The importance of place and space. *International Journal of Sport & Society, 2*(2), 41–48.

research that support some preventive measures that may give you some ideas for positive interventions:

- Frail and non-frail elderly who participated in an exercise-training group demonstrated significant improvement in physical capacity, cognitive performance, and quality of life. Benefits were equivalent between frail and nonfrail participants (Langlois, Vu, Chassé, et al., 2012). One study found that for obese frail older persons, a combination of weight loss and exercise therapy improved their physical status (Villareal, Chode, Parimi, et al., 2011).
- Malnutrition, impaired mobility, and care dependency are potential reversible factors related to falls (Meijers, Halfens, Neyens, et al., 2012). Sixty-seven frail elders who lived alone were provided Internet access. They maintained physical and cognitive status, whereas the control group declined significantly in both (Tomita, Mann, Stanton, et al., 2007).

Advise caregivers and older adults to take the following measures that are thought to prevent or slow the progression of frailty (National Health Information Center, 2012):

- Engage in daily physical activity to the extent possible: walking and weights to build aerobic fitness, build muscle, and improve joint stiffness and pain.
- Eat a balanced diet, including enough protein, fiber, and fluids.
- If you smoke, stop.
- Get regular checkups.
- Keep the mind active by socializing, working puzzles, reading, or playing games.

Interventions for All Older Adults

Some interventions are appropriate for all older adults.

Preserving Functional Abilities Focus on preserving functional abilities, including the ability and motivation to function in the patient's own environment. Look for simple things you can do to promote better functioning. For example, if the patient cannot see to sort his medications, you might try turning on more lights, or having a brighter light installed. For all interventions and interactions, ask yourself, "Does this promote the client's dignity and self-esteem?"

✚ Teaching for Safety Teach older adults about age-related changes and what these changes mean for their daily routine. For example, age-related changes diminish stamina, conditioning, reflexes, and the speed of processing information. Therefore, when multitasking or performing seemingly non-thinking physical activities, older adults need to be very purposeful in their actions and attend to the details of the task or activity. Failing to do so could result in missteps, injury, or exhaustion.

Illness Prevention Although the risks for disease and disability increase with age, poor health need not always occur. Known prevention measures can help older adults avoid many illnesses and disabilities associated with chronic diseases. Stress the importance of a healthy lifestyle (e.g., healthy eating; regular physical activity; avoiding tobacco use; screening for breast, cervical, and colorectal cancers). Older adults who engage in progressive aerobic training can maintain their independence longer and delay the aging process perhaps by as much as 10 years (Shephard, 2008).

Immunizations Health-promotion activities for all older adults include teaching and facilitating immunizations for varicella, influenza, pneumonia, herpes zoster (shingles), and tetanus/diphtheria/pertussis (Fig. 10-4).

Empowerment Many older adults have Internet savvy. You can empower them by suggesting Web sites offering resources to help them understand and cope with the unknowns of their situation. Some good resources include the following:

www.nihseniorhealth.gov—Developed by the National Institute on Aging and the National Library of Medicine, this site provides up-to-date information on a variety of topics, such as arthritis, depression, and exercise. It includes videos and quizzes. New topics are added regularly.

http://www.alz.org/we_can_help_we_can_help.asp—The Alzheimer's Association designed this site to help families find care for family members with Alzheimer's disease. Use of the site is free.

www.lotsahelpinghands.com—This is an online service to help family caregivers to organize and communicate with other family members and significant others to coordinate visits and help with meals, transportation, and so on.

Communicating With Older Adults

Many normal changes of aging affect communication. For example, older adults tend to process information more slowly, so speak slowly and allow time for the patient to form an answer.

Until you know there is no hearing deficit, look at the patient as you speak to allow for lip reading. But do not assume that all older adults are deaf or that they do not understand the meaning of your communication. And remember, you need to speak slowly, not loudly. Of course you should check for sensory deficits at the beginning of your interaction.

You will need to rely on body language more than usual. Notice nonverbal communication, such as fidgeting, hand-wringing, tearfulness, or quivering lips. Memory deficits make it difficult for some older adults to find the words to express what they mean.

Appropriate speech may be accompanied by inappropriate affect. For instance, a client may speak coherently and make sense while telling you that she was able to walk to the bathroom today, and then begin crying for no apparent reason. Nevertheless, the information about her ambulation may be credible.

Recommended Adult Immunization Schedule—United States - 2013
Note: These recommendations must be read with the footnotes that follow containing number of doses, intervals between doses, and other important information.

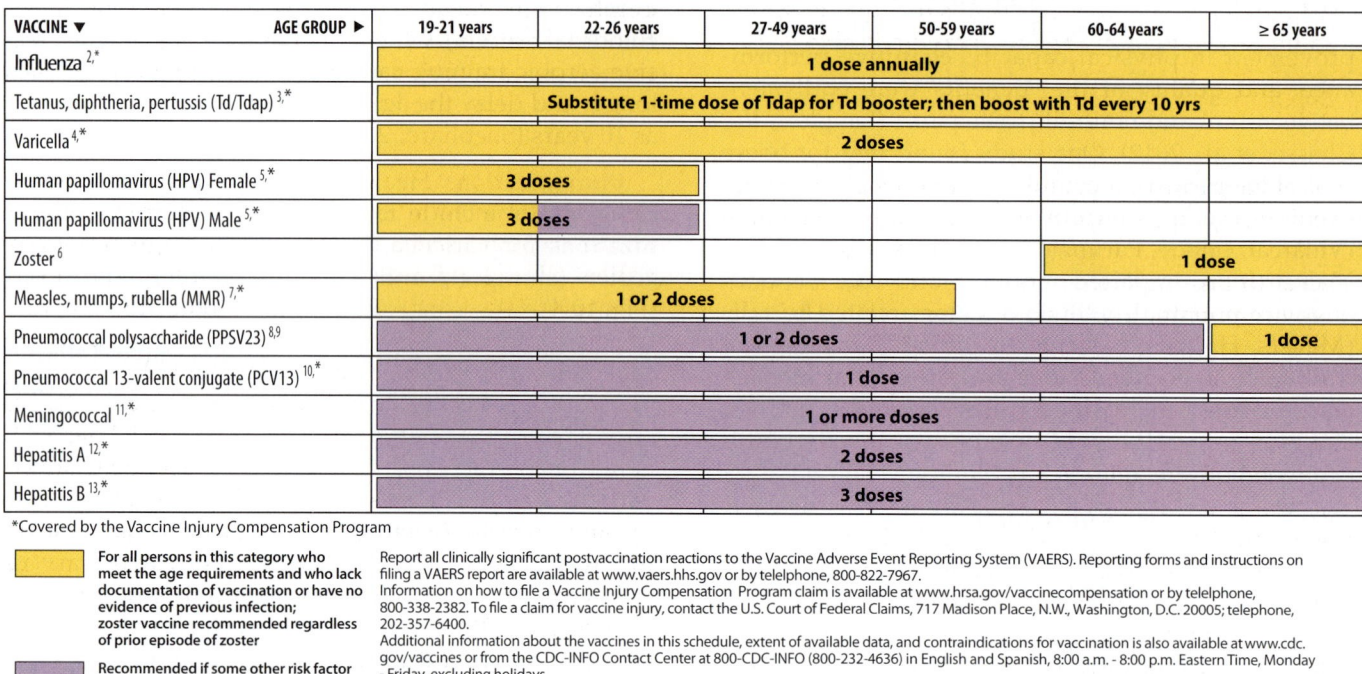

VACCINE ▼ AGE GROUP ▶	19-21 years	22-26 years	27-49 years	50-59 years	60-64 years	≥ 65 years
Influenza [2,*]	1 dose annually					
Tetanus, diphtheria, pertussis (Td/Tdap) [3,*]	Substitute 1-time dose of Tdap for Td booster; then boost with Td every 10 yrs					
Varicella [4,*]	2 doses					
Human papillomavirus (HPV) Female [5,*]	3 doses					
Human papillomavirus (HPV) Male [5,*]	3 doses					
Zoster [6]					1 dose	
Measles, mumps, rubella (MMR) [7,*]	1 or 2 doses					
Pneumococcal polysaccharide (PPSV23) [8,9]	1 or 2 doses					1 dose
Pneumococcal 13-valent conjugate (PCV13) [10,*]	1 dose					
Meningococcal [11,*]	1 or more doses					
Hepatitis A [12,*]	2 doses					
Hepatitis B [13,*]	3 doses					

*Covered by the Vaccine Injury Compensation Program

(yellow box)	For all persons in this category who meet the age requirements and who lack documentation of vaccination or have no evidence of previous infection; zoster vaccine recommended regardless of prior episode of zoster
(purple box)	Recommended if some other risk factor is present (e.g., on the basis of medical, occupational, lifestyle, or other indication)
(white box)	No recommendation

Report all clinically significant postvaccination reactions to the Vaccine Adverse Event Reporting System (VAERS). Reporting forms and instructions on filing a VAERS report are available at www.vaers.hhs.gov or by telephone, 800-822-7967.

Information on how to file a Vaccine Injury Compensation Program claim is available at www.hrsa.gov/vaccinecompensation or by telephone, 800-338-2382. To file a claim for vaccine injury, contact the U.S. Court of Federal Claims, 717 Madison Place, N.W., Washington, D.C. 20005; telephone, 202-357-6400.

Additional information about the vaccines in this schedule, extent of available data, and contraindications for vaccination is also available at www.cdc.gov/vaccines or from the CDC-INFO Contact Center at 800-CDC-INFO (800-232-4636) in English and Spanish, 8:00 a.m. - 8:00 p.m. Eastern Time, Monday - Friday, excluding holidays.

Use of trade names and commercial sources is for identification only and does not imply endorsement by the U.S. Department of Health and Human Services.

The recommendations in this schedule were approved by the Centers for Disease Control and Prevention's (CDC) Advisory Committee on Immunization Practices (ACIP), the American Academy of Family Physicians (AAFP), the American College of Physicians (ACP), American College of Obstetricians and Gynecologists (ACOG) and American College of Nurse-Midwives (ACNM).

FIGURE 10-4 Recommended Adult Immunization Schedule, United States, 2013. (*Source:* Centers for Disease Control and Prevention (CDC), Department of Health and Human Services. Retrieved September 18, 2013, from http://www.cdc.gov/vaccines/schedules/downloads/adult/adult-schedule.pdf.)

Conversely, inappropriate affect and incoherent speech do not always indicate lack of understanding. For example, a client may laugh appropriately at something funny, but not be able to speak clearly or find the words to ask you what time it is.

Be aware that some older adults are confused at one time and not another. A client may begin by giving you credible information, but as the conversation progresses, he may lose track of the topic or talk about something irrelevant. When a client seems confused, use focused assessment to determine his mental status. If you conclude that his communication is unreliable, you can always finish the talk later, when he is less confused.

Key Point: *The ability to speak does not always reflect the person's ability to understand; and what the patient says may or may not match what she is feeling.*

Interventions for Example Problem: Dementia
Dementia is an irreversible, progressive decline in mental abilities. Individuals with moderate to severe dementia or Alzheimer's disease often require special care, including supervision (sometimes 24 hours a day), specialized communication techniques, and management of difficult behavior. They may need help with ADLs such as bathing, eating, getting out of bed to a chair or wheelchair, toileting, and other personal care.

Most often this care falls on a family member or caregiver in the home (see the section Providing Caregiver Support later in the chapter).

Communicating With Persons With Cognitive Deficit.
In addition to the normal changes of aging, many older adults have more severe problems with memory and at least one other cognitive ability (e.g., judgment, thinking, language, or coordination). Because of their decline in mental abilities, people with dementia have difficulty speaking and understanding. In addition to the general approaches for all older adults, the following are some ideas to help you communicate with people with cognitive deficits:

- Use simple, short sentences, with one idea at a time: "Where does it hurt?" rather than "Please describe the quality and location of your pain."
- Avoid vague comments (e.g., "I see," "Um-hmm," "Yes, yes, okay"). The patient will not be able to interpret these responses. Instead, echo the patient's comment and state your response directly and simply: "You are hungry. I will bring your lunch."
- If the patient doesn't understand what you say, repeat your words exactly. Under other circumstances, you

usually rephrase your sentences when someone doesn't understand, but for patients with dementia, giving new information just adds to their confusion.

- Try to understand that the patient's reality is distorted and he is behaving in the only way he is able. When the patient is conversing superficially and seems comfortable, it may seem he is competent.

Promoting Independence and Maintaining Function

Focus your care on maximizing independent activity and enhancing function. Often this will involve helping older adults to adapt and develop new skills so they can continue to take part in activities they enjoy. Consider any environmental modifications that might aid independence, including assistive technology. Facilitate and encourage physical exercise in order to help improve continence and help prevent further loss of mobility. Exercise also improves strength, balance, and endurance, and aids in falls prevention.

Electronic technology is increasingly being used to deliver care "remotely" and support older adults in their own homes. *Telehealth technologies* involve such things as electronic reminder systems, video conference visiting, and remotely controlled security sensors (Gellis, Kenaley, McGinty, et al., 2012; Stall, Nowaczynski, & Sinha, 2013; Young, Foster, Silander, et al., 2011).

Promoting Cognitive Function

The National Institute for Health and Clinical Excellence (NICE) (2006) identified a link between improving cognitive symptoms and ability to maintain day-to-day functioning. You can promote cognitive function by providing older adults with activities and materials that are engaging and involve some degree of cognitive processing (e.g., reading, playing board games, playing a musical instrument, dancing). Activities should be person-centered and appropriate to the age group. An emphasis on social activities will improve participation. In addition, reality orientation, life review, and reminiscence are simple interventions that can be used to promote cognitive functioning.

Providing Caregiver Support

A diagnosis of dementia can be traumatic and devastating. Family members are often the primary caregivers (either through choice or necessity). Caregivers of any patient are more likely than noncaregivers to be at risk for depression, heart disease, high blood pressure, and other chronic illnesses, even death. Caring for a person with dementia puts them at even higher risk.

Most caregivers of those suffering from dementia are also older adults who themselves have special needs. It is not uncommon for the caregiver to feel abandoned and unsupported, not only by services but also by family and friends. Exhaustion and despair can quickly follow. In order to assist and support caregivers the following approaches are suggested (Brodaty, Green, & Koschera, 2003):

- education about dementia
- supportive counseling
- psychotherapy
- rapid support in crisis
- support from other caregivers (respite)
- faith-based spiritual assistance

Interventions such as these can contribute to physical and psychological well-being, help maintain hope, and reduce caregiver burden.

Toward Evidence-Based Practice

Smith, G. E., Lunde, A. M., Hathaway, J. C., et al. (2007). Telehealth home monitoring of solitary persons with mild dementia. *American Journal of Alzheimer's Disease and Other Dementias, 22*(1), 20–26.

Quantitative and qualitative outcome data were collected from eight persons with mild dementia. Two-way interactive video technology was used to monitor medication compliance and findings revealed that medication compliance was 81% in the video-monitored group compared with 66% in the control group. Video-monitored participants' compliance remained stable while unmonitored patients' compliance fell 12 percentage points, consistent with expectations for older adults with dementia. Qualitative interviews with the caregivers found that there was a strong feeling that the intervention prevented relocation of the patient to extended care facilities.

Chumbler, N. R., Mann, W. C., Wu, S., et al. (2004). The association of home-telehealth use and care coordination with improvement of functional and cognitive functioning in frail elderly men. *Telemedicine Journal & E-Health, 10*(2), 129–137.

Investigators evaluated the extent to which home-telehealth technology use was associated with improvement in functional and cognitive status for 176 male elderly veterans as compared with a group of 226 frail elderly men not receiving home-telehealth. Over a 12-month period, the investigators found greater improvements in both IADL and ADL independence in the home-telehealth group than in the control group. Elders in the home-telehealth group also experienced significantly greater improvements in cognitive status. This evidence suggests that the use of home-telehealth has the potential to improve the functional and cognitive status of frail older individuals.

1. What ideas does each study give you for ways in which you might help an older adult with dementia who is living at home?

2. What benefits does the use of home telehealth technology provide for caregivers of patients with dementia?

ThinkLike a Nurse 10-5

What factors contribute to a community of functionally active older adults?

PUTTING IT ALL TOGETHER

Recall Ethel Higginbotham, in the Meet Your Patient scenario. She is very thin and frail and refuses to eat. She says, "I just want to die." Do you feel ready to plan her nursing care now?

You might diagnose Ms. Higginbotham with Adult Failure to Thrive. An appropriate *NOC outcome* would be Will to Live. An *individualized goal* might be "Ms. Higginbotham will gain 1 pound and participate in at least one daily group activity by the first of next month." Interventions depend on the diagnosis and its etiology.

Ms. Higginbotham will need care that helps her adjust to widowhood, provides adequate nutrition, and offers activities that provide interaction with others. *NIC interventions* appropriate for Ms. Higginbotham are as follows: Coping Enhancement, Hope Instillation, Self-Care Assistance, Spiritual Support.

Individualized interventions for Ms. Higginbotham include grief counseling, nutritional support, and working with her and her family to determine whether it is appropriate for her to continue to live independently.

As a full-spectrum nurse, you should assess the developmental stage of each of your clients. In maternity and pediatric care, this is a routine part of nursing care.

However, growth and development continue to be important throughout the life span. To assess growth and development you must gather data such as the client's age, height, and weight; activities the client engages in; and the client's communication skills. You should also perform age-specific assessments, such as those discussed in previous sections.

 To explore learning resources for this chapter,

Go to Davis*Plus* at DavisPl.us/Wilkinson3.

Chapter Resources for Chapter 10:

    Response Sheets for all learning activities

    Resources for Caregivers and Health Professionals

    Reading More About Life Span: Older Adults (suggested readings)

    Concept Map of chapter content

Interactive Case Studies

NCLEX-Style and Chapter Review Questions

Chapter Overview Podcasts

For references cited in this chapter,

 Go to Volume 2, **References Cited.**

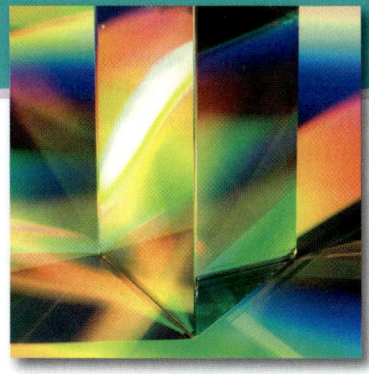

CHAPTER 11

Experiencing Health & Illness

Learning Outcomes

After completing this chapter, you should be able to:

➤ Explore the concepts of health and illness from a holistic perspective.

➤ Compare and contrast three models of health and illness.

➤ Describe the various ways that people experience health and illness.

➤ Identify factors that disrupt health.

➤ Describe the five stages of illness behavior.

➤ Differentiate between acute and chronic illness.

➤ Identify factors that influence individuals' responses to illness.

➤ Apply the concepts presented in this chapter to a variety of patient care situations.

➤ Explain what the concepts in this chapter mean to you as you work toward becoming a full-spectrum nurse.

Key Concepts

Health

Health experience

Illness

Illness experience

Related Concepts

See the Concept Map on DavisPlus.

Meet Your Patient

Evelyn is 87 years old and has lived in a long-term care facility for the last 5 years. She suffers from congestive heart failure, hypertension, diabetes, macular degeneration resulting in near blindness, a severe hearing deficit, urinary incontinence, and immobility resulting from a hip fracture.

Evelyn was married nearly 60 years to Lloyd, who died 6 years ago. They have 5 children, 17 grandchildren, and 14 great-grandchildren. In these last few years, she has experienced the loss of her husband, home, vision, hearing, mobility, and bladder control. Despite these limitations, she keeps current in the lives of all of her extended family and friends.

She is the confidante of the facility staff and knows about their children, their romances, and the gossip around the institution. She is an avid Minnesota Twins fan and also keeps track of the televised high school basketball tournaments. Whenever there is an election, she makes sure that she votes. She "reads" every talking book she can get her hands on. Recently Evelyn was admitted to the hospital in severe congestive heart failure. She told her pastor, "I don't want to die yet. I'm having too much fun!"

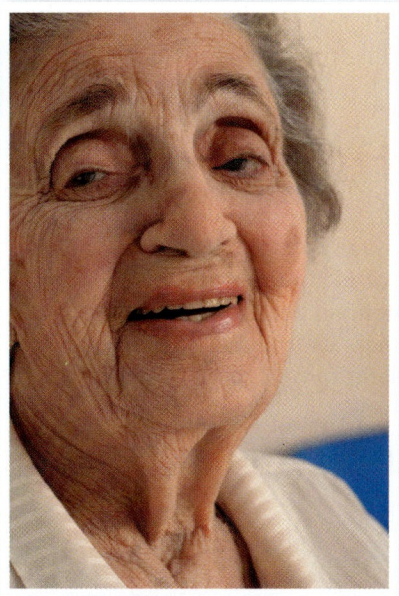

Evelyn's situation is a far cry from what most people would picture as "good health." However, as you consider the ideas of health presented in this chapter, you might conclude that she is a reasonably healthy person from many standpoints.

Theoretical Knowledge
knowing why

Every day there is something in the news about health or illness. Politicians talk about their desire to improve our health and reorganize healthcare. Schools want students to eat healthy, exercise, and receive regular immunizations. In an attempt to reduce health insurance claims, employers open on-site fitness centers and employ nurses and counselors to work with employees to improve employee health. Everyone says they want to be healthy.

As a nursing student, you have probably already cared for clients in various stages of health and illness. But have you ever considered what those terms mean? Our understanding of health and illness is influenced by our family, culture, health history, and a host of other factors. As you evolve as a nurse, you'll find that your understanding of these concepts evolves, too. Here we examine some ways that you and your clients might define health and illness and some ways that full-spectrum nurses have come to understand these terms through their thinking, doing, and caring.

You may find this chapter a little different from other chapters in this book and other textbooks. That is because the goal of the chapter is not so much to help you learn facts about health and illness, but to understand how people experience them. Even the language of the chapter is designed for that purpose. Relax and flow with the chapter. Instead of agonizing over each detail, read it in a way that will help you see the "big picture."

ABOUT THE KEY CONCEPTS

You will need to understand the abstract concepts of **health** and **illness** to help you appreciate the **experience of health and illness**, as lived by real, not abstract, people. Strive for an overview of factors that are disruptive to health and factors that nourish health. Try to understand the subconcept of hardiness as it relates to patients, and healing presence as it relates to your work as a nurse.

HOW DO WE UNDERSTAND HEALTH AND ILLNESS?

First let's examine the key concept, **health**. What is your image of health? Here are some ideas.

The "Body Beautiful" Being a "picture of health" can depend on whether you were born in the right era—or in the right country. Styles of beautiful bodies come and go. For instance, much Indian, African, Greek, and European art portrays ideal women as well-rounded creatures. The perfect body view of health also denies the possibility of health to people who use wheelchairs, prosthetics, or even eyeglasses and hearing aids. Yet many full-spectrum nurses working with disabled clients would indeed describe their clients as healthy.

Not Having an Illness In describing healthy people, would you disqualify someone with a cold, dandruff, or athlete's foot? What about diabetes, heart disease, or cancer? Doing so would reflect another view of health: that is, not having an illness. This view unfairly and unrealistically restricts health to those who do not have some kind of physical impairment.

Something You Can Buy Another popular view is that health is something you can buy: an exercise bicycle, membership in a health club, medicine, liposuction, coronary bypasses, and so on. In this view, health does not come from within. It's something "out there" that is available if you have enough money or insurance.

Ideal Physical and Mental Well-Being Health can also be described as an ideal state of physical and mental well-being: something to strive for, but never to attain. In this view, good health is never actually reached, because there is always something more to be achieved. Health is the goal itself, the end instead of one of the means to fulfilling life's purposes.

The Ability of the Soul to Cope Theologian Jürgen Moltmann (1983) described health in a different way: "True health is the strength to live, the strength to suffer, and the strength to die. Health is not a condition of my body; it is the power of my soul to cope with the varying condition of that body" (p. 142). Similarly, novelist and poet Robert Louis Stevenson wrote of health, "It is not a matter of holding good cards, it's playing a poor hand well." For more traditional definitions of health, refer to Box 11-1.

Nurses Understand Health and Illness as Individual Experiences

If you were the nurse caring for Evelyn in the Meet Your Patient scenario, would you understand health as a perfect body or the absence of disease? Probably not. **Key Point:** *Nurses understand health and illness as individual experiences, emerging from each patient's unique responses. The person with an illness rarely perceives the experience as a medical diagnosis. Instead, people describe their illness in terms of how it makes them feel.*

Think back to the last time you were ill. How did you feel? Did you feel pain, sadness, fatigue, loss? Did you feel overwhelmed? These responses are disruptions to health and, as such, constitute the lived experience of illness. **Lived experience** is unique to each patient: Just as Evelyn might describe herself as "raring to go," another patient who is 10 years younger and on half as many medications may describe herself as "exhausted all the time" and "just waiting to die." In short, nurses honor the client's understanding of his or her state of being. For many years, nurses have recognized that, like Evelyn, some clients strive to maintain a state of optimal health even when coping with chronic and even terminal disease. Many experience this state as wellness: "a way of life oriented toward optimal health and well-being in which

BOX 11-1 ■ What Do the Experts Say About Health?

- *The World Health Organization (WHO)* initially defined health as "a state of complete physical, mental and social well-being and not merely the absence of disease or infirmity" (WHO, 1948).

- *In 1986 WHO* redefined health as "a resource for everyday life, not the objective of living. Health is a positive concept emphasizing social and personal resources, as well as physical capacities" (The Ottawa Charter for Health Promotion, 1986).

- *Traditional Chinese medicine* considers health to be a balance between the opposite energy forces of *yin* and *yang*.

- *Ayurveda*, an ancient Indian medical system, describes health as the trinity of body, mind, and spiritual awareness (Sheinfeld-Gorin & Arnold, 2006).

- *Florence Nightingale* believed that health was prevention of disease through the use of fresh air, pure water, efficient drainage, cleanliness, and light (1859/1992).

- *Nursing theorist Jean Watson* (1979) believes that health implies at least three elements: (1) a high level of overall physical, mental, and social functioning; (2) a general adaptive–maintenance level of daily functioning; and (3) the absence of illness (or the presence of efforts that lead to its absence). To Watson, health is a matter of perception. Even an individual with a terminal illness may be considered healthy if he has a high level of functioning, is coping with the diagnosis, and is actively making efforts to improve his status.

body, mind, and spirit are integrated by the individual to live more fully within the human and natural community" (Myers, Sweeney, & Witmer, 2000, p. 252). This perspective acknowledges the influence of attitude and lifestyle choices on the client's state of being. It also implies that nursing interventions in support of wellness are important for clients who are illness free, but also for those who are experiencing disease, or even facing death.

Think**Like a Nurse** 11-1

What qualities are essential to your own personal definition of health? How do you define illness?

KnowledgeCheck 11-1

- Provide at least two common definitions of health.
- Explain how full-spectrum nurses define health and illness.
- Define *wellness* in your own words.

Nurses Use Conceptual Models to Understand Health and Illness

You can use a variety of models to understand health and illness. Each emphasizes somewhat different aspects of these complex experiences. Nurses have found the following models particularly useful.

The Health–Illness Continuum

Most of us recognize that our health status changes frequently. For example, although today I feel pretty good and yesterday I was exhausted, I believe I was healthy on both of those days. I know that my exhaustion was related to staying up late enjoying the company of good friends. My medical record states that I have diabetes and hypertension, but I keep both diseases in control. I take multiple medications, read food labels, exercise aerobically 5 days a week, and lift weights 3 days a week. Am I healthy, ill, or a health nut?

The preceding example illustrates the complex and dynamic nature of human health. In an effort to describe this complex state, many theorists speak of a **health–illness continuum**, that is, they see health and illness as a graduated spectrum that cannot be divided—except arbitrarily—into parts. A person's position moves back and forth on the continuum with physiological changes, lifestyle choices, and the results of various therapies. As shown in Figure 11-1, the number 1 represents a state of being gravely ill, and 10 represents excellent health, a person in peak form. Notice, however, that a client like Evelyn (Meet Your Patient) may view herself at various points on this continuum according to how she feels on any particular day. In other words, the continuum is personal and dynamic: Health changes over the course of time.

Dunn's Health Grid

Dunn (1959) created a health grid that plots a person's status on the health–illness continuum against environmental conditions (Fig. 11-2). Many nurses use this grid to help them predict the likelihood that a client will experience a change in health status. For example, Evelyn (Meet Your Patient) has several health problems. On a scale of 1 to 10, an observer who does not know Evelyn

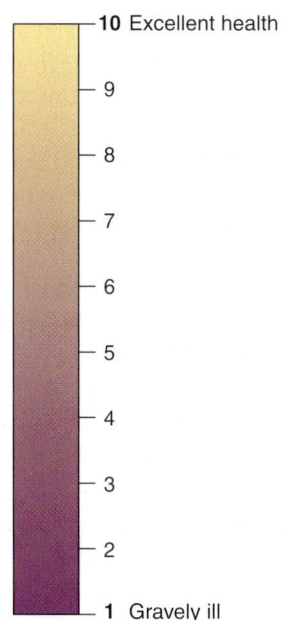

FIGURE 11-1 Over a lifetime, an individual moves up and down on the health–illness continuum.

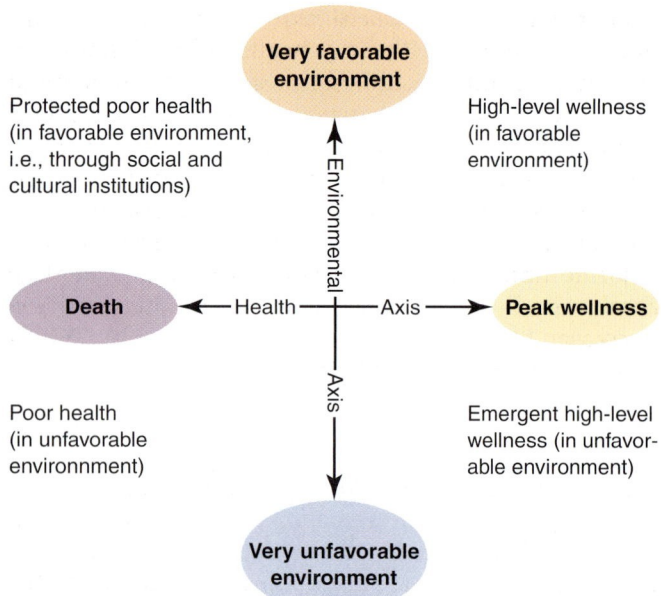

FIGURE 11-2 Dunn's health grid: Health is affected by an individual's status on the health–illness continuum as well as environmental conditions. (*Source:* Adapted from Dunn, H. L. (1959). High level wellness for man and society. *American Journal of Public Health, 49*(6), 786–788.)

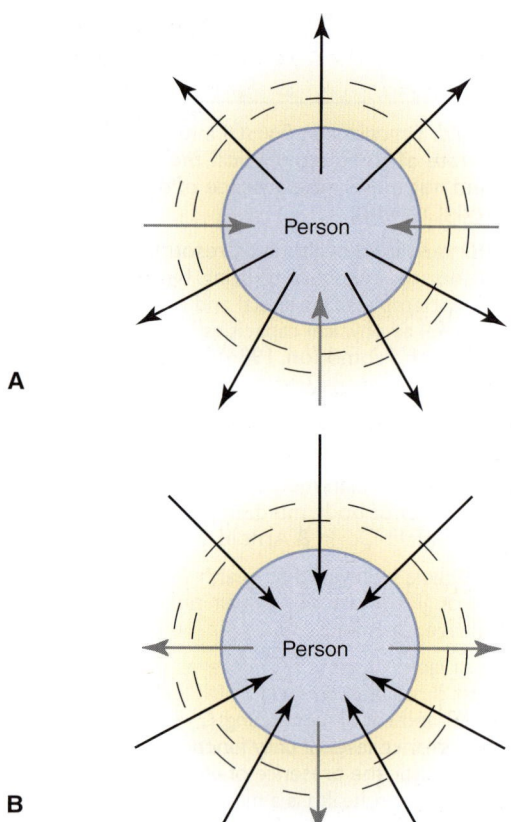

FIGURE 11-3 Neuman's continuum: A balance of input and output. *A,* When energy output exceeds input, illness results. *B,* Wellness occurs when more energy is generated than is expended. (*Source:* Neuman, B. (1995). The Neuman systems model. In B. Neuman, *The Neuman systems model* (3rd ed., pp. 3–61). East Norwalk, CT: Appleton & Lange.)

well might rate her health as a 3. However, Evelyn has a positive outlook and tells her pastor, "I don't want to die yet. I'm having too much fun!" She also has excellent support from her friends, family, and the facility staff. Clearly, Evelyn is in a favorable environment. This positive setting protects her from harm and provides a good quality of life. On Dunn's grid, Evelyn would probably fall in the area of "protected poor health."

Neuman's Continuum
Nursing theorist Betty Neuman (2002) views health as an expression of living energy available to an individual. The energy is displayed as a continuum with high energy (wellness) at one end and low energy (illness) at the opposite end (Fig. 11-3). The person is said to have varying levels of energy at various stages of life. When more energy is generated than is expended, there is wellness. When more energy is expended than is generated, there is illness—possibly death. Although Evelyn (Meet Your Patient) has several clearly identified health problems, she is engaged in life and active with her family, friends, and long-term care facility staff. We might not all agree on where to place her on Neuman's continuum, but certainly her activity and energy counterbalance her physical frailty.

HOW DO PEOPLE EXPERIENCE HEALTH AND ILLNESS?
In envisioning health and illness as a continuum, full-spectrum nurses promote wellness regardless of the circumstances a client faces now or in the future. This

approach requires the holistic understanding that health is multidimensional. The following are some of the many dimensions of health that we experience along the health–illness continuum. An understanding of these dimensions should broaden your concept of health.

Biological Factors
Although biological factors are not entirely within our control, most people consider them when they describe themselves as "well" or "ill." A healthy genetic makeup and freedom from debilitating age-related changes are certainly desired states, and they tip the scale toward the wellness end of the health–illness continuum.

Genetic Makeup For example, the risk of breast cancer increases dramatically in women who have a family history of a mother, sister, or daughter with breast cancer. Recently, a genetic marker for this type of breast cancer has been discovered—that is, some people inherit a tendency to develop breast cancer.

Gender Many diseases occur more commonly in one gender than in another. For example, rheumatoid arthritis, osteoporosis, and breast cancer are more common in women, whereas ulcers, color blindness, and bladder cancer are more common in men.

Age and Developmental Stage Age and developmental stage influence the likelihood of becoming ill. Certain health problems can be correlated to developmental stage. For example, more than 75% of new breast cancer cases are diagnosed in women older than age 50. As another example, adolescent boys have much higher rates of head injury and spinal cord injury than the general public because of their tendency toward risk-taking behaviors. For further discussion of growth and development, see Chapters 9 and 10 in this book. Developmental stage influences coping ability and perceptions, hence their experience of health and illness.

- **Developmental influences on coping ability.** Developmental stage influences a person's ability to cope with stressors that tend to move him toward the illness end of the continuum. Infants or children who are ill, frightened, or hurt have a limited repertoire of experiences, communication ability, and understanding to help them in their responses. As we progress through the stages of development, we develop understanding and skills to help us deal with illness.
- **Developmental influences on perceptions.** When disease, loss, or other disruptions occur at a younger age than expected, they change our perception of the event and may present a greater challenge to our coping skills than disruptions that are expected. For example, a child's death may seem more tragic than that of an older adult. It is important, though, not to discount the impact of disruptions that occur during the period of a person's life when they might be expected.

For example, the death of a spouse is no less traumatic for an older adult than it would be for a young spouse. Losing someone with whom one has spent most of one's life is an incredible loss, whether or not it is "expected" at that stage of life.

Nutrition

Health requires nourishment, and the most obvious form of nourishment is food. The influence of diet on human health is undeniable: Nutrient-deficiency diseases, such as scurvy and night blindness, are unknown in people who consume a nutritious diet. In addition, many chronic diseases, such as type 2 diabetes mellitus and heart disease, are influenced by our diets, and nutrition appears to play at least a moderate role in a variety of other diseases, such as osteoporosis and some forms of cancer (Thompson & Manore, 2012). As more studies look at the protective properties of some foods (e.g., antioxidants) and the hazards of others (e.g., refined carbohydrates, *trans*-fatty acids), the phrase "You are what you eat" seems more accurate each day. Chapter 27 discusses nutrition in greater detail.

Physical Activity

Healthy people are usually active people. When they are unable to maintain previous levels of activity, they may perceive themselves as less healthy. Studies support the benefit of moderate physical activity in reducing the risk of chronic disease and promoting longevity (Thompson & Manore, 2012). As little as 30 minutes of gardening or 15 minutes of jogging on most days of the week can lead to these benefits. In addition, certain types of exercise have been shown to reduce the risk of specific diseases, such as osteoporosis and heart disease. For example, weight training has been shown to increase bone density and reduce the risk of osteoporosis in women older than age 40, and aerobic activity, such as walking, decreases the risk of heart disease. Physical activity is discussed more fully in Chapter 32.

Sleep and Rest

Sleep nourishes health. Most of the body's growth hormone, which assists in tissue regeneration, synthesis of bone, and formation of red blood cells, is released during sleep. Sleep is also important to mental health because it provides time for the mind to slow down and rejuvenate. In controlled studies, people kept awake for 24 hours experienced difficulty concentrating and performing routine tasks. With increasing levels of sleep deprivation, sensory deficits and mood disturbances occurred. Outside the laboratory, mild but chronic sleep deprivation is common, particularly among students, mothers of infants and young children, and people in pain. Sleep and rest are discussed in more detail in Chapter 34.

Meaningful Work

Many people find that work is a healthy way to cope with stressors. Psychologist Victor Frankl, who survived internment in a Nazi concentration camp, observed in *Man's Search for Meaning* (1959, 1962, 1984, 2004) that engaging in meaningful work promotes health and, even in the midst of horrific stressors, can defend against physical and mental breakdown. The definition of meaningful work varies, but many share the view offered by Morrie Schwartz in *Tuesdays With Morrie*: "You know what really gives you satisfaction? Offering others what you have to give. . . . [D]evote yourself to your community around you, and . . . to creating something that gives you purpose and meaning. You notice, there's nothing in there about a salary" (Albom, 1997).

People also experience meaningful work as a dimension of wellness. For many people, volunteering, pursuing hobbies, and engaging in pleasurable activities can be forms of meaningful work. For example, some find that singing, playing a musical instrument, or listening to music is particularly healing. For others, it may be literature, art, playing basketball, knitting, gardening, hiking in the wilderness, or even shopping. Remember that being healthy is not all about denying yourself the pleasure of ice cream and French fries. Healthful activities can be fun, too. By supporting clients' life work, hobbies, and personal interests, you help them nourish their health in their unique way.

Lifestyle Choices

People who consider themselves healthy are usually those who make healthy lifestyle choices. They are aware of the threats to health created by cigarette smoking, alcohol consumption, drug abuse, unprotected sex, and other risky behaviors. Consider the following examples:

Tobacco Tobacco use increases recovery time from other illnesses, injuries, and surgery. Smoking also increases the risk of diabetes, infertility, low birth weight and preterm babies, and perinatal death.

Alcohol Studies have indicated that drinking a glass of red wine each day can reduce the risk of heart disease and slow bone loss. In contrast, excessive alcohol consumption damages the brain, liver, pancreas, intestines, and neurological system and can lead to malnutrition. It has also been implicated in several forms of cancer and in fetal alcohol syndrome in newborns.

✚ Finally, excessive alcohol consumption is implicated in about half of all motor vehicle accidents and other injuries.

Other Substances Abuse of alcohol and illicit drugs leads to deterioration in health, functioning, and relationships. Even prescription drugs can be abused. Substance abuse is a risk factor in many diseases. For example, people who inject illegal drugs are at increased risk of hepatitis and HIV.

You will learn more about effects of lifestyle choices on wellness and safety in Chapters 9, 24, and 42.

Personal Relationships

Living in a healthy family is an important dimension of wellness. Moreover, the family influences a person's view of himself as well or ill. Look at Table 11-1. Of the five pairs of families listed there, which family in each pair would you expect to experience a higher level of wellness?

Especially when clients are coping with life-threatening disease, family relationships can provide critical sustenance

and preserve optimal wellness during the experience. Weeks before his death from amyotrophic lateral sclerosis (ALS), a neurological disease, sociologist Morrie Schwartz stated, "It's become quite clear to me as I've been sick. If you don't have the support and love and caring and concern that you get from a family, you don't have much at all." (Albom, 1997, p. 91). You will learn more about the role of family in human health in Chapter 14.

When illness occurs, some people prefer to be totally independent, priding themselves on never asking for or accepting help. But the reality is that during times of disruption, support from others (e.g., family, friends, coworkers, pastors, counselors) is crucial, even for rugged individualists. Knowing that support is available, and being willing to accept the support, can greatly affect a person's response to disruptions.

Culture

The healthcare culture has traditionally responded to illness with specific therapies aimed at treating a biophysical disorder, whereas nursing, as part of the culture of holism, responds to the physical, emotional, mental, and spiritual dimensions of illness. The culture of a region, a neighborhood, a school or work environment, affluence or poverty, or a religious group, can also influence individual and family health. Culture affects the experience of illness in the following ways:

- **It influences health decisions, behaviors, perceptions, and view of self as well or ill.** For example, the cultural group may share health-promoting values, such as a nutritious diet or regular physical activity. This is not to say that individuals can be "defined" by their culture. Some, either consciously or unconsciously, decide to break away from culturally conditioned responses.
- **It influences responses to illness.** Our response to illness is also partly determined by our culture. For example, people who belong to fundamentalist religions may interpret illness as a punishment from God and may bear their symptoms stoically (i.e., hide their

Table 11-1 ➤ Family Personal Relationships		
Which family would likely experience a higher level of wellness?		
Family A: Places a high priority on health promotion	OR	**Family B:** Responds to health issues only in times of serious illness
Family C: Encourages adventure and risk taking	OR	**Family D:** Emphasizes caution in new situations
Family D: Is very open about expressing feelings and disagreements	OR	**Family E.** Squelches personal feelings to avoid conflict in the family
Family F: Views the family as capable and successful	OR	**Family G:** Views them as powerless victims
Family H: Teaches good negotiation skills, builds a network of family support, while encouraging the development of independence	OR	**Family I:** Parents do not have a large repertoire of coping and communication skills to share with their children

symptoms) to try to pay for their sins (retribution). People who identify themselves with the New Age movement may believe that illness is a lesson we give ourselves to teach us something we need to learn for our spiritual evolution. If you need more information about the influence of culture on health and illness, see Chapter 15.

Religion and Spirituality

Religion and spirituality are closely tied to culture, and clients' religious beliefs and practices can influence their healthcare choices. For example, some people believe that spiritual beliefs influence the mind–body connection to promote wellness and healing. A dramatic example is seemingly spontaneous recovery after a religious rite, as when, for example, a Native American with crippling arthritis is visited by the "false faces" (shamans wearing masks depicting spirits) and then recovers enough to walk across the room. When healing is not possible because of terminal illness or external circumstances beyond our control, spiritual reserves can help maintain our view of ourselves as "well." You will learn more about the influence of spirituality on health in Chapter 16.

Environmental Factors

The environment can also nourish wellness. For institutionalized clients, a little corner of the room that is uniquely "theirs," with photos and other mementos, can be healing. Other clients may be soothed by the quietness of a chapel, a walk in the park, or even a trip to a shopping mall. Spending time in any place where they feel harmony and peace and draw strength can promote clients' health.

On the other hand, environmental pollutants are a common cause of illness. For example, exposure to secondhand smoke causes an estimated 3,000 deaths from lung cancer among American adults each year (Centers for Disease Control and Prevention [CDC], 2010a). Carbon monoxide and lead poisoning, mold, radon, chemicals (e.g., insecticides), and other pollutants also cause serious disease. See Chapter 24 for more information about environmental pollutants.

Finances

It is often said that money doesn't buy happiness. Certainly this is true. However, money does buy access to healthcare and healthcare choices and thus nourishes wellness. In the United States, health insurance is often tied to employment or income level, and health insurance dictates which providers you have access to and what services are available to you. Even in countries with national health programs, such as Canada and some European countries, the standard care available may not include all the services or medications a person desires. The same is true in the United States, for example with Medicare.

Sometimes healthcare providers wonder why people do not take advantage of services that are available to them. Why do they let things go so long before seeking help—or fail to follow up with recommended treatment plans? **Key Point:** *A client's apparent lack of concern or lack of compliance to a treatment regimen may be, in reality, a problem of access to healthcare. Any one or more factors may keep individuals and families from getting the help that they need (e.g., distance from the resources, knowledge of available resources, trust in the available resources, financial status, and lifestyle adjustments such as a change in employment).*

 Think**Like a Nurse** 11-2

- In what ways could you improve your eating, exercise, and sleep habits?
- How might a hospitalized patient get away from the routine and find peace and harmony?

WHAT FACTORS DISRUPT HEALTH?

We spend much of our lives trying to maintain good health—eating, sleeping, keeping our bodies at a comfortable temperature—in general, tending to our high-maintenance bodily needs. It's a continual process because of the many disruptions to health we face. Not all of these disruptions are incapacitating, but all challenge our ability to function and enjoy our everyday lives, and they tend to move us toward the illness end of the health–illness continuum. What are **health disruptions**? Let's explore the concept by learning about some specific examples.

Physical Disease

Disease disrupts our lives in so many ways. It may reduce our ability to perform our life roles effectively or to engage in activities we enjoyed before the illness. The diagnosis of a chronic or life-threatening disease may bring shock, fear, anxiety, anger, or grief: Will I become disabled? How will I support my family? What did I do to deserve this? And finally, it may also cause clients to question the meaning and purpose of their lives, to become more inwardly focused, or to embrace life even more fully. When she first learned of her diagnosis of breast cancer at age 36, Treya Killam Wilber wrote, "Strange things happen to the mind when catastrophe strikes. . . . I was so stunned that it was as if absolutely nothing had happened. A tremendous strength descended on me, the strength of being both totally jolted and totally stupefied. I was clear, present, and very determined" (Wilber, 2000).

Injury

Injury can cause the same symptoms and emotions as disease, but perhaps its most disruptive aspect is its suddenness. In *Still Me*, actor Christopher Reeve (Superman) described his thoughts in the first days after he recovered consciousness following his cervical spinal cord injury: "The thought that kept going

Quality and Safety Education for Nurses

Chronic Illness and Self-Management Through Telehealth

Chapter Key Concepts: *Health, Illness*

Competency: *Informatics (knowledge, skills, attitudes)**

Background: Telehealth encourages patients to be in more control of their health and to take ownership of their condition (Pearce, 2012). Healthcare is transitioning to a focus on patient self-management. Telecommunication provides a strategy for self-management by empowering patients and helping them feel more secure in monitoring and managing their care (Kim, Kim, Kim, et al., 2012). In chronic conditions there is a window of opportunity for remote monitoring to detect health changes sooner and to initiate earlier interventions (Kim, Kim, Kim, et al., 2012).

Scenario: A patient with long-standing chronic obstructive pulmonary disease (COPD) frequently experiences exacerbations requiring hospital admission. Because the patient lives in a remote rural area he often delays seeking healthcare. At the last clinic visit the nurse provided the patient with home monitoring devices that connected him to telehealth services.

Think about it:

➤ What advantages can telehealth provide for a patient with chronic illness?

➤ How might telehealth increase the patient's self-care management of COPD?

➤ Discuss how informatics (specifically telehealth) can impact an individual's position on the health–illness continuum.

 Go to the QSEN Web site at http://qsen.org/ competencies/pre-licensure-ksas/

*As reference for your QSEN log box, the QSEN KSA that is most pertinent is: *Describe examples of how technology and information management are related to the quality and safety of patient management.*

---

through my mind was: I've ruined my life. I've ruined my life, and you only get one. There's no counter you can go up to and say, 'I dropped my ice cream cone; could I please have another one?'. . . . Why isn't there a higher authority you can go to and say, 'Wait a minute, you didn't mean for this to happen to *me*'" (Reeve, 1998).

Mental Illness

Clients with mental illness and their families experience a level of pain, suffering, and chronic sorrow that is difficult for healthy people to fully appreciate (Godress, Ozgul, Owen, et al., 2005; Kokanovic, Petersen, & Klimidis, 2006). In addition, if the illness affects work ability, they experience loss of income and altered role relationships, accompanied by the costs of various therapies.

Mental illness carries with it a stigma that may be diminishing slowly, but is highly visible to those who suffer from its effects (Townsend, 2012). This stigmatization can also disrupt the health of family members. Families must adjust to a major upheaval in their lives, as they experience the pain associated with the loss of a once promising child or relative to the spiral of mental illness (Townsend, 2012). Family members may also live in constant fear that their loved one hurt herself or even commit suicide.

Pain

Whether mild or severe, temporary or long lasting, pain is a disruption. It's not that we can't live with pain—many people do, every day of their lives. However, pain disrupts the smooth operation of our lives; it can change personality, erode coping skills, and interfere with healthy communication. It's hard to concentrate on what we are trying to accomplish when pain is competing for our attention. Pain can interfere in life at all levels, particularly when it is chronic or severe.

Pain that is easily remedied with over-the-counter (OTC) medications or that is short lived serves only as a minor disruption in our lives. However, pain that is all-encompassing permeates a person's entire existence. Sometimes that pain is physical, sometimes psychological. One young mother of a profoundly mentally disabled 14-year-old girl spoke of "hurting so bad that my bones hurt."

As you know, some of our nursing interventions inflict pain. We ask patients to turn, deep-breathe, and cough after surgery, even though it hurts—a *lot*! We put needles in them, catheterize them, and get them out of bed when they would rather sleep. We pull off tape. We invade their physical personal space. We ask them questions about personal things, such as their bowel movements. It is a challenge to be a comforting, healing presence when we have to do things that cause discomfort.

Loss

Loss is a disruption that cuts to the core of who we are—whether the loss of a job; the end of a romantic relationship; the death of a loved one; or the loss of youth, beauty, functioning, or identity. Most of us cling to a unique identity, which usually does *not* include gaining weight or getting wrinkles and gray hair, let alone being a "patient" or losing major bodily functions. When such a loss occurs, the resulting period of significant disintegration may continue until the person either finds a way to cope with the loss or succeeds in reinterpreting the loss in a meaningful way. Toward the end of her battle with cancer, Treya Killam Wilber lost her near vision. One way she coped with this loss was by replacing her passion for reading with sitting at her window contemplating the mountains beyond (Wilber, 2000).

Loss of Sense of Self Many have written about the indignities people suffered in concentration camps, including nakedness, exposure to human excrement, and being treated like children, incapable of thoughtful judgment (Bettelheim, 1979; Frankl, 1959, 1962, 1984,

2004; Valladares, 2001). Those three indignities are crucial threats to a person's sense of self. Sadly, patients in healthcare institutions may also suffer those indignities. Think how patients feel who have to don a hospital gown and allow their body to be exposed for various tests or procedures, or how it feels to lose control of bladder or bowel function. One woman who was paralyzed as the result of a lesion on her spine indicated that one of the toughest things she had to deal with was having her daughter give her enemas and clean her up as if she were a baby. **Key Point: *As healthcare providers, we may easily forget how humiliating such "routine procedures" may be for the patient. You can help relieve the disruption of disease and injury when you respect patients' dignity, provide for privacy, and allow them to make choices regarding their care.***

Permanent Loss If temporary losses are difficult, what about those that are permanent? C. S. Lewis (1961) wrote about his response to the death of his wife: "I know that the thing I want is exactly the thing I can never get. The old life, the jokes, the drinks, the arguments, the lovemaking, the tiny, heartbreaking commonplace" (p. 22). As nurses, we would like to "fix" everything. Though we can't "fix" the holes that are left when a person suffers a loss, we can be open and sensitive to his heart's cry.

Impending Death

It is easy for most of us to ignore that we have a 100% chance of dying and live as though death were only a remote possibility. Lifton and Olson (1974) state that during middle age, even without the presence of life-threatening illness, people tend to become more aware of the compelling reality of death: "One's life is suddenly felt to be limited. . . . It also becomes apparent that . . . there will not be time for all one's projects" (p. 63).

As a nurse, you will care for clients who are living in disruptions of the shadow of death. Some may be aware of their condition; others may choose to deny it, ignore it, or "fight it to the end" by trying a series of conventional and alternative therapies. Caring for dying clients makes us painfully aware of our own frailty and is one of the most difficult experiences you will face as a nurse. Chapter 17 provides further discussion of loss, grieving, and dying.

Competing Demands

Even in the normal flow of life, there are many competing demands. Taken independently, they may be easy to handle. Taken together, the cumulative effect wears us down. In times of illness, the other competing demands continue. Children need to be cared for. Aging parents may need care. Bills still need to be paid. Job responsibilities press in. One man with depression reported, "[T]he whole thing bundled together—one caused the other which caused more and it was just a degenerative loop. . . . [O]ne thing feeds another which

feeds another and so forth until you just constantly go down" (Smith, 1992, p. 104).

Sometimes people ignore health issues because the competing demands are too great. Symptoms may even go unnoticed because attention is scattered in so many directions and there is not enough time and energy to research one's symptoms, schedule a doctor's appointment, or follow through with treatments.

When an illness is acute, such as a broken bone, the stress is usually bearable because it usually lasts for a set amount of time. Bettleheim (1979) states: "The worst calamity becomes bearable if one believes its end is in sight" (pp. 3–4). But when the illness is chronic, the competing demands can take a heavy toll. One woman who took care of her husband who lived at home on a respirator recounted the overwhelming burden she felt when, after 2 years, he was "no better and no worse. This could go on forever!" Although people came in to help, she felt she had to maintain constant alertness in case something went wrong with his ventilator, and she still had to meet many other demands and challenges each day.

As nurses, we sometimes find it easy to criticize how people deal with their situations. But it is so important to realize that the short amount of time that you spend with someone in a hospital or clinic or in a home visit is only one tiny fragment of the cumulative experience that patients and their families experience, sometimes unrelentingly for years on end.

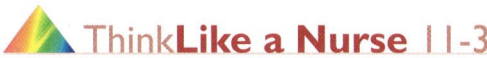

ThinkLike a Nurse 11-3

How might you assist your patient to maintain normalcy in spite of illness?

The Unknown

Even normal life changes present challenges. For example, most parents bringing their first baby home from the hospital are in for plenty of surprises. With some unknowns, there is time to investigate the potential problem and prepare. For example, if an expectant couple learns via amniocentesis (a prenatal test) that their child has a genetic defect, then during the remaining months of pregnancy they can read about the disorder and meet with other parents who have had children similarly affected. But injuries and illnesses can happen abruptly, with no chance to prepare ourselves for new realities. A woman described her experience of finding out she had cancer of the lung with metastasis: "It was on a . . . Friday—I got to feeling kind of bad—kind of like you had the flu or something, you know? . . . so I went to the doctor. . . . And he sent me to the hospital. . . . they started doin' tests on me—all kinds of tests—and found out I had cancer" (Smith, 1992, p. 107).

Imbalance

Our sense of justice tells us that when we are good, good things should happen. When we are bad, bad things should happen. The Buddhist concept of karma suggests that there is a fair balance between what one gives to life and what one receives. Thus, when we perceive that life has violated this rule, we experience that as a disruption, as in these examples:

- **Death of a child.** Our sense of balance is perhaps most dramatically disturbed by the death of children. Such deaths are sometimes referred to as "out of order" because children (of any age) "should" not die before their parents.
- **Treatment failure.** Balance is also disrupted when patients, expecting that their painful and harrowing treatments "should" help them get better, do not get better. One young woman under treatment for advanced cancer described it like this: "It's just—you've been working hard . . . . you're doin' what you're supposed to be doin' and focusing and all this and that—and your body is still not responding" (Smith, 1992, p. 111).

Have you seen the bumper sticker "Life is hard. And then you die"? Cynical perhaps, but we do not have to live long before we realize that as much as we would like for everything to be fair, it is not going to happen. Knowing this intellectually, however, does not necessarily reduce the disruptive effect of the imbalance.

Isolation

How many times have you thought, "No one knows what I'm going through!"? A sense of isolation or aloneness seems to accompany suffering. C. S. Lewis (1961) states, "You can't really share someone else's weakness, or fear or pain" (p. 13). Vanauken (1977), in writing about the death of his young wife, reveals that it was not only suffering his loss, but having to go through the experience *without* her that made it so difficult: "Along with the emptiness . . . I kept wanting to *tell* her about it. We always told each other—that was what sharing was—and now this huge thing was happening to me, and I couldn't tell her" (p. 181).

The sense of aloneness reported by seriously ill clients is related in part to their actual physical separation from loved ones during treatments, hospitalizations, or clinic visits. But it also stems from their feeling that there is no one who is really "in their world." Having someone physically present does not necessarily remove the sense of aloneness:

> When I lay here it's lonely—very, very lonely. Because [my daughter] can't just sit here and talk to me all the time. She's got wash to do, fold and all that stuff. And then the kids to worry about. . . . The worst thing I've found about this whole disease is the loneliness. . . . Because your family can be with you and if they don't come and sit down and talk to you about different things, you're lonely. It's the loneliness that makes you sad inside. . . . It's like everybody's afraid of you or something. They're afraid that maybe they're gonna catch what you got or something. (Smith, 1992)

KnowledgeCheck 11-2

Identify at least four factors that disrupt health.

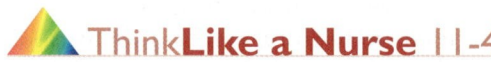 **Think**Like a Nurse 11-4

- What impact do disruptions have on your life?
- How could you apply the information about disruptions to the health of a community? To the health of a nation?

WHY DO PEOPLE EXPERIENCE ILLNESS DIFFERENTLY?

Earlier in this chapter, we mentioned that people vary greatly in terms of their response to life situations. Why is this so? Why do some people react to seemingly insurmountable problems with calmness and grace, while others fall apart over seemingly "small" disruptions? The human experience is so complex and interactive that it is impossible to make neat little categories that we might add up to determine a score predicting how a person will respond to a given situation. There are several factors, however, that may influence an individual's responses to illness. Focus now on the concepts of illness stage; acute and chronic illness; hardiness; and the intensity, duration, and multiplicity of the disruption.

Stages of Illness Behavior

Illness can be viewed as a social role, in which both the patients and caregivers have duties and expectations that are shaped by the society in which they live. Therefore, how people react to an illness depends in part on their illness stage. Suchman (1972) identified five stages of illness behaviors that people move through as they cope with disruptions to health: experiencing symptoms, sick role behavior, seeking professional care, dependence on others, and recovery.

Experiencing Symptoms Symptoms are a signal that illness has begun. If the symptoms are recognizable, such as a runny nose, sneezing, and a cough, you may identify the problem as a common cold and turn to previously used remedies. Common problems rarely progress beyond this stage. However, if the symptoms are unusual, severe, or overwhelming, you may progress to the next stage.

Sick Role Behavior When you have identified yourself as ill, you assume the sick role. The sick role relieves you of normal duties, such as work, school, or tasks at home. In Western biomedical culture, the prevailing view is that sick persons are not responsible for their illnesses and that a curative process outside the person is needed to restore wellness. We believe that the sick person has the duty to try to get well, to seek healthcare, and to cooperate with the care providers (Cockerham, 2011). The severity of the symptoms and anticipated length of illness determine whether you will progress further along the stages of illness.

Seeking Professional Care The next stage is seeking professional care. To reach this stage, you must determine that you are ill and that professional care is required to treat the illness. Persons who seek professional care are asking for validation of their illness, explanations for their symptoms, appropriate treatment, and information about the anticipated length of illness. Healthcare professionals often bypass this stage, relying on themselves to identify and treat the problem. This is not always the best course of action because it is difficult to be objective when examining yourself.

Dependence on Others When you accept the diagnosis and treatment of the healthcare provider you typically also accept the need to depend on others. The severity of the illness and the type of treatment determine the extent of dependence. This may be limited to listening to the provider's instructions, filling the prescription, and following directions given in the office. However, illness that requires hospitalization is often associated with dependence on nursing staff and hospital personnel for activities of daily living (ADLs), medications, and treatments. Some people easily make the transition to dependence; others remain as independent as possible even in the face of severe illness. Personal characteristics and values play a large role in determining how each of us will respond to the challenges of being dependent.

Recovery The final stage of illness is called **recovery**. The person gradually resumes independence and returns to normal roles and functioning. In minor illness, this is usually a return to the status quo. Severe illnesses may require a newly defined level of optimal function. The greater the change, the more difficult this transition will be. Learning to manage a chronic illness is the equivalent of a cure in an acute illness (Parsons, 1975). Both represent the recovery stage.

The Nature of the Illness

The nature of the illness (e.g., whether the illness is chronic or acute) affects the way persons react to disruptions and respond to illness.

Acute Illness An **acute illness** occurs suddenly and lasts for a limited amount of time. Acute illnesses, such as a cold, flu, or viral infection, may be minor and require no formal healthcare. Some acute illnesses, such as strep throat, may require a visit to a healthcare provider for treatment or even hospitalization or surgery, as in cholecystitis (gallbladder inflammation secondary to gallstone formation) or pyelonephritis (infection of the kidney). Although hospitalization and surgery can be quite traumatic, in each case the person is expected to recover. In acute illness, a person may experience the disruptions of pain, competing demands, and the unknown. However, an end is in sight. Relief is expected.

Chronic Illness In contrast, **chronic illness** lasts for a long period of time, usually 6 months or more, often for a lifetime. Chronic illness requires the person to make

life changes. These changes might be regular visits to the clinic or hospital, daily medications, or lifestyle modifications such as a low-fat diet or smoking cessation. Common chronic illnesses include AIDS, diabetes mellitus, rheumatoid arthritis, and hypertension. Because of the lengthy period of illness, people with chronic disease often experience periods of remission or exacerbation. A **remission** occurs when symptoms are minimal to none. An **exacerbation** ("flare-up") occurs when symptoms intensify. Clients with chronic illness often complain about the unrelenting nature of their health problems. A person with chronic illness may experience virtually all of the disruptions identified earlier. Box 11-2 identifies some interesting facts about chronic conditions.

Hardiness

Why does one client who drinks, smokes, overeats, and avoids exercise live into his 90s, yet another client who

---

BOX 11-2 ■ Facts About Chronic Conditions

- More than 90 million Americans live with chronic conditions.
- Chronic conditions account for about 70% of all deaths in the United States.

- About 80% of older adults have at least one chronic condition; 50% have at least two.
- Approximately 6% of adults older than age 65 have a diagnosable depressive illness.

- The top three risks for functional decline are cognitive impairment, depression, and disease burden.
- The largest declines in functional abilities are associated with these physical conditions: arthritis of the hip or knee; sciatica; and chronic pulmonary diseases.
- Arthritis affects 1 in 5 U.S. adults; for more than 40% of those, arthritis limits their activities.
- About 32% of the adult population and 17.1% of children and adolescents were obese in 2003–2004.
- In a large sample of Medicare beneficiaries, the following were the most frequent chronic physical conditions:

Hypertension (56%)	Depression (13%)
Hyperlipidemia (47%)	Osteoporosis (12%)
Ischemic heart disease (32%)	Atrial fibrillation (8%)
	Alzheimer's disease (11%)
Diabetes (27%)	Any cancer (other than skin cancer) (7%)
Arthritis (21%)	
Heart failure (18%)	Emphysema, asthma, or COPD (11%)
Chronic kidney disease (13%)	Stroke (5%)

Sources: Centers for Disease Control and Prevention (CDC) (2002, 2010a, n.d.); Centers for Medicare & Medicaid Services (2011); Peikes, D., Chen, A., Schore, J., et al. (2009); Wiktorsson, S., Runeson, B., Skoog, I., et al. (2010); Stuck, A. E., Walthert, J. M., Nikolaus, T., et al., 1999.

"follows all the rules" dies of a sudden heart attack at age 39? Our bodies do not react to the same stressors in the same way. One factor that may contribute to this difference is the person's hardiness.

Will to Live Hardiness has been described as developing a very strong positive force to live—and enjoying the ride (Fig. 11-4)! A man with heart problems said, "I guess everybody that's in the situation, who has to fight to live, and has learned the mental wizardry of it, you know, to make yourself want to live on. But if you want to, you develop this—this very, very strong positive force to make it go" (Smith, 1992, p. 131). Seigel (1986) reported a study by London researchers that revealed a 10-year survival rate of 75% "among cancer patients who reacted to the diagnosis with a 'fighting spirit,'" compared with a 22% survival rate "among those who responded with 'stoic acceptance' or feelings of helplessness or hopelessness" (p. 25).

Adapting to Change Another aspect of hardiness is the willingness to draw on resources within oneself or from others to break out of old patterns of living when life situations change. When disruption hits, some people don't have the cognitive, communicative, creative, and spiritual resources they need to make life changes, and they just give up. Hardy individuals are willing to seek out information and take initiative in dealing with life situations rather than sitting back and letting someone else control their lives. Ironically, some people survive and thrive during times of adversity. Those who see themselves as hardy tend to approach changes with an "I can deal with this" attitude.

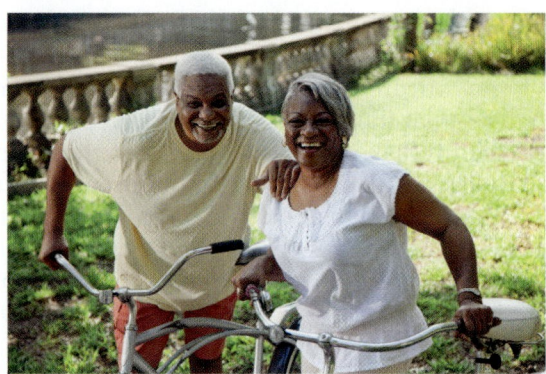

FIGURE 11-4 Hardiness has been described as developing a very strong positive force to live—and enjoying the ride!

The Intensity, Duration, and Multiplicity of the Disruption

Everyone has limits. For healthcare providers, too many demands over too long a period of time can lead to "burnout," a feeling of being overwhelmed and demoralized. For clients and their families, dealing with the cumulative effect of illness and other life disruptions can break down what might otherwise be excellent coping skills. Therefore, their responses may not be typical of what they usually have demonstrated.

KnowledgeCheck 11-3

- Identify the factors that affect how a person responds to the disruptions of illness.
- Define *hardiness*.

Toward Evidence-Based Practice

Rodin, D., & Stewart, D. E. (2012). Resilience in elderly survivors of child maltreatment. *SAGE Open, 2*(2), 1–9.

This study of older adults was conducted to better understand the factors that contribute to resilience (positive adaptation of individuals, despite exposure to adversity) in the elderly population. In this qualitative study of nine survivors of childhood abuse, resilience was found to be high, despite earlier trauma and the subsequent challenges of old age. The authors found that active engagement in relationships and in valued activities were the most often mentioned contributors to resilience.

Jaser, S. S., & White, L. E. (2011). Coping and resilience in adolescents with type 1 diabetes. *Child: Care, Health and Development, 37*(3), 335–342.

Thirty adolescents between the ages of 10 and 16 with type 1 diabetes and their mothers completed questionnaires on adolescents' coping strategy use, competence, and quality of life. Greater use of coping strategies (such as problem-solving and emotional expression) was associated with higher social competence scores, better quality of life, and better metabolic control. Adolescents who reported a lack of coping strategies (instead using withdrawal or denial) reported lower social competence and poorer metabolic control of their diabetes.

1. How do the results of these studies apply to the concept of health as presented in this chapter?

2. Identify ways in which the methods and findings could be applied to other populations.

 Go to Chapter 11, **Toward Evidence-Based Practice Suggested Responses,** on Davis*Plus*.

Practical Knowledge
knowing **how**

In the preceding section, you have learned how people experience health, wellness, and illness. In this section, we look at how this information can be applied to your nursing practice.

USING THE NURSING PROCESS TO PROMOTE HEALTH

Throughout this textbook, you will learn to use the nursing process to help clients deal with a variety of health problems. But how does the nursing process relate to the broader aspects of health and illness described in this chapter? Overall, it involves helping clients—regardless of the type of health problem—to look within themselves to develop creative ways to deal with the realities they are facing.

Patients may fail to comply with a proposed healthcare regimen if healthcare providers develop a plan of care that has no cultural or personal relevance for the patient (or family). Perhaps the plan does not consider the knowledge level of the patient or caregiver; or perhaps it is not feasible in terms of available support, time, energy, finances, or location. Patients may leave a hospital setting *against medical advice* (AMA), thereby endangering their chances of recovery. They may believe that the treatment offered them will not help or that the illness is preferable to the proposed treatment. Noncompliance often occurs because the effort, inconvenience, or pain involved with a therapeutic plan of care is too much for them to handle.

Remember that people probably do not refuse to carry out a plan of care simply out of stubbornness, hostility toward healthcare providers, or wanton disregard for their own welfare. The challenge for nurses is to develop an individualized plan of care in collaboration with patients, based on mutual goals and respect.

ASSESSMENT

In looking at an individual's health status, it is easy to focus on the measurable aspects. Physical needs obviously are crucial, but competing issues may be present and cause the client to view the therapeutic interventions as irrelevant or even disruptive.

What Does It Mean to Communicate Care and Concern?

Key Point: *Obtaining data about the psychosocial, emotional, and spiritual aspects of health requires a level of communication that goes beyond a neat list of skills. Communicating genuine care, concern, and sensitivity comes from who you are as a person, not from assuming a*

professional persona (putting on your "nurse's hat"). The following are aspects of a high level of communicating:

Settling In Your initial approach to a patient creates a climate that determines the level of communication that takes place. The patient is probably in a new environment, and your tone, words, and facial expressions can bring comfort and ease. Nurses can be in new situations too, and taking a few moments to settle in to the situation can be helpful in establishing a therapeutic relationship and facilitating communication.

Attuning Being maximally attentive is another key factor in facilitating communication. Most people are hungry for someone to listen to them. So often, listeners are so busy thinking about what they want to say that they fail to really listen. Try to focus on what the patient or family has to say instead of thinking ahead to what you want to ask next.

Acceptance Another vital aspect of communicating is acceptance—acceptance of appearance, lifestyles, ways of coping, and values. You might ask, "How can I be accepting when there are aspects of this person that go against my entire value system?" Accepting is not the same as "agreeing with." You can accept people as valued, creative, unique individuals, despite their differences from your own ways of being. This view of acceptance does not mean that people will not be held accountable for their actions, for example, in cases of domestic violence and child abuse. It does mean, though, that in your role as a caregiver, you must convey an attitude of accepting the intrinsic value of life—in whatever form that life takes.

Enjoying Perhaps even more difficult than accepting is enjoying. You will come into contact with a wide array of individuals, many of whom are different from people you have grown up around and have come to know and enjoy. A challenge for you is to broaden the repertoire of people you enjoy: to see and enjoy commonalities among individuals seemingly so different and to recognize and appreciate the pathos of suffering in the unique experience of each person.

How Can I Be a Better Communicator?

Settling in, attuning, respecting, and enjoying—certainly this is not a step-by-step process, but each is vital to creating a climate for the openness and communication needed for assessment.

Take Time to Communicate You might argue that the healthcare environment does not allow time for such a high level of attentiveness. Consider, though, how much time is spent in delivering nursing care. As a full-spectrum nurse, you will assess patients continually while thinking, doing, and caring for your patients. In fact, the physical contact involved in carrying out nursing procedures seems to break down barriers of communication. Nurses hold a unique opportunity in "being with" individuals during difficult life situations. Indeed, Benner and Wrubel (1989) state that expert nurses call this the "privileged place of nursing" (p. xi).

Identify the Patient's Main Concern One way to approach assessment, whether in outpatient, acute care, long-term care, or home settings, is to ask the patient, "What is the biggest concern you are dealing with today?" You may have a plan of care that addresses areas that you know to be important, but it may fall far short of meeting your patient's needs if you have not addressed the concern that is fundamental to your patient.

Develop Your Observation Skills In addition to communicating, developing your observation skills will enable you to assess your patients more fully. Watching your patient's responses to you and your care; observing the presence or absence of visitors and the effect on your patients; and observing signs of religious or cultural practices that have significance all provide important information about your patient's strengths and needs.

ANALYSIS/NURSING DIAGNOSIS

Several of the nursing diagnosis labels identified by NANDA International relate to health issues discussed in this chapter. Some examples are Anxiety, Caregiver Role Strain, Deficient Knowledge, and Spiritual Distress. An analysis of the assessment data that you gather should also provide the information needed to describe related causal factors, such as Spiritual Distress related to fear of impending death, or Situational Low Self-esteem related to loss of job secondary to frequent absences for chemotherapy.

KnowledgeCheck 11-4
Compare and contrast attuning, acceptance, and enjoying.

PLANNING OUTCOMES/EVALUATION

Goals and outcomes should be both realistic and valued by the patient and family. When you set goals in the broader dimension of health and illness (as in this chapter), it is much harder to be specific in describing expected outcomes and time frames. As a nurse, your role is to help the patient (or family member) envision acceptable outcomes and to set smaller, realistic goals so that the patient recognizes progress. For example, an older woman caring for a spouse with Alzheimer's disease may have a nursing diagnosis of Caregiver Role Strain related to care of spouse with dementia. Together you would establish acceptable goals and break them down into realistic steps. You also would identify outcomes to indicate that the caregiver actually experiences a reduction in strain, such as being able to sleep or having time to pursue meaningful activities.

PLANNING INTERVENTIONS/IMPLEMENTATION

The ideal approach is to draw on patient and family strengths to help achieve the desired outcomes. In the preceding example of the older adult caregiver, you would discuss with her the options available to provide support, but she would identify which options were acceptable to her and her spouse. In the stress of illness, patients and families may not recognize the strengths and creative abilities that they bring to a situation. **Key Point:** *Part of the art of nursing is to envision strengths and potential in patients and families, just as an artful teacher might recognize a "spark" in a child and encourage that child to learn and grow.*

 ThinkLike a Nurse 11-5

- How can you use the concepts of health when you are admitting a patient to a hospital setting? To a clinic? To an emergency department? To a rehabilitation or long-term care setting? In initiating home care?
- What questions can you ask or what observations can you make to help you gain information about individuals' health strategies, disruptions to health, and factors contributing to their responses to disruptions?
- How would you consider health concepts in planning for patients' discharge from healthcare settings?

How Can I Honor Each Client's Unique Health/Illness Experience?

As a nurse, you can be an instrument of healing in a hurtful world. However, being an instrument of healing does not come automatically with your nursing license. Nor does it allow you the luxury of learning just one approach and applying it to every client. It means cultivating a healing presence by listening, being maximally attentive, being aware of your own gifts and limitations of communication, being willing to learn from those in your care, recognizing and respecting others' ways of coping, and enjoying others for who they are.

Patients may be impressed by your skill and knowledge and amazed by the healthcare technology used to diagnose and treat their illnesses. However, what they most often remember, perhaps through the rest of their lives, is that person who connected with them in a very special way. One man, quadriplegic for 26 years following a car accident in his teens, spoke of a senior nursing student who cared for him during his initial hospitalization. He said that after 26 years, he not only still remembered her, but also still could sense the warmth of her caring presence.

During times of vulnerability, people seem acutely attuned to those who are helpful to them and also to those who slight them in hurtful ways, whether intentionally or not. What a challenge this creates for a nurse! In this section, we discuss steps you can take to prepare yourself for responding to your clients in ways that are meaningful and healing to them.

Examine Life's Uncertainties

Wellness is a balancing act between living in the mostly known present and the mostly unknown future. Encourage your clients to make active decisions that positively affect their future. You do not have control over a drunk driver who sails across the median and hits you head-on, but you do have control over getting the brakes on your car fixed or wearing your seat belt. Likewise, you do not know whether you will develop cancer or heart disease, but you can take responsibility for learning and practicing prevention and detection of problems.

Making health-promoting lifestyle choices is important, but it cannot protect us from risk. Significant life experiences, such as getting married, having children, investing in friendships, venturing into business, and selecting a profession all involve risk. Making a commitment to *anything* is a risk. Each person has a different "risk–comfort range." Some are willing to risk little, have fewer disappointments, and less sparkling achievements. To others, security is not as important, and they are comfortable taking greater risks.

In *A Severe Mercy*, Sheldon Vanauken (1977) writes about finding and losing a great love. He reasons: "The joy would be worth the pain—if, indeed, they went together. If there were a choice . . . between, on the one hand, the heights and the depths and, on the other hand, some sort of safe, cautious middle way, he, for one, here and now chose the heights and the depths" (p. 9). He did, indeed, find a great love, and when he lost his wife at an early age, he was able to accept their time together as one of his life's greatest blessings. As a nurse, you will face many uncertainties and dilemmas. You will certainly face new experiences and challenges, situations you thought *you* never would have to deal with. You will observe pain, suffering, and death. You may never understand the apparent unfairness of it all. But often life brings new meaning when it takes a different direction from the one planned. For example, a couple formerly embittered over their third miscarriage found joy in adopting two children with disabilities.

You will also be privileged to witness many joys. Some might even qualify as minor triumphs: a patient taking his first steps after major surgery, a pathology report that isn't as bad as feared, or even a peaceful death that brings closure to a grieving family. As you move from novice to expert, you may find that such witnessing causes you to stop questioning life's uncertainties and instead to start treasuring them.

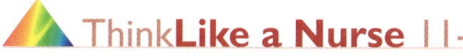

ThinkLike a Nurse 11-6

- What uncertainties have you struggled with?
- What approaches have proved effective for you in dealing with uncertainties?

Envision Wellness for Your Clients and Yourself

Wherever there is a dream, there is someone there to tell you it can't be done, or at least not by you. There is something to be said, however, for "envisioning" wellness for your clients and yourself. Remember Evelyn (Meet Your Patient)? If her nurses had labeled her as debilitated and close to death, how would that have affected her? In contrast, their acceptance of her vision of herself as well and full of life supports her and aids her healing. In the same way, think of how you view your own health. Is the life you envision for yourself characterized by zest and vigor? What are your family relationships like? What are your values? Does your work give meaning and purpose to your life? The wellness that you envision for yourself can be the blueprint for what you want to become. The skeptic in you might say, "What if I do everything that I know to do to maintain a healthy life and still have a heart attack at 45?" As we have seen, life is full of uncertainties. That does not mean that you have to stop envisioning. Instead, use *flexible envisioning*, adjusting your goals and dreams to each new reality. Health does not mean always getting your first choice. Part of health is being able to dream a new dream, starting over if you need to, but always envisioning that there is something worth striving for.

Establish Trust at Your First Patient Contact

When patients are admitted to a hospital or ambulatory care facility, you will need to support them in their transition from wellness to illness, in dealing with the unknown, and in adjusting to a new environment. The relationship and trust you establish in your first contact with patients can go a long way toward relieving their anxiety and preserving the energy needed for healing. Take time to get to know your client. Try to set a tone of caring, respect, and understanding.

You can make the transition smoother for patients if you are prepared. The following activities should be incorporated into your nursing care.

- *Prepare the room.* A room that is prepared for the client conveys a message of acceptance. Room preparation depends on the type of unit or facility, the client's needs, and the anticipated treatment.

 Go to Chapter 11, **Clinical Insight 11-1: Preparing the Room for an Admission,** in Volume 2.

- *Greet the client.* Gather basic information ahead of time, such as name, diagnosis, and anticipated length of stay. Imagine how it might feel if you were a new patient and you heard the staff say, "Who's this? I didn't know we were getting an admission. How am I supposed to take care of this one, too?"
- *Introduce yourself to the client and family.* Explain who you are. Don't be afraid to tell a client that you are a nursing student. Many clients are aware that students have more time to spend with them.
- *Orient the client to the room and the unit.* Make sure the client knows how to use the bed, the call light, and any equipment that you expect him to use. Show the client the location of the restroom. If you will be measuring the client's intake and output, tell him so during your orientation. If the client is alert, he may be able to assist you with these measures. Remember that one of the disruptions associated with illness is anxiety

about the unknown. If you tell your client what to expect, you help to minimize his anxiety.

- *Gather a health history.* In Chapter 3, you learned about assessment. Chapter 22 provides a step-by-step approach to physical assessment. Be sure to include in your health history the client's expectations and concerns.
- *Establish a relationship with the client.* Take time to get to know your client. Try to set a tone of caring, respect, and understanding.

For detailed directions on how to admit a client to a hospital unit,

 Go to Chapter 11, **Procedure 11-1: Admitting a Patient to a Nursing Unit,** in Volume 2.

Provide a Healing Presence

Part of what you do as a healing presence will never show up in a written care plan. However, your healing presence may be the most important aspect of care that you have to offer. A statement by a young woman undergoing chemotherapy illustrates the difference the healing presence of a nurse made:

> *The nursing care I got was in response to the physical symptoms I showed. If I was not feeling good, they were sympathetic with me, you know. . . . But it was nothing further than that. There was no exploration of feelings or anything like that.*
>
> *Some of them were—seemed to be very caring. I remember [one nurse] . . . but she was just a really nice person. And I remember one time that I was throwing up dreadfully. . . . I rang for her and I said, "I'm sorry," and she was almost crying and she said, "No, I'm sorry you have to do this—you must feel awful." And she was just very empathetic with it, and I felt like, you know, I wasn't infringing upon her to make her empty my emesis basin or anything like that. (Smith, 1992, pp. 233–234)*

Maintain Trust During Transitions

Just as you help patients transition into illness, your support is important in helping them transition to other units within the agency, other agencies, or home. As discussed in Chapter 5, planning for discharge begins with the admission assessment and continues until the patient is well enough to go home or is transferred to another unit or facility.

Handoffs and Transfers

Patients may transfer from one unit to another when their health status changes. For example, a patient on a general nursing unit may be transferred to an intensive care unit when he develops sepsis (a generalized, systemic infection that is often fatal). Patients may transfer from hospital to a long-term care facility or rehabilitation center when they no longer require an acute care hospital or when their changed health status means that family members will not be able to care for him at home. A patient residing in a long-term care facility may be transferred to a hospital when he becomes acutely ill. A patient residing in a long-term care facility may be transferred to a hospital when he becomes acutely ill.

When the patient is transferred, he must adjust to a new environment, new routines, and new caregivers. This is yet another disruption for the patient and family. You can help by ensuring the transition is smooth and that there is continuity of care. Ensure the patient's comfort and safety, provide for teaching needs, and communicate with the agency or unit sending or receiving the patient. The process at time of transfer is similar. For detailed information on transfer reports (e.g., "SBAR"), see Chapter 18. Also refer to the accompanying Highlights of Procedures box and,

 Go to **Procedure 11-2, Transferring a Patient to Another Unit in the Agency, and Procedure 11-3, Transferring a Patient to a Long-Term Care Facility,** in Volume 2.

Discharge From the Healthcare Facility

As much as patients usually look forward to being discharged, this, too, is a disruption. Patients are discharged when the outcomes of care are met. However, they are often dependent on family members for care and treatments they cannot manage alone. Inability to assume self-care can be stressful and anxiety producing. Successful discharge planning must begin at first patient assessment, on admission to the facility. The same conditions that require a formal discharge plan frequently also indicate the need for referrals for posthospital care in the community. Review Discharge Planning in Chapter 5, as needed.

Procedures for discharge vary among agencies. There may be a discharge planner or case manager to coordinate the transition to another agency or to home, but often you will need to manage the discharge. You can help by communicating and coordinating care and services, and by teaching the patient and caregivers about the continuing care the patient needs. For more information, see the accompanying Highlights of Procedures box and,

 Go to **Procedure 11-4, Discharging a Patient From the Healthcare Facility; Forms, Discharge Assessment/Instructions; and Patient Education Form,** in Volume 2.

KnowledgeCheck 11-5

Explain how you can promote patient trust during admissions, transfers, and discharges.

Is a Healthy Life Attainable?

The concepts suggested in this chapter as ways to live a healthy life did not come from people who had easy lives. These themes were teased from literature, autobiographies, and interviews with people who were dealing with life situations that would be viewed as difficult from anyone's standpoint. However, in the midst of their circumstances, they were very much involved in

For steps to follow in all procedures, refer to the Universal Steps for All Procedures found on the inside back cover of Volume 2. Go to the full procedures in Volume 2 to practice and learn the skill. Use these Procedure Highlights later to help you review key steps.

Procedure 11-1 Admitting a Patient to a Nursing Unit

➤ Begin the admission: Introduce yourself, assist the patient into a hospital gown, weigh him, assist him into the bed.

➤ Validate patient identity.

➤ Obtain a translator, if needed.

➤ Complete the nursing assessment, including vital signs; validate the admission list of medications.

➤ Provide information: Room, equipment, routines, Health Insurance Portability and Accountability Act (HIPAA), nurse call system, and advance directives.

➤ Answer any questions.

➤ Provide printed information.

➤ Complete nursing admission paperwork according to agency policy.

➤ Complete or ensure that admission orders have been completed.

➤ Inventory the patient's belongings; send home or lock up valuables.

➤ Finish the admission process.

　➤ Ensure patient comfort (water, positioning, pain).

　➤ Make one last safety check: call light, bed position, siderails.

　➤ Ask: "Is there anything else I can do for you?"

Procedure 11-2 Transferring a Patient to Another Unit in the Agency

➤ Make a final, brief, focused assessment.

➤ Plan ahead the amount of help needed.

➤ Schedule time of the transfer.

➤ Make appropriate notifications.

➤ Gather and label patient medications.

➤ Gather the patient's belongings, supplies, and treatment equipment.

➤ Bring the transfer vehicle to the bedside.

➤ Transfer the patient to the new room.

➤ Give oral handoff report and make final nursing notes entry.

Procedure 11-3 Transferring a Patient to a Long-Term Care Facility

➤ Plan in advance: Notify the patient and family of the impending transfer.

➤ Prepare the patient's records; copy for the new facility if needed.

➤ Pack personal items and treatment supplies.

➤ Coordinate the transfer with the receiving facility and other hospital departments.

➤ Make the final assessment; document and sign.

➤ Move the patient to the transportation vehicle.

➤ Give an oral or telephone report to the receiving nurse; use standardized form if available.

➤ Notify the long-term care facility if the patient is colonized or infected with methicillin-resistant *Staphylococcus aureus* (MRSA) or other contagious microorganisms.

Procedure 11-4 Discharging a Patient From the Healthcare Facility

➤ Notify the patient and family well in advance of the discharge.

➤ A day or two before discharge:

Arrange for or confirm: transportation and services and equipment needed at home.

Make referrals.

Provide teaching about the patient's condition and medications.

Provide training in use of equipment.

Ask the caregiver to bring clothing for the patient to wear home.

➤ Day of discharge:

Make and document final assessments.

Confirm that the patient has house keys, heat is turned on, and food is available.

Make final notifications (community agencies, transportation).

Gather and pack the patient's personal items and treatment supplies.

Label and give take-home medications to the patient.

Give the patient prescriptions, instruction sheets, and appointment cards.

Review discharge instructions with the patient.

Answer questions.

Document the final nursing note and complete the discharge summary.

Accompany the patient out of the hospital.

Notify Admissions of the discharge.

Ensure records are sent to the medical records department.

living. Ripples or even waves of disruption or despair came into their lives, but through it all they evolved an overriding sense of life worth pursuing. This can be true for you as a nurse and also for those privileged to be under your care.

As a nurse, you offer your personal health and strength to your patients and their families every day. If you barely have enough physical, emotional, and spiritual strength to manage your own stressors, you will not have much available to offer others who are depleted. This is why it is so important for you to nurture yourself in all aspects of your life, to balance learning how to care for others with caring for yourself, to develop yourself as a healing presence in this world.

To explore learning resources for this chapter,

 Go to Davis*Plus* at DavisPl.us/Wilkinson3.

Chapter Resources for Chapter 11:
   Response sheets for all learning activities
   Resources for Caregivers and Health Professionals
   Reading More About Experiencing Health & Illness (suggested readings)
   Concept Map of chapter content
Interactive Case Studies
NCLEX-Style and Chapter Review Questions
Chapter Overview Podcasts

For references cited in this chapter,

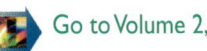 Go to Volume 2, **References Cited.**

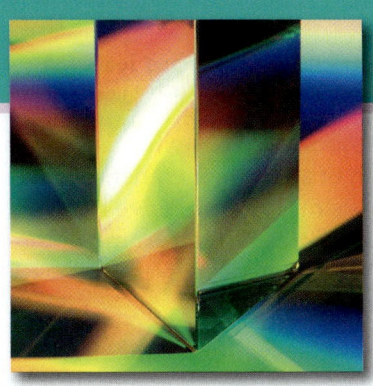

CHAPTER 12

Stress & Adaptation

Learning Outcomes

After completing this chapter, you should be able to:

➤ Define *stress*.
➤ Explain the difference between adaptive and maladaptive coping strategies.
➤ Explain the relationship between stressors, responses, and adaptation.
➤ Describe physical changes occurring during the three stages of Selye's general adaptation syndrome (GAS).
➤ Explain how Selye's local adaptation syndrome (LAS) is different from the GAS.
➤ Discuss the inflammatory response: What triggers it, and what physiological changes occur?
➤ Explain how anxiety, fear, and anger relate to stress.
➤ Provide examples and definitions of specific ego defense mechanisms.

➤ Describe the effects of prolonged stress and unsuccessful adaptation on the various body systems.
➤ Briefly describe: hypochondriasis, somatization, somatoform pain disorder, and malingering.
➤ Compare and contrast crisis and burnout.
➤ State three ways in which you could assess for each of the following: (1) stressors and risk factors, (2) coping methods and adaptation, (3) physiological responses to stress, (4) emotional and behavioral responses to stresses, (5) cognitive responses to stress, and (6) adequacy of support systems.
➤ Describe several interventions or activities for preventing and managing stress.

Key Concepts

Adaptation
Anxiety
Coping
Fear
Stress

Related Concepts

See the Concept Map on DavisPlus.

Meet Your Patients

Gloria and her husband, John, live in a residential community from which John commutes to work in a nearby city. Gloria runs an accounting business from their home. They have two teenage boys who are active in sports, church activities, Boy Scouts, and the school band. The boys need transportation to activities. Gloria and John teach Sunday school and are Boy Scout leaders. Gloria's mother needs knee replacement surgery and so cannot take care of Gloria's father, who has early-stage Alzheimer's disease. In addition to her own home responsibilities, Gloria must go to her parents' home to prepare meals and to provide care for them during the day. Gloria's sister comes at 8:00 p.m. to sleep in the parents' home during the night.

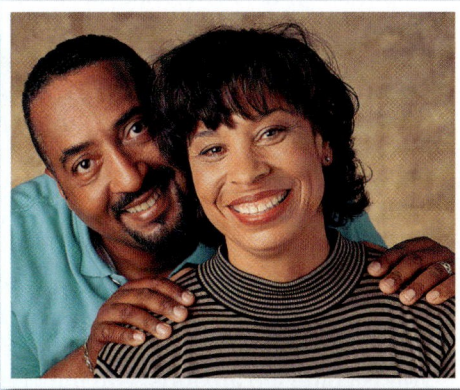

Theoretical Knowledge
knowing why

Everyone experiences stress as a part of daily life, but we each perceive and respond to stress in our own unique way. Our responses are holistic—that is, physical, psychological, spiritual, and social. Stress has been directly linked to heart disease (Richardson, Shaffer, Falzon, et al., 2012), stroke, injury, suicide, and homicide. Indirectly, it is also linked to cancer (Ohio State University, 2013), chronic liver disease, chronic bronchitis, and emphysema (Quick, Saleh, Sime, et al., 2006). As a nurse, you need to understand stress to help your clients cope effectively and adapt to the stressors of illness and caregiving. In addition, you will encounter many stressful situations in your career, so you must develop healthful ways of responding.

ABOUT THE KEY CONCEPTS

The two overarching concepts for this chapter are *stress* and *adaptation*. To help you grasp those concepts, we will present definitions and examples, as well as numerous sub-concepts that relate to health and illness in various ways. Another important concept is *coping*. The stressors of illness and caregiving include *anxiety* and *fear*. As a nurse, you need to understand stress and related concepts in order to help your clients cope effectively with anxiety and fear.

WHAT IS STRESS?

Stress is any disturbance in a person's normal balanced state. A **stressor** is a stimulus that the person perceives as a challenge or threat; it disturbs the person's equilibrium by initiating a physical or emotional response. When stress occurs, it produces voluntary and involuntary **coping responses** aimed at restoring equilibrium (balance, or homeostasis). The changes that take place as a result of stress and coping are called **adaptations**. We can also define adaptation as an ongoing effort to maintain external and internal equilibrium, or **homeostasis**.

Stress is not necessarily bad. It can keep you alert and motivate you to function at a higher performance level. On the one hand, when you are preparing for an examination, your desire to succeed can create just enough anxiety to motivate you to study. On the other hand, if you become too anxious, you may be unable to focus on the task or think clearly.

Types of Stressors

The sources of stress are infinite; however, stressors are commonly categorized in the following ways:

Distress/Eustress Distress threatens health, and **eustress** (literally "good stress") is protective. A passionate kiss can produce as strong a stress response as a slap in the face. On the Holmes–Rahe stress scale, for example,

marriage and divorce receive similarly high scores. To see this scale,

 Go to Chapter 25, **Assessment Guidelines and Tools, The Holmes–Rahe Social Readjustment Scale,** in Volume 2.

External/Internal Stressors may be **external** to the person, for example, death of a family member, a hurricane, or even something as simple as excessive heat in a room. Stressors may also be **internal**, for example, diseases, anxiety, nervous anticipation of an event, or negative self-talk.

Developmental/Situational Developmental stressors are those that can be predicted to occur at various stages of a person's life. For example, most young adults face the stress of leaving home and beginning a career, and many middle-aged adults must adjust to aging parents and accepting their own physical changes. In a sense, developmental stressors may be easier to cope with because they are expected and the person has some time to prepare for them. For theoretical knowledge about developmental stages, refer to the theories of Erikson and Havighurst in Chapter 9 of Volume 1. Also see Box 12-1 for examples of developmental stressors.

Situational stressors are unpredictable. For example, you cannot predict if you will experience an automobile accident, a natural disaster, or an illness. Situational stressors can occur at any life stage and can affect infants, children, and adults equally.

Physiological/Psychosocial Physiological stressors are those that affect body structure or function. You can categorize them as follows; a few examples are given for each category.

- Chemical—poison, medications, tobacco
- Physical or mechanical—trauma, cold, joint overuse
- Nutritional—vitamin deficiency, high-fat diet
- Biological—viruses, bacteria
- Genetic—inborn errors of metabolism
- Lifestyle—obesity, sedentary lifestyle

Psychosocial stressors are external stressors that arise from work, family dynamics, living situation, social relationships, and other aspects of our daily lives. The Holmes–Rahe Scale in Volume 2 contains examples of psychosocial stressors.

KnowledgeCheck 12-1

Refer to the Meet Your Patients scenario.
- What are Gloria's stressors? Classify each of them as follows: (1) Are they physiological or psychosocial? (2) Are they developmental or situational?
- What are John's stressors?

Models of Stress

Some theorists conceptualize stress as a complex, dynamic, and reciprocal transaction between person and environment. Other theorists view stress solely as a

Toward Evidence-Based Practice

Hamer, M., Kivimaki, M., Stamatakis, G., et al. (2012, June 18). **Psychological distress as a risk factor for death from cerebrovascular disease.** *Canadian Medical Association Journal.* doi:10.1503/cmaj.111719. Retrieved September 6, 2012, from http://www.cmaj.ca/content/early/2012/06/18/cmaj.111719.full.pdf+html

Researchers found psychological distress influences not only coronary disease but also other types of cardiovascular (CV) diseases, such as stroke. They obtained data from 68,652 adults with no know CV disease. Data showed the risk of death from ischemic heart disease was 59% greater in patients with psychological distress, including anxiety, depression, and sleep disturbance. The risk for stroke was even higher (69%) as compared with those without psychological distress and after controlling for confounders, such as body mass index (BMI), blood pressure, and diabetes.

Slopen, N., Glynn, R. J., Lewis, T. T., et al. (2012, July 18). **Job strain, job insecurity, and incident cardiovascular disease in the women's health study: Results from a 10-year prospective study of America.** *PLoS One, 7*(7), e40512. Retrieved September 6, 2012, from http://www.ncbi.nlm.nih.gov/pmc/articles/PMC3399852/?tool=pubmed

In a large study of more than 22,000 women healthcare workers over a period of 10 years, researchers looked for associations between job strain and job insecurity and cardiovascular disease (CVD) among women. They found women with high stress in the workplace were 38% more likely to experience a non-fatal CVD event, such as myocardial infarction, as compared with women who reported low levels of job strain. No evidence supported an association between job insecurity and long-term CVD risk.

Fagundes, C. P., Glaser, R., Johnson, S. L., et al. (2012, June). **Basal cell carcinoma: Stressful life events and the tumor environment.** *Archives of General Psychiatry, 69*(6), 618–626. doi:10.1001/archgenpsychiatry.2011.1535

This retrospective study examined the effect of stress on the immune system's response in either progressing or regressing tumors among 91 adults with a history of basal cell carcinoma (BCC). Researchers found that people who were emotionally maltreated by parents (especially mothers) in childhood and who also had a recent, severe life event had a poorer immune response to the BCC tumor as compared with those did not experience these stress triggers.

1. Hans Selye (1974, 1976) found that physical, emotional, psychological, and spiritual stressors, or the anticipation of stressors can initiate a physiological stress response. What might the underlying mechanism be linking psychological stress and researchers' findings of stroke and nonfatal myocardial infarction in people experiencing high levels of stress?

2. What other physiological response to emotional distress was demonstrated in the study conducted by Fagundes and associates?

 Go to Chapter 12, **Toward Evidence-Based Practice Suggested Responses**, on Davis*Plus*.

PICOT

Stress and Multiple Responsibilities

Situation: The nurse is preparing to meet with a mother who has two children: one a 9-year-old with some behavior problems at school, and another a 5-year-old with Down syndrome. The mother reports she and her husband work alternate work shifts, although she also has total responsibility for childcare and household responsibilities.

PICOT Components:

P Population/client	=	Siblings of Down syndrome children
I Intervention/indicator	=	Parents with less satisfactory relationships
C Comparator/control	=	Parents with psychosocial well-being
0 Outcome	=	Behavior problems
T Time	=	During school

SEARCHABLE QUESTION: Do _____ (P) who receive/are exposed to _____ (I) demonstrate _____ (O) as compared with _____ (C) during _____ (T)?

Example of Evidence: Healthcare providers caring for families with a Down syndrome child look to the literature to gain understanding about ways to improve sibling adaptation. While reports show there seems to be greater intimacy among siblings of children with DS, there are other factors that influence sibling adaptation negatively. One study associated the degree of adaptation in two groups of siblings (DS, TD) to the level of parental distress. Parents who were depressed and had less satisfactory marital relationships tended to have less well-adapted children than those with psychosocial well-being. These children were more likely to show deviant behavior problems both at home and in school.

Choi, H., & Riper, M. (2013). Siblings of children with Down syndrome: An integrative review. *MCN, The American Journal of Maternal/Child Nursing, 38*(2), 72–78.

BOX 12-1 ■ Stressors Throughout the Life Span

The following are common developmental stressors. Of course not everyone will experience these stressors.

Childhood

School-age children may also experience stressors at school or among peers; however, children's stressors occur primarily in the home:

- Absence of parental figures
- Failure of parents to meet needs for safety, security, love, and belonging
- Failure of parents to meet basic physiological needs for oxygen, food, elimination, rest, and cleanliness

Adolescence

- Exposure to an expanded environment and a wider circle of friends and acceptance by peers
- Rapid changes in body appearance
- Need for academic achievement, sports performance, or demonstration of other talents
- Peer pressure
- Maintaining self-esteem while searching for identity
- Decisions about the future in the areas of school, work, and relationships
- Conflicts between standards for behavior and the sex drive
- Decisions about and involvement with alcohol and drugs

Young Adult

- Separation from family, starting college or a job
- Making the transition from youth to adult responsibilities
- Preparing for careers: graduation from college, learning a trade
- Establishing career goals and planning how to achieve success and career stability
- Financial stressors around relationships and providing a home for self or family
- Parenting children
- Conflicts between responsibilities for work and family or other relationships

Middle Age

- Concern with career achievement and continuing career challenges
- Continuation of child rearing; marriage of the children; grandparenting
- Changes in appearance and health due to aging
- Dealing with too many responsibilities: e.g., children, work, elderly parents, community activities
- Empty-nest syndrome when the children leave home
- Being "sandwiched" between caring for aging parents as well as children or grandchildren
- "Mid-life crisis" (wanting to escape from one's present life): The person regresses and unrealistically tries to recapture youth, for example, by buying a new sports car that is too small to hold the entire family, making a geographic move, taking an exotic vacation that strains the budget, engaging in an affair, daydreaming excessively about the ideal life in retirement, "partying" and overuse of alcohol and illicit drugs, engaging in "workaholic" behavior, or unhealthy "addiction" to cosmetic surgery. Any one of these behaviors does not necessarily signal mid-life crisis, but they are all examples of behaviors someone might use as an escape.

Older Adults

- Loss of family and friends due to illness or death, resulting in loneliness and isolation
- Changes in physical appearance and functional abilities, including mobility
- Major life changes (e.g., retirement, loss of life partner)
- Health problems (e.g., chronic diseases) with accompanying discomfort or pain
- The cost of healthcare
- Learning to live on a fixed, perhaps inadequate, income
- Adjusting to loss of independence
- Reduction in social status
- Alcohol abuse or dependence symptoms is a problem for about 12% of adults age of 50 to 64, and 7% of those older than 65 years (Wang & Andrade, 2013). These adults are more likely to engage in binge drinking and prescription drug misuse (Blazer & Wu, 2011).

---

stimulus that causes psychological or physiological responses that in turn increase vulnerability to disease. This chapter uses the **response-based model** of Hans Selye (1974, 1976), and our distinction between *stressors* and *stress* stems from this model. Selye found that physical, emotional, psychological, and spiritual stressors, or the anticipation of a stressor (as in anxiety), can initiate nonspecific physiological *responses*. Selye defined these responses as stress.

For more information about the transaction and stimulus models of stress,

 Go to Chapter 12, **Supplemental Materials: Models of Stress**, on *DavisPlus*.

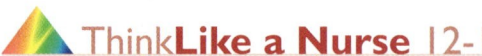

ThinkLike a Nurse 12-1

- Make a list of your own stressors in the following areas: work, school, family, and living situation.
- What physiological stressors do you have?

HOW DO COPING AND ADAPTATION RELATE TO STRESS?

Coping strategies are the thinking processes and behaviors a person uses to manage stressors. Some examples are problem-solving, daydreaming, making changes in lifestyle (e.g., exercising more, eating less), sleeping, and consulting others for support or advice. Coping strategies can be adaptive or maladaptive.

Adaptive (effective) coping consists of making healthy choices that reduce the negative effects of stress (e.g., exercising to relieve tension, engaging in a favorite hobby, consulting others for support or advice). Sometimes the difference between effective and ineffective coping is in the degree to which a technique is used (for examples, see the section Ego Defense Mechanisms later in this chapter).

Maladaptive (ineffective) coping does not promote adaptation. Unhealthful coping choices include overeating, working too much, excessive sleeping, and substance abuse. Although a maladaptive behavior may temporarily relieve anxiety, it may have other harmful effects. For example, a person who smokes to relieve the tensions of a stressful work situation may experience an immediate decrease in anxiety. However, the person is doing nothing to change or adapt to the stressful situation, and, over time, is increasing her risk of cardiorespiratory disease.

Three Approaches to Coping Are Commonly Used

People use three approaches to cope with stress, at different times and in various combinations:

Altering the Stressor In some situations, a person takes actions to remove or change the stressor. For example, Gloria (Meet Your Patients) might remove one of her stressors by resigning her position as a Scout leader.

Adapting to the Stressor It is not always possible to remove or change a stressor. Adapting involves changing one's thoughts or behaviors related to the stressor. Gloria cannot change the fact that her father needs ongoing care and her mother needs surgery, but as she gains experience as a caregiver, she may find easier, more efficient ways to care for her parents. This would give her a little more time to relax or attend to other responsibilities.

Avoiding the Stressor Sometimes it is healthful to avoid a stressor. For example, you may find that being with a certain person is stressful for you, even though you have tried many times to change the dynamics of the relationship. In that case, it may be best to minimize or end your relationship with the person. In other situations, avoidance may be maladaptive. For example, a woman who discovers a lump in her breast becomes anxious that she may have cancer. She copes with her anxiety by putting it out of her mind and avoids seeking medical care. As a result, if the lump is cancerous, it would not be treated at an early stage.

The Outcome of Stress Is Either Adaptation or Disease

Stress results in either adaptation or disease. Successful adaptation allows for normal growth and development and effective responses to changes and challenges in daily life. The outcome depends on the balance between the strength of the stressors and the effectiveness of the person's coping methods (Fig. 12-1). In the following equation, **E** is the event (stressor), **R** is the person's response (which is determined in part by past experiences, perception of the stressor, and coping methods used), and **O** is the outcome.

$$E \quad + \quad R \quad = \quad O$$

| stressful event | response (experience, perception, coping methods) | outcome (adaptation or disease) |

Some events produce more stress than others. However, a person with good coping skills can usually adapt to a single stressful event, even a demanding one. But suppose several stressors occur in a short period of time. Gloria (Meet Your Patients) has many stressors, so her coping abilities may be taxed to the limit. When there are many stressors or when stressors continue for a long period of time, adaptation is more likely to fail.

Personal Factors Influence Adaptation

Why do some people succumb to overwhelming stress while others adapt and thrive? Fortunately, successful adaptation does not depend entirely on being able to alter or avoid stressors. Various personal factors also influence the outcome:

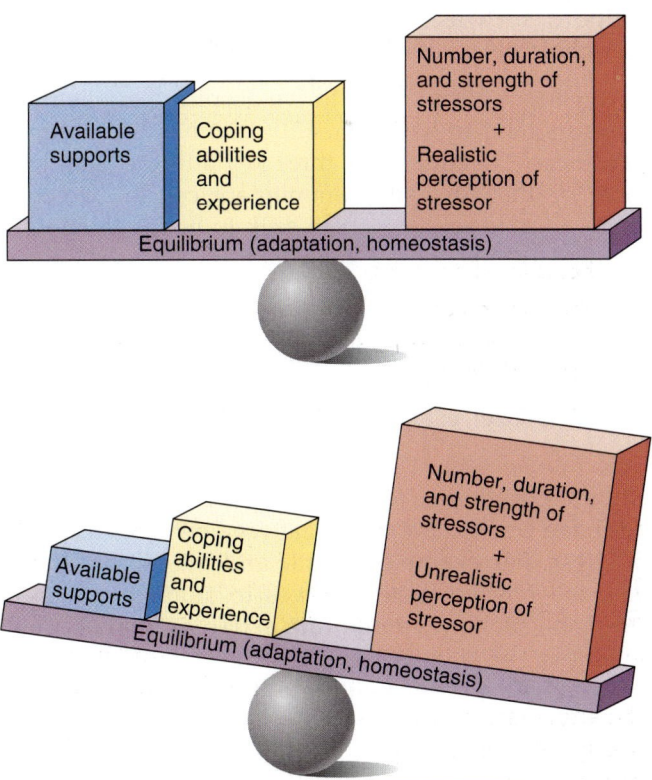

FIGURE 12-1 Adaptation occurs when a person has supports and coping abilities adequate to enable him to deal with the stressors. A realistic perception of the stressful event promotes adaptation, whereas an unrealistic perception makes adaptation more difficult.

Perception of the Stressor A person's perception may be realistic or exaggerated. Suppose two women with similar coping skills and support systems both must have a mastectomy. Mrs. King thinks, "Yes, I am losing a part of my body, but I am more than just a breast. This will be a difficult adjustment, but I am so grateful to be alive." Mrs. Alan thinks, "I will be so ugly. My husband won't want to touch me. I won't be much of a woman now. This is the worst thing that could ever happen." Which woman do you think is more likely to adapt successfully to this change in her body?

Overall Health Status On the one hand, stressors may actually cause a healthy person to engage in constructive adaptive behaviors that improve health. A person who has just discovered that he has hypertension may react by modifying his diet and exercising to lower his blood pressure and prevent complications. On the other hand, if a person with hypertension also has been coping for years with pain and immobility from arthritis, he may be too overwhelmed and exhausted to take any actions to lower his blood pressure.

Support System A **support system** may include friends, family, counseling groups, church groups, or other like-minded people who share common interests. A good support system can help a person adapt to stress, provide emotional support, encourage expression of feelings, and help the person solve problems. It may also provide financial and other concrete types of support, such as a place to live, meal preparation, household help, child care, and transportation.

Hardiness People who thrive despite overwhelming stressors tend to have a quality that has been termed **hardiness**. They maintain three key attitudes that help them weather adversity: commitment, control, and challenge. *Commitment* lets them seek to be involved with ongoing events, rather than feeling isolated. *Control* enables them to struggle and try to influence outcomes instead of becoming passive and feeling powerless. *Challenge* allows them to perceive stressful changes as opportunities for learning (Maddi, 2002; Maddi, Koshaba, Fazel, et al., 2009).

Other Personal Factors Age, developmental level, and life experiences (e.g., learning which coping methods have worked for you) all affect a person's response to stress. For example, infants and the very old may lack the physiological reserves to adapt to physical stressors, such as temperature extremes, dehydration, or illness.

Even with a positive attitude and good coping skills, excessive amounts of stress can lead to maladaptation and disease. Some people succumb to illness after experiencing only a few stressors, whereas others seem to adapt to multiple, intensely difficult stressors. Each person has a different ability to tolerate stress, but everyone has a breaking point at which stress becomes overwhelming.

KnowledgeCheck 12-2

- True or false: The difference between adaptive and maladaptive coping is that maladaptive coping does not relieve stress.
- In addition to avoiding the stressor, what are two other approaches to coping?
- (Complete the sentence.) The outcome of stress (adaptation or disease) depends on the balance among the strength, number, and duration of the stressors and _____.

HOW DO PEOPLE RESPOND TO STRESSORS?

Although Selye's (1974, 1976) response-based model acknowledges physical, emotional, psychological, and spiritual *stressors*, his ideas about responses (*stress*) are primarily physiological. As you know, the body has various homeostatic mechanisms for regulating its internal environment to maintain homeostasis. In Selye's theory, physiological responses to stress are described by the general adaptation syndrome (GAS) and the local adaptation syndrome (LAS).

The General Adaptation Syndrome Includes Nonspecific, Systemic Responses

Would you be surprised to know that a near-miss automobile accident and kicking the winning field goal at a football game would both produce the same general body responses? It is true. Regardless of the specific stressor, the responses involve the whole body, especially the autonomic nervous system and the endocrine system. The **general adaptation syndrome (GAS)** is Selye's name for the group of nonspecific responses that all people share in the face of stressors. The GAS has three stages: (1) the initial alarm stage, (2) resistance (adaptation), and (3) the final stage of either recovery or exhaustion (Fig. 12-2).

Alarm Stage—"Fight or Flight"

Imagine yourself in this situation: It is dark. You are alone, walking to your car, when you hear footsteps behind you. You stop and look around and see no one. As you begin walking again, the footsteps return. You walk faster; the footsteps are faster. Stop reading, shut your eyes, and use your imagination. How do you feel? Pay attention to your physical and emotional reactions. If you are not feeling a response to this imaginary situation, think back to a time when something similar happened to you—when something frightened you. Is your heart pounding? Are you breathing fast? Is there a flutter in your stomach? What is the physical sensation in your muscles? Do you feel frightened? What are your emotions? Are you straining to hear the footsteps? Do you want to run away, or are you "frozen"? If someone were to walk into the room where you are studying right now, would it startle you?

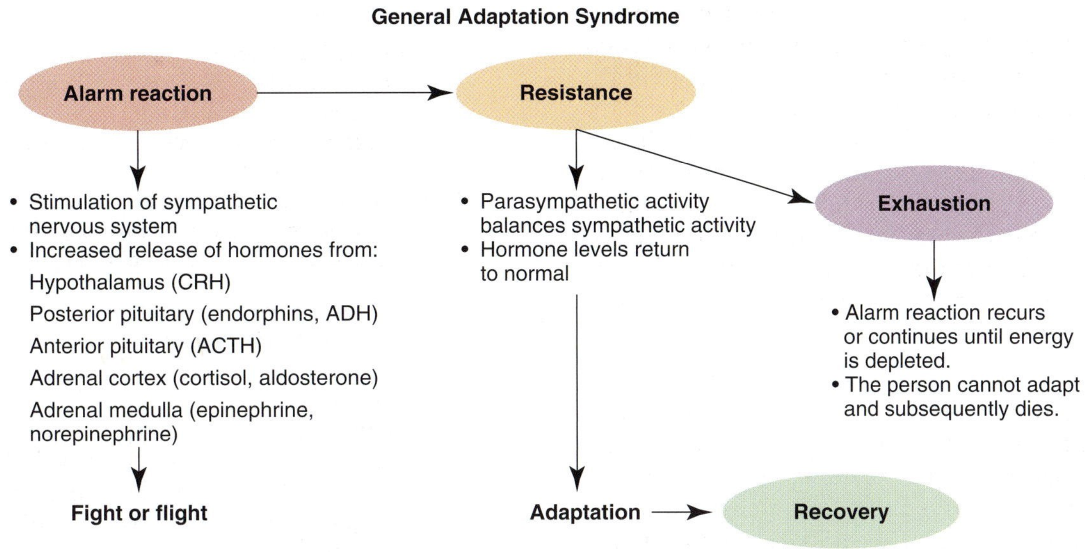

General Adaptation Syndrome

Alarm reaction → Resistance → Exhaustion

Alarm reaction:
- Stimulation of sympathetic nervous system
- Increased release of hormones from:
  Hypothalamus (CRH)
  Posterior pituitary (endorphins, ADH)
  Anterior pituitary (ACTH)
  Adrenal cortex (cortisol, aldosterone)
  Adrenal medulla (epinephrine, norepinephrine)

Fight or flight

Resistance:
- Parasympathetic activity balances sympathetic activity
- Hormone levels return to normal

Exhaustion:
- Alarm reaction recurs or continues until energy is depleted.
- The person cannot adapt and subsequently dies.

Adaptation → **Recovery**

FIGURE 12-2 The stages of Selye's general adaptation syndrome (GAS) are (1) *alarm* (also called "fight or flight"); (2) *resistance* (or adaptation), in which the body enacts physical and psychological adaptive mechanisms to maintain homeostasis; and (3) either *recovery* or *exhaustion* (which usually ends in disease or death).

This scenario should help you to imagine the experience of the alarm stage, during which the body prepares for *"fight or flight."* The alarm stage has two phases: shock and countershock. The **shock phase** begins when the cerebral cortex first perceives a stressor and sends out messages to activate the endocrine and sympathetic nervous systems. Epinephrine (adrenaline) and various other hormones prepare the body for fight or flight. The shock phase does not last long—usually less than 24 hours, and sometimes only a minute or two. In the **countershock phase**, all the changes produced in the shock phase are reversed, and the person becomes less able to deal with the immediate threat.

Endocrine System Responses

In response to a perceived stressor, the following endocrine responses occur:

1. The *hypothalamus* releases corticotropin-releasing hormone (CRH).
2. *CRH*, together with messages from the cerebral cortex, directs the pituitary gland to release adrenocorticotropic hormone (ACTH) and antidiuretic hormone (ADH).
3. *ACTH* stimulates the adrenal cortex to produce and secrete glucocorticoids (especially cortisol) and mineralocorticoids (especially aldosterone).
   Cortisol, in general, has a glucose-sparing effect. It increases the use of fats and proteins for energy and conserves glucose for use by the brain. Cortisol also has an anti-inflammatory effect. See Figure 12-3 for the effects of cortisol during the alarm reaction of the GAS.
   Aldosterone promotes fluid retention by causing the kidneys to reabsorb more sodium. In that way, it helps to increase fluid volume and maintain or increase blood pressure.

4. *ADH* also promotes fluid retention by increasing the reabsorption of water by kidney tubules. See Figure 12-4 for the effects of aldosterone and ADH.
5. *Endorphins,* secreted by the hypothalamus and posterior pituitary, act like opiates to produce a sense of well-being and reduce pain.
6. *Thyroid-stimulating hormone (TSH)* is secreted by the pituitary gland to increase the efficiency of cellular metabolism and fat conversion to energy for cell and muscle needs.

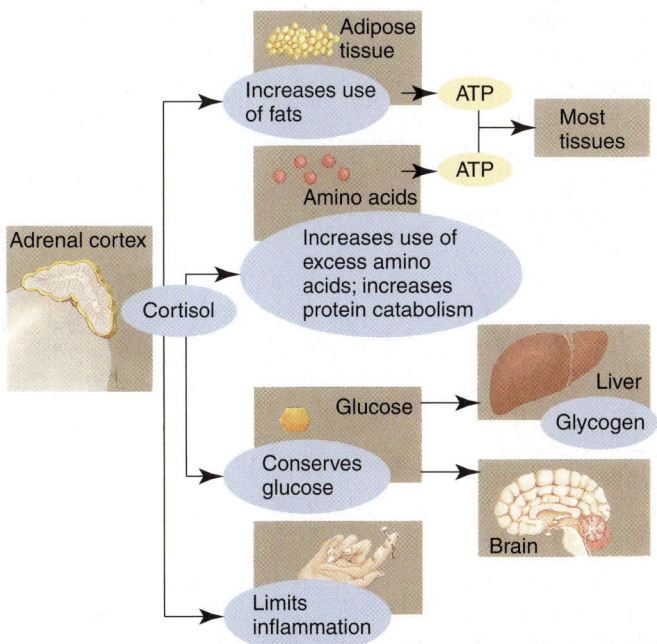

FIGURE 12-3 Functions of cortisol during the alarm stage of the GAS. (From Scanlon, V., & Sanders, T. (2011). *Essentials of anatomy and physiology* (6th ed.). Philadelphia: F. A. Davis, p. 241.)

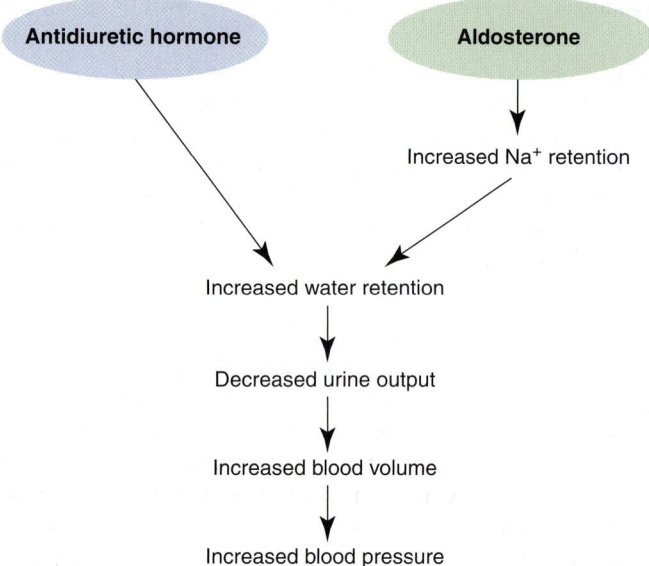

FIGURE 12-4 The release of ADH (from the posterior pituitary gland) and aldosterone (from the adrenal cortex) leads to sodium and water retention, increases blood volume, and increases blood pressure.

Sympathetic Nervous System Responses

The cerebral cortex also sends messages via the hypothalamus to stimulate the sympathetic nervous system. The sympathetic nervous system then stimulates the adrenal glands to secrete adrenaline and norepinephrine, which increase mental alertness. This allows the person to assess the situation and aids in a decision to stand and fight or run away in flight. Adrenaline also increases the ability of the muscles to contract and causes the pupils to dilate, producing greater visual fields. See Figure 12-5 for the effects of adrenaline during the alarm reaction of the GAS.

Other Body System Responses in the Alarm Stage

The following are some body system responses that occur in the alarm stage as a result of endocrine and sympathetic nervous system activity. Refer to Figures 12-2 through 12-5 to see how these changes are produced.

- *Cardiovascular system.* The heart rate and contraction force increase. Peripheral and visceral vasoconstriction increase blood flow to vital organs (e.g., brain, lungs) and to muscles preparing for flight. Blood volume and blood pressure also increase, and the blood clots more readily.
- *Respiratory system.* The bronchioles dilate, thereby increasing the depth of respiration and tidal volume. This makes oxygen available for diffusion to muscle, brain, and cardiac cells.
- *Metabolism.* The metabolic rate increases. The liver converts more glycogen to glucose (*glycogenolysis*), making it available for energy. Except in the brain, the body uses less glucose for energy. The use of amino acids and the mobilization of fats for energy (*lipolysis*) increase.

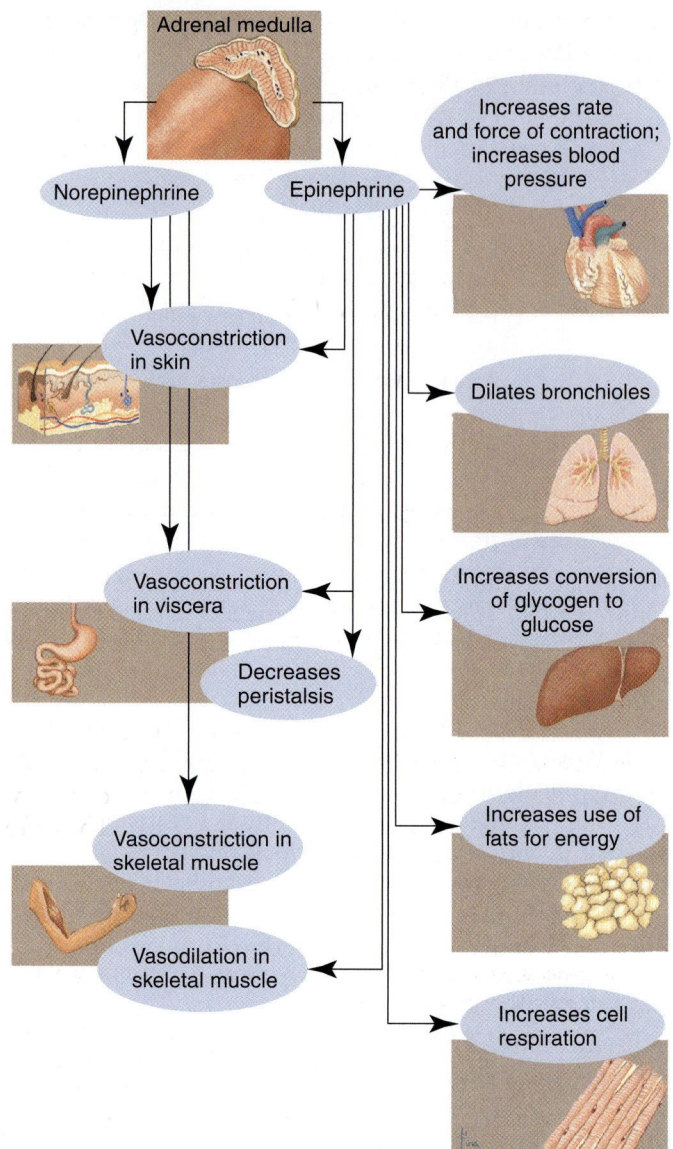

FIGURE 12-5 Functions of epinephrine and norepinephrine during the alarm stage of the GAS. (From Scanlon, V., & Sanders, T. (2011). *Essentials of anatomy and physiology* (6th ed.). Philadelphia: F. A. Davis, p. 239.)

- *Urinary system.* Blood flow to the kidneys decreases, and they retain more sodium and water. The kidneys secrete renin, which produces *angiotensin*. In turn, angiotensin constricts the arterioles and tends to increase blood pressure.
- *Gastrointestinal system.* Peristalsis and secretions of digestive enzymes decrease. The blood glucose level increases to fuel the energy needed for fight or flight.
- *Musculoskeletal system.* Blood vessels dilate, increasing flow of blood (and thus oxygen and energy) to skeletal muscles.

Resistance Stage—Coping With the Stressor

During the second stage of the GAS, **resistance** (or *adaptation*), the body tries to cope, protect itself against the stressor, and maintain homeostasis. Stabilization involves the use of physiological and psychological coping mechanisms. Psychological defense mechanisms for coping are discussed shortly. Physical adaptations help the heart rate, blood pressure, cardiac output, respiratory function, and hormone levels return to normal. If the person adapts successfully or if the stress can be confined to a small area (as in the inflammatory response, also discussed shortly), the body regains homeostasis. If the stress is too great (as in serious illness or severe blood loss), defense mechanisms fail, and the person enters the third phase of the GAS.

Exhaustion or Recovery Stage—Final Effort to Adapt

If stress continues and adaptive mechanisms become ineffective or are used up, a person enters the final stage, **exhaustion**. Physiological responses in this stage include vasodilation, decreased blood pressure, and increased pulse and respirations. Physical adaptive resources and energy are depleted. The body is unable to defend itself and cannot maintain resistance against the continuing stressors. Exhaustion usually ends in injury, illness, or death.

In contrast, if adaptation is successful, the final stage is **recovery**. For example, after a miscarriage, a couple participates in a support group and begins to focus more deeply on their relationship with each other. They are able gradually to resolve their grief.

KnowledgeCheck 12-3

- In general, what is the difference between the alarm stage and the resistance stage of the GAS?
- Name the gland that releases each of the following hormones in response to stress, and name each hormone's function: corticotropin-releasing hormone (CRH), antidiuretic hormone (ADH), adrenocorticotropic hormone (ACTH), aldosterone, cortisol, epinephrine, and norepinephrine.
- In the alarm stage of the GAS, what are the effects of the sympathetic nervous system on each of the following: heart, brain, glycogen stores, and skeletal muscle?
- What is the effect of Selye's resistance stage on the cardiovascular and respiratory systems? On hormone levels?

The Local Adaptation Syndrome Involves a Specific Local Response

Whereas the GAS is a whole-body response to a stressor, the **local adaptation syndrome (LAS)** is a localized body response; that is, it involves only a specific body part, tissue, or organ. It is a short-term attempt to restore homeostasis. As a nurse, the two most common LAS responses you will deal with are the reflex pain response and the inflammatory response (others include blood clotting and pupil constriction in response to light).

Reflex Pain Response

When you perceive a painful stimulus, especially in one of your limbs, you immediately and unconsciously withdraw from the source of pain. If you've ever accidentally touched a hot stove, you certainly didn't stop to ponder, "Hmmm, I think I will withdraw my hand." You pulled your hand away before you could even think about it. This is a protective **reflex** (an involuntary, predictable response). Pain receptors send sensory impulses to the spinal cord, where they synapse with the spinal motor neurons. The motor impulses travel back to the site of stimulation, causing the flexor muscles in the limb to contract. This is a local, rather than a whole-body, response.

Inflammatory Response

The **inflammatory response** is a local reaction to cell injury, either by pathogens or by physical, chemical, or other agents (Box 12-2). Regardless of the injuring agent (stressor), its mechanisms are the same, and they produce the classic symptoms of inflammation: pain, heat, swelling, redness, and loss of function. The inflammatory process includes a vascular response, a cellular response, formation of exudate, and healing.

Vascular Response Immediately after injury, blood vessels at the site constrict (narrow) to control bleeding. After the injured cells release histamine, the vessels dilate, increasing blood flow to the area (**hyperemia**). Under the influence of kinins released by the dying cells, the capillaries become more permeable, allowing movement of fluid from capillaries into tissue spaces. The tissue becomes **edematous** (swollen). After **leukocytes** (white blood cells) move into the area, localized blood flow again decreases to keep them in the area to fight infection.

Cellular Response Specialized white blood cells (**phagocytes**) migrate to the site of injury and engulf bacteria, other foreign material, and damaged cells and destroy them. Sometimes they form a "wall" around an

---

BOX 12-2 ■ Agents Causing Inflammatory Responses

The following agents stimulate the inflammatory response by causing cell injury:

- Autoimmune disorders
- Antigen–antibody responses
- Body substances (e.g., digestive enzymes leaking into the abdomen; accumulation of uric acid crystals in joints)
- Chemical injury (e.g., acid or alkali burns)
- Ischemia
- Neoplastic growth (i.e., cancer)
- Pathogens (e.g., bacteria, viruses)
- Physical agents:
  Heat or cold
  Radiation
  Electrothermal injury
  Mechanical trauma (e.g., abrasion, contusion, laceration, puncture, incision, fractures, sprains)

invading pathogen. The accumulation of dead white cells, digested bacteria, and other cell debris in the presence of infection is called *pus.*

Exudate Formation The fluid and white blood cells that move from the circulation to the site of injury are called **exudate.** The nature and quantity of exudate depend on the severity of injury and the tissues involved. For example, a surgical incision may ooze serosanguineous (clear or pinkish) exudate for a day or two.

Healing Healing is the replacement of tissue by regeneration or repair. **Regeneration** is replacement of the damaged cells with identical or similar cells. However, not all cells can regenerate (e.g., some central nervous system neurons and cardiac muscle cells cannot regenerate). Most injuries heal by **repair,** wherein scar tissue replaces the original tissue. You will find a thorough discussion of wound healing in Chapter 35.

The inflammatory response is adaptive in that it protects the body from infection and promotes healing. However, chronic inflammation, as in arthritis, is itself a stressor.

Do not confuse inflammation with infection. Inflammation is a mechanism for eliminating invading pathogens; therefore, you always see inflammation when there is infection. However, inflammation is stimulated by trauma as well as by pathogens (as in the example of a sprained ankle); thus, it can occur when there is no infection.

KnowledgeCheck 12-4
- What are four characteristics of the LAS?
- Name two LAS responses.
- What are the classic symptoms of the inflammatory process?

Psychological Responses to Stress Include Feelings, Thoughts, and Behaviors

Health professionals understand most human health disorders to be *biopsychosocial* in nature (Alford, 2007). That is, they consist of interactions among biological, psychological, and social factors. Recall that stress responses are holistic. That means we respond and adapt to stress physically, mentally, and behaviorally, and many would add spiritually.

Psychological responses are both emotional and cognitive, and they include feelings, thoughts, and behaviors (Box 12-3). They may be fleeting, as in a flash of anger that is gone in seconds; or long term, as in the avoidance of relationships by an adult whose needs for love and security were not met as a child.

As with physical responses, psychological responses can be adaptive or harmful. Consider this example case:

Both Mr. Laslow and Mr. Harvey have had heart attacks and are both anxious about the future. To relieve his anxiety, Mr. Laslow takes a problem-solving approach, learning about diet, exercise, and lifestyle changes that he must make. Mr. Harvey uses denial;

BOX 12-3 ■ Psychological Responses to Stressors

Cognitive Responses
Difficulty concentrating
Poor judgment
Decrease in accuracy (e.g., in counting money)
Forgetfulness
Decreased problem-solving ability
Decreased attention to detail
Difficulty learning
Narrowing of focus
Preoccupation, daydreaming

Emotional Responses
Adjustment disorders
Anger
Anxiety
Depression
Fear
Feelings of inadequacy
Low self-esteem
Irritability
Lack of motivation
Lethargy

Behavioral Responses
Academic difficulties
Aggressiveness
Crying, emotional outbursts
Dependence
Nightmares
Poor job performance
Substance use and abuse
Sleeplessness (or sleeping too much)
Change in eating habits (e.g., loss of appetite, overeating)
Decrease in quality of job performance
Preoccupation (i.e., daydreaming)
Illnesses
Increased absenteeism from work or school
Increased number of accidents
Strained family or social relationships
Avoiding social situations or relationships
Rebellion, acting out

he cannot even accept that he has "really" had a heart attack. He says, "I'm not an invalid. I feel fine. I could follow all those rules and still get hit by a truck and die tomorrow." Both of these responses may relieve the person's anxiety. Which one do you think is more adaptive in the long term?

Common emotional responses to stress include anxiety, fear, anger, and depression.

Anxiety and Fear

Anxiety is diffuse and not easily defined. NANDA International (2012, p. 344) defines it as a "vague, uneasy feeling of discomfort or dread accompanied by an autonomic response (the source often nonspecific or unknown to the individual); a feeling of apprehension caused by anticipation of danger. . . ." Notice that the response is not to a danger but to the *anticipation* of danger—to imagining it. An anxious person worries; feels nervous, uneasy, and fearful; may be tearful; and often has physical symptoms, such as nausea, trembling, and sweating.

Fear is an emotion or feeling of apprehension (dread) from an identified danger, threat, or pain. The danger may be real or imagined. Anxiety and fear produce similar responses; however, some experts differentiate them as follows:

- Fear is a cognitive response, whereas anxiety is an emotional response.
- Fear is related to a present event, whereas anxiety is related to a future (or anticipated) event.
- The source of fear is easily identifiable, whereas the source of anxiety may not be identifiable.
- Fear can result from either a physical or a psychological event; anxiety results from psychological conflict rather than physical threat.

Mild to moderate anxiety may be adaptive because it motivates and mobilizes the person to action. However, severe anxiety consumes energy and interferes with the person's ability to focus on and respond to what is really happening. See Chapter 13 to refresh your theoretical knowledge of anxiety and fear, including levels of anxiety.

Anxiety and fear initiate the release of epinephrine, which stimulates the sympathetic nervous system and prepares the person for fight or flight. Therefore, living with anxiety can be physically, emotionally, and spiritually exhausting.

 ## ThinkLike a Nurse 12-2

Read the following two scenarios.

1. You are a student assigned to a 6-hour day in the clinical area. Each time you have a clinical day coming up, you feel anticipation and look forward to working in the clinical area. However, you do not know what to expect. You think: "What will my patients be like? How will the day go? Do I know enough to handle it? Do I need to practice any procedures?" It is hard to answer these questions until you are actually on the unit and see your patients.

2. Given the same situation, suppose that when you begin your clinical day, your clinical instructor tells you that he will be in the agency asking questions, supervising, evaluating your performance—and, perhaps from your perspective, making your life miserable.

   In which situation are you most likely to feel fear rather than anxiety? Explain your reasoning.

Ego Defense Mechanisms When faced with a stressful situation, the ego defense systems may kick in to diminish the inner tension associated with the stressors. **Ego defense mechanisms** are unconscious mental mechanisms that make a stressful situation more tolerable by decreasing the inner tension associated with the stressors. Just as the body responds physiologically to stressors, it has psychological responses that protect the person from anxiety and assist with adaptation. When used sparingly, and for mild to moderate anxiety, defense mechanisms can be helpful. When overused, however, they become habits that give us the false illusion that we are coping. If psychological defense mechanisms (Table 12-1) are inadequate to diminish the threat and restore equilibrium, the person may develop an anxiety disorder.

Anger and Depression

Anger is a strong, uncomfortable feeling of animosity, hostility, extreme indignation, or displeasure. A person who cannot control stressors may become apprehensive (anxious about what may happen) and respond with anger. Thus, moderate anger is often a first protective response against anxiety. As anxiety increases and the person recognizes fear, he feels more threatened and may resort to bullying behavior to increase the personal feeling of power, control, and self-esteem.

Anger may be expressed in screaming or shouting, throwing things, or hitting, or more subtly with sarcastic, caustic remarks. Some people attempt to hide their emotions and soften their hurtful remarks, or make them more socially acceptable, through the use of humor and joking. When anger involves destructive behaviors such as physical or verbal abuse, it is called **hostility**. When expressed appropriately and clearly (i.e., verbally), anger can be adaptive, because it temporarily releases the person's feelings of tension. When the anger is out in the open, both parties can deal with it. Nevertheless, even verbal expressions of anger can be destructive if the anger continues after the person expresses it.

Depression is sometimes associated with unresolved anger and may result from stress. It is normal to feel depression in response to any loss or a traumatic event, but long-term depression is a reason for concern. Review Chapter 13 for information about anger and depression.

KnowledgeCheck 12-5

- In addition to ego defense mechanisms, name four common emotional responses to stress.
- Explain how mild to moderate anxiety can be adaptive.
- True or false: One difference between anxiety and fear is that the danger in anxiety may be imagined, whereas in fear the danger is real.
- What are ego defense mechanisms?

Spiritual Responses to Stress Are Multifaceted

Spiritual responses vary among individuals—as do all human responses. Many people depend on a higher power or religious community for support when coping with stress. Some search for a larger meaning in the

Table 12-1 ▶ Psychological Defense Mechanisms

DEFENSE MECHANISM	EXAMPLES	EXAMPLES AND CONSEQUENCES OF OVERUSE
Avoidance—Unconsciously staying away from events or situations that might open feelings of aggression or anxiety	"I can't go to the class reunion tonight. I'm too tired; I have to sleep."	The person becomes socially isolated because of the tension he feels when around other people.
Compensation—Making up for a perceived inadequacy by developing or emphasizing some other desirable trait	A small boy who wants to be on the football team instead becomes a great singer	Use of drugs or alcohol to gain courage to enter a social situation
Conversion—Emotional conflict is changed into physical symptoms that have no physical basis. The symptoms often disappear after the threat is over.	Feeling back pain when it is difficult to continue carrying the pressures of life; developing nausea that causes the person to miss a major exam	Laryngitis, inability to speak on the anniversary of father's death. Continued anxiety can lead to actual physical disorders, such as gastric ulcers.
Denial—Transforming reality by refusing to acknowledge thoughts, feeling, desires, or impulses. This is unconscious; the person is *not* consciously lying. Denial is usually the first defense learned.	A student refuses to acknowledge that he is barely passing anatomy, does not withdraw from the class, and is now failing a nursing course. An alcoholic states, "I can quit any time I want to."	Overuse can lead to repression and dissociative disorders (e.g., dual personalities, selective amnesia).
Displacement—"Kick the dog." Transferring emotions, ideas, or wishes from one original object or situation to a substitute inappropriate person or object that is perceived to be less powerful or threatening	Husband loses his job, goes home, and yells at his wife. (This mechanism is rarely adaptive.)	In extreme situations, this mechanism leads to verbal and physical abuse.
Dissociation—Painful events are separated or dissociated from the conscious mind.	A person who was sexually abused as a child describes the events as though they happened to a sibling.	May result in a dissociative disorder, such as multiple personality disorder.
Identification—A person takes on the ideas, personality, or characteristics of another person, especially someone that the person fears or respects.	Children play cowboy, police, firefighter, or mommy.	Assumes mannerisms, wears clothing, and arranges hair and physical appearance to match those of the other person.
Intellectualization—Cognitive reasoning is used to block or avoid feelings about a painful incident.	When her husband dies, the wife relieves her pain by thinking, "It's better this way; he was in so much pain." A person says, "I think" rather than, "I feel."	"My husband loves me, so he doesn't like it when another man talks to me; that's why he beats me."
Minimization—Not acknowledging or accepting the significance of one's own behavior, making it less important	"It doesn't matter how much I drink. I never drive when I'm drinking."	Person engages in unhealthy or antisocial behavior; there is no motivation to change behavior
Projection—Blaming others. Attributing one's own personality traits, mistakes, emotions, motives, and thoughts to another; "finger pointing."	"The clinical instructor makes me nervous, so I cannot do well." "I forgot to bake cookies because you did not tell me that cookies were due at school today."	Person cannot see his own responsibility for a situation, so he cannot make adaptive behaviors. Person criticizes habits in others that are the same as one's own bad habits.

Table 12-1 ➤ Psychological Defense Mechanisms—cont'd

DEFENSE MECHANISM	EXAMPLES	EXAMPLES AND CONSEQUENCES OF OVERUSE
Rationalization—Use of a logical-sounding excuse to cover up or justify true ideas, actions, or feelings. An attempt to preserve self-respect or approval or to conceal a motive for some action by giving a socially acceptable reason. Similar to intellectualization, but uses faulty logic.	"It was God's will that this happened to me." "If I didn't have to work, I would be a better wife."	This mechanism can lead to self-deception.
Reaction formation—Similar to compensation, except the person develops the exact opposite trait. The person is aware of her feelings but acts in ways opposite to what she is really feeling.	"It's OK that you forgot my birthday" (when it really is not OK).	Overuse can cause failure to resolve internal conflicts.
Regression—Using behavior appropriate in an earlier stage of development to overcome feeling of insecurity in a present situation	Prepares and eats a comfort food (e.g., hot fudge sundae). A 60-year-old divorcee dresses and acts like a teenager.	Can interfere with perception of reality
Repression—Unconscious "burying" or "forgetting" of painful thoughts, feelings, memories, ideas; pushing them from a conscious to an unconscious level. It is a step deeper than denial.	Having no memory of sexual abuse by sibling or father An adolescent forgets to put out the trash because being "bossed" makes him angry, but he feels guilty if he consciously chooses not to do it.	Flashbacks, post-traumatic stress syndrome, and amnesia
Restitution (undoing)—Making amends for a behavior one thinks is unacceptable, to reduce guilt	Giving a treat to a child who has been punished for wrongdoing	May send double messages. Relieves the person of the responsibility for honesty about the situation
Sublimation—Unacceptable drives, traits, or behaviors (often sexual or aggressive) are unconsciously diverted to socially accepted traits.	Anger is expressed by aggression when playing sports. A person who chooses to not have children runs a day-care center.	The "acceptable" behavior might reinforce the negative tendencies, and the person may still show signs of the undesirable trait or behavior. For example, a person indulges in child pornography to obtain sexual gratification.

Source: Adapted from Neeb, K. (2006). *Fundamentals of mental health nursing* (3rd ed.). Philadelphia: F.A. Davis.

illness or other stressor. Others may view stress as a test, a punishment, or a challenge.

Often, a first response during the alarm stage is to pray or ask for help (e.g., healing, coping). Prayer, meditation, and religious affiliation can also help during the second stage (adaptation). In the final stage, spiritual resources may be exhausted, leaving the person feeling abandoned, helpless, and hopeless. If your own spiritual life is healthy, you will be better equipped to support patients who are experiencing spiritual challenges.

For more information about spiritual responses to stress, see Chapter 16.

WHAT HAPPENS WHEN ADAPTATION FAILS?

Living with continual stress strains adaptive mechanisms. This strain can lead to exhaustion and disease, which in turn can lead to more stress. Once established, this type of positive feedback loop is difficult to break. Three types of disorders that can develop when adaptation fails are stress-induced organic responses, somatoform disorders, and psychological disorders.

Stress-Induced Organic Responses

As a result of repeated central nervous system stimulation and elevation of certain hormones, continual stress brings about long-term changes in various body systems. People who use maladaptive coping strategies (e.g., overeating, substance abuse) create additional stress on the body, further contributing to disease (Table 12-2).

Somatoform Disorders

Somatoform disorders are conditions characterized by the presence of physical symptoms with no known organic cause. They are believed to result from unconscious denial, repression, and displacement of anxiety. Certain people seem predisposed to somatoform disorders—for instance, those who suffer from personality disorders and major psychiatric illness, those who do not handle anxiety well, and those who are dependent, emotionally needy, frustrated, and resentful (Neeb, 2006). The physical symptoms allow the person to avoid a situation that, if confronted, would provoke extreme anxiety. The following are examples of somatoform disorders:

- **Hypochondriasis.** The person is preoccupied with the idea that he is or will become seriously ill. The person is abnormally concerned with his health and interprets his real or imagined symptoms unrealistically, fearing that they will get worse or become incurable. The person is not "faking it"; anxiety about his health may trigger the physical sensations.
- **Somatization.** In this disorder, anxiety and emotional turmoil are expressed in physical symptoms, loss of physical function, pain that changes location often, and depression. The patient is unable to control the symptoms and behaviors, and complaints are vague or exaggerated.
- **Pain disorder.** Previously called *somatoform pain disorder*, this is emotional pain that manifests physically. Pain is the main focus of the person's life. The level of pain the person states is inconsistent with the physical condition—that is, the physical cause is either disproportionate to the pain or cannot be found at all. The pain does not change location.
- **Malingering.** Malingering is different from the other disorders because it is a *conscious* effort to escape

Table 12-2 ➤ Organic Disorders Brought About by Failure of Adaptive Mechanisms	
BODY SYSTEM	**PHYSIOLOGICAL RESPONSE**
Cardiovascular System	Continued secretion of epinephrine may cause cardiovascular disorders including angina, myocardial infarction, cardiomegaly, and congestive heart failure, all of which lead to decreased cardiac output. As cardiac output decreases, less oxygen circulates to meet cellular metabolic demands, and the body becomes fatigued. Prolonged secretion of epinephrine and renin result in vasoconstriction, causing hypertension. ADH, aldosterone, ACTH, and cortisol create electrolyte imbalance and retention of sodium and water, thus promoting peripheral edema.
Endocrine System	Continuing high levels of blood glucose and insulin can cause diabetes. Metabolic disorders of hyperthyroidism or hypothyroidism can result as persistent demands for thyroid hormone production cause a rebound failure of the gland. Even prenatal stress can cause adaptive changes in fetal endocrine and metabolic processes that impact later adult health (Sullivan, Hawes, Winchester, et al., 2008).
Immune System	Stress reduces the ability of the body's immune cells to differentiate between self and nonself. Thus, the immune cells begin to attack body tissues, producing autoimmune illness. Common autoimmune illnesses include rheumatoid arthritis, lupus, cancer, and allergies. Research has linked stress to suppression of the immune system and even to viral replication in HIV patients (e.g., Davidson, Kabat-Zinn, Schumacher, et al., 2003; McCain, Gray, Elswick, et al., 2008).
Gastrointestinal System	The gastrointestinal system may respond to central nervous system stimulation with constipation or diarrhea, gastroesophageal reflux, colitis, or irritable bowel syndrome. Continued secretion of hydrochloric acid produces gastric hyperacidity and erosion of the gastrointestinal tract, especially in the presence of Helicobacter pylori (H. pylori).
Musculoskeletal System	Constant readiness for fight or flight produces muscle tension and pain in various body sites. Tension headache and temporomandibular joint pain result from prolonged muscle tension in the head, neck, and spine.
Respiratory System	Epinephrine and circulating hormones dilate the bronchial tubes and increase the rate of respiration. Hyperventilation can produce symptoms of alkalosis, including dizziness, tingling hands and feet, and anxiety. Distress in the respiratory system can exacerbate existing asthma, hay fever, and allergies.

unpleasant situations. The patient merely pretends to have the symptoms for personal or tangible gain (e.g., calling in sick because the person does not want to go to work).

KnowledgeCheck 12-6

- Name and describe three stress-induced organic or systemic responses to stress.
- Name and describe at least three somatoform disorders.

Stress-Induced Psychological Responses

Even if coping mechanisms are effective initially, with long-term stress, exhaustion sets in and the mechanisms begin to fail. The person may then try maladaptive ways to cope. As work and personal relationships deteriorate, the person loses self-esteem. Prolonged stress can eventually result in crisis and burnout (Fig. 12-6). More severe responses include psychiatric illnesses, such as anxiety disorders, clinical depression, and post-traumatic stress disorder (PTSD). Anxiety and depression are discussed in Chapter 13.

Crisis

A **crisis** exists when (1) an event in a person's life drastically changes the person's routine and he perceives it as a threat to self, and (2) the person's usual coping methods are ineffective, resulting in high levels of anxiety and inability to function adequately. Such events are usually sudden and unexpected (e.g., serious illness or death of a loved one, serious financial losses, an automobile accident, rape, and natural disasters) (Fig. 12-6).

Each person has a different tolerance for stress; an event that creates a crisis for one may be just a minor nuisance for another. Nevertheless, most experts agree that people experiencing crisis go through five phases (Neeb, 2006; Stuart, 2012).

1. *Precrisis.* In response to the event and the anxiety, the person uses her usual coping strategies; has no symptoms; denies feeling stress; and may even report a sense of well-being.
2. *Impact.* If the usual strategies are not effective, anxiety and confusion increase. The person may have trouble organizing her personal life and may feel the stress but minimize its severity.
3. *Crisis.* The person experiences more anxiety and tries new ways of coping, such as withdrawal, rationalization, and projection (refer to Table 12-1). The person recognizes the problem but denies that it is out of control.
4. *Adaptive.* The person redefines the threat and perceives the crisis in a realistic way. She begins to think rationally and does some positive problem-solving, regains some self-esteem, and is able to begin socializing

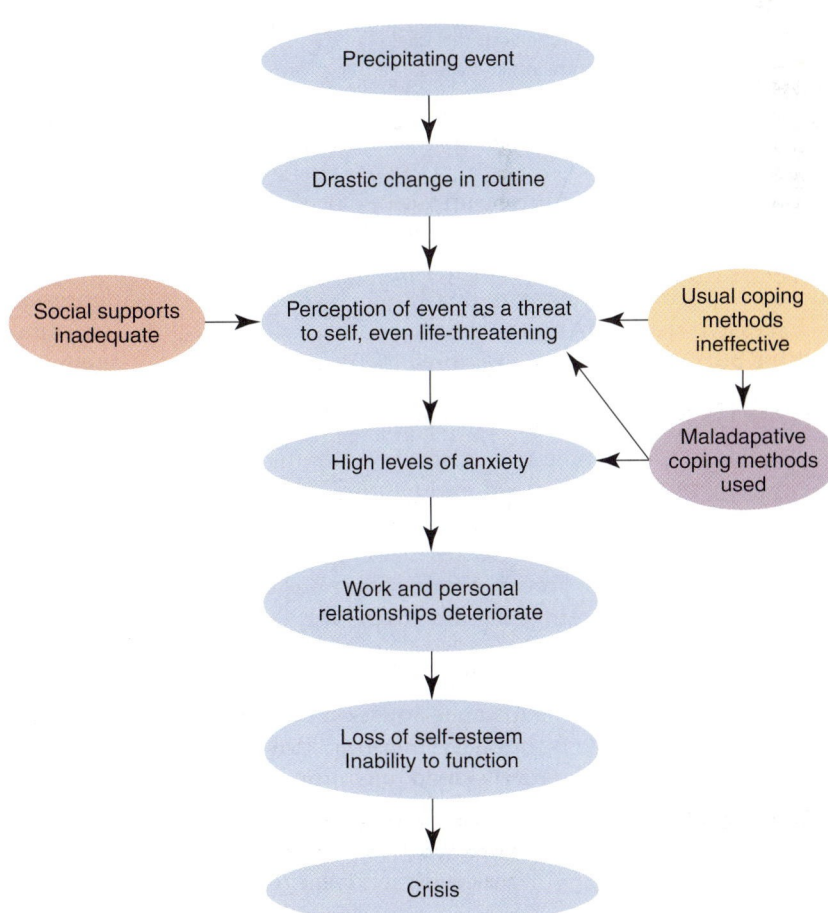

FIGURE 12-6 How a crisis develops.

again. Adaptation is more likely if the person can use effective coping strategies and if situational supports are available.

5. *Postcrisis.* The aftermath of a crisis may have both positive and negative effects on functioning. The person may have developed better ways of coping with stress. Or she may be critical, hostile, and depressed, and may use maladaptive strategies (e.g., overeating or substance abuse) to deal with what has happened.

People in crisis are at risk for physical and emotional harm, so intervention is essential (see Crisis Intervention later in the chapter).

ThinkLike a Nurse 12-3

Suppose you are the charge nurse on a 30-bed surgical unit. In addition, you must assume care of three patients because another nurse called in sick. It is a normal, busy day with seven postoperative patients and eight discharges. In addition, a patient went into cardiac arrhythmia and was transferred to the coronary care unit. Because the sick nurse was supposed to work a 12-hour shift and no replacement has been found, you are told you must stay and work 4 hours overtime. You had plans to have dinner with your spouse this evening because it is your anniversary. Now you will surely not be home before 8:00 p.m., and you will be exhausted.

- What would be the stressors for you in this situation?
- What thoughts and feelings would you have?
- What physical responses would you probably notice?
- What are some psychological responses that you would use to help you adapt and cope with this day?
- How would you probably react if the same thing were to happen on the following day?

Burnout

Burnout occurs when nurses and other professionals cannot cope effectively with the physical and emotional demands of the workplace. You will find examples of stressors specific to nursing in Box 12-4.

Excessive demands by an employer serve as a catalyst for burnout. In some situations, the nurse receives no respect and little support from the employer or coworkers. Filled with feelings of injustice for treatment received, the nurse may respond with anger and frustration, feel overwhelmed and helpless, and suffer low self-esteem and depression. Some nurses experience grief reactions, moral distress, and guilt feelings because the situation prevents them from performing as well as they believe they should (Badger, 2008). As a result, a nurse may develop a physical illness, a negative attitude, or may use maladaptive coping techniques such as smoking, substance abuse, or distancing from patients—"going through the motions" but not really interacting with patients in a meaningful way. Many nurses with these feeling may give up and leave nursing. You will find suggestions for preventing burnout later in the chapter.

BOX 12-4 ■ Stressors That Can Lead to Burnout

- Dealing with difficult personalities (e.g., patient, supervisors, physicians)
- Working 12-hour shifts with minimal breaks for food, water, or rest
- Frequent rotating shifts that upset the circadian rhythm of the body and lower the immune system response
- Mandatory overtime
- Being "floated" to an unfamiliar unit (e.g., a maternity nurse may be "floated" to an orthopedic unit)
- Workload: low staffing ratio (one nurse to many patients)
- Frustration with patients (e.g., who do not follow therapeutic routines)
- Need to constantly anticipate patients' needs and cope with the unexpected
- Feeling helpless against a patient's disease process or lack of healing
- Dealing with death and dying
- Lack of rewards (both intrinsic and extrinsic)
- Lack of participation in decision making
- Inability to delegate responsibilities
- Organizational philosophy that conflicts with personal philosophy

---

Post-Traumatic Stress Disorder

Post-traumatic stress disorder (PTSD) is a specific response to a violent, traumatizing event, (e.g., earthquake, flood, or other natural disaster) or to physical or emotional abuse, such as rape, torture, or war. The victim experiences anxiety and flashbacks that may last for months or years. Other symptoms include social withdrawal, feelings of low self-esteem, changes in existing relationships, difficulty forming new relationships, irritability and outbursts of anger for no obvious reason, depression, and chemical abuse or dependence.

Counseling, special interventions, and stress management are needed to help the person cope with and recover from the impact of the traumatic event (Bisson & Andrew, 2007).

KnowledgeCheck 12-7

Define *crisis*, *burnout*, and *post-traumatic stress disorder*.

PracticalKnowledge
knowing **how**

People under stress may not be thinking clearly or able to communicate effectively; therefore, it is important to intervene to relieve their immediate anxiety as much as possible, demonstrate empathy, and develop rapport before beginning an assessment. Focus the patient by asking short, direct questions and then proceeding to open-ended questions that will provide you with as much information as possible (see Chapter 21 if you need to review questioning techniques).

ASSESSMENT

Assessment should explore subjective and objective data about the person's stressors, risk factors, coping and adaptation, support systems, and stress responses (psychosocial and physiological).

Assess Stressors, Risk Factors, and Coping and Adaptation

Data about the patient's stressors and risk factors should help you to:

- Determine whether the client has a realistic or an exaggerated perception of the stressors
- Identify factors that increase risk for future stress
- Identify interventions to reduce current stress and to provide anticipatory guidance to prevent future stress

You might begin gathering these data by having the patient complete a stress inventory, such as the Holmes–Rahe Social Readjustment Scale. Then follow up with questions such as those in Assessment Guidelines and Tools in Chapter 12, Volume 2. You will also find questions to help you obtain information about patients' coping methods and adaptation in those guidelines.

 Go to Chapter 12, **Assessment Guidelines and Tools, the Holmes–Rahe Social Readjustment Scale** and **Assessing for Stress: Questions to Ask,** in Volume 2.

Assess Responses to Stress

When assessing responses to stress, recall that stress responses are holistic. Therefore, you will need to assess physiological, emotional, cognitive, and behavioral indicators of stress. For examples of questions to ask,

 Go to Chapter 12, **Assessment Guidelines and Tools, Assessing for Stress: Questions to Ask,** in Volume 2.

Assessing Physiological Responses Because the GAS is nonspecific, you must obtain data from all body systems (for physical examination techniques, see Chapter 22). A check of vital signs for elevations in pulse, respiration, and blood pressure will indicate whether the fight-or-flight response is present. In your general survey, or overview, of the patient, you should note hygiene, grooming, facial expression, and ability to make eye contact. Box 12-5 summarizes physiological responses that indicate stress. If coping is successful, clinical signs and symptoms of stress may not be present.

Assessing Emotional and Behavioral Responses Assess for the emotional and behavioral responses to stress that are described in Box 12-3. As the client answers questions, note posture, facial expression, body tension,

---

BOX 12-5 ■ Physiological Responses to Stressors

- Dilated pupils
- Muscle tension
- Stiff neck
- Headaches
- Nail biting
- Skin pallor
- Skin lesions (e.g., eczema)
- Diaphoresis, sweaty palms
- Dry mouth
- Nausea
- Weight or appetite changes
- Increased blood glucose
- Increased heart rate
- Cardiac dysrhythmias
- Hyperventilation
- Chest pain
- Water retention
- Increased urinary frequency or decreased urinary output
- Diarrhea or constipation
- Flatulence

---

and other nonverbal behaviors. Also note mood and affect. Does the client seem angry, anxious, or depressed? Check the client's records, and observe for and ask the client about destructive behaviors (e.g., drug abuse, anger). The client may or may not be aware that the feelings or behaviors are related to stress.

Assessing Cognitive Responses You can assess the client's cognitive functioning as you assess other functional areas. See Box 12-3 to review examples of cognitive responses. Notice whether the person has difficulty focusing and responding to your questions. When you ask the client to describe and rate the intensity of the stressors, you can begin to assess whether he perceives the stressors realistically or in an exaggerated way. The client's responses concerning any coping strategies will give you an idea of his problem-solving abilities.

Assess Support Systems

Recall that support systems such as family, friends, and coworkers are important to the success of a client's coping strategies. Conversely, these people may be affected by the same stressors or by the client's responses to them. For these reasons, you should determine the supports available and their ability to assist the client—that is, do the significant others have the sensitivity and skills to be supportive? For examples of questions to ask,

 Go to Chapter 12, **Assessment Guidelines and Tools, Assessing for Stress: Questions to Ask,** in Volume 2.

ThinkLike a Nurse 12-4

Review the scenario of Gloria and John (Meet Your Patients). How much does it really tell you about the clients' situation?

- Which aspect of stress do you have the most information about: their stressors, their coping methods and adaptation, their responses to stress, or their support systems?
- What facts do you have about either Gloria's or John's physiological responses to their multiple stressors? What can you infer their responses might be?
- What facts do you have about the clients' emotional and behavioral responses to their stressors?
- What information do you have about how well they are adapting to stress?
- What data do you have about their support systems? What information do you need?

ANALYSIS/NURSING DIAGNOSIS

Stress is nonspecific, so there is almost no limit to the number of nursing diagnoses that could be stress induced. Your theoretical knowledge of the holistic nature of stress should lead you to identify diagnoses in the physical, behavioral, cognitive, emotional, interpersonal, and spiritual domains. The following are some examples.

Physical	Constipation r/t decreased peristalsis secondary to stress
Behavioral	Ineffective Health Maintenance r/t use of denial as an ego defense mechanism to relieve anxiety
Cognitive	Impaired Short-Term Memory r/t overwhelming number and severity of stressors
Emotional	Anxiety r/t uncertainty about the future and ineffectiveness of usual coping mechanisms
Interpersonal	Impaired Parenting r/t maladaptive use of alcohol to cope with recent stress of divorce
Spiritual	Hopelessness r/t perceived lack of support and ability to change the present situation

For a more extensive list of stress-related nursing diagnoses,

 Go to Chapter 12, **Standardized Language, NANDA-I Nursing Diagnoses Associated With Stress,** in Volume 2.

It is important to correctly identify the etiology of the diagnosis so that you can choose interventions to remove or modify the stressor. For example, if you believe a patient's Diarrhea is being caused by stress, you would intervene by modifying the stressor, helping the patient to perceive the stressor differently, and so on. If, instead, the Diarrhea were being caused by a gastrointestinal virus, your interventions would not have been helpful.

KnowledgeCheck 12-8

- How might you identify and assess Gloria and John's stressors (Meet Your Patients)?
- List three questions you could ask to find out how Gloria is coping and adapting to stress.
- List three questions you could ask to assess Gloria's physiological responses to stress. What observations might you also make?
- List three questions you could ask to assess Gloria's emotional and behavioral responses to stress.
- How might you determine whether stress is affecting Gloria's cognitive functioning?
- You know Gloria's sister is providing some support. How could you find out more about the extent of Gloria and John's support system?

PLANNING OUTCOMES/EVALUATION

NOC standardized outcomes are outcomes that if achieved demonstrate resolution of the problem stated by the nursing diagnosis. For example, if you make a diagnosis of Anxiety related to the client's perception that he will not be able to fulfill family responsibilities, you might use the NOC outcome Anxiety Control. For a list of NOC outcomes to use for stress diagnoses,

 Go to Chapter 12, **Standardized Language, Standardized Outcomes and Interventions for Stress-Related Nursing Diagnosis,** in Volume 2.

Individualized goal or outcome statements are also specific to each nursing diagnosis. Broad, general goals for clients experiencing stress are to (1) reduce the strength and duration of the stressor, (2) relieve or remove responses to stress, and (3) use effective coping mechanisms. Examples of specific outcome statements you might write include the following:

- Reports (or physical exam reveals) reduction in physical symptoms of stress.
- Demonstrates less physical tension in facial expression and other muscle groups.
- Verbalizes increased feelings of control in the stressful situation.
- Uses problem-solving and anxiety-reducing techniques.
- Demonstrates relaxation and stress-reducing strategies.

PLANNING INTERVENTIONS/IMPLEMENTATION

NIC standardized interventions for stress may be linked to both the problem and the etiology of the nursing diagnosis. Using the preceding example of Anxiety related to the client's perception that he will not be able to fulfill family responsibilities, some interventions may focus on supporting the client's ability to fulfill family roles; others may focus on general techniques for relieving anxiety (e.g., Anxiety Reduction, Calming Technique). For other stress-related NIC interventions,

 Go to Chapter 12, **Standardized Language, Standardized Outcomes and Interventions for Stress-Related Nursing Diagnoses,** in Volume 2.

Specific nursing activities will be individualized on the basis of the patient's needs and the etiologies of the nursing diagnoses. As you implement stress-reduction interventions, it is essential to consider compliance. Will the patient adhere to or cooperate with therapeutic suggestions? Does the person wish to use complementary or alternative care measures? How open is he to deviating from traditional Western therapies? Confer and collaborate with patients to determine what will fit most comfortably into their lifestyle. Those are the interventions that will be most effective.

Most stress-relieving interventions work by one or more of the following means:

- Removing or modifying the stressor(s)
- Supporting coping abilities (e.g., changing the person's perception of the stressor)
- Treating the person's responses to stress (e.g., symptoms such as anxiety or diarrhea)

As you read through the following interventions, see whether you can identify the rationale for the action. Look back at the list above as you need to.

Health Promotion Activities

People cannot always control the occurrence of a stressful event, and there are no high-tech treatments for coping with stress. However, a healthy lifestyle can prevent some stressors and improve the ability to cope with others. Chapter 42 provides an in-depth discussion of wellness promotion. The following suggestions are a brief guide to a healthy lifestyle.

Nutrition Nutrition is important for maintaining physical homeostasis and resisting stress. For example, adequate nutrition is essential to maintain the integrity of the immune system; and proteins are needed for tissue building and healing. In addition, overweight and malnutrition are stressors that may lead to illness. See Chapter 27 if you need detailed information about nutrition. To summarize, you should advise clients to:

- Maintain a normal body weight.
- Limit the intake of fat (especially animal fat) to no more than 30% of daily calories.
- Limit the intake of sugar and salt.
- Eat more fish and poultry and less red meat.
- Eat smaller, more frequent meals to aid digestion.
- Consume 25 grams of fiber (fruits, vegetables, and whole grains) daily to promote bowel elimination.
- Consume no more than one or two alcoholic beverages per day.

Exercise Regular exercise promotes physical homeostasis by improving muscle tone and controlling weight. It also improves the functioning of the heart and lungs and reduces the risk of cardiovascular disease. Exercise also improves emotional homeostasis by promoting relaxation and reducing tension. During exercise, the brain releases endogenous opioids (e.g., endorphins), which create a feeling of well-being. To achieve any health benefits, the client needs to exercise for at least 300 minutes per week (U.S. Department of Health and Human Services, 2008). See Chapter 32 for more specific physical activities to manage stress.

- Advise clients who are obese, chronically ill, or who have always been sedentary to consult a primary caregiver before beginning a new exercise program.
- Suggest that the client identify a variety of physical activities that he enjoys (e.g., swimming, bicycling, walking, sports) and, if possible, schedule regular sessions with one or more exercise "buddies." These strategies help the client adhere to the exercise routine.

Sleep and Rest Sleep and rest restore energy levels, allow the body to repair itself, and promote mental relaxation. Most people need 7 or 8 hours of sleep a day; however, the amount of sleep varies among individuals. Stress, pain, and illness may interfere with the ability to sleep, so some clients may need help identifying and implementing techniques for relaxing and going to sleep (see Chapter 34 for more information on sleep, as needed).

Leisure Activities Compared with exercise, which not everyone enjoys, leisure activities are any activities that provide joy and satisfaction. They may involve physical activity (after all, many people do enjoy exercising), or they may be sedentary activities, such as reading, painting, and even watching television. Leisure activities are a form of rest and, as such, are restorative.

Time Management People who manage their time efficiently and organize their life routines feel more in control and, therefore, less stressed. If clients feel overwhelmed, you can help them to prioritize tasks and make "to do" lists. It is also important that they learn to delegate responsibilities and set boundaries on the use of time. For example, a working couple with three children may need to assign each child mealtime tasks, such as setting the table, drying the dishes, and so forth. Or they may need to limit the amount of time they spend cooking, reserving elaborate meals for weekends.

Time management also includes learning to say no. Out of a need to be liked or a strong sense of responsibility to others, people sometimes try to make everyone happy by agreeing to every request for assistance: from spouse, children, parents, friends, church, school, and the community. Prompt clients to identify how much they can realistically accomplish—what is essential to do, and what would be "nice" to do.

KnowledgeCheck 12-9

Name and discuss at least four aspects of a healthful lifestyle that can help prevent or relieve stress.

Relieving Anxiety

Because anxiety is a common response to illness, medical tests, and treatments, you will use anxiety-relief interventions every day of your professional life. For example, when you tell patients what to expect before you perform a procedure or ask them to take deep breaths during a painful treatment, you lessen anxiety. If you have developed a therapeutic, trusting relationship, your very presence will help to ease the patient's anxiety. You will find specific interventions for anxiety in Chapter 13, and many of the interventions in the following sections provide anxiety relief as well (see Complementary & Alternative Modalities [CAM]: Using CAM for Stress Reduction).

Anger Management

Anger is a common response to stress. However, clients usually do not openly say, "I am angry." In fact, they may not even recognize that they are angry. Instead, they engage in angry behaviors. For example, they may become hypercritical of family members or caregivers, become verbally abusive, or become demanding. By now you have probably heard stories from nurses about the client who is "on the call light constantly." Unfortunately, such behaviors often provoke frustration or anger in others—even nurses. Be aware of how you are responding to stressed-out clients. Are you relieving your own stress, or are you relieving the client's stress? If you respond angrily to relieve your own stress, you may provoke further negative emotion in the client and even escalate the situation to the point of violence. Not only that, but anger also blocks communication and can lead to poor patient care and reduced patient satisfaction. For other tips on managing anger, refer to Box 24-8, Dealing With Violence, and

 Go to Chapter 12, **Clinical Insight 12-1: Dealing With Angry Patients,** in Volume 2.

Stress Management Techniques

It is important to teach your clients about relaxation and other stress management techniques. Most such techniques focus on discharging tension or simplifying one's life to modify stressors or control stress responses. **Relaxation** is a state of reduced physical and mental arousal. It is an important intervention because it reverses some stress responses. By elongating muscle fibers, relaxation reduces neural impulses sent to the brain and decreases the activity of the brain and other body systems. Blood pressure, heart rate, respiratory rate, and oxygen consumption decrease, while peripheral skin temperatures and brain alpha wave activity increase.

Many of the techniques in this section are complementary or alternative therapies that require special training, and which are discussed in detail in other chapters. If you would like to have detailed information about CAM, refer to Chapter 46. For 12 weeks of daily suggestions for coping with stress,

 Go to Chapter 12, **Tables, Boxes, Figures: ESG Box 12-1,** on DavisPlus.

Exercise   Exercise is used to treat, as well as prevent stress. It reduces stress because it releases tension held in muscles, improves muscle tone and posture, expresses emotions, and stimulates the secretion of endorphins, thus creating a feeling of well-being and relaxation.

Relaxation Techniques   Relaxation techniques involve teaching the patient to relax individual muscle groups. **Progressive relaxation** in a quiet meditation state or lying in bed, relaxing and contracting muscle groups is much less traumatic and damaging to fragile joints and muscles than active exercise. Therefore, it may be used even by people who are not in good health. **Passive relaxation**, in which the person relaxes the muscle groups without first contracting them, is even less traumatic and requires even less energy.

Meditation   Managing stress through meditation involves heightening one's attention or awareness. Regular

Complementary & Alternative Modalities (CAM)

Using CAM for Stress Reduction

Barrett, B., Muller, H. M., Ward, A., et al. (2012). Meditation or exercise for preventing acute respiratory infection: A randomized controlled trial. *Annals of Family Medicine, 10(4),* 337–463.

In a study designed to evaluate the potential preventive effects of meditation or exercise, 154 adults 50 years and older were randomized to one of three groups: (1) those who received an 8-week training course in mindful meditation to reduce stress; (2) a matched group involved in an 8-week training course in moderate-intensity and sustained exercise; and (3) an observational group. Researchers found fewer episodes and reduced severity of acute respiratory infection (ARI) in the meditation and exercise groups.

Gaylord, S. A., Paisson, O. S., Garland, El. L., et al. (2011). Mindfulness training reduces the severity of irritable bowel syndrome in women: Results of a randomized controlled trial. *The American Journal of Gastroenterology, 106(9),* 1678–1688.

This article reports on the successful use of alternative and complementary therapies as adjunct therapies to decrease the severity of symptoms during episodes of irritable bowel syndrome in women, often triggered by stress. Researchers found that women who trained for 8 weeks in mindfulness meditation rated their IBS symptoms as less than did women who participated in an IBS support group. The groups did not differ in quality of life, psychological stress, or anxiety related to GI sensations.

Kiecolt-Glaser, J. K., Christian, L., Preston, H., et al. (2010). Stress, inflammation, and yoga practice. *Psychosomatic Medicine, 72(2),* 113–121.

Researchers interested in the benefit of yoga to cope with stress studied the body chemistry of women practicing yoga at least twice weekly. They found markers for inflammation to be five times higher in yoga novices or those not performing yoga. Yoga experts had lower heart rates when facing stress events than did those learning yoga. Mood was also more positive in both yoga novice and expert groups than in those using other interventions (walking, video).

meditation increases harmony among mind, body, and spirit, thereby reducing anxiety and giving the person control. See Chapter 42 for further information. For a script to lead a client through a guided meditation to reduce stress,

 Go to Chapter 12, **Tables, Boxes, Figures: ESG Box 12-2, Script for Visualization,** on Davis*Plus*.

Visualization or Imagery Visualization (imagery) techniques are often used to complement the effects of relaxation techniques. They are explained in Chapter 46.

Biofeedback Techniques of biofeedback use electronic instruments to measure neuromuscular and autonomic nervous system activity and provide information about those responses to the person. The immediate feedback helps the person become aware of and learn how to voluntarily control certain physiological responses, such as those produced by stress (Olson, 2003). Biofeedback practitioners require special training, and most are credentialed in biofeedback. For more information, see Chapter 46.

Acupuncture Acupuncture involves insertion of a needle into "meridian points" to regulate the flow of energy or life force throughout the body. It can modify pain perception and restore normal physiological functions (e.g., decrease the heart rate). Special training is required to use this intervention (see Chapter 31).

Chiropractic Adjustment Misalignment of the vertebrae is thought to lead to pain, loss of function, and illness. Chiropractic adjustment is the manual realignment of the vertebrae to free energy, release muscle tension, and improve body function and health. Chiropractors undergo special education and training before they are qualified to perform adjustments. See Chapter 46 for more information.

Touch Therapies Healing touch, Reiki, and **therapeutic touch** are focused on energy modulation. Healing energy is channeled through a practitioner's hands to improve well-being, reduce pain, and accelerate healing. Further studies are needed for use in children and conditions other than pain (So, Jiang, & Qin, 2008, online 2012, August 15). See Chapters 31 and 46 for more information.

Massage Through manipulation of the soft tissues, massage relaxes muscles, releases body tension, improves circulation, and allows energy and blood to flow through muscles and soft tissues more readily. See Chapters 31 and 42 for more information. For instructions on how to give a back rub,

 Go to Chapter 34, **Procedure 34–1: Giving a Back Massage,** in Volume 2.

Reflexology Reflexology is the application of pressure to specific points on the feet, hands, or ears, which are thought to correspond with certain organs of the body. The goal is to relieve blockage, promote the flow of energy, and reduce tension—thus, reflexology may be helpful in treating stress-related illnesses. Reflexology requires special training. See Chapter 46 for more information.

The following are simpler activities you can recommend to most clients to aid in relaxation and stress reduction:

- **Humor.** Laughter releases endorphins and relieves feelings of stress (Fig. 12-7). It enhances respiration and circulation, oxygenates the blood, suppresses the stress-related hormones in the brain, and activates the immune system. Some medical centers have begun implementing in-house humor programs (Bennett & Lengacher, 2007; Cousins, 1979; du Pré, 1998; Johnson, 2002).
- **Listening to Music.** Music soothes and relaxes when its vibrations are in harmony with body frequencies. Listening to tranquil music can also relax the mind.
- **Engaging in Art Activities.** Painting, working with clay, and engaging in other art activities help to express emotions and release endorphins.
- **Dance and Sports.** Like other forms of exercise, movement and physical activity release pent-up physical tension and emotions. Steady-state exercises, such as running or swimming at a consistent pace, offer stress relief in a meditative manner through sustained deep breathing and repetitive motion. Physical activity can also enhance self-esteem and help people feel better by the simple act of accomplishing a personal goal.
- **Journal Writing.** Expressive writing can help a person reduce stress and anxiety by venting emotion and reflecting on experiences. Journaling can provide insights into causes of stress and ways to modify stressors.

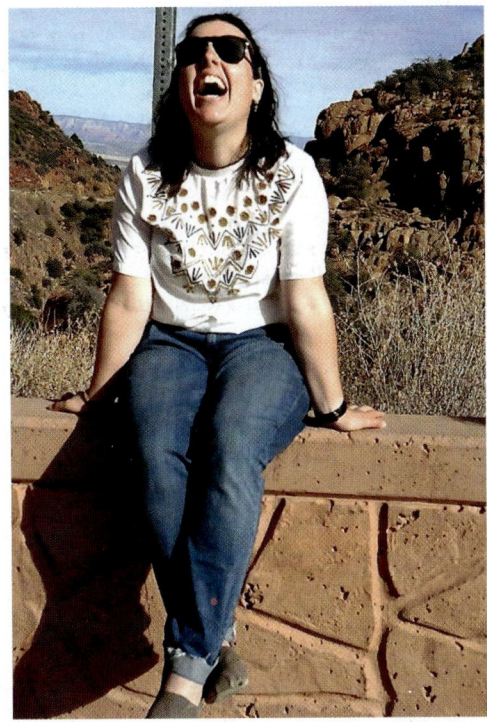

FIGURE 12-7 Laughter releases endorphins and helps relieve stress.

Changing Perception of Stressors or Self

Recall that altering one's perception is one way to improve adaptation to stress. For clients who have an unrealistic perception of the stressor and can imagine only negative outcomes, a technique, called **cognitive restructuring**, may be helpful. With this technique, you help clients to recognize their negative focus and to restructure their thinking in more positive and realistic ways. For example, you might encourage a working mother with demanding family members to take a single positive step, such as saying no to someone at least once a day.

You can also help clients to identify positive aspects of themselves and their coping abilities. This promotes self-esteem and helps them to recognize and use the resources they have for coping with their stressors. **Positive self-talk** is another method for increasing self-esteem. Each time you hear negative self-talk, stop the client, and ask him to rephrase the statement so that it is positive.

Identifying and Using Support Systems

You can facilitate successful adaptation by helping clients to identify and contact people and groups who offer various supports (e.g., listening, encouragement, advice, problem-solving, help with household tasks, financial support). Be aware of the groups available in your community (e.g., Weight Watchers, Alcoholics Anonymous, Parents Without Partners, Reach for Recovery). You may need to teach socialization skills to clients who are socially isolated so that they can begin to build a support system.

Reducing the Stress of Hospitalization

Illness and hospitalization are stressful for patients and their families. In addition to being sick, patients find themselves in unfamiliar surroundings, with little privacy, and a certain loss of control. Promote patient-centered care in the healthcare agency as much as you can. Involving patients and families actively in their care helps them adapt to the stressors of hospitalization. Teach patients what to expect from hospitalization, and give them a few tips to help plan ahead to minimize the stress they experience (See Self-Care: Teaching Clients How to Reduce the Stress of Hospitalization).

Providing Spiritual Support

In addition to helping clients obtain spiritual support from church groups and clergy, you can help to strengthen the client spiritually. You may wish to:

- Pray for or with clients, if they desire, and if you are comfortable doing so. Prayer can help reduce their feelings of powerlessness and loneliness.
- Help clients to define their values and set boundaries that honor themselves and uphold those values.
- Teach clients to silently recite an affirming mantra (e.g., on inhalation, say, "I am free." Exhale and say, "Stress, leave me.")

For other ways to provide spiritual support, see Chapter 16.

Self-Care

Teaching Clients How to Reduce the Stress of Hospitalization

Share the following tips with clients, preferably before hospitalization:

- ➤ Bring what you need from home. Make a list of necessities and pack carefully before you go. For example, bring your own soap, toothpaste, lotion, pajamas, and slippers—or your favorite tea bags and sweetener. Having familiar things can make your stay more pleasant for you.

- ➤ If you will feel well enough, bring your computer, reading material, crossword puzzles, or whatever you like to do that can help prevent boredom and depression. You might want to bring a few family photos for your nightstand.

- ➤ Bring a notepad and pencils so that you can take notes about what your primary care providers tell you (e.g., about diagnostic tests, instructions for care, and so on).

- ➤ Do *not* bring jewelry, cash, credit cards, or other valuables.

- ➤ Do not bring clothing that is not washable or that is uncomfortable or tight.

- ➤ Do not allow family or friends to visit if they are ill.

- ➤ It helps to ask family or friends to stay at the bedside, particularly when the physician is "making rounds." They can advocate for you and help you feel confident that everything will go well. You may not feel well enough to ask for what you need, but a family member can do that for you.

- ➤ Your family members or friends can also help you interpret and remember information and instructions that you will receive from nurses, physicians, and other care providers. There may be 30 people in your room each day, and when you are ill or taking certain medications it is hard to keep track of everything.

- ➤ Keep a bottle of hand sanitizer by your bed or insist visitors, including family members and care providers, use a hand hygiene product at the door when entering the room, just as you do.

- ➤ Know the name of your primary nurse (or nurses) on each shift, and ask as many questions as you need to.

- ➤ Even though some things seem to not make sense (e.g., taking your temperature at 3 a.m.), there is likely a medical reason for it. Try to be as patient and cheerful as possible.

Crisis Intervention

As an entry-level nurse in acute and ambulatory care settings, you are more likely to see patients in the first three phases of crisis and not be present for the adaptive and postcrisis stages. The goals of crisis intervention at an entry level of practice include the following (Brammer & MacDonald, 2003; Neeb, 2006):

1. Assess the situation.
2. Ensure the patient's safety.
3. Defuse the situation.
4. Decrease the person's anxiety.
5. Determine the problem.

6. Decide on the type of help needed.
7. Return the person to precrisis level of functioning.

For further explanation and to learn how to intervene when a patient is in crisis,

 Go to Chapter 12, **Clinical Insight 12-2: Crisis Intervention Guidelines,** in Volume 2.

Crisis centers often rely on telephone counseling ("hotlines"). If telephone counseling is not adequate, or if observations of the home environment are needed, home visits may be necessary.

KnowledgeCheck 12-10
- Describe at least five specific interventions for dealing with an angry person.
- What is cognitive restructuring?
- What is the purpose of positive self-talk?
- List the seven steps of crisis intervention.
- Why is relaxation an important stress intervention?

Stress Management in the Workplace
You will need to pay attention to your feelings, your body, and your personal responses to stress. Do you notice that you are eating more than usual or have lost your appetite? Are you feeling edgy or impatient with family or coworkers, or not sleeping well? Check your body. Do you feel tired or often have headaches or gastrointestinal distress? Are the muscles in your face and shoulders tense? Do you often take work home with you? Are you unable to stop thinking about work, even when you are at home? Do concerns about finances or personal situations consume your thinking and create a sense of doom? If so, you probably need to start managing your stress. You can better manage workplace stress and avoid burnout by following the advice you give your patients. For some tips,

 Go to Chapter 12, **Tables, Boxes, Figures: ESG Box 12-1,** on DavisPlus.

When stressors arise from the workplace, the following actions are especially important:

- Set realistic expectations of yourself and others. Don't be overcritical; most people, including you, are doing the best they can.
- Ask for help. Seeking the support of others does not indicate weakness or incompetence. It can even make others feel good by giving them an opportunity to practice collegiality.
- Offer support to colleagues who need help with tasks or with their feelings. This adds to the overall good feeling on a unit and improves the efficiency of performing many tasks.
- Be proactive about the things you can change and accept the things that you cannot change. Get involved in constructive efforts to change a particular stressor (e.g., staffing, overtime, and safety practices). If you cannot effect the changes, and if you cannot accept

things as they are, you may need to think about removing yourself from the situation. Complaining and negative talk add to your own stress and that of others.
- Join and support professional organizations that address workplace issues (e.g., the National Student Nurses Association [NSNA] and the ANA).
- Strive for balance in these six key areas: family, financial responsibilities, health, social contributions, career, vocation or education, and spirituality or faith. Focus on the most important items and task; remember, work affects life, but your life also affects your work.
- Obtain counseling for stress that exceeds your ability to cope.

Making Referrals
This chapter has presented many assessments and interventions for reducing stress. Remember, though, you are not yet an expert nurse and no one, not even an experienced nurse, is an expert in all areas. It is important not to "get in over your head" with clients who are under stress and showing maladaptive coping. You can help by recognizing your limitations and by referring the client to the appropriate professionals as needed (e.g., a spiritual leader, a counselor, a social worker, a practitioner of complementary therapies, a physician, a psychologist, or a psychiatrist).

 ThinkLike a Nurse 12-5

Sally is an RN seeking employment at a local nursing home. She left her previous employer because of stress and frustration with agency policy, for which the bottom line was financial gain rather than quality patient care. What can Sally do to help ensure that she will not experience the same problem in the new agency?

 To explore learning resources for this chapter,

 Go to DavisPlus at **DavisPl.us/Wilkinson3.**

Chapter Resources for Chapter 12:
    Response sheets for all learning activities
    Resources for Caregivers and Health Professionals
    Reading More About Stress & Adaptation (suggested readings)
    Concept Map of chapter content
Interactive Case Studies
NCLEX-Style and Chapter Review Questions
Chapter Overview Podcasts

For references cited in this chapter,

 Go to Volume 2, **References Cited.**

 Bibliography: Go to Volume 2, **Bibliography.**

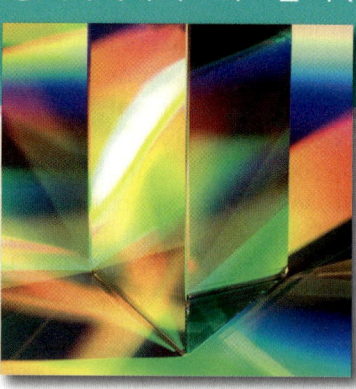

CHAPTER 13

Psychosocial Health & Illness

Learning Outcomes

After completing this chapter, you should be able to:

➤ Explain the relationship of psychosocial factors to overall health and development.

➤ Identify the factors that influence the development and stability of self-concept.

➤ List the four interrelated components of self-concept.

➤ Develop a nursing care plan for patients exhibiting disturbances in self-concept and self-esteem.

➤ Identify nursing diagnoses, outcomes, and interventions specific to body image disturbance.

➤ Describe interventions for preventing depersonalization.

➤ List the psychological and physiological effects of anxiety.

➤ Recognize the levels and symptoms of anxiety that are severe enough to merit referral to a mental health professional.

➤ Devise a nursing care plan for the nursing diagnosis of Anxiety.

➤ Differentiate between mild depression and that which should be referred to a mental health professional.

➤ Assess older adults for manifestations of depression.

➤ Plan outcomes and nursing interventions for patients who are depressed.

➤ Plan outcomes and nursing interventions for patients with a diagnosis of Risk for Suicide.

Key Concepts

Anxiety

Depression

Psychosocial health

Self-concept

Related Concepts

See the Concept Map on Davis*Plus*.

Example Problems

Anxiety

Depression

Self-concept disturbances

Low self-esteem

Meet Your Patient

You are caring for a 16-year-old patient named Karli who is suffering from fractures to both arms and several ribs, as well as extensive first- and second-degree burns to 30% of her body, following a motor vehicle accident. Karli was driving her parents' car home from her part-time job when she lost control of the car and crashed into a wall. The car exploded in flames. A passerby quickly reported the accident, and fast action by the emergency response team saved Karli's life.

Karli is suffering from a moderate amount of shock and pain. She alternates among outbursts of anger, self-directed sarcasm, and despondence. She tells you that she cannot understand how the accident happened, that one moment she was adjusting the car radio, and the next moment she awoke in the hospital. Then suddenly she explodes. "It's not fair! I just took my eyes off the road for a second; that's all!"

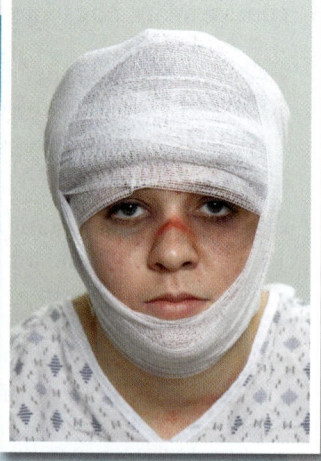

She bursts into tears. Picking at her bandages, she sobs, "No one will ever love me the way I'm going to look. My life is over. I hate myself! You take her hand. "I used to be pretty," she says, "but now I'll look like a freak! What did I do to deserve this? I know plenty of kids who drive drunk or high all the time. I wasn't doing anything wrong! Why did this happen to me?"

Before reading on, jot down a list of the multiple physical, psychological, and social issues that you would need to consider in developing a comprehensive care plan for Karli. You can revisit your list throughout this chapter to compare your answers.

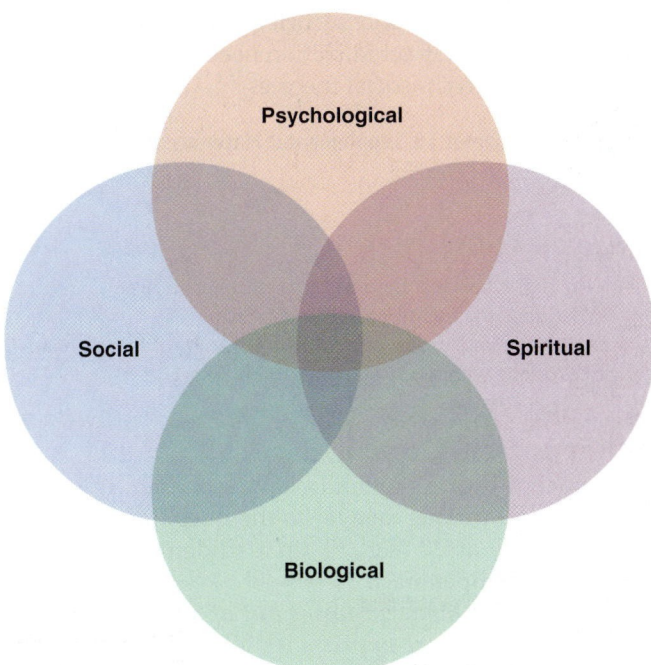

FIGURE 13-1 In the biopsychosocial view of health, biological, psychological, social, and spiritual factors interact to contribute to health.

ThinkLike a Nurse 13-1

Review Chapter 9 as needed.

- What theoretical knowledge about Karli's developmental stage will assist you in determining nursing diagnoses, interventions, and outcomes?
- Considering that Karli will need a significant amount of assistance for activities of daily living (ADLs) because of her fractures and burns, how might you use the time to develop your therapeutic relationship?

ABOUT THE KEY CONCEPTS

This chapter introduces you to the key concepts of **psychosocial health, self-concept, anxiety,** and **depression**. As you study the related topics and terms in the chapter, you will gain a more complete understanding of the four key concepts. All of these will help you organize the content in your memory.

Theoretical Knowledge
knowing why

This chapter is designed to help you provide basic psychosocial care for patients in general practice settings.

PSYCHOSOCIAL HEALTH

The interactions of the mind and body are continuous and complex. One of the strengths of nursing is that we can go beyond a *biomedical* (disease-oriented) focus to care for the whole person. Nurses recognize that patient responses to illness are influenced not only by the physical pathology but also by the person's psychosocial health and its relationship to her overall wellness.

The term *psychosocial* encompasses both psychological and social factors: A person's psychological state interacts with his social development and position within society to contribute to his overall—or biopsychosocial—well-being (Fig. 13-1). Figure 13-2 illustrates the interlocking psychosocial influences on health and personal development.

Keep in mind that any human dimension may dominate health needs at a given time. For example, a patient suffering from a severe flare-up of psoriasis (a skin disease characterized by red, scaly patches) may require physiological interventions during the acute stage. He may not be ready to deal with body image issues (psychological dimension) until his skin lesions are better. Remember, though, that your patients' psychosocial needs are just as important as, for example, their dietary requirements or their level of pain.

What Is Psychosocial Theory?

You can think of **psychosocial theory** as a method of understanding people as a combination of psychological and social events. Of the many theories of psychosocial

development, the works of the German psychologist Erik Erikson (1902–1994) are foremost. Using Erikson's theory, you can assess for successful completion of developmental tasks. Refer to Chapter 9 for more information about Erikson's theory. For a summary of developmental tasks,

 Go to Chapter 13, **Tables, Boxes, Figures: ESG Table 13-1**, on *DavisPlus*.

Chapter 12 presents another important psychosocial theory that is relevant for healthcare providers: psychologist Abraham Maslow's theory of self-actualization and self-transcendence. Maslow (1968) developed a widely accepted hierarchy of human needs and motivations, in which essential needs (e.g., air, water, and food) must be met before higher needs (e.g., learning, creating, understanding, and self-fulfillment). Recall that, in order from most basic to highest need, Maslow's hierarchy includes

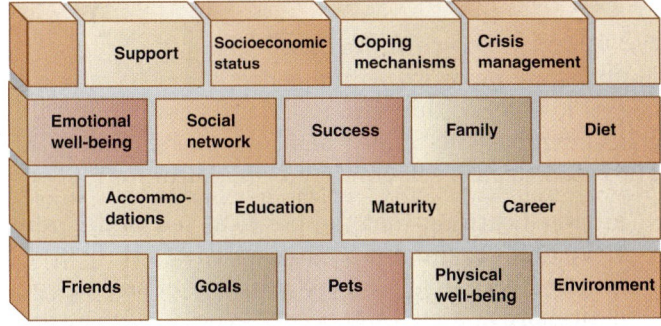

FIGURE 13-2 Interlocking psychosocial influences.

physiological, safety and security, love and belonging, self-esteem, and self-actualization needs. For more information about psychosocial theories,

 Go to Chapter 13, **Supplemental Materials: Psychosocial Theory,** on Davis*Plus*.

KnowledgeCheck 13-1

- Why is psychosocial theory relevant to healthcare?
- What does the term *biopsychosocial* mean?
- Explain the implication of Maslow's hierarchy of human needs for working with a homeless man with gangrene.

What Is Self-Concept?

Self-concept is one's overall view of oneself. It is your complete and unique answer to the question, "Who do you think you are?" (e.g., "I am a student"; "I am successful and competent").

Key Point: *Self-concept forms out of a person's evaluation of his physical appearance, sexual performance, intellectual abilities, success in the workplace, friendship and approval from others, problem-solving and coping abilities, unique talents, and so on. A person with a healthy self-concept has a mostly positive perception of these evaluations of self.*

Self-concept both influences and is influenced by social functioning. For example, Karli's self-concept is that she is no longer pretty and that she "looks like a freak." If this self-concept continues, it may cause her to withdraw from social interaction and make it difficult to form new relationships (social functioning). Equally, if others—for example, prospective employers—*do* see her as hideously ugly, she may have difficulty finding a place in society.

The "Dynamic Self" The self forms and changes in response to our environment.

Anthropologist Margaret Mead (1934) states that we discover who we are through a lifelong process of differentiating from and comparing our self to others. As we experience life events, we continually reconstruct and develop our understanding of who we are. Dickstein (1977) called this idea the **dynamic self,** meaning that who we are (the self) is subject to change through social and environmental influence. But if our concept of self is changeable, what factors cause it to change? Can it be harmed, and how? And how does it first develop? These questions are explored next.

How Is Self-Concept Formed?

Humans are not born with a concept of self; rather, it begins to develop during infancy and childhood as the child interacts with family members, peers, and others. The broad steps of self-concept formation are as follows:

- Infant—Learning that the physical self is different from the environment: "me; not me."
- Child—Internalizing others' attitudes about the self, primarily parents and peers: "Who do *they* say that I am?"

Child and adult—Internalizing standards of society: "How do I compare to others?"
Adult—Self-actualization and self-adjustment: "This *is* who I am and who I will continue to be."

Change occurs gradually, and the steps overlap. Also, the age at which the stages occur varies widely among individuals. For a summary of the growth of self-concept through the various developmental stages,

 Go to Chapter 13, **Tables, Boxes, Figures: ESGTable 13-2,** Development of Self-Concept on Davis*Plus*.

 ## ThinkLike a Nurse 13-2

- Explain how each of Maslow's five basic needs is related to psychosocial development; that is, how might each of the needs affect psychosocial health if met or not met?
- To what extent do social relationships help or hinder a person in meeting each need?

What Factors Affect a Person's Self-Concept?

Some factors affecting a person's self-concept cannot be changed, for example, gender and developmental level. Others, such as socioeconomic status and family relationships, can be changed to a degree, but are not fully under the person's control—and certainly not during childhood, when the self-concept is forming. Understanding that such factors are not within a patient's control may help you provide more sensitive, compassionate care to patients experiencing impaired self-concept.

Gender

Certain aspects of self-concept differ by gender. Some of the differences appear to be related to the role expectations of boys and girls rather than any actual difference in ability. For example,

Girls typically rate teamwork and cooperation as important to their sense of self, whereas most boys place a higher value on individual achievement.
Physical appearance seems more important to girls, and they may be less satisfied and more self-conscious throughout life because of this.
As role expectations and career choices for both men and women expand, these gender-based differences in self-concept may fade.

Developmental Level

As we mature, our self-concept becomes more inner-guided. That is, others (e.g., friends, the media) have less influence on our ideas about who we are. We become less likely to view our failures and shortcomings as evidence of worthlessness and more likely to see them as challenges common to humans everywhere.

Family and Peer Relationships

The family strongly influences a child's developing self-concept. As an infant's sense of self permanence develops and becomes stable, categories of self begin to emerge. These include notions of gender, values, and a sense of having a distinct "place" among family members (Feiring & Taska, as cited in Bracken, 1996). Social identity is first fostered by interactions between infants and their parents and broadens in toddlerhood through relationships with siblings, grandparents, and extended family members. For older children, peers become more important than family in this respect.

Locus of Control

Whereas the preceding external influences contribute to the *formation* of our self-concept, internal influences help us to *moderate* it. For example, biochemical brain processes influence perceptual acuity, interpretation abilities, and level of insight and judgment.

- **Internal Locus of Control.** People who allow their inner "voice" to influence their self-concept have what is called an **internal locus of control**. Such people feel they can exert control over their lives. They take appropriate responsibility for their life experiences and for their responses to them. This enables them to interpret unexpected adverse events (e.g., injuries and illnesses) in a more positive light.
- **External Locus of Control.** In contrast, people who have an **external locus of control** attribute control of their situation to factors outside themselves, including other people, institutions, and God. They may feel they lack the ability to change what happens to them.

KnowledgeCheck 13-2

- When does self-concept become stable?
- What factors have been determined to have an impact on our self-concept?

What Are the Components of Self-Concept?

Self-concept embraces four interrelated components: body image, role performance, personal identity, and self-esteem.

Body Image

How often do you hear someone say something like the following?

"Look at the muscles on that man. He looks good!"
"Look at her pigging out. She needs that candy like I need a hole in my head."

You probably grew up overhearing similar statements. Such preoccupations with food, weight, and appearance have led to a prejudice against people who do not have perfect bodies. No wonder people engage in unhealthy behaviors in order to be thin or that patients like Karli have difficulty coping with disfiguring accidents or with surgeries such as limb amputation and mastectomy.

Body image is your mental image of your physical self, including physical appearance and physical functioning. Both cognitive understanding and sensory input influence body image. Our cognitive understanding is in turn influenced by family, social, ethnic, and cultural norms; education; and exposure to alternative values. The American media portray the ideal male as young, tall, and muscular; nevertheless, many older, short, slender men maintain a positive body image because their cognitive understanding indicates they are in good health, are attractive to their partners, and so on.

Ideal, Perceived, and Actual Body Image People do not always see their own bodies as objectively as others see them. Some psychological disorders interfere with the ability to interpret sensory data objectively. For example, people with the eating disorders anorexia nervosa and bulimia nervosa see themselves as fat even when their mirror reflects, and other people see, a normal or even an emaciated body. The closer the match between a person's ideal body image and sensory input about his or her body (perceived body image), the more positive the person's body image is likely to be.

For Janalee, thick, luxurious hair is an important component of her ideal body image. Amy hardly thinks about her hair at all; she keeps it very short so that it is easy to care for. Both women have been receiving chemotherapy to treat their cancer, and both are experiencing severe hair loss. Which person do you think will be more likely to experience body image disturbance because of this?

Appearance and Function Influence Body Image Not surprisingly, a physical disability, such as blindness, deafness, or paraplegia, can interfere with the development of a positive body image. Children born with a physical disability are at risk for poor self-concept and depression. Risks are partially created by social values and the child's resulting difficulty in forming adequate social relationships, but it may also relate to the person's perception that he has low social value. In contrast, an attractive appearance and superior functioning, whether in a career, sports, or academics, make it easier to develop a positive body image. Nevertheless, cognitive understanding can increase self-concept even in people who are average in appearance or achievement. For instance, people of average appearance who learn to value integrity, honesty, teamwork, and other social values equally with physical attractiveness or success in sports are less likely to suffer from body image disturbance.

Gradual Versus Sudden Body Changes Gradual changes in physical appearance occur naturally throughout life as the body matures and grows old. Most people adapt to such changes relatively easily, especially because their friends and colleagues are aging, too. In contrast, when changes in appearance or functioning occur abruptly (e.g., following an acute illness or an accident, as happened to your patient, Karli), they are much more difficult to accept. Denial, anger, self-hatred, and despair are a few of many reactions that can follow such an abrupt change in body image.

Influence of Body Image on Health Body image influences health and health behaviors. A negative body image has been associated with:

- Depression (Cargill, Clark, Pera, et al., 2012; McCabe & Ricciardelli, 2012; Muehlenkamp, & Brausch, 2012)
- Initiation of smoking among adolescents (Cargill, Clark, Pera, et al., 2012)
- Increased risk for unintended pregnancy and sexually transmitted infections, including HIV infection (Larson, Clark, Robinson, et al., 2012; Woertman & van den Brink, 2012)
- Increased incidence of being bullied (Brixval, Rayce, Rasmussen, et al., 2012)

In contrast, a positive body image was found to be a major contributor to overall life happiness in adult women (Walters-Brown & Hall, 2012). There is not yet enough evidence to determine how much of the effect is due to body image alone and how much to body image in combination with other psychosocial issues.

Role Performance

Before you began your nursing program, what were your expectations? What activities did you imagine yourself engaged in, and what behaviors did you think would be expected of you? Together, these expectations make up your conception of the *role* of nursing student. In addition to being a student, you probably play several roles, such as parent, sibling, friend, breadwinner, caregiver, volunteer, and so on.

Role performance can be defined as the actions a person takes and the behaviors he demonstrates in fulfilling a role. Instead of expectations, role performance is the reality. If you expected that you would sail through your nursing program and instead you find yourself so overwhelmed that lately you have begun to skip classes, then you are experiencing **role strain**, a mismatch between role expectations and role performance. In addition, your ideas about how to perform the nursing student role may be very different from those of your instructors. When that type of mismatch occurs, you are experiencing an **interpersonal role conflict**. Other types of role conflict are also common. For instance, what if you are a single parent and your child's sudden illness causes you to miss a week of classes and clinicals? When two roles make competing demands on an individual, **interrole conflict** occurs.

Personal Identity

How would you describe yourself to others? Make a list of 10 words or short phrases that describe who you are (e.g., student, motorcycle rider, woman). Then list them in order, with the most important one first. Are you happy with your list? Are you satisfied with who you are? Compare your list with a friend's list. Could you identify her based on her list of identifying labels? Could she identify you?

Your **personal identity** is your view of yourself as a unique human being, different and separate from all others. Identity develops over time, beginning in childhood when you identified with your parents, and then later with teachers, peers, and others. Unlike body image, which is expected to change over time, personal identity is relatively constant and consistent. It is culturally determined and learned through socialization.

People with a strong sense of personal identity are less likely to compare themselves to others or to be unduly influenced by them. They tend to appreciate the unique perspective and contributions of others, yet value their own perspectives and contributions. In contrast, people with a weak sense of personal identity have difficulty distinguishing their boundaries from those of others. They may interpret events in the environment personally, or they may interpret their personal experiences as belonging to everyone. For example, a patient with a weak personal identity may insist that a breakdown in the hospital's air-conditioning system is a punishment for his complaint that his room was too cold.

Patients may experience an impaired sense of identity when they are challenged by a serious or chronic illness (e.g., cancer, AIDS, or rheumatoid arthritis). They then place too many limitations on their activities or interpret the responses of others in light of their illness. For instance, a woman with osteoporosis (loss of bone density) might say, "I used to enjoy going bird-watching, but I don't go anymore because I might trip and fall."

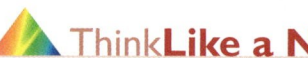

ThinkLike a Nurse 13-3

Think about Karli in the Meet Your Patient scenario. If you asked Karli to list 10 labels to identify herself, what do you think they would be? (You may not have enough information to come up with 10, but think of as many as you can.)

Self-Esteem

Self-esteem is, in the simplest terms, how well a person likes himself. It is the difference between the "ideal self" and "actual self," that is, between "what I think I ought (or want) to be" and "what I really am." The area of overlap in Figure 13-3 illustrates the extent of self-esteem. The more overlap there is, the higher the self-esteem.

The balance between our self-expectations and our true abilities can be precarious. When we succeed beyond our ambitions, we experience a high sense of self-esteem; but when we aim for an ideal self beyond our capabilities, we risk loss of self-esteem.

It is not difficult to imagine how a sudden, disfiguring accident such as Karli's might provoke a crisis in self-esteem, because Karli's ideal self is currently out of her reach. Even mild illnesses and minor setbacks can cause some people to question their self-worth. This is especially true if the problem is interpreted as one incident in a continuing pattern—for example, a couple hoping to become parents who experience a third pregnancy loss.

As another example, if as a nursing student you find that you are more successful than you expected to be when you enrolled in your nursing program, that is a

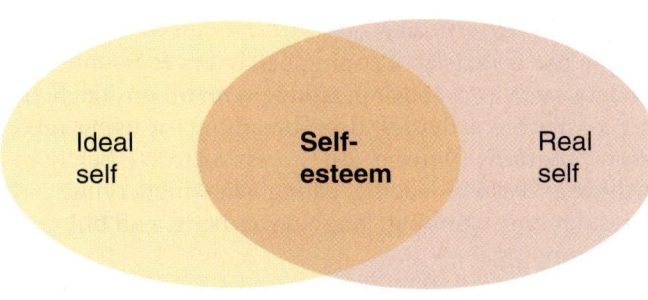

Ideal self: expectations and aspirations; "what I ought to be," "what I wish I were"

Real self: current skills, attributes, and successes; "what I really am"

FIGURE 13-3 Self-esteem is determined by the relationship between an individual's ideal self and real self.

boost to your self-esteem. If, however, your expectations of being a skillful nurse outweigh your current abilities, then lower self-esteem is likely.

 Think**Like a Nurse** 13-4

What if a person does not have any aspirations to success, but is content to meet each day as a learner, vitalized by her daily discoveries? How do you think a high score on an exam would affect her self-esteem? How do you think a poor score on a clinical skills test would affect her self-esteem?

KnowledgeCheck 13-3

- What four components contribute to an individual's self-concept?
- What is self-esteem?

PSYCHOSOCIAL ILLNESS: ANXIETY AND DEPRESSION

Think about the advertisements you've seen recently on TV or in newspapers and magazines. How many times do you recall seeing an ad for a medication for anxiety or depression? These two problems are not confined to mental health settings. They are woven into the fabric of our everyday lives. As a nurse, you should be prepared to recognize and provide care for anxious and depressed patients in all practice settings.

Example Problem: Anxiety

I wake up in the middle of the night with a knot in my stomach and thinking about work. I go over and over my day and worry about my decisions and what I should have done instead. I replay the meetings in my head and think, "I know what that person said, but what did she mean by that?" I wonder whether I can handle the responsibility. My neck and shoulders are so tense that I get headaches. But when I try to relax and watch TV, I can feel my heart racing, and I feel shaky. I can't concentrate well enough to read.

Anxiety is a common emotional response to a stressor. It is a "vague, uneasy feeling of discomfort or dread accompanied by an autonomic response (the source often nonspecific or unknown to the individual); a feeling of apprehension caused by anticipation of danger. It is an alerting signal that warns of impending danger and enables the individual to take measures to deal with threat" (NANDA International, 2012 p. 344). An anxious person worries; feels nervous, uneasy, and fearful; may be tearful; and often has physical symptoms such as nausea, trembling, and sweating. Anxiety and fear produce similar responses; however, some experts differentiate them as follows:

Fear is a specific, cognitive response to a known threat. It is related to a present event, either physical *or* psychological.

Anxiety is a vague, emotional response to a known or unknown threat. It is related to anticipation of a future event and is the result of psychological conflict rather than physical threat.

Key Point: *Anxiety is so common that mild anxiety is considered normal and even necessary for our survival. No matter what area of nursing you work in, nearly every patient you meet will have at least some degree of anxiety. Chronic anxiety has been associated with physical problems, such as the risk of heart attack (Compare, Germani, Proietti, et al., 2011; Wittstein, 2010).*

Patients encounter anxiety-producing situations in healthcare settings because of threats to their basic needs (Stuart, 2012). Consider the following examples:

- Physiological—anxiety in anticipation of or in response to a diagnosis of cancer
- Safety and security—an upcoming surgery or diagnostic test, such as cardiac catheterization
- Love and belonging—anxiety over potential or actual loss of a loved one
- Esteem—anxiety over potential or actual loss of ability or appearance
- Self-actualization—anxiety over lack of self-fulfillment

Levels of Anxiety

Anxiety ranges from normal to abnormal, depending on its **intensity** and **duration**—how much anxiety is present and how long it has been present.

- **Normal anxiety** is an essential reaction to a realistic danger or threat to our physical or psychological integrity. In other words, it enables us to survive and, when the threat is no longer present, to move on. For example, anxiety when hiking on a rocky and narrow mountain trail heightens your awareness and quickens your responses, thereby reducing the likelihood of falls.
- **Abnormal anxiety** is out of proportion to the situation and lasts long after the threat is over, perhaps causing the person to alter her lifestyle. For example,

after breaking her ankle in a fall down a short flight of stairs, a young woman moves to a ground-floor apartment. Five years later, she still refuses to use stairs.

You should determine a patient's level of anxiety as accurately as possible because each requires different nursing actions. Peplau (1963) described the four levels found in Table 13-1.

Coping With Anxiety

People use a variety of coping behaviors to relieve mild anxiety, such as exercising, talking with others, engaging in pleasurable activities, deep-breathing, or using relaxation programs (Bourne, 2011). Less adaptive behaviors include excessive sleeping, eating, smoking, crying, pacing, fidgeting, drinking, laughing, cursing, nail biting, or finger tapping.

Table 13-1 ➤ Levels of Anxiety

DEFINITION OR DESCRIPTION	SYMPTOMS
Mild Anxiety	
This is normal anxiety, experienced in response to the events of day-to-day living. It heightens perception, sharpens the senses, enhances learning, and enables the person to function at his optimal level.	If present, symptoms may include muscle tension, restlessness, irritability, and a sense of unease. The person usually does not experience distress.
Moderate Anxiety	
As anxiety increases, the perceptual field narrows, and the person begins to focus on self and the need to relieve his discomfort.	■ Less alert to environmental events ■ Distracts easily ■ Shorter attention span ■ May need help with problem-solving but can attend to his needs with direction ■ Physical symptoms may include: 　Increased heart and respiratory rates 　Increased perspiration 　Gastric discomfort 　Increased muscle tension ■ Rapid, loud, and higher pitched speech
Severe Anxiety	
Perceptual field is so narrow that the person can focus on only one particular detail or may shift focus to many extraneous details. Focus is totally on self and the need to relieve the anxiety.	■ Concentration and attention span are severely limited, so the person has difficulty completing simple tasks. ■ Anxiety prevents problem-solving and learning. ■ May report feelings of dread, confusion, and other unpleasant emotions. ■ Physical symptoms may include headaches, palpitations, tachycardia, insomnia, dizziness, nausea, trembling, hyperventilation, urinary frequency, and diarrhea.
Panic Anxiety	
The person becomes unreasonable and irrational and is unable to focus on even one detail in the environment. He may misperceive environmental cues or lose contact with reality (e.g., experience hallucinations or delusions).	■ May react wildly (e.g., shouting, screaming, running about, clinging to something) or withdraw completely. ■ Cannot function or communicate effectively (e.g., may speak incoherently or be unable to speak). ■ May feel terror and impending doom, believe he has a life-threatening illness, or that he is "going crazy." ■ Physical symptoms include dilated pupils, labored breathing, severe trembling, sleeplessness, palpitations, diaphoresis, pallor, and muscular incoordination (Townsend, 2010).

When anxiety is more severe, the person attempts to counteract the anxiety in some way. Each person develops unique patterns of coping with anxiety, called **defense mechanisms**, which are used consciously or unconsciously to relieve the anxiety. Examples of defense mechanisms are **denial** (refusing to acknowledge the existence of a real situation or associated feelings) and **displacement** (transferring feelings from one target to another that seems less threatening—for example, kicking the dog when you are angry at your boss). See Chapter 12 for further discussion of defense mechanisms.

When overused, defense mechanisms can be maladaptive and lead to psychological disorders such as phobias, obsessive–compulsive disorders, and dissociative disorders (e.g., amnesia). Excessive or unrelieved anxiety may also contribute to **psychosis**, which is a loss of ability to differentiate self from nonself or by impaired reality testing (that is, knowing what is real and what exists only in one's mind), often accompanied by hallucinations and delusions. Examples of psychotic responses to anxiety include schizophrenia and delusional disorders. These disorders are beyond the scope of this book. If you need more information, refer to a mental health text.

KnowledgeCheck 13-4

- What is anxiety?
- When is anxiety a normal response to life?
- Identify at least three healthcare scenarios that might trigger anxiety in patients.

Example Problem: Depression

Others imply that they know what it is like to be depressed because they have gone through a divorce, lost a job or broken up with someone. But these experiences carry with them feelings. Depression, instead, is flat, hollow, and unendurable.
—Kay Redfield Jamison (1997, p. 218), An Unquiet Mind

The term **depression** is commonly used to describe a feeling of sadness or "the blues." But to psychologists, nurses, and other healthcare professionals, it refers to a specific condition with characteristic symptoms and often devastating consequences if left untreated (Steptoe, 2007; Suls & Howren, 2012). Depression occurs in all age groups, even in very young children. It affects about 9.1% of the adult population in the United States, and is one of the top three risks for functional decline. The incidence is higher in women than in men (*Morbidity and Mortality Weekly Report*, October 1, 2011). See Table 13-2 for common truths and myths about depression.

Criteria established by the American Psychiatric Association (APA) (2013) for **major depressive disorder** include:

- Depressed mood most of the day nearly every day for at least 2 weeks, typically accompanied by markedly diminished interest or pleasure in activities the person previously enjoyed

Table 13-2 ➤ Depression: Truths and Myths	
TRUE	**FALSE**
Depressive disorders are more common among women than men (2:1).	"Getting on with life" will cure depression.
Spiritual distress is associated with depression.	Everyone likes to talk about how they feel.
Depression can be defined as a maladaptive emotional response.	Medication is the answer to depression.
Low socioeconomic circumstances and social isolation correlate with depression.	Once depression has been cured, it does not return.

- Insomnia or hypersomnia
- Loss of energy
- Feelings of worthlessness
- Diminished ability to concentrate
- Recurrent thoughts of death (APA, 2013)

Unlike the feeling of true sadness, such as might accompany a divorce, death, or other loss, the depressed mood is typically marked by a sense of emptiness. This contributes to the depressed person's tendency to withdraw from social contacts and also explains the characteristically flat affect (Fig. 13-4).

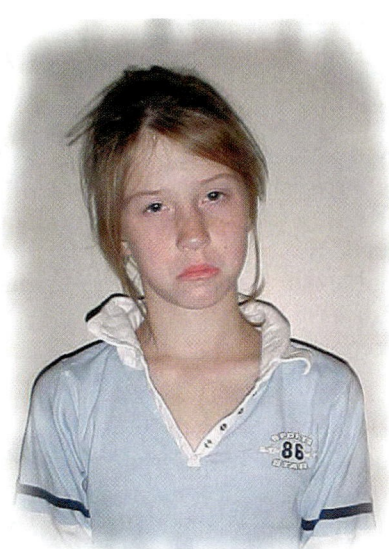

FIGURE 13-4 Depressed affect.

Depression in Older and Middle Adults

The incidence of depression is slightly higher for older adults than for the population as a whole. Of adults 65 to 74 years old, 10% reported that they had feelings associated with depression (sadness, hopelessness, worthlessness, and feeling that everything is an effort) "all or most of the time." For adults 75 and older, this was 12%. The incidence is much higher if you count the people who reported having those feelings only "some of the time" (Schiller, Lucas, Ward, et al., 2012, Table 14).

We typically think of older adults as being at higher risk because of their many losses and multiple physical illnesses (Touhy & Jett, 2009). However, at least one recent large, international study found that people in their late 40s are approximately twice as likely to be taking antidepressants as individuals—with the same characteristics—who are under the age of 25 or over the age of 65 (Blanchflower & Oswald, 2012), and that happiness and sense of well-being reach their lowest in the 40s. This study remains controversial, and more research is needed, but the findings are interesting.

What Causes Depression?

Are our genes responsible for the development of depression? Is depression "anger turned inward"? Depression theories fall into four groupings:

- *Physiological theories* relate depression to biochemical imbalances stemming from hormonal, neurological, or genetic factors.
- *Psychodynamic theories* relate depression to loss, abandonment, and emotional detachment and to diurnal and seasonal mood variations.
- *Cognitive theory* relates depression to negative thinking.
- *Social/environmental theories* relate depression to poor family relationships, difficult interpersonal relationships, and socioeconomic and political factors.

  Research has shown that the following factors increase the risk for depression:
  Family history of depression
  Hormonal or nutritional imbalance
  Inability to externalize anger
  Low self-esteem
  Negative thinking
  Learned helplessness and hopelessness
  Prior success or failure in coping mechanisms
  Traumatic loss
  Catastrophic stressors (e.g., unemployment)
  Chronic disease
  Female gender

How Is Depression Treated?

People who are clinically depressed cannot just "snap out of it." If untreated, the symptoms may continue for weeks or even years. The physiological theory of depression predominates in the medical community, and current evidence shows that biochemical processes determine moods, thought, cognition, and perception. Therefore,

treatment of serious depression relies more heavily on antidepressant medication than on psychotherapy. However, the medications have a number of unpleasant, and even serious, side effects, and some patients say that they do not effectively elevate their mood. Psychotherapists acknowledge that individual tolerance of symptoms, coping resources, education, and social support networks all have an important effect on outcomes and treatment.

Of course, you will not be conducting psychotherapy with depressed patients in your general practice. However, you *will* care for patients who are taking antidepressant medications and who have situational or even clinical depressions. Even without being a "psych nurse," there is much you can do to make your care of these patients more effective.

KnowledgeCheck 13-5

- What distinguishes clinical depression from feelings of sadness?
- How might a child manifest depression?
- Why is the nurse–patient (therapeutic) relationship important when caring for depressed individuals?

PracticalKnowledge
knowing how

Practical knowledge in this chapter consists of planning, implementing, and evaluating care to promote clients' mental health and provide support when they experience psychosocial and psychological problems. Remember, the physical body is only one dimension of a person. What patients are thinking and feeling may be equally important to their healing process.

As a nurse generalist, your independent role is to assess and document the patient's behavioral state as it relates to his medical-surgical condition, rather than to diagnose and treat mental illnesses. Clients who are anxious, for example, may not understand or recall instructions for self-care; and those who are depressed may not have the energy or motivation to follow a medical regimen or keep appointments with their healthcare providers.

NURSING CARE TO PROMOTE PSYCHOSOCIAL HEALTH

Physical illness may be particularly stressful when it occurs in combination with psychosocial issues. For example, think of Karli (Meet Your Patient). Might her condition have been less complicated if (1) she had no disfiguring injuries or (2) she were an older adult at a developmental stage when appearance is generally less crucial?

ASSESSMENTS: PSYCHOSOCIAL

No matter what the patient's medical diagnosis, you need to perform accurate and ongoing psychosocial assessments to develop holistic nursing diagnoses and interventions. Most admission assessment forms have a few questions to screen psychosocial status. If any of the answers indicate risk for a problem, you may need to conduct a more comprehensive special needs (or system specific) assessment. For an example of a psychosocial assessment tool,

 Go to Chapter 13, **Tables, Boxes, Figures: ESGFigure 13-1,** on Davis*Plus.*

A comprehensive psychosocial assessment should include the following categories:

- Biological details
- Recent life changes or stressors (both positive and negative)
- Lifestyle and relationships with the wider social environment
- History of psychiatric disorders
- Functional abilities (behavioral performance)
- Self-efficacy (the belief that you can influence your own behaviors and outcomes)
- Family relationships
- Social resources and network
- Usual coping mechanisms
- Interpersonal communication
- Understanding about current illness
- Major issues raised by current illness
- Health priorities
- Spirituality (see the HOPE assessment tool in Chapter 16)

After interviewing the patient, assess her *personality style*. That is, identify any personality traits that may affect her care or compliance, such as a tendency to be dependent, hostile, dramatic, or critical (Gorman & Sultan, 2008).

Psychosocial information is personal and sometimes sensitive. To encourage patients to share this information, you will need to use your developing communication skills. For example:

- Be aware of your own biases and discomforts that could influence your assessment.
- Use active listening through eye contact and verbal response. Be sensitive, though; eye contact is uncomfortable for some people.
- Proceed from general details ("How do you get along with your parents?") to the specific ("Does your mother ever hit you?").
- Use an open and positive voice tone, facial expression, and body language (e.g., avoid frowning, criticizing, or expressing shock).
- Keep the focus on the patient.
- Be respectful and sensitive to cultural and gender-specific details.
- Use open-ended questions (questions that cannot be answered with a yes or no).
- Follow the patient's cues by using reflection and restating.
- Be flexible and use humor as appropriate.
- Provide empathetic feedback and touch as appropriate.

You will learn more about interviewing and communication skills in Chapter 21.

 ### Think**Like a Nurse** 13-5

Psychologically, Karli is worried about the unfairness of her situation, and is probably struggling with body image issues. In addition, what do you think her *social* concerns might be?

ANALYSIS/NURSING DIAGNOSIS: PSYCHOSOCIAL

Psychosocial issues involve nearly all areas of patient functioning, so there is overlap between what we are calling "psychosocial" diagnoses and those used in the rest of the chapter to describe the more specific problems of self-concept, anxiety, and depression. That is, you may use some of these psychosocial diagnoses for clients who have problems of self-concept, anxiety, and depression. It would be impossible to list every possible psychosocial diagnosis; the following are but a few.

- *Family Coping [Compromised and/or Disabled].* Usual support (comfort and assistance) from a significant other is either compromised (insufficient or withdrawn) or disabled (competing or maladapted), causing a significant health challenge.
- *Parental Role Conflict.* A parent shows significant role confusion and/or conflict in response to crises.
- *Ineffective Coping.* The patient fails to comprehend and effectively judge stressors, when he perceives incorrect or dangerous life choices as normal, and when there is an inability to use available resources. Inability to identify strengths and resources may be secondary to low self-esteem.
- *Post-Trauma Syndrome.* There is a maladaptive learned response to a traumatic and distressing event.
- *Risk for Loneliness.* The person is separated from persons, culture, objects, or environments to which a person may have ongoing attachments.
- *Social Isolation.* The person experiences significant aloneness that has a negative impact on health, or perceives the isolation as a threat to health.
- *Risk for Other-Directed Violence.* Situations in which a person threatens or uses aggression or violence to harm others. The intention of harm may not be limited to physical harm.

Psychosocial issues can be a problem, a symptom of a problem, or the etiology of a problem. It is important for you to determine what is cause and what is effect, although this can be hard to unravel at times. What you identify significantly affects your choice of goals and nursing activities (Table 13-3).

PLANNING PSYCHOSOCIAL OUTCOMES/EVALUATION

As always, the outcomes you identify will serve as guidelines for ongoing assessment and as criteria for evaluation of your patients' responses to care.

Individualized goal/outcome statements will depend on the nursing diagnoses used, client input, and realistic

Table 13-3 ➤ Implications of Identifying a Psychosocial Issue as Problem, Etiology, or Symptom

	AS PROBLEM	AS ETIOLOGY	AS SYMPTOM
Nursing Diagnosis	**Interrupted Family Processes** r/t tumult from parental divorce	Delayed Development r/t lack of stimulation **secondary to Interrupted Family Processes** (parental divorce)	Ineffective Individual Coping (Mother) r/t poor judgment and impaired reality perception, **as manifested by Interrupted Family Processes** and risk-taking behaviors
Sample Goals (based on problem)	*NOC Outcome* Family Functioning	*NOC Outcome* Child Development: 4 years	*NOC Outcomes* Coping, Decision Making, Role Performance, Social Support, Impulse Control
	Goals Members perform expected family roles. Family cares for dependent members.	*Goals* Child demonstrates age-appropriate motor activities. Child uses four- and five-word sentences.	*Goals* Identifies coping strategies that have been effective in the past. Discusses the implications of decision alternatives with family.
Sample Interventions and Activities (based on etiology)	*NIC Interventions* Family Integrity Promotion Family Process Maintenance Normalization Promotion	*NIC Interventions* Developmental Enhancement: Child Parent Education Health Screening	*NIC Interventions* Coping Enhancement Decision-Making Support Impulse Control Training Family Involvement Promotion Support Group Support System Enhancement
	Specific Activities Promote parental involvement in healthcare. Assist the family with skills and education of conflict resolution, coping skills, and problem-solving. Link the individual and family to the appropriate support and education services.	*Specific Activities* Establish time for one-on-one care. Provide for creative play (e.g., clay, blocks, painting). Teach parents appropriate stimulation. Teach parents about developmental milestones and expected behaviors. Assess changes in family processes.	*Specific Activities* Identify and discuss alternative behaviors. Encourage delaying decision-making when under stress. Help the mother solve problems constructively. Assist her to evaluate her own behavior. Identify and discuss past successful coping behaviors she has used.

expectations of what the client can achieve and agrees to. For example, for Compromised or Disabled Family Coping, examples of goal statements are, "Involves family members in decision making" and "Expresses feelings and emotions freely." If the nursing diagnosis is Impaired Social Interaction, goal statements may call for the client to develop the skills of "engagement, assertiveness, compromise, confrontation, and consideration."

The Psychosocial Health domain of the NOC taxonomy includes approximately 30 *NOC standardized outcomes* to describe psychological well-being, psychosocial adaptation, self-control, and social interaction. The following are a few examples:

Abusive Behavior Self-Restraint
Coping
Child Adaptation to Hospitalization
Psychosocial Adjustment: Life Change
Role Performance
Social Interaction Skills

Examples from other domains include Family Coping, Family Functioning, and Family Resiliency.

Other NOC domains also include useful psychosocial outcomes. The following are only a few examples (Moorhead, Johnson, Maas, et al., 2013):

Family Coping
Family Functioning
Family Participation in Professional Care
Family Resiliency

PLANNING PSYCHOSOCIAL INTERVENTIONS/ IMPLEMENTATION

Psychosocial nursing interventions and activities will be determined by the nursing diagnoses you identify, especially by the etiologies.

NIC standardized interventions for psychosocial diagnoses are found primarily in the Behavioral and Family domains of the NIC system. The following are some examples from the Behavioral domain:

Anger Control Assistance
Anxiety Reduction
Coping Enhancement
Decision-Making Support
Socialization Enhancement

The following are examples of interventions from the Family domain:

Family Involvement Promotion
Family Support
Family Therapy
Parenting Promotion (Bulechek, Butcher, & Dochterman, 2012)

Specific, individualized nursing activities used to help patients maintain a sense of personhood are discussed in the following section, Preventing Depersonalization. For nursing activities in which the nursing goal is to provide conflict mediation, enhance socialization, or strengthen the family,

 Go to Student Resources: Chapter 13, **Supplemental Materials, Psychosocial Nursing Interventions,** on Davis*Plus*.

Preventing Depersonalization

Illness, and especially hospitalization, can have a depersonalizing effect that alters the self-concept. The ill person may feel that she has become an object to be examined, poked, prodded, and discussed. You can help patients maintain a sense of personhood by using a caring approach:

- Introduce yourself if the patient does not know you.
- Address the patient by her preferred name each time you enter the room, and always speak respectfully.
- Listen actively when the patient speaks.
- Do not talk *about* the patient to others in the room (e.g., do not say, "He seems to be better today, don't you think?"). Speak *to* the patient.

- Use eye contact and touch, keeping in mind that people vary in their desire to be touched.
- Always offer an explanation before beginning a procedure, and warn the patient before you touch him ("I'm going to touch your leg now").
- Move, turn, and position the patient gently.
- Provide for privacy when performing procedures or discussing something personal or sensitive.

Nursing Care for Example Problems Self-Concept Disturbance and Low Self-Esteem

As is true for psychosocial issues, self-concept and self-esteem issues are a part of the holistic care of well and ill patients in all settings.

ASSESSMENT: SELF-CONCEPT AND SELF-ESTEEM

Psychological tests are typically administered by a clinical psychologist or licensed social worker. However, if you were working in a mental health agency, you might collect in-depth information regarding self-concept by using a psychological measurement tool, to be interpreted by a clinical psychologist or licensed social worker. For an all-purpose assessment you might use screening in any setting,

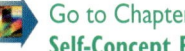 Go to Chapter 13, **Clinical insight 13-1: Assessing Self-Concept Problems,** in Volume 2.

Observe for behaviors and comments specifically associated with low self-esteem. People with low self-esteem tend to avoid eye contact and have a stooped posture. They may move slowly and have poor grooming. Their verbal behaviors include speaking hesitantly, being overly critical of others and of self ("I never do anything right."), not accepting positive comments about self ("Oh, anybody could have done it."), apologizing frequently, and verbalizing feelings of powerlessness ("Whatever you say is fine with me."; "It doesn't matter what I do; it won't change anything."). To assess specifically for the self-esteem dimension of a person's self-concept, you can

 Go to Chapter 13, **Clinical Insight 13-2: Performing a Self-Esteem Inventory,** in Volume 2.

Key Point: *If you suspect serious problems with self-concept, document the patient's responses in your nursing notes and refer the patient for appropriate psychological testing.*

 ### Think**Like a Nurse** 13-6

In the Meet Your Patient scenario, Karli perceives herself as unlovable "looking this way." You should not assume that you know exactly what Karli means by this. Also from the scenario: Picking at her bandages, she sobs that no one will love her looking as she does, that her life is over, and that she hates herself. "You take her hand. 'I used to be pretty,' she says, 'but now I'll look like a freak!'"

- Which of her words do you need to clarify with her?
- What might you say to her to get her to provide more information about the psychosocial meaning of her statement?

ANALYSIS/NURSING DIAGNOSIS: SELF-CONCEPT AND SELF-ESTEEM

Psychosocial and self-concept issues can be a problem, a symptom of a problem, or the etiology of a problem. It is important for you to determine what is cause and what is effect, although this may not always be clear. As you can see in Table 13-3, your analysis significantly affects your choice of goals and nursing activities.

When analyzing data for self-concept problems, keep the following two guidelines in mind:

- *Avoid seeking simplistic cause-and-effect relationships.* Instead, recognize the complexity of human responses. For example:

    Molly, a 19-year-old student, has just been admitted to your unit and is presenting with clinical depression and low self-esteem. Is Molly depressed because she has low self-esteem? Or is longstanding low self-esteem causing her to feel depressed? Or are the two interrelated?

- *Avoid confusing low self-concept with clinical emotional and/or behavioral psychiatric diagnoses.* There is no recognized diagnosis describing self-concept disorder in the APA's *Diagnostic and Statistical Manual of Mental Disorders,* 5th ed., Text Revision (*DSM-5,* 2013). Self-concept (particularly self-esteem) plays a secondary role in a number of disorders but is not a primary disorder itself.

Self-Concept or Body Image as a Problem

You can diagnose a body image or self-concept problem when it is the result of a particular condition and might not exist if not for the condition (e.g., a profoundly deaf adolescent develops self-worth problems). The following nursing diagnoses may be useful for patients with either low overall self-concept or difficulties in specific domains of self-concept (e.g., self-esteem):

Chronic Low Self-Esteem The person expresses ongoing and longstanding overall self-dissatisfaction and negative self-appraisal (i.e., wide differences between "ideal" and "actual" or "perceived" self). *Etiologies* include but are not limited to depression, mismatch in ideal and perceived self, dysfunctional family, anxiety, or failure to adapt to a change in physical appearance or functioning.

Situational Low Self-Esteem The person exhibits self-disapproval and negative self-evaluations as a specific reaction to loss or change. *Etiologies:* See Chronic Low Self-Esteem, preceding.

Disturbed Personal Identity Negative and incorrect assessment of self-identity and inability to determine boundaries between self and others. *Etiologies* include but are not limited to distorted perceptions of self, such as occur in certain mental illnesses; loss of health, limb, physical appearance, or functioning; or dysfunctional family.

Ineffective Role Performance A person experiences or perceives difficulty in fulfilling a usual role, or there is a mismatch between role expectations and role performance (either perceived or societal expectations). *Etiologies* include but are not limited to job demands exceeding abilities, inadequate resources or support system, family conflicts, domestic violence, unrealistic role expectations, lack of a role model, substance abuse, cognitive deficits, illness or disease, low self-esteem, pain, fatigue, and cognitive deficits.

Disturbed Body Image An individual has a confused image of his physical self or negatively evaluates his body or an aspect of it. *Etiologies* include but are not limited to loss of functioning or appearance (e.g., acne, scars, breast removal, amputation), eating disorder, gender conflict, or personality disorder.

ThinkLike a Nurse 13-7

- Refer to Karli in Meet Your Patient. Look at the preceding five NANDA-I labels for self-concept problems (Chronic Low Self-Esteem, Situational Low Self-Esteem, Disturbed Personal Identity, Ineffective Role Performance, Disturbed Body Image). Which one most clearly applies to Karli? Explain your thinking.
- Write a nursing diagnosis (problem r/t etiology) for the problem you chose.

Self-Concept or Body Image as Etiology

Self-concept problems are an etiology when they precede a condition such as depression and play a central role in the condition (e.g., low self-esteem causing and maintaining depression or leading to an anxiety disorder). The following are examples of nursing diagnoses with self-concept (e.g., self-esteem) as the etiology:

- *Impaired Adjustment* should be used where a patient experiences difficulties adapting perception and evaluation of self after changes in health status.
- *Complicated Grieving* may develop in anticipation of or following body changes (e.g., hysterectomy) or loss of key roles (e.g., resulting from death of a spouse).
- *Deficient Knowledge* of a healthcare situation may occur because of low self-esteem and lack of confidence in ability to learn or to manage care. Low self-esteem diminishes the motivation to learn.
- *Hopelessness* may occur because of overwhelming role demands, external locus of control, or lack of confidence in abilities.
- *Impaired Social Interaction* may occur when the person's low self-esteem and external locus of control cause him to fear criticism or lack of acceptance from others.

- *Ineffective Health Maintenance* may occur as a result of low self-esteem: not perceiving one's self as capable, or feeling there is no point to making the effort.
- *Sexual Dysfunction* or *Ineffective Sexuality Pattern* may result from negative body image brought about by changes in body structure or function (e.g., pregnancy, medications, surgery, trauma, diseases such as arthritis, or treatments such as radiation).

PLANNING OUTCOMES/EVALUATION: SELF-CONCEPT AND SELF-ESTEEM

You will choose outcomes based on the client's specific nursing diagnosis. For example:

> *Nursing Diagnosis*: Chronic Low Self-Esteem
>   *NOC Outcome:* Quality of Life
>   *Individualized Outcome:* Expresses pleasure in participating in activities

> *Nursing Diagnosis:* Disturbed Body Image
>   *NOC Outcome:* Body Image
>   *Individualized Outcome:* Verbalizes positive aspects of body

To see a more extensive list of *NOC standardized outcomes* and indicators for selected self-concept problems, as well as *individualized goal/outcome statement* examples,

 Go to Chapter 13, **Standardized Nursing Language, Self-Concept Diagnoses: Selected Standardized and Individualized Outcomes,** on Davis*Plus.*

When self-concept is the etiology of other problems (e.g., Sexual Dysfunction related to negative body image), choose outcomes based on the problem label (e.g., Sexual Abuse Recovery, Sexual Functioning, Body Image). The overall goal, in all cases, is that the patient's self-concept (or some aspect of it) will improve.

PLANNING INTERVENTIONS/IMPLEMENTATION: SELF-CONCEPT AND SELF-ESTEEM

Common NIC standardized interventions for self-concept and self-esteem diagnoses include Anticipatory Guidance, Behavior Modification, Decision-Making Support, and Self-Esteem Enhancement. For a more extensive list, along with examples of nursing activities,

 Go to Chapter 13, **Standardized Nursing Language, Self-Concept Diagnoses: Selected NIC Interventions and Nursing Activities,** on Davis*Plus.*

Although not all-inclusive, those examples should give you an idea of the types of care needed to support self-concept.

Specific, individualized nursing activities used frequently for patients with psychosocial and self-concept diagnoses are discussed in the text that follows. They include supportive measures to promote self-esteem, self-concept, positive body image, and role satisfaction.

Promoting Self-Esteem and Self-Concept

The dependence that often accompanies illness and aging can bring about loss of self-esteem. Although the foundation for self-esteem is laid in childhood and affected by many sociocultural variables, your nursing approach can help preserve and enhance a patient's self-esteem. Your efforts to preserve self-worth of course promote self-esteem.

Identifying Patient Strengths It is important to help the client identify past achievements and areas of strength. One way to do that is to point out areas of strength that you observe, such as the following:

> *Emotional strengths* might include the ability to express emotions, to "feel" for others.
> *Relationship strengths* include being sensitive to others' needs and being a good listener.
> *Spiritual strengths* may include faith in God and participation in church activities.

Evaluate the client's sense of humor, which can also be a strength—and be sure the client considers special aptitudes, such as cooking, arts and crafts, sports, work, and education.

It is important to help the client identify past achievements and areas of strength. One way to do that is to point out areas of strength that you observe. Be sure the client considers special aptitudes, such as cooking, arts and crafts, sports, work, and education. Other emotional strengths might include the ability to express emotions, to "feel" for others, to give and receive affection. Relationship strengths include being sensitive to others' needs, being a good listener, and making people feel comfortable.

Other Interventions The following are other nursing actions specific to self-esteem:

- Establish a therapeutic nursing relationship emphasizing trust, consistency, honest communication, and unconditional positive regard.
- Encourage the client to be as independent as possible (e.g., by performing self-care).
- Monitor for and discourage self-criticism and negative self-talk.
- Teach the client to substitute positive self-talk for negative self-talk. For example, the client says, "I know my blood sugar is high, but I can't seem to stay on my diet. I ate way too much again today." You might remind the client that she exercised today and has been following her exercise program religiously. Eventually, she should learn to cue herself.
- Use positive and reaffirming language.
- Be supportive and accepting, but do not invade the client's personal space.
- Help the client develop realistic goals that provide achievable challenges (no-fail situations).
- Encourage the client to take part in activities that offer opportunities for success.

- Role-model communications skills that will help the person develop interpersonal relationships. Provide opportunities for practice.
- Refer to self-help and support groups, as needed.
- When possible, ask the client's advice (e.g., "How do you usually do this dressing change?")
- Point out good health practices and healthy aspects of the client's body functions.
- Refer to the Self-Care box for suggestions about teaching parents about promoting self-esteem in their children.

Promoting Positive Body Image

You can help parents promote a positive body image in their children, and you can help patients develop a different attitude toward their body. The following suggestions may be useful.

- Examine your own attitudes about what constitutes a healthy body, and pay attention to the messages you convey to others.
- Encourage patients to discuss body changes resulting from their illness, surgery, or trauma.
- Provide the opportunity to interact with people who have had similar body changes.

Teach clients the following, some of which are the same as for developing self-concept and self-esteem.

Healthy Does Not Mean Perfect Help clients to accept that healthy bodies come in a wide range of shapes and sizes. Fashion magazines portray an ideal body that is unrealistic and unhealthy for most people. If they make you feel bad by comparison, don't read them!

Focus on Activity and Healthy Eating Encourage clients to be active and focus on healthy eating rather than starving and depriving themselves to lose weight.

Don't Make Negative Comments About Your Body Monitor for negative comments about body functions, weight, or size. Advise the client not to talk negatively about body weight, size, or deformity. Urge clients to be kind to themselves, and point out when they are being unrealistically critical of their body.

Keep a List Suggest that the client keep a list of things he likes about his body and refer to it when he is feeling down.

Accept Compliments Provide the client with practice in accepting positive comments about his appearance. Coach his responses as needed (e.g., say, "Thank you" after a compliment).

Challenge Critical Comments Teach the client to challenge critical comments from others about her appearance.

Surround Yourself With Positive People Support the client in surrounding herself with positive people who support the changes she is trying to make in her image of her body, and avoid people who are critical.

Use a Counter Suggest that the client buy a counter and click it each time he makes a deliberate effort to accept positive feedback about his body or engages in positive body behaviors.

To see a Care Plan and Care Map for Disturbed Body Image,

 Go to Chapter 13, **Care Plan and Care Map,** on Davis*Plus.*

 Think**Like a Nurse** 13-8
- Which of the preceding body image interventions would be most appropriate for Karli's nursing diagnosis?
- For the interventions you did not choose, explain why.

Self-Care

Teaching Parents to Promote Self-Esteem in Children

Demonstrate love and acceptance by doing the following:
- ➤ Spending some one-on-one time with the child as often as possible: read, play, or just be together
- ➤ Being free with touches: a hug, a pat on the back
- ➤ Refraining from frequent negative criticism
- ➤ Providing nearly total acceptance of the child

Provide security by:
- ➤ Having clearly defined limits and consequences for breaking rules
- ➤ Being firm and consistent in applying the rules
- ➤ Being sure the rules are reasonable
- ➤ Allowing some latitude for individual actions within defined limits
- ➤ Treating the child with respect

- ➤ Establishing routines, such as bedtime activity, homework before play, dressing for school before breakfast in the morning, and so on
- ➤ Clearly defining every family member's role

Promote competence by:
- ➤ Setting realistic expectations about behaviors
- ➤ Assigning a few chores that are within the child's capability (e.g., picking up toys, making the bed)
- ➤ Role-modeling values, such as respect for others, honesty, and responsibility
- ➤ Providing positive feedback
- ➤ Helping the child accomplish goals
- ➤ Providing a stimulating and responsive environment
- ➤ Providing support in meeting challenges

Facilitating Role Enhancement

Sometimes the difficulty with self-concept centers on an inability to fulfill one's usual or desired role. Specific actions to enhance role satisfaction include the following:

- Help the client distinguish between ideal and actual role performance.
- Help the person to identify her past, present, and future roles. For older adults, encourage reminiscence.
- Discuss boundaries, expectations, and management defined by lifestyle and family networks.
- Facilitate communication between client and significant other regarding the sharing of role responsibilities to accommodate role changes of the ill person.
- Help the client describe realistic roles and expectations tailored to specific health changes.
- Compare realistic roles with previous and less functional roles.
- Help the client examine the difference between previous roles and current role by providing education and a learning environment that focuses on positive and supportive change.
- Help the client identify and role-play behaviors needed in new roles.

KnowledgeCheck 13-6

Without looking back at the preceding material, see whether you can:

- List three interventions for preserving self-worth.
- List three interventions for promoting self-esteem.
- List three interventions for fostering positive body image.
- List three interventions for promoting role enhancement.

Nursing Care For Example Problem: Anxiety

In general practice, the focus of nursing care for clients with anxiety is (1) to differentiate between mild anxiety and that which is severe enough to require referral to a mental health professional and (2) to provide interventions to relieve anxiety.

ASSESSMENT FOR EXAMPLE PROBLEM: ANXIETY

Your patient assessment should identify the *presence*, *level*, and *cause* of anxiety. It should include data about the following:

- **Observable behaviors**—poor eye contact, restlessness (e.g., pacing, wringing the hands, fidgeting, shuffling the feet), crying, trembling, rapid speech
- **Cognitive changes**—confusion, difficulty concentrating, forgetfulness
- **Objective physical data**—sweating, rapid pulse and respirations, dilated pupils
- **Subjective data**—shortness of breath, nausea, insomnia, worry

As we have said, most ill patients will have at least some level of anxiety. Anxiety becomes a problem when it escalates to a level that interferes with the ability to meet basic needs. You must determine whether the anxiety is normal and adaptive or whether it is severe enough to require nursing interventions, consultation, or referral to a mental health professional. For a checklist to help you make this determination,

 Go to Chapter 13, Assessment Guidelines and Tools, **Focused Assessment: Anxiety Assessment Guide,** in Volume 2.

Severe Anxiety If you suspect severe or disabling anxiety, document the patient's responses in your nursing notes, and refer the person to a physician or mental health clinician. Involve a mental health professional immediately (same day) if you discover any of the following:

- Suicidal thoughts and/or plans that make you uncertain of the patient's safety
- Assaultive or homicidal thoughts and/or plans that make you uncertain about the safety of the patient or others
- Loss of touch with reality (psychosis)
- Significant or prolonged inability to work and care for self or family

Physical Assessment Consider a comprehensive physical assessment for anxious patients, to rule out underlying disease or disorders. For example, a patient who suffers from heart palpitations when anxious may be found to have significant cardiac arrhythmias. Other medical conditions that may mimic anxiety symptoms include hormone imbalance, nutritional deficiencies, electrolyte imbalance, and central nervous system disorders. Most anxious patients, even those with diagnosed obsessive–compulsive disorder or panic attacks, are not admitted to the hospital just for their anxiety. You will encounter them more often in community settings or when they are hospitalized for other illnesses.

ANALYSIS/NURSING DIAGNOSIS FOR EXAMPLE PROBLEM: ANXIETY

For severe anxiety (neuroses, psychoses), medical treatment includes anti-anxiety medications and perhaps psychotherapy. The following five NANDA-I labels represent anxiety problems for which nursing interventions may be effective:

- *Anxiety* is a vague, uneasy feeling of discomfort or dread, accompanied by some of the symptoms listed in the preceding Assessment section. Anxiety may be unconscious; that is, the patient may not recognize that he is anxious (e.g., "My heart is pounding, and I can't seem to get my breath. What is wrong?").
- *Death Anxiety* is apprehension, worry, or fear related to death or dying.
- *Decisional Conflict* describes a person who is uncertain about what action to take when the choice among

the alternatives involves risk, loss, or challenge to personal life values.

- *Fear* is a response to a perceived threat that is consciously recognized as a danger (e.g., "My father died of this same surgery. Truly, I'm scared to death."). Fear is difficult to differentiate from Anxiety because many of the symptoms are similar.
- *Ineffective Denial* occurs when the person consciously or unconsciously rejects the knowledge or meaning of an event (e.g., a client having a heart attack says or thinks, "They have made a mistake. It's just sore muscles or pleurisy. I'll go back to work this afternoon.").

Anxiety can be the etiology or a symptom of many other nursing diagnoses, such as Deficient Knowledge, Self-Mutilation, Ineffective Sexuality Pattern, or Insomnia.

KnowledgeCheck 13-7

- List five NANDA-I labels you could use to describe a problem of anxiety.
- List four observations that would alert you that anxiety is severe enough to merit referral to a mental health professional.

▰ PLANNING OUTCOMES/EVALUATION FOR EXAMPLE PROBLEM: ANXIETY

You will use outcomes developed in the planning stage as criteria for evaluating patient progress and the success of your nursing interventions. Whether anxiety is a symptom, a problem, or the cause or etiology of a problem, one of the desired outcomes is that the anxiety will be relieved.

For selected NOC standardized outcomes and indicators for anxiety-related diagnoses,

 Go to Chapter 13, **Standardized Nursing Language, Anxiety-Related Diagnoses: Selected NOC Outcomes and NIC Interventions,** in Volume 2.

Individualized goal/outcome statements should relate the patient's specific nursing diagnosis, stating behaviors that will indicate that the problem is resolving. The following are some examples.

For Anxiety:
Plans coping strategies for anxious situations.
Uses relaxation techniques as required.
Reports absence of physical and psychological manifestations of anxiety.

For Death Anxiety:
Reports feeling less fearful.
Discusses funeral arrangements with family.

For Decisional Conflict:
Identifies relevant information about the decision and its consequences.
Recognizes how various alternatives conflict with others' desires.

For Fear:
Uses effective coping strategies.
Maintains social relationships and control over life.

For Ineffective Denial:
Verbalizes understanding of the complications that may occur if the disease is not treated.
Follows prescribed regimen for treatments and medications.

 ## ThinkLike a Nurse 13-9

 Go to Chapter 13, **Standardized Nursing Language, Anxiety-Related Diagnoses: Selected NOC Outcomes and NIC Interventions,** in Volume 2.

Notice that Anxiety Control is listed as a possible outcome for each of the nursing diagnoses. Explain how anxiety relates to each of the diagnoses: Is it a problem, a symptom, or an etiology?

▰ PLANNING INTERVENTIONS/IMPLEMENTATION FOR EXAMPLE PROBLEM, ANXIETY

Interventions for anxious clients will depend on the cause of the anxiety; however, for *all* anxious clients, regardless of the etiology, the nursing goals in most situations are to help the client to:

- *Recognize that the client is anxious.* Because the symptoms may be varied, subtle, and physical, a person may demonstrate anxious behaviors without even realizing why he is doing so. Or he may attribute his symptoms to a physical illness.
- *Identify the source of the client's anxiety.* This may require a more extended relationship than you might have with a hospitalized client, because it involves the uncovering of emotional conflicts. Nevertheless, a more permanent relief can be obtained once the client recognizes the conflict and can use his conscious, rational mind to deal with it.
- *Deal with the symptoms of the client's anxiety.* For example, you may use massage, relaxation techniques, and so forth.

For *NIC standardized interventions* and selected activities for anxiety-related diagnoses,

 Go to Chapter 13, **Standardized Nursing Language, Anxiety-Related Diagnoses: Selected NOC Outcomes and NIC Interventions,** in Volume 2

Specific nursing activities for reducing anxiety include the following:

- Provide a calm and safe environment, including a quiet, reassuring approach to communication and nursing activities. This will help the person remain centered and focused.
- Establish a relationship of trust, caring, and unconditional positive regard (i.e., don't make promises you

can't keep; don't make any "judgment" statements such as, "You ought to . . ." or "You shouldn't . . .").

- Be present and stay with the individual to help allay fears, create trust, and promote safety.
- Help the person identify triggers and situations that create anxiety.
- Use clear and factual knowledge tailored to the individual's circumstances.
- Explain and, if necessary, explore details of all health-care procedures.
- Develop coping strategies and behavior modification techniques.
- Encourage enjoyable, nonstressful activities to give the person an opportunity to think about something other than the anxiety-producing situation.
- Advise regular physical exercise unless contraindicated by a physical condition.
- Control the environment by removing anxiety-provoking equipment and people.
- Administer and monitor anti-anxiety medication when required.
- Assist the patient in relaxation methods, such as biofeedback, meditation, and therapeutic touch. For specific information about these methods,

 Go to **Chapter 46, Holistic Healing,** on DavisPlus.

- In addition, interventions specific for Death Anxiety include the following (also refer to Chapter 17):
    Stay physically close to the patient when he is fearful.
    Obtain spiritual support for the patient and family, as needed.
    Inquire about the patient's and family's specific requests for care.

Nursing Care For Example Problem: Depression

The nurse–patient relationship is vital when you work with a depressed person. Whereas an anxious patient may actively seek your assistance, a depressed person is likely to avoid your approach and may even feel unworthy of your time and effort. Establishing a nurse–patient bond requires a specific, empathetic approach involving warmth, acceptance, and understanding (unconditional positive regard) even in the face of an unresponsive, even angry, patient response.

ASSESSMENT FOR EXAMPLE PROBLEM: DEPRESSION

You should be alert for risk factors and signs and symptoms of depression in all healthcare settings. If cues are present, you will need to perform a more thorough screening or comprehensive assessment, such as the following:

 Go to Chapter 13, **Depression Assessment Guide: Patient Health Questionnaire (PHQ-9),** in Volume 2.

Risk Factors Specific to Older Adults For older adults, risk factors for depression include dementia, cancer, alcohol and substance abuse, stroke, myocardial infarction, functional disability, being widowed, being a caregiver, and social isolation (Kurlowicz, 2008). Presence of risk factors should alert you to the need for a system-specific (or special needs) assessment to determine whether depression is present.

Symptoms of Depression

Because there are so many symptoms, categorizing them may help to you to remember them. Depression is expressed by changes in feelings, cognition, and behaviors, as well as physical symptoms and changes in lifestyle. Symptoms may differ in some ways in children and older adults. When assessing for depression, observe for symptoms in the following areas:

Feelings (Affect) Depression is characterized by a flat affect; difficulty concentrating; and **anhedonia,** a loss of interest or pleasure in previously enjoyable activities (Steptoe, 2007). Finally, the person may feel worthless, guilt-ridden, or suicidal. Observe for anger, anxiety, guilt, helplessness, powerlessness, hopelessness, sadness; verbalizing lack of feeling; inability to enjoy previously enjoyable activities, low self-esteem, and worthlessness.

Cognition (Thoughts) The person may be preoccupied with loss (e.g., of job, of function); may experience self-blame, ambivalence, guilt, confusion, inability to make decisions; or blame others. You may observe, or the person may report, slowed thinking, poor concentration, preoccupation with bodily changes, and inability to accept positive comments,

Behavior The person may be unable to sleep, or sleep too much, dreading the moment when he has to get out of bed and face family members or responsibilities. Some people lose interest in eating and, therefore, lose weight; others eat frequently but without pleasure in an attempt to keep their "emptiness" at bay. Some people become agitated and restless; others experience slowed thinking and lethargy. Many experience fatigue or feelings of exhaustion throughout the day. Depression may be expressed in children by irritability, tantrums, or not eating. Look for persistently sad expression, poor eye contact, tearfulness, regression, restlessness, agitation, psychomotor retardation, withdrawal, poor grooming/hygiene, decreased sexual interest, past or current alcohol or substance abuse, and past history of suicide attempts.

Lifestyle Effects Social isolation is common. Depression may be masked by attempts to "self-medicate" with alcohol, over-the-counter (OTC) drugs, or illegal substances; or by disordered eating, participation in dangerous sports, or other forms of reckless behavior. In children, depression may manifest in skipping school or difficulty with relationships with others.

Physiological Effects Like all mental illnesses, depression carries a social stigma; thus, patients who are unwilling to admit—even to themselves—that they might be depressed may present with a physical complaint such as persistent fatigue or a fear of cancer. In such cases, skillful psychosocial assessment is critical. Physical conditions that might accompany depression include dizziness, headache, migraines, joint aches and pains (e.g., back pain), stomach ulcers and digestive upsets, chest pain, lethargy, constipation, sleep deprivation or hypersomnia, fatigue, anorexia or overeating, and weight changes.

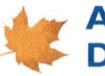

Assessing Older Adults: Depression, Dementia, or Delirium?

Unfortunately for older adults, cognitive difficulty and depression continue to be under-recognized and undertreated. You will find more information about dementia in Chapter 10.

Delirium Also called *acute confusion*, **delirium** is an acute and potentially reversible disturbance of consciousness and cognition in response to underlying medical or mental illnesses, drug toxicity, and a variety of other causes. An estimated 30% to 40% of cases of delirium are preventable (Fong, Tulebaev, & Inouye, 2009). In fact, the Agency for Healthcare Research and Quality (2003, reaffirmed July, 2012) identified delirium as a marker of quality of care and patient safety. Many aspects of the care you will be providing, such as medication administration, evaluation of complications, and assessment of dehydration, nutrition, and sleep, are factors that can be modified to prevent the development of delirium.

Dementia **Dementia** is an irreversible decline in mental abilities. APA (2013) defines dementia as part of **neurocognitive disorders (NCDs),** a group of disorders in which the primary clinical deficit is in cognitive function. NCDs are acquired rather than developmental and may be associated with Alzheimer's disease; vascular disease; Parkinson's disease; traumatic brain injury; HIV infection; or substance/medication-induced NCD. Dementia affects about 22% of adults 71 years and older. Dementia prevalence increases with age: The rate is about 40% in those older than age 85. Confusion may be present in patients with depression, as well as those who have dementia or delirium.

The Geriatric Depression Scale is especially useful in screening for depression in older adults. It requires minimal training to use, and will help you decide whether the patient needs further assessment.

To see a short form of the Geriatric Depression Scale,

Go to Chapter 13, **Tables, Boxes, Figures: ESG Figure 13-2,** on Davis*Plus*.

For a comparison of the symptoms of depression and dementia,

Go to Chapter 13, **Assessment Guidelines and Tools, Differentiating Depression and Dementia,** in Volume 2.

When Should I Refer the Patient to a Mental Health Specialist?

Because depression is so common, many of the patients you see (e.g., medical-surgical, maternity, clinics) will have at least some degree of depression. It will be important for you to differentiate among temporary, situational sadness, low energy, and a psychiatric diagnosis (clinical depression). Figure 13-5 illustrates the continuum of mild to severe depression incorporating aspects of mood, behavior, thoughts, and physical symptoms.

The presence of any of the following should alert you to make a referral. If you suspect severe depression, document the patient's responses in your nursing notes, and refer the patient to a mental health specialist.

- Personal history of recurrent depression or bipolar disorder
- Family history of recurrent depression or bipolar disorder
- Personal history of recurrence of depression within 1 year after stopping effective treatment
- Episode of major depression before age 20
- Severe, sudden, or life-threatening depressive episode (i.e., suicide attempt). If you believe there is a risk for suicide, make the referral immediately (Box 13-1).

For two alternative methods you can use to identify patients who should be referred to a mental health specialist for evaluation and/or treatment of depression,

Go to Chapter 13, **Clinical Insight 13-3: Identifying Depressed Patients Who Should Be Referred for Evaluation,** in Volume 2.

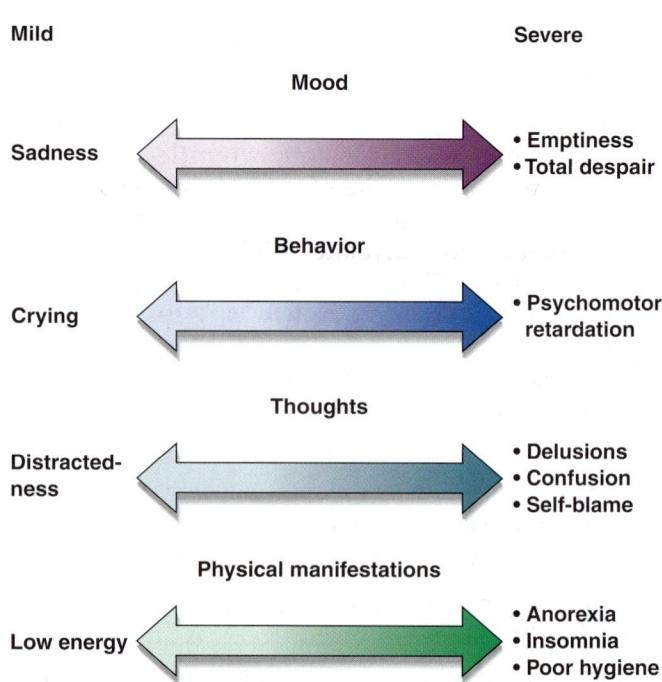

FIGURE 13-5 Depression assessment continuum incorporating mood, behavior, thoughts, and physical state.

BOX 13-1 ■ Cues Indicating a Possible Risk for Suicide

Risk Factors

- Alcohol substance abuse
- Family history of mental disorders or substance abuse
- Family history of suicide
- Firearms in the home
- Family violence, including physical or sexual abuse
- A significant medical illness, such as cancer or chronic pain
- Compulsive gambling
- Recent losses: Physical, financial, personal
- Age, gender, race (elderly or young adult, unmarried, white, male, living alone)
- Recent discharge from an inpatient psychiatry unit

Warning Signs

Patients with risk factors who exhibit any of the following warning signs clearly raise a red flag and merit immediate referral.

- Withdrawal from social contact
- Desire to be left alone

- Preoccupation with death and dying, or violence
- Risky or self-destructive behavior, such as drug use or unsafe driving
- Changes in routine, sleeping patterns
- Changes in eating habits
- Giving away belongings or getting affairs in order
- Personality changes, such as becoming very outgoing after being shy
- Saying goodbye to people as if they won't be seen again
- Talking about suicide (e.g., "I'm going to kill myself," I wish I were dead," or "I wish I hadn't been born.")

Source: Maybury, B. C. (2008, March 10). Suicide prevention: Every nurse's responsibility. Nurse.com. Retrieved January 10, 2013, from http://news.nurse.com/article/20080310/NY02/80305017

ANALYSIS/NURSING DIAGNOSIS FOR EXAMPLE PROBLEM: DEPRESSION

Depression is a psychiatric diagnosis, so you will not make that diagnosis. Nevertheless, you will need to describe associated problems that are appropriate for nursing intervention. The NANDA-I taxonomy does not have a specific diagnosis that uses the term *depression;* however, the following nursing diagnoses may be useful in describing the feelings and moods of patients who are depressed:

- *Hopelessness* may apply to a person who is unable to seek or comprehend opportunities, options, and alternatives because of a distressed emotional and unmotivated state. Note that research shows hopelessness to correlate highly with suicide (Cheung, Law, Chan, et al., 2006; Goldston, Reboussin, & Daniel, 2006; Nekanda_Trepka, Bishop, & Blackburn, 2011).
- *Powerlessness* may be diagnosed when a person's perception of control over situations and life events is significantly impaired and externally based.

Risk for Suicide must always be considered when a patient is depressed, especially when the person has a history of prior attempts or is verbalizing the desire to die or the intent to kill himself.

Remember that depression can cause a variety of physical and behavioral problems, such as the following:

Activity Intolerance
Adult Failure to Thrive
Constipation

Imbalanced Nutrition: Less than Body Requirements

Imbalanced Nutrition: More than Body Requirements
Impaired Social Interaction
Ineffective Health Maintenance
Ineffective Therapeutic Regimen Management

Insomnia
Noncompliance
Self-Care Deficit (Bathing/Hygiene, Dressing/ Grooming)
Self-Neglect

The diagnoses of Situational and Chronic Low Self-Esteem are also useful because depressed clients often experience low self-esteem. These diagnoses were presented in the preceding section, Analysis/Nursing Diagnosis: Self-Concept and Self-Esteem.

PLANNING OUTCOMES/EVALUATION FOR EXAMPLE PROBLEM: DEPRESSION

You will use outcomes developed in the planning stage as criteria for evaluating the patient's progress and the success of your nursing interventions.

For selected NOC standardized outcomes and indicators for depression-related diagnoses,

 Go to Chapter 13, **Standardized Nursing Language, Depression-Related Diagnoses: Selected NOC Outcomes and NIC Interventions,** in Volume 2.

Individualized goal/outcome statements should relate to the patient's specific nursing diagnosis, stating behaviors

that will indicate that the problem is resolving. The following are some examples:

For Depressed Mood:
Affect is appropriate to the situation.
Reports feeling less sadness and depression.
Interacts willingly and appropriately with others.
Eats a well-balanced diet to prevent weight loss.
Bathes, washes and combs hair, dresses—maintains grooming and hygiene.

For Hopelessness:
Expresses positive belief in self, others, and meaning of life.
Demonstrates interest in life/activity.
Maintains spiritual belief system or religious affiliation.

For Powerlessness:
Participates in healthcare decisions to the extent possible.
Sets realistic goals for self.

For Risk for Suicide:
Verbalizes any suicidal ideas to staff.
Trusts staff enough to disclose any specific plans for suicide.

▦ PLANNING INTERVENTIONS/IMPLEMENTATION FOR EXAMPLE PROBLEM: DEPRESSION

For *NIC standardized interventions and selected activities* for depression-related diagnoses,

 Go to Chapter 13, **Standardized Nursing Language, Depression-Related Diagnoses: Selected NOC Outcomes and NIC Interventions,** in Volume 2.

Individualized nursing activities for depression-related diagnoses focus on altering the problem etiologies and relieving symptoms of depression. In general, care of the depressed person involves (1) developing a therapeutic relationship through effective communication and (2) promoting nutrition, exercise, and personal hygiene.

- Use therapeutic communication:
   Be honest and open.
   Be patient.
   Be consistent.
   Do not use false reassurance ("You'll feel better soon").
   Avoid phrases such as "Cheer up" or "Think how lucky you are to have a good family."
   Do make comments such as, "I like the way you look in that dress."
   Do not be overly cheerful.
   Encourage the client to express feelings, including anger.
   Be accepting and nonjudgmental when the client expresses feelings.
   Encourage communication that explores reality, grief, and personal loss.
- Promote activity. Activities in small groups can help build self-esteem.

- Promote and teach good nutrition and hydration.
- Provide support as needed for self-care and decision making, while promoting as much independence as possible.
- Assess for and provide information about use of complementary and alternative therapies for depression (see Complementary & Alternative Modalities (CAM): Depression & Anxiety: Teaching for CAM Use).

- ✚ Monitor for suicide risk. Ask directly: "Have you thought about harming yourself? If so, what do you plan to do?"

- Institute measures to build self-esteem (see Promoting Self-Esteem and Self-Concept in this chapter).
- Provide information on support and educational groups.
- Encourage the person to maintain his religious affiliations.

🍁 Nursing Interventions for Older Adults

Remember that depression is not a normal part of aging. As mentioned previously, it is important to identify depression in older adults and not mistake it for dementia or "signs of old age."

Team Communication If you identify signs of depression, be certain to communicate that to other members of the staff and to the primary care provider. You and the other nurses may be the only ones who have repeated contact with the patient, so you might be able to observe cues that are missed by other providers.

✚ **Medications** Because metabolism changes with aging, the risk of adverse medication effects is high for older adults. Closely supervise patients being treated with antidepressants because severe side effects are possible. When a patient is admitted to a hospital there is a risk that self-administered medications may be overlooked. If one of those medications is an antidepressant, missed doses combined with a physical illness may cause depression symptoms to worsen.

Reminiscence Use reminiscence and life review as an intervention. Encourage the patient to talk about significant positive and negative experiences that have occurred during her life.

Suicide Risk **Key Point:** *Keep in mind that depression is a significant predictor of suicide in older adults.*

As an example, the suicide rate among white men age 85 and older is almost double that of the U.S. general population (National Institute of Mental Health, 2010). Older adults often succeed in their suicide attempts. To illustrate: Among adults older than age 75 years, there is one suicide for every four attempts; among young adults, there is one suicide for every 100 to 200 attempts (Centers for Disease Control and Prevention [CDC], 2012a).

Complementary & Alternative Modalities (CAM)

Depression & Anxiety: Teaching for CAM Use

Many people use herbal therapies to relieve symptoms of anxiety and depression. Patients may self-treat, or herbal therapies may be prescribed by CAM practitioners. You should assess for CAM use to be sure the method is not contraindicated and that the patient has informed the primary care provider about its use.

DEPRESSION

Ginkgo Biloba

Can take 6–8 weeks for patient to feel any better.

Mixing with some fruits and nuts could produce poison ivy–like reaction.

Patients using anticoagulants must use with caution.

Should not be used by patients with peptic ulcer disease, children, or women who are pregnant or breastfeeding.

Ginseng

There are many kinds of ginseng; patient should look up the specific type he is using.

Should not be used by patients who are anticoagulated or who have hypertension, hypotension diabetes, cardiovascular disease; or by women who are pregnant or breastfeeding.

Kava

May experience symptom relief within 1 week.

Significant adverse reactions may occur.

Kava enhances the effects of alcohol and central nervous system (CNS) medications (e.g., alprazolam and CNS depressants).

Should not be used by women who are pregnant or breastfeeding.

Because of liver toxicity, the CDC has cautioned consumers against using kava (CDC, 2002). Its use is severely limited and regulated in Australia (Therapeutic Goods Administration, 2005).

St. John's Wort

Patients who are depressed should not take this herb without medical supervision.

Should not be taken by children or women who are pregnant or lactating, nor by those who use monoamine oxidase inhibitors (MAOIs), selective serotonin reuptake inhibitors (SSRIs), alcohol, or OTC cold and flu medications.

S-Adenosyl Methionine (SAMe)

Patients with bipolar disorder should not use this supplement unless under direct supervision of their physician.

Use enteric-coated forms to decrease gastric irritation.

ANXIETY

Kava

See Depression, preceding. Not recommended for use.

Source: Adapted from Hulisz, D.T. (2008). Top herbal products: Efficacy and safety concerns. Medscape Nurses. ©2007. Retrieved January 18, 2013, from http://www.medscape.org/viewprogram/8494; and Neeb, K. (2005). *Fundamentals of mental health nursing* (3rd ed.). Philadelphia: F.A. Davis, pp. 365–378.

For more in-depth information about CAM use for depression and anxiety,

 Go to Chapter Resources: Chapter 13, **Tables, Boxes, Figures: CAM Box. Teaching for Patients Who Use CAM for Depression and Anxiety,** on Davis*Plus*.

Professional Help Encourage the patient to seek professional help. Older adults are likely to try to "handle it themselves," or even not think of depression as a health problem. Many think that it is normal to be depressed as they grow older

Suicide Prevention Interventions

It is not only patients on psychiatric units who commit suicide. They may be the same patients you care for on a medical-surgical unit or in their homes. Illnesses such as advanced cancer and AIDS are often accompanied by uncontrolled pain and delirium. Because of the suffering and dependency they cause, they are associated with higher suicide rates.

Key Point: *Your most important intervention is assessment. Be alert for risk factors and warning signs that may indicate the possibility of suicide (see Box 13-1).*

Remember that about 80% of those who attempt suicide give some prior verbal or indirect cues.

- Evaluate the patient's medications (e.g., certain antihypertensive agents, steroids, cancer chemotherapeutic agents, and amphotericin-B can cause depression).
- If risk factors are present, put them prominently on the care plan and report them to other caregivers.
- Do not avoid the patient because you fear saying the wrong thing. Talking about suicide does not increase the risk.
- Be aware of your personal feelings and anxieties regarding suicide.
- If the patient mentions suicide specifically, be direct. Ask whether he is having thoughts of harming himself.
- If he answers yes, do not leave him. Have someone contact his primary care provider so that a psychiatric consult can be ordered, and possibly transfer to a psychiatric unit if the patient is physically stable.

- Ask if the patient has a plan for suicide, and if so, what it is.
- Remove items that might be used for self-harm (e.g., razor blades and other sharp objects, shoelaces, belts, intravenous tubing, telephone cords, pills, and glasses). Search the room and the bathroom.
- Make sure the windows cannot be opened.

- Follow agency policy for continuous monitoring, moving to a room close to the nurses' station, and so on. (Gorman & Sultan, 2008; Maybury, 2008; Valente, 2010).

Key Point: Most of all, never attempt to work with a suicidal patient by yourself. Involve other members of the team immediately.

Toward Evidence-Based Practice

(Study A) Piderman, K., Lapid, M., Stevens, S., et al. (2011). Spiritual well-being and spiritual practices in elderly depressed psychiatric inpatients. *Journal of Pastoral Care & Counseling: JPCC*, 65(1–2), 3–31.

Researchers studied 45 elderly psychiatric inpatients to examine associations among spirituality, depression, and quality of life (QOL). They found that patients with spiritual well-being reported a higher QOL and those with poor spiritual well-being had a higher incidence of depression. During hospitalization, participants with increased spiritual well-being reported peacefulness and reduced hopelessness, worthlessness, and guilt.

(Study B) Judson, P., Dickson, E., Argenta, P., et al. (2011). A prospective, randomized trial of integrative medicine for women with ovarian cancer. *Gynecologic Oncology*, 123(2), 346–350.

This pilot trial evaluated the usefulness of complementary or integrative medicine (CM-IM) in women with ovarian cancer and evaluated its effects on QOL, chemotherapy toxicity, and immunological profiles. Forty-three women with newly diagnosed ovarian cancer requiring chemotherapy were randomized to the experimental group who received hypnosis, therapeutic massage, and healing touch with each cycle of chemotherapy and the control group who received chemotherapy without complementary or integrative therapy.

The researchers concluded that women who received CM-IM demonstrated no improvement in QOL or chemotherapy toxicity.

(Study C) Lin, P. C., Lin, M. L., Huang, L. C., et al. (2011). Music therapy for patients receiving spine surgery. *Journal of Clinical Nursing*, 20(7–8), 960–968.

This study compared the effects of music therapy with a quiet, uninterrupted rest period on pain intensity, anxiety,

and physiological parameters after spinal surgery. A total of 60 patients receiving spinal surgery were randomly assigned to listen to selected music from the evening before surgery to the second day after surgery. The control group did not listen to music. Researchers found that patients who listened to music experienced a significant reduction in anxiety and pain, but that there was no effect on blood pressure, heart rate, or cortisol levels. They concluded that patients recovering from spinal surgery may benefit from music therapy.

1. To help you with your analysis for the following questions, complete this table.

	STUDY A	STUDY B	STUDY C
Intervention			
Type of patient			
Result/conclusion			

2. Which of the studies tested an intervention?

3. Which of the interventions was most successful in relieving anxiety? Explain your thinking.

4. Think about the study that did not test an intervention. What, if anything, is its value to nurses or patients?

 Go to Chapter 13, **Toward Evidence-Based Practice Suggested Responses**, on *DavisPlus*.

To explore learning resources for this chapter,

 Go to Davis*Plus* at **DavisPl.us/Wilkinson3.**

Chapter Resources for Chapter 13:
> **Response sheets for all learning activities**
> **Resources for Caregivers and Health Professionals**
> **Reading More About Psychosocial Health & Illness (suggested readings)**
> **Concept Map of chapter content**

Interactive Case Studies

NCLEX-Style and Chapter Review Questions

Chapter Overview Podcasts

For references cited in this chapter,

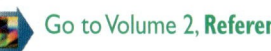 Go to Volume 2, **References Cited.**

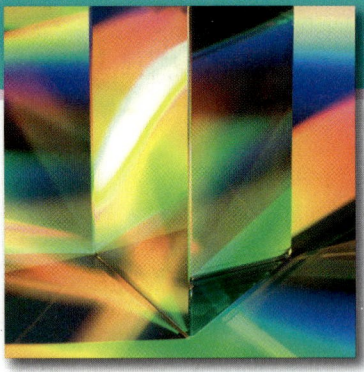

CHAPTER 14

The Family

Learning Outcomes

After completing this chapter, you should be able to:

➤ Distinguish among different family structures.

➤ Describe approaches to working with various types of families to provide optimal care to both well and ill clients.

➤ Explain how family theories provide a framework to understand family functioning.

➤ Identify family risk factors in five different stages of the family life span.

➤ Discuss how economic factors influence nursing practice, family care, and access to services.

➤ Present ways that chronic, life-threatening illness can affect families.

➤ Identify populations most at risk for homelessness.

➤ Demonstrate an understanding of family violence.

➤ Conduct a family assessment.

➤ Identify common health beliefs and communication patterns among families.

➤ Identify appropriate nursing interventions when a family member is ill.

➤ Review how risk factors, such as illness and death, substance abuse, violence, mental health disorders, financial hardship, unemployment, and other issues, can change a family's structure, communication, and coping strategies.

➤ Discuss the sandwich generation and assessment and intervention strategies for caregiver burnout.

Key Concepts

Family
Family nursing

Related Concepts

See the Concept Map on Davis*Plus*.

Example Problem

Caregiver role strain

Meet Your Patient

J. B. is an 80-year-old man who is hospitalized for end-stage renal disease. His wife died 4 years ago. His remaining family includes two married daughters and four grandchildren. J. B. has several siblings, but they live far away and rarely phone or visit.

J. B. has lived in the same neighborhood for more than 55 years. When he and his wife, Pamela, first moved into the neighborhood, they lived across the street from Mike and Lena. The two couples socialized, raised their children, and enjoyed many holidays and festivities together. After the children were grown, the two couples sold their homes and each moved into a townhouse near the center of town. They lived next door to each other and continued to spend time together. A year after Pamela died, Mike's wife, Lena, died from liver cancer.

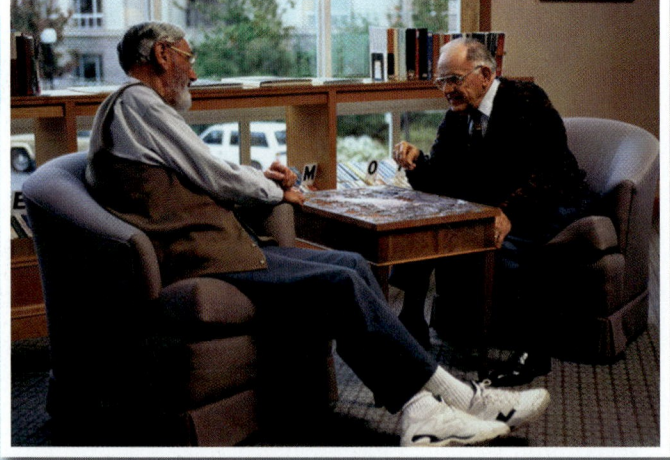

Theoretical Knowledge
knowing why

ABOUT THE KEY CONCEPTS

This chapter is about contemporary families and how they differ from those of the past. As you study the chapter, you will begin to see how **family, family nursing,** and other related concepts apply to J. B. and Mike (Meet Your Patient). The key concepts are the basis of the theoretical knowledge to which you will apply the nursing process and your nursing judgment, as you learn to meet the challenges of family health as a full-spectrum nurse.

WHAT IS A FAMILY?

Traditionally, people have thought of a family as consisting of a husband, wife, and their children. However, with increasingly cultural diversity and changes in social traditions and lifestyles, the concept of family has become broader. A family is formally defined as two or more people related by birth, marriage, or adoption residing in the same household (Lofquist, Lugaila, O'Connell, et al., 2012). A more holistic definition of **family** is "two or more individuals who provide physical, emotional, economic, or spiritual support to each other." They may or may not be related by blood, but maintain involvement in each other's lives. Most often, people who consider themselves to be family live in the same household; however, adult children living apart from their parents continue to be part of a family unit, which may also include siblings, aunts, uncles, and cousins. In short, families come in many forms, living arrangements, and emotional connections.

Changes in Family Structures

We continue to see significant changes in the living arrangements of families in the United States as a result of socioeconomic factors, an aging population, cultural influences, increasing average age at first marriage, high divorce rates, improvements in the health and financial status of the older population, and changing residential preferences. Although family householders (the householder, his/her spouse, and children) accounted for 87% of the population, the number of nonfamily households increased 16% from 2000 to 2010. During this time, we also saw an 18% increase in female householders with no spouse, a 31% increase in male householders with no spouse, a 41% increase in unmarried couple households, and an increase in the number of multigenerational households (Lofquist, Lugalia, O'Connell, et al., 2012). Conversely, the number of husband–wife households, in relation to the total number of households, continues to show a downward trend, from 55.2% in 1990 to 48.4% in 2010.

Traditional Families In the past, the majority of American families consisted of married couples with at least one child, the husband in the labor force, and a wife not employed outside the home. U.S. Census Bureau data collected in 2010 show that 20.2% of American households consisted of a husband–wife household with children as compared with 23.5% in 2000. Asian children are more likely to live in a two-parent household (87%), followed by White non-Hispanic (75%). Black children were least likely to live with both parents (37%), followed by Hispanic children (67%) (Kreider & Ellis, 2011). The vast majority of "stay-at-home" parents are still women (5.0 million) while only 154,000 fathers "stay at home" (U.S. Census Bureau, 2012).

Grandparent Families When parents are unable or unwilling to assume the parenting role, grandparents will raise their grandchildren to prevent them from going to foster care or other alternate placement. In households without a parent, 64% of Black, 61% of Hispanics, 55% of White, and 35% of Asian children live with grandparents (Kreider & Ellis, 2011).

Married Adults Without Children Once only a small number in American society, this group now accounts for 28% of households (Lofquist, Lugaila, O'Connell, et al., 2012).

Dual-Earner Families A dual-earner family has both parents in the workforce. Parents of older children (6–11 years) were more likely to have jobs (1.9 million) than parents with younger children under 3 years of age (1.4 million) (U.S. Census, 2012b).

Single-Parent Families Single-parent families result from divorce, from the death of a partner, or from partners who choose not to marry or live together. In 2009, 27% of children lived with one parent. Most single-parent families are headed by women (15.3 million); however, the number of men raising children without a spouse has increased in recent years to 5.8 million in 2010. The percentage of single-parent households in the United States varies among geographic areas and ethnic groups.

Blended and Stepfamilies A **blended family** is established when single parents marry and either or both have children from a previous relationship. The nonbiological partner becomes the stepparent and a stepfamily is created. Blended families can include stepsiblings, half-siblings, or stepparents (Kreider & Ellis, 2011). Commonly, biological parents who are not living together in the child's home alternate the responsibilities and the child will have two mother or father figures (biological and step).

Extended Families In many cultural groups, it is not unusual for extended family members (e.g., grandparents, aunts, uncles, cousins) to live within a single dwelling or in close proximity and be considered immediate family. A less formal view of extended family incorporates close friends and other non-relatives. Consider, for example, the Meet Your Patient scenario. Although J. B.'s siblings are members of his extended family, they do not live with him, and he would not view them as his immediate family because his emotional bond and daily involvement is with Mike.

Sandwich Families The growing number of older adults has created **sandwich families** (Petrovich, 2008; Schumacher, MacNeil, Mobily, et al., 2012), in which middle-aged adults who still have children at home must care for and share their household with aging parents. The more affluent adults (household income > $100,000/year) and Hispanics are more likely to be in sandwich families (Parker & Patten, 2013). Although competent in the caregiver role, they feel personally overwhelmed and emotionally conflicted, but report being as happy as the non-sandwiched families.

Other Family Structures In addition to families bound by marriage and bloodlines, increasingly other family types exist, such as *heterosexual individuals* who may reside in a common household, or *gay and lesbian couples with or without children*. Although *individuals or couples who adopt children* are not biologically related, nonetheless, they are very much a family as they are emotionally attached and participate in the care and experiences in each other's lives. **Cohabiting adults** choose to live together and not marry or live together as a "trial run" prior to marriage. Cohabiting couples who marry have a higher rate of separation than their counterparts who do not live together before marriage, although this trend is declining (Copen, Daniels, Vespa, et al., 2012).

Recall that a family is a group of individuals who provide support and assistance to each other. In the

Meet Your Patient scenario, J. B. and Mike are not blood relatives, yet they provide strong support for each other. Many refer to this type of bond as **kith**, persons with a kinship bond. For some people, this bond is stronger than those created through bloodline.

Approaches to Family Nursing

Family nursing refers to nursing care that is holistically directed toward the whole family as well as to individual members (Fig. 14-1). Knowing the family unit is affected by acute or chronic illness, hospitalization, or healthcare interventions, the nurse best cares for the family by involving them in patient care decisions. For J. B. (Meet Your Patient) the nurses would support Mike's daily visits, and Mike is listed on the Health Insurance Portability and Accountability Act (HIPAA) form for communication of patient information. The staff would involve Mike and J. B.'s adult children in his care, discharge planning, and follow-up care at home. They would also teach Mike about J. B.'s medications and treatments so that he can assist J. B. in his activities of daily living (ADLs).

Three perspectives on family nursing include the family as (1) context, (2) unit of care, and (3) system. Family nursing is a specialty; to work with the family as a unit of care or as a system, you may need additional preparation.

Family as the Context for Care As a graduate nurse, you should be prepared to work, at least, with the family

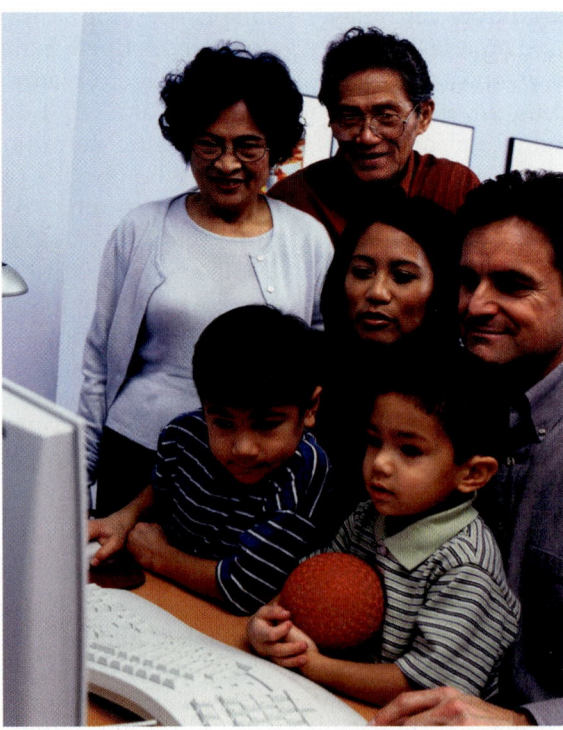

FIGURE 14-1 Family nursing refers to nursing care that is holistically directed toward the whole family as well as to individual members.

as the context for care of an individual person. Your focus in this approach is on the ill individual. From this perspective, you view the family as either a resource or a stressor to your patient. Using this knowledge, you would recognize the importance of J. B.'s friend and roommate, Mike, who is J. B.'s primary source of support. Before discharge, you would ask J. B., "Will Mike or will your daughters be able to help you when you go home?"

Family as the Unit of Care A slightly more complex approach views the family as the unit of care. Wellness of each member is critical to promoting family health. In this approach, you would view the family as the sum of all individual members and provide assessment and care for all family members; however, you might direct interventions to individual family members rather than the family as a whole. For example, you might provide teaching on nutrition and physical activity to all family members to promote their health. Or, to use our earlier example, you might check Mike's blood pressure when he visits J. B.

Family as a System The third perspective is the family as a system. In this approach, you focus on the family as a whole and as an interactional system. Using this perspective, you direct your assessment and intervention to communications and interactions between family members. The systems approach sees the family as embedded in and interacting with a larger community. Using this approach, you might ask, for example, "How has your family's relationship within the senior's group at your townhouse complex changed since your illness?"

KnowledgeCheck 14-1

- Name at least three types of family structures.
- What are two topics that the nurse can discuss with the family as a unit?

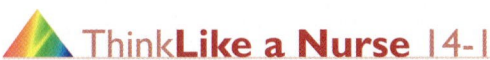 ThinkLike a Nurse 14-1

- How can you promote family cohesion for a family whose members live great distances from each other?

WHAT THEORIES ARE USEFUL FOR FAMILY CARE?

Several theories have been proposed to help us understand family functioning. Four such theories are general systems theory, structural–functional theories, family interactional theory, and developmental theory.

General Systems Theory

General systems theory (see Chapter 8) focuses on interactions between systems and the changes that result from these interactions. The family is considered an open system because the members function as individuals, are interdependent, and operate as a family unit (a *whole*, in systems language). Interaction can occur between members of the family or between multiple families. Healthy families strive to maintain a balance between external stress and internal relationships.

Changes in the behaviors or attitudes of an individual member affect the family unit, and changes in family structure and functioning affect individual members. It may help to think of a system as a mobile; if one piece of the mobile is moved, that movement sets the whole mobile in motion.

Other systems surround the family unit (e.g., the community, the city, the state, the healthcare system). Because these systems are broader than the family, they are referred to as **suprasystems.** Smaller components that fit within the family system (e.g., the mother, the marital couple) may be viewed as **subsystems.** Each system has a particular function. For example, one family member might be viewed as the decision maker, another as the peacekeeper, and yet another, the worker, and another as the disciplinarian for the children.

Structural–Functional Theories

Structural–functional family theories are based on the developmental theories of Freud, Erikson, and Havighurst (see Chapter 9 for review) and include the concepts of family roles and interactions. According to Parsons and Bales (1955), the structural–functional approach includes the following assumptions:

- A family is a social system with functional requirements.
- A family is a small group possessing certain features common to small groups.
- The family accomplishes functions that serve both the individual and society.
- Individuals act according to internalized norms that are learned through socialization.

Although they view the family as a social system, structural–functional theories, unlike systems theory, focus on *outcome* rather than process. You would use this theory to assess how well the family functions, both internally among family members and externally with outside systems. Examples of family functions include socialization of children; meeting the physical, financial, and emotional needs of family members; caring for older members; and being productive members of society.

Family Interactional Theory

Family interactional theory views the family as a unit of interacting personalities (Hill & Hansen, 1960). The major emphasis is on family roles. This approach to understanding families de-emphasizes the influence of the external world on what occurs within the family. Nurses working from an interactional perspective focus family healthcare on the interaction and communication between family members; their roles and power; family coping; and relationships with other people outside the direct family unit.

Developmental Theories

Developmental theories focus on the stage of family development. Theorists typically identify eight stages in the family life cycle according to the ages of the children and parents: beginning family, childbearing family, family with preschool children, family with school-age children, family with teenagers and young adults, family launching young adults, postparental family, and aging family. Each stage is associated with developmental tasks the family needs to achieve. Most family development theories do not identify stages and tasks for families who remain childless throughout their lives. To learn about developmental tasks associated with family stages, including those for families without children,

 Go to Chapter 14, **Assessment Guidelines and Tools, Assessing Family Developmental Tasks,** in Volume 2.

Generally the stages follow one another in a linear progression; however, some families may be in more than one stage at a time or may revert to previous stages. This overlap or reversion is most common in families that have children spaced far apart, in blended families, and in stepfamilies. See Chapter 9 for developmental theories applicable to individual family members.

KnowledgeCheck 14-2

- Which type of theory focuses on interactions among families, family members, and groups in the environment?
- What is the name of the theory that views families as a social system with a focus on outcomes?
- What are some examples of family functions as defined by structural–functional theories?

ThinkLike a Nurse 14-2

- Using systems theory, you could view J. B., his siblings, his children, and his grandchildren as a system. Refer to the section on family structures—how would you categorize this family structurally?
- Again using systems theory, what or who are the subsystems in the family system described in the preceding question?
- Considering J. B. alone, at what developmental stage is his "family"?

WHAT ARE SOME FAMILY HEALTH RISK FACTORS?

Many health risk factors are the same for families as for individuals, and they are similar across age groups and family types. Basically, destructive behaviors remain destructive behaviors, regardless of who is performing them. For a more complete discussion of this topic,

 Go to Chapter 14, **Supplemental Materials: What Are Some Family Health Risk Factors?** on DavisPlus.

For specific topics as they relate to families, also see Chapters 9 and 10 covering growth and development, Chapter 12 on stress and adaptation, Chapter 19 on teaching clients, and Chapter 21 on communication.

Childless and Childbearing Couples

Adapting to new roles within the home creates stress for newly married couples, couples who are trying to become pregnant, and new parents who are inexperienced in the challenges and responsibilities of raising a healthy, happy, and safe child (Fig. 14-2). Use of maladaptive coping mechanisms can lead to health problems and deterioration in relationships. For example, someone who uses alcohol to deal with stress is at risk for addiction, self-injury, and liver disease, and the family may possibly suffer the harmful effects of neglect and family violence. In addition to health risks related to pregnancy (e.g., miscarriage), abuse of alcohol could lead to congenital malformations and genetic defects in the child.

Families With Young Children

Finding safe, nurturing, and affordable childcare can be a major source of family stress for parents working outside the home. Common parenting concerns center on the child's development, socialization, education, discipline, nutrition, sleeping, toileting, and safety. In addition, the demands of work and child rearing mean less time is available to nurture the couple's relationship, leaving them at increased risk for marital discord.

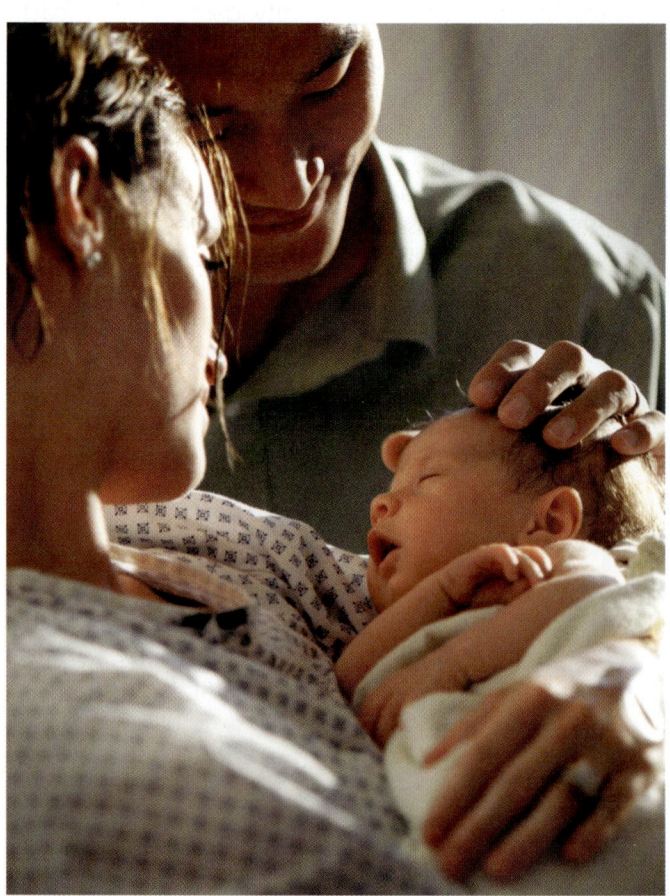

FIGURE 14-2 Newly married couples, couples who are trying to become pregnant, and new parents are vulnerable to stress as they adapt to new roles.

Injuries and illness create risks to family health. For example, those receiving group childcare or attending school are exposed to other children who might have contagious diseases that can spread to other family members. To reduce the risk for serious infectious diseases (e.g., mumps or hepatitis B), parents need to be aware of the importance of adhering to the recommended childhood immunization schedule. Research shows that the percentage of parents who refuse immunizations for their children continues to increase each year. Parents report various concerns, including personal perceptions and healthcare system issues (Luthy, Beckstrand, Callister, et al., 2012). For families who live with a chronic illness (e.g., asthma or type 1 diabetes) or a developmental or learning disability (e.g., autism), the stress related to compromised health, falling behind in school, financial burdens, and even day-to-day living can become overwhelming.

Families With Adolescents

Families with adolescents are often concerned about teen risk-taking behaviors. Some specific risk-taking behaviors include using tobacco, alcohol, and other illicit drugs; engaging in extreme stunts and accepting dares; rebelling against authority; and being sexually promiscuous.

Adolescents may participate in risky behaviors to impress others, to feel cool or important, or to experience a feeling of power. Developmentally, adolescents typically do not feel the threat of real danger. Other contributing factors include family expectations of not completing school and being in a large family (Homer, Rew, & Brown, 2012).

Families with adolescents may also be dealing with aging parents or grandparents (Fig. 14-3). Parents may become "sandwiched" between the needs of the growing adolescents and the needs of their aging parents. Women are particularly at risk for stress in these situations because they are usually the ones who provide the additional care for older relatives.

Families With Young Adults

Young adults commonly move out of the parental home as their school years end, taking on full-time jobs, many for the first time. This is a time when many marry and begin childbearing and rearing. Some confront such problems as tight finances, inability to find meaningful work, nontherapeutic personal relationships, or other life challenges.

Financial strain might influence a young adult, alone or with a newly formed family, to move back with his parents until he can "get back on his feet." This return to the nest, although sensible, can nonetheless be a stress on the family. Role strain and poor communication are common. Although young adults returning to the home of origin can represent a new opportunity for family attachment, the presence of another person in the household commonly changes family dynamics.

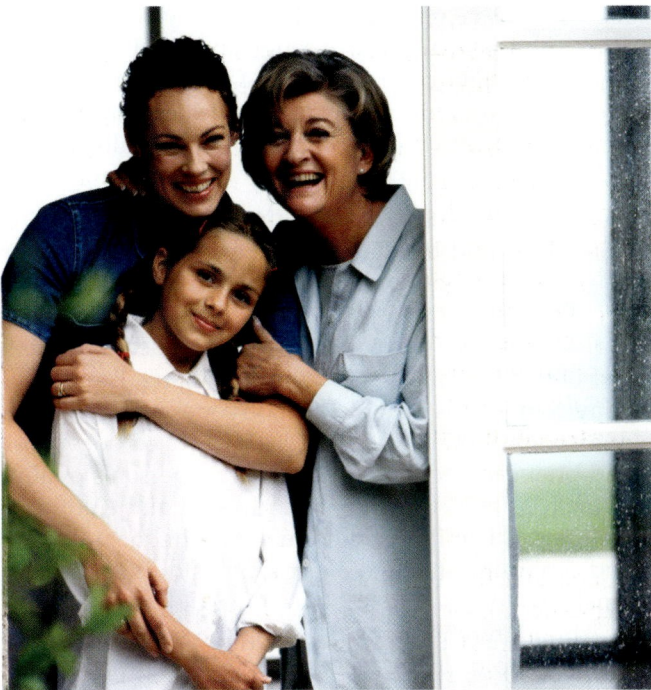

FIGURE 14-3 In families with adolescents or young adults, the parents may become "sandwiched" between the needs of the growing adolescents and the needs of their own parents.

Not every transition is a permanent accomplishment or marker of social success. Newly found autonomy and independence is exhilarating for some and anxiety-provoking for others. The boundary between adolescence and adulthood is blurred by societal forces (e.g., a contracting economy, changing labor force expectations, and expanding opportunities for women). As this continues, roles within the family will evolve and families will need to find healthy ways to adapt.

Families With Middle-Aged Adults

The middle years are a time of examining life goals and coping with aging and the empty nest. This can be a satisfying time of role fulfillment, career success, financial security, and social comfort. The quality of the spousal relationship might take on a new importance. The middle-aged adult may experience a new sense of freedom and need for self-exploration and personal growth. Without the time demands of raising children, adults have more time available to pursue other personal interests or professional paths.

The middle years can also be a time of self-doubt triggered by the changes of aging, menopause, an empty nest, care or death of parents, heightened career demands, or change in career life or relationships, all of which can cause emotional strain. Some adults suffer a **mid-life crisis**, which is a period of intense questioning about the meaning and direction in life, asking what brings personal fulfillment. Adults battling mid-life crisis might display signs of depression, anxiety, or rebellion from the status quo.

The effects of long-standing unhealthy behaviors often become apparent in middle adulthood. For example, people who have used tobacco for many years may now begin to notice an increase in cough and chest congestion or those who have consumed high-fat diets may develop high blood pressure or elevated cholesterol levels. Remember, individual health impacts family health.

Families With Older Adults

Falls and trauma are a common health risk for families with older adults. For more information about this, see Chapters 10 and 24. Older adults are also at risk for social isolation and loneliness because of the loss of relationships that occurs with aging. Family dynamics change as the older person copes with the death of a spouse, sibling, friends, or other loved ones. Loss and grief can deeply affect an elderly person's quality of life, clarity of thinking, and physical and emotional well-being. Families should maintain frequent contact and communications to offset feelings of isolation and loneliness.

Although retirement can bring the simpler life that many people desire, retired individuals must deal with the loss of daily contact with colleagues in the workplace and, for some, a reduced sense of responsibility or purpose. Friends can be a significant source of support (Fig. 14-4), but functional losses may cause the person to limit physical activity, volunteer work, church attendance, and other social activities. Elderly adults have an increased risk for depression.

Maintaining good nutrition and hydration becomes more difficult as a person ages, particularly for the frail elderly. The following are situations that may compromise the nutrition of older adults:

- Forgetting to eat (especially those who live alone)
- Inadequate or unreliable transportation to shop for food
- Lack of money to buy food
- Physical changes that alter taste (e.g., reduced sensitivity in the taste buds and less saliva for taste and swallowing)
- Loss of appetite
- Poorly fitting dentures
- For more information about nutrition, see Chapter 27.

Memory and problem-solving abilities change with aging. Forgetfulness and confusion can pose risks to safety for older adults, particularly for those living alone or with other aging adults whose mental status is compromised. When older adults, and especially frail elderly, lose their ability to reason, they are vulnerable to physical harm. The demands of keeping the aging adult safe can lead to caregiver role strain and family stress.

It is easy to understand from the above scenarios the cascading effect that one deficit, such as lack of transportation, can have on the health of an older adult and her family. Be sure to educate them about the availability of community resources, such as Meals on Wheels and home health aides, as many may not be aware that help is available.

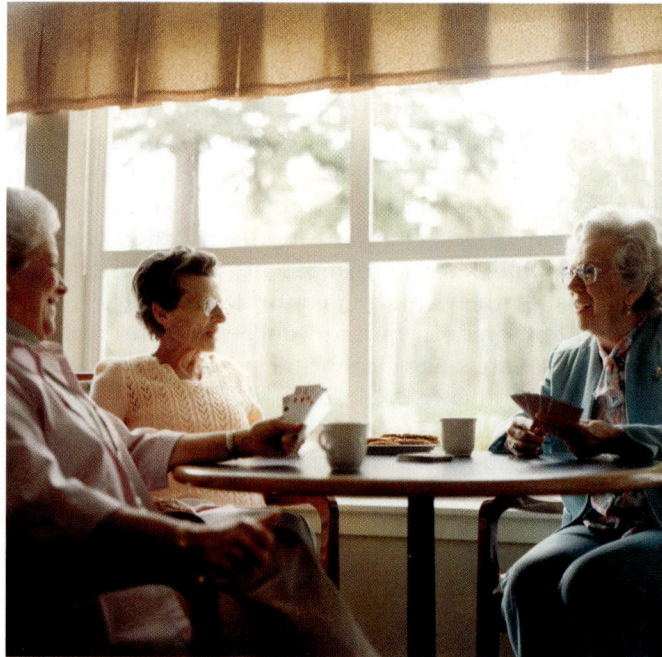

FIGURE 14-4 Friends play an important role in the support system of older people.

 Think**Like a Nurse** 14-3

- What developmental stage is your family in? How do you know?
- What basic attitudes, values, or beliefs influenced you in your childhood family?
- How were decisions made in your childhood family? Were people's feelings and individuals' needs considered?
- Can you remember good times and laughter that bonded you together as a family? In your present family life, how often do you laugh together?
- In the Meet Your Patient scenario, what health risks do J. B. and Mike face, considering their age and health?

WHAT ARE SOME CHALLENGES TO FAMILY HEALTH?

We have already mentioned the effects of some demographic changes, such as an aging population, on families. This section examines other regional and national trends that affect families.

Poverty and Unemployment

When the economy takes a downturn, families may struggle to provide for basic needs (e.g., food and shelter) and healthcare. In 2010, 50.0 million people in the United States did not have health insurance (DeNavas-Wall, Proctor, & Smith, 2012). The Affordable Care Act, passed in 2010, has provisions to provide healthcare coverage for people who cannot obtain private or employment-funded insurance. In 2011, however, the number of uninsured people decreased to 48.6 million. Seven million children under age 18 did not have health insurance. Children in poverty had an uninsured rate of 13.8% compared with 9.4% for all children.

Families with no or inadequate health insurance do not seek preventive medical care and often come to the emergency room with acute medical conditions.

Teenage pregnancy is strongly associated with poverty, unemployment, and health risks. While teen birth rates declined in 2009, and again in 2011 (to 329,797), they still remain higher than in other developed countries (Centers for Disease Control and Prevention [CDC], 2010, updated 2012, November 21; Pazol, Warner, Gavin, et al., 2011). Infants born to teen mothers are more likely to have health problems at birth as a result of numerous factors, including late or no prenatal care. Thirty-four percent of pregnant females under age 20 failed to obtain first-trimester prenatal care compared with 28% of women between the ages of 20 and 24. In addition to the economic costs ($11 billion in 2008), teenage mothers have greater health disparities, are more likely to drop out of schools, have high unemployment rates, and their children have higher involvement in the juvenile justice system. Because of the numerous and long-lasting problems associated with teenage pregnancy, the CDC has partnered with the federal Office of the Assistant Secretary for Health (OASH) to launch a campaign aimed at reducing teenage pregnancy and addressing health disparities in teen pregnancy and birth rates (CDC, 2010, updated 2012, November 21).

Families in all socioeconomic levels can experience difficulties in an economic downturn, especially those with low reserves. Single-parent and low-income families are hardest hit. Most people who are living at or below the federal poverty level are workers with minimum-wage or seasonal jobs. In a sluggish economy, nonessential jobs may be eliminated; and many sectors of business and service suffer. This means that not only family income is compromised, but also, on a larger level, fewer workers are paying taxes. Thus, government programs supporting families in need may be underfunded. Although some people find creative solutions to family poverty (e.g., a woman who is laid off assumes childcare for another family whose members remain employed), many families experience extreme hardships when the economy is suffering.

Middle-income families are also affected by corporate downsizing or stock market fluctuations. Both skilled and unskilled laborers suffer when consumer spending and housing economies decline. Even families who were living in seeming prosperity may not have sufficient funds to cover a period of unemployment or economic recession. Many people in the United States carry significant credit card debt, a first and possibly second mortgage, car payments, a variety of insurance premiums, and perhaps school or other loans.

KnowledgeCheck 14-3
- Which socioeconomic group of families is hardest hit during poor economic periods?
- How are middle-income families affected by poor economic times?
- What concerns are associated with teenage pregnancies?

Infectious Diseases
Family health may be affected by any number of new or resistant pathogens, such as severe acute respiratory syndrome (SARS), methicillin-resistant *Staphylococcus aureus* (MRSA), West Nile virus, and H1N1 virus. The 2009 H1N1, also called swine flu, caused illness in humans, especially young children, pregnant women, people 65 years and older, and those with certain chronic diseases. Influenza A (H3N2), 2009 H1N1, and influenza B viruses were associated with the 2012–2013 seasonal flu, which caused widespread illnesses and several deaths in persons across the lifespan (CDC, 2012).

HIV infection is a devastating event that significantly impacts the family. In addition to the obvious physical and financial stressors, women who infect their infants and partners who infect the other partner with HIV bear a tremendous burden of guilt. The populations at highest risk for contracting HIV are men who have sex with men (whites, blacks, and Hispanics), followed by heterosexual black women, black males, Hispanic women, and white women (Prejean, Song, Hernandez, et al., 2011). When compared with their white counterparts, the number of new HIV cases is seven times higher for black males and 20 times higher for black females (CDC, n.d.). Some families keep the diagnosis a secret and blame each other, whereas other families support each other and manage the illness as best they can.

Advances in treating HIV infection and preventing its spread have been made through public and patient education, vaccination, antiviral therapy, and other antimicrobial treatments for HIV-related complications. The nurse should emphasize the use of proper protective precautions to minimize the spread of the disease.

Even "old" diseases, once thought to be eradicated, can threaten family health. In recent years, diseases once controlled by immunization are making a comeback (e.g., pertussis [whooping cough], polio, mumps, and smallpox). Many families either refuse or fail to comply with immunizations schedules. As a result, *herd immunity* is reduced. The outcome is high physical, social, and economic costs from illness, absent schooldays or workdays, doctor and hospital visits, and even premature deaths (CDC, 2007, updated 2012, November 21).

KnowledgeCheck 14-4
- What gender groups are experiencing the fastest rate of growth in new HIV cases?
- Name two previously eradicated diseases that have become a threat again.

Chronic Illness and Disability
Chronic illness and disability profoundly change the way families function. Family members' roles evolve over time, especially for the caregiver. Many people with chronic illness and disability require assistance with ADLs, such as getting around the home, feeding, bathing, dressing, toileting, and getting in and out of a

chair or bed. Many are not able to work or generate family income, often creating financial strain or poverty. Long-term illness and disability cause mental, emotional, or physical limitations that affect family communication patterns. In addition, relationships within the family may be difficult due to caregiver strain and issues related to dependency. Long-term care of a family member may increase the risk for abuse and neglect, including maltreatment of frail elderly family members.

The Americans with Disabilities Act (ADA) Amendments Act of 2008 defines one component of disability as a physical or mental impairment that substantially interferes with a person's ability to engage in major life activities (U.S. Equal Opportunity Commission, 2008). Individuals have a disability if they meet criteria involving limitations in mobility/ambulation, hearing, vision, learning, cognitive, self-care, or independent living, to name a few. In the United States:

- 38 million (12%) of noninstitutionalized people reported one or more disabilities in 2011.
- The prevalence of disability was lowest for children under age 5 years (0.8%) and highest for those 65 years and older (36.8%).
- 6.5 million (32.6%) of noninstitutionalized people with disabilities were employed.
- The poverty rate was 31% for persons with a work disability, 28.8 % for those with a broad disability, and 28.6% for persons with both work and broad disabilities.
- Among the various types of disabilities, 10.2 million were people with ambulatory disabilities while the lowest group was those with vision disability at 3.5 million (1.8%) (Rehabilitation Research and Training, 2012).

🍁 Disabilities and other mobility limitations can lead to poor health outcomes in older adults because of limited ability to access needed resources such as fresh food and medical care. It is essential that nurses collaborate with social work/case management to ensure that older adults have the resources needed to remain independent as long as possible. Independence is associated with better long-term health outcomes.

Homelessness

Homelessness is a growing problem in many U.S. cities, not only for individuals but for also for families. Many homeless people sleep on the streets, although others live temporarily with relatives or in mission shelters. Homelessness is far more complex than lack of housing. This problem might be explained by a number of factors, such as financial crises, socially dysfunctional relationships, unemployment, lack of job skills, substance abuse, healthcare expenses, or the inability or lack of desire to live within the socially accepted norms of society. In the United States, deep poverty and homelessness often result from mental illness, disability, or misfortune.

Homeless families are often socially isolated. Many homeless children do not attend school, and those who do tend to perform poorly. Often, homeless families do not seek care for significant health problems, primarily because they don't know how to access the healthcare system and qualify for healthcare services. Homelessness threatens family relationship and emotional and physical health. The focus is on meeting basic needs of food and shelter, which according to Maslow's Hierarchy of Needs theory (Chapter 4), must be met before the family can grow.

Single women, members of minority groups, and single-parent families are particularly vulnerable to homelessness and poverty (Fig. 14-5). It is not uncommon for divorced women to end up with less income than their ex-husbands. In addition, many women also might have sole custody of their children, which creates additional expenses for them. In many states, social service departments are underfunded and unable to enforce child support laws. Some biological fathers struggle to pay child support while maintaining their own living expenses. Others may be incarcerated or their whereabouts unknown.

Violence and Neglect Within Families

Domestic violence—including physical, emotional, and sexual abuse—occurs throughout all strata of our society, among all racial, social, and economic groups. As many as one in every four women will be a victim of violence during her lifetime, and more than 3 million children each year are reported to child protective services agencies as alleged abuse victims. The National Child Abuse and Neglect Data Systems reported that 676,569 children were victims of child abuse and neglect in 2011, which represents 9.1 victims per 1,000 children (Children's Bureau, 2012). Race and ethnic data showed that 43.9% of victims were white, followed by Hispanics (22.1%) and African Americans (21.5%). The highest rate of victimization occurred in younger children (21.2%). The majority of the child victims were neglected (78.5%), followed by physical abuse (17.6%) and sexual abuse (9.1%). Children ages 12 to 14 had the highest percentage of sexual abuse (26.3%), followed by ages 15 to 17 (21.8%), and 9 to 11 (18.5%). Children age 2 and

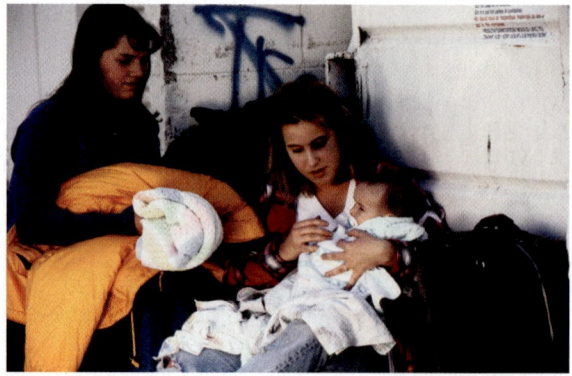

FIGURE 14-5 Many homeless people are single women and children.

younger were the most frequent victims of fatalities (73.8%) from abuse and neglect (Children's Bureau, 2012). These children are the most vulnerable for many reasons, including their dependency, small size, and inability to defend themselves.

Any type of violence is likely to have long-lasting effects on the victims and on the family. It may result in the disintegration of the family relationships and structure (e.g., sending the children to foster care, escaping to a battered women's shelter, living with others). Health issues related to domestic violence include physical injury from the assault itself, as well as chronic health problems that emerge either as a complication of traumatic injury or as a physical response to the ongoing stress from violence or neglect. Families experiencing domestic violence have more unintended pregnancies, miscarriages, abortions, and low-birth-weight babies. They also have more sexually transmitted infections and higher rates of depression, post-traumatic stress syndrome, substance abuse, and suicide. And even though the emotional and physical pain may stop when the victim leaves the family environment, often there are long-term effects involving emotional injury, marred self-esteem, or poor-quality relationships. Victims of family violence learn patterns of ineffective coping that can be repeated in successive generations.

KnowledgeCheck 14-5

- Name two causes of homelessness.
- Name two groups of individuals who are vulnerable to homelessness.
- Name two types of violence.
- Among children, which age group is the most vulnerable to abuse and neglect?
- Describe the effects of family violence that generally endure after the physical injury has healed.

PracticalKnowledge
knowing how

A holistic view of family health integrates the biological, social, cultural, and spiritual aspects of life and refers to individual members as well as the whole family. Nurses play a vital role in promoting family wellness across the life span. When working with families, you will encourage them to take responsibility for their own family health. Your interactions with families can empower them to practice behaviors that will aid in healing and maintaining good health.

ASSESSMENT

Health assessment for the family is similar to that for individuals. Gather all essential assessment information for each family member. Ensuring family privacy is essential for obtaining an accurate and comprehensive family health assessment. (See Chapter 22 for additional information on physical assessment.) In addition to the individual factors, assess the health of the family unit. For an example of a family assessment form used by a community health agency,

 Go to Chapter 14, **Tables, Boxes, Figures: ESG Figure 14-1,** on Davis*Plus.*

In general, a family assessment should include the following:

- Relevant medical data, social and family history for individuals within the family
- Family composition
- Family genogram showing health issues
- Family history and developmental stage
- Description of the home environment and surroundings
- Family structure, including communication patterns and power and role structures
- Family functions
- Health beliefs, values, and behaviors
- Family strengths
- Family stressors and coping
- Abuse and violence within the family. To see an abuse assessment,

 Go to Chapter 9, **Procedure 9-1: Assessing for Abuse,** in Volume 2.

For a more complete description of the context of a family assessment,

 Go to Chapter 14, **Clinical Insights 14-1: Conducting a Family Assessment,** and the assessment tool, **Assessing Family Developmental Tasks,** in Volume 2.

The following sections discuss in more detail the assessment of family health beliefs, communication patterns, coping processes, and caregiver role strain.

Assessing the Family's Health History

The family history can provide clues about a person's health and susceptibility for disease. Genetic linkages have been discovered for common, complex diseases, such as breast cancer, Alzheimer's' disease, diabetes, macular degeneration, seizures, inflammatory bowel disease, lupus, and heart disease, to name a few.

Genomics is the study of human genes and their function, including the interactions among other genes and the environment. Simply said, it is about the interplay between a person's genetic makeup, and food and environmental factors such as lifestyle and stress.

How Can Genomics Be Useful? Genomics can be used to personalize a patient's plan of care by:

- Identifying at-risk individuals for certain conditions so more effective preventive care can be provided
- More accurately detecting illness, even before symptoms appear

- Tailoring healthcare to the individual, while reducing a trial-and-error approach
- Evaluating a person's response to the care, considering multiple factors

Genomics helps us to understand how people respond differently to particular drugs and medical treatments. For example, one client with a genetic predisposition for high cholesterol can benefit from a change in diet and exercise to decrease the likelihood that the genetic risk will be expressed. Another person may not respond to lifestyle measures and require cholesterol-reducing drugs.

How Is a Genogram Constructed? When assessing the family history, you can use a pictorial tool, called a **genogram**, to display the relationship of family members with pertinent health-related information (Fig. 14-6). This type of family tree can provide a quick and useful context in which to evaluate an individual's health risks.

To construct a genogram, you will note the causes of death, genetically linked diseases, and other important health problems. Use a three-generation (or more) genogram to also show environmental (e.g., toxin) and mental health issues (e.g., depression, alcohol abuse, suicide), occupational diseases (e.g., asbestos), infections (e.g., MRSA), and obesity among family members. When developing a genogram, use symbols and abbreviations

to denote family members, including a key for interpretation (Box 14-1).

Assessing the Family's Health Beliefs

Health beliefs can vary widely among families and among individuals within families. The differences can be especially great among different generations of a family (e.g., between grandparents and their grandchildren). Some common health beliefs are expressed in such adages as "An apple a day keeps the doctor away," "Doctor knows best," and "Feed a cold, starve a fever." Some families may have an intense skepticism or mistrust of medical care and hospitals and may seek treatment only when absolutely necessary (e.g., when the pain becomes unbearable). Many of these beliefs are passed on from generation to generation.

Even if one family member does not share all of the beliefs of the family, you need to be aware of the family's beliefs because they may influence the individual's decision making. To illustrate this point, consider a family caring for a member who is frail elderly, confused, and immobile. Suppose one family member believes quality of life issues are more important than quantity. Yet another family member who is giving care has a fundamental disagreement with this belief and supports the right of the older adult to receive whatever care is needed for physical safety, emotional fulfillment, and

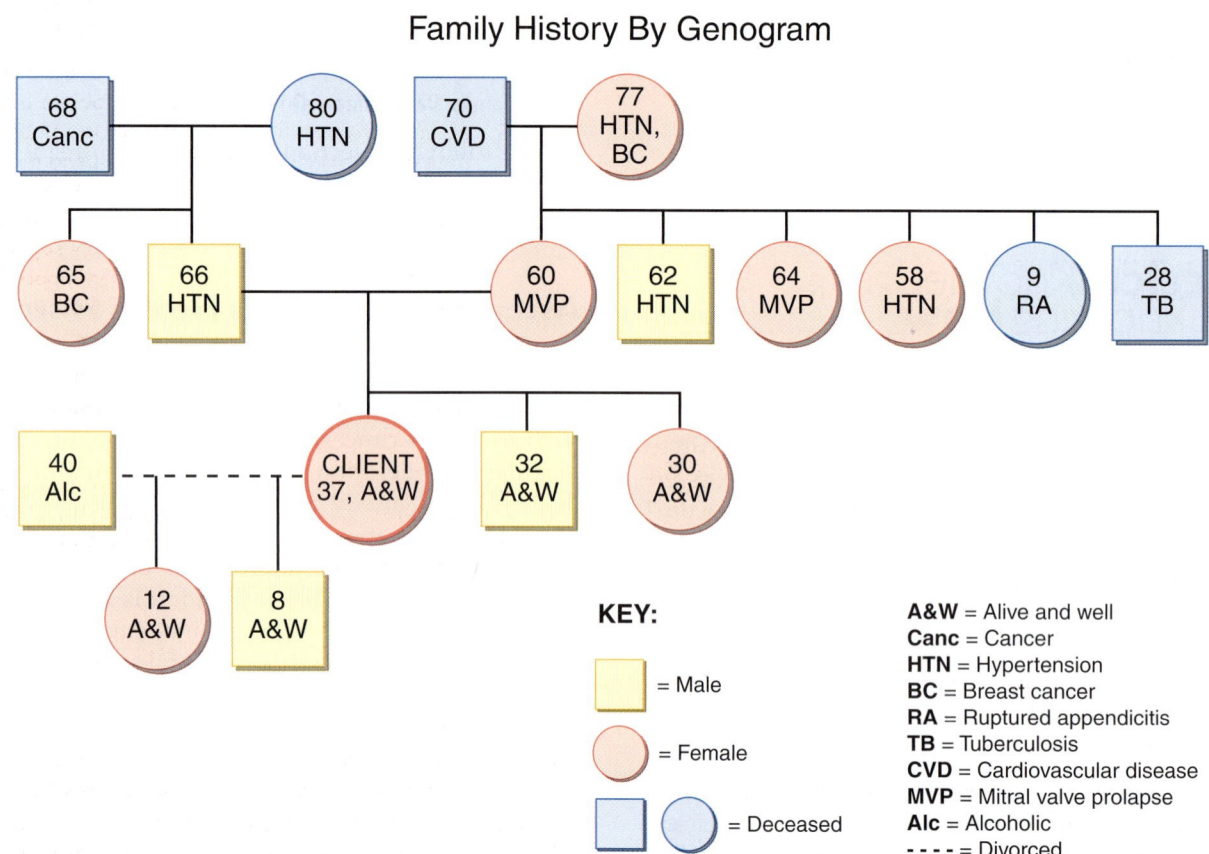

FIGURE 14-6 Family history by genogram.

BOX 14-1 ■ Family History by Listing Family Members

The following history is for a 37-year-old female patient.

Patient: Age 37, alive and well

Spouse: Age 40, divorced, alcoholism

Daughter: Age 12, alive and well

Son: Age 8, alive and well

Brother: Age 32, alive and well

Sister: Age 30, alive and well

Father: Age 66, hypertension (HTN)

Mother: Age 60, mitral valve prolapse (MVP)

Paternal aunt: Age 65, breast cancer

Maternal uncle: Age 62, HTN

Maternal uncle: Deceased age 28, tuberculosis (TB)

Maternal aunt: Age 64, MVP

Maternal aunt: Age 58, HTN

Maternal aunt: Deceased age 9, ruptured appendix

Paternal grandfather: Deceased age 68, cancer

Paternal grandmother: Age 80, HTN

Maternal grandmother: Age 77, HTN, breast cancer

Maternal grandfather: Deceased age 70, cardiovascular disease (CVD)

spiritual well-being for any length of time. In a situation like this, the family is at risk for interpersonal conflict, impaired communication, and caregiver strain. If you would like more information on health beliefs, see Chapter 42.

ThinkLike a Nurse 14-4

- As a nurse, how can you promote overall wellness in a family with a critically ill member?
- What health beliefs would you ask J. B.'s family about?

Assessing the Family's Communication Patterns

To assess family communication patterns, you will need to interview the family and also carefully observe the interactions between family members. Try to uncover the following information:

- Who is the primary decision maker in the family?
- How are family decisions made: by one individual or by family conference?
- What is the most frequent type of communication among family members (e.g., visits to the home, telephone, texting, e-mail)?

Family members who participate in dysfunctional communication patterns may not come to scheduled family meetings and may not be present during the initial interview. Additionally, when relationships among family members are strained or dysfunctional, they may distort the information they provide about a home situation or another family member.

Key Point: *Do not rely solely on the information provided by the family members during the interview process. Families usually want to "put on the best face" for healthcare providers, so they may be careful to give socially desirable responses. Carefully observe the words people use and other cues involved in communication, such as body language, direct eye contact, and other nonverbal expressions, particularly among family members.*

PICOT

Alcohol Treatment and Family Support

Situation: The nurse is meeting with a family prior to the discharge of the husband/father from alcohol treatment. The teenage daughter asks the nurse whether her father will ever drink again.

PICOT Components:

P Population/client	=	Alcoholic adults
I Intervention/indicator	=	Family Support
C Comparator/control	=	No family support
O Outcome	=	Decreased risk of relapse
T Time	=	Over time

Searchable Question: Do _____ (P) who receive/are exposed to _____ (I) demonstrate_____ (O) as compared to _____ (C) during _____ (T)?

Example of Evidence: Alcohol abuse is a common social, family, and individual health problem. Inpatient alcohol treatment has been a common solution. Research indicates that clients who spend more time in treatment and subsequent time in an abstinence-related group home, as well as having overall family support are less likely to relapse. Family support did not need to be alcohol related; rather, support for the client in general was shown to have a positive effect on the client's sustained sobriety.

Practice Change: The nurse made certain to assess family relationships and support for this and future clients.

Reference: Groh, D., Jason, L., Davis, M., et al. (2007). Friends, family, and alcohol abuse: An examination of general and alcohol-specific social support. *American Journal on Addictions, 16*(1), 49–55. doi:10.1080/10550490601080084

Assessing the Family's Coping Processes

The physiological manifestations of stress (e.g., anxiety, increased pulse rate) may decrease the effectiveness of interventions and negatively affect a client's health. Family members who are not coping effectively may cause the client to become stressed or anxious or have problems sleeping. Assessing family coping is a first step to helping the family develop more effective coping patterns. Observe for physical indications of stress, anxiety, or loss of sleep in the client and for relationships and communication patterns among family members. As a nurse, you can assess whether family members are irritable and "snap at" (speak harshly or curtly to) one another. Pay attention to who is visiting. Family members who are not coping well may avoid coming to visit the patient, so this may be an indicator of who is coping and who is not.

KnowledgeCheck 14-6

- Why is it important for you to ask about family health beliefs?
- What factors may impede a family's ability to cope with an individual's illness?
- What is the significance of a genogram?

Assessing for Caregiver Role Strain

Conflicts between caregiving and other responsibilities can produce tremendous family stress. The physical, emotional, and time demands involved in caring for family members who are chronically ill, disabled, or frail can create difficulties among family members and compromise relationships. Financial stress can also be a factor in family functioning. When these stressors add up, family caregivers might suffer from what NANDA-I terms Caregiver Role Strain. This is present when a person has difficulty in performing adequately in the family caregiver role.

To assess for caregiver burnout, observe for dysfunctional communication, such as abusive language and aggression. Look for physical injury to the patient, which may occur when caregivers are overwhelmed and overstressed. Alternatively, you might see the caregiver withdrawing emotionally, which could result in emotional neglect and isolation. Caregivers experiencing role strain might exhibit emotional distress, including depressive symptoms and apathy.

■ ANALYSIS/NURSING DIAGNOSIS

Recall in the diagnostic process you must analyze the data for cues (data that deviate from norms). Therefore, you should be familiar with the characteristics of a healthy family so you can use them as your basis for comparison (Box 14-2). For individual family members, of course, any NANDA-I diagnosis may be appropriate for describing a client's health status. **Family diagnoses,** however, are meant to describe the health status of the family as a whole. The following are examples:

Caregiver Role Strain (actual and risk for)
Family Coping: Compromised
Family Coping: Disabled
Dysfunctional Family Processes
Impaired Home Maintenance
Impaired Parenting (actual and risk for)
Ineffective Family Therapeutic Regimen Management
Ineffective Role Performance
Interrupted Family Processes
Readiness for Enhanced Family Coping

BOX 14-2 ■ Characteristics of a Healthy Family

A healthy family requires more than merely the absence of family dysfunction or disease in an individual member. Characteristics of a healthy family are listed, following:

State of family well-being

Sense of belonging and connectedness

Clear boundaries between family members where the responsibilities of adults are clear and separate from responsibilities of growing children

Sense of trust and respect

Honesty and freedom of expression, including different opinions or viewpoints

Spending time together, sharing rituals and traditions

Relaxed body language, physical touch, and frequent eye contact

Flexibility: adaptability and ability to deal with stress, openness to change

Commitment: working together to maintain the family

Spiritual well-being

Respect for privacy of individual members

Balance of giving and receiving

Positive, effective communication

Accountability, including acceptance when mistakes are made

Appreciation and affection for each other

Responding to the needs and interests of all members

Health-promoting lifestyle of individual members

Readiness for Enhanced Parenting
Relocation Stress Syndrome
Risk for Impaired Attachment
Social Isolation

For standardized definitions and terminology to describe nursing diagnoses, outcomes, and interventions for families,

 Go to Chapter 14, **Standardized Language, NOC Family Health Outcomes,** and **NIC Family Interventions,** on DavisPlus.

■ PLANNING OUTCOMES AND EVALUATION

NOC outcomes specifically for families as units are found in the NOC domain Family Health, which includes the classes Family Coping, Family Health Status, Family Integrity, and Parenting Performance. Outcomes from other domains may apply as well, depending on the nursing diagnosis you have made. You will find these on DavisPlus, as mentioned just above.

Individualized goals/outcome statements you might write for a family include the following examples, which represent some of the traits of healthy families in Box 14-2. The family:

Teaches respect for others within and outside the family.

Observes rituals and traditions (e.g., celebrates birthdays).

Respects the privacy of each member.

Communicates effectively and openly.

Remember the outcomes you develop for the care plan serve as the criteria for evaluating your patient's responses to nursing interventions.

PLANNING INTERVENTIONS/IMPLEMENTATION

NIC interventions for families as units are found in the NIC domain Family Integrity Promotion, which includes the classes for the Childbearing Family. Interventions from other domains may apply as well, depending on the nursing diagnosis you have made. You will find NIC family interventions on Davis*Plus,* as mentioned above.

Individualized nursing actions you might use with families include the following examples (other interventions are described in succeeding sections):

- Collaborate with family in problem solving and decision making.
- Refer the family to support groups of other families dealing with similar problems.
- Monitor current family relationships.
- Assist with family with conflict resolution.

- Encourage family to maintain positive relationships.
- Establish trusting relationship with family members.
- Counsel family members on additional effective coping skills for their own use.
- Refer for family therapy, as indicated.
- Tell family members it is safe and acceptable to use typical expression of affection when in a hospital setting.
- Encourage family members to verbalize their concerns, fears, and perceptions.

Promoting Family Wellness

Encouraging families to value and incorporate health promotion into their lifestyles will also affect the health of individual members. Health-promotion behaviors are typically learned within the family. You can promote family wellness by addressing both individual and family needs. It is important to identify both strengths and basic weaknesses of the family to adequately meet healthcare needs.

Involving the family in each phase of the nursing process promotes positive health outcomes and helps establish trust between you and the family. Wellness interventions may include contracting, health teaching, anticipatory guidance, and promoting family cohesion during a crisis (e.g., hospitalization of a family member). For specific health promotion activities, see Chapter 42.

Toward Evidence-Based Practice

Backhouse, J., & Graham, A. (2012). Grandparents raising grandchildren: Negotiating the complexities of role-identity conflict. *Child & Family Social Work, 17*(3), 306–315.

A qualitative study was conducted to identify common themes from the experiences of 27 grandmothers and 7 grandfathers who were raising their grandchildren ranging in ages from 1 to 17 years. Some of the pain and challenges described by the subjects were feelings of grief and loss regarding their children's situations, emotional and financial costs of dealing with the legal and welfare systems, inability to meet the physical activity needs of their grandchildren, and the thought of dying before the grandchildren reached adulthood. Nevertheless, the positive experiences dominated the relationships. These included the emotional bond and attachment with the grandchildren, the satisfaction of providing them with security and stability, and having more tolerance and patience with child raising experiences.

Conway, F. (2011). Emotional strain in caregiving among African American grandmothers raising their grandchildren. *Journal of Women & Aging, 23*(2), 113–128.

Researchers examined the emotional and role strain experienced by 88 African American grandmothers, ages 33 to 88, who were raising their grandchildren. Results showed that younger grandmothers experienced more emotional and caregiving strain than their older counterparts. In

addition, unmarried grandmothers had more emotional and caregiving strain than married grandmothers.

Huges, M. E., Waite, L. J., LaPierre, T. A., et al. (2007). All in the family: The impact of caring for grandchildren on grandparents' health. *The Journals of Gerontology Series B: Psychological Sciences and Social Sciences, 62,* S108–S119.

Researchers were interested in knowing the effects of caring for grandchildren on the physical and psychological health of older adults. Using a sample of 12,872 grandparents ages 50 through 80, researchers found no evidence that caring for grandchildren negatively affects grandparents' health and mental well-being. In contrast, grandparents who babysit had higher levels of physical health and emotional benefits. Only a small number of grandparents may have had their health compromised by having children in the home, likely the result of infections. The findings were different when parental involvement was low: Grandmothers were more likely to experience poor health behaviors, depression, and lower self-rating of overall health. The study highlights the benefits of grandparents caring for their grandchildren.

1. Based on this research, if you were the nurse, what kinds of information would you want to gather from families in which grandparents provided custodial care to grandchildren?

2. What ways can you think of to support grandparents who assume major roles in rearing grandchildren?

Interventions When a Family Member Is Ill

When a family member is ill or hospitalized, the other family members experience a range of emotions—especially when the illness is severe or of sudden onset. Family members may display signs of stress in a variety of ways, for example, by arguing with each other or with healthcare providers, by insisting on immediate care for their loved one, by avoiding the client's room, by being critical of the care provided, or by frequently asking that information be repeated. These are normal reactions; do not take them personally.

The patient and family need to understand the medical diagnosis, the plan of care, and the recovery process. In addition, it is often the nurse who provides extensive discharge instructions to the client and family before they leave the hospital. For interventions to help the family members manage stress when a family member is ill, see Box 14-3.

Interventions for Caregiver Role Strain

Interventions specific to caregiver role strain center include the following:

Assessing the caregiver for degree of impaired functioning (e.g., difficult sleeping, weight loss)

Assessing for safety issues that exist for the care receiver

Identifying causes of caregiver strain (e.g., lack of knowledge, frail client with around-the-clock care needs, complex treatments, or conflicts between caregiver and care receiver)

Helping the caregiver to identify and express feelings, including negative ones (e.g., by use of statements such as "This must be hard for you." Or, "I hear you saying you feel angry and confused.")

Supporting the caregiver's ability to manage the situation (e.g., by helping identify community supports, finding someone to share housekeeping activities)

Providing information about and demonstrating caregiving skills and techniques (e.g., dealing with the client's pain)

For a list of NIC interventions for Caregiver Role Strain,

 Go to Chapter 14, **Standardized Language, NOC Outcomes and NIC Interventions,** in Volume 2.

Interventions When There Is a Death in the Family

Death of a close family member is one of the most devastating life experiences. A family needs sensitive and compassionate care during this time, and such care is an appropriate focus for family-centered nursing. Interventions include facilitating the grieving process, encouraging communication, providing spiritual support, and providing compassionate care of the body after death. For more in-depth information about care of the family of a dying patient, see Chapter 17.

 To explore learning resources for this chapter,

 Go to DavisPlus at **DavisPl.us/Wilkinson3.**

Chapter Resources for Chapter 14:
    Response sheets for all learning activities
    Resources for Caregivers and Health Professionals
    Reading More About The Family (suggested readings)
    Content Map of chapter content
Interactive Case Studies
NCLEX-Style and Chapter Review Questions
Chapter Overview Podcast

For references cited in this chapter,

 Go to Volume 2, **References Cited.**

BOX 14-3 ■ Interventions to Help the Family Coping With Hospitalization

Provide written materials explaining the client's diagnosis or condition.

Actively involve the family in team meetings.

Promptly follow up with family concerns or questions.

Encourage the family to go home and rest.

Encourage the family to call for updates when they cannot be present.

Suggest ideas for stress-reducing activities (e.g., walking, meditating).

Inform the family about on-site availability of a chaplain or chapel.

Encourage the family to participate in care activities as appropriate.

Keep the family informed of the client's progress.

Help the family to identify sources of stress and develop strategies to work through and dissolve the root cause.

Provide anticipatory guidance regarding outcome and expectations for discharge.

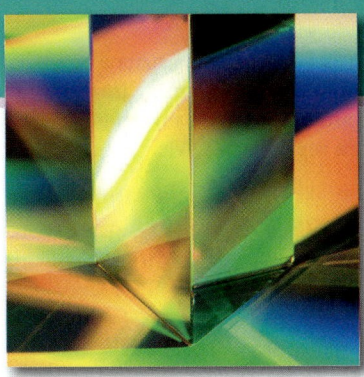

Culture & Ethnicity

Learning Outcomes

After completing this chapter, you should be able to:

➤ Explain why cultural competence is important for nurses.

➤ Explain what is meant by *culture* and *acculturation.*

➤ Discuss concepts pertaining to cultural diversity in nursing.

➤ Identify vulnerable populations in the United States.

➤ Define and give an example of culture universals and of culture specifics.

➤ Differentiate between cultural archetypes and cultural stereotypes.

➤ Describe the culture of the North American healthcare system, including professional subcultures.

➤ Identify the phenomena of culture, including how they can affect the nursing care needs of clients and families.

➤ Discuss the differing views of culturally diverse clients, including biomedical, holistic, and alternative health systems, such as folk medicine.

➤ Explain guidelines for performing a transcultural assessment, including a cultural assessment model.

➤ Recognize the cultural implications inherent in nursing diagnoses.

➤ Describe nursing strategies that promote delivery of culturally competent care to clients and their families.

➤ State some techniques for communicating with clients when there is a language barrier.

Key Concepts

Culture
Cultural competence

Related Concepts

See the Concept Map on Davis*Plus.*

Meet Your Patients

Your clinical assignment is to spend the day in a walk-in clinic with a primary care provider. Your initial job is to greet the clients and help them complete a health history form. These are the first patients you greet:

▪ Romano Salvatore points to his head and moans. When you ask him what is wrong, he makes a gesture to convey to you that he does not understand what you are saying. He speaks a foreign language that sounds to you like Italian.

▪ Rosanna is a frantic young mother, carrying her son, José, a 4-year-old who is crying and coughing. Rosanna informs you that José complains of a sore throat and has a fever. She also tells you that she has been to her *curandero,* but José is not getting any better. You notice that José is wearing a heavy coat and knit hat although it is quite warm outside. When you question Rosanna about the child's clothing, she says that José is cold.

▪ Lee Chan, an elderly Chinese American man, is accompanied by eight family members. Because the waiting area is small, all except his daughter Kim are asked to wait outside. Mr. Chan

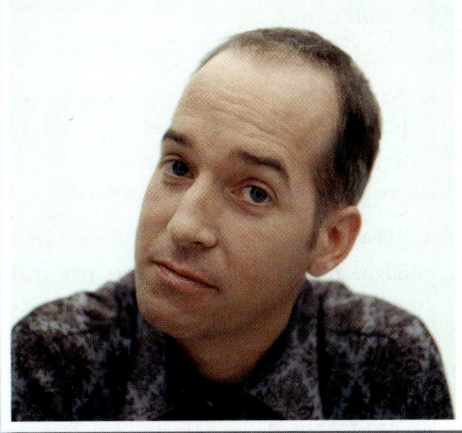

is quiet and does not make eye contact with you. His daughter Kim explains that her father has stomach cancer and is in a lot of pain because of disharmony. When you ask him to rate his pain, he just shakes his head and looks away. Would you wonder what *disharmony* means?

Theoretical Knowledge
knowing why

Try to answer the following questions about the patients you have just met. You may not have the theoretical knowledge to answer them all—you will acquire that in this chapter—but do your best based on the background you now have.

 ## Think Like a Nurse 15-1

- Think about Romano Salvatore.
  If you could speak Italian, what would you ask him?
- Think about Rosanna and her child.
  One question that might spring immediately to your mind is, "What is a *curandero*?" How could you find out this information?
  Why do you think that the child is dressed more warmly than you would expect for the weather?
- Think about Mr. Chan and his family.
  How would you feel about so many of his family members coming with Mr. Chan to the clinic?
  Why do you think he is not looking at or speaking to you?
  How could you communicate with Mr. Chan? Would you assume that he does not speak your language? Explain your reasoning.

ABOUT THE KEY CONCEPTS

The overarching concepts for this chapter are **culture** and **cultural competence**. The concept of cultural competence helps clarify why the concept of culture is important for nurses to understand. Related concepts, such as assimilation and culture universals, will broaden your understanding of culture and cultural competence. When you have studied the chapter, you should be able to see how all these concepts are linked to each other.

WHY LEARN ABOUT CULTURE?

The following are some reasons for nurses to learn about culture and cultural competence.

The Population Is Diverse In your practice, you will almost certainly care for patients who are not from your culture. The United States is a multicultural society. We continue to see a trend of increasing immigration from Asian and Spanish-speaking nations. The population saw a net increase of 3.4 million Asians and 13.1 million Hispanics between 2000 and 2009 (U.S. Census, 2012a). Box 15-1 shows projection data to year 2060.

Minorities will increase from 37% of the U.S. population in 2012 to 57% by 2060. Projections indicated that the United States will "become a majority-minority nation for the first time in 2043, . . . [and] no group will make up a majority" (U.S. Census, 2012b).

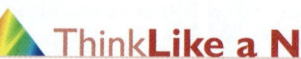 ## Think Like a Nurse 15-2

- With what cultural groups do you identify?
- In the neighborhood where you live, identify the cultural or ethnic groups that are different from your own. How many are there?
- In the school you are now attending, how many different cultural or ethnic groups are represented? What are they?

Health Disparities Exist Among Racial and Ethnic Groups A *Healthy People 2020* overarching goal is to eliminate disparities and improve the health of all groups (Healthy People 2020, n.d.a.)

- **Health status.** One disparity is that minority groups experience higher rates of illness and death and, in general, poorer health status compared with the white, non-Hispanic population. For example, the infant death rate among Black Americans, American Indians, and Alaska Natives is significantly higher.
- **Quality of care.** Disparities among racial groups are common. When compared with whites, blacks received worse care on 41% of quality measures; Hispanics, 39%; and Asians, American Indians, and Alaska Natives, 30% (Agency for Healthcare Research and Quality [AHRQ], 2012). For example, in nursing homes, use of physical restraints is higher among Asians than among non-Hispanic whites (AHRQ, 2012).
- **Access to care.** Lack of access to preventive healthcare and language barriers can account for differences in the health status of racial and ethnic groups (Hicks, 2012). For example, when compared with their white counterparts, black females experienced a higher rate of advanced stage breast cancer and maternal deaths. Black children received inadequate preventive asthma care, resulting in significantly higher rates of emergency room visits than other groups. Similarly, Pacific Islanders and Native Hawaiians had the highest rate of uncontrolled diabetes and hypertension when compared with white groups (AHRQ, 2012), which can lead to complications such as strokes and heart attacks. Improving access to care is one way to decrease healthcare disparities and improve health outcomes.

If you are interested in learning more about health disparities,

 Go to Chapter 15, **Resources for Caregivers and Health Professionals,** on DavisPlus.

Nursing Is Challenged to Provide Culturally Competent Care In North America, the healthcare culture reflects the dominant or European American culture. However, as you saw in the Meet Your Patients scenarios, nurses care for patients from many different races and cultures. Nursing care that is appropriate for the dominant cultural group may be ineffective and inappropriate for people who have a different cultural heritage. Of course, it is impossible to know about every culture, but it is important to learn about the ones you will encounter most often in your practice. A good understanding of culture

BOX 15-1 ■ Population Projections per Racial Group, 2012–2060

Group	2012 Population (in millions)	2060 Projections (in millions)
Non-Hispanic Whites	197.8	179.0
Hispanic	53.3	128.8
Black/African American	41.2	61.8
Asian	15.9	34.4
American Indian & Alaska Natives	3.9	6.3
Native Hawaiian & Other Pacific Islander	706 (thousand)	1.4

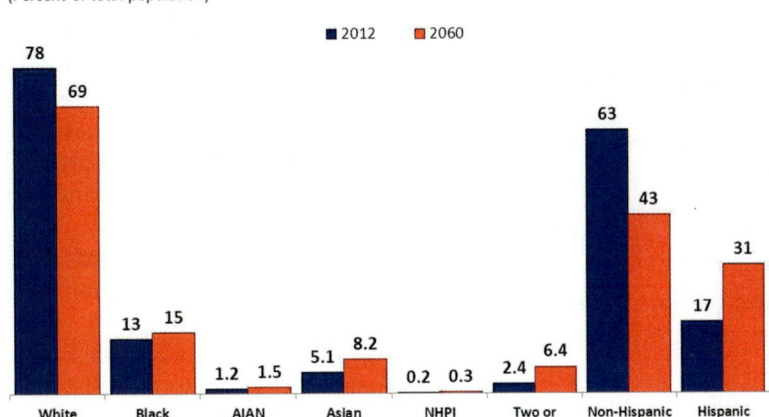

Population by Race and Hispanic Origin: 2012 and 2060
(Percent of total population)

AIAN=American Indian and Alaska Native; NHPI=Native Hawaiian and Other Pacific Islander

Source: Adapted from U.S. Census Bureau (2012b). U.S. Census Bureau Projections show a slower growing, older, more diverse nation a half century from now. Retrieved February 8, 2013, from http://www.census.gov/newsroom/releases/archives/population/cb12-243.html

and ethnicity will help you in providing direct care, teaching, supervising, delegating, and role-modeling culturally competent care to other care providers.

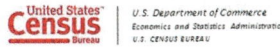KnowledgeCheck 15-1

- What do recent demographic trends in North America indicate?
- Why should nurses know more about the culture and ethnicity of clients?

WHAT IS MEANT BY CULTURE?

To provide care in a culturally diverse population, you need to understand the concept of *culture*. We know that culture is both *universal* (everyone has it) and *dynamic* (active). In simple terms, **culture** is what people in a group have in common and it changes over time. Formally defined, **culture** is "the totality of socially transmitted behavior patterns, arts, beliefs, values, customs, lifeways, and all other products of human work and thought characteristics of a population of people that

guides their worldview and decision making" (Purnell & Paulanka, 2008, p. 404). For other definitions of culture,

 Go to Chapter 15, **Supplemental Materials: Definitions of Culture,** on Davis*Plus.*

Characteristics of Culture

When you are trying to determine what is meant by *culture* or *cultural,* keep in mind the following characteristics:

- **Cultural beliefs provide identity and a sense of belonging for its members.** They do so as long as they do not conflict with the dominant culture and continue to satisfy its members.
- **Cultures consist of common beliefs and practices.** Most members of a culture share the same beliefs, traditions, customs, and practices as long as they continue to be adaptive and satisfy the members' needs. Some members of the group may deviate from cultural norms, but for a norm to be considered cultural, many members must follow it.

- **Culture exists at many levels.** Culture exists as both the material (art, writings, dress, or artifacts) and the nonmaterial (customs, traditions, language, beliefs, and practices) levels. See Figure 15-1.
- **Culture is learned and taught.** Cultural values, beliefs, and traditions are passed down from generation to generation. Learning occurs through life experiences shared with other members of the culture, either formally (e.g., in schools) or informally (e.g., in families). Some generations totally adopt the values, beliefs, and traditions of their elders; others partially accept the teachings; and some generations completely reject them.
- **Culture is dynamic and adaptive.** Cultural customs, beliefs, and practices are not static. They change over time and at different rates. Cultural change occurs with adaptation in response to the environment.
- **Culture is complex.** Reread the Purnell and Paulanka (2008) definition to review the many aspects of culture. Cultural assumptions and habits are unconscious and thus may be difficult for members of the culture to explain to others or to identify as different from another culture.
- **Culture is diverse.** Culture demonstrates the variety that exists among groups and among members of a particular group.
- **Culture is all-encompassing.** Culture can influence everything its members think and do.

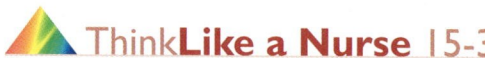 **ThinkLike a Nurse** 15-3

Figure 15-1 depicts an example of ways members of particular cultural groups express their cultural uniqueness in dance. Can you think of other ways that people express their culture?

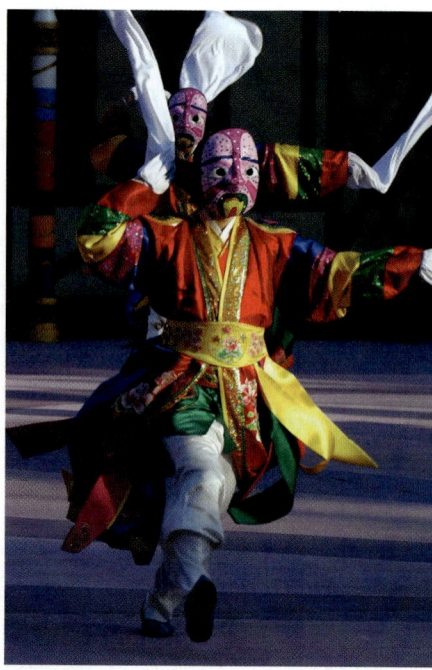

FIGURE 15-1 Traditional lunar New Year dancer in South Korea.

Ethnicity, Race, and Religion

People sometimes use the terms *culture*, *ethnicity*, and *race* interchangeably, but in fact they have separate, specific meanings. Distinctions between culture, ethnicity, race, and religion might seem confusing, but think of it this way: You are a member of the subculture of nursing, but you are also a member of an ethnic group (e.g., Portuguese Americans from the Azores), a racial group (e.g., white), and a religion (e.g., Roman Catholicism), each with its own sets of beliefs and values. So, your culture is a blend of all of those.

Ethnicity

Ethnicity is similar to *culture* in that it refers to groups whose members share a common social and cultural heritage that is passed down from generation to generation. Ethnicity is also similar to *subculture* in that the members of an **ethnic group** have some characteristics in common (e.g., race, ancestry, physical characteristics, geographic region, lifestyle, religion) that are not shared or understood by outsiders. Examples of ethnic groups include French Canadians, Roman Catholics, Hmongs, and Latinos.

Ethnicity may include race and Hispanic origin, but the two are separate and distinct concepts. To demonstrate, the U.S. Census Bureau (2012a) has numerous categories for *race* (see the next section). In addition, two categories are identified for *ethnicity*: (1) Hispanic, Latino, or Spanish and (2) *Not* Hispanic, Latino, or Spanish.

- **Hispanic** Americans are people who originally came from any Spanish-speaking country (e.g., Mexico, Spain). Sixty-five percent of the Hispanic population in the United States are of Mexican origin.
- **Latino**, strictly speaking, refers only to people from Central or South America.
- **Spanish** implies an origin in Spain.

If you know a client's country of origin, it is more accurate to use it when referring to the client's ethnicity (e.g., Mexican American, Colombian American) than to use either of the terms *Hispanic*, *Latino*, or *Spanish*.

Race

Unlike ethnicity, **race** is strictly related to biology. *Race* refers to the grouping of people based on biological similarities, such as skin color, blood type, or bone structure (Purnell & Paulanka, 2008; Purnell, 2012). The terms *race* and *ethnicity* overlap somewhat, because race can be a characteristic of a specific ethnic group. The U.S. Census Bureau asks people to choose the race with which they identify and divides the population into the list of racial categories following:

- White
- Black, African American, or Negro
- American Indian or Alaska Native
- Korean
- Vietnamese
- Other Asian

- Asian Indian
- Chinese
- Filipino
- Japanese
- Native Hawaiian
- Guamanian or Chamorro
- Samoan
- Other Pacific Islanders

People of Hispanic, Latino, or Spanish origin may be of any race, because the U.S. Census Bureau includes Hispanic/Latino/Spanish as a sociocultural, rather than a race category. For an explanation of each of the categories,

 Go to Chapter Resources, Chapter 15, Tables, Boxes and Figures, **ESG Table 15-1, Racial Categories, Origins and/or Self-Identified Entries,** on DavisPlus.

Can you determine a person's race by his appearance? Frequently not. So, then, is race determined by heredity? What race is someone whose father is African American and whose mother is white? Historically, most North Americans would say that the person is African American. In some other countries (e.g., most of South America), that same person would be categorized as white. Although we commonly think of race as being based on biological characteristics, many, including the U.S. Census Bureau, believe that race is socially rather than biologically determined. As a culturally sensitive nurse, you will ask people what race they identify with and what name they prefer to use for it. For more information on race as a social construct,

 Go to Chapter 15, **Supplemental Materials: Race as a Social Construct,** on DavisPlus.

We tend to group and categorize data to make them meaningful and useful, but we must be careful to avoid using these categories as the basis for interacting with people or providing care. When you need to designate a name for a group, be as specific as possible (e.g., Syrian American instead of white).

Religion

Religion may be confused with ethnicity because people within an ethnic group may share the same religion. For example, the Jewish culture overlaps with the Jewish faith community. **Religion** refers to an ordered system of beliefs regarding the cause, nature, and purpose of the universe, especially the beliefs related to the worship of a God or gods (Andrews & Boyle, 2007). In many cultures, religion is a high priority (Fig. 15-2).

Concepts Related to Culture

The concept **bicultural** describes a person who identifies with two cultures and integrates some of the values and lifestyles of each into his life. The person uses more of one cultural base over another when situations call for it. Consider a Jewish man who marries an Italian Catholic woman. Their bicultural children may choose to follow Jewish tradition while still holding some of the values and beliefs of their Italian heritage. A bicultural

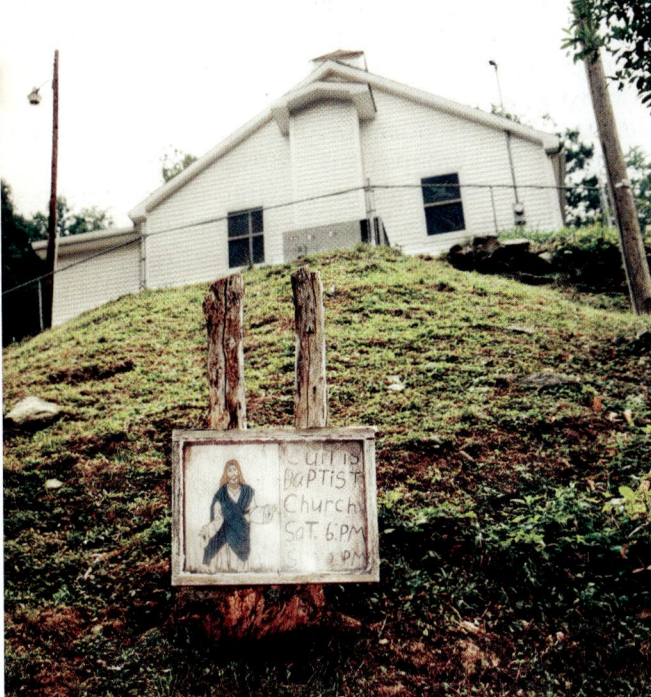

FIGURE 15-2 Even in this tiny community of rural Appalachia, people have built a place for worship.

person may experience divided loyalties or enjoy the best of both cultures.

In this chapter, **multicultural** refers to many cultures and is used to describe groups rather than individuals. Many regions of the United States are multicultural, meaning that the region is populated by individuals from many different cultural groups. The same can be said about workplace environments. Remember that culture does not always refer to the ethnicity of a group. Think of a hospital: Caregivers may be members of various ethnic, racial, and religious groups, and the nurses, physicians, physical therapists, and students each make up a different subculture. Thus, a hospital is multicultural setting.

Socialization, Acculturation, and Assimilation

Socialization is the process of learning to become a member of a society or a group. A person becomes socialized by learning social rules and roles, by learning the behaviors, norms, values, and perceptions of others in the same group or role. Your education program is socializing you into the role of a professional nurse. Families, schools, churches, peer groups, and the media are also agents of socialization and foster their members' identification with the culture.

Immigrants (new members of a group or country) assume the characteristics of that culture through a learning process called **acculturation.** A person who is acculturated accepts both his own and the new culture, adopting elements of each. Acculturation is the outgrowth of the minority group's need to survive and flourish in the new culture. Many experts theorize that it takes several years, perhaps three generations, for an immigrant group to become acculturated. Acculturation is viewed as a social determinant of health and its understanding is essential to address healthcare disparities among cultural groups (Baker, 2011).

Cultural assimilation occurs when the new members gradually learn and take on the essential values, beliefs, and behaviors of the dominant culture. Assimilation is complete when the newcomer is fully merged into the dominant cultural group. A person becomes assimilated by, for example, learning to speak the dominant language, marrying a member from the new (host) culture, and making close, personal relationships with members of the new group. For example, if you emigrated from your home in the United States to Mexico, you would take with you your own language and food preferences. But over time, you would gradually begin to eat more of the local foods and learn to speak Spanish.

Dominant Cultures, Subcultures, and Minority Groups

What do you think is the dominant culture of the United States? If you said white or Caucasian or European American, you would be only partially correct. The ancestors of most white Americans emigrated from Europe, and many were of Protestant or other Christian religions. Thus, the dominant culture in the United States and Canada is considered white Anglo-Saxon Christian of European descent. A **dominant culture** is the group that has the most authority or power to control values and reward or punish behaviors. It is usually, but not always, the largest group.

Because the white culture has been dominant in North America, most white people have been around others similar to themselves. When asked about their culture, they may reply, "I don't know; I don't think I have one." They have not been aware of their culture because they did not see it in contrast to other ways of being. Or, if they did see differences, they assumed their ways were the norm and that everyone else was culturally different.

Ethnocentrism is the tendency to think that your own group (cultural, professional, ethnic, or social) is superior to others and to view behaviors and beliefs that differ greatly from your own as somehow wrong, strange, or unenlightened. The tendency to ethnocentrism exists in all groups, not just in the dominant culture.

Subcultures are groups within a larger culture or social system that have some characteristics (e.g., values, behaviors, ancestry, ways of living) that are different from those of the dominant culture. People in subcultures have had different experiences from those in the dominant group because of status, residence, gender, sexual orientation, ethnic background, education, or other factors that unify the group (Purnell, 2012). You may be able to recognize subcultures by their speech patterns, dress, gestures, eating habits, lifestyles, and so

on. Some examples of subcultures are street gangs, physicians, nurses, women, older adults, persons with disabilities, gays and lesbians, people of Appalachian heritage, rural Midwesterners, and people who abuse certain drugs.

Key Point: *Nursing subcultures within hospitals can impact quality of care and thus patient outcomes. Nurses in specialty subcultures (e.g., intensive care units, emergency rooms) had greater control over their practice, which was associated with better quality of patient care and fewer adverse events when compared with the medical subculture (Mallidou, Cummings, Estabrook, et al., 2011).*

Minority groups are also made up of individuals who share race, religion, or ethnic heritage. They are viewed as subordinate to and usually have fewer members than the majority group. Depending on the type of group, they may or may not share beliefs, practices, or physical characteristics. The term *minority* is sometimes used to refer to a group of people who receive different and unequal treatment from others in society. You should consider that this term may be offensive to some people because it suggests inferiority and marginalization.

KnowledgeCheck 15-2

- Define *culture*.
- Give an example of each: ethnic group, race, religion.
- How does culture provide identity for an individual?
- Give an example of acculturation.

Vulnerable Populations as Subcultures

Vulnerable populations are groups that are more likely to develop health problems and experience poorer outcomes because of limited access to care, high-risk behaviors, and/or multiple and cumulative stressors (e.g., the homeless [Fig. 15-3], poor, or mentally ill; people with physical disabilities; the very young; and older adults). Some ethnic and racial minority groups are also

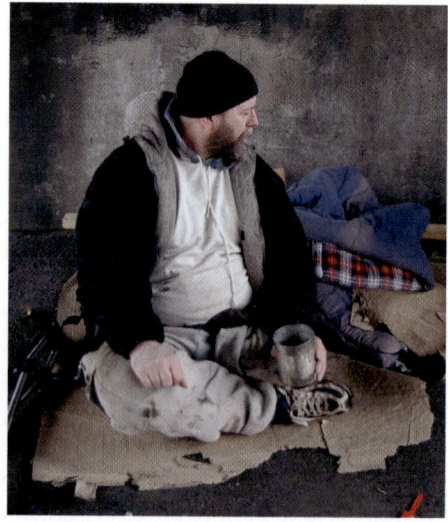

FIGURE 15-3 A homeless man sits on his cardboard, begging for spare change.

vulnerable. For example, among American Indians and Native Alaskans, there is a higher incidence of diabetes, notably type 2 diabetes in those under 20 years of age, which results in higher mortality rates (Centers for Disease Control and Prevention [CDC], 2011a, updated 2013, 2011b). Vulnerable populations can be considered subcultures of all of the major cultural groups.

Socioeconomic vulnerability is particularly important. Vulnerability is not limited to a particular cultural or ethnic group. People of various socioeconomic classes are found in all ethnic groups. In fact, the subculture of poverty can be found throughout the world. When caring for patients from vulnerable populations, it is important that you focus on their strengths and resources, not exclusively on their difficulties and risks.

The public health initiative *Healthy People 2020* addresses the care of vulnerable populations (Healthy People 2020, n.d.b). One of its overarching goals is to achieve health equity, eliminate disparities, and improve the health of all groups. Nursing research and literature address these inequities, such as the following:

- Oral health disparities in vulnerable populations (Carrion, Castañeda, Martinez-Tyson, et al., 2011; Lester, Henderson, & Taylor, 2012)
- Overweight and obesity among children of different ethnic groups (Long, Mareno, Shabo, et al., 2012)
- Neighborhood disparities in access to healthy foods (Hilmers, Hilmers, & Dave, 2012).

Gender as a Subculture

It should come as no surprise that some behaviors are considered acceptable for men but not for women, and vice versa; and that there are values and responses considered more typical of one sex than of the other. For example, in the dominant culture it is more acceptable for women to cry out in pain than for men to do so, who are supposed to "be strong." As another example, the U.S. culture tends to view caring and nurturing as the province of women. For this reason, historically, males were excluded from the nursing profession. Today, the number of males nurses continue to increase and research shows that they are well integrated and accepted by their peers and given fair, if not preferential, treatment in career advancement (McMurry, 2011).

Old Age as a Subculture

Older adults, especially the very old, can be thought of as a vulnerable population in some respects. You should assess for elder abuse in all cultures and not assume that indicators of abuse are a result of cultural practice. Researchers used *Promotores* (local Spanish-speaking Latinos) to assess for elder abuse among low-income Latino immigrants. Results reveal a variety of abuses, including psychological (25%), physical (11%), sexual (9%), financial (17%), and caregiver neglect (12%). Failure to report abuse may be due to mistrust of the system, protecting the family, and/or language barriers (Deliema, Gassoumis, Homeier, et al., 2012).

HOW DO CULTURAL VALUES, BELIEFS, AND PRACTICES AFFECT HEALTH?

Values are important because they help shape health-related beliefs and practices. Do you know what values are? Think for a minute about what you "value" in your own life. What are the five ideals, principles, or things that are most important to you?

You may name, for example, learning, family, independence, faith, and cleanliness. Or you may have said something entirely different. Simply put, a personal value is a principle or standard that has meaning or worth to an individual. An example is cleanliness. In contrast, a belief is something that one accepts as true (e.g., "I believe that germs cause disease"), and a practice is a set of behaviors that one follows (e.g., "I always wash my hands before preparing food"). Do you see how values, beliefs, and practices are related?

Cultural values, beliefs, and practices are the principles, standards, ideas, and behaviors that members of a cultural group share. Some values of the dominant U.S. culture are youth, beauty, success, independence, and material belongings. You should not assume a client shares your values, beliefs, and practices—nor those of the dominant culture.

Key Point: *Remember, also, that individuals within an ethnocultural group vary widely and that learning commonalities is no substitute for careful assessment of each person.*

What Are Culture Universals and Specifics?

Culture universals are the values, beliefs, and practices that people from *all* cultures share. Leininger and McFarland (2006) refer to these as culture commonalities. In contrast, **culture specifics** (culture diversities in Leininger's theory) are those values, beliefs, and practices that are special or unique to a culture. Let's look at an example. All cultures celebrate the birth of a new baby in some way (a culture universal), but different cultures celebrate "birth rites" in different ways (a culture specific). In Belize, a baby is christened before visitors are allowed, a practice carried out to prevent the *evil eye* (bad spells cast by others); in Greece, *amulets* (objects or charms worn to protect against evil spirits) may be placed on the baby; and in Israel, Jewish male infants are circumcised on the eighth day of life. Similarly, people from all cultures practice marriage rituals in elaborate rituals that are culture specific (Fig. 15-4).

Archetype or Stereotype?

At about this point in your efforts to be culturally sensitive you might be thinking: "Wait a minute. I went to a Chinese wedding, and it was no different from my own wedding"; or "I know plenty of Greek people who don't put amulets on their babies." Of course you are correct. However, acknowledging that there are commonalities

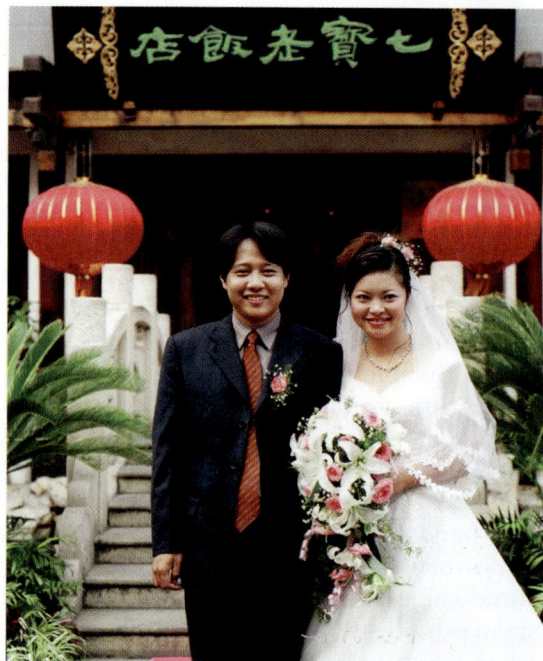

FIGURE 15-4 People of all cultures practice marriage rituals.

within a group is not the same as saying that *all* people in the group have those characteristics. And that is, more or less, the difference between an archetype and a stereotype.

A **cultural stereotype** is a widely held but oversimplified and unsubstantiated belief that all people of a certain racial or ethnic group are alike in certain respects. Stereotypes are not always negative. Someone may think, for example, that people of a particular heritage are "naturally intelligent" or "naturally athletic." A **cultural archetype** is similar to a model, which you learned about in Chapter 8. An archetype is an *example* of a person or thing—something that is recurrent—and it has its basis in facts. Therefore, as a symbol in your mind, it may help you to remember some of the culture specifics. Unlike stereotypes, archetypes are usually not negative. For example, you might think of Mexican Americans as having brown eyes, or of European Americans as having light-colored skin. There is nothing negative about eye color or skin color.

Remember, there is probably more variation among people *within* an ethnic or cultural group than there is *between* the groups, and that much variation stems from socioeconomic differences or regional origin as much as from race or ethnicity.

Key Point: *The general principle that should guide your practice is that each person must be seen as unique—as a member of an ethnic group, influenced by his heritage, but not defined by it.*

How Do Culture Specifics Affect Health?

Just as they influence our celebrations of births and weddings, culture specifics affect our health beliefs and behaviors. Thus, knowledge of the culture specifics of groups in your community will help explain why clients from different cultures have different expectations of healthcare. Ultimately, it will help you to provide culturally competent care. In the following sections, we will explore six culture specifics that influence health: communication, space, time orientation, social organization, environmental control, and biological variations (Giger, 2012). We will also briefly discuss several other culture specifics: religion and philosophy, politics and law, the economy, and education.

Communication

Communication is an exchange of information, ideas, and feelings. It includes verbal and nonverbal language (i.e., spoken language, gestures, eye contact, and even silences). Think how difficult it would be if you became ill in a foreign country and did not speak the language. How would you tell the caregivers your symptoms? How would you know what they were going to do to treat your illness? Language differences present one of the most difficult obstacles to providing care. Even when you and the client speak the same language, culture influences how feelings and thoughts are expressed and which verbal and nonverbal expressions are appropriate to use. Also see Chapter 21 for more on communication strategies.

Space

Space refers to a person's personal space, or the boundary lines that determine how close another person can come. A person's comfort level is related to space. A similar concept, **territoriality**, means the geographical space a person views as owned or claimed, such as an area or room (Spector, 2013). Both of these concepts are influenced by culture. If you are invading a person's personal space, a common reaction is for the person to move away from you. When personal space is protected, a person feels secure and safe, less anxious, and in control. The following are some examples of culturally influenced attitudes toward personal space (Purnell & Paulanka, 2008; Purnell, 2012):

- Americans, Canadians of Northern European ancestry, and the British keep at least 18 inches of space between themselves and the person with whom they are conversing.
- Arabs and others from the Middle East typically stand quite close when talking. They tend to keep steady eye contact, but not between men and women
- Germans usually require a great deal of space, and consider even looking into a room an invasion of privacy.

Within all cultural groups, personal space varies depending on the relationship between the people speaking: intimates versus acquaintances, people of the same versus opposite sex, and people of a different position within the social hierarchy.

Time Orientation

Time orientation varies among people of different cultures. Some persons tend to be past-, present- or future-oriented. Groups from the Far East tend to be past-oriented and value traditions and relationships over time and deadlines. In contrast, European Americans tend to be future-oriented, and Latin Americans and Filipinos are more present-oriented and enjoy living in the moment. Differences in time orientation can be important as you plan nursing interventions. For example, clients who are past-oriented may show up late (or not at all) for follow-up appointments; therefore, you should provide a written or telephone reminder of their appointment.

 ### ThinkLike a Nurse 15-4

- Suppose you say to a client, "You will need to exercise and follow a low-calorie diet to lose weight and control your diabetes." What kind of time orientation would a client most likely have in order to follow your directions?
- Suppose a client says, "I know I need to lose weight, but I work so much, and the children take so much time. I just don't have time to shop for and cook the right foods or to exercise." What time orientation does this illustrate?

Social Organization

Social organization includes the family unit (e.g., nuclear, single-parent, or extended family) and the wider organizations (e.g., community, religious, ethnic) with which the individual or family identifies (Spector, 2013).

- *A close social organization can be found in all cultures; however, the specifics vary.* For example, in Middle Eastern and Latino cultures, the man is likely to be the dominant family member and the woman the homemaker. But many African American families are matriarchal; that is, the decision maker and family leader is a woman.
- *The social organization of your clients' cultures can provide clues as to how they will act during such life events as birth, death, illness, grieving, and mourning.* For example, imagine a patient who does not trust large institutions or government agencies, but must depend on Medicaid to pay for her healthcare. She is likely to use home remedies and delay seeing a conventional medical physician.
- *Kinship and social ties also determine who receives healthcare, and in what priority.* In the United States, for example, someone of high status (e.g., a celebrity or political figure) is likely to receive better care than a poor person who is unknown in the community. In some cultures, men receive care before women and children.

Environmental Control

Environmental control refers to a person's perception of his ability to plan activities that control nature or direct environmental factors (Spector, 2013). A person's health and illness beliefs and practices are directly related to this concept. For example, if a person does

not believe he can do anything to "change things," this would negatively affect his decision to seek medical care, to take his medications, to exercise, and to eat properly. Environmental control is also illustrated in Asian Americans' perception and tolerance of pain. They do not view circumstances as something to be "controlled"; therefore, they tend to accept pain stoically, and not demand relief. Think again about Mr. Chan (Meet Your Patients). Why do you think he just shakes his head and looks away when asked to rate his pain?

Biological Variations

Biological variations are the ways in which people are different genetically and physiologically. They include body build and structure, skin color, vital signs, enzymatic and genetic variations, and drug metabolism (Purnell, 2012; Spector, 2013). Biological variations create susceptibility to certain diseases and injuries and explain differences in responses to treatment. For example, African Americans have poorer responses to certain categories of antihypertensive drugs when compared with their white counterparts (Gupta, 2010). Consequently, clinical trials (drug studies) now recommend incorporating biological variations. For more information about assessing biological variations,

 Go to Chapter 15, **Clinical Insight 15-1: Assessing for Biological Variations,** in Volume 2.

To read more about biological susceptibility to diseases,

 Go to Chapter 15, **Supplemental Materials: Disease Risks for Each of the Major Cultural Groups of the United States,** on Davis*Plus*.

Other Culture Specifics

The following may also be culture specifics. The first two, religion/philosophy and education, vary among subcultures in the United States, whereas technology, politics/law, and the economy exert broader effects that can be seen among different countries, but less so among subcultures within a country.

- **Religion and Philosophy.** A person's religion may determine what healthcare is acceptable to him. For example, some religions (e.g., Jehovah's Witnesses) do not accept blood transfusions, and many religions forbid abortion.
- **Education.** Education influences the perception of wellness and illness and the knowledge of options that are available for healthcare. These, in turn, affect the person's expectations for care.
- **Technology.** The availability of supplies and equipment determines what is used in the healthcare setting and what becomes culturally expected. Nurses in most of North America, for example, assume they will have bed linens, water, electricity, necessary medications, and technology such as

electrocardiography and x-ray imaging. In many parts of the world, however, these items are not available or even expected.

- **Politics and the Law.** Government policies affect healthcare, as seen in the Affordable Care Act. They determine what programs will be funded, reimbursement for providers, and acceptable functions and standards. Review Chapter 1 for an overview of governmental healthcare programs.
- **Economy.** The condition of the economy directly affects the availability of funds for publicly funded services. It also affects the individual's ability to pay for healthcare.

For more information about each of those dimensions of culture,

 Go to Chapter 15, **Tables, Boxes, Figures: ESG Table 15-2,** on Davis*Plus.*

 Think**Like a Nurse** 15-5

Consider this example: Mrs. Miyagi, a Japanese American, has been admitted to your care from the postanesthesia care unit (PACU), having undergone a major surgical procedure. She refuses pain medicine, although she appears to be in pain. As the hours pass, Mrs. Miyagi continues to refuse pain medication, so eventually the nurses stop asking.

- Do you assume that she is experiencing no pain?
- Are you or the other nurses stereotyping her for her cultural response to pain?
- What would you do?

KnowledgeCheck 15-3

- Explain the difference between an archetype and a stereotype.
- Identify at least six culture specifics affecting health.
- How could you use this information about culture specifics to provide better care to your clients?

WHAT IS THE "CULTURE OF HEALTHCARE"?

In any culture, two healthcare systems usually exist side by side: indigenous and professional (Leininger & McFarland, 2002, 2006). Each has its own culture.

Indigenous Healthcare System The **indigenous healthcare system** consists of *folk medicine* and *traditional healing methods,* which may include over-the-counter (OTC) and self-treatment remedies. Different groups have different folk practices (Table 15-1), but all cultural groups probably use a professional healthcare system to some degree.

Professional Healthcare System In contrast, the **professional healthcare system** is run by a set of professional healthcare providers who have been formally educated and trained for their appropriate roles and responsibilities. In North America, professional healthcare is dominated by a biomedical healthcare

system that combines Western biomedical beliefs with traditional North American values of self-reliance, individualism, and aggressive action. This system is also known as Western medicine and allopathic medicine. Table 15-2 summarizes the norms of the North American professional healthcare system.

The professional healthcare system also includes practitioners formally trained in alternative healthcare, such as diet therapy, mind–body control methods, therapeutic touch, acupressure, reflexology, naturopathy, kinesiology, and chiropractic. If you would like more information about alternative healthcare, see Chapter 46 on Holistic Healing.

Conflicts may occur when the professional healthcare provider does not understand the beliefs and practices of the indigenous healthcare systems and traditional healers. The professional provider views the indigenous beliefs and practices as uncivilized and based on the supernatural, and believers in indigenous methods view the professional healthcare culture with distrust. This type of thinking benefits no one. As a nurse, you should become aware of and understand a variety of health beliefs and practices so that you can meet the needs of your clients and families.

What Are Health and Illness Beliefs?

To provide evidenced-based culturally competent care, you need to know how people in various cultural groups understand life processes, how they define health and illness, their health-seeking behaviors, and what resources are available to promote health and treat illness (Transcultural Nursing Society, 2010). Generally speaking, people follow one of three major health belief systems: scientific, magico-religious, or holistic (Andrews & Boyle, 2011). You are probably familiar with the scientific or biomedical health system. Belief in supernatural (mystical) forces dominates the magico-religious system, which is considered "alternative" or "indigenous" in the United States. One example is voodoo, which is practiced in some developing nations in Africa, Latin America, and the Caribbean, and which considers the lion a spiritual symbol (Fig. 15-5). The holistic belief system can be similar to magico-religious, but it focuses more on the need for harmony and balance of the body with nature.

 Think**Like a Nurse** 15-6

- What do you do to keep yourself healthy?
- What do you do to treat minor illnesses when you do not want to see a healthcare provider?

What Are Health and Illness Practices?

In addition to knowing the values and beliefs of different cultures, you need to know what people in various cultural groups do to maintain wellness.

Table 15-1 ➤ Folk Healers and Practices

FOLK HEALERS	FOLK PRACTICES
White, European American	
Nurse Physician Chiropractor Acupuncturist Massage therapist Physical therapist Occupational therapist Respiratory therapist	Medicines (OTC and prescribed) Therapeutic or modified diets Exercise Religious healing rituals (including prayer) Sleep Cleanliness Amulets Herbal therapy Naturopathy Massage Spinal adjustment Aromatherapy
Hispanic	
Curandero/curandera *Espiritualista* (spiritualist) *Partera* *Yerbero* (herbalist) *Sabador*	"Hot" and "cold" therapies Medals and amulets Prayers Herbs and herbal teas Massage Jewelry to ward off the "Evil Eye"
African American	
"Old lady" healer Spiritualist *Hougan*, or voodoo priest or priestess	Herbs Oils and poultices Talismans and amulets (worn or carried to ward off evil) Religious rituals ("laying on of hands")
Native American, Eskimo, and Aleut	
Shaman Crystal gazer Hand trembler Medicine woman or man	Herbs, incantations, and prayers Rituals and healing ceremonies Blessed medicine bundles or other dried plants or flowers, or burning of dried plants Stargazing and sandpainting
Asian and Pacific Islander	
Herbalist Acupuncturist Physician Priest	"Hot" and "cold" foods Herbs Meditation Acupuncture (inserting needles into meridians or life energy pathways) Acupressure Energy (Qi) to restore *yin, yang* balance

Sources: Adapted from Andrews, M., & Boyle, J. S. (2011). *Transcultural concepts in nursing care* (6th ed.). Philadelphia: Lippincott Williams & Wilkins; Giger, J., & Davidhizar, R. (2008). *Transcultural nursing: Assessment and intervention* (5th ed.). St. Louis, MO: C.V. Mosby; Purnell, L. (2012). *Transcultural health care: A culturally competent approach* (4th ed.). Philadelphia: F.A. Davis; and Spector, R. (2013). *Cultural diversity in health and illness* (8th ed.). Upper Saddle River, NJ: Pearson Education, Inc..

Think about Mr. Chan (Meet Your Patients). If he or his daughter asked for a Chinese priest to come to his room and perform a ceremony to restore his harmony, do you think this ceremony would be harmful or helpful to him? Would you support or discourage this? What about Rosanna's dressing her child in a heavy coat and knit hat although it is quite warm outside? Is this harmful or helpful to them? Would you support or discourage this? As you think about those questions,

keep in mind that cultural health practices can be any of the following (Giger & Davidhizar, 2008):

Efficacious (helpful)
Neutral (neither helpful nor causing harm)
Dysfunctional (harmful)
Uncertain (not known)

You should encourage practices that could be helpful and discourage those that may cause harm. We will

Table 15-2 ➤ Summary of Cultural Norms of the North American Healthcare System	
NORM	**EXAMPLES**
Beliefs and Values	Standardized definitions of *health* and *illness*
	Significance of technology
	Reliance on the biomedical system
	Desire to conquer disease
	Defines health as absence or minimization of disease
Practices	Maintaining health and preventing disease through such practices as immunizations and avoidance of stress
	Annual physical examinations and diagnostic tests
Habits	Handwashing
	Use of jargon (e.g., "take your vitals")
	Use of problem-solving methods
	Documentation
Likes	Punctuality
	Neatness and organization
	Compliance (e.g., with medical "orders")
Dislikes	Tardiness
	Disorganization
	Messiness, lack of cleanliness
Customs	Use of procedures (e.g., circumcision, last rites) surrounding birth and death
	Professional respect and observance of hierarchy found in autocratic and bureaucratic systems
	Adherence to a set of ethical standards and codes of conduct
Rituals	Annual physical examination
	The surgical procedure

Sources: Adapted from Giger, J., & Davidhizar, R. (2008). *Transcultural nursing: Assessment and intervention* (5th ed.). St. Louis, MO: C.V. Mosby; Munoz, C., & Luckmann, J. (2005). *Transcultural communication in healthcare.* Clifton Park, NY: Thomson Delmar; Purnell, L. (2012). *Transcultural health care: A culturally competent approach* (4th ed.). Philadelphia: F.A. Davis; and Spector, R. (2013). *Cultural diversity in health and illness* (8th ed.). Upper Saddle River, NJ: Pearson Education, Inc.

discuss this more in the section on Nursing Strategies for Providing Culturally Competent Care.

KnowledgeCheck 15-4

- List three types of alternative healthcare that are delivered by formally trained practitioners as a part of the professional healthcare system.

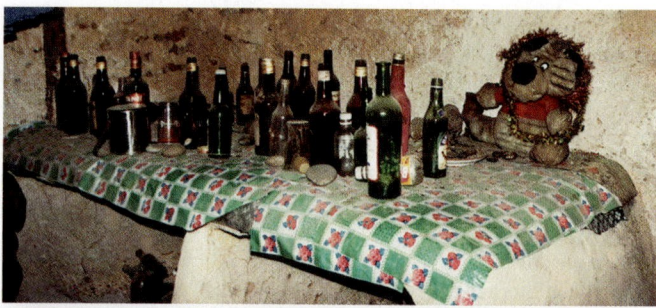

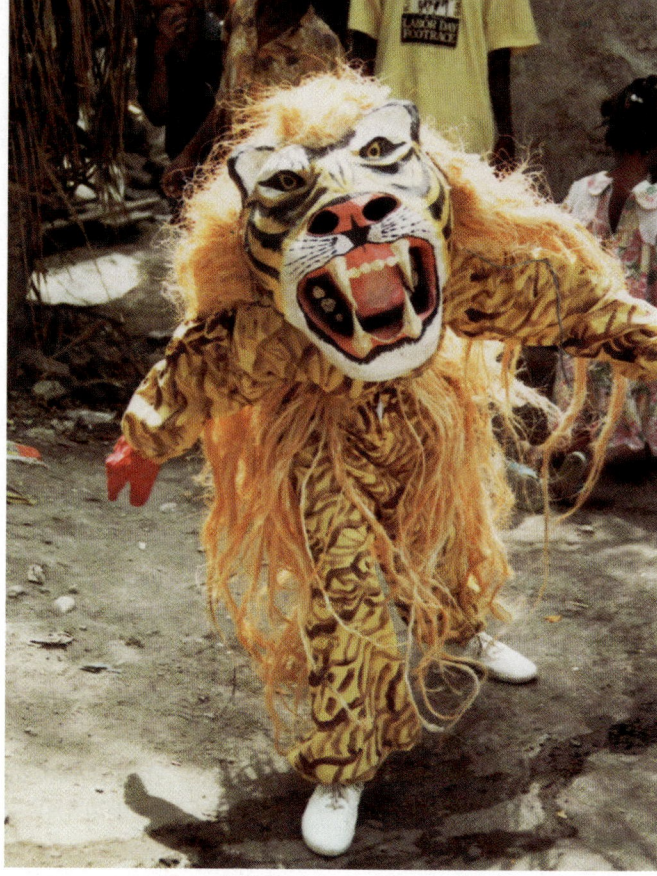

FIGURE 15-5 Voodoo is an example of a magico-religious belief system. *Top,* A Haitian voodoo shrine (notice the lion). *Bottom,* A Haitian man costumed for carnival as the spirit of the lion.

- What are magico-religious belief systems?
- As a nurse, in which of the following cultural health practices would you support your client: efficacious, neutral, dysfunctional, uncertain? Why?
- Refer to the Meet Your Patients feature. Identify an efficacious practice.

 ThinkLike a Nurse 15-7

What aspects of the indigenous and professional systems have you used for yourself or your family? Give examples.

Nursing and Other Professional Subcultures

Members of the biomedical healthcare system in the United States belong to a culture with its own set of norms. That culture can be further divided into subcultures, such as those of physicians, nurses, respiratory therapists. Nursing is the largest subculture within the healthcare culture. Leininger (1978) defines the **culture of nursing** as the learned and transmitted lifeways, values, symbols, patterns, and normative practices of members of the nursing profession that are not the same as those of the mainstream culture. The nursing subculture's beliefs and values have been formed in part by the society at large, which historically has been dominated by white Anglo-Saxon Protestants. Nursing values include, in addition to those listed in Table 15-2, the following:

- Silent suffering as a response to pain
- Objective reporting and description of pain, but not an emotional response
- Use of the nursing process
- Nursing autonomy
- Caring

In this book, we add *knowledge* and *critical thinking* to the list of nursing values. Although these values may not be consistently rewarded in practice, we believe that a steadily increasing number of nurses realize their importance—that nursing is "knowledge work" and that the nurse's knowledge and thinking are essential to the well-being of patients.

As you become more socialized into the nursing culture, you should continue to examine professional values to see how strongly you identify with them and how they affect your work with patients. For example, if you value silent suffering in response to pain, how might that cause you to respond to a woman in very early labor who is screaming and crying even though her contractions are very mild on palpation? Would you dismiss her for being a "whiner"? Or scold her ("You can't be hurting that badly this early in labor")? You must be careful not to lose the ability to understand health and illness from the patient's point of view.

Review the case of Rosanna and José (Meet Your Patients). After a positive strep test, the primary care provider prescribes an antibiotic for José's fever and sore throat. You observe that Rosanna does not seem to be happy with the medicine, so you stress to her the importance of buying the medicine right away to make him better. On her way out of the clinic, Rosanna throws the prescription in the trash. Why do you think she threw away the prescription?

If you had difficulty thinking of possible answers to the question, see Table 15-3.

Also,

 Go to the **Hispanic Health Cultural Specifics** in **ESG Table 15-2 (Culture Specifics Affecting Health),** on Davis*Plus.*

Some people of Mexican heritage believe that illness is caused by the body's imbalance of "hot" and "cold" (not related to temperature). The scenario doesn't tell you for sure, but it could be that Rosanna did not believe the medication would help her son, so she decided not to spend money on it. This problem could have been prevented if you or the primary care provider assessed Rosanna's health beliefs and practices and involved her in José's care by discussing treatment options with her. For example, if she considered his throat infection to be "hot," then the provider might have been able to explain that the prescribed medication would get rid of the heat and pain that José is experiencing from the infection, or perhaps find another medication that Rosanna would consider to be "cold."

This is an example of what can happen when healthcare providers are so rigidly grounded in the beliefs of the professional healthcare culture that they fail to recognize and understand the health beliefs and practices of their clients. As you may guess, this way of practicing is a barrier to culturally competent care.

KnowledgeCheck 15-5

How do the cultural norms of the North American healthcare system differ from those of other cultural groups? Refer to Tables 15-2 and 15-3 in this chapter as needed.

Traditional and Alternative Healing

As a part of your culturally competent care, you need to know how healers from various cultures cure and care for members of their group. All cultures think of their healthcare system and beliefs as "traditional"; however, we use *traditional* in this chapter to refer to alternative beliefs, those that are not of the Western, North American, biomedical, or professional healthcare systems (previously discussed). You have already learned about different healthcare beliefs and practices clients may have (e.g., biomedical or scientific, holistic, magico-religious). The following section focuses on the types of healing systems that are used in different cultures.

Folk Medicine

When you feel as if you're getting a cold or the flu, what do you do? If you said that you take aspirin or vitamin C or eat chicken soup, then you are practicing folk medicine. You most likely do what your mother or some other relative did for you in similar situations. In North America there is a "pill" for almost everything, and virtually everyone self-medicates with OTC medicines. For many cultures, folk medicine involves natural medicines, such as herbs, plants, minerals, and animal substances. Magico-religious folk medicine involves the use of charms, holy words, rituals, and holy actions for preventing and treating illnesses (Spector, 2013).

Folk medicine is defined as the beliefs and practices that the members of a cultural group follow when they are ill, as opposed to more conventional (i.e., biomedical or professional) standards (Andrews & Boyle,

Table 15-3 ➤ Values and Health and Illness Beliefs and Practices for Selected Ethnocultural Groups in North America

GROUP	DOMINANT VALUES	HEALTH AND ILLNESS BELIEFS	HEALTH AND ILLNESS PRACTICES
Native American	Bonding to family or group Acceptance of nature (Mother Earth) Tradition Sharing Belief in a spiritual power Respect of elders	Health means living in harmony with nature. Surviving under difficult circumstances Body treated with respect Illness is associated with disharmony or evil spirits. Illness is caused by an action that should not have been performed.	Rituals and ceremonies Chanting Purification Meditation Herbs
Asian and Pacific Islander	Extended family Respect for elders Group orientation Subordination to authority Conformity Self-respect and self-control Love of the land	Health is a state of physical and spiritual harmony. Illness is disharmony of basic principles: yin and yang.	Acupuncture Amulets Moxibustion Meditation Herbs
Black or African American	Family bonding Matrifocal Spiritual orientation Present-oriented	Health is harmony with nature (mind, body, and spirit). Illness is the result of disharmony or failure to eat proper foods.	Prayer Laying on of hands Magic rituals Voodoo Herbs
Hispanic or Latino	Extended family Group emphasis Fatalistic Faith and spirituality	Health is good luck or a reward for good behavior, a gift from God. Illness is body imbalance (hot or cold, wet or dry) or punishment.	Prayer Belief in miracles Wearing of religious metals or amulets Religious relics in home Herbs and spices Rituals "Hot" and "cold" therapy
White or European American	Independence Individuality Wealth Comfort Cleanliness Achievement Youth and beauty	Health is a state of physical and emotional well-being. Illness is contagion or contamination that is hereditary, psychosomatic, or supernatural	Biomedical care Home remedies Religious traditions Diet and exercise

Note: Most people in North America use a combination of biomedical and traditional (specific to their culture) healthcare practices.
Sources: Adapted from Andrews, M., & Boyle, J. (2011). *Transcultural concepts in nursing care* (6th ed.). Philadelphia: Lippincott; Giger, J., & Davidhizar, R. (2008). *Transcultural nursing: Assessment and intervention* (5th ed.). St. Louis, MO: C.V. Mosby; Munoz, C., & Luckmann, J. (2005). *Transcultural communication in healthcare.* Clifton Park, NY: Thomson Delmar; Spector, R. (2013). *Cultural diversity in health and illness* (8th ed.). Upper Saddle River, NJ: Pearson Education, Inc.; and Purnell, L. (2012). *Transcultural health care: A culturally competent approach* (4th ed.). Philadelphia: F.A. Davis.

2011). All cultures throughout the world use folk medicine. Knowledge of these treatments is passed down from generation to generation by oral, and sometimes written, tradition. Folk medicine includes both self-treatment and use of folk healers.

Why would someone want to see a folk healer rather than a professional healthcare provider? In the dominant North American culture, the folk healer *is* the professional healthcare provider (i.e., the nurse practitioner, physician, certified nurse midwife, and so on). People of other cultures may seek out folk healers because they speak their native language, share their values and beliefs, charge less money, are readily available, or make house calls. If people perceive that the professional healing system cannot meet their needs, they are likely to seek care from the folk healers within their cultures and avoid the professional system.

Key Point: *Many folk healing traditions (see Table 15-1) are guided not only by cultural practices but also by religious beliefs and rituals. Religious rituals are often associated with births (e.g., circumcision) and deaths (e.g., who is allowed to wash the body and prepare it for burial). Although, there is a strong association between culture and religious beliefs, you should never assume that because your patient is a member of a certain culture he will also be of a certain religion. You should always ask as a part of your cultural assessment.*

Complementary and Alternative Medicine

Complementary medicine is the use of rigorously tested therapies that are outside of the mainstream medical or nursing care *to complement* those of conventional medicine (Andrews & Boyle, 2011; Buchan, Shakeel, Trinidade, et al., 2012). Examples include chiropractic care, biofeedback, and the use of certain supplements. In contrast, **alternative medicine** is defined as therapies used *instead of* conventional (i.e., biomedical) medicine, and whose reliability has not been validated through clinical testing in the United States. Examples of alternative therapies include iridology, aromatherapy, and magnet therapy.

Some complementary and alternative modalities (CAMs) are derived from the ancient and indigenous healthcare systems of people of other countries, such as traditional Chinese medicine (TCM), and **ayurveda**, the traditional healthcare system of India. Certain CAMs require a healer specially trained in their use (e.g., chiropractic, reflexology, massage therapy) and are licensed by the state (e.g., massage therapists). For a more thorough discussion on CAMs,

 Go to Chapter 46, Holistic Healing, on Davis*Plus*.

KnowledgeCheck 15-6

- What is folk medicine?
- What are some common folk medicine practices?
- Why might members of some cultural groups seek out the local folk healer rather than the conventional healthcare provider?

WHAT IS CULTURALLY COMPETENT CARE?

The terms *cultural awareness, cultural sensitivity,* and *cultural competence* are often used interchangeably; however, they are different.

- **Cultural awareness** refers to an appreciation of the external signs of diversity.
- **Cultural sensitivity** relates to personal attitudes and being careful not to say or do something that might be offensive to someone from a different culture (Purnell & Paulanka, 2008).
- **Cultural competence** is attained on a continuum ranging from cultural destructiveness (most negative) to cultural proficiency (most positive) (Cross, Bazron, Dennis, et al., 1989) or incompetent to competent (Purnell & Paulanka, 2008). You cannot achieve cultural competence overnight because it is a developmental process. As you become more aware of and sensitive to the needs of individuals from various ethnocultural groups, you will move forward on the journey toward cultural competence: being able to use knowledge and sensitivity in practice. The following are some ideas from nursing organizations and theorist about cultural competence.

The American Nurses Association (ANA)

The American Nurses Association's publication *Nursing: Scope and Standards of Practice* (2010) states that the registered nurse should provide holistic care that does the following:

- Addresses the needs of diverse populations.
- Is provided within the context of culturally sensitive interpersonal relationships.
- Includes providing cultural assessments and formulating individualized and culturally appropriate expected outcomes and nursing interventions to foster healing.

Quality and Safety Education for Nurses (QSEN)

Several of the QSEN competencies speak to culturally competent care. For example, from the patient-centered care competency, the graduate nurse should be prepared to:

- Provide patient-centered care with sensitivity and respect for the diversity of human experience.
- Seek learning opportunities with patients who represent all aspects of human diversity.
- Recognize personally held attitudes about working with patients from different ethnic, cultural, and social backgrounds.

Purnell and Paulanka

The Purnell model for cultural competence stresses teamwork in providing culturally sensitive and competent care to improve outcomes for individuals, families, and communities (Purnell, 2000, 2002, 2012; Purnell & Paulanka, 2008). In the context of nursing, Purnell's model defines **cultural competence** as "having the knowledge, abilities, and skills to deliver care congruent with the client's cultural beliefs and practices" (Purnell & Paulanka, 2008, p. 404). The pie-shaped wedges in Figure 15-6 depict the issues all societies and humans share (e.g., pregnancy, nutrition, high-risk behavior, family organization, and death) that are expressed in ways specific to the culture. These domains provide the organizing framework for the model. The center of the model is empty and represents that which is unknown about a cultural group.

Quality and Safety Education for Nurses

How Cultural Competency Improves Patient Outcomes

Chapter Key Concepts: *Cultural Competency, Patient Outcomes, Quality Improvement*

Competency: *Quality Improvement (Knowledge, skills, attitudes)**

Background: The QSEN competency of quality improvement is applicable to culturally competent care. Cultural competence encompasses more than just ethnicity and race; it requires sensitivity to vulnerable populations and the disparities within the healthcare system (Clingerman, 2011). Kersey-Matusiak (2012) claims that becoming culturally competent is an ongoing, lifetime process requiring skill development, thoughtful reflection, and self-awareness. Furthermore the author reports that cultural competency promotes better nurse–patient communication. This contributes to a cultural partnership and sensitivity, which results in the following:

➤ Both nurse and patient better understand the disease process and treatment management.

➤ The patient is more likely to adhere to the treatment protocols.

➤ Patient outcomes are improved (Kersey-Matusiak, 2012).

Think about it:

What is the relationship between cultural competence and healthcare disparities?
How can cultural competence by healthcare providers impact patient outcomes?

As reference for your QSEN log box, the QSEN KSA that is most pertinent is:

Recognize that students of nursing and other health professions are parts of systems of care and care processes that affect outcomes for patients and families.

Sources: Clingerman, E., (2011); Kersey-Matusiak, G. (2012).
*For specific Knowledge, Skills, and Attitudes,

 Go to the QSEN Web site at http://qsen.org/
competencies/pre-licensure-ksas/

The model identifies levels of several levels of cultural competence. Think about the meaning of each level:

Unconsciously incompetent
Consciously incompetent
Consciously competent
Unconsciously competent

Increasing one's consciousness of cultural diversity improves the possibilities for healthcare practitioners to provide culturally competent care.

Leininger

Although Madeline Leininger does not use the specific term *cultural competence*, her theory fits with that concept (Leininger, 2007; Leininger & McFarland, 2006). The goal of her theory is to guide research that will assist nurses to provide *culturally congruent care* using her three modes of nursing care actions and decisions (to be explained later in the chapter). Nurses can achieve this goal by:

■ Discovering cultural care and caring beliefs, values, and practices
■ Analyzing the similarities and differences of these beliefs among the different cultures

For more information on Leininger's theory of culture care diversity and universality,

 Go to Chapter 15, **Supplemental Materials: Leininger's Theory, and Tables, Boxes, Figures: ESG Figure 15-1, Leininger's Sunrise Model,** on DavisPlus.

Deardorff

Based on a recent study, Deardorff (2006, 2009) categorized intercultural competence into the following five categories:

■ *Attitudes*—The key attitudes include respect, openness, and curiosity, which imply the ability to move beyond your own comfort zone.
■ *Knowledge*—This includes cultural self-awareness, understanding others' perspectives, and culture-specific knowledge.
■ *Skills*—These skills address the processing of knowledge. They include observation, listening, evaluating, interpreting, and relating. You need to obtain and process information; you cannot rely on knowledge alone.
■ *Internal Outcomes*—"Outcome" implies change. Using your attitudes, knowledge, and skills should make you more flexible, adaptable, and empathetic. Ideally, you will be able to see from others' perspective and care for them in the ways that meet their needs.
■ *External Outcomes*—External outcomes describe the ways in which you behave and communicate as a result of the preceding four categories. They answer the question of how effective and appropriate you are in intercultural situations.

WHAT ARE SOME BARRIERS TO CULTURALLY COMPETENT CARE?

Your ability to provide culturally competent care may be hampered by various prejudices, attitudes and language barriers. Self-knowledge and critical thinking are essential in helping you identify and manage them. You should avoid the following in your practice:

■ **Bias**, one-sidedness: a tendency to "lean" a certain way, a lack of impartiality. A bias can be either positive or negative.
■ **Ethnocentrism** is the tendency of people to be biased toward their own culture, believing their own beliefs and values are right and that those of other cultures are wrong (or at least bizarre). If you take this attitude,

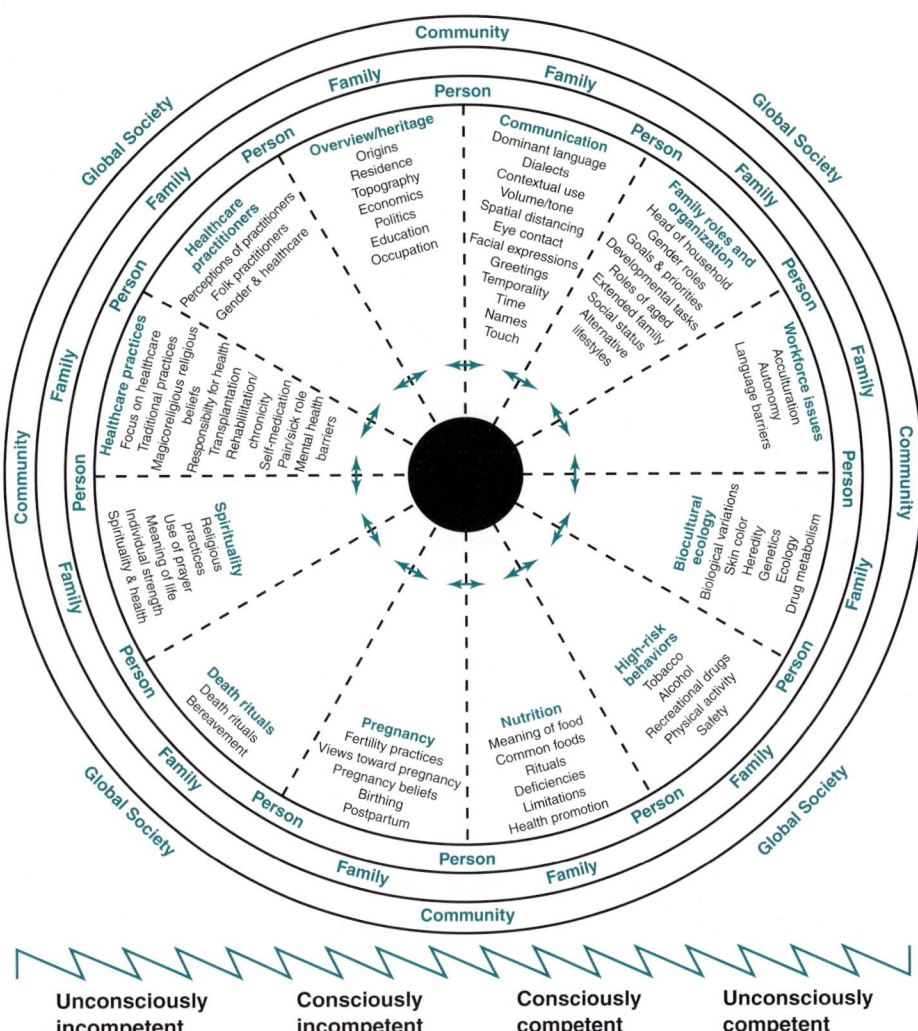

FIGURE 15-6 Purnell's model for cultural competence. (*Source:* From Purnell, L., & Paulanka, B. (2008). *Transcultural health care: A culturally competent approach* (3rd ed.). Philadelphia: F. A. Davis, p. 21. Reprinted with permission.)

your patient may feel that you disapprove of him or that you don't understand or respect him.

- **Cultural stereotyping** is the unsubstantiated belief that all people of a certain racial or ethnic group are alike in certain respects. Similar to biases, a stereotype may be positive or negative.
- **Prejudices** are negative attitudes toward other people based on faulty and rigid stereotypes about race, gender, sexual orientation, and so on.
- **Discrimination** is the behavioral manifestations of prejudice. For example, before the 1960s many U.S. hospitals refused treatment to African Americans. Slightly more subtle discrimination against minority groups still exists in housing, banking, the job market, and other areas of life.

Racism

Racism is a form of prejudice and discrimination based on the belief that (a) race is the principal determining factor of human traits and capabilities and (b) that racial differences produce an inherent superiority (or inferiority). The word *race* evokes powerful emotional responses for people who feel that they or their ancestors have been oppressed or exploited, and equally for those who deny

such a responsibility. In the United States, the history of discrimination against non-whites has created a focus on differences and racial divisiveness. As a nurse, you must recognize that unconscious racism and the use of words considered "racist" can play a major role in your ability to communicate with people of other races.

Sexism

Sexism is the assumption that members of one sex are superior to those of the other sex. For example, women have been viewed as more emotional and less rational than men. Assertiveness, a trait considered positive in men, is viewed as aggressiveness and an undesirable quality in women. Similarly, male nurses must combat sexism, mainly that it is "unnatural" for men to engage in caring behaviors. Thus, male nurses may initially be rejected by their female peers and some patients.

Male chauvinism (assumption of male superiority) is common in many cultures and in healthcare settings. It may be overt or subtle. The assumption of equality, by either party, changes the way people communicate. When you have the opportunity to do so, observe a conversation between a male nurse and a male physician. You may note that the male nurse communicates more directly and uses more eye contact than female nurses do with this same physician. We are not assuming all physicians (or nurses) are chauvinistic; we are simply stating that you will probably be able to observe this kind of interchange among some professionals.

Language Barriers

About 55 million people in the United States speak a language other than English at home. Another 24.5 million speak English poorly or not at all (Shin & Kominski, 2010). Language barriers will obviously affect your ability to communicate with clients. Language barriers can involve foreign languages, dialects, regionalisms (words or pronunciation particular to a specific region), street talk, and jargon.

Recall Mr. Salvatore, in Meet Your Patients. Suppose it is found that he has a brain tumor and needs immediate surgery. You would need to get his consent for surgery even though he and his family do not speak English. You might get a certified interpreter. However, the interpreter can have difficulty understanding Mr. Salvatore completely if he uses a different dialect or slang. This is not an unusual situation. In such a case, you would need to explore the policies of your healthcare facility to obtain additional resources. If there were no other options for translation help, you would have to temporarily resort to nonverbal language and pictures to communicate. If a consent issue is involved, the hospital must ensure adequate resources to comply with informed consent requirements.

Street Talk, Slang, and Jargon These can be as challenging as a foreign language. Their meaning changes and not everyone has the same interpretations. For example, the word *bad* can mean bad or good. Ebonics (also called African American Vernacular English, or AA-VE) is a type of English that has, in the past, been spoken primarily by African Americans, but many youths of other races, enamored with hip-hop culture, now embrace Ebonics as a way to connect with street culture. Texting can be another form of jargon. Not everyone understands the abbreviations used in texting.

Healthcare Jargon Words or expressions used by a subculture, including nursing and medicine, are called jargon. In healthcare, we use our peculiar terminology and abbreviations so often we may forget that our clients do not understand them. For example, you may frighten some patients if you say to them, "I'm going to take your vitals" before assessing their blood pressure. And many patients will not know what you mean if you ask, "Have you voided today?" Even worse, patients may hesitate to ask for clarification because they don't like admitting that they don't understand a certain word. This can both distress and isolate the patient.

Other Barriers

Lack of knowledge about the cultural and ethnic values, beliefs, and behaviors of people within their community is not unusual among healthcare providers. It can cause them to misinterpret a client's behaviors. *Emotional responses,* such as fear and distrust (both yours and the client's), can arise any time members of different cultural groups meet. If you are aware this may happen, you may be able to avoid this barrier and communicate with your clients effectively. Self-knowledge is essential in removing barriers.

KnowledgeCheck 15-7
- Define *cultural competence.*
- How do the barriers of ethnocentrism and language impede nursing care of diverse populations?

PracticalKnowledge
knowing **how**

Each phase of the nursing process presents an opportunity to provide culturally sensitive, congruent, and competent care. Regardless of the patient's cultural group, it is important to establish rapport before beginning data collection.

◼ ASSESSMENT

Various regulating bodies (e.g., The Joint Commission and the Office of Minority Health) require healthcare organizations to integrate cultural data into a patient's health records. Cultural assessment consists of an interview and a physical assessment. When you perform a cultural assessment, you should gather data directly from your client, but if this is not possible, you may ask a friend or family member of the client to assist you.

Key Point: *When an interpreter is needed, because of privacy concerns and legal guidelines you should not rely on a family member.*

The Health History

Regardless of the patient's cultural group, it is important for you to establish rapport before beginning data collection, especially for sensitive or personal information. To encourage clients to talk about themselves, you must convey empathy, show respect, build rapport, establish trust, listen actively, and provide appropriate feedback (Munoz & Luckmann, 2005). Ask open-ended questions when beginning a cultural assessment.

✚ Always ask clients about their use of alternative medicine and folk remedies so their effects on traditional biomedical medications and treatments can be evaluated. Some remedies may interfere with traditional treatments; others can be dangerous. Many people use folk remedies, but they may be reluctant to tell you because they fear ridicule or disapproval.

You will not need to perform an in-depth cultural assessment on every client, but you will need to recognize situations in which this is needed. For a list of questions to help you gather essential information for a cultural assessment,

Toward Evidence-Based Practice

> **Reneau, M. (2013). Teaching nurses sight unseen: Comparing the cultural competency of online and on-campus BSN faculty.** *Journal of Transcultural Nursing, 24*(1), 78–85.

The researcher compared the levels of cultural competency between 222 online and on-campus faculty. Results found that those teaching both online and on-campus had the highest level of cultural competency, followed by online educators. Faculty teaching on-campus had the lowest level of cultural competency. Recent cultural training was correlated with higher cultural competency scores.

> **Starr, S., & Wallace, D. (2011). Client perceptions of cultural competence of community-based nurses.** *Journal of Community Health Nursing, 28*(2), 57–69.

Clients assessed the cultural competency of their community-based nurses in the areas of communication, interpersonal style, and decision making. The nurses self-assessed their own cultural competency. Nurses were rated by the clients as very high in all three areas. Nurses reported encountering multiple racial/ethnic groups in their practice and considered themselves as "very culturally competent."

> **Musolino, G., Burkhalter, S., Crookston, B., et al. (2010). Understanding and eliminating disparities in health care: Development and assessment of cultural competence for interdisciplinary health professionals at the University of Utah—a 3-year investigation.** *Journal of Physical Therapy Education, 24*(1), 25–36.

A 3-year study tested the pre- and post-cultural competency learning outcomes of 2,124 Interdisciplinary Health Science students (medicine, physical therapy, nursing, pharmacy) who enrolled in a Cultural Competency and Mutual Respect course. The course consisted of four modules that focused on working and learning relationships involving different cultures. Results revealed students showed progression in the area of cultural competency for the constructs of attitudes, knowledge and skills, but did not achieve the constructs of cultural desires and cultural encounters.

> **Sequist, T., Fitzmaurice, G., Marshall R., et al. (2010). Cultural competency training and performance reports to improve diabetes care for black patients: A cluster randomized, controlled trial.** *Annals of Internal Medicine, 152*(1), 40–46.

Increasing clinicians' awareness of racial disparities may improve communication and outcomes in patients. Researchers examined the effect of an intervention consisting of cultural competency training. Monthly reports of race stratified data on 2,699 blacks and 4,858 white diabetic patients. Primary care clinicians who received the intervention were more aware of racial differences and disparities in diabetic care among black patients, although the overall clinical outcomes did not improve.

Instructions: Staff nurses have expressed concerns that nursing students are not incorporating cultural differences in the patients' plans of care. They have asked that students receive more education on cultural care in their nursing program of study. Answer the following questions:

1. Which studies or results support the belief that education and learning activities on culture will improve cultural competence?

2. What is the importance of encounters with clients from various cultures on acquiring cultural competency?

3. Which study provides the best evidence for including cultural education in the nursing program of study?

 Go to Chapter 15, **Toward Evidence-Based Practice Suggested Responses,** on Davis*Plus* at **DavisPl.us/ Wilkinson3.**

 Go to Chapter 15, **Assessment Guidelines and Tools, Focused Assessment: Obtaining Minimal Cultural Information,** in Volume 2.

Physical Assessment

Physical assessment may reveal biocultural variations. To assess and evaluate clients accurately, you need to know the normal physiological variations among healthy members of selected populations (e.g., body proportions, vital signs, general appearance, skin, musculoskeletal system, illness, and laboratory values).

Assessing the Skin You will need to know about biocultural variations in skin because of the importance of assessing for pallor, cyanosis, jaundice, erythema, and petechiae, which may be more difficult to evaluate in dark-skinned persons, challenging you to be more observant. For helpful suggestions and for more information about assessing the skin, see Chapter 35, and

 Go to Chapter 15, **Clinical Insight 15-1: Assessing for Biological Variations,** in Volume 2.

Assessing for Pain Culture influences the patient's responses to pain. Because pain and comfort are subjective responses, you need to quantify your client's pain as objectively as possible by using a pain measurement scale. Regardless of the literature descriptions of cultural responses, it is essential to investigate the meaning of pain to each individual and what they view as acceptable ways to express or cope with pain. For descriptions of some cultural responses to pain,

 Go to Chapter 15, **Clinical Insight 15-2, Pain Perception in Selected Cultural Groups,** in Volume 2.

Cultural Assessment Models and Tools

Some agencies have special tools for in-depth cultural assessments. If yours does not, you can structure your assessments using any culture model, such as the following examples.

- Purnell Model for Cultural Competence (2002)
- Andrews and Boyle Transcultural Nursing Assessment Guide (2011)
- Spector's Heritage Assessment Model (2004). Instead of assessing culture specifics, this tool assesses heritage consistency: the degree to which a person's lifestyle reflects his traditional culture (country of origin, race, or ethnic group). This assessment tool also reveals the degree to which the client still identifies with his cultural origins.
- Giger and Davidhizar's Transcultural Assessment Model (2008)

For more information on the preceding cultural assessment models,

 Go to Chapter 15, Tables, Boxes, Figures: ESG Figures 15-2 and 15-3, and ESG Box 15-1 and ESG Table 15-3, on DavisPlus.

For another example of a focused cultural assessment,

 Go to Chapter 15, Assessment Guidelines and Tools, Focused Assessment Cultural Assessment Using the Transcultural Model, in Volume 2.

ANALYSIS/NURSING DIAGNOSIS

There are no NANDA-I diagnoses that specifically address culture. However, cultural factors can be the etiology of various problems. Any of the NANDA-I diagnostic labels can be used for patients of any culture, provided that the defining characteristics are present. Some possible examples include the following:

- **Risk for Imbalanced Nutrition: Less Than Body Requirements** might apply to a patient who is hospitalized and cannot obtain foods prepared in the traditional way of his ethnic group.
- **Impaired Parenting** could occur if the patient's traditional methods of discipline are not acceptable or appropriate in the dominant culture.
- **Powerlessness** might occur when the patient is unable to make healthcare personnel understand the importance of his cultural rituals or healthcare practices.
- **Impaired Verbal Communication** is sometimes used for patients who do not speak or understand the nurse's language. However, this diagnosis is of questionable value in such circumstances. In a classic study, Geissler (1991) found that Impaired Verbal Communication related more to cultural differences between the patient and healthcare provider than to

the inability to communicate. The patient and nurse are equally "verbally impaired"—that is, communication is as much a problem for the nurse as it is for the patient. It is probably better to use Impaired Verbal Communication as the etiology of other diagnoses, such as Deficient Knowledge.

- **Noncompliance** can be used for clients and/or caregivers who do not follow a health-promoting or therapeutic plan the healthcare provider believes they agreed to. For example, the plan may not "fit" with the client's perception of the cause of his illness, as in the following scenario:

> *Example: Suppose that a 60-year-old woman who works as a hotel maid is repeatedly admitted to your hospital for uncontrolled hypertension. You know that she does not take her medication, and you diagnose Noncompliance (failure to take prescribed medication). But do you know that a month's supply of antihypertensive medication can cost more than $100? Perhaps your patient is raising her grandchildren and paying for food, shelter, and clothing consumes her entire income. Or perhaps she believes that herbs, diet, and other practices will reduce her blood pressure.*

You should use the Noncompliance diagnosis cautiously and only after completing a cultural assessment. Geissler (1991) found that additional defining characteristics are needed before Noncompliance can be appropriately applied to clients not of the dominant U.S. culture. In fact, Geissler suggests the nurses use the term *Nonadherence* instead of *Noncompliance*.

The preceding example illustrates that standardized nursing diagnoses are not always culturally sensitive and therefore may not apply accurately to patients who are not from the dominant culture. Nursing diagnoses should describe responses that *patients* see as problematic. A nurse and patient who are from different cultures will likely have different perceptions of health and illness. This can lead to misdiagnosis. The nurse may either diagnose a problem that doesn't exist for the patient or diagnose a "real" problem but fail to describe it accurately (Wilkinson, 2011).

The following are a few examples of NANDA-I nursing diagnoses that could be interpreted differently by people from different cultures. Undoubtedly there are others.

Acute Pain	Impaired Social
Anxiety	Interaction
Decisional Conflict	Ineffective Coping
Readiness for Enhanced	Ineffective Role
Breastfeeding	Performance
Imbalanced Nutrition: More	Noncompliance
Than Body Requirements	Powerlessness

The point is to use all labels carefully and to validate nursing diagnoses with the patient to be sure that the statement describes her health status as *she* sees it.

PLANNING OUTCOMES/EVALUATION

The outcomes you choose (whether standardized or individualized) depend on the nursing diagnoses you have identified. If the diagnoses are culturally sensitive, the outcomes should be as well. However, you must involve the patient in order to be certain. For example, suppose your patient is dying. You and the patient agree that her diagnosis is Acute Pain, but your goals may be different. You might want the patient to be free from pain. However, the patient's goal may be to stay alert enough to interact with her family, even if it means she must endure some pain. When your cultures differ, it is even more important to validate the goals with the patient. Some individualized goal/outcome statements associated with cultural differences might include the following:

- Agrees to take prescribed analgesic (pain medication) before bedtime and after family leaves for the evening.
- Talks to her spiritual adviser about the possibility of a treatment plan that conflicts with her religious beliefs.
- Freely shares information about folk practices and OTC medications with the primary care provider.

PLANNING INTERVENTIONS/IMPLEMENTATION

You should become familiar with the cultural groups that are dominant in your area and that you will encounter in your nursing practice to plan culturally appropriate care.

NIC standardized interventions related to culture and the provision of culturally competent care include the following examples:

Active Listening (for Impaired Verbal Communication)
Mutual Goal Setting (for Impaired Parenting)
Self-Responsibility Facilitation (for Powerlessness)
Culture Brokerage (for Noncompliance)

Culture Brokerage, a Nursing Intervention Classification (NIC) intervention, is defined as "the deliberate use of culturally competent strategies to bridge or mediate between the patient's culture and the biomedical healthcare system" (Bulechek, Butcher, & Dochterman, 2013, p. 136).

Individualized nursing activities and focused assessments are important for all patients. However, patients from different cultural and ethnic groups may have unique needs that can be met by some of the activities included in the following discussion regarding culturally competent care.

Nursing Strategies for Providing Culturally Competent Care

When planning care for your clients, information about their cultural values, beliefs, and practices will help you identify interventions that will support these practices and incorporate them into their care as much as possible (Wilkinson, 2011). For example, when you are teaching about a specific treatment regimen ordered by the primary care provider, you should find out whether it conflicts with any of the patient's folk beliefs or alternative treatments so you can suggest necessary modifications. Remember also to identify educational methods that are most appropriate for your client's needs (e.g., translated materials and/or diagrams) and to make community referrals as necessary.

KnowledgeCheck 15-8

- Describe, in general, how the nursing process can help you provide culturally competent care.
- How can nursing diagnoses cause bias in the planning of care for clients from different cultures?

How Should I Respond to a Client's Cultural Health Practices?

Theorists describe different situations in which nursing decisions and actions are needed regarding a client's cultural health practices. A practice may be helpful, harmful, or neutral; or the effects may be unknown (Giger, 2012; Leininger, 1991; Leininger & McFarland, 2006). See Table 15-4.

Negotiation The client's perspective may differ from yours about the effects of a particular practice. Negotiation acknowledges that gap. You must negotiate when folk or traditional practices might be harmful to the client.

Example: The nurse negotiates with the client to continue seeing the curandero, but to come to the clinic every 6 weeks to have his blood pressure checked. If the client refuses all biomedical or nursing interventions, the only avenue still open is to continue monitoring the client to identify changes in his health status. If a health crisis occurs, it may be possible to renegotiate the care.

Repatterning/Restructuring This means that you attempt to change your actions or the client's lifestyle (Leininger, 1991; Leininger & McFarland, 2006). You would support and encourage the client to greatly modify his behaviors and to adopt new, different, and beneficial health behaviors, while still respecting his cultural values and beliefs.

Example 1. Change in the nurse's actions. When the client absolutely refuses to take the prescribed pain medication, the nurse uses massage, distraction, and other nonpharmacological techniques to help relieve his pain.

Example 2. Modification of the client's behaviors. A client refuses to see a biomedical doctor for her family's needs. However, when the folk healer is unsuccessful in treating her child's illness and the child becomes critically ill, the nurse convinces the client to bring the child to the emergency department.

Table 15-4 ➤ Possible Effects of a Patient's Cultural Health Practices

THE EFFECTS ARE:	EXAMPLE	NURSING APPROACH
Efficacious (Helpful)	Bringing ethnic foods that are appropriate for the client's prescribed diet.	Encourage practices that will likely improve client health and help her preserve cultural values related to health.
Neutral (Neither Helpful nor Harmful)	People of Arab heritage associate good health with eating properly and fasting to cure disease. Some may treat illness with prayers or simple foods such as dates, honey, salt, and olive oil (Purnell & Paulanka, 2008; Purnell, 2012).	There should be no harm in allowing a patient to continue a neutral health practice. You would not want to interfere with these neutral practices.
Uncertain (Unknown by You)	A client drinks a daily smoothie that consists of certain herbs and spices such as ginger, cinnamon, and basil for "good health."	You can neither encourage nor discourage these practices until you obtain more information about them. Do this as soon as possible.
Dysfunctional (Harmful)	A client may refuse to give prescribed medication to her child.	Discourage folk practices that may cause harm. In such instances, you should support and enable the client to adapt to biomedical therapies (repatterning/restructuring) or negotiate with the client to achieve satisfying outcomes.

How Do I Communicate With Clients Who Speak a Different Language?

Communicating with clients who do not speak your language can be especially challenging. The Internet and computer software allow patients to type information in their native language and translate it into English as a way to communicate with providers. However, the best way to provide culturally competent care to such clients is to use a professional medical interpreter or translator. An **interpreter** is specially trained to provide the meaning behind the words, whereas a **translator** just restates the words from one language to another. An interpreter can serve as a cultural broker by conveying the client's responses to questions and by providing general information about the client's culture. Both must meet predetermined standards to participate in translation services. Do not use family or friends as interpreters except if requested by the patient. For guidelines when using an interpreter and when an interpreter is not available,

 Go to Chapter 15, **Clinical Insights 15-3: Communicating With Clients Who Speak a Different Language,** in Volume 2.

CLAS Standards

Healthcare facilities must provide language assistance services by, in order of preference, bilingual staff, face-to face interpretation by trained persons, or telephone interpreters. Healthcare interpreters should be used to obtain informed consent and to assist the patient to understand the treatment plan (U.S. Department of

Health and Human Services, Office of Minority Health, 2001; Wilson-Stronks, Lee, & Cordero, 2008).

Research shows that many hospitals do provide patients with information on their rights to receive language services; however, the information is provided in English. In addition, the majority of hospitals continue to use untrained or family members as interpreters, contrary to CLAS standard 6 (Diamond, Wilson-Stronks, & Jacobs, 2010). Only 13% of hospitals surveyed met all four language-related standards. Hospitals with a diverse inpatient population, not-for-profits hospitals, and those located in affluent and competitive markets had a high degree of cultural competency (Weech-Maldonado, Elliott, Pradhan, et al., 2012). You should advocate for your clients to ensure the goal of cultural competence is met. For a complete listing of the CLAS standards,

 Go to Chapter 15, **Supplemental Materials: CLAS Standards,** on DavisPlus.

Developing Strategies

There are several strategies for you to consider and many resources to help you develop strategies specific to various cultural groups (Box 15-2). Consider the following as you move forward on your journey toward cultural competence:

Reflect and Know Yourself

- Understand your own cultural values and practices and appreciate how they may differ from those held by people of other cultures.

BOX 15-2 ▪ Being Considerate of Cultural Specifics

Consider verbal and nonverbal communication.

- Know, or find out, whether touch (e.g., a handshake) is expected or prohibited.
- Know, or find out, whether eye contact is expected or avoided. Avoiding eye contact, for some, is a sign of respect.
- Ask the client how he wishes to be addressed.
- Know, or find out, the ways people welcome each other.

Consider the person's need for personal space.

- Know the person's cultural and religious customs regarding touching and contact.
- Know the usual comfortable distance for conversing in the client's culture.

Consider body language.

- Gestures that are acceptable in one culture may be taboo in another. Know what is acceptable to the client.
- Be aware that smiling does not universally indicate friendliness.

Consider time orientation.

- Tell clients when you are coming, and be on time.
- Avoid surprise visits.
- Share your own expectations about time.
- Ask clients what they expect regarding time, appointments, and so on.
- Be sure you know the times for and meanings of the client's religious and ethnic holidays.

Consider social organization.

- Know which person in the family is the leader or decision maker.
- Know what dates are important and whether gifts are expected or not.
- Know how special events, such as births and funerals, are celebrated, whether certain colors have meaning, and what the expected rituals are.

Consider the person's perspective on environmental control.

- Find out what the client's health traditions and practices are.
- Know whether the person believes she has any ability to "change things."
- Know the general influence of the culture on perception and tolerance of pain.
- Know what foods are forbidden, what foods may or may not be eaten together, and what and how utensils are used.

- Recognize your own biases about people and groups, and consider how they may affect the care you provide.
- Learn from your mistakes, and don't make them again.

Keep Learning

- Learn as much as you can about the cultural groups in your community and work area.
- Study nursing theories and principles pertaining to culture.
- Take advantage of every opportunity to interact with persons from different cultural groups.

Accommodate and Negotiate

- Make an effort to incorporate beliefs and practices from various cultures into your nursing care and teaching materials.
- Encourage helpful or neutral cultural practices, and discourage those that are dysfunctional (harmful).
- Suggest alternatives to harmful practices.
- Accommodate cultural dietary practices when possible. For inpatients, some dietary departments can make special foods, and you can encourage families to bring food from home. In all situations, help patients and families adapt cultural foods to therapeutic diets.

Collaborate

- Work with the folk medicine practitioner in the interest of the client.
- Advocate for all of your clients, but especially for those not from the dominant culture.
- Consider the cultural role of the family member who makes the primary decisions. To ignore this person is to doom your interventions to failure.

Respect

- Consider each client as a unique individual, influenced but not defined by his culture.
- Respect your clients regardless of cultural background, and never force, pressure, manipulate, or coerce them to participate in care that conflicts with their values and beliefs.

This is by no means an exhaustive list. Most likely, you can think of other strategies. It may help you to "take a trip to BALI":

Be aware of your own cultural heritage.
Appreciate that the client is unique: influenced, but not defined by his culture.
Learn about the client's cultural group.
Incorporate the client's cultural values/behaviors into the care plan.

KnowledgeCheck 15-9

- List five factors to consider to help you develop strategies to become more culturally competent.
- What does the acronym "BALI" stand for?

How Can I Become Culturally Competent?

Of course you can't become culturally competent just by reading. People acquire cultural competence gradually, progressing through the following stages:

Unconscious incompetence—not being aware that you lack knowledge about another culture

Conscious incompetence—being aware that you lack knowledge about another culture

Conscious competence—learning about the client's culture, verifying generalizations about the culture (e.g., archetypes), and providing culture specific interventions

Unconscious competence—automatically providing culturally congruent care to clients of diverse cultures (Purnell & Paulanka, 2008, p. 6)

Theoretical knowledge can increase your awareness and appreciation of cultural differences, but you can achieve cultural competence only if you are motivated and even then only by interacting with people from cultures different from your own (Musolino, Burkhalter, Crookston, et al., 2010). Carballeira (1997) sums up this process with the LIVE and LEARN model for culturally competent family services:

Like		**L**isten
Inquire		**E**valuate
Visit	and	**A**cknowledge
Experience		**R**ecommend
		Negotiate

Key Point: *If there were only one intervention you could use to improve your cultural competence, it should be to routinely ask patients what matters most to them in their illness and treatment.*

No matter how busy you are, you can find time to do that. You can then use that information to incorporate cultural needs into the client plan of care.

 Think**Like a Nurse** 15-8

What kind of knowledge do you need to become culturally competent (theoretical, practical, self, ethical)? Explain your answer.

 To explore learning resources for this chapter,

 Go to Davis*Plus* at **DavisPl.us/Wilkinson3.**

Chapter Resources for Chapter 15:

Response sheets for all learning activities

Resources for Caregivers and Health Professionals

Reading More About Culture & Ethnicity (suggested readings)

Concept Map of chapter content

Interactive Case Studies

NCLEX-Style and Chapter Review Questions

Chapter Overview Podcasts

For references cited in this chapter,

 Go to Volume 2, **References Cited.**

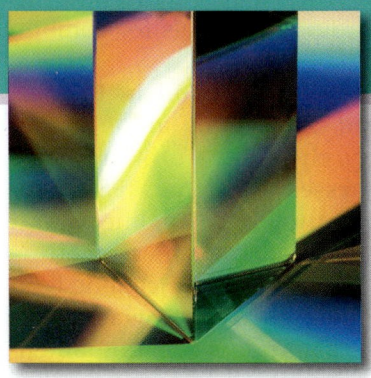

CHAPTER 16

Spirituality

Learning Outcomes

After completing this chapter, you should be able to:

➤ Describe the differences and similarities between religion and spirituality.

➤ Discuss what is meant by *spirituality*.

➤ For each of the religions briefly covered in this chapter, describe its major beliefs and their implications for nursing care.

➤ Identify five barriers to spiritual care.

➤ Perform a spiritual assessment.

➤ Recognize the differences between spiritual care diagnoses and those that

may serve as etiologies of other nursing diagnoses.

➤ Plan nursing interventions based on the data obtained in a spiritual assessment.

➤ Examine your own level of comfort in terms of performing spiritual interventions.

➤ Describe collaborative efforts to ensure the spiritual care of the patient or family.

Key Concepts

Spirituality

Religion

Spiritual care

Related Concepts

See the Concept Map on Davis*Plus*.

Meet Your Patient

Charles Johnson is a 75-year-old African American man with newly diagnosed lung cancer. He began smoking at age 15. His physicians want to start chemotherapy to try to increase his life span. He is unsure whether he wants to have chemotherapy.

Mr. Johnson was brought up in the Baptist Church, but has fallen away from practicing his faith over the years. He has been a heavy drinker all of his adult life and, as a young man, has distanced himself from church. He explains: "Church folks are all a bunch of hypocrites, if you ask me. I choose not to be a part of any of that." Nevertheless, he says that he tries to be kind to and tolerant of others. "I've messed up my life, so I figure I don't have any business telling other people how to live. I guess I just figure that how a person lives is between him and God."

Mr. Johnson has one surviving relative, a sister, who is concerned about him. His sister is a devout Jehovah's Witness, and she has tried several times to talk to Mr. Johnson about the importance of Jehovah in her life. She continually leaves religious pamphlets and materials in his mailbox to encourage him to think about religion again.

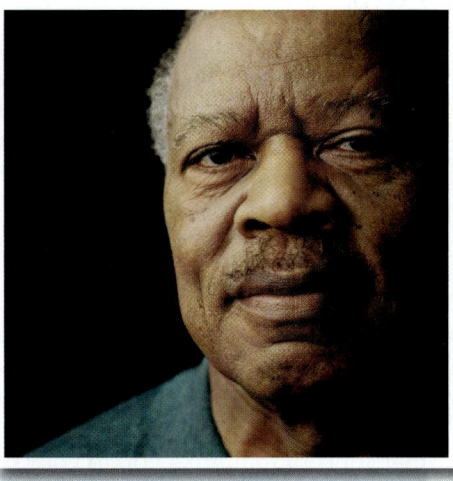

Mr. Johnson's wife divorced him 20 years ago because of his drinking behaviors, and he has alienated his two middle-aged children, so he rarely sees his grandchildren. He lives alone, is retired, and is having some trouble making ends meet financially. He has one avid hobby: He loves to go out in a boat and fish all day with his buddy, Jim.

■ Mr. Johnson clearly has some physical and psychosocial difficulties. Can you identify them?

■ Assess Mr. Johnson's support system. Whom can he rely on for help?

■ How might you help Mr. Johnson to add some spiritual supports to his available resources?

Theoretical Knowledge
knowing **why**

Spirituality in nursing has multiple layers. The following layers of competing concerns must be properly balanced to minimize your confusion, frustration, and avoidance of spiritual care.

- **Spirituality of the Nurse.** Each nurse's spirituality serves as part of the guiding framework for her practice.
- **Spirituality of the Patient and Family.** Spirituality will be understood in different ways by your patients and their families. Their spirituality may be deeply ingrained or totally separate from formal religion.
- **Effects of Nursing Education.** The emphasis placed on spiritual care interventions will vary among the various nursing programs; however, many teach students to avoid imposing their spiritual beliefs, or lack of, on patients.
- **Demands of Nursing Practice.** Time constraints imposed by the day-to-day patient care activities in healthcare environments can be viewed as negatively impacting your ability to meet your patients' spiritual needs. Rely on your communication and assessment skills to establish a therapeutic nurse–patient relationship that is the foundation for meeting your patients' spiritual needs (Biro, 2012).

This chapter presents a holistic interpretation of spirituality—one that views spirituality as a component of every person's life. It also encourages you to engage your own spirituality to improve your patients' health and wholeness. It should help you to answer some of the questions posed for Mr. Johnson.

ABOUT THE KEY CONCEPTS

As you study this chapter, try to relate what you are reading to the key concepts of **spirituality** and **religion**, and try to understand how those two concepts relate to each other. This will provide you a foundation from which to work with the concept of **spiritual care**. It is that concept that links you to your patients.

HISTORY OF SPIRITUALITY IN NURSING

Through the ages, nurses and other caregivers have demonstrated deep concern for the spiritual as well as the physical and psychological needs of those who are sick and infirm.

In the pre-Christian era, caring for the sick was an expression of the values of hospitality and charity. People prayed to the god(s) for healing and as an adjunct for primitive medical procedures.

In the early Christian era, nursing the sick was honored and respected because it was one of Jesus Christ's primary teachings. Caring for the sick was a vital component of loving one's neighbor. Gradually, religious communities of women and men in the 4th through 12th centuries provided models for combining the healing arts with religious care.

During the post-Reformation period in Europe, nursing orders continued to flourish, among them the Daughters of Charity, the Sisters of Mercy, and the Kaiserswerth Deaconesses (Donahue, 1985). Florence Nightingale trained under Pastor Fliedner at his Deaconess School in Kaiserswerth, as well as under the Daughters of Charity of St. Vincent de Paul in France. For Nightingale, spirituality was at the very heart of human nature and thus was fundamental to healing. Nightingale instilled this value in her nurses, particularly during their missions in the Crimea where "the lady with the lamp" brought comfort and relief to the sick and the dying (Dolarno, 2010; McDonald, 2002).

By the mid-20th century, nursing in the United States had begun to see spiritual care as less important. As science continued to develop and expand, and as more nurses studied in university settings, nursing joined ranks with the scientific disciplines: Its spiritual underpinnings were replaced by what could be "seen and tested" by the scientific method. Only recently has nursing (and the broader health community) reclaimed the spiritual dimension as a vital part of its identity and recognized its power to influence health.

Key Point: *Today, spiritual care cannot be the "overlooked" area of nursing practice. Professional standards of care make clear that meeting patients' spiritual needs is essential to provide holistic nursing care.* The Joint Commission (2010) has established standards for spiritual care. In addition, the American Nurses Association's (ANA) Code for Nurses (2010) states that nurses should consider each patient's lifestyle, value system, and religious beliefs in planning care; and that nursing care measures should enable the patient to live with as much physical, emotional, social, and spiritual well-being as possible.

WHAT ARE RELIGION AND SPIRITUALITY?

Spirituality and religion are related, yet they are two distinct and different concepts, as identified in Table 16-1. For example, atheists and agnostics have no religious foundation, but may have spiritual needs (Sessana, Finnell, Underhill, et al., 2011). One way to distinguish religion from spirituality is to think of religion as a map and spirituality as a journey.

What Is Religion?

You may use a map to get to a certain location. The "map" of religion tells you what to believe and what values are essential. It provides codes of conduct that integrate beliefs and values into a way of living. The

The Impact of Nurse Self-Awareness on Patient Spiritual Care

Chapter Key Concepts: Spirituality, Patient-Centeredness, Nurse Self-Awareness

Competency: Patient-Centered Care (Knowledge, skills, attitudes)*

Background: Holistic nursing care includes addressing the patient's physical, psychosocial and spiritual needs. Spirituality isn't always linked with religion. Rather, spirituality is what the individual professes it to be (Schaefer, Stonecipher, & Kane, 2012). The QSEN competency of patient-centered care recognizes "the patient as the source of control and full partner in providing compassionate and coordinated care based on respect for patient's preferences, values, and needs" (Cronenwett, Sherwood, Barnsteiner, et al., 2007). To provide holistic care the nurse must understand the meaning of spirituality and have a self-awareness of her own spirituality. An awareness of one's own spirituality contributes to the ability to relate meaningfully with patients and to provide care to support patients' spiritual needs (Lee & Higgens, 2010).

Think about it:

➤ Describe nursing interventions that would meet the spiritual needs of the patient.

➤ How does providing patient-centered care attend to the spiritual needs of the patient?

➤ Discuss how spiritual self-awareness by the nurse might influence the spiritual care provided for the patient.

Sources: Cronenwett, L., Sherwood, G., Barnsteiner, J., et al. (2007); Lee, D., & Higgens, P. (2010); Schaefer, J., Stonecipher, S., & Kane, I. (2012).

As reference for your QSEN log box, the QSEN KSA that is most pertinent is:

Respect and encourage individual expression of patient values, preferences and expressed needs.

*For specific Knowledge, Skills, and Attitudes,

 Go to the QSEN Web site at **http://qsen.org/ competencies/pre-licensure-ksas/**

Quality and Safety Education for Nurses

Table 16-1 ➤ Comparison of Religion and Spirituality

RELIGION (THE MAP)	SPIRITUALITY (THE JOURNEY)
A "roadmap" that defines: Beliefs Values Code(s) of conduct and ethics	One's journey through life; a personal quest to define meaning, fulfillment, and satisfaction in life; a will to live; a belief in self; an exploration of who you are
A tradition or system of worship that provides: Rituals Answers Norms Connection with God	A dynamic relationship with that which transcends; a capacity to know and be known (a sense of openness, expectation); connectedness with self, others, nature, and a higher power (Cavendish, Konecny, Mitzeliotis, et al., 2003); belief in a divine being, or infinite source of energy (Beckman, Boxley-Harges, Bruick-Sorge, et al., 2007).
The roadmap and tradition define: What is to be believed How beliefs affect life Self-image and identity	A lifelong process of growth (which may involve joy and/or struggle); a constant process of taking in "truth" and then adding individual insight to arrive at a way of perceiving and acting in the world
Issues: Faith, belief, trust, the nature of good and evil, the meaning of suffering, judgment, or enlightenment	Issues: Faith, hope, love

map itself may be in the form of a religious tradition (e.g., Christianity) or denomination (e.g., Baptist), which provides an identity and a "lens" for reading the world. The rituals, symbols, sacraments, and holy writings associated with religions serve as bases of authority and provide diverse ways to transcend the physical and access the divine (e.g., God) (Fig. 16-1). Regardless

of their differences, many of the world religions have the following in common:

- **Theology**—that is, discussions and theories related to God and God's relation to the world
- Sacred writings that are regarded as authoritative and/or reveal the nature of the divine in some way

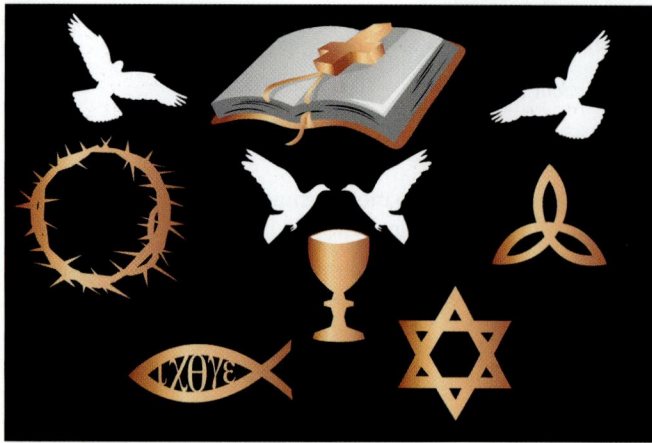

FIGURE 16-1 Associated with religion are various symbols and holy writings, such as this cross and Bible representing Christianity.

- Notion of created order and purpose
- Definition of *human being* that includes important life events
- Notion of sin (primarily in Western religions)
- Explanation of the origin of evil and the nature of suffering
- Conception of either salvation (in Judeo-Christian religions) or enlightenment (in Eastern religions)
- **Eschatology**, or doctrines about the human soul and its relation to death, judgment, and eternal life (primarily a Western concept)
- Explanation of the nature of reality, the higher Self or soul, the relationship between humans and the divine, and the purpose of human existence

What Is Spirituality?

If religion serves as the map, spirituality is the day-to-day, moment-by-moment journey in life and living. Like a journey, spirituality involves personal subjective experiences that take place over time. Many life events that prompt spiritual growth are fulfilling and joyful, but growth often results from painful life events that cause great internal upheaval, struggle, and challenge.

Like religion, spirituality allows various ways and means to experience the divine in our daily lives, to transcend the physical world, or simply to be still and introspective. You can also think of spirituality as the insight, value, purpose, and meaning of life derived from accumulated life experiences. They may agree or conflict with traditional religious values and cultural teachings. For example, after studying a variety of religions and traveling in Asia for several years, an American raised in the Episcopal Church may develop a spirituality that is both universal and highly individual and may feel "at home" in any place of worship in the world.

One Western model of spirituality asserts that we learn to "read" the spiritual in everyday events only when we attain a new "level of literacy." Life then is a process of recognizing everyday signs of an active Spirit in the world and understanding its meaning. This model states that we can engage this Spirit through such sources as nature, animals, leisure, creativity, and service (Brussat & Brussat, 1996).

It is critical for you to recognize and respect the different ways that patients understand religion and spirituality. You need to understand that most people are comfortable with their beliefs (or lack thereof) and that in providing spiritual care your primary goal is to support their healing, not convert them to a different view. You must also be able to recognize situations when patients may be experiencing spiritual distress and may need referral to professionals with more specialized training. These aspects of spiritual care are discussed later in this chapter.

KnowledgeCheck 16-1

- Regardless of their differences, what do many world religions have in common?
- Which can be compared to a journey: religion or spirituality?
- True or false? Both religion and spirituality allow a person various ways to access the divine.
- What is Mr. Johnson's religion (Meet Your Patient)?
- What is his sister's religion?

ThinkLike a Nurse 16-1

- What do you know, or what can you speculate, about Mr. Johnson's (Meet Your Patient) spirituality?

What Are the Core Issues of Spirituality?

By now you know that spirituality has many dimensions. We limit discussion here to three core issues. In his first letter to the Corinthians in the New Testament of the Bible, Saint Paul identified "three things that last": faith, hope, and love. Following in this tradition, a manual for nursing care of the dying (Aspen Reference Group, 2002) identifies this same trio as the three core issues of spirituality.

Faith

Faith is an evolving pattern of believing that guides and grounds us, helps us make sense of the world, and confront the challenges we face (Dyess, 2011). It allows us to trust and to maintain an optimistic perspective on life events and to find purpose in life. Like spirituality, faith represents a set of beliefs developed over time, through events that cause us to suffer and those that enable us to rejoice.

Faith struggles are common among people who experience illness and significant loss. People experiencing faith struggles might feel anger, guilt, self-judgment, and worthlessness. C. S. Lewis, a devout Christian, reveals that after the death of his wife, his grief caused him to doubt whether God exists at all, or if so, whether He is perhaps a "Cosmic Sadist" (1961, p. 35) who deliberately tortures us. Finally, Lewis came to understand that such shattering experiences are "one of the marks of His presence" (Lewis, 1961, p. 76).

People who are experiencing the *joys of faith* exhibit a sense of self, as well as insights into their gifts and talents. In his book *Callings,* Gregg Levoy (1997, p. 65) observes that our joy and our enthusiasm move us "toward a kind of divine presence because, through our passions, we are utterly present. . . . We hitch ourselves to something bigger."

Hope

Hope is a dynamic process that reflects a positive orientation towards future outcomes. It includes our basic human need to achieve, create, and to shape something of our life that will endure. If faith is expressed in terms of belief, then hope is rooted in purpose—who am I, what is my purpose, and why have I been created? People who are confronting a debilitating or terminal illness often lose hope. Research shows that support systems, attitudes of healthcare providers, and skilled nursing care are important in fostering hope in patients who experienced traumatic injuries (Warwick, 2012). After suffering a near-fatal spinal cord injury, actor Christopher Reeve struggled with hope; yet, he wrote in an essay, "Hope . . . is different from optimism or wishful thinking. When we have hope, we discover powers within ourselves we may have never known—the power to make sacrifices, to endure, to heal, and to love. Once we choose hope, everything is possible" (Reeve, 2002, p. 176).

Love

Although it is better defined as a strong affection for another, many view love as a trade: We extend our love because we hope to find that love is returned in some way. But relationships can be a source of pain. Even when our love is shared, we must inevitably face separation at our death or the death of our loved ones. Thus, while active loving in human relationships opens us up to joy and can give life meaning and purpose, it also carries with it the certainty of heartbreak (e.g., when a loved one dies).

Illness and sudden injury can prompt "struggles with love." For example, when a man with a debilitating disease loses his ability to work and requires increasing levels of caregiving, he may see himself as a "burden" and question whether his loved ones would be "better off" if he were to die. Family members are invaluable in showing their unconditional love to help restore the patient's inner integrity and self-worth. Reeve stated that the most powerful words his wife spoke to him in the first days after his injury, "the words that saved my life," were, "You're still you. And I love you" (Reeve, 1998, p. 32). This support, combined with the compassionate love transmitted by healthcare providers, can help patients to overcome negative states, increase healing, and promote better-quality outcomes (Posadzki, 2010).

Cures, Miracles, and Spiritual Healing

The patient or family may request a prayer asking God for a cure when your expertise tells you that all curative measures have been exhausted. You should not say that a cure is impossible; however, it is equally important to avoid exposing the patient and family to false hope. In such cases, it may be possible for you, as care provider and companion on the spiritual journey, to offer a way to reframe the situation. Perhaps, healing does not necessarily have to imply the elimination of all types of suffering or of the disease. Rather, it may mean a transformation in a patient's thinking or feeling or acknowledging the patient's belief in the spirit. In such instances, various forms of healing can occur, and the person may experience it as a miracle.

A **miracle** is anything that allows for the presence of the transcendent (e.g., God, a Higher Being, the experience of one's angel, or any brush with the divine). We typically think of miracles as events that break with the natural order of things; however, miracles may proceed according to natural law. After the death of her patient, a physician described the patient's long-resisted acceptance of his impending death as the miracle, which prevented fruitless interventions and unnecessary suffering (La Madrid, 2012). What makes events miracles is that they far exceed our expectations. For instance, an elderly woman, bitter for decades over the death of her daughter during childhood, "feels" her daughter's presence and dies in peace. As you can see, miracles do not always involve physical cures. Miracles can also be spiritual phenomena. As such, they are mysterious and difficult to define, explain, and comprehend. In one sense, miracles can be viewed as perfectly ordinary events; in another, they can only be explained as the act of a "deity" (McGrew, 2013). For example, a blind person suddenly can see, with no treatment or explanation.

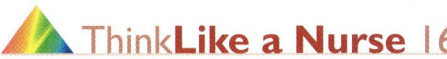

ThinkLike a Nurse 16-2

Faith is a constant search for comprehension and meaning. What are some of your struggles with faith, and what are some of the "joys" of your faith?

How Might Spiritual Beliefs Affect Health?

Religion and spirituality have been presented as two separate and distinct constructs; however, current research on their influence on health tends to combine them into one concept, namely, religion or religious involvement. Research findings are varied in terms of the relationship of religion and/or spirituality on health outcomes and behaviors.

- One study found that religious involvement was instrumental in decreasing anxiety and depression and increasing overall quality of life (Huang, Hsu, & Chen, 2012).
- Another study found that African Americans and Hispanic Americans had a greater rate of religiosity; however, they did not experience greater mental health

benefits. In addition, only White Americans experienced better mental health benefits from attending religious services (Sternthal, Williams, Musick, et al., 2012).

■ Other researchers investigated the effect of religious beliefs on health disparities (Jun & Oh, 2013). The impact of the religious/cultural belief of *fatalismo* among Hispanics and fatalism among Asians was shown to have a negative effect on compliance with preventive cancer screening. Fatalism, which is rooted in Buddhism, views fatal diseases as destined by nature and acceptance as a sign of wisdom and maturity. Likewise, *fatalismo*, with roots in Christianity, views diseases as predetermined with a predictable outcome. Both groups had high pessimistic perceptions that preventive screening would lower their risk of getting cancer.

In research on spirituality, the variables studied tend to be broadly stated and nonspecific. Most use broad measures, such as self-reports of one's own religiousness, denominational affiliation, church attendance or membership (e.g., "On a scale of 1 to 5, how religious are you?" "How often do you attend church?"). Thus, they do not allow for researchers to examine whether there might be potential harmful effects of religion. For a list of other recent studies,

 Go to Chapter 16, **Reading More About Spirituality,** on Davis*Plus.*

Although some research suggests that religion has a positive influence on healthcare outcomes, it does not yet answer *how* or *why* religion has this effect. However, there is growing awareness that religion and spirituality are complex variables involving cognitive, emotional, behavioral, interpersonal, and physiological dimensions. For a description of recent research testing more specific variables (e.g., religion as a factor to live a healthy lifestyle),

 Go to Chapter 16, **Supplemental Materials: Religion and Health: Recent Research Areas,** on Davis*Plus.*

Toward Evidence-Based Practice

Grudzen, C., Stone, S., Mohanty, S., et al. (2011). "I want to be taking my own last breath": Patients' reflections on illness when presenting to the emergency department at the end of life. *Journal of Palliative Medicine, 14*(3), 293–296.

Interviews were conducted with 13 patients with advanced illness who presented to the emergency department for palliative care. While many were comforted by their faith in God, they did not view themselves as controlling their fate. Although they preferred to die at home surrounded by their family, they had not discussed this with their physician. The nurse's role of advocacy will ensure that patients' wishes are known and communicated appropriately.

Yanez, B., Edmondson, D., Stanton, A., et al. (2009). Facets of spirituality as predictors of adjustments to cancer: Relative contributions of having faith and finding meaning. *Journal of Consulting and Clinical Psychology, 77,* 730–741.

In two longitudinal studies of breast cancer patients (Study 1, N = 418 breast cancer patients; Study 2, N = 165 cancer survivors), meaning/peace and faith and their interactions were examined to determine the effect on psychological adjustment. Higher meaning/peace scores were associated with a decline in depressive symptoms, an increase in vitality, improved mental health, and lower cancer-related distress. The ability to find meaning and peace in life was found to be the most influential contributor to favorable adjustment during cancer survivorship.

Buck, H., Overcash, J., & McMillan, S. (2009). The geriatric cancer experience at the end of life: Testing an adapted model. *Oncology Nursing Forum, 36*(6), 664–673.

Researchers found that the majority of variability (67%) in the quality of life factor in 403 hospice homecare patients was due to severity of symptoms and spiritual experiences. Increases in quality of life were related to increases in the spiritual experience.

Astrow, A., Wexler, A., Texeira, K., et al. (2007). Is failure to meet spiritual needs associated with cancer patients' perceptions of quality of care and their satisfaction with care? *Journal of Clinical Oncology, 25*(36), 5753–5757.

Researchers administered religion and spiritual belief and needs questionnaires to 369 outpatients at a cancer treatment facility. Results revealed an inverse relationship between fulfillment of spiritual needs and quality and satisfaction with care. Patients whose spiritual needs were not meet had lower ratings on satisfaction with and quality of care.

---

1. For which of the following do these studies, taken as a whole, provide the stronger support for the premise:
   a. Spirituality has a positive effect on physical factors.
   b. Spirituality has a positive effect on psychosocial or emotional factors.

Explain your reasoning.

2. Suppose you are a nursing home administrator in an institution where the focus is almost entirely on physical care. You are thinking about a program to teach and encourage your staff to integrate spiritual interventions into their care. Evaluate the findings from each of the studies to see how useful it would be in supporting your idea. Explain your thinking.

 Go to Chapter 16, **Toward Evidence-Based Practice Suggested Responses,** on Davis*Plus.*

KnowledgeCheck 16-2

- What are some of the ways that religion might positively influence health?

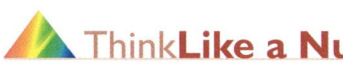

ThinkLike a Nurse 16-3

- How might religion negatively influence health?
- Has there been a pivotal moment in your life, a moment of crisis or despair that eventually provided an opportunity for spiritual growth?

Major Religions: What Should I Know?

The more you know about the differences and similarities among the world's major religions, the more you will be able to offer comprehensive and compassionate care to patients. Of course, learning about other religions requires you to be open and nonjudgmental. When you care for a patient from a known religious background, you will need to think about how the person's beliefs affect her ideas of health, healing, hospitalization, and the experience of dying. To help you make these connections, the following brief descriptions of several of the world's major religious traditions provide you with several different "worldviews." To learn about the influence of various religions on end-of-life care, see Chapter 17. For more detailed information about each religion,

 Go to Chapter 16, **Supplemental Materials: Major Religions: What Should I Know?** and **Reading More About Spirituality,** on DavisPlus.

Judaism

Judaism is one of the Western world's oldest religions and the foundation on which Christianity and Islam were built. The Jewish Law is set down in the collective writings of the Torah. Judaism is based on the worship of one God (monotheism), obeying the Ten Commandments, and practicing charity and tolerance toward others. The degree to which Jews celebrate rituals and holy days depends on whether the person identifies with the Orthodox, Liberal, Conservative, or Reconstructionist beliefs (Oxtoby & Segal, 2007; Pawlikowski, 1990).

Jews celebrate the Sabbath from sunset on Friday to sunset Saturday evening. For Orthodox Jews, work is prohibited on the Sabbath. This includes writing, traveling, and switching on lights and appliances. During Passover (in March or April), some Jewish patients may require special foods, dinnerware, and utensils. The Day of Atonement, or Yom Kippur (in September or October), is the holiest day of the Jewish calendar. It is a special day of fasting, but fasting is not required if it would be a danger to the patient. A Jewish patient will normally wish to keep that day to pray and rest. For Orthodox patients, you might offer alternatives to oral medication (e.g., injections or suppositories).

Conservative Jews observe strict dietary laws: Only kosher foods are accepted. **Kosher foods** have been prepared under strict guidelines for how animals are slaughtered and do not contain pork, certain types of seafood, or combinations of dairy and meat. Meals are also double-packaged if kosher foods are heated in nonkosher heating units (Noble, Rom, Newsome-Wicks, et al., 2009). If possible, consult a rabbi or dietitian who is knowledgeable about Jewish dietary laws for assistance in planning dietary and activity modifications.

Orthodox Jewish women prefer to have their bodies and limbs covered. They may also prefer to keep their hair covered with a scarf and often wear a wig. Orthodox men keep their head covered with a hat or skullcap (*kappel*). Some Orthodox Jewish sects forbid contraception unless the woman's health is at risk. Nearly all Jewish boys are circumcised, usually 8 days after birth. Orthodox Judaism usually forbids organ transplants, but opinions vary and decisions may rest with the rabbinic authority.

Both Reconstructionist and Reform Judaism incorporate current societal values. Reconstructionist Judaism was founded in the 1920s by Rabbi Mordecai Kaplan and is based on Western ideas of democracy, equality, and spirituality. Followers viewed Judaism, not as a religion with rituals mandated by God, but as a spiritual path with unity and connections developed among persons (Bronstein, 2012). Likewise, followers of Reform Judaism adhere to the traditional tenets, but practice inclusion, such as the acceptance of non-Jews, members of the Gay, Lesbian & Transgender community, and women as rabbis (Union for Reform Judaism, 2011).

Christianity

Christianity is the world's largest religion. Christians worship Jesus Christ and believe that his death atoned for their sins by granting them forgiveness from God, which allows for eternal life. Their sacred text, the Bible, includes the Judaic Old Testament and the New Testament relating to the life of Christ. The many denominations within Christianity include Roman Catholicism (with allegiance to the pope in Rome), Orthodoxy (with allegiance to the patriarch of Constantinople), Protestant denominations (e.g., Lutheran, Baptist, United Methodist), and others (e.g., Jehovah's Witnesses, Christian Scientists). Rituals and practices vary among the Christian denominations.

- Many practice baptism, which is a sign of moral cleansing and correlates to being born again. The baptism of an infant, also known as "christening," indicates that the child will be raised with Christian values and influences, so when infants or children are very ill, baptism should be offered.
- Christians usually have no special dietary requirements, although some choose to abstain from eating meat on Fridays and/or during Lent and some abstain from alcohol. Others fast (abstain from food) to become closer to God, to pray for blessings, or before receiving Holy Communion. Most Christians do not

object to blood transfusion or organ transplantation. Perspectives vary on family planning using artificial birth control methods; however, natural family planning methods (e.g., rhythm) are widely accepted.

Roman Catholicism

In Roman Catholicism, the **sacraments** are a means to obtain grace. A Roman Catholic who is seriously ill might wish to receive the sacrament of *anointing the sick*. This sacrament, once known as the last rites, can be repeated if the person recovers and then becomes ill at a later time. Only a priest can hear the *sacrament of reconciliation* (confession), during which God, through the agency of the priest, grants forgiveness for past sins. The *Eucharist* (communion bread), consecrated at the *mass* (a religious service), may be brought to hospitalized patients by a priest, deacon, or designated lay Eucharistic minister. Other denominations within Christianity (e.g., Episcopalians and Lutherans) observe certain sacraments as well, although the meaning and details of the rituals may vary.

Christian Science

The Christian Science faith, established in 1879, is a unique form of Christianity. Christian Scientists believe that illness is caused by faulty thinking, is evil, and is not a part of God's plan, for God is good (Waldman, Perlman, & Chaudhry, 2010). Therefore, followers practice a reliance on God and prayer for healing. Although they may not believe in immunizations and vaccinations, they will follow the laws of the state (Christian Science, 2013). Although adults will probably not accept a blood transfusion, parents usually consent to transfusions and other medical care for their child if doctors consider it essential or the law so requires. You will most likely encounter followers as patients only after accidents or because of family or legal pressures.

While Christian Scientists do not oppose Western medicine, it is usually not their first choice to promote health and prevent illness. They advocate proper nutrition, adequate sleep/rest, and avoidance of alcohol and tobacco. Strict Christian Scientists may not drink tea or coffee.

Jehovah's Witnesses

Many Jehovah's Witnesses adhere to the commands of God as written in both the Old and New Testaments of the Bible. A practice that can create medical concerns is their refusal to accept blood transfusions or blood products, which they view as morally wrong. Patients who adhere to this faith would accept death rather than accept blood (Dyer, 2012; Lindstrom & Johnstone, 2010). The Jehovah's Witnesses faith also does not permit autologous blood transfusions or donation or receipt of an organ through which blood flows. If blood is not involved (e.g., corneal transplants) they may accept transplantation. Consistent with this practice, meat is not acceptable if an animal has been strangled or shot and not bled properly. Some Jehovah's Witnesses do not eat raw or any meat at all. Jehovah's Witnesses abstain from tobacco and other recreational drugs. They may drink alcohol but do not condone drunkenness. Jehovah's Witnesses do not celebrate birthdays or holidays, except for the anniversary of the death of Christ. This date usually corresponds with the Christian Easter or Jewish Passover.

Mormonism

The Church of Jesus Christ of Latter-Day Saints (LDS) is commonly called the Mormon Church. Mormons believe in Jesus and one God and adhere to the sacred writing the Book of Mormon (which Joseph Smith translated from ancient records written on gold plates in 1830). Mormons follow a strict health code, known as the Word of Wisdom, which advises healthful living and prohibits the use of tea, coffee, alcohol, and tobacco. Many believe in life before and after death; thus, death represents the passage into another life phrase (Waldman, Perlman, & Chaudhry, 2012).

Some Mormons (both men and women) wear a sacred undergarment (temple garments) that is "an outward expression of an inward commitment to follow the Savior" (The Church of Jesus Christ of Latter-Day Saints, 2013). The garments are only removed for purposes such as hygiene, elimination, or being intimate in marriage. Nurses may also remove it before surgery, but it must at all times be considered intensely private and be treated with respect (Keddington, 2007).

Seventh Day Adventism

The Seventh Day Adventist Church is distinguished mostly by observance of Saturday, the original seventh day of the Judeo-Christian week, as the Sabbath, a day of rest and worship. To keep the Sabbath holy, Adventists do no secular work or unnecessary business on Saturday. Adventists usually practice communion, which begins with a foot-washing ceremony, four times a year. Some members believed that a healthy mind and body are an essential element of faith and worship and that both spiritual health and physical health are enhanced by good nutrition (Nath, 2010). The church also emphasizes culturally conservative principles and many Adventists refrain from body piercing, tattoos, and wearing jewelry. The following are other principles and practices:

- The church recommends a vegetarian diet and adherence to the kosher laws in the Old Testament of the Bible, which includes avoidance of pork, shellfish, and other "unclean" foods. Some Adventists, however, do eat meat.
- Most avoid alcohol, tobacco, illegal drugs, and beverages containing caffeine.
- Although the church is generally anti-abortion, in cases of serious dilemmas (e.g., threat to the woman's life or pregnancy resulting from rape or incest), women are counseled to make their own decisions. Birth control is permitted for married couples.
- The Adventist church is officially against active euthanasia but permits a passive form through withdrawal of medical support to allow the patient to die. Death is akin to sleep and the person is viewed as being in an unconscious state (Taylor & Carr, 2009).

Islam

Islam was the third monotheistic religion to emerge, following Judaism and Christianity and is now the second largest (Abdel-Khalek, 2011). The word *Islam* means submission. In particular, a Muslim is one who submits to Allah (God). Muhammad is the founder of Islam and a respected deity among Muslims. The sacred book of authority in Islam, the Koran (Holy Qu'ran), is the result of messages from the angel Gabriel sent from God to the prophet Muhammad. It contains the one common message of all faiths: There is a Supreme Being whose sovereignty is acknowledged in worship and whose teaching and commandments must be obeyed.

Muslims are forbidden to eat pork. They may eat other meat, but it has to be *halal* meat, that is, killed in a special manner stated in Islamic law. Fish and eggs are allowed, but not if they are cooked near pork or non-halal (*haram*) meat. During the month of Ramadan, a Muslim fasts between sunrise and sunset; however, those who are sick are not expected to fast. Essential drugs and medicines are allowed at all hours during Ramadan.

Muslims always wash their hands before eating and it is customary to eat with the right hand (unless prevented by injury). Patients prefer to wash in free-flowing water, so tub baths are considered unhygienic. If a shower is not available, provide a pitcher to use in the bath.

Women prefer to be treated by female staff. Some women may refuse vaginal examination by a male nurse or physician because they are forbidden to expose their bodies to or be touched by any man other than their husband. Women may wear a locket containing religious writing around the neck in a small leather bag. These are kept for protection and strength, so you should never remove them. After the birth of a baby, prayers are whispered in the baby's ear so the first thing heard are words of prayer.

There is no specific religious rule prohibiting blood transfusion or organ transplantation; however, strict Muslims will not usually agree to organ transplants. Orthodox Muslims do not approve of contraception; however, individuals vary widely in their practices. Abortion is frowned on but may be tolerated for medical reasons.

Hinduism

Hinduism, which many religious scholars believe is the oldest major religion still practiced today, does not embrace a single body of beliefs and practices. Nor does it maintain the existence of a single deity, believing that no one manifestation of God can possibly capture the limitless nature of God. Thus, Hindus may worship several or even hundreds of gods and goddesses. Even elements in the natural world, such as rivers, fire, and so forth, are considered aspects of God. Sacred Hindu texts include the *Vedas*, the *Bhagavad Gita* (Song of the Blessed One), and the *Ramayana*, the story of the life of the god Rama. Despite commonly held beliefs and texts, Hindu religious practices vary a great deal, depending on areas of origin. Hindus believe in the core concepts of Karma, Dharma, and Reincarnation (Wilkins & Mailoo, 2010). Karma teaches that every action has or causes an effect. A person who does not fulfill his destiny or given purpose in life (Dharma) will have bad karma. After death, persons begin a new life in a different body or spiritual form (Reincarnation).

Hindus practice **ayurvedic medicine**, which encompasses all aspects of life, including diet, sleep, elimination, and hygiene. Some believe in the medicinal properties of "hot" and "cold" foods—"hot" and "cold" having nothing to do with either temperature or spicy qualities. Although some Hindus will eat eggs and even chicken, most are lacto-vegetarians, consuming milk but no eggs. Many will not eat beef and avoid bovine-derived medication because of the reincarnation of certain Gods (Wilkins & Mailoo, 2010). Fasting, which may mean eating only "pure" foods such as fruit or yogurt, is common during major festivals but is not expected of the sick. Tobacco and alcohol may or may not be accepted.

Hindus prefer to wash in free-flowing water (e.g., a shower instead of a tub bath). If a shower is not available, provide a jug of water for the person to use in the bath. Women are modest and usually prefer to be treated by female medical staff. Jewelry often has a religious or cultural significance. Some Hindus wear "sacred thread" or religious jewelry around the body or wrist. Do not remove or cut these without permission from the patient or next of kin. Some Hindus may consider touching a person's feet or touching them on the head a sign of disrespect. You should always do a careful religious assessment (Wilkins & Mailoo, 2010). There is no religious objection to contraception, blood transfusion, or organ donation, as a rule.

Buddhism

The Buddha, or the "Awakened One," is revered not as a god, but as an example of a way of life (Fig. 16-2). Siddhartha Gautama was born into a royal family in 624 BCE in a part of northern India that is now in Nepal, gained enlightenment at the age of 35, and then began to teach others how to attain liberation from suffering for themselves and others.

One of the Buddha's core teachings is that suffering can be ended by following the eightfold path: right understanding, right intention, right speech, right action, right livelihood, right effort, right mindfulness, and right contemplation (Bodhi, 2007; Knierim, n.d.). **Nirvana**, similar to the Christian concept of heaven, can be attained only through an absence of desire, the achievement of perfection, and the lack of a unique identity. Buddhism is about finding spirituality within one's self. Like Hindus, Buddhists believe in karma and reincarnation.

Food is an essential component of maintaining spiritual focus, meditation, and interactions with others (Nath, 2010). Many Buddhists follow a vegetarian diet; in some cases, the diet may include both milk and eggs. Fasting customs vary by tradition. Buddhists accept

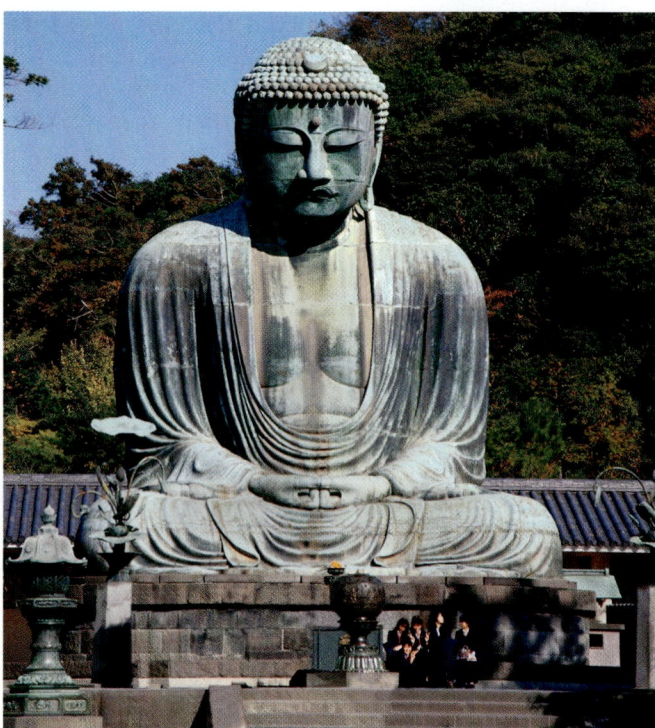

FIGURE 16-2 The Buddha is revered as an example of a way of life.

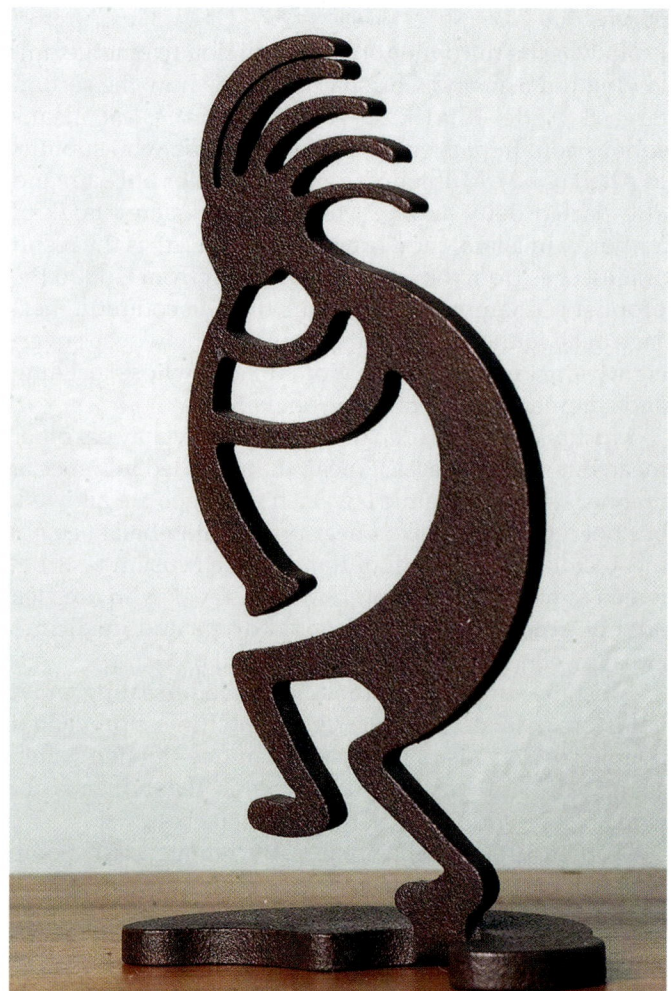

FIGURE 16-3 Kokopelli, the humpbacked flute player, has been a sacred figure to Native Americans of the Southwest for thousands of years. He is a legendary symbol of fertility who brought well-being to the people.

contraception but typically condemn abortion and active euthanasia. They will usually accept blood transfusion and organ transplantation.

Native American Religions

There are more than 400 federally recognized Native American nations or tribes in the United States. Although each has its own traditions and cultural heritage, some general beliefs underlie the more specific tribal ideas. The Earth is considered to be a living organism, the body of a higher individual, and humankind has an intimate relation with this organism through nature. Thus, rather than having a designated sacred place to worship, Native Americans place value in the land, mountains, rivers, and meadows (Fowler, 2009). When the Earth is harmed, humankind is harmed, and vice versa. The land belongs to life, life belongs to the land, and the land belongs to itself (Boyd, 1974).

Health is a state of harmony with nature. Whenever disharmony exists, disease or illness can occur. The traditional healer is the medicine man or woman who is wise in the interrelationships of land, humankind, and the universe. Many Native Americans believe that the treatments they receive from medicine men and women and traditional healers are far better than those rendered by the dominant healthcare establishment, which often treats Native Americans with scorn or disrespect (Fig. 16-3). You should know that for some tribes, note taking by the professional is forbidden; when you take a history or perform an exam, you must rely on your memory to record findings later. Native Americans tend to converse in a low

tone of voice and may maintain long periods of silence. Be sure the setting is quiet enough to allow you to hear the patient because it is impolite to indicate that you did not hear the communications.

Rastafarianism

Rastafarianism is a personal religion that emphasizes dignity and a deep love of God. The authoritative writings include the Old and New Testaments of the Bible, but as a rule Rastafarians do not consider themselves to be Christian. There are no churches, services, or official clergy.

Rastafarians do not eat pork and shellfish, some are completely vegetarian, and some do not drink milk or coffee. Many prefer alternative therapies (e.g., herbalism, marijuana, or acupuncture), do not believe in contraception, and avoid any treatment that will contaminate the body. They will accept blood transfusion, but may require reassurance about its safety. The women dress modestly; however, wearing secondhand clothing is taboo, so the patient may be unwilling to wear hospital gowns that have been worn by others. You may need to provide a disposable gown or allow the person to wear her own personal nightclothes.

Atheism

Atheists do not believe in the presence of God or supernatural deities. Rather than receiving directives on living from external sources, atheists have their own personal moral code that is derived from their value systems, beliefs, and life experiences. They can be spiritual and even religious, but focus on the humanistic, secular perspectives. A nurse recalls a patient's comment that he regretted putting "Atheist" on his admission paperwork, because he would have welcomed the presence of a chaplain to discuss where he was spiritually (Mais, 2010).

Key Point: *This comment does not imply that all atheists would react in the same way as this one. It does, however, reinforce the importance of a thorough assessment of patient needs instead of relying on categories and labels.*

KnowledgeCheck 16-3

- Which major religion believes in the anointing of the sick or dying?
- Which denomination or religion does not believe in blood transfusions?
- In terms of Native American beliefs and healthcare, who is the traditional healer or the person to be consulted in the event of "illness"?
- True or false: Most Hindus are vegetarian.

ThinkLike a Nurse 16-4

What are some ways that world religions might influence nursing care?

SelfKnowledge
what every nurse should
know

As you have seen, your patients' spiritual and religious backgrounds may be diverse and may involve ways of thinking and doing that seem strange to you or that you do not fully understand. Before trying to understand your patients' religious or spiritual experience, you must give considerable thought to your own religious or spiritual journey. Attaining self-knowledge is an important aspect of becoming a full-spectrum nurse. This section will help you in your reflections.

What Are Your Personal Biases?

We each carry our own perspectives with us at all times. We tend to view the world through lenses we acquired in childhood, adolescence, and early adulthood. In addition, our religious education is sometimes taught with a certain flavor of "upmanship"; that is, we are taught that our religious beliefs and practices are superior to all others. When you view your own experience as the norm or as the preferred way of organizing the world, you tend to limit the range of care you provide to the patient who believes differently. Spiritual care demands nonjudgmental attitudes and an open manner of thinking that invites rather than excludes.

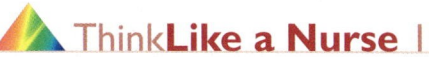 ThinkLike a Nurse 16-5

Consider the following examples. For each person, what moral/spiritual judgments should the nurse avoid?

- A nurse is caring for a gay man who is hospitalized with end-stage AIDS.
- A woman has come to the clinic to be treated for gonorrhea (a sexually transmitted disease). She says she has had at least six sexual partners this year.
- A man comes to the emergency department (ED) at least once a month to ask for morphine to treat his back pain. He is known to abuse drugs and to visit other EDs for the same purpose.

If you are aware of your biases, it will be easier to avoid abuses of spiritual care, such as the following:

- **Attempting to convert others to your beliefs.** For example, if a patient is near death, he and his family might be offended if their nurse inquires whether they are "saved" Christians. By remaining focused on the patient's need to talk about meaning, salvation, or other end-of-life issues, you provide full-spectrum spiritual care. In Meet Your Patient you notice that Mr. Johnson's sister seems very close to imposing her religion on him. This may alienate him further if he perceives that he is being "pushed."
- **Trying to be all things to all people,** regardless of their background or the extent of spiritual care needed. Clearly, there are times when you should refer to others with more knowledge and experience in religion and spirituality, with the patient's permission, of course. In addition, whenever a patient requests the services of a rabbi, priest, or other spiritual adviser, you should relay that request to the agency's chaplain so that all disciplines remain informed.

In summary, to work effectively with a diverse population, you must first obtain a greater degree of self-knowledge by (1) being open to the many possibilities for diverse thinking, (2) welcoming challenging experiences that allow for personal growth, and (3) taking time to think about how your actions and biases might affect the care of others. The more you know about yourself, the more effectively you care for others.

What Are Some Barriers to Spiritual Care?

Although most nurses would acknowledge that patients have a spiritual dimension, few actually identify spiritual problems or provide spiritual interventions. This may be a result of economic constraints, poor staffing, and high-tech care, which force nurses to focus only on physical needs, or the inconsistencies in the meaning of spirituality (Cavendish, Konecny, Mitzeliotis, et al., 2003; Nardi & Rooda, 2011; Swinton & Pattison, 2010). You may judge these nurses less harshly after you understand more about the barriers to spiritual interventions by nurses.

Lack of General Awareness of Spirituality

A greater awareness of spirituality in general will help you tune into the spiritual needs of patients and improve your comfort in communicating about spiritual matters. Research consistently reveals the need for more education on spiritual care. McSherry and Jamieson (2011) identified that many nurses felt inadequately trained and educated in addressing the spiritual needs of patients. One study showed that nurses could not define spirituality and related it to end-of-life care needs (Smyth & Allen, 2011). Another showed that patients at risk for spiritual distress are not identified (Blanchard, Dunlap, & Fitchett, 2012) or are inaccurately assessed (Highfield, 1992).

Lack of Awareness of Your Own Spiritual Belief System

To feel comfortable making spiritual interventions, you will need more than just theoretical knowledge. You will need introspection and an awareness of your own spiritual journey to integrate the spiritual domain into patient care. Nurses who are aware of their own spirituality are better able to incorporate spiritual care in their practice (Chan, 2010). Several steps can be taken to enhance your spiritual growth (Baldacchino, 2011; Lane, 1987):

1. Understand the differences between religion, spirituality, and spiritual care.
2. Develop an awareness of your own spirituality and how it is applied (or not) in meeting the patient's spiritual needs.
3. Open yourself by being totally present with the patient, including being an active listener.
4. Allow the patient to share his feelings and emotions without reserve and reflect in your attitude and demeanor that you care and have the time to listen.

Activities to heighten your awareness of your own spirituality, gain a broader view of spirituality, and increase sensitivity to others' spiritual needs include the following (Beckman, Boxley-Harges, Bruick-Sorge, et al., 2007):

- Increase your knowledge about spirituality.
- Develop your critical and reflective thinking abilities.
- Explore your own spirituality (e.g., reflection, discussing with others). One technique is to write your own epitaph: one or two lines summing up how you would like to be remembered.
- Reflect on your thoughts and feelings about end-of-life issues. Imagine you have only a few weeks to live; think how you would feel.

- Reflect on your personal experience with grief and loss. For example, what is the first death you can remember? What were your feelings at the time? How do you usually cope with loss? What actions by others comforted you?

You must find ways to take care of and nurture your own spiritual needs; otherwise, providing this aspect of care can be emotionally draining.

Differences in Spirituality Between Nurse and Patient

Patients and nurses can be at different levels in terms of spirituality. When a patient's spiritual beliefs are very different from your own, you must be careful not to impose your beliefs on the patient or discount the importance of the patient's beliefs and rituals. When the patient's views or beliefs are similar to yours, take care not to make false assumptions about his spiritual needs. Although you share some commonalities, this does not mean you will have the same perspectives or needs in all areas of spirituality or religion.

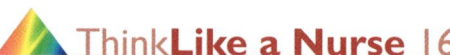 Think**Like a Nurse** 16-6

- How does your religion or spirituality differ from Mr. Johnson's (Meet Your Patient)?
- How is it similar?
- Can you think of problems these differences and similarities could cause you in caring for him?

Fear That Your Knowledge Base Is Insufficient

Nurses sometimes avoid giving spiritual care because they believe they lack knowledge of spirituality or of the patient's religion. This is a realistic concern. In several studies, nurses were found to be unsure of what constituted spiritual problems and spiritual interventions (Blanchard, Dunlap, & Fitchett, 2012; Smyth & Allen, 2011). In some cases they did not identify the spiritual dimension of care, or they took religious aspects into account but did not place them into a broader spiritual perspective. Your ability to incorporate spiritual care into practice will increase with experience. Ronaldson and colleagues (2012) found that the spiritual care practices of RNs working in palliative care were more advanced than those of their RN counterparts working in acute care. While both groups identified insufficient time as a barrier to spiritual care, the acute care group also identified lack of patient privacy. The palliative care RNs were older and more experienced. The good news is that spiritual care has never been more welcomed by patients. You now know the importance of and can provide care to meet your patient's spiritual needs.

Older adults, for example, have identified their spiritual needs in healthcare settings as understanding their spiritual practices; relationship with God; hope, meaning, and purpose of life; interpersonal connection; and therapeutic professional staff interactions (Hodge, Horvath, Larkin, et al., 2012).

Fear of Where Spiritual Discussions May Lead

Many nurses fear that inquiring into the spiritual domain might cause harm to the patient. For example, what if a patient asks, "Do you think active euthanasia is morally wrong? Would it jeopardize my salvation?" Here are some fears that may arise:

- You may not feel prepared to answer the questions.
- You might have an answer based on your personal religious beliefs but fear the patient may think you are imposing your beliefs on him.
- You might wonder whether communicating your own beliefs (e.g., if you favor active euthanasia) might jeopardize the patient's spiritual life if your ideas turn out to be "wrong."

The following are some ideas that may help counter your fears. Most important, the patient addressing this concern with you indicates his recognition that you are open to spiritual matters and offers an opportunity to address his spiritual domain of care. Second, the patient is concerned with issues related to euthanasia. This could lead to discussions about the patient's fears of pain, dependence, being a burden on family members, and dying alone. Third, this is an area for which you should seek collaboration with a chaplain, who is more prepared to deal with specific religious issues. You should realize that being open to the spiritual realm and assessing the patient's need for spiritual intervention does not mean that you must be a chaplain or have the extraordinary ability to deal with all spiritual or religious questions or requests. The Practical Knowledge section will provide a more detailed understanding of your role in spiritual care.

KnowledgeCheck 16-4

- What qualities can you demonstrate that may help you improve the quality of spiritual care you provide?
- What common barriers to spiritual interventions do nurses encounter?
- True or false: No matter how nonjudgmental and open we may think of ourselves, we all carry our own unique biases and prejudices that have the potential to affect patient care.

 ThinkLike a Nurse 16-7

- What are some possible errors made by nurses related to spiritual care?
- What are some ways that you can develop a greater awareness of the "spirit within the self"?
- Discuss ways that nurses and patients can nurture their own spiritual needs.

PracticalKnowledge
knowing how

Most hospital admission forms include a place to record the patient's religious preferences, and most nursing assessment forms even include questions such as, "What religious rituals do you practice?" Unfortunately, some nurses believe that by completing such forms, they have addressed the patient's spiritual needs. They may be relieved because they don't feel competent to deal any further with spirituality or because they are afraid to be perceived as imposing their own religion on the patient. However, armed with your basic theoretical knowledge of spirituality and your growing spiritual self-knowledge, you should be able to provide a level of support that extends beyond paperwork to compassion and caring.

To see a care plan and care map for a client with Spiritual Distress,

 Go to Chapter 16, **Chapter Resources, Nursing Care Plan: Spiritual Distress, and Care Map: Spiritual Distress,** on Davis*Plus*.

 ## ASSESSMENT

People of the same religion often vary greatly in the degree to which they follow religious practices. It is not enough to "fill in the religion blank" on an assessment form. You must assess each person individually to determine religious needs and practices, keeping in mind that this may be a sensitive area for some persons.

It may be difficult to obtain meaningful information on the initial admission assessment due to time constraints in completing the paperwork, collaboration with the healthcare team, and the stresses involved in getting the patient introduced to the healthcare setting. For this reason, you must at that time obtain the essential data of the patient's church preference, name of clergy, whom to call in case of emergency, dietary requirements/restrictions, and any religious implications for medical care (e.g. refusal of blood transfusions). As you have further interactions with the patient and family, trust will develop, and you will be able to obtain more sensitive, complex, and meaningful spiritual/religious information.

Sources of Spiritual Data

You can acquire information about a patient's spirituality from a variety of sources other than interviews:

- **Patient's environment.** Observe the patient's environment for hints about her spirituality (e.g., pictures of family and/or pets, the presence of sacred texts or reading materials, articles used in worship [a crucifix, rosary beads, religious medals, statues], or copies of church bulletins/sermon tapes).
- **Patient's questions.** The patient may ask questions that are indicative of spiritual comfort, longing, or distress. For example, the patient may ask if you attend church and if so, whether it provides you with a sense of comfort and meaning.
- **Patient's behaviors, moods, and feelings.** Emotional behaviors give a clear and certain indication that the patient is struggling with issues that have spiritual overtones. These warrant further assessment and nursing intervention. For example, a patient may ask you if you have ever really felt guilty about something you did as a child.

- **Nonverbal communication.** Body language may indicate hopeful or distressing times. For example, you may observe a patient praying; or when asking about spirituality, you may see the patient rolling his eyes, shaking his head, and demonstrating muscle tension.

Spiritual Assessment Tools

Some healthcare agencies have focused spiritual assessment tools tailored to their particular setting. Several others have been developed.

HOPE　An easy-to-use screening method is use of the HOPE questions. Although not validated by research, they do allow for an open-ended exploration of spiritual resources and concerns (Gowri & Hight, 2001). HOPE is a mnemonic, as follows:

H—sources of Hope
O—Organized religion
P—Personal spirituality/Practices
E—Effects on medical care and end-of-life issues

JAREL　The JAREL spiritual well-being scale was developed and is commonly used by nurses (Hungelmann, Kenkel-Rossi, Klassen, et al., 1996). Cutting across religious and atheistic belief systems, it assesses three key dimensions: (1) faith/belief, (2) life/self-responsibility, and (3) life-satisfaction/self-actualization.

SPIRIT　The comprehensive spiritual assessment tool developed by Highfield (2000) involves an interview that is concerned with six key areas designated by the acronym SPIRIT:

SP—**Sp**iritual/religious belief system
I—**I**ntegration within a spiritual community
R—**R**itualized practices and restrictions
I—**I**mplications for medical care
T—**T**erminal events planning.

To see a copy of a spiritual assessment based on this model, and for questions to use for the HOPE approach,

 Go to Chapter 16, **Assessment Guidelines and Tools,** in Volume 2.

You can use the SPIRIT model with the JAREL tool and the combined assessment tool and plan of care in the ESG. To find these tools,

 Go to Chapter 16, **Tables, Boxes, Figures: ESG Figures 16-1 and 16-2,** on DavisPlus.

 Go to Chapter 16, **Assessment Guidelines and Tools,** in Volume 2.

KnowledgeCheck 16-5

What are the six areas for spiritual assessment summarized in Highfield's (2000) acronym SPIRIT?

 Think**Like a Nurse** 16-8

Complete the SPIRIT assessment on yourself. Discuss it with your classmates.

ANALYSIS/NURSING DIAGNOSIS

When analyzing spiritual assessment data, you must consider the person's developmental stage. People progress through stages of spiritual development in much the same way as they develop physically and cognitively. Spiritual behaviors that seem problematic in one stage may not be so in an earlier stage. To review developmental stages, refer to Chapters 9 and 10.

Spirituality Diagnoses

Box 16-1 contains NANDA-I diagnostic labels that specifically deal with religion and spirituality. The following are examples of full diagnostic statements for spiritual problems:

- *Spiritual Distress* related to overwhelming anxiety associated with the need to have a surgical procedure that is not accepted by her religion
- *Risk for Spiritual Distress* related to unremitting pain and loss of hope for relief, as manifested by patient's question about the usefulness of prayer ("God has forgotten about me.")

A Non-NANDA–I Diagnosis　Millspaugh (2005) has suggested *Spiritual Pain* as a diagnosis. When a person experiences a combination of awareness of death, loss of relationships, loss of self, loss of purpose, and loss of control, Spiritual Pain may occur. However, this combination of negative experiences can be balanced by having a life-affirming and transcending purpose and an internal sense of control (Fig. 16-4). The presence and quality of Spiritual Pain is determined by the degree to which the person is experiencing each component, and by the relationship of the components to each other.

 Think**Like a Nurse** 16-9

Which of these nursing diagnoses would you use for Mr. Johnson (Meet Your Patient): Spiritual Distress, Risk for Spiritual Distress or Readiness for Enhanced Spiritual Well-Being? Why?

Spirituality as Etiology

In the spiritual realm, it is difficult sometimes to determine what is the problem and what is the etiology. Does the patient experience Spiritual Distress because of pain and hopelessness? Or did the patient first lose faith in God, which led to hopelessness and anxiety? Either way, spiritual support is needed.

Several of the NANDA-I diagnoses relate to spirituality as the problem, etiology, or symptom. Examples include Anxiety, Chronic Sorrow, Death Anxiety, Decisional Conflict, Hopelessness, Interrupted Family Processes, Noncompliance, Powerlessness, and Social Isolation. Non–NANDA-I problems include anger or resentment; feelings of guilt, shame, inadequacy, abandonment, or distrust; depression or sadness; and the inability to find meaning in life. The following are examples of diagnostic statements with spiritual etiologies:

Anxiety related to inability to reconcile decision to use birth control with religious proscriptions

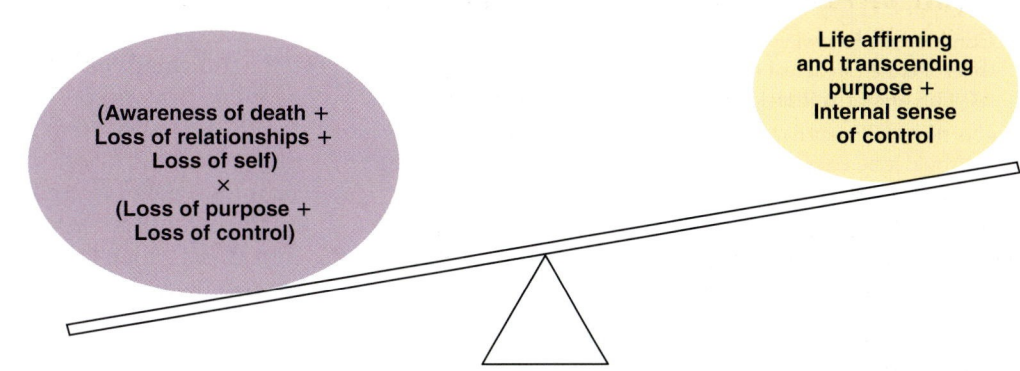

FIGURE 16-4 Components of spiritual pain. (Based on: Millspaugh, C. D. (2005). Assessment and response to spiritual pain: Part II. *Journal of Palliative Medicine*, 8(6), 1110–1117.)

Decisional Conflict related to confusion about the religious implications of the decision to forego heroic treatment measures

Hopelessness related to lack of belief in a power outside self, combined with overwhelming lack of energy

Noncompliance (with treatment regimen) related to the belief that the illness is "God's will" and that healing will occur (without treatment) for the same reason

---

BOX 16-1 ■ NANDA-International Spirituality Diagnoses

Moral Distress	Experienced when the person makes an ethical or moral decision, but then is unable to carry out the chosen action. Defining characteristics include anguish, powerlessness, guilt, frustration, anxiety, self-doubt, and fear over the inability to act on the moral choice.
Impaired Religiosity	Difficulty in exercising or impaired ability to exercise reliance on beliefs or to participate in rituals of a faith tradition (e.g., go to church, take communion).
Readiness for Enhanced Religiosity	The ability to increase reliance on religious beliefs and/or participate in rituals of a particular faith tradition. The patient is not experiencing a problem, but wishes to make a satisfactory situation even better.
Readiness for Enhanced Spiritual Well-Being	Describes healthy spirituality. "A pattern of experiencing and integrating meaning and purpose in life through connectedness with self, others, art, music, literature, nature, and/or a power greater than oneself that is sufficient for well-being and can be strengthened" (NANDA-I, 2012, p. 394). It is the opposite of Spiritual Distress, so you will see positive expressions of faith, hope, love, courage, acceptance, and peace; healthy connections with others and with art, music, literature, and nature; and prayer and other expressions of a connection with a power higher than oneself.
Risk for Impaired Religiosity	Occurs when risk factors are present, but symptoms are not. Risk factors may be categorized as developmental, environmental, physical, psychological, sociocultural, or spiritual. Specific examples include life transitions, lack of transportation, pain, depression, social isolation, and suffering.
Risk for Spiritual Distress	Related to unremitting pain and loss of hope for relief, as manifested by patient's question about the usefulness of prayer ("God has forgotten about me.")
Spiritual Distress	"Impaired ability to experience and integrate meaning and purpose in life through connectedness with self, others, art, music, literature, nature, and/or a power greater than oneself" (NANDA International, 2012, p. 410). Defining characteristics (signs and symptoms) of this diagnosis include the following.

- *Connections to self:* Expressing a lack of hope, love, courage, acceptance, or peace; a lack of meaning and purpose in life; inability to forgive self; feelings of anger or guilt

- *Connections with others:* Refusing to see clergy; refusing to interact with family or friends; reporting lack of support system; expressions of alienation

- *Connections with art, music, literature, nature:* No interest in nature; decrease in previous interest in music, writing, art; no interest in spiritual reading

- *Connections with power greater than self:* Inability to pray, inability or refusal to participate in religious activities, feelings of abandonment by God or other deity, expressions of anger toward God or other deity, requests to see a religious leader, sudden changes in spiritual practices (increased or decreased)

Source: Adapted from NANDA International. (2012). *Nursing diagnoses: Definitions and classification 2012–2014.* Philadelphia: Wiley-Blackwell.

KnowledgeCheck 16-6

Consider the following statement: A nursing diagnosis that reflects either an actual or a potential problem may reflect religious and/or spiritual dimensions of the human condition.

- Is this statement true?
- Would it be true for a *physical* diagnosis (e.g., Disturbed Sleep Pattern)? Explain your thinking.

PLANNING OUTCOMES/EVALUATION

The outcomes you establish in the planning stage of the nursing process serve as the criteria for your evaluation of the patient's progress and the success of the nursing interventions.

NOC standardized outcomes associated with spirituality diagnoses include, but are not limited to, the following: Anxiety Level, Comfortable Death, Comfort Status: Psychospiritual, Dignified Life Closure, Hope, Loneliness Severity, Personal Resiliency, Personal Well-Being, Quality of Life, Spiritual Health, and Will to Live (Moorhead, Johnson, Maas, et al., 2013).

Individualized goals/outcome statements you might write for spiritual diagnoses include the following:

- **For Risk for Spiritual Distress**—Exhibits no signs or symptoms of spiritual distress (e.g., finds meaning in life, expresses hope and faith, follows usual religious practices).
- **For Spiritual Distress**—Returns to previous state of spiritual well-being and comfort (e.g., expresses a sense of peace, asks to see religious adviser).
- **For Readiness for Enhanced Spiritual Well-Being**—Experiences a higher level of connectedness with self, others, higher power, and/or nature.

PLANNING INTERVENTIONS/IMPLEMENTATION

Spiritual interventions are those used to treat and prevent spiritual problems related to the patient's illness. You will direct some nursing activities to resolving the problem, others at removing the etiology, and still others at relieving symptoms. You will, of course, base your nursing activities on the patient's symptoms and the problem etiologies. However, there are some nursing interventions that address spiritual problems in general.

Standardized (NIC) Spirituality Interventions

To see Nursing Interventions Classification (NIC) interventions and selected activities for the spirituality and religiosity diagnoses discussed in the preceding text.

 Go to Standardized Nursing Language, **Using Selected NIC Interventions and Activities to Support Spirituality,** in Volume 2.

A few NIC standardized interventions to promote spirituality are discussed in this section. The evidence base for these is specific to older adults (Gaskamp, Sutter, & Meraviglia, 2006); however, they would seem to be indicated for other age groups, as well.

When you are performing interventions of a spiritual nature, remember that you absolutely must follow the patient's lead and be caring and respectful without inserting your own beliefs into the conversation. Choose your language carefully—words similar to *saved*, *repentance*, and *born again*, which may be a part of everyday conversation for people who follow religion, may cause some patients to feel pressured or uncomfortable. Try to mirror, and not go beyond, the patient's religious terminology. It requires knowledge, skill, and practice to provide religious support without imposing your own beliefs. The safest course of action, of course, is to offer to contact a chaplain for the patient. However, patients cannot always—or may not always want to—wait for a chaplain.

Active Listening (NIC)

The Active Listening intervention allows the nurse to establish a trusting relationship and to hear, understand, and interpret what the client is saying. Listening actively involves four NIC interventions, and one non-standardized activity.

Presence (NIC) Presence means to be with patient and family in meaningful ways. This requires not only your actual presence at the bedside, but also being open to issues and concerns of the patient and allowing the patient to lead discussions rather than setting the agenda or controlling the conversation. It involves sincere communication and being fully available to the client, and might include listening to the patient's "stories" about his illness.

Touch (NIC) Caring touch, such as hand holding or touching an arm or shoulder, facilitates communication. It conveys concern, comfort, and acceptance, especially during stressful experiences. At least one study has shown touch to improve life satisfaction and faith. Some people prefer not to be touched, so carefully observe the patient's responses.

Exploring Meaning (non-NIC) Meaning refers to a clear understanding of the illness or loss (e.g., loss of independence). It also refers to the concepts of finding meaning and purpose in life, or a sense of personal worthiness. You can facilitate the patient's search for meaning by asking probing questions, providing explanations, and reframing maladaptive interpretations of life events.

Reminiscence Therapy (NIC) Reminiscence is the recalling and sharing with another person's past life events. It promotes meaning-making through rethinking and clarifying previous experiences. As the patient reminisces, he may make spiritual links by expressing personal beliefs that helped him live through difficult life events. This intervention is more effective within a long-term relationship.

Spiritual Support (NIC)

NIC defines Spiritual Support as "assisting the patient to feel balance and connection with a greater power" (Bulechek, Butcher, Dochterman, et al., 2012, p. 353). Effective Spiritual Support is based on a focused spiritual assessment, including the person's belief system. It may include assisting with forgiveness, encouraging hope, praying, and reading scriptures or other texts the patient requests.

Forgiveness Facilitation (NIC) **Forgiveness** is the act of pardoning or being pardoned for an offense, debt, or obligation. Letting go of the resentment felt for another promotes constructive changes in a person's life, as well as a sense of renewal and reconciliation with God, church, and one's inner being. To provide this intervention, you must first assess the patient's needs for reconciliation with self, others, and God. If, like Mr. Johnson (Meet Your Patient), the patient has lost contact with family members because of disagreements, you could collaborate with the social worker and chaplain about ways to facilitate a meeting.

Forgiveness is one aspect of love. People have a spiritual need to forgive others and to be forgiven. When a person cannot forgive others, it separates him from them and interferes with giving and receiving love. When a person cannot forgive himself, he may feel the pain of shame, guilt, and anger. Or the person may be hurting because he wants forgiveness from someone he has wronged or from God. Many people interpret their illness as punishment for sins.

Some find it difficult to seek forgiveness and to believe that they have been forgiven, but this is important to achieving spiritual peace. You can help by listening when the person expresses self-doubt or guilt, providing guidance, praying with the patient if he requests it, inquiring if he is ready to forgive someone else, or offering to contact his chosen spiritual leader if intensive spiritual support is needed.

Hope Inspiration (NIC) **Hope** is a subjective state of confidence in the possibility of a better future. It includes a positive orientation, faith, and will to live. **Hopelessness** is a state in which the person perceives limited or no alternatives or personal choices. To intervene effectively, it is important to know the source of the person's hope and the factors underlying the feelings of hopelessness. As a nurse, you can encourage spiritual growth, which is thought to facilitate hope, and you can refer your patient to a support group to help in stress reduction, coping, and hope.

Prayer (Non-NIC) Prayer is an integral component of almost every religion. Research shows that the percentage of adults who use prayer for health concerns increased from 42% to 49% over a 5-year period (Wachholtz & Sambamoorthi, 2011). A recent study found that patients who received intercessory prayer had a significant improvement in spiritual and emotional well-being (Olver & Dutney, 2012). Prayer has been found "very helpful" by 69% of adults in the United States (McCaffrey, Eisenberg, Legedza, et al., 2004). So, it is quite possible that a patient or a family member may ask you to pray for him or with him.

At least 49 million older adults pray for health. African Americans and Hispanic older adults are more likely to pray for health than whites. Women are considerably more likely (97%) to pray than men and older adults at the lower income level and with chronic conditions are more likely to pray for health (Tait, Laditka, Laditka, et al., 2011). Prayer is used by older adults as a form of complementary healing treatment (84%) and to cope with stress (96%) (Dunn & Horgas, 2000). Spiritual nursing care is an integral component of quality patient care.

It is important to distinguish between *praying with* and *praying for*. If the patient asks you to pray *with* him, you must determine whether he simply wants you to be present while he or another person leads the prayer. You should ask whether he wants you to begin the prayer or whether he wants to begin the prayer. If a patient asks you to pray *for* him, assess what it is that he wants you to pray for. Often the patient is merely asking you to pray for him on your own time, as frequently as your schedule allows.

Regardless of the situation, if you feel comfortable doing so, then you should enter the experience of prayer with confidence; after all, the patient or family member has asked you to be present because he feels at ease with you and trusts in your abilities. However, if you feel at all uncomfortable about offering prayer, then you should state those feelings and offer to find someone who is comfortable with prayer. For example, you might say either of the following to the patient or family, "Thank you for asking me to pray with you; there is another nurse on the floor who is better at this than I am. May I have your permission to seek that person out for you?" Or, you might reply as follows: "I am confident that the chaplain can help you in many ways with your request. May I make a referral to the chaplain for you?"

If you do wish to pray with patients, understanding the different types of prayer may help. **Prayer** consists of those ways that we respond to and interact with the Supreme Being, whether by words, thoughts, or actions (e.g., the painting in Fig. 16-5). People tend to think of prayer in its narrowest sense as being requests for something (intercession), and this is an important and useful type of prayer. However, there are at least six other types of prayer, including adoration, praise, thanksgiving, penitence, offering, and petition (*Book of Common Prayer*, 1979). For the various types of prayers,

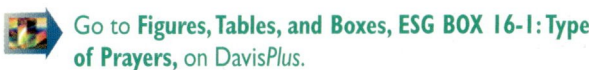

Go to **Figures, Tables, and Boxes, ESG BOX 16-1: Types of Prayers,** on Davis*Plus*.

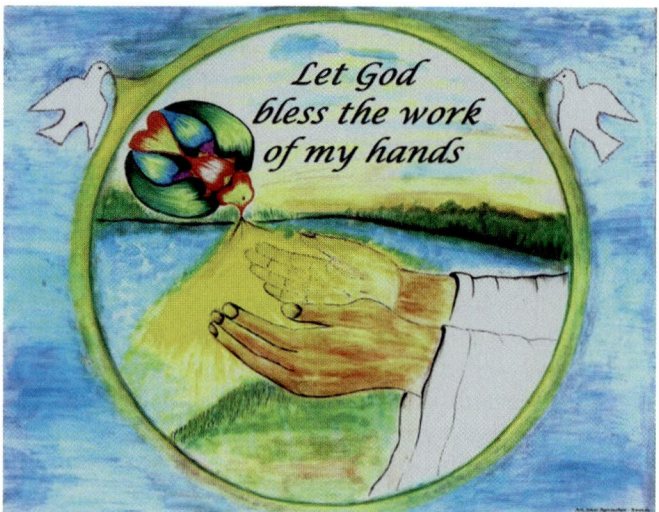

FIGURE 16-5 This painting may be an expression of prayer.

The following is an excerpt from an aunt's e-mail to a distribution group of her family and friends. It movingly demonstrates a belief in the powerful nature of prayer, and is an example of the research findings that many people rely on intercessory prayer during illness.

Example: I would really appreciate your prayers . . . for my nephew . . . who is newly diagnosed with Hodgkin's lymphoma. We go to the clinic at 10 a.m. to get his labs and then [to] the Children's Hospital to start his chemotherapy. . . . He is very sad and scared. His chest symptoms have increased . . . [and] we know the mass is still growing. Please pray . . . for wisdom and communication with the doctors and nurses. Pray all who come in contact with my nephew give peace, comfort, and soothing touch. Pray the side effects . . . are minimal. More than anything, . . . pray the chemo targets every cancerous cell . . . and specifically for greater than 70% shrinkage. [Pray also for] no more . . . fever, night sweats, weight loss, [and] chest pain. God truly can work miracles in times of trial and we are trusting fully in Him at this great time of need. (D. Wojcik, personal communication, March 1, 2013)

Prayer has a variety of purposes, expressions, and meanings to patients and their families, as well as to nurses. Prayer may provide for periods of intimacy with God, reveal the presence and love of God, and serve as a powerful source of comfort and hope.

 Go to **Clinical Insight 16-1: Praying With Patients,** in Volume 2.

Other Nursing Activities

Spiritual care involves you in relationships with people who have come face-to-face with a significant life event that calls forth a new sense of meaning and purpose. Specific nursing activities, to be individualized to each client's needs, are discussed, following.

- **Make Referrals When Needed.** There are times when you should refer a patient to others with more

Complementary & Alternative Modalities (CAM)

Intercessory Prayer

Many people pray when they are ill, and prayer seems to have positive effects. But what about the effects of *intercessory prayer*—the prayers of people for *others* who are ill? How useful is intercessory prayer? The following studies provide little support for the use of intercessory prayer as a CAM. However, this is not an exhaustive list of studies of intercessory prayer, and research is ongoing.

- **Schlitz, Hopf, Eskenazi, et al. (2012).** Researchers explored the efforts of distant healing intention (DHI) (also known as intercessory prayer, spiritual healing, etc.) on wound healing of 72 postoperative women. The results showed that DHI did not affect wound healing or self-reported postoperative emotional or physical health. However, the women who knowingly received prayer had a significantly longer length of surgery. The groups that believed in and knowingly or unknowingly received DHI had worse physical and self-reported well-being outcomes.

- **Roberts, Ahmed, Hall, et al. (2011).** Selecting 10 trials from the literature that randomized more than 7,800 participants, researchers concluded that there was not a significant difference in outcomes for those receiving intercessory prayer and those who did not. However, researchers noted that in a trial on high risk of death, people in the intercessory group who were at a high risk of death were significantly more likely to live. Another trial found that some specific complications were significantly more likely to occur in the non-intercessory prayer group, but "certainty of receiving prayer was associated with a lower incidence of complications."

- **Benson, Dusek, Sherwood, et al. (2006).** In patients recovering after coronary artery bypass graft (CABG) surgery, this study found that intercessory prayer itself had no effect on complication-free recovery from CABG, but "certainty of receiving intercessory prayer was associated with a lower incidence of complications (p. 940)."

- **Palmer, Katerndahl, & Morgan-Kidd (2004).** Researchers studied 86 community-dwelling persons, ages 18 to 88 years. Intercessory prayer was used for 1 month to intervene with a life concern or problem the participant disclosed at the beginning. No effect on problem resolution was found. Prayer did effectively reduce a subject's level of concern, but only if the subject initially believed that the problem could be resolved. Also, better physical functioning was observed among those who had a high belief in prayer.

knowledge and experience in religion and spirituality. For example, a patient may be experiencing Spiritual Distress because he believes he needs forgiveness for a past act, or a patient may refuse medical treatment because she thinks her church would not approve. For hospitalized and hospice patients, you can usually ask the chaplain's office to refer the patient and family to clergy or religious counselors in the community. If you are working in a home or community setting, use the Internet or telephone directory to find resources for you and the patient, such as local churches, priests, ministers, rabbis, or other spiritual advisers.

- **Encourage Expression of Feelings.** The best way to do this is simply to ask the patient how he is feeling or what he thinks about a particular situation.
- **Help the Patient Identify Feelings of Guilt.** You might ask the following after a patient has voiced a concern: "How do you feel about that?" or "You seem to feel sad about saying/doing that."
- **Help Significant Others Understand the Patient's Feelings and Needs.** Encourage family members to talk with the patient or simply to have a seat at the bedside. Periods of silence often lead into the most therapeutic of discussions.
- **Maximize the Patient's Comfort.** This is one of the most important spiritual activities a nurse can perform. A patient cannot think about spiritual issues when plagued with physical pain or discomfort.
- **Listen to the Patient's "Stories."** These tell the life history surrounding the person's illness and spiritual comfort or distress.
- **Assess the Patient's Needs for Reconciliation.** This may include reconciliation with self, others, and God. If, like Mr. Johnson (Meet Your Patient), the patient has lost contact with family members because of disagreements related to past events, you could collaborate with the social worker and chaplain about ways to facilitate a meeting.
- **Explore With the Client the Possible Meanings of Healing, Miracle, and Cure.** Refer to the discussion of miracles earlier in this chapter.

- **Collaborate With the Dietary Department.** Provide foods compatible with the person's religious needs. Encourage family members to bring foods from home, as appropriate.
- **Respect the Patient's Dress (and other) Requirements as Determined by His Religion.** This may include wearing religious icons, jewelry, or special clothes.
- **Do Not Make Assumptions About the Patient's and Family's Beliefs.** When a patient dies, for example, a seemingly harmless statement such as "He's gone to a better place" assumes the family believes in an afterlife. If they ask, you can briefly share your beliefs, but reflect their questions back to them (e.g., "Tell me what *you* think happens after death").

KnowledgeCheck 16-7

- What is prayer?
- What are ways can you support a patient's prayer needs?
- When a patient asks you to pray for him, what might be your most effective first response?

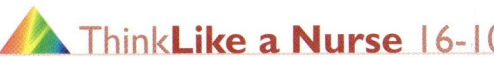 ThinkLike a Nurse 16-10

- A patient dying of lung cancer asks you to pray with him early one morning. You agree and ask him what he would like you to pray for. He responds: "That I may be cured of my cancer and go back home." He is on oxygen therapy, has pain medications given as prescribed, and is in a room by himself. Construct a prayer that might be meaningful and helpful.

Return to the scenario for Charles Johnson (Meet Your Patient). See whether you can answer the three questions more completely now after reading this chapter.

Spiritual Care

Complementary & Alternative Modalities (CAM)

Spiritual interventions, especially prayer, are a frequently used CAM:

➤ **Bekke-Hansen, Pedersen, Thygesen, et al. (2012)**—A recent study found that 76% of adult patients with acute coronary syndrome rated CAM treatments as having a positive influence on their quality of life. The most prevalent types of CAM used were dietary and exercise counseling and dietary and nutritional supplements.

➤ **Ben-Arye, Schiff, Vintal, et al. (2012)**—In this study researchers found that oncology patients with a higher spiritual quest had an increased use of CAM and higher expectations that providers integrate CAM into their care.

➤ **Ellison, Bradshaw, & Roberts (2012)**—When compared with spiritual-only, participants who were both spiritual and religious were more likely to use body–mind therapies when it included the CAM of prayer, meditation,

or spiritual healing and less likely (44%) when these CAMs were removed. Religious-only participants were not inclined to use CAM.

➤ **Trinkaus, Burman, Barmala, et al. (2011)**—Of the 123 patients with advanced cancer on a palliative care unit, 85% had used CAM; 42% used it for curative intent. The use of CAM for cure was associated with increased spiritual faith, but low existential well-being.

➤ **Johannessen (2011)**—Nurses reported in interviews that self-realization and development of self were core issues in holistic nursing. They also related these to psychological and spiritual well-being.

➤ **Wu, Weber, Kozak, et al. (2009)**—Neurosurgeons reported acupuncture, herbs, massage therapy, prayer, and yoga as the most common CAM used by their patients. At least 38% indicated they pray for their patients and 42% believed that prayer and spirituality can affect surgical outcomes.

To explore learning resources for this chapter,

Go to Davis*Plus* at DavisPl.us/Wilkinson3.

Chapter Resources for Chapter 16:
   Response sheets for all learning activities
   Resources for Caregivers and Health Professionals
   Reading More About Spirituality (suggested readings)
   Concept map of chapter content
Interactive Case Studies
NCLEX-Style and Chapter Review Questions
Chapter Overview Podcasts

For references cited in this chapter,

Go to Volume 2, **References Cited.**

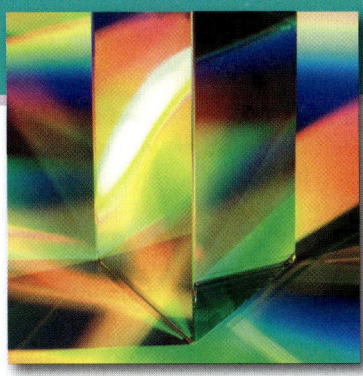

CHAPTER 17

Loss, Grief, & Dying

Learning Outcomes

After completing this chapter, you should be able to:

- ➤ Name and describe at least four types of loss.
- ➤ Identify the stages of grief as described by Engel, Worden, Rando, and Bowlby.
- ➤ Compare and contrast four types of grief.
- ➤ List and discuss at least five factors that affect grieving.
- ➤ Define *death* according to the Uniform Determination of Death Act.
- ➤ Give a definition of *higher-brain death*.
- ➤ Create a time line of the dying process, indicating the physiological signs and symptoms common to each stage.

- ➤ List and describe the Kübler-Ross stages of dying and grief.
- ➤ Define *end-of-life care*, *hospice care*, and *palliative care*.
- ➤ Identify the legal and ethical issues involved in death and dying.
- ➤ Assess, diagnose, plan, and implement care of dying patients and their families.
- ➤ Describe the responsibilities of the nurse regarding postmortem care.
- ➤ Identify nursing interventions to help clients who are grieving.

Key Concepts

Loss
Grief
Death/dying
End-of-life care

Related Concepts

See the Concept Map on Davis*Plus*.

Meet Your Patient

Thomas Manning is a 47-year-old man who is in the oncology unit with end-stage cancer of the pancreas. He is married and has three children, ages 18, 15, and 13. His oldest daughter has been away at college for only 6 months. Mr. Manning's father died 3 months ago from complications of alcoholism, and his mother has been withdrawn and grieving. His wife, Mary, tells you that Thomas "just wants to die" and does not want anyone trying to revive him or "pushing on his chest" if he dies. Mary is distressed and wants him to "keep fighting."

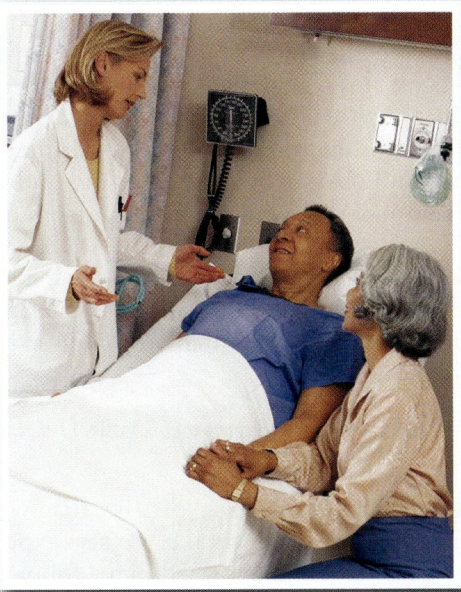

Theoretical Knowledge
knowing why

Throughout your nursing career, you will care for patients coping with loss—of youth, beauty, previous health, functioning, or quality of life. Many of your patients, like Thomas Manning, will be confronting their own approaching death, while family members will be facing loss of their loved one. As their nurse, you can help these people cope with their losses and grieve in a way that is healing, even transformative. But to do so, you need to know how to assess each patient's response to loss, plan appropriate outcomes, and intervene with skill and compassion. As a foundation, you must understand your own feelings and attitudes about loss, grief, and dying. We encourage you to increase your self- knowledge as you work through this chapter.

ABOUT THE KEY CONCEPTS

In order to provide care for patients experiencing loss, you will need to understand the key concepts of **loss, grief, death and dying,** and **end-of-life care.** Related concepts, such as stages of death, depression, and grief education, will expand the way you think about the key concepts. As you study the chapter, think often about how all the specific "parts and pieces" are related to the key concepts.

WHAT IS LOSS?

What is the first thing that comes to mind when you think of *loss*? Many people think of losing a loved one through death. Loss, however, is a daily occurrence. Our losses begin at birth when we lose the warmth and security of the womb, and end with the ultimate loss, the death of self. Loss can be defined as the undesired change or removal of a valued object, person, or situation.

Can you think of the first time you experienced a loss and what that felt like? What other losses have you undergone as you matured? For losses that are common at different developmental stages,

 Go to Chapter 17, Tables, Boxes, Figures: ESG Table 17-1, on the DavisPlus.

Whenever there is change, there is loss. Because we experience many changes throughout life, we also experience much loss. Loss can be categorized in the following ways:

- **Actual versus perceived loss. Actual loss** includes the death of a loved one (or relationship), theft, deterioration, destruction, and natural disaster. Actual loss can be identified by others, not just by the person experiencing it (e.g., hair loss during chemotherapy). In contrast, **perceived loss** is internal; it is identified only by

Quality and Safety Education for Nurses

Respecting Patient and Family Needs

Chapter Key Concepts: *Loss, grief, dying, end-of-life care*
Competency: *Patient-Centered Care (Skills, Attitudes)**

Situation. Karen Litvak is a 64-year-old woman who has lived her entire life with her mother, who is 86 years old. The mother is hospitalized with pneumonia. Karen spends each day at her side. "I don't know how to help her," Karen says to the nurse. "She always took care of me." When her mother stopped breathing, a code was called and doctors, nurses, and therapists ran into the room and began aggressive resuscitation (CPR). Karen stood out of the way but did not leave the room. The chaplain asked her to come out into the hallway with him, but she refused. The chaplain continued to urge her until she said forcefully, "No, I want to stay." Karen looked to the nurses, who nodded yes, she could stay.

The CPR efforts were not successful. The nurses asked Karen if she would like to come closer while they cleaned her mother. Karen talked about her mother as the nurses washed the mother's face and hands, put a clean hospital gown on her, and folded a clean sheet up to her waist. Karen thanked the nurses and turned to go. The nurses asked her where she would go and whether she had anyone to stay with her. She said she had a sister and would stay with her for a while.

Think about it: Patient-centered care means showing respect for the patient's significant other's values and needs and the diversity of human experience.

➤ Should the nurses have allowed the daughter to stay during CPR? Why or why not?

➤ How did the nurses show respect for Karen?

➤ How would you describe the daughter's values and needs?

 Go to the QSEN Web site at **http://qsen.org/ competencies/pre-licensure-ksas/**

the person experiencing it (e.g., a woman diagnosed with a sexually transmitted infection may perceive herself as having lost her purity).

- **Physical loss versus psychological loss. Physical loss** includes (1) injuries (e.g., when a limb is amputated), (2) removal of an organ (e.g., hysterectomy), and (3) loss of function (e.g., loss of mobility). **Psychological losses** challenge our belief system. They are commonly seen in the areas of sexuality, control, fairness, meaning, and trust. Some losses may be mixed. For example, after removal of a prostate gland, a man may feel both the physical and psychological loss of sexuality.
- **External versus internal loss. External losses** are actual losses of objects that are important to the person because of their cost or sentimental value (e.g., jewelry, a home). These losses can be brought about by

theft, destruction, or disasters such as floods and fire. **Internal loss** is another term for perceived or psychological loss.

- **Loss of aspects of self.** These losses include physical losses such as body organs, limbs, body functions, and/or body disfigurement. Psychological and perceived losses in this category include aspects of one's personality, developmental change (as in the aging process), loss of hopes and dreams, and loss of faith.
- **Environmental loss.** This loss involves a change in the familiar, even if the change is perceived as positive. Examples include moving to a new home, getting a new job, and going to college. These losses can be perceived or actual.
- **Loss of significant relationships.** This type of loss includes, but is not limited to, actual loss of spouses, siblings, family members, or significant others through death, divorce, or separation (e.g., military deployment).

 ThinkLike a Nurse 17-1

Which kinds of loss do you think Thomas Manning is experiencing?

Why is it important to recognize loss?

WHAT IS GRIEF?

Whenever there is loss, there is grieving. Grieving requires energy, so it can interfere with health and delay healing. However, grieving is positive in the sense that it is essential to psychological healing after a loss. Consider the following losses and the different reactions of the women involved.

Both Mrs. Smith and Mrs. Jones have lost a dog. Mrs. Smith's son left his dog with her when he went away to college last year. It has died of old age. Mrs. Jones's dog has been with her for 10 years and has been her only companion since her husband died 5 years ago. Her dog was killed by a car today as they were on their morning walk. Which woman do you think will grieve her loss more? Why? Discuss this situation with a classmate. Do you both have the same opinion about this?

This exercise demonstrates that it is really impossible to decide who would feel "more" grief.

Key Point: *The intensity of the grief depends on the meaning the person attaches to the loss.*

Both women probably felt sad. However, the meaning of and attachment to the dog are different for each one. You might have thought Mrs. Smith's loss was minor; however, her dog was owned by her son and may have represented him in her mind. Mrs. Jones's dog was a companion and a protector and may have represented security and friendship. Each woman must grieve what the loss represents to her. This is true for everyone, whether the losses are actual or perceived, physical or psychological.

Grief is the physical, psychological, and spiritual responses to a loss. **Mourning** consists of actions associated with grief (e.g., crying, wearing black clothing). These processes are normal and natural responses to a loss. The mourning and adjustment time after a loss is the period of **bereavement**. Although each person may express grief differently, some aspects of grief are shared by almost everyone.

KnowledgeCheck 17-1

What types of losses commonly occur in our lives?

Stages of Grief

There is no single, correct way to grieve, nor do people move neatly from one stage or step of grief to the next. Rather, grieving is a fluid, ongoing process. There is constant movement among stages, including recurrences of phases the bereaved person thought were resolved. The following are four major stage theorists in the field

George Engel (1961) Engel believed that uncomplicated grief has a clear onset and a predictable course, modified mainly by the abruptness and significance of the loss and how well the bereaved person was prepared for it. Uncomplicated grief is universal and does not require treatment.

John Bowlby (1982) Drawing on attachment theory, Bowlby suggested that grief occurs when the bereaved learn that the object of their attachment is lost. Some experts assert that Bowlby's theory does not take into account the individual nature of grief and that it implies loved ones can be replaced. Nevertheless, our understanding of grief is broadened by his idea that grief is a mature way of dealing with loss of attachment. He also provides a slightly different perspective on the stages of grief.

Theresa Rando (1984, 1986, 1993, 2000) Rando identified three processes of grieving (Table 17-1). Rando's (1984) stages are commonly described as the six R's of grieving:

1. *R*ecognizing the loss (awareness)
2. *R*eacting to the separation (feeling the emotions)
3. *R*ecollecting memories of the deceased (remembering, reliving)
4. *R*elinquishing the old attachment (new ways of living without the deceased)
5. *R*eadjusting to the new environment (new coping skills)
6. *R*einvesting self (energy once turned inward on grief begins to be focused outward again).

William Worden (2002) Worden described the tasks a grieving person must achieve. They progress from an initial numbness or denial through experiencing and working through pain and grief and eventually moving on with life.

Table 17-1 ➤ Theories of Grief. A Comparison

STAGES	DESCRIPTION
George Engel (1961)—Three Stages of Grief	
Shock and disbelief	Initial phase. The sufferer denies the loss in an attempt to protect himself against the shock of reality.
Developing awareness of the loss	The sufferer experiences painful feelings of sadness, guilt, shame, helplessness, hopelessness, loss, and emptiness. The person may lose interest in usual activities and experience impaired work performance. She may also experience loss of appetite, sleep disturbances, and even physical symptoms of pain or other discomfort.
Restitution and recovery	The final phase, which is prolonged and gradual. The person carries on the work of mourning and overcomes the trauma of the loss, and a state of health and well-being is reestablished.
John Bowlby (1982)—Phases of Grief	
Shock and numbness	Initial stage, in which the person experiences disorientation and feelings of helplessness
Yearning and searching	The grieving person yearns to be reconnected with the deceased and searches for connections
Disorganization and despair	The permanence of the loss becomes real. The person feels the pain and emotions of grief to their fullest and feels there is no hope of reconnection.
Reorganization	Adjusting to life without the deceased (or lost object); developing new coping skills
Theresa Rando (1984, 1986, 1993, 2000)—Three Processes of Grieving	
Avoidance	Includes shock, disbelief, denial, anger, and bargaining
Confrontation	The person actually begins to face the loss; a very emotional and upsetting time, when the person feels the grief most acutely
Accommodation	The person begins to live with the loss, feel better, and resume some routine activities
William Worden (2002)—Four Tasks of Grieving	
Accepting the reality of the loss	*Realizing that the loved one (or object) is gone.* In the hours and days after a significant loss, the grieving person typically feels numb and unable to accept the fact of the loss. This numbness is thought to be a helpful form of denial, which allows the person to "take in" only what the psyche is capable of handling at that time. So, the task of realizing the loved one or object is gone may take several days or, in the case of a sudden death, weeks.
Working through the pain and grief	*Feelings and emotions that surface are intense and can change rapidly.* This makes the person feel "out of control." People in this stage may say they feel as if they are "going crazy." This is usually the longest phase for two reasons. First, because none of us likes to be in pain; we become expert at finding ways not to feel it. We overeat, overmedicate, overwork, and drink to excess to avoid feeling the pain, and we thereby prolong the process of grief. Second, caring people do not like to see their loved ones in pain, so they make attempts to remove the pain (e.g., by distraction) rather than letting the person experience it. Like avoidance, this well-meaning behavior also prolongs the process.
Adjusting to the environment in which the deceased is missing	*Adjusting to the environment without the deceased.* This may mean performing alone activities and tasks, such as going for walks or shopping, that were once shared. Or it may include taking on roles and responsibilities that the deceased previously held. Such experiences can be extremely sad, frustrating and challenging, or very rewarding. However, once the person has established the new pattern, he or she typically feels satisfaction and increased self-esteem.
Emotionally relocating the deceased and moving on with life	*Investing emotional energy.* Initially all energy is focused on the deceased: thinking about the person, talking about him/her, reliving memories, and so on. It is nearly impossible to think of anything else. Concentration is difficult, so the grieving person finds it hard to engage in activities such as reading. When the person's energy begins to flow toward others or to different or former interests (e.g., working, socializing), the healing process is in progress.

Sources: Bowlby, J. (1982). *Attachment and loss.* 3 vols. New York: Basic Books; Engel, G. L. (1961). Is grief a disease? A challenge for medical research. *Psychosomatic Medicine, 23*(1), 18–22; Rando, T. (1984). *Grief, dying and death: Clinical interventions for caregivers.* Champaign, IL: Research Press; and Worden, J. W. (2002). *Grief counseling and grief therapy: A handbook for the mental health practitioner* (3rd ed.). New York: Springer.

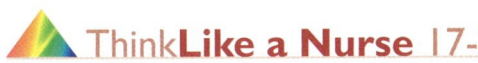

ThinkLike a Nurse 17-2

What are some of the similarities you see in the four theories described?

Grieving as Reconstructing Meaning

Some theorists are moving away from stage models of grieving toward the idea of grieving as a process of reconstructing meaning. For example, many recognize that the sorrow of loss is always present (Boss & Carnes, 2012; Florczak, 2008), whether in the foreground or the background of a person's life. However, the meaning of the loss is constantly changing for the bereaved. The sorrow becomes "remembered" sorrow, which sometimes resurfaces and at other times sinks in to the background of other sorrows, joys, and everyday life.

Factors Affecting Grief

To begin thinking about factors affecting grieving, consider the following exercise.

ThinkLike a Nurse 17-3

Mr. Klein is an 86-year-old man whose wife died of heart disease 2 months ago. He has two adult children who regularly visit him. He also has a very supportive pastor, Mr. Owens, who meets him in the park to share stories. Mr. Owens is 30 years old and has been raising his 5-year-old daughter alone after the sudden death of his wife 6 months ago in an automobile accident. His parents and siblings live out of state. Both of these men are missing their wives very much.

■ What factors do you think play a role in each man's grief?
■ Who do you think will "get over it" faster?
■ What are some issues that may make each man's grief uniquely difficult?

No two people ever grieve in the same manner because there are so many factors that play a role in the grieving process. They include the following:

■ **Significance of the Loss.** The meaning the person has attached to the person or object lost will be different for each person. The greater the attachment, the more difficult is the grief.
■ **Support System.** People with strong emotional and psychosocial support typically have less complicated grief.
■ **Unresolved Conflict.** An unresolved conflict at the time of death may cause prolonged grief. For example, if a couple had an argument just before one partner's sudden death, the remaining partner's grief may be complicated by guilt.
■ **Circumstances of the Loss.** Specifically, was there an opportunity to prepare for it? Was this a sudden, unexpected death, or had the person been suffering from a chronic illness? Was the death a suicide or homicide? Was the death in any sense avoidable? Was the person in pain? Is it an "ambiguous loss" or open-ended loss that occurs with the sudden disappearance of a loved one? If the circumstances

of the loss leave the bereaved feeling guilty or responsible, his grieving process may be impeded. This may occur in losses other than death (e.g., loss of a job).
■ **Previous Loss.** If the person has sustained more than one loss in a short period of time, the grieving process can become more complicated. In the hospital, you will frequently care for patients experiencing multiple losses. For example, consider a patient who has suffered a stroke and loss of mobility and moves to a nursing home. The patient has the compounded loss of health and functioning, independence, and the familiar surroundings of his home.
■ **Spiritual/Cultural Beliefs and Practices.** Spirituality and religious beliefs can help or hinder the grieving process. One person might believe the deceased is in a place of contentment and happiness, where all suffering is over. Another may believe that the deceased person will be reborn into another form. Yet another may believe that death is final and there is no afterlife. How do you think these beliefs might influence the grieving process? Most cultures engage in rituals (e.g., funerals) that help the bereaved begin the grieving process by openly expressing their emotions and pain (Fig. 17-1). Some cultures may emphasize keeping emotions more subdued and limiting expressions of grief to private settings.
■ **Timeliness of the Death.** The death of a child or a young person is almost universally more difficult to accept than the death of an older person. In addition to loss of the person, there is a sense of unfairness because of the loss of *potential*—of what the child might have become or achieved. You may hear someone ask,

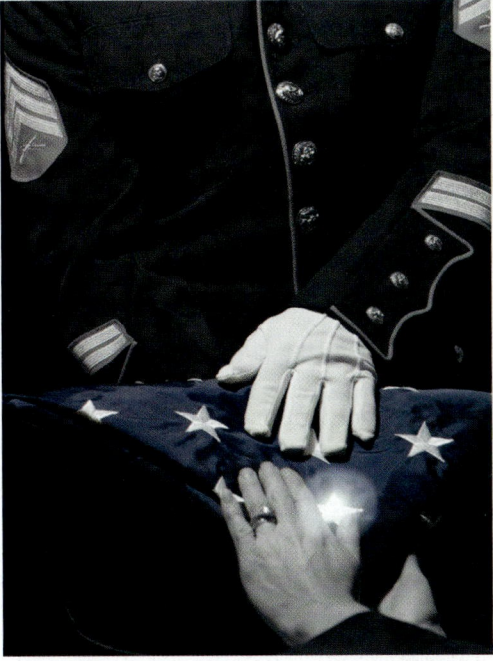

FIGURE 17-1 Rituals are used to facilitate grieving.

"Why was her life cut short?" or state, "He had so much going for him, but God didn't give him a chance."

Research shows that support groups are effective in reducing the severity of grief in widowed older adults, while religious support was most effective in the reduction of grief severity (Ghesquiere, Shear, & Duan, 2013). Your care plan should incorporate support groups to minimize complicated grief and depression in older adults.

Developmental Stages and Grief

Based on Erik Erikson's stages of psychological growth, we all must achieve certain psychological milestones during a lifetime. Grief can affect the healthy development of life stages, and in turn, the person's stage of development can affect the grieving process. If you need to review Erikson's theory, review Chapter 9.

Childhood Because cognitive development is not yet complete, preschool children do not understand that death is final. They believe that death is temporary and reversible, as with cartoon characters that "die" and then "come to life" again. During early childhood, children begin to understand that death is permanent, but believe that it will never happen to them or anyone they know. Between ages 8 and 11, children recognize that death can happen to them and may be fearful (Brown, 2009).

Young children believe they are the cause of what happens around them. This is known as *magical thinking*. Such thinking may cause them to feel guilt when there is a death of someone close to them. Other responses include regressing to a previous developmental stage: "acting like a baby," demanding food and attention, becoming incontinent, and talking "baby talk."

During the weeks after a death, a child may feel immediate grief, may or may not display sadness, or may continue to believe the person is still alive. These are normal reactions.

Adolescence The bereavement and emotions felt by adolescents along with confusion regarding their identity and role can create major uncertainty. The adolescent struggles to learn who he is as a person as he breaks away from parental control. An adolescent who experiences the loss of a parent while "pushing the parent away" may feel a sense of guilt and unfinished business.

At the same time, the bereaved teen also faces psychological, physiological, social, and academic pressures. Although teens may look mature, they often lack emotional maturity. Teens are often expected to be "grown up" and support a surviving parent or younger siblings. When they feel this responsibility, they do not have the opportunity, or the permission, to mourn. Adolescents may turn to those outside of the family to discuss their feelings (Brown, 2009).

Research shows that bereaved youths who have lost a parent have a higher frequency of engaging in health risk behaviors (Hamdan, Mazariegos, Melhem, et al., 2012). Adult caregivers must be alert to these behaviors and take appropriate interventions to meet the bereavement and safety needs of children and adolescents.

Adulthood Adults are cognitively able to understand the nature of death, and they have usually experienced other types of loss by this time. Over time, they perceive loss as a normal part of living. How they respond to loss depends on factors such as the person's self-esteem and the availability of supports.

Older Adulthood A special difficulty for older adults is the cumulative effects of the many losses that they experience. Most deaths occur among older adults, so they are likely to lose friends and siblings in rapid succession, along with physical and functional losses and the loss of independence. In addition, they began the process of preparatory grief in anticipation of their own death (MacKenzie, 2011). The emotional effects may be devastating.

Research reveals that elderly adults who have suffered the loss of a child experience significant and sometimes irreparable mental and physical outcomes, accelerated disabilities, and loss of the ability to function independently. To minimize these negative outcomes, caregivers should use listening skills and metaphors and promote storytelling (Smith, Kerr, Galligan, et al., 2011).

KnowledgeCheck 17-2

- What are the main tasks of the grieving process?
- What factors affect the grieving process?

ThinkLike a Nurse 17-4

Refer to Thomas Manning and his wife (Meet Your Patient). Apply each of the preceding factors affecting grief to Thomas and to Mary (they may be different for each spouse). If the scenario does not provide enough information for you to comment, say so and then describe how you would obtain the data you need.

Types of Grief

Grief can be categorized in several ways, most of which have to do with timing and intensity.

Uncomplicated Grief (normal grief) is the natural response to a loss. The bereaved person experiences the feelings, behaviors, and cognitions that are expected in light of his culture, social status, and relationship to the lost person or object. The emotions are intense but gradually diminish over time (several months to several years). Some emotions will always be present, but the intensity will change.

Complicated Grief, also known as prolonged acute grief, is characterized by its length of time and intensity of emotion. The person's responses last longer than 6 months and are maladaptive, dysfunctional, unusually prolonged, or overwhelming (Germain, Shear, Walsh, et al., 2013). For example, the bereaved may become severely depressed, violent, or suicidal; become a "workaholic"; become socially isolated; or demonstrate addictive behavior. Or after several years the person may still be experiencing as much pain and disruption as in the first months after the loss. Complicated grief has been associated with depression, suicidal ideation, and hypertension and can be very distressing and disabling (Prigerson, Frank, Kasl, et al., 1995; Prigerson, Horowitz, Jacobs, et al., 2009). Risk factors for complicated grief include previous loss, exposure to trauma, sudden death of a significant other, emotional instability, and lack of social support (Lobb, Kristjanson, Aoun, et al., 2010). Chronic, masked, and delayed grief all are examples of complicated grief:

- **Chronic grief** begins as normal grief but continues long term, with little resolution of feelings and inability to rejoin normal life.
- **Masked grief** occurs when the person is grieving, but expressing the grief through other types of behavior. For example, a man whose wife has died may begin drinking heavily, or a couple whose child has died may find themselves engaging in violent arguments with each other. This change in behavior is part of their grief response, but they don't recognize it as such.
- **Delayed grief** is grief that is put off until a later time (e.g., "I'll think about it later; right now, I'm busy trying to keep a roof over our heads and care for my children").

Typically, complicated grief results when the grieving process has been impeded for some reason (e.g., something keeps the person "stuck" in the grief process). Usually the bereaved benefits from the assistance of a grief counselor to help establish and work through the problem areas.

Disenfranchised Grief is experienced in connection with a loss that is not socially supported or acknowledged by the usual rites or ceremonies. Some examples include a couple who experienced a miscarriage, the unplanned termination of a child's foster placement, a mistress whose lover dies, or a bereaved partner in a homosexual relationship (Lang, Fleiszer, Duhamel, et al., 2011; Riggs & Willsmore, 2012). In each of these instances, the bereaved person lacks the familial or communal support that is helpful in grieving.

Anticipatory Grief is experienced before a loss occurs. A wife caring for her husband through a long illness may grieve as she sees the vibrant man she once knew change before her eyes as she anticipates his death. Family members experience anticipatory grief as they watch the mental capacity diminish in a loved one with Alzheimer's disease and realize that the person they once knew is becoming progressively removed from them. The potential negative outcome of anticipatory grief is that the survivor may detach from a dying person too early in the dying process, leaving the person without emotional support during that period. This does not always happen, of course.

 ThinkLike a Nurse 17-5

Thomas Manning (Meet Your Patient) had a strained relationship with his father for most of his life. His father was an alcoholic and constantly fought with his mother while Thomas was growing up. A few months ago, his father was hospitalized for the third time for complications of alcoholism, and Thomas visited him. He confronted his father regarding his drinking and the problems and pain it had caused him and the family. The confrontation ended in an argument. That night, Thomas's father slipped into a coma. He died a few days later, without recovering consciousness.

- What issues does Thomas have to deal with?
- Why might this be a complicated grief process?

DEATH AND DYING

Death is the ultimate loss. The dying person faces the loss of physical control and function, independence, relationships, possibilities, and ultimately life itself. In mainstream North American culture, death is not seen as a natural part of life, but rather as something to avoid at all costs. People even avoid talking or thinking about it.

How Is Death Defined?

Historically, *death* was defined as the cessation of the flow of vital bodily fluids. This evolved into the traditional definition of **heart–lung death**: the irreversible cessation of spontaneous respirations and circulation. This was later replaced with **whole-brain death**: the irreversible cessation of all functions of the brain, including the brainstem. Spontaneous respirations cannot continue once the brainstem stops functioning; however, the heart may continue to beat until it becomes oxygen starved from cessation of respirations.

In the 1970s, many practitioners began using the term **higher-brain death**, which defines death as the irreversible cessation of all "higher" brain functions (e.g., cognitive functioning, consciousness, memory, reasoning, and so on). By this definition, the brainstem can still be functioning, so both respiratory and cardiac activity may continue even though the person does not make purposive responses to external stimuli; cephalic reflexes are absent; and the electroencephalogram shows no activity.

Under those definitions, it was technically possible to keep a person "alive" indefinitely by using a mechanical ventilator. In 1981, the President's Commission for the Study of Ethical Problems in Medicine proposed the **Uniform Determination of Death Act** (Box 17-1) that provides a highly reliable means of declaring death for respirator-maintained bodies—loss of brainstem function (DeSpelder & Strickland, 1996, p. 328). For criteria for assessing brainstem functioning,

 Go to Chapter 17, **Supplemental Materials: Some Criteria for Assessing Brainstem Functioning,** on DavisPlus.

What Are Coma and Persistent Vegetative State?

A **coma** is a prolonged, deep state of unconsciousness lasting days or even years. The patient cannot be aroused and may or may not have decreased brainstem reflexes.

Persistent vegetative state (PVS) sometimes follows a coma, but can also occur after any event that affects cerebrovascular flow. In PVS, the person does not purposefully respond to stimuli, is unaware of the environment, and has no cognition or affective mental functions. However, the person has lost only the higher cerebral functions (see the preceding definition of higher-brain death) and so continues to have a sleep–wake cycle, may have some spontaneous movements, and may open her eyes in response to external stimuli. The person cannot speak or obey commands. Patients in a PVS may look somewhat normal and may occasionally grimace, cry, or laugh. The family may believe that the patient is responding to the environment and thus not want to give up hope for recovery. Because they cannot work through the grieving process, they continue to grieve each day.

What Are the Stages of Dying?

To help dying patients and their families understand the dying process, your theoretical knowledge base must include information on both physiological and psychological processes.

Physiological Stages of Dying

The dying process is unique to each person. However, people experience many similar symptoms as they approach the end of life. Fewer than 10% of patients die suddenly and unexpectedly, as in an accident or massive heart attack. Ninety percent die after a long illness, progressively deteriorating until an active dying phase at the end (Emanuel, Ferris, von Gunten, et al., 2008). The following time line describes the physiological responses of that group (Karnes, 1995).

One to Three Months Before Death The dying person begins to withdraw from the world and people. Sleep increases; it becomes difficult for the body to digest food, especially meats; and appetite and food intake decrease. Liquids are preferred. Anorexia and the resulting ketosis may be protective, as they can diminish pain and increase the person's sense of well-being.

One to Two Weeks Before Death A host of physical changes indicates the body is beginning to lose its ability to maintain itself. Cardiovascular deterioration brings reduced blood pressure, changes in pulse and skin color (e.g., a yellowish pallor), and extreme pallor of the extremities. Temperature fluctuates and perspiration increases. Respiratory rate may increase or decrease; during sleep, the dying person may experience brief periods of apnea. Congestion may cause a rattling sound and/or a nonproductive cough.

Days to Hours Before Death Often a surge of energy brings mental clarity and a desire to eat and talk with family members. However, as death approaches, patients tend to become dehydrated and have difficulty swallowing, which results in decreased blood volume. The tissues of the tongue and soft palate sag, and the gag reflex declines, so secretions accumulate in the oropharynx and/or bronchi. Often the mucous membranes become dry and tacky and lips become cracked. Dehydration during the last hours of dying is thought not to cause distress, and perhaps to stimulate endorphin release (Emanuel, Ferris, von Gunten, et al., 2008).

Breathing may be shallow, rapid, or irregular: Periods of apnea may lengthen to 10 to 30 seconds before breathing resumes. Congestion causes a "death rattle" that can be quite loud. **Cheyne-Stokes respirations** may occur. This is a cyclic pattern consisting of a 10- to 60-second period of apnea and then a gradual increase in depth and rate of respirations. Respirations gradually become slow and shallow, and then the cycle begins again with apnea.

Peripheral circulation decreases, and the person perspires and feels "clammy." The blood pressure decreases, and the pulse may be hard to detect. The extremities become cool and mottled, and the underside of the body may be much darker. Decreased circulation also results in reduced kidney function and decreased urinary output.

Muscles throughout the body relax, causing the face to "droop." As peristalsis slows, the patient may retain feces. Urine output decreases and urine often becomes more concentrated and foul smelling. Sphincters relax, and bowel and bladder incontinence can occur. Vision blurs; the eyes may be open or partially open, but unseeing. Instead, the patient may see things that are not visible to others.

In the final hours of life, many patients become restless and agitated. This response may be caused by medications, liver failure, cerebral hypoxia, renal failure, stool impaction, distended bladder, increased pain, or unresolved emotional or spiritual issues. Near to the time of death, some people unexpectedly become more coherent and energized for a time. Others become less communicative, quiet, and withdrawn (Pitorak, 2003). Fatigue is common.

Moments Before Death The dying person does not respond to touch or sound and cannot be awakened. Typically, there is a short series of long-spaced breaths before breathing ceases entirely and the heart stops beating (Karnes, 1995; National Caregiver Library, n.d.).

Psychological Stages of Dying

Perhaps the best known author on the psychology of dying is Dr. Elisabeth Kübler-Ross (1969). She felt that if people understood what dying patients are experiencing, they would be more competent in caring for them. From her research with dying patients, she observed that people tend to experience one or more of five psychological stages during the period from the terminal diagnosis to the actual death (Box 17-2). Her theory has become a classic for professional and lay readers alike, and has been applied to losses other than death. When you study the Kübler-Ross stages, it is important to understand that dying people:

- May not go through *every* stage.
- May not go through the stages in a linear fashion, but rather in random order.

BOX 17-2 ■ Kübler-Ross: Stages of Dying and Grief

Stage	Defining Characteristics
Denial	■ "Not me." "This cannot be happening." "I don't believe it." Usually the person is in a state of shock. Denial is not necessarily negative; it gives the person a chance to prepare psychologically for accepting the news.
Anger	■ "Why me?" "Why is this happening?" Anger can be obvious or subtle. It is the person's response to the feeling that the situation is unfair. The person may take his anger out on people who are "safe" (e.g., family, spouse) or from whom there will be no reprisals (e.g., nurses, physician).
Bargaining	■ "If only I can live until . . ." "Yes me, but . . ." Usually this takes the form of a bargain with God or a Higher Power, in which the person asks to live to see a birth, graduation, wedding, and so forth.
Depression	■ A withdrawn sadness, not to be confused with clinical depression. This is a response to the current loss as well as to any accumulated and/or future losses.
Acceptance	■ Not necessarily *wanting* death (or the loss), but coming to terms with it and ceasing to fight it. The person may seem almost devoid of feelings.

Source: Adapted from Kübler-Ross, E. (1969). On death and dying. New York: Macmillan.

- Do not necessarily complete one stage and move on to the next.
- May experience two or three stages simultaneously.

Key Point: *Remember that it is not the nurse's responsibility to move people to the next stage so that dying patients accept death. It is our responsibility to accept and support people "where they are" and help them to verbalize their feelings. We need to understand patients, not change them.*

What Is End-of-Life Care?

When, precisely, is the end of life? There is no set, agreed-upon definition or set of criteria. A recent set of guidelines provides a working definition that includes the following three situations:

- The patient has a fatal condition.
- Death is likely with the next exacerbation of disease.
- The patient acknowledges the seriousness of the situation (Qaseem, Snow, Shekelle, et al., 2008).

In an effort to humanize healthcare, organizations such as the Institute of Medicine (2013), the American Association of Colleges of Nursing (2010, updated 2013), and the Robert Wood Johnson Foundation (2012) have undertaken initiatives to ensure that end-of-life care is delivered with compassion, sensitivity, and competency. Some of these competencies include the following (Bednash & Ferrell, 2000; End-of-Life Nursing Education Consortium [ELNEC], 2012):

- Holistic assessment of patients and families (i.e., physical, psychological, social, and spiritual)
- Acknowledging diversity in patients' beliefs and customs
- Using both traditional and complementary approaches
- Incorporating essential communication strategies that meet spiritual and cultural needs
- Applying legal and ethical principles to end-of-life care
- Demonstrating respect for the patients' views and wishes during end-of-life care
- Assessing patient, family, colleagues, and one's own success in coping with suffering, grief, loss, and bereavement at the end of life
- Providing quality postmortem care

For end-of-life nursing care competencies recommended by the American Association of Colleges of Nursing (AACN),

 Go to Chapter 17, **Tables, Boxes, Figures: ESG Box 17-1,** on Davis*Plus*.

End-of-life care includes palliative care and hospice care, which are similar in that both may involve caring for dying patients, and neither focuses on cure. Some people use the terms interchangeably; however, there are subtle differences.

End-of-Life Care

Complementary & Alternative Modalities (CAM)

> **Hodgson (2013)** studied the effects of reflexology and Swedish massage on pain reduction and symptoms of agitation in 60 end-stage dementia patients. Results revealed that both CAMs promoted palliation of symptoms and pain reduction.

> **Heath, Oh, Clarke, et al. (2012)** interviewed parents of children who had died of cancer to determine the perceived efficacy of CAM and its effect on the overall end-of-life experience. The primary types of CAM used were organic foods, faith healing, and homeopathy, with 44% of respondents using more than one type. The majority (78%) reported a significant benefit from CAM use.

> **Kraft (2012)** reviewed research studies and reviews to determine the effect of CAM on depression, anxiety, grief, and other symptoms in advanced palliative care patients. Although short lived, yoga, acupuncture, aromatherapy, and some massage techniques had a positive effect on depression. These therapies also successfully treated anxiety, as did music therapy and mindfulness-based stress reduction. Acupuncture had a positive benefit on fatigue.

> **Rahim-Jamal, Sarte, Kozak, et al. (2011)** found that 81% of 49 hospice patients expressed an interest in CAM for pain relief, relaxation, and enhanced well-being. Of those, 79 % had used CAM prior to entering the hospice setting.

Palliative Care

When patients reach a stage in their illness in which cure is no longer possible, or when they refuse further treatment, they may be eligible to receive "comfort care"—meaning that no further efforts will be made to stop the disease process or prevent the patient from dying. However, the patient will receive treatment to minimize unpleasant symptoms, (e.g., nausea, pain). The correct interpretation of the term *comfort care* is, "Nothing more *can* be done to cure your loved one." However, family members sometimes interpret it to mean "Nothing more will be done." In this situation, the term *palliative care* may be more acceptable. As a specialty, palliative care is provided by a holistic team of professionals. However, many patients receive palliative care from their general practice provider, and even in acute care hospitals, especially if staff are comfortable and skilled with pain management and end-of-life care.

Palliative care is actually aggressively planned, holistic comfort care. General issues for most end-of-life care patients include the following:

- Supporting families and caregivers
- Ensuring continuity of care
- Ensuring respect for persons
- Ensuring informed decision making
- Attending to emotional and spiritual concerns
- Supporting function and survival duration
- Managing symptoms (e.g., pain, dyspnea, depression)

A patient does not necessarily have to be "actively dying" to receive palliative care. It is also provided over a long period of time for those who have slowly progressive diseases. Palliative care should not be seen as merely limiting life-sustaining treatment or allowing death. It should result in increased patient satisfaction, improved symptom control, and cost savings for hospitals (Owens, Eby, Burson, et al., 2012; Qaseem, Snow, Shekelle, et al., 2008).

Hospice Care

The hospice movement was set in motion in England by Dame Cicely Sanders, who founded the first modern-day hospice within a London hospital in 1968. More than 5,000 hospice providers in the United States alone served 1.6 million patients in 2011 (National Hospice and Palliative Care Organization, 2011). **Hospice care** focuses on holistic care of patients who are dying or debilitated and not expected to improve. For a patient to be eligible for hospice insurance benefits, a physician must certify that the patient is likely to die within 6 months. This is a primary difference between palliative care and hospice.

Hospice care is based on two key premises: (1) The quality of life is as important as the length of life, and (2) those who are terminally ill should be allowed to face death with dignity and surrounded by the comfort of their homes and families. Although you may think of hospice as "home" care, hospice is a *way* of caring rather than a setting. Some hospitals are able to devote some inpatient beds to hospice care, and freestanding hospices also exist. The purpose of admitting a patient is to provide a family with some respite for a period of time or to stabilize a patient who requires symptom management, or to care for a patient who is in the end stage of a disease (e.g., AIDS or cancer) and needs a level of expert care that family members cannot provide at home. Treatment is holistic, addressing the patient's emotional, spiritual, and physical needs. Physical care is primarily palliative, involving symptom management. For example, pain management is considered crucial because patients must be relatively free from pain to make the most of their remaining time.

An interdisciplinary team plans care with the patient and family. Family members are encouraged to be active in the team to the extent they are able. Nursing support is available 24 hours a day and families are taught what to expect as the disease progresses. Psychosocial and spiritual care have high priority. As the patient nears death, hospice workers remain as long as necessary. After the patient dies, there is follow-up bereavement care for the families.

Legal and Ethical Considerations at End of Life

The technology of life support makes it possible to prolong bodily functions almost indefinitely, leaving patients and families struggling to decide whether prolonging life is appropriate. More clients depend on nurses for education regarding patient rights and end-of-life care choices. Each situation is unique, and you should be able to explore with clients the various options available. See Chapters 44 and 45, for more information about the ethical and legal aspects of each of the following topics.

Advance Directives

An advance directive is a group of instructions (written or oral) stating a person's wishes regarding his healthcare if he were incapacitated or unable to make that decision. An ordinary power of attorney does not give another person the right to make healthcare decisions for the patient; only a durable power of attorney for healthcare decisions can do that.

The **Patient Self-Determination Act (PSDA),** passed by Congress in 1990, requires that all healthcare providers who receive Medicare funds (e.g., hospitals, home care agencies, hospices, nursing homes) must educate staff and patients and provide an opportunity for all patients to complete an advance directive (see Chapter 45 if you want more information). The Joint Commission (2008) also requires institutions to address the wishes of the patient regarding end-of-life decisions. Laws in each state vary regarding advance directives. It is important for you to understand the federal and state laws and the policies of your institution. Two types of advance directives serve different purposes.

- A **living will** is a document that provides specific instructions about the kinds of healthcare the person would wish or would wish *not* to have in particular situations. For example, it might specify that the person does not want to be maintained on a ventilator or receive tube feedings.
- A **durable power of attorney (DPOA),** or **healthcare proxy**, exists when another person is identified to make decisions for the individual regarding healthcare choices when he is unable to do so based on circumstances (e.g., irreversible coma, terminal illness). The individual should provide specific instructions about his desires regarding hydration, feeding tubes, medication, resuscitation, and mechanical ventilation. Since this is a legal document, it should be properly prepared (executed) and can be changed or canceled at any time by the patient. For an example of an advance directive,

 Go to Chapter 17, **Tables, Boxes, Figures: ESG Figure 17-1,** on Davis*Plus*.

For details of the Patient Self-Determination Act,

 Go to Chapter 17, **Supplemental Materials: Patient Self-Determination Act,** on Davis*Plus*.

Some people fear that once an advance directive is signed, no further care will be provided. It is important to explain to families and patients that these directives ensure that they will get as much or little care as *they* wish. Remind them that everyone should get advance

directives while they are healthy. Such explanations are independent nursing activities, for which you are responsible.

Orders for DNAR

A **DNAR order** is an order to *not* attempt resuscitation of the patient in the event of cardiac or respiratory failure. Formerly known as *DNR (do not resuscitate),* a DNAR must be prescribed by a physician. Some are recommending the acronym **AND** (allow natural death) to replace DNAR (Breault, 2011), because the word *death* in the acronym makes clear the intent of the provider's order (American Nurses Association [ANA], 2012). Regardless, you must pay careful attention to these orders, agency policies, and advance directives to be prepared if the patient suffers a cardiopulmonary arrest. For an example of a DNAR (DNR, AND) order,

 Go to Chapter 17, **Forms, Do Not Resuscitate Orders,** in Volume 2.

In many healthcare settings, cardiopulmonary resuscitation (CPR) is performed almost automatically. This practice may be slowly changing, however, as the AHA provides guidance on the appropriate use of CPR. For example, in considering whether DNAR (DNR, AND) is appropriate, emphasis is placed on the efficacy of CPR attempts, balancing the benefits and burdens and therapeutic goals (ANA, 2012).

You should carefully explain to patients and families what CPR involves and their available options. They should know that the physician cannot write a DNAR order without their permission. They have the right to refuse CPR and may request the physician to write a DNAR (AND) order. The American Nurses Association (ANA, 2004, 2012) recommendations regarding DNAR (AND) are summarized in Box 17-3. For a complete list of the ANA recommendations,

 Go to Chapter 17, **Tables, Boxes, Figures: ESG Box 17-2,** on Davis*Plus*.

There is growing evidence that strategies, such as formal and informal family meetings, daily team consensus processes, palliative care team case finding, and ethics consultation, improve communication about end-of-life decisions (Boyle, Miller, & Forbes-Thompson, 2005).

Assisted Suicide

Assisted suicide means making available that which is needed for the patient to end his own life (e.g., pharmacological agents or weapons). The patient is physically capable of ending his own life, has expressed the intention to do so, and has turned to the healthcare provider merely to supply the means. Although physician-assisted suicide is legal in a few states, the ANA (1994a, 1994b, 2013) continues to oppose assisted suicide. "ANA prohibits nurses' participation in assisted suicide and euthanasia because these are in direct violation of *Code of Ethics for Nurses With Interpretive Statements* . . . , the ethical traditions and goals

BOX 17-3 ■ Highlights of ANA Recommendations Concerning DNAR/AND

- The competent patient's choices have highest priority when there is conflict.

- When the patient is not competent, give highest priority to advance directives or the surrogate decision makers.

- DNAR orders should be discussed explicitly with the patient and significant others.

- DNAR orders must be documented, reviewed, and updated.

- DNAR does *not* mean "discontinue care" or substandard care!

- Nurses should be aware of and have an active role in developing DNAR policies in the institutions where they work; they should participate in interdisciplinary mechanisms for resolving disputes among patients, families, and healthcare practitioners concerning DNAR orders.

- Nurses should consider the acronym AND (allow natural death) because the word *death* makes the intent clear.

- Nurses have a responsibility to avoid participation in "slow codes" or "partial codes."

- Nurses have a duty to educate patients and families about technologies and termination of treatment decisions, and to encourage them to think about end-of-life preferences and make their wishes known in advance.

- Nurses have a duty to communicate relevant information and to advocate for a patient's end-of-life preferences to be honored.

Source: Adapted from American Nurses Association (ANA). (2004). Position statement: Nursing care and do-not-resuscitate decisions. Retrieved from http://ana.nursingworld.org/MainMenuCategories/EthicsStandards/Ethics-Position-Statements/Copy%20of%20dnr0414405.aspx; American Nurses Association (ANA). (2012). Revised position statement: Nursing care and Do Not Resuscitate (DNR) and Allow Natural Death (AND) decisions. Retrieved April 19, 2013, from http://www.nursingworld.org/dnrposition

---

of the profession, and its covenant with society" (ANA, 2013). Assisted suicide violates the ethical principle of nonmaleficence (Friend, 2011).

Some advocate the use of continuous sedation until death as an alternative to assisted suicide (Raus, Sterckx, & Mortier, 2011). The Hospice and Palliative Nurses Association promotes **palliative sedation** as the "controlled and monitored use of non-opioid medications intended to lower the patient's level of consciousness to the extent necessary, for relief of awareness of refractory and unendurable symptoms" (Hospice and Palliative Nurses Association, 2011, pg. 1).

Euthanasia

The term **euthanasia** comes from the Greek word *euthanatos*, which means "good death." It refers to the deliberate ending of the life of someone suffering from a terminal or incurable illness. **Active euthanasia** occurs as a result of a direct action (e.g., giving an overdose of

medication). Active euthanasia can be *voluntary* (patient consents); *involuntary* (patient refuses); or *nonvoluntary* (patient is unable to consent, or someone else makes the decision and the patient is unaware of it). Active euthanasia goes a step further than assisted suicide. In assisted suicide, the person assisting makes available the means for the person to take his own life; in euthanasia, the assistant also serves as the direct agent of death (e.g., administers the medication).

Passive euthanasia occurs as a result of a *lack* of action (e.g., withholding medications or food necessary to sustain life). Honoring the patient's refusal of treatments is not generally considered passive euthanasia and can be ethically and legally permissible. For more information about the ethical and legal issues surrounding euthanasia, see Chapters 44 and 45, respectively.

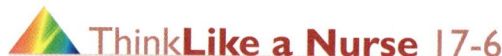 ### ThinkLike a Nurse 17-6

What are your feelings about assisted suicide, continuous sedation, and euthanasia? Focus on your feelings, not on principles, explanations, and rationales.

Autopsy

An autopsy is a medical examination of the body to determine the cause of death. Autopsies have also provided relevant data about disease processes and causes. The pathologist performs a detailed internal and external evaluation of the body, removes body organs, and extracts sample tissues for further examination. The organs are then replaced in the body, and the body cavities are closed with sutures. An autopsy requires signed permission from the next of kin, except in cases in which autopsy is required by law (e.g., suspicious or unwitnessed deaths).

Organ Donation

The Uniform Anatomical Gift Act (UACA) provides guidance on tissue, eye, and organ donation (National Conference of Commissioners on Uniform State Laws, 2009). The new act specifically added language that would prevent others from overriding an individual's prior decision regarding organ donation. However, there remain ethical concerns that the new UAGA might result in donors being maintained on life support against their family's wishes.

Key Point: *A conflict between a potential organ donor's advance directives and measures to ensure the viability of his organs (e.g., life support) must be resolved as soon as possible, by one of the following, in this order: (1) the donor (if able), (2) the surrogate decision maker, or (3) another person as authorized under state law. Until resolution, maintaining the suitability of the organs has the highest priority. You should advocate that your patient's advance directives are clear on end-of-life care and organ donation.*

The UAGA has been adopted in all but four states (as of May 2013). In general, the UAGA states the following:

- As a rule, general donors must be at least 18 years of age or an emancipated minor.

- Next of kin can donate organs when a person dies, unless an objection is known.
- Relatives cannot revoke a person's donation, even after death.
- The person making the gift can amend or revoke it at any time.

To see the UAGA major provisions in greater detail,

 Go to Chapter 17, **Tables, Boxes, Figures: ESG Box 17-3, Major Provisions of the Uniform Anatomical Gift Act,** on *DavisPlus.*

Many states issue identification cards or allow driver's licenses to be amended to identify a person as an organ donor. However, even though donor cards are legal in all states, many institutions will not procure organs from the deceased if there is strong family objection (Fig. 17-2). Therefore, if a patient is planning to donate organs or tissues, be sure that he discusses these wishes with family members. If death is imminent, a healthcare team member (physician or nurse) should ask whether the patient has agreed to be an organ donor, has a donor card, or is registered with the state's donor database. In many institutions, a transplant coordinator contacts the family and makes the request for organ and tissue donation.

KnowledgeCheck 17-3

- What are advance directives?
- What is the ANA's position on assisted suicide?

PracticalKnowledge
knowing **how**

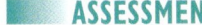

ASSESSMENT

When a patient is dying or has experienced a loss, you must carefully assess the patient and significant others for the common physical, emotional, behavioral, and cognitive grief reactions. For a list of these, along with guidelines to follow when assessing dying and grieving patients,

 Go to Chapter 17, **Assessment Guidelines and Tools,** in Volume 2.

Other important areas to assess include knowledge base, history of loss, coping patterns and abilities, meaning of the loss or illness, and support systems. For dying patients, you should also make the following assessments:

- When the client and family are ready, encourage them to talk about the client's wishes for burial or cremation or tasks that the client would like taken care of (e.g., giving away valuables, calling family members).
- Determine whether the dying client has advance directives (e.g., living will, durable power of attorney for healthcare).

Is It Grief or Depression?

When you are performing a focused assessment for grief or loss, you will need to distinguish between grief and depression. Sadness and depression are an integral part of grief. However, depression that lingers beyond what is expected may be a sign that the stress of grieving has triggered a major depressive episode (Ferszt & Leveillee, 2006; Widera & Block, 2012). Although grief and depression have several symptoms in common (e.g., sadness, insomnia, poor appetite, and weight loss), grief tends to come and go—to be triggered, for example, by a holiday. For help in differentiating them,

 Go to Chapter 17, **Assessment Guidelines and Tools, Assessing Grief and Loss,** in Volume 2.

KnowledgeCheck 17-4

What assessments should you make for your terminally ill patient and his or her family?

ANALYSIS/DIAGNOSIS

When you are analyzing patient data, keep in mind that most grief is normal, not complicated or dysfunctional. You must determine whether loss and grieving are the problem or the etiology, because the etiology will influence your interventions. Also note that the same diagnoses can be used in the context of death, dying, grief, or loss.

Loss and Grieving as Problem Various nursing diagnoses may be appropriate for a person who is dying or grieving. The two most obvious ones are Grieving and Complicated Grieving. Do not use a Complicated Grieving diagnosis for every person who is grieving a loss. Complicated Grieving is disabling pain and grief, characterized by long-term grieving (perhaps years), functional impairment, and/or intense emotions. The person may deny or have difficulty expressing feelings of loss or may experience physical symptoms as a result of suppressing feelings.

Organ/Tissue Donor Card

I wish to donate my organs and tissues. I wish to give:

☐ any needed organs and tissues   ☐ only the following organs and tissues:

_____

Donor
Signature _____ Date _____
Witness _____
Witness _____

FIGURE 17-2 **Example of an organ donor card.** (*Source:* U.S. Department of Health and Human Services. Retrieved May 20, 2013, from http://dying.about.com/od/livingafteradeath/ss/organdonate_3.htm)

Other diagnoses may include Ineffective Denial, Hopelessness, Powerlessness, Chronic Sorrow, Spiritual Distress, Self-Neglect, Constipation, and many other physiological diagnoses. To see the defining characteristics of NANDA-I diagnoses representing emotional responses to loss or impeding death,

 Go to Chapter 17, **Standardized Language, NOC Outcomes and Interventions for Loss and Grieving Diagnoses,** on DavisPlus.

 Think**Like a Nurse** 17-7

Refer to the table in Standardized Nursing Language, NOC Outcomes and Interventions on DavisPlus. Answer the questions in the table. Also refer to a nursing diagnosis handbook and NIC and NOC manuals, if needed.

Loss and Grieving as Etiology Loss, grief, and dying are an etiology when they create problems in other areas of patient or family function. The following are examples of such nursing diagnoses.

- Situational or Chronic Low Self-Esteem related to inability to change the event for self or significant other; or related to dying while having "unfinished business"
- Anxiety related to inability to cope with the loss; or related to unknown outcome of situation
- Death Anxiety (or Fear) related to impending death
- Decisional Conflict related to end-of-life treatment measures (e.g., concern about the expense of "useless" procedures or their effect on the family; knowledge that the treatment may lengthen life but decrease the quality of life)
- Deficient Knowledge related to the new experience of caring for a terminally ill person
- Fatigue related to demands of caring for a dying loved one
- Spiritual Distress related to loss of trust in a loving God

PLANNING OUTCOMES/EVALUATION

Encourage the patient and family to play an active role in planning care. Involving family members helps facilitate their acceptance of the diagnosis and may put the patient more at ease. Questions such as the following will help to elicit the patient's goals for end of life (Matzo & Sherman, 2009; Weissman, Quill, & Arnold, 2010):

- "What do you still want to accomplish or do?"
- "What are the things you wish you could still do?"
- "Whom would you like to see?"
- "What would make you 'medically comfortable'?"
- "If you have pain, what would be an acceptable level for you, on a 0 to 10 scale?"
- "Where do you want to spend the rest of your life? Where are you most comfortable?"
- "If spiritual peace is important to you, what would help you achieve it?"

NOC standardized outcomes are determined by the diagnostic label you use. For examples,

 Go to Chapter 17, **NOC Outcomes and NIC Interventions for Loss and Grieving Diagnoses,** on DavisPlus.

Individualized goals/outcome statements you might write for a grieving or dying person include the following examples. The patient and/or family will:

- Communicate openly among themselves and health-care providers (e.g., express fear, concerns, pain)
- Obtain satisfactory pain relief and symptom management
- Use all resources available to assist with coping
- Exercise control in the management of care to the extent possible

As always, you will use the goals set in the planning stage as criteria for evaluating the patient's or family's health status.

Knowledge Check 17-5

- List three nursing diagnosis labels you might consider when dying or grieving is the primary problem.
- List three nursing diagnosis labels that might occur as a result of dying or grieving.

PLANNING INTERVENTIONS/IMPLEMENTATION

NIC standardized interventions associated with death, dying, and bereavement are found on DavisPlus.

 Go to Chapter 17, **NOC Outcomes and NIC Interventions for Loss and Grieving Diagnoses,** on DavisPlus.

Specific nursing activities are determined by the nursing diagnosis, especially by the etiology. Your ability to help someone who is grieving or dying is largely determined by your attitude. A compassionate approach is essential but may be challenging. Watching patients struggle with pain, loss, grief, and death may stir our own deepest doubts and fears, and we may reject the challenge to respond from the heart. We may be aware that employers usually reward nurses for what they *do* rather than who they *are* as people, so it is easy to rationalize that we have other tasks to accomplish that may be equally important. When we do that, we ignore the real gift we have to offer the suffering patient is our willingness to "walk the walk" with them, if even for a short time. Full-spectrum nurses combine their psychomotor and thinking skills with compassion in ministering to those who are suffering.

Some important nursing interventions, including therapeutic communication, facilitating grief work, helping families, and specific activities involved in care of the dying person, are discussed in the following sections. Also see the Nursing Care Plan and Care Map for Grieving.

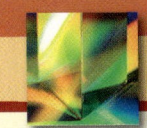

Nursing Care Plan

Client Data

Wilma Peterson is caring for her son, Henry, who has AIDS. Henry is 20 years old; his older brother, William, died at home of AIDS-related pneumonia 2 years earlier at age 24. William had left home at 18 to live in Miami and returned to his home in rural Alabama when he became too ill to manage on his own. Henry stayed home to help his mother care for William and learned he was HIV-positive just before his brother died. Henry did not tell his mother of his diagnosis until he was hospitalized for the first time with cytomegalovirus (CMV) infection. Since then, he has not followed nutritional and medical advice and has continued to stay out late and party when he feels well enough. His health has steadily declined.

You are participating in a special Caring for the Caregiver program set up by the public health nurse in your community. In this program, registered nurses visit primary caregivers to assess their needs and offer support services as needed. You are assigned to Wilma Peterson.

Ms. Peterson is initially cordial when you visit but tells you, "This is a mother's responsibility. I don't stop being his mother because he's grown up. I'm always his mother." As your discussion continues, Ms. Peterson wistfully talks about when William and Henry were boys. She says, "I didn't really understand this awful disease until William got so sick. Now, I look at Henry and I know what's waiting for him. I know we are going to lose him. Sad . . . just so sad. . . ." Her voice trails off as tears well in her eyes.

Nursing Diagnosis

Grieving related to the client's anticipating the loss of a second son, as evidenced by her previous experience caring for her other son who died at home of AIDS and by the client's stating, "I know what's waiting for him."

NOC Outcomes	Individualized Goals / Expected Outcomes
Family Coping (NOC 2600) Psychosocial Adjustment: Life Change (NOC 1305)	*(Short-term goals) At the end of the initial home visit, Ms. Peterson will:* 1. Identify community resources available to help her care for Henry at home during acute illnesses. 2. Begin to feel comfortable discussing her concerns with the nurse. *(Long-term goals) Within 6 weeks, Ms. Peterson will:* 1. Explore activities she would like to participate in once she is no longer caring for Henry. 2. Talk with Henry to learn what type of funeral he would like.

(continued on next page)

Nursing Care Plan (continued)

NIC Interventions*

Anticipatory Guidance (NIC 5210)
Coping Enhancement (NIC 5230)
Grief Work Facilitation (NIC 5290)

Nursing Activities	Rationales
1. Encourage Ms. Peterson to talk about her experiences caring for William before he died.	1. Grieving often occurs in the context of repeated caregiving (Boyle, Bunting, Hodnicki, et al., 2001) or in situations in which the caregiver has other types of previous experience with the same or a similar terminal illness. Supportive communication allows for asking questions, sharing information, and ultimately coming to terms with the loss (Ostler, 2010).
2. Ask her to relate similarities and differences between care for William and care for Henry.	2. Asking the client to discuss previous experiences allows the nurse to validate the nursing diagnosis (O'Connor & Lunney, 1998) and provides an opportunity for the client to discuss her specific needs (Kelly, Malloy, Munevar, et al., 2010).
3. Ask Ms. Peterson to describe the elements of Henry's care and to identify which she considers to be the most important.	3. Clients are holistic and consider more than just medical treatment in the care of a family member. Their actions are often based on care needed, cultural and religious beliefs, and previous experiences instead of a medically based care plan. Clients may operate on a different, parallel track from that of the healthcare providers (Boyle, Bunting, Hodnicki, et al., 2001). By asking Ms. Peterson how she prioritizes and provides Henry's care, the nurse can learn from the client rather than making assumptions based on the healthcare perspective. By showing respect for her experience as a caregiver, the nurse can build a stronger relationship with Ms. Peterson, which will facilitate future nursing interventions and anticipatory guidance (Reinhard, Given, Petlick, et al., 2008).
4. Talk with Ms. Peterson to find out what community resources she used when she cared for William and whether she has accessed them now in caring for Henry.	4. Isolation and loneliness are risk factors for sole caregivers at home. By assessing community resources, the nurse can determine whether Ms. Peterson is "connected" or isolating herself. Isolation and previous loss put her at risk for Complicated Grieving (Lobb, Kristjanson, Aoun, et al., 2010). Many community resources provide a sense of belonging and enhance and support coping strategies as well.
5. Promote shared decision making if this is acceptable to Henry Peterson.	5. Informing both Ms. Peterson and Henry about the disease, prognosis, treatment, and comfort options allows them to retain some control over their lives together, which is essential for effective palliative care (Teno, Casey, Welch, et al., 2001; Wilson, Gott, & Ingleton, 2013). Henry's permission must be obtained to preserve his autonomy.
6. Provide nonjudgmental emotional support to Ms. Peterson, and support healthy coping activities she is using.	6. Establishing a comfortable and emotionally safe environment will allow Ms. Peterson to share her concerns without fear of being judged because of her son's diagnosis (Boyle, Bunting, Hodnicki, et al., 2001; Milberg & Strang, 2011).

---

*Interventions are only a sample of those linked to this diagnosis by *NIC*. Activities should be individualized for each client.

Nursing Care Plan (continued)

Evaluation

Review the initial short-term outcomes and goals. Reassess your client to determine whether the goals are achieved in the stated time frame. In this case, long-term goals will fluctuate based on the progression of Henry's illness. The following occurred as the care plan was implemented:

- Ms. Peterson cried as she described the deterioration in William's health before he died. She worries that Henry will suffer and does not want him to lose his dignity the way she believes William did.

- Ms. Peterson's greatest concern is that Henry is not eating enough. Much of her self-value as a mother arises from her ability to prepare homemade meals to feed her family, and Henry doesn't have much of an appetite. This is very distressing to her.

- She has not contacted community agencies. She is holding off, hoping Henry will not be "so sick for so long. With these new drugs, he can get better."

- She remains involved in her church, which is the same one she attended as a little girl. However, she will not tell her church group that Henry has AIDS. "They talk too much," she says. Instead, she says he has leukemia.

Only one short-term goal is met at this visit—establishing a comfort level between the client and the nurse. Ms. Peterson has not identified community resources related to caring for Henry at this time.

Plan for Further Evaluation

Additional supportive visits will be needed to help Ms. Peterson understand that contacting community agencies does not mean Henry will die sooner. An important coping mechanism for Ms. Peterson is denying the need for community help; however, it is not affecting her ability to care for her son. If his condition worsens, this issue will need to be promptly addressed.

References

Boyle, J. S., Bunting, S. M., Hodnicki, D. R., et al. (2001). Critical thinking in black mothers who care for adult children with HIV: A cultural analysis. *Journal of Transcultural Nursing, 12*(3), 193–202.

Bulechek, G., Butcher, H., & Dochterman, J. M. (2013). *Nursing interventions classification (NIC)* (6th ed.). St. Louis, MO: C. V. Mosby.

Johnson, M., Moorhead, S., Bulechek, G., et al. (2013). *NOC and NIC Linkages to NANDA-I and clinical conditions* (3rd ed.). St. Louis, MO: C. V. Mosby.

Kelly, K., Malloy, P., Munevar, C., et al. (2010). Beyond bad news: communication skills of nurses in palliative care. *Journal of Hospice and Palliative Nursing, 12*(3), 166–174.

Lobb, E., Kristjanson, L., Aoun, S., et al. (2010). Predictors of complicated grief: A systematic review of empirical studies. *Death Studies, 34*(8), 673–698.

Matzo, M., Shermann, D., Sheehan, D., et al. (2003). Teaching strategies from the ELNEC curriculum. *Nursing Education Perspectives, 21*(1), 176–183.

Milberg, A., & Strang, P. (2011). Protection against perceptions of powerlessness and helplessness during palliative care: The family members' perspective. *Palliative & Supportive Care, 9*(3), 251–262.

Moorhead, S., Johnson, M., Maas, M., et al. (2013). *Nursing outcomes classification (NOC)* (5th ed.). St. Louis, MO: C. V. Mosby

O'Connor, L., & Lunney, M. (1998). Care of the caregiver—family member with a chronic illness. *Nursing Diagnosis, 9*(4), 152.

Ostler, T. (2010). Grief and coping in early childhood: The role of communication in the mourning process. *Zero to Three, 31*(1), 29–35.

Reinhard, S., Given, B., Petlick, N., et al. (2008). Supporting family caregivers in providing support. In R. Hughes (Ed.), *Patient safety and quality: An evidence-based handbook for nurses* (Chapter 14). Rockville, MD: Agency for Healthcare Research and Quality. Retrieved April 25, 2013, from http://www.ncbi.nlm.nih.gov/books/NBK2665/

Teno, J. M., Casey, V. A., Welch, L. C., et al. (2001). Patient-focused, family-centered end-of-life medical care: Views of the guidelines and bereaved family members. *Journal of Pain and Symptom Management, 22*, 738–751.

Wilson, F., Gott, M., & Ingleton, C. (2013). Perceived risks around choice and decision making at end-of-life: A literature review. *Palliative Medicine, 27*(1), 38–53.

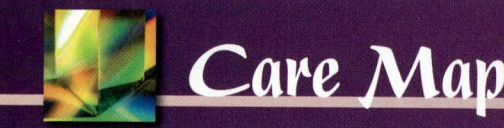

Care Map

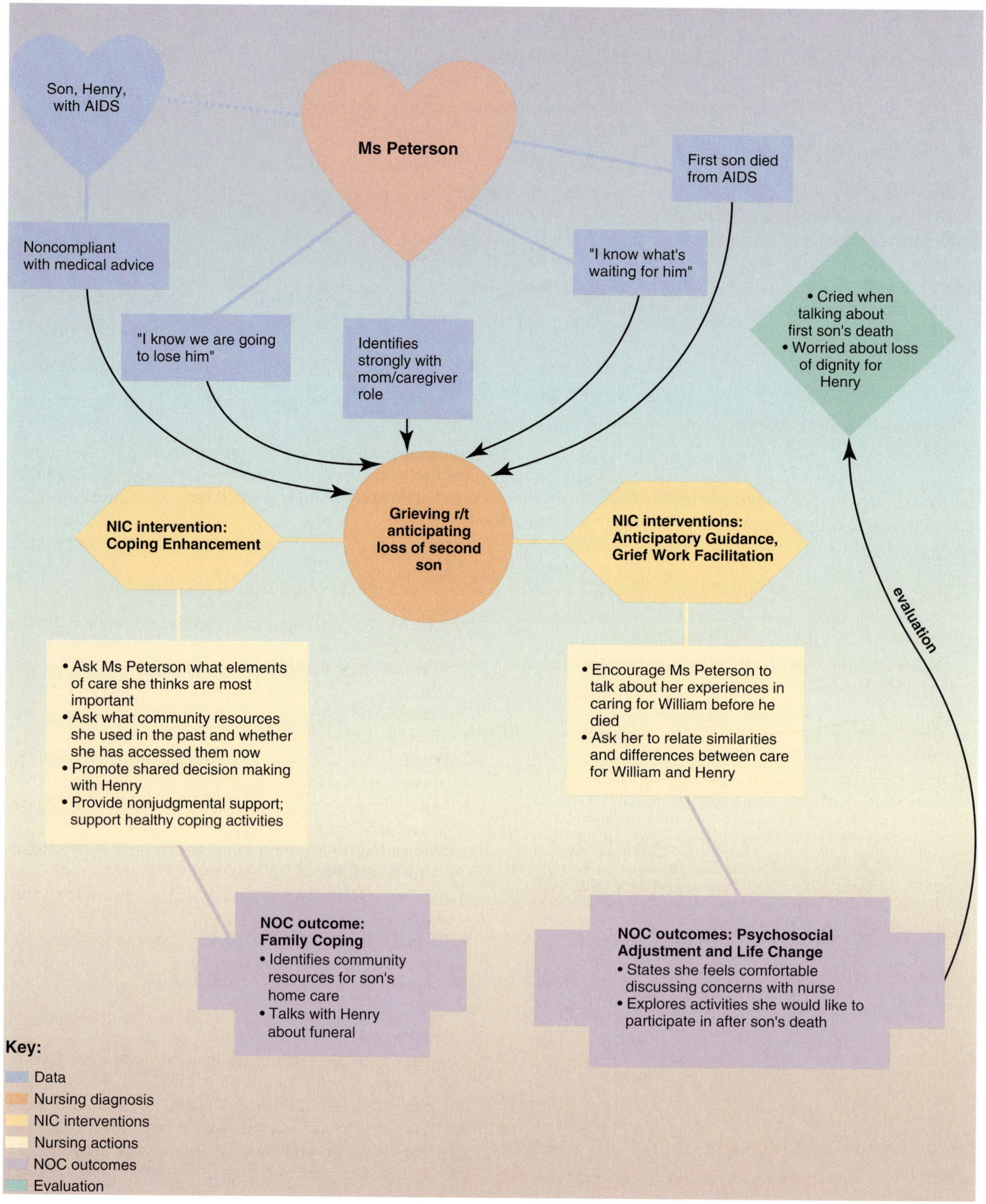

Son, Henry, with AIDS

Ms Peterson

First son died from AIDS

Noncompliant with medical advice

"I know what's waiting for him"

• Cried when talking about first son's death
• Worried about loss of dignity for Henry

"I know we are going to lose him"

Identifies strongly with mom/caregiver role

Grieving r/t anticipating loss of second son

NIC intervention: Coping Enhancement

NIC interventions: Anticipatory Guidance, Grief Work Facilitation

evaluation

• Ask Ms Peterson what elements of care she thinks are most important
• Ask what community resources she used in the past and whether she has accessed them now
• Promote shared decision making with Henry
• Provide nonjudgmental support; support healthy coping activities

• Encourage Ms Peterson to talk about her experiences in caring for William before he died
• Ask her to relate similarities and differences between care for William and Henry

NOC outcome: Family Coping
• Identifies community resources for son's home care
• Talks with Henry about funeral

NOC outcomes: Psychosocial Adjustment and Life Change
• States she feels comfortable discussing concerns with nurse
• Explores activities she would like to participate in after son's death

Key:

Data

Nursing diagnosis

NIC interventions

Nursing actions

NOC outcomes

Evaluation

Therapeutic Communication

Therapeutic communication is critical to building a trusting relationship with the dying or **grieving** patient and their significant others (Fig. 17-3). It is most important to listen to the dying patient and to be alert for and respond to nonverbal cues. Encourage patients and family members to express their feelings, and reassure them that their feelings are normal and not "wrong." In discussions about DNAR (AND) or withholding or withdrawing treatments, it is important to find out why the patient is seeking that option: Does she wish to avoid suffering, or does she fear being a burden to loved ones?

Physicians and nurses should always work to improve their communication skills because they are essential for achieving better outcomes at end of life (Boyle, Miller, & Forbes-Thompson, 2005; Galushko, Romotzky, & Voltz, 2012). See Box 17-4 for some barriers to end-of-life communication. For tips on communicating with people who are dying or bereaved,

 Go to Chapter 17, **Clinical Insight 17-1: Communicating With People Who Are Grieving,** in Volume 2.

If you need more information on communication and therapeutic relationships, refer to Chapter 21.

Facilitating Grief Work

Whether grief results from a loss of health, from an impending death, or from some other loss, you can help patients and families work through their grief by helping them express their feelings, recall memories, and find meaning in their lives. Later in this chapter, we discuss interventions for helping families after the death of a loved one. This section focuses more generally on grieving *any* loss.

Expressing Feelings

It is the family, not just an individual patient, who grieves a death or loss. Grief is a normal process, and for people and to deal with it in a healthy way they must

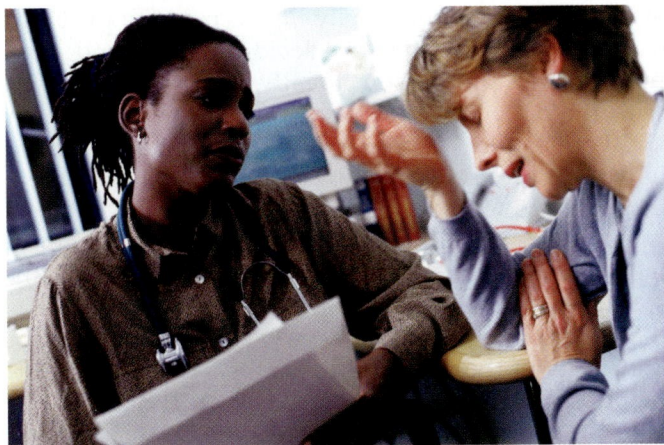

FIGURE 17-3 The nurse encourages and accepts expression of feelings.

BOX 17-4 ■ Barriers to End-of-Life Communication

- Fear of one's own mortality
- Unresolved personal grief issues (e.g., the loss of one's own parent)
- Lack of experience with death and dying
- Fear of expressing emotion (i.e., crying)
- Fear of not knowing the answer to a question
- Not knowing whether to give an honest (and possibly unwelcome) answer to a question
- Not understanding the family's culture
- Keeping physical distance (e.g., standing away from the person or avoiding eye contact)
- Insensitivity: interrupting communication, patronizing, giving false reassurance

Sources: Malloy, P., Virani, R., Kelly, K., et al. (2008). End-of-life care: Improving communication skills to enhance palliative care. *Medscape*. Retrieved April 27, 2013, from http://www.medscape .org/viewprogram/12632; Matzo, M., Shermann, D., Sheehan, D., et al. (2003). Teaching strategies from the ELNEC curriculum.

---

communicate their feeling. Sometimes people are uncomfortable expressing their feeling and will hold them in. These self-contained emotions will interfere with their grief resolution, so you may need to facilitate the process, using your therapeutic communication skills (refer to Chapter 21 as needed). The following are some ways to facilitate expression of feelings:

- Encourage questions, and respond to them within a reasonable time.
- Sit beside the head of the bed; do not appear rushed.
- When you observe the patient or family member expressing feelings, either verbally or nonverbally, encourage them to continue.
- Expect and accept a wide range of feelings, including anger, fear, and loneliness.
- Ask, "How would you like me to help?" "What do you need?"
- Be sure that everyone on the healthcare team understands and follows the care plan.
- Ask yourself what you would do if this were your family member.
- Do not compare another person's loss with your own experience. Avoid comments such as "I know how you feel." Instead, say, "Tell me how you feel."

Recalling Memories

Grieving patients and family members may need to recall memories, both good and difficult. One way to encourage recall is to go through photo albums with them and ask questions about the people in the pictures. Also look for objects of sentiment (e.g., a family heirloom) in the environment and ask the dying or bereaved person to share their significance.

Finding Meaning

Another way to facilitate grief work is to help the patient or family find meaning in their lives or in their past. Talking through this meaning is a healthy way to cope. Facilitating life review is one technique to help the patient and/or family recognize the unique contributions this person has made to family, friends, and society. You can begin by asking about the various aspects of the patient's life (e.g., "What were some of his favorite hobbies/activities?"), commenting on pictures in the room, or picking up on verbal cues that are expressed.

Bibliotherapy

Bibliotherapy is a counseling technique used when grief therapy is indicated. It uses guided reading of self-help literature or fiction to increase client awareness and understanding and promote healing. Poems, novels, and essays can help produce new insights, either as the client retells the story or is guided to discuss his feelings and thoughts about the characters in the story (Briggs & Pehrsson, 2008; Songprakun & McCann, 2012).

 ### ThinkLike a Nurse 17-8

- What would you say to Mrs. Manning (Meet Your Patient) if you walked into a room and found her sitting in a chair and softly weeping while Mr. Manning sleeps?
- What response would you make when Mr. Manning waves his hand in the air and says, "I'm not taking any more of those damn pills" as you bring him his medications?
- A young woman approaches you in the hall and says, "I want to visit Mom and stay with her, but I just can't stand to see her like that. I feel guilty for wanting to leave." What would be your therapeutic response?

Helping Families of Dying Patients

When a patient is dying, it is important to view the family as your unit of care. If the patient is unresponsive, you may find yourself spending most of your care time with the family. This time should be spent providing education, support, and a listening ear. Observing their loved one dying can leave family members feeling confused, angry, helpless, and even devastated. Sensitive, compassionate nursing care is always essential, especially during this time. You can use the interventions in the preceding sections as you help family members to understand that what they see may be very different from what the patient is experiencing. For more specific interventions for helping families of dying patients,

 Go to Chapter 17, **Clinical Insight 17-2: Helping Families of Dying Patients,** in Volume 2.

KnowledgeCheck 17-6

- Describe four ways to facilitate the grief work of a grieving or dying person.
- List two specific interventions, in addition to facilitating grief work, for helping grieving families.

Caring for the Dying Person

To effectively care for terminally ill patients, you must meet their physiological, psychological, social, sexual, and spiritual needs. Most hospitals and hospice facilities have an interdisciplinary team to provide holistic care to dying patients and their families. This team may be made up of a physician, nurse, social worker, pastoral care worker, nutritionist, physical therapist (and sometimes occupational and speech therapists), and volunteers.

Meeting Physiological Needs

Active dying usually occurs over a period of 10 to 14 days (although it can take as little as 24 hours). The "final hours" refers to the last 4 to 48 hours of life, in which failure of body systems results in death (Brennan, Prince-Paul, & Wiencek, 2011; Pitorak, 2003). In the last hours of life, most patients need skilled care around the clock. Physiological needs during this time include mobility, oxygenation, safety, nutrition, fluids, elimination, personal hygiene, and control of pain and symptoms (nausea, vomiting).

 Research shows that older adults with refractory dyspnea from conditions such as heart failure or chronic obstructive pulmonary disease are not getting adequate symptom management because of fear of hastening death or other concerns. Nurses should work with members of the interdisciplinary healthcare team to ensure that patients receive the "most effective pharmacological treatment for the palliation of refractory dyspnea" (Lowey, Powers, & Xue, 2013, p. 50).

See the previous discussion of the physiological stages of dying to review signs of impending death. For specific interventions and guidelines to use when caring for a dying patient,

 Go to Chapter 17, **Clinical Insight 17-3: Caring for the Dying Person: Meeting Physiological Needs,** in Volume 2.

Meeting Psychological Needs

When a patient is terminally ill, the primary provider is usually responsible for deciding what and how much to tell the person. Ideally, everyone involved with the patient should have input into this decision and you should know exactly what he and the family have been told. Most patients want to know their prognosis as soon as possible so that they can put personal affairs in order, share their feelings with family members, and come to terms with their life and death. A systematic review of research suggests that rather than protecting patients, efforts to shield patients from the reality of their situation usually create greater difficulties for them (Hancock, Clayton, Parker, et al., 2007). A "conspiracy of silence" causes fear, anxiety, and confusion, and denies people the opportunity to make needed life adaptations. However, culture may determine which family members are to be informed and how much, if any, information is given to the patient. You should seek guidance for the proper balance between cultural influences and the patient's autonomy. Also, many patients realize without being told that they are dying. For specific interventions to help meet the psychological needs of dying patients,

 Go to Chapter 17, **Clinical Insight 17-4: Caring for the Dying Person: Meeting Psychological Needs,** in Volume 2.

KnowledgeCheck 17-7

- Describe six nursing interventions to use in meeting the physiological needs of a dying person.
- Describe six nursing interventions to use in meeting the psychological needs of a dying person.
- What should be the focus of your interventions when the patient is very near death?

Addressing Spiritual Needs

When a person is terminally ill, his spirituality may become very important as he searches for meaning in the illness and suffering. The person may be looking for forgiveness and/or acceptance or be reaching out to feel connected. Ways to address this need include (but are not limited to) empathetic listening, contacting pastoral care or clergy if the patient asks for this service, special rituals, praying with the patient, music, meditation, or special readings.

Information about specific religious practices may help you provide appropriate interventions at end of life. For example, after the death of an Orthodox Jewish patient, you should handle the body as little as possible if you are not Jewish. Most Christian denominations will not object to your washing and preparing the body. Remember, though, that there are wide individual differences and that you must assess each patient and family to determine how closely they adhere to the rituals of their religion. Review Chapters 15 and 16, as needed. For detailed information about a variety of religious practices surrounding death,

 Go to Chapter 17, **Supplemental Materials: Addressing Spiritual Needs,** on DavisPlus.

Toward Evidence-Based Practice

Hancock, K., Clayton, J. M., Parker, S. M., et al. (2007). Truthtelling in discussing prognosis in advanced life-limiting illnesses: A systematic review. *Palliative Medicine, 21,* 507–517.

This was a systematic review of 46 studies related to truthtelling in discussing prognosis with patients with progressive, advanced life-limiting illnesses and their caregivers. Results revealed the following:

- Many health professionals expressed discomfort at having to inform the patient and family of limited life expectancy. Although the majority thought that patients and their caregivers should be told the truth, many either withhold information about prognosis or avoid discussing it.
- Reasons for not telling the truth include perceived lack of training, stress, no time to attend to the patient's emotional needs, fear of a negative effect on the patient, uncertainty about the prognosis, requests from family to withhold information, and feeling inadequate because further curative treatment was not available.

Fine, E., Reid, C., Shengelia, R., et al. (2010). Directly observed patient–physician discussions in palliative and end-of-life care: A systematic review of the literature. *Journal of Palliative Medicine, 13(5),* 595–603.

Researchers reviewed 20 studies that used direct observations in end-of-life/palliative communications. Several common themes emerged. Physicians tended to dominate the discussions and focused more on medical/technical aspects. Emphasis was not placed on emotional or quality of life issues. Patient satisfaction was associated with supportive behaviors by physicians.

Gramling, R., Norton, S., Ladwig, S., et al. (2013). Direct observation of prognosis communication in palliative care: A descriptive study. *Journal of Pain & Symptom Management, 45(2),* 202–412.

Researchers audio-recorded the initial visit of 71 seriously ill patients and their families who were referred for discussions of end-of-life decision making or goal clarification. Results identified these major themes: (1) Patient-focused quality of life discussions occurred more frequently than did survival discussions focused on the general population. (2) Pessimistic cues regarding prognosis occurred more often than did optimistic ones.

1. Based on these research results, do you think health professionals should inform patients when they have an advanced life-limiting (terminal) illness? What should be the focus of the communication? Explain your thinking.

2. Health professionals feared a negative effect on patients of telling them the truth about their condition. What sorts of negative effects do you think they might be anticipating?

3. What should be the goal of communications between health professionals and terminally ill patients related to end-of-life care?

 Go to Chapter 17, **Toward Evidence-Based Practice Suggested Responses,** on DavisPlus.

Addressing Cultural Needs

Cultural values can influence a person's openness to discussions regarding death and his end-of-life healthcare preferences. Researchers found that regardless of ethnicity or gender, end-of-life concerns important to most people include comfort, physician communication, having responsibilities taken care of, support, hope and optimism, and honoring spiritual beliefs. Other concerns were being cared for, love and compassion, expressing feelings, fixing relationships, saying goodbye, having choices, making plans, not being in pain or unable to breathe, and being "ready to go" (Duffy, Jackson, Schim, et al., 2006; Valente, 2010).

There is some overlap between religious and cultural practices. For example, most cultural groups engage in some type of religious ceremony that helps the bereaved begin the grieving process (Fig. 17-4). Nevertheless, some death rituals and expressions of grief may be culture based but not necessarily involve religion. For example:

- Some cultures may emphasize keeping emotions more subdued and limiting expressions of grief to private settings, whereas others gauge the value of the deceased by the amount of wailing and crying (Fig. 17-5).
- Blacks and Hispanics may be reluctant to withdraw life-sustaining treatment or to use a hospice, whereas Arab Muslims may be reluctant to prolong life unnecessarily (Duffy, Jackson, Schim, et al., 2006; Health Care Chaplaincy, updated 2013).

Despite the commonalities among groups, there are some culture-specific differences. To provide culturally sensitive care at end of life, you will need some information about specific cultural practices surrounding death. For this information,

 Go to Chapter 17, **Supplemental Materials: Addressing Cultural Needs**, on DavisPlus.

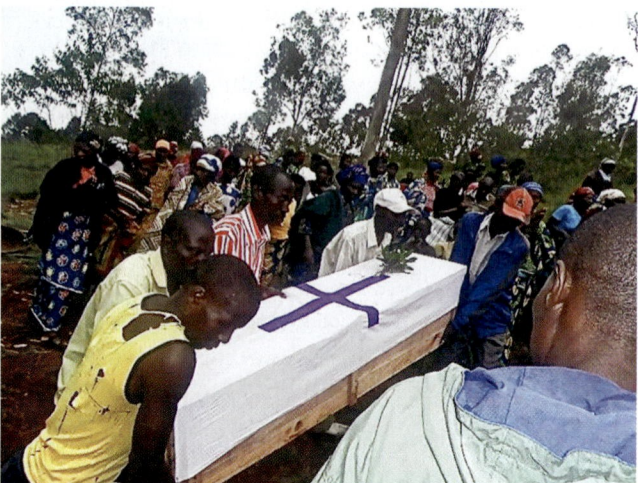

FIGURE 17-4 After death, rituals (e.g., this Rwandan burial) are viewed as respect for the deceased and help friends and family bring closure.

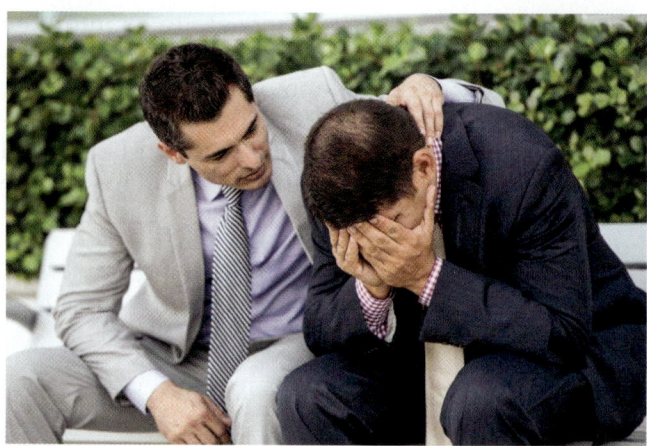

FIGURE 17-5 Family openly expressing grief.

Key Point: *As with spiritual care, remember that you cannot assume that a person follows the practices of her cultural group; you must assess to be sure.*

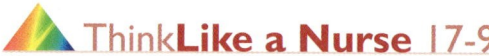 ThinkLike a Nurse 17-9

Reflect on this reading by Theresa Rando in *The Gift of Presence*:

It is one of the most difficult things in the world to do to sit and listen while another's heart is breaking with grief, to hold the hand of a dying patient who cries silently while staring into space. The gift of presence, the gift of being with those in pain, is the only gift we can give. It is the sole armor patients have against the anguish. The very most we can do for dying patients is to make it better, with our presence and concern, than it would be if we were not there. . . . We cannot "do" anything that can get rid of the psychic pain of impending loss and death. (Rando, 1984, p. 272)

Close your eyes and visualize yourself sitting quietly beside a dying patient and holding her hand. Visualize the patient crying silently. Can you still your mind and remain silent, or do you feel you must say something to make the patient feel better?

Providing Postmortem Care

Postmortem care includes care of the patient's body after death and fulfilling any legal obligations, such as arranging transportation to the morgue or funeral home and determining the disposition of the patient's belongings. You will follow agency policies and respect cultural and spiritual preferences, along with the care that is commonly provided. In most states, the physician must pronounce death; in some areas, however, a coroner or a nurse may also perform this task.

- **Rigor mortis** (the stiffening of the body after death) is caused by contraction of the muscles from a lack of adenosine triphosphate (ATP). It occurs about 2 to 4 hours after death. Rigor mortis begins in the involuntary muscles (e.g., the heart). It appears next in the head, neck, and trunk, and finally in the extremities. It disappears about 96 hours after death.

- **Algor mortis** occurs when the blood stops circulating. The body temperature drops about 1.88°F (1°C) per hour until it reaches room temperature.
- **Livor mortis** occurs when the dependent parts of the body appear bluish and mottled. That happens when the blood stops circulating and the red blood cells break down, releasing hemoglobin.

If the family wishes to be alone with the body, straighten the bedcovers, remove all tubes (unless contraindicated), and make the patient look as natural as possible. Give family members whatever time they need before you prepare the body. Ideally, you will have already established a relationship with the family and will have begun to facilitate their grieving during the patient's dying period. And you will have prepared them as the death becomes imminent. For specific guidelines for care of the body and other immediate postmortem interventions to support family members,

 Go to Chapter 17, **Clinical Insight 17-5: Providing Postmortem Care,** in Volume 2.

KnowledgeCheck 17-8

- Why is it important to position the body with a pillow under the head and shoulders soon after death?
- Why is it important to close the eyes and mouth of the deceased and position the body within at least 2 to 4 hours after death?

Providing Grief Education

Sometime after the immediate postmortem period, explain the stages of grief and point out that it may take months or even years to resolve. Explain that grief may become more intense on the anniversary of the death (or other loss) and on significant dates (e.g., birthdays).

Recall that once the bereaved person accepts that the loss is real, his feelings may be so intense that he may wonder whether he is losing his sanity. The grieving person may be fatigued from not sleeping, may be disoriented or unable to concentrate, and have numerous other symptoms. Reassure the person that such responses are expected and that there is no single right way to grieve (Egan & Arnold, 2003; Holtslander & McMillan, 2011). Also assure him that although the grief process takes time, the symptoms won't last forever.

Helping Children Deal With Loss

Some families may need information about helping children deal with grief, especially when there is a death in the family. You may need to explain that children perceive death differently from adults. See the accompanying Self-Care box for teaching surviving relatives how to help children deal with grief.

Taking Care of Yourself

When caring for dying patients, you will confront your own feelings of mortality. It is important to understand

Helping Children Deal With Loss

Teach surviving adult relatives the following:

- ➤ If a child is frightened about attending a funeral, do not force him to go. It is important, however, to include the child in some service or observance, such as lighting a candle, saying a prayer, or visiting the gravesite, at a later time.
- ➤ Spend as much time as possible with the child, making it clear that the child has permission to show her feelings openly or freely.
- ➤ Be prepared for intermittent expressions of sadness and anger from the child, over a long period of time.
- ➤ Be prepared for the possibility of regression to earlier developmental stages (e.g., talking "baby talk").
- ➤ Assure the child that he was in no way responsible for the death.
- ➤ The following warning signs may indicate the need for professional help, especially if they are prolonged:

  An extended period in which the child loses interest in daily activities and events

  Inability to sleep

  Loss of appetite

  Fear of being alone

  Extended regression

  Repeated statements about wanting to join the dead person

  Withdrawal from friends

  Refusal to attend school

  Sharp drop in school performance

your own attitudes, fears, and beliefs concerning death, so think about these before you encounter dying patients. This will enable you to deal in a more healthy way with patients and their families. In addition, suppressing feelings associated with death of patients can take a heavy toll on you emotionally.

When you become involved with dying persons and their families at such an intimate time in their lives, you become connected to them. There is nothing wrong with this emotional involvement; it helps you to be effective in your work. But just as you care for these families, you need also to care for yourself during these times.

- Recognize that feelings of grief and loss are normal.
- Talk with other colleagues about your feelings. Nurses are known for being able to take care of everyone but themselves! Don't be afraid to ask for what you need.
- Do not be afraid to confront grief. Some nurses feel they have to be strong and tend to deny their feelings. They overwork in caring for others and underwork in caring for themselves. If you use this approach, the feelings will accumulate and begin to wear you down physically and emotionally.

- If you wish, it is appropriate for you to attend calling hours and/or funeral services when one of your patients dies. This helps you diffuse some of your feelings of loss. It also is very meaningful to family members to know that you took the time to remember them and their loved one.
- Learn how to get support for yourself and how to support your colleagues when they experience the death of a patient. One idea is a nurses' support group, or grief team, that meets regularly to talk about the feelings and to remember those who have died. If you need or want a facilitator, pastoral care workers and social workers may be available for these services.
- Do some nice things for yourself on a regular basis (e.g., facial, quiet bubble bath, massage, a sports event). Try to set aside a special spot in your home that is only for relaxation; decorate it with items that help you focus on peaceful thoughts (e.g., candles, pictures, religious objects).

Caring for the dying can be very rewarding but is also emotionally draining. To be effective in your practice, learn to care for yourself as well.

To explore learning resources for this chapter,

   Go to DavisPlus at DavisPl.us/Wilkinson3.

Chapter Resources for Chapter 17:
   Response sheets for all learning activities
   Resources for Caregivers and Health Professionals
   Reading More About Loss, Grief, & Dying (suggested readings)
   Concept Map of chapter content
Interactive Case Studies
NCLEX-Style and Chapter Review Questions
Chapter Overview Podcast

For references cited in this chapter,

   Go to Volume 2, **References Cited.**

Essential Nursing Interventions

CHAPTER 18

Documenting & Reporting

Learning Outcomes

After completing this chapter you should be able to:

➤ Explain the purposes of documentation.

➤ Compare and contrast the differences between electronic and written documentation.

➤ Identify a variety of charting formats and their purposes.

➤ Describe guidelines for written and electronic documentation in the clinical setting.

➤ Identify approved abbreviations to use in charting.

➤ Follow documentation guidelines to accurately record patient health status, nursing interventions, and patient outcomes.

➤ Discuss the key elements of giving an oral patient report.

➤ Explain the process for verifying or questioning a medical order.

Key Concepts

Documentation
Oral reporting

Related Concepts

See the Concept Map on DavisPlus.

Meet Your Patient

Steven Stellanski is a 16-year-old male who has just been released from the post-anesthesia care unit (PACU) after an emergency appendectomy. You are to admit him to your unit. Steven is groggy but moaning in pain. "Help me, help me," he whispers. He is holding his abdomen and grimacing. The PACU nurse tells you that Steven has Down syndrome and functions at an elementary school–age level.

Steven's vital signs are as follows: tympanic membrane temperature 99.9°F (37.7°C); pulse, 104 beats/min; respirations, 24 breaths/min; and blood pressure 104/68 mm Hg. An intravenous (IV) bag of lactated Ringer's solution is infusing at 125 mL/hr. The dressing on Steven's right lower abdomen is dry and intact. An indwelling catheter is draining pale yellow urine.

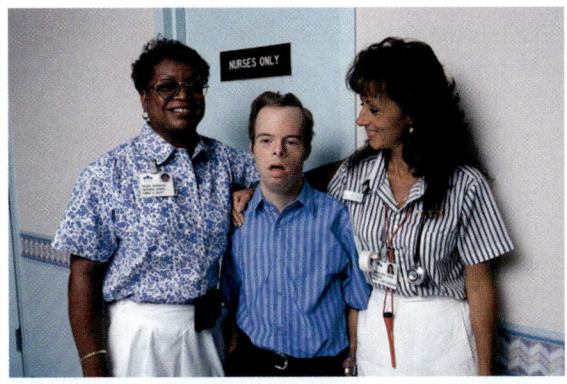

The provider has prescribed a patient-controlled analgesia (PCA) pump that will deliver morphine sulfate at 1 mg every 15 minutes, up to 4 mg per hour. Steven is to remain NPO (nothing by mouth) for now. His postoperative dressing is to be changed tomorrow morning and the nurses are to institute progressive ambulation as tolerated.

Theoretical Knowledge
knowing why

When you imagine yourself working as a nurse, what do you think of? Most people picture themselves at the bedside working with patients. When you look at ads for nursing jobs, they often show a nurse hanging an IV bag, listening to heart sounds, or perhaps teaching a patient. Photos rarely show the nurse charting or orally reporting care. Yet healthcare professionals rely on these two methods of communication to coordinate patient care. In this chapter, we discuss paper, electronic, and oral communication.

ABOUT THE KEY CONCEPTS

Documentation and **oral reporting** are the two broad concepts to which all other concepts in this chapter are linked. As you read, think: "What does this have to do with documentation?" and "How does this relate to oral reporting?"

DOCUMENTATION

Documentation is the act of recording patient status and care in written or electronic form, or in a combination of the two forms. Documentation is not limited to "writing nursing notes," but is the act of making a written record. The terms *documenting, recording,* and *charting* are often used to mean the same thing. Oral communication about a patient's status is called **reporting**—that is discussed later in this chapter.

Historically, the collection of documentation, orders, and other care information for a patient had been called the **medical record** or **chart**. However, with the present emphasis on health promotion, the medical record is now more commonly referred to as the **health record**. A patient's health record permanently documents:

- Care, in chronological order, provided by all healthcare providers
- The patient's responses to interventions and treatments
- Important facts about a client's health history, including past and present illnesses, examinations, tests, treatments, and outcomes

As a nurse, you are responsible for managing and implementing the interdisciplinary plan of care. That responsibility includes documenting the care provided and the progress made toward goals. Research shows that nurses routinely spend 15% to 25% of their workday documenting the care they give, and in some cases considerably more (Yee, Needleman, Pearson, et al., 2012).

How Do Healthcare Providers Use Documentation?

Clear, complete, concise, comprehensive and correct documentation in a client health record serves the following purposes:

Communication One important function is communication. Members of the interdisciplinary team use the health record to communicate about the patient's status and care. For example, if it is not possible to speak directly to the respiratory therapist on your shift, you can at least review the progress notes. Documentation enables healthcare professionals to plan and evaluate treatment and monitor health status over time.

Continuity of Care Communication promotes continuity of care. For example, if you are concerned that the patient is at high risk for developing an infection, you can include a nursing diagnosis of Risk for Infection on the written or electronic interdisciplinary plan of care. You would then initiate nursing orders for other nurses to regularly observe for and document signs of infection.

Quality Improvement Healthcare organizations and other agencies perform **manual chart audits** (directed reviews of client medical records) of written documentation. In electronic health record (EHR) systems, reports are run to analyze large amounts of data. Results are used to formulate strategies to improve care, decrease length of stay, control costs, and identify knowledge and practice gaps that can be addressed through inservice and continuing education. Accrediting agencies, such as The Joint Commission, review written and electronic records to ensure delivery of quality care and public safety.

Planning and Evaluation of Patient Outcomes Documentation enables physicians, nurses, and other healthcare professionals to plan and evaluate treatment and monitor health status over time.

Legal Documentation The health record will be scrutinized by legal experts if a dispute about a client's care arises. In court, the health record is legal evidence of the care given to a client, and is used to judge whether the interventions were timely and appropriate. Expert reviewers look for documentation of the client's baseline status, changes in status, interpretation of the changes, interventions implemented, and the client's responses to those interventions.

Professional Standards of Care The American Nurses Association (ANA) *Scope and Standards of Practice* (2nd ed.) (2010) includes documentation in many of its standards. By the ANA standards and competencies, the registered nurse:

- *Documents relevant data* in a retrievable format. (Standard 1, Assessment)

- *Documents diagnoses* or issues in a manner that facilitates the determination of the expected outcomes and plan. (Standard 2, Diagnosis)
- *Documents expected outcomes* as measurable goals. (Standard 3, Outcomes Identification)
- *Documents the plan* in a manner that uses standardized language or recognized terminology. (Standard 4, Planning)
- *Documents implementation* and any modifications, including changes or omission, of the identified plan. (Standard 5, Implementation)
- *Documents the coordination of the care.* (Standard 5a, Coordination of Care)
- *Documents the results of the evaluation.* (Standard 6, Evaluation)
- *Communicates effectively* in a variety of written, spoken and technological formats. (Standard 11, Communication)
- Cooperates in *creating a documented plan* focused on outcomes and decisions related to care and delivery of services that indicates communication with patients, families, and others. (Standard 14 Collaboration)

Reimbursement and Utilization Review Insurance companies, government and third-party payers, budget managers, and organization billing staff use client health records to determine the cost of care. They also use the health record for **utilization review**, the determination of whether the medical treatments and interventions were necessary and appropriate.

Education and Research As a student, you are well aware that the health record provides a snapshot of what is going on with the client, enabling you to research unfamiliar diagnoses, orders, and treatments before beginning direct care. This helps you to deliver safe care.

The health record is also used to gather data for clinical research. The increasing use of EHRs enables rapid analysis of large numbers of health records. Use of large samples of health records and clinical data sets is an essential step toward better understanding the cause and progression of disease, treatment methods, and outcomes across varied populations and diseases.

Why Are Standardized Nursing Languages Important?

Nurses have long understood the need for a standardized vocabulary for describing what nurses do and patient outcomes that result. As healthcare costs escalated, it became necessary to measure nursing's contribution to care and demonstrate the value of nursing. Standardized nursing terminology helps do that by making nursing care and its effect on patient outcomes more visible in patient records.

The ANA (2010) recommends that documentation systems use ANA-recognized terminology (e.g., NANDA-I, NIC, NOC). Standardized terminologies allow researchers to retrieve nursing data for aggregation and analysis. Through the use of standardized languages in nursing documentation, a standard for evidence-based nursing care delivery has now been established. This is a step toward closing the gap between what research shows to be the best nursing practices and the interventions nurses actually use in practice.

Standardized languages are especially important in EHR systems because computers require standardized information that can be converted to numerical codes. Several standardized nursing language models are used in nursing documentation, such as NANDA International (NANDA-I), Nursing Interventions Classification (NIC), and Nursing Outcomes Classification (NOC). To review using standardized nursing language models in your own practice, see the standardized language sections in Chapters 4, 5, and 6.

How Are Health Records Systems Organized?

A **health records system** is the overall process by which all patient records are created, stored, and retrieved in an organization. In a sense, it consists of all the EHRs in an organization. Each healthcare agency determines the health record system that is used. The nursing leaders in each organization usually determine the documentation forms that nurses will use within the records system.

Source-Oriented Record Systems

Patients in hospitals and long-term care facilities receive care from a variety of disciplines, so these institutions commonly use **source-oriented records**. Members of each discipline record their findings in a separately labeled section of the chart. In paper records, nurses chart in the nurses' notes and graphic data sections. A typical source-oriented record includes the following sections:

- *Admission data*—demographic information, insurance data, contact information
- *Advance directive*—information on client's wishes for the extent of care and medical support that should be given in the event of a life-threatening event
- *History and physical*—a detailed summary of the current health problem; past medical, surgical and social history; medications taken; allergies; review of systems, and physical examination data
- *Provider's orders*—orders for medications, treatments, and activities
- *Progress notes*—chronological charting by healthcare team members including patient exams, problem identification, and patient's response to therapy
- *Diagnostic studies*—reports detailing the findings of tests that have been performed, such as x-ray exam, ultrasound, or pulmonary function tests

- *Laboratory data*—results from diagnostic tests, such as complete blood count (CBC)
- *Nurses' notes*—documentation of patient care and response to treatment recorded by nurses (usually chronological)
- *Graphic data*—numerical data collected over time and displayed visually to allow analysis of trends. Examples include intake and output records, vital sign flowsheets, rating scales, and checklists regarding patient activity, dietary intake, and activities of daily living (ADL) tasks.
- *Rehabilitation and therapy notes*—chronological charting by therapists (e.g., physical, occupational, respiratory) about assessments, treatment plan, and patient response to therapy.
- *Discharge planning*—includes data from utilization review, case managers, or discharge planners on anticipated client needs after discharge

Advantages In source-oriented records, you can easily find the care provided by each discipline and the results of laboratory and diagnostic tests.

Disadvantages A drawback of this system is that data may be fragmented and scattered throughout the patient's record. That means that you need to review all sections of the chart to fully understand the client's condition and care. It is especially difficult with source-oriented records to track the treatments and client outcomes associated with a particular problem. For example, suppose a client with congestive heart failure is retaining fluids, causing her to be short of breath on exertion. To find the interventions for the problem, you would need to look (1) in the primary care providers' (PCP) orders to see whether cardiac drugs or diuretics were prescribed to help with the fluid retention, (2) in the respiratory therapist's notes for breathing treatments and the client's response, (3) in the nursing notes to see whether the client is being positioned with the head of the bed elevated to facilitate breathing, and (4) in the graphic section to evaluate urinary output in response to the diuretic.

Problem-Oriented Record Systems

Problem-oriented records (PORs) are organized around the patient's problems. There are no separate sections for each discipline. The POR consists of four parts: database, problem list, plan of care, and progress notes.

- The **database** consists of demographic data, the history and physical, nursing assessment data, and family and social history. As the patient's condition changes, the database is updated to reflect the patient's current status.
- The **problem list** is a concise listing of problems that have been identified from the database. Once a problem is resolved, it is noted on the problem list. If a problem changes or is redefined, the problem list is updated to reflect the change. See Figure 18-1 for an example of a problem list.

Problem number	Date entered	Date resolved	Client problem
1	mm/dd/yyyy	mm/dd/yyyy	Abdominal pain (unknown etiology) Redefined mm/dd/yyyy
1A	mm/dd/yyyy		Appendicitis resulting in emergency appendectomy
1B	mm/dd/yyyy		Acute pain r/t abdominal incision 2 appendectomy
2	mm/dd/yyyy		Down syndrome — functions at school-age level
3	mm/dd/yyyy		Risk for constipation r/t opioid use for pain control and h/o appendicitis

FIGURE 18-1 A problem list for Steven Stellanski (Meet Your Patient). Note that problem 1 has been redefined now that the cause of Steven's pain has been determined. Note also that the list contains both medical and nursing diagnoses.

- The **plan of care** includes the PCP's orders and the nursing care plan to address the identified problems. Other disciplines may also contribute to the plan.
- **Progress notes** are organized according to the problem list. Each discipline charts on shared notes. Charting is labeled according to problem number.

Advantages A common problem list allows for input from all disciplines, making it is easy to monitor the patient's progress. Because each problem is readily identified in the notes, each discipline has ready access to the findings of the other members of the health team, which promotes greater collaboration.

Disadvantages To work well, the POR system requires a cooperative spirit among health providers as well as diligence in maintaining a current database and problem list.

Charting by Exception

Charting by exception (CBE) is more than a format; it is a system of charting in which only significant findings or exceptions to standards and norms of care are charted. To use the CBE system effectively, you must know and adhere to professional, legal, and organizational guidelines for nursing assessments and interventions.

CBE uses preprinted flowsheets to record most aspects of care. CBE assumes that all standards have been met and the patient has responded normally, unless a separate entry is made (an *exception*). Normal responses for various assessments are defined on the front or back of the form. Each flowsheet has entries for expected aspects of care and thus can vary by specialty areas or diagnosis.

Advantages CBE reduces the amount of time spent on documentation, reduces repetitive charting of routine care, provides a record that is easily read and understood, and clearly highlights any variations from the expected plan of care. In many organizations, CBE records are kept at the bedside, which promotes timely documentation.

Disadvantages Inadvertent omissions are the main problem associated with CBE. Omissions may result from disagreement over what constitutes a significant variation. Research shows that some participants used either a deviation from patients' baseline or normal physiological standards to define when a finding is not "within normal limits" (WNL) (Kerr, 2013). Critics of CBE believe it: (1) requires nurses to be overly familiar with the organization's documentation standards and policies; (2) makes it difficult to capture the skilled judgment of nurses; and (3) reduces care to such rote repetitions that you may forget to chart an exception to the established standards.

CBE can lead to errors because nurses may conclude that care has been completed, when in fact it was not done. This system requires you to carefully assess and validate care provided.

Here is an example of what part of a CBE flowsheet for your patient, Steven Stellanski, might look like. Notice in the first section that the day-shift nurse merely initials that she has made an assessment or taken one of the listed actions at each of the designated times:

DATE: 04/11/16				
Hour	0800	0900	1000	1100
ACTIVITY				
Bedrest		LP		
Ambulate	LP*			
Sleeping				
BRP				
HOB elevated	LP	LP		

	DAY	EVENING	NIGHT	
Neurological		√		
Cardiovascular		√		
Pulmonary		√		
Gastrointestinal		*		Vomited 3×1,100 mL clear yellow fluid at 0730. Given Compazine 1 mg IV with relief.

Key: √ = normal findings, * = significant finding

Notice also the second table (with the checkmarks) is a summary for the day shift. This is where the nurse describes and discusses any of the significant findings noted at the individual assessment times.

Electronic Health Record Systems

The EHR consists of records that are entered via computer. EHRs typically combine source-oriented and problem-oriented record styles, although the source-oriented system is most common. For example, a client's EHR often contains orders, clinical documentation, laboratory and other test and procedure results, as well as an interdisciplinary plan of care (IPOC), a problem and diagnosis list, and progress notes entered by physicians, nurses, respiratory therapists, and other professional providers.

Figure 18-2 is a section of an electronic form for recording intake and output in source-oriented format. As you can see, the intake and output (I&O) screen records numerical data. It also allows the nurse to add brief narrative comments in each field. Figure 18-3 is an electronic IPOC in problem-oriented format. The IPOC can be updated at the times specified by the organization, and the I&O data can be entered at any time. Both exist within the same electronic records system.

Advantages of Electronic Health Records

- **Enhanced communication and collaboration.** Communication is improved among healthcare providers.
- **Improved access to information.**
    Multiple healthcare providers can access the same information at the same time.
    Authorized persons can access information remotely (e.g., from a patient's home).
    EHRs integrate client information between multiple departments so that one area can immediately see information from another. For example, when the laboratory enters a critical result, such as a clotting time, you do not need to wait for the lab to phone or to send a paper result to the nursing unit.
- **Time savings.**
    Nurses spend up to 25% less time charting.
    Information is stored and retrieved quickly and easily.
    Reports can be created quickly because of the computer's ability to aggregate data (e.g., a 24-hour graph of the patient's vital signs).
    Repetition and duplication are reduced.
- **Improved quality of care.**
    The system can use protocols to automatically enter orders based on the client's condition. For example, most organizations have policies for making falls prevention assessments. Some EHR systems will automatically enter an order to observe and document risk of falls more often when a patient's "falls score" exceeds a certain level.
    Embedded protocols enhance caregiver knowledge and the ability to follow clinical practice guidelines.

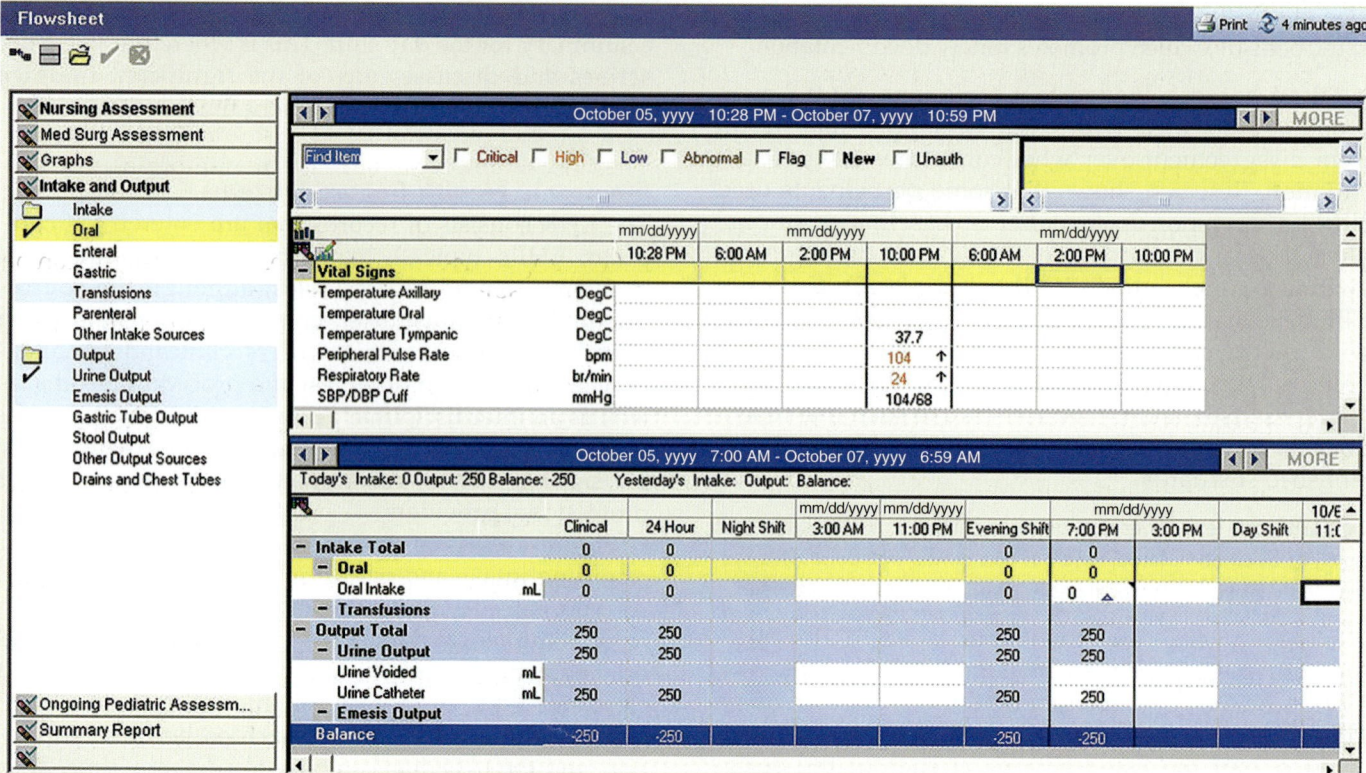

FIGURE 18-2 An electronic intake and output (I&O) entry form. (Courtesy of Cerner Corporation, Kansas City, MO.)

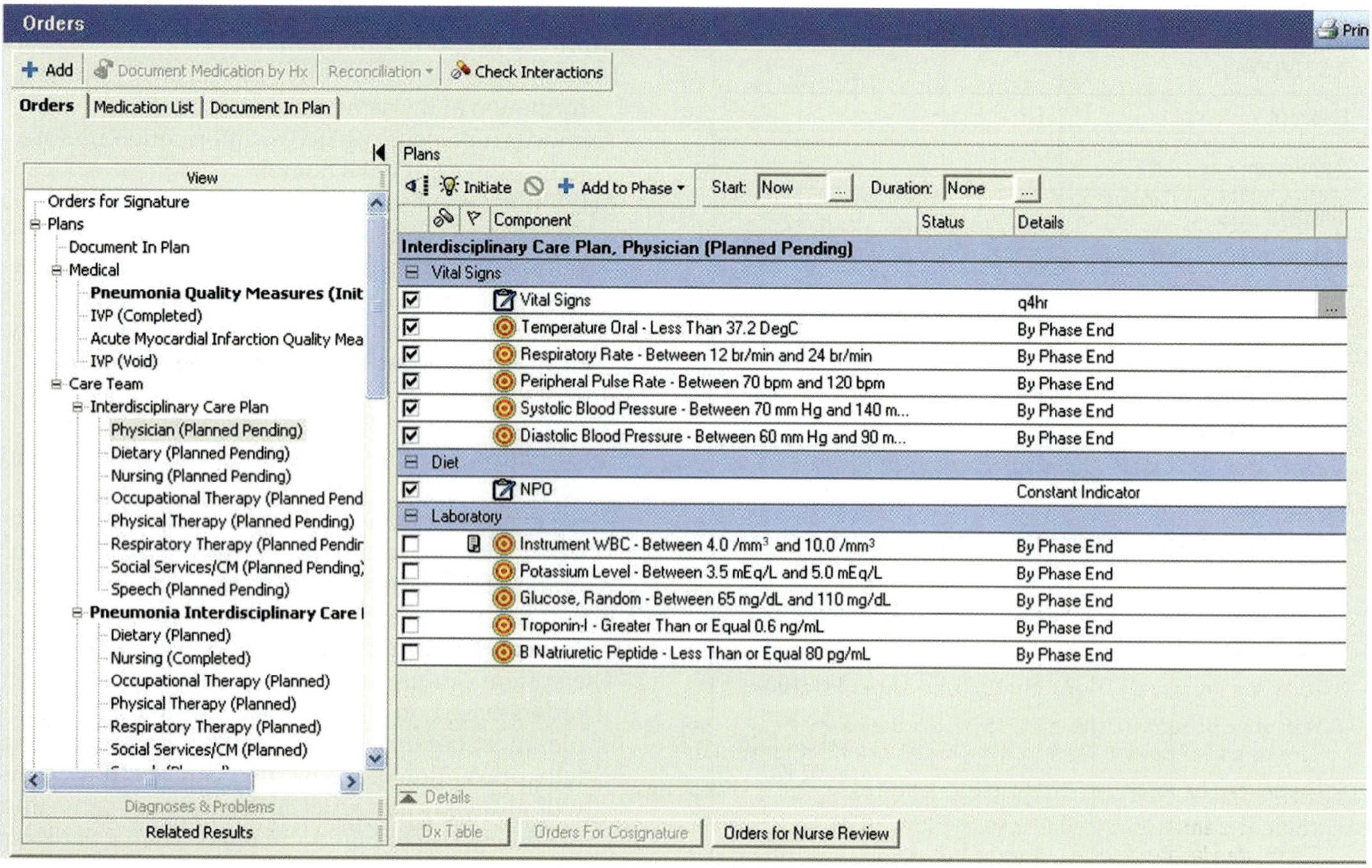

FIGURE 18-3 A portion of an electronic interdisciplinary plan of care (IPOC) form. (Courtesy of Cerner Corporation, Kansas City, MO.)

For example, suppose there is a medical prescription to administer insulin on the basis of a patient's blood glucose results. In some EHR systems, the nurse can activate an immediate link to the tables of information needed to decide how much insulin to give to the patient.

Medical errors are minimized by programmed alerts that are automatically displayed when a care provider takes an action that could be harmful (e.g., when a provider prescribes a drug to which a patient is allergic or calls for a dose that exceeds the safe range).

Data can be analyzed at the time of collection, making immediate nursing decision making possible.

EHRs facilitate evidence-based practice by making it possible to analyze thousands of records in ways that cannot be done with paper forms. With aggregated data, nursing practice can be compared across populations and geographic locations to support nursing decisions and guide professional and organization quality improvement.

- **Information is private and safe.**

Information is permanently stored and not likely to be lost.

Confidentiality of client information is enhanced by tracking everyone who accesses the healthcare record, proper security clearances, unique passwords, restricted access, and using front-view screen protectors.

Disadvantages of Electronic Health Records

- **Expense:** Electronic documentation systems are expensive.
- **Downtime:** Downtime processes must be in place for times when parts of the EHR are not available (e.g., because of power outages, severe weather, and system upgrades).
- **Difficulties associated change:**

Learning to use some documentation systems can be challenging and time consuming.

Some healthcare providers resist the change from paper to EHR.

It is not easy to capture narrative nursing content from paper charting into an electronic format.

Some EHRs are not user-friendly (e.g., difficult to quickly find information needed to make care decisions).

Some systems do not control redundancy well, requiring caregivers to ask the patient for the same information over and over.

- **Lack of integration:** Most EHRs are not integrated across the different departments.

This means sometimes a person with a legitimate reason to enter the chart cannot see entries made by other departments and must then request verbal, e-mail, or paper reports (e.g., lab results).

Advantages and Disadvantages of Paper Records

For a summary of the advantages and disadvantages of paper health records, see Box 18-1.

BOX 18-1 ■ Advantages and Disadvantages of a Paper Health Record

ADVANTAGES
- Care providers are comfortable with it because it is familiar. There is little "learning curve."
- Paper records do not require large databases and secure networks to function.
- There is no downtime for system changes, weather, and so on.
- It is relatively inexpensive to create new forms and update old ones.

DISADVANTAGES

Access may be delayed. Only one care provider can access the record at a time; and the provider must be in the same location as the chart.

Retrieving information may be slow.
- Healthcare providers may need to search through multiple pages to find needed information.
- Specific documentation is difficult to retrieve when needed, especially when files are archived in another part of the building.

Documentation is time consuming.
- Documentation may take more time because handwriting is slower than computer entry.
- Documentation is often redundant and repetitive.
- Paper records require manual audit of many charts to create reports and collect client data. This is time and resource intensive.

There is a relatively high risk for patient care error.
- Narrative documents are hard to read if the handwriting is illegible or messy. This means nurses have to take time from patient care to contact providers to clarify handwritten prescriptions.
- Papers can be lost from the chart or damaged, leading to duplicate assessments or medication errors.
- There is tremendous inconsistency in how the same client information is documented, even within the same organization. Often standardized terminology is not used.

Storage of paper records is expensive.

Confidentiality is difficult to protect. There is no way to know who may have access to the paper health record without proper authorization.

KnowledgeCheck 18-1

- Identify the purposes of the client health record.
- What are the key differences in the organization of source-oriented records, problem-oriented records, electronic documentation systems, and CBE systems?
- What are three advantages of paper health records?
- What are three advantages of EHRs?

For more information on the transition to electronic health record systems,

 Go to Chapter 18, **Supplemental Materials,** on Davis*Plus.*

Documentation and the Nursing Process

The goal of all nursing documentation is a clear, concise and complete representation of the client's healthcare experience that is easily accessible and understood by all members of the healthcare team. Effective documentation allows you to help clients to make sound health decisions. It also enables use of current and consistent data, problem statements, diagnoses, goals, and strategies to support continuity of care. However, research continues to identify insufficient documentation of the steps in the nursing process (e.g., inadequate assessment information, lack of decisions based on a nursing diagnoses, inadequate evaluation and revisions in the plan of care) (Blair & Smith, 2012; Wang, Hailey, & Yu, 2011). Regardless of the type of documentation that is used, you must use or refer to the nursing process as a guideline when charting.

- **Assessment:** Chart signs and symptoms that may indicate actual or potential client problems. At an initial assessment, document comprehensive data about all client systems.
- **Diagnosis/Analysis**: After analyzing assessment data, document your clinical nursing judgment about the client's response to actual or potential health conditions or needs.
- **Outcomes/Planning:** Document a measurable and achievable short-term and long-term plan of care with goals directed at preventing, minimizing, or resolving identified client problems or issues.
- **Implementation:** After putting the plan of care into effect, record the specific interventions that were used.
- **Evaluation:** Document client responses to nursing care; chart whether the plan of care was effective in preventing, minimizing or resolving the identified problems; and then modify the plan as needed.

What Are Some Common Formats for Nursing Progress Notes?

Nursing documentation can take many forms, including paper charts, computerized electronic documents, audio or video files, e-mails, faxes, scanned paper documents, electronically stored photographs, x-ray findings, and other images. Depending on the documentation model your organization selects, you may use one or more of the following charting formats. Choice of format is also influenced by whether your nursing documentation is written on paper, captured and stored electronically, or a blend of the two. In all formats, you must learn to use abbreviations appropriately.

Use of Abbreviations

Recall the case of Steven Stellanski (Meet Your Patient). Below is a brief admission note using narrative charting format. Underline any words or entries that you do not understand:

> *4/11/16   1600   Pt received on unit from PACU. VSS. TM temp 99.9°F (37.7°C), P 104, and BP 104.68. LOC unstable. Arouses when name called but quickly drifts off to sleep. PERRLA. Moaning, grimacing, holding abd, whispers "Help me. Help me." LR at 125 mL/hr infusing in R forearm. Urinary catheter in place, draining pale yellow urine. Drsg dry & intact. Morphine sulfate PCA ordered. Will initiate. ——*
> *———————————————————— Ron Allen, RN.*

You can see from this entry that nurses use many abbreviations in their paper record charting. Every healthcare institution has a list of approved abbreviations that may and may not be used in documentation. Be sure to consult your organization's list before you chart. For a list of commonly used abbreviations in healthcare and another list of abbreviations that pertain to medication administration,

 Go to Chapter 18, **Abbreviations Commonly Used in Healthcare,** in Volume 2.

 Also go to Chapter 26, **Medication-Related Abbreviations,** in Volume 2.

The Joint Commission (2012a) created a "do not use" list that directs medical personnel in healthcare organizations to write out certain words, rather than use the abbreviations (see Table 18-1).

In consideration of furthering The Joint Commissions Patient Safety Goals, some institutions also:

- Write out "greater than" or "less than"—rather than using the symbols ">" or "<".
- Write drug names in full—rather than using abbreviations.
- Use metric units—instead of apothecary units.
- Write "at" or "each"—rather than use the "@"symbol.
- Write "mL" or "milliliters"—in place of the "cc" abbreviation.
- Write "mcg" or "micrograms"—instead of the "µg" abbreviation.

These actions minimize many common errors that occur in healthcare organizations.

Table 18-1 ➤ Joint Commission "Do Not Use" List

DO NOT USE THIS ABBREVIATION	WRITE OUT THE WORD OR DOSE
"U" or "u"	Unit
"IU" for	International Unit
Q.D., QD, q.d., qd	Daily
Q.O.D., QOD, q.o.d., qod	every other day
MS, MSO4, and MgSO4	either morphine sulfate or magnesium sulfate
The trailing zero for medications (X.0 mg)	X mg (e.g., 10 mg)
Lack of leading zero (.X mg)	0.X mg (e.g., 0.1 mg)

Narrative

Narrative format is used with written source-oriented and problem-oriented charts. The **narrative chart entry** tells the story of the patient's experience in a chronological format (i.e., in the order that it happens). It provides information on the details of the client's care—client status, activities, nursing interventions, psychosocial context, and response to treatment. The goal is to track the client's changing health status and progress toward goals. Narrative charting is especially useful when attempting to construct a timeline of events, such as a cardiac arrest or other emergency situations. It highlights critical thinking and captures the true art of nursing (Spoerner, 2009).

Disadvantages of narrative charting are that it may be time consuming, disorganized, contain multiple and sometimes duplicate entries, requires you to read the entire note or multiple notes to find client responses and outcomes to interventions, and does not readily identify problems and trends. Blair and Smith (2012) believe that narrative charting is not ideal in today's healthcare environment.

Problem–Intervention–Evaluation (PIE)

The Problem–Intervention–Evaluation (PIE) system organizes information according to the patient's problems and requires keeping a daily assessment record and progress notes. This eliminates the need for a separate care plan and provides a nursing-focused rather than medical-focused record.

Problem: Use data from your original assessment to identify appropriate nursing diagnoses.

Intervention: Record the nursing actions you take for each nursing diagnosis.

Evaluation: Document the patient's response to interventions and treatments.

Problems are identified from the admission assessment. Subsequent entries begin with identification of the problem number. This type of charting establishes an ongoing care plan. A PIE charting entry for Steven Stellanski (Meet Your Patient) might look like this:

4/11/16   1630

P: 1B

I: Pt c̅ 1 mg doses up to 4 mg morphine/hr. Pt groggy yet c/o pain. Has not triggered PCA independently. Rates pain as 8 on scale of 1–10. PCA use reviewed with pt. Demonstrated use c̅ 1st dose at 1615.

E: Pt still moaning & grimacing. Has not initiated another dose via PCA. 2nd dose given as additional demo. Will reevaluate in 1 hr. May need continuous infusion if pt unable to use to control pain. ——————————————— Ron Allen, RN

This style of charting tends to focus only on the listed problems and not on the client as a whole. However, the primary disadvantage of PIE charting is that it does not document the planning portion of the nursing process. There is no seamless flow of client data, nursing diagnosis, and interventions, such as seen in a nursing care plan.

SOAP/SOAPIE/SOAP (IER)

The SOAP format is often used to write nursing and other progress notes. It can be used in source-oriented, problem-oriented, and electronic health records. The acronyms SOAP, SOAPIE, and SOAP(IER) are explained below.

- **S***ubjective data*—What the patient or family members tell you about the client's signs and symptoms and the reason they are seeking healthcare. Typically this is recorded by quoting the actual words said.
- **O***bjective data*—Factual, measurable clinical findings such as vital signs, test results, and quality of breath sounds. Refer to Chapter 3 to review subjective and objective data.
- **A***ssessment*—Conclusions drawn from the subjective and objective data, usually patient problems or nursing diagnoses. **Key Point:** *SOAP terminology is different from nursing process terminology. In the nursing process chapters we referred to conclusions about data as inferences or problems, and stated that assessment does not include conclusions about data. When using SOAP, you should chart your conclusions about the data under "A."*

- **P***lan*: Short-term and long-term goals and strategies that will be used to relieve the patient's problems.
- **I***nterventions*: Actions of the healthcare team that are performed to achieve expected outcomes.
- **E***valuation*: An analysis of the effectiveness of interventions.
- **R***evision*: Changes made to the original care plan.

Recall that a POR is organized according to specific patient problems, and has five components: database, problem list, initial plan, progress notes, and a discharge summary. You will refer to and use the following four parts when charting in SOAP format.

Problem List A numbered list of the patient's current problems in chronological order is compiled so that you can refer to the number when entering your notes.

Initial Plan This includes expected outcomes and plans for further care interventions and teaching. There is only one initial plan so you must update and change the plan in subsequent progress notes.

Progress Notes This is where you record the SOAP(IER) information. As a rule, you enter a note for each current problem every 24 hours or when the patient's condition changes.

Discharge Summary At discharge, each problem on the list is covered and a notation made about whether it was resolved. Unresolved problems, with plans for each, are included when communicating with the patient, other facilities, and home health agencies.

Following is an example of SOAP progress notes using the admission data of Steven Stellanski (Meet Your Patient). In the previous section, these same data were used to create a narrative note. Notice that the data are similar; however, the narrative note is organized by data source. Steven's SOAP(IER) charting entry related to his postoperative nausea and pain could look like this:

04/11/16	0830	#1 – Nausea related to anesthesia
		S – Pt states "I feel sick to my stomach. Help me."
		O – Pt vomited 100 ml clear, light yellow fluid.
		A – Pt is nauseated secondary to anesthesia.
		P – Monitor nausea and give antiemetic as needed.
		I – Pt given Compazine 1 mg IV at 0830.
	0900	E – Pt states he feels less sick to his stomach.—Ron Allen, RN
04/11/16	0830	#1B – Acute pain related to abdominal incision 2° appendectomy
		S – States, "Help me, help me." Moaning and grimacing.

		O – Moaning and grimacing; holding abd. Drsg dry & intact. BP 104/68, P 104, Resp 24, and TM temp 99.9°F. PERRLA.
		A – Postoperative pain
		P – Give analgesic as needed.
		I – Morphine PCA initiated at 0835. Pt. instructed in use. 1st dose (1 mg) administered as demonstration.
	0900	E – Still moaning & grimacing even after 2nd dose given as additional demo. Still has not initiated additional PCA dose.———— Ron Allen, RN
	0930	R – Still no pain relief; still has not used PCA independently. Discussed w/ Dr. Jadu. Continuous infusion begun at 2 mg/hr. Will supplement up to 4 mg/hr prn.————————Ron Allen, RN

Disadvantages of SOAP(IE) charting are that it can be inefficient and ineffective. You may find the same interventions and responses repeated in more than one section for clients with overlapping problems. You may also find that nurses write a complete narrative rather than a single problem entry. The use of SOAP has also been shown to shift the focus from the patient to the disease, thus promoting a medical model instead of the nursing process (Blair & Smith, 2012).

Focus Charting®

The term *focus* is used to encourage you to view the client's status from a positive, rather than problem-oriented, perspective. **Focus Charting®** uses assessment data to evaluate client care concerns, problems, or strengths. It also identifies necessary revisions to the care plan as you record each entry.

The focus is often identified as a nursing diagnosis (e.g., Ineffective Breathing Pattern), a sign or symptom (e.g., shortness of breath), a client behavior (e.g., inability to follow inhaler instructions), a special need (e.g., non-English speaking), an acute change in condition (e.g., sudden appearance of chest pain), or a significant event (e.g., surgery). Focus Charting® works well in acute care settings and in areas where the same care and procedures are repeated frequently.

The first column contains the time and date. The second column identifies the focus or problem addressed in the note. The third column contains charting in a DAR format. DAR is an acronym for *data, action,* and *response.*

Data Subjective and objective information that supports the focus. This aspect reflects the assessment phase of the nursing process and includes other data, such as laboratory results or other diagnostic testing.

Action Describe interventions performed, such as administering medications or making calls to the physician. This aspect reflects the planning and implementation phases of the nursing process.

Response The patient's response to your interventions reflects the evaluation phase of the nursing process.

Focus Charting® is attractive because it addresses the client's concerns holistically. However, the lack of a common problem list may lead to inconsistency in labeling the focus of notes and cause difficulty in tracking patient progress. The following is an example of a Focus® note.

| 04/11/16 1800 | Focus:

developmental delay | **D:** 16 y.o. rec'd on unit at 1600 from PACU post-appendectomy. Pt w/ Down syndrome. Morphine PCA initiated. Pt unable to use PCA to control pain. Continuous infusion at 2 mg/hr begun at 1745. PERRLA. Alert, drifting in & out of sleep. PACU RN reports pt functions at elementary school–age level.

A: Will discuss pt status w/ parents and adjust plan of care accordingly.————
————————*Ron Allen, RN* |
| 1830 | | **R:** Met w/ parents, who report that pt has significant developmental delays & needs supervision w/ all ADLs. Pt comfortable on 2 mg/hr infusion of morphine. Use of PCA for supplementary pain control reviewed with parents. Parents demonstrated understanding and that they will assist pt w/ PCA if add'l meds are needed.——
———————— *Ron Allen, RN* |

FACT System

Noted for its individual elements, the FACT documentation model incorporates many charting-by-exception (CBE) principles and includes four key elements:

*F*lowsheets individualized to specific services
*A*ssessment features standardized with baseline parameters

*C*oncise, integrated progress notes and flowsheets documenting the client's condition and responses
*T*imely entries documented when care is given

FACT documentation includes only exceptions to the norm or significant information about the patient. It eliminates the need to chart normal findings. The disadvantages of the FACT system are the same as for CBE. The following is a FACT example for Steven Stellanski (Meet Your Patient).

DATE/TIME	04/12/16 0900	04/12/16 1330
Neurological Alert and oriented to time, place, and person. PERRLA. Symmetry of strength in extremities. No difficulty with coordination. Behavior appropriate to situation. Sensation intact without numbness or paresthesias.	√	√
Orient patient		
Refer to neurological flowsheet		
Pain No report of pain. If present, include pain scale intensity choice by patient (0–10) with location, description, duration, radiation, precipitating and alleviating factors.	Abdominal incision pain – score 10	√
Location	RLQ	
Description	Dull, constant	
Relief measures	Percocet 1 tablet by mouth	
Pain relief: Y = yes / N = no	Y	
Cardiovascular Apical pulse 60 to 100. S_1 and S_2 present. Regular rhythm. Peripheral pulses (radial, pedal) present bilaterally. No edema or calf tenderness. Extremities pink, warm, moveable within patient's ROM.		
IV Solution and Rate	lactated Ringer's at 125 mL/hr	lactated Ringer's at 125 mL/hr

Electronic Entry

The Health Information Technology for Economic and Clinical Health (HITECH) Act has been instrumental in the widespread conversion from paper to electronic health records. Electronic clinical information systems streamline documentation processes, make them more accurate and efficient, and reduce the risk of human error. This frees you to do the expert work that only nurses can do. Electronic documentation requires a shift in how you record your work.

- EHRs change documentation formats from paper to electronic.
- Documentation is done at the bedside, instead of at the nurse's station.
- Decision-making processes change from gradual to immediate.

As a nurse, you will almost certainly need to have computer skills (Fig. 18-4). You will play a crucial role in the development and evaluation of effective EHR systems that make sense to nurses. You may even participate directly in the design–implementation–redesign cycle of the EHR system in your organization.

Electronic documentation forms and flowsheets (such as Fig. 18-2) include the information that your organization has decided is important to record. Reminders to document specific kinds of information, such as overdue medications and overdue nursing interventions, display automatically to help ensure your charting is accurate. Also, the extensive use of clearly named data entry fields, drop-down menus, check boxes, and specially created templates allows you to enter your nursing documentation quickly and efficiently, usually with minimal keyboard typing.

Depending on the EHR system used and the associated charting form, progress notes may be entered electronically in prebuilt note formats. In some electronic systems, you may still need to write progress notes on lined paper, in narrative, SOAP, PIE, Focus®, or FACT formats. Transitioning from paper to electronic documentation can be challenging for some people. It usually takes a few days to know where to document your nursing care and feel confident that you haven't overlooked anything. However, EHR software is becoming more logical and user-friendly. Many organizations have printed information, classes, webinars, or Web-based tutorials that provide information about electronic documentation. Take advantage of opportunities to build your knowledge when they arise.

KnowledgeCheck 18-2

Summarize the characteristics of each of the different kinds of nursing documentation formats (narrative, PIE, SOAP, Focus®, CBE and FACT, and electronic entry).

 ThinkLike a Nurse 18-1

Compare the documentation examples (narrative, PIE, SOAP, Focus®, CBE and FACT, and electronic documentation). If you have had experience with charting in the clinical setting, apply this experience as well. With which charting format do you feel most comfortable? Why?

What Forms Do Nurses Use to Document Nursing Care?

Documentation forms vary by purpose, institution, and unit. However, regardless of the system or forms used, nursing documentation reflects the nursing process. You record assessments, diagnoses, planning, implementation (what you actually did), and evaluation of client responses. This section discusses the most commonly used paper and electronic forms that are used in addition to the nursing progress notes discussed in the preceding sections.

Nursing Admission Data Forms

A separate nursing admission form or a combined interdisciplinary form is completed at the time the patient enters the healthcare system. A baseline assessment is essential because it: (1) may be used as a benchmark to monitor change; (2) provides information about the client's support system and helps forecast future needs; (3) contains critical information (e.g., presenting illness or reason for admission, vital signs, allergy information, current medications, activities of daily living (ADL) status, physical assessment data, and discharge planning information). For examples of a paper admission form,

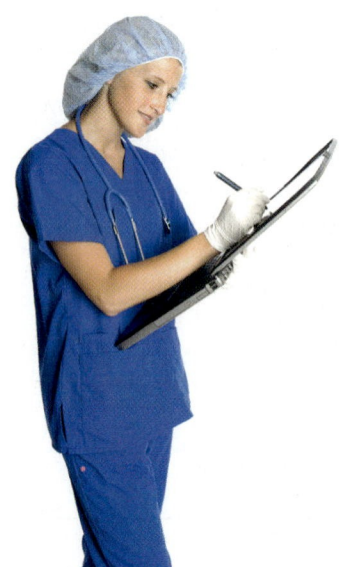

FIGURE 18-4 Many healthcare institutions are adopting computerized patient records.

 Go to Chapter 3, **Nursing Admission Data Form,** and

Go to Chapter 18, **Tables, Boxes, Figures: ESG Figure 18-1 (Adult Inpatient Admission Assessment),** on DavisPlus.

To see part of an electronic nursing admission data form,

 Go to Chapter 18, **Charting Forms, Adult Admission History Electronic Screen,** in Volume 2.

You will use admission forms in all settings, for example, in ambulatory clinics and long-term care facilities that contain the same or similar sections. Admission forms for long-term care are similar to hospital admission forms. An ambulatory care admission form includes demographic data, allergy information, current medications, family health data, social history, and the client's past medical history. The form completed by Nam Nguyen (in Volume 2) at his first clinic visit is an example of an ambulatory care admission form. To see Mr. Nguyen's completed form,

 Go to **Meet the Nguyens** at the beginning of Volume 2.

Discharge Summary

Discharge data are obtained with the admission assessment, but are often recorded on a separate form. **Key Point:** *A general principle in nursing is that discharge planning begins on admission. Therefore, discharge needs should be evaluated when the patient first enters a healthcare facility, especially in acute care facilities.* Ask yourself what this patient would need if he were to go home in the next few days. For example,

would he need help with food preparation? Does he understand how to use his medicines?

A **discharge summary** is the last entry made in the paper chart. In the electronic chart, the discharge summary can be started any time after admission and revised throughout the hospitalization. A summary is completed when the patient is transferred within the same organization, to another facility, or discharged to home. The discharge summary may be a multidisciplinary document or each discipline may write a separate summary. The forms are different in each organization, but they contain similar data. For examples of electronic and paper discharge summaries, respectively, see Figure 18-5 and

 Go to Chapter 11, **Forms, Discharge Assessment/ Instructions,** in Volume 2; also refer to **Procedure 11-4, Discharging a Patient From the Healthcare Facility,** in Volume 2.

As you can see in Figure 18-5, there is a drop-down menu in which the Nursing Discharge Note is located. It is important to clearly document the patient's condition on discharge because the discharge summary serves as baseline data for the healthcare professionals who will provide discharge care.

Flowsheets and Graphic Records

You will use flowsheets and graphic records to document assessments and care that are performed frequently, on a recurring schedule, or as a part of unit routines. For

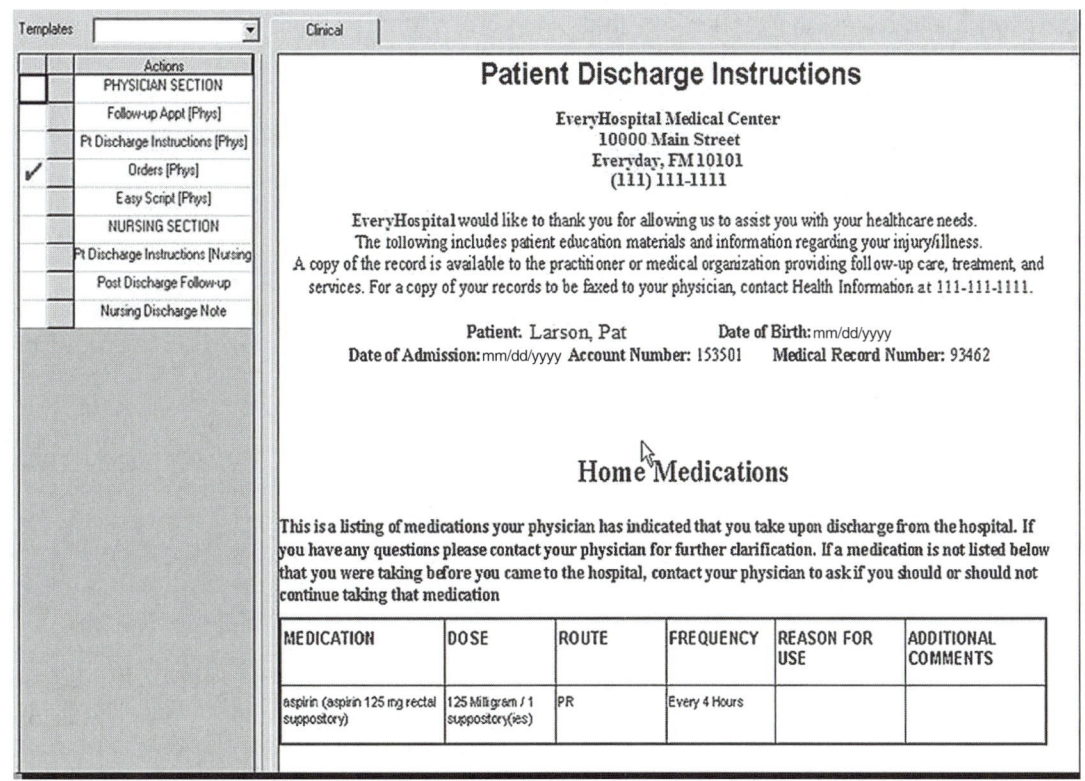

FIGURE 18-5 A portion of an electronic discharge planning form. (Courtesy of Cerner Corporation, Kansas City, MO.)

example, most hospital units require that vital signs be taken every 8 hours for all patients. How often you perform and document care activities depends on your patient's condition and the unit policy. In the first hour after surgery, for example, you would probably record vital signs every 15 minutes; then every 30 minutes for 1 hour; and then every hour for 4 hours.

The simplest paper forms are organized with time in columns across the top and the activities or patient assessment parameters in rows down the side. On electronic forms, the areas (fields) to enter the time and activities are arranged close together. Flowsheets and graphic records allow you to see patterns of change in patient status. For instance, you may view a steady increase in the line representing a patient's blood pressure compared to his pain score on an electronically generated graph. On a paper form, you may scan across a row to see that your patient has not had a bowel movement for several days. Other types of information recorded on flowsheets include intake and output (I&O), weight, hygiene measures, ADLs, and medications administered. For examples of a paper graphic record and an electronic flowsheet, see Figure 3-4 (paper) and Figure 18-2 (electronic).

To see a flowsheet for long-term care,

 Go to Chapter 18, **ESG Figure 18-5,** on DavisPlus.

Checklists

Assessments and care may also be recorded on paper and electronic checklists. Common normal and abnormal findings are usually organized according to body systems. Figure 18-6 is an example of a paper checklist.

Using a paper form, the nurse checks the box that reflects the current assessment findings. Some checklists include nursing actions, such as wound care, treatments, or IV fluid administration. Essentially these forms are comprehensive charting documents. Exceptions, patient care activities, and patient responses are recorded in the narrative note section of the paper form.

Using an electronic field-based checklist, the nurse enters values or text in the appropriate fields and saves the documentation. Electronic flowsheets typically contain content similar to paper checklists, but also include a greater range of potential documentation areas that can be opened as needed. This allows for a more comprehensive record of a patient's assessment, treatments, IV fluid administration, and many other parameters.

Intake and Output Records

You will sometimes use separate intake and output (I&O) paper records to document data about the patient's fluid balance. Electronic systems have flowsheet sections or I&O forms to enter I&O and save it into the patient's EHR (see Fig. 18-2). Usually these documentation forms contain data totaled by shift and by 24-hour periods. Paper forms must be totaled manually, whereas electronic systems usually automatically total I&O figures for you. For a paper I&O record,

 Go to Chapter 18, **Charting Forms, Intake and Output Sheet,** in Volume 2.

I&O paper graphics may be kept at the bedside. If your patient or a family member is able to assist with measuring his I&O, teach him how to record data on the paper form. You might also complete electronic I&O documentation at the bedside using a portable or stationary computer. When appropriate, patients can still track their own intake and output on paper, but you will need to enter the patient's I&O data into the EHR. Chapter 28 provides detailed information about monitoring intake and output.

Medication Administration Records

Medication administration records (MARs) contain information about the medications that have been prescribed for the client. The information and format vary by setting, with significant differences between outpatient and inpatient facilities.

- **Inpatient facilities:** Inpatient medication records not only contain a list of prescribed medications, but also track medication administration and usage for the agency. For a comparison of the content of inpatient and outpatient MARs, see Table 18-2.
- **Outpatient facilities** (e.g., include clinics, primary care offices, and treatment facilities). Because patients do not stay at the facility, usually the MAR primarily contains information about how the patient is to use the medications prescribed. Patients retain responsibility for administering their own medications either independently or with the help of family or caregivers.

Some electronic MARs allow care providers to look up detailed information about the medication, including indications, contraindications, expected and adverse effects, and safe dosage ranges based on routes of administration. Figure 18-7 is a portion of an electronic medication record. Figure 26-7 is a paper MAR.

Terminology for Medication Administration Times.

You will document medications according to the times they are given: scheduled, unscheduled, continuous, prn, STAT, and so on.

- **Scheduled medications** are medications that are to be given on a regularly scheduled basis.
- **Unscheduled medications** are medications that are to be given on call at the appropriate time. An example of an unscheduled medication is a preoperative medication to be administered immediately before the patient goes to the surgical holding area.
- **Continuous infusions** are IV fluids that are running consistently unless stopped for a blood transfusion or to give an IV medication that is not compatible with the IV fluid running.

DATE / /

PHYSICAL ASSESSMENT - SHIFT _____

NEURO

LOC	ORIENTATION	SPEECH
❏ ALERT	❏ X3 ❏ FOR AGE	❏ APPROPRIATE
❏ SEDATED	❏ PERSON	❏ APHASIA
❏ LETHARGIC	❏ PLACE	❏ SLURRED
❏ UNRESPONSIVE	❏ TIME	❏ RAMBLING

SENSATION	FONTANELS	
❏ INTACT	❏ FLAT	❏ NA
❏ NUMBNESS	❏ SUNKEN	
❏ TINGLING	❏ BULGING	

CARDIOVASCULAR

RHYTHM	PULSE	EDEMA	CAP. REFILL
❏ REGULAR	❏ STRONG	❏ ABSENT	❏ < 3 SEC.
❏ IRREGULAR	❏ WEAK	❏ _____	❏ > 3 SEC.
❏ MURMUR	❏		

MONITOR RHYTHM

RESPIRATORY

EFFORT		BREATH
		LU LL SOUNDS RU RL
❏ NORMAL	❏ DYSPNEA	❏❏ CLEAR ❏❏
❏ LABORED	❏ COUGH	❏❏ CRACKLES ❏❏
❏ NASAL FLARING	❏ SPUTUM	❏❏ RHONCHI ❏❏
❏ RETRACTIONS	❏ CRYING	❏❏ WHEEZING ❏❏
❏ IRREGULAR		❏❏ DIMINISHED ❏❏
		❏❏ ABSENT ❏❏

GASTROINTESTINAL

ABDOMEN		
❏ FLAT	❏ FIRM	❏ NAUSEA
❏ ROUNDED	❏ TENDER	❏ VOMITING
❏ DISTENDED	❏ NON-TENDER	
❏ SOFT		
❏ GIRTH_____ CM		

BOWEL SOUNDS	STOOL	
❏ ACTIVE	❏ REGULAR	LAST BM
❏ ABSENT	❏ CONSTIPATED	
❏ HYPER	❏ DIARRHEA	
❏ HYPO	❏ INCONTINENT	_____

SUCTION
❏ INTERMITTANT   ❏ CONSTANT   ❏ CLAMPED

❏ FEEDING TUBE   ❏ PATENT
❏ NG   ❏ PLACEMENT ✔

DRNG COLOR:

GU

URINE		❏ CATHETER
❏ CLEAR, YELLOW / AMBER ❏ QS		❏ PAIN
❏ OTHER _____	❏ FREQUENT	
	❏ RETENTION	❏ INCONTINENT

MUSCULOSKELETAL

MOBILITY	MUSCLE TONE	ROM
❏ NORMAL	❏ GOOD	❏ FULL
❏ ASSIST X _____	❏ OTHER	❏ LIMITED
❏ AMBULATORY		
❏ BED REST		
❏ OTHER	❏ P.T. CONSULT	

SKIN

CONDITION	TURGOR	MUCOUS MEM
❏ WARM, DRY INTACT	❏ ADEQUATE	❏ MOIST
❏ BREAKDOWN	❏ DECREASED	❏ DRY

COLOR ❏ NORMAL
❏ PALE ❏ CYANOTIC ❏ FLUSHED ❏ _____

WOUND/INCISION/ DRESSING

LOCATION/CONDITION/DRAINAGE	HEALING NO S/S INFECTION
_____	❏
_____	❏
_____	❏

TUBES/DRAINS

LOCATION/CONDITION/DRAINAGE	GRAVITY	SUCTION
_____	❏	❏
_____	❏	❏
_____	❏	❏

IV'S

IV SITE / CONDITION	PATENT, NO REDNESS OR SWELLING	PUMP
_____	❏	❏
_____	❏	❏
_____	❏	❏

PAIN
❏ ABSENT   PAIN SCALE _____
❏ PRESENT   LOCATION _____
❏ CONTROLLED

PSYCHOSOCIAL

EYE CONTACT   ❏ YES ❏ NO

❏ APPROPRIATE	❏ RESTLESS	❏ COMBATIVE
❏ FLAT AFFECT	❏ AGITATED	❏ BELLIGERENT
❏ UNCOOPERATIVE	❏ CRYING	❏ ODOR
❏ ANXIOUS	❏ SUBSTANCE USE	

DISCHARGE

DISCHARGE PLAN

❏ NA	❏ ONGOING	❏ COMPLETED
❏ D.P. CONSULT	❏ O.T CONSULT	❏ H.H. CONSULT

EQUIPMENT

❏ BED ALARM	❏ CARDIAC MONITOR
❏ CPM	❏ FEEDING PUMP
❏ IV PUMP X_____	❏ K - PAD
❏ OXIMETER	❏ PCA PUMP
❏ PASSPORT	❏ POLAR ICE
❏ SUCTION	❏ TELEMETRY
❏ _____	❏ _____
❏ _____	❏ _____

SIGN

SIGNATURE X_____   TIME_____

REASSESSED BY X_____   TIME_____

OBSERVATION / INTERVENTION / EVALUATION

(TIME & INITIAL ENTRIES)

PHYSICAL ASSESSMENT - SHIFT _____

NEURO

LOC	ORIENTATION	SPEECH
❏ ALERT	❏ X3 ❏ FOR AGE	❏ APPROPRIATE
❏ SEDATED	❏ PERSON	❏ APHASIA
❏ LETHARGIC	❏ PLACE	❏ SLURRED
❏ UNRESPONSIVE	❏ TIME	❏ RAMBLING

SENSATION	FONTANELS	
❏ INTACT	❏ FLAT	❏ NA
❏ NUMBNESS	❏ SUNKEN	
❏ TINGLING	❏ BULGING	

CARDIOVASCULAR

RHYTHM	PULSE	EDEMA	CAP. REFILL
❏ REGULAR	❏ STRONG	❏ ABSENT	❏ < 3 SEC.
❏ IRREGULAR	❏ WEAK	❏ _____	❏ > 3 SEC.
❏ MURMUR	❏		

MONITOR RHYTHM

RESPIRATORY

EFFORT		BREATH
		LU LL SOUNDS RU RL
❏ NORMAL	❏ DYSPNEA	❏❏ CLEAR ❏❏
❏ LABORED	❏ COUGH	❏❏ CRACKLES ❏❏
❏ NASAL FLARING	❏ SPUTUM	❏❏ RHONCHI ❏❏
❏ RETRACTIONS	❏ CRYING	❏❏ WHEEZING ❏❏
❏ IRREGULAR		❏❏ DIMINISHED ❏❏
		❏❏ ABSENT ❏❏

GASTROINTESTINAL

ABDOMEN		
❏ FLAT	❏ FIRM	❏ NAUSEA
❏ ROUNDED	❏ TENDER	❏ VOMITING
❏ DISTENDED	❏ NON-TENDER	
❏ SOFT		
❏ GIRTH_____ CM		

BOWEL SOUNDS	STOOL	
❏ ACTIVE	❏ REGULAR	LAST BM
❏ ABSENT	❏ CONSTIPATED	
❏ HYPER	❏ DIARRHEA	
❏ HYPO	❏ INCONTINENT	_____

SUCTION
❏ INTERMITTANT   ❏ CONSTANT   ❏ CLAMPED

❏ FEEDING TUBE   ❏ PATENT
❏ NG   ❏ PLACEMENT

DRNG COLOR:

GU

URINE		❏ CATHETER
❏ CLEAR, YELLOW / AMBER ❏ QS		❏ PAIN
❏ OTHER _____	❏ FREQUENT	
	❏ RETENTION	❏ INCONTINENT

MUSCULOSKELETAL

MOBILITY	MUSCLE TONE	ROM
❏ NORMAL	❏ GOOD	❏ FULL
❏ ASSIST X _____	❏ OTHER	❏ LIMITED
❏ AMBULATORY		
❏ BED REST		
❏ OTHER	❏ P.T. CONSULT	

SKIN

CONDITION	TURGOR	MUCOUS MEM
❏ WARM, DRY INTACT	❏ ADEQUATE	❏ MOIST
❏ BREAKDOWN	❏ DECREASED	❏ DRY

COLOR ❏ NORMAL
❏ PALE ❏ CYANOTIC ❏ FLUSHED ❏ _____

WOUND/INCISION/ DRESSING

LOCATION/CONDITION/DRAINAGE	HEALING NO S/S INFECTION
_____	❏
_____	❏
_____	❏

TUBES/DRAINS

LOCATION/CONDITION/DRAINAGE	GRAVITY	SUCTION
_____	❏	❏
_____	❏	❏
_____	❏	❏

IV'S

IV SITE / CONDITION	PATENT, NO REDNESS OR SWELLING	PUMP
_____	❏	❏
_____	❏	❏
_____	❏	❏

NURSING ASSESSMENT   PATIENT NAME

FIGURE 18-6 A portion of a nursing assessment checklist.

Table 18-2 ➤ Comparison of Content of MARs for Inpatient and Outpatient Facilities

INPATIENT MARS	OUTPATIENT MARS
■ Drug name	■ Drug name
■ Dosage	■ Dosage
■ Route of administration	■ Route of administration
■ Frequency	■ Number of pills, patches, and so on to be dispensed at each prescription refill
■ Duration	■ Number of refills ordered
■ Scheduled times of administration	■ Directions for using the medication, including frequency and duration
■ Charting of medication administration	■ Historical information about prescriptions, pharmacies used, and refills authorized
■ Signatures (written or electronic) of nurses administering medication	

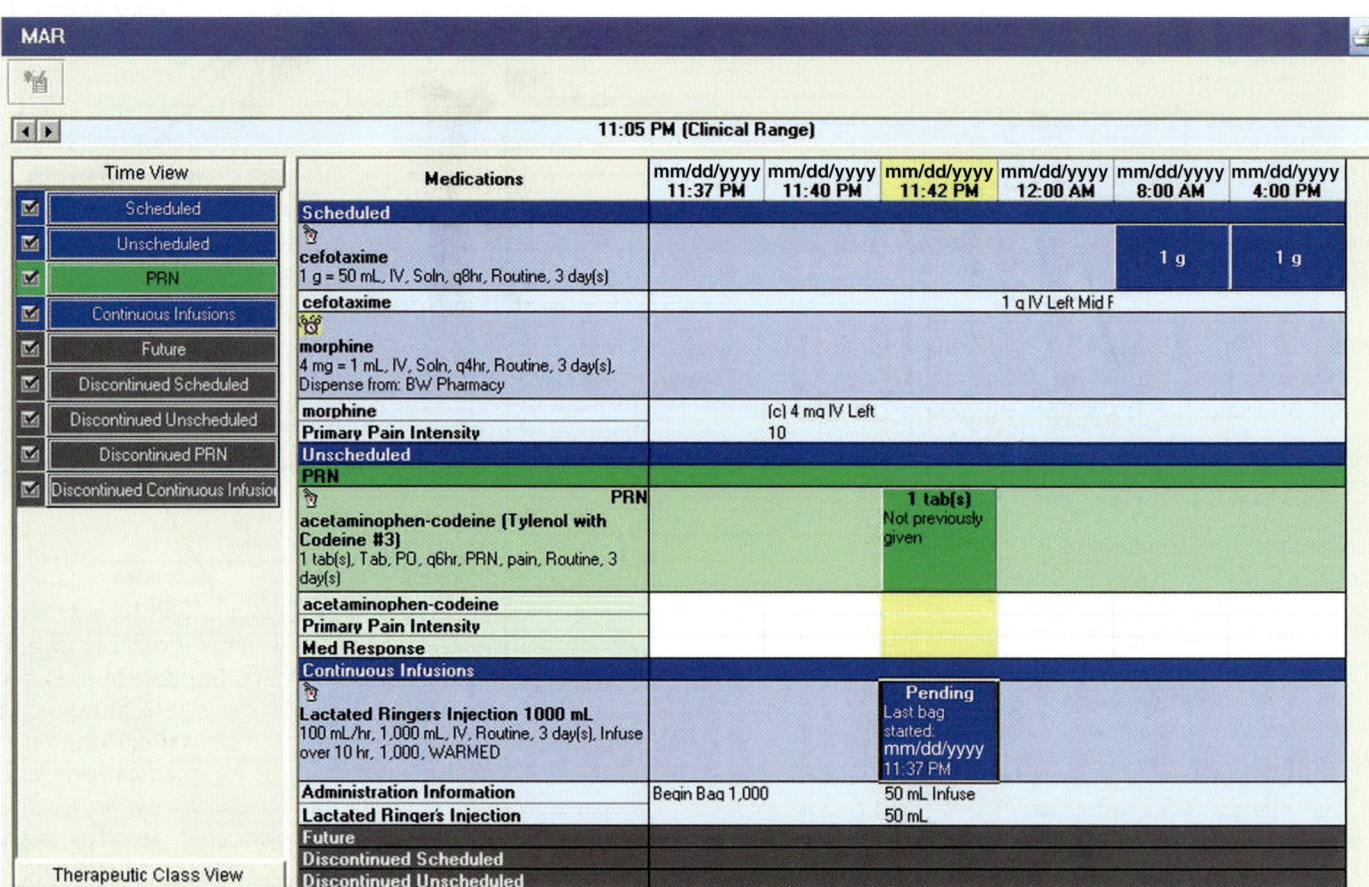

FIGURE 18-7 A portion of an electronic medication administration record. (Courtesy of Cerner Corporation, Kansas City, MO.)

■ **Prn** means "as needed." It is an abbreviation of the Latin term *pro re nata*. Medications administered prn are given only when the patient meets certain conditions that were established in the medication prescription. Typically, medications are prescribed prn for relief of pain, fever, nausea, and constipation. You should administer a prn medication when you assess that the patient needs it or when the patient requests it. Document immediately after you administer the medication.

■ A **STAT** medication is given and charted immediately and only once.

■ A **single-order** medication is given once at a prescribed time, but not necessarily immediately.

Charting Additional Information About Medications. For scheduled medications, you may only have to initial and make a checkmark in the column that corresponds with the preprinted times at the top. In the circumstances following, you will often need to record additional information on the MAR and sometimes even in the Progress Notes.

- **Injections.** If you administer an injection, you must chart the type and the site of administration to protect the patient from repeated injections in the same location.
- **Assessment Required Before Administration.** Some medications require you to make a specific assessment before administering the drug, to ensure that it is safe to give it. You must document that assessment data on the MAR, along with the time of administration and other required information (see Chapter 26). As an example, most protocols instruct you to not give digoxin (a cardiac medication) if the heart rate is below 60 beats/min., so you must auscultate the rate before giving the drug. Blood pressure and pain medications, insulin, and anticoagulants also require assessments before administration.

- ✚ **Drug Allergies.** Drug allergies are always noted on the paper or electronic MAR. This makes them easily visible for caregivers who are prescribing or administering medication. If the patient has an allergic reaction to a medicine, you must record this response on the MAR and in the nurses' notes. Of course you would also report this to the prescriber, as discussed later in this chapter.

- **STAT, prn, Unscheduled, and Single-Order Medications.** Enter on the MAR the time the medication is given. Make a narrative note of your assessment findings and the patient's response to the medication in the appropriate location on the paper or electronic MAR. Some documented data, such as the pain score before administration of an analgesic, may automatically migrate from other documentation sources to become visible on the MAR.

  You may occasionally see a prn order that provides a range of medication to be given based on your assessment of the patient, for example, "Titrate morphine 2–3 mg IV every 1–2 hours to achieve pain control."

✚ In the electronic MAR system, medication range orders (e.g., 1 to 2 mg) are difficult to order, so The Joint Commission and most agency protocols no longer allow dosage range orders.

- **Patient Refusal.** If the patient refuses a medication, note the refusal on the paper or electronic MAR. Your organization's policy will determine how this is recorded. On paper, you might draw a circle around the scheduled time of administration. When documenting electronically, you can click on an option offered in the MAR, such as Not Given, and then select *Patient Refused* from a drop-down field listing multiple reasons why a medication is not given.
- **Omitted Medication or Delayed Administration.** If the patient is not available or is experiencing health changes that require immediate interventions, it may be necessary to withhold a medication or delay its administration. On the paper MAR, some organizations

provide a boxed section at the bottom, with a code to indicate why the medication was withheld or given at a different time. Circle the scheduled time and fill in the symbol. You will also have to chart the omission or delay in your nurses' notes. However, in the electronic MAR, often it is possible to reschedule administration times for a single dose or permanently going forward. Many systems will require you enter the reason and the action taken.

Kardex or Patient Care Summary

As discussed in Chapter 5, the Kardex is a special kind of paper form or folding card that briefly summarizes a patient's status and plan of care. Paper Kardex and electronic patient care summaries typically pull patient data from multiple areas of the health record (medical and nursing diagnoses, orders, treatments, results). Figure 18-8 is an example of an electronic patient care summary screen. To see a paper Kardex,

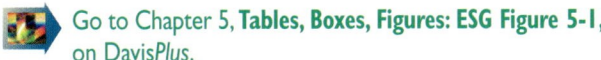

Go to Chapter 5, **Tables, Boxes, Figures: ESG Figure 5-1,** on Davis*Plus*.

Paper Kardexes are usually kept together in a portable file in a central location in the nurses' station to allow all team members access to patients' summary information. Each patient has a separate screen in an electronic summary. All authorized members of the care team can access the electronic care summary at the same time, even if they are away from the patient or outside the organization in a remote location, depending on the institution's permission for access. Neither the paper Kardex nor the electronic care summary is a permanent part of the patient's health record.

Integrated Plan of Care

Integrated plans of care (IPOCs) are a combined charting and care plan form. They exist in both paper and electronic formats. An IPOC maps out day-by-day patient goals, outcomes, interventions, and treatments for a specific diagnosis or condition from admission to discharge. Lab work, diagnostic testing, medications, and therapies are all included in the pathway, as well as standardized interventions captured in the plan. IPOCs help administrators predict length of stay, monitor costs of care, and can assist with staffing. They also eliminate duplicate charting, increase team effort, and enhance the nurse's teaching about what the patient can expect during the hospital stay. Figure 18-3 is an example of an electronic IPOC. For examples of complete printed IPOCs,

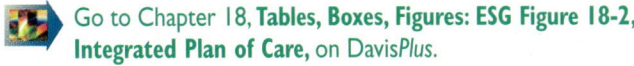

Go to Chapter 18, **Tables, Boxes, Figures: ESG Figure 18-2, Integrated Plan of Care,** on Davis*Plus*.

Multiple patient diagnoses can be captured easily in an electronic IPOC. However, in special situations, you may need to individualize the paper IPOC by commenting on special issues in the space provided for narrative

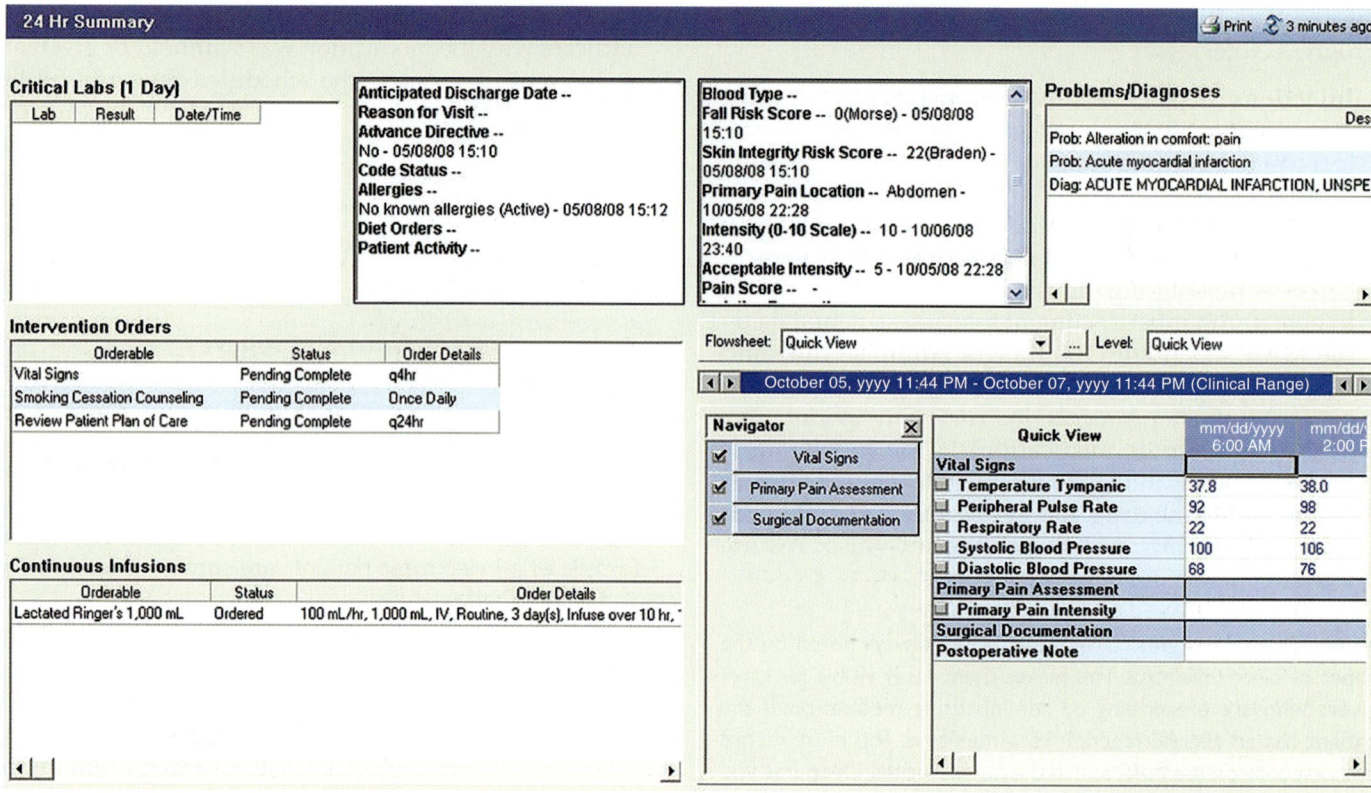

FIGURE 18-8 A portion of an electronic patient care summary screen. (Courtesy of Cerner Corporation, Kansas City, MO.)

comments (e.g., developmental delay with our patient Steven Stellanski).

Occurrence Reports

An **occurrence report**, or incident report, is a formal record of an unusual occurrence or accident. This is an organizational report that is used to analyze the event, identify areas for quality improvement, and formulate strategies to prevent future occurrences. The overall goal is to create safer processes and procedures for clients and staff. **Key Point:** *An occurrence report is not part of the client's health record and thus should never be referenced in the nurses' notes or in other sections of the health record.* The paper report should be sent to risk management, according to agency protocol, while the electronic form is completed on the organization's secure internal network. See Box 18-2 for examples of events that require the completion of an occurrence report.

You should report all errors, even if there was no adverse impact on the client. This is important from a safety standpoint for improving your institution's quality of care and from a legal perspective to provide defensible information. When completing an occurrence form, be sure to clearly identify the client, date, time, and location. Briefly describe the incident in objective terms. Quote the client or persons involved if possible. Identify any witnesses to the event, equipment involved, and environmental conditions. Avoid drawing conclusions or placing blame. You should document actions taken and the patient response to the

BOX 18-2 ■ Events Requiring an Occurrence Report

- Patient fall or other injury
- Medication error
- Incorrect implementation of a prescribed treatment
- Needlestick injury or other injury to staff
- Loss of patient belongings
- Injury of a visitor
- Unsafe staffing situation
- Lack of availability of essential patient care supplies
- Inadequate response to emergency situation

interventions. Chapter 45 provides additional information on occurrence reports.

KnowledgeCheck 18-3

- Identify at least five types of paper documentation forms.
- What should you document after administering a prn medication?
- What is the purpose of an occurrence report?
- Identify four events in which you will need to complete an occurrence report.
- Identify the following abbreviations (see Volume 2):

abd	OOB	NKDA
BRP	pc	tid
DM	prn	q
fx	STD	LUQ

What Is Unique About Documentation in Home Healthcare?

Although you will perform many of the same assessments and interventions in home care that you do in other areas of healthcare, the documentation is unique. The Centers for Medicare & Medicaid Services (CMS) guidelines govern home healthcare documentation. Among the requirements for care are (1) certification of home-bound status, (2) a plan of care, and (3) ongoing assessment of the need for skilled care.

The most commonly used paper home health documentation form is known as OASIS—the Outcome and Assessment Information Set. Because of a federal government mandate that Medicare providers convert to electronic e-prescribing, many home health agencies have electronic documentation systems or plans to adopt a system. Home health nurses can use laptop computers to retrieve patient data and record progress notes in the home. The computer also allows the nurse to conveniently order needed supplies for home care and to coordinate scheduling of follow-up visits.

In home care, a monthly summary describing the patient's status and ongoing needs is required. The patient's PCP signs this form, which is submitted for reimbursement. Chapter 43 provides further information about home care.

Home health documentation includes the following:

- Your assessment highlighting changes in the client's condition
- Interventions performed (wound care, dressing changes, teaching, and other treatments)
- The client's response to interventions
- Any interaction or teaching that you conducted with caregivers
- Any interaction with the patient's PCP

If you would like to see an OASIS form,

Go to Chapter 18, **Tables, Boxes, Figures: ESG Figure 18-3, Outcome and Assessment Information Set (OASIS),** on Davis*Plus.*

 ThinkLike a Nurse 18-2
Why do you think it is essential to document homebound status and the ongoing need for skilled care?

What Is Unique About Documentation in Long-Term Care?

Documentation requirements for long-term care depend on the level of care the client requires. All clients in long-term care facilities must have a comprehensive assessment at admission. Federal law requires that a resident be evaluated using the Minimum Data Set for Resident Assessment and Care Screening (MDS) within 14 days of admission. The MDS must be updated every 3 months and with any significant change in client condition. For an example of an MDS form,

Go to Chapter 18, **Tables, Boxes, Figures: ESG Figure 18-4, Minimum Data Set,** on Davis*Plus.*

Legal requirements to protect older adults mandate that you report changes in a client's condition to the PCP and to the client's family. Chart your reports in narrative notes on paper or in the appropriate areas of electronic forms. If you are caring for a client receiving Medicare-reimbursed services, such as IV therapy, wound care, or rehabilitation services, documentation is required with each shift. In addition, a summary written by a nurse must be recorded weekly. The weekly summary for adult clients must include the following:

- A summary of the client's condition
- An evaluation of the client's ability to perform ADLs
- The client's level of consciousness and mood
- Hydration and nutrition status
- Response to medications
- Any treatments provided
- Safety measures (e.g., bed rails, bed alarm, wander guard)

Long-term care facilities also provide intermediate-care services for clients who need assistance with medications, nutrition, and ADLs. These clients require a nursing care summary every 2 weeks. For a nursing assessment flowsheet used in long-term care,

Go to Chapter 18, **Charting Forms, A Flowsheet Used in Long-term Care,** in Volume 2.

KnowledgeCheck 18-4
How do home care and long-term care documentation differ from hospital-based documentation?

 ThinkLike a Nurse 18-3
Why do long-term care clients require less frequent charting than clients in acute care settings?

ORAL REPORTING

The purpose of giving an oral report is to maintain continuity of care. The oral report provides an opportunity for professional communication that assists in organizing your work, and also for learning, building team relationships, and collaborating to improve patient care. Whether the source of the information shared is from a written report form, a paper Kardex, or a summary in the EHR, the quality of the report you give and receive influences how you and others plan the day's (or night's) work. Restrict your oral reports to patient-focused discussion and limit unimportant details and social conversation.

How Do I Give a Handoff Report?
The purpose of a **handoff report** (sometimes called a *change-of-shift report* or *handover report*) is to promote continuity in care. The receiving nurse is alerted to the

client's status or recent changes in the client's condition; planned activities, tests, and procedures; or concerns that require follow-up. A handoff report may be given at the bedside or in a conference room, using paper notes or a mobile or desktop EHR device.

Handoff reports are usually given orally, although some organizations use written or audio-recorded reports. As a student nurse, you will receive report from either the nurse completing the shift or from the nurse assigned to the client during the shift you will be working. Report any changes to the nurse assigned to the client during your shift, and always give a report before leaving the unit.

- **A bedside report**, sometimes known as "walking rounds," allows you to observe important aspects of care, such as patient appearance, IV pumps, and wounds. With a bedside report, the outgoing nurse can introduce you to the patient and you can begin your assessment. If the patient is alert, give him the opportunity to participate in the report and ask questions. This type of report encourages continuity of care, team collaboration, and patient/family communication. Previously criticized as time consuming, Nelson and Massey (2010) reported that using an electronic template and process at the bedside decreased the time spent in change of shift report. **Key Point: *Ensure that the patient's privacy rights are protected when using bedside reports.***

- **A face-to-face oral report**, may involve only the outgoing and oncoming nurse or may include the entire oncoming shift. When given in a conference room, an oral report does not let you directly observe the patient, but it is time efficient and still allows interaction between nurses.

- **An audio-recorded report**, is a convenient, but sometimes time-consuming, way to transmit information. The outgoing nurse audio-records a report on the clients under her care. This method can be time-consuming, especially if you must listen to the entire unit report before hearing about your own assigned patients. A major disadvantage of an audio-recorded report is that the oncoming nurse has limited opportunity to ask questions about the client. Occasionally, audio quality is poor and the report is not clear. An advantage of this method is that the outgoing nurse continues to provide patient care while the incoming nurse receives report.

To minimize communication errors, the outgoing and incoming nurses should speak directly to each other to update information or answer any questions about the patients care. This complies with The Joint Commission Center for Transforming Healthcare (2010) recommendation that a handoff system allows for questioning between the giver and receiver of the information.

Standardized Report Formats. In more than 3,000 root-cause analyses of patient errors, communication was a primary contributor in 65% to 70% of the events (Triplett & Schuveiller, 2011). Other data indicate that "an estimated 80 percent of serious medical errors involve miscommunication between caregivers when patients are transferred or handed-off" (The Joint Commission, 2012b). No matter where or how the handoff report is given, nurses should use a consistent, structured (standardized) process that contains critical key items.

- The **PACE** format is one example of a standardized approach developed specifically to organize patient data in handoffs. The acronym stands for Patient/Problem, Assessment/Actions, Continuing/Changes, and Evaluation (Schroeder, 2006).

- The **SBAR** (Situation–Background–Assessment–Recommendation) is an easy-to-remember, concrete acronym useful for framing any conversation. Because nurses and physicians communicate in very different ways, SBAR is useful for interdisciplinary communication, especially critical situations requiring a clinician's immediate attention and action. SBAR allows for an easy and focused way to set expectations for what will be communicated and how between members of the team. The SBAR technique can be adapted for handoff reports.

For additional information about communicating with SBAR and PACE,

Go to Chapter 21, **Clinical Insight 21-3, Communicating With SBAR,** and Chapter 18, **Clinical Insight 18-1, Giving Oral Reports,** in Volume 2.

Regardless of the format used, to prepare to give a handoff report, you need to collect the following information:

- Client progress made during your shift
- Therapies and treatments administered
- Teaching done
- Consultations done or planned with other disciplines
- Status of identified desired outcomes
- Any changes in client status
- Progress made on discharge planning

Knowledge Check 18-5

- What data should be included in a handoff report?
- What are the types of handoff reports?

What Is a Transfer Report?

Transfer reports are given when a patient is transferred from unit to unit or from facility to facility. For information to include in an oral transfer report,

Go to Chapter 18, **Clinical Insight 18-1: Giving Oral Reports,** in Volume 2.

If the patient is being transported to another unit in the same facility, you will need to transport a paper chart with the patient. If both units are using an EHR documentation system, then the receiving unit can access the client record

Quality and Safety Education for Nurses

Handoff Reporting: Decreasing Risks for Miscommunication

Chapter Key Concepts: *Documentation, Oral reporting*

Competencies: *Safety (Knowledge, Skills, and Attitudes); Teamwork and Collaboration (Knowledge, Skills, and Attitudes)**

Think about it: How do the chapter key concepts relate to the QSEN competencies? Think about the number of patient handoffs per day among nurses and other professionals (e.g., physicians). Then consider some risks to patient safety that have been caused by miscommunication:

➤ Errors that have occurred because of poor *physician handoff reporting* include amputating the wrong leg, removing a healthy adrenal gland, failing to obtain serum sodium levels from a patient with diabetes insipidus, failing to act on stroke symptoms, and failing to correct electrolyte imbalances. All of these errors resulted in death or permanent brain damage.

➤ Potential harms in nursing *shift change handoffs* include delays in initiating critical medications or obtaining specimens; failing to initiate new treatments, communicate change in patient status, or report critical lab results; and repeating outdated information.

Causes. Factors contributing to poor quality handoffs include lack of a standardized protocol or form, relying on memory,

varying levels of experience, and lack of dedicated time for reporting.

Actions. Collaborate with others in your facility to suggest the following strategies for improving quality of care, teamwork, and patient safety:

➤ Standardize the information (e.g., SBAR) to be conveyed but avoid giving too much or too little information.

➤ Include "if . . . , then . . ." statements for current problems (e.g., *if* the glucose level is still elevated, *then* call physician for insulin orders).

➤ Develop an electronic form or other tool to reinforce and clarify the transfer of knowledge and responsibility.

➤ Conduct training sessions to lessen the chance of reporting errors.

For specific Knowledge, Skills, and Attitudes

 Go to the QSEN Web site **at http://qsen.org/ competencies/pre-licensure-ksas/**

Source: Collins, S., Stein, D., Vawdrey, D., et al. (2011); Kitch, B., Cooper, J., Zapol, W., et al. (2008); Riesenberg, L., Leisch, J., & Cunningham, J. (2010).

---

electronically. Detailed information about the patient's health history can be communicated between healthcare professionals or transmitted before transfer. For transfers to other facilities, your organization will have a policy on what is to be copied and how materials should be transmitted to the receiving facility.

Research shows that older adults are vulnerable to errors in care when transitioning from one healthcare facility to another. Medication errors were dominant, resulting in increased hospital readmissions, injuries, or death. MBAR—**M**edication–**B**ackground–**A**ssessment–**R**ecommendation—was developed to provide a structured, standardized handoff that promotes medication reconciliation during handoffs and transfers (Blank, Benyo, & Glover, 2012).

For a review of transfers and discharges, see Chapter 11 in this volume and

 Go to Chapter 11, **Procedures 11-2, 11-3, and 11-4,** in Volume 2.

How Do I Receive and Document Verbal and Telephone Orders?

Although licensed nurses may find it necessary to accept verbal or telephone orders on occasion, verbal and telephone orders increase the risk of hearing or writing the order incorrectly. The Joint Commission recommends the person to validate a

verbal order or report of critical test results using a written and read-back process before taking any action (The Joint Commission, 2011). SBAR-R is a revised version that adds the read-back component to minimize errors and failures in communication between the nurse and provider.

Telephone Orders

Telephone orders can lead to error because of differences in pronunciation, dialect, or accent; background noise; poor reception; and unfamiliar terminology. Taking a telephone order may be acceptable when there has been a sudden change in your patient's condition and the client's PCP is not in the hospital, or the physician does not have access to placing orders electronically. Verbal or telephone orders are also acceptable in a life-threatening emergency, but you must apply the document and "read-back" safeguard. Faxes, text messages, and e-mail have reduced the need for telephone orders; however, their use may never disappear entirely.

For guidelines to use when taking telephone orders,

 Go to Chapter 18, **Clinical Insight 18-2: Receiving Telephone and Verbal Orders,** in Volume 2.

The following is an example of a telephone order transcribed to a paper order sheet:

08/27/16 0805 Morphine 2 mg IV push once for pain now.————————TO Dr. Kent/S. Hogan RN

If the telephone order is entered electronically, the date/time and order remain the same, the order is marked as an electronic entry, and will go to the selected physician, Dr. Kent, for his signature.

Verbal Orders

Verbal orders are spoken directions for patient care given to you in person, usually during an emergency. Providers should never use verbal orders as a routine method of communicating orders. When recording a verbal order, include the date, time, and the written text of the order or the electronic entry of the order. If you are writing the order on an order sheet, an indicator "VO" designating verbal orders is then followed by the provider's name and your name. If you are entering the order electronically, then the order will be designated as a verbal order and be routed to the selected physician for co-signature. Follow The Joint Commission safety guidelines, above, and

 Go to Chapter 18, **Clinical Insight 18-2: Receiving Telephone and Verbal Orders,** in Volume 2.

KnowledgeCheck 18-6

- What important factors should you document when receiving a telephone order?
- What is the purpose of a verbal order? When should it be used?

How Do I Question an Order?

If you feel uncertain about an order, you must question it. As a student, you will first want to discuss your concerns with your clinical instructor or the nurse you are working with during your clinical time. Remember, the goal is to provide safe care. If you have concerns, do not remain quiet—act on them.

As a nurse, you will follow your organization's policy for clarifying orders. If an order is written illegibly on a paper order sheet or is entered into the EHR missing details or order components, contact the provider directly to seek clarification. Generally, you should contact the provider who wrote the order. If the provider leaves the order as-is and you still don't feel comfortable with it or believe there is an error, you may refuse to carry it out. Inform the chain of command at your organization about your refusal. Usually you will speak with the charge nurse, who may then contact the nurse manager or nursing supervisor. The nature of the order will determine how the situation is handled.

As a new nurse, you may feel uncomfortable about questioning an order. Even experienced nurses sometimes feel uneasy with this challenge. If you are uncertain how to proceed, you can discuss your concerns with your colleagues, the charge nurse, or the supervisor before contacting the provider. Your efforts to clarify the orders help to protect your patient. If you do refuse an order, you must document your refusal and the actions you took to clarify the order.

Key Point: *If you believe an order is inappropriate or unsafe, you are legally and ethically required to question the order.*

PracticalKnowledge
knowing **how**

To document care effectively, you need to be familiar with the forms and requirements of your institution. Chart routine nursing actions (e.g., skin care) on the designated paper or electronic flowsheets or forms; and record your assessments, interventions, and patient responses to care in the format approved by your organization. It is important to chart accurately, completely, and consistently so that the patient's progress can be tracked and appropriate care given.

Remember that the patient's health record is permanent and that information contained in the chart is confidential. As a student, you are granted access to a client's charts for educational purposes. You have a duty to keep the information private and confidential. The Health Insurance Portability and Accountability Act (HIPAA) regulations affect access, storage, transfer, and discussion of patient information. For more information about privacy, confidentiality, and HIPAA, refer to Chapters 44 and 45.

ThinkLike a Nurse 18-4

You note that your client with asthma is having increasing difficulty breathing. You call the physician, who gives you a telephone order for an asthma medication, and then hangs up. When you enter the order electronically as a verbal order, you find out the medication is a nonformulary medication that your pharmacy does not carry.

- Is this an acceptable reason to take a verbal order?
- The physician gets irritated when you call back and says, "I prescribed what I wanted." How would you handle this situation?
- You entered the order electronically after the physician hung up. How could this situation have been avoided?

GUIDELINES FOR DOCUMENTING CARE

Key Point: *Your documentation should convey the care that you provided to the patient during your shift.*

Thus, if you read your documentation 3 years later, as in the case of malpractice lawsuits, it should attest that the care you provided to the patient adhered to minimum standards of nursing practice. For a brief set of documentation tips, see Box 18-3. For detailed guidelines for documentation,

 Go to Chapter 18, **Clinical Insight 18-3,** in Volume 2.

Guidelines for Paper Health Records

To comply with HIPAA requirements, paper health records need to be stored in designated areas to which only healthcare providers have access. To ensure your

BOX 18-3 ■ Documentation ABCs

Accurate
Bias-free
Complete
Detailed
Easy to read
Factual
Grammatical
Harmless (legally)

written paper documentation is effective, the forms used must be efficient, comprehensive, and relevant to the patient's healthcare needs. The forms should guide you to document appropriately according to your organization's policies and procedures. The following guidelines will further assist you in documenting appropriately.

- **Maintain confidentiality.** Do not provide written or verbal information to anyone not involved in the direct care of the patient without the patient's consent.
- **Ensure you have the correct form (e.g., I&O sheet, graphic record) before you begin writing.**
- **Check that the chart and documentation forms are clearly marked with the patient's name and identification number.**
- **Write legibly, neatly, and in an organized manner.** This enables others to read your entries and use them to make clinical decisions. Sloppy or illegible handwriting creates errors or, at least, leads to poor communication.
- **Always use black ink for handwritten notes (some agencies do permit blue ink).** Inks other than black or blue are not legible when a chart is photocopied. Do NOT use green or red pen. Remember that the chart is a legal document.
- **Do not leave blank lines in the narrative notes.** If you need to leave space for clarity, draw a straight line through the area and begin on the next line. Open areas leave an opportunity for later tampering.
- **Draw a line through the incorrect charting and initial it.** Never use a correction fluid, "ink over," or otherwise cover up written notes.
- **Sign all your paper charting entries with your first name, last name, and professional credentials, such as Judy Long, RN.**
- **Don't write in "shorthand" or your own abbreviated symbols.**
- **Use only abbreviations that are approved by your organization.**

Guidelines for Electronic Health Records

Well-designed nursing documentation forms and systems help you organize your work, manage your care plans, track client diagnoses and outcomes, and support decision making by healthcare providers.

How Can I Document Efficiently and Effectively?

To ensure your documentation in the EHR is most efficient and effective, keep the following in mind:

- **You must have basic computer, mouse, and software skills** to document effectively in the EHR.
- **If you are uneasy or more stressed using computers**, or unfamiliar with the software it may take you longer to make the transition to documenting in the EHR.
- **Help keep patient rooms clutter-free** so that you have a place to use a portable computer in the room for direct charting.

What Is Unique About Entering the Data?

- **Before Charting.** Before opening charting forms, you must ensure that the patient's name, identification number, and any other unique health record identifiers are correct.
- **Saving Documentation.** If your EHR allows you to save partially completed documentation before signing it, do complete the documentation and sign it as quickly as possible. In most EHR systems, saved documentation cannot be seen by others until it is signed.
- **Checklists.** Electronic forms and flowsheets are often built in a format similar to a checklist. This can make it more difficult to capture detailed patient changes and findings.
- **Errors.** If you make an error (e.g., make entries on the wrong chart or enter and sign the wrong information), you can correct it. The entry can never be completely deleted, but only the corrected information will be visible to anyone viewing the chart.

What Happens If the Computer Doesn't Work?

EHR systems can have periodic downtimes due to scheduled maintenance or network or interface problems. Client care does not stop, so you need to know the processes and procedures to follow when the EHR is offline and inaccessible. Follow organization policies regarding the amount of time the EHR needs to be "down" before you begin documenting on paper form.

How Do I Maintain Confidentiality and Data Security?

Although the specific risks to and safeguards of confidentiality differ in detail between paper and electronic records, confidentiality is equally important in both. The following safeguards are specific to EHRs:

- *When moving away from the open EHR*, close the screen and temporarily or permanently log off to ensure confidentiality and privacy. Most computer stations will automatically log-off after a specified period of inactivity. This helps keep unauthorized viewers from having access to patient information.
- *Privacy filters*—Some computer screens are equipped with privacy filters to protect patient information from the view of non-authorized viewers.

- *Create a secure password*—not something obvious, such as your birth date, Social Security number, or family members' names. Instead, you might choose a password that is at least six characters long and includes at least one capital letter (if the system is case sensitive), one number, and (if allowed by the system) one symbol. The system you are using will determine the specifications.
- *Change your password at regular intervals* even if your organization does not require it. Some systems will lock you out of the system if your password is not changed as required.
- *Do not share your personal username or password* with anyone. You are responsible for the data recorded and saved using your electronic identity. If someone else enters data or accesses charts under your identity, you will be held responsible for those actions if the patient initiates legal action.
- *Do not leave patient data displayed on the screen where others can see it.*
- *Do not leave the computer unattended after you have logged on.* This allows others access to confidential data, and to document under your name.
- *Do not leave a portable device (e.g., a laptop or PDA) unattended in a public location,* such as on a countertop in the nurses' station. This increases the possibility of theft or unauthorized access to secured patient information.
- *Never access client health records that you have no professional reason to view.* This is a severe breach of client

privacy rules. Know your state and federal laws consequences for privacy violations.
- *Become familiar with your organization's policies* regarding network and patient health record information security and confidentiality.

KnowledgeCheck 18-7

 Refer to **Clinical Insight 18-3, in Volume 2,** to help you answer the following questions.

- What aspects of care should be documented?
- When should care be documented?
- How is documentation on paper different from documentation in an EHR or on an electronic digital form?

ThinkLike a Nurse 18-5

You are caring for two clients on a medical-surgical unit. One of your clients is short of breath and complaining of chest pain. Your other client is recovering from abdominal surgery. He is alert, stable, and free from pain at this time. After stabilizing your first client, you realize you are 45 minutes late administering a medication to the abdominal surgery patient. You are not sure how to proceed.

- What theoretical knowledge do you need?
- You give the medicine as soon as you can (60 minutes late). How and where should you chart the medication administered?
- If you had been aware that you were going to be late with the medication, what might you have done to be sure it was given on time?

Toward Evidence-Based Practice

Cherry, B., Ford, E., & Peterson, L. (2011). Experiences with electronic health records: Early adopters in long-term care facilities. *Health Care Management Review, 36(3),* 265–274.

The implementation of electronic health records in 10 long-term care facilities revealed that administrators, nurses, managers, nurses, certified nurse aides, and other system users indicated that EHRs (1) were cost effective in improved quality of care, (2) increased documentation accuracy and implementation of evidence-based practices, (3) improved access to resident information, (4) reduced nursing overtime, and (5) resulted in an overall positive attitude among personnel working with the system.

Huryk, L. (2010). Factors influencing nurses' attitudes toward healthcare information technology. *Journal of Nursing Management, 18(5),* 606–612.

A systematic review of 13 articles on nurses' attitudes toward healthcare information technology (HIT) revealed that more positive attitudes were associated with (1) increased computer

experience, (2) perceptions that HIT will enhance patient care or safety, (3) positive attitude of administrators, and (4) user-friendly and well-integrated systems. Less positive attitudes were associated with (1) perceptions of dehumanizing patient care, and (2) technological system issues/flaws. A theme of not returning to paper charting was dominant.

Kossman, S., & Scheidenhelm, S. (2008). Nurses' perceptions of the impact of electronic health records on work and patient outcomes. *CIN: Computers, Informatics, Nursing, 26(2),* 69–77.

This study addressed 46 medical-surgical and intensive care unit nurses' use of electronic health records (EHR) and their views of the impact of such records on job performance and patient outcomes. Results indicated that nurses (1) preferred EHR to paper charts and were comfortable with technology; (2) thought use of EHR impaired critical thinking, decreased interdisciplinary communication, and created a high demand on work time (73% reported spending at least half their shift

Toward Evidence-Based Practice—cont'd

using the records); (3) believed that EHR improved organization, efficiency, and information access (e.g., helpful alert screens); and (4) thought the use of EHR enabled them to provide safer care but decreased the quality of care.

1. Compare the advantages given in Advantages of Electronic Health Records with the findings in the above studies. Which EHR advantage is *not* supported by either of these studies? What is the

statement in each study that conflicts with the advantages reported in your text?

2. Which study disagrees with the statement that EHR improves communication between healthcare providers? What does the study say about that?

 Go to Chapter 18, **Toward Evidence-Based Practice Suggested Responses,** on the Davis*Plus*.

Can I Delegate Charting?

In some facilities, each member of the team is responsible for documenting care provided to the client. Nursing assistants or other nursing assistive personnel (NAP) often chart ADLs, activity, and I&O on graphic records. You are responsible for documenting the nursing care you provide. Never chart the actions of others as though you performed them. If an action is crucial to a chain of events, you may document that action on paper or in the EHR, referring to the person who did the action clearly. For example, "Became dizzy; assisted to chair by Nora Roverdale, NAP."

KnowledgeCheck 18-8

- Can charting be delegated?
- You are a student nurse on a medical-surgical unit. You review your client's chart and notice that the physician entered prescriptions that do not appear to be appropriate for your client. The physician is still in the area. How would you handle this situation?

 To explore learning resources for this chapter,

 Go to Davis*Plus* at **DavisPl.us/Wilkinson3.**

Chapter Resources for Chapter 18:

Response sheets for all learning activities

Resources for Caregivers and Health Professionals

Reading More About Documenting & Reporting (suggested readings)

Concept Map of chapter content

Interactive Case Studies

NCLEX-Style and Chapter Review Questions

Chapter Overview Podcasts

For references cited in this chapter, Go to Volume 2, References Cited.

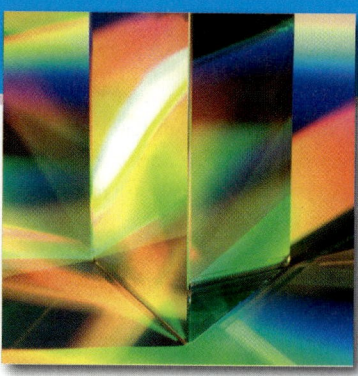

CHAPTER 19

Teaching & Learning

Learning Outcomes

After completing this chapter, you should be able to:

➤ Present three factors contributing to the expanding role of teaching in professional nursing.

➤ Describe the concepts of teaching and learning.

➤ Name, define, and give one example of each of Bloom's three domains of learning.

➤ Discuss how each of the following factors can affect learning: motivation, readiness, physical condition, emotions, timing, active involvement, feedback, repetition, environment, scheduling of the teaching session, amount and complexity of the content, communication, special needs (e.g., learning disability), developmental stage, culture, and literacy.

➤ List at least six barriers to teaching and learning.

➤ Describe some strategies for motivating learners.

➤ Develop strategies for working with clients with cultural or learning differences.

➤ Describe the content of a learning assessment.

➤ Discuss correct and incorrect uses of the nursing diagnosis Deficient Knowledge.

➤ Develop teaching plans for clients.

➤ List four methods for evaluating the outcomes of teaching and learning.

➤ Document teaching content, methods, and patient responses to learning.

Key Concepts

Learning

Health literacy

Learning environment

Teaching

Related Concepts

See the Concept Map on DavisPlus.

Meet Your Patients

You are the student nurse assigned to Heather, a 20-year-old mother, and her 4-year-old preschooler. They have come to a family practice clinic for a well-child checkup. During the healthcare visit, you notice that the child speaks only in one- or two-word phrases. The mother's tone to her daughter is impatient and she repeatedly tells her to "stop using that baby talk."

Heather says, "I don't know what I'm doing wrong. All her friends are taller and talking more. She was even small when she was born, so I suppose it's my fault."

Your assessment shows the child is below the 5th percentile for height and weight. What health teaching could you provide that might help resolve this problem? Your nursing instructor tells you to assess for teaching needs and provide anticipatory guidance to the mother. How would you begin to address Heather's learning needs without reinforcing her feelings of self-blame?

Your anticipatory guidance should include information about safety measures for a 4-year-old, nutrition for pre-school-age children, and expected growth and development. How can you evaluate whether or not the teaching has been effective and further promote Heather's retention of this new information?

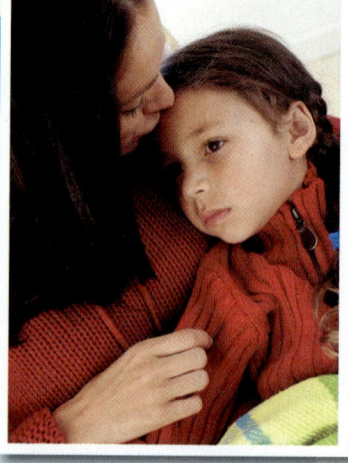

By the time you finish working through this chapter, you should be able to answer these questions and provide teaching to meet the unique needs of other patients you encounter.

ABOUT THE KEY CONCEPTS

This chapter covers concepts that underlie how people take in and offer information within the healthcare environment. The overarching concepts of **teaching** and **learning** provide a "hook" on which you can hang what you learn about all the other concepts in this chapter. A firm grasp of these and other key concepts will allow you to call to mind the information you need to apply in your professional role as a patient teacher.

Theoretical Knowledge
knowing why

Nurses have been teaching patients since Florence Nightingale taught both nurses and patients about the value of good nutrition, fresh air, exercise, and personal hygiene (Nightingale, 1860/1992). Since that time, teaching has become progressively more important due in part to the following:

Patients Participate in Healthcare Decisions Patients are taking responsibility for their own healthcare. Primary care providers expect patients to take an active role in making decisions about their health; patients and families need information so that they make *informed* decisions. You can help patients get answers to their questions, find resources, recognize problems, and develop self-care behaviors.

Hospital Stays Are Brief A great deal of complex care is being given in homes and the community. Patients are often sent home still needing medications, dressing changes, and skilled procedures, such as urinary catheterization. Nurses have a responsibility to teach family members how to provide care and to teach patients to care for themselves as they are able.

Healthcare Is Expensive Patient education can help to decrease the overall cost of healthcare. It does so by helping to increase patient compliance with medical and nursing regimens, which can shorten hospital stays and decrease frequency of medical treatments and admissions (Bastable, 2008).

As you might conclude from the foregoing discussion, the basic purpose of teaching and learning is to provide information that will empower clients and families to (1) perform self-care, and (2) make informed decisions about their healthcare options. Like other interventions, you can use teaching to promote wellness; prevent or limit illness; restore health; adapt to changes in body function; and facilitate coping with stress, illness, and loss.

WHO ARE THE LEARNERS?

As a nurse, your learners are clients, families, and others who care for the client. You will often provide informal one-to-one teaching while performing other nursing interventions. For example, as you give a medication, you will teach about its therapeutic and side effects. Or you may do more formal teaching to groups of people. You might demonstrate a baby bath to a class of expectant parents.

You will find your learners wherever you work: hospital, an ambulatory setting, home care, or in the community. As a community health nurse, you would be more likely to teach large groups of people; for example, you might teach a healthy lifestyles class to a group of teens.

As nurse, you will also be responsible for teaching healthcare workers whom you supervise. For example, you may instruct nursing assistive personnel (NAP) when you observe an error in technique for measuring blood pressure. Or you may help a new nurse learn how to use new equipment on the unit. Nurses in practice are also involved in clinical instruction of nursing students, new graduates, and other members of the healthcare team. Most of this teaching may be informal, although you might also present specific topics at unit meetings and conferences. For example, if there is a change in the agency's documentation system, you might teach a class to the nurses on your shift to learn the new system.

WHAT ARE MY TEACHING RESPONSIBILITIES?

Teaching is a major component of clinical practice skills and is an independent nursing function. In many states, nurses' teaching role and responsibility is defined in the Nurse Practice Act.

The American Nurses Association (ANA) The *ANA Code of Ethics for Nurses with Interpretive Statements* (2001) says that nurses are responsible for promoting and protecting health, safety, and rights of patients. Patient teaching is essential in fulfilling that responsibility.

ANA standards of practice (2010), Standard 5B, states, "The registered nurse employs strategies to promote health and a safe environment." The following are the specific measurement criteria for that standard:

- Provides health teaching that addresses such topics as healthy lifestyles, risk-reducing behaviors, developmental needs, activities of daily living, and preventive self-care.
- Uses health promotion and health teaching methods appropriate to the situation and the patient's values, beliefs, health practices, patient's developmental level, learning needs, readiness and ability to learn, language preference, spirituality, culture, and socioeconomic status.
- Seeks opportunities for feedback and evaluation of the effectiveness of the strategies used.
- Uses information technologies to communicate health promotion and disease prevention information to the healthcare consumer in a variety of settings.
- Provides healthcare consumers with information about intended effects and potential adverse effects of proposed therapies.

The Joint Commission Hospital accreditation standards require educators in healthcare organizations to consider the literacy, developmental and physical limitations, financial limitations, language barriers, culture, and religious practices of every patient. Teaching must also include any person who will be responsible for the patient's care (The Joint Commission, 2010, 2013).

The American Hospital Association (AHA) The AHA Patient Care Partnership (previously the Patient's Bill of Rights) that describes in simple language the right of patients to receive high-quality care. Patient rights include a clean and safe environment; protection of privacy; complete and current information about disease/condition, diagnosis, treatment, and prognosis; information communicated in ways patients can understand; and the right to be informed of hospital policies and practices that relate to them (American Hospital Association [AHA], 2003).

WHAT ARE SOME BASIC LEARNING CONCEPTS AND PRINCIPLES?

The educational process involves the concepts of teaching and learning. **Teaching** is an interactive process that involves planning and implementing instructional activities to meet intended learner outcomes or providing activities that allow the learner to learn (Bastable, 2008). Teachers must have effective communication skills to (1) adequately convey information, (2) assess verbal and nonverbal feedback, and (3) accommodate various learning styles. In patient education, nurses can use teaching, counseling, and behavioral modification together to achieve effective client learning.

Learning is a change in behavior, knowledge, skills, or attitudes. It occurs as a result of planned or spontaneously occurring situations, events, or exposures. *Conscious, goal-oriented learning* is intended and deliberate. It involves motivation to learn. Learning can occur in a rote manner, informally by circumstance, by formal instruction, or by a combination of approaches. It is not enough for the teacher to give the person written or verbal information; information alone will not change behaviors. Box 19-1 summarizes some basic principles of learning and provides a quick check for planning teaching sessions. For information about learning theories (social learning theory, behavioral learning theory, cognitive theory, and humanism),

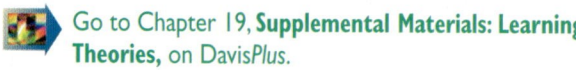 Go to Chapter 19, **Supplemental Materials: Learning Theories,** on DavisPlus.

KnowledgeCheck 19-1

- Identify at least three reasons nurses have a responsibility to teach clients.
- Define *teaching*.
- Define *learning*.

BOX 19-1 ■ Five Rights of Teaching

When you are making a teaching plan, you can use this as a checklist to ensure that you consider each of the five "rights" of teaching in the plan.

Right Time
- Is the learner ready, free of pain and anxiety, and motivated?
- Have you and the learner developed a trusting relationship?
- Have you set aside sufficient time for the teaching session?

Right Context
- Is the environment quiet, free of distractions, and private?
- Is the environment soothing or stimulating, depending on the desired effect?

Right Goal
- Is the learner actively involved in planning the learning objectives?
- Are you and your client both committed to reaching mutually set goals of learning that achieve the desired behavioral changes?
- Are family or friends included in planning so that they can help follow through on behavioral changes?
- Are the learning objectives realistic and valued by the client; do they reflect the client's lifestyle?

Right Content
- Is the content appropriate for the client's needs?
- Is it new information or reinforcement of information that has already been provided?
- Is the content presented at the learner's level?
- Does the content relate to the learner's life experiences or is it otherwise relevant to the learner?

Right Method
- Do the teaching strategies fit the learning style of the learner?
- Do the strategies fit the client's learning ability?
- Are the teaching strategies varied?

Learning Occurs in Three Domains

People learn in three ways, or *domains*: cognitive, psychomotor, and affective (Bloom & Krathwohl, 1956). You should include each of these domains, involving thinking, doing, and feeling/caring, when writing objectives and planning teaching and evaluation strategies, which are discussed later in this chapter. Table 19-1 provides examples of client learning in each of the domains. For a more detailed version of this table, which identifies levels of behavior associated with each domain,

 Go to Chapter 19, **Tables, Boxes, Figures: ESG Table 19-1,** on DavisPlus.

Table 19-1 ➤ Bloom's Domains of Learning

DOMAIN AND LEVELS OF BEHAVIOR	EXAMPLES
Cognitive (thinking)	
Includes memorization; recall; comprehension; and ability to analyze, synthesize, apply, and evaluate ideas.	A client is able to report the names and doses of the three medications he is taking.
	A client explains the expected effect of the medication she has been prescribed.
	A client designs a planned schedule for dressing changes for a wound on her leg.
	A client describes how to distinguish between normal inflammation and signs of infection in a wound.
	A client recognizes the need for behavioral changes to decrease the chance of recurrence of infection.
Psychomotor (skills)	
Includes sensory awareness of cues involved in learning, as well as imitation and performance of skills and creation of new skills.	A client identifies that he needs to read directions before starting a project.
	A client brings personal equipment to a teaching session.
	A new mother follows the instructor who is demonstrating diapering of her newborn, imitating her movements.
	A new father is observed diapering his newborn after observing a demonstration.
	A client independently changes her complex dressing. The wound heals with no signs of infection.
	A client with limited vision creates a new approach to giving his daily injections.
Affective (feelings)	
Includes receiving and responding to new ideas, demonstrating commitment to or preference for new ideas, and integrating new ideas into a value system.	An adolescent makes eye contact with the nurse as she explains the admission process.
	A client asks questions about what to expect during a procedure he is to undergo.
	A parent of a child who has just been admitted to the hospital expresses commitment to staying with her child after the nurse explains the impact of hospitalization.
	A client who has overcome drug addiction chooses to present his story to high school groups.

Adapted from Bloom B. S., & Krathwohl, D. R. (1956). Taxonomy of educational objectives: The classification of educational goals. *Handbook I: Cognitive domain.* New York: Longmans, Green; and Bloom, B. S., Mesia, B. B., & Krathwohl, D. R. (1964). Taxonomy of educational objectives (Vol. 1: *The affective domain* and Vol. 2: *The cognitive domain*). New York: David McKay.

Anderson and Krathwohl (2001) adapted Bloom's model describing learning using a more outcomes-based approach, including the following domains:

Remember
Understand
Apply
Analyze
Evaluate
Create

Cognitive Learning

Cognitive learning includes storing and recalling information in the brain. Ranging from simple to complex processes, it encompasses six levels of behavior: memorization, recall, comprehension and analysis, synthesis, application, and evaluation of ideas (see Table 19-1). Strategies and tools to support teaching cognitive-type content include lectures, reading materials, panel discussions, audiovisual materials, programmed instruction, computer-assisted instruction (CAI), and problem-based learning (e.g., case studies and care plans).

Psychomotor Learning

Psychomotor learning involves learning a skill that requires both mental and physical activity. It requires the learner to accept and value the skill (the affective domain) as well as know about the skill (the cognitive domain). Strategies and tools used to teach psychomotor skills include demonstration and return demonstration, simulation models, audiovisual materials (e.g., DVDs, streaming video), journaling and self-reflection, and printed materials, especially with photographs and illustrations.

Affective Learning

Affective learning involves changes in feelings, beliefs, attitudes, and values. It is considered the "feeling domain." Strategies and tools for promoting affective learning include role modeling, group work, panel discussion, role playing, mentoring, one-to-one counseling and discussion, audiovisual materials (e.g., DVDs, streaming video, interactive computer-based modules, movies), computer and printed materials. Levels of affective behavior are shown in ESG Table 19-1, on Davis*Plus*.

KnowledgeCheck 19-2

- What are the three domains of learning?
- What strategies and tools are used to promote learning within each of the three domains of learning?
- Give an example of each of the domains of learning.

 ## ThinkLike a Nurse 19-1

By now, you have probably already learned how to assess a patient's blood pressure (BP).

- Think about how you were taught to perform that *skill*. What would have been the best way for *you* to learn to take a BP? To read a book and look at the photos closely? To watch a DVD? To have someone tell you how to do it? To have someone demonstrate the skill? Perform the blood pressure measurement yourself? Some other way?
- Now think about the *principles* involved with BP (e.g., normal ranges, the physiological regulation of the BP). What, for you, would have been the best way to learn the principles? Read a book? Listen to a lecture? Physically obtain a BP reading for a patient? Work a case involving BP? Some other way?
- From your answers to the two preceding questions, what (if anything) can you conclude about different domains of learning and the kinds of activities to use in teaching and learning in each domain?

Many Factors Affect Client Learning

Because learning is complex, many factors can either enhance or interfere with it. An understanding of the following factors will help you to design effective teaching interventions and promote client learning.

Motivation

Motivation is desire from within. It is created by an idea, a physical need, an emotion, or some other kind of force. Without motivation, little learning can occur. Motivation is greatest when clients recognize the need for learning, believe it is possible to improve their health, and are interested in the information

they are being given. Think about classes you have taken. Have you studied harder in some than in others? What motivated you? Was it because you were intrigued by the information, wanted to earn a good grade or the approval of the instructor, or had other incentives?

Motivation may be based on physical and social needs, the need for task mastery or success, and health beliefs. In your teaching, try to apply the following principles for motivating learners:

- Conveying your interest in and respect for the learner and the learning process helps to motivate the learner.
- Creating a warm, friendly environment can enhance social needs motivation, as can your enthusiasm.
- You can sometimes motivate clients by helping them identify a physical need. For example, Heather (Meet Your Patient) may not be aware that her child is at risk for accidents and injury from home hazards. Helping her to understand the normal behavior of a 4-year-old may help her to see the need for child-proofing her home.
- The need for achievement and competence is related to task mastery and self-efficacy. When a person succeeds at a task, he is usually motivated to continue learning. Rewards and incentives can provide this type of motivation.
- The client will be motivated to learn only if she believes that health is important. For example, Heather may understand that a 4-year-old likes to explore and may recognize there are safety hazards in the home; however, she will not be motivated to learn safety measures if her attitude is that "it is no big deal."

Many of the following factors also provide motivation as well as contributing in other ways to learning.

Readiness

Readiness is the demonstration of behaviors that indicate the learner is both *motivated* and *able* to learn *at a specific time.* For instance, a client may not be "ready" for teaching right before scheduled diagnostic tests or invasive treatments because anxiety makes it difficult to focus on the material. In addition, readiness for learning includes the physical and emotional capacity to take in, process, and recall information.

Physical Condition Physical and intact cognition contribute to a patient's readiness to learn. You must consider them in your planning. For example:

- Pain interferes with the ability to concentrate on the material the nurse presents.
- The client needs adequate strength, coordination, energy, and mobility to demonstrate psychomotor learning.
- You will need to adapt your teaching and evaluation strategies to accommodate clients with impaired cognition, hearing, or vision.

Emotions Emotions such as severe anxiety, stress, and emotional pain interfere with the ability to learn. In addition, the learning itself, and the idea that behaviors must be changed, can create anxiety. However, a mild level of anxiety can enhance learning by providing motivation. For example, a client newly diagnosed with diabetes may not be experiencing physical complications related to the disease, so he may not be interested in learning about diabetes. You may be able to motivate him (i.e., create some anxiety) by pointing out the potential and serious complications (e.g., blindness, kidney damage) of uncontrolled diabetes. Provoke mild anxiety carefully so the client does not interpret your words as a threat or excessive negativity.

Timing

You must present information at a time when the learner is open to learning. Timing is therefore related to readiness, and it is important in the following ways, as well:

- People retain information better when they have an opportunity to use it soon after it is presented. For example, a student reads about insulin in her textbook and takes a test on the content 2 weeks later. Another student reads the same information and during the 2 weeks also administers different types of insulin to several patients. The second student will have an advantage at test time.
- For some concepts, the learner might need more time to absorb and apply information, especially when more complex thinking is required.

Active Involvement

Learning is more meaningful when the client is actively engaged in the planning and the learning activities. Learners retain 10% of what they read, but they retain 90% of what they speak and do (London, 1999). Passive listening is not typically as effective for processing and retaining information as activities involving more than one style of learning. For instance, a demonstration with a return demonstration and a patient education brochure is often an effective way to teach patients how to perform a new skill. Demonstration is particularly effective for kinesthetic learners (which most adults are). Can you think of other examples of learning that involve multiple senses?

Feedback

Feedback is information about the learner's performance. For example, a test grade is feedback for students, conveying the message, "You need to work on that content some more," or "You have successfully mastered the lesson." Feedback in the clinical setting or skills lab might be, "You consistently maintained sterile technique."

Key Point: *Positive feedback encourages learners and boosts morale when it comes to tackling difficult content or devoting the time and effort needed to get the most out of the educational process. This is especially critical when significant behavioral changes are required to be a successful learner.*

Patients, too, tend to respond well to positive interaction while learning. For example, the patient teaching experience reinforces the patient with a new ostomy who successfully changes her appliance or a patient with diabetes who learns to correctly draw up an insulin dose. Sometimes you may need to act like a coach, encouraging the learner with frequent feedback and praise or by suggesting alternatives. At other times, you may need to point out errors; but try to do so in a positive way. Be careful not to seem judgmental when clients are learning a new skill or are giving home care. Fear of failure or judgment can be a serious barrier to learning at what could be the patient's most teachable moment.

Repetition

The client is more likely to retain information and incorporate it into his life if the content is repeated. Each time the learner hears the information, the likelihood of retention increases. For example, often patients forget what medication is prescribed for certain conditions. Repeating the name of the drug can help patients better remember it. This is especially true for learning psychomotor skills. Do you remember the first time you counted a radial pulse? Even that simple skill may have been difficult at first. By now it is probably very easy for you.

 ThinkLike a Nurse 19-2

Use examples from your own experience, if you can. Do not use examples you have read in the preceding sections.

- Give an example to illustrate the importance of relevance in learning.
- Give an example to illustrate the importance of repetition in learning.
- Give an example to illustrate the importance of timing in learning.

Learning Environment

Have you ever tried to concentrate on a lecture right after lunch when you were sitting in a warm, stuffy room? Or when someone is talking or texting you via cell phone? Keep in mind, though, that some learners are best motivated and engaged when teaching occurs in a group situation. Social learners can be distracted from the task when alone in a quiet space.

When you are planning a teaching session, provide lighting and comfortable seating that is conducive for conversations. Have your teaching materials ready at hand to avoid gaps in the teaching session. If you have an area that is set aside for teaching, try to use inspirational or motivational accessories (e.g., photographs, posters).

A quiet, private space, free of distractions, is ideal for teaching. If none is available, at least try to find a quiet corner, pull the bed curtain shut, close the door, or sit close to the client so that you can talk softly (Fig. 19-1). Make the best of what you have to work with.

Did you recognize how the concept of learning environment is related to the concepts of teaching and learning?

Scheduling the Session

Plan for uninterrupted time to allow you to adequately assess and understand the client. The teaching time doesn't always need to be long, just uninterrupted. Based on the client's condition (e.g., activity intolerance, attention span, fatigue, pain), shorter teaching sessions may be best for comprehension and retention. Finding suitable time to teach can be a challenge, but a moment can be a teaching session, as shown in Box 19-2.

Amount and Complexity of the Content

The more complex or detailed the content, the more difficult it is for most people to learn and retain, as you

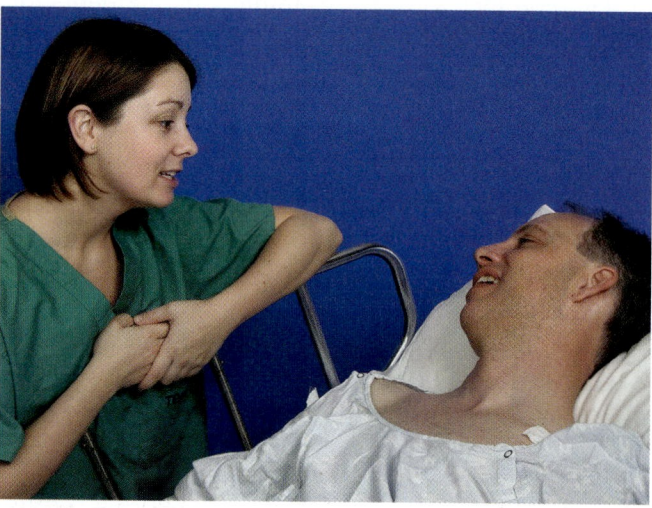

FIGURE 19-1 To provide privacy, sit or stand close to the patient so that you can talk privately.

BOX 19-2 ■ Teachable Moments

This week in class a student nurse has been studying patient teaching. Her instructor has informed the students that she expects them to incorporate teaching into each clinical day. While caring for the patient, the student ponders, "I am way too busy to find time to teach. What am I going to do?" Later in the day, she asks the nurse who is co-assigned to her client for suggestions. The nurse questions the student: "Did you take the patient's blood pressure?" When the student answers that she did, the nurse says, "Did you explain why you were doing that and what the BP readings mean?" Again the student says, "Yes." The nurse asks, "When you gave your patient his medications, did you explain why you were giving each one and the common side effects?" The student begins to understand that almost every patient contact presents an opportunity for teaching and doesn't have to take a long time.

---

probably know from your own learning experiences. For example, imagine teaching parents about the need for isolation precautions for their newborn who has just been diagnosed with an immune disorder. In comparison, teaching parents how to diaper their healthy newborn would be far less challenging.

In addition, the greater the change, the greater will be the challenge for both teacher and client. For example, a client rehabilitating after a stroke who has to relearn using eating utensils, swallowing, and other basic tasks for daily hygiene and self-care will experience a more demanding learning challenge than one who has to learn only a daily schedule for taking medications.

Communication

Communication is central to the teaching and learning process in which teachers and learners communicate information, perceptions, and feelings. Barriers to communication include pain, anxiety, fatigue, illness, hunger, dysfunctional relationships, language differences, vision and hearing impairment, cultural factors, and various environmental issues, such as noise and distraction. Attend carefully to verbal and nonverbal feedback that the client gives; it can tell you whether or not the learner is attentive and focusing on the learning activities. For more information about communication, see Chapter 21.

 ThinkLike a Nurse 19-3

A client who has a brain injury needs to learn how to administer insulin. Another learner who must learn to change a wound dressing has attention deficit-hyperactivity disorder (ADHD).

- How do you think these clients' health status might affect:
    1. Their motivation to learn?
    2. Their ability to be actively involved in the learning?
- What approaches or changes might you need to make in:
    1. The learning environment?
    2. The timing of the teaching session?
    3. The use of repetition?
    4. Your communication?
    5. The amount and complexity of content presented in a session?
    6. Your use of feedback?
    7. The amount of teacher support?

Special Populations

For clients who have special needs (e.g., those with learning disabilities, ADHD, mental illness, affective or communication disorders, mental illness, or brain injury) you must plan carefully to ensure that you use appropriate strategies to maximize learning. Consider a variety of teaching approaches—one size does not fit all. For example, you may need to use brief, frequent learning sessions or pay special attention to minimizing distracting stimuli in the environment. Or you may need to present information slowly, use repetition, and be satisfied with slower progress. The adaptations you make will depend on the nature of the special need, so if you are not familiar with the patient's condition, you must acquire theoretical knowledge of it. Include a family member, caregiver, or other significant person in the teaching to reinforce the learning and act as a safety net for implementing the information.

Developmental Stage

An understanding of intellectual development will help you to gear your teaching strategies and content to the level of the learner. When teaching psychomotor skills, you will need to assess the person's fine and gross motor development. For example, a young child may not have adequate fine motor skills to complete a skill such as tying shoes without assistance (Fig. 19-2). If you would like to review an extensive discussion of intellectual development, including Piaget's theory (1966), see Chapter 9.

Stages of Cognitive Development

Piaget identified three stages of cognitive development that are especially important in client teaching in the cognitive domain:

- **The Preoperational Stage** (2 to 7 years old), in which the child begins to acquire language skills and find meaning through use of symbols and pictures.
- **The Stage of Concrete Operations** (7 to 11 years old), in which the child learns best by manipulating concrete, tangible objects and can classify objects in two or more ways (e.g., identify a shape as a triangle and also as green). Logical thinking begins, and the child can understand the relationship between numbers and the idea of reversibility. He also can begin to recognize and adapt to the perspective of others.
- **The Formal Operational Stage** (age 11 years or older), in which the person can use abstract thinking and deductive reasoning. The person can relate general concepts to specific situations, consider alternatives, begin to establish values, and try to find meaning in life. Not everyone reaches this stage, including some adults.

Always assess cognitive development. For clients who have not achieved the stage of formal operations, use examples instead of definitions; use concrete rather than abstract terms.

Teaching Older Adults

When teaching older adults, consider the numerous factors that can adversely affect the teaching. Possible barriers include vision and hearing impairments, illness, pain, reduced social interaction, reduced mobility, dementia, medication effects, sensory deficit, sociocultural factors, and a noisy or chaotic environment. Allow extra time for teaching, and stop occasionally for rest periods. Assess for sensory deficits (e.g., hearing and vision) and adapt your style according to any restrictions. Use large print for the visual aids, and repeat information as necessary. Refer to Table 19-2 for some learning principles that apply to older adults, as well as tips for effectively teaching older adults.

Teaching Children

When you work with children, use strategies to gain trust, reduce their anxiety, promote cooperation, and enhance their emotional readiness to learn. For instance, for a child who needs surgery, schedule a tour of the hospital at least 1 week before the admission date, and introduce the child to staff members and other patients of the same age (if possible). Have the child practice breathing exercises or other aspects of tests or treatments that he will be involved in. With the parents' permission, provide the child with ice cream or other food, game, or material "reward," and give the child a coloring book or other item about the upcoming surgery to take home.

If you are teaching a child in the preoperational stage or an adult with limited intellectual development, you will need to simplify the content and use pictures and concrete examples. For example, there is little point in going into detail with a preschooler regarding the rationale for taking an antibiotic. Instead, tell the child that the medicine will keep her from getting sick; use pictures of a child drinking from a medicine cup, or provide a calendar that the child can mark each time she takes a dose. A reward system is often an effective way of improving compliance.

Cultural Factors

Awareness of norms, values, communication, social structure, time orientation, and cultural identification are important in planning teaching (see Chapter 15 to review these concepts). If English is not the client's primary language, you may need to use an interpreter.

Key Point: *Cultural sensitivity involves respect for clients' identity and needs, regardless of who they are, where they're from, how they speak, how old they are, what if any religion they practice, whether they are disabled, how much wealth or poverty they experience, how much they weigh, how socially popular they are, or any other aspect that can lead to unfair treatment.*

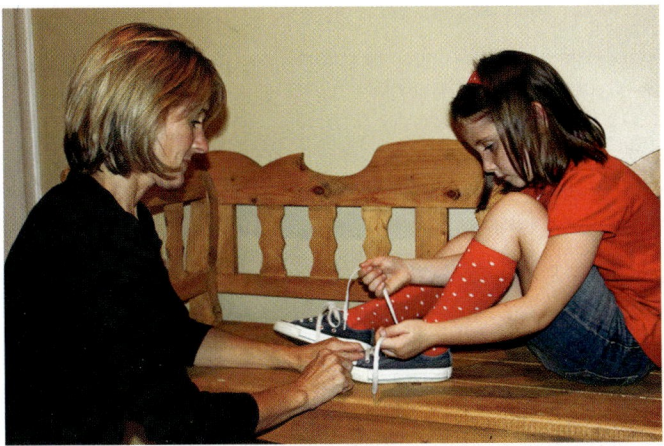

FIGURE 19-2 When teaching psychomotor skills, consider the person's gross and fine motor development.

Table 19-2 ➤ Incorporating Principles of Adult Learning Into the Teaching of Older Adults

CHARACTERISTICS OF ADULT AND OLDER ADULT LEARNERS	TIPS FOR TEACHING ADULTS
Attitudes	
Adults are independent and self-directed learners.	Help them to identify their own learning needs.
Adults must recognize the need to learn before they become willing to learn.	Explain why the information or new skill is important. Be sure to include materials with practical tips and realistic goals for learning.
Some adults may be afraid of the learning process because of (1) fear of failure, (2) past unsatisfactory experiences with educational processes, (3) not having participated in formal education for many years, or (4) feeling that "being taught" is for children.	Present content in a nonthreatening environment, where there is no risk of judgment or embarrassment in front of peers. Offer feedback (evaluation) simply to improve important skills and not for the sake of a grade. Remember the intent of patient education is to improve clinical outcome. Privacy is often necessary.
Adults are more motivated to learn if they think they will be able to use the information or skills immediately.	Plan the teaching session at the time of greatest need. That is, hold the teaching session close to the time the patient will need the information or need to perform a new skill.
Adults prefer to be partners in the learning process—to have some control over what they learn and how they learn it.	Encourage learners to tell you first what they intend to gain from the educational session. You might spell out the goals of your session in advance and allow the learner to customize it.
Some adults may feel threatened by the need to learn new information. They may feel, "I've gotten along just fine all these years without needing to know that; why should I learn it now?" Or they may believe that they are "too old to learn." These attitudes may be defenses to avoid failure or to resist change.	Work with the learner to establish the "need to know" at the onset of the program. Involve the learner in defining what he or she intends to gain from the educational session. Reassure the learner about the importance of the information and encourage the learner to tackle a little at a time.
Older adults may be socially less active and might perceive bias, ageism, or isolation.	As for any group of people, it is essential to honor cultural backgrounds, local customs and practices, and personal preferences.
Experience	
Adults have previous life experiences that can enhance learning.	Relate new content to past experiences and knowledge and have learners use their experiences to solve problems. Encourage older adults to share life experiences.
Messages are best received when they are part of the real-life experience.	In the teacher role, model the message you are conveying to your audience. "Walk the walk" and not just "talk the talk."
Learning Environment	
Many adult learners do well when a hands-on approach is used. Older adults must practice a new skill, or rehearse new information, in order to learn it.	Offer active participation and opportunities for interaction with instructor and other learners. Demonstrations and practical tips are useful for adult learners, particularly older adults.
Many older adult learners need to review new information away from the initial learning environment in order to retain it. It might not be until later that information sinks in.	Use take-home materials, such as colorful posters, table tents, and tip sheets, and patient-friendly brochures to reinforce information.
Older adult learners can be distracted and annoyed by cell phones and other electronic devices.	Request phones, radios, or other electronic devices be turned off for the educational session. Turn off your own phone's ringer, as well.
Many older adults were raised in an era when learning occurred primarily through the reading, discussion, and retelling of stories. Technology was not as prevalent as it is today.	Use informal teaching sessions that include storytelling. Tie the patient's past experiences to what you are teaching. To elicit stories, you must be a patient and empathetic listener. Keep your stories short. Ask open-ended questions and be willing to wait for the answer. Convey your genuine interest in your learners before sharing personal stories. Allow more time for older adults, especially those with chronic illness, to tell their own stories.

Table 19-2 ➤ Incorporating Principles of Adult Learning Into the Teaching of Older Adults—cont'd	
CHARACTERISTICS OF ADULT AND OLDER ADULT LEARNERS	**TIPS FOR TEACHING ADULTS**
Older individuals may bring family members or other caregivers to the teaching session to help interpret or remember information presented. Sometimes the extra people in the room can be noisy and distracting to the patient's learning situation.	If they are distracting, it may be helpful to ask others in the room to minimize other conversations, or in some circumstances to leave the room for a time.
Some older adults learn better when they are not overwhelmed with multiple needs, topics, or skills at one time.	Introduce only a few topics at a time. Usually tackling one to three new topics or skills is enough. Identify what is the most important information for your learner to walk away with. Define those topics and cover them well. Remember, slow and steady wins the race, especially when it comes to learning information that is essential to the patient's health.
Sensory and Physical	
Changes in visual distance, depth, acuity, and light perception occur with aging, thus diminishing the ability to take in information. Older adults experience increased sensitivity to glare and reduced color perception with aging. Processing of sensory information is also slower in the latter decades of life.	(1) Avoid colors such as blue, green, and lavender, because they are difficult for older adults to differentiate. (2) Remove physical barriers that could compromise the field of vision, such as projector position, tables, and so on. (3) In teaching materials, choose fonts that are bold, black, and a minimum size of 18-points. Fancy lettering is harder to decipher. (4) A nonglare background without a stylized pattern is easier to see and process than complex designs. (5) For those who cannot read or who have severe visual impairment, consider recording instructional material.
Reduced hearing acuity is common in older adults. Auditory perception for various tones and filtration of extraneous noise also diminish with age.	(1) Speak slowly, using a normal tone of voice. If you must speak more loudly than normal, be careful not to sound demeaning as though speaking to a child. You don't want learners to perceive annoyance in your tone. (2) Many older adults do some lip reading, although they may be unaware of it. You can facilitate lip reading by not distorting your facial features by exaggerated pronunciation. (3) Provide a quiet setting and reduce background noise. Close the door or windows if outside noise interferes with the teaching/learning experience.
Because of some short-term memory loss that occurs with aging, some older adults learn better when they have a source of supplemental information or support.	Reinforce your teaching with follow-up opportunities and connections to the community for information and support in grasping new information or acquiring a new skill.
Older adult learners can be particularly affected by fatigue, illness, medication, pain, stress, and other personal factors.	Be sure to plan the teaching session when the patient is well rested, pain-free as possible, and comfortable.

Box 19-3 highlights key concepts of teaching with a culturally competent approach.

Health Literacy

Health literacy is the capacity to obtain, process, and understand basic health information and services needed to make appropriate healthcare decisions (Nielsen-Bohlman, Panzer, & Kindig, and the Institute of Medicine of the National Academies, 2004; Ratzan & Parker, 2000). It does not refer simply to a person's ability to read and write but rather the way a person can apply language skills to understanding instructions on a medication bottle, or fully understanding explanations regarding a medical procedure to provide informed consent, for instance. On the contrary, **health illiteracy** occurs when the language spoken is not the patient's preferred language (i.e., limited English proficiency). Or perhaps the format through which the information is communicated is not suited to the patient. For example, if the patient has a hearing impairment and discharge teaching is done verbally, then a communication gap can occur. A gap in health literacy results when a healthcare provider uses medical terminology that is unfamiliar or misunderstood by the patient, thus resulting in an unintended message or lack of meaningful information. Limited health literacy is more common among the medically underserved community, minority populations, and older adults.

Patients with low health literacy are not as likely to understand the connection between risky behavior and

BOX 19-3 ■ Culturally Competent Teaching

Assessments

- Inquire or observe interactions among family members to decide who is the decision maker and how decisions are made. Include the family in the planning and teaching.
- Assess for customs or taboos that may conflict with the information you plan to present.
- Observe verbal and nonverbal communication patterns.
- Assess whether the family is past, present, or future oriented.
- Determine if the patient and/or family prefers a same-sex nurse to teach a client about personal topics, such as birth control and sexually transmitted infections. Different cultures have different ideas about what is appropriate for discussion between men and women.
- Determine whether the client's values and wishes are in congruence or conflict with the family.

Self-Knowledge

- Admit unfamiliarity with the culture, but express willingness to learn.
- Find sources of information that can help you learn about the culture and its healthcare practices.

Caring

- Respect, accept, and validate the client's beliefs.
- Find ways to incorporate the client's current healthcare practices and beliefs into the plan of care unless there is potential for harm.

Interventions

- Allow the patient to include cultural practices in the plan of care.
- Speak slowly and clearly; avoid slurring syllables.
- Do not use slang expressions.
- Use short sentences and concrete rather than abstract words. Present only one idea in each sentence.
- Use pictures and other visual aids to help communicate your meaning.
- Provide teaching materials in the client's language. If you cannot read it, have it translated so that you can judge its appropriateness.
- Avoid using humor; jokes often do not translate well because of connotations, jargon, and culture-specific context.

Feedback

- Obtain feedback carefully. Do not assume that a client who smiles, nods, and says yes really understands what you are teaching. The client may be embarrassed to ask questions or may feel that it will embarrass you.
- Encourage the client to ask questions; stop often to evaluate client understanding.

health. The following are some of the problems they encounter:

- Difficulty taking medication as prescribed (Berkman, Sheridan, Donahue, et al., 2011)
- Difficulty managing complex or chronic health problems (Osborn, Paasche-Orlow, Bailey, et al., 2011).

- Higher rates of ED visits, hospitalization, rehospitalization, and death (Mitchell, Sadikova, Jack, et al., 2012; Murray, Wu, Tu, et al., 2009).

 Older adults, especially, are less likely to recall information after a clinic visit (Kessels, 2003).

Inability to read or write English is a growing problem in the United States with regard to health literacy. One in five do not speak English at home (Sarkar, Karter, Liu, et al., 2010). Patients with limited reading proficiency in English might not be able to grasp information in health-related brochures or printed discharge instructions. To enhance understanding between you and your patients, refer to Box 19-4, which presents tips for promoting health literacy.

Barriers to Teaching and Learning

As you gain experience in teaching, you will learn to recognize the factors we have just discussed (e.g., timing, the environment) and to manipulate those that can be changed to enhance the teaching and learning experience. At the same time, take care to avoid factors that act as outright barriers to teaching/learning In a traditional, on-site classroom, for example, transportation, class schedule, time, childcare, didactic-style instruction are a few of the barriers. The most common barriers to effective teaching are identified in Box 24-5.

When learning outside the traditional classroom, one of the highest rated problems is the lack of social interactions. Poor learner motivation, diverse learning styles, time issues, and technical problems also contribute to

BOX 19-4 ■ Promoting Health Literacy With Patients

- Ask questions that involve "how" and "what" rather than "yes" and "no".
- Assist patients in completing forms and/or health histories as needed.
- Organize information so the most important material stands out and is repeated for emphasis and clarity.
- Present information in three to five "chunks" at a time.
- Write out instructions and appointments using plain language while avoiding medical jargon and technical terms.
- For those with low health literacy, printed materials should have words with three or fewer syllables and sentences with fewer than 15 words. However, paragraphs made of short, simple sentences can make information too basic and therefore, may not accurately communicate complex information (Badarudeen & Sabharwal, 2010).
- Speak using simple words, short sentences, and structuring sentences with active rather than passive voice. For example, instead of saying, "The pill should be taken every 8 hours," say "Take the pill every 8 hours."
- Use as many drawings and photographs as possible to illustrate your statements.
- For those with Limited English Proficiency (LEP), provide information in primary language, use online or software translation tools, or seek an interpreter to translate.

BOX 19-5 ■ Barriers to Effective Teaching and Learning in the Healthcare Environment

Barriers for the Teacher

- Competing demands on the nurse's time
- Limited opportunity to prepare for teaching
- Conflicting schedules between the nurse's available time for teaching and patient's available time to learn (e.g., sleep, procedures, physical therapy)
- Lack of space and privacy
- Teaching not seen as a priority (either by the nurse or the organization)
- No third-party reimbursement for teaching
- Frustration with the amount of documentation needed
- Lack of coordination by various healthcare providers

Barriers for the Learner

- Illness, fatigue, and personal stress
- Physical condition
- Anxiety
- Low literacy
- A negative environmental influence
- Lack of time to learn
- Overwhelming amount of behavioral change needed
- Lack of support and ongoing positive reinforcement
- Lack of willingness to take responsibility
- The complexity of the healthcare system, which can lead to discouragement or abandonment
- Communication gap resulting from language barrier
- Teaching not adapted to the learner's preferences and learning style
- Provider who uses excessive jargon and technical terminology
- Lack of perceived need for the information taught

dissatisfaction with the online learning environment. Access to the Internet can be problematic for some people (Muilenburg & Bergeb, 2005). When deciding whether online learning is best suited to your learners, consider learners' technical and health literacy (Sarkar, Karter, Liu, et al., 2010). For more information about barriers to online learning,

 Go to Chapter Resources, Chapter 19, **ESG Box 19-1, Barriers to Technology-based Learning Environment,** on DavisPlus.

KnowledgeCheck 19-3

- List and define six factors that affect the learning process.
- What is one strategy you could use to motivate a client who seems uninterested in learning?
- What are some aspects of the environment that can enhance or interfere with learning?
- What two strategies might you use with a learner functioning with low cognitive ability?

 ## ThinkLike a Nurse 19-4

- List some actions you can take to avoid each of the barriers for the teacher.
- Give an example of each of the barriers to the learner. Take the example of stress of illness: A patient is frightened after having a heart attack, fearing death or serious, long-term impairment; worried about the cost of the medical treatment; and concerned about not being able to go to work. Therefore, he cannot concentrate on the health information you are presenting to him.

Note: These questions may be difficult, depending on your knowledge base and experience. Work with others to answer the questions, as necessary.

PracticalKnowledge
knowing **how**

The teaching process parallels the nursing process. You will assess learning needs and readiness, make educational diagnoses, write learning objectives, plan and implement teaching strategies, and evaluate client learning. Effective client teaching begins with assessment of learning needs.

ASSESSMENT

A learning assessment will help you to determine the right setting for the teaching, the necessary content to cover, learning goals, and teaching strategies. Your initial assessment consists of general information about the amount of time and resources available for your teaching. Also be clear about your intended audience. For example, with Heather (Meet Your Patient) assess the following:

Learning Needs To understand her child's behaviors, Heather needs to learn about normal growth and development and nutritional needs of 4-year-olds. She will need safety and health instructions for the next year because her child may not return for another checkup until age 5.

Client's Knowledge Level You need to identify Heather's current expectations of her preschooler as well as her understanding of how the child has developed up to this point. You should also find out what Heather knows about preschooler nutrition and language development.

Health Beliefs and Practices Determine Heather's (and her daughter's) current healthcare practices as well as trust and investment in the healthcare system. For example, what kinds of meals does she offer the preschooler?

Physical Readiness Is Heather able to sit and listen to the information presented? You may need to provide appropriate play materials for her preschooler so that she will require less attention from her. Some interruptions are likely, because 4-year-olds have short attention spans.

Emotional Readiness In the case of Heather, emotional maturity is a factor in her readiness to learn. Heather has expressed concern that her child is so small, which offers you an opportunity to begin the teaching based on her interest in her child's progress and health. However, she may have trouble focusing on her responses to the care provider during the healthcare visit if her child is restless or if she has limited time for her appointment.

Ability to Learn During the interview, you can begin to assess Heather's ability to learn, based on her responses to questions. You can also ask about her educational level.

Literacy Level You might ask Heather to read a short statement or paragraph related to the topic you're teaching. Then ask questions to determine if Heather understood the printed information.

Neurosensory Factors By observing Heather's interactions with her preschooler, you can assess her vision, hearing, and manual dexterity. Observe her response to visual and auditory clues that are given by her child or healthcare providers. Watching her manipulate a pen, pencil, or toy could help you determine manual dexterity.

Learning Styles Ask Heather how she learns best. Understanding that she probably doesn't have extensive blocks of time or focused attention to read or listen, you might give her single-page handouts, videos, or pamphlets instead of books or more detailed booklets.

For guidelines and questions to ask when conducting a learning assessment,

 Go to Chapter 19, **Assessment Guidelines and Tools, Learning Assessment Guidelines,** in Volume 2.

ANALYSIS/NURSING DIAGNOSIS

Deficient Knowledge is the most frequently used (and perhaps misused) nursing diagnosis for a teaching plan. It may be either a problem or the etiology of a problem.

Deficient Knowledge as the Primary Problem

Key Point: *You should use Deficient Knowledge only if you believe that the lack of knowledge is the **primary** problem. Use it to describe conditions in which the "patient needs new, additional, or extensive knowledge.*

Identify the specific knowledge deficit as the problem, and follow with the etiology and related signs and symptoms. For example:

Deficient Knowledge (diabetic foot care) related to lack of prior experience, as manifested by anxiety and many questions about foot care

Deficient Knowledge as the Etiology

Deficient Knowledge is probably most useful as the etiology of other nursing diagnoses, such as the following:

- Ineffective Health Maintenance related to (r/t) Deficient Knowledge of immunizations

- Risk for Impaired Parenting r/t Deficient Knowledge of child developmental stages and needs for stimulation
- Ineffective Self-Health Management r/t Deficient Knowledge of the procedure for drawing up and injecting insulin
- Risk for Imbalanced Nutrition: Less Than Body Requirements r/t the pregnant woman's Deficient Knowledge about additional calories and nutrients needed during pregnancy and her fear of "getting fat"

Wellness Diagnoses

Teaching is the primary intervention for wellness diagnoses, such as Readiness for Enhanced Breastfeeding, Readiness for Enhanced Communication, and the almost 30 other NANDA-I labels beginning with the phrase "Readiness for Enhanced."

Incorrect Uses of Deficient Knowledge

Beware of routine or premature diagnosing. It is easy to see that a patient lacks information, label it as a Deficient Knowledge problem, and try to solve the problem by giving information—which may not be what the patient needs at all. Always look beyond the knowledge deficit to see what problematic *responses* it produces.

Do not use Deficient Knowledge routinely as a problem label for all patients (Jarrell, Alpers, & Wotring, 2011). There are information needs associated with almost every medical and nursing diagnosis. However, you cannot assume a particular patient needs to be taught that information. For example, a person with a foot ulcer secondary to long-standing diabetes may already know more than you do about foot care. For most nursing diagnoses (e.g., Anxiety, Imbalanced Nutrition), you can merely write a nursing order to provide the informal teaching needed instead of writing a Deficient Knowledge diagnosis.

Do not use Deficient Knowledge for problems involving the client's *ability to learn*. To accurately describe such situations, use non-NANDA-I diagnoses such as:

- Impaired Ability to Learn r/t fear and anxiety
- Impaired Ability to Learn r/t delayed cognitive development
- Lack of Motivation to Learn r/t feelings of powerlessness

PLANNING OUTCOMES

Before making a teaching plan, educators contract with the learner for what they want to accomplish together. **Contractual agreements** are statements of understanding between teacher and learner about how to achieve mutually set goals. The contract usually describes the responsibilities of both teacher and learner, time frame for the teaching, content to be included, and expectations of all participants. Learning contracts increase commitment by the learner to reach the teaching and behavioral goals. They are usually informal.

Teaching goals are broad in scope and set down what is expected as the final outcome of the teaching and learning process. They should address all three domains of learning. In contrast, **learning objectives** are single, specific, one-dimensional behaviors that must be completed to accomplish the goal. They are short term and ideally are accomplished in one or two sessions. Similar to patient outcomes in the nursing process, learning objectives/goals should include an action verb, an activity that can be measured or observed, the circumstances of the learner's performance, and how learning will be measured. For example:

> *Goal:* Client will demonstrate ability to perform newborn care in 3 days.
>
> *Learning Objectives:* (1) Client changes infant's diaper, making sure that umbilical cord remains outside the diaper. (2) Client demonstrates bathing baby while maintaining newborn's axillary temperature of greater than 98.5°F (36.9°C).

See Table 19-3 for examples of active verbs for each domain of learning. See Chapter 5 for a review of goals and outcomes.

NOC standardized outcomes for Deficient Knowledge depend on the content that needs to be taught. *Nursing Outcomes Classification (NOC)* (Moorhead, Johnson, Maas, et al., 2013) has identified more than 60 Health Knowledge outcomes for specific topics, for example, Knowledge: Diabetes Management and Knowledge: Infant Care.

 Go to Chapter 19, **Standardized Language, NOC Outcomes for Health Knowledge,** on Davis*Plus.*

If you use Deficient Knowledge as the etiology of another diagnosis (e.g., Imbalanced Nutrition) then you would use NOC outcomes linked to that diagnosis (e.g., Knowledge: Diet, or Nutritional Status).

Individualized goals/outcome statements you might write for a client with a diagnosis of Deficient Knowledge include examples such as the following:

- For Deficient Knowledge (Breastfeeding): After demonstration and teaching, mother will position infant correctly at breast.
- For Deficient Knowledge (Child Physical Safety): After demonstration and explanation, parents will fasten preschooler safely and securely in infant car seat.
- For Deficient Knowledge (Diabetes Management): After reading pamphlets, client will explain the relationship of carbohydrate intake and exercise to blood sugar.

As you can see, choice of outcome is directly related to the area in which the client lacks knowledge or information.

The outcomes you choose depend on whether you have used Deficient Knowledge in the problem clause or the etiology clause of the nursing diagnosis. For example, if your nursing diagnosis for Heather (Meet Your Patient) was Deficient Knowledge (Preschooler Nutrition) related to lack of experience and family support,

Table 19-3 ➤ Active Verbs for Domains of Learning		
COGNITIVE DOMAIN	**AFFECTIVE DOMAIN**	**PSYCHOMOTOR DOMAIN**
Compare	Cry	Adapt
Define	Choose	Apply
Describe	Defend	Arrange
Design	Discuss	Assemble
Differentiate	Display	Begin
Explain	Form (e.g., an opinion)	Change
Give examples	Express	Construct
Identify	Give	Create
List	Help	Demonstrate
Name	Initiate	Draw up (e.g., medication)
Plan	Justify	Inject (e.g., medication)
State	Relate	Manipulate
Summarize	Revise	Move
	Select	Organize
	Share	Show
	Smile	Start
	State a feeling	Take
	Use	Work
	Value	

then one outcome might be, "Heather will plan nutritious meals for her child, based on the MyPlate recommendations." If, however, your diagnosis for the child was Risk for Impaired Nutrition: Less Than Body Requirements related to the mother's Deficient Knowledge about nutrition, then one outcome might be, "Preschooler will gain weight so that she is in at least the 10th percentile for weight by September of this year."

 ThinkLike a Nurse 19-5

A client has just been diagnosed with diabetes mellitus. He must monitor and record his blood glucose three times a day. The two of you establish a goal that he will be able to perform glucose testing independently within 1 week. What objectives would you need to write to achieve this goal?

 PLANNING INTERVENTIONS/IMPLEMENTATION

In Chapters 5 and 6, you learned about creating a nursing care plan. For clients and families with learning needs, you will create individualized teaching plans. The teaching plan is often one part of the client's complete nursing care plan. For an example, see the teaching plan at end of this chapter.

Creating Teaching Plans

The process of creating a teaching plan differs from that of creating a nursing care plan in two key ways. First, in a teaching plan, the interventions are actually teaching strategies. Second, when planning teaching, you will plan content, sequencing, and the types of instructional materials to be used.

Let's apply these aspects of a teaching plan, using the Heather (Meet Your Patient) scenario. You have assessed the need for anticipatory guidance regarding safety for

her 4-year-old. Your nursing diagnosis is Deficient Knowledge (safety for a 4-year-old) related to the mother's inexperience.

Teaching Strategies are the method used to present content. For Heather, they might include one-to-one instruction and printed information. You must use plain language always. The Joint Commission (2007) recommends "teach back" and "show back" techniques to assess and ensure patient understanding. You may use drawings, models, or devices to demonstrate your teaching message. Build feedback points into the plan where you will encourage your patients to ask questions to avoid misunderstanding.

Content includes the information the learner must understand to reach the desired goal. It can include facts, skills, or emotions. For Heather, the content of your informal teaching might include the following:

- Poison control and prevention—Curiosity and lack of ability to understand danger puts the preschooler at greater risk.
- Accident prevention—This would include the need for car seats, increased supervision when exploring, and the use of a helmet when the child rides a tricycle.
- Risk of choking—Foods that are hard to swallow or chunky (e.g., hot dogs) are a concern for a 4-year-old.
- Need for immunizations and physical checkup during the next year.

Scheduling and Sequencing refer to how you organize the information, that is, in what order to present the topics. As a general rule, you should present simple before complex topics and nonthreatening topics before more controversial ones. You must also determine when the teaching session(s) should be scheduled based on the client's and teacher's needs. When extensive content is involved, it is best to schedule a teaching session in advance; the teacher and learner are then committed and prepared for the session. Using small amounts of time can be effective if teaching is brief and organized.

For example, you could teach Heather (Meet Your Patient) about poison control and accident prevention in the lobby while she and her preschooler are waiting for the child to be examined. During the child's examination, you could review immunizations and the need for an annual checkup. At the end of the examination, when discussing the child's nutrition, you might include a discussion of foods that are a choking hazard, such as a hot dog.

Instructional Materials are used to introduce information and reinforce learning. You might give Heather printed handouts about poison control (including the Poison Control Center [PCC] telephone number) and about accident prevention (e.g., how to properly install a child car seat). The child's immunization record would list current immunizations and the schedule for further immunizations may be printed on it. To involve the child, you might include a coloring book and stickers about one of the topics.

Patient Teaching

General Tips for Effective Patient Teaching

Create a conducive learning environment.

➤ **Provide private space to talk** with your patient and other designated family members. Be sure the setting allows for privacy and is free of distractions and interruptions.

➤ **Time the session when the patient is in the best state of mind to concentrate** on what you are saying. For example, you will want to be sure the patient has pain under control but is not drowsy from pain relievers. Anxiety, depression, and fatigue also interfere with learning.

➤ **Help your patient decide who should be involved in the teaching session.** Caregivers assisting in the care after discharge would benefit from the learning process. On the other hand, some patients may not want others to be present because of modesty or cultural practices.

Plan and communicate information according to your patient's needs.

➤ **Be considerate of cultural, religious, or other issues** that might influence the way your patient receives information.

➤ **Developmental delays or cognitive impairment can also hamper learning.** Adjust learning style and level of complexity accordingly. Likewise, modify teaching approach for those with visual or hearing deficits. Also, consider limited English proficiency when communicating with patients.

➤ **Find out what your patient needs to know before making a teaching plan.** Involve him in the learning process. This not only improves your patient's motivation to learn, but also helps your patient to get more out of the education.

➤ **Be sure you provide the vital information needed for home care.** As time, staffing, and resources are limited in the healthcare setting, decide what is most important and set that as priority teaching (Alsbaugh, n.d.).

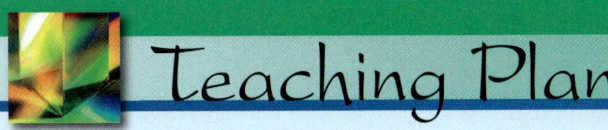

Teaching Plan

Client Data

Emily O'Connor is the advanced practice nurse (APN) in charge of the student health center on campus at State University. A research project by one of her nursing students last semester revealed that 60% of students surveyed on campus reported they spent 300 minutes per week of moderate intensity exercise, which was consistent with a study examining compliance with the *Physical Activity Guidelines for Americans* (Tucker, Welk, & Beyler, 2011). However, researchers found 62% adherence by self-report but only 10% when measured via accelerometer. Thus, Emily decides to teach students and interested campus staff members about the importance of physical activity for physical and emotional well-being. To reinforce the content, Ms. O'Connor develops colorful brochures with photos and charts to make the information more visually appealing, and an interactive teaching session to capture learners' attention. She also provides food, so people will have additional motivation to attend.

Nursing Diagnosis

Possible Deficient Knowledge (health behaviors) about physical activity as evidenced by campus-wide survey results showing that less than two-thirds of students comply with the U.S. Department of Health and Human Services recommendation for physical activity.

NOC Outcome

Knowledge: Health Behavior (1805)

NIC Intervention

Teaching: Group (5604)

Teaching Environment

1. Provide an environment conducive to learning. Promote comfort by making personal introductions and offering refreshments during break time.

   Rationale: When adult learners are in an environment in which they feel comfortable, they are less distracted and more able to learn. Physical and emotional comfort of the participants is important for creating a positive atmosphere for adult learning. The environment influences a learner's interest level and actual motivation to acquire new knowledge (Edutopia, 2011).

Overall Strategy / Approach

1. Focus on real-world problems.
2. Emphasize application of content to everyday life.
3. Relate content to life experience.
4. Explain how the education will solve a problem.
5. Involve learners in the educational process.
6. Use a variety of methodologies.

   Rationale: Utilizes principles of adult learning. Using a variety of methodologies is important because different people learn in different ways.

Instructional Materials

1. Printed materials (brochures, fact sheets)

   Rationale: Print materials at an appropriate reading level (usually 6th to 7th grade) for the target audience allow participants to review information when it is convenient for them (U.S. Department of Health and Human Services, 2013). In a study looking at the effectiveness of five different types of media (print materials, online PDF, audio files, audio with text Web page, and streaming video demonstration) for improving patient's learning, findings show that although participants preferred multimedia presentations, patients retained information using supplementary materials regardless of form the content was presented in (Wilson, Makoul, Bojarski, et al., 2012).

2. Video (DVD) demonstrating types of exercises

   Rationale: In a study investigating the effectiveness of video for patient education, findings indicate patients using streaming video reported video as better than text for presenting health information (Hoffman, Salzman, Garbaccio, et al., 2011).

(continued)

Teaching Plan (continued)

3. Flash, streaming video, or other interactive multimedia (animation, narration, and text) on computer, to accompany PowerPoint slides

   Rationale: In a study examining the effectiveness of streaming video on medical student learning, researchers found a positive effect on learning when it was used to complement other in-class methods and multimedia sources (Bridge, Jackson, & Robinson, 2009).

Learning Objective	Schedule / Sequence	Content	Teaching Strategy
By the end of the first educational session, participants will be able to explain why physical activity is important.	April 1–8	1. Determine date, time, and content of class to be held.	Advertise the educational session by using posters on campus, the campus newspaper, newsletter, social networking sites, school's web-calendar, and text and e-mail blasts.
	April 9 6:30–7:00 p.m.	2. Social hour. Healthy snacks and beverages. Get acquainted.	
	7:00–7:30 p.m.	3. Identify barriers to engaging in at least 300 minutes of moderate intensity or 150 minutes of vigorous intensity physical activity per week.	Lecture with PowerPoint slides, including photos
	7:30–7:50 p.m.	4. Describe how physical activity helps to promote health, prevent illness, control weight, and enhance overall quality of life.	Projected information (e.g., PowerPoint, YouTube)
	7:50–8:00 p.m.	5. Provide thorough instruction for proper technique for exercises to build strength, improve balance, and increase flexibility.	Live or videotaped demonstration of different types of exercises, with participant demonstration of techniques
	8:00–9:00 p.m.	6. Promote awareness and track activity recorded in fitness logs in follow-up contact with participants.	Questions and answers
		7. Provide access to group fitness classes at the local community center.	Handout printed passes or URL for downloading them from the community center's Web site, if available.

Rationale: Content is based on the Health Belief Model, designed by the U.S. Public Health Service. It identifies four key factors that promote health-seeking behavior (adapted for this setting): (1) Person perceives she is at risk for disease (low activity level). (2) Person perceives poor fitness is harmful and has serious consequences. (3) Person believes the suggested intervention (300 min/week of physical activity) will improve health and. (4) Person believes treatment (physical activity) effectiveness is worth overcoming barriers (Boston University School of Public Health, 2013).

Teaching Plan (continued)

Evaluation

Eighteen women and twenty men attended the session. When Emily O'Connor began the educational session, the participants were seated in chairs facing the front of the room, where the screen was set up for a YouTube video presentation. She distributed the printed handout materials and provided a short introduction. Before she began teaching, two women began talking about their battle with obesity and difficulty getting out to exercise. Three women shared stories about friends and family members who had suffered poor health and immobility. One had a question about sports-related injuries. During this discussion, the participants turned their chairs to face each other and talked among themselves.

Ms. O'Connor realized that learning takes place when participants share stories with facilitation by the group leader. Teaching does not have to be led exclusively by the facilitator. Even though she had a teaching plan, she was flexible enough to modify the plan to meet participants' needs. She turned off the PowerPoint, turned on the lights, and, instead of lecturing or showing videos from the CDC Web site, she shared information by answering questions and guiding the discussion.

During this process, Ms. O'Connor realized she had made assumptions about the participants' goals for this educational program and their educational needs. She learned that the women who attended came to the program with an understanding of the benefits of exercise and consequences of low levels of physical activity; they knew that exercise is important for health and fitness. They wanted to talk about their obstacles, concerns, and questions; they wanted to separate myths from facts; and they wanted to learn proper technique and how they could maintain motivation to perform at least 300 min/week of moderate intensity physical activity

After the session, Ms. O'Connor realized that she needed to revise her plan and offer a second session in a week or two. Her assumption that a lack of knowledge was responsible for the low number of people adhering to the Physical Activity Guidelines for Americans was not confirmed by discussion with the participants. She developed new goals for the second session:

1. By the end of the educational intervention, participants will:
   a. State that questions pertaining to weekly physical fitness have been addressed.
   b. Identify the factors that act as a barrier to engaging in physical activity.
   c. Share strategies for overcoming barriers to engaging in physical activity.
   d. Suggest at least five ways to perform at least 300 minutes of moderate intensity physical activity per week.
   e. List steps to follow if an injury occurs while engaging in physical activity
2. At the 1-year follow-up visit, participants will report that they increased physical activity by 60 minutes per week during the last 12 months.

References

Boston University School of Public Health. (2013); Edutopia (2011); Tucker, Welk, & Beyler (2011; U.S. Department of Health and Human Services (2013); Wilson, Makoul, Bojarski, et al. (2012).

Selecting NIC Interventions

NIC standardized interventions related to patient learning depend on the nursing diagnoses you have identified. The *Nursing Interventions Classification (NIC)* (Bulechek, Butcher, Dochterman, et al., 2013) lists 30 patient education interventions from which to choose, depending on the content being taught. An example is Health Education and Teaching: Disease Process. To see the entire list,

 Go to Chapter 19, **Standardized Language, NIC Interventions for Patient Education,** on Davis*Plus*.

Selecting Specific Teaching Strategies

Several different types of teaching strategies are currently available. Before selecting one, consider the learner's differences, needs, learning style, and advantages and disadvantages of each method. For a comparison of advantages and disadvantages of each of the teaching formats discussed following, see Table 19-4. For more information about other teaching strategies, such as audiovisual materials, simulation, role-playing, self-instruction, distance learning, computer assisted instruction, online coursework, gaming, case method, and concept mapping,

 Go to Chapter 19, **Supplemental Materials, General Teaching Strategies,** on Davis*Plus*.

The nurse may reinforce material taught by various methods by asking, "What questions do you have?" However, when asking "Do you understand?" some patients are likely to answer "yes" out of embarrassment or a need to cooperate.

Key Point: *A patient's lack of questions does not necessarily mean that she understands what's been taught; it could in fact mean the opposite (Dickens & Piano, 2013).*

Demonstration and Return Demonstration

In this method, the teacher explains and demonstrates a skill or task. The learner then demonstrates comprehension by returning the demonstration. Return demonstrations should be scheduled close to the initial teaching of the skill. This format allows for targeted questions and answers and practical matters, rather than theory. This method requires the demonstrator to have specialized expertise if highly technical tasks are involved. Mannequins are being used more and more in clinical teaching (Fig. 19-3).

One-to-One Instruction and Mentoring

In one-to-one instruction, generally one teacher presents information to an individual learner. They mutually formulate objectives at the beginning of the session. Often the learner receives printed or audiovisual materials to reinforce the information presented. As a nurse, you will often use this method for patient teaching. Mentoring involves a more personal interaction between teacher and learner, involving not only the exchange of information but also role modeling and problem-solving. It

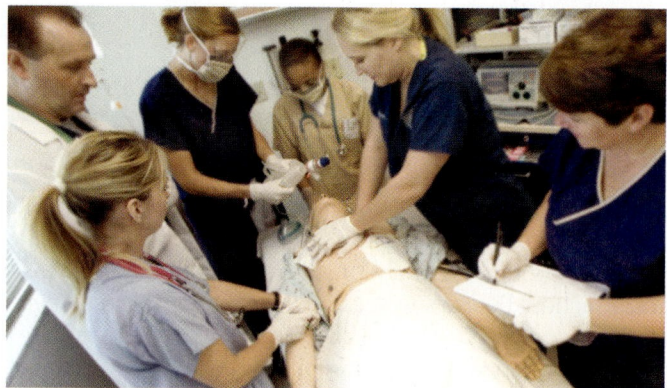

FIGURE 19-3 Simulation mannequins can offer realism and relevance to the educational experience.

offers an opportunity to directly observe and offer feedback on the learner's performance. Mentoring often involves learners in a clinical practice.

Printed Materials

Printed materials may be available in the form of fact sheets, discharge instructions, printed pamphlets, or detailed booklets. When teaching children, you might use age-appropriate printed books, coloring books, and activity books with mazes and other games. To be sure the clients understand the information, you must provide an opportunity for them to ask questions after they have read the materials. You will usually use printed materials to supplement other teaching strategies.

When you are creating your own teaching materials, remember the tips for ensuring readability in the Health Literacy section of this chapter (see Box 19-4). Many standard word processing programs allow you to check the reading level of materials you create. However, keep in mind that health-related information often contains medical terminology, which tends to have more syllables. Reading levels computed based on the syllable count can falsely indicate a higher-grade for reading level than what is reflected predominantly in the document. Figure 19-4 is an example of a patient teaching fact sheet written at the level of grade 6.8.

Include specific step-by-step actions you want them to take. Avoid abstract words in the instructions. Be sure the materials do not contain jargon, abbreviations, or acronyms, as readers might not be familiar with these. Create printed materials in an easy-to-read font (e.g., Arial, Helvetica, Times Roman). Active voice and action verbs are clearer than the passive form. To reinforce what you want patients to remember, phrase directions positively (e.g., say "do" rather than "don't" or "never").

Provide your clients with a take-home summary of the main points you want them most to remember after the teaching session. Having something clients can put their hands on to refer to at a later time can be invaluable for reinforcing important information.

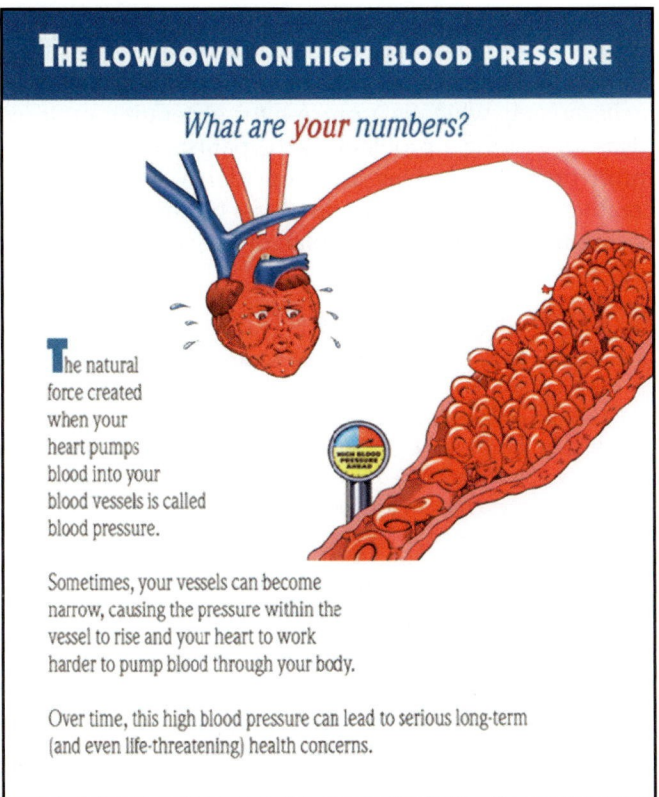

THE LOWDOWN ON HIGH BLOOD PRESSURE

What are *your* numbers?

The natural
force created
when your
heart pumps
blood into your
blood vessels is called
blood pressure.

Sometimes, your vessels can become
narrow, causing the pressure within the
vessel to rise and your heart to work
harder to pump blood through your body.

Over time, this high blood pressure can lead to serious long-term
(and even life-threatening) health concerns.

FIGURE 19-4 Reading level of this patient teaching aid is grade 6.8.

Role Modeling

In role modeling, the instructor teaches by example, demonstrating the behaviors and/or attitudes that learners should adopt. Role modeling is even more effective when the teaching point corresponds with the role model's action. Role modeling is integral to mentoring relationships in which students or patients learn by seeing, hearing, and doing. Be aware that learning occurs unconsciously as well as intentionally. Therefore, you must consider what you are communicating. Role models must connect the learning to the objectives. Role modeling is more successful when the teaching point is made apparent to learners during the learning experience.

Many experienced pediatric nurses find that role modeling using a puppet or a child's own doll or stuffed animal can be helpful in reducing the child's anxiety and enhancing the child's learning. For instance, you can suggest that the child be "the nurse" and "feel Miss Bunny's pulse," or have a puppet "suggest" to a child, "When I get a shot, I say, 'Ouch!' real loud, and then it's all over!"

Digital Sources of Information

Learners can obtain extensive information and support geared toward the lay public as well as healthcare professionals via the Internet through electronic mailing lists and credible Web sites (e.g., Centers for Disease Control and Prevention [CDC], the Joanna Briggs Institute [Best Practice], Hartford Geriatric Nursing Initiative). Electronic learning platforms offer education

---

Quality and Safety Education for Nurses

Teaching Clients Through Collaborative Partnership

Chapter Key Concepts: *Teaching, Learning*

Competency: *Patient-Centered Care; Teamwork and Collaboration (Knowledge, skills, attitudes)**

Background Often patients with chronic illnesses or multiple comorbidities have learning needs related to their medical conditions. Successfully attending to the learning needs of patients requires the nurse to actively engage and empower the patient. Collaboration with the patient as a full partner in care empowers the patient and potentially improves health outcomes (Hain & Sandy, 2013). Effective patient teaching should increase patient knowledge and should facilitate health decision-making by the patient. In order to effectively teach patients, one must utilize a patient-centered, collaborative approach. Collaboration requires the nurse to engage the patient in the entire teaching/learning process, establish a partnership with the patient as the core member of the healthcare team, and empower the patient to make informed health decisions.

Think about it: Using a patient-centered, collaborative approach, what should be your first step in order to teach effectively?

➤ Discuss how you would engage the patient in the teaching/learning process.

➤ Discuss how patient partnership and empowerment has the potential to change health behaviors.

➤ Describe how you would arrive at the desired outcomes for a teaching/learning session?

Reference: Hain, D., & Sandy, D. (2013).

*For specific Knowledge, Skills, and Attitudes,

 Go to the QSEN Web site at **http://qsen.org/competencies/pre-licensure-ksas/**

---

through multimedia, search engines, electronic libraries, content portals, and social networking sites and blogs. Learners can connect with others in similar situations through electronic mailing lists, which are online communities sharing a common focus or interest. Through blogs, electronic mailing lists, and other threaded discussions, participants exchange information; express opinions; offer support; inquire about topics of interest to the greater community; promote special interests; and network with others for personal or professional intent.

Mobile technology with applications (apps) for smartphones, tablet computers, and electronic book readers offers learners convenient access to a variety of engaging learning tools and gaming opportunities. For example, smartphone and tablet apps are designed with customizable medication reminders, rewards systems for healthy behaviors, and educational components.

Audiovisual materials (e.g., streaming video or Flash format, computer animations, audio clips online or per CD/DVD, film, slides, or computer-generated material) can be effective supplements to other methods, especially if the teaching session is followed by a question-and-answer session, a discussion of the content, a test, or printed materials to expand understanding.

Lecture

Lecture is a traditional method in which one or more presenters orally share information while learners listen. It can be enhanced by including discussion and question-and-answer periods for clarifying content and by use of computer-projected slide presentation, streaming video, flip charts, transparencies, posters, brochures, models, and other audiovisual formats. Teachers can engage learners with an attention-getting opening and by supporting teaching points with stories, quotes, images, analogies or metaphors, and humor.

Group Discussion

In a group discussion, several participants discuss topics, exchanging information and presenting their points of view. The teacher acts as a facilitator to achieve objectives shared with the group at the beginning of the session. Effective group discussion requires an atmosphere of trust that encourages everyone to participate. Openness to new ideas and confidentiality of the content expressed are essential for participation. One type of group discussion is *brainstorming*, which is a process for generating multiple ideas for solving a problem. Participants suggest a maximum number of ideas and consider a wide array of creative ideas; then they analyze options, identify a best solution, and develop a plan of action.

KnowledgeCheck 19-4

- True or false: When a patient has a learning disability, you should use a non-NANDA-I diagnosis (e.g., Impaired Ability to Learn) to describe the problem.
- True or false: Learning objectives are short term and ideally should be accomplished in one or two teaching sessions.
- List and state the advantages and disadvantages of at least six teaching strategies.

EVALUATION OF LEARNING

As with all nursing interventions, evaluation is central to the educational process—that is, patient learning is an outcome that is achieved or not. Evaluation of the effectiveness of the teaching plan is essential to improving the quality of instruction. You should evaluate the entire nursing

---

Toward Evidence-Based Practice

Free, C., Phillips, G., Galli, L., et al. (2013). The effectiveness of mobile-health technology-based health behavior change or disease management interventions for health care consumers: A systematic review. *PLoS, 10*, e1001363. Retrieved August 14, 2013, from http://www.ncbi.nlm.nih.gov/pmc/articles/PMC3548655/

A rigorous scientific review of 75 controlled trials examined the effectiveness of mobile technology for healthcare consumers.

- Text messaging improved education adherence for low-income patients receiving antiretroviral therapy as well as for a smoking cessation group in a high-income setting. Text messaging also showed short-term benefit in glucose management as well as physical activity and psychological support for patients with diabetes. Attendance for vaccination was increased with text reminders and information.
- PDA-based education also increased scores for confidence in self-care for patients with lung transplantation.

Deniard-Thompson, N. R., Steven, S. S., & Wofford, J. L. (2012). iPod technology for teaching patients about anticoagulation: A pilot study of mobile computer-assisted patient education. *Primary Health Care Research and Development, 13*(1), 42–47. doi: 10.1017/S146342361100034X

Researchers interested in knowing whether education modules using a handheld, multimedia computer (iPod) are beneficial for office-based patient education found the mobile devices to be a practical and sustainable strategy. Ninety percent of subjects reported the content, audio, and visual display as high in quality. More patients preferred the educational experience using the mobile technology as compared with print materials. The iPod method also standardized the educational content, improved clinic efficiency, and contributed to higher numbers of patients receiving patient education. None of the equipment was lost, stolen, or broken during the study period.

1. In the first article discussing mobile technology for patient education and compliance, why do you think text messaging for conveying health information and reminders was more effective for patient teaching than traditional methods?

2. Based on the results of the second study, why do you think mobile devices might be an effective method of instruction for office- or clinic-based healthcare or even inpatient care?

3. Have you experienced use of tablet computer from your healthcare provider as part of your own patient education? Was it beneficial to you for learning new information or reinforcing information you received prior to your visit? Why or why not?

 Go to Chapter 19, **Toward Evidence-Based Practice Suggested Responses,** on Davis*Plus*.

process (as you may recall from Chapter 7). Was your assessment adequate, or did you fail to notice that the patient was physically uncomfortable and therefore not ready to learn? Was your nursing diagnosis accurate? Were your learning objectives realistic? When evaluating the teaching, consider the type of strategy you used, the timing of the teaching, the content, the amount of information, and the teaching materials. The client is your best source for feedback. He can tell you whether the materials and methods were helpful, or uninteresting, and so on.

Table 19-4 ➤ Formats for Patient Teaching: Advantages and Disadvantages

Lecture

Advantages. An efficient and cost-effective way to impart information, especially to large groups. Is useful for conveying basic concepts and information that serve as the foundation for higher-level, critical thinking later. The presenter can use media-rich formats within the lecture in order to reach learners with auditory and visual learning styles. Lectures may be recorded for future use.

Limitations

- Does not allow for individualization of teaching.
- Passive-learning technique that for most learners is not suited for optimal retention of information.
- May not be geared to the level of the learner.
- Not effective for teaching in the psychomotor or affective domains.
- Can lead to oversaturation if too much information is presented in too short a time frame.
- Boredom is common.
- Not a good strategy for promoting critical thinking.
- Little opportunity for assessment of learner comprehension.

Group Discussion

Advantages. A learner-centered and effective method for teaching in the affective and cognitive domains. Many students enjoy a learning environment with opportunities for interaction with peers. Social involvement can enhance content.

Limitations

- Less effective with large groups.
- The teacher must be comfortable with less structure and with unpredictable learner responses.
- Managing group discussion requires good leadership skills of the instructor.
- Group discussion is not well suited for teaching in the psychomotor domain.
- The quality of group work can be negatively affected by "group think"—a force that stifles creativity by succumbing to the subtle pressure of agreeing with the group even though affirmation doesn't reflect the learner's individual opinion.
- Brainstorming fails when participants are distracted or fail to contribute ideas because of fears of rejection or ridicule by peers. Some might even hold back with brainstorming when anticipating the ideas to be unpopular with the instructor. Individuals who dominate can be equally problematic when crowding out less confident participants. Those who are disruptive or intentionally sabotage the activity can interfere in successful group discussion.

Demonstration and Return Demonstration

Advantages. Is most effective in teaching psychomotor skills (e.g., use of equipment, self-injection, dressing changes). It can be used in small groups if enough equipment is available. When the task or skill is performed correctly, return demonstration can increase self-confidence.

Limitation.

- Does not work well with large groups or for those who do not learn best by observing others.
- May not be well suited for participants who learn at different rates; some might need repeated demonstration or slow enactment of steps, while others do not.
- Time consuming and labor intensive.
- Involves preparation time to set up equipment.
- Space must be suitable for the demonstration format.

(continued)

Table 19-4 ➤ Formats for Patient Teaching: Advantages and Disadvantages—cont'd

One-to-One Instruction and Mentoring

Advantages. Gives the teacher the opportunity to establish a relationship with a learner; convey interest in his learning needs; and tailor the teaching to the learner's needs as the session proceeds. Mentoring allows reluctant learners to more readily ask questions. It enables the teacher to obtain frequent feedback so that material can be repeated and clarified as needed. The method is useful for teaching in all three domains: affective, psychomotor, and cognitive. It provides an opportunity for learners to build skills and problem-solve in situations with expert supervision, guidance, and feedback.

Limitations

- Can be labor intensive and reaches the fewest numbers of learners.
- May be overwhelming to learners because of the large quantity of information given in a short period of time, and therefore may not promote retention.
- One-on-one instruction tends to isolate the learner from others who may share the same learning needs and who could provide support.
- Can be hampered by personality conflicts.
- Relies heavily on the instructor, preceptor, or nurse being a good role model and having effective teaching skills.

Printed Materials

Advantages. Allows for standardized information to be presented to each client, but with some room for individualization. Hard-copy documents are an excellent way to reinforce material taught in lecture, demonstration and return demonstration, or one-to-one instruction. Handouts allow the teacher to cover just the main ideas while using the time more efficiently for face-to-face instruction. Printed materials are portable, so people can read the information when it most convenient.

Limitations

- Assumes literacy, motivation to read the content, organization to keep track of materials, and visual acuity to decipher the print.
- Materials must be written at a 5th grade reading level with words that most people understand.

Role Modeling

Advantages. Allows the learner to identify with the teacher. It can be a subtle but powerful method to increase motivation and ability to perform a desired behavior. It tends to generate high learner interest, and doesn't usually require additional preparation on the part of the role model.

Limitations

- Learners need to be aware and receptive to this type of teaching.
- A role model who does not effectively represent desired behaviors can send the wrong message.

Online Sources of Information

Advantages. The Internet makes a vast amount of information readily available. The easily available health-related information makes it possible for consumers to participate in self-care and make informed decisions. Patients feel empowered when they have access to relevant and understandable information. They often cope better and experience less uncertainty when health information is available.

Using audiovisual materials is a stimulating method because it engages both sight and hearing, and can accommodate large groups.

Limitations

- The teacher has little control over the quality of information learners access via the Internet. Before recommending particular Web sites to a patient, you need to read it yourself to be sure the information is accurate and the format and reading level are best suited to your patient. See Chapter 41 for information about evaluating materials you obtain from a Web site.
- Audiovisual hardware and software can be expensive and must be replaced when they become outdated.

The following methods are commonly used for outcomes evaluation (client learning):

- *Oral questions/interviews/questionnaires/checklists* allow clients to evaluate their own progress and determine future learning needs. You may obtain more information by talking with the client; however, you may obtain more honest responses by using written questions and providing for anonymous completion of the evaluations.
- *Direct observations of client performance* are anecdotal, descriptive notes that you make of the learner's performance. They will help you in providing feedback to the client either to reinforce accurate learning or to

correct misinformation. Provide feedback as soon as possible after you observe performance.

- *Reports and client records.* Clients and/or families can keep records of performance and results. You can then evaluate the data and give feedback accordingly. Documentation of performance is best when following criteria or other clear expectations. You can make plans for further teaching when you analyze the data and determine the learners' knowledge deficits.

- *Tests, checklists, and written exercises* can be used to measure retention and progress toward meeting cognitive objectives. This method requires the learner to be actively involved and have adequate literacy skills.

Clients will not remember everything you teach them. That is normal. If you start to question your effectiveness as a teacher, think about one of the courses you took last semester. Did you score 100% on every test? How much of the material presented in that course do you remember now? Repetition, reinforcement, and practice are necessary for retention; and so is information made memorable.

Documentation of Teaching and Learning

As is true for all nursing interventions (as you learned in Chapter 18), it is important to record the responses of the client and family to teaching interventions. Documentation also provides legal evidence that teaching was done and communicates the information to other health professionals. Write objective statements about what was taught and the client skills and behaviors that demonstrate learning. For informal teaching that occurs during other care activities, you may simply record in the nursing notes. For planned teaching that is provided frequently for a particular population of clients, many agencies provide special documentation forms. For an example of a patient education record,

Go to Chapter 19, **Tables, Boxes, Figures: ESG Figure 19-1,** on Davis*Plus*.

To explore learning resources for this chapter,

Go to DavisPlus at DavisPl.us/Wilkinson3.

Chapter Resources for Chapter 19:
  Response sheets for all learning activities
  Resources for Caregivers and Health Professionals
  Reading More About Teaching & Learning (suggested readings)
  Concept Map of chapter content
Interactive Case Studies
NCLEX-Style and Chapter Review Questions
Chapter Overview Podcasts

For references cited in this chapter,

Go to Volume 2, **References Cited.**

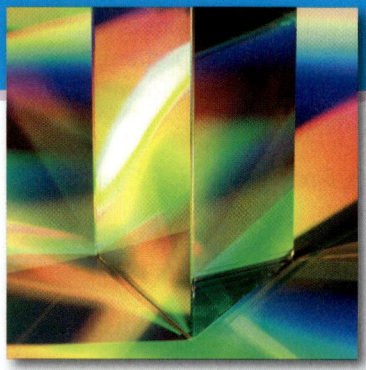

CHAPTER 20

Measuring Vital Signs

Learning Outcomes

After completing this chapter, you should be able to:

- ➤ Describe the physiological processes involved in regulating body temperature, pulse, respirations, and blood pressure.
- ➤ Convert between the Fahrenheit and centigrade temperature scales.
- ➤ For different patient situations, choose the best procedure for measuring temperature, pulse, respiration, and blood pressure, including site and equipment.
- ➤ Discuss the concept of a "normal" temperature.
- ➤ Describe nursing interventions for the patient with temperature alterations.
- ➤ Given a client's age, differentiate between normal vital signs findings and those that should be referred to the primary healthcare provider.
- ➤ State at least one nursing diagnosis that might be used to describe a problem for each of the vital signs: temperature, pulse, respirations, and blood pressure.

- ➤ Define *arterial oxygen saturation*, *hypoxia*, *hyperventilation*, and *hypoventilation*.
- ➤ Discuss nursing interventions for the client with impaired respiratory status.
- ➤ State the normal temperature, pulse, respiration, and blood pressure ranges for the average adult.
- ➤ Explain why it is important to interpret a client's blood pressure pattern rather than relying on a single reading.
- ➤ Discuss the importance of cuff size when obtaining a blood pressure reading.
- ➤ Define *hypotension*, *hypertension*, *essential hypertension*, and *secondary hypertension*.
- ➤ Identify nursing interventions for the client with hypertension.
- ➤ Demonstrate correct technique for measuring temperature, pulse, respiration, and blood pressure.

Key Concepts

Vital signs
Thermoregulation
Perfusion (pulse, blood pressure)
Oxygenation (respirations)

Related Concepts
See the Concept Map on Davis*Plus*.

Example Problems
Pyrexia (fever)
Hyperthermia
Hypothermia
Hypertension
Hypotension

Meet Your Patients

Your instructor has scheduled a clinical day at a local community health fair for students to answer health-related questions, administer flu vaccines, check blood sugar levels, and take vital signs: temperature, pulse, respirations, and blood pressure. You have been asked to check vital signs.

Jason. The first person who arrives at the booth is Rosemary, a young mother, with Jason, her 2-year-old son. She tells you he has been eating poorly and is very irritable. The child's skin is warm and dry and he is flushed. Rosemary explains that she does not have a thermometer, and she would like you to take her son's temperature. Jason's axillary temperature is 101.8°F (38.8°C).

Now it is time to think like a nurse! What could this temperature reading mean? What, if any, additional data should you collect? How will you explain your findings to Rosemary? What action would you advise Rosemary to take? You may not yet have all the theoretical knowledge you need to answer these questions, but try to do so anyway, based on your present knowledge base and your life experiences.

Ms. Sharma. The next person to arrive at the booth is Ms. Sharma, an active 80-year-old woman who works part-time in a local literacy program and walks 3 miles four times per week. Ms. Sharma notes that she has "lost a little pep. I don't feel sick, but I'm tired lately." Her pulse is difficult to feel. The rhythm is irregular, and the strength of the pulse is uneven—some beats are strong, while others are weak. What might this finding mean? What questions do you have for Ms. Sharma? What, if any, additional data should you collect? How will you explain your findings to Ms. Sharma? What action would you advise her to take?

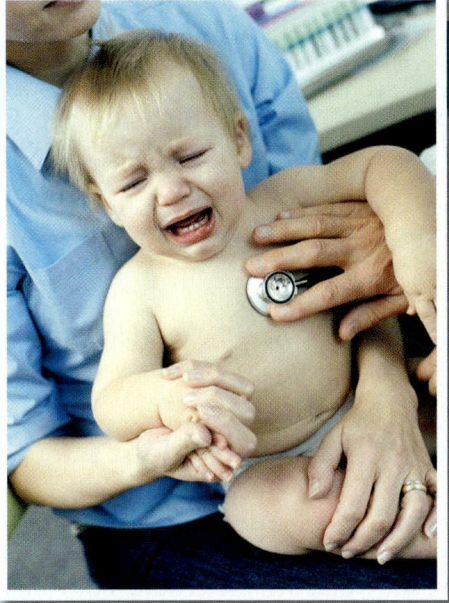

Mr. Jackson. As Mr. Jackson sits down next to you, you notice he is short of breath. His respiratory rate is 28 breaths/min, and he appears to be struggling to breathe. What do you think this respiratory rate means? What should be your next action? What would you say to Mr. Jackson?

Lucas. The next client to arrive is Lucas, a 35-year-old accountant who works for a firm in a nearby office building. Lucas tells you he has been under a lot of stress and is worried about his blood pressure. You measure his blood pressure as 150/98 mm Hg. Is this an acceptable blood pressure? What does this reading mean? What should you discuss with Lucas? What advice should you offer?

You will gain the theoretical knowledge you need to answer the preceding questions as you work through this chapter and learn more about vital signs.

ABOUT THE KEY CONCEPTS

All of the content in this chapter pertains to the concept of **vital signs**. The key concepts of **thermoregulation, perfusion,** and **oxygenation** pertain to specific vital signs you will learn about (temperature, pulse, respirations, and blood pressure). A grasp of these underlying concepts will help you understand and remember the rationale for what you do when measuring vital signs.

WHAT ARE VITAL SIGNS?

The term **vital signs (VS)** suggests assessment of vital or critical physiological functions. Variations in temperature (T), pulse (P), respirations (P), or blood pressure (BP) are indicators of a person's state of health and function of the body systems. Therefore, these four measurements are among the most frequent assessments you will make as a nurse. Because of their importance, your accurate measurements and documentation of each vital sign is a top priority.

Do not become complacent when a client's vital signs are within normal limits. Although stable vital signs *indicate* physiological well-being, they do not *guarantee* it. Vital signs alone are limited in detecting some important physiological changes; for example, vital signs may sometimes remain stable even when there is moderately large blood loss. Evaluate the vital signs in the context of your overall assessment of the client.

Other Vital Signs Some experts have recommended that other factors that affect patient care and outcomes be added to the four traditional measures of physiological status, for example:

- *Pain* is widely regarded as the fifth vital sign. See Chapter 31.
- *Oxygen saturation* obtained by pulse oximetry provides important information on arterial blood oxygen concentration.
- *Smoking status* has been assessed by some providers as a VS during the initial patient encounter (Lockwood & Conroy-Hiller, 2004; Rothemich, Woolf, Johnson,

et al., 2008), although it does not fit with the traditional concept.

- *Emotional distress* is recommended by some as a vital sign.

Rather than being overly concerned about whether or not these parameters should be referred to as vital signs, we recommend that nurses include them in all of their ongoing assessments of patients: temperature, pulse, and respirations (TPR); blood pressure (BP); pain; pulse oximetry; emotional status; and (on initial encounter) smoking status.

The rest of this chapter explains the meaning of each of the traditional vital signs and how to assess them.

When Should I Measure a Patient's Vital Signs?

In the Meet Your Patients scenario, clients asked you to take their vital signs. However, in many clinical settings you and other care providers will determine how often to measure and document VS. The following are common occasions for assessing vital signs:

- On admission to the hospital
- For inpatients, at the beginning of a shift
- At a visit to the healthcare provider's office or clinic
- Before, during, and after surgery or certain procedures
- To monitor the effects of certain medications or activities
- Whenever the patient's condition changes

The optimal frequency for assessing vital signs depends on the patient's condition and the events taking place (Schulman & Staul, 2010). Also, agency policies usually require that nurses monitor and record vital signs regularly. The frequency varies by setting. Below are commonly used frequencies. However, one recent study suggests that low-risk patients might be allowed to rest instead of waking them up for routine vital signs during the night (Jordan, Yoder, Yuen, et al., 2013).

- In the hospital: once every 4 to 8 hours
- In the home health setting: at each visit
- In the clinic: at each visit
- In skilled nursing facilities, also known as convalescent hospitals: weekly to monthly

It is up to the nurse to decide whether vital signs need to be monitored more frequently than the primary care provider has prescribed. Initially, you will measure VS to establish the patient's baseline.

Key Point: *A baseline is important because (1) a change in vital signs may be caused by a disease state, the effect of therapies, or merely by changes in activity and environment; and (2) there are normal variations in vital signs among individuals.*

Table 20-1 shows average or normal findings for adults, but it is important to remember that each person has his or her own baseline for "normal." If a patient's vital signs vary from established norms, compare the finding to that person's baseline to determine the degree and severity of the variation. When a client's VS vary

Table 20-1 ➤ Vital Signs: Average Normal Findings for Adults	
Mean Adult Temperature	
Oral	98°F (36.7°C)*
Rectal	98.6°F (37°C)*
Pulse	
Normal range	60–100 beats/min
Average	80 beats/min
Respirations	
Normal range	12–20 breaths/min
Blood Pressure	
Normal range	100–119 systolic and 60–80 diastolic
Prehypertensive	120–139 systolic and 80–89 diastolic
Average	110/70 (the middle of the "normal" range) (Joint National Committee on Prevention, Detection, Evaluation, and Treatment of High Blood Pressure, 2004)

*This is revised downward from the traditional norms to reflect more recent research (Mackowiak, Wasserman, & Levine, 1998) and a systematic review of the literature (Sund-Levander, Forsberg, & Wahren, 2002). The systematic review reported the following mean normal temperatures: Oral 97.3°F (36.3°C), Rectal 98.3°F (36.9°C). The traditional Wunderlich (1871) average normal temperature is 98.6°F (37.0°C) to 99.5°F (37.5°C), depending on measurement site.

from their baseline, you should assess and document them more frequently, perhaps every 5 to 15 minutes. As a beginning practitioner, you should validate your clinical assessments with a more experienced nurse.

How Do I Document Vital Signs?

Most agencies have special flowsheets for documenting vital signs. If the VS are not within normal limits, you will also record them in the nurses' notes, along with any associated symptoms (e.g., cyanosis [blue-gray skin] with abnormal respirations). Nurses are required to take appropriate actions based on their assessment finding. Therefore, you must document your interventions as well (e.g., elevating the head of the bed when the patient has shortness of breath). For an example of a graphic flowsheet for documenting vital signs,

 Go to Chapter 20, **Forms**, in Volume 2.

BODY TEMPERATURE

Body temperature is the degree of heat maintained by the body. It is the difference between heat produced by the body and heat lost to the environment.

Theoretical Knowledge
knowing **why**

Although the focus in this chapter is on body temperature, you must understand the concept of "thermoregulation" to assess and support regulation of body temperature at a professional level. You will learn the normal temperature range, how heat is produced by and lost from the body, and factors that influence body temperature.

What Is a Normal Temperature?

No single number can be considered "normal," because body temperature varies among individuals as a result of differences in metabolism. Furthermore, each person's temperature fluctuates with age, exercise, and environmental conditions. However, the body does function optimally within a narrow temperature range.

There is little definitive evidence about what, exactly, is a normal temperature. You may see different values in the many sources you read. We can at least conclude that the traditional belief of 98.6°F (37°C) for an average normal reading is too high, based on available research. A systematic review of the literature found a mean normal oral temperature of 97.3°F (36.3°C) (Sund-Levander, Forsberg, & Wahren, 2002). See Table 20-1. Research findings are inconsistent as to whether older adults have lower body temperatures (Lu & Dai, 2009) and recommend that body temperature be evaluated based on individual variability (Sund-Levander, Grodzinsky, Loyd, et al., 2004).

Pregnant women run higher baseline body temperatures. For age-related variations for all vital signs, including temperature,

 Chapter Resources: Chapter 20, **Tables, Boxes, Figures: ESG Table 20-1, Comparison of Normal Vital Signs for Various Ages,** on Davis*Plus.*

An adult's normal internal temperature, called the **core temperature**, ranges from about 97°F to 100.8°F (36.1°C to 38.2°C). Most research and clinical practice situations do not report core body temperature because it is not convenient to measure. The core temperature is typically 1°F to 2°F (0.6°C to 1.2°C) higher than surface (skin) temperature. Rectal and tympanic membrane measurements are used to represent core temperatures; oral and axillary measurements reflect surface temperatures.

Temporary, slight variations of temperature above or below normal usually are not significant. Greater variations indicate a disturbance of function in some system or region of the body (Fig. 20-1). However, the degree of temperature elevation does not always indicate the seriousness of the underlying disease or condition. For example, some acute, even fatal, infections may cause only a mild temperature elevation. However, a continuous elevation, even if slight, is cause for concern and indicates a need for further evaluation.

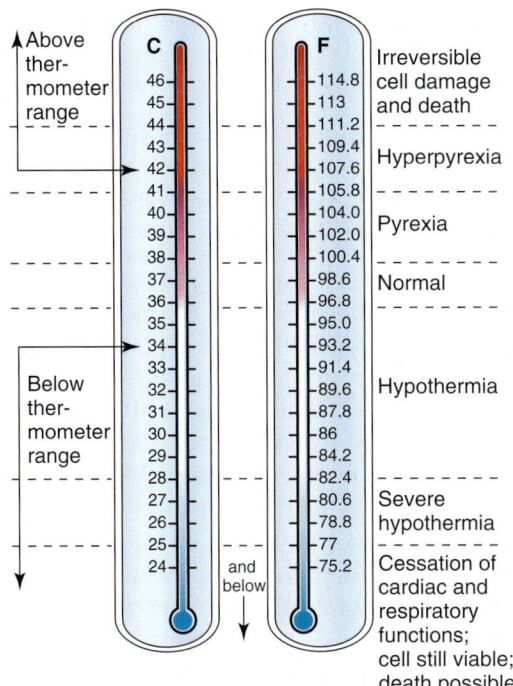

FIGURE 20-1 Ranges of normal and altered body temperatures.

What Is Thermoregulation?

Thermoregulation is the process of maintaining a stable temperature. To keep the body temperature constant, the body must balance heat production and heat loss. This balance is controlled by the hypothalamus, located between the cerebral hemispheres of the brain. Similar to a thermostat, the hypothalamus recognizes even small changes in body temperature that are sent to it by sensory receptors in the skin.

Decreasing the Body Temperature When heat sensors in the hypothalamus are stimulated, they send out impulses to reduce the body temperature. This activates compensatory mechanisms, such as peripheral vasodilation, sweating, and inhibition of heat production. **Vasodilation** (increase in the diameter of the blood vessels) diverts core-warmed blood to the body surface, where heat can be transferred to the surrounding environment.

Increasing the Body Temperature When the sensors in the hypothalamus detect cold, they send out impulses to increase heat production and reduce heat loss. To produce heat, the body responds with shivering and the release of epinephrine, which increases metabolism. To reduce heat loss, the blood vessels constrict. **Vasoconstriction** (narrowing of the blood vessels) conserves heat by shunting blood away from the periphery (where heat is lost) to the core of the body, where the blood is warmed. **Piloerection** (hairs standing on end) also occurs, but it is not an important heat-conserving mechanism in humans.

Behavioral Control of Temperature In addition, body temperature is under our behavioral control. When people feel cool, they can turn up the thermostat, put on more clothing, or move to a warmer place. When they feel too warm, they can turn on an air conditioner, remove some clothing, or take a cool shower.

How Is Heat Produced in the Body?

The body produces heat through the interaction of three factors: metabolism, the movement of skeletal muscles, and nonshivering thermogenesis.

Metabolism

Metabolism is the sum of all physical and chemical processes and changes that take place in the body. Metabolism uses energy and generates heat. The **basal metabolic rate (BMR)** is the amount of energy required to maintain the body at rest. Body size, lean muscle mass, and numerous hormones influence BMR. For example, hyperthyroidism (an increase in the thyroid hormone **thyroxine**) increases the BMR. Clients with hyperthyroidism often complain of feeling warm even when in a cool environment. By contrast, when the thyroxine level is low (hypothyroidism), less heat is produced, and clients commonly report feeling cold. Epinephrine and norepinephrine, produced from stimulation of the sympathetic nervous system, also increase BMR and heat production.

Skeletal Muscle Movement

Skeletal muscles are used in all body movements. Muscles need fuel to function. The breakdown (**catabolism**) of fats and carbohydrates in muscle produces energy and heat. It requires very little muscle activity to sit and read this text. However, if you were to go for a run, you would use more skeletal muscles. After your run, your body temperature would be higher, perhaps as high as 101°F to 104°F (38.3°C to 40°C). In contrast, if you were to go outside without a coat when the temperature was 35°F (1.6°C), you would begin to feel cold. Your hypothalamus would sense a drop in body temperature and you would begin shivering. This mechanism is so efficient that body heat production can rise to about four times the normal rate in just a few minutes.

Nonshivering Thermogenesis

Nonshivering thermogenesis is the metabolism of brown fat to produce heat. It is used by infants because they cannot produce heat through shivering, as do adults and children. This mechanism disappears in the first few months after birth.

How Is Heat Exchanged Between the Body and the Environment?

Heat moves from an area of higher to an area of lower temperature; that is, cool air and objects "pick up" heat from warmer ones. The mechanisms that affect the exchange of heat between the body and the environment are radiation, convection, evaporation, and conduction (Fig. 20-2).

Radiation is the loss of heat through electromagnetic waves emitting from surfaces that are warmer than the surrounding air. If the uncovered skin is warmer than the air, the body loses heat through the skin. This is why a cool room warms by radiation when it is filled with many people. In contrast, a person can acquire heat by turning on a heat lamp or being in the sunlight. Radiation accounts for almost 50% of body heat loss.

Convection is the transfer of heat through currents of air or water. Nurses use this principle to intentionally effect changes in a patient's body temperature. Immersion in a warm bath may raise body temperature for a hypothermic client. In contrast, the currents of cool air produced by a fan can help reduce a fever. Together, the processes of convection and conduction account for approximately 15% to 20% of all heat loss to the environment.

Evaporation occurs when water is converted to vapor and lost from the skin (as perspiration) or the mucous membranes (through the breath). Evaporation causes cooling. Water loss by evaporation is called **insensible loss.** Evaporation is affected by the relative **humidity** (moisture in the environment). If the air already contains much humidity, then less moisture evaporates from the skin and less cooling occurs.

Conduction is the process whereby heat is transferred from a warm to a cool surface by direct contact. Suppose that a patient's temperature is 98.6°F (37°C) while he is fully dressed in the examination room. If he dresses in a thin, hospital gown and lies on a cool metal radiology table, his temperature will drop, perhaps as much as a full degree Fahrenheit in the first hour.

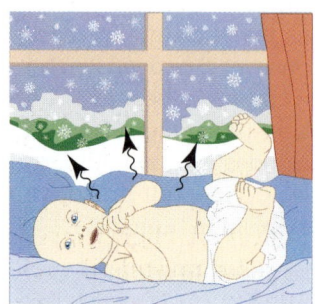 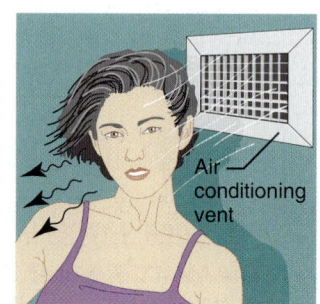 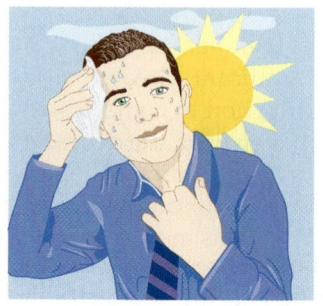 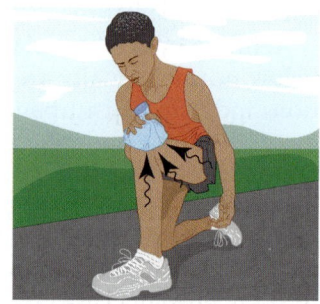

FIGURE 20-2 Mechanisms of heat exchange with the environment: Radiation, convection, evaporation, and conduction.

What Factors Influence Body Temperature?

The following are some examples of internal and external factors involved in the delicate balance of body temperature:

Developmental Level Infants and older adults are most susceptible to the effects of environmental temperature extremes. Infants lose approximately 30% of their body heat through the head, which is proportionally larger than the rest of the body compared to adults. This places them at increased risk for decreased body temperature. Body temperature begins to stabilize during early childhood and remains relatively stable until older adulthood.

 Older adults have difficulty maintaining body heat because of slower metabolism, decreased vasomotor control, and loss of subcutaneous tissue. In a recent study, older adults (age 85 years and older) had mean body temperatures lower than 98.6°F (37°C) (Lu & Dai, 2009). Temperatures ranged from 94°F (34.4°C) to 99.6°F (37.6°C), but few ever reached 98.6°F (Gomolin, Aung, Wolf-Klein, et al., 2005). You can think of the average normal temperature for older adults as about 95°F to 96.8°F (35°C to 36°C).

For a comparison of normal VS for various ages,

Go to Chapter Resources: Chapter 20, **Tables, Boxes, Figures: ESG Table 20-1,** on Davis*Plus.*

Environment The environment strongly influences body temperature. For example, warm room temperatures, high humidity, or hot baths can increase body temperature. Very high external temperatures can significantly increase internal temperatures, causing heat stroke. In contrast, cold environments, especially with strong air currents, can lower body temperatures and, in severe cases, lead to hypothermia.

Gender A woman's body temperature varies (as much as 1°F, or 0.6°C) with her menstrual cycle and pregnancy. Body temperature is lower when progesterone levels are low and increases as progesterone levels increase. Hormonal fluctuations during menopause, when menses stop, often cause temperature fluctuations commonly known as *hot flashes,* which can produce episodes of intense body heat and sweating. Research studies have found differences in the range of normal body temperatures for women and men (Lu & Dai, 2009; Sund-Levander, Forsberg, & Wahren, 2002).

Exercise Because it increases metabolism, hard work or strenuous exercise can increase body core temperature to 101°F to 104°F (38.3°C to 40°C). The sweat that is produced during exercise evaporates and helps to cool the body.

Emotions and Stress Emotional stress, excitement, anxiety, and nervousness stimulate the sympathetic nervous system, causing production of epinephrine and norepinephrine. These biochemical agents trigger an increase in the metabolic rate, which in turn increases body temperature.

Circadian Rhythm Circadian rhythm is a cyclical repetition of certain physiological processes (e.g., changes in temperature and blood pressure) that occurs every 24 hours. Temperature fluctuates 1°F to 2°F (0.6°C to 1.2°C) over the course of 24 hours. It is usually lowest in the early morning hours and highest in late afternoon or early evening.

ThinkLike a Nurse 20-1

- You notice the following temperature readings in your client's medical records:
  0400: 97.4°F
  0800: 97.9°F
  1200: 98.4°F
  1600: 99.6°F
  2000: 100.9°F
  When you assess the client's temperature at midnight, it is 101.2°F. What do you notice about the pattern of the temperature readings?
- What is important in this scenario?
- As a nursing student, what should you do?

KnowledgeCheck 20-1

- Which age groups are most susceptible to thermoregulation problems, and why?
- List five factors that affect body temperature.
- What are the compensatory mechanisms for decreasing body temperature?
- What are the compensatory mechanisms for increasing body temperature?

Example Problem: Fever (Pyrexia)

Fever, or **pyrexia**, is a temperature above the person's usual range of normal. Traditionally we have thought of fever as an oral temperature higher than 100°F (37.8°C), or a rectal temperature of 101°F (38.3°C) in an adult. But remember that many people, especially older adults, have lower normal body temperatures and that a person's normal body temperature changes by as much as 1°F (0.6°C) throughout the day. So it follows that many people, especially older adults, experience fever at a temperature lower than our traditional definition. A person with a fever is said to be **febrile**; one without fever is **afebrile**. A single high reading may not indicate fever. You need several readings at different times of the day, as well as the person's usual normal reading.

A moderate fever (up to 103°F, or 39.5°C) may be uncomfortable, and it may signal an underlying problem (e.g., influenza or other infection). However, the fever itself does not pose a threat to most clients and is the body's natural defense against infection. Higher fevers can damage body cells and cause delirium and seizures. **Hyperpyrexia** is fever above 105.8°F (41.0°C). Hyperpyrexia is dangerous and requires intervention.

Fever occurs in response to **pyrogens** (fever-producing substances). When bacteria or other foreign substances invade the body, they stimulate **phagocytes** (specialized white blood cells), which ingest the invaders and secrete pyrogens (e.g., interleukin-1). Pyrogens induce secretion of **prostaglandins** (substances that reset the hypothalamic thermostat at a higher temperature). The reset value is called the **set point**. The body's heat-regulating mechanisms then act to bring the core temperature up to this new setting. When the stressor is removed, the set point resets at normal.

Fever occurs in three phases:

1. *The initial phase (febrile episode or onset):* The period during which body temperature is rising but has not yet reached the new set point. The onset of fever may be sudden or gradual, depending on the condition causing it. The person usually feels chilly and generally uncomfortable and may shiver.
2. *The second phase (course):* The period during which body temperature reaches its maximum (set point) and remains fairly constant at the new higher level. The person is flushed and feels warm and dry during this phase, which may last from a few days to a few weeks.
3. *The third phase (defervescence or crisis):* The period during which the temperature returns to normal. The person feels warm and appears flushed in response to vasodilation. Diaphoresis occurs, which assists with heat loss by evaporation. This phase is commonly referred to as the fever's "breaking."

The following are four important ways to describe a fever:

- **Intermittent fever:** Temperature alternates regularly between periods of fever and periods of normal or below-normal temperature without pharmacological intervention; or the temperature returns to normal at least once every 24 hours.
- **Remittent fever:** Fluctuations in temperature (greater than 3.6°F, or 2°C), all above normal, during a 24-hour period.
- **Constant (sustained) fever:** Temperature may fluctuate slightly (less than 1°F, or 0.55°C) but is always above normal.
- **Relapsing (or recurrent) fever:** Short periods of fever alternating with periods of normal temperatures, each lasting 1 to 2 days.

At some time in your life, you most likely have taken acetaminophen (Tylenol) or ibuprofen (Advil, Motrin) for a fever. Can you think of a reason it may or may not always be a good idea to do that at the first signs of a fever? Why should you think carefully before administering **antipyretic** (fever-reducing) medications to a client?

The answer is that fever, up to a point, is beneficial (for most people). High temperatures (up to 102.2°F, or 39°C) enhance the immune response because they (1) kill or inhibit the growth of many microorganisms, (2) enhance phagocytosis, (3) cause the breakdown of lysosomes and self-destruction of virally infected cells, and (4) cause the release of interferon, a substance that protects cells from viral infection.

This does not mean that you should *never* administer, or take, antipyretic medications. They may be needed to promote comfort and keep the temperature from becoming dangerously high. Temperatures of 105.8°F (41.0°C) and above can damage cells throughout the body, especially in the brain, causing agitation, confusion, stupor, or coma. Vascular collapse may follow, producing cerebral edema, shock, and death. Death usually results if body temperature becomes higher than 109°F to 112°F (43°C to 44°C) (McCance & Huether, 2010). Note that certain patients (e.g., those with epilepsy) are especially sensitive to even slight temperature elevations, so antipyretics might be used at the first sign of temperature elevation.

Example Problem: Hyperthermia (Heat Exhaustion, Heat Stroke)

Hyperthermia, like hyperpyrexia (fever), is a body temperature above normal. However, in hyperthermia, the elevated body temperature is higher than the set point. The hypothalamic regulation of body temperature is overwhelmed and does not reset the set point as it does in fever. Hyperthermia occurs because the body cannot promote heat loss fast enough to balance heat production or high environmental temperatures. **Heat exhaustion** and **heat stroke** are common examples. With overexposure to high temperatures and inadequate fluid replacement, the body loses its ability to sweat and is unable to cool down.

Heat Exhaustion may occur with a core temperature of 98.6°F (37°C) to 103°F (39.4°C). Warning signs of heat exhaustion vary, but may include weakness, nausea, vomiting, syncope, tachycardia, tachypnea, muscle aches, headache, diaphoresis (heavy sweating), and flushed skin.

Heat Stroke occurs when the body's temperature regulation fails, usually when the hyperthermia progresses to a temperature above 103°F (39.4°C). Symptoms include rapid, strong pulse; throbbing headache; delirium; confusion; impaired judgment; lethargy; red, hot, dry skin; dizziness; seizures; and coma. The body is unable to sweat. Temperatures of 106°F (41.1°C) and higher may be reached. If emergency treatment is not given, heat stroke can result in permanent disability and death (Centers for Disease Control and Prevention [CDC], 2010b).

Example Problem: Hypothermia

The CDC (2010a) defines **hypothermia** as an abnormally low core temperature, less than 95°F (less than 35°C). You must know the person's usual normal range of temperature because some people, especially older adults, have a normal temperature of less than 95°F. As the body temperature drops, metabolic processes slow. Prolonged exposure to the cold is no longer correctable by shivering and may prove fatal (CDC, 2010a).

Hypothermia may be associated with surgery, extreme weather conditions, immersion in cold water, or lack of shelter and clothing. Hypothermia is sometimes deliberately induced under close monitoring to decrease the need for oxygen in body tissues (e.g., during cardiac or neurological surgery).

- **Early signs of hypothermia** include shivering, cyanosis of lips and fingers, and poor coordination. The person first feels cold, then may feel some pain in the extremities. As body temperature continues to fall, the person experiences mental impairment, confusion, disorientation, slowing of the heart rate and respirations, and inability to take precautions from the cold.
- **Severe hypothermia** occurs when the body temperature drops below 82.4°F (28°C). The person becomes unconscious and stops shivering. The pulse and respirations are irregular and difficult to detect. Although survival has been known to occur at a core temperature of 60.8°F (16°C), death usually results when body temperature falls below 70°F to 75°F (21°C to 24°C).

PracticalKnowledge
knowing **how**

Now that you understand the concept of thermoregulation, you are ready to gain the practical knowledge of how to assess and support a patient's body temperature.

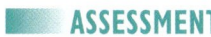 ASSESSMENT

In our daily routines, we commonly assess temperature by touch. For example, when you remove a blanket from a warming unit, you can feel that it is warm; however, you probably could not pinpoint the exact temperature of the blanket. The same is true of body temperature. Although some research has shown that people can use simple touch to detect fever, they cannot differentiate *degrees* of fever. Because vital signs are used as indicators of a client's health status, it is essential to have an accurate measure. To see the sequence of steps to take when measuring a patient's temperature,

 Go to **Procedure 20-1: Assessing Body Temperature,** in Volume 2.

The Home Care section of Procedure 20-1, in Volume 2, will assist you in teaching clients how to check their temperature at home.

Temperature Measurement Scales: Fahrenheit and Centigrade

Two scales are used for recording temperature: Fahrenheit and centigrade (or Celsius), a metric scale. Most people in the United States are familiar with the Fahrenheit scale;

however, some healthcare agencies use centigrade. Electronic and tympanic membrane thermometers can usually measure temperature in either scale; often all you need to do is to flip a switch. Some types of thermometers may read only one scale (Fig. 20-3 shows both scales, for comparison), so you may need to convert a reading from one scale to the other. For example, you may have obtained a centigrade reading for a child and plan to explain its significance to the mother, who is familiar only with Fahrenheit. For a chart to use to convert between Fahrenheit and centigrade readings,

 Go to Chapter 20, **Centigrade–Fahrenheit Conversion Chart,** in Volume 2.

You will probably have access to a conversion chart in clinical settings, but if not you may need to convert mathematically. To convert from Fahrenheit to centigrade, subtract 32 from the Fahrenheit temperature and multiply by ⁵⁄₉. For example:

A client has a temperature of 102°F. What is his temperature as measured in centigrade?

$$(102 - 32) \times \tfrac{5}{9} = (70 \times 5) \div 9 = 39°C$$

To convert a centigrade reading to Fahrenheit, multiply the centigrade temperature by ⁹⁄₅, and add 32. As a cross-check we can verify the preceding example:

Client temperature = 39°C
$$(39 \times \tfrac{9}{5}) + 32 = (351 \div 5) + 32 = 102°F$$

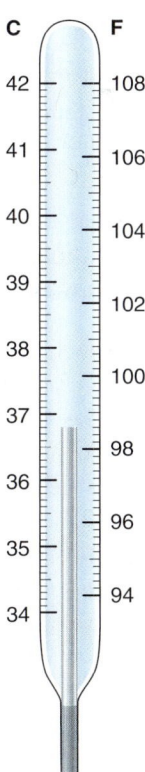

FIGURE 20-3 Thermometers are available with degree markings in Fahrenheit or centigrade. *Left,* Centigrade scale. *Right,* Fahrenheit scale.

For steps to follow in *all* procedures, refer to the Universal Steps for All Procedures found on the inside back cover of Volume 2. Go to the full procedures in Volume 2 to practice and learn the procedure steps. Use these procedure highlights later to help you review key points.

Procedure 20-1: Assessing Body Temperature

➤ Clean thermometer before and after using if it is not disposable.

➤ Select the appropriate site and thermometer type.

➤ Turn on or otherwise ready the thermometer.

➤ Insert the thermometer in its sheath, or use a thermometer designated only for the patient.

➤ Insert and leave an electronic thermometer in place until it beeps; for other thermometers use the recommended times.

➤ Cleanse and store in recharging base (store glass thermometers safely to prevent breakage).

➤ For an oral temperature, obtain a reading 20 to 30 minutes after the patient consumes hot or cold food or fluids or smokes.

➤ Hold a rectal thermometer securely in place, and never leave it unattended.

Procedure 20-2: Assessing Peripheral Pulses

➤ Make sure the client is resting while you assess the pulse.

➤ Count for 15 or 30 seconds if the pulse is regular; count for 60 seconds if it is irregular.

➤ Note pulse rate, rhythm, and quality.

➤ Compare pulses bilaterally.

Procedure 20-3: Assessing the Apical Pulse

➤ Position the patient supine or sitting.

➤ Palpate and place the stethoscope at the 5th intercostal space at the midclavicular line.

➤ Count for 60 seconds.

➤ Note pulse rate, rhythm, and quality and the S_1 and S_2 heart sounds.

Procedure 20-4: Assessing for an Apical-Radial Pulse Deficit

➤ Palpate and place stethoscope over apex of the heart.

➤ Palpate the radial pulse.

➤ Have two nurses carry out the procedure, if possible.

➤ Count for 60 seconds, simultaneously.

➤ Compare the pulse rate at both sites; calculate the difference.

Procedure 20-5: Assessing Respirations

➤ Count unobtrusively (e.g., while palpating the radial pulse).

➤ Count for 30 seconds if respirations are regular; count for 60 seconds if they are irregular.

➤ Observe the rate, rhythm, and depth of respirations.

Procedure 20-6: Measuring Blood Pressure

➤ If possible, place the patient in a sitting position, with the feet on the floor and the legs uncrossed.

➤ Measure BP after the patient has been inactive for 5 minutes.

➤ Support the patient's arm at the level of the heart.

➤ Use a cuff of the appropriate size.

➤ Wrap the cuff snugly.

➤ Inflate the cuff while palpating the artery. Inflate to 30 mm Hg above the point at which you can no longer feel the artery pulsating.

➤ Place the stethoscope on the artery, and release pressure at 2 to 3 mm Hg per second.

➤ Record systolic/diastolic pressures (first and last sounds heard—e.g., 110/80).

➤ Wait at least 2 minutes before remeasuring.

What Equipment Do I Need?

Nurses measure temperature with various kinds of thermometers. Each type has advantages and disadvantages, shown in Table 20-2, so you need to think critically about the type of thermometer best suited for each patient situation.

Glass Thermometers

Historically, the thermometer was a glass mercury-filled tube marked in degrees Fahrenheit or centigrade and read visually. Researchers at Children's Hospital Boston found that children under 4 years suffered broken glass to the mouth or rectum, exposure to mercury, and/or required imaging to detect foreign objects in the body associated with the use of glass thermometers (Aprahamian, Lee, Shannon, et al., 2009).

Because of such dangers, the U.S. Environmental Protection Agency and the American Hospital Association now advise against use of equipment containing mercury (U.S. Environmental Protection Agency [EPA], 2012).

Many healthcare facilities have replaced glass thermometers with electronic digital thermometers or with glass or plastic thermometers containing other liquids, such as alcohol or gallium–indium–tin (galinstan). However, you may find some patients still using them at home.

Electronic Thermometers are rechargeable units consisting of an electronic probe attached to a portable unit by a thin wire. A beep sounds when the peak temperature is reached. Disposable plastic sheaths are used to cover the probe. To prevent transmission of infection, you discard the sheath after each use. Most units have a separate probe for rectal and oral temperatures, color-coded red and blue, respectively, to be certain the correct probe is used.

Electronic Infrared Thermometers are rechargeable units that contain a sensor that detects heat in the form of infrared energy given off by the body, for example, at the tympanic membrane or at the temporal artery. The thermometer does not actually touch the tympanic

membrane. A beep sounds when the peak temperature is reached.

Disposable Chemical Thermometers are a thin plastic strip, patch, or tape containing a matrix of chemicals that produce color changes at a designated body temperature. Most are used once for an oral or axillary reading, and then discarded. Another form consists of temperature-sensitive tape containing liquid crystals that change color in response to temperature. The tape is

---

Table 20-2 ➤ Advantages and Disadvantages of Various Thermometers

ADVANTAGES	DISADVANTAGES
Glass Thermometer	
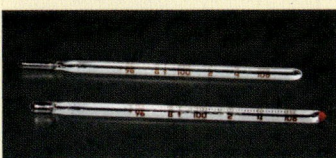	➕ Do not use glass thermometers containing mercury. If you find one, recommend that it be replaced immediately. Avoid using glass thermometers when possible; some patients do still use them at home.
▪ Flexibility of use: Can be used for measuring oral, rectal, or axillary temperature. ▪ Inexpensive initial cost ▪ Accuracy, as indicated by several studies ▪ Easily disinfected	▪ Easily broken, so there is ongoing cost of replacement and risk for injury ▪ Slow: It takes 3–8 min to obtain an accurate reading, depending on the site. ▪ Difficult for some people to read accurately
Electronic Thermometer	
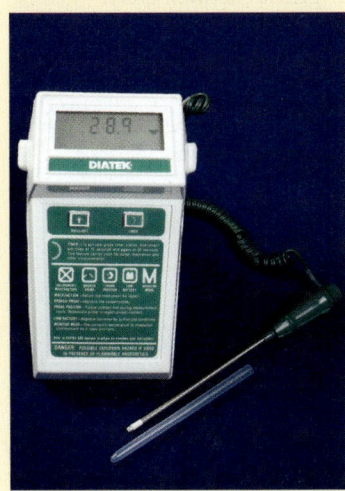	▪ Expensive initial cost ▪ Requires regular inspection and maintenance to ensure accuracy. ▪ Data are conflicting regarding their accuracy compared to other types of thermometer. ▪ Need to be kept charged.
▪ Flexibility of use: Can be used for measuring oral, rectal, or axillary temperature. ▪ Ease of use ▪ Rapid measurement: It takes 2–60 sec to obtain reading, depending on the unit.	

(continued)

Table 20-2 ➤ Advantages and Disadvantages of Various Thermometers—cont'd

ADVANTAGES	DISADVANTAGES
Electronic With Infrared Sensor	

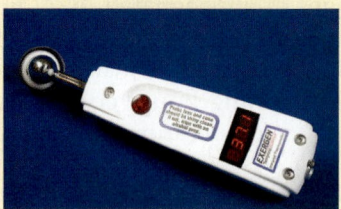

A, Temporal scanner

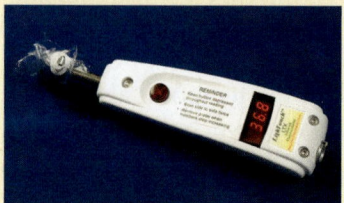

B, Otic thermometer

ADVANTAGES	DISADVANTAGES
■ Ease of use	■ Expensive initial cost.
■ Rapid measurement: It takes 2–5 sec to measure the temperature.	■ Less accurate than electronic or glass/plastic thermometers when used for tympanic membrane temperatures, as some studies indicate.
■ May be the most cost-effective method because of time and labor savings from their rapid reading capabilities.	■ Requires regular inspection and maintenance to ensure accuracy.
■ Low rate of operator error	■ Batteries require recharging.

| **Disposable Chemical Thermometer** | |

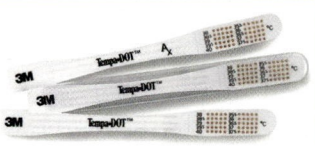

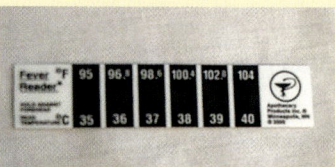

ADVANTAGES	DISADVANTAGES
■ Ease of use; requires no special training.	■ Less reliable than glass or plastic thermometers.
■ Equally as accurate as the electronic thermometer.	■ The skin must be dry.
■ Less expensive than purchasing supplies for and maintaining an electronic thermometer.	■ Indicates only body surface temperature; does not reflect core.
■ Because it is disposable, it may prevent spread of infection among patients.	■ Guidelines presently recommend only for pediatric patients.
■ Recommended for measuring axillary temperature among pediatric patients over the age of 2 years (Cincinnati Children's Hospital Medical Center, 2011).	

applied to the skin of the forehead or abdomen and left for a time specified by the manufacturer (e.g., 15 seconds). Recent guidelines conclude that measurements done on children are as accurate as those done with electronic thermometers (Cincinnati Children's Hospital Medical Center, 2011). However, there is conflicting research regarding the accuracy of the temperature readings with disposal chemical thermometers (Barnason, Williams, & Proehl, 2012; Farnell, Maxwell, Tan, et al., 2005; Washington & Matney, 2008). Disposable thermometers are useful in the home and for patients in protective isolation.

Other Types of Thermometers For special uses, devices have been created to take measurements from the nasopharynx, the pulmonary artery, the bladder, and the skin. A wireless intestinal temperature monitoring system in the form of a pill and an external receiver is sometimes used, for example, during cardiac surgery. Infrared devices have also been used to take thermal measurements of skin surface temperature.

What Sites Should I Use?

Temperatures in the pulmonary artery, esophagus, and bladder accurately measure core temperature. These sites are used in surgery and intensive care, but they are invasive, expensive, and impractical for most clinical settings. Pulmonary artery temperature is considered the "gold standard" to which other sites are compared. A device is placed in the pulmonary artery, and readings are continuously displayed on a monitor.

The usual sites for intermittent measurements are the mouth, rectum, axillae, tympanic membrane, and skin over the temporal artery. These sites allow the thermometer to contact body tissues that are well supplied with blood vessels. This is essential for accurate measurement. Each site has advantages and disadvantages, so you must choose the safest, most accurate, and most reliable site for each client (Table 20-3).

Temperature readings vary depending on the site used. Be aware that research on site differences is conflicting, for example:

- Temporal artery temperature is usually about the same as rectal temperature (Hebbar, Fortenberry, Rogers, et al., 2005).
- Some researchers report tympanic membrane temperatures to be higher than oral measurements (Fadzil, Choon, & Arumugam, 2010); however, others have found them to be similar.

From lowest to highest readings, the sites are generally thought to be as follows: axillary, oral, tympanic membrane, rectal, and temporal artery. For oral, axillary, and rectal temperatures, there is an approximately 0.8°F or 0.4°C difference between each site and the next higher one. For convenience, nurses tend to round the fraction up to a full 1°F (0.5°C). For example, an axillary temperature of 98.1°F is similar to an oral reading of 99.1°F or a rectal reading of 100.1°F. Use this *only* to help you understand your patient's data. You cannot reliably convert temperatures mathematically between sites. When you measure a temperature, record the value you obtain and the site used.

ThinkLike a Nurse 20-2

- Convert the following temperatures and analyze the readings. What might they mean?
  - a. 38.5°C _____ °F
  - b. 96.5°F _____ °C
  - c. 37.0°C _____ °F
- Rank the expected early evening temperatures of the following individuals from lowest to highest.
  - a. A 22-year-old college athlete
  - b. A 5-year-old kindergarten student
  - c. An 88-year-old nursing home resident

ANALYSIS/NURSING DIAGNOSIS

Fever and hypothermia may be medical diagnoses, nursing diagnoses, or symptoms of other problems. The following nursing diagnoses may be used when they describe a *client problem* and not just a symptom of an illness or other problem (e.g., fever may be a symptom of problems such as Deficient Fluid Volume, or dehydration). Notice that the nursing diagnosis of Hyperthermia can be used both for temperature elevation from fever (hyperpyrexia) and from heat exhaustion (hyperthermia).

- *Hyperthermia* is diagnosed when a person's body temperature is above normal. Defining characteristics are convulsions, flushed skin, tachycardia, tachypnea, and warmth to touch.

- *Hypothermia* is diagnosed when a person's body temperature is below normal range. Defining characteristics include cool skin, cyanotic nailbeds, elevated blood pressure, pallor, piloerection, shivering, slow capillary refill, and tachycardia.
- *Ineffective Thermoregulation* applies when a person's temperature fluctuates above and below the normal range.
- *Risk for Imbalanced Body Temperature* is used when the temperature is normal but the client is at risk for failure to maintain body temperature within the normal range (e.g., newborns and the frail elderly). As you can see, this diagnosis can also apply to risk for either hypothermia or fever.

PLANNING OUTCOMES/EVALUATION

Associated NOC standardized outcomes for NANDA-I diagnoses pertaining to body temperature include the following: Thermoregulation, Thermoregulation: Newborn, and Vital Signs. For other NOC outcomes you might use for alterations in temperature regulation,

Go to Chapter Resources: Chapter 20, **Standardized Language,** on Davis*Plus*.

Individualized goals/outcome statements you might write for a client with Hyperthermia include the following:

- Oral temperature of less than 97.6°F (less than 36.4°C) (client's usual normal temperature)
- No clinical signs of fever present (e.g., no chills or flushing)
- Pulse and respiratory rates within normal range for patient

For a client with Hypothermia, the following are examples of goal statements:

- Oral temperature greater than 97.6°F (greater than 36.4°C) (client's usual normal temperature)
- No clinical signs of Hypothermia present (e.g., no disorientation, no decrease in urine output)
- Pulse and respiratory rates within normal range

Use the goals set in the planning outcomes stage to evaluate client responses to interventions.

PLANNING INTERVENTIONS/IMPLEMENTATION

Overall care of the patient depends on the cause of the fever or hypothermia, and on specific orders from the primary provider. Nevertheless, there are nursing interventions and activities that address fever and hypothermia, regardless of the cause.

Interventions for Example Problem: Hyperthermia

NIC standardized interventions for Hyperthermia and Ineffective Thermoregulation include Fever Treatment, Malignant Hyperthermia Precautions, Newborn Care,

Table 20-3 ➤ **Disadvantages and Contraindications of Various Sites for Measuring Temperature**

ADVANTAGES	DISADVANTAGES	CONTRAINDICATIONS
Temporal Artery		
■ Most accurate representation of core temperature. ■ Fast. Most scanners provide a reading in about 3 sec. ■ No discomfort is associated with the procedure. ■ Safe. Can be used even for those who cannot follow instructions (e.g., infants). ■ Less prone to error than tympanic thermometer.	■ Requires special scanning thermometer. ■ Any covering, hat, hair, etc., prevents heat from dissipating and causes the reading to be falsely high. This is also true for the side of the head lying on a pillow.	
Rectal		
■ Accurately represents core (internal) body temperature. ■ Use for clients who are unable to follow directions for oral temperature monitoring, or in situations where accuracy is crucial.	■ Most clients find this method objectionable or embarrassing. ■ ✚ Not recommended as the first choice of site because of the risk for injury to the rectal mucosa, especially infants. ■ Requires special positioning of the client. ■ Does not reflect changes in core temperature as rapidly as the oral method. ■ Presence of stool may cause inaccurate reading.	■ ✚ Clients who may be injured by this method (e.g., clients who have a rectal disease, severe diarrhea, or rectal surgery; newborns, whose rectal mucosa is fragile). ■ Because it can slow the heart rate by stimulating the vagus nerve, this method is sometimes contraindicated for clients with cardiac surgery and some heart conditions. ■ Clients with hemorrhoids. ■ Immunosuppressed clients or those with clotting disorders.
Oral		
■ Simple, convenient. ■ Comfortable for most patients. ■ Safe for adults and children who are old enough to follow simple directions	■ ✚ Glass thermometers can break if bitten. ■ Slow; requires up to 8 min to ensure an accurate reading (if glass or plastic thermometer used). ■ Patient must keep her mouth closed for several minutes (glass or plastic thermometers). ■ Eating, drinking (e.g., ice water, hot tea), and smoking in the 30 minutes before measurement affect the accuracy of the reading. ■ Bradypnea may create false temperature elevations.	■ ✚ Clients who cannot cooperate with the instructions or who might be injured (e.g., infants and small children; patients who have had oral surgery, breathe through the mouth, have chills, or are confused or unconscious). When possible, avoid using a glass thermometer for all patients.
Axillary		
■ Safe ■ Easy to use ■ Can be used for children and for uncooperative or unconscious clients.	■ Not reflective of core temperature ■ Considered one of the least accurate sites. ■ Diaphoresis (sweating) can affect the reading.	■ Clients who are perspiring heavily ■ Does not accurately diagnose fever. If fever is suspected, confirm with measurement from another route.

Table 20-3 ➤ Disadvantages and Contraindications of Various Sites for Measuring Temperature—cont'd

ADVANTAGES	DISADVANTAGES	CONTRAINDICATIONS
■ Recommended over rectal site for routine measurements.	■ Thermometer may need to be left in place for a long time (8 minutes if glass or plastic is used).	
Tympanic Membrane		
■ Fast (2–5 sec). ■ Can be used for children and for uncooperative or unconscious clients.	■ Requires a special thermometer, a relatively expensive initial purchase. ■ More variable than oral and rectal sites. ■ Must be carefully positioned to ensure accuracy; prone to caregiver measurement errors. ■ Presence of cerumen (earwax) may affect accuracy. ■ Significant differences have been found between readings in left and right ear of same patient. ■ Risk of injury to tympanic membrane if not positioned carefully to avoid touching it. ■ May be uncomfortable for the client. ■ Chemical thermometers (skin temperatures) have been found to be more accurate and reliable than tympanic membrane instruments. ■ Hearing aids must be removed.	■ ✚ Clients who have had recent ear surgery. ■ Contraindicated in the presence of ear infection.
Skin (e.g., forehead)		
■ Safe, convenient. ■ Easy to use for nonprofessionals. ■ Can be used when other sites are contraindicated. ■ Inexpensive (chemical paper or tape is used).	■ Forehead skin temperature is generally 2–4°F (1–2°C) less than core temperature; if marked deviations in skin temperatures are detected, the readings must be confirmed via a more reliable route.	■ Should not be used when accurate, reliable readings are required (e.g., in the presence of hypothermia or heatstroke). ■ However, at least one study has shown skin temperatures to be accurate and reliable when obtained with an infrared skin thermometer (DeCurtis, Calzolari, Marciano, et al., 2008).

Temperature Regulation, Temperature Regulation: Intraoperative, and Vital Signs Monitoring. For other NIC labels you might use,

 Go to Chapter Resources: Chapter 20, **Standardized Language, NOC Outcomes and NIC Interventions Associated With Abnormal Vital Signs,** on Davis*Plus.*

Specific nursing activities for clients with fever and/or nursing diagnoses of Hyperthermia or Ineffective Thermoregulation include the following:

Provide Focused Assessments such as the following:

■ *Help determine the cause of the fever.* For example, you may collect specimens from various body sites for culture.

■ *Monitor the temperature and other VS at least every 2 hours,* and more often if the temperature is rising rapidly or if the clinical symptoms are changing. Recall that the increased metabolism accompanying a fever also increases the pulse and respirations. When you suspect fever, it is wise to verify the reading obtained from the infrared tympanic thermometer or disposable thermometer by taking a rectal reading with a different type of thermometer for comparison. Obtain an oral reading if the rectal site is contraindicated.

■ *Observe for the clinical signs that accompany a fever.* Symptoms vary, depending on the phase of the fever. The characteristic symptoms include flushed face; dry, hot skin; eyes that appear bright and somewhat apprehensive; rapid, shallow respirations; increased heart rate; unusual thirst; loss of appetite; headache; and complaints of nausea. If the fever is extreme, urine may be concentrated and decreased in volume. Seizures, confusion, or delirium can also be associated with very high fevers.

Provide Collaborative Care to Treat the Underlying Cause of the Fever

For example, you may administer antibiotics that a provider prescribes to treat a bacterial infection.

Use Nonpharmacological Measures to Reduce Fever

- Some measures are likely to produce shivering, which produces heat; therefore, they can actually raise instead of lower the patient's temperature. When using the following interventions, be careful not to cause your patient to shiver.
  Cooling blankets that circulate water
  Cloth-covered ice packs or cool washcloths to the groin, neck, or axillae
  Circulating fan in the room
  Instruct the client to use minimal bed covers
  Alcohol or tepid baths

   Although alcohol baths may be effective to reduce temperature, the topical application of large amounts of isopropyl alcohol can cause alcohol poisoning and toxicity in children and older adults (Smitherman, Janise, & Mathur, 2005; Thompson & Kagan, 2011).

- **Provide emergency treatment, if necessary.** Heat stroke is a medical emergency because death can occur rapidly. Cooling blankets or cool water baths can be used successfully if the surface temperature is not lowered too quickly. Rapid lowering of the surface temperature causes vasoconstriction, which delays core cooling.

Provide Supportive Measures for Associated Symptoms

- **Provide oral or intravenous fluids.** This replaces fluids lost through diaphoresis. They help prevent dehydration or hypovolemia (fluid deficiency) secondary to the fever.
- **Provide nutritional support.** Food is essential to meet the increased energy needs created by the high metabolic rate accompanying fever. However, lack of appetite often accompanies fever, so food must be made appealing to the patient.
  - **Provide special mouth care.** Apply a water-soluble lip lubricant. Lips may become dry and **cracked, the tongue may be s**wollen, and sores may be present.
- **Keep clothing and bed linens dry.** This promotes comfort and helps prevent chilling. Recall that diaphoresis occurs during defervescence.

Provide teaching for self-care such as the following.
- **Teach emergency treatment for hyperthermia and hyperpyrexia at home.** Immediately move the person to a shady area if he is outdoors. Cool the victim by placing him in a tub of cool water or a cool shower, or sponging with cool water.

  - **Advise older adults to stay in air-conditioned buildings** when the outside temperature is extremely high; to take cool baths and showers; to limit physical activity; and to drink plenty of nonalcoholic and noncaffeinated fluids.
- **Advise family to check on elderly neighbors and family members** at least twice a day, and make sure they have an electric fan.

Interventions for Example Problem: Hypothermia

NIC standardized interventions recommended for Hypothermia and Ineffective Thermoregulation include Hypothermia Treatment, Newborn Care, Temperature Regulation, Temperature Regulation: Intraoperative, and Vital Signs Monitoring. For other NIC labels,

Go to Chapter Resources: Chapter 20, **Standardized Language, NOC Outcomes and NIC Interventions Associated With Abnormal Vital Signs,** on *DavisPlus*.

Specific nursing activities include the following:

Provide Focused Assessments for Hypothermic Patients

- Monitor the temperature and other VS frequently. Hypothermia causes vasoconstriction, coagulation in the microcirculation, and tissue ischemia (lack of oxygen). In the heart, this can lead to dysrhythmias.
- Observe for the following symptoms of hypothermia:
  Body temperature less than 95°F (less than 35°C)
  Decreased or irregular pulse, respirations, and blood pressure
  A subjective feeling of being cold
  Severe shivering (only initially)
  Pale, cool, shiny skin
  Decreased urine output
  Disorientation and/or drowsiness

Institute Warming Measures

- Provide warm, dry clothing, warm drinks, warm blankets, and a warm environment. For mild cases of Hypothermia, this may be enough to restore normal temperature.
- For patients with a temperature below 86°F (30°C), also use warmed intravenous fluids, heating pads or heating blankets, and/or warm baths.
- Give warm, sweet drinks if the person is conscious. Avoid alcoholic and caffeinated drinks.

■ ✚ Rewarm a patient who is severely hypothermic gradually to prevent complications, such as shock or dysrhythmias (abnormal heartbeats) and to ensure core, as well as surface, warming.

Don't use electric blankets. Vasoconstricted skin burns easily.

Don't apply pulse oximetry probes to a vasoconstricted finger.

🍁 ### Teach Older Adults Ways to Prevent Hypothermia

Examples include the following tips (National Institutes for Health, n.d., last reviewed 2014):

■ Keep your home warm enough, at least 68 to 70 degrees. Even mildly cool indoor temperatures of 60 to 65 degrees can lead to hypothermia in older adults.
■ Wear socks and slippers, long underwear under your clothes. Wear a hat or cap indoors.
■ Cover your legs and shoulders with a blanket or afghan to keep warm.

Wear a hat, scarf, and gloves or mittens when going outdoors in the cold. This helps prevent loss heat through your head and hands. A large portion of body heat can be lost through the head, so the cap is important. Dress in several layers of warm loose clothing. This traps warm air between the layers and keeps body head in.

🌈 ## ThinkLike a Nurse 20-3

Recall the clients in the Meet Your Patients scenario. Two-year-old Jason's axillary temperature was 101.8°F (38.8°C) and his skin was warm, dry, and flushed. His mother told you that he had been eating poorly and was very irritable.

■ What changes in behavior alert you that something is wrong?
■ Do you have enough theoretical knowledge or patient information to know what is going on?
■ What, if any, additional information about the patient situation do you need?

Toward Evidence-Based Practice

Paes, B., Vermeulen, K., Brohet, R., et al. (2010). Accuracy of tympanic and infrared skin thermometer in children. *Archives of Disease in Childhood*, 95(12), 974–978.

Researchers evaluated the accuracy of the tympanic and infrared skin thermometer as alternatives to rectal temperature readings. In 100 hospitalized pediatric patients, the tympanic thermometer was less accurate than the rectal thermometer, but more accurate than the infrared skin thermometer.

Frommelt, T., Ott, C., & Hays, V. (2008). Accuracy of different devices to measure temperature. *MedSurg Nursing*, 17(3), 171–182.

Using 86 postoperative adult patients, researchers measured oral, tympanic, and temporal artery temperature using different devices. The researchers found significant differences from the referenced oral thermometer and the oral disposable, tympanic, and temporal artery thermometers. The tympanic thermometry had the greatest variation (least accurate) from the oral thermometry.

Lawson, L., Bridges, E. J., Ballou, I., et al. (2007). Accuracy and precision of noninvasive temperature measurement in adult intensive care patients. *American Journal of Critical Care*, 16(5), 485–496.

Over a period of 6 months, researchers took repeated measurements at various sites, including the gold standard pulmonary artery catheter, from 60 adults with cardiopulmonary disease in intensive care. They found oral and temporal artery measurements to be the most

accurate and precise. Axillary measurements were less accurate, and ear measurements were the least accurate and precise.

Heusch, A. I., & McCarthy, P. W. (2005). The patient: A novel source of error in clinical temperature measurement using infrared aural thermometry. *Journal of Alternative & Complementary Medicine*, 11(3), 473–476.

Researchers used an infrared tympanic thermometer to measure the temperatures of 132 subjects, ages 18 to 48 years, who were asymptomatic with no known pathological problems. Temperatures were measured in both ears. There was a significant difference in the temperature in the left compared with the right ear. Also, at temperatures below 36.7°C, the left ear registered a lower temperature than the right. At temperatures above 36.7°C, the left ear registered a higher temperature than the right ear. Researchers suggested that averaging the temperature in both ears might increase the reliability of infrared tympanic thermometers.

Farnell, S., Maxwell, L., Tan, S., et al. (2005). Temperature measurement: Comparison of non-invasive methods used in adult critical care. *Journal of Clinical Nursing*, 14(5), 632–639.

Researchers took 160 sets of temperature measurements from 25 adult intensive care patients, using a chemical (Tempa·DOT) and a tympanic thermometer. Patients' temperatures were also being measuring with the gold standard pulmonary artery catheter. They found the chemical thermometer to be more accurate and reliable

(continued)

CarePlanning & MappingPractice

For Care Planning/Care Mapping practice,

 Go to Chapter Resources, **Care Planning & Care Mapping Practice,** on Davis*Plus*.

PULSE

The concept of **perfusion** refers to the continuous supply of oxygenated blood through the blood vessels to the vital organs. The **pulse** is the rhythmic expansion of an artery produced when a bolus of oxygenated blood is forced into it by contraction of the heart. How do you think the pulse affects perfusion; how might perfusion affect the pulse?

TheoreticalKnowledge
knowing **why**

To assess and support regulation of a client's pulse, you will need to understand the concept of perfusion, know the normal pulse range, how the pulse is produced and regulated, and factors that influence pulse rate. An important reason to assess the pulse is to identify when more advanced monitoring is required.

What Is a Normal Pulse Rate?

Pulse rate is measured in beats per minute. The normal range for healthy young and middle-aged adults is 60 to 100 beats/min, with an average rate of 70 to 80 beats/min. Table 20-1 identifies average pulse rates for adults. For average pulse rates for other age groups,

 Go to Chapter 20, **Tables, Boxes, Figures: ESG Table 20-1,** on Davis*Plus*.

When the heart rate is of concern, you will most likely use a cardiac monitor to determine not only the rate, but also the rhythm and intensity of the pulse.

How Does the Body Produce and Regulate the Pulse?

The pulse wave begins when the left heart ventricle contracts and ends when it relaxes. Each contraction forces blood into the already filled aorta, increasing pressure within the arterial system. The intermittent pressure and expansion of the arteries causes the blood to move along in a wavelike motion toward the capillaries. You can palpate a light tap at the peak of the wave, when the artery expands. The trough (low point) of a pulse wave occurs when the artery contracts to push the blood along its way. The peak of the wave corresponds to **systole**, or the contraction of the heart; the trough corresponds to **diastole**, or the resting phase of the heart.

Stroke volume is the quantity of blood forced out by each contraction of the left ventricle. You will not usually know your patient's actual stroke volume, though it averages 70 mL in most healthy adults. If stroke volume decreases (as in a large blood loss, or *hemorrhage*), the body tries to maintain the same cardiac output by increasing the pulse rate. The **cardiac output** is the total quantity of blood pumped per minute. It is expressed in liters per minute and calculated as follows:

Cardiac output = stroke volume × pulse (heart) rate

For a person with a pulse of 80 beats/min and an average stroke volume (70 mL), the cardiac output would be about 5,600 mL (or 5.6 liters) per minute.

The autonomic nervous system regulates the heart rate. Sympathetic stimulation increases the heart rate (and thus the cardiac output); parasympathetic stimulation decreases it. We discuss this in more detail in Chapter 37.

What Factors Influence the Pulse Rate?

In a healthy adult, the peripheral pulse rate is the same as the heart rate. Therefore, taking the pulse is a quick and simple way to assess the condition of the heart, blood vessels, and circulation. The pulse changes in response to changes in the volume of blood pumped through the heart, variations in heart rate, changes in the elasticity of the arterial walls, or any condition that interferes with heart function. Because the heart and blood vessels are regulated by the nervous system, conditions that interfere with normal functioning of the nervous system also affect the pulse. Other factors that may cause variations in pulse rate, rhythm, or quality include the following:

- *Developmental level.* Newborns have a rapid pulse rate. The rate stabilizes in childhood and gradually slows through old age. Although resting heart rate increases with age, variability decreases (Chester & Rudolph, 2011). Thus, you should not rely solely on changes in the pulse rate of older adults to detect their response to external stressors.

- *Gender.* Adult women have a slightly more rapid pulse rate than do adult men.

- *Exercise.* Muscle activity normally increases the pulse rate. After exercise, a well-conditioned heart returns to normal more quickly than does a nonconditioned heart. Also, people who are well conditioned have lower heart rates, both before and during exercise, than do those who are not.

- *Food.* Ingestion of food causes a slight increase in pulse rate for several hours.

- *Stress.* Stress triggers the fight-or-flight sympathetic nervous system response, which increases both pulse rate and strength of the heart contractions (stroke volume).

- *Fever.* The pulse rate tends to increase about 10 beats/ min for each degree Fahrenheit of temperature elevation. The reasons are that (1) the metabolic rate increases and (2) the body attempts to compensate for the decrease in blood pressure produced by the peripheral vasodilation that occurs with fever.

- *Disease.* Diseases, such as heart disease, hyperthyroidism, respiratory diseases, and infections, are generally associated with increased pulse rates. Hypothyroidism is associated with decreased pulse rates.

- *Blood loss.* Small blood loss is generally well tolerated and produces only a temporary increase in pulse rate. Theoretically, a large blood loss stimulates the sympathetic nervous system, bringing about an increase in pulse rate to compensate for the decreased blood volume. However, some studies suggest that VS are limited in their ability to detect large blood losses and that a stable pulse and blood pressure alone do not ensure that there has been no blood loss. Research to detect early blood loss using sensors and smartphone technologies is being conducted (Worcester Polytechnic Institute, 2012).

- *Position changes.* Standing and sitting positions generally cause a temporary increase in pulse rate and decrease in blood pressure as a result of blood pooling in the veins of the feet and legs. This decreases blood return to the heart, decreasing blood pressure and subsequently increasing heart rate.

- *Medications.* Stimulant drugs (e.g., epinephrine) increase pulse rate. Cardiotonics (e.g., digitalis) and opioids (e.g., narcotic analgesics) or sedative drugs decrease pulse rate.

Practical Knowledge
knowing **how**

Now that you understand some of the concepts and factors that produce and affect the pulse, you are ready to learn the practical knowledge of how to assess and support this aspect of physical functioning.

■ ASSESSMENT

Assess the pulse by **palpation** (feeling) or **auscultation** (listening with a stethoscope). To palpate the pulse, select the pulse site and lightly compress the client's artery against the underlying bone with the index and middle finger of one of your hands. When a client's pulse is difficult to palpate, you may need to use a Doppler device, which has an ultrasound transducer that transmits the pulse sounds to an audio unit. For a summary of the steps for assessing a client's peripheral pulse, see the Highlights of Procedures box. For the full procedure,

 Go to **Procedure 20-2: Assessing Peripheral Pulses, in** Volume 2.

What Equipment Do I Need?

To count the pulse, you need a watch or clock with a second hand or digital display. To auscultate the pulse, you will use a stethoscope. The stethoscope does not magnify sounds, but rather blocks out noise so that you can hear blood pressure and other faint sounds. A **stethoscope** consists of a sound-transmitting device (bell and diaphragm) that is attached to earpieces by rubber tubing and hollow metal tubes (Fig. 20-4). With the earpieces in place, you can use the bell to hear low-frequency sounds (e.g., certain heart sounds). Use the diaphragm to assess high-frequency sounds (e.g., lung sounds).

Stethoscopes can be either single lumen or double lumen. A single-lumen stethoscope has one tube connected to the chestpiece; a double-lumen stethoscope has two tubes attached to the chestpiece. Double-lumen stethoscopes are more sensitive than single-lumen instruments.

Most stethoscopes come with soft earpieces that help seal your ear canal to block room noise from interfering with the sound. Stethoscopes have varying lengths of tubing. Short tubing requires you to be close to the patient and to bend more, but the sound may be a bit better than with longer tubing, which is more likely to rub against the body or clothing. Some stethoscopes are made to work effectively through clothing; however, unless you know you are using that type you should place the instrument directly on the skin. Digital stethoscopes are also available, to provide sound clarity in noisy environments, with obese patients, and for care providers who have impaired hearing.

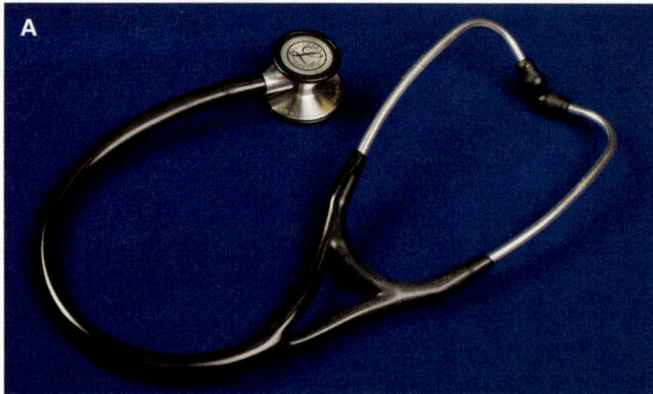

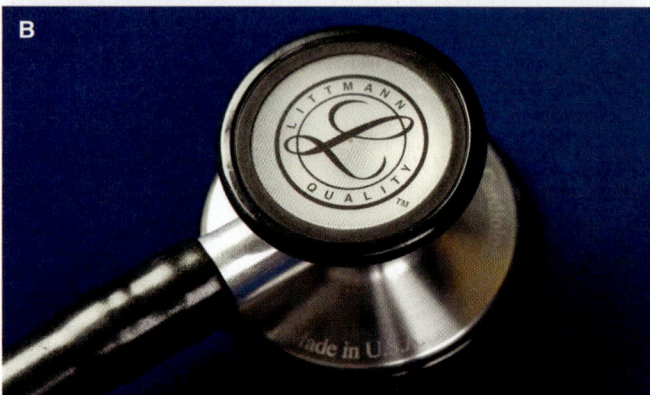

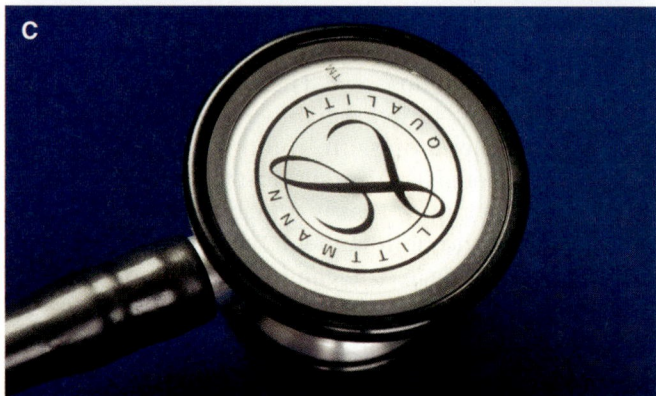

FIGURE 20-4 *A,* A stethoscope. *B,* The bell, for low-frequency sounds. *C,* The diaphragm, for high-frequency sounds.

✚ To prevent cross-contamination, always clean your stethoscope before and after using it to examine a patient. Use a 70% alcohol or benzalkonium chloride wipe. Bacteria colonize on most stethoscopes, although only a small percentage are pathogenic. Cleaning can reduce the bacterial count by 94% to 100% (CDC, 2008; Kennedy, Dreimanis, Beckingham, et al., 2003; Rutala & Weber, 2004). Researchers found that the mean skin flora colony forming on stethoscopes decreased from 27 prior to cleaning to 1 after cleaning (Mitchell, DeAlwis, Collins, et al., 2010). Similarly subjects in the precleaning group had bacterial growth on their stethoscopes compared with no bacterial growth in the postcleaning group (Russell, Secrest, & Schreeder, 2012). Antimicrobial stethoscope covers have been developed to prevent

surface contamination; however, research has associated them with higher colony counts (Wood, Lund, & Stevenson, 2007). A few agencies have wall-mounted "single-swipe" sterilizers for sterilizing stethoscopes.

To prevent injury, do not wear a stethoscope around your neck.

What Sites Should I Use?

Nurses assess the pulse at the apex of the heart **(apical pulse)** or at a place where an artery can be pressed by the fingers against a bone **(peripheral pulses).** Peripheral sites are shown in Figure 20-5.

The choice of pulse site depends on the reason for assessing the pulse and/or the accessibility of a site. To measure a peripheral pulse, you would, for example, use the:

- *Radial artery* for routine assessment of vital signs. This is the most commonly used site because it is easily found and readily accessible.
- *Brachial artery* when performing cardiopulmonary resuscitation of infants.
- *Carotid artery* when performing CPR of inpatient adults and for assessing circulation to the brain.

✚ Palpate only one side of the neck at a time to avoid interrupting circulation to the head. Palpate lightly so that you don't occlude the artery; and don't massage the area because that can decrease the heart rate and blood pressure. Lay persons should not check the carotid pulse.

- *Temporal artery*—when assessing circulation to the head or when other sites are not easily accessible.
- *Dorsalis pedis* (also called *pedal pulse*) and *posterior tibial arteries* for assessing peripheral circulation.
- *Femoral artery* to determine circulation to the legs, in cases of cardiac arrest, and for children.
- *Popliteal artery* for assessing circulation to the lower leg.

🔺 Think**Like a Nurse** 20-4

- If you obtain a very slow radial pulse, how might you check to be sure your count is accurate?
- What kind of nursing knowledge does this require (i.e., theoretical, practical, self, or ethical knowledge)?

When Should I Take an Apical Pulse?

The apical pulse reading is the most accurate of the pulses. In a healthy person, the apical and peripheral pulses should be about the same. However, in some cardiovascular diseases, they can differ. If the heartbeat is weak, for example, some beats may be too weak to feel in a peripheral site. In this case, you would obtain a lower count for the radial than for the apical pulse. The apical pulse would accurately reflect the heartbeat. Use the apical site when:

- The radial pulse is weak or irregular.
- The rate is less than 60 beats/min or greater than 100 beats/min.

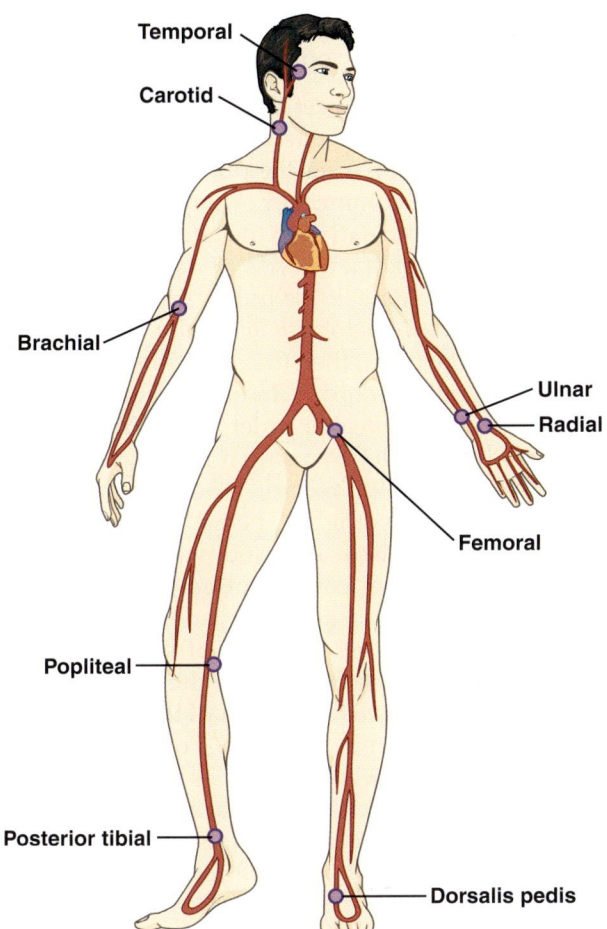

FIGURE 20-5 Sites commonly used for assessing a pulse.

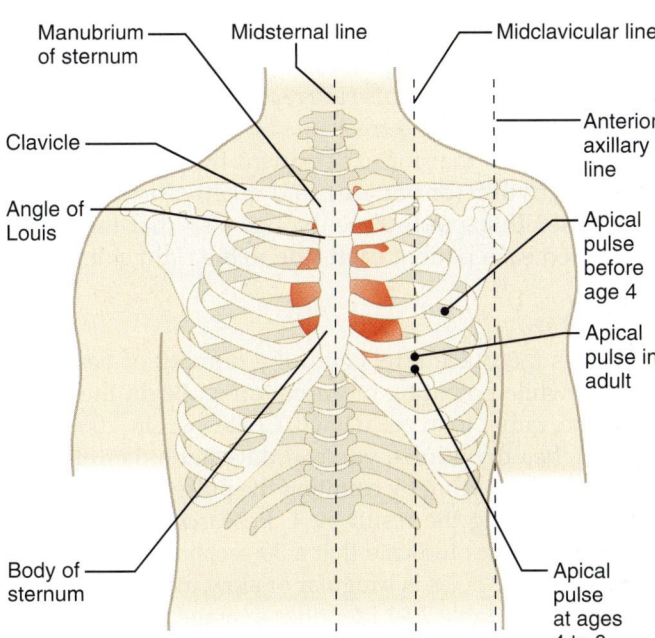

FIGURE 20-6 Location of apical pulse for adults and children.

You may detect a pulse deficit in conditions that interfere with peripheral perfusion, such as atrial fibrillation. You should report pulse deficits promptly to the primary care provider. See the Highlights of Procedures box for a summary, and

 Go to **Procedure 20-4: Assessing for an Apical-Radial Pulse Deficit,** in Volume 2.

KnowledgeCheck 20-2

For each of the following, would you expect the pulse rate to be greater or less than the normal adult rate of 80 beats/min?

- A healthy professional tennis player
- A newborn infant
- An adolescent who has just finished running track
- A client who has just undergone a painful procedure
- A client with a fever
- An accident victim who is hemorrhaging
- A 90-year-old man

What Data Should I Collect?

A nurse has documented the following data for five patients:

Patient A: Radial pulse 80 beats/min, strong, regular, and equal bilaterally (the same in both arms)

Patient B: Pedal pulse 96 beats/min, regular, moderate volume, but stronger in the left ankle than the right

Patient C: Brachial pulse 86 beats/min in both arms, slightly irregular; skips about every fifth beat; weak but stronger in left arm

Patient D: Apical pulse 60 beats/min, slightly irregular; heart sounds clearly auscultated

Patient E: Radial pulse 92 beats/min, irregular—beats in triplets—weak, equal bilaterally

- The patient is taking cardiac medications (e.g., digitalis).
- The patient is an infant or a child up to age 3 (because peripheral pulses may be difficult to palpate).

To assess the apical pulse, auscultate and count the number of heartbeats at the apex of the heart. For an adult, this site is on the anterior chest at 3 inches (8 cm) or less to the left of the sternum, at the 4th, 5th, or 6th intercostal space at the midclavicular line. For children, the location is different, depending on age (Fig. 20-6). You will hear two sounds, "lub" and "dub," as the heart valves close. Count each pair of sounds ("lub-dub") as one heartbeat. For step-by-step instructions, see the summary in the Highlights of Procedure box and

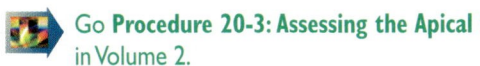 Go **Procedure 20-3: Assessing the Apical Pulse,** in Volume 2.

When Should I Take an Apical-Radial Pulse?

You will sometimes need to obtain a radial and apical pulse reading at the same time to assess for heart function or the presence of heart irregularities. A difference between the two counts **(pulse deficit)** indicates that not all apex beats are being transmitted or felt at the radial artery. As you are listening at the apical site, you will hear a beat without feeling a pulse at the radial artery.

What types of information has the nurse gathered about these patients' pulses? (At least three different characteristics of the pulse are represented in the nurse's charting; look for patterns.)

Did you see that for each patient the nurse recorded the rate, rhythm (or pattern), and quality (or volume) of the pulse? If so, well done. Notice also that the nurse compared each patient's left side to the right side.

Pulse Rate

To assess the pulse **rate**, count the number of beats per minute while palpating or auscultating. Begin the count with one, rather than zero (Hwu, Coates, & Lin, 2000). For normal, healthy adults, you can determine the rate of a regular heart rhythm by counting the pulse for 15 seconds and multiplying the result by 4. Research is conflicting, but some studies indicate that a 30-second count is more accurate. If the pulse is irregular or slow, always count for 1 full minute. Table 20-1 identifies average pulse rates for adults. For average pulse rates for other age groups,

 Go to Chapter 20, Tables, Boxes, Figures: **ESG Table 20-1, Comparison of Normal Vital Signs for Various Ages,** on DavisPlus.

Rates below 60 beats/min are known as **bradycardia** (*brady* = slow, *cardia* = heart). Rates over 100 beats/min are known as **tachycardia** (*tachy* = rapid, *cardia* = heart).

Pulse Rhythm

The intervals between heartbeats establish a pulse pattern known as the **rhythm**. Normally, the heart beats at regular intervals, much like a metronome. When the intervals between beats vary enough to be noticeable, the rhythm is abnormal **(dysrhythmia).** Abnormal rhythms may be single beats that occur too early or too late, or a group of irregular beats that form a pattern. When assessing an irregular pulse, it is important to determine whether the beat is *regularly irregular* (an irregular rhythm that forms a pattern) or *irregularly irregular* (an unpredictable rhythm). To make this distinction, you must count the rate for one full minute. An irregular heart rhythm can be very serious and may require additional assessment by **electrocardiogram (ECG),** a procedure that traces the electrical pattern of the heart.

Pulse Quality

The **quality** of the pulse is assessed by determining the pulse volume and bilateral (both sides) equality of pulses. **Pulse volume** refers to the amount of force produced by the blood pulsing through the arteries. Normally, the pulse volume for each beat is the same. The following terminology refers to the characteristics of the pulse volume; the numbers are assigned on a scale of 0 to 3.

0—Absent: Pulse cannot be felt.
1—Weak or thready: Pulse is barely felt and can be easily obliterated by pressing with the fingers.
2—Normal quality: Pulse is easily palpated, not weak or bounding.

3—Bounding or full: Pulse is easily felt with little pressure; not easily obliterated.

Bilateral equality is useful in determining whether the blood flow to a body part is adequate. Assess bilateral equality by comparing the pulses on both sides of the body for equal volume. For example, if you are concerned about the circulation to the left hand, assess both the right and left radial arteries to determine whether the volume is the same. If the pulses feel the same, they are said to be *equal in strength bilaterally*. If one pulse is stronger than the other, then the pulses are *unequal bilaterally*. You would record, "Radial pulses unequal in strength bilaterally; weaker in left arm." You may also document the equality by using a pulse volume scale. For example, you might record, "Radial pulses unequal in strength bilaterally; Right 2, Left 1."

If a peripheral pulse is absent or weak, it may be because the circulation is compromised in that extremity. If this is the case, then pallor or cyanosis may be present. **Pallor** refers to the paleness of skin in one area when compared to another part of the body. **Cyanosis** is a bluish or grayish discoloration of the skin resulting from deficient oxygen in the blood. For example, when circulation to the lower extremities is compromised, the feet often appear pale in comparison to the trunk or arms, the dorsalis pedis and/or posterior tibial pulses may be weak or absent, and the feet may feel cool to the touch.

ANALYSIS/NURSING DIAGNOSIS

An abnormal pulse may present as weak, thready, bounding, irregular, or absent. Pulse changes are symptoms, not problems. Therefore, nursing diagnoses are useful for describing the condition that is *causing* the pulse changes. By itself, a change in pulse (e.g., weak and thready) is not adequate to support the following diagnoses. Other symptoms must also be present.

- **Ineffective Tissue Perfusion (Peripheral)** can be used when a pulse is absent or weak and cool, pale skin is present.
- **Risk for Impaired Skin Integrity** and **Risk for Impaired Tissue Integrity** may be used as secondary diagnoses when Ineffective Tissue Perfusion is present. If tissue is not adequately perfused, tissue ischemia and *necrosis* (death of tissue) may occur.
- **Deficient Fluid Volume** may cause the pulse to be weak and thready.
- **Excess Fluid Volume** may cause the pulse to be bounding and full.
- **Decreased Cardiac Output** may cause tachycardia, bradycardia, or changes in pulse volume.

PLANNING OUTCOMES/EVALUATION

NOC standardized outcomes include the following:

- Vital Signs Status is the only outcome that directly pertains to assessing the pulse.

- Other outcomes depend on the nursing diagnosis causing the pulse changes. For example, Ineffective Peripheral Tissue Perfusion can be monitored with the NOC label of Circulation Status.

Some *individualized goal/outcome statements* you might write for pulse status follow:

- Apical pulse will be 60 to 80 beats/min when at rest.
- Pedal pulses will be 80 to 100 beats/min, 2 (on a scale of 0 to 3), and equal bilaterally.

 Think**Like a Nurse** 20-5

Did you notice that the pulse rates in the preceding two goals are not the same as the full normal range shown in Table 20-1? What do you think might be a reason for this?

PLANNING INTERVENTIONS/IMPLEMENTATION

NIC standardized interventions include the following:

- Dysrhythmia Management, which applies to monitoring an abnormal pulse.
- Vital Signs Monitoring, which may be used for general evaluation of clients who do not have an identified problem with the pulse,

 Go to Chapter 20, **Standardized Language, NOC Outcomes and NIC Interventions Associated With Abnormal Vital Signs,** on Davis*Plus.*

Specific nursing activities and focused assessments for a patient with a dysrhythmia depend on the cause of the problem and on specific orders from the physician. For example, a client with a pulse rate of 50 beats/min is usually considered to have bradycardia. However, such a slow resting heart rate would be perfectly normal for a well-trained athlete. Some dysrhythmias are *benign*; that is, they are not dangerous to the client, and they require no interventions. Nursing strategies that address dysrhythmias, regardless of cause, include the following:

- *Closely monitor the patient's VS.* A reduced heart rate may alter blood pressure and tissue perfusion. The extent of intervention depends on the effect of the dysrhythmia on the client's other vital signs.
- *Monitor the patient's activity tolerance.* The degree of activity, orientation, and level of fatigue while the dysrhythmia is present are indicators of the patient's ability to tolerate the dysrhythmia.
- *Collect and assess laboratory data as prescribed.* Cardiac function depends on normal electrolyte balance, particularly potassium, calcium, and magnesium levels. If a client is receiving medications that affect cardiac rhythm, serum levels of these medications must be checked periodically.
- *Help determine the cause of the dysrhythmia.* Determine when the client experiences the dysrhythmia. Are there precipitating or alleviating factors?
- *Administer antidysrhythmic medications.* These are prescribed to control the heart rhythm.

- *Provide emotional support.* The client experiencing a dysrhythmia may be frightened by the experience. Explain all procedures to the client and family members, and maintain a calm presence.

 Think**Like a Nurse** 20-6

- Which of the following findings should be referred to the primary healthcare provider so that an electrocardiogram (ECG) can be ordered? Why?
  Patient A, who has a radial pulse of 100 beats/min, regular, and equal bilaterally
  Patient B, who has a regular apical pulse of 100 beats/min
  Patient C, who has a very irregular apical pulse of 78 beats/min
- Recall the clients in the Meet Your Patients scenario. Ms. Sharma is an active 80-year-old woman who works part-time and exercises four times per week. She is complaining of feeling tired. You find that her pulse is irregular and uneven.
  What other patient data do you need to know? How would you go about getting this additional information?
  What actions should you consider taking while meeting with Ms. Sharma?
  What theoretical knowledge (rationale) supports your beliefs and actions?

RESPIRATION

Respiration is the exchange of oxygen and carbon dioxide in the body. The process of respiration consists of two aspects: mechanical and chemical.

- **Mechanical.** The mechanical aspects of respiration involve the active movement of air into and out of the respiratory system. This is known as **pulmonary ventilation** or, more commonly, breathing.
- **Chemical.** The chemical aspects of respiration include the following:
  External respiration—The exchange of oxygen and carbon dioxide between the alveoli and the pulmonary blood supply
  Gas transport—The transport of these gases throughout the body
  Internal respiration—The exchange of these gases between the capillaries and body tissue cells

This chapter focuses on the mechanical aspects of respiration. Chapters 36 and 37 explore gas exchange and transport throughout the body. For an animated visual explanation of respiration,

 Go to Student Resources, **Animations: Cardiovascular/ Pulmonary Animations, Carbon Dioxide/Oxygen Transport,** on Davis*Plus.*

Theoretical Knowledge
knowing **why**

To assess and support clients' respirations, you will need to know the normal range of respiratory rates, how respiration is regulated, the mechanics of breathing, and factors that affect respiration.

What Is a Normal Respiratory Rate?

Respiratory rate normally varies with age, exertion, emotions, and other factors. Normal adult respirations are identified in Table 20-1. For normal respiratory rates at other developmental stages,

 Go to Chapter 20, **Tables, Boxes, Figures: ESG Table 20-1,** on Davis*Plus.*

How Does the Body Regulate Respiration?

Special respiratory centers in the medulla oblongata and pons of the brain, along with nerve fibers of the autonomic nervous system, regulate breathing in response to minute changes in the concentrations of oxygen (O_2) and carbon dioxide (CO_2) in the arterial blood. The primary stimulus for breathing is the level of CO_2 tension in the blood.

- **Central chemoreceptors**, located in the respiratory centers, are sensitive to CO_2 and hydrogen ion (pH) concentrations. Minor increases in either stimulate respirations.
- **Peripheral chemoreceptors** are located in the carotid and aortic bodies. The partial pressure of oxygen in arterial blood (PaO_2) is normally between 80 and 100. When the PaO_2 falls below normal, peripheral chemoreceptors stimulate respirations.

Usually breathing is an involuntary action that requires little effort. However, it is possible to exert conscious control over respiration (e.g., a young child holding his breath during a temper tantrum; a person holding her breath when swimming).

What Are the Mechanics of Breathing?

Pulmonary ventilation depends on changes in the capacity of the chest cavity (Fig. 20-7).

Inspiration In response to impulses sent from the respiratory center along the phrenic nerve, the thoracic muscles and the diaphragm contract. The ribs move upward from midline ½ to 1 inch (1.2 to 2.5 cm), the diaphragm moves downward and out about 0.4 inch (1 cm), and the abdominal organs move downward and forward, expanding the thorax in all directions. As expansion causes airway pressure to decrease below atmospheric pressure, air moves into and expands the lungs. This stage of respiration (drawing air into the lungs) is termed **inspiration**.

Expiration When the diaphragm and thoracic muscles relax, the chest cavity decreases in size, and the lungs recoil, forcing air from the lungs until the pressure within the lungs again reaches atmospheric pressure. This stage, which involves the expulsion of air from the

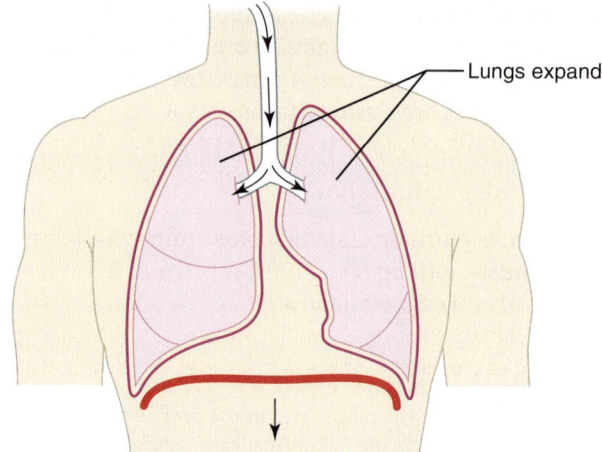

A During inspiration (diaphragm contracting)

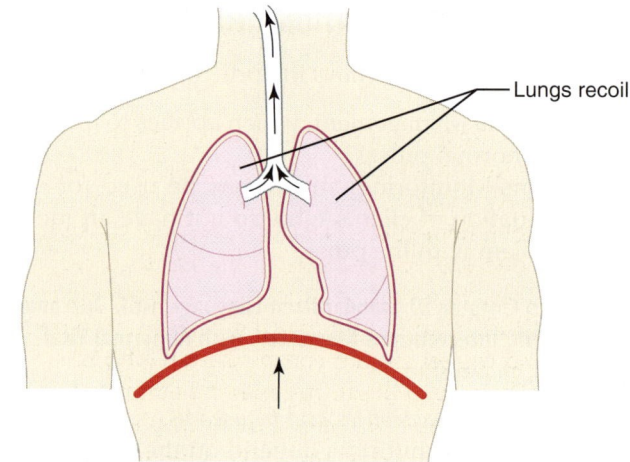

B During expiration (diaphragm relaxing)

FIGURE 20-7 Changes in thoracic cavity during inspiration and expiration. *A,* During inspiration. *B,* During expiration.

lungs, is called **expiration**. Expiration is passive and normally takes 2 to 3 seconds, compared to 1 to 1.5 seconds for inspiration. During normal breathing, the chest wall and abdomen gently rise and fall.

KnowledgeCheck 20-3

- Which two gases are exchanged through respiration?
- Which respiratory process involves the movement of air into and out of the lungs?
- What is external respiration?
- What is the primary stimulus for breathing?
- What mechanical forces allow the lungs to expand?

What Factors Influence Respiration?

To interpret the meaning of your client's respiratory data, you need to be aware of factors that influence breathing.

- *Developmental level.* A newborn's respiratory rate usually ranges from 40 to 60 breaths per minute. However, some references give an upper limit of 90 breaths/min so long as it is for a short period of time (transient tachypnea). The rate gradually decreases until it reaches the normal adult rate of 12 to 20 breaths per minute. The respiratory rate decreases slightly in older adults.

- *Exercise.* Muscular activity causes a temporary increase in respiratory rate and depth so as to increase oxygen availability to the tissues and to rid the body of excess carbon dioxide.
- *Pain.* Acute pain causes an increase in respiratory rate, but a decrease in depth.
- *Stress.* Psychological stress, such as anxiety or fear, may markedly influence respiration as a result of sympathetic stimulation. The most common change is an increase in rate.
- *Smoking.* Chronic smoking increases resting respiratory rate as a result of changes in airway compliance (elasticity).
- *Fever.* When heart rate increases because of fever, respiratory rate also increases. For every 1°F (0.6°C) the temperature rises, the respiratory rate may increase up to 4 breaths/min.
- *Hemoglobin.* Respiratory rate and depth increase as a result of anemia (reduced hemoglobin), sickle cell anemia (abnormally shaped red blood cells), and high altitudes. When hemoglobin is decreased or abnormal, the rate and depth of respirations, as well as the heart rate, may increase to maintain adequate tissue oxygenation. High altitudes inhibit the binding of oxygen to hemoglobin and trigger similar compensation efforts.
- *Disease.* The rate of breathing may be increased or decreased by various diseases. For example, brainstem injuries and increased intracranial pressure may interfere with the respiratory center, inhibiting respirations or altering respiratory rhythm.
- *Medications.* Central nervous system depressants, such as morphine or general anesthetics, cause slower, deeper respirations. Caffeine and atropine can cause shallow, fast breathing.
- *Position.* Standing up maximizes respiratory depth; lying flat reduces respiratory depth. Slumping (sitting with shoulders forward, and the back curved in a C) prevents chest expansion, which impedes breathing.

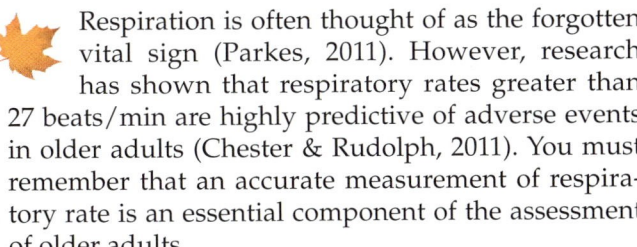 Respiration is often thought of as the forgotten vital sign (Parkes, 2011). However, research has shown that respiratory rates greater than 27 beats/min are highly predictive of adverse events in older adults (Chester & Rudolph, 2011). You must remember that an accurate measurement of respiratory rate is an essential component of the assessment of older adults.

ThinkLike a Nurse 20-7

Consider the following client situations. What effect would each have on respirations?

- A client with four fractured ribs
- A woman who is 9 months pregnant
- A young child excited at her birthday party
- An adult who has consumed alcoholic beverages

PracticalKnowledge
knowing **how**

Although you may assess the adequacy of external and internal respiration in various ways, it is pulmonary ventilation (breathing) that you assess as a vital sign. Accurate assessment of respirations depends on your ability to recognize normal breathing, abnormal breathing, and factors that affect breathing. This chapter discusses only assessment of respirations. For nursing diagnoses, outcomes, and interventions for respiratory problems, see Chapter 36.

ASSESSMENT

Because people can control their breathing rate, it is best to count respirations when the client is unaware of what you are doing. One way to do this is to palpate and count the radial pulse, and then count the respirations before removing your fingers from the client's wrist. For a summary of this procedure, see the Highlights of Procedures box. For the entire sequence of steps,

 Go to **Procedure 20-5: Assessing Respirations,** in Volume 2.

What Equipment Do I Need?

The only equipment you need for measuring respiratory rate is a watch with a second hand or digital display. You will need a stethoscope if you auscultate respirations. Many electronic thermometers have counter displays and signals that indicate 15-, 30-, and 60-second time intervals for counting respirations.

What Data Should I Obtain?

In addition to measuring the respiratory rate, you will also observe indicators of overall respiratory function, including depth, rhythm, effort, and others. For additional information on respiratory assessment, see Chapter 22 and

 Go to Chapter 22, **Procedure 22–12: Assessing the Chest and Lungs,** in Volume 2.

Respiratory Rate

The **respiratory rate** is the number of times a person breathes (or completes a cycle of inhalation and exhalation) within one full minute. You can easily count and observe respirations by:

- Placing your hand on the client's chest (palpation) or observing (inspection) the number of times the client's chest or abdomen rises (inspiration) and falls (expiration)
- Placing your stethoscope on the client's chest (auscultation) and counting the number of inhalation and exhalation cycles

For a new patient or when you need to ensure accuracy, you must count for 60 seconds (Morton & Rempher, 2009; Vital Signs, 1999). In some situations, for example, for a patient you know well and for whom respiratory rate is not directly relevant to the assessment, you may count for only 30 seconds and multiply by 2. If respirations vary from normal ranges, you should count for a full minute by auscultation. Normal adult respiratory rates are identified in Table 20-1.

Respiratory rate is a measure of the client's general condition, but rate alone is not a good indicator of the adequacy of respiration. You must also assess other characteristics of the respirations. If oxygenation must be carefully monitored, use a pulse oximeter (see Chapter 36). A person can tolerate **apnea**, cessation of breathing, for only a few minutes. If apnea continues for more than 4 to 6 minutes, brain damage and even death can occur. See Table 20-4 for terminology to describe respiratory rhythms.

Respiratory Depth

Tidal volume is the amount of air taken in on inspiration—about 300 to 500 mL for a healthy adult. Specialized equipment is required to measure tidal volume. However, you can estimate the adequacy of tidal volume by observing the depth of a client's respirations. This is a subjective evaluation of how much or how little the chest or abdomen rises during breathing. Respiratory depth is described as *deep* (taking in a very large volume of air and fully expanding one's chest or abdomen), *shallow* (when the chest barely rises and is difficult to observe), or *normal* (falling between shallow and deep).

Respiratory Rhythm

Rhythm is assessed simply as *regular* or *irregular*. Generally, the period between each respiratory cycle is the same, and there is a regular breathing pattern (see Eupnea, in Table 20-4). Infant breathing rhythms are more likely to be irregular than adult rhythms. An abnormal breathing pattern may indicate other healthcare problems and deserves further assessment. Two abnormal breathing patterns, Cheyne-Stokes and Biot's breathing, are discussed in Chapter 36.

Respiratory Effort

Respiratory effort refers to the degree of work required to breathe. Normal breathing is effortless. When diseases such as asthma or pneumonia are present, the person must work harder to breathe. Increased effort with breathing is called **dyspnea** or labored breathing. It is uncomfortable for the client and frequently produces fatigue and fear. **Orthopnea** is difficulty or inability to breathe when in a horizontal position. You will observe this in some clients with respiratory or cardiac conditions.

Table 20-4 ➤ Respiratory Rates and Rhythms		
TYPE	**DESCRIPTION**	**ILLUSTRATION**
Eupnea	Normal respirations, with equal rate and depth, 12–20 breaths/min	
Bradypnea	Slow respirations, < 10 breaths/min	
Tachypnea	Fast respirations, > 24 breaths/min, usually shallow	
Kussmaul's Respirations	Respirations that are regular but abnormally deep and increased in rate	
Biot's Respirations	Irregular respirations of variable depth (usually shallow), alternating with periods of apnea (absence of breathing)	
Cheyne-Stokes Respirations	Gradual increase in depth of respirations, followed by gradual decrease and then a period of apnea	
Apnea	Absence of breathing	

Breath Sounds

You will use a stethoscope to listen for breath sounds. Normal respirations are quiet. Abnormal (adventitious) sounds include the following:

- **Wheezes** are high-pitched, continuous musical sounds, usually heard on expiration. Wheezes are caused by narrowing of the airways. Wheezes can often be heard without a stethoscope.
- **Rhonchi** are low-pitched, continuous gurgling sounds caused by secretions in the large airways. They often clear with coughing.
- **Crackles** are caused by fluid in the alveoli. They are discontinuous sounds usually heard on inspiration, but they may be heard throughout the respiratory cycle. They may be high-pitched, popping sounds or low-pitched, bubbling sounds, and have been described as similar to the sound made by rubbing strands of hair together with the fingertips.
- **Stridor** is a piercing, high-pitched sound that is heard without a stethoscope, primarily during inspiration, in infants who are experiencing respiratory distress or in someone with an obstructed airway.
- **Stertor** refers to labored breathing that produces a snoring sound. It is common with mouth breathing due to nasal congestion. The "death rattle" is a type of stertorous breathing.

See Chapter 22 for further discussion of abnormal breath sounds. To listen to the sounds,

 Go to **Sound File, Breath Sounds,** on *DavisPlus.*

Chest and Abdomen Movement

The chest or abdomen normally rises with inspiration and falls with expiration in a gentle and rhythmic pattern. When a person is having difficulty moving air into or out of the lungs, respiratory patterns change. **Intercostal retraction** refers to the visible sinking of tissues around and between the ribs that occurs when the person must use additional effort to breathe. **Substernal retraction** exists when tissues are drawn in beneath the sternum (breastbone), and **suprasternal retraction** exists when tissues are drawn in above the clavicle (shoulder girdle).

Associated Clinical Signs

When you assess respiration, it is important to assess for clinical signs of oxygenation. Signs of **hypoxia** (inadequate cellular oxygenation) include pallor or cyanosis, restlessness, apprehension, confusion, dizziness, fatigue, decreased level of consciousness, tachycardia, tachypnea, and changes in blood pressure. When evaluating cyanosis, the tongue and oral mucosa are the best indicators of hypoxia. Cyanosis of the nails, lips, and skin may be caused by hypoxia, but may also be related to cold or reduced circulation in that area. Chronic hypoxia causes **clubbing** (loss of the nail angle) of the fingers.

A **cough** is a forceful or violent expulsion of air during expiration. Coughs may be *constant* (occurring frequently and consistently) or *intermittent* (occurring occasionally). If secretions are expectorated (coughed up), the cough is *productive*. If no secretions are produced, the cough is *nonproductive* or *dry*. A *hacking cough* is a series of dry coughs that occur together, whereas a *whooping cough* is a sudden, periodic cough that ends with a whooping sound on inspiration. Coughs may be symptoms of allergic reactions, lung disease, respiratory infection, or heart conditions.

KnowledgeCheck 20-4

- How can you estimate a client's tidal volume?
- What is the range of normal for an adult's respiratory rate?
- Besides the rate, what other characteristics of a client's respirations should you observe?
- What are some common clinical signs associated with poor oxygenation?

Arterial Oxygen Saturation

The rate, quality, and depth of the respirations are indicators of the general health of the respiratory system. However, they do not measure the amounts of oxygen and carbon dioxide present in the blood—information that is essential for evaluating the effectiveness of respiratory effort. Two methods exist to measure O_2 and CO_2 blood levels. One method is invasive; the other is not.

- **Arterial blood gas (ABG) sampling** directly measures the partial pressures of oxygen and carbon dioxide and blood pH, in other words, the gases in the arterial blood. This method requires the puncture of an artery followed by laboratory testing of the sample. It provides comprehensive data, but is invasive, painful, time consuming, and relatively expensive. If you need more information about this diagnostic test, consult a medical-surgical nursing or laboratory tests text.
- **Pulse oximetry** is a noninvasive method of monitoring respiratory status with a device that measures **oxygen saturation** (an indication of the oxygen being carried by hemoglobin in the arterial blood). The oximeter emits light, and a photosensor placed on the client's finger or earlobe measures the light passing through the site and calculates a pulse saturation (SpO_2) that is a good estimate of arterial oxygen saturation. The only risk in pulse oximetry is that clinicians may become too dependent on it or trust erroneous readings. Do not neglect the other aspects of holistic respiratory assessment. In many situations, oxygen saturation is monitored routinely along with the other vital signs. To learn how to apply a pulse oximeter,

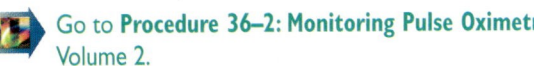 Go to **Procedure 36–2: Monitoring Pulse Oximetry,** in Volume 2.

ThinkLike a Nurse 20-8

- Mrs. Dowell has smoked two packs of cigarettes per day for 45 years. She has recently been diagnosed with pneumonia—an infection of the lungs. What VS assessments would be important for Mrs. Dowell, and why?
- Recall the clients in the Meet Your Patients scenario. Mr. Jackson is short of breath and struggling to breathe. His respiratory rate is 28 breaths/min. What else do you need to know about the patient situation? What is important and what is not important in this scenario? What is probably least important?

 ANALYSIS/NURSING DIAGNOSIS

As noted earlier, *hypoxia* refers to inadequate cellular oxygenation. It results from decreased oxygen intake, decreased ability of tissues to remove oxygen from blood, impaired ventilation or perfusion, impaired gas exchange between the blood and alveoli, or inadequate levels of hemoglobin. The following are two common alterations in respiration:

- **Hyperventilation** occurs when rapid and deep breathing result in excess loss of CO_2 (*hypocapnia*). A client who is hyperventilating may complain of feeling lightheaded and tingly. Causes of hyperventilation include anxiety, infection, shock, hypoxia, drugs (e.g., aspirin, amphetamines), diabetes mellitus, or acid–base imbalance.
- **Hypoventilation** occurs when the rate and depth of respirations are decreased and CO_2 is retained or alveolar ventilation is compromised. Hypoventilation may be related to chronic obstructive pulmonary disease (COPD), general anesthesia, impending respiratory failure, or other conditions that result in decreased respirations.

Two nursing diagnoses commonly used to describe various respiratory problems are Impaired Gas Exchange and Ineffective Breathing patterns. For a more complete list, see Chapter 36.

BLOOD PRESSURE

Blood pressure (BP), an important indicator of overall cardiovascular health, is the pressure of the blood as it is forced against arterial walls during cardiac contraction. **Systolic pressure** is the peak pressure exerted against arterial walls as the ventricles contract and eject blood. **Diastolic pressure** is the minimum pressure exerted against arterial walls, between cardiac contractions when the heart is at rest.

Blood pressure is measured in millimeters of mercury (mm Hg) and is recorded as systolic pressure over diastolic pressure (e.g., 110/74 mm Hg). The pulse that can be palpated to determine heart rate is due to the difference between the systolic and diastolic pressures. This difference is known as the **pulse pressure**. The pulse pressure for a BP of 120/80 mm Hg is 40 mm Hg. The pulse pressure is an indication of the volume output of

the left ventricle. Generally, the pulse pressure should be no greater than one-third of the systolic pressure, as in the example of a BP of 120/80, with a pulse pressure of 40 ($\frac{1}{3} \times 120 = 40$).

KnowledgeCheck 20-5

- For a client whose BP is 150/80, what is the pulse pressure?
- Is that normal? If so, explain. If not, what should the pulse pressure be?

TheoreticalKnowledge
knowing **why**

To assess and support clients' blood pressure, you will need to understand how it contributes to the concept of **perfusion**. An adequate BP is necessary to ensure that tissue perfusion is maintained. Contraction of the heart (systolic pressure) forces a bolus of oxygenated blood into the arterial circulation to provide a continuous supply of oxygen to all body cells. The heart then rests and refills with blood (diastolic pressure), which is pumped out to the tissues. Any factor that interferes with this cycle can cause impaired tissue perfusion.

You will also need to know, and will learn in this section, what constitutes a normal reading for a client, how the body regulates blood pressure, and what factors affect the blood pressure.

What Is a Normal Blood Pressure Reading?

For many years, a BP of less than 120 to 129 systolic and less than 80 to 84 diastolic was considered "optimal" for adults; and up to 130 systolic and 85 diastolic was considered "normal" for adults. More recently, an expert panel has classified "normal" as systolic BP below 120 and diastolic BP below 80 (Table 20-5) (Joint National Committee on Prevention, Detection, Evaluation, and Treatment of High Blood Pressure, 2004).

How Does the Body Regulate Blood Pressure?

Blood pressure regulation is a highly complex process. It is influenced by three factors: cardiac function, peripheral vascular resistance, and blood volume. The body constantly regulates and adjusts arterial pressure to supply blood to body tissues via perfusion of the capillary beds. For in-depth discussion, see Chapter 37.

Cardiac Function

Recall that *cardiac output* is the volume of blood pumped by the heart per minute, and that it reflects the functioning of the heart. An increase in cardiac output causes an increase in BP; a decrease in cardiac output causes a decrease in BP (if all other factors remain the same). A

Table 20-5 ➤ Classification of Adult Blood Pressure*

CATEGORY	SYSTOLIC (MM HG)		DIASTOLIC (MM HG)	FOLLOW-UP
Normal	< 120	and	< 80	Encourage lifestyle modification if there are risk factors. Recheck in 1–2 yr or sooner if there are risk factors.
Prehypertension	120–139	or	80–89	Encourage lifestyle changes; recheck in 1 yr or sooner if indicated. Antihypertensives are prescribed only with compelling indications, such as renal disease.
Stage I Hypertension	140–159	or	90–99	Encourage lifestyle modification. Follow up with primary care provider in 1–2 mo. (Most patients will be started on thiazide-type diuretics.) Newer (JNC 8) guidelines recommend treating older adults only when the B/P is 150/90.
Stage II Hypertension	≥ 160	or	≥ 100	Encourage lifestyle modification. Refer for care within 1 wk, or immediately if warranted. (Most patients will be given a two-drug combination therapy, e.g., thiazide-type diuretics with angiotensin-converting enzyme [ACE] inhibitors.)

Source: Data from the Joint National Committee on Prevention, Detection, Evaluation, and Treatment of High Blood Pressure. (2004). *JNC 7 Complete Report. The seventh report of the Joint National Committee on Prevention, Detection, Evaluation, and Treatment of High Blood Pressure.* Bethesda, MD: National Institutes of Health. Retrieved January 3, 2013, from http://www.nhlbi.nih.gov/guidelines/hypertension/index.htm; James, Oparil, Carter, et al. (2014), "Evidence-based guideline for the management of high blood pressure in adults. Report from the panel members appointed to the eighth Joint National Committee (JNC8)." *JAMA, 311*(5), pp. 507–520.

*For adults age 18 and older, based on the average of two or more readings taken at each of two or more visits after an initial screening.

change in either stroke volume or heart rate alters cardiac output.

Stroke Volume Conditions that *increase cardiac output* by increasing stroke volume include:

- Increased blood volume (as occurs during pregnancy, for example).
- More forceful contraction of the ventricles (as occurs during exercise, for example).

Conditions that *decrease cardiac output* by decreasing stroke volume include:

- Dehydration
- Active bleeding
- Damage to the heart (as seen after myocardial infarction, or heart attack)

Heart Rate Up to a point, an increase in heart rate increases cardiac output. However, a very rapid heart rate limits the time allotted for the ventricles to fill, resulting in decreased stroke volume and, ultimately, decreased cardiac output.

Peripheral Resistance

Peripheral resistance refers to arterial and capillary resistance to blood flow as a result of friction between blood and the vessel walls. Increased peripheral resistance creates a temporary increase in BP. The amount of friction or resistance depends on blood **viscosity** (thickness), arterial size, and arterial **compliance** (elasticity). The walls of the veins are thin and very distensible, so they have little influence on peripheral resistance and BP.

Blood Viscosity Blood viscosity influences the ease with which blood flows through the vessels. Viscosity is determined by the **hematocrit** (the percentage of red blood cells in plasma). Any disorder that increases hematocrit (e.g., dehydration) increases blood viscosity and, therefore, BP. Conversely, a low hematocrit, as seen in anemia, lowers viscosity and may reduce BP.

Arterial Size The smaller the radius of a blood vessel, the more resistance it offers to blood flow. Constricted arteries prevent the free flow of blood and, subsequently, increase BP. Dilated arteries allow unrestricted flow of blood, thereby reducing blood pressure. The sympathetic nervous system controls vasoconstriction and vasodilation.

Arterial Compliance Arteries with good elasticity can distend and recoil easily and adequately. When age- or disease-related changes in arterial structure cause a loss of elasticity, peripheral resistance, and possibly BP, increase. **Arteriosclerosis** (hardening of the arteries) is a common contributor to increased BP in middle-aged and older adults.

Blood Volume

The normal volume of blood in the body is about 5 liters (5,000 mL). A significant volume decrease, as occurs with hemorrhage or other fluid losses, reduces vascular volume, and BP falls. When vascular volume is increased above the norm, as occurs with renal (kidney) failure and fluid retention, BP increases.

What Factors Influence Blood Pressure?

Blood pressure normally changes from minute to minute with changes in activity or in body position. Therefore, you must establish *BP patterns* rather than relying on individual BP readings when determining whether a client's BP is normal or abnormal. This is even more important for older adults because their BP tends to fluctuate even more. The following are some factors that affect the BP:

Developmental Stage An average newborn has a systolic BP of about 60 to 80 mm Hg and a diastolic BP of 40 to 50 mm Hg (Lowdermilk, Perry, Cashion, et al., 2012). It increases gradually throughout childhood. A child or adolescent's BP depends on body size; therefore, a smaller child or adolescent has a lower blood pressure than does a larger child.

Both systolic and diastolic BP continue to increase with age as a result of decreased arterial compliance and changes in the left ventricular wall. These normal aging process changes can lead to cardiovascular instability (Lange, 2012).

For BP normal ranges for various age groups,

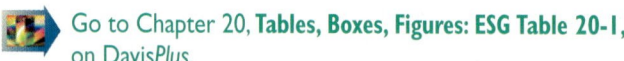 Go to Chapter 20, **Tables, Boxes, Figures: ESG Table 20-1,** on Davis*Plus*.

Gender The average BP for men is slightly higher than that for women of comparable age, although the difference is not considered significant. After menopause, a woman's BP tends to increase, possibly due to a decrease in estrogen.

Family History A family history of hypertension markedly increases the likelihood of an individual's developing hypertension.

Lifestyle Increased sodium consumption, smoking, and consumption of three or more alcoholic drinks per day have been shown to elevate BP. Caffeine may raise BP for a short while after ingestion, but it has no long-term effect on the BP.

Exercise Physical fitness has been shown to reduce BP in many individuals. However, muscular exertion temporarily increases BP as a result of increased heart rate and cardiac output. You should, therefore, wait about 30 minutes before you assess the BP of someone who has been physically active.

Body Position BP is higher when a person is standing than when sitting or lying down. Readings are higher if taken with the client's arm above heart level or if the arm is unsupported at the client's side. Seated readings are higher if the client's feet are dangling rather than resting on the floor or if the legs are crossed at the knees.

Stress Fear, worry, excitement, and other stressors cause BP to rise sharply because of sympathetic nervous system stimulation (fight-or-flight response). One example of this is "white-coat hypertension." This occurs

when a patient's BP is elevated in the physician's office or clinic—a situation in which he is likely to experience stress—but not at other times. However white-coat hypertension may indicate what happens during other times of stress, so if it is consistently displayed, treatment may be indicated.

Pain Pain often causes the BP to increase. However, severe or prolonged pain can significantly decrease BP.

Race African Americans have a higher rate of hypertension than do European Americans, and they have a higher incidence of complications and hypertension-related deaths (McCance & Heuther, 2010).

Obesity As a rule, obesity increases BP. This increase is related to the additional vascular supply required to perfuse the large body mass and the resultant increase in peripheral resistance.

Diurnal Variations Generally, BP varies according to the person's daily schedules and routines. BP is lower while the person is sleeping and when he first gets up, rising during the day and dropping again toward bedtime.

Medications Many medications alter BP. This effect may be intended, as with antihypertensive medications, or unintended, such as the drop in BP that often results when a client receives pain medication. Many over-the-counter preparations, herbal products, and illicit drugs can affect BP.

Diseases Diseases that affect the circulatory system or any of the major organs of the body (e.g., the kidneys) may affect BP.

Genetic Variations/Genes Researchers used the recognized 29 genetic variants known to influence systolic and diastolic blood pressure to develop a genetic risk score. Twenty-nine percent of people with the top 10% of genetic risks had hypertension compared with 16% in the lowest risk groups (National Institute of Health, 2011).

ThinkLike a Nurse 20-9

- Evaluate the following adult blood pressures. Are they high, low, or normal?
  116/90 mm Hg
  80/50 mm Hg
  184/102 mm Hg
  140/90 mm Hg
  40/0 mm Hg
- What theoretical knowledge did you use in evaluating the blood pressures?

PracticalKnowledge
knowing **how**

Now that you understand the concept of perfusion and how blood pressure is maintained and regulated, you are ready to gain the practical knowledge of how to assess and support this aspect of physical functioning.

ASSESSMENT

Blood pressure may be assessed directly or indirectly.

Direct Measurement   In the *direct method*, a catheter is threaded into an artery under sterile conditions and attached to tubing that is connected to an electronic monitoring system. The pressure is constantly displayed as a waveform on the monitor screen. Although the direct method of measuring BP is very accurate, its use is confined to critical care areas and surgery because of the risk of sudden arterial blood loss.

Indirect Measurement   Usually you will measure BP via the *indirect*, or *noninvasive*, *method*. This is an accurate estimate of arterial BP that can be performed in any clinical or community setting. For a summary of a procedure for noninvasive blood pressure monitoring, see the Highlights of Procedures box. For the complete procedure,

 Go to **Procedure 20-6: Measuring Blood Pressure,** in Volume 2.

For an animated visual explanation of blood pressure readings,

 Go to Student Resources **Animations: Reading Blood Pressure,** on Davis*Plus*.

What Equipment Do I Need?

You will need a stethoscope, a blood pressure cuff and sphygmomanometer, or an electronic blood pressure monitor to assess blood pressure. Electronic monitoring is gradually replacing the stethoscope and sphygmomanometer in inpatient settings. However, a common stethoscope and sphygmomanometer are generally sufficient to hear most clients' blood pressures. When blood pressure is weak, ultrasonic stethoscopes are useful for magnifying sound waves occurring during systole.

Evidence-based guidelines suggest that using the bell of the stethoscope enables you to hear blood pressure sounds more accurately, especially at diastolic pressures (Perloff, Grim, Flack, et al., 1993; Shindler, 2007; Vital Signs, 1999). However, most people use the diaphragm because it is easily placed and because some stethoscopes do not have a bell (see Fig. 20-4). The key to clarity of sound is to use a high-quality stethoscope with short tubing.

A **sphygmomanometer** consists of a vinyl or cloth cuff, a pressure bulb with a regulating valve, and a manometer (Fig. 20-8). Blood pressure cuffs contain an inflatable rubber bladder.

The cuff is attached to a gauge or manometer and a valved pressure bulb that inflates the bladder (Fig. 20-9). Cuffs can be placed on either the upper arm or midthigh and are supplied in various sizes.

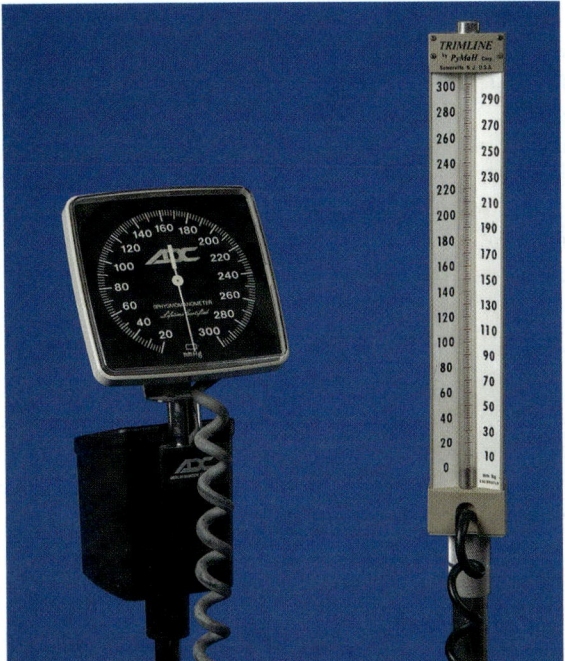
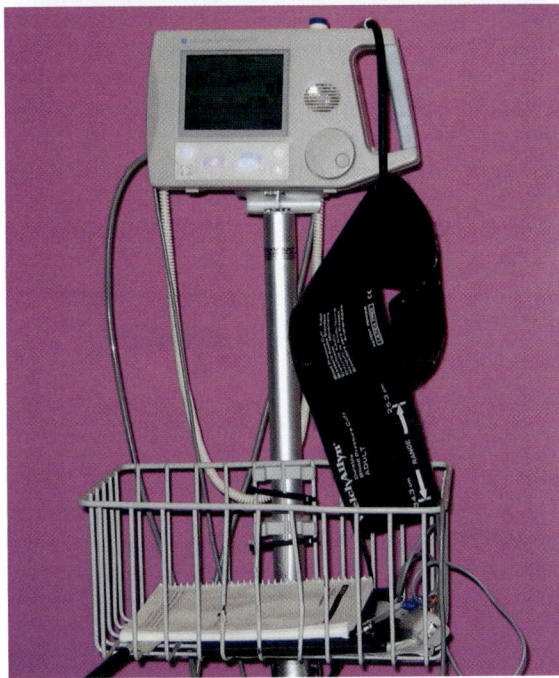

FIGURE 20-8 Types of manometers: *top left*, aneroid; *top right*, mercury; *bottom*, electronic.

Sphygmomanometers are either aneroid or mercury. **Aneroid** manometers have dials that register BP by pointers attached to a spring. **Mercury** manometers measure BP using a calibrated upright tube containing mercury (see Fig. 20-8, top). As the bladder of the cuff is inflated, the pressure pushes the column of mercury up the tube. The column of mercury falls as the cuff is deflated. Mercury manometers are not as popular as aneroid manometers because they pose a health hazard if the mercury tube is broken. They are however, easier to maintain and more accurate than aneroid manometers, which

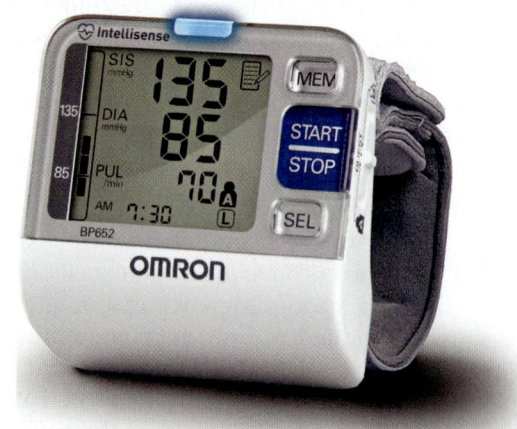

FIGURE 20-9 A blood pressure cuff showing placement of bladder within the cuff.

require frequent calibration. In 1998, the American Hospital Association and the EPA recommended that the healthcare industry eliminate mercury-containing waste by the year 2005 (EPA, 2001, 2012). Most healthcare agencies have committed to or phased out the use of mercury-containing products (Mercury-Free Health Care, n.d.).

Electronic blood pressure monitors use either microphones to sense sounds or sensors that detect pressure waves as blood flows through arteries (Fig. 20-8, bottom). They can be set to monitor and record BP at timed intervals and do not require the use of a stethoscope. They measure systolic, diastolic, and mean arterial pressures. Electronic monitors are useful when you must monitor BP frequently (e.g., during surgery or when a client is critically ill). However, some evidence suggests that they may be less accurate than auscultated blood pressures (Bern, Brandt, & Mbelu, 2007; Nelson, Kennedy, & Regnerus, 2008), so you should auscultate a baseline BP before initiating automatic monitoring (Pickering, Hall, Appel, et al., 2005).

Many clients use a version of the electronic BP monitor in their homes. These devices can be purchased in grocery stores and pharmacies. They are useful for screening, but clients should seek follow-up care when readings are not within their normal range. The accompanying Home Care box identifies teaching topics for clients using electronic BP monitors.

What Cuff Size Should I Use?

The *width* of the bladder of a properly fitting cuff will cover approximately two-thirds of the *length* of the upper arm (or other extremity) for an adult, and the entire upper arm for a child (Fig. 20-10) (National Heart, Lung, and Blood Institute, 1996, revised 2005, 2007). Alternatively, you can check that (1) the *cuff width* is 40% of the arm circumference and (2) the *length* of the bladder encircles 80% of the arm in adults (Tomlinson, 2010).

Using a cuff or bladder of the incorrect size can result in a measurement error of as much as 30 mm Hg. If the cuff is too narrow, your reading will be too high; if it is too wide, the reading will be too low. Although cuffs are manufactured in various sizes, in practice, you will

---

Home Care

Teaching Your Client Self-Monitoring of Blood Pressure

Various models of common, acceptable BP devices are available for self-monitoring using the upper arm (finger monitors are inaccurate) (American Heart Association, 2012).

A wrist monitor for blood pressure.

- With a portable home device, the client simply pushes a button, and the cuff inflates and deflates automatically. The device provides an electronic digital readout of the BP. Because these devices are sensitive, arm movement or improper cuff placement can cause inaccurate readings. Also, these devices must be recalibrated at least every 6 to 12 months.

- Some grocery stores, fitness clubs, and other public places have stationary automatic BP devices for public use. The person places his arm in the cuff, which fits over his clothing. The machine gives a visual display of the BP reading. The accuracy of these machines varies.

Benefits of Self-Monitoring

- May detect high BP in those who have not previously had a problem (screening).

- Allows for observation of the BP *pattern* over time, rather than a one-time office reading. The results can be analyzed to distinguish "white-coat hypertension" from actual hypertension.

- For clients with hypertension, self-monitoring increases participation in treatment and may improve compliance with treatment.

Teaching Your Client Self-Monitoring of Blood Pressure—cont'd

Disadvantages of Self-Monitoring

■ Possible incorrect use of the BP device

■ Needless anxiety over a single elevated reading

■ Clients with hypertension may make adjustments to their medications based on the BP readings without consulting their care provider.

Nursing Implications

■ Teach proper use of the self-measurement devices.

■ Periodically evaluate the client's technique.

■ Teach the meaning of BP readings and the need to look for patterns from multiple readings, not just a single reading.

■ Explain the need for calibration of the home-monitoring device at least once a year or according to the manufacturer's instructions.

■ Have the client bring the home-monitoring device to clinical visits so that readings can be compared with simultaneously recorded auscultatory readings.

■ Teach the client to have abnormally high or low readings (occurring on more than one occasion) rechecked by a healthcare provider. Home readings of 135/85 or higher should be considered elevated.

■ Advise the client to keep a written record of BP readings, including the date and time for each, and bring it to each clinic or office visit.

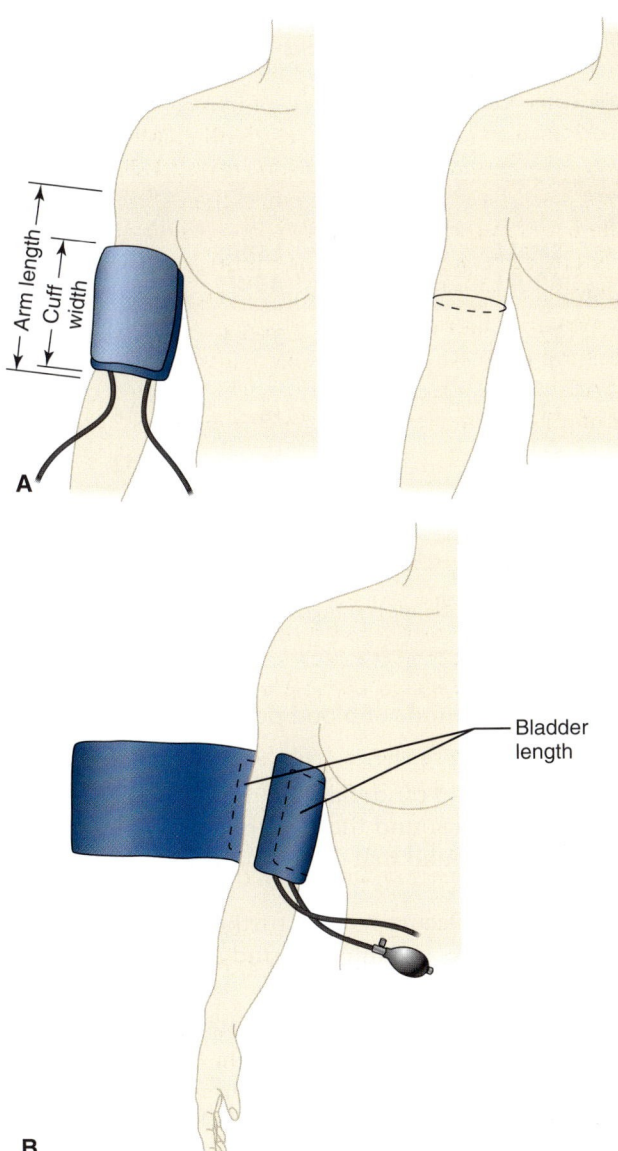

FIGURE 20-10 Determining correct BP cuff size. A, The cuff width should be two-thirds of the length of the upper arm, or should encircle 40% of the arm. B, The length of the bladder should encircle 80% of the upper arm.

probably have access to only two or three different adult sizes. If you must use a cuff of the improper size, (1) it is better to use one that is too large than one that is too small, and (2) be sure to document the cuff size along with the BP reading. Even if you do have a cuff of the proper size, it is helpful to document the size anyway: (1) for consistency, and (2) because it provides evidence of accuracy in making treatment decisions.

Refer to Table 20-6 for information about cuff sizes in centimeters; also,

 Go to **Clinical Insight 20-1, Choosing a Blood Pressure Cuff Size,** in Volume 2.

Which Site Should I Use?

You usually use the *brachial artery* for assessing BP. However, the condition of the client's arm as well as other factors can interfere with accurate BP measurement. Avoid assessing blood pressure in an arm that has an intravenous access device, renal dialysis fistula, or skin graft; that is paralyzed, diseased, or has extensive trauma; that has a cast or dressings; or that is on the same side of breast or shoulder surgery. In these and similar instances, you can use the forearm, thigh, or calf. Systolic pressure may be 20 to 30 mm Hg higher in the lower extremities than in the arms, but diastolic pressures are similar. Also, forearm and upper arm readings may not be interchangeable. Document the site used. For a summary of the procedure for measuring blood pressure, see the Highlights of Procedures box. For the entire procedure,

 Go to **Procedure 20-6: Measuring Blood Pressure,** in Volume 2.

Also refer to the QSEN Box, Using Evidence to Support Clinical Practice.

Auscultating Blood Pressure

Blood pressure can be measured indirectly by auscultation or palpation. The preferred, and most commonly used, method is auscultation; however, palpation is

Quality and Safety Education for Nurses

Using Evidence to Support Clinical Practice

Chapter Key Concept: *Perfusion (blood pressure)*

Competency: *Evidence-Based Practice (Knowledge, skills, attitudes)**

Background: It is essential to measure blood pressure accurately for appropriate treatment and management (Turner, Burns, Chaney, et al., 2008; Elliott & Coventry, 2012). Accuracy and reliability of blood pressure measurement are improved by proper patient position, arm position, and timing. Research shows a correlation between increased readings and timing of the measurement, positioning of the patient (standing, versus sitting in a chair, versus sitting on examining table) and positioning of the arm at the level of the heart (Pickering, Hall, Appel, et al., 2005; Tomlinson, 2010; Turner, Burns, Chaney, et al., 2008).

Scenario: A 70-year-old obese patient is seen at the ambulatory care setting with a history of hypertension and peripheral vascular disease. You are assessing the vital signs to provide data for medication management. Prior to taking the patient's blood pressure you obtain an aneroid

sphygmomanometer and then request she sit in a chair and extend one arm while supporting the arm at level of the heart. Another nurse states, "You don't need to do all that."

Think about it:

- What factors could influence the accuracy of the blood pressure assessment in this patient?

- What evidence will you give the other nurse for your actions and how will you locate best evidence to support your response?

- What other actions should you institute to maintain accuracy in blood pressure measurement?

*For specific Knowledge, Skills, and Attitudes,

 Go to the QSEN Web site at **http://qsen.org/ competencies/pre-licensure-ksas/**

The QSEN KSA that is most pertinent is: *Locate evidence reports related clinical practice topics and guidelines.*

Table 20-6 ▶ Blood Pressure Cuffs: Acceptable Bladder Sizes*

CUFF TYPE——>	NEWBORN	INFANT	CHILD	SMALL ADULT	ADULT	LARGE ADULT	ADULT THIGH
Arm circumference at midpoint (cm)**	< 6	6–15	16–21	22–26	27–34	35–44	45–52
Bladder width (cm)	3	5	8	12	16	16	16
Bladder length (cm)	6	15	21	22	30	36	42

Sources: Perloff, Grim, Flack, et al. (1993); Pickering, Hall, Appel, et al. (2005).
*The National Heart, Lung, and Blood Institute states that practically speaking, "correct cuff size equals the largest cuff that will fit on the upper arm with room below for the stethoscope head" (2007).
**Arm circumference is half the distance from the acromion to the olecranon process. If correct size not available, use next larger (rather than smaller) size.

---

useful in certain situations. When auscultating BP, place your stethoscope over an artery, inflate the cuff, and listen for sounds as you deflate the cuff.

As you *inflate* the cuff, the artery is occluded as the pressure of the cuff exceeds the pressure in the artery. At that point, blood flow through the artery is halted, and no sound can be heard. As you *deflate* the cuff, blood begins to flow rapidly through the partially open artery, producing turbulence that you will hear through the stethoscope as a tapping sound.

- *The first sound* you hear when the cuff is slowly deflated is the systolic pressure.
- *The disappearance of sound* identifies the diastolic BP. When the artery is no longer compressed, blood flows freely, and no sound is heard.

The sounds you listen for when you assess BP are called **Korotkoff sounds.** These sounds, described by Russian neurologist Nicolai Korotkoff in 1906, are used

to describe the sounds of blood pulsating through arteries (Fig. 20-11).

1st sound—As you deflate the BP cuff, you will initially hear a sound that occurs during systole. It is a tapping sound that corresponds to the pulse (systolic BP).

2nd sound—Occurs as you further deflate the cuff. It is a soft, swishing sound caused by blood turbulence.

3rd sound—Begins midway through the BP and is a sharp, rhythmic tapping sound.

4th sound—Like the third sound, but softer and fading.

5th sound—Silence; it corresponds with diastole (diastolic BP).

You will not always be able to identify each of the five sounds. In some clients the sounds are distinct, but in others you will note little difference between beginning and ending sounds. To hear these sounds,

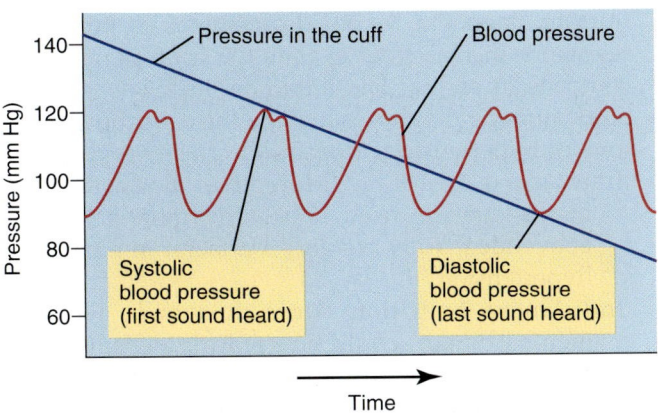

FIGURE 20-11 Relationship of blood pressure to changes in cuff pressure and the first and fifth Korotkoff sounds (BP 120/80).

 Go to **Sounds, Blood Pressure Sounds,** on Davis*Plus.*

 Also go to Chapter Resources, **Chapter 20, Resources for Caregivers and Health Professionals: Sounds,** on Davis*Plus.*

Palpating Blood Pressure

When the BP is difficult to hear (e.g., in shock, or other conditions that compromise circulation) you can use palpation alone. You can usually palpate only the systolic BP, because diastolic pressure is difficult to feel. To learn this technique,

 Go to **Procedure 20-6, Variation D, Palpating the Blood Pressure,** in Volume 2.

Using Palpation With Auscultation

You should use palpation with auscultation for calculating the proper cuff inflation pressure before auscultating the BP and for detecting an auscultatory gap, to be discussed shortly.

Calculating Proper Inflation Pressure

The first time you measure a client's BP, you do not know what the systolic BP will be. Should you pump the cuff to 200 mm Hg, just to be sure you don't miss the first sound? The answer is NO. If you overinflate the cuff, the patient will feel discomfort. However, if you underinflate it (e.g., stop inflating at 110 mm Hg), you may miss the first sound and obtain an incorrect reading.

You can use palpation with auscultation to estimate the systolic BP. This helps ensure that you inflate the cuff to the proper level to obtain an accurate reading. To learn how to perform this method,

 Go to **Procedure 20-6, Measuring Blood Pressure,** in Volume 2

Recognizing an Auscultatory Gap

If the client has hypertension, as you auscultate the BP during deflation of the cuff you may note the loss of sounds for as much as 30 mm Hg, followed by the return of sound. This loss and later return of sound is referred to as an **auscultatory gap**. Palpating first and then auscultating (as described in the preceding paragraphs) ensures that you will not miss the isolated first sound. You should record the range of pressures in which the gap occurs (e.g., BP left arm, sitting, 170/90 with an auscultatory gap from 170 to 140). Failure to recognize an auscultatory gap can result in a serious misreading of the systolic BP. For tips that will help ensure the validity of your BP measurements,

 Go to Chapter 20, **Clinical Insight 20-2: Taking an Accurate Blood Pressure,** in Volume 2.

KnowledgeCheck 20-6

- Which of the Korotkoff sounds would you record as the systolic pressure?
- Which of the Korotkoff sounds would you record as the diastolic pressure?
- A nurse is auscultating a BP. He hears the first sound at 170 mm Hg. The sound disappears immediately. At 150 mm Hg, the sound appears again and continues until there is silence at 80 mm Hg. The pressures were taken in the client's right arm while the client was lying down.
  How should the nurse record these pressures?
  How do you explain what happened?

■ ANALYSIS/NURSING DIAGNOSIS

Hypotension and hypertension are medical diagnoses or, more commonly, symptoms rather than nursing diagnoses. However, they may be the etiology of nursing diagnoses—for example, Risk for Falls related to orthostatic hypotension.

Example Problem: Hypotension

Hypotension is diagnosed when systolic blood pressure is less than 100 mm Hg. A low blood pressure is usually not considered a problem. However, further evaluation is always called for if:

- The client is also experiencing dizziness, fatigue, concentration problems, activity intolerance, or shortness of breath, or
- The low blood pressure is of sudden onset.

Hemorrhage and heart failure are two causes of hypotension. Very low BP (hypovolemic shock) is a medical emergency. If you need more information on hypovolemic shock, consult a medical-surgical nursing text.

Orthostatic, or postural, hypotension occurs when a person's BP drops suddenly on moving from a lying position to a sitting or standing position. Orthostatic hypotension is defined as a decrease of 10 mm Hg in standing blood pressure when associated with dizziness and/or fainting (Joint National Committee, 2004). Postural hypotension results from peripheral vasodilation without a compensatory increase in cardiac output. It is most likely to occur in older adults, pregnant women, clients on prolonged bed rest, and clients with decreased blood volume (e.g., from dehydration or recent blood loss).

The following are examples of nursing diagnoses with hypotension as the etiology.

- Risk for Falls related to dizziness secondary to postural hypotension
- Fear of falling related to fainting secondary to postural hypotension

Example Problem: Hypertension

A transient elevation in BP is a normal response to physiological or psychological stress (e.g., after eating, after exercise). **Prehypertension** is a BP reading of 120 to 139 mm Hg systolic or 80 to 89 mm Hg diastolic, obtained with two readings taken 6 minutes apart, with the patient sitting. **Hypertension** is a persistently higher than normal BP. It is diagnosed when BP is above 140 mm Hg systolic or above 90 mm Hg diastolic on two or more separate occasions. Physiologically, hypertension is related to thickening of the arterial walls and decreased elasticity of the arteries.

Hypertension is a major cause of illness and death in the United States. Hypertension increases the stress on the heart and blood vessels, and if untreated, it may lead to heart attack, heart failure, peripheral vascular disease, kidney damage, or stroke (American Heart Association, n.d.a). The severity of the disorder is directly related to the degree of elevation; however, the latest guidelines (Joint National Committee, 2004) recommend that even prehypertension be treated by lifestyle modifications to prevent coronary artery disease. The diagnosis of hypertension is often delayed because symptoms are mild or absent. Those who experience symptoms may complain of early morning suboccipital headaches, fatigue, and visual changes.

Primary, or **essential**, **hypertension** is diagnosed when there is no known cause for the BP elevation. Essential hypertension accounts for at least 90% of all cases of hypertension. Although no single cause is identified, family history, age, race, obesity, diet, heavy alcohol consumption, smoking history, high cholesterol levels, and stress all contribute to the development of essential hypertension.

Secondary hypertension occurs when there is a clearly identified cause for the persistent rise in BP. A variety of renal and endocrine disorders may lead to secondary hypertension. Several prescription and non-prescription drugs can also cause BP elevation (e.g., nonsteroidal anti-inflammatory drugs [NSAIDs], oral contraceptives, some decongestants, and adrenal steroid hormones). Nicotine and caffeine cause transient (temporary) BP increases. Other causes of hypertension include use of cocaine, amphetamines, and other illicit drugs, as well as chronic overuse of alcohol. Treatment is directed at eliminating the underlying cause.

Hypertension is not a nursing diagnosis; it is a medical diagnosis. However, there are nursing diagnoses associated with it, as in the following examples:

- Risk for Decreased Cardiac Output occurs as a response to hypertension (i.e., hypertension is the etiology of this nursing diagnosis). As blood pressure rises, peripheral resistance increases. Over time the heart is unable to compensate, and cardiac output declines.
- Some nursing diagnoses may be the contributing factors for hypertension, for example:

  Imbalanced Nutrition: More than Body Requirements may be used if obesity (more than 20% above ideal body weight) is a factor in a patient's hypertension.

  Imbalanced Nutrition: More than Body Requirements (for salt) could be used for a client whose high dietary sodium intake is contributing to hypertension.

- Hypertension may be a defining characteristic (symptom) of some nursing diagnoses, for example: Anxiety and Pain may cause an increase in BP.
- Hypertension may create a diagnosis of Deficient Knowledge related to the need to make lifestyle changes.

PLANNING OUTCOMES/EVALUATION

You may need goals for overall blood pressure monitoring, but more likely you will use them for problems related to hypotension and hypertension.

Outcomes for Example Problem: Hypotension

The *NOC outcomes and goals* you use depend on the nursing diagnosis (the problem caused by the hypotension). For Risk for Falls, you might use NOC's Falls Occurrence. You might write *an individualized goal* such as, "Patient will have no falls while walking."

Outcomes for Example Problem: Hypertension

The NOC standardized outcome for assessing the blood pressure is Vital Signs Status. If it becomes necessary to monitor cardiac output, you could use the labels of Cardiac Pump Effectiveness and Circulation Status.

Individualized goals/outcome statements are developed from the nursing diagnosis. For example, for Decreased Cardiac Output, goals might be, "BP will be at least 110/80," and "Extremities will be warm to the touch with quick capillary refill." If the nursing diagnosis were Imbalanced Nutrition: More Than Body Requirements, the desired outcomes would address the target weight for the client and the ideal number of calories to be consumed.

 Also go to Chapter Resources for Chapter 20, **Standardized Language, NOC Outcomes and NIC Interventions Associated With Abnormal Vital Signs**, on Davis*Plus*.

PLANNING INTERVENTIONS/IMPLEMENTATION

NIC standardized interventions for monitoring VS include the following:

Vital Signs Monitoring applies to monitoring an abnormal blood pressure.

Hemodynamic Regulation would be used to evaluate Decreased Cardiac Output.

 Go to Chapter Resources for Chapter 20, **Standardized Language,** on Davis*Plus*.

Interventions for Example Problem: Hypotension

NIC standardized interventions will be determined by the nursing diagnosis you use. For example, for Risk for Falls related to orthostatic hypotension, you might use the following: Fall Prevention; Self-Care Assistance: Transfer; and Surveillance: Safety.

Specific nursing activities, regardless of the nursing diagnosis, must address the etiology. For example, when you detect orthostatic hypotension:

1. Help the client lie down.
2. Next, obtain *orthostatic vital signs*—that is, take the pulse and BP with the client supine, sitting, and standing. Take each reading 1 to 3 minutes after the client changes position. Notify the provider or nurse in charge of the measurements.
3. When documenting orthostatic vital signs, record the client's position in addition to the pulse and BP measurements (e.g., supine P = 80, BP = 150/90; sitting P = 84, BP = 140/84; standing P = 90, BP = 104/60).

Interventions for Example Problem: Hypertension

Specific nursing activities for the patient with hypertension depend on whether hypertension is primary or secondary and on specific orders from the physician. Nursing activities and focused assessments that address hypertension, regardless of its cause, include the following:

Focused Assessments

- *Monitor all VS.* An elevated BP may affect the client's other VS. Watch for increases in pulse and respiratory rate.
- *Monitor the patient's activity tolerance.* The patient's degree of involvement in care, orientation, and level of fatigue while experiencing hypertension are all important indicators of decreased cardiac output.
- *Accurately measure intake and output.* If intake is appreciably greater than output, the increased blood volume will cause the BP to rise further. Pay attention to free fluids as well as fluid in food sources. Also monitor for edema, which is an indicator of fluid retention.
- *Weigh the client regularly.* Weight loss of as little as 10 lb (4.5 kg) lowers BP in many overweight persons with hypertension. Weight gain may signal poor compliance with the treatment plan and/or indicate fluid retention.
- *Collect and assess laboratory data as ordered.* Blood urea nitrogen (BUN), creatinine, electrolytes, hemoglobin, hematocrit, and lipid levels must all be assessed regularly.

Administering Medications

Administer antihypertensive medications as prescribed to control blood pressure. Unless the healthcare provider instructs otherwise, antihypertensives may best be taken at bedtime. Research has found that taking at least one antihypertensive medication at night decreases the risk of cardiovascular disease (Keller, 2011).

 Assess the client's attitude and beliefs about taking antihypertensive medications. Research shows that older adults with negative beliefs about their medication are more likely to be noncompliant in maintaining the medication regime (Ruppar, Dobbels, & Geest, 2012). You should help the client understand and gain realistic expectations regarding the medication therapy.

Teaching for Self-Care

- *For self-monitoring of BP,* see the box Home Care: Teaching Your Client Self-Monitoring of Blood Pressure. One study has found that self-monitoring better predicted clinical outcomes than single office measurements (Ransome, 2005).
- *For client teaching regarding hypertension,* see the box Self-Care: Teaching Your Client About Hypertension.
- *Teach stress management and relaxation techniques.*

 Such training has been effective in helping older adults with systolic hypertension to eliminate at least one antihypertensive drug and reduce their BP to target levels (Dusek, Hibberd, Buczynski, et al., 2008).

- *Teach and encourage self-management of behaviors;* provide positive feedback when the patient makes lifestyle changes.
- *Certain alternative therapies may help lower blood pressure* (see the box Complementary & Alternative Modalities).

Complementary & Alternative Modalities (CAM)

Alternative Therapies for Lowering Blood Pressure

According to a recent American Heart Association Scientific statement, some alternative methods reduce blood pressure—particularly aerobic exercise and resistance training—can be considered adjunctive to the medical therapies of diet and medication. Biofeedback techniques (isometric handgrip exercise and device-guided slow breathing) are likely to reduce blood pressure by a small amount, but the evidence is not as strong. Evidence is insufficient to support use of the following as adjunctive treatments for hypertension: meditation, yoga, relaxation therapy, stress-reduction techniques, and acupuncture.

Source: Brook, R., Appel, L., Rubenfire, M., et al. (2013). AHA scientific statement. Beyond medications and diet: Alternative approaches to lowering blood pressure. *Hypertension, 61* (6), 1360–1383. Retrieved on April 23, 2013, from http://hyper.ahajournals.org/content/61/6/1360.long

KnowledgeCheck 20-7

- Which of the following patients has hypertension? One with a BP of:
  150/80 on two separate occasions
  180/100 on one occasion
  138/88 on two occasions

- Which of the following client(s) has/have *primary* hypertension?
  Client A, who is obese and has a high sodium intake
  Client B, who is in renal failure
  Client C, who has hypertension induced by pregnancy
  Client D, who has a family history of hypertension

Self-Care

Teaching Your Client About Hypertension

Teach the client and family about lifestyle changes for preventing and managing hypertension.

➤ Limit salt intake to 1 teaspoon per day (2,400 mg of sodium).

➤ Consume a diet high in potassium (e.g., fresh fruits and vegetables, such as bananas, potatoes, yogurt, and acorn squash).

➤ Consume a diet high in calcium (e.g., milk and milk products, sardines, molasses, tofu).

➤ Limit alcohol intake to 1 or 2 drinks per day for men; 1 for women. (One drink is a can of beer, one jigger of liquor, or a glass of wine. Wine is preferred.)

➤ Maintain ideal body weight; lose weight if overweight.

➤ For overall cardiovascular health, reduce saturated fat and cholesterol intake.

➤ Eliminate smoking.

➤ Engage in aerobic exercise (30 to 45 minutes, several days a week, or a total of 150 minutes per week).

➤ Try to reduce stress and stressful situations.

➤ Teach the client that even one lifestyle change has effects similar to treatment with a single antihypertensive drug. More than one change has an even more positive effect on the BP.

Teach the client about monitoring his blood pressure at home.

➤ Monitor blood pressure at home to determine whether lifestyle modifications and/or medications are effective.

➤ Keep a record of your BP readings that contain the date, time, systolic and diastolic numbers, and any information that you want your provider to know.

➤ Take your BP whenever you experience symptoms such as headaches, dizziness, etc.

➤ Use an upper arm or wrist BP monitor that has been validated.

➤ Take your BP equipment when you visit your healthcare provider to check your monitor for accuracy.

➤ Follow the researchers' and manufacturer's guidelines for arm position and recalibration. This is especially true for wrist monitors (Dourmap, Girerd, Marquand, et al., 2010; Zeng, Huang, Sheng, et al., 2012).

Teach the need for follow-up assessments.

For BP of:			Teaching Points
Systolic		**Diastolic**	**Analysis and Client Action**
<120 mm Hg	and	<80 mm Hg	Normal Blood Pressure Recheck at each healthcare encounter or at least every 2 years.
120–139 mm Hg	Or	80–89 mm Hg	Prehypertension Review lifestyle modifications and make follow-up visits as your primary healthcare provider advises. If you have not seen a provider, consult one within 1 to 2 months.
140–159 mm Hg	Or	90–99 mm Hg	High Blood Pressure—Stage 1 (Note: This may differ slightly for older adults.) Review lifestyle modifications and schedule follow-up with a healthcare provider within 1 to 2 months.
160 or higher mm Hg	Or	100 or higher mm Hg	High Blood Pressure—Stage 2 Consult the primary care provider within 1 week, or immediately if the clinical situation warrants.

Source: The Joint National Committee on Prevention, Detection, Evaluation, and Treatment of High Blood Pressure. (2004). *JNC 7 Complete Report. The seventh report of the Joint National Committee on Prevention, Detection, Evaluation, and Treatment of High Blood Pressure.* Bethesda, MD: National Institutes of Health. Retrieved January 3, 2013, from http://www.nhlbi.nih.gov/guidelines/hypertension/index.htm

ThinkLike a Nurse 20-10

Recall the clients in the Meet Your Patients scenario. Lucas is 35 years old. He has been under a lot of stress. His blood pressure is 150/98.

- To evaluate his BP, what else do you need to know about Lucas's situation (the context)?
- What possible actions should you consider while meeting with Lucas?
- What is the theoretical knowledge (rationale) to support your decisions?

PUTTING IT ALL TOGETHER

In the hospital setting, you will usually take a complete set of VS on patients at regular intervals. In ambulatory care settings, the VS you measure may vary according to the client's chief complaint. Regardless of setting, you will need to use clinical judgment about which VS to measure and how often to measure them.

Evaluating Vital Signs

You should evaluate the client's VS on the basis of known norms as well as the particular client's trends. Suppose your client's BP has consistently been 150 to 160/90 over the past 3 days. This afternoon his BP is 108/60. Although this BP is theoretically normal, it is significantly different from his norm. Therefore, you must evaluate the cause of the change. Has there been a change in the other VS? Has there been a change in the client's medications or condition? How does the client feel? Has his activity level been altered by the change in BP? This change may be positive or negative. You must put all the VS and other clinical signs together to determine your course of action.

A high fever can cause BP to drop precipitously. Suppose this client's temperature is 103.5°F (39.7°C). In that case, in addition to his drop in BP, you should also anticipate a rise in pulse and respiratory rate. What should you do? Your action depends on the client's condition and the context. What else is going on in the situation? If medication for the fever has been prescribed for the client, you would administer the medication and evaluate the VS again at frequent intervals. If the VS do not improve, you would then notify the primary care provider.

Now change the context slightly. Add to your preceding data that the client has undergone a surgical procedure and is not taking any antibiotics. Now what should you do? If your answer is to notify the primary care provider, you are correct. Always evaluate all the VS as a unit. A sudden change in the client's condition requires you to thoroughly assess the client and report your findings to the primary care provider.

A change in a client's VS may also be a positive sign. For instance, if the client has been in severe pain for 3 days and has finally obtained pain relief, a decrease in BP probably indicates that the current medication regimen has provided better control of the pain. You would still need to monitor the VS at more frequent intervals, however, to ensure that the BP does not continue to fall.

Delegating Vital Signs

In many healthcare settings, several providers interact with the clients. VS may be obtained by nursing assistants or other unlicensed personnel.

 When working with complex or critical patients, you should carefully consider whether to delegate VS to a NAP. The significance of the VS results must be analyzed in relation to other assessment data.

If you are working in a team nursing model as the registered nurse (RN), you are responsible for reviewing and interpreting the findings of all NAPs. This includes evaluating the technique of NAPs and the accuracy of their measurements. The professional nurse *never* relinquishes the responsibility for interpretation of VS trends and decisions based on abnormal VS findings. As a student nurse, you are responsible for functioning within your scope of knowledge. If you are unsure how to interpret the meaning of a patient's VS, you must discuss the findings with your instructor and/or the nurse assigned to care for your client. Even though you are participating in the client's care, the assigned nurse maintains responsibility for client oversight.

 To explore learning resources for this chapter,

Go to DavisPlus at DavisPl.us/Wilkinson3.

Chapter Resources for Chapter 20:
   Response sheets for all learning activities
   Resources for Caregivers and Health Professionals
   Reading More About Vital Signs (suggested readings)
   Concept Map of chapter content
Interactive Case Studies
NCLEX-Style and Chapter Review Questions
Chapter Overview Podcasts

For references cited in this chapter,

 Go to Volume 2, **References Cited.**

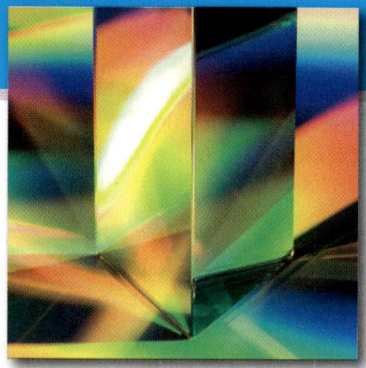

CHAPTER 21

Communication & Therapeutic Relationships

Learning Outcomes

After completing this chapter, you should be able to:

➤ Define communication.

➤ Identify the three basic levels of communication.

➤ Discuss the elements of the communication process.

➤ List the characteristics of verbal and nonverbal communication.

➤ Analyze factors that influence the communication process.

➤ Describe the elements of collaborative professional communication.

➤ Explain how relationships and roles influence communication.

➤ Describe the role of communication in each of the four phases of the therapeutic relationship.

➤ Compare and contrast techniques that enhance communication to techniques that hinder communication.

➤ Communicate with clients with impaired hearing, speech, or cognition.

➤ Communicate with clients whose culture or language is different from yours.

➤ Write a nursing care plan for a client experiencing impaired communication.

Key Concepts

Communication
Communication techniques
Therapeutic relationships

Related Concepts

See the Concept Map on Davis*Plus*.

Meet Your Patient

You have been assigned to care for John Barker, a 56-year-old man admitted to the hospital with bleeding in the lower gastrointestinal tract. When you approach Mr. Barker to introduce yourself, you find him in his room with his wife at the bedside. They are holding hands, and clearly both have been crying. You begin by saying, "Good afternoon, Mr. Barker, I am a nursing student from the nearby university. I've been assigned to care for you tomorrow." Mr. Barker swallows hard and says, "I don't think you'll be able to do anything for me!" His wife says, "Don't take it personally. It's not a good time right now. Please just leave us alone."

You leave the room unsure how to respond. When you go to the unit station to review the chart, the charge nurse says, "Oh my! You've been assigned to him? I hope you've got a lot of experience." As you review the chart, you realize that Mr. Barker was just informed that he has metastatic colon cancer and probably has only a few months to live.

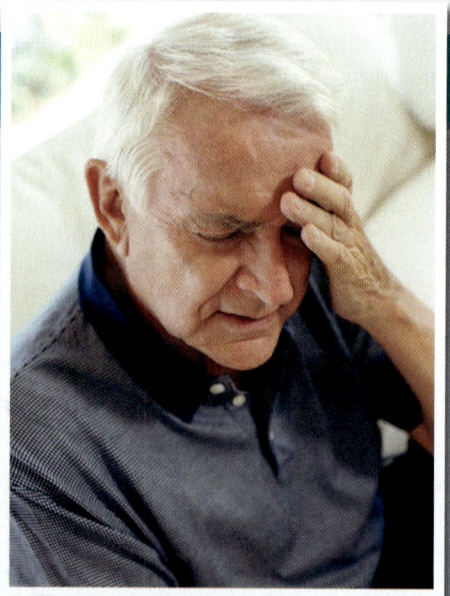

TheoreticalKnowledge
knowing **why**

As a resource to you while you are learning what it means to care for patients in difficult situations such as Mr. Barker's, you might look to the following professional and regulatory agencies that stress the importance of good communication:

- ✚ **Quality and Safety Education for Nurses (QSEN).** To provide for patient safety, nurses need to effectively communicate their concerns about hazards and errors to patients, families, and the healthcare team (Cronenwett, Sherwood, Barnsteiner, et al., 2007).
- **The Joint Commission (2013).** The Joint Commission National Patient Safety Goal 2, aims to improve patient safety by improving communication among caregivers.
- **The Joint Commission (2010b).** Performance standards state that patients have the right to receive effective, understandable information.

As you read this chapter, you will gain theoretical and practical knowledge to help you to communicate effectively with patients, families, and other members of the healthcare team.

ABOUT THE KEY CONCEPTS

In this chapter you will learn how **communication techniques** link to the concept of **communication**, and how they both help you to form **therapeutic relationships**. With an understanding of these and the related concepts, you will be able to communicate more effectively with patients, families, and members of the healthcare team.

WHAT IS COMMUNICATION?

Communication is a dynamic, two-way process of sending and receiving messages. The messages may be verbal, nonverbal, or both, and they may involve two or more people. As such, communication forms the basis for sharing meaning and building effective working relationships among individuals, families, and the healthcare team. Successful communication occurs when providers understand and use information shared by their patients when devising a plan for care. Likewise, patients must also be able to accurately comprehend information in a way that enables them to participate responsibly in their own care (The Joint Commission, 2010a, 2010b).

Communication is more than the act of talking and listening (Box 21-1). It is a basic function of human life. From the first cry of a newborn to the whisper of a patient who is dying, the primary purpose of communication is to share information and obtain a response. People use communication to meet their physical, psychosocial, emotional, and spiritual needs.

BOX 21-1 ■ What Is Communication?

Communication is ...

- Sharing or transmitting thoughts or feelings
- A way to meet physical, psychosocial, emotional, and spiritual needs
- A process—the act of sending, receiving, interpreting, and responding to a message
- Content—the actual subject matter, words, gestures, and substance of the message

---

Communication Occurs on Many Levels

When we think about communication, we usually imagine a dialogue between two individuals. But communication actually occurs on any of many levels.

Intrapersonal Communication is conscious internal dialogue, sometimes known as self-talk. Constructive affirmations, or positive self-talk (e.g., "This will work! I can do it"), promote success in a task. In contrast, negative self-talk (e.g., "I can't do this, it is too difficult") may adversely affect a person's ability to complete a task. Nurses often engage in intrapersonal communication. For example, if you enter a room and notice that your patient is pale, diaphoretic, and moaning, you may ask yourself, "What's happened? This client appears to be in a lot of pain."

Interpersonal Communication occurs between two or more people. Face-to-face conversation between two people is the most frequent form of interpersonal communication. Nurses use interpersonal communication to gather information during assessment, to teach about health issues, to explain care, and to provide comfort and support. In addition to communicating directly with clients, professional nurses communicate with other nurses and healthcare team members to provide comprehensive care for clients. Because professional nurses are accountable for appropriate delegation of activities, they must also communicate effectively with nursing assistive personnel (NAP).

Group Communication is interaction that occurs among several people. *Small-group communication* occurs when you engage in an exchange of ideas with two or more individuals at the same time. Examples of small-group communication include staff meetings, committee meetings, educational groups, self-help groups, and family teaching sessions. Working with groups requires effective communication skills and a basic understanding of group processes—discussed later in the chapter.

Public Speaking is a unique form of group communication. Generally, the speaker addresses a dozen to hundreds of people, with varying degrees of interaction. Speakers may deliver a speech, talk directly with a small group of audience members, or have open discussion with the group. Nurses engage in public speaking to educate groups of people about health issues, to lobby for health legislation, and to address colleagues at professional conferences.

Communication Involves Content

Communication has two major components: content and process. Both are important for effective communication. The **content** of communication describes the actual subject matter, words, gestures, and substance of the message. It is the message that everyone may hear or see. For example, suppose your client said, "I slept through lunch." This statement is open to interpretation. We cannot tell—without also observing him, knowing his history, and so on—whether he thinks this is a good thing because he wanted or needed rest, or a bad thing because he is so exhausted, or a complaint about the staff because they did not wake him for lunch, or an apology and request for a late lunch. As you can see, the words are just a part of communication. You must also consider the process.

Communication Is a Process

Process refers to the act of sending, receiving, interpreting, and reacting to a message. The communication process has five elements: sender, message, receiver, feedback, and channel. Figure 21-1 illustrates the relationship among these elements.

- The **sender** begins the conversation to deliver a message (content) to another person. The sender, also called the *source* or the *encoder,* uses verbal and nonverbal methods to transmit the message.

- **Encoding** refers to the process of selecting the words, gestures, tone of voice, signs, and symbols used to transmit the message. For example, as a beginning nursing student, you might feel anxious about caring for Mr. Barker (Meet Your Patient). How could you communicate your concerns to your instructor? You might directly state, "It makes me nervous to be assigned to him"; or you might avoid eye contact with your instructor and tell her, "I'm going to need some help today." Both styles communicate your anxiety, but they are encoded differently. Encoding is affected by the situation, the nature of the message, the mood of the sender, and the relationship between sender and receiver.

- The **message** is the verbal and/or nonverbal information the sender communicates. It might be content of a conversation, a speech, a gesture, a letter, and so forth. Effective messages are complete, clear, concise, organized, timely, and expressed in a manner that the receiver can understand. The message must be appropriate for the situation and for the developmental level of the person receiving the message.

- The **channel** is the medium used to send the message. Face-to-face communication is a commonly used channel. Nurses frequently use touch as a nonverbal way to communicate caring and concern. Other channels include written pamphlets, audiovisual aids, recordings, telephone and text messages, and the Internet. When choosing the best channel for communicating, consider the type of message, its purpose,

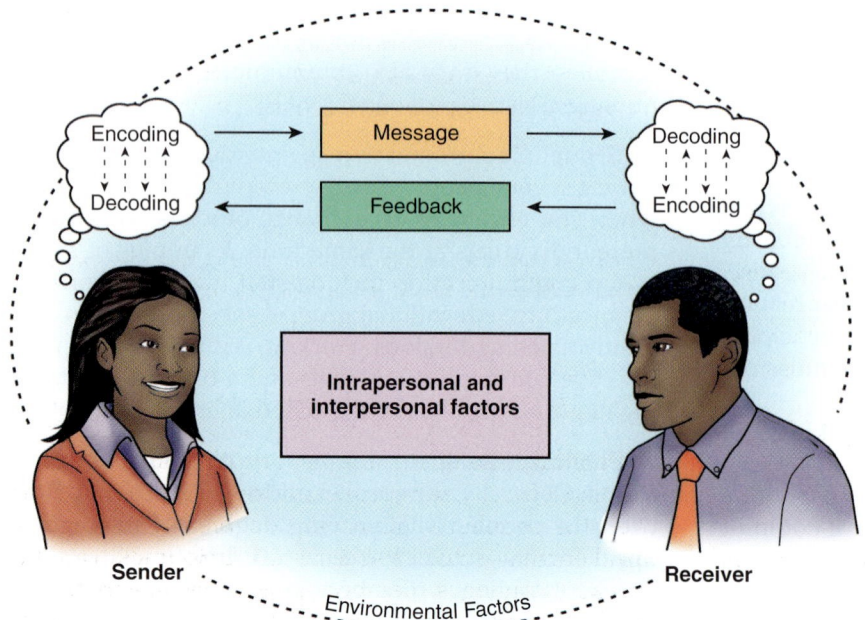

FIGURE 21-1 Communication: A sender encodes and transmits a message to a receiver, who decodes it and transmits feedback.

and the size of the audience. In Mr. Barker's case (Meet Your Patient), for example, touching his hand while remaining silent might send a clearer message of caring than any words you could say.

- The **receiver** is the observer, listener, and interpreter of the message. **Interpretation**, also called **decoding**, refers to relating the message to your past experiences to determine the sender's meaning. The receiver uses visual, auditory, and tactile senses to decode the message. If the decoded meaning matches the intended meaning, then the message was effective. However, messages are sometimes misinterpreted, especially when the receiver is not physically or emotionally ready to receive the message. For example, if you approached your instructor to discuss your concerns about Mr. Barker when she was assisting with an emergency, she might be unable to receive your message.
- **Feedback** may be verbal, nonverbal, or both. Once the receiver has received and interpreted the message, he may be stimulated to respond by providing feedback to the sender. Feedback validates that the receiver received the message and understood it as the sender intended. Verifying the message avoids confusion.

KnowledgeCheck 21-2

Using the Meet Your Patient scenario, identify at least one sender, one message, one receiver, one channel, and one example of feedback.

Verbal Communication

People send and receive messages both verbally and nonverbally. The two forms of communication occur spontaneously and simultaneously. **Verbal communication** is the use of spoken and written words to send a message. It is influenced by such factors as educational background, culture, language, age, and past experiences. Verbal communication is generally a conscious act in which the sender is able to select the most effective words to communicate a message. When delivering a verbal message, the goal is that the receiver will understand both your words and your meaning. Many factors, including the following, affect how a message is received.

Vocabulary

Healthcare workers have a large vocabulary of technical terms and jargon. However, laypersons are often unfamiliar with healthcare language and find its use intimidating, or at best puzzling. Consider the following example, in which a nurse says:

"You are scheduled for surgery tomorrow. You need to be NPO after 2400. I'll be in to prep the op site at about 8. You'll need to void before your pre-med. After that we'll move you to a gurney and transfer you to the holding area."

Do you think most clients would understand this message? Do *you* understand all the words? For various reasons (e.g., being embarrassed at not knowing), many clients hesitate to ask questions to clarify what said the healthcare provider says. How much better it would be if the nurse had said:

"Your surgery will be tomorrow morning. You will not be able to eat or drink anything after midnight. I'll come in about 8 in the morning to clean your hip and get it ready for the operation. Then you'll need to urinate before I give you some medicine to relax you. After that, we'll put you on a cart and roll you up to the operating area."

Key Point: *It is your responsibility to deliver messages that the client can understand; therefore, use medical terms only when you are certain the listener understands them.*

When encoding a message, consider the receiver's age, knowledge, education, and any cultural differences, including primary language spoken. (These factors are discussed shortly.) Encourage feedback to be sure that the receiver understood the message as you intended.

Denotative and Connotative Meaning

Denotation is the literal (dictionary) meaning of a word. In contrast, **connotation** is the implied or emotional meaning of the word. Consider the following examples:

A mother says to her infant, "Don't cry, baby."
A 40-year-old man says to his nurse, "Would you rub my back, baby?"
A 10-year-old boy says to another boy, "You're a baby!"

The denotative meaning of *baby* is a very young child who is not yet able to walk. However, the connotative meaning is different in each example. In the first example, the connotative meaning is the same as the denotative meaning. In the second example, the nurse might interpret it as a sexist remark; and in the last example, the 10-year-old boy undoubtedly meant *baby* as an insult. As you can see, words are often value-laden or biased. The situation, qualities of the participants, and the words they choose all affect interpretation. Use terms that provide clear, objective data and are not open for misinterpretation.

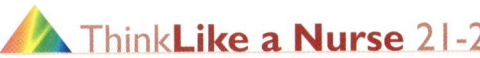 ### ThinkLike a Nurse 21-2

Think of two other examples in which the connotative meaning may be different from the denotative meaning.

Pacing

What happens when a professor talks very slowly during a lecture? Do you find your mind wandering: "I need to take the dog to the vet. . . . What shall we have for dinner? . . ." The pace and rhythm of the delivery can alter the receiver's interpretation of the message. A rapid pace does not allow the receiver to track what the speaker is saying, so the receiver may become frustrated and lose interest. The pace must be slow enough for the receiver to interpret one thought before the sender moves on to the next thought, but must also be fast enough to maintain the listener's interest. Pausing at intervals gives the listener time to respond.

Intonation

Tone of voice, or **intonation**, reflects the feeling behind the words. We get a sense of a person's intonation by listening to the *pitch* (high or low), *cadence* (rising and falling of the pitch), and *volume* (soft or loud). For example, experiment with the variety of ways you might say, "Your test results are in."

Pitch, cadence, and volume can either reinforce or contradict the message. When spoken at a moderate pitch and volume, with a falling cadence, the words, "I understand that I am to report at noon," can be a simple confirmation that the person has received the message while conveying emotions. People tend to lose interest when someone speaks in a monotone (does not vary the pitch, cadence, and volume). Before presenting lengthy information, whether to an individual or to a group, experiment with these variables to ensure that the listener remains engaged with your topic.

When electronic messaging is used, the receiver does not have the advantage of intonation or body language. This may lead to miscommunication. People sometimes insert *emoticons* (symbols such as "smiley faces"), uppercasing, and punctuation, such as exclamation marks, to provide cues to the emotional tone of a message.

Clarity and Brevity

Clarity in communication requires that you select words that convey the intended meaning and that you make sure your spoken words and the nonverbal language send the same message. You can achieve brevity by using the fewest words possible. A conversation that is clear and brief holds the interest of all parties and effectively conveys the intended messages.

Timing and Relevance

Timing is crucial. Before starting a conversation, assess your client. A person who is distracted by pain, hunger, or other physiological needs will not receive the message as you intended it. Similarly, a client attempting to cope with stressors, such as limited finances, an upcoming surgery, or a terminal diagnosis, may be unable to listen effectively.

- **Consider the presence of others.** Asking a client about a personal issue in a public corridor may inhibit his response. You will receive a different response if you ask the same question in a more private setting. In contrast, if you are instructing a client about a recommended diet, be sure that the person who is responsible for shopping and cooking is also present. If your client does neither in his household, he may pay little attention to your instruction—it will not be relevant to him.

- **Communication is effective when both parties value the interaction and find the discussion relevant.** To teach your client about his medicines, choose a time when he is alert, pain-free (or with a manageable pain level), and not distracted. Begin by reminding him of the purpose of the discussion: "I'm going to teach you how to take this medication so that it effectively controls your pain."

- **The interaction must allow time for response.** A rapid flow of questions or one-sided conversation inhibits interaction.

Credibility

Clients judge the **credibility** (or believability) of the message by the trustworthiness of the sender. Your credibility depends on a pattern of honest and timely response to patient concerns, as well as congruence between your verbal and nonverbal communication.

- **Give information only if you are certain of the facts.** As a nurse, you will be called on to provide information on a wide range of topics. Give information only if you are certain of the facts. A response such as, "I don't know, but I'll find out and let you know" is far more credible than an incorrect answer or a guess.

- **If a situation makes you uncomfortable, it is better to acknowledge your discomfort than to risk loss of credibility.** For example, you may feel uncomfortable talking to Mr. Barker (Meet Your Patient) about his recent diagnosis. You may be tempted to say, "Maybe the test results are wrong," or "The timeline is just a guess. I think you can beat this." This approach avoids uncomfortable discussion and may make the patient feel better temporarily. However, a more honest approach would be to tell Mr. Barker that you would like him to talk with a counselor or hospital chaplain.

- **Always be open and honest with patients.** Deceiving patients can take many forms, but it always destroys trust. Trust in their care providers helps patients feel less vulnerable. If you tell the patient you will be right back with pain medication but forget to return until she reminds you an hour later, she may doubt your credibility. False reassurance (e.g., telling him that the procedure won't hurt or everything will be okay) also reduces your credibility and conveys to the patient that he can't trust you to tell him the truth.

- **To be credible, your nonverbal communication must match your spoken words.** For example, if your client asks you whether his wound is "ugly," he will pay attention to your facial expressions as well as your spoken response. If you respond that "the wound looks good," but frown or fail to make eye contact, the client will most likely believe that you are not being completely honest. This may jeopardize future interactions.

Humor

Laughter can create physiological changes that contribute to well-being and provide an emotional release in a tense situation, thus positively influencing the patient's attitude and healing. Humor is highly subjective and personal; and it also depends on cultural norms. Use humor cautiously, and never direct humor at the client, disease process, or treatment team. Misused humor can have a negative effect on self-esteem, self-confidence, or the client's confidence in the treatment team. Consider the different effects the following uses of humor might have. Imagine that your patient has had vomiting and diarrhea for the past 8 hours. When you enter the room you jokingly say, "Oh my! You look like you had too much to drink last night." Although the intent was to lighten the mood, this statement may offend your patient. In contrast, imagine that you notice that an older patient thoroughly enjoys visits from his young grandchildren. You might consider sharing with him an amusing story about your own children.

Nonverbal Communication

Nonverbal communication (or body language) is the exchange of messages without the use of words. Verbal communication is a highly conscious activity in which we choose words to communicate. Nonverbal communication occurs on a more unconscious level. Because nonverbal language emerges from how the sender is feeling, it more accurately conveys the true meaning of a message. It may thereby reinforce or contradict the spoken message. For example, Mr. Barker (Meet Your Patient) uses few words. However, he is tearful and distressed. That body language gives you valuable insight into how he is adjusting to the news of his cancer. Let's look at some nonverbal messages.

Facial Expression

Expressions of the face and especially the eyes are some of the most obvious forms of nonverbal communication. Facial expressions communicate joy, anger, sadness, concern, or fear. Raised eyebrows, staring, squinting, or darting eyes all convey meaning.

Smiling is one expression that everyone understands. In contrast, the interpretation of many other facial expressions is culturally dependent. For example, downcast eyes may indicate sadness, poor self-esteem, a desire to avoid the conversation, respect, powerlessness, or submissive behavior. In Western cultures, eye contact usually indicates an interest in the conversation and a willingness to communicate; however, in Eastern cultures, the amount of eye contact considered acceptable varies. Chapter 15 discusses cultural variations.

A mismatch between your verbal message and facial expression may cause the client to doubt your credibility (Fig. 21-2). For example, suppose that a patient states, "I just had my pain pill. Why is my pain still so bad?" You answer, "The medication should take effect within a few more minutes. If it doesn't, call me." Imagine the

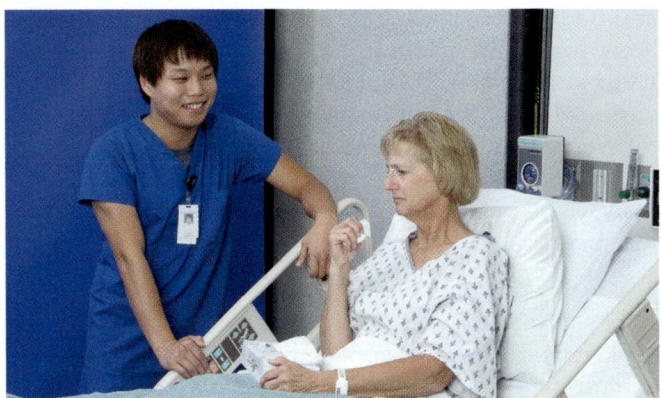

FIGURE 21-2 The nurse's facial expression is not appropriate because the patient appears to be in distress.

different effect this reply would have if you were smiling, frowning, raising one eyebrow, or avoiding eye contact.

Posture and Gait

Body position, gait, and posture offer clues to a person's attitudes, emotions, physical well-being, and self-concept. When you see someone with an erect posture, head held high, and a quick gait, what do you think? In Western culture, these are nonverbal indicators of health and a sense of self-assuredness. In contrast, a slow, shuffling gait may signify someone who is ill, has pain, is depressed, or has poor self-esteem.

Personal Appearance

Clothing and personal appearance provide clues to a person's feelings, socioeconomic status, culture, and religion. A person who is ill, tired, or depressed may lack energy for hygiene and grooming. Lack of attention to personal appearance is especially significant in a person who typically engages in meticulous grooming. As with all nonverbal data, you need to investigate the meaning of personal appearance to avoid drawing erroneous conclusions.

Dress and accessories are powerful cultural clues. Does the patient dress in a style that differs from local custom? Are pieces of jewelry or religious medallions visible? These are clues to the patient's values, as well as the patient's socioeconomic status. Pay attention to these clues, but do not make assumptions from them. A person who wears an elaborate religious medal may like the ornamentation but not espouse the beliefs that are attached to the symbol.

Key Point: *Have you thought about what your own personal appearance conveys to your patients and colleagues?*

Most people express their individuality through their clothing, hairstyle, and so on. Nurses, however, must also consider how patients perceive them and whether their appearance helps or hinders their patient relationships. Issues of safety and cleanliness are also essential for nurses, when choosing clothing, hairstyles, and body adornment (e.g., jewelry, nail polish, tattoos, body piercings). The traditional white nursing uniform has been almost completely replaced by scrubs of various colors, which makes it difficult for patients to differentiate nurses from the rest of the healthcare team. To counteract this, some agencies are assigning colors for various personnel (e.g., blue for physicians, purple for nurses).

Gestures

Hand and body gestures emphasize and clarify the spoken word. They are good indicators of the feeling tone behind the conversation. Imagine that your client says, "I'm okay." What might it mean if he accompanies his statement with a broad grin and raised arms? What might it mean if, instead, he lowers his head to his hands?

Gestures vary widely among individuals and cultures, so use them with caution. For example, consider the gesture of a "V" made with the second and third fingers of the hand. To some people, this is a peace sign; to others, it also represents the number two; and still others may attach no meaning to it at all. Gestures can help you communicate with individuals with impaired verbal communication, but only if you and the patient agree on the meaning of the gestures.

Touch

Touch can convey affection, caring, concern, and encouragement (Fig. 21-3). Avoid using touch when dealing with someone who is angry or mentally disturbed because the touch may be misinterpreted (e.g., as a sign of aggression or sexual attraction). Although touch can be highly effective, use it with sensitivity to the situation, environment, culture, and receptivity of the patient.

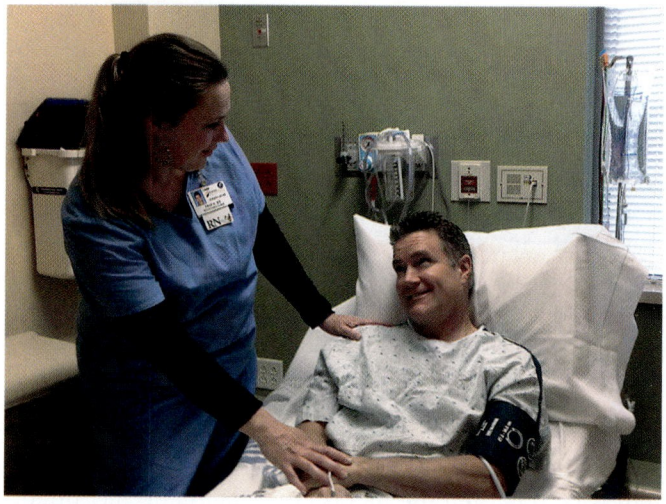

FIGURE 21-3 The nurse conveys genuine caring using touch.

For examples of therapeutic nonverbal behaviors and how patients may interpret them,

 Go to **Clinical Insight 21-1: Enhancing Communication Through Nonverbal Behaviors,** in Volume 2.

KnowledgeCheck 21-3

- Identify the components of verbal and nonverbal communication.
- What action should you take when there is a discrepancy between the client's spoken word and nonverbal body language?

Toward Evidence-Based Practice

Cousin, G., Mast, M. S., Roter, D., et al. (2012). Concordance between physician communication style and patient attitudes predicts patient satisfaction. *Patient Education and Counseling, 87(2),* 193–197.

This study investigated the impact of physicians' communication style on patient satisfaction. In a study of patients with recurrent headaches, researchers found that a high caring physician communication style led to higher satisfaction than a low caring one.

Griffiths, J., Speed, S., & Keeley, P. (2012). A caring professional attitude: What service users and carers seek in graduate nurses and the challenge for educators. *Nurse Education Today, 32(2),* 121–127.

Researchers compared the qualities emphasized in a nursing curriculum and those valued by patients. A diverse sample of patients expressed value in technical competence, knowledge, and willingness to seek information. Additionally, they overwhelmingly prioritized caring professional attitude,

which included empathy, communication skills, and nonjudgmental, patient-centered care.

1. Suppose you are a graduate nurse working in an intensive care unit of a large teaching hospital. You are providing care to the following three patients. What are some ways you would communicate caring to these patients and their families? List at least three strategies for each patient.
   a. 65-year-old man 3 hours post-op after repair of an abdominal aortic aneurysm. Your patient is intubated and breathing with the assistance of a mechanical ventilator. He is fully alert and responsive after surgery.
   b. 88-year-old frail woman with delirium receiving a blood transfusion for a lower GI bleed.
   c. 3-year-old child with an acute epiglottitis whose parents are not in the unit.

2. What pitfalls in communicating would you avoid in caring for your patients?

ThinkLike a Nurse 21-3

- Observe an interaction between family members or your fellow students. Look for congruence between verbal and nonverbal communication. Strategize what you would say to validate the intended meaning when the two modes of communication are not in agreement.
- Recall the brief interaction with the charge nurse in the Meet Your Patient scenario. What might you say or do in response?

WHAT FACTORS AFFECT COMMUNICATION?

The following is a discussion of the major factors, in addition to verbal and nonverbal language, that affect communication.

Environment

Communication is most successful in an environment that is quiet, private, free of unpleasant smells, and at a comfortable temperature. As a beginning student, you are aware of the noises and distractions in the clinical setting. However, experienced nurses become accustomed to such distractions. Be sensitive to how the environment is affecting your client. Background noise is distracting, interferes with hearing, and can create confusion. Being around others in pain or distress creates anxiety and fear; lack of privacy may cause embarrassment. All of those feelings may prevent your patient from sharing personal information.

Think creatively to secure the most comfortable environment possible for communicating with patients and families. Hospital chapels, foyers, and activity rooms may be ideal locations for conversation. To discuss private matters, consider talking with the patient in a conference room rather than a shared room. If none of these is possible, at least close privacy curtains and turn off the radio or television.

Developmental Variations

Physical and cognitive development, language skills, level of education, and maturity influence the communication process. Thus, you will need to modify your communication strategies to fit your client's developmental level. By the time you enter nursing practice, your goal should be to communicate effectively, respectfully, and compassionately with patients at all developmental stages.

- *Infants and young toddlers* with limited language skills communicate nonverbally. Your response may combine verbal and nonverbal communication. For example, if a hospitalized 1-year-old cries out for his mother, you might cuddle the child with his favorite toy and reassure him saying "Mama will be back very soon."
- *Older toddlers and preschoolers* have more verbal ability. Although they may prefer to have a parent present, they are likely to talk with you and answer questions.
- *School-age children* are usually quite comfortable interacting verbally. Pay attention to their vocabulary as they speak, and be sure to match it to the extent possible, using words and phrasing the child will understand.
- By the time children reach *adolescence*, most can process abstract concepts. As a result, they are usually able to understand disease processes, treatments, and other health issues. Bear in mind that children with chronic health problems that have required frequent interventions are often more knowledgeable than would be expected for their age.

Older adults may be affected by **sensory alterations**, such as hearing loss or vision changes, or any of a variety of healthcare problems that affect cognition, such as dementia. Communication strategies for these situations are discussed in the Planning Interventions/Implementation section of this chapter.

Gender

Males and females communicate differently and may interpret the same communication differently. Women tend to communicate to form connections and establish relationships (Tannen, 2001). In contrast, male communication styles typically focus on goals, tasks, and maintaining independence and favorable positions in a hierarchy.

These communication patterns have their roots in early socialization differences. Traditionally, boys are socialized to participate in competitive team sports. Through this play, they learn how to compete, strategize, and win or lose. In contrast, young girls are more likely to engage in one-on-one or fantasy play that requires cooperation and focuses on fairness and negotiation. This early socialization is carried over into communication patterns. Men are more likely to be comfortable in situations that result in a win or loss, whereas women are more likely to attempt to reach consensus. Male communication tends to be purpose driven: more about conveying information and accomplishing a goal, whereas female communication is more relationally driven.

Gender differences in communication are important to nurses because male and female patients may communicate their needs very differently. Similarly, the gender of the nurse may affect the response to the patient's requests. For example, a female patient might state, "I feel so lousy today." A female nurse may interpret this as a desire to talk. In contrast, a male nurse may discuss pain control.

Personal Space

People vary in the amount of physical space they are comfortable with when communicating. The distance they maintain between one another is influenced by the relationship of the individuals, the nature of the conversation, the setting, and cultural influences (Fig. 21-4). Also see Chapter 15 for cultural preferences for personal space. Hall (1992) describes four distinct distances influencing communication: intimate distance, personal distance, social distance, and public distance.

Intimate Distance is the area immediately surrounding people that they define as their "private space." People prefer to maintain intimate distance between themselves and others during interactions. In Western cultures, intimate distance is within 18 inches of the other person. Within this distance, people can sense each other's smell and body heat and usually can hear each other speaking at a low volume. It is also at this distance that body contact occurs. As a nurse, you invade a client's intimate distance to perform assessments and procedures. You even breach a client's intimate distance when touching a hand or shoulder to offer support. This may make some clients uncomfortable.

Key Point: *Before providing nursing interventions in the client's intimate distance, discuss what you are about to do. It is best to ask the client's permission, even for gentle touch, if you are in the slightest doubt about his receptivity.*

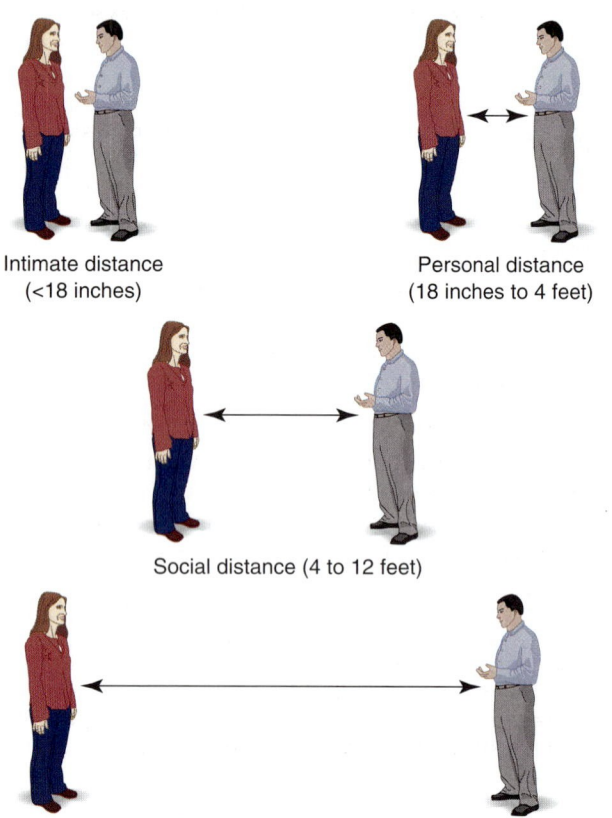

Intimate distance
(<18 inches)

Personal distance
(18 inches to 4 feet)

Social distance (4 to 12 feet)

Public distance (12 feet)

FIGURE 21-4 The distance that individuals who are engaged in communication maintain between one another is influenced by their relationship, the nature of the conversation, the setting, and cultural influences.

Personal Distance is a distance of 18 inches to 4 feet. Your interactions with clients and healthcare team members will commonly occur in this range. This distance facilitates sharing of feelings or personal thoughts and is appropriate to maintain when communicating caring or concern.

Social Distance is a distance of 4 to 12 feet. It is used in more formal interaction or when communicating with a group of individuals at the same time. At this distance, individuals are not within range to be physically touched. The volume of the spoken words may be loud enough for others to overhear, so people share personal feelings and thoughts less often at this distance. For example, if you stand by a client's door and ask how she is feeling, you will likely receive a more impersonal response than if you were to ask the same question at her bedside.

Public Distance is considered to be beyond 12 feet. This distance requires loud and clear enunciation for communication. This distance is characterized by a lack of individuality and a greater focus on the group or community.

Territoriality

Territoriality refers to the space and things that an individual identifies as belonging to him. Territories may be bounded and visible to others or may be defined by the individual in a way not noticeable to others. In a hospital setting, many clients consider everything within the curtain boundary to be their territory. Clients may be offended if you change, rearrange, or interfere with this territory by moving furniture, discarding objects, or borrowing items from the room, even if they are institutional property. To establish trust, you must request permission to rearrange the client's territory. Also recognize that hospitalized clients are not in their "home" territory and are therefore, likely to be less at ease during interactions.

Sociocultural Factors

Culture and socioeconomic status strongly influence communication. Facial expressions, nonverbal communication, and even the selection of whom to interact with are affected. For example, in some cultures it would be unacceptable for a male nurse to address and provide care to a female patient.

Social status also plays a role in communication. Have you ever been present while a physician explained a treatment plan to a patient? Often the patient asks no questions or nods approval, yet barrages you with questions when the physician leaves. This may be because many clients perceive less social distance between themselves and the nurse. Social distance can also play a role in how health professionals view patients. For example, you may see impoverished patients being treated with less respect than wealthy members of the community, although this is obviously unethical.

Roles and Relationships

Think of the way you interact with your instructor. Compare this with the way you interact with your class-mates. What are the differences? The roles and relationships of the sender and receiver affect the choice of vocabulary, tone of voice, use of gestures, and distance associated with the communication.

Many patients have stereotyped notions about nurses. Some may view you as an authority figure. Others may perceive nursing as a lowly occupation limited to matters of comfort and hygiene, and may not choose to have conversation with you. Still others become confused by the fact that many healthcare workers, such as medical assistants and nursing assistive personnel (NAPs), call themselves nurses in spite of the fact that they cannot legally use the title. If you are working with NAPs or other team members, be sure to clarify their roles with the patient so he can communicate his questions and concerns to the appropriate healthcare provider.

KnowledgeCheck 21-4

- What are the major factors that affect communication?
- In what distance(s) do most nurse–client interactions occur?

WHAT IS COLLABORATIVE PROFESSIONAL COMMUNICATION?

Communication is essential to collaborative practice among nurses, physicians, and health professionals from other disciplines. Each of you shares the common goal of providing optimal patient care. This goal guides the manner in which you communicate—at the bedside, at the nurse's station, in care conferences, or via the patient record. Nurses also communicate with peers and colleagues in order to contribute to their professional development. See Box 21-2 for statements from professional organizations about collaborative communication.

Think of communication styles as a continuum from passive, through assertive, to aggressive. A **passive**

BOX 21-2 ■ Collaborative Professional Communication

American Nurses Association (ANA) (2010)

Standards of professional performance stress the importance of communication to collegiality, leadership, and collaboration. The following are some of the competencies for these standards. The registered nurse:

Standard 11. Communication

- Assesses communication format preferences of healthcare consumers, families, and colleagues.
- Assesses his or her own communication skills in encounters with healthcare consumers, families, and colleagues.
- Seeks continuous improvement of communication and conflict resolution skills.
- Conveys information to healthcare consumers, families, the interprofessional team, and others in communication formats that promote accuracy.
- Questions the rationale supporting care processes and decisions when they do not appear to be in the best interest of the patient.
- Discloses observations or concerns related to hazards and errors in care or the practice environment to the appropriate level.
- Maintains communication with other providers to minimize risks associated with transfers and transition in care delivery.
- Contributes her or his own professional perspective in discussion with the interprofessional team.

Standard 12. Leadership

- Develops communication and conflict resolution skills.
- Communicates effectively with the healthcare consumer and colleagues.

Standard 13. Collaboration

- Communicates effectively with the healthcare consumer, the family, and healthcare providers regarding healthcare consumer care and the nurse's role in the provision of care.

- Applies group process and negotiation techniques with healthcare consumers and colleagues.

Standard 14. Professional Practice Evaluation

- Provides peers with formal or informal constructive feedback regarding their practice or role performance.

American Association of Critical-Care Nurses (AACN)

Skilled communication is necessary to a healthy work environment. Nurses must be proficient in communication skills. Critical elements of communication include the following:

- Focusing on finding solutions and achieving desirable outcomes
- Seeking to protect and advance collaborative relationships among colleagues
- Inviting and hearing all relevant perspectives
- Striving for goodwill and mutual respect
- Building consensus and arriving at common understanding
- Achieving congruence between words and actions, and holding others accountable for doing so
- Developing proficiency with communication technologies (AACN, 2005)

Quality and Safety Education for Nurses (QSEN)

Communication is essential for teamwork and collaboration. On graduation from nursing school, you should be able to analyze differences in others' communication style preferences and describe the impact of your own communication style on others (Cronenwett, Sherwood, Barnsteiner, et al., 2007).

The Joint Commission (2013)

The 2013 National Patient Safety Goals added Goal 2.03.01, which calls for getting important test results to the right staff person on time. The broad Goal 2 calls for improving the effectiveness of communication among caregivers.

approach avoids conflict and allows others to take the lead. It tends to be submissive, helpless, indecisive, apologetic, or whining. "Whatever you want. I don't want you to change anything for me," is an example of a passive approach. In contrast, an **aggressive approach** forces others to lose. The goal is to win and be in control. "My way is the correct way. You don't know what you're talking about" typifies an aggressive approach. Other aggressive characteristics include being bossy, arrogant, opinionated, sarcastic, manipulative, intolerant, or overbearing.

Why might you adopt a **nonassertive style**? As you have learned, men and women tend to communicate differently. The same is true when communicating with persons of higher or lower status. When speaking to physicians, some nurses still communicate their needs in a style that assures physicians that they are not telling them what to do (e.g., "Do you think Mrs. King's heart rate is a little fast today?" instead of "Mrs. King's heart rate was 120 beats per minute at 0800." This has been referred to as the "doctor–nurse game" (Stein, Watts, & Howell, 1990). Such unclear, indirect communication contributes to errors and poor patient outcomes.

Communicating Assertively

Assertive communication is the expression of a wide range of positive and negative thoughts and feelings in a style that is direct, open, honest, spontaneous, responsible, and nonjudgmental. Assertiveness recognizes your rights while still respecting the rights of others. It allows you to take responsibility for your own thoughts and actions without blaming others, encourages feedback, and enables you to find mutually satisfying solutions to conflict by confronting people constructively.

✚ Effective communication and teamwork are essential for the delivery of high-quality, safe patient care. To avoid communication failures that can lead to unanticipated adverse events in patients, nurses must speak up when they have concerns and take the necessary steps to communicate assertively and collaboratively with the healthcare team.

A study exploring nurses' perception of their ability to speak up and be heard in the workplace environment found open communication leads to better patient care, improved safety, and better staff satisfaction (Garon, 2012). To advocate for clients, you must question care decisions that don't seem right to you, and assertively discuss errors or poor clinical judgment with coworkers.

So how do you communicate assertively?

- *Question care decisions openly and honestly.* Refuse to play the doctor–nurse game. Avoid beginning your statements with self-effacing statements that fail to take credit for your contributions (e.g., "You may disagree with this, but . . ."). Be frank, but be flexible and open-minded.

- *Use "I" statements.* An "I" statement should include the elements of behavior (or facts), feeling, and effect (on you). For example, instead of saying, "Why haven't you ordered Mrs. Johnson's pain medications yet?" you might say, "I telephoned you this morning about Mrs. Johnson's lack of pain relief, but I don't see a change in her analgesic order. I am concerned about her discomfort and the effect it may have on her willingness to ambulate."

- *Focus on the issue, not the participants.* For example, "I think this approach might be the best, but I'd like to hear your thoughts."

- *Use effective nonverbal language.* Your body and verbal language should be congruent. Eye contact demonstrates interest and shows sincerity. Use a calm, well-modulated voice tone, and add appropriate gestures for emphasis.

- *Don't invite negative responses.* For example, say, "I would really appreciate it if you could help me weigh Mr. Max on the bed scale," rather than, "Can you help me weigh him?"

- *Use "fogging" to help you accept criticism without becoming anxious or defensive.* Acknowledge that there may be some truth to it, but remain the judge of your own action Suppose Mrs. Johnson's physician says, "Are you playing pharmacist today?" You might respond, "I agree that I may not be a pharmacist and that I do not know everything there is to know about analgesics. However, Mrs. Johnson needs pain relief and I need your assistance with pain medication."

- *Use negative inquiry.* You might choose, in the preceding situation, to use negative inquiry. You would reply, "So you believe that I do not have adequate knowledge to discuss Mrs. Johnson's pain control?"

- *Strive for a workable compromise*, but not if it affects patient well-being or your feelings of self-respect. Suppose an administrator comes to a patient's room while you are inserting a nasogastric tube and says, "I need to see you right now. Come to the desk immediately." An example of a workable compromise would be to say, "I understand that you need to talk to me right away, and I need to finish what I am doing. So what about meeting you at the desk as soon as I finish, in about 10 minutes?"

- **Key Point:** Use "critical (CUS) language." *Remember the words* **C***oncerned,* **U***ncomfortable, and* **S***afety—as in, "I'm concerned, I'm uncomfortable, this is unsafe, or I'm scared" (Leonard, Graham, & Bonacum, 2004). Some organizations identify a code phrase for themselves, for example, "I need clarity." When anyone there says, "I need clarity," the receiver of the request must stop and listen attentively while the sender asserts the issues that need to be clarified (Amer, 2013).*

It may help to practice ahead of time how you want to look and sound before attempting assertive communication. Assertiveness is a learned skill. Role-playing with a colleague can build your confidence.

For a summary of assertive communication techniques, see Box 21-3. Also,

 Go to Chapter 21, **Clinical Insight 21-2, Techniques for Assertive Communication,** in Volume 2.

Using Standardized Communication Tools

Doctors and nurses often have different communication styles. Nurses are taught to be more descriptive of clinical situations, whereas physicians learn to be very concise. Standardized communication tools are quite effective in overcoming differences in nurse–physician communication styles, and conveying key information clearly and concisely. Structured communication tools not only ensure accuracy but also create an environment for individuals to speak up and express concerns, thus improving interdisciplinary communication and patient outcomes.

A well-known and highly effective method for team communication and collaboration is the **SBAR** model. The acronym represents **S**ituation, **B**ackground, **A**ssessment, **R**ecommendation. For a summary of this model,

 Go to Chapter 21, **Clinical Insight 21-3, Communicating With SBAR,** in Volume 2.

If you need other information about giving a verbal report, also see Chapter 18.

Using the Patient Rounds Approach

Patient rounding is a collaborative approach in which physicians and nurses gather at the patient's bedside to discuss goals for care and/or changes in the plan of care and to answer the questions of the patient, family, and healthcare staff. Meeting for rounds allows the nurse to provide input, which results in improved nurse and physician working relationships and professional satisfaction (Chapman, 2009).

BOX 21-3 ■ Five Steps for Assertive Communication

1. Get the person's attention.
2. Express your concern.
3. State the problem.
4. Propose an action.
5. Reach a decision.

Source: Leonard, M., Graham, S., & Bonacum, D. (2004). The human factor: The critical importance of effective teamwork and communication in providing safe care. *Quality and Safety in Health Care, 13*(Suppl.), 85–90.

WHAT IS THE ROLE OF COMMUNICATION IN THERAPEUTIC RELATIONSHIPS?

Caring is integral to a therapeutic nurse–patient relationship, which according to Benner (1984) is the hallmark of nursing practice. She uses the terms of connectedness and involvement to describe nursing. These terms are also the foundation of meaningful communication (Alpers, Jarrell, & Roxena, 2013). In today's demanding environment, nurses multitask and function with many competing priorities. Because of this, they run the risk of conveying a rushed, noncaring attitude to patients. This can be frustrating to patients and exhausting for nurses.

A **therapeutic relationship** focuses on improving the health of the client, whether an individual or community. The client gains information and knowledge and works through issues, concerns, and problems related to health status, treatments, and nursing care. **Therapeutic communication** is client-centered communication directed at achieving client goals. It is used to establish the therapeutic relationship, provide and obtain healthcare information, and express interest, concern, and caring for the client and family.

Communication Is Essential to All Phases of the Therapeutic Relationship

The therapeutic relationship consists of four phases. As you read about each phase, notice the fundamental role of client-focused communication.

Pre-interaction Phase Even before you meet the client, the pre-interaction phase is established. You begin establishing communication by gathering information about the client, but the nurse and client do not have direct communication. As a student, you initiate this phase as you prepare for clinical days. The client also experiences a pre-interaction phase when she identifies the need for healthcare.

Orientation Phase The phase begins when you meet the client and introduce yourself and your role in the relationship. You then address him by his preferred name and/or title. In the orientation phase before collecting personal or health information, inform the client that pertinent information will be shared with the healthcare team (Nurses Association of New Brunswick, 2011).

The goal of this phase is to establish rapport and trust through the use of verbal and nonverbal communication. When rapport is established, patients are more likely to express their concerns openly and seek emotional support (Joanna Briggs Institute, 2011). As patients may not be immediately ready to communicate, it is important to be sensitive to the patient's mood, past experience, and overall physical and psychological state. Try to understand the cause of the client's behavior, comments, and attitudes, and respond with patience and wisdom. Orientation ends when the relationship has been defined.

Working Phase The bulk of therapeutic communication occurs in the **working phase**, the active part of the relationship. During this phase, the nurse communicates caring, the patient expresses thoughts and feelings, mutual respect is maintained, and honest verbal and nonverbal expression occurs. Key communication goals are to assist the client to clarify feelings and concerns. A professional relationship is courteous, competent, trustworthy, and confidential, and accomplished by active listening and other techniques of therapeutic communication presented later in this chapter.

Termination Phase The conclusion of the relationship marks the **termination phase**, whether at the end of the nurse's shift or on the client's discharge from the unit, facility, or service. Reviewing and summarizing help to bring the relationship to a comfortable conclusion. If communication has been effective, the termination phase prepares the nurse and client for future interactions. Unsuccessful communication may affect the client's health outcomes or understanding of his disease process, as well as affect the nurse's job satisfaction.

 Think**Like a Nurse** 21-4

Recall the scenario of Mr. Barker (Meet Your Patient).

■ What phase of the therapeutic relationship is illustrated in the scenario?

■ How might the interaction between you and Mr. Barker change if it occurred in a different phase of the therapeutic relationship?

■ What could you have done differently?

Therapeutic Communication Has Five Key Characteristics

The therapeutic relationship requires conscious use of your knowledge and skills to effect change in the patient. This is often called the *therapeutic use of self*. Therapeutic use of self requires some practice for you to recognize the boundaries of a therapeutic relationship and to keep the focus on the patient rather than on your own feelings and experiences. Five qualities characterize communication in the therapeutic relationship: empathy, respect, genuineness, concreteness, and confrontation. Box 21-4 identifies skills associated with these qualities. Later, the chapter presents specific strategies for enhancing communication, as well as barriers to therapeutic communication. Look for these techniques and barriers in any conversation you analyze.

Empathy The desire to understand and be sensitive to the feelings, beliefs, and situation of another person is called **empathy**. Empathy is more than sharing of information. Empathy requires you to be willing to adapt your style, tone, vocabulary, and behavior to create the

---

Quality and Safety Education for Nurses

Limits and Boundaries of Therapeutic Relationships

Chapter Key Concept: *Therapeutic Relationships*

Competency: *Patient-Centered Care (Knowledge, Skill)**

What are boundaries? Boundaries define personal space and allow people to communicate comfortably. This box illustrates the effects of boundaries on the competency, Patient-Centered Care, and the key concept, therapeutic relationships. Therapeutic (professional) relationships have stricter boundaries than personal relationships: Questions and comments made to friends may be inappropriate between colleagues or with clients. Moreover, boundaries between patients and care providers are not equal and are not always clear. Patients are asked intimate details of their lives, are physically exposed, and are often dependent on the care provider. Behaviors that suggest you might have boundary issues include:

➤ Thinking about or socializing with the patient while away from work.

➤ Disclosing personal information.

➤ Engaging in physical contact, flirting, or discussing sexual attraction, including by texting or online messaging.

Think about it: How do those factors make patients vulnerable? What Knowledge and Skills do you need to develop trust-based therapeutic relationships with patients

and families? What can you do to help them maintain their dignity?

Actions: In developing professional and therapeutic boundaries, try to achieve the "zone of helpfulness." That is, find a balance between under-involvement on one end and over-involvement on the other (National Council of State Boards of Nursing [NCSBN], 2009). The NCSBN calls for nurses to:

➤ Show respect for human dignity.

➤ Avoid personal gratification at the patient's expense.

➤ Never interfere in the patient's personal relationships.

➤ Promote patient autonomy and self-determination.

➤ Understand that the nurse–patient relationship is based on trust.

Nurses have a moral duty to protect patients from inappropriate relationships. Patient-centered care is only possible when boundaries are respected and patients and their families feel safe.

Sources: Hall, K. (2011); Hanna, A., & Suplee, P. (2012); Holder, K., Schenthal, S. (2007); NCSBN (2007).
*For specific Knowledge, Skills, and Attitudes

 Go to the QSEN Web site at http://qsen.org/ competencies/pre-licensure-ksas/

BOX 21-4 ■ Skills Needed in a Therapeutic Relationship

The ability to:

- Appreciate experiences and beliefs that differ from your own.
- Recognize and interpret verbal and nonverbal messages.
- Guide the interaction to accomplish goals.
- Determine *whether* communication is taking place.
- Speak when appropriate and remain silent when appropriate.
- Adapt to the pace, tone, and vocabulary of the client.
- Evaluate your own participation in an interaction.

best approach for each client situation. It is relatively easy to have empathy for people who are like you and who are likeable. It is more difficult to connect with people you see as "difficult" or "different." To empathize with a client, you must look beyond outward appearance or behavior and put yourself, mentally and emotionally, in the client's place. This will help you appreciate the uniqueness of the client and better understand his needs.

Respect   In the therapeutic relationship, you communicate **respect** by valuing the client and being flexible to meet the client's needs. As a nurse, you must be willing to adjust to your client rather than expecting the client to adjust to you, the healthcare environment, or hospital routines. Most healthcare experiences strip the client of power—clothes are removed, roles are discontinued or altered, people are separated from loved ones and familiar surroundings, and schedules are changed. When a relationship is grounded in respect, both parties maintain power and self-esteem. You show your respect for clients in the way you address them, the words and intonation you choose, and in your acknowledgment of their strengths and needs. Making even minor adjustments, such as delaying breakfast for an hour to allow the client to sleep, communicates that you respect the client's wishes.

Genuineness   When interviewing clients, we expect them to respond truthfully. After all, many healthcare decisions are based on the client's responses. Similarly, clients have a right to expect truthful responses from healthcare providers as well. **Genuineness** is the ability to respond honestly. If you are unable to answer a client's question, do not offer guesses. Be honest. Tell the client you need assistance before you can answer the question. Genuineness also involves willingness to self-evaluate. How well did I communicate? Did I handle that situation appropriately? How could I improve my communication?

Concreteness and Confrontation   In a therapeutic relationship, you must offer understandable responses to a client's questions and concerns. To do so requires you to express in concrete, specific terms what you mean. The message must be constructed and delivered in a manner that is suitable for the client. Communication is a reciprocal process. If your client is unable to express his thoughts clearly, you must be willing to confront her to request clarification. Similarly, you must be willing to be confronted if you are unclear.

Communication Is Important in Group Helping Relationships

Most of our previous discussion focused on one-on-one communication. However, nurses frequently communicate with groups. Group communication occurs when you interact with a family, a community, or a committee. Groups can enhance problem-solving and creativity, generate understanding and support, enhance morale, and provide affiliation.

Task Groups are formed to address a task or fulfill a need. Members are chosen based on ability to complete the task or defined project. Short-term groups dissolve once the task is completed. *Short-term groups* might include a task force to address holiday scheduling or a panel to critique response to a disaster drill. Because the time together is limited, the focus of communication is on the task at hand. Often, time to develop rapport or relationships is limited. Direct verbal communication with congruent nonverbal communication allows the group to function most effectively.

Ongoing Groups address issues that are recurrent. Committees are a form of task group. Common ongoing committees in healthcare organizations include quality assurance, infection control, and discharge planning. A committee has a chairperson who may be elected from within or appointed. Members have designated roles within the groups (e.g., recorder, time keeper). In small groups, all members have an opportunity to communicate their opinions. In larger groups, patterns of communication form; some members voice their opinion regularly, whereas others are often silent. When not all members speak, it is essential to examine nonverbal behavior to determine whether the nonspeaking members are in agreement.

Self-Help Groups are voluntary organizations composed of individuals with a common need. Alcoholics Anonymous may be the most widely recognized self-help group. Other well-known self-help groups include Weight Watchers, Narcotics Anonymous, and Reach for Recovery (for women with breast cancer).

Nurses may be members, facilitators, or consultants for self-help groups. Members are encouraged to share experiences and seek support from other members of the group. Members who have met the goals of the group often serve as the group facilitator by leading the interactions, or simply arranging meeting logistics. Healthcare professionals or experts in the field may be consulted to offer guidance or education to the group. Self-help groups most often have face-to-face meetings; but may also participate through social networking or blog groups, or receive information via newsletters. Communication of shared interests or needs is the link that holds these groups together.

Therapy Groups are organized to help individual members cope with challenging personal issues or stressful life events, such as divorce, death of a spouse, or new motherhood. Therapy groups may also address ways improve relationships and improve communication between or among people. These groups are also called self-awareness or growth groups. They may be ongoing or have a designated length of operation.

Community, public health, and psychiatric nurses sometimes facilitate therapy groups. Group facilitators arrange the time and place of the group and often introduce topics for discussion.

Work-Related Social Support Groups help members of a profession cope with the stress associated with their work. Social support groups provide an opportunity to share concerns and offer mutual support through formal meetings with a facilitator or informal drop-in events.

Formation of a group does not guarantee its success. To be successful, a group must have characteristics that allow the group to function and achieve its goals (Box 21-5).

KnowledgeCheck 21-5

- Identify and describe the phases of the therapeutic relationship.
- What are the five characteristics of therapeutic communication?
- Describe the difference between a task group and a self-help group.
- Compare and contrast the role of a therapy group with a work-related support group.

BOX 21-5 ■ Characteristics of a Successful Group

A successful group has:

- Clearly defined purpose
- Shared set of guidelines under which the group functions
- Sense of shared responsibility
- Shared leadership
- Mutual trust
- Comfort among members
- Climate that is cohesive but does not stifle individuality
- Members who are willing to share feelings, concerns, or beliefs
- Flexibility to change what is not working

 ThinkLike a Nurse 21-5

Review the local newspaper, hospital bulletin board, Internet search engines, and the school intranet. Identify at least three group helping experiences available. How might you learn more about these organizations? How would you determine whether they are resources that you might make available to your patients?

PracticalKnowledge
knowing **how**

Therapeutic communication is used throughout the nursing process. In the next few sections we will explore communication problems as well as therapeutic interventions.

ASSESSMENT

Assessment is essential to effective communication. You should assess for factors that alter a client's ability to receive, process, or transmit information, such as the following:

- *Language barrier.* Imagine how difficult it would be if you became ill while traveling in a country where you were unable to speak or read the language. How would you communicate that you were nauseated or in pain; how would you tell a care provider the point at which the symptom started or what makes it worse? Also consider your client's education and literacy. You cannot assume that everyone has an extensive vocabulary, nor that they can read and write.
- *Cognitive skills.* Difficulty understanding or engaging in communication may signal cognitive impairment. Developmental delays and pathology or injury of the central nervous system affect language and cognitive skills.
- *Sensory perceptual alterations.* Assess hearing and vision. Assess for **aphasia** (a difficulty expressing or interpreting messages that may develop after cerebrovascular accident [stroke] or neurological disease). Drug or alcohol intoxication can also interfere with perception and the ability to perceive or receive accurate information.
- *Physiological barriers.* These may include respiratory problems, loose-fitting dentures, or cleft palate, which may interfere with speaking.

For guidelines for a focused communication assessment,

 Go to Chapter 21, **Assessment Guidelines and Tools,** in Volume 2.

ANALYSIS/NURSING DIAGNOSIS

Communication can be the problem or the etiology of a nursing diagnosis. The following NANDA-I diagnosis labels describe communication problems. Note that communication problems may involve the inability to receive, interpret, or express spoken, written, and non-verbal messages.

- *Readiness for Enhanced Communication* is appropriate when the client expresses willingness to enhance communication that is already effective.
- *Impaired Verbal Communication* is an appropriate diagnosis if the client has (1) expressive aphasia or a physiological problem such as dyspnea, stuttering, or laryngeal cancer that impairs the ability to speak; or (2) receptive aphasia or sensory deficits that impair the ability to receive messages.
- *Impaired Communication* is the preferred diagnosis if the client is unfamiliar with the dominant language or has some other difficulty receiving and sending messages. Note that this is not a NANDA-I label.

Etiologies of Communication Diagnoses

Your assessment data will help you determine whether communication impairment is the primary problem or whether it is a result of other health problems. Some nursing diagnoses may cause or contribute to communication problems. For example:

- Clients with Acute or Chronic Confusion often have difficulty expressing or receiving verbal and nonverbal messages. Confusion may be related to physical or mental health problems, or may be a side effect of medications or sleep deprivation.
- Mental health problems can also lead to communication problems. For example, Anxiety impairs the ability to deliver and receive messages, and Chronic or Situational Low Self-Esteem often results in limited interaction with others.

Communication as Etiology of Other Nursing Diagnoses

Impaired Verbal Communication may be the etiology of other nursing diagnoses, for example:

- Anxiety r/t inability to communicate needs
- Social Isolation r/t difficulty maintaining relationships secondary to Impaired Verbal Communication
- Impaired Social Interaction r/t inability to carry on conversation
- Chronic Low Self-Esteem r/t fear of conversing with others secondary to stuttering

▰▰▰ PLANNING OUTCOMES/EVALUATION

NOC standardized outcomes associated with Impaired Verbal Communication include Communication, Communication: Expressive, and Communication: Receptive. To see selected indicators for those outcomes,

Go to Chapter 21, **Standardized Language, Selected NOC Outcomes and NIC Interventions for Impaired Verbal Communication,** on DavisPlus.

Using NOC indicators with the outcomes, you can develop goals for clients' communication problems.

Individualized client outcomes and goals depend on the nursing diagnosis you identify. For example, for Impaired Verbal Communication, you might write the following desired outcomes. The client:

- Uses alternative methods of communication (e.g., writing, picture board, gestures) effectively (specify time frame).
- Demonstrates minimal frustration with communication difficulties (specify time frame).
- Communicates effectively using a translator or interpreter.
- Interprets messages accurately, as evidenced by appropriate verbal or nonverbal feedback.

▰▰▰ PLANNING INTERVENTIONS/IMPLEMENTATION

Examples of *NIC standardized interventions* for Impaired Verbal Communication are Active Listening; Communication Enhancement: Hearing Deficit, Speech Deficit; Dementia Management; and Environmental Management. For other NIC interventions and selected nursing activities,

Go to Chapter 21, **Standardized Language,** on DavisPlus.

Specific nursing activities for communication problems depend on the etiology of the problem and on the goals selected. The focus of nursing interventions is to facilitate communication and to resolve or reduce the factors interfering with it.

Enhancing Therapeutic Communication

The following are techniques and activities you can implement immediately to improve your communication with patients and others.

Active Listening

People often think of listening as a passive activity. If you have ever been in a one-sided conversation, you are certainly aware that listening can be passive. In contrast, an active listener uses all senses to focus on the sender's message. An active listener gives full attention and allows the sender the opportunity to complete comments without interruption. To listen actively, pay attention to verbal and nonverbal communication and look for congruence. If a message is unclear, seek clarification through use of probing questions or reflective comments, such as "Tell me more," or "When you say . . . what do you mean?"

You can demonstrate active listening by facing your client, making eye contact, and focusing the conversation on issues of importance to the client (Fig. 21-5). If you must take notes during the conversation, record only key words to stimulate your memory at another time. Taking extensive notes distracts you from active

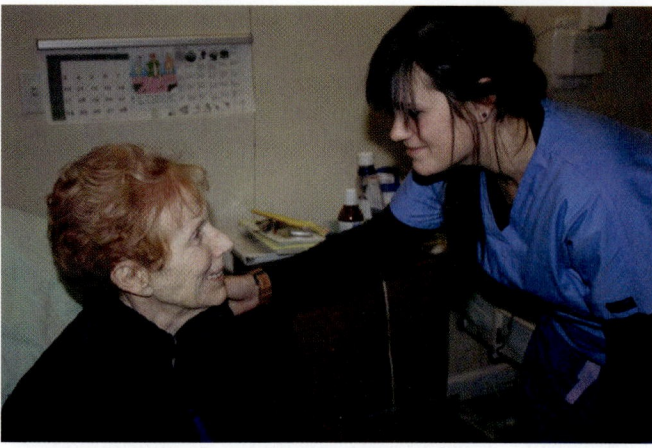

FIGURE 21-5 Active listening using full attention, direct eye contact, and caring touch.

Source: Adapted from Leebov, W. (2011, July 11). Nursing communication: How to make sure patients feel our caring. Retrieved May 5, 2013, from http://allnurses.com/showthread.php?t=378288

BOX 21-6 ■ Communicating With Care

- Keep your attention in the moment and on the patient.
- While the patient is sharing personal information, tune in and do not multitask.
- Face the person. Lean in. Pay attention.
- Maintain eye contact while listening.
- Do not interrupt the patient.
- Avoid glancing at your cell phone or watch. And never text while the patient is talking.
- Do not casually talk with coworkers while the patient is waiting.

listening. Active listening behaviors convey caring; signal a willingness to listen; and provide a comfortable environment for the client to share his concerns (Box 21-6).

Failure to listen to your client will result in missed messages or misinterpretation. Consider this example:

Patient:	I guess I'm going to surgery tomorrow.
Nurse:	[*Checking the IV fluids and hanging a medication*] Uh-huh.
Patient:	The surgeon says I'll be in intensive care for a few days.
Nurse:	[*Looking at the drainage in the urine collection bag*] Okay. Your urine looks good.
Patient:	I guess this is pretty risky surgery.
Nurse:	[*Recording on the flowsheet*] Yep.

How do you think the patient must feel in this situation? The patient is clearly expressing concern about his upcoming surgery and seems to want to talk about it with the nurse. However, the nurse is busy with a variety of tasks and is not paying attention to the conversation. Undoubtedly, the patient will continue to feel anxious. In fact, his unsuccessful attempts to communicate may even increase his anxiety. If the nurse were listening, this would be an excellent opportunity to discuss the patient's concerns, provide preoperative teaching, and help the patient ease his anxiety.

Establishing Trust

Mutual trust is an essential component not just of professional communication, but also of therapeutic communication because it facilitates disclosure and honesty. As you and the client establish trust, the client can more easily relay information and share feelings. To establish trust, always greet the client by name, listen actively, respond honestly to the client's concerns, and provide care competently and consistently.

Being Assertive

An assertive person is one who is able to express himself effectively and directly communicate his point of view while still respecting the viewpoint and beliefs of others. Because assertive communication is based on mutual respect, the therapeutic relationship is a safe place for clients to convey their needs and concerns without feeling judged. As needed, review assertiveness and collaborative professional communication, earlier in this chapter (e.g., Box 21-3).

Restating, Clarifying, and Validating Messages

Restating means using your own words to summarize the message you received from the client. This demonstrates concern, active listening, and understanding of what the patient has said. Below is an example:

Client:	I'm so worried about this diabetes. I have young kids. I want to see them grow up. Every diabetic I've known has died young.
Nurse:	Diabetes is a serious disease. I understand your worry about its effects on you. However, we want to focus on becoming well controlled so that you can avoid complications.

Clarifying messages helps ensure that you have accurately interpreted the information. For instance, you might state, "I'm not sure what you mean when you say you're so worried about your diabetes." Or, "When you say you're worried, what do you mean?"

To **validate** the message, ask the client whether you are making a correct interpretation: "When you say you're worried about your diabetes, do you mean you are afraid you will die soon?" These techniques help to identify client concerns and focus communication. They are especially helpful if the client is unclear or vague with a message.

Interpreting Body Language and Sharing Observations

Be attentive to what the patient says and how she says it. Note the tone of voice, rate of speech, distance, eye movement, facial expressions, and gestures. Look for congruence between the spoken message and the nonverbal message. If there is inconsistency, share your observations with the patient. You can share your observations by describing the patient's body language or tone of voice. For example, you might state, "I know you said you feel well, but your voice and hands are trembling. How can I help you?" Or more simply, "You're frowning. Has something upset you?"

Exploring Issues

Ask open-ended questions to obtain a clear understanding of an issue and follow your client's thoughts (see Chapter 3). Probing comments, such as "Tell me more," or "What does that mean to you?" encourage your client to share information.

Using Silence

Learn to be comfortable with silence. When you remain attentive, silence demonstrates acceptance and allows clients to organize their thoughts and so provide further information. It is especially effective if your client is emotionally upset.

Summarizing the Conversation

At the end of the conversation, summarize what you have heard. For example, you might say, "Today we talked about diet, exercise, and medications for high blood pressure. Your job now is to review the handouts and start taking your medication every morning. I'll see you in 2 weeks when you return for your follow-up visit." Summarizing demonstrates active listening and allows the client to clarify any misunderstandings.

Process Recordings

Therapeutic communication requires practice. A strategy commonly used to improve communication skills is called *process recording*. In **process recording**, two people converse while a third records the conversation. Afterward, the participants analyze the interaction. Audio recording can facilitate process recording. It effectively captures the words and intonation of the conversation, but must be supplemented by notes describing the nonverbal communication. Videotaping allows participants to examine both verbal and nonverbal communication. As you examine an interaction, look for communication skills discussed in Box 21-4.

Barriers to Therapeutic Communication

As you learn to communicate therapeutically, you may find yourself thinking, doing, or saying things that seem to close down your conversation. If so, acknowledge your error and return to therapeutic patterns. The following sections describe the most common barriers to therapeutic communication.

Asking Too Many Questions

Asking questions at the appropriate time is important. However, asking too many questions, especially closed questions (requiring only a yes or no answer), can make clients feel they are being interrogated. Excessive questioning may suggest insensitivity or lack of respect for the client's issues, as in the following dialogue:

Patient:	I feel lousy today.
Nurse:	Didn't you sleep well?
Patient:	No, hardly at all.
Nurse:	Did you take anything to help you sleep?
Patient:	No.
Nurse:	Do you think you should have taken something?
Patient:	I guess.
Nurse:	Why didn't you tell the night nurse you needed something?
Patient:	I don't know.

As you can see, this approach controls the range and nature of responses that the client provides. In contrast, open-ended questions stimulate conversation and exploration. Contrast the preceding conversation with the conversation below.

Patient:	I feel lousy today.
Nurse:	Lousy? Tell me more.
Patient:	Well, my back and neck hurt, and I hardly slept at all. I thought it would go away, but I just lay in bed last night worrying.
Nurse:	What kind of things are you worrying about?
Patient:	I'm worried about . . .

In the second conversation, the nurse asked open-ended questions. These prompts encouraged the patient to discuss his concerns.

Asking Why

In many health situations, we want to learn why a patient acted or responded as he did. However, directly asking for reasons suggests criticism to some people. If you ask, "Why did you stop taking your medication?" the patient may become defensive and stop talking. A more subtle approach is usually more comfortable for the patient. You might ask, "What concerns do you have about your medicines?" or "Tell me more about your experience with the medication." Both of these approaches will help you gather more information about the client's concerns, without suggesting criticism. Review the first dialogue in the previous section, Asking Too Many Questions, for another example of the effect of "why" questions. How do you think this patient felt?

Fire-Hosing Information

Sometimes a healthcare provider might meet with a patient or family and deliver an overwhelming amount of information. The patient or family members might understand what the provider said, but afterward remember only a fraction of it. Or they might feel stunned, confused, intimidated, and helpless. Instead, engage your patient in a *dialogue* in which you give important information while your patient shares his own concerns and questions. You can then ask him how he understands what has been shared and clarify when needed.

Changing the Subject Inappropriately

Abruptly changing the topic of discussion makes you seem uninterested. This often occurs when the nurse is intent on one issue and the patient is focused on another. For example, imagine that you want to tell the patient about a change in the scheduling for a diagnostic test before you forget. As you enter the room, your patient says, "I am having a lot of pain in my knee today." This situation requires you to address the patient's concern first and postpone discussing the schedule change until the patient can be receptive to the information. In an ongoing dialogue, changing the subject can stop the flow of conversation cold. Both patients and nurses sometime use this tactic to avoid discussing sensitive topics. The following is an example:

Nurse:	This must be a tough time for you. Your wife is very sick. How are you handling this?
Patient's husband:	Yes, it's tough, but I went out to a movie last night. Have you seen that new movie with the avatars? The special effects . . .

Your relationship with the patient's husband and the facts of the patient situation would determine whether you would redirect this conversation back to the original subject or allow him to wander. You may choose to give the husband more time to be comfortable with you before approaching this topic again.

Failing to Probe

Failing to probe can result in incomplete assessment and affect the quality of your care. A thorough assessment requires you to explore issues in detail. Review the following conversations.

Patient:	I'm having a lot of discomfort in my back.
Nurse:	How much does it hurt?
Patient:	Quite a bit. I had trouble sleeping last night.
Nurse:	I'll get you something for pain.

Compare that conversation with the next example, in which the nurse gathers additional data.

Patient:	I'm having a lot of discomfort in my back.
Nurse:	Tell me about the discomfort.
Patient:	It hurts a lot. I had trouble sleeping last night.
Nurse:	When did you first notice this pain?
Patient:	It started in the middle of the night.
Nurse:	What does it feel like?
Patient:	I feel sore. I'd like to turn over to my side, but I can't because of this heavy cast.
Nurse:	Let me help you turn. (*Assists patient to turn and uses pillows to hold the patient on her side*)
Patient:	Oh, that feels better!
Nurse:	How is the discomfort now?
Patient:	It's pretty much gone.
Nurse:	I'm glad you're feeling better. Would you like something for pain as well?
Patient:	I think I'm okay now.

In the second example, the nurse followed her original question with additional probing questions. A few additional questions helped clarify what the patient needed and led to immediate comfort.

Expressing Approval or Disapproval

Although it may be appropriate with friends and family, you should be cautious about offering approval or disapproval within the nurse–patient relationship. Although it may seem supportive, expressing approval can inhibit further sharing—it puts you in the position of being the judge of what is "right." This often prompts the patient to continue to seek approval. He thinks, "I'd better be careful; she may not approve of the next thing I was going to tell her. She expects me to be *this* way." Consider instead offering recommendations and allowing the patient to choose. Read the following exchange.

Patient:	I've decided I'm going to have the surgery.
Nurse:	That's great. I think you made the right choice.

Compare that conversation with the following example.

Patient:	I've decided I'm going to have the surgery.
Nurse:	Tell me about your decision.
Patient:	Well, my shoulder has been bothering me for several months now. I know I said I wanted to put off surgery, but I think I'll have a faster recovery if I just get the surgery done now.
Nurse:	So your choices are to do a trial of physical therapy and anti-inflammatory medicines, to try a steroid injection, or to have surgery.

Patient: Right. But there's a good chance I'll still need surgery even if I try the therapy or medicines. The only thing that will actually fix the problem is surgery. The others don't guarantee improvement.

Can you see how different the conversation becomes if the nurse does not express approval? By allowing the patient to discuss the choices, the nurse has empowered the patient to make his own healthcare decisions.

Offering Advice

Offering an opinion is rarely helpful. Avoid statements such as, "If I were you . . ." or, "You should . . ." These statements impose your opinion on your clients. In effect, your statements function as approval if they agree with the client's thoughts or disapproval if they do not. As with other forms of approval or disapproval, conversation halts. If the client asks, "What should I do?" help clarify the options, and provide her with information about the choices. Giving the client your solution negates the client's opportunity to participate as a mutual partner in the decision-making process.

Providing False Reassurance

Providing reassurance helps to ease concern, offers comfort, and communicates empathy. So it is an appropriate and therapeutic action—if the reassurance is warranted. For example, consider the client who comes to the emergency department (ED) for treatment of an acute episode of asthma. Because anxiety exacerbates asthma, it is certainly therapeutic to reassure the client that he will be cared for promptly and effectively. In contrast, false reassurance is a barrier to therapeutic communication. When clients or family members ask for information or tell you that they are worried, it is easy to reassure them that everything will be okay. However, such responses are uninformed, inaccurate, and may feel dismissive—even condescending—to the receiver. Examine the following scenario:

You are a nurse working at the triage station in the local ED. Your role is to evaluate the condition and prioritize the care of all clients on their arrival. An ambulance arrives with a man complaining of severe chest pain. He is ashen and short of breath. He tells you his pain is "crushing." Suspecting a heart attack, you immediately move him to the critical care bay of the ED and request urgent evaluation. Several minutes later his wife arrives by private car and approaches the triage station. She anxiously asks, "How is my husband?" How would you respond?

It may feel natural to offer a response such as, "Don't worry, everything will be all right." But do you really know that will be the case? A better approach is to provide accurate information: "I had him immediately taken in for treatment. I'll get you in to see him as soon as I can. Please have a seat, and I'll check on him." This comment is accurate, calming, and avoids misleading the person.

Stereotyping

As discussed in Chapter 15, racial, cultural, religious, age-related, or gender stereotypes distort assessment and prevent you from recognizing the patient's uniqueness. Examples of statements reflecting a stereotype include "He's old, he won't remember anything you tell him," and "Men are always the biggest crybabies about pain." Such comments may shut down communication and escalate tension. Avoid their use with patients and colleagues.

Stereotypes may be blatant or subtle. Blatant examples, such as those above, are easily recognized and may create an intense reaction. Subtle stereotypes, however, may be equally disruptive to care. Subtle stereotypes common in healthcare include the following:

- Believing a patient will be calm and know what to expect because he has had previous hospitalizations for the same diagnosis, has had previous surgeries or other procedures, or was given information about his condition
- Assuming that patients will understand their healthcare because of their educational level or work experience, for example, expecting that a physician who has suffered a heart attack needs no explanation of her care
- Expecting all patients with the same surgery or diagnosis to experience similar responses

Using Patronizing Language

Patronizing language communicates superiority or disapproval. Statements such as, "You know better than that," are patronizing and offensive to the client. Condescending approaches, such as, "You should have used the call button before you got up. You're lucky you didn't hurt yourself," do not communicate respect for the client.

Have you heard staff call clients "Sweetie," "Dearie," or "Mama"? The term *elderspeak* describes ways that healthcare workers may unintentionally show disrespect to elderly patients by using such phrases and speaking to them in a high-pitched, slow, repetitive, childlike voice. Staff may also alter pronouns, saying, for example, "Are we ready for our bath?" Although the intent is to communicate caring, many patients are offended because it sounds as though you are speaking to a child. Research indicates mentally competent nursing home residents are irritated by elderspeak, and that people with moderate Alzheimer's disease become more agitated and resistant to care if they are addressed in this manner (Williams, Herman, Gajewski, et al., 2008).

Key Point: *When you first meet your client, use a formal title—Mr., Ms., Dr. and so on. In the orientation phase of the relationship, ask your patient how he would prefer to be addressed.*

If the patient is unable to respond, ask family members how to address the patient. This conveys respect, which is essential to a therapeutic relationship.

KnowledgeCheck 21-6

Identify at least five barriers to communication.

Enhancing Communication With Clients From Another Culture

Healthcare facilities should provide interpretation (including translation) services as necessary (The Joint Commission, 2010b). Many health facilities have in-house translation services available for communication with non-English-speaking patients. Translators may also be available through telephone contact; a few are linked via computer to a healthcare interpreter network to enable video teleconferencing.

Use relatives as translators only if there are no other options. It is often culturally unacceptable to have family members ask personal questions. As a result, translations may be altered or questions remain unasked. See Chapter 15 for additional information on the use of translators.

Non-English-speaking patients are increasingly more common in the healthcare setting. If you do not speak the primary language of the patient, many hospitals employ translators: however, it is good to learn a few key words to help you communicate until a translator arrives. Additionally, Internet and mobile technologies offer applications for translating English into various other languages. For a list of a few useful Spanish terms, for examples, and for guidelines for communicating with clients from other cultures,

 Go to Chapter 21, **Clinical Insight 21-4: Communicating With Clients From Another Culture,** in Volume 2.

Enhancing Communication With Clients Who Have Impaired Hearing or Speech

For guidelines to help you communicate with clients who have speech, visual, or hearing deficits, respectively,

 Go to Chapter 21, **Clinical Insight 21-5: Communicating With Clients Who Have Impaired Speech,** in Volume 2.

 Go to Chapter 30, **Clinical Insight 30-2: Communicating With Visually Impaired Clients,** in Volume 2.

 Go to Chapter 30, **Clinical Insight 30-3: Communicating With Hearing-Impaired Clients,** in Volume 2.

Enhancing Communication With Clients With Impaired Cognition or Decreased Level of Consciousness

Communicating with cognitively impaired clients can be difficult, time consuming, and frustrating for even the most experienced healthcare provider. This might be a patient with acute illness or neurological injury, a patient with congenital abnormality, a person with sensory or language deficits, or an older adult with dementia. In the hospital setting, impairments are heightened as a result of the effect of illness, changed routines and environment, and medication. As a result, the patient may be unable to understand explanations, follow directions, ask for help, or report symptoms (Zembrzuski, 2013, revised).

Key Point: *It is critical that you make every effort to communicate whether or not the client can understand you.*

For guidelines to help you communicate with clients with impaired cognition or consciousness,

 Go to Chapter 21, **Clinical Insight 21-6: Communicating With Clients Who Have Impaired Cognition or Consciousness,** in Volume 2.

 To explore learning resources for this chapter,

 Go to Davis*Plus* at DavisPl.us/Wilkinson3.

Chapter Resources for Chapter 21:
  Response sheets for all learning activities
  Resources for Caregivers and Health Professionals
  Reading More About Communication & Therapeutic Relationships (suggested readings)
  Concept Map of chapter content
Interactive Case Studies
NCLEX-Style and Chapter Review Questions
Chapter Overview Podcasts

For references cited in this chapter,

 Go to Volume 2, **References Cited.**

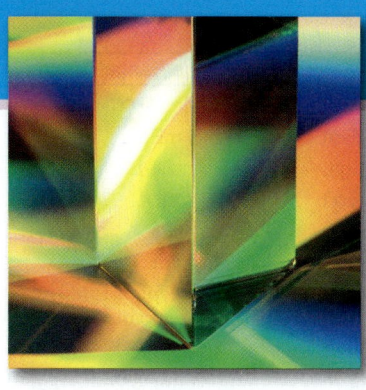

CHAPTER 22

Health Assessment

Learning Outcomes

After completing this chapter, you should be able to:

➤ Identify the purposes and components of a physical examination.

➤ Discuss the differences among a comprehensive, focused, and ongoing physical examination.

➤ Describe how to prepare for a physical examination.

➤ Demonstrate the skills used in physical examination.

➤ Explain adaptations that may be required when you examine clients of various ages.

➤ Identify the components of the general survey.

➤ Conduct a full physical examination of a client.

➤ Discuss the expected findings of a physical examination.

➤ Document the findings of a physical examination.

➤ Perform a brief bedside physical examination.

Key Concepts

Health assessment
Nursing assessment
Physical assessment

Related Concepts

See the Concept Map on Davis*Plus*.

Meet Your Patient

Nam Nguyen is scheduled for a comprehensive physical exam at the family health center at 1400 today. As you recall, he has previously been seen and evaluated by Zach Jackson, RN, FNP. Mr. Nguyen has medical diagnoses of hypertension, degenerative joint disease, obesity, and heavy tobacco use. During his earlier visit, Zach instructed Mr. Nguyen on a low-salt, low-fat diet and advised him to lose weight and quit smoking. Zach also ordered lab work to establish a baseline for wellness and detect abnormalities that might indicate illness. Review the results of Mr. Nguyen's lab work that follow.

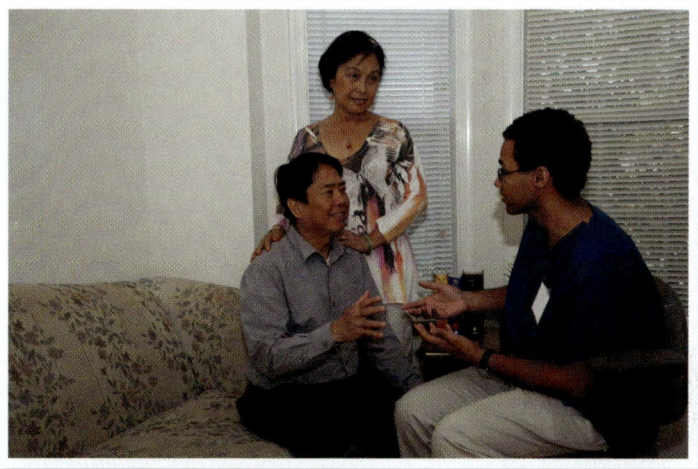

At today's visit, Zach will perform a comprehensive physical examination of Mr. Nguyen and review his lab results. After Nam's appointment, Yen Nguyen will also have a comprehensive exam.

Laboratory Data for Nam Nguyen

Name: Nam Nguyen	**DOB:** 7/12/50	
Acct#: K00205412	Family Medicine Center, J. Miller	

Test	Result	Reference Range*
CBC/Differential		
WBC	5.6 x 10^3/mm^3	5–10 x 10^3/mm^3
Hemoglobin	14.8 g/dL	M: 14–18 g/dL F: 12–16 g/dL
Hematocrit	45.1%	M: 42–52% F: 37–47%
RBC count	5.1 million/mm^3	M: 4.7–5.14 million/mm^3 F: 4.2–4.87 million/mm^3
MCV	84 mm^3	85–95 mm^3
MCH	29 pg	28–32 pg
MCHC	34%	33–35%
Neutrophils	57%	59%
Lymphocytes	30%	34%
Monocytes	5%	4%
Eosinophils	2.5%	2.7%
Basophils	0.7%	0.5%
Platelet count	197,000/mm^3	150,000–400,000/mm^3

Test	Result	Reference Range*
Comprehensive Metabolic Panel		
Sodium	138 mEq/L	135–145 mEq/L
Potassium	4.3 mEq/L	3.5–5.0 mEq/L
Chloride	101 mEq/L	97–107 mEq/L
Carbon dioxide	27 mEq/L	23–29 mEq/L
BUN	16 mg/dL	10–31 mg/dL
Creatinine	0.8 mg/dL	M: 0.6–1.2 mg/dL F: 0.5–1.1 mg/dL
Glucose	156 mg/dL	75–110 mg/dL
Albumin	4.0 g/dL	19–60 years: 3.2–4.8 g/dL
Total protein	7.2 g/dL	6.8–8.0 g/dL
ALT (alanine aminotransferase, also called SGPT)	18 units/L	M: 10–40 units/L F: 7–35 units/L
ALP (alkaline phosphatase)	43 units/L	M: 35–142 units/L F: 25–125 units/L
AST (aspartate aminotranspeptidase, also called SGOT)	26 units/L	M: 19–48 units/L F: 9–36 units/L
Bilirubin, total	0.7 mg/dL	0.3–1.2 mg/dL
Calcium	8.5 mg/dL	8.2–10.2 mg/dL

Test	Result	Reference Range*	
Lipid Panel**			
Total cholesterol	201 mg/dL	<200 200–239 >240	-Desirable -Borderline high -High
LDL cholesterol (Primary target of therapy)	140 mg/dL	<100 mg/dL 100–129 mg/dL 130–159 160–189 >190	-Optimal -Near optimal/ above optimal -Borderline high -High -Very high
HDL cholesterol	34 mg/dL	<40	-Low
Triglycerides	196 mg/dL		

**To interpret lipid panel results, follow the most recent guidelines of the National Cholesterol Education Program (NCEP) Expert Panel on Detection, Evaluation, and Blood Cholesterol in Adults available at www.nhlbi.nih.gov/guidelines/cholesterol/atglance.pdf. The reference range figures in this table will undoubtedly be revised (and lowered) by NCEP in the near future.

Also, the norms for an individual patient's lipid panel depend on the calculation of risk factors. Nam is hypertensive, is obese, and has an elevated blood sugar. His norms reflect high risk for coronary heart disease; they would be about <160 for total cholesterol, <100 for triglycerides, <100 for LDL, and >45 for HDL.

Test	Result	Reference Range*
Urinalysis		
Appearance	Clear	Clear
Color	Amber	Light yellow to amber
Odor	Aromatic	None–aromatic
pH	6.0	5.0–9.0
Specific gravity	1.012	1.001–1.035
Leukocyte esterase	Negative	Negative
Nitrites	Negative	Negative
Ketones	Negative	Negative
Protein	5 mg/dL	<20 mg/dL
Crystals	None	In acid urine: uric acid, calcium oxalate, amorphous urates In alkaline urine: triple phosphate, calcium phosphate, ammonium biurate, calcium carbonate, amorphous phosphates
Casts	None	None, except rare hyaline
Glucose	Negative	Negative
WBC	1/hpf	<5/hpf
RBC	1/hpf	<5/hpf
PSA (prostate-specific antigen)	2.8 ng/mL	<4 ng/mL
Fecal occult blood screen		
Sample #1 — negative Sample #2 — negative Sample #3 — negative		

*For most studies, each laboratory establishes its own reference range.

Theoretical Knowledge
knowing **why**

In this chapter, theoretical knowledge consists mostly of information about the key concepts. You will see how an understanding of the key concepts will prepare you and the client for the examination, and help you to modify your assessments for different age groups.

ABOUT THE KEY CONCEPTS

Health assessment is a comprehensive assessment of the physical, mental, spiritual, socioeconomic, and cultural status of an individual, group, or community. **Nursing assessments** focus on the client's functional abilities and physical responses to illness and other stressors. In contrast, medical assessments focus on disease and pathology. As a nurse practitioner, Zach Jackson combines the nursing and medical approaches. **Physical assessment**, or physical examination, consists of the techniques used to gather objective data about the body.

PHYSICAL EXAMINATION

A complete health assessment includes both a nursing history and a physical examination. In addition to physical examination, you will also ask questions to obtain subjective data about each body system or area. This may be done in a separate nursing interview or as you perform the physical examination. Both the interview and the exam require tact and sensitivity.

What Are the Purposes of a Physical Examination?

A physical examination is performed for any of several reasons:

- *To obtain baseline data.* Data about the patient's physical status and functional abilities serve as a baseline for comparison as the patient's health status changes.
- *To identify nursing diagnoses, collaborative problems, and wellness diagnoses.* Problem statements form the basis for the plan of care and help you to address the patient's nursing care needs.
- *To monitor the status of a previously identified problem.* For example, Mr. Nguyen has already begun treatment for hypertension. Today's examination will be linked to the lab results to further explore the status of his hypertension.
- *To screen for health problems.* Regular checkups can help to identify health problems at early stages. Because Mr. Nguyen has an enlarged prostate, a prostate-specific antigen (PSA) test was done to screen for prostate cancer.

The type of physical examination you perform will depend on the client's health status, the nature of the client encounter, and the setting. For example, at an outpatient appointment for an annual physical, on a client's admission to an inpatient setting, or at the initial home health visit, you would perform a **comprehensive physical assessment**, which includes a health history interview and a complete head-to-toe examination of every body system. In an emergency situation, your assessment will be rapid and focused on the presenting problem. A **focused physical assessment** pertains to a particular topic, problem, body part, or functional ability rather than overall health status, and it adds to the database created by the comprehensive assessment. A **system-specific assessment** is a focused assessment limited to one body system (e.g., the lungs, the peripheral circulation). The following are examples of focused and system-specific physical assessments, respectively:

- Assessing bowel sounds when a client has abdominal pain
- Listening to breath sounds, counting respirations, and obtaining pulse oximetry readings to assess a patient's respiratory status

Ongoing assessment is performed as needed, after the initial database is completed, and, ideally, at every interaction with the patient. For example, on a medical–surgical unit, each nurse who provides care to a client conducts a brief ongoing assessment to determine changes in the client's status and evaluate client outcomes. For more details on the types of assessment, see Chapter 3. For a form to use in making a brief bedside assessment,

 Go to Chapter 22, **Procedure 22-20, Brief Bedside Assessment,** in Volume 2.

How Do I Prepare to Perform a Physical Examination?

You should develop a systematic approach and follow the same order each time you perform a physical exam. This will help you recall the steps and include all important data. A **head-to-toe approach** starts at the head and neck and progresses down the body, examining the feet last. A **body systems approach** examines each system in a predetermined order (e.g., musculoskeletal, cardiovascular, neurological). Whatever the approach, prepare yourself, the environment, and the client before you begin.

Prepare Yourself

Preparing for a physical examination requires theoretical knowledge of anatomy and physiology, examination equipment and techniques, therapeutic communication, and documentation. Self-knowledge is also important. How comfortable are you when performing an examination? What skills do you need to review or practice? Will you need assistance to perform some aspects of the exam? Will you need help documenting your findings?

Honestly evaluate your strengths as well as areas that need improvement. Be sure to seek help from your instructor, an experienced nurse, fellow students, or other healthcare providers as needed.

Before approaching the patient, familiarize yourself with his situation. What are the patient's main health concerns? What is the purpose of your exam? For instance, if you are doing a focused assessment of a client's wound, you will need to learn about the wound being examined. Is there a dressing over the wound? What supplies will you need to remove and replace the dressing? Has the patient required pain medication before exams in the past? Reviewing previous findings helps you work efficiently and to formulate any questions you might want to ask the patient.

Finally, unless this is an initial assessment, review the nursing plan of care and keep it in mind as you examine the patient. Your assessment data may lead to modification or updating of the care plan.

Prepare the Environment

Key Point: *Physical examination requires you to observe and touch the client's body, so privacy is essential.*

You will need a room with curtains or a door to shield the client from view. For additional privacy, drape your client and uncover only the area you are examining. For convenience you may use bed linens and/or a gown to drape. Disposable paper drapes are also available.

Because you will need to hear the patient and listen to a variety of sounds during the exam, turn off the television, radio, or other media. You will need good lighting to observe subtle changes in skin and body contours. Adjust the temperature of the room according to patient comfort.

Determine the instruments and equipment you will need. Take everything you need so that you will not have to leave the client to obtain supplies. To see commonly used equipment,

 Go to the box, **Equipment Needed for Physical Examination,** in Procedure 22-1, of Volume 2.

Prepare the Client

In most clinical settings, you must examine a client often to evaluate a changing status, and timing will be decided by the client's condition rather than by convenience. However, when possible, select a time when the client is comfortable and receptive to the exam. Avoid conducting the exam when the client is in pain or is hungry, tired, anxious, or unwilling to cooperate in the assessment.

Take the time to establish rapport with the client, to help him relax and cooperate fully in the assessment. Introduce yourself, ask the client how he wishes to be addressed, and explain what you will be doing. Ask the client to void before the examination; this promotes relaxation and also makes it easier to palpate the abdomen. Always alert the client before touching him.

For example, before you start to palpate the neck for lymph nodes, say, "I'm going to feel your neck now." Proper positioning during the exam also promotes comfort (see the following section). Pay attention to the pace of your exam, being careful not to prolong it and tire the client.

Key Point: *Consider developmental and cultural differences. For example, some clients may wish to have a family member present during an exam; some may require a same-sex clinician. If you and the client do not speak the same language, arrange to have an interpreter present.*

Quality and Safety Education for Nurses

Health Assessment and Cultural Adaptation

Chapter Key Concept: *Health Assessment (related concept: Developmental Stages)*

Competency: *Patient-Centered Care (Knowledge, skills, attitudes)**

Background: When performing a health assessment, adaptation for the developmental age of the client is a widely accepted nursing practice. It is also important to adapt for the client's culture. In order to engage diverse clients and respond to their preferences and values, culturally competent communication must be an integral component when initiating the health assessment according to Chircop, Edgecombe, Hayward, et al. (2013). The QSEN competency of patient-centered care promotes the same principle. Four areas that demonstrate cultural adaptation in the health assessment are eliciting client preferences regarding: (1) comfort with touch, (2) comfort with exposure (modesty), (3) need for personal space, (4) and need for the presence of a support person (Chircop, Edgecombe, Hayward, et al., 2013).

Scenario: A client who speaks Portuguese requires an interpreter while hospitalized. You are assigned to complete the initial health assessment.

Think about it: (1) To whom does the nurse direct the questions and make eye contact with when obtaining the history, the interpreter or the client? Discuss how your response supports cultural adaptation. (2) Formulate questions for the nursing history to elicit client preferences regarding comfort with touch, comfort with exposure, personal space, and the presence of a support person.

Sources: Chircop, A., Edgecombe, N., Hayward, K., et al. (2013).

As reference for your QSEN log box, the KSA that is most pertinent is: *Elicit patient values, preferences and expressed needs as part of clinical interview, implementation of care plan and evaluation of care.*

For specific Knowledge, Skills, and Attitudes,

 Go to the QSEN Web site at **http://qsen.org/ competencies/pre-licensure-ksas/**

KnowledgeCheck 22-1

- What are the purposes of a physical examination?
- Describe how you would prepare for a physical exam.

ThinkLike a Nurse 22-1
- The nurse conducts a physical assessment for Nam and Yen Nguyen (see Meet Your Patient) at an outpatient clinic. Discuss the differences between their planned experience and a focused physical exam of a hospital inpatient.
- Identify a plan to practice and improve your assessment skills.

How Do I Position the Client for a Physical Examination?
The client will need to assume a variety of positions during a comprehensive physical examination. To begin the examination, seat the client on the side of the bed or examination table. Face the client, and establish eye contact. This helps to build rapport and put the client at ease. If your client is unable to sit, assist him to a position on his back with the head of the bed elevated. An upright position allows the client to expand his lungs fully and is useful for assessing vital signs, the head and neck, the heart and lungs, the back, and the upper extremities.

As you place your client in positions that allow you to best observe the body system you are examining, be alert to special needs that call for you to modify the position. For example, a patient with a cervical spine problem would need a neck roll when lying supine. Table 22-1 illustrates and describes the major positions you will need to use.

KnowledgeCheck 22-2
Identify the best position for examining the lungs, heart, pulses, and abdomen.

Table 22-1 ▶ Positioning the Client

POSITION AND DESCRIPTION	COMMENTS
Standing	
Upright posture with both feet flat on the floor **posture with both feet flat on the floor**	Use to examine the musculoskeletal and neurological systems and to assess gait and cerebellar function. Clients who are weak or who have poor balance may not be able to assume this position.
Sitting	
Sitting upright at side of bed or exam table 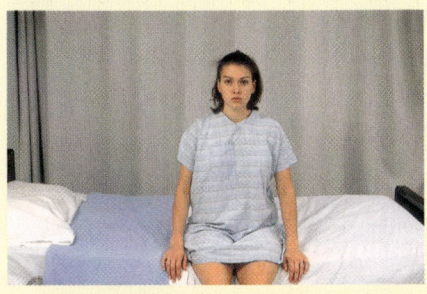	Use to assess vital signs, head and neck, chest, cardiovascular system, and breasts. If your client is weak, he may need assistance to maintain this position.
Supine	
(Including Fowler's and semi-Fowler's positions) Lying flat on the back with arms and legs fully extended 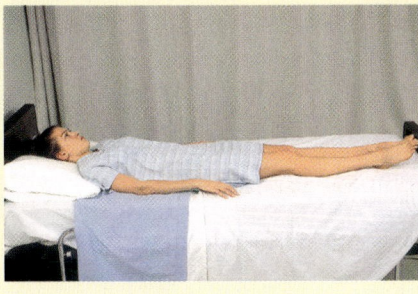	Use to assess the abdomen, breasts, extremities, and pulses. If your client becomes short of breath, raise the head of the bed (HOB). In Fowler's position, the head is elevated 60°. In semi-Fowler's position, the head is elevated only 30°–45°.

Continued

Table 22-1 ➤ Positioning the Client—cont'd

POSITION AND DESCRIPTION	COMMENTS
Dorsal Recumbent	
Supine with knees flexed 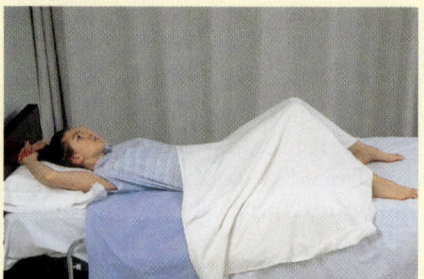	Use for abdominal assessment if your client has abdominal or pelvic pain. Flexing the knees promotes relaxation of the abdominal muscles.
Lithotomy	
Dorsal recumbent position at end of table with feet in stirrups, legs flexed, and widely open 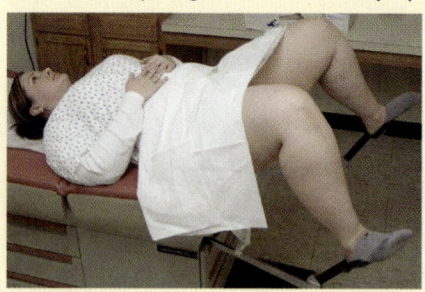	Use for a female pelvic exam; provides maximum exposure of genitals. Older patients may need support to assume and maintain this position. The patient's legs are exposed here to illustrate position. To see a privacy drape refer to Procedure 25-4, Providing Perineal Care.
Sims'	
Flexion of the hip and knees in a side-lying position 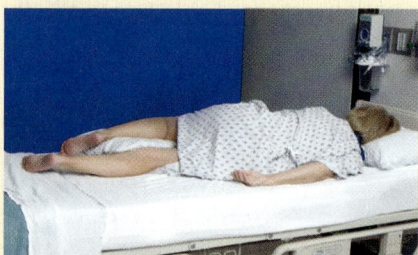	Use to examine the rectal area. Use for a female pelvic exam if the patient is unable to assume the lithotomy position. Do *not* use if the client has had total hip replacement.
Prone	
Lying on stomach (A small pillow under the abdomen makes this position more comfortable.) 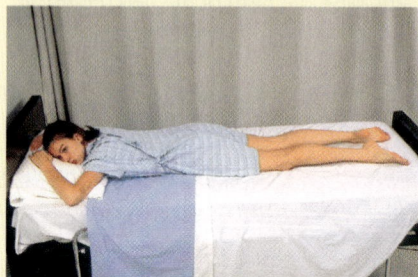	Use to examine the musculoskeletal system, especially hip extension; may also be used to examine the back and buttocks. May be difficult to assume by clients with respiratory problems.

Table 22-1 ➤ Positioning the Client—cont'd

POSITION AND DESCRIPTION	COMMENTS
Lateral Recumbent	
Lying on the side in a straight line 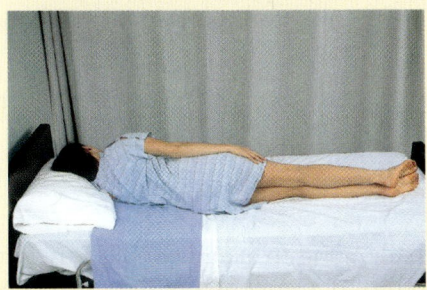	Left lateral recumbent is used to evaluate heart murmur or during a thorough cardiovascular assessment. This position brings the heart closer to the chest wall. If the client cannot assume this position, listen to the heart with the client seated and bending forward.
Knee–Chest	
On hands and knees with head down and buttocks elevated 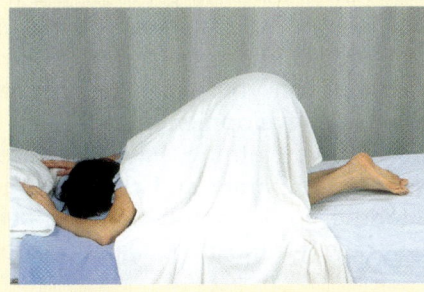	Provides good visualization for examining the rectal area. However, it is not used often because it is embarrassing and uncomfortable for the client.

What Techniques Do I Need to Perform a Physical Examination?

The skills used in physical examination include inspection, palpation, percussion, auscultation, and sometimes olfaction. You will use these skills in that order, with one exception: When performing an abdominal assessment, perform auscultation before percussion and palpation to avoid disturbing the abdominal sounds.

Inspection is the use of sight to gather data. You begin to use **inspection** the moment you meet the client and continue as you observe the person's gait, personal hygiene, affect, and behavior during the general survey. You will also use inspectiand such abnormalities as edema, masses, or areas of tenderness. As you begin and move through the assessment of each body system, always inform the client that you are about to touch him, and use a gentle approach. Be certain your hands are warm. Begin with light pressure to detect surface characteristics. Then move to deep palpation to assess the underlying structures. Examine last any areas of discomfort or sensitivity. Following is a list of the most common palpation techniques, using different parts of the hand.

- *Fingertips:* Use for fine tactile discrimination, including assessment of skin texture, swelling, and specific locations of pulsations and masses.

- *Dorsum of hand:* Use for temperature determination.
- *Palmar surface of hand:* Use for locating general area of pulsations.
- *Grasping with fingers and thumb:* Use to detect the position, shape, and consistency of a mass.

Percussion is tapping your fingers on the skin using short strokes. Tapping (**percussing**) produces vibrations, and the resulting sound allows you to determine location, size, and density of underlying structures. Percussion is especially useful when assessing the abdomen and lungs. Percussion takes practice. To learn more about percussion, including direct and indirect percussion and terminology for the notes you may hear,

 Go to Chapter 22, **Clinical Insight 22-1: Performing Percussion,** in Volume 2.

A quiet environment allows you to perceive the subtle differences in percussion notes. To listen to some percussion sounds,

 Go to Student Resources, **Sound Files: Percussion Sounds,** on Davis*Plus*.

Auscultation is the use of hearing to gather data. **Direct auscultation** is listening without using an instrument. If

you have heard wheezing or chest congestion without the use of a stethoscope, you have already performed direct auscultation. **Indirect auscultation** is listening with the help of a stethoscope. The stethoscope has two end pieces, the diaphragm and the bell.

- Use the diaphragm to listen to high-pitched sounds that normally occur in the heart, lungs, and abdomen. Press the diaphragm hard enough to produce an obvious ring on the patient's skin.
- Use the bell to hear low-pitched sounds, such as extra heart sounds (murmurs) or turbulent blood flow, known as bruits. Apply the bell lightly with just enough pressure to produce an air seal with its entire rim.

    To improve your skill in indirect auscultation,

 Go to Chapter 22, **Clinical Insight 22-2: Performing Auscultation,** in Volume 2.

Olfaction is the use of the sense of smell to gather data. Some clinicians may not consider **olfaction** a formal assessment skill; however, you will certainly use this skill in the clinical setting. Olfaction adds information to the data you collect through the other techniques. Consider these examples:

- If a client is slurring his words, you will want to look for data that reveal the cause of the problem. Slurred speech might be caused by a stroke or by sedative medications. However, if the client smells of alcohol you would first investigate recent alcohol use as a probable cause for the slurred words.
- If an older client smells of urine, you would want to assess for problems with leakage of urine or inability to perform self-care.
- If the client's breath has a "fruity" or "acetone" odor, you would suspect ketoacidosis (which may accompany diabetes). You would know to assess the urine for ketones and contact the primary care provider if necessary. You would also ask the client about dietary patterns, because a high-protein, high-fat, low-carbohydrate diet can cause a buildup of ketones in the blood.

KnowledgeCheck 22-3

- Identify five physical assessment skills.
- In what order are these skills performed?

 ThinkLike a Nurse 22-2

Think about olfaction as an assessment technique. Give two or three additional examples of data you might collect through the use of smell.

How Do I Modify Assessment for Different Age Groups?

The basic techniques of physical assessment remain the same for all age groups. However, your approach will vary according to the developmental stage of your patient.

Infants

Use the assessment as an opportunity to teach the parent about normal growth and development. Infants usually feel most secure if a parent holds them during the examination, either against the chest or, for older infants who can sit without support, on the parent's lap. Otherwise, position an infant on a padded examination table.

✚ If there are siderails, raise them to prevent falling. Do not leave the infant's side or turn your back on the infant.

Toddlers

Toddlers can be challenging to examine. They are interested in exploring the environment, but they also like to stay close by a parent, often in the parent's lap. Because they may be fearful of invasive procedures such as examination of the oral cavity or inner ear, perform these procedures last. Most toddlers enjoy making choices, so use this characteristic to promote the toddler's cooperation. For example, you might provide a choice by saying, "Should I listen to your chest first, or should we see how much you weigh?" Allow the child to show you his developmental skills. If he needs assistance to remove clothing, have the parent help, and observe how the parent and child interact. Always praise the toddler for his abilities and cooperation. This sets the stage for positive feelings about healthcare.

Preschoolers

Preschool children are developing initiative and, as a result, usually cooperate with an examination. However, children of this age have fantasies and fears that may arise during the examination. For example, they may object to a noninvasive procedure because they believe it will cause pain or injury, or they may refuse to step on the scale because to them it resembles a monster. In such cases, it may be helpful to demonstrate the procedure on a doll or have the parent step on the scale before you approach the child.

As appropriate, allow the preschool child to sit in a parent's lap if she wishes. By age 5, most children will be comfortable enough to lie on the examination table if a parent is present. Let the child help with the exam. For example, have her hold equipment or remember her height and weight. Give reassurance as you go through the examination: for example, "Your lungs sound very healthy." Always compliment the child on her cooperation.

School-Age Children

The school-age child has a rapidly expanding vocabulary and usually seeks approval of parents, teachers, and healthcare providers. Develop rapport by asking the child about his favorite school or play activities. Allow the child to undress himself and get up and down from the exam table. Demonstrate your equipment before you use it. The school-age child will be interested in how his body works, so use this opportunity for teaching.

Adolescents

The adolescent is self-conscious and introspective and may wish to be examined without parents or siblings present, at least during the more personal aspects of the exam. Offer this choice. Adolescents often worry about the "normalcy" of their changing bodies and appreciate respect for their privacy. Be certain to discuss the normal physiological changes that accompany puberty. If you need to review those changes, see the section on adolescence in Chapter 9.

Adolescent behavior may be strongly influenced by peer values, so emphasize lifestyle habits that promote wellness, including a healthful diet; adequate rest and exercise; and avoidance of tobacco, alcohol, and other drugs. Also discuss sexually transmitted infections and cancer, particularly testicular cancer and human papillomavirus. The first pelvic examination and breast examination usually take place in the teen years. Because suicide is the third leading cause of death among adolescents, you should also use this opportunity to screen for depression and suicide risk (see Chapter 13 for a review of depression and suicide).

Young and Middle Adults

Most young and middle adults are able to cooperate during a physical examination and do not require a modified approach. Modifications may be required if the client has acute or chronic illness or cannot understand or follow instructions.

Older Adults

Older adults are adjusting to changes in physical abilities and health. As part of a comprehensive exam, assess the client's support system and ability to perform activities of daily living. Observe your client's energy level during the physical examination and provide rest periods if needed. If the client tires easily, arrange the exam sequence to limit position changes. Also be aware that stiff muscles and arthritic joints may make it impossible for the client to assume certain positions. Older adults may have impaired vision or hearing, so you may need to adapt your techniques to compensate for this. Obtain feedback to be sure the patient is seeing and hearing you adequately.

The acronym SPICES will help you to remember common problems of the elderly that require nursing intervention (Fulmer, 1991, 2007) and to focus your assessment as you perform a comprehensive physical examination:

S—Sleep disorders
P—Problems with eating or feeding
I—Incontinence
C—Confusion
E—Evidence of falls
S—Skin breakdown

KnowledgeCheck 22-4

What exam modifications, based on developmental stage, should you consider for the following clients (Meet Your Patient)?

- Nam Nguyen
- Nam's 3-year-old grandson, Kim Phan
- Nam's elderly mother, Mai Nguyen

PracticalKnowledge
knowing how

The remainder of the chapter discusses each of the components of a comprehensive physical examination. The Highlights of Procedures box near the end of this chapter summarizes the entire comprehensive physical assessment, including a summary of the general survey. For a step-by-step approach to perform each assessment,

 Go to Chapter 22, **Procedures,** in Volume 2.

As you perform your physical assessments, you may wish to refer to laboratory tests associated with each of the systems you are assessing. You can find some normal lab values in the Laboratory Data for Nam Nguyen (Reference Ranges) at the beginning of this chapter. For a list of laboratory tests,

 Go to Chapter 22, **Supplemental Materials: Laboratory and Diagnostic Tests by System,** on Davis*Plus.*

THE GENERAL SURVEY

The general survey is your overall impression of the client. It begins at first contact and continues throughout the exam. When you discover a deviation from normal in the general survey, you will explore it further during focused assessment of that body system. For example, if on meeting the patient you notice a drooping eyelid (**ptosis**) on one side of her face, you will keep that in mind as you perform the neurological assessment. Ptosis may be caused by a stroke or neurological injury. For a step-by-step approach,

 Go to Chapter 22, **Procedure 22-1: Performing the General Survey,** in Volume 2.

The following are aspects of the general survey.

Appearance and Behavior

Observe the client's general characteristics. Are his speech and behavior appropriate for his developmental stage? Look for indications of his mood and mental status—for instance, does he make eye contact with you? Notice any signs of distress, either physical or emotional. Observe the condition of your client's face, and note the quality of the visible skin. For example, excessive wrinkling of the skin from sun exposure, tobacco use, or illness may make the client appear older than his stated age. Be sure to consider cultural background, because this may influence your findings and interpretation.

Body Type and Posture

Next, observe your client's body size, build, and gait. As you introduce yourself and greet him, assess his muscle strength, mobility, and skin temperature and texture. Posture is also a clue about overall health status. A slumped position may indicate fatigue, depression, osteoporosis, or pain. If your client is immobile, observe his ability to move from side to side and change positions in the bed. Are the client's body movements smooth and coordinated? Does he use a cane or other assistive device? An unsteady gait may be associated with joint, muscle, or neurological disorders. Focused assessments in the remainder of the exam will help to reveal the exact meaning of such cues.

Speech

As you speak with the client and ask health-related questions, look for clues offered by his speech.

- Inappropriate or illogical responses may be associated with psychiatric disorders.
- Difficulty speaking or changes in voice quality may indicate a neurological problem.
- Rapid speech may be a sign of anxiety, hyperactivity, or use of stimulants.
- Hoarseness could indicate inflammation in the throat from infection, overuse, a foreign body, or perhaps a tumor or other obstructive material.
- Slow speech may be due to depression, sedation from medications, or neurological disorders.
- Vocabulary and sentence structure provide information about the client's educational level and comfort with the language.
- A foreign accent with hesitancy and/or sparse verbalization may signal a language barrier and a need for an interpreter.

Dress, Grooming, and Hygiene

A client's ability to dress and perform personal hygiene is affected by physical and emotional well-being. An unkempt appearance may reflect chronic pain, fatigue, depression, or low self-esteem. Poor hygiene may indicate a self-care deficit of physical or mental origin, or lack of easily accessible bathroom facilities.

Mental State

Mental state includes level of consciousness and capacity to interact. If the client has an altered mental status, ask a family member about the onset of the change.

 Keep in mind that many medications, especially in older adults, may contribute to confusion or other changes in mental status.

- Bizarre responses may signal a psychiatric problem.
- Lethargy may be due to medications; depression; or a neurological, thyroid, liver, kidney, or cardiovascular disorder.
- Confusion and irritability may indicate hypoxia or medication side effects.
- Inability to provide a health history or to recall information may indicate a neurological disorder.

Vital Signs

You should assess vital signs as a part of the general survey and with subsequent assessments. Analyze for trends. See Chapter 20 for a complete discussion of vital signs, if needed.

Height and Weight

Height and weight provide valuable information about your client's growth and development, nutritional status, overall general health, and risk for various diseases such as diabetes and heart disease. These data are important for proper dosing of medication. For adults who can stand, measure height and weight using a platform scale with a sliding ruler (Fig. 22-1). When possible, the client should wear minimal clothing (gown) and no shoes. If the client cannot stand safely, use a bed scale. To measure an infant's length, use a stationary measure. Because children have frequent changes in growth, their measurements are documented on growth charts for easy monitoring and comparison to age- and gender-related standards. For growth charts for males and females from birth to 20 years of age,

 Go to Chapter 22, **Supplemental Materials: Growth Charts,** on Davis*Plus.*

Body mass index (BMI) evaluates the relationship between height and weight. You can calculate the BMI for adults using a BMI calculator or table. For a BMI table,

 Go to Chapter 22, **Procedure 22-1: Performing the General Survey,** in Volume 2.

Because the proportion of fat to muscle affects BMI calculation, the BMI is not useful for athletes (who have a larger proportion of muscle), for pregnant and

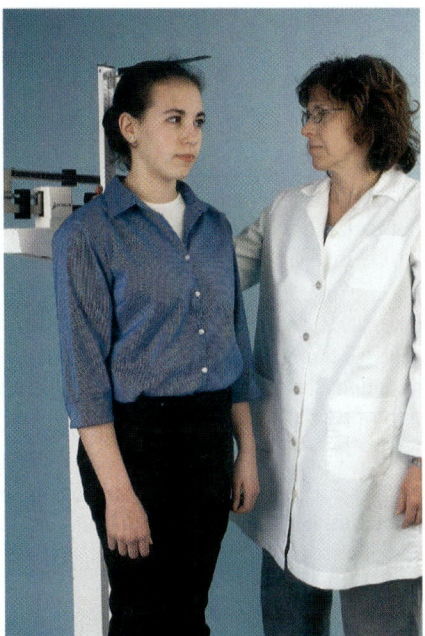

FIGURE 22-1 For adults, measure height with the client's back to the platform scale.

lactating women (who have a larger blood and tissue volume), for growing children, or for frail and sedentary older adults.

Once you have completed your general survey of the client, you can begin to focus on each body system. Whether you are doing a complete or focused physical assessment, remember that all body systems are interrelated. A problem in one system may affect or be affected by other systems.

THE INTEGUMENTARY SYSTEM

The integumentary system consists of the skin, hair, and nails. In a comprehensive exam, you assess this system briefly in the general survey, and then in greater detail as you move to examine other areas of the body. This allows the client to remain draped as long as possible.

The Skin

To perform a skin assessment, observe skin color, lesions, and other characteristics. Also notice unusual odors. An unpleasant body odor may be a sign of poor hygiene, the presence of a wound, or underlying disease. Excessive sweating may be related to activity (e.g., if the client has just finished exercising), thyroid problems, or overactive sweat glands. An odor of urine or stool may indicate a nursing diagnosis of Self-Care Deficit or Bowel or Urinary Incontinence.

For a summary of skin assessment, refer to the Highlights of Procedures box near the end of this chapter. For step-by-step instructions,

 Go to Chapter 22, **Procedure 22-2: Assessing the Skin,** in Volume 2.

Skin Color

Skin color varies according to age and race, although each person's skin color is fairly uniform. Exposed areas, such as the hands, face, and neck, are often darker than unexposed areas, whereas the palms, soles, and nailbeds are lighter than the rest of the skin. In people with dark skin, the lips are also usually lighter than surrounding skin. Variations in skin color commonly seen in neonates and infants include the following:

- **Mongolian spots** are benign, blue-black birthmarks that occur on the lower back and buttocks of black, Hispanic, Native American, and Asian babies. They are the result of pigmented cells in the deeper areas of skin. Most fade by age 2 but can persist until early adolescence.
- **Capillary hemangiomas**, sometimes known as "stork bites," are small, irregular pink-red areas that are often seen around the face and nape of the neck in newborns. They typically disappear in infancy although they can persist until age 5.
- **Café-au-lait spots** are light brown birthmarks that can occur anywhere on the body. The name of these birthmarks is French for "coffee with milk" because of their light-brown color. Most often café-au-lait spots are not associated with medical problems, although they can sometimes signal a genetic disorder.

Table 22-2 discusses the significance of other skin color variations that may be seen in clients of any age.

Skin Characteristics

As does color, the temperature, texture, and turgor of the skin offer clues to the client's health status. Although it is not technically a skin characteristic, you should also check for edema while you are assessing the skin.

Skin Temperature Use the dorsum of the hand or fingers to assess skin temperature. Compare the temperature of the hands with that of the feet, and compare the right side of the body with the left. The skin should feel warm, but keep in mind that the temperature should be consistent with the room temperature and the patient's activity level. Be sure to check the temperature of the skin over any area of erythema. When accompanied by warmth, erythema may indicate infection or inflammatory changes.

If the patient's skin feels excessively warm, validate your data: Check her temperature to determine whether she has a fever. Hyperthyroidism stimulates the metabolism and may also elevate skin temperature. Excessive coolness may be due to poor peripheral circulation, shock, exposure to cold, or hypothyroidism.

Table 22-2 ➤ Common Skin Color Variations

COLOR VARIATION AND DESCRIPTION	SIGNIFICANCE
Pallor	
In light-skinned clients: extreme paleness; skin appears white; loss of pink or yellow tones. In dark-skinned clients: a loss of red tones	May be related to poor circulation or a low hemoglobin level (anemia). Best sites to assess for pallor include the oral mucous membranes, conjunctiva, nailbeds, palms, and soles of feet.
Cyanosis	
A blue-gray coloration of the skin, often described as ashen	If seen in the lips, tongue, mucous membranes, and facial features, it is known as *central cyanosis* and is associated with hypoxia. **Acrocyanosis**, which is bluish discoloration of palms and soles in the first few hours to days of life, is normal in newborns.
	Cold causes the lips to turn blue but the tongue is not affected. Cyanosis may also be seen in the extremities, especially hands and feet, after exposure to extreme cold.
Jaundice	
A yellow-orange cast to the skin	Often associated with liver disorders. Best sites to assess for jaundice include the sclera, mucous membranes, hard palate of the mouth, palms, and soles. Jaundice in the newborn is a normal finding in the first few weeks of life unless there is blood incompatibility or a congenital disorder.
Flushing	
A widespread, diffuse area of redness	Generalized redness of the face and body may occur as a result of fever, excessive room temperature, sunburn, polycythemia (an abnormal increase in red blood cells), vigorous exercise, or certain skin conditions, such as rosacea.
Erythema	
A reddened area	Associated with rashes, skin infections, prolonged pressure on the skin, or application of heat or cold.
Ecchymosis	
Bruised (blue-green-yellow) area	May be seen anywhere on the body. The color will vary based on the age of the injury. May indicate physical abuse, internal bleeding, side effect to medication, or bleeding disorder. To review assessing for abuse, refer to Procedure 9-1, Assessing for Abuse, in Volume 2. Also,
	Go to Chapter 9, **Example Problem: Abuse, Neglect, and Violence**, in Volume 1.
Petechiae	
Tiny, pinpoint red or reddish-purple spots	Visible in the skin due to extravasation (leakage from vessels) of blood into the skin. May be associated with a variety of disorders and medications.
Mottling	
Bluish marbling	Occurs in light-skinned clients, especially when cold. In newborns mottling indicates overstimulation of the autonomic nervous system.

Skin Moisture Normally the skin is warm and dry. Excessive moisture may result from hyperthermia, thyroid hyperactivity, anxiety, or **hyperhidrosis** (excessive sweating). Oily skin is often seen with acne. Dry skin may result from dehydration, chronic renal failure, hypothyroidism, excessive exposure, or overzealous hygiene.

Skin Texture Normal skin is smooth and soft. The following factors affect skin texture:

- *Exposure.* Exposed areas tend to be drier and coarser in texture, as do the elbows and knees.
- *Age.* The skin of infants and young children is very smooth because of lack of exposure to the environment.

- *Hyperthyroidism and other endocrine disorders.* These may cause the skin to become coarse, thick, and dry.
- *Impaired circulation.* Peripheral arterial insufficiency is associated with smooth, thin, shiny skin with little to no hair. In contrast, venous insufficiency leads to thick, rough skin that is often hyperpigmented.

Skin Turgor refers to the elasticity of the skin, which provides data about hydration status. Poor turgor, or **tenting** (skin that tends to stay pinched for a few seconds), may be a sigh of dehydration. Elasticity decreases with age, so tenting may also be seen with normal aging. Edema or scleroderma creates tension in the tissues preventing the skin from being pinched up.

Edema, an excessive amount of fluid in the tissues, is an abnormal finding. It is common in clients with congestive heart failure, kidney disease, peripheral vascular disease, or low albumin levels. A client with edema may tell you his skin feels "tight" or say, "My shoes don't fit any more." Swollen tissue may feel tender to the touch. Edema is not actually a condition of the skin, but it is convenient to assess for it while assessing the skin. Table 22-3 provides a grading system for edema.

Skin Lesions

Any **lesion**, variation in pigment, or break in continuous tissue requires assessment. Lesions considered to be normal variations and not harmful include:

- **Milia.** White raised areas on the nose, chin, and forehead of newborns. These lesions, which resemble "whiteheads," are due to retention of sebum in the maturing sebaceous glands. They disappear during infancy.
- **Nevi (moles), freckles, birthmarks.**
- **Skin tags.** Tiny tags or buds of skin usually around skin creases, in middle and older adults
- **Striae.** Silver-to-pink "stretch marks" in pregnant women, women who have had children, and anyone who has experienced significant weight fluctuations.

Abnormal lesions are classified as primary or secondary.

- **Primary skin lesions.** Develop as a result of disease or irritation. The pustules of acne are an example.
- **Secondary skin lesions.** Develop from primary lesions as a result of continued illness, exposure, injury, or infection, such as the crusts that form from ruptured pustules.

When you observe a lesion, evaluate it for size, shape, pattern, color, distribution, texture, surface relationship, exudate, tenderness, pain, or itching. The table, Describing Skin Lesions, at the end of Procedure 22-2 should help you to categorize lesions. Also see the Abnormal Atlas at the end of Chapter 22 in Volume 2 to view abnormal lesions associated with particular conditions such as cellulitis and scabies.

 Go to Chapter 22, **Procedure 22-2: Assessing the Skin, and Abnormal Atlas, Skin Lesions,** in Volume 2.

Evaluate all skin lesions for the possibility of malignancy, especially those located in a site exposed to chronic rubbing or other trauma. Ask the client whether he has any newly developed moles or skin lesions or whether there has been any change in the appearance of existing lesions. You can remember the warning signs of malignant lesions by thinking of the letters ABCDE:

Asymmetry
Border irregularity,
Color variation,
Diameter greater than 0.5 cm
Elevation above the skin surface.

KnowledgeCheck 22-5

- What aspects of the skin should you assess?
- What assessments should you perform if you find a lesion?
- What warning signs lead you to suspect a malignant lesion?

The Hair

When assessing the hair, inspect and palpate for color, texture, and distribution, as well as the condition of the scalp. The hair should be clean and free of debris. A client who does not properly groom her hair may need help with other self-care tasks.

Color There is a wide range of naturally occurring hair color. Age-related graying of the hair varies among individuals according to their genetic background. White hair accompanied by very pale skin is seen in a condition known as **albinism**, or lack of pigment.

Texture Normal hair texture varies from fine to coarse. However, hair that is exceptionally dry and coarse hair may be a sign of hypothyroidism; very fine, silky hair may indicate hyperthyroidism.

Table 22-3 ➤ Assessing Edema	
SCALE	**DESCRIPTION**
Trace	Minimal depression with pressure.
+1	2 mm depression; rapid return of skin to position.
+2	4 mm depression that disappears in 10–15 seconds.
+3	6 mm depression that lasts 1–2 minutes. Area appears swollen.
+4	8 mm depression that persists for 2–3 minutes. Area is grossly edematous.

Distribution Generally the hair is evenly distributed on the scalp, and fine body hair is present over the body. Men often have more hair on the face, chest, and back. Alterations in hair distribution may be signs of disease.

- **Alopecia** (hair loss) along the temples and in the center of the scalp is considered a normal balding pattern in men and is largely genetically based. Diffuse alopecia can be caused by chemotherapy for the treatment of cancer, by nutritional deficiencies, or by endocrine disorders. Thinning hair can also occur in the perimenopausal period when hormone levels are fluctuating. Patchy hair loss may be caused by fungal infections of the scalp, hair pulling, constant wearing of caps, or **alopecia areata**, a benign autoimmune disorder.
- **Hirsutism** (excess facial or trunk hair) may be due to endocrine disorders or steroid use.

Scalp Normally the scalp is smooth, firm, symmetrical, nontender, and without lesions. Common deviations include an asymmetrical or bumpy scalp due to trauma or lesions, and scaly flakes or patches due to fungal infection (e.g., dandruff), dermatitis, or psoriasis. Tenderness may indicate a localized infection or trauma. In newborns, **cradle cap**—scaly white patches over the scalp due to secretion of sebum—is common. It can be removed with washing and gentle scrubbing.

Pediculosis In addition, the hair should be free of debris and **pediculosis** (head lice infestation). Head lice are tiny, very mobile, and difficult to see. You may find it easier to see the eggs, or **nits**, that are deposited on the hair shaft close to the scalp. For a step-by-step description of assessing the hair, see the Highlights of Procedures box near the end of this chapter, and

 Go to Chapter 22, **Procedure 22-3: Assessing the Hair,** in Volume 2.

The Nails

Healthy nailbeds are level, firm, and similar to the color of the skin. The nail is smooth and uniform in texture. Examine nails on both hands and feet. However, you may defer examination of the toenails until you are assessing the peripheral circulation. Variations in color, shape, or texture may indicate health problems. For illustrations of nail variations and for a step-by-step description of nail assessment, see the Highlights of Procedures box near the end of this chapter, and

 Go to Chapter 22, **Abnormal Atlas,** and **Procedure 22-4: Assessing the Nails and Abnormal Atlas,** respectively, in Volume 2.

Nail Color

Pink nails with rapid capillary refill indicate circulation to the extremities. Pale or cyanotic nailbeds are seen in clients with circulatory or respiratory disorders that result in anemia or hypoxia. Other color abnormalities that you may encounter include the following:

- *Half-and-half nails,* in which a distal band of reddish-pink covers 20% to 60% of the nail. These occur in clients with low albumin levels or renal disease.
- *Mees' lines,* which are transverse white lines in the nailbed. They are seen in clients who have experienced severe illnesses or nutritional deficiencies.
- *Splinter hemorrhages,* which are small hemorrhages under the nailbed. They are associated with bacterial endocarditis or trauma.
- *Black nails,* resulting from blood under the nail, are seen after local trauma. Nails can also drop after blunt trauma.
- *White spots* may indicate zinc deficiency.

Nail Shape

A change in nail shape may indicate underlying disease. Figure 22-2 illustrates the typical nail plate angle of 160°. Clubbing, in which the nail plate angle is 180° or more, is associated with long-term hypoxic states, such as occur with chronic lung disease (see Procedure 22-4, in Volume 2). Spoon-shaped nails may result from iron deficiency.

Nail Texture

Nails are normally smooth in texture. You may see the following indications of problems:

- Thickened nails may result from poor circulation.
- A thick nail with yellowing is an indication of fungal infection known as *onychomycosis.*
- Brittle nails are seen with hyperthyroidism, malnutrition, calcium and iron deficiency, and repeated use of harsh nail products.
- Soft, boggy nails are seen with poor oxygenation.

The tissue surrounding the nail should be smooth epidermis. Chronic nail-picking results in callus formation

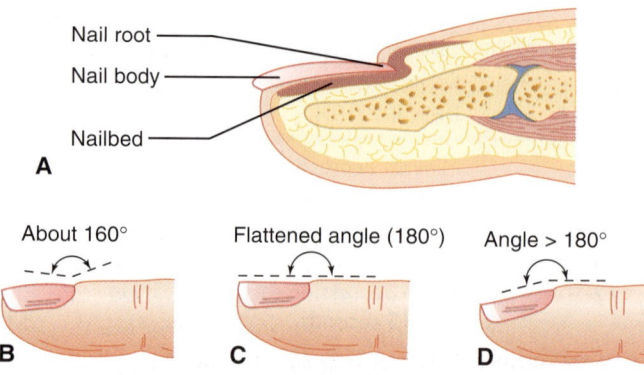

FIGURE 22-2 Nails. *A,* Parts of the nail. *B,* The normal nail plate angle is 160°. *C,* A nail plate angle of 180° or more is known as clubbing. *D,* Late clubbing from long-term hypoxia.

around the nail. Occasionally the surrounding skin becomes inflamed. This condition, known as *paronychia*, is painful and may require drainage if infection is present.

ThinkLike a Nurse 22-3

You are caring for a woman who has no hair on her head. How might you determine the cause of her hair loss? What other assessments should you perform?

THE HEAD

Assessment of the head is often referred to by the acronym HEENT: head, eyes, ears, nose, and throat. You will use all the assessment techniques—inspection, palpation, percussion, and auscultation—in the HEENT exam.

The Skull and Face

Taking individual variation into account, on inspection the skull should be rounded and the face symmetrical in appearance and movement. Inspect head size; if it seems unusual, measure it.

- A large head in an adolescent or adult may be associated with **acromegaly**, a disorder associated with excess growth hormone. Head size is familial, as well.
- **Microcephaly,** an abnormally small head size, is seen in clients with certain types of mental retardation.

Also inspect for shape and symmetry of the head:

- Asymmetry may be the result of trauma, surgery, neuromuscular disorder, paralysis, or congenital deformity.
- In infants, abnormal shape or flattening of the skull may result from trauma during a vaginal birth or placing the baby in the same position for several hours every day.
- In infants and children, a head that is growing disproportionally faster than the body may be a sign of **hydrocephalus** (an accumulation of excessive cerebrospinal fluid).
- Facial appearance that is inconsistent with gender, age, or racial/ethnic group may indicate an inherited or chronic disorder, such as Graves' disease, hypothyroidism with myxedema, or Cushing's syndrome.

Palpate the skull. It should be smooth to palpation, with no unusual contours or bulges. Contour abnormalities, bulging, or tenderness may be a result of trauma, congenital anomalies, or surgery. Irregular jaw movement or cracking of the jaw may indicate **TMJ (temporomandibular joint) syndrome.**

The Highlights of Procedures box near the end of this chapter summarizes the assessment of the face. For the entire procedure, and an Abnormal Atlas of facial abnormalities,

Go to Chapter 22, **Procedure 22-5: Assessing the Head and Face,** in Volume 2.

The Eyes

In examining the eyes, you will inspect and palpate the external eye structures, assess vision, and examine the internal eye structures. The Highlights of Procedures box near the end of this chapter summarizes the eye exam. For step-by-step instructions,

Go to Chapter 22, **Procedure 22-6: Assessing the Eyes,** in Volume 2.

For convenience, you may wish to perform some cranial nerve testing along with the eye exam (e.g., corneal reflex, pupillary reaction, accommodation, and extraocular movements). For instructions on performing a cranial nerve examination,

Go to Chapter 22, **Procedure 22-16: Assessing the Sensory-Neurological System,** in Volume 2.

External Structures

To review the structure of the external eye, see Figure 22-3. Normal eyelid margins are moist and pink with short lashes that are evenly spaced and curl outward. The lower eyelid margin appears at the bottom edge of the iris, and the upper eyelid covers half the upper iris. The conjunctiva is smooth, glistening, and peach in color, with minimal blood vessels present. There should be no pallor, dryness, or edema.

Eyelids The following are common abnormal findings on the eyelids:

- Crusting, scales, or swelling of the lid is associated with infection of the eyelids or eyelashes.
- A **pterygium** is a growth or thickening of conjunctiva from the inner canthus toward the iris.
  - **Ectropion**, an everted eyelid, is commonly seen in older adults secondary to loss of skin tone. It can lead to excessive dryness of the eyes.
- **Entropion**, an inverted eyelid, can lead to corneal damage.
- **Ptosis**, or drooping of the lid, may be seen in clients who have experienced a stroke (cerebrovascular accident [CVA]) or Bell's palsy (paralysis of the facial nerve). To see ptosis and other abnormalities,

Go to Chapter 22, **Procedure 22-5: Assessing the Head and Face,** and **Abnormal Atlas,** in Volume 2.

Sclera and Conjunctiva Associated disorders may include infection, allergies, injuries, and liver disorders. For example, yellow (**icteric**) sclera may be seen with an elevated bilirubin. Blood visible in the sclera is known as a **subconjunctival hemorrhage** and may be related to trauma or hypertension.

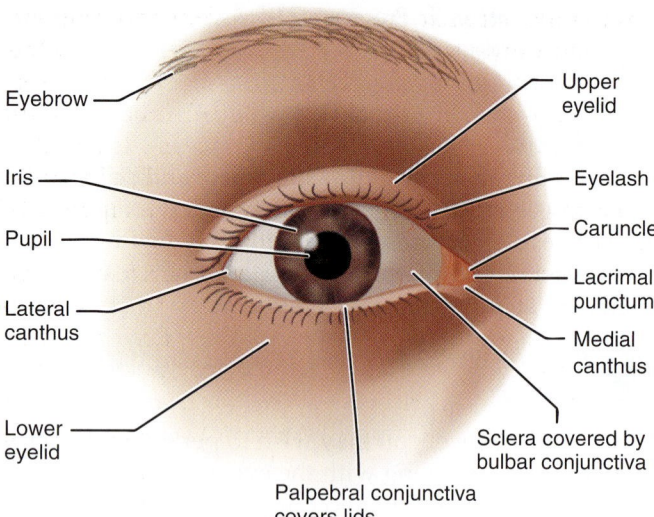

Eyebrow
Iris
Pupil
Lateral canthus
Lower eyelid

Upper eyelid
Eyelash
Caruncle
Lacrimal punctum
Medial canthus
Sclera covered by bulbar conjunctiva

Palpebral conjunctiva covers lids

FIGURE 22-3 The external eye and eyelid.

Lens and Cornea The lens and the **cornea**, or outermost layer of the eyeball, are transparent, smooth, and moist. Roughness or irregularity of the cornea is seen with trauma or a corneal abrasion.

 Lens opacities, known as **cataracts**, are frequently seen in older adults and may impair vision.

Pupils The **pupils** should be uniform in color, equal in size, and round. They should **accommodate** equally; that is, the pupils constrict and the eyes converge (cross) as a person attempts to focus on an object moving toward him. This is typically charted as PERRLA: pupils equal, round, reactive to light and accommodation. The following are common pupillary abnormalities:

- Sluggish accommodation may be caused by anticholinergic drugs or advanced age.
- Failure of one or both pupils to accommodate may reflect a cranial nerve III problem or **exophthalmos** (associated with hyperthyroidism).
- Congenital cataracts, although rare, may be seen in infants and are checked during an eye exam using the "red reflex." Congenital cataracts cause "lazy eye" or amblyopi and can lead to other eye problems such as nystagmus, strabismus and inability to fix a gaze upon objects.

 - Cloudy pupils, a finding related to cataracts, are commonly seen in older adults.

- **Mydriasis** (enlarged pupils) may be seen with glaucoma, an increase in intraocular pressure.
- Many medications affect pupil size (e.g., *mydriatics* are used to dilate the pupil to allow better visualization of the internal eye during examination.
- **Miosis** (constricted pupils) often results from medications to treat glaucoma.
- **Anisocoria** (unequal pupils) may be seen with central nervous system disorders such as stroke, head

trauma, or cranial nerve injuries. In some individuals, anisocoria may be normal.

Visual Acuity

Visual acuity is a measure of the eye's ability to detect the details of an image. When testing visual acuity, you will assess distant, near, peripheral, and color vision. Nurses usually perform screening tests of visual acuity. Other testing is performed by nurses in advanced or specialty practice or by an optometrist or ophthalmologist as needed.

Distance Vision

Use the Snellen chart from a distance of 20 feet to assess distance vision. Assess each eye separately, and then assess both eyes together. Normal vision is a measure of clear vision at 20 feet (20/20) in the right eye, left eye, and both eyes. If a patient hesitates when reporting the letters or symbols he sees on the Snellen chart, document "with hesitation." If the person misses one or two items in a line, record the number of items missed.

Myopia, or diminished distant vision, is associated with a smaller fraction. For example, 20/100 vision means that to see text a person with normal vision can read at 100 feet, the client has to stand just 20 feet from the Snellen chart. A child's distance vision does not reach 20/20 until around 6 or 7 years of age.

Near Vision

Test near vision by having the client read newsprint from a distance of 35.5 cm (14 in.). A client with normal near vision will be able to read the newsprint without hesitation with either eye and both eyes. With **hyperopia**, or diminished near vision, the client must hold the paper more than 35.5 cm (14 in.) away. As we age, the lens of the eye naturally loses some ability to accommodate to near objects. In clients older than 45 years of age, diminished near vision is known as **presbyopia**.

Color Vision

Color vision is the ability to detect color. **Color blindness** may be genetically inherited (usually seen in males), or it may result from macular degeneration or other diseases that affect the cones of the eye. Use the color bars at the base of the Snellen chart to test color vision. *Ishihara cards* are specialized cards that enable thorough testing for color blindness. They contain embedded figures within a field of color. A person with normal color vision will be able to successfully identify the figures in the cards or the bars on the base of the Snellen chart; one who is color blind will not. To see Snellen chart and Ishihara cards,

 Go to Chapter 22, **Procedure 22-6: Assess the Eyes,** in Volume 2.

Visual Field

Visual field is the area the eye is able to observe. It is related to peripheral vision and extraocular muscle (EOM) function. Visual field abnormalities may be caused by problems with cranial nerves III, IV, and VI or with the retina. Poorly controlled diabetes, cataracts, macular degeneration, and advanced glaucoma are other disorders that limit the visual field. **Peripheral vision** describes the boundaries of the visual field while the eye is in a fixed position. The common phrase, "I see you out of the corner of my eye," refers to peripheral vision.

The EOMs control the movement of the eye and eyelids and allow you to track movement. Three cranial nerves (CN) innervate the EOM. They are CN III (oculomotor), CN IV (trochlear), and CN VI (abducens). CN III also works together with CN II (optic) to control the pupillary reaction to light. Figure 22-4 illustrates the eye positions affected by the EOM and the corresponding cranial nerves.

Strabismus (crossed eye) is a condition in which one or both eyes deviate from the object they are looking at. It is normal during the first 1 or 2 months of life. After that, it may be caused by weak intraocular muscles or a lesion on the oculomotor nerve. Constant strabismus of one eye may result in **amblyopia** ("lazy eye"), in which the brain does not fully acknowledge the images seen by the amblyopic eye. This creates reduced vision in that eye, not correctable by glasses or contact lenses.

Internal Structures of the Eye

Use an ophthalmoscope to visualize the internal structures of the eye (the optic disc, physiological cup, retinal vessels, retinal background, and macula). This is an advanced assessment technique; however, advanced practice nurses and registered nurses on specialty units do perform it with training. Advanced practice nurses use this technique to gain information about certain diseases that affect the eye, such as hypertension and diabetes.

KnowledgeCheck 22-6

- What are the major components of an eye assessment?
- Identify the cranial nerves involved with eye movement and function.

The Ears and Hearing

The ears are involved in both hearing and equilibrium. The **external ear** collects and conveys sound waves to the middle ear. It protects the middle ear from environmental factors such as humidity and temperature and prevents entry of foreign matter. The **middle ear** contains the tympanic membrane and cavity, the eustachian tube, and the **ossicles** (the small bones of the middle ear: the malleus, incus, and stapes). The middle ear conducts sound waves to the inner ear. The **inner ear** is responsible for hearing and equilibrium. Figure 22-5 illustrates the structures of the ear.

Nurses are usually responsible only for screening the ears and making referrals. However, in some settings nurses perform advanced assessments. For procedure steps and guidelines for using the otoscope and tuning fork, as well as for other aspects of ear examination, see the Highlights of Procedures box near the end of this chapter and

 Go to Chapter 22, **Procedure 22-7: Assessing the Ears and Hearing,** in Volume 2.

Examining the External and Middle Ear

On inspection, the ears should be of equal size and similar appearance. Normally the pinna is level with the corner of the eye and within a 10° angle of vertical position (shown in Procedure 22-7 in Volume 2). Altered placement of the ear may be a sign of hearing deficit or genetic disorders, including Down syndrome. There should be no lesions or drainage. Bloody drainage may result from trauma. Purulent drainage may be seen with infection.

On palpation, the external structures of the ear are smooth, nontender, pliable, and without nodules. A painful auricle or tragus may be associated with **otitis externa** (an outer ear infection), whereas tenderness behind the ear is seen with **otitis media** (a middle ear infection).

Otoscopic Examination As you begin the otoscopic examination, you may notice that the external auditory canal contains **cerumen** (wax), which protects the middle ear from excessive drying. However, it should not completely obstruct the ear canal. Cerumen may be

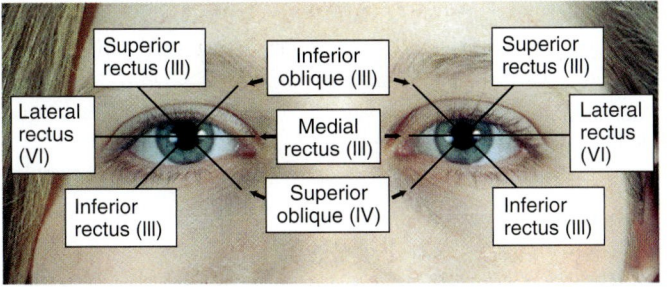

FIGURE 22-4 Cranial nerves and the extraocular muscles.

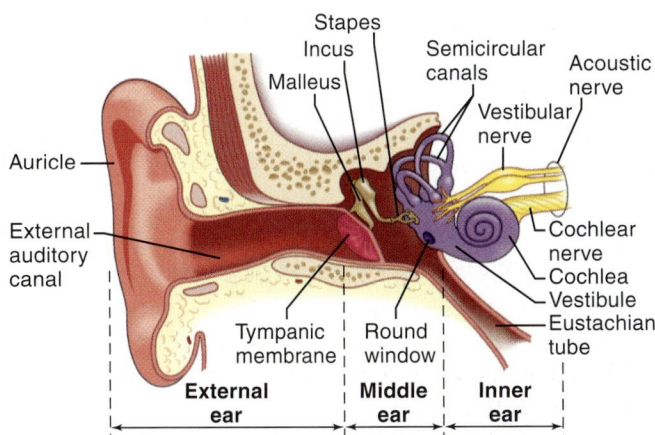

FIGURE 22-5 Cross section of the ear.

black, dark red, yellowish, or brown in color and waxy, flaky, soft, or hard, with no odor; all are normal variations. Be careful as you manipulate the otoscope, because the inner two-thirds of the canal can be tender with the pressure and manipulation of the otoscope head.

Normally the **tympanic membrane (TM)** is pearly gray, shiny, and translucent. The structures of the middle ear should be visible through the membrane. Changes in its appearance arise from abnormalities such as otitis media (which causes a red, bulging TM) and the presence of pressure equalization tubes in young clients with chronic ear infections.

Assessing Hearing

To assess hearing, you will need a quiet room and a tuning fork. Gross hearing ability includes the ability to hear both high- and low-pitched tones. A client who hears low tones will be able to hear and repeat words whispered from 1 to 2 feet behind him. The client can hear high tones if he is able to hear a watch ticking at 5 inches (12 to 13 cm) from each ear.

The Weber and Rinne Tests

Hearing involves transmission of sound vibrations and generation of nerve impulses along CN VIII. The **Weber test** assesses both aspects. When you place a vibrating tuning fork on the center of the client's head, he should be able to sense the vibration equally in both ears. Record a positive Weber test if the vibration is louder in one ear.

If the Weber test is positive, you will need to perform the Rinne test to assess the type of hearing problem. The **Rinne test** also uses a tuning fork to compare air conduction (AC) and bone conduction (BC). Normally AC is twice as long as BC. For step-by-step instructions for performing the Weber and the Rinne tests,

 Go to Chapter 22, **Procedure 22-7: Assessing the Ears and Hearing,** in Volume 2.

The Romberg Test

Along with the cerebellum and midbrain, *vestibular cells* in the ear are responsible for maintaining equilibrium. To assess equilibrium, perform the Romberg test. The client should be able to stand with feet together and eyes closed, and maintain balance with minimal swaying. Swaying and moving (positive Romberg) may indicate a vestibular or cerebellar disorder. You may prefer to perform the Romberg test with examination of the neurological system instead of with the ears.

KnowledgeCheck 22-7

Your client has a negative Weber test. What further testing is required?

ThinkLike a Nurse 22-4

What type of symptoms would you expect a client to be experiencing if he had a positive Romberg test?

The Nose

The nose and sinuses (Fig. 22-6) are part of the respiratory system and are the organs of smell. Vaporized molecules sniffed into the upper nasal cavities trigger receptors that generate impulses along the olfactory nerve (CN I) that travel to olfactory centers in the temporal lobes.

 The sense of smell diminishes in older adults because of a gradual decrease in and atrophy of the olfactory nerve fibers.

See the Highlights of Procedures box near the end of this chapter for a summary of the examination steps. For the complete procedure, along with expected findings,

 Go to Chapter 22, **Procedure 22-8: Assessing the Nose and Sinuses,** in Volume 2.

The Mouth and Oropharynx

The structures of the mouth include the lips, tongue, teeth, **gingiva** (gums), uvula, hard and soft palate, and salivary glands and ducts (Fig. 22-7). On external

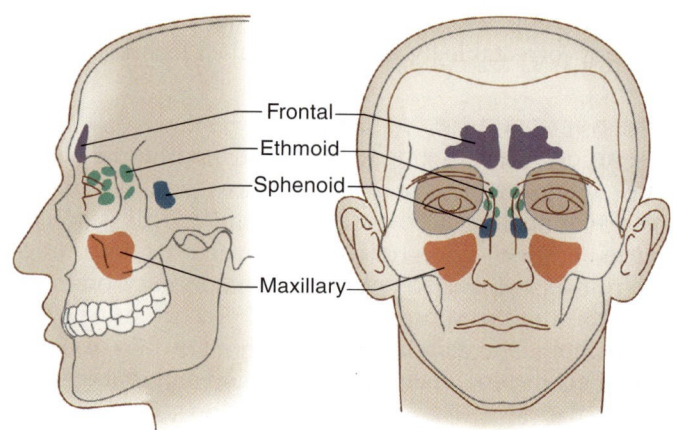

FIGURE 22-6 Paranasal sinuses: frontal, ethmoid, sphenoid, and maxillary.

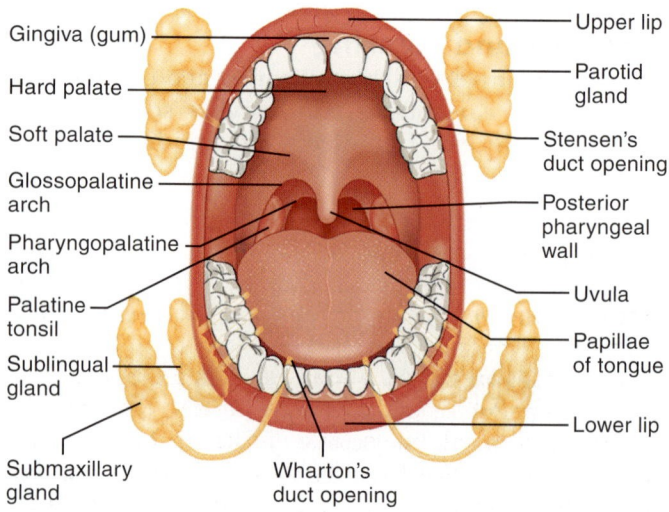

FIGURE 22-7 Structures of the mouth.

inspection, the mouth and lips should be symmetrical and without lesions, swelling, or drooping. For an illustration of structures of the mouth, illustrations of abnormal conditions, and instructions for examining the mouth and oropharynx,

 Go to Chapter 22, **Procedure 22-9: Assessing the Mouth and Oropharynx,** in Volume 2.

Also see the Highlights of Procedures box near the end of this chapter.

The Lips, Buccal Mucosa, and Gingiva

The lips, **buccal mucosa** (mucous membrane of the cheeks), and gums should be smooth, moist, and pink in color. Increased pigmentation (e.g., bluish or dark patches) occurs in dark-skinned clients. No lesions should be present. The following are abnormal findings:

- Pallor may indicate anemia or inadequate oxygenation.
- **Gingivitis** is a sign of periodontal disease. You will see red, swollen, or spongy, bleeding gingiva and receding gum lines. The gums may be tender.
- **Parotitis** is an inflammation of the parotid salivary gland.
- **Stomatitis** is inflammation of the oral mucosa.
- **Leukoplakia** (thick, elevated white patches) that do not scrape off may be precancerous lesions; white, curdy patches that scrape off and bleed indicate **thrush** (a fungal infection).
- Redness or abrasions of the gingiva may be caused by poorly fitted dentures.
- **Aphthous ulcers** are small, painful vesicles with a reddened periphery and a white or pale yellow base. **Canker sores** are a benign type of aphthous ulcer believed to be caused by viral infection, allergies, stress, or trauma. So-called "major" aphthous ulcers may be caused by herpes simplex virus, human immunodeficiency virus, and bacterial infections.

When inspecting the mouth, be sure to ask your client about use of tobacco, either smoked or chewed. Both forms are associated with increased risk for oral cancer.

The Teeth

Healthy adults typically have 28 teeth, or 32 if the wisdom teeth are present. The teeth should be fixed to the gum and without obvious debris or darkening that may indicate caries. Tooth decay and periodontal (gum) disease are common. Poor oral hygiene is a major contributing factor for both. As you examine the mouth and teeth, talk to the patient about his oral care. Recommend tooth brushing after each meal, daily flossing, and dental checkups every 6 months. See Chapter 25 for a more complete discussion of oral hygiene and prevention of periodontal disease.

The Tongue

When inspecting the mouth, carefully examine all aspects of the tongue: dorsal, ventral, and lateral. The **tongue** should be moist, symmetrical, slightly rough, smooth, pink, and freely movable. The following are abnormal findings:

- Limited mobility of the tongue
- Deviation from the midline, which may be caused by damage to the hypoglossal nerve (CN XII)
- **Glossitis** (inflammation of the tongue)
- A dry, furry tongue, which is associated with dehydration
- A black, "hairy" tongue, which is associated with fungal infections
- Reddened mucosa, ulcerations, and absence of papillae which may indicate allergy, inflammation, or infection
- Swelling, nodules, or ulcers
- A smooth, red tongue, which may occur in clients who have a deficiency of iron, vitamin B^{12}, or vitamin B^3

The Hard and Soft Palates and Oropharynx

The hard palate, soft palate, and oropharynx should be pink, moist, and intact. No lesions, swelling, erythema, or discharge should be present. If the tonsils are present, they should be symmetrical, small in size, and free of exudate in a healthy person. The uvula is midline and should rise on **phonation** (vocalization).

THE NECK

The neck has components of the musculoskeletal, neurological, vascular, respiratory, endocrine, and lymphatic systems. The sternocleidomastoid and trapezius muscles form the landmarks of the neck, known as the **anterior and posterior triangles**. The symmetrical neck muscles center and coordinate movement of the head. Asymmetrical head position may result from damage to the muscles, swelling, or masses. Painful or erratic movement may be due to a benign condition, such as muscle spasm, or to significant problems, including meningitis, neurological injuries, or chronic arthritis.

The trachea, thyroid gland, anterior cervical nodes, and carotid arteries are positioned in the anterior triangle; the posterior cervical nodes are in the posterior triangle. You will palpate the tracheal rings and the cricoid and thyroid cartilage in the midline of the anterior neck. For a summary of assessment step, see the Highlights of Procedures box near the end of this chapter. For the complete procedure and for illustrations of structures of the neck,

 Go to Chapter 22, **Procedure 22-10: Assessing the Neck,** in Volume 2.

The Thyroid Gland

Normally the thyroid is smooth, firm, and nontender. It is often nonpalpable. Thyroid abnormalities are common. An enlarged thyroid may be associated with either hypothyroidism or hyperthyroidism. Thyroid tenderness usually results from inflammation. Thyroid masses may be malignant but are usually benign.

The Cervical Lymph Nodes

The cervical lymph nodes occur in three chains. The anterior chain is in the anterior triangle, the posterior chain in the posterior triangle. There is a deep cervical chain under the sternocleidomastoid muscle. The lymph nodes are generally not palpable, although occasionally nodes can be felt, especially in young children. Normal nodes are small in size (less than 1 cm), mobile, soft, and nontender. You should describe enlarged nodes (greater than 1 cm in diameter) according to their location, size, shape, consistency, mobility, and tenderness. Enlarged or tender nodes may be caused by infection, malignancy, and other diseases. For illustrations and step-by-step instructions, see Procedure 22-10.

 ThinkLike a Nurse 22-5

A client complains of sore throat, fever, chills, and runny nose. What assessments should you perform?

THE BREASTS AND AXILLAE

The breasts consist of glandular, adipose, and connective tissue; smooth muscle; and nerves (Fig. 22-8). The functions of the female breast are sexual stimulation and milk production for nourishing offspring. Breast size and shape vary among women, and commonly one breast is slightly larger than the other. At puberty, the ovaries produce estrogen and progesterone, which stimulate the breasts to develop. The menstrual cycle, pregnancy, and breastfeeding also enlarge breast tissue. Although breasts are thought of as female organs, men also have breasts. However, because of limited estrogen and progesterone levels, male breasts develop only minimally.

Breast tissue and lymph drainage for the breast extend up into the axilla. The majority of breast tumors are found in the tail of Spence, in the axilla. A breast exam therefore always includes an exam of the axillae. Many women have breast reconstruction, either after breast removal as a result of cancer or breast augmentation for cosmetic reasons. These women should not omit breast examination, and it is performed in exactly the same way as for natural breasts.

Clinical Breast Examination You should perform a breast exam for the woman if she cannot do it herself, and demonstrate the procedure as part of client teaching for self-care. Clinical breast exams should be done annually for women aged 40 and older, and every 1 to 3 years

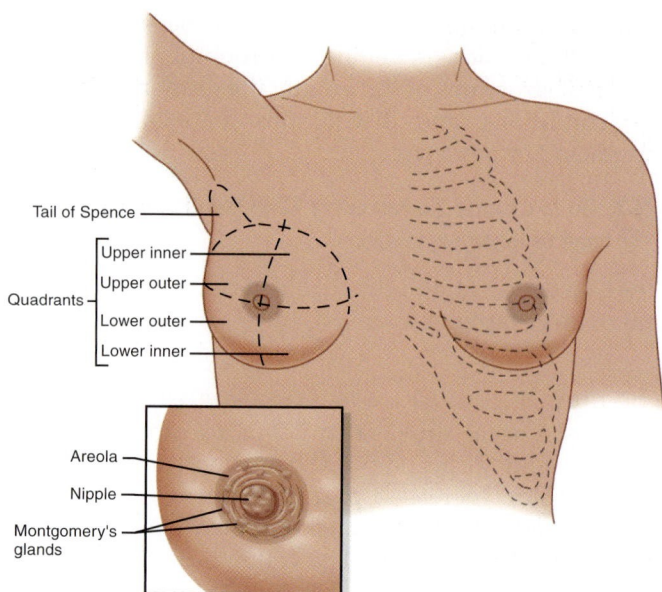

FIGURE 22-8 Breast tissue extends up into the axilla.

for women aged 20 to 39 (American Congress of Obstetricians and Gynecologists [ACOG], 2011). Guidelines vary as to the age at which women should start having clinical breast exams (CBE) and mammograms to screen for breast cancer.

Key Point: *Researchers agree that patients who perform a breast self-exam (BSE) should be trained in proper technique in order to avoid falsely negative findings (ACOG, 2009; Smith, Cokkinides, Brooks, et al., 2011; Smith, Duffy, & Tabár, 2012).*

Chapter 42 includes a thorough discussion of teaching your client how to perform a breast self-exam.

Mammography and Thermography Annual or biennial mammograms or breast thermography most commonly begin after age 40, or at a younger age and more often for those at high risk. ACOG recommends annual mammograms (ACOG, 2011; American Cancer Society, n.d., last revised 2013a, n.d., last revised 2013b).

Controversy exists about whether women should continue to have mammograms after age 74 (refer to Chapters 10 and 42).

For a summary of breast examination, see the Procedure Highlights box at the end of this chapter. For a step-by-step guide to examining the breasts and axillae,

 Go to Chapter 22, **Procedure 22-11: Assessing the Breasts and Axillae,** in Volume 2.

 ThinkLike a Nurse 22-6

What strategies might encourage more women to regularly perform breast self-examination, if your agency has decided to promote that measure?

THE CHEST AND LUNGS

The chest, or thorax, is the bony cage that protects the heart, lungs, and great vessels. The ribs, sternum, and vertebrae form the chest. Be systematic in your assessment: Always assess the areas of the chest and lungs in the same order. To learn how to assess the chest and lungs,

 Go to Chapter 22, **Procedure 22-12, Assessing the Chest and Lungs**, in Volume 2.

For a summary, see the Highlights of Procedures box near the end of this chapter.

Chest Landmarks

Before beginning the thoracic exam, review the following important landmarks that will help you visualize the underlying structures and perform an accurate assessment.

- *Anterior chest*—Identify positions vertically on the anterior chest in relation to the ribs. For example, the space between the 5th and 6th ribs is known as the 5th intercostal space (5th ICS). You can easily palpate the ribs and count the spaces if you remember that the 1st rib is tucked up next to the clavicle (Fig. 22-9A).
- *Anterior chest*—Use a series of imaginary vertical lines (Fig. 22-9B) with the rib spaces to further aid in identifying locations on the anterior chest. For instance, the apex of the heart is usually located in the 5th intercostal space at left midclavicular line (5th ICS MCL).
- *Posterior chest*—Identify positions vertically in relation to the vertebra (Fig. 22-10B). The prominent vertebra at the base of the neck is the 7th cervical vertebra (C7). The next one down is T1 (1st thoracic). Counting down to about T9 should be adequate.
- *Lateral and posterior chest*—Use imaginary lines on the lateral and posterior chest as well. Figure 22-10, parts A and C, illustrates the location of these lines. Notice

that the anterior axillary line can be used to locate sounds on both the anterior and lateral chest.

Chest Shape and Size

The normal adult chest is symmetrical and rises and falls with respirations. The chest diameter expands up to 3 inches (7.6 cm) with deep inspiration. The anteroposterior diameter of the chest (side view) is about half the size of the lateral diameter (front or back view). This is written as AP: Lateral = 1:2). In young children, the chest is apple-shaped. This change is also seen, regardless of age, in clients who have chronic obstructive pulmonary disease (COPD), a disorder associated with long-term smoking. Figure 22-11 illustrates the normal chest ratio and the barrel chest appearance that develops with COPD, in which the anteroposterior and lateral diameters may be equal.

Spinal alterations, such as **kyphosis** (excessive curvature of the thoracic spine) and **scoliosis** (lateral curvature of the spine) alter the shape of the thoracic cage.

Osteoporosis, a common disorder associated with aging, is associated with increased porosity of the vertebrae. As a result, vertebrae may compress or collapse, shortening the length of the spine and pushing the ribs forward and downward.

Breath Sounds

Listen to breath sounds in a quiet room by auscultating one full respiratory cycle at each site. Directly apply the stethoscope to the client's skin. Compare breath sounds bilaterally. Three types of breath sounds are heard (Fig. 22-12).

- **Bronchial breath sounds** are loud, high-pitched, tubular sounds; expiration is of longer duration than inspiration. Air moving through the trachea produces these sounds, which you will hear best over the

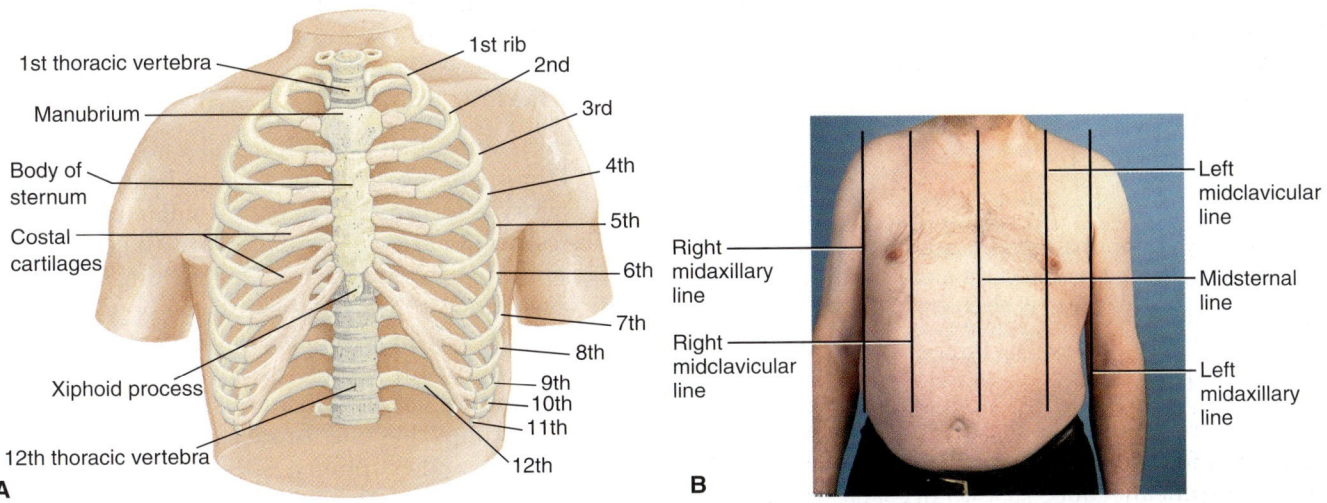

FIGURE 22-9 *A,* The anterior thoracic cage and the bony landmarks. *B,* A series of imaginary vertical lines is used to describe locations on the chest.

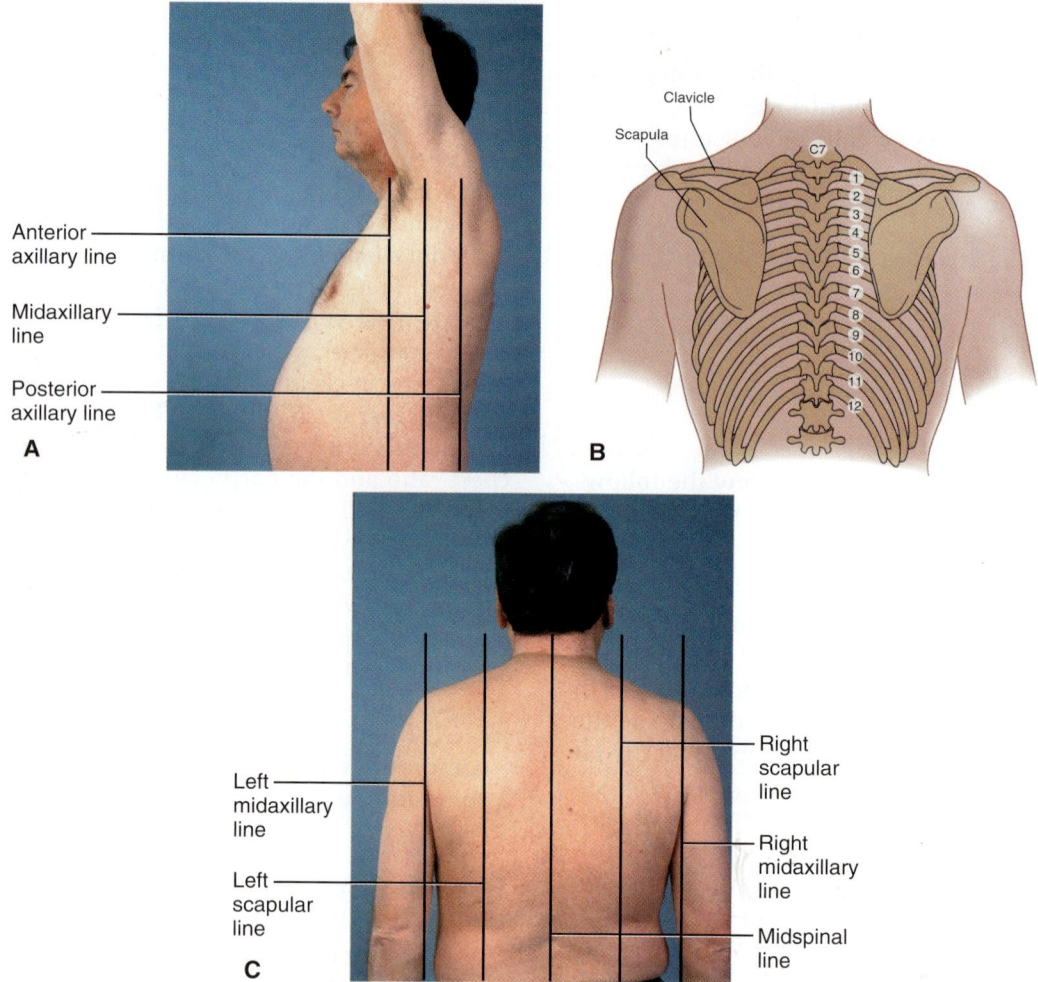

FIGURE 22-10 *A*, Lateral chest landmarks. *B*, The vertebrae are the landmarks on the posterior chest. *C*, Landmark lines on the posterior chest.

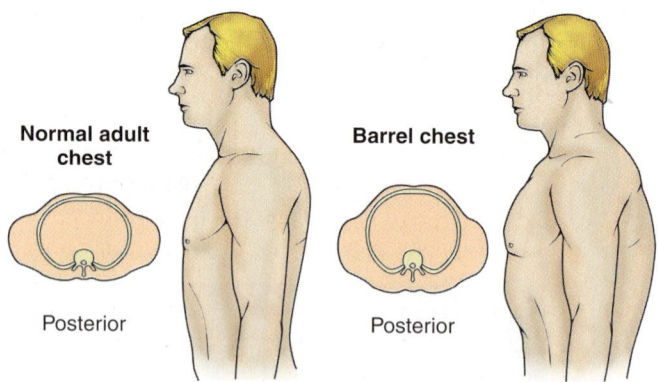

FIGURE 22-11 The normal anteroposterior to lateral ratio is 1:2. The lateral aspect of the chest increases dramatically with COPD, leading to a barrel chest appearance.

trachea on the anterior chest and below the nape of the neck on the posterior chest.

- **Bronchovesicular breath sounds** are medium-pitched with an equal inspiratory and expiratory phase. Air moving through the large airways of the bronchi produces these sounds, which you will hear best over the 1st and 2nd ICS adjacent to the sternum on the anterior chest and between the scapula on the posterior chest.

- **Vesicular breath sounds** are soft, low-pitched, breezy sounds with a lengthy inspiratory phase and a short expiratory phase. Air moving through the smaller airways produces these sounds, which you will hear best over the lung fields.

Breath sounds that differ from those above are abnormal. **Diminished breath sounds** are heard with poor inspiratory effort, in the very muscular or obese, or with restricted airflow. **Misplaced breath sounds** (e.g., bronchial breath sounds heard over the lung fields) indicate constriction of flow. **Adventitious breath sounds**, such as wheezes, rhonchi, and rales, are sounds heard over normal breath sounds. If an abnormal sound is heard, have the client cough and listen again. Other abnormal findings include **bronchophony**, **whispered pectoriloquy**, and **egophony**. These are abnormal voice sounds that result from consolidation of lung tissue. To find a discussion of these and to listen to normal and adventitious breath sounds,

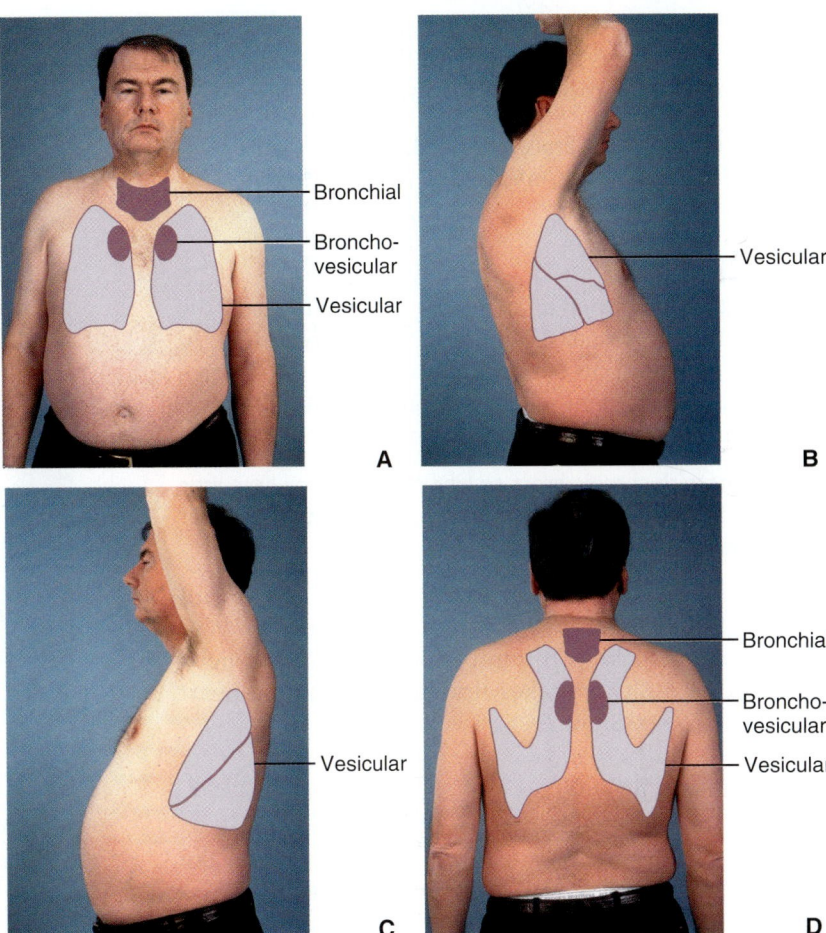

FIGURE 22-12 Normal breath sounds. *A,* Anterior. *B,* Right lateral. *C,* Left lateral. *D,* Posterior.

 Go to Chapter 22, **Supplemental Materials: Abnormal Voice Sounds,** and the various **sound files** for normal and abnormal breath sounds in the Student Resources, on Davis*Plus.*

For more information about the respiratory system, see Chapter 36. The Highlights of Procedures box at the end of this chapter summarizes respiratory assessment. For a table describing abnormal breath sounds and the procedure for performing a respiratory assessment,

 Go to Chapter 22, **Procedure 22-12, Assessing the Chest and Lungs,** in Volume 2.

KnowledgeCheck 22-8

- List and describe the location of the horizontal and vertical landmarks of the anterior chest.
- List and describe the location of the horizontal and vertical landmarks of the posterior chest.
- List and describe the location of the vertical landmarks of the lateral chest.

THE CARDIOVASCULAR SYSTEM

The cardiovascular system consists of the heart and the blood vessels. The heart is a muscle that pumps blood throughout the body. In a healthy adult, it is about the size of a clenched fist. The blood vessels, which make up the vascular system, have two main networks: the pulmonary circulation and the systemic circulation. See Chapter 37 if you need to review the anatomy of the cardiovascular system.

Oxygen-depleted blood circulates from the heart into the lungs, where it is oxygenated, then back to the heart. This system is known as the **pulmonary circulation**. From the heart, the blood enters the **systemic circulation**. The left ventricle is the largest chamber of the heart. It pumps blood into the systemic circulation via the arterial system. The arteries subdivide many times, becoming smaller and smaller until they separate, in the tissues and organs, into capillaries. It is at the capillary level that oxygen is delivered to the tissues. The venous system collects the oxygen-depleted blood and returns it to the right atrium of the heart to begin the circuit again. **Coronary circulation**, which circulates blood through the heart itself, is a part of the systemic circulation. For further discussion on pulmonary circulation and oxygenation, see Chapter 37. For animated presentations of the circulatory system and oxygen transport,

 Go to Student Resources, **Animations: Blood Flow and Carbon Dioxide/Oxygen Transport,** on Davis*Plus.*

The Highlights of Procedures box at the end of this chapter summarizes assessment of the heart and vascular system. For a complete step-by-step procedure,

 Go to Chapter 22, **Procedure 22-13: Assessing the Heart and Vascular System,** in Volume 2.

The Heart

The heart is positioned at an angle on the left side of the chest in the 3rd, 4th, and 5th intercostal spaces (ICS). To facilitate auscultation of specific heart sounds, perform the cardiac assessment with the client in three positions: sitting, supine, and left lateral recumbent.

Clients with chronic heart or lung problems may have little cardiac reserve, so minimize position changes to conserve your client's energy.

Be systematic. To keep from missing important parts of the exam, always listen in the same order to all the areas. To help minimize your client's anxiety, explain that it always takes time to examine the heart and circulatory system.

The Cardiac Cycle

During a cardiac cycle, the atria and ventricles alternately contract and relax to fill and empty; while the atria are contracting (emptying), the ventricles are relaxing (filling), and vice versa. **Systole** refers to the contraction, or emptying, of the ventricles. **Diastole** refers to the relaxation, or filling, phase of the ventricles.

Inspecting and Palpating the Heart

Begin with the client sitting (Fig. 22-13). Observe the **precordium**, the area of the chest over the heart, for visible pulsations. A small pulsation at the 5th ICS midclavicular line, also known as the **point of maximal impulse (PMI)**, is normal. Other visible pulsations on the precordium, known as **heaves** or **lifts**, are associated with an enlarged ventricle.

Palpate for vibrations. A **thrill** is a vibration or pulsation palpated in any area except the PMI. A thrill is associated with abnormal blood flow and usually has an accompanying **murmur** (additional heart sound).

Auscultating the Heart

Auscultate to establish cardiac rate and rhythm and to identify normal and abnormal heart sounds. A quiet room is essential. You can hear heart sounds from any location on the anterior chest wall. However, the four sites located over the heart valves are the preferred listening areas. Table 22-4 and Figure 22-13 describe these locations. To learn more about auscultating the precordium,

 Go to Chapter 22, **Procedure 22-13, Assessing the Heart and Vascular System,** in Volume 2.

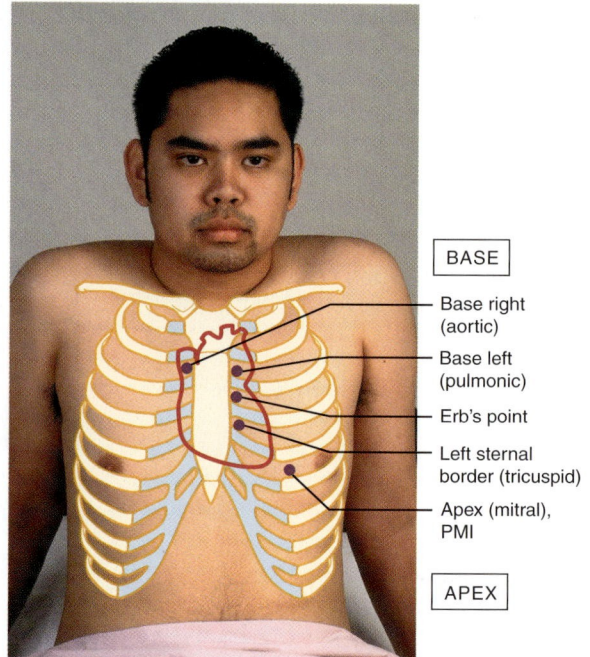

FIGURE 22-13 Cardiac auscultation sites.

Table 22-4 ▶ Locations for Assessing the Heart		
TITLE	**STRUCTURE ASSESSED**	**LOCATION**
Base Right	Aortic valve	2nd ICS right sternal border
Base Left	Pulmonic valve	2nd ICS left sternal border
Left Lateral	Tricuspid valve	4th ICS left sternal border
Apex	Mitral valve	5th ICS MCL

Auscultate in an orderly fashion. Start at the aortic area, and move gradually through each landmark. The following is a mnemonic you may use to recall the order of the heart sound landmarks:

*A*unt	Aortic
*P*olly	Pulmonic
*T*akes	Tricuspid
*M*eds	Mitral

Listen carefully at each site to each component of the heart sounds.

First Heart Sound The first heart sound (S_1, or "lub") results from the closure of the valves between the atria and ventricles. S_1 ("lub") is a dull, low-pitched sound, loudest over the mitral and tricuspid areas. S_1 marks the beginning of systole.

Second Heart Sound The second heart sound (S_2, or "dub") corresponds to closure of the semilunar valves (between the ventricles and the great arteries exiting the heart). "Dub" is higher in pitch and shorter than the S_1 "lub." The S_2 is loudest at the aortic and pulmonic areas. S_2 marks the beginning of diastole. Normally, the mitral and tricuspid valves and the aortic and pulmonic valves close within a fraction of a second from each other. This near simultaneous closure results in a singular S_1 and S_2 sound. However, a split sound may occur, at either S_1 or S_2, if there is a delay in closure of one of the valves.

Third Heart Sounds A third heart sound (S_3), heard immediately after S_2, has a gallop cadence that follows the rhythm of the word "KenTUCKy." It is best heard at the apical site with the client lying on his left side. An S_3 is normal in young children and adolescents when they are sitting or lying, but it disappears when they stand or sit up. It is also a normal variant in the third trimester of pregnancy. In adults, an S_3 that does not disappear with position change is abnormal and represents heart failure or volume overload.

Fourth Heart Sounds A fourth heart sound (S_4), heard immediately before S_1, has a rhythm that follows the word "FLOrida." S_4 is best heard at the apical site, using the bell of the stethoscope, with the client lying on his left side. An S_4 is normal in athletes and some older clients. It may also be heard in adults with coronary artery disease, hypertension, and pulmonic stenosis. To listen to heart sounds,

 Go to Student Resources, **Sound Files, Heart Sounds,** on Davis*Plus*.

Murmurs Murmurs are additional sounds produced by turbulent flow through the heart. Some murmurs are "innocent," but others represent pathology such as alteration in valve structure. Identifying and classifying a murmur are advanced skills that require practice. To learn more about assessing murmurs, see the Highlights of Procedures box, and

 Go to Chapter 22, **Procedure 22-13: Assessing the Heart and Vascular System,** in Volume 2. Also go to Chapter 22, **Supplemental Materials: Heart Murmurs,** and **Tables, Boxes, Figures: ESG Table 22-1,** on Davis*Plus*.

 ThinkLike a Nurse 22-7

What findings would you anticipate when assessing Mr. Nguyen's (Meet Your Patient) thorax?

The Vascular System

The vascular system is a network of arteries and veins that transport oxygen, carbon dioxide, and nutrients to the cells of the body. Arteries carry blood away from the heart: The pulmonary arteries carry oxygen-depleted blood from the right ventricle to the lungs, whereas the systemic arteries carry oxygenated blood from the left ventricle to the body periphery. Veins carry blood toward the heart: The pulmonary veins transport oxygenated blood from the lungs to the left atrium, whereas the systemic veins return oxygen-depleted blood from the periphery to the right atrium of the heart.

The Central Vessels

The carotid arteries and internal jugular veins run alongside the sternocleidomastoid muscle on both sides of the neck (Fig. 22-14). These central vessels provide circulation to the brain.

The Carotid Arteries

Because the carotid arteries are large and close to the heart, you can easily feel a pulse over the carotid artery even when it is difficult to palpate a peripheral pulse.

 Never palpate both carotid arteries at the same time because bilateral pressure may impair cerebral blood flow. Palpate very lightly and avoid massaging the carotid artery, because pressure on the carotids will cause the pulse rate to drop, and can even lead to cardiac arrest. As a general rule, avoid palpating the carotids except during cardiopulmonary resuscitation or when it is necessary to assess them for a specific reason (such as in a comprehensive physical exam, or when an underlying pathology makes it necessary to establish that circulation to the head is adequate).

Turbulent blood flow through the carotid artery produces a whooshing sound known as a **bruit**, which you can auscultate using a stethoscope. The following conditions cause turbulence: **carotid stenosis** (narrowing from plaque), increased cardiac output secondary to fluid overload, use of stimulants, and hyperthyroidism. If you hear a bruit, lightly palpate the neck for thrills (pulsations or vibrations), which further confirm turbulent flow.

Bruits are common among older adults.

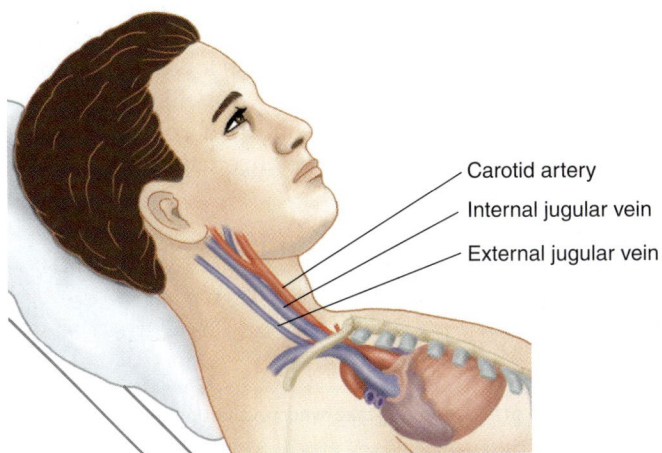

FIGURE 22-14 The central vessels.

Carotid artery
Internal jugular vein
External jugular vein

The Jugular Veins

The jugular veins return blood from the brain to the superior vena cava. The external jugular veins are superficial; the internal jugular veins are deep. Normally the jugular veins are flat when the client is in an upright position and distend when the client lies flat. Jugular venous distention (JVD) is seen when the right side of the heart is congested because of inadequate pump function. The best position for assessment of JVD is semi-Fowler's (30° to 45° angle)

The Peripheral Vessels

The peripheral vessels supply blood to all the body cells. The **arteries** are a high-pressure system with several palpable pulse sites. The **veins** are a low-pressure system with valves to prevent backflow caused by gravity. The veins return blood to the heart via the continuing pressure from the arterial system and pumping action of the adjacent skeletal muscles. If you were to lay out all the blood vessels in the peripheral system of an average sized person, you would find more than 60,000 miles of arteries, arterioles, capillaries, and venules.

You will assess the peripheral vascular system by:

- *Measuring the blood pressure* (see Chapter 20), usually at the start of the exam as part of the general survey.
- *Palpating the peripheral pulses* (see Chapter 20). In a healthy individual, pulses will be regular, strong, and equal bilaterally. Weak, absent, or asymmetrical pulses may indicate partial or complete occlusion of the artery. Other signs of arterial occlusion include pain, pallor, cool temperature, paresthesia, or paralysis.
- *Inspecting and performing tests for adequate perfusion.*

The data you obtain when inspecting and palpating the integumentary system provide some information about peripheral tissue perfusion. Recall that when an area is not adequately oxygenated, the skin may be pale, cyanotic, cool, and shiny; hair growth may be sparse; and there may be clubbing of the nails. Inadequate tissue oxygenation may be a result of chronic pulmonary problems; however, it can also result from impaired central or peripheral circulation.

Also assess the veins for signs of distention. Superficial spiderlike veins, especially on the lower extremities, may occur with normal aging. Ropelike distended veins, or **varicosities**, may be painful. If a client has varicosities, assess for valve competence using the **manual compression test**. To see that,

 Go to Chapter 22, **Procedure 22-13, Assessing the Heart and Vascular System,** in Volume 2.

KnowledgeCheck 22-9

Identify the precautions to take when evaluating the carotid arteries.

THE ABDOMEN

The method most commonly used to identify the location of assessment findings is the four-quadrant method, which divides the abdomen into four sections by "drawing" a line vertically from the xiphoid process to the symphysis pubis and a horizontal line at the level of the umbilicus (Fig. 22-15).

For the rarely used nine-region method,

 Go to Chapter 22, **Tables, Boxes, Figures: ESG Table 22-2, The Nine Regions of the Abdomen;** and **ESG Figure 22-1, The Nine Regions of the Abdomen,** on *DavisPlus.*

Examination of the abdomen differs in sequence from all other body systems. Percussion and palpation stimulate the bowel and may alter bowel sounds. Therefore, you should inspect and auscultate before performing percussion and palpation. To promote comfort, ask the client to empty his bladder before the examination. Have the client assume a supine position with flexed knees. This relaxes the abdominal muscles and is usually the most comfortable position. If the client has a painful area, examine that area last to minimize discomfort during the rest of the exam.

Inspecting the Abdomen

The skin over the abdomen is usually paler than that over other parts of the body. The abdomen should be symmetrical with a rounded contour and sunken umbilicus. You may be able to see peristalsis and aortic pulsations on a very thin client, but in most clients usually you will see no movement. In clients with abdominal distention, the skin appears taut. Distention may be

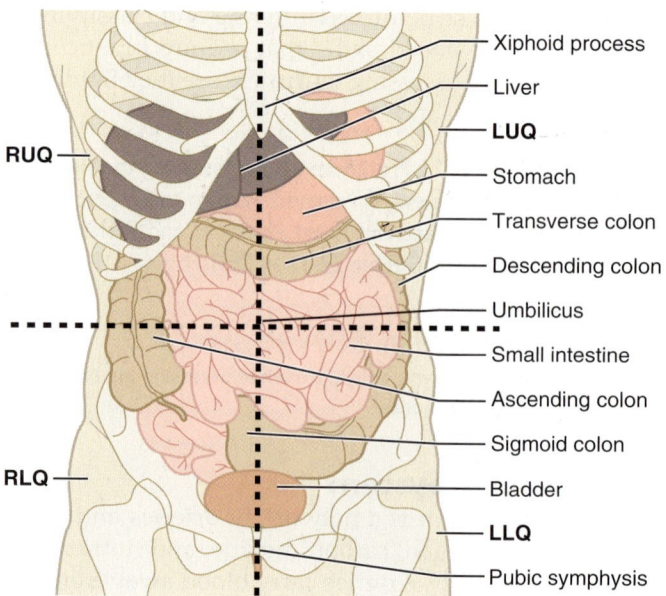

FIGURE 22-15 The four abdominal quadrants.

normal, as with pregnancy, or it may be due to gas or fluid retention or to bowel obstruction. See Figure 22-16 for normal variations in abdominal shape.

Auscultating the Abdomen

Proceed in an organized manner, listening in several areas in all four quadrants. Use the same pattern for every examination so that it becomes a habit.

First Auscultate Bowel Sounds Bowel sounds are high-pitched, irregular gurgles or clicks lasting one to several seconds and occurring every 5 to 15 seconds (or 5 to 30 times per minute) in the average adult. If the client has a nasogastric (NG) tube that is attached to suction, discontinue the suction or clamp off the tube while listening for bowel sounds. Otherwise, you may mistake the sound of suction in the stomach for bowel sounds. Bowel sounds may be:

- **Normal.** Audible, occurring every 5 to 15 sec (or 5–30 times per min) in a healthy adult.
- **Hyperactive (hyperperistalsis).** Loud, rushing sounds occurring every 2 or 3 sec (or more than 30 per min); may indicate diarrhea, early bowel obstruction, or gastroenteritis (infection of the GI tract).
- **Hypoactive (hypoperistalsis).** Very faint and infrequent (fewer than 5 sounds per min); may occur after abdominal surgery or with bowel obstruction, infection, or problems of innervation.
- **Absent.** None after listening for 5 min.

To hear some bowel sounds,

 Go to **Sound Files: Bowel Sounds,** on DavisPlus.

Next Auscultate the Major Arteries Major arterial vessels lie in the abdomen below the intestines. Listen over the aorta and the renal, iliac, and femoral arteries for the presence of bruits.

Percussing the Abdomen

Use indirect percussion to assess for fluid, air, organs, or masses. Normally there is generalized tympany over the bowels (due to the presence of gas) and the abdomen is nontender, soft, and without masses. You will hear dullness when percussing organs, masses, or fluids. Some

practitioners include percussion of the kidney with the abdominal examination.

Palpating the Abdomen

Begin with light palpation to put the patient at ease. Palpate for tenderness and guarding in all four quadrants. Palpation of the liver and spleen is an advanced technique not usually performed by staff nurses, except perhaps in some specialty areas. The Highlights of Procedures box at the end of this chapter summarizes abdominal assessment. For the complete procedure,

 Go to Chapter 22, **Procedure 22-14: Assessing the Abdomen,** in Volume 2.

KnowledgeCheck 22-10

- What strategies can you use to make the client more comfortable during an abdominal assessment?
- Identify the sequence of assessment for the abdominal exam.

THE MUSCULOSKELETAL SYSTEM

The musculoskeletal system consists of bones, muscles, and joints. Bone is complex living tissue that responds to nutrition, stress, and illness. The bones include *long bones,* such as the humerus and tibia; *flat bones,* such as the sternum and ribs; and *irregular bones,* such as the vertebrae and pelvis. Tendons, ligaments, and cartilage serve as connecting structures. **Bursae,** small disc-shaped, fluid-filled sacs, act as cushions to reduce friction between the joint and the tendons that cross over the joint (Fig. 22-17). The musculoskeletal system provides shape and support to the body, allows movement, protects internal organs, produces red blood cells in the bone marrow, and stores calcium and phosphorus.

Assessment of the musculoskeletal system includes evaluation of the client's posture, gait, bone structure, muscle function, and joint mobility. The procedure is summarized in the Highlights of Procedures box at the end of this chapter. For step-by-step instructions,

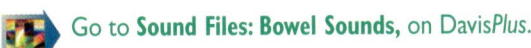 Go to Chapter 22, **Procedure 22-15: Assessing the Musculoskeletal System,** in Volume 2.

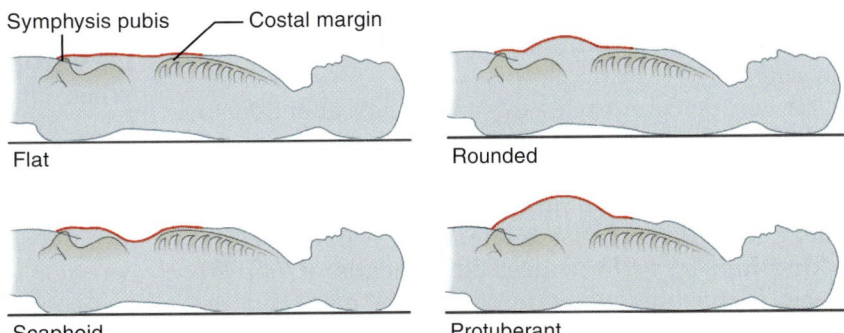

FIGURE 22-16 Normal variations in abdominal contour.

Symphysis pubis — Costal margin

Flat

Rounded

Scaphoid

Protuberant

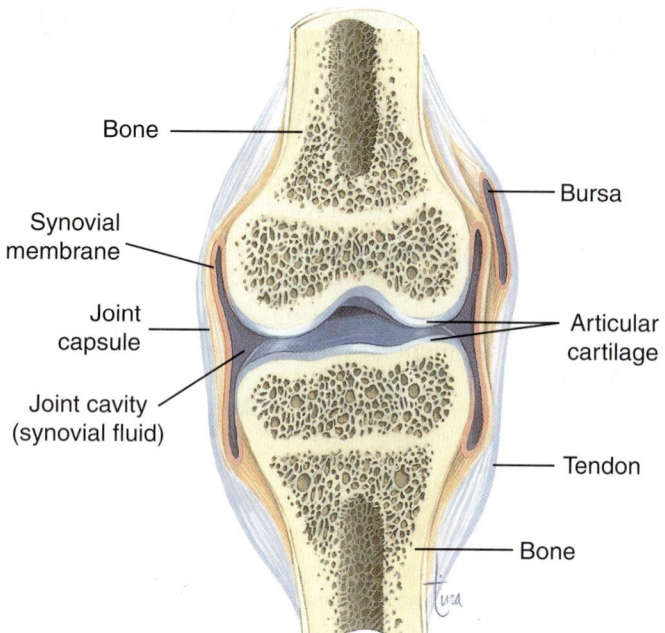

Bone

Synovial membrane

Joint capsule

Joint cavity (synovial fluid)

Bursa

Articular cartilage

Tendon

Bone

FIGURE 22-17 Many synovial joints have bursae that act as cushions against friction.

Body Shape and Symmetry

To assess bone structure, examine body shape and symmetry. Major deformities in bone structure affect posture and gait. The client should be able to stand upright with the neck and head midline. There are four normal curvatures of the spine (see Procedure 22-15). The cervical and lumbar are concave, and the thoracic and sacral are convex. Commonly seen abnormalities include **kyphosis** (accentuated thoracic curve), **scoliosis** (lateral "S" deviation of the spine), and **lordosis** (accentuated lumbar curve).

Balance, Coordination, and Movement

Walking is a complex task involving balance, coordination, and movement. Pay attention to the *base of support* and *stride* as the client walks. A wide base of support or shortened stride may indicate a balance problem. If the client has an altered gait, try to identify the specific portion of the gait that is abnormal. Abnormal gait may be caused by muscle hypertonicity (e.g., from stroke or brain tumor), lumbar disc problems, muscle atrophy, nerve damage, Parkinson's disease, cerebral palsy, multiple sclerosis, or spinal tumors. If you need additional information on gait, see Chapter 32.

As you perform each assessment, pay attention to the client's stability and level of comfort. Do not attempt movements that may produce pain or cause the client to fall. For example, recall that Mr. Nguyen (Meet Your Patient) has bilateral knee pain. Before asking him to perform deep knee bends or hop in place, you would want to assess his pain and its triggers.

Joint Mobility and Muscle Function

Any joint deformity requires investigation. Color changes in a joint indicate inflammation or infection. If you see erythema or swelling, investigate further by feeling for warmth. Determine any effect the deformity has on function.

Joints should move freely and without pain or **crepitus** (clicking or grating at a joint). To assess function, test range of motion (ROM) and muscle strength. **Active ROM** requires the client to move the joint through its full ROM. **Passive ROM** is used when the client is unable to exercise each joint independently. Instead, you support the body and move each joint through its ROM. Assess **muscle strength** along with movement by asking the patient to perform ROM while you apply resistance to the part being moved. For more information about the musculoskeletal system, see Chapter 32.

 ThinkLike a **Nurse** 22-8

As you recall, Mr. Nguyen (Meet Your Patient) is obese and has been having pain in both of his knees.

- What history questions would you ask him to assess his knee pain?
- What would you do to examine his knees?

THE NEUROLOGICAL SYSTEM

The neurological system controls or affects the function of all body systems and allows interaction with the external world. Its work is carried out through the transmission of chemical and electrical signals between the brain and the rest of the body. The basic functions of the nervous system are cognition, emotion, memory, sensation and perception, and regulation of homeostasis.

A comprehensive neurological assessment takes hours to complete and is usually reserved for clients with symptoms of neurological problems. As a staff nurse in general practice, you usually perform only portions of a neurological exam. In the next few sections, we look at the components of a focused neurological exam. For a summary, see the Highlights of Procedures box at the end of this chapter. For the complete procedure,

 Go to Chapter 22, **Procedure 22-16: Assessing the Sensory-Neurological System,** in Volume 2.

Developmental Considerations

When interpreting a neurological exam, consider the following developmental changes and modifications:

Infants Reflexes present at birth include rooting, sucking, palmar grasp, tonic neck reflex (fencing), and Moro. These reflexes disappear during infancy. With neurological injury, as may occur with stroke or trauma, these reflexes may return, indicating severe neurological problems. To review these reflexes, refer to Chapter 9.

Young Children Because language skills and motor development are age-dependent, the Denver Developmental Screening Test (Denver II, 1990) is used as a neurological screen for young children. The Denver II examines motor, language, and coordination skills. It requires specialized training to administer and evaluate.

For toddlers and older children, you can usually perform a comprehensive neurological exam with age-appropriate modifications. For example, when testing for smell, use materials that a young child knows, such as bananas or apples.

Older Adults With advanced age, changes commonly observed are slower reaction time, a decreased ability for rapid problem-solving, and slower voluntary movement. The number of functioning neurons decreases. However, intelligence, memory, and discrimination do not change with normal aging. Neurological deficits in older adults are usually the result of adverse effects of medications or medication interactions, nutritional deficits, dehydration, cardiovascular changes that alter cerebral blood flow, diabetes, degenerative neurological conditions (e.g., Parkinson's disease or Alzheimer's disease), alcohol or drug use, depression, or abuse.

Cerebral Function

Cerebral function refers to the client's intellectual and behavioral functioning. It includes level of consciousness, orientation, mental status and cognitive function, and communication.

Level of Consciousness

Decreased level of consciousness is often the first sign of neurological deterioration. **Level of consciousness (LOC)** includes arousal and orientation. Arousal may range from alert to deeply comatose. Arousal is classified based on the type of stimuli (auditory, tactile, or painful) required to produce a response from the client. An alert client responds to *auditory stimuli* (e.g., verbal communication or noise).

Key Point: *Remember, if your client does not speak your language he may not respond to questions or commands.*

If the client does not respond to auditory stimuli, try *tactile stimuli.* Begin with gentle touch to awaken the client and capture attention. Be aware that many clients who have hearing deficits lip-read to compensate. If you catch the client's attention by touching her hand, she may be able to respond to the combined auditory and visual stimuli. If still no response is obtained, use *painful stimuli* (e.g., squeezing the trapezius muscle). Clients who respond to painful stimuli withdraw when pressure is applied.

Document LOC by describing the client's response or by using the Glasgow Coma Scale (GCS) to grade eye, motor, and verbal responses. The GCS evaluates eye opening, motor responses, and verbal responses. Its limitations are that it relies heavily on vision and verbal interaction, and does not evaluate brainstem reflexes. A systematic review of evidence suggests that best practice should include use of the GCS plus other evaluation of brainstem reflexes, eye examination, vital signs, and respiratory assessment. A newer tool, the Full Outline of UnResponsiveness (FOUR), provides additional information beyond that of the GCS. Both scales are included in Volume 2 for you to use in clinical settings.

 Go to Chapter 22, **Procedure 22-16: Assessing the Sensory–Neurological System, Glasgow Coma Scale, and Full Outline of UnResponsiveness Scale,** in Volume 2.

If you are not using the GCS, use the following terms to describe LOC.

- **Alert.** Follows commands in a timely fashion.
- **Lethargic.** Appears drowsy, easily drifts off to sleep.
- **Stuporous.** Requires vigorous stimulation before responding.
- **Comatose.** Does not respond to verbal or painful stimuli.

Although those terms are widely used, a thorough description is preferable. Look at the following two chart entries:

Example 1. Pt lethargic.
Example 2. Pt responds to repeated tactile and verbal stimulation. Quickly drifts off to sleep if stimulation is discontinued.

As you can see, the second charting entry provides significantly more information than the first.

Orientation

Orientation refers to the client's awareness of time, place, and person.

- **Time orientation** includes awareness of the year, date, and time of day. Older adults who become disoriented to time usually think it is an earlier date. If a client offers a bizarre time or futuristic date, consider psychiatric concerns as the cause of disorientation. Hospitalized patients are subjected to lights and noise around the clock; are roused in the middle of the night for medications or time-sensitive treatments; and are given anesthesia and pain medications that alter their sense of awareness, so they easily become disoriented to time.
- **Orientation to place** involves awareness of surroundings. The patient should know that he is, for example, in the hospital and not in church. Patients who have been moved (e.g., from the emergency department to a ward bed) may not recall their room number but are easily reoriented.
- **Orientation to person** involves recognition of familiar persons and self-identity. The client should be able to

state her name or identify people in photographs at the bedside. Because a client may meet many health professionals during a hospitalization, she may not be able to recall your name unless you have had repeated encounters with her.

Mental Status and Cognitive Function

Mental status and cognitive function include behavior, appearance, response to stimuli, speech, memory, communication, and judgment. By this point in the exam, you would have already interviewed the client and talked with him while performing the exam, so you would have a good deal of information about his mental status and cognitive function. You would have already assessed posture, gait, motor movements, dress, and hygiene through the general survey and the musculoskeletal exam; and you would be aware of the client's mood based on his tone of voice, actions, and statements.

Many clinicians choose to screen for mental status and cognitive function by asking questions of the client as they assess other body systems. This type of informal assessment helps relax the client. If you choose this method, observe for clarity of thought, appropriate content, concentration, memory, and ability to perform abstract reasoning. Normal findings include the ability to express and explain realistic thoughts with clear speech;

speak with a smooth, natural pattern; follow multistep directions; listen; answer questions; and recall significant past events.

Cranial Nerve Function

Cranial nerve assessment is a key component of the neurological exam. The cranial nerves control a variety of sensory and motor functions (Table 22-5 and Fig. 22-18).

Reflex Function

Deep tendon reflexes (DTRs) are automatic responses that do not require conscious thought from the brain. A reflex produces a rapid, involuntary response that occurs at the level of the spinal cord (Fig. 22-19). Because the brain is not involved, muscle response is instantaneous. Intact sensory and motor systems are required for a normal reflex response. Each DTR corresponds to a certain level of the cord and is graded on a 0 to 4+ scale. To see the scale,

 Procedure 22-16, Assessing the Sensory-Neurological System, in Volume 2.

You can elicit **superficial reflexes** by swiftly and lightly stroking a body part (e.g., with the reflex hammer). Superficial reflexes are graded as positive or negative.

Table 22-5 ➤ Cranial Nerves		
CRANIAL NERVE NUMBER & NAME	**TYPE OF NERVE**	**FUNCTION OF NERVE**
I. Olfactory	Sensory	Smell
II. Optic	Sensory	Visual acuity, visual fields, and ocular fundi
III. Oculomotor	Motor	EOM, pupil constriction
IV. Trochlear	Motor	EOM
V. Trigeminal: 3 branches	Sensory and motor	Corneal reflex; scalp, teeth, and facial sensation; and jaw movement
VI. Abducens	Motor	EOM
VII. Facial	Motor and sensory	Facial movement, sense of taste
VIII. Auditory	Sensory	Hearing and equilibrium
IX. Glossopharyngeal	Motor and sensory	Swallowing, gag response, tongue movement, taste, secretion of saliva
X. Vagus	Motor and sensory	Sensation of pharynx and larynx; motor activity of swallowing and vocal cords; sensory in cardiac, respiratory, and blood pressure reflexes; peristalsis; digestive secretions
XI. Spinal accessory	Motor	Head movement and shoulder elevation; motor to larynx (speaking)
XII. Hypoglossal	Motor	Tongue movement

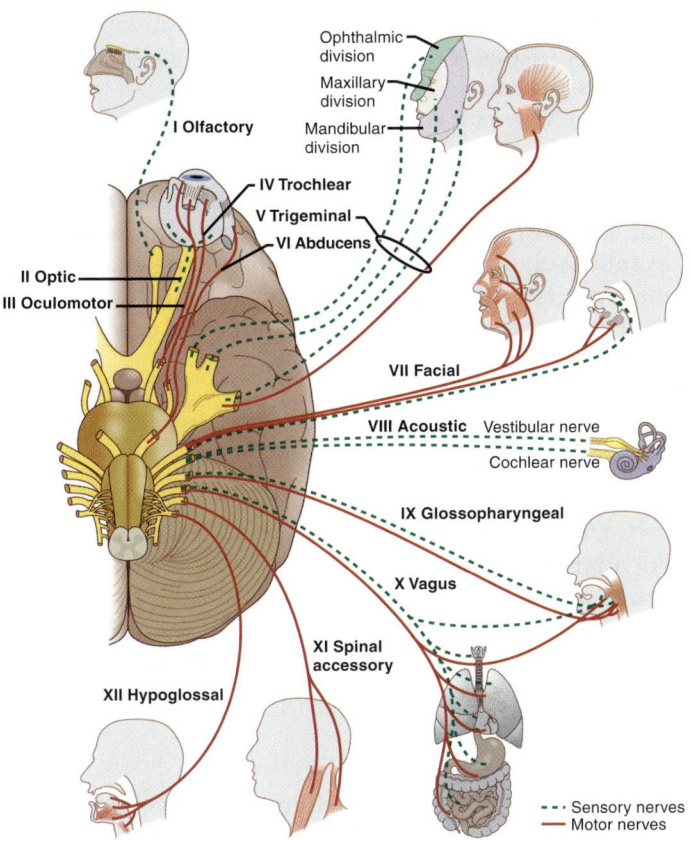

FIGURE 22-18 Origin of cranial nerves.

Sensory Function

To assess sensory function, ask the client to keep his eyes closed as you apply various stimuli. Ask him to indicate when he feels a sensation. Vary your location and approach so that you test sensation, not pattern recognition. If you notice an area of altered sensation, systematically assess the area to define the border of the change. Usually you will limit your testing to the upper and lower extremities and the trunk. If the client has known or suspected deficits, you should test at numerous other sites. For techniques for assessing reflexes and sensory function,

 Go to Chapter 22, **Procedure 22-16: Assessing the Sensory-Neurological System,** in Volume 2.

Motor and Cerebellar Function

The neurological system coordinates the function of the skeleton and muscles. Motor pathways transmit information between the brain and muscles and the muscles control movement of the skeleton. The cerebellum helps coordinate muscle movement, regulate muscle tone, and maintain posture and equilibrium. The cerebellum is also largely responsible for **proprioception**, or body positioning. Disorders of motor and cerebellar function result in pain or problems with movement, gait, or posture. Thus, when you assess the musculoskeletal system, you also assess the motor functions of the neurological system.

KnowledgeCheck 22-11

- Identify and describe the components assessed in the neurological exam.
- What approach to assessment should you take if:
  Your client has no neurological problems but you are performing a comprehensive exam?
  Your client is hospitalized for a documented cerebrovascular accident?
  Your client has been admitted with an acute head injury and the extent of neurological injury is unknown?

THE GENITOURINARY SYSTEM

In most practice settings, nurses assess only the patient's external genitalia and inguinal lymph nodes. Nurse practitioners and physicians perform comprehensive examinations of the female and male reproductive and urinary systems, as do nurses working in specialty areas. However, even as a novice nurse you may assist with exams or just be present as a witness or to provide emotional support to the client.

The genitourinary system includes both the reproductive system and the urinary system (Figs. 22-20 and 22-21). Because assessment focuses on elimination and sexual and reproductive function, it might be embarrassing or uncomfortable for many people. A competent, professional approach is needed. Your confidence and ease with these topics will help the client to feel more relaxed.

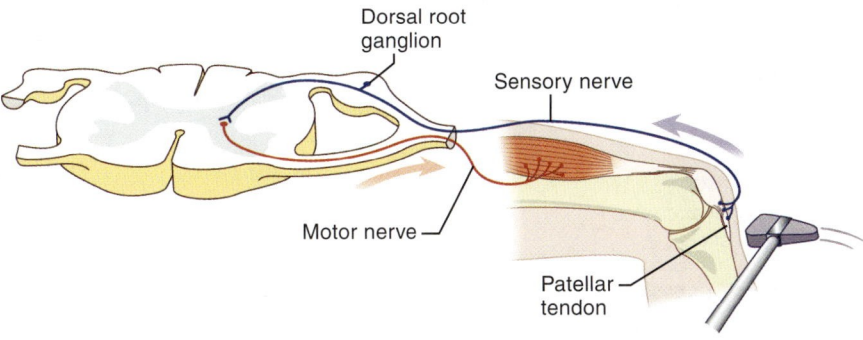

FIGURE 22-19 Reflex arc.

The Male Genitourinary System

A complete examination includes assessment of the external genitalia, evaluation for hernias, and a rectal exam for prostate screening. The penis and scrotum are examined by inspection and palpation. You will assess some of the urinary system organs when examining the back (kidneys, ureters) and the abdomen (bladder); the prostate gland is palpated during the exam of the rectum and anus (discussed later in this chapter). For steps to follow in examining the male genitourinary system, see the summary in the Highlights of Procedures box at the end of this chapter and

 Go to Chapter 22, **Procedure 22-17: Assessing the Male Genitourinary System,** in Volume 2.

As a result of the scarcity of clear, scientific evidence, the American Academy of Pediatrics no longer recommends newborn male **circumcision** (excision of the foreskin of the penis) as a routine practice. However, circumcision is tied to some religious and cultural beliefs (e.g., among Jews and Muslims), so it is still common.

A **hernia** is a protrusion of the intestine (or other organ) through the wall that contains it. In men, this is most likely to be a protrusion of the intestine either through the abdominal wall (**direct hernia**) or into the inguinal canal and possibly into the scrotum (**indirect hernia**). A hernia may be a small protrusion or it may cause pain and distention as a loop of bowel extends into the scrotum. An **umbilical hernia** (fairly common in infants) is an outward bulging due to delayed closure around a small muscle around the umbilicus (belly button). For an illustration of an umbilical hernia,

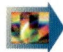 Go to **Procedure 22-14: Assessing the Abdomen,** in Volume 2.

KnowledgeCheck 22-12

- What assessment techniques are used when examining the male genitourinary system?
- What is the most common hernia occurring in men?

The Female Genitourinary System

You may be called upon to assist with a comprehensive examination. For a procedure for inspecting external female genitalia and palpating inguinal lymph nodes, see the Highlights of Procedures box at the end of this chapter and,

 Go to Chapter 22, **Procedure 22-18: Assessing the Female Genitourinary System,** in Volume 2.

External Examination

For adolescents and young women who are not sexually active, an external GU examination includes the inspection of the amount and distribution of pubic hair, the skin of the pubic area, and the external genitalia; and palpation of the inguinal lymph nodes.

Internal Examination

Women who are sexually active; who have abnormal findings on external examination; who have abdominal, pelvic, or genitourinary complaints; or who are on hormone therapy require an internal genital examination. The exam includes the following:

- Palpation of Bartholin's glands and Skene's ducts (Fig. 22-21).
- Assessment of vaginal muscle tone and pelvic musculature
- Speculum examination
- Bimanual examination, wherein the examiner palpates the cervix, uterus, and adnexal tissues using one or two fingers within the vagina and the other hand

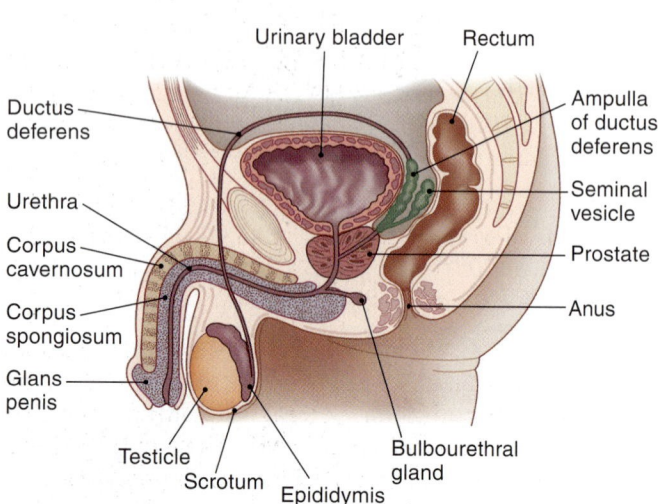

FIGURE 22-20 The male genitourinary system.

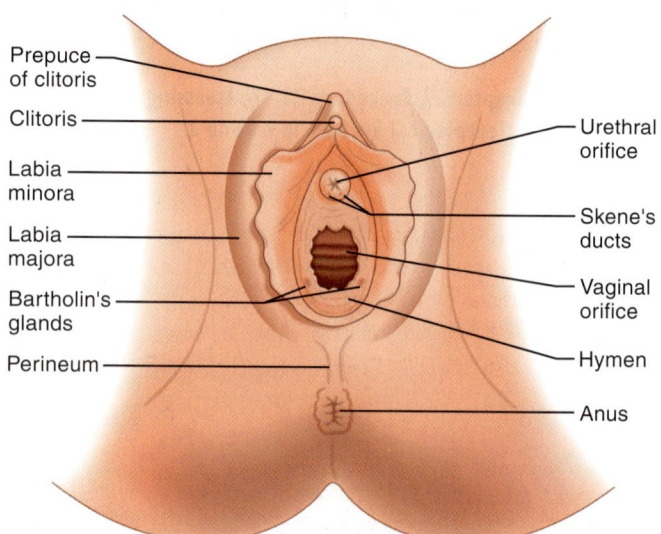

FIGURE 22-21 External female genitalia.

on the outside to help bring the inner structures toward the two hands.

Pap Smear Recent changes to major guidelines recommend, in general, less frequent routine Papanicolaou tests (Pap smears) to screen for cervical and uterine cancer. They recommend the following for women:

- Younger than age 21: Do not be screen, regardless of whether they are sexually active or have other risk-taking behaviors.
- Ages 21 through 29: Screen every 3 years.
- Ages 30 to 65: Screen every 3 to 5 years (and follow the advice of their provider).
- Older than age 65: Do not routinely screen unless they are at high risk. However, a recent study states that the cancer incidence rates used for guidelines do not account for high prevalence of hysterectomy in the United States. This has the largest impact on older, black women. Authors recommend that the risk and screening guidelines be reconsidered (Rositch, Nowak, and Gravitt, 2014)
- Those with certain vulnerabilities (e.g., weakened immune system, HIV-positive) should have a Pap test every year (Agency for Healthcare Research and Quality [AHRQ], 2005, last revised 2013; American Cancer Society, n.d.b, revised 2013)

Key Point: *National screening guidelines vary, and they change frequently.*

Additional cultures or screens may be done if there is unusual discharge or risk of sexually transmitted infection. A **speculum examination** is performed to collect specimens and assess the cervix. To learn about assisting with a speculum exam, see Clinical Insight 22-3,

 Clinical Insight 22-3, Assisting with a Speculum Exam, in Volume 2.

KnowledgeCheck 22-13

What are the responsibilities of the nurse during an internal exam of the female genitourinary system?

The Anus, Rectum, and Prostate

Examining the rectum and anus is the last aspect of a comprehensive examination. For the female client, this exam is usually performed at the end of a bimanual pelvic examination while the client is still in the lithotomy position. Usually a male client assumes the Sims' position, and you perform the exam after completing your examination of the genitals. For a summary of this procedure, see the Highlights of Procedures box at the end of this chapter. For a step-by-step procedure,

 Go to **Procedure 22-19: Assessing the Anus and Rectum,** in Volume 2.

Inspect the anus and rectum for skin condition and hemorrhoids and palpate for muscle tone, masses, and tenderness. Skin irritation and erythema are common in clients who have diarrhea and infants and toddlers who wear diapers. **Hemorrhoids** (dilated, usually painful, anal vessels) may be seen in clients with a history of constipation. Many women develop hemorrhoids with pregnancy and childbirth.

A comprehensive examination for a man should include a digital rectal examination to assess for prostate enlargement. An enlarged prostate may indicate benign enlargement of the prostate, which is common in men older than age 50; or it may indicate prostatitis. A hard nodule or multiple nodules may indicate prostate cancer.

 ThinkLike a Nurse 22-9

How will examination of the rectum and anus differ for Nam and Yen Nguyen (Meet Your Patient)?

DOCUMENTING PHYSICAL ASSESSMENT FINDINGS

Zach Jackson has completed his physical assessment of Nam Nguyen (Meet Your Patient). Below is his charting entry. Recall that Zach is an advanced practice nurse and has performed a comprehensive physical assessment. Therefore, this examination and charting entry are more extensive than what would be expected of a staff nurse. Keep in mind that you should use only abbreviations on your clinical agency's approved list.

General Survey 56-year-old obese man presents to the clinic for a physical exam in no apparent distress. Pt appears stated age; is well dressed and groomed; and alert and oriented to time, place, and person. Speech is clear, response and affect appropriate. Moves all extremities well, gait steady and balanced. Smells of cigarettes.

Height	5 ft 4 in.
Weight	185 lb (84 kg)
BP	166/100
Pulse	88 beats/min
RR	22 breaths/min
Temp	98.5°F (36.9°C), oral
BMI	33

Integumentary Skin even in color, warm & dry, good turgor, no suspicious lesions. Well healed scar in right inguinal area. Hair clean, coarse, evenly distributed. Some graying. Nails pink, brisk capillary refill, no clubbing.

Head & Neck Normocephalic, erect, midline. Scalp mobile, no lesions, tenderness, or masses. Facial features symmetrical. Thyroid gland symmetrical and not enlarged; cervical lymph nodes not palpable or tender.

Eyes Snellen = right eye 20/100, left eye 20/100, both eyes 20/100. Color vision intact. Difficulty noted with near vision. Visual fields normal by confrontation. Extraocular movements intact. PERRLA at 3 mm by direct and consensual. Eyes clear and bright, + blink, no lid lag or abnormalities. Anterior chamber clear. Cornea & iris intact. Sclera white, conjunctiva clear. Lacrimal glands and ducts nontender. + red reflex bilateral, discs flat with sharp margins, vessels intact, retina & macula even in color.

Ears, Nose, & Throat Skin intact, no masses, lesions, or discharge. Position WNL. External ears nontender to palpation. + whisper test. Weber—no lateralization. External canals clear without redness, swelling, lesions, or discharge. Tympanic membranes intact, light reflex and bony landmarks visible; frontal and maxillary sinuses nontender. Nares patent, able to distinguish familiar odors, mucosa pink, no discharge, septum intact with no deviation.

Mouth Lips, oral mucosa, gingivae pink with no lesions. All teeth present and in good repair. Pharynx pink, tonsils absent, palate intact. Symmetrical rise of the uvula, + gag and swallow reflex. Tongue smooth, pink, symmetrical, mobile, without lesions, taste intact (correctly identified sweet, salty, and sour).

Respiratory Respirations 22 breaths/min and unlabored. Trachea midline, AP < transverse chest diameter. Chest expansion symmetrical. No tenderness, scars, masses, or lesions. Diaphragmatic excursion 5 cm. Lungs clear to auscultation.

Cardiovascular PMI @ MCL at 5th ICS, P 85, regular, no murmurs, gallops, or thrills present; pulses +2, no bruits or thrills, no varicosities; jugular venous pulsation 2 cm at 45°. Carotids without bruits.

Breasts Symmetrical. No masses, lymphadenopathy, or discharge.

Abdomen Abdomen soft, rounded, no masses or pulsations. Surgical scar R inguinal area. + bowel sounds, + tympany throughout.

Musculoskeletal Normal spinal curvature. Joints and muscles symmetrical, no deformity. + Bilateral knee pain (right more than left). Full ROM in upper and lower extremities, + 5 muscle strength, moderate crepitus right knee.

Neurological Awake, alert, and oriented to time, place, and person. CN I–XII intact. Gait steady and coordinated; negative Romberg; unable to do deep knee bends due to pain. Point-point localization, superficial and deep sensation intact, + 2 deep tendon reflexes.

Genitourinary Circumcised male; penis nontender, no masses, urethral meatus midline, no discharge; testicles descended bilaterally, nontender, inguinal and femoral canals free of masses, prostate small, smooth, mobile, nontender. Rectal wall smooth, no masses, stool hemoccult negative.

Highlights of Procedures 22-1 through 22-20

 For steps to follow in *all* procedures, refer to the Universal Steps for All Procedures found on the inside back cover of Volume 2. Go to the full procedures in Volume 2 to practice and learn the skill. Use these procedure highlights later to help you review key steps.

Note: Throughout the assessment, compare findings on both sides of the body.

Procedure 22-1: Performing the General Survey

➤ Observe the patient's apparent age, sex, race, facial expression, body size and type, posture, movements, speech, grooming, dress, hygiene, mental state, and affect.

➤ Identify any signs of distress.

➤ Measure vital signs.

➤ Measure height and weight, and calculate body mass index (BMI).

➤ Consider the client's cultural/ethnic background, gender, and developmental stage.

➤ Review history data that may influence general survey findings, including usual state of health, current health problem, allergies, and unexplained changes in weight.

 ➤ Perform functional and SPICES assessments for older adults.

➤ Note verbal and nonverbal responses throughout exam.

Procedure 22-2: Assessing the Skin

➤ Techniques: Inspection, palpation, and olfaction

➤ Assess both exposed and unexposed areas.

➤ Inspect skin color; note any unusual odors.

➤ Inspect and palpate any lesions. Describe their size, shape, color, distribution, texture, surface relationship, and exudate.

➤ Evaluate the lesions for possible malignancy, remembering the mnemonic ABCDE.

➤ Use dorsal aspect of your hand to palpate skin temperature.

➤ Check skin turgor.

➤ Palpate skin for texture, moisture, and hydration.

➤ Review history that may influence skin findings.

Procedure 22-3: Assessing the Hair

➤ Techniques: Inspection and palpation

➤ Assess scalp hair and body hair.

➤ Inspect hair for color, quantity, distribution, condition of scalp, and presence of lesions or pediculosis.

➤ Palpate the texture of the hair.

➤ Palpate the scalp for mobility and tenderness.

Procedure 22-4: Assessing the Nails

➤ Techniques: Inspection and palpation

- ➤ Inspect the nails for color, condition, and shape.
- ➤ Palpate the texture of the nails.
- ➤ Assess capillary refill.
- ➤ Assess factors that may alter nail assessment findings (e.g., a cold environment may slow capillary refill).
- ➤ Examine nails on both hands and feet.
- ➤ You may defer examination of the toenails until you assess peripheral circulation.

Procedure 22-5: Assessing the Head and Face

- ➤ Techniques: Inspection, palpation
- ➤ Inspect the head for size, shape, symmetry, and position.
- ➤ Compare side to side throughout the exam.
- ➤ Inspect the face for expression and symmetry.
- ➤ Palpate the head for masses, tenderness, and scalp mobility.
- ➤ Palpate the face for symmetry, tenderness, muscle tone, and TMJ function.

Procedure 22-6: Assessing the Eyes

- ➤ Techniques: Inspection and palpation
- ➤ Assess distance vision using a Snellen chart.
- ➤ Test near vision by measuring the client's ability to read newsprint at a distance of 14 inches (35.5 cm).
- ➤ Test color vision by using color plates or the color bars on the Snellen chart.
- ➤ Assess peripheral vision by determining when an object comes into sight.
- ➤ Assess EOMs by examining the corneal light reflex, observing the six cardinal gaze positions, and performing the cover/uncover test.
- ➤ Inspect the external eye structures.
- ➤ Test the corneal reflex with a cotton wisp, if appropriate.
- ➤ Check pupil reaction for direct and consensual response.
- ➤ Assess accommodation by having the patient focus on an approaching object.
- ➤ Palpate the external eye structures.

Procedure 22-7: Assessing the Ears and Hearing

- ➤ Techniques: Inspection and palpation
- ➤ Inspect the external ear for placement, size, shape, symmetry, and the condition of the skin.
- ➤ Palpate the external structures of the ear for skin condition and tenderness.
- ➤ Inspect the tympanic membrane and bony landmarks.
- ➤ Assess gross hearing with the whisper and watch-tick tests.
- ➤ Perform the Weber test to assess hearing loss.
- ➤ Perform the Rinne test to identify whether hearing loss is conductive or sensorineural.

Procedure 22-8: Assessing the Nose and the Sinuses

- ➤ Techniques: Inspection and palpation
- ➤ Insert the speculum about 1 cm, and then open it as much as possible.
- ➤ Inspect the external and internal structures of the nose.
- ➤ Transilluminate and palpate the sinuses.
- ➤ Palpate the external structures of the nose.

Procedure 22-9: Assessing the Mouth and Oropharynx

- ➤ Techniques: Inspection and palpation
- ➤ Inspect the lips, oral mucosa, gums, teeth, and bite.
- ➤ Inspect the hard/soft palate, tonsils, and uvula.
- ➤ Inspect the tongue and frenulum; inspect under the tongue.
- ➤ Palpate the lips and tongue for tenderness and muscle tone.
- ➤ Test the gag reflex by touching the back of the soft palate with a tongue blade.

Procedure 22-10: Assessing the Neck

- ➤ Techniques: Inspection and palpation (auscultation as needed)
- ➤ Inspect the neck. Note symmetry, ROM, and the skin condition.
- ➤ Palpate the cervical lymph nodes. Note the size, shape, symmetry, consistency, mobility, tenderness, and temperature of any palpable nodes.
- ➤ Palpate the thyroid. If it is enlarged or if there is a mass, auscultate.

Procedure 22-11: Assessing the Breasts and Axillae

- ➤ Techniques: Inspection and palpation
- ➤ Inspect the breasts and axillae for skin condition, size, shape, symmetry, and color.
- ➤ Inspect the nipples for discharge. Culture any discharge, if present.

➤ ✚ If you notice an open lesion or nipple discharge, wear procedure gloves to palpate the breasts.

- ➤ Palpate the breasts using the vertical strip method, pie wedge method, or concentric circles method.
- ➤ Palpate the nipples, areolae, and lymph nodes.

Procedure 22-12: Assessing the Chest and Lungs

- ➤ Techniques: Inspection, palpation, percussion, auscultation
- ➤ Assess respirations by counting the rate and observing the rhythm, depth, and symmetry of chest movement.
- ➤ Inspect the chest for anteroposterior to lateral ratio, costal angle, spinal deformity, respiratory effort, and skin condition.
- ➤ Palpate the trachea.
- ➤ Palpate the chest for tenderness, masses, or crepitus; chest excursion, and tactile fremitus.
- ➤ Percuss the chest; percuss diaphragmatic excursion.
- ➤ Auscultate breath sounds.

(Continued)

Procedure 22-13: Assessing the Heart and Vascular System

➤ Techniques: Inspection, palpation, auscultation

➤ If possible, work from your patient's right side.

➤ Inspect the neck for pulsations.

➤ Measure jugular venous pressure (JVP).

➤ Inspect the precordium for pulsations.

➤ Palpate the carotid arteries.

➤ Palpate the precordium for pulsations, lifts, heaves, or thrills.

➤ Auscultate the carotid arteries with the bell of the stethoscope.

➤ Auscultate the jugular veins with the bell of the stethoscope.

➤ Auscultate the precordium at the apex, left lower sternal border, base left, and base right. Use the bell and then the diaphragm of the stethoscope.

➤ Palpate the peripheral pulses. Any abnormalities require further evaluation.

Procedure 22-14: Assessing the Abdomen

➤ Techniques: Inspection, auscultation, percussion, palpation (in that order)

➤ Have the client void before the exam.

➤ Position the client supine with the knees slightly flexed.

➤ Inspect the abdomen.

➤ Auscultate the abdomen for bowel sounds and bruits.

➤ Use indirect percussion to assess at multiple sites in all four quadrants.

➤ Using your fist or blunt percussion, percuss the costovertebral angle bilaterally to assess for kidney tenderness.

➤ Lightly palpate throughout the abdomen by pressing down 1 to 2 cm in a rotating motion. Identify surface characteristics, tenderness, muscle resistance, and turgor.

➤ Use deep palpation to palpate organs and masses.

Procedure 22-15: Assessing the Musculoskeletal System

➤ Techniques: Inspection and palpation

➤ Compare bilaterally during the assessment.

➤ Assess posture, body alignment, and symmetry.

➤ Assess the spinal curvature.

➤ Examine the gait by assessing the base of support, stride, and phases of the gait.

➤ Assess balance through tandem walking, heel-and-toe walking, deep knee bends, hopping, and the Romberg test.

➤ Assess coordination by testing finger–thumb opposition, rhythmic movements of lower and upper extremities, and rapid alternating movements.

➤ Test the accuracy of movements by having the client touch his finger to his nose with his eyes closed.

➤ Measure limb length and circumference.

➤ nspect muscle symmetry.

➤ Perform range of motion of all joints.

➤ Assess muscle strength by having the client perform ROM against resistance.

Procedure 22-16: Assessing the Sensory-Neurological System

➤ Assess behavior.

➤ Determine level of arousal.

➤ Determine level of orientation.

➤ Assess memory.

➤ Assess mathematical and calculation skills.

➤ Assess general knowledge.

➤ Evaluate thought processes.

➤ Assess abstract thinking.

➤ Assess judgment.

➤ Assess communication ability.

➤ Test cranial nerves.

➤ Test superficial sensations; begin with most peripheral part of the limb.

➤ Test deep sensations: vibratory and kinesthetic.

➤ Test discriminatory sensations: stereognosis, graphesthesia, two-point discrimination, point localization, and sensory extinction.

➤ Test deep tendon reflexes: biceps, triceps, brachioradialis, patellar, and Achilles.

➤ Test superficial reflexes.

➤ Assess for dementia in institutionalized older adults.

Procedure 22-17: Assessing the Male Genitourinary System

➤ Techniques: Inspection and palpation

➤ Inspect the external genitalia, including color, discharge, and the pattern of hair distribution.

➤ Palpate for lumps, masses, hernias, or enlarged lymph nodes.

Procedure 22-18: Assessing the Female Genitourinary System

➤ Techniques: Inspection and palpation

➤ Inspect the external genitalia, including hair distribution; skin, mucosa; urethral meatus; and vaginal introitus, color, discharge, and lesions.

➤ Palpate Bartholin's and Skene's glands.

➤ Assess vaginal and pelvic muscle tone.

➤ Palpate lymph nodes and possible hernia sites.

Procedure 22-19: Assessing the Anus and Rectum

➤ Inspect the external anal area, sphincter tone, and stool for occult blood.

Highlights of Procedures 22-1 through 22-20

➤ Palpate the anus and rectum for muscle tone and masses.

➤ For women, assessment of the anus and rectum is usually performed at the end of the internal pelvic exam; for men, it is done after the genitourinary exam.

Proedure 22-20: Brief Bedside Assessment

➤ Modify the procedure to fit the patient's health status.

➤ Observe the environment and the patient's general appearance.

➤ Measure vital signs, pain status, and pulse oximetry.

➤ Use a systematic (e.g., head-to-toe) approach.

➤ Assess the integument (hair, nails, and skin).

➤ Assess the head and neck (ears, eyes, lips, tongue and oropharynx, carotids)

➤ Assess the back with patient sitting (including breath sounds).

➤ Assess the anterior chest (heart and lungs).

➤ Assess the abdomen with patient supine.

➤ Assess urinary status.

➤ Assess upper extremities, including edema and capillary refill.

➤ Assess lower extremities, including edema and capillary refill.

➤ Assess for spinal deformities with patient standing.

➤ Assess balance, coordination, ROM, and gait.

➤ Check Babinski and Homan's reflexes.

 To explore learning resources for this chapter,

 Go to DavisPlus at DavisPl.us/Wilkinson3.

Chapter Resources for Chapter 22:

> **Response sheets for all learning activities**
>
> **Resources for Caregivers and Health Professionals**
>
> **Reading More About Health Assessment (suggested readings)**
>
> **Concept Map of chapter content**

Interactive Case Studies

NCLEX-Style and Chapter Review Questions

Chapter Overview Podcasts

For references cited in this chapter,

 Go to Volume 2, **References Cited.**

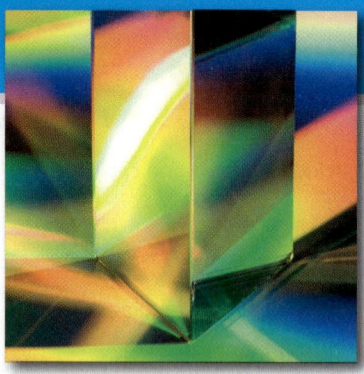

Promoting Asepsis & Preventing Infection

Learning Outcomes

After completing this chapter, you should be able to:

➤ Discuss the six links in the chain of infection.

➤ Describe the stages of a typical infectious process.

➤ Describe four processes involved in primary, secondary, and tertiary defenses.

➤ Identify activities that promote immune function.

➤ Discuss the factors that place an individual at increased risk for infection.

➤ Explain why it is important to be aware of emerging infectious diseases.

➤ Explain why multidrug-resistant pathogens are of special concern in healthcare.

➤ Use standard precautions to prevent transmission of infection through blood and body fluids.

➤ Describe additional precautions that must be taken when there is concern about contact, droplet, or airborne disease transmission.

➤ Compare and contrast methods of preventing infection by breaking the chain of infection.

➤ Implement measures to prevent healthcare-related infections.

➤ Use medical asepsis when providing care to clients.

➤ Discuss infection prevention and control measures in the home and community.

➤ Implement sterile technique in selected patient care activities.

➤ Discuss the nurse's role in recognizing, preventing, and helping to contain the spread of a biological epidemic.

Key Concepts

Infection

Medical asepsis

Surgical asepsis

Body defenses

Infection prevention and control

Related Concepts

See the Concept Map on DavisPlus.

Example Problems

Drug-Resistant Pathogens

Meet Your Nursing Role Model

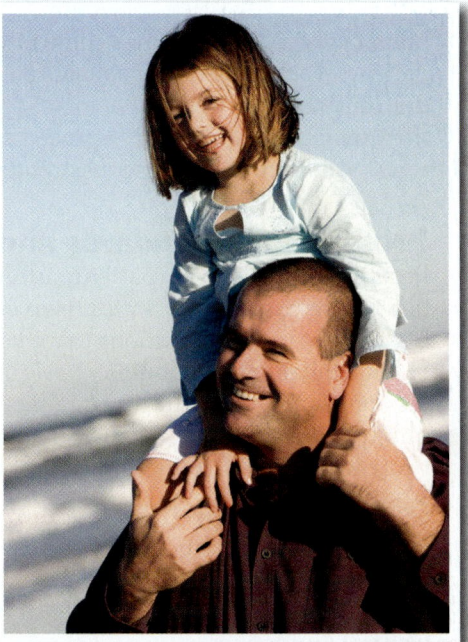

Stephanie Sergi is the 7-year-old daughter of Jason Sergi. Jason works as a nurse on a busy labor and delivery unit in a major medical center. One night at the dinner table, Stephanie asks, "Daddy, what was the most important thing you did at work today?" Jason takes a few minutes to consider his reply. Finally Jason answers, "I washed my hands—a lot."

Jason tells his daughter that he also assisted in the births of five infants, resuscitated one of the infants who was initially struggling for breath, and identified several problems that prevented complications or even death of mothers in labor. "Daddy, I don't understand why you think washing your hands was so important," Stephanie protested. "Look at all the *really* important things you did today!"

As you read this chapter, think back to Jason's discussion with his daughter. Perhaps you will someday say the same thing to your child or anyone who asks about your day.

ABOUT THE KEY CONCEPTS

A grasp of the broad concept of **infection** will enable you to promote biological safety for your clients, using **infection prevention and control** activities. Those activities include **medical and surgical asepsis** and interventions to support patients' body defenses.

Theoretical Knowledge
knowing **why**

Research continues to lead to the discovery of new infectious microorganisms. Researchers are currently investigating the role of viruses in the development of cancer and other diseases. For example, virally induced cancers include Hodgkin's disease, Kaposi's sarcoma, and cervical cancer. Other research is investigating the role that certain species of bacteria play in burn treatment and healing (Peral, Huaman Martinez, & Valdez, 2009).

WHY MUST NURSES KNOW ABOUT INFECTION PROCESSES?

The goals of infection prevention and control discussed in this section are to:

- Protect patients from healthcare-related infections. Healthcare-associated infections will affect 1 out of every 20 hospitalized patients (Centers for Disease Control and Prevention [CDC], n.d.a).
- Meet professional standards and guidelines.

- Protect yourself from diseases. You must know how to avoid contact with infectious material and exposure to diseases such as AIDS, hepatitis B and C, and drug-resistant tuberculosis, as well as the many common illness-producing microorganisms you will encounter.
- Help lower the cost of healthcare. Healthcare-associated infections are responsible for between $28 and $33 billion dollars annually (Agency for Healthcare Research and Quality [AHRQ], 2012a).

In this chapter, you will learn how infections occur and about measures to prevent them. We will discuss healthcare-associated infections and related professional standards and guidelines.

Healthcare-Associated Infections

The term **healthcare-associated infections (HAIs)** refers to infections associated with healthcare given in any setting (e.g., hospitals, home care, long-term care, and ambulatory settings). The term **nosocomial infections** refers more specifically to hospital-acquired infections. Healthcare-associated infections aggravate existing illness and lengthen hospital stay and recovery time. HAIs are the leading complication of hospital care and one of the 10 leading causes of death in the United States (AHRQ, 2011; Klevens, Morrison, & Nadle, 2007; Siegel, Rhinehart, Jackson, et al., 2007) and are preventable (Cardo, Dennehy, Halverson, et al., 2010). Approximately 1 out of every 20 hospitalized patients will contract an HAI (CDC, n.d.a). You may be surprised at these facts. After all, healthcare workers are supposed to cure, not harm, people. But when people come to hospitals (and other facilities) for care, they come into contact with many personnel and patients. Ill patients are vulnerable to infection, and they are a source of infection for others. In addition, they undergo invasive procedures (e.g., injections), which can introduce infectious organisms into their body.

Professional Standards and Guidelines

Because HAIs lead to patient suffering and increased healthcare costs, many states have enacted laws requiring healthcare organizations to make information about HAIs available to the public. Various government, professional, and accrediting organizations have created quality-control guidelines for healthcare agencies and professionals. The following are important examples:

The Centers for Disease Control and Prevention (CDC), a federal agency, has an extensive Web site devoted to infection control and prevention in healthcare settings. To access this site and retrieve Infection Control Guidelines,

 Go to http://www.cdc.gov/hai/

Among the U. S. Department of Health and Human Services (2011) goals for the healthcare setting are to:

- Reduce catheter-associated adverse infections by 50%.
- Reduce targeted antimicrobial-resistant bacterial infections by 50%.
- Reduce surgical site infections by 25% over the course of five years.
- Reduce catheter-associated urinary tract infections by 25%.

The Agency for Healthcare Research and Quality (AHRQ) has a Web site featuring links to information, tools, and resources on HAIs. The site contains resources for healthcare providers and consumers, and highlights AHRQ-funded research and initiatives to reduce HAIs. To access this site,

 Go to http://www.ahrq.gov/qual/hais.htm

The Joint Commission is a quality oversight agency. Their standards of performance include extensive criteria describing what healthcare organizations must do to minimize the risks of infection. In addition, Goal 7 of their National Patient Safety Goals for 2012 is to "reduce the risk of health care associated infections" (The Joint Commission, 2012). The Infection Control Initiatives present strategies for healthcare providers to prevent infection in inpatient and community-based settings. To read these initiatives,

 Go to http://www.jointcommission.org/assets/1/6/2011_ NPSGs_HAP.pdf

Quality and Safety Education for Nurses (QSEN) is a group of educators that was formed to address the challenge of preparing nurses with the competencies

necessary to improve the quality and safety of their places of work—competencies that you should have on completing your nursing education. Safety is one of the six competencies you should have on completing your nursing education. Although QSEN does not specifically say that safety includes being safe from infection, they make several broad statements regarding knowledge, skills, and attitudes about safety that do apply to infection. For example, you should be able to:

- Demonstrate knowledge of basic scientific methods and processes (e.g., infectious process, inflammatory process).
- Minimize risk of harm to patients and providers (e.g., infectious diseases) through both system effectiveness and individual performance.
- Demonstrate effective use of technology and standardized practice (e.g., CDC guidelines for infection control) that support safety and quality (Cronenwett, Sherwood, Barnsteiner, J., et al., 2007).

To access the QSEN Web site,

 Go to http://www.qsen.org

American Nurses Association (ANA) Using the same broad understanding as for the QSEN competencies, you should assume that the following criteria from Standard 5 of *Nursing: Scope & Standards of Practice* (2010) apply to infection prevention and control:

- Partners with the person/family/significant others/caregiver to implement the plan in a safe and timely manner.
- Implements the plan in a timely manner in accordance with the patient safety goals.

HOW DOES INFECTION OCCUR?

Imagine that your clinical instructor alerts you to an outbreak of infectious disease in the hospital where you have your assignment. The hospital census is currently more than 200 patients. So far, 14 have become infected, and one has died. Have you ever wondered how infections are spread and why they seem to affect some people more than others?

Infections Develop in Response to a Chain of Factors

The process by which infections spread is commonly referred to as the **chain of infection**. It is made up of six links, all of which must be present for the infection to be transmitted from one individual to another (Fig. 23-1). Here we describe each of the six links. Later in the chapter we discuss how to interrupt the chain to limit the spread of infection. For information about common disease-producing microorganisms and their transmission,

 Go to Chapter Resources, **ESG Table 23-1, Common Pathogens,** on Davis*Plus*.

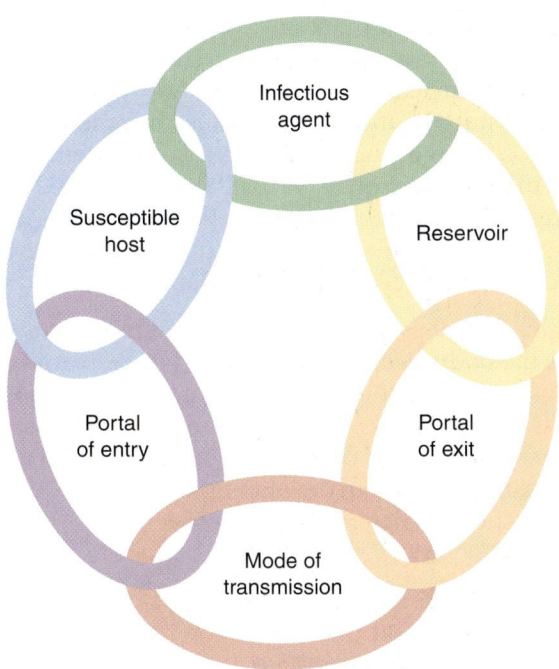

FIGURE 23-1 All of the six links in the chain of infection must be present for infection to be transmitted from one person to another.

Infectious Agent

Some microorganisms live on or in the human body without causing harm. For instance, the *Staphylococcus* bacteria growing on human skin are usually harmless. Other microorganisms are beneficial or even essential for human health and well-being. They are referred to as **normal flora.** Normal flora in the intestine aid in digestion and synthesize vitamin K, and release vitamin B_{12}, thiamine, and riboflavin when they die. In addition, they limit the growth of harmful bacteria by competing with them for available nutrients.

Flora There are two types of normal flora: transient and resident. **Transient flora** are normal microbes that a person picks up by coming in contact with objects or another person (e.g., when you touch a soiled dressing). You can remove these with handwashing. **Resident flora** live deep in skin layers, where they live and multiply harmlessly. They are permanent inhabitants of the skin, and cannot usually be removed with routine handwashing. They are not usually harmful unless they enter the deep tissues (e.g., as through an open wound) or unless the patient is especially vulnerable to disease.

Pathogens These microorganisms are capable of causing disease. The largest groups of pathogenic microorganisms are bacteria, viruses, and fungi (which include yeasts and molds). Less common pathogens are protozoa, helminths (commonly called worms), and *prions*, which are infectious protein particles that cause certain neurological diseases. In addition, normal flora may become pathogenic if disease or injury permits them to enter

body regions they do not normally inhabit. For instance, rupture of the bowel through trauma or disease allows intestinal microbes to enter the abdominal cavity or bloodstream, where they cause infection.

Once a pathogen gains entry into a host, four factors determine whether the person develops infection:

- **Virulence** of the organism (its power to cause disease)
- Ability of the organism to survive in the host environment
- Number of organisms (the greater the number, the more likely they are to cause disease)
- Ability of the host's defenses to prevent infection

Reservoir

A **reservoir** is a source of infection: a place where pathogens survive and multiply. The human body is the most common reservoir for pathogens. Animals, insects, and humans are other living reservoirs. Nonliving reservoirs include soil, water, food, and environmental surfaces. Examples include contaminated water, stagnant ponds, garbage, soiled diapers, wound dressings, and raw sewage. In healthcare facilities, many surfaces act as reservoirs. Microorganisms have mass, and they eventually fall to the floor or onto bedside tables, chairs, or equipment. Other surfaces, such as sinks, toilets, bed rails, and bed linens, may also become reservoirs because of their proximity to patients, family members, and healthcare providers harboring pathogens, such as *Legionella* spp. In this manner, some hands-free faucets are reported to have higher levels of disease-carrying bacteria (e.g., *Legionella* spp.) than conventional, manually operated faucets (American Society for Healthcare Engineering [ASHE] and the Association for Professionals in Infection Control & Epidemiology [APIC], 2011), although there are controversial reports of design flaws with some hands-free faucets in the flow of water, resulting in contamination with hazardous bacteria (Johns Hopkins Medicine, 2011).

Some people are capable of defending themselves from active disease but harbor the pathogenic organisms within their bodies. These individuals, called **carriers**, have no symptoms of disease, yet they serve as reservoirs and can pass the disease to others.

Most pathogens prefer a warm, moist, dark environment. To live and thrive in humans, microbes must be able to use the body's precise balance of food, moisture, nutrients, electrolytes, pH, temperature, and light. Food, water, and soil that provide these conditions may serve as nonliving reservoirs, as well.

Nutrients Bacteria can rapidly multiply in food left at room temperature. For example, the species *Salmonella enteritidis*, which causes salmonellosis ("food poisoning"), can multiply in raw and undercooked meat and eggs. To prevent the growth of pathogens, many foods are cooked at high temperatures and stored in a cool environment. Alternatively, many foods are prepared with a concentration of solutes that inhibits the growth of pathogenic microbes. This concept underlies the salting of meats and the production of fruit jellies, jams, and preserves.

Moisture Pathogens require moisture for survival, for example, the moist environment of wounds, the genitourinary tract, the throat, and airways. However, the spores formed by some bacteria allow them to live without water (e.g., the *Bacillus* and *Clostridium* species, both of which cause foodborne disease).

Temperature For most pathogens, the ideal temperature for existence is 95°F (35°C). Environments that are either too hot or too cold for a particular species will slow its growth or even kill the entire population. In part, the microbes that are pathogenic to humans are so because they thrive at about the same temperature as the human body. Thus, a fever in response to infection can inhibit and even kill invading pathogens.

Oxygen Many bacteria and most protozoa and fungi are **aerobic**. That is, they must have oxygen to live and grow. For example, the yeast *Candida albicans* causes infections in the oral mucosa ("thrush") and the vaginal mucosa. **Anaerobic organisms** do not require oxygen for growth and may even be killed in its presence. One example is *Clostridium tetani*, a spore-forming bacterium, which causes tetanus when a spore enters the body through an open wound.

pH and Electrolytes To live in humans, pathogens need the body's precise balance of moisture, sugars, pH (acidity), and electrolytes. Most prefer a pH range of 5 to 8. Therefore, they cannot survive in the highly acidic environment of the stomach. When patients take antacids, stomach pH increases and removes this defense. The organisms multiply and can then cause infection in other systems, such as the lungs. Microbes that have a higher or lower pH and electrolyte concentration than the human body are not pathogenic to human beings. That's why, for example, the bacteria that thrive in the Great Salt Lake would not cause infection on your skin.

Light Microbes grow best in dark environments (e.g., inside the body, deep in wounds, and under dressings). Ultraviolet light is sometimes used to remove pathogens such as *Staphylococcus*, *Salmonella*, and viruses from surgical instruments and other objects. It is also used to disinfect drinking water in developing countries to prevent diseases such as cholera and typhoid fever.

KnowledgeCheck 23-1

- What is a pathogen?
- What is the role of normal flora?
- Identify at least five reservoirs of infection.

Portal of Exit

A contained reservoir is only a potential source of infection. For infection to spread, a pathogen must exit the reservoir. In the case of human or animal reservoirs, the most frequent **portal of exit** is through body fluids, including blood, mucus, saliva, breast milk, urine, feces, vomitus, semen, or other secretions. The body's natural response to foreign materials, including pathogens, is to

---

PICOT

Situation: The handoff report has been concluded in an ICU. The Unit Manager alerted the staff that there has been an increase in enterococci-related urinary tract infections (UTIs) on the unit, and the infection control team will be following several of the unit's clients. The primary nurse is preparing to bathe a client in the intensive care unit (ICU), and notices that the basin is wet from the previous bath. Knowing that bacteria need a damp environment to grow, she wonders whether the bath basin might be a reservoir for enterococci. What question might the nurse ask to guide her in a search for evidence?

PICOT Components

P	Population/client	= Intensive care unit patients
I	Intervention/indicator	= Basin bath
C	Comparator/control	= Absence of hospital associated urinary tract infection
O	Outcome	= Enterococci urinary tract infection
T	Time	= During ICU stay

Searchable Question: How do _____(P) who receive/are exposed to _____(I) develop _____ (O) as compared to _____(C) during _____(T)?

Example of Evidence: Hospital-associated infections (HAIs) are linked to a high number of client deaths every year. It is important to identify possible reservoirs for pathogen colonization, and minimize the client risk of infection. Johnson, Lineweaver, and Maze (2009) cultured 92 bath basins at three acute care hospitals, including three ICUs. Of the samples cultured, 98% grew some form of bacteria. The most common organisms identified were enterococci, *Staphylococcus aureus*, vancomycin-resistant enterococci, methicillin-resistant *S. aureus*, *Pseudomonas aeruginosa*, *Candida albicans*, and *Escherichia coli*. Although this sample is small, it clearly indicates that bath basins are a reservoir for bacteria, and nurses need to be aware that the basin is a potential source of HAI, especially in the at-risk client.

Practice Change: As a result of her findings in the literature, the nurse resolved to dry bath basins well after using them and to talk to colleagues about doing the same. She also suggested to the Unit Manager that the unit should look into the feasibility of using disposable bath basins.

Source: Johnson, D., Lineweaver, L., Maze, L. M., (2009). Patients' bath basins as potential sources of infection: A multicenter sampling study. *American Journal of Critical Care*, *18*(1), 31–38, 41. doi:10.4037/ajcc2009968

try to expel them. If you have a pathogen in the respiratory system, you cough and sneeze. If it is in the gastrointestinal system, you vomit or experience intestinal cramping and diarrhea. Microbes responsible for sexually transmitted infections can exit via semen, vaginal secretions, or blood that is present during sex.

Cuts, bites, and abrasions also provide an exit for body fluid. Blood and pus seeping from a wound help transport pathogens away from the broken skin but become a portal by which infection may be transmitted to others. In healthcare-related infections, puncture sites, drainage tubes, feeding tubes, and intravenous lines commonly serve as routes for pathogens to exit the body.

Mode of Transmission

Contact, either direct or indirect, is the most frequent **mode of transmission** of infection. **Direct contact** between two people usually involves touching, kissing, or sexual intercourse. Animals commonly transmit infection via scratching and biting as well. **Indirect contact** involves contact with a **fomite**, a contaminated object that transfers a pathogen. For example, suppose that while you are charting you begin to sneeze or cough. If you cover your nose and mouth with your hand and then resume charting, you may transmit pathogens to the pen, paper, and chart (or keyboard). Shoes, eyeglasses, stethoscopes, and other items we wear also commonly serve as fomites, as do contaminated needles. Some microbes can live only a few seconds on fomites; others can live for years. It depends on the type of microorganism and the environment.

Droplet Transmission Infection is passed when the pathogen travels in water droplets expelled as an infected person exhales, coughs, sneezes, or talks. It may also occur during suctioning and oral care. The usual method of transmission is for the droplet to be inhaled or enter the eye of a susceptible person. Although droplets can travel only a few feet from the infectious person, within that distance they may readily contaminate fomites that then transmit the organism by contact.

Airborne Transmission Microorganisms that float considerable distances on air currents can pass infection to vulnerable hosts. Airborne pathogens can travel through heating and air-conditioning systems to infect large numbers of people. Sweeping a floor or shaking out contaminated bed linens can stir up airborne microorganisms and launch them on air currents—imagine a flying magic carpet (of pathogens). The agents of measles and tuberculosis, as well as many fungal infections, are commonly transmitted in this manner.

Vector This is an organism that carries a pathogen to a susceptible host, typically by biting or stinging, creating another portal of entry into the body. The mosquito is a common vector for diseases, including malaria, yellow fever, and the West Nile virus. Ticks, fleas, mites, and other insects also carry various diseases.

Portal of Entry

Pathogens can enter the body through various **portals of entry**. Normal body openings, such as the conjunctiva of the eye, the nares (nostrils), mouth, urethra, vagina, and anus are potential portals of entry, as are abnormal openings, such as cuts, scrapes, and surgical incisions. Vectors, such as mosquitoes, create portals of entry when they bite through the skin. In healthcare settings, common portals of entry include wounds, surgical sites, and insertion sites for tubes or needles.

Susceptible Host

A **susceptible** (or *compromised*) **host** is a person who is at risk for infection because of inadequate defenses against the invading pathogen. Various factors can increase susceptibility to infection, among them: age (the very young or very old), compromised immune system (as in those receiving immune suppression for organ transplantation or treatment of cancer or chronic illness), and immune deficiency conditions (e.g., HIV, leukemia).

KnowledgeCheck 23-2

- Identify the six links in the chain of infection.
- What kinds of microbes favor the human body as a reservoir of infection?

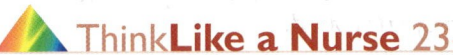

ThinkLike a Nurse 23-1

You are working as a nurse on a medical-surgical unit. What roles might you play in the chain of infection?

Infections Can Be Classified in Various Ways

Infections are classified according to their location in the body, whether it is the patient's first infection, where it was acquired, and how long it lasts.

Local or Systemic Some infections cause harm in a limited region of the body, such as the upper respiratory tract, the urethra, or a single bone or joint. Such infections are said to be **local**. In contrast, **systemic** infections occur when pathogens invade the blood or lymph and spread throughout the body. **Bacteremia** is the clinical presence of bacteria in the blood, whereas **septicemia** is symptomatic systemic infection spread via the blood.

Primary or Secondary A **primary infection** is the first infection that occurs in a patient. Especially in immunocompromised patients, one or more **secondary infections** may follow a primary infection. For example, a frail client infected with pneumonia may develop herpes zoster (shingles, a viral infection related to past infection with varicella) related to the stress of illness.

Exogenous or Endogenous Healthcare providers need to determine the source of pathogens in a patient infected while he is in the facility. In **exogenous healthcare-related infections**, the pathogen is acquired from the healthcare environment. In **endogenous healthcare-related infections**, the pathogen arises from the patient's normal flora, when some form of treatment (e.g., chemotherapy or antibiotics) causes the normally harmless microbe to multiply and cause infection. For example, a yeast infection may develop in a client receiving antibiotics after surgery.

Acute or Chronic Infections that have a rapid onset but last only a short time, such as the common cold, are said to be **acute**. In contrast, **chronic infections** (e.g., an abscess) develop slowly and last for weeks, months, or even years. Some chronic infections, such as relapsing fever, recur after periods of remission. **Latent infections** cause no symptoms for long periods of time, even decades. Tuberculosis and human immunodeficiency virus (HIV) are examples. HIV typically causes an initial, brief illness that is then followed by about 10 years of latency before the patient begins to experience symptoms of AIDS.

Infections Follow Predictable Stages

Many infections follow a fairly predictable course of events, although the precise duration and intensity of symptoms in each stage vary from one individual to another:

- **Incubation** is the stage between successful invasion of the pathogen into the body and the first appearance of symptoms. In this stage, the person does not suspect that he has been infected but may be capable of infecting others. This stage may last only a day, as with the influenza virus, or as long as several months or even years, as with tuberculosis.
- The **prodromal stage** is characterized by the first appearance of vague symptoms. For example, a person infected with a cold virus may experience a mild throat irritation. Not all infections have a prodromal stage.
- **Illness** is the stage marked by the appearance of the signs and symptoms characteristic of the disease. If the patient's immune defenses and medical treatments (if any) are ineffective, this stage can end in the death of the patient.
- **Decline** is the stage during which the patient's immune defenses, along with any medical therapies, successfully reduce the number of pathogenic microbes. As a result, the signs and symptoms of the infection begin to fade.
- **Convalescence** is characterized by tissue repair and a return to health as the remaining number of microorganisms approaches zero. Convalescence may require only a day or two or, for severe infections, as long as a year or more.

Why Should Nurses Be Aware of Emerging Pathogens and Diseases?

An **epidemic** is an outbreak of a disease that suddenly affects a large group of people in a geographic region (e.g., a city or state) or in a defined population group (e.g., children, healthcare workers). A **pandemic** is an exceptionally widespread epidemic—that is, one that affects a large number of people in an entire country or worldwide. Examples of pandemics are H1N1 influenza ("swine flu") and malaria.

You should also know the term *emerging infectious disease*. Although there are various definitions, you can think of **emerging infectious diseases** as:

- Newly identified diseases caused by an unrecognized microorganism (e.g., the virus causing AIDS was unknown before 1980) or a known organism (e.g., enterovirus D68, *Streptococcus* infection causing toxic shock syndrome)
- Diseases occurring in new geographic areas (e.g., 2014 ebola pandemic originating from western Africa, West Nile virus in the Western hemisphere) or settings, such as *Clostridium difficile*, which was primarily a hospital-acquired infection and now occurs in the community
- Microorganisms in animals that extend their host range to begin infecting humans (e.g., avian influenza, or "bird flu"; and the H1N1 virus).
- Microbes that evolve to become more virulent (e.g., a strain of *Escherichia coli*, which now causes severe illness)
- Known diseases that dramatically increase in incidence (e.g., mumps and pertussis, also known as whooping cough)
- Organisms that are deliberately altered for bioterrorism (e.g., the contamination of some mail in the United States with *Bacillus anthracis* [anthrax] in 2001).
- Most emerging pathogens are viruses. For a brief discussion of some important emerging infections,

 Go to **Supplemental Materials: Emerging Infectious Diseases,** and **Reading More About Promoting Asepsis & Preventing Infection,** on Davis*Plus*.

Continental and intercontinental travel contributes to the spread of emerging pathogens throughout the world. Air travel enables a person to infect people headed for widespread locations, often before the reservoir person shows symptoms of the disease. Cooperative efforts among many disciplines and organizations worldwide are required to limit the spread of infectious diseases. To this end, the World Health Organization (WHO) has chosen as the first "global patient safety challenge" the reduction of HAIs. More than 15,000 healthcare facilities in 169 countries have registered for the WHO's "Save Lives: Clean Your Hands" program (World Health Organization, 2011, 2012). Also, The Joint Commission (2012b) requires hospitals to have an emergency management plan for responding to large numbers of infectious patients who might need to be treated as a result of an epidemic.

Example Problem: Drug-Resistant Pathogens

Some microorganisms, mostly bacteria, have mutated to develop resistance to one or more classes of antimicrobial drugs. These organisms are said to be **drug-resistant or multidrug-resistant**. Today antibiotic resistance is one of the most significant challenges in treating patients with severe infectious diseases. During the last several decades, the prevalence of multidrug-resistant organisms (MDROs) in U.S. hospitals and medical centers has increased steadily. MDROs are a serious problem because options for treating MDRO infections are limited. Furthermore, they are associated with serious illness, increased mortality, and increased hospital lengths of stay and costs.

A variety of risk factors are associated with MDRO infections (CDC, n.d.b, n.d.f; Siegel, Rhinehart, Jackson, et al., 2006). Among them are the following:

- Severe illness
- Previous exposure to antimicrobial agents (e.g., antibiotics)
- Underlying diseases or conditions that make it difficult for the person to fight infection (in particular, chronic renal disease, insulin-dependent diabetes mellitus, peripheral vascular disease, dermatitis, skin lesions)
- Invasive procedures and devices, such as dialysis, urinary catheterization, and intravenous lines
- Repeated contact with the healthcare system, especially acute care facilities, and especially intensive care units (where infection rates tend to be highest)
- Advanced age

MDROs are transmitted by the same routes as other microorganisms. A major factor, though, is transmission in healthcare settings via the hands of healthcare workers, especially for methicillin-resistant *Staphylococcus aureus* (MRSA), *C. difficile*, and vancomycin-resistant enterococci (VRE), discussed following. Other significant MDROs include multidrug-resistant tuberculosis (MDR-TB), penicillin-resistant *Streptococcus pneumoniae*, multidrug-resistant *E. coli*, and *Klebsiella pneumoniae*. If you need more information about diseases caused by those organisms, consult a medical-surgical textbook or,

 Go to **Supplemental Materials: What Are Drug-Resistant Pathogens?,** on Davis*Plus*.

Methicillin-Resistant Staphylococcus aureus (MRSA)

Staphylococcus aureus lives on the skin and in the nose, usually without causing problems. If a person does have a "staph" infection it is normally treated with methicillin, but methicillin-resistant *S. aureus* (MRSA) can't be killed by this drug. More than a million hospitalized patients acquire MRSA infection each year in the United States (APIC, 2010); it can be fatal. The organism is spread by skin-to-skin contact, and by living in crowded conditions. Control of MRSA has become a national priority.

✚ Because MRSA can survive on hands, clothing, environmental surfaces, and equipment, it is easily spread to vulnerable patients in healthcare settings. Healthcare institutions are targeting MRSA with staff education, aggressive handwashing and use of alcohol-based handrubs for 20 to 30 seconds for hand hygiene before touching a patient, increased use of protective gloves and gowns, and targeted screening (Klevens, Morrison, Nadle, et al., 2007; Upshaw-Owens & Bailey, 2012).

Vancomycin-Resistant Enterococci

Enterococci, normal residents in the intestines and the female genital tract, also occur in the environment. Most VRE infections occur in hospitals. Their spread is attributed to failure to follow infection control measures (Rice, 2001). VRE are a leading cause of healthcare-acquired bacteremia (bacteria in the blood), surgical wound infection, and urinary tract infection. Risk factors include previous long-term antibiotic treatment, weakened immune system, surgical procedures, long-term devices (e.g., urinary catheters), or colonization by VRE (CDC, 2011).

Clostridium difficile

inflammation of lg. intestine "flu-like" symptoms

About 3% of healthy adults carry a harmless version of *C. diff.* However, it can become harmful when antibiotics destroy healthy bacteria that normally protect against the disease. The newer *C. diff.* strain is resistant to nearly all antibiotics and virulent enough to cause sepsis, lasting intestinal damage, the need for colon removal, and even death. It thrives in hospital environments, so the federal government is pressuring physicians and hospitals to better enforce sanitation standards and to prevent the overprescription of antibiotics. However, because spores survive for days on surfaces such as doorknobs and toilet seats, at least 10% of *C. diff.* infections are acquired outside the hospital (CDC, 2012). Prevention of transmission in a healthcare facility focuses on the following:

Application of contact precautions for patients with diarrhea
Accurate identification of patients
Rigorous cleaning of patient rooms and equipment
Consistent hand hygiene, using soap and water rather than alcohol-based handrubs for mechanical removal of spores
✚ A bleach-containing disinfectant for environmental disinfection

Handwashing with soap and water. Alcohol-based handrubs are not effective because they do not destroy *C. diff.* spores.

 Think**Like a Nurse** 23-2

Why are emerging infections of special concern in healthcare?
Why are MDROs of special concern in healthcare?

WHAT ARE THE BODY'S DEFENSES AGAINST INFECTION?

The human body has three "lines of defense" against infectious disease:

- Primary defenses—Certain anatomical features limit the entry of pathogens.
- Secondary defenses—Protective biochemical processes fight pathogens that do enter.
- Tertiary defenses—The presence of pathogens activates immune responses against specific, recognized invaders.

The primary and secondary lines of defense are nonspecific; that is, they have no means of adapting their response to each specific invader. Instead, they act in precisely the same way against any and all intruders, from a simple cold virus to deadly fungal spores.

Primary Defenses

The "soldiers" in the first line of defense are the structural barriers of the human body. These **primary defenses** prevent organisms from entering the body. The normal flora of the body provide one such defense. Any treatment that disturbs the balance between the normal flora and other microorganisms can increase the client's risk of developing disease. For example, when broad-spectrum antibiotics are used to treat infection, they may eliminate normal flora in addition to those causing the infection. This allows other kinds of pathogens to multiply, producing a **superinfection**. Other primary defenses are as follows:

- *Skin.* The surface of intact, healthy skin is tough and resilient and prevents entry of many pathogens. The normal flora of the skin inhibit multiplication of other organisms, including pathogens, that land on the skin.
- *The respiratory tree.* The nares, trachea, and bronchi are covered with mucous membranes that trap pathogens, which are then expelled. The nose contains hairs that filter the upper airway; and the nasal passages, sinuses, trachea, and larger bronchi are lined with cilia, tiny hairlike cells that sweep microorganisms upward from the lower airways. Coughing and sneezing forcefully expel organisms from the respiratory tract.
- *Eyes.* The lacrimal glands produce tears that contain lysozyme, an antimicrobial enzyme. This means that tears help the body to wash infective organisms from the eyes.
- *The mouth.* The mouth normally has a large number of pathogenic microorganisms, but saliva, like tears, contains lysozyme and helps continually wash microbes from the teeth and gums. The rich blood supply of the mouth swiftly transports defensive blood cells (discussed later in this section) that keep the microorganisms in check. In addition, normal flora of the mouth compete for nutrition with invading organisms, thereby limiting the number of pathogens.
- *The gastrointestinal tract.* Many pathogens that reach the stomach are destroyed in its acidic environment. Those that successfully enter the small intestine face the antimicrobial action of bile. Simple peristalsis as well as diarrhea and vomiting are other first-line defense mechanisms for pathogens that invade the gastrointestinal tract. In addition, normal flora in the intestine secrete antibacterial substances.
- *The genitourinary tract.* Like the respiratory tree, the genitourinary tract is protected with mucous membranes. The epithelial cells lining the urethra and anus secrete mucus, which adheres to pathogens to promote their excretion through urine and stool. Urine itself is highly acidic and contains lysozyme. Mucous membranes lining the vagina also help keep pathogens from establishing colonies there. In addition, the high acidity and normal flora of the vagina keep pathogens in check.

Secondary Defenses

Pathogens that dodge the primary defenses and gain entry into the body begin to release wastes and secretions and to cause the breakdown of cells and tissues. The presence of such chemicals activates a set of **secondary defenses**.

- **Phagocytosis**—the process by which phagocytes (specialized white blood cells [WBCs]) engulf and destroy pathogens directly is called phagocytosis. Phagocytic WBCs include neutrophils, monocytes, and eosinophils. Table 23-1 summarizes the types of white blood cells and their roles in defending against infection.
- **The complement cascade**—a process by which a set of blood proteins, called complement, triggers the release of chemicals that attack the cell membranes of pathogens, causing them to rupture. Complement also signals basophils (WBCs) to release histamine, which prompts inflammation.
- **Inflammation**—a process that begins when histamine and other chemicals are released either from damaged cells, or from basophils being activated by complement. With inflammation blood vessels dilate and become more permeable, which increases the flow of phagocytes, antimicrobial chemicals, oxygen, and nutrients to the affected area. The classic signs and symptoms of inflammation are localized warmth and erythema (redness), which develop as blood flow is increased. In addition, fluid leaking from the more permeable blood vessels accumulates in the surrounding tissue, causing edema, which in turn prompts pain as pressure is exerted on nerve endings (Bauman, Machunis-Masuoka, & Tizard, 2006).
- **Fever**—a rise in core body temperature that increases metabolism, inhibits multiplication of pathogens, and triggers specific immune responses (discussed

Table 23-1 ▶ Types and Functions of White Blood Cells

TYPE	FUNCTION
Granular	
Basophils: 0.5%–1% of total WBCs	Release histamine and heparin granules as part of the inflammatory response. Percentage normal during infections.
Eosinophils: 1%–3% of total WBCs	Destroy helminths; mediate allergic reactions; have limited role in phagocytosis. Percentage increases in parasitic infections.
Neutrophils: 55%–70% of total WBCs	Phagocytize pathogens
Agranular	
Lymphocytes: 20%–35% of total WBCs	T cells—responsible for cell-mediated immunity; recognize, attack, and destroy antigens.
	B cells—responsible for humoral immunity; produce immunoglobulins to attack and destroy antigens. Percentage of total lymphocytes increases in viral infection and chronic bacterial infection; decreases in sepsis.
Monocytes: 3%–8% of total WBCs	Able to phagocytize directly as well as to differentiate into macrophages, which help clean up damaged or injured tissue. Percentage increases in tuberculosis, protozoal, and rickettsial infections.

Note: Laboratory values alone are not adequate for diagnosing infection. Presence of clinical signs (e.g., fever, pain, swelling) must be assessed.

shortly). Believing that low-grade fevers are a necessary natural defense mechanism, many clinicians do not treat a fever unless it's greater than 102°F (38.9°C).

Tertiary Defenses

Immunity against an infection is achieved through the presence of antibodies that neutralize or destroy toxins or disease-producing organisms. **Active immunity** occurs when the body makes its own antibodies or T cells to protect the body against a pathogen. Immunity can also be achieved when a person is given antibodies to a pathogen rather than producing them through her own immune system, called **passive immunity** (Box 23-1).

Why is it that people who recover from an infectious disease like measles or chickenpox never get the disease again, even if they are repeatedly exposed to the virus? The reason is **specific immunity**: the process by which the body's immune cells "learn" to recognize and destroy pathogens they have encountered before.

The cells involved in specific immunity are white blood cells called **lymphocytes**, which are produced from stem cells in the red bone marrow. Lymphocytes that grow to maturity in the bone marrow are designated *B lymphocytes,* or *B cells,* whereas those that mature in the thymus are designated *T lymphocytes,* or *T cells.*

Key Point: *Remember that* **T** *cells mature in the* **Thymus;** *and* **B** *cells mature in Bone marrow.*

After they have matured, most B cells and T cells travel to the lymph nodes, spleen, and other sites of lymphatic tissue. From all of these locations, lymphocytes seek out foreign cells and other matter to target for destruction. Lymphocytes recognize foreign substances by the molecules present on their surfaces. These molecules that trigger a specific immune response are called **antigens**. The two types of specific immunity involving B cells and T cells are discussed next.

Humoral Immunity

The humoral immune response (or antibody-mediated response) protects the body by circulating antibodies to fight against pathogens. The body's defense system acts by producing specialized white blood cells (leukocytes) to seek out and destroy invaders by any of the following methods (Fig. 23-2; Box 23-2):

- *Phagocytosis.* Antibodies do not phagocytize directly, but instead signal leukocytes (macrophages and neutrophils) to attack the pathogens to which the antibodies are bound.
- *Neutralization.* By binding to a pathogen's attachment sites, antibodies disable the pathogens by adhering to the invading body cells. Thus, although they are not destroyed, the pathogens become ineffective.
- *Agglutination.* Antibodies have two attachment sites; therefore, each antibody can attach to two pathogenic cells in a population. This quality causes the cells to clump together (agglutinate), reducing the cells' activity and increasing the likelihood that the group will be detected by leukocytes and phagocytized.

BOX 23-1 ■ Four Types of Immunity

Natural active immunity—After a person becomes ill with an infection, the body produces its own antibodies to fight the disease-causing organism and protect from infection in the future (e.g., influenza).

Natural passive immunity—Immunity results when natural antibodies are passed from one body to another, such as from mother to baby through the placenta, or through breast-feeding.

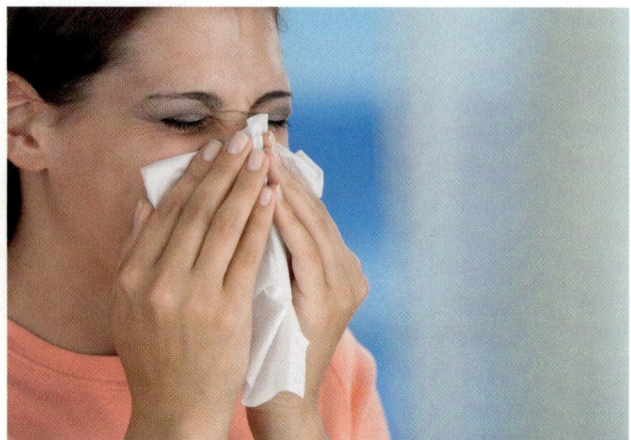

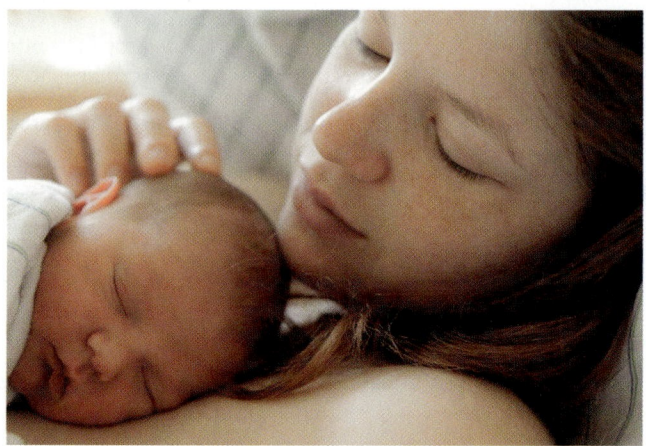

Artificial active immunity—An immune response occurs when the body is exposed to weakened or dead pathogens in a vaccine. The body then makes T cells or antibodies to keep from actually developing the illness (e.g., tetanus, measles). This type of immunity offers long-lasting or even lifetime protection.

Artificial passive immunity—Protection from infection is achieved when a person receives serum from another person or animal that has already produced antibodies against the pathogen (e.g., serum for treatment of rabies or botulism).

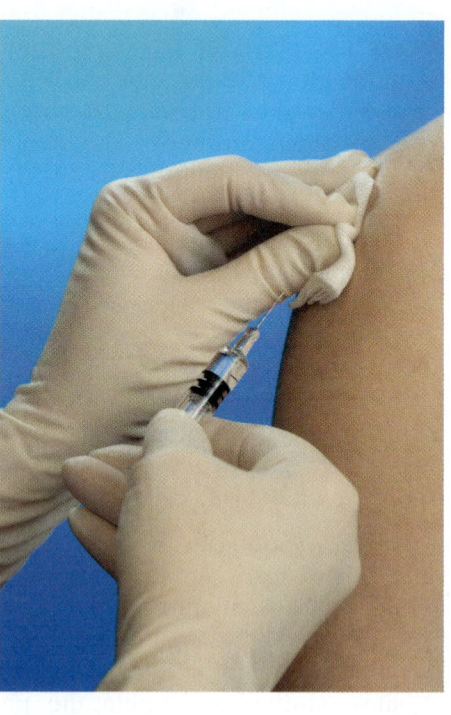

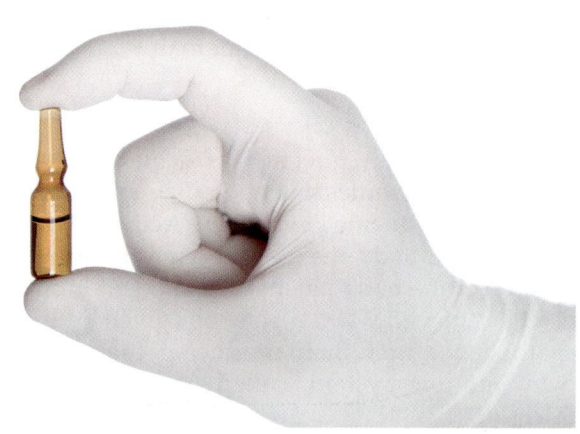

■ *Activation of complement and inflammation.* Antibodies trigger the complement cascade and stimulate the release of inflammatory chemicals to destroy the antigen.

Cellular Immunity

Cellular (cell-mediated) immune response acts directly to destroy pathogens (i.e., viruses, fungi, protozoans, cancers) without using antibodies but rather activating

phagocytes and T and B cells. Four types of T cells play a role in fighting infection (Fig. 23-3):

■ *Cytotoxic (killer) T cells* directly attack and kill body cells infected with pathogens.
■ *Helper T cells* play a supportive role in cell-mediated responses by secreting **interleukin**, which attracts infection-fighting white blood cells.

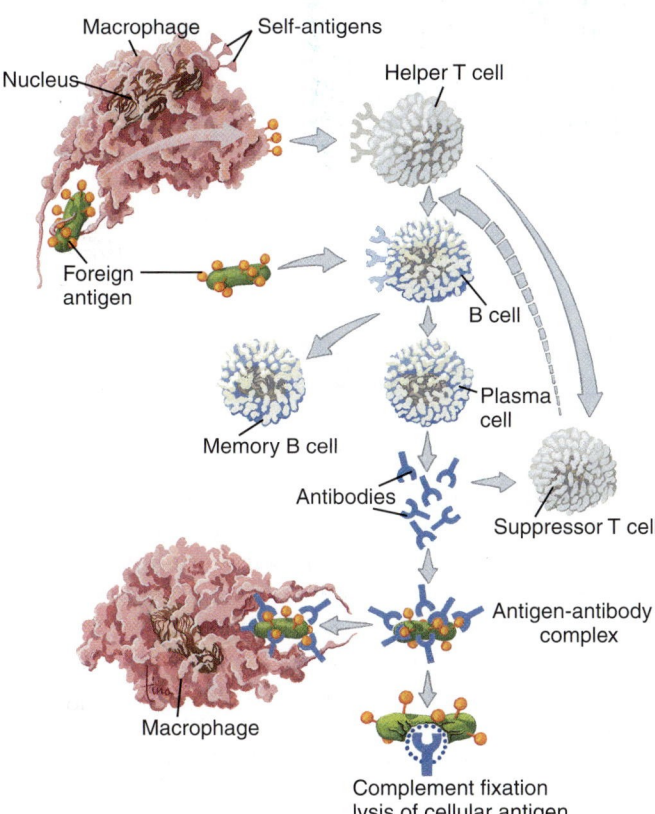

FIGURE 23-2 The humoral immune response produces antibodies to destroy antigens.

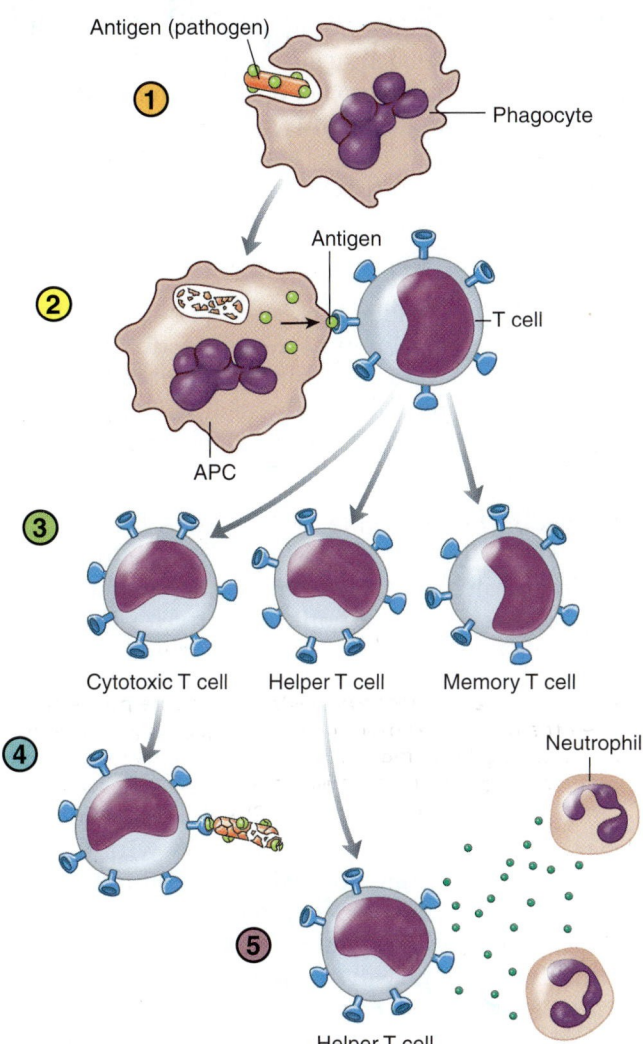

FIGURE 23-3 The cell-mediated immune response causes white blood cells to attack antigens.

BOX 23-2 ■ Immunoglobulin (Ig) Classes

- **IgM** is the first antibody to appear when an antigen (e.g., pathogen) is encountered. It is also involved in agglutination with incompatible blood types.

- **IgG** is the most common immunoglobin in the body. It takes at least 10 days for IgG to be produced in response to an initial infection. IgG is the only immunoglobulin that can cross the placenta to provide temporary immunity to the fetus/infant.

- **IgE** is the immunoglobulin primarily responsible for the allergic response.

- **IgA** is found in mucous membranes in the intestines, respiratory and urinary tracts, saliva, tears, and breast milk. IgA provides additional immune protection by secreting around the body openings.

- **IgD** forms on the surface of B cells and traps the potential pathogen to prevent it from replicating and causing disease.

For a more extended explanation of immunoglobulins,

 Go to Chapter 22, **Supplemental Materials, Humoral Immunity,** on Davis*Plus*.

- *Memory T cells.* The first time an antigen invades the body, T cells form that respond to that specific antigen. With subsequent infections, the memory T cells are able to increase the speed and amount of the T-cell response.

- *Suppressor T cells* are thought to stop the immune response when the infection has been contained (also see Fig. 23-2).

KnowledgeCheck 23-3

- Identify and describe the purpose of the body's three major lines of defense against infection.
- If a patient's lab work reveals that IgM, but not IgG, is present in the blood, what could you conclude about this infection?

WHAT FACTORS INCREASE HOST SUSCEPTIBILITY?

Anything that weakens the defenses makes a person more susceptible to infection. In addition, any factors that increase the person's exposure to pathogens, such as working at a day-care center or being a nurse, increase the risk for infection. Some of the most common factors are discussed below.

Developmental Stage Young children are vulnerable because their immune systems are immature and have had limited exposure to pathogens. Children frequently begin to have more infections when they start interacting with people outside their family (e.g., when they begin day care or start school). With exposure, the body's natural defense systems turn on to protect from infection. This is a natural process known as acquiring **active immunity**.

Older adults are also susceptible hosts because the immune response declines with aging. Skin, a primary defense, becomes less elastic and more prone to breakdown with aging. Elders also tend to be less active, and their nutrition may be inadequate.

Breaks in the First Line of Defense A break in the skin, whether caused by a surgical procedure, skin breakdown, an insect bite, or insertion of an intravenous device, creates a portal of entry for infectious microorganisms.

Illness or Injury Recuperation from infection or injury limits the physical resources available to combat a new pathogen.

Tobacco Use Smoking is a major risk factor for pulmonary infections. Smoking interferes with normal respiratory functioning, including the ability to move the chest, cough, sneeze, or have full air exchange. Chemicals in tobacco paralyze cilia; thus, secretions pool in the lower airways, creating a favorable environment for bacterial growth. Although tobacco users are most profoundly affected by these changes, people exposed chronically to secondhand smoke (e.g., bartenders, children of smokers) are also affected by these changes and are at increased risk for infection.

Substance Abuse Alcohol curbs hunger because it contains many calories. As a result, many chronic alcohol users do not consume an adequate diet. Alcohol is also toxic to the liver and to the cells lining the intestinal mucosa. Inhaled substances, such as marijuana and cocaine, affect respiratory cilia in a manner similar to tobacco. Any substances that affect orientation and energy level will diminish food intake, activity, rest, and hygiene—factors that support host defenses. Injecting substances leads to breaks in skin integrity, further increasing the risk of infection.

Multiple Sexual Partners The number of sexual partners is directly related to the risk of sexually transmitted infections and cervical cancer.

Environmental Factors Increased exposure to pathogens in one's work situation (e.g., kindergarten teacher, healthcare worker), living situation (e.g., nursing home, parents with young children who are in preschool), and other environmental factors increase one's risk for infection.

Chronic Disease Many chronic diseases diminish the body's ability to fight infection. Diseases that impair peripheral circulation, such as uncontrolled hypertension (high blood pressure) and diabetes mellitus, make the patient prone to infection in the extremities. Poor circulation prevents antibodies and T cells from reaching the pathogens and damages tissue, making it easier for pathogens to enter. Leukemia, a form of cancer of the blood, increases the production of abnormal white blood cells, but these cells are ineffective in combating infection. Because HIV infects T cells, a patient with AIDS has a reduced ability to fight off secondary infections.

Medications Some medications are given for the purpose of reducing the immune response, for example, to patients receiving organ or tissue transplants. For most patients, however, decreased immunity is an unwanted side effect of treatment. Even common medications, such as nonsteroidal anti-inflammatory agents (NSAIDs) (e.g., ibuprofen), decrease the immune response. As a side effect, some medications, such as chemotherapeutic agents, decrease the production of white blood cells or cause the cells produced to be abnormal. Even antibiotics can increase the risk for infection. For example, an antibiotic given for a respiratory infection may cause a vaginal yeast infection because it destroys colonies of normal vaginal flora, allowing the harmful microbes to thrive. Such **superinfections** (opportunistic growth of harmful transient pathogens that are normally kept in check) can be extremely challenging to treat.

Invasive Nursing and Medical Procedures Several procedures are associated with an increased risk of infection. For example, urinary catheterization may injure the fragile urethral mucosa, provide a direct pathway for pathogens into the bladder, and prevent the normal flushing of the urethra. Also, an IV line inserted to infuse an antibiotic may serve as a portal of entry for pathogens to enter a patient's body.

KnowledgeCheck 23-4

What factors increase a client's risk for infection?

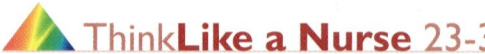

ThinkLike a Nurse 23-3

Consider your current lifestyle. How would you evaluate your ability to support your body's defenses?

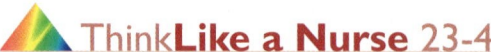

ThinkLike a Nurse 23-4

Recall the scenario of Jason Sergi, the labor and delivery nurse, and his daughter (Meet Your Nursing Role Model). Why did Jason say that handwashing was the most important thing he did at work that day? Explain your answer by referring to all of the links in the chain of infection.

Practical Knowledge
knowing **how**

As a nurse you will have direct contact with patients who are infected with a variety of pathogens or who are at increased risk for infection. The remainder of this chapter provides practical information for preventing infection in your clients and for caring for clients with infection.

ASSESSMENT

Some elements of the nursing history and physical assessment focus specifically on the risk factors and symptoms of infection.

Nursing History

To elicit information related to infection, ask the client about the following:

- Any exposure to pathogens in the environment, including at work, recent or international travel, contact with people who are ill, and unprotected sexual behavior
- If the patient is febrile ask, "Have you recently traveled outside the country?"
- Any unusual foods or products ingested
- Past and present disease or injury history
- Medications, over-the-counter preparations, herbal products, alcohol intake, and any substances currently in use
- Current level of stress
- Immunization history
- Symptoms of illness

Physical Assessment

Observe the patient's general appearance: Does he seem fatigued? Is he diaphoretic? Is he wrapped in blankets or complaining of feeling chilled? Does the patient appear well nourished? Are the mucous membranes dry? Does the skin have normal elasticity (turgor)? Physical assessment includes a thorough examination of the skin. Look for signs of local infection evidenced by pain, redness, swelling, and warmth. Note the presence or absence of any rashes, along with any breaks or reddened areas of the skin. Patients with poor peripheral circulation often have various skin discolorations, rather than signs of inflammation, when experiencing an infection. Swollen lymph nodes indicate the possible presence of an infection in the area that drains into the nodes. Elevated temperature and pulse rate are classic signs of an infection.

It is important to remember that the presence of one infection does not eliminate the risk for an additional infection. For example, a patient being treated with IV medications for a wound infection is at risk for infection at the IV site, as well as for a superinfection or an infection related to insufficient immunizations. For a list of tests commonly used to evaluate evidence of or risk for infection,

 Go to Chapter 23, **Diagnostic Testing, Common Tests for Evaluating the Presence of or Risk for Infection,** in Volume 2.

Each specific test should be evaluated based on the patient's condition, age, and coexisting conditions.

ANALYSIS/NURSING DIAGNOSIS

The following two NANDA-I diagnoses directly pertain to infection:

Readiness for Enhanced Immunization Status This is a wellness diagnosis, used to describe a person who is already following the local, national, and/or international standards of immunization, but who wants to enhance behavior to prevent infectious disease, and learn more about providers of immunizations, possible problems associated with immunizations, knowledge of standards, and record keeping.

Risk for Infection Virtually any patient in a healthcare setting is at Risk for Infection due to exposure to pathogens in the environment. Use this diagnosis only for patients who are at higher than usual risk (e.g., those with poor nutritional status) and who need nursing interventions to help prevent infection. Do not use it for the generic assessments you do routinely for all patients (e.g., assessing temperature, routine examination of surgical incision). Patients with actual infection are managed collaboratively with the healthcare team. Examples of appropriate use of this diagnosis include the following:

- Risk for Infection r/t altered immune response secondary to corticosteroid therapy
- Risk for Infection r/t impaired skin integrity and poor nutritional status

Infection may be a medical diagnosis or the etiology of other nursing diagnoses, such as Fatigue, Risk for Imbalanced Body Temperature, or Pain. Patients with infection may experience other health problems due to their infected status. For example:

- Social Isolation r/t communicable disease (e.g., tuberculosis [TB])
- Deficient Diversional Activity r/t inability to leave room secondary to protective isolation

Other diagnostic statements may apply, depending upon the patient's condition, treatment ordered, and the patient's response to illness. For a care plan and care map for Risk for Infection,

 Go to Chapter 23, **Care Plan** and **Care Map,** on Davis*Plus.*

PLANNING OUTCOMES/EVALUATION

For NOC standardized outcomes for Risk for Infection,

Go to Chapter 23, **Standardized Language,** on Davis*Plus*.

Individualized goals/outcomes statements depend on the specific nursing diagnosis and etiology. For example, for an undernourished woman, if the nursing diagnosis is Risk for Infection r/t intravenous puncture site and probable invasive procedures secondary to active labor, an appropriate goal would be:

Patient will show no signs of localized infection at the infusion site, as evidenced by the absence of swelling, redness, excessive warmth, pain, or drainage.

You will evaluate the nursing care plan by examining the extent to which such goals have been met.

PLANNING INTERVENTIONS/IMPLEMENTATION

When caring for a patient at risk for infection, nursing activities are aimed at breaking the chain of infection at every possible link. Some of the most common reasons patients are diagnosed with Risk for Infection are exposure to pathogens, compromise to their normal defense mechanisms, increased physiological stress, or inadequate immune response. Direct nursing care toward these concerns, and provide the following broad interventions:

- Reduce exposure to pathogens through the use of aseptic technique (discussed shortly).
- Maintain skin integrity and support natural defenses against infection.
- Reduce stress.
- Promote immune function through collaborative care.
- Provide supportive measures to decrease the length of time that invasive devices, such as intravenous lines and urinary catheters, are needed by a patient.

For NIC standardized interventions for Risk for Infection:

Go to Chapter 23, **Standardized Language,** on Davis*Plus*.

Specific nursing activities will be based on the unique situation of the client, as described in the etiology of the diagnostic statement. For example:

- For clients who have had surgery and general anesthesia or who are at risk for pneumonia, promote coughing and deep breathing on a regular basis.
- For clients being mechanically ventilated, provide special oral care designed to prevent ventilator-associated pneumonia. (See the accompanying QSEN box for an example.)
- For older adults, especially those who or frail or in a debilitated state and those living in a group residence, encourage immunizations that can help them to acquire immunity from some communicable diseases, such as influenza.

- Healthcare workers can also benefit from immunizations to protect them from HAIs.
- Community health nurses can limit disease transmission through surveillance of the community, tracking of disease patterns, and initiation of prompt treatment.
- For clients who have breaks in the skin or incision sites, provide regular assessment for infection status and follow appropriate medical or surgical asepsis guidelines.
- For all clients at risk for infection, provide care that is based on principles of medical asepsis.

Other preventive nursing activities are discussed in the following sections. They include providing client teaching, supporting host defenses, and practicing medical and surgical asepsis.

Providing Client Teaching

Clients and caregivers in their own homes are usually at less risk for infection than they are in the hospital. The client and caregiver share the same potential pathogens and antibodies, and there is limited exposure to others with illness. Nevertheless, to protect their own health and the health of others, clients need to understand basic principles of medical asepsis, personal hygiene, and infection control. You should also teach them to recognize signs and symptoms of infection; and for those who have an infection, help them to understand that particular organism and disease process. For information about teaching infection control in the home and community, see Home Care: Preventing Infection in the Home and Community. To help clients avoid acquiring or spreading community-acquired MRSA (CA-MRSA), see Self-Care: Teaching Your Patient About Preventing the Spread of CA-MRSA.

Promoting Wellness to Support Host Defenses

Efforts to promote wellness help break the chain of infection by strengthening a person's defenses against invading pathogens. Lifestyle factors essential for promoting host defenses are healthful nutrition, adequate hygiene, rest and exercise, stress reduction, and immunizations.

Nutrition An acute infection depletes the body's nutritional stores. Therefore, it is important to monitor and support client nutrition, including protein, vitamins, minerals, and water. Nutrients are required to replace lost stores, to maintain production of white blood cells, and to repair damaged tissues. Fever and increased secretions of mucus, which are common defenses against infection, increase water loss. Additional water is needed to supplement the lost fluid and to support the increased metabolic rate that occurs with a fever. Chapter 27 further discusses the importance of adequate nutrition.

Hygiene is crucial for maintaining intact skin, a primary host defense. Encourage frequent handwashing, as well as regular showering or bathing, to decrease the bacterial count on the skin. However, be aware that overzealous cleanliness diminishes the skin's natural oils and may lead to cracking of the skin. Chapter 25

Quality and Safety Education for Nurses

Successful QI Project: Improving the Rate of Ventilator-Associated Pneumonia (VAP)

Key Concept: *Infection prevention and control*

Competency: *Quality Improvement (Knowledge, Skills, Attitudes)**

You and your colleagues have the privilege and opportunity to become partners in improving the quality of patient care. Think about the following project and consider what Knowledge, Skills, and Attitudes were required for its success and how they relate to the key concept.

Situation: Nurses and physicians at the Mercy Medical Center Critical Care Unit in Springfield, Maine, wanted to decrease their rate of ventilator-associated pneumonia (VAP). They

collected data to establish the existing rate of 12.6 cases per 1,000 ventilator days.

Intervention developed: Nurses provided oral care with cetylpyridinium chloride (Oral-B) using a suction toothbrush every 4 hours. After that, they cleaned each patient's mouth with a hydrogen peroxide–treated suction swab, performed deep oropharyngeal suctioning, and applied mouth moisturizer.

Result: Incidence of VAP declined 72%, and after changing the tooth cleanser to chlorhexidine gluconate, by an impressive 90%!

Time Frame	Intervention	Cases/1,000 Vent Days	% of Decline
2004	Usual care	12.6	
5/2005–12/2005	Oral care protocol introduced	4.12	67%
2006	Oral care protocol maintained	3.57	72%
2007	Oral care protocol maintained; tooth cleanser changed to chlorhexidine gluconate (Peridex)	1.3	90%

Think about it:

➤ What QSEN Knowledge and Attitudes did the nurses and team members need before changing the care of patients on ventilators?

➤ How is a meaningful and measurable outcome an essential Skill for effective quality improvement interventions? Is the outcome a direct result of the care?

➤ What is your attitude about the significance of the team's work? How will the team's efforts affect patients?

Source: Hutchins K., Karras, G., Erwin, J., et al. (2009).

*To learn about specific Knowledge, Skills, and Attitudes,

 Go to the QSEN Web site at **http:www.qsen.org.ksas_prelicensure.php**

Self-Care

Teaching Your Patient About Preventing the Spread of CA-MRSA

As measures to prevent community-acquired MRSA, everyone should:

➤ Take antibiotics as prescribed. Complete the course of medication as recommended until it is finished.

➤ Contact your healthcare provider if the infection doesn't improve after a few days of taking an antibiotic.

➤ Never use antibiotics prescribed for someone else; and do not give your medication to others.

➤ Follow your healthcare provider's recommendations for influenza and pneumonia vaccinations. Preventing respiratory infections decreases antibiotic use.

➤ Make sure your healthcare providers clean their hands before they touch you. This is one of the most important infection prevention and control measures.

➤ Wash your hands often with soap and water. Wash for 15 to 30 seconds, or as long as it takes to sing the "Happy Birthday" song.

➤ Use alcohol-based hand sanitizer if soap and water are not available or hands are not visibly soiled. Sanitizer should have at least 60% alcohol.

➤ Avoid sharing personal items (e.g., towels, makeup, combs, clothing).

➤ Pay attention to symptoms that may indicate an infection (e.g., drainage from or inflammation of a wound), and contact your healthcare provider immediately.

➤ Cough and sneeze into your elbow and wash your hands after using a tissue.

Clients who have MRSA on their skin or who are infected with MRSA should be taught to:

➤ Keep all sores and cuts clean and covered with bandages.

➤ When changing a bandage:

Don't touch the sore with your bare hands. Wear gloves.

(Continued)

Self-Care

Teaching Your Patient About Preventing the Spread of CA-MRSA—cont'd

Immediately discard the soiled bandage and gloves in a trashbag where no one else can touch them.

Wash your hands after removing the gloves.

➤ Avoid touching other people's cuts or bandages.

➤ Avoid close-contact activities until your skin infection is healed, unless you can ensure that your sore will not come in contact with another person (e.g., if your sore can be well covered by a bandage and clothing).

➤ Shower daily, using antibacterial soap if your healthcare provider advises it.

➤ Wash your clothing, towels, and bedding separately from other family members' items. Use warm or hot water and bleach, if possible. Use warm or hot setting on the dryer.

➤ Wash exercise clothes after each use.

Sources: Adapted from CDC (n.d.e), *Antibiotic/antimicrobial resistance.* Retrieved November 2012, from http://www.cdc.gov/drugresistance/about.html; Polcomo, A. A. (2008). MRSA infections. *Nursing2008, 38(8),* 33; Leung-Chen, P. (2008). Emerging infections. Everybody's crying MRSA. *American Journal of Nursing, 108*(8), 29–31.

Home Care

Preventing Infection in the Home and Community

➤ To disinfect the home environment, use and teach caregivers to create a dilute bleach solution. Mix 1 part regular-strength bleach to 50 parts water. The mixture may be stored for a month in an opaque container.

✚ NEVER mix the solution with other household cleaners.

➤ Procedures performed using sterile technique in the hospital (e.g., urinary catheterization) are often performed by clean procedure in the home because of the decreased risk of infection.

➤ Washing dishware and eating utensils in a dishwasher with hot water and detergents is sufficient decontamination.

➤ Healthcare workers in the home are a potential source of pathogens and should use caution to avoid infecting the client.

➤ If the client or family member is capable and willing to perform the required treatment, provide the necessary teaching; the client will have less exposure to pathogens than he would should a healthcare provider came to the home to provide care.

➤ Assess for subtle signs of infection: temperature increase, fatigue, lymph gland enlargement, delayed healing of wounds, fever, chills, or drainage.

➤ Instruct clients and family members in the signs and symptoms of infection and how and when to contact their primary care provider to report these findings.

➤ Advise those planning international travel to get their vaccinations before departing, especially for travel to Africa, South-Central Asia, or Central America, where they may contract malaria, dengue, rickettsiosis, and influenza.

➤ Teach clients and family members basic hygiene and infection prevention measures in the home, including:

The importance of handwashing before preparing food, before eating, after going to the bathroom, blowing the nose, and before putting the hands near the face.

Keeping the home environment clean to create an optimal environment for care

Safe food preparation and storage (see Chapter 27)

Not sharing personal care items (e.g., towels, washcloths, toothbrushes, combs)

➤ Teach clients and family members actions they can take to help prevent infection when they are outside the home, including:

Washing hands and not touching surfaces in a public bathroom

Carrying and using antibacterial hand gel, as needed while in public places

Using a wet-wipe on the receiver and mouthpiece of public phones before making a call

Washing hands upon returning home (e.g., from shopping)

Asking healthcare providers to wash their hands before physical contact, if they have not done so

Using tongs, not fingers, to get food from serving trays in grocery stores and restaurants

➤ For additional information on home care practices, see Chapter 43.

---

focuses on the importance of hygiene for health. Also see the Home Care box.

✚ For the immunocompromised or bed-bound hospitalized patient, the American Association of Critical-Care Nurses (AACN) (2013) advocates daily bedside baths using filtered tap water and disposable basins, including prepackaged bathing products. Nurses should use disposable cloths with 2% chlorhexidine gluconate (CHG) to reduce colonization of specific bacteria and infections with MDROs.

Rest and Sleep Rest and sleep renew the body and mind and conserve strength. Sleep needs vary, and there is really no "correct" amount or pattern of sleep. However, sleep of 6 to 9 hours per night is considered fully restorative for most people.

Exercise and Activity Research demonstrates that exercise is just as important as rest and sleep. Too little activity causes circulation to slow and the lungs to supply less oxygen. Excessive exercise leads to fatigue and joint injury. Chapters 32 and 34 provide in-depth discussion on rest, sleep, activity, and exercise.

Stress Reduction Whether physical or mental, stress decreases the body's immune defenses. Numerous studies demonstrate a correlation between increased stress and increased disease (Cousins, 1979; Franco, de Barros, Nogueira-Martins, et al., 2003; Schneider, Alexander, Staggers, et al., 2005; Tegethoff, Greene, Olsen, et al., 2011). Laughing, in contrast, increases oxygenation, promotes body movement, and increases immune responses. See Chapter 12 for further details on the effects of stress, if you wish.

Immunizations Immunization via vaccination can protect against several infectious diseases (e.g., measles, mumps, and other childhood diseases; pneumonia; influenza; smallpox; shingles). Unfortunately, some pathogens, such as the virus that causes the common cold, mutate too rapidly for an immunization to be developed. Encourage clients to follow recommendations for immunizations. For most diseases, at least 85% of the population must be immunized in order to protect the entire population from the disease. If you need specific recommended immunizations throughout the life span and their role in health promotion, see Chapters 9 and 10 for various age groups, and

 Go to Chapter 9, **ESG Figures 9-1, 9-2,** and **9-3** on Davis*Plus.*

Also

 Go to Chapter 10, **ESG Figure 10-4,** on Davis*Plus.*

KnowledgeCheck 23-5

What actions improve host ability to prevent infection?

PRACTICING MEDICAL ASEPSIS

Asepsis is a term that means absence of contamination by disease-causing microorganisms. **Medical asepsis** ("clean technique") refers to procedures that decrease the potential for the spread of infections. You probably already practice medical asepsis in other settings without realizing it. For example, at home you wash your hands before and after handling foods. Before chopping food, you make sure the cutting board and utensils you use are clean. After using it, you wash the board with hot, soapy water. In the healthcare setting, medical asepsis includes hand hygiene, environmental cleanliness, standard precautions, and protective isolation.

✚ The effectiveness of these measures, and the patient's safety, depend on nurses' rigorously and consistently following the principles of asepsis. When you are hurrying, you may be tempted to take shortcuts or forget to follow a guideline. Remember: You are putting your patient, and possibly yourself, at risk for an infection that could cause serious illness. Assume every patient is potentially infected or colonized with an organism that could be transmitted to others.

Maintaining Clean Hands

Key Point: *Hand hygiene is the single most important activity for preventing and controlling infection.*

The WHO has chosen as the first "global patient safety challenge" the reduction of HAIs, with the theme, "clean care is safer care." They have made hand hygiene the cornerstone strategy because it is simple, standardized, low cost, and based on solid scientific evidence.

Although you may think you already know how to wash your hands, remember that in healthcare settings you are coming in contact with pathogens that are potentially dangerous to you and your patients. Decisions about the type of hand hygiene to use, how long to wash, when to wash, and so on are based on the amount of contact you have with patients or contaminated objects, as well as the patient's infection status and susceptibility to infection. Handwashing involves five key factors: time, water, soap, friction, and drying (Fig. 23-4). The following briefly summarizes the CDC recommendations for these factors (Boyce & Pittet, 2002). For more specific details and guidelines to use when making handwashing decisions,

 Go to **Clinical Insight 23-1: Guidelines for Hand Hygiene,** in Volume 2.

- *Time.* In a nonsurgical setting, wash the hands vigorously for at least 15 seconds, longer if hands are visibly soiled. In a surgical setting wash for 2 to 6 minutes, depending on the soap or other product used.
- *Water.* Use warm water and rinse off soap completely. Hot water and soap increase the potential for skin breakdown.

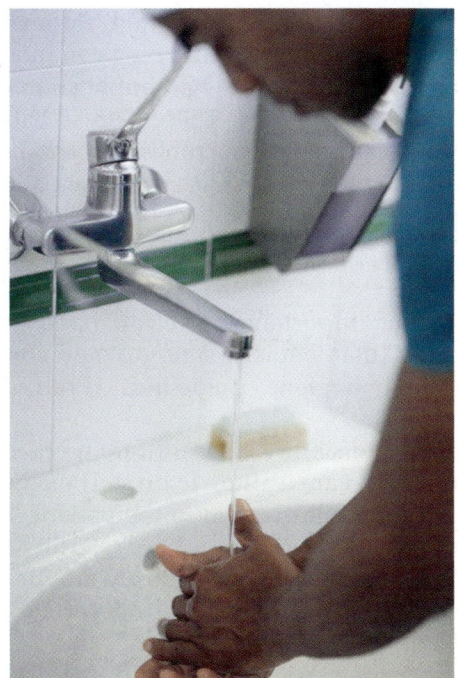

FIGURE 23-4 Clean hands reduce the risk of transmitting infection.

- *Soap.* Use agency-approved soap. The CDC (2002) recommends using a 60% alcohol-based solution (rubs, sprays, gels) for routine hand cleansing, and plain or antimicrobial soap and water when hands are visibly dirty. Iodine compounds are also effective, but usually too irritating for regular hand hygiene.

 If there is a potential for contact with bacterial spores (e.g., when caring for a client with a *C. diff.* infection), you must wash your hands with soap and water; alcohol-based solutions are not effective against spores.

If you are interested in a comparison of the effectiveness of various hand-hygiene antiseptic agents,

 Go to Chapter 23, **DP Table 23-2,** on Davis*Plus.*

- *Friction.* Rub all surfaces of the hands and wrists vigorously, including the backs of the hands and between the fingers. Remove jewelry and clean areas underneath. Clean underneath the fingernails using an orangewood stick.
- *Drying.* Use single-use towels or hand dryers to remove all moisture after washing the hands. If using antimicrobial hand gels, apply and rub hands until dry.

For a step-by-step procedure on hand hygiene,

Go to Chapter 23, **Procedure 23-1: Hand Hygiene,** in Volume 2.

In addition to handwashing, you should keep your fingernails short. According to the CDC (2002), long nails, artificial nails, nail extenders, fingernail polish, watches, and rings with stones can harbor microorganisms. Even shorter nail length of 2 mm or less is preferred (Association of periOperative Registered Nurses [AORN], 2004; Boyce & Pittet, 2002; Pratt, Pellowe, Wilson, et al., 2007; Rupp, Fitzgerald, Puumala, et al., 2008). Drying, chaffing, and chapping commonly occur with frequent handwashing and application of petroleum-based skin products. These skin irritations and interruptions can harbor microbes that can be passed from one person to another.

 The most important aspect of medical asepsis is hand cleanliness. Clean hands markedly decrease the transmission of infection.

Despite the importance of clean hands, research demonstrates that clinical staff do not consistently observe hand hygiene guidelines (Pratt, Pellowe, Wilson, et al., 2007).

It is the responsibility of healthcare workers to perform standard of care. Failure to do so is medical negligence and can result in harm to the patient. Breaks in sterility or even witnesses to errors in sterility may lead to patient neglect. In 2008, Medicare stopped paying for patient complications arising from certain hospital-acquired infections, which in many cases result from poor handwashing. You can help improve clinical practice by serving as a role model for good hand hygiene.

Maintaining a Clean Environment

A clean environment includes the surfaces in a patient's room, as well as supplies, equipment, and other objects brought into the room. An object is contaminated if it becomes unclean—that is, if you suspect it may contain pathogens. The floor, soiled dressings, used tissues, sinks, commodes, and bedpans are other examples of contaminated items. Agency policies determine whether a reusable item is cleaned, disinfected, or sterilized, based on how the item is used.

Cleaning

Cleaning is the removal of visible soil (organic and inorganic) from objects and surfaces. It normally is accomplished manually or mechanically using water with detergents or enzymatic products. A goal of medical asepsis is to keep all public and patient care areas within the facility clean and free from dust, debris, and contamination. Any spilled liquids, dirty surfaces, or potentially contaminated areas should be cleaned immediately. In your home, you use hot water and general cleaning supplies. However, healthcare facilities use special techniques and cleaning solutions formulated to inhibit microbial growth. Items must be cleaned thoroughly before they can be disinfected or sterilized.

Disinfecting

Disinfection removes virtually all pathogens on inanimate objects by physical or chemical means, including steam, gas, chemicals, and ultraviolet light. Disinfection reduces microbial populations, but it does not guarantee that all pathogens are eliminated, because certain viruses, other pathogenic microbes, and spores can remain (Bauman, Machunis-Masuoka, & Tizard, 2006). Chemical germicides can achieve three levels of disinfection. *High-level disinfection* kills all organisms except high levels of bacterial spores. *Intermediate-level disinfection* kills mycobacteria, most viruses, and bacteria. *Low-level disinfection* kills some viruses and bacteria. Disinfection is used for semicritical and noncritical items:

- **Semicritical items** are those that contact mucous membranes or nonintact skin. This category includes reusable devices, such as flexible endoscopes and respiratory therapy and anesthesia equipment. They must be free of all microorganisms except bacterial spores, so they must at least be disinfected, and sometimes sterilized.
- **Noncritical items** are supplies and equipment that come in contact with intact skin but not mucous membranes. They do not carry a high risk of infection transmission, and they can be decontaminated where they are used. Examples of noncritical patient care items are bedpans, stethoscopes, and blood pressure cuffs. Examples of noncritical environmental surfaces include floors, food utensils, bed linens, and bed rails (CDC, 2008). Disinfection is adequate for noncritical items.

Sterilizing

Sterilization is the elimination of all microorganisms (except prions) in or on an object. The most common sterilizing methods used in hospitals are (1) autoclaving with moist heat, (2) ethylene oxide gas at low heat, (3) dry heat, and (4) low temperature hydrogen peroxide gas (AORN, 2012). Sterilization is used when absolute purity of an object or surface is critical.

- **Critical items** are ones that pose a high risk for infection if they are contaminated with any microorganism. Critical items include those that enter the vascular system or sterile tissue, or through which blood flows. Examples are intravenous catheters, needles for injections, urinary catheters, surgical instruments, some wound dressings, and chest tubes.

If you need more specific information on methods for disinfection and sterilization of patient-care items and environmental surfaces,

 Go to Chapter 23, **ESG Table 23-3, Methods for Disinfection and Sterilization of Patient-Care Items and Surfaces,** on Davis*Plus.*

Specially trained personnel carry out disinfection and sterilization in most agencies. As a nurse, you must be familiar with the agency's policies and procedures for cleaning, handling, and transporting items to be disinfected and sterilized, and for working collaboratively with other departments (e.g., the housekeeping department) to keep the patient care area as clean and free of clutter as possible. Clients and caregivers are usually at less risk for infection in their own homes than they are in the hospital. They share the same potential pathogens and antibodies, and there is limited exposure to others with illness and to care providers carrying unusual pathogens, so levels of disinfection and sterilization may differ.

For more specific information about maintaining a clean environment in institutional and home care,

 Go to Chapter 23, **Clinical Insight 23-2, Providing a Clean Patient Environment,** in Volume 2.

CDC Guidelines for Preventing Transmission of Pathogens

In addition to handwashing and maintaining a clean environment, you should follow other precautions to protect yourself and your patients. CDC guidelines provide for two tiers of protection.

- **Standard precautions,** the first tier of protection, apply to care of all patients.
- **Transmission-based precautions,** the second tier of protection, outline precautions to be taken based on the mode of transmission of the infection (Siegel, Rhinehart, Jackson, et al., 2007). Recall from the discussion on the chain of infection that pathogens may be transmitted by contact, droplet, or air. Each mode

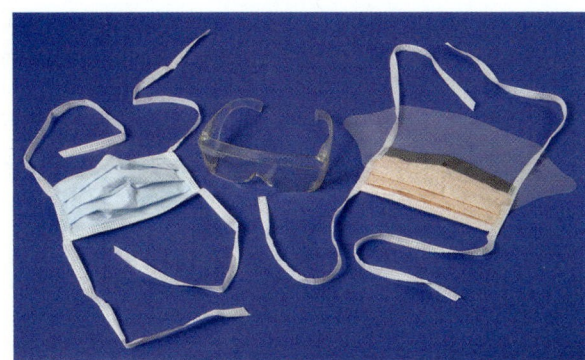

FIGURE 23-5 Several types of face masks and eye shields are available.

of transmission requires a different approach to prevent infection.

Table 23-2 provides a summary comparison of standard and transmission-based precautions. For detailed guidelines to aid you in following both types of precautions,

 Go to Chapter 23, **Clinical Insight 23-3, Following CDC Standard Precautions,** and **Clinical Insight 23-4, Following Transmission-Based Precautions,** in Volume 2.

Personal Protective Equipment The CDC recommends and the U.S. Occupational Safety and Health Administration requires employers to provide personal protective equipment (PPE) for healthcare workers (e.g., gloves, gowns, face masks, and eye protection) (U.S. Department of Labor, n.d.). This equipment is to be used in standard precautions as well as transmission-based precautions. Figure 23-5 provides examples of face masks and eye protection equipment. Procedure Highlights 23-2 through 23-8 summarize the steps for donning and removing PPE. For complete instructions,

 Go to **Procedure 23-2: Donning Personal Protective Equipment (PPE),** and **Procedure 23-3: Removing Personal Protective Equipment (PPE),** in Volume 2.

KnowledgeCheck 23-6

Under what circumstances are standard precautions used?

Intervention for Example Problem: Preventing MDROs

Evidence suggests that MDROs are carried from one person to another via the hands of healthcare personnel.

✚ To prevent MDROs, you must adhere strictly to published recommendations for hand hygiene, glove use, and isolation precautions; and for performing invasive procedures such as intravenous and urinary catheterization and care of central venous ports.

Table 23-2 ▶ Comparison of CDC Standard and Transmission-Based Precautions	
STANDARD PRECAUTIONS	**TRANSMISSION-BASED PRECAUTIONS**
Tier 1 Precautions	Tier 2 Precautions
Use with all clients, in all settings, regardless of suspected or confirmed presence of infection.	Use for patients known or suspected to be infected or colonized with infectious agents.
Principle: All blood, body fluids, secretions, excretions except sweat, nonintact skin, and mucous membranes may contain pathogens.	*Principle:* Routes of transmission for some microorganisms are not completely interrupted using standard precautions alone. Used *in addition to* standard precautions.
Include: Hand hygiene; use of gloves, gown, mask, eye protection, or face shield (depending on expected exposure); and safe injection practices.	Three categories of precautions:
Does not completely protect against microorganisms spread by contact, droplets, or through the air.	*Contact Precautions*—For organisms spread by direct contact with the patient or his environment. This is the most common form of transmission.
New Elements of Standard Precautions	*Droplet Precautions*—For pathogens spread through close respiratory or mucous membrane contact with respiratory secretions (e.g., sneezing, coughing, talking); pathogens that do not remain infectious over long distances.
Added for protection of patients more than of healthcare personnel. They include:	
Respiratory hygiene and cough etiquette	*Airborne Precautions*—For pathogens that are very small and remain infectious over long distances when suspended in the air; and easily transmitted through air currents (e.g., fanning linens, ventilating systems).
Safe injection practices	
Wearing a mask when performing special lumbar puncture procedures	

Source: Siegel, J. D., Rhinehart, E., Jackson, M., et al. (2007). *2007 guideline for isolation precautions: Preventing transmission of infectious agents in the healthcare setting.* Retrieved November 12, 2012, from http://www.cdc.gov/hicpac/2007IP/2007isolationPrecautions.html

For a list of actions you can take to help prevent MDROs,

 Go to **Clinical Insight 23-5, Preventing Multidrug-Resistant Organism Infections,** in Volume 2.

Protective Environment in Special Situations

Patients who are immunosuppressed (e.g., receiving chemotherapy) may be placed in a special form of isolation, called protective isolation or reverse isolation. However, the CDC states that standard and transmission-based precautions are adequate protection for most of those patients. They recommend a "protective environment" only for a special class of stem cell transplant patients who are neutropenic (have a low white blood cell count secondary to chemotherapy). Most of the recommendations are engineering and environmental services rather than nursing measures. If you are interested in learning the details of maintaining a protective environment,

 Go to **Clinical Insight 23-6, Maintaining a Protective Environment in Special Situations,** in Volume 2.

Patients with compromised immunity are more likely to become infected by pathogens harbored in their own bodies than from pathogens transmitted by other people

(Siegel, Rhinehart, Jackson, et al., 2007). Therefore, except for the special situation described, standard and transmission-based precautions should protect even unusually vulnerable patients from organisms brought in by healthcare workers and visitors.

Nevertheless, you may see what has been called **protective isolation** being used for clients with low WBC counts, clients undergoing chemotherapy, or clients with large open wounds or weak immune systems. Protective isolation usually includes following standard precautions, placing the patient in a private room; restricting visitors; wearing a mask, gown, and gloves for patient care; and special cleaning or disposal of the patient's equipment and supplies. Some units, such as neonatal intensive care units, burn units, and labor and delivery suites, may follow some aspects of protective isolation all the time. Most of these precautions are described by standard and transmission-based precautions.

Control of Potentially Contaminated Equipment and Supplies

Whenever possible, use disposable equipment in an isolation room. Nondisposable equipment and supplies require special handling.

- **Protective Isolation** If a client is in protective isolation, be sure that equipment has been disinfected *before*

Toward Evidence-Based Practice

Labeau, S. O., Witdouck, S. S., Vandijck, D. M., et al. (2010). Nurses' knowledge of evidence-based guidelines for the prevention of surgical site infection. *Worldviews on Evidence-Based Nursing, 7(1),* 16–24.

The purpose of this study was to evaluate intensive care unit (ICU) nurses' specific knowledge of surgical site infection prevention guidelines preparatory to developing an online infection prevention education module. Survey data were collected from 650 intensive care nurses who attended the Flemish Society for Critical Care Nurses Congress regarding their knowledge of the current evidence-based CDC recommendations for prevention of surgical site infection. The study results concluded that ICU nurses' knowledge of surgical site infection prevention can be substantially improved through ongoing education and training.

Broex, E. C. J., van Asselet, A. D. I., & Bruggeman, C. A. (2009). Surgical site infections: How high are the costs? *Journal of Hospital Infection, 72,* 193–201.

The authors reviewed 16 studies from hospitals throughout the world published between 2004 and 2008. They examined the effects of facility-acquired infections on patients' length of stay, hospital costs, and societal costs, including effects on patients and their families. The study authors concluded that surgical site infection (SSI) is responsible for a significant increase in healthcare-related costs: up to two times the cost of a patient without an SSI.

Bailey, R. R., Stuckey, D. R., Norman, B. A., et al. (2011). Economic value of dispensing home-based preoperative chlorhexidine bathing cloths to prevent surgical site infection. *Infection Control and Hospital Epidemiology, 32(5),* 465–471.

The objective of this research was to examine the economic value of providing preoperative chlorhexidine bathing cloth kits for home use by orthopedic patients, with the goal of preventing surgical site infection (SSI). The study results indicated that even with low (50%) patient compliance, routine distribution of preoperative

chlorhexidine bathing cloth kits is a cost-effective strategy to prevent SSI.

Kamel, C., McGahan, L., Polisena, J., et al. (2012). Preoperative skin antiseptic preparations surgical site infections: A systematic review. *Infection Control and Hospital Epidemiology, 33(6),* 608–617.

A systematic review of literature published between January 2011 and June 2011 was conducted examining data from 20 randomized and nonrandomized controlled trials of preoperative skin antisepsis. Results indicated that preoperative surgical showers using an antiseptic preparation effectively reduces skin flora and bacterial colonization and may reduce surgical site infection (SSI) rates.

Jakobsson, J., Perlkvist, A., & Wann-Hansson, C. (2011). Searching for evidence regarding using preoperative disinfection showers to prevent surgical site infections: A systematic review. *Worldviews on Evidence-Based Nursing, 8(3),* 143–152.

The purpose of this study was to determine how many preoperative showers using a disinfecting agent are needed to effectively reduce bacteria on the skin and decrease the risk of surgical site infection (SSI). Data from 10 studies on preoperative disinfection showers published in the United States and Europe between 1987 and 2008 were analyzed. The analysis did not reveal consistent data on the optimal number of preoperative showers with a disinfecting agent.

1. From these abstracts, what do you know about the purpose of these studies?

2. What do the Jakobsson and Kamel studies conclude about preoperative disinfective showers to surgical sites?

3. In what way do the data in the study conducted by Labeau support the other studies? What were the limitations of this study?

 Go to Chapter 23, **Toward Evidence-Based Practice Suggested Responses,** on Davis*Plus*.

---

it is taken into the room. Take linens and dishes directly to the protective isolation room, and hand them to someone wearing the required protective garb.

- **Transmission-based Isolation** If the client is in transmission-based isolation, disinfect the equipment *on removal* from the room. When removing linens or nondisposable items from a room with contact, droplet, or airborne isolation, place them in special isolation bags.

Disposing of Used Isolation Supplies Place contaminated disposable equipment and materials containing body fluids in special isolation bags. This process requires two healthcare workers. The worker inside the room wears protective clothing and handles only contaminated items. The second worker stands at the door and holds the isolation bag open. The first worker places items inside the bag without touching the outside of the bag. If the bag contains linens, the isolation bag is closed and placed in a laundry hamper. Securely close an isolation trash bag, and place it in a special isolation trash container. Special disposal methods are used to prevent these objects from going into a landfill, where they could become a reservoir of infection. Because this trash is much more expensive to process, take care to put *only* contaminated materials in the contaminated trash.

Sharps Disposal   Always place disposable needles, syringes, and other sharp items, such as broken glass, in special disposable sharps containers immediately after their use. Never recap a contaminated needle. Refer to Chapters 24 and 26 for further information on preventing needlestick injuries.

Laboratory Specimens   Laboratory specimens contain blood and body fluids and are always considered contaminated. Label the specimen container in a clean area before taking it to the patient. Have the specimen collected by a healthcare worker wearing appropriate protective clothing. Once the specimen is collected, place it in a special transport bag. Do not allow the outside of the bag to touch any contaminated item, including your gloves.

For specific guidelines on care of contaminated equipment and supplies,

 Go to Chapter 23, **Clinical Insight 23-2, Providing a Clean Patient Environment; Clinical Insight 23-3, Following CDC Standard Precautions;** and **Clinical Insight 23-4, Following Transmission-Based Precautions,** in Volume 2.

Supporting the Psychological Needs of Patients in Isolation

Remember, isolation precautions are designed to prevent the spread of disease. It is the disease that is being isolated, *not* the person who has the disease. Patients who are in isolation continue to have a need for human contact. In fact, isolation may produce anxiety and increase the desire for human contact. When caring for a client in isolation, search for ways to reassure and maintain contact with the patient. Possible solutions include the following:

- When wearing the required protective equipment, touch the patient.
- Organize the time you spend in the patient's room to include time for discussion about how the client is coping with isolation.
- If the patient is in droplet isolation, remember that the danger area is 3 feet from the patient. You can go to the door of the room and speak to the patient without a mask.
- Reassure the patient that precautions are temporary.
- Explain that the precautions and the PPE protect you and the patient, as well as family members and other patients.

KnowledgeCheck 23-7
- If you needed to disinfect a sink in a client's home, what would you use?
- List at least three actions clients can take to help avoid infection when they are out in the community.

PRACTICING SURGICAL ASEPSIS
Sterile means "without life." If an object is sterile, it contains no life and therefore no infectious organisms. The exception is *prions*, the protein particles that cause severe neurological degeneration in animals and humans, such as in bovine spongiform encephalopathy (BSE, also known as "mad cow disease") in cattle and Creutzfeldt-Jakob disease (CJD) in humans. Researchers

---

 For steps to follow in *all* procedures, refer to the Universal Steps for All Procedures found on the inside back cover of Volume 2. Go to the full procedures in Volume 2 to practice and learn the procedure steps. Use these procedure highlights later to help you review key points.

Highlights of Procedures 23-1 through 23-8

Procedure 23-1: Hand Hygiene
If using alcohol-based handrubs:
1. Use alcohol-based handrubs when hands are not soiled.
2. Cover all surfaces of fingers and hands.
3. Rub together until dry.

Procedure 23-2: Donning Personal Protective Equipment (PPE)
➤ Before exposure, don appropriate PPE according to standard precautions or transmission guidelines.
➤ Wear an N-95 respirator mask for airborne isolation.
➤ Wear a surgical mask for droplet isolation.

Procedure 23-3: Removing Personal Protective Equipment (PPE)
➤ Remove PPE at doorway before leaving patient room, or in an anteroom.
➤ Avoid contaminating self, others, or environment when removing equipment.
➤ Considered contaminated: front areas, sleeves, head cover, mask, and gloves of the PPE.
➤ Considered clean: the inside of the gown, gloves, and head cover; the ties on the mask; and ties in the back of the gown.
➤ Always remove gloves first when removing PPE, unless gown ties in front.

Procedure 23-4: Surgical Handwashing: Traditional Method

➤ Don surgical shoe covers, cap, and face mask before the scrub.

➤ Use warm water.

➤ Perform a prewash, using soap and water.

➤ Clean under your fingernails under running water.

➤ Wet the scrub sponge, and apply a generous amount of antimicrobial soap.

➤ Using a circular motion, scrub all surfaces of nails, hands, and forearms at least 10 times, or the length of time specified by agency policy.

➤ Rinse hands and arms by keeping your fingertips higher than your elbow.

➤ Grasp a sterile towel, and back away from the sterile field.

➤ Thoroughly dry your hands before donning sterile gloves.

Procedure 23-5: Surgical Handwashing: Brushless System

➤ Don surgical shoe covers, cap, and face mask before the scrub.

➤ Use warm water.

➤ Perform a prewash, using soap and water.

➤ Clean under your nails under running water.

➤ Apply a generous amount of antimicrobial soap.

➤ Using a circular motion, scrub all surfaces of nails, hands, and forearms at least 10 times, or the length of time specified by agency policy.

➤ Rinse hands and arms by keeping your fingertips higher than your elbow.

➤ Grasp a sterile towel, and back away from the sterile field.

➤ Thoroughly dry your hands before donning sterile gloves.

Procedure 23-6: Sterile Gown and Gloves (Closed Method)

➤ Put on shoe covers, hair covers, and mask before scrub

➤ Perform surgical scrub.

➤ Grasp the gown at the neckline, and slide your arms into the sleeves without extending your hands through the cuffs.

➤ Have a coworker pull the shoulders of the gown up and tie the neck tie.

➤ Don gloves using the closed method by keeping your hands covered at all times, first with the gown cuffs, and then with the sterile gloves.

➤ Secure the waist tie on your gown by handing it to a coworker and turning to receive it.

➤ Keep your hands within your field of vision at all times.

➤ Do not turn your back to a sterile field.

Procedure 23-7: Sterile Gloves (Open Method)

➤ Remove all jewelry, including rings and watches.

➤ Place the glove package on a clean, dry surface.

➤ Open the inner package so that the cuffs are closest to you.

➤ Apply the glove of your dominant hand first by touching only the inside of the glove (the folded-over cuff) with your nondominant hand.

➤ Apply the second glove by touching only the outer part of the glove with your already-gloved hand; keep your sterile thumb well away from your bare skin.

➤ Do not touch the gloves to any unsterile items.

Procedure 23-8: Sterile Fields

➤ Prepare the sterile field as close as possible to the time of use.

➤ Do not cover the sterile field once established.

➤ Do not turn away from the sterile field.

➤ Inspect for package integrity, inclusion of sterile indicator, and/or expiration date. Do not use outdated items.

➤ Clear a space and prepare the patient before setting up the sterile field.

➤ Establish the sterile field with a sterile drape or sterile package wrapper.

➤ Add items to the sterile field by gently dropping them onto the sterile field.

➤ Pour sterile solutions into a sterile bowl or receptacle without touching the bowl or splashing onto the sterile field.

➤ Don sterile gloves and perform the procedure.

---

have not yet determined what types of antimicrobial techniques are successful in destroying prions. Inanimate objects, such as surgical equipment, gauze dressings, or wound irrigation fluid, may be sterile. However, humans will always have microorganisms in and on their bodies; and researchers have not yet determined what types of techniques, if any, can destroy prions.

Surgical asepsis, or **sterile technique,** requires creation of a sterile environment and use of sterile equipment. It differs from medical asepsis in that it is more complex and it is not required for use with all patients. Sterilization can be accomplished through the use

of special gases or high heat. Surgical equipment and implanted devices are examples of materials that must be sterilized. If you need more information about sterilization processes,

Go to Chapter 23, **ESG Table 23-3, Methods for Disinfection and Sterilization of Patient-Care Items and Surfaces,** on DavisPlus.

To create a sterile area, housekeeping personnel perform extensive cleaning using special solutions and procedures. All health personnel working in the area must wear appropriate surgical attire and perform a surgical hand scrub.

Levels of Asepsis Recent guidelines suggest using modified sterile technique for many bedside procedures that have traditionally used sterile technique (e.g., tracheostomy care and wound care).

- **Sterile technique** is the use of sterile gloves and sterile supplies (e.g., drapes, wound dressings, instruments, water).
- **Modified sterile technique** is the use of nonsterile procedure gloves with sterile supplies.
- **Clean technique** is the use of clean hands or nonsterile gloves and clean, rather than sterile, supplies (e.g., tap water).

Performing a Surgical Scrub

A surgical scrub is a modification of the handwashing procedure described earlier (see Table 23-3 for a comparison). It traditionally involves an extended scrub of the hands using a sponge, nail cleaner, and a bactericidal scrubbing agent. A newer method uses a brushless scrub, using a bactericidal scrubbing agent. All methods require a prewash before the surgical scrub. For a summary of the steps involved, see the Highlights of Procedures box for Procedures 23-4 and 23-5. For the full procedures,

 Go to **Surgical Handwashing: Traditional Method** and **Surgical Handwashing: Brushless System** procedures, in Volume 2.

Donning Surgical Attire

Burn units; labor and birth units; and some surgical wards, intensive care units, nurseries, and oncology wards require surgical attire for patient caregiving. In each of these units, nurses care for clients who are at increased risk for infection or are undergoing an invasive procedure that places them at increased risk. The goal on all of these units is to protect the patient from infection transmitted by healthcare workers.

All personnel on these units don *clean* surgical attire, or scrub suits, when they arrive on the unit. These scrub suits should not be worn outside the unit. If you must transport a patient to another area or leave the unit to gather supplies, wear a covering over the scrub suit. Remove the covering on your return to the unit. Additional precautions include a disposable hat to cover the hair, shoe coverings, and face masks.

Personnel engaged in surgery or certain invasive procedures must dress in *sterile* surgical attire. As a beginning student, you will soon find yourself in such a situation. Initially your role will be limited to observation, but you will need to be prepared for these experiences.

First you will change into a scrub suit, apply shoe coverings, and put on a disposable hat. Wash your hands, and apply a face mask. If there is potential for spray of fluids, wear a face mask with eye shield. Be sure to adjust the mask so that it is comfortable to breathe through. Once you have adjusted the mask, perform the surgical scrub. If a surgical gown is required, don it after the hand scrub.

If you are applying full surgical attire, you will need to apply gloves using a closed method, after you have put on your gown. Once you don sterile gloves, you may touch only sterile items. The Highlights of Procedures box pertains to donning sterile attire. For complete instructions,

 Go to **Procedure 23-6: Donning Sterile Gloves and Gown (Closed Method)** and **Procedure 23-7, Sterile Gloves (Open Method)**; in Volume 2.

You will often wear sterile gloves for procedures that do not require full surgical attire. Open the glove packaging slowly. Avoid fanning the wrapping or touching the gloves. Put the first glove on your dominant hand (Fig. 23-6). This is the open method of gloving.

✚ A general rule to consider when applying the second glove is to touch glove-to-glove and skin-to-skin. The already-gloved hand may touch any of the sterile surfaces of the second glove.

	HAND HYGIENE	SURGICAL SCRUB
No visible soil	Use alcohol-based handrub or soap (plain or antimicrobial) and water.	1. Perform handwashing with soap and water. 2. Then perform the surgical scrub using either an FDA-approved antimicrobial scrub product or an antiseptic handrub that is FDA-approved for surgical hand asepsis.
Hands visibly soiled	Wash with soap (plain or antimicrobial) and water.	Surgical scrub steps remain the same, even with visible soil.

Table 23-3 ➤ A Comparison of Hand Hygiene and Surgical Scrub

Sources: AORN (2010b); Boyce & Pittet (2002); Garbutt (2011).

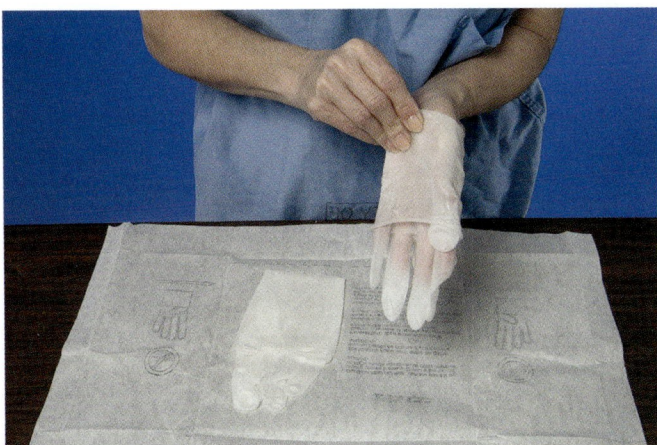

FIGURE 23-6 When applying the first glove, touch only the inside cuff of the glove.

The second hand may touch only the inside of the glove—the portion that will have contact with the skin. Figure 23-7 illustrates the hand positions used to apply the second glove. Although this process sounds awkward, you will develop comfort with practice. The box Highlights of Procedures 23-1 Through 23-8 contains a summary of the open method of gloving. For complete instructions,

 Go to **Procedure 23-7: Sterile Gloves (Open Method),** in Volume 2.

Using Sterile Technique in Nursing Care

Healthcare providers use sterile technique to perform a variety of procedures. Some of the procedures require full surgical attire; others do not. The following procedures, for example, use both sterile technique and principles of medical asepsis: administering an injection, starting an IV line, and performing a sterile dressing

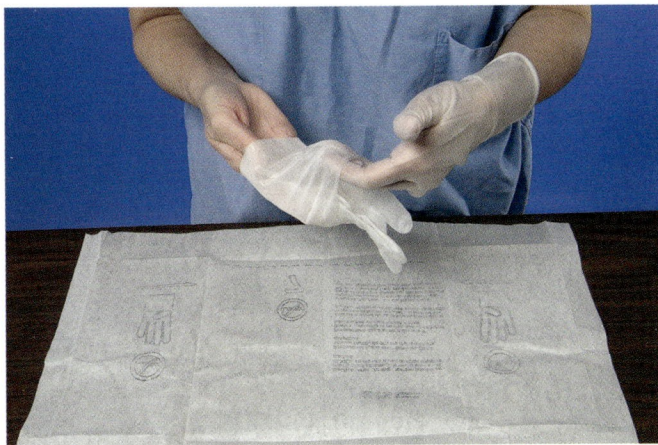

FIGURE 23-7 When applying the second glove, consider this general rule: glove-to-glove, skin-to-skin.

change. To clarify, when administering an injection, you prepare the patient, cleanse the injection site, and remove the needle cap using standard precautions. You do not don sterile gloves, but for the rest of the procedure you observe sterile technique by taking care not to touch or otherwise contaminate the exposed needle.

Before performing a sterile procedure, determine what supplies you will need and whether you will need assistance. If the patient is unable to maintain a position required for the procedure, you will need a helper to hold the patient during the procedure. Wash your hands before gathering materials from the sterile supply area, and then gather the other required supplies and equipment. Check the expiration date on each package. Check the package to make sure it is intact. If it has paper or cloth wrapping, be sure there are no indications that it has ever been wet.

For guidelines related to sterile technique and preparing and maintaining sterile fields,

 Go to **Clinical Insight 23-7: Guidelines for Observing Sterile Technique,** in Volume 2.

Preparing and Maintaining Sterile Fields

There are some variations in how you might set up sterile fields. Sometimes it is as simple as opening a package of supplies wrapped in a sterile disposable cover. The inside of the cover becomes your sterile field; the supplies on it are sterile, as well. At other times, you may work with a larger, reusable or disposable sterile drape (wrapped in an outer wrapping). In that situation, you open the outer wrapping, then pick up the sterile drape grasping only the corners, and allow it to fall open to create a sterile field, perhaps to entirely cover a table surface or to create a sterile field on the patient's bed.

In any sterile field, only the horizontal plane (e.g., the table top) is considered sterile. Consider nonsterile any material that drapes over the horizontal plane. A 1-inch margin around the edges of the sterile field is also considered unsterile because it is in contact with contaminated surfaces.

The box Highlights of Procedures 23-1 Through 23-8 contains a summary of how to prepare and maintain a sterile field, as well as add supplies and sterile liquids to it. For complete procedural steps,

 Go to **Procedure 23-8A: Setting Up a Sterile Field,** in Volume 2.

Adding Supplies to a Sterile Field

Some supplies (e.g., urinary catheter kits) are packaged in a wrapper that can form a sterile field. The outside of these packages is considered clean, and the inside is sterile. You must open these packages in a way that does not contaminate the inside of the wrapping. Be cautious when adding supplies to the sterile field. If they are light and small, gently add them to the sterile field by separating the package flaps and allowing them to fall onto the field. If the object is large, such as an irrigation bowl, slowly unwrap the packaging and, touching only the outside wrapper, place the bowl on the field. If any object falls only partly on the field, it is no longer sterile. For detailed instructions on how to add supplies to a sterile field,

 Go to **Procedure 23-8B: Adding Supplies to a Sterile Field,** in Volume 2.

Adding Sterile Solutions to a Sterile Field

Add sterile liquids to a sterile field by gently pouring them into a container on the field. Some sterile drapes contain an impermeable membrane between layers. This membrane serves as a barrier to moisture and prevents wicking. With this type of drape, you may pour sterile liquid directly on gauze pads on the field. Pour only an amount of liquid that is sufficient to make the gauze pads damp. Excess fluid may run off the field, causing the field to become contaminated—a wet field is not sterile because it does not provide a barrier to microorganisms on the unsterile surface under the drape. For step-by-step instruction in how to add sterile solutions to a sterile field,

 Go to **Procedure 23-8C: Adding Sterile Solutions to a Sterile Field,** in Volume 2.

KnowledgeCheck 23-8

- When will you need to don sterile gloves using the closed method?
- (True or false) Some procedures require both standard precautions and sterile technique.
- What part(s) of a sterile field are considered to be unsterile?

INFECTION CONTROL AND PREVENTION FOR HEALTHCARE WORKERS

It is critical that you learn how to protect yourself from infections. You want not only to avoid personal illness, but also to avoid becoming a reservoir for infection. Nurses and other patient care workers are at great risk of acquiring infections because they come in contact with a large number and variety of pathogens. Skin contact, mucous membrane contact, and puncture wounds often serve as portals of entry.

Nursing assistive personnel (NAP), ancillary personnel, and housekeeping and maintenance workers are often present on nursing units. Visitors, volunteers, and family are also on the unit. It is essential that you protect them from potential hazardous exposure as well as protect yourself and patients from possible microorganisms brought into the unit. As a nurse, you need to monitor other healthcare workers, patients, and visitors for breaks in infection control and prevention.

BOX 23-3 ■ Common Breaks in Sterility

To avoid common breaks in sterility:

- Never reach across a sterile field.
- Make sure your clothing or lab coat never touches any part of the sterile field.
- Keep your fingernails short and clean. Avoid nail polish and artificial nails.
- Avoid wearing jewelry that dangles or can fall into the sterile field.
- Keep long hair pulled back, or covered by a head covering designed for sterility.
- Change your gown or reinforce with additional sterile drapes if it is soaked through.
- Avoid splashing any kind of solution onto the sterile field.
- Keep doors closed so turbulent airflow does not contaminate a sterile area with airborne microbes.
- Make sure you are opening equipment packaged with labels indicating it has been sterilized properly.
- Clean wounds and prep sterile sites from clean to dirty.
- When witnessing someone else contaminate a sterile field or object, identify the break and cover the area with sterile drapes or replace with a new sterile setup, gown, or gloves.

Source: Adapted from Simko, L. (2012). Breaking sterility: Procedural violations in healthcare. *Nursing 2012, 42*(8), 22–26.

What Role Does the Infection Preventionist Nurse Play?

The task of the infection prevention nurse is to minimize the number of infections in the healthcare facility. Because it is not possible to provide absolute protection all the time, the nurse must balance the risks for infection with the costs of protective measures and the benefits of various strategies. Infection preventionists must keep current with information about pathogens, antibiotic resistance, and infection control. The nurse also functions as an epidemiologist, tracking down the source of HAIs and strengthening measures to prevent their recurrence. Finally, all members of the infection prevention team enforce compliance with federal, state, and local regulations related to infection control and prevention.

What Should I Do If I Am Exposed to Bloodborne Pathogens?

Exposure to blood, body secretions, or body tissues containing blood or secretions requires immediate action. See Box 23-4 for complete instructions. The first step is to minimize the exposure by washing the area thoroughly. Then notify the appropriate people, complete an injury report, and seek medical attention.

Anyone exposed to bloodborne pathogens should have baseline lab work done to check for hepatitis and HIV. If the patient source is known, the infection preventionist

BOX 23-4 ■ If You Are Exposed to Blood or Other Body Fluids

 If you are stuck by a needle or other sharp, or get blood or other potentially infectious materials in your eyes, nose, mouth, or on broken skin:

1. Immediately flood the exposed area with water and clean any wound with soap and water or a skin disinfectant if available.

2. Report the exposure immediately to the appropriate person in the agency. If you are a student, also report immediately to your instructor.

3. Seek immediate medical attention. Consent to testing and follow-up treatment as advised.

4. Complete an incident or injury report.

5. Attend counseling sessions provided by the agency.

Source: Occupational Safety & Health Administration. U.S. Department of Labor. (n.d.). Bloodborne pathogens and needlestick prevention. Post-exposure evaluation. Retrieved January 21, 2013, from http://www.osha.gov/archive/SLTC/bloodbornepathogens/postexposure.html

will arrange to have the patient tested. Subsequent testing and possible preventive treatment are based on the type of exposure and what is known about the source and the injured person. To limit risks from the exposure, the infection prevention team will provide counseling and recommendations as soon as possible after the event. Chapters 24 and 26 present information on preventing needlestick injuries.

How Can I Minimize the Effects of Bioterrorism and Epidemics?

Bioterrorism is the intentional release, or threatened release, of disease-producing organisms or substances for the purpose of causing death, illness, harm, economic damage, or fear. Five diseases with recognized bioterrorism potential are anthrax, botulism, pneumonic plague, smallpox, viral hemorrhagic fevers, and tularemia. The U.S. government has recently funded development of drugs to treat three of these diseases (anthrax, plague, and tularemia).

Recognize an Outbreak Should a biological event occur, either as a result of bioterrorism or a naturally occurring epidemic, a key factor in minimizing its effects is the ability to quickly recognize unusual disease patterns and detect the presence of infectious diseases. Some electronic patient record systems include special pattern identification programs. The use of these systems supplements, but does not replace, clinical observation skills. Nurses need to assess not only the individual patient's condition, but also clusters of symptoms. Hospital, emergency department, and clinic nurses are in key positions to recognize outbreaks because they see

patients from multiple primary care providers. Nurses must keep the following questions in mind:

- Am I seeing an unexpected number of infectious diseases, or diseases possibly caused by infectious organisms?
- Am I seeing similar cases that are not responding to medical treatment?
- Are healthcare workers who come in contact with infectious patients becoming ill?

Notify the Safety Officer After identifying a suspicious pattern, you should notify the institution's interventionist or safety officer as soon as possible. Appropriate cultures will be needed, and the federal and state health departments should be notified. If the infectious organism is unknown, samples must be preserved for future analysis.

Institute Appropriate Level of Standard Precautions In the event of an epidemic, the essential principles of hand hygiene and standard precautions will be the core of your infection prevention and control measures. Patients with similar symptoms should be cared for by a minimum number of healthcare personnel, and those personnel must use appropriate isolation precautions. If the etiology and transmission route of the causative organism are unknown, standard, contact, and airborne precautions should be implemented as needed. The Occupational Safety and Health Administration (OSHA) defines types of personal protective equipment and situations in which you are required to wear it (U.S. Department of Labor, n.d.).

Prepare Clients for a Pandemic Teach clients that preparing for pandemic disease is similar to preparing for other general kinds of emergency preparedness, such as power outages and natural disasters (see Self-Care: Teaching Your Patient About Preparing for a Pandemic Disease Outbreak).

Summary

After studying this chapter, you should be armed with the basic knowledge you need to protect yourself and your clients from infection. However, knowledge is not enough. Research continues to show that healthcare professionals too often fail to comply with guidelines for infection prevention, especially the seemingly simple measures such as hand hygiene and standard precautions. Although healthcare workers must wash their hands, patients do not necessarily feel comfortable asking them to do so (Ottum, Sethi, Jacobs, et al., 2012). Your role as a nurse is to integrate the best current evidence with your clinical expertise and, through your own individual performance, to minimize harm to patients and others. This includes using technology and standardized practices that support patient safety and quality.

Wash your hands! Follow standard precautions!

If you would like to know more about microbiology,

Go to **Student Resources, A Brief Introduction to Microbiology,** on DavisPlus.

Self-Care

Teaching Your Patient About Preparing for a Pandemic Disease Outbreak

➤ Make a preparedness plan with your family and others in the community (e.g., school, business, church groups). Help organize local response planning and be available to help if there is an outbreak. Participate in emergency planning at work and get training if it is available.

➤ Talk with family members about what will be needed to care for them in your home if someone becomes ill.

➤ Expect that usual community services may be disrupted—for example, banks, stores, post offices, and even hospitals and public buildings may be closed

➤ Store a 2-week supply of bottled water and food. Keep extra nonperishable foods. Examples of food and nonperishables include:

Ready-to-eat canned meats (e.g., ham, tuna)

Canned fruits, vegetables, beans, soups

Protein or fruit bars

Dry cereals

Peanut butter or nuts

Dried fruit and nuts

Crackers

Canned juices

Canned baby food and formula, if an infant is in the home

Pet food, as needed

➤ Periodically check your regular prescription drugs to keep a continuous supply on hand.

➤ Have nonprescription drugs and health supplies on hand. Examples include:

Medical supplies, such as blood pressure and glucose monitors

Medicines for fever (e.g., acetaminophen, ibuprofen)

Thermometer

Soap and water or alcohol-based, antibacterial hand gel

Antidiarrheal medication

Vitamins

Fluids with electrolytes

➤ Keep a 2-week supply of other emergency supplies on hand, such as a flashlight, batteries, portable radio, manual can opener, trash bags, tissues, toilet paper, and disposable diapers.

➤ Keep your family's health information up to date, organized, and accessible.

➤ Make sure you have more than one method to communicate (e.g., telephone and e-mail) and that you can get information from the outside world (including by battery-powered radio).

➤ Be sure everyone in the family washes hands frequently and properly and covers coughs and sneezes with tissues.

➤ Teach family members to stay away from others as much as possible if they are sick. Stay home from work and school if sick.

➤ Get an annual seasonal influenza vaccination.

➤ Explore the possibility of working by telecommuting during a pandemic to avoid unnecessary exposure.

Sources. Davey, V. (2007). Disaster care. Questions and answers on pandemic influenza. American Journal of Nursing, 107(7), 50–57; Flu.gov. (n.d.). Pandemic awareness. Retrieved February 9, 2013, from http://www.flu.gov/pandemic; New York State Department of Health Influenza Pandemic (March 2011). Retrieved January 21, 2013, from http://www.health.ny.gov/diseases/communicable/influenza/pandemic; Plan to Protect You and Your Family. Retrieved January 21, 2013, from http://www.ready.gov/emergency-planning-checklists; U.S. Department of Health & Human Services. (n.d.a). Pandemic flu planning checklists for individuals and families. Retrieved January 21, 2013, from http://www.gchd.us/Services/GeneralPrograms/EmergencyPreparedness/Pandemic%20Flu%20Checklist.pdf; U.S. Department of Health & Human Services (n.d.b). Flu pandemics. Retrieved September 23, 2012, from http://www.flu.gov/individualfamily/about/pandemic/index.html

To explore learning resources for this chapter,

 Go to DavisPlus at DavisPl.us/Wilkinson3.

Chapter Resources for Chapter 23:

Response sheets for all exercises and learning activities

Resources for Caregivers and Health Professionals

Reading More About Promoting Asepsis & Preventing Infection (suggested readings)

Concept Map of chapter content

Interactive Case Studies

NCLEX-Style and Chapter Review Questions

Chapter Overview Podcasts

References Cited:

    Go to Volume 2, **References Cited.**

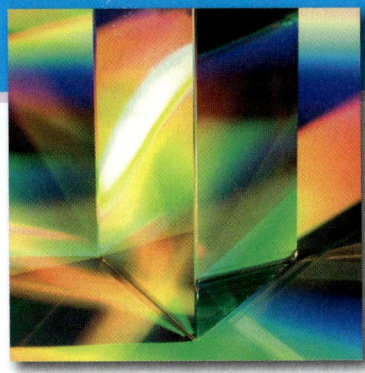

CHAPTER 24

Promoting Safety

Learning Outcomes

After completing this chapter, you should be able to:

➤ List the three leading causes of accidental death in the United States.

➤ Discuss developmental and individual factors that create safety risks.

➤ Identify at least five safety hazards in the home environment and interventions to prevent injury from them.

➤ Discuss the steps to follow when you suspect that a client has ingested a poisonous substance.

➤ Describe the choking rescue maneuver, and identify instances when it is appropriate to use it.

➤ Describe the four main physical hazards that are found in the community and interventions to prevent injury from them.

➤ Describe and give examples of hazards that we encounter in the healthcare agency.

➤ Identify four interventions to prevent falls in the healthcare agency.

➤ Discuss the appropriate use of siderails in the healthcare agency.

➤ Properly apply restraints and discuss measures to prevent injury in clients who are restrained.

➤ Discuss at least one data collection instrument that is used to assess the client who is at risk for falls.

➤ Formulate a nursing diagnosis in relation to preventing injury in the environment.

➤ Write an individualized goal for clients with a nursing diagnosis of Risk for Falls.

Key Concepts

Safety
Patient safety

Related Concepts

See the Concept Map on Davis*Plus*.

Example Problem

Falls

Meet Your Patient

1. **Alvin Lin.** Alvin Lin is a 79-year-old man who was just transferred from a long-term care facility to your medical unit. His admitting diagnosis is dehydration and pneumonia. In the morning report you were told that he had rested well during the night and was alert and oriented. When you enter his room, he is confused and does not know where he is. He is becoming combative and is trying to get out of bed. How should you respond to the situation?

2. **Teresa.** Suppose you are a nurse making a home visit to Teresa, who lives in a rural area. Teresa is 20 years old and has a 2-year-old daughter. She is also responsible for caring for her elderly grandmother, who is recovering from a hip fracture. Teresa states that it is getting more difficult to keep up with her toddler, who is "into everything," and to care for the needs of her grandmother. Her grandmother has a fear of falling and is reluctant to do anything for herself.

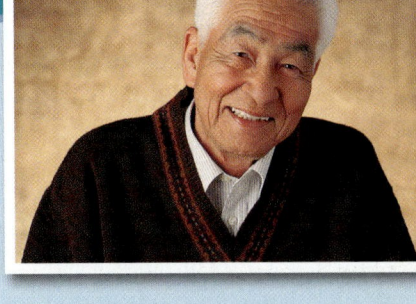

TheoreticalKnowledge
knowing **why**

This chapter will increase your ability to recognize safety hazards in the home, community, and healthcare facility, and to plan interventions that promote safety for clients of all ages, such as the two in the Meet Your Patients scenario. Many accidental injuries can be prevented by being aware of hazards and taking reasonable precautions.

ABOUT THE KEY CONCEPTS

Safety is a basic human need, second only to survival needs such as oxygen, nutrition, and fluids. As a nurse, the concept of safety is fundamental to providing high-quality care to your clients. A contribution of nursing to **patient safety**, in any setting, is the ability to coordinate and integrate the multiple aspects of quality within the care directly provided by nursing, and across the care delivered by others in the setting. You must also be concerned with your own safety and the safety of other care providers. Many accidental injuries can be prevented by being aware of hazards and taking reasonable precautions.

IMPORTANCE OF SAFETY

According to the National Safety Council (NSC), accidents, or unintentional injuries, are the fifth leading cause of deaths in the United States. More than 118,000 people die each year as a result of accidents (NSC, 2011). Expressed another way, one person dies from an accident every 5 minutes. Poisoning is now listed as the number one cause of unintentional death, followed by motor vehicle accidents, firearms, falls, drowning, and fires. Of course, the death rate is not the only significant number: In 2008, approximately 26 million people received injuries that disabled them beyond the day of injury (NSC, 2010) (see Table 24-1). Many healthcare organizations are campaigning for safer patient care in an effort to reduce the cost of healthcare and the burden of suffering. The following are examples:

- **The Joint Commission**, the accrediting body for healthcare facilities, each year publishes National Patient Safety Goals. For example, in 2013 the goals included improving the accuracy of patient identification, improving the safety of medication use, reducing the risk of healthcare-associated infections, and preventing mistakes in surgery. For a link to the 2013 National Patient Safety Goals,

 Go to Chapter 24, **Resources for Caregivers and Healthcare Professionals,** on Davis*Plus.*

- **Institute of Medicine's (IOM)** report, *To Err Is Human: Building a Safer Health System,* brought public attention to patient safety. It stated that it is simply not acceptable for patients to be harmed by the same healthcare

Table 24-1 ➤ Leading Causes of Unintentional Deaths in the United States.	
MECHANISM OF INJURY	**TOTAL ANNUAL DEATHS, ALL AGE GROUPS**
Poisoning and exposure to noxious substances	41,592
Motor vehicles	34,485
Firearms	31,347
Falls	25,562
Drowning	3,517
Fires, flames, and smoke	2,756

Source: Kochanek, K. D., Xu, J., Murphy, S. L., et al. (2012). Deaths: Final data for 2009. *National Vital Statistics Reports, 60*(3). Hyattsville, MD: National Center for Health Statistics. Retrieved May 20, 2013, from http://www.cdc.gov/nchs/data/nvsr/nvsr60/nvsr60_03.pdf

system that is supposed to offer healing and comfort. The report identified five critical principles to ensure safe healthcare systems: provide leadership, recognize human limits in process design, promote effective team functioning, anticipate the unexpected, and create a learning environment (IOM, 2001). To learn what is meant by a "culture of safety" in the healthcare setting, read the accompanying QSEN box.

- **American Nurses Association (ANA).** The ANA's *Health System Reform Agenda* (2010) recommends six major public policy changes that can raise the quality of healthcare. Quality Aim 1 is safe healthcare.

- **Quality and Safety Education for Nurses (QSEN Institute).** This task force to improve nursing education identified and described six competencies that all nursing students should have by graduation. Safety is one of those competencies (Cronenwett, Sherwood, Barnsteiner, et al., 2007; Cronenwett, Sherwood, & Gelmon, 2009). For a list of the essential features that demonstrate the safety competence,

 Go to Chapter 24, **ESG Table 24-1, QSEN Safety Competency,** on Davis*Plus.*

- **Medicare.** This federal agency has identified **"never events"** or hospital-acquired conditions (HAC): costly errors that cause serious injury or death, and that are mostly preventable (e.g., falls, injury from restraints). Medicare will no longer pay institutions for care required to treat the effects of such errors (Centers for Medicare & Medicaid Services, 2006a, modified 2011).

WHAT FACTORS AFFECT SAFETY?

To promote client safety, you will need theoretical knowledge about developmental stages and individual risk factors that affect clients' ability to avoid accidental

Creating a Culture of Safety

Chapter Key Concept: Safety

Competency: Safety (Knowledge, Skills, Attitudes)*

Background: Until recently the healthcare industry assumed that correct (safe) actions would be performed by all dedicated practitioners and that people who made mistakes were "bad apples" to be fired. Mistakes were hushed up. This culture of secrecy and blame still exists, with a high cost to society and a huge impact of medical mistakes on patients and their families.

The Institute of Medicine (IOM) has called for healthcare organizations to work to dismantle the culture of secrecy and blame and to create a culture of safety. It calls for nurses to be leaders in these efforts. The Quality and Safety Education for Nurses (QSEN) competencies were created specifically to help prepare nurses for these roles.

Think about it: Although people make the mistakes, it is system factors that create a mistake-prone environment. Understanding the types of errors that occur in your facility should suggest baseline knowledge and skills you need to acquire. It is equally important to determine what systems need to be in place to build the culture of safety. Some critical features include:

➤ All staff members providing care are formally encouraged to communicate their concerns to the team. **Why do you**

think nurses or junior doctors might not communicate concerns?

➤ All information needed to appropriately manage the patient across shifts, units, facilities or after other handoffs is available at all times. **What types of errors can occur during handoffs?**

➤ Facility adopts a nonpunitive response to error and uses strategies such as root cause analysis to identify system issues. **What effect might a punitive culture have on error reporting?**

➤ Facility recognizes both individual and system causes of error but emphasizes a systems approach to error reduction. **Describe one system that can break down and make error more likely.**

➤ Each person providing care acknowledges own potential for error and values own role in preventing errors. **What can you do to help prevent errors?**

Sources: IOM (Institute of Medicine (IOM) (2001, 2011).

*To learn about specific QSEN Safety Knowledge, Skills, and Attitudes,

 Go to the QSEN web site **at http://qsen.org/ competencies/pre-licensure-ksas/**

---

injury. This chapter discusses specific risk factors and describes hazards in three environments: the home, the community, and the healthcare agency.

Developmental Factors

The type and incidence of accidents vary among age groups. You will find interventions for all age groups integrated into the topics throughout this chapter. Keep in mind that the descriptions given for each age group are characteristics common to most people in that group. However, individuals progress through developmental stages at their own pace, so there will always be some people who do not fit the group description closely. For supplemental discussion of safety needs during different developmental stages, review Chapter 9.

Infant/Toddler Drowning is the leading cause of death for children ages 1 to 4, followed by motor vehicle accidents (*Morbidity and Mortality Weekly Report,* April 16, 2012). Falls, choking, sudden infant death syndrome (SIDS), and ingesting poisons are other critical safety concerns. Infants and toddlers are completely dependent on others for their care. They are able to walk and manipulate objects before they have the judgment to recognize dangers such as falling. In addition, infants and toddlers are curious and tend to explore the environment by putting objects in their mouth. This is why the incidence of choking is highest between 6 months and 3 years of age. As mobility continues to improve, toddlers gain

more freedom, and their curiosity leads them to explore cupboards, stairs, open windows, swimming pools, and other hazards (Centers for Disease Control and Prevention [CDC], 2012).

Preschooler Motor vehicle injuries are a major cause of accidental death, along with drowning, fires, and poisoning. Falls are the primary cause of nonfatal injuries. After age 3, children are a little less prone to falls because their gross and fine motor skills, coordination, and balance have improved. However, as they begin to play more outside (playgrounds, pools, front yards, and so on) there are additional safety concerns. Although preschoolers are more aware of dangers and limitations, adult supervision continues to be essential.

School-Age Child Motor vehicles continue to be the leading cause of accidental death in this age group. Falls are the leading cause of nonfatal injuries. School-age children have developed more refined muscle coordination and control, and improved decision-making skills. However, because they become more involved in activities outside the home, bone and muscle injuries are common. Injuries are often related to sports, skateboarding, bicycle riding, and playground injuries. Most school-age children are less fearful than are toddlers, and are ready to try any new skill with or without practice or training. Exposure to the wider school and neighborhood environment also increases the risk for injury inflicted by people outside the home (e.g., abduction).

Adolescent The leading cause of death in this age group is motor vehicle accidents, followed by homicide— both frequently associated with alcohol and drug use. Sports and recreational injuries, including diving and drowning incidents are also common, especially when drinking and drug use are involved. Peak physical, sensory, and psychomotor abilities give teenagers a feeling of strength and confidence, yet they lack the wisdom and judgment of adults. This combination, along with feelings of being indestructible, makes them more likely to participate in risk-taking behavior, and in turn, more prone to injury.

Adult Among people 35 to 64 years old, unintentional poisoning causes more deaths than motor vehicle accidents (CDC, 2010a). Workplace injury may also be a significant concern. Other injuries to adults are related to lifestyle (e.g., excessive alcohol use), stress, carelessness, abuse, and decline in strength and stamina. For many, work and family responsibilities often leave little time for regular physical activity, increasing the risk of musculoskeletal injury in the so-called weekend athlete.

Older Adult Although many older adults have intact senses that enable them to continue to enjoy life as they age, physiological changes do occur (e.g., reduced muscle strength and joint mobility; slowing of reflexes; decreased ability to respond to multiple stimuli; and sensory losses, particularly hearing and vision). These changes increase the older adult's risk for falls, burns, car accidents, and other injury. Falls are the most common cause of accidental death for adults age 65 and older (CDC, n.d.a).

Individual Risk Factors

In addition to developmental stage, individual factors also influence a person's risk for unintentional injury. These include lifestyle, cognitive awareness, sensoriperceptual status, ability to communicate, mobility status, physical and emotional health, and awareness of safety measures (Table 24-2).

KnowledgeCheck 24-1

- What are some important developmental considerations when providing a safe environment for a preschool child?
- What is the main cause of injuries during the adolescent period?
- What are some ways that the aging process makes the older adult more prone to injury?
- Based on your theoretical knowledge and the scant patient data you have, why do you think Teresa's toddler (Meet Your Patients) is at risk for accidents? What about Teresa's grandmother?

SAFETY HAZARDS IN THE HOME

What safety issues in the home environment would you need to assess with regard to Teresa's toddler and grandmother (see Meet Your Patient)? If you cannot already answer the question about Teresa's family and home, you should be able to do so after reading this section which provides an overview of safety hazards in the home.

Except for motor vehicle accidents, most fatal accidents occur in the home. The leading causes of death in the home are poisonings, falls, fires and burns, and choking. For children, having older siblings, maternal age, financial difficulties, and maternal mental health problems are associated with less safe homes (Myhre, Thoresen, Grøgaard, et al., 2012).

Poisoning

Poisoning death rates have more than quadrupled in the past 20 years. Although young children are frequent victims, the increase has been mainly among adults. In many cases, the person does not die but becomes ill or suffers other effects. Poisoning exposure accounts for about 2,000 emergency department visits per day (CDC, 2010b).

- *Young children* are poisoned mostly because of improper storage of household chemicals, medicines and vitamins, and cosmetics. Box 24-1 lists poisonous agents commonly ingested by children.

Table 24-2 ➤ Individual Risk Factors for Injury	
RISK FACTORS	**BEHAVIOR MANIFESTATION**
Lifestyle	Smoking, alcohol abuse, risk-taking behaviors
Cognitive awareness	Confusion due to stress and loss of short-term memory
Sensory and perceptual status	Loss of senses (e.g., vision, hearing, pain), which provide first line of defense
Impaired communication	Language barriers and hearing and speech impairment related to disease processes
Impaired mobility	Impaired strength with accompanying problems in mobility, balance, and endurance
Physical and emotional well-being	Reduced physical stamina and depression, with feelings of loss of control and helplessness
Safety awareness	Reduced cognitive awareness (e.g., of older adult) and immature development of the child

- Household cleansers, including oven cleaner, drain cleaner, toilet bowl cleaner, and furniture polish
- Medicines, including cough and cold preparations, vitamins, pain medications, antidepressants, anticonvulsants, and iron tablets, which to children may look like candies
- Indoor house plants, including poinsettia, Dieffenbachia, philodendron, and many others
- Cosmetics, hair relaxer, nail products, mouthwash
- Pesticides
- Kerosene, gasoline, lighter fluid, paint thinner, lamp oil, antifreeze, windshield washer fluid, lighter fluid, and other chemicals
- Alcoholic beverages
- Wild plants and mushrooms
- Pesticides, rodent poisons

The use of lead in paint has been banned since 1978, but lead-based paint can still be found in older homes and toys produced in some foreign countries. Some soil (which young children often put in their mouth) contains high levels of lead. In the United States, poor, urban, and immigrant populations are at higher risk for lead exposure than other groups.

- **Older children and adolescents** may attempt suicide by overdosing with medicines or be poisoned accidentally when experimenting with recreational or prescription drugs intended for adults. In adults, most poisonings occur as a result of illegal drug use or misuse or abuse of prescription drugs, especially narcotic medications, tranquilizers, and antidepressants.
- **Deaths from prescription painkillers** have reached epidemic levels in the past decade, now greater than deaths from heroin and cocaine combined. A big part of the problem is nonmedical use of prescription painkillers—using drugs without a prescription, or using drugs just for the "high" they cause. In 2010, about 12 million Americans (age 12 or older) reported nonmedical use of prescription painkillers in the past year (CDC, 2011a).
- **Treatment choice** depends on the poison ingested. For most poisonings, the most effective intervention is professional administration of activated charcoal orally or via gastric tube. However, charcoal is not effective for ethanol, alkali, iron, boric acid, lithium, methanol, or cyanide. Depending on the situation, other options for medical treatment include gastric lavage, dialysis, administration of antidotes, and forced diuresis. For a list of medical treatments for commonly ingested poisons,

Go to Chapter 24, **Tables, Boxes, Figures: ESG Table 24-2,** on DavisPlus.

Never induce vomiting when the ingested material is acidic or caustic to the esophagus. Although the American Academy of Pediatrics no longer recommends inducing emesis (e.g., with syrup of ipecac), some practitioners may still do so. The National Capitol Poison Center does not support the routine stocking of ipecac in households with young children. The organization states that it should be given only on specific recommendation from a poison center or qualified medical personnel (National Capitol Poison Center, n.d.).

Carbon Monoxide Exposure

Carbon monoxide (CO) is a colorless, tasteless, odorless toxic gas. Exposure can cause headaches, weakness, nausea, and vomiting; prolonged exposure leads to seizures, dysrhythmias, unconsciousness, brain damage, and death. Each year in the United States, CO poisoning causes approximately 500 unintentional deaths (Bronstein, 2011). Most CO exposures occur at home and most often involve females, children under age 17 years, and adults aged 18 to 44 years. It accounts for a majority of deaths at the scene of fires, and is also a relatively common method of suicide. Many CO deaths occur during cold weather among older adults and the poor who seek nonconventional heat sources (e.g., gas ranges and ovens) to stay warm.

Scalds and Burns

The following are common causes of scalds and burns:

- **Scald injuries** (e.g., from hot water, steam, or grease) are the most common cause of burns in children younger than age 3. Scalding burns (especially on both feet or both hands) and cigarette burns in children and vulnerable older adults should always prompt you to assess for abuse (see Procedure 9-1).
- **Warming food or formula in the microwave** may cause the food to become hotter than intended, leading to burns in infants and young children.
- **Sunburn** can cause a first- or second-degree burn.
- **Contact burns** may occur from contact with metal surfaces and vinyl seats when cars are parked in the sun. The risk of contact burns in all age groups is greater in the presence of such heating devices as kerosene heaters, wood-burning stoves, and home sauna heating elements. People may use these as heat sources when they cannot afford the cost of traditional furnace fuels.
- **Chemical agents**, such as acid, alkali, or other organic compounds, can also cause localized burns.

Fires

Home fires are a major cause of death and injury. Older adults and children younger than age 5 years have the greatest risk of fire death. Most *fatal* home fires occur while people are asleep, and most fire-related deaths occur from smoke inhalation. The following are common causes of fire in the home:

- *Cooking fires* are the number one cause of home fires and home fire injuries.
- *Smoking* (e.g., cigarettes) is the leading cause of fatal home fires, but during the winter months, *heating equipment* is equally responsible.
- *Home oxygen administration equipment* is also a hazard. In 75% of the home fires involving oxygen, smoking materials are the ignition source; cooking and candles are other common factors. When more oxygen is in the air, items such as hair, plastic, skin oils, clothing, and furniture catch fire at lower temperatures, so any fire that starts will burn hotter and faster. Other causes of fire include unsupervised children playing with matches, improper use of candles, and faulty wiring.

Example Problem: Falls

Falls are the third leading cause of injury-related deaths—the leading cause for older adults. An average of 4 in 100 people experience a nonfatal fall for which they seek medical advice. The rate triples for adults older than age 75 (Adams, Martinez, Vickerie, et al., 2011). More than half of all falls occur in the home, and about 80% of home falls involve people age 65 years and older. Health issues that increase the risk for falls include poor vision, hypotension (low blood pressure), a history of falls, dizziness, pain, alcohol use, cognitive impairment, polypharmacy, arthritis, gait or balance deficits, and age greater than 80 years (Akyol, 2007; Malafarina, Úriz-Otano, Iniesta, et al., 2012).

Firearm Injuries

Gun ownership is a controversial issue. Some people keep guns in the home for protection and/or recreation (e.g., hunting, target shooting). However, guns are a source of unintentional injury and death. Gun safety and security are especially important when there are children in the home or someone with a substance abuse problem. Household access to firearms has been implicated as a risk factor for youth suicide and domestic homicide, as well as unintentional injury (Hizel, Ozcebe, Sanli, et al., 2008; Lewiecki & Miller, 2013). Because of the frequency and severity of unintentional firearm injuries involving children, the American Academy of Pediatrics and other groups have mounted efforts to educate parents about firearm safety.

ThinkLike a Nurse 24-1

- What are some initial questions you might ask Teresa regarding her home environment?
- What are some basic interventions you might suggest to Teresa to help child-proof her home? To answer this question, you will need to recall information about:
  Safety hazards that we encounter in the home
  Developmental and lifestyle factors that affect safety

Specific nursing activities that can be used to prevent accidents or injuries related to the environmental hazards (e.g., firearms)

Suffocation/Asphyxiation

Suffocation by smothering is the leading cause of death for infants younger than 1 year. Suffocation may also be caused by drowning, choking on a foreign object, or inhaling gas or smoke. Suffocation of infants is often related to bed or crib hazards, such as excess bedding or pillows, or toys hung from long ribbons inside the infant's crib. Infants can become entangled in cords from window blinds or in the ribbon or string used to hang a pacifier around an infant's neck.

Drowning is an important cause of accidental death in children 1 to 18 years old. **Key Point:** *Children up to age 4 are especially at risk for drowning and should never be left unattended in or near a bathtub, hot tub, swimming pool, or other source of water. Even wading pools, toilets, and mop buckets hold enough water to drown a small child.*

Food items, including hot dogs, raw vegetables, popcorn, hard candies, nuts, and grapes, are responsible for most nonfatal choking incidents. Nonfood items, such as latex balloons and plastic bags, cause the majority of suffocation deaths in young children.

KnowledgeCheck 24-2

- What are the most common poisonous agents ingested by children?
- Name one source of carbon monoxide (CO) poisoning.

Take-Home Toxins

Take-home toxins are hazardous substances transported from the workplace to the home. The National Institute for Occupational Safety and Health (NIOSH) reports that pathogenic microorganisms, asbestos, lead, mercury, arsenic, pesticides, caustic farm products, and dozens of other agents cause significant morbidity and mortality in workers' homes (NIOSH, 2004). These toxins are most likely transported to workers' homes on the workers themselves, on their clothing, or on objects brought from the workplace. In the home, contamination occurs via any of three sources:

- Direct skin-to-skin contact, or direct contact with contaminated clothing
- Arthropod vectors, such as ticks that are responsible for Lyme disease
- Transmission on dust particles that are inhaled (e.g., anthrax spores, arsenic in mine and smelter dust)

SAFETY HAZARDS IN THE COMMUNITY

Hazardous agents in the community are a major contributor to illness, disability, and death worldwide. This section discusses four major topics of concern: motor vehicle accidents, pathogens, pollution, and electrical storms.

Motor Vehicle Accidents

Motor vehicle accidents (MVAs) are a leading cause of accidental death in American adults and children older than 1 year of age. They account for about 34% of all accidental deaths (CDC, n.d.b). The risk of being injured or killed in a car crash increases for older drivers. Every day, on average, 500 people over age 65 are injured in an automobile accident.

Failure to use seat belts and proper child car seats continues to be the major contributing factor. Severe injuries and death also occur from air bag deployment when young children are improperly placed in the front passenger seat. Other risk factors for MVAs and related injuries and deaths include speed, alcohol, and nonuse of helmets. More recently, driver distraction, particularly due to cell phone use, has become an emerging concern. Although laws exist curtailing or banning their use in almost all states, a recent survey of drivers reported cell phone use while driving at least once in the past 30 days ranged from 21% in the UK to 69% in the United States; the prevalence of drivers who had read or sent text or e-mail messages while driving at least once in the past 30 days ranged from 15% in Spain to 31% in Portugal and the United States (*Morbidity and Mortality Weekly Report*, March 15, 2013).

Pathogens

A **pathogen** is any microorganism capable of causing an illness. Pathogens can enter the body through several sources in the environment: food, mosquitoes and other insects, rodents and other animals, and unclean water.

Foodborne Pathogens

Food poisoning is a nonspecific term that describes illness caused by ingesting bacteria and other microorganisms, or their toxins, in food. Improper food storage and preparation are a major cause of food poisoning. Raw foods are commonly associated with foodborne illness, for example, raw meat, poultry, eggs, shellfish, raw fruits and vegetables, and unpasteurized milk and fruit juice. Poisonous chemicals in the environment, such as mercury, arsenic, zinc, and potassium chlorate, may also contaminate foods. Education is an important intervention for preventing food poisoning. See the section Intervention: Teaching for Safety Self-Care in the Community, and the Self-Care box Food Safety, later in the chapter.

Vectorborne Pathogens

Vectors are organisms that transmit pathogenic bacteria, viruses, and protozoa from one host to another. The following are examples:

Mosquitoes The severity of the reaction to a mosquito bite depends on the degree of allergy to the mosquito's saliva. In addition to the discomfort caused by their bites, infected mosquitoes can transmit diseases, such as West Nile virus and malaria. They can also transmit parasites to domestic animals (e.g., dog heartworm, equine encephalitis).

Other Insects Other insects, such as roaches, fleas, sand flies, lice, and ticks (which are, technically, arachnids and not insects) can also transmit serious diseases and produce a wide variety of allergens. Allergic sensitivity to cockroaches, for example, is a predictive factor for asthma severity (Page, 2012).

Animals Rodents and other animals can also act as vectors and allergens. For example, rabies can be spread through the bite of a rabid animal, some fungal diseases can spread via the inhalation of bird droppings, and mouse proteins have been implicated in the occurrence of asthma. Structural defects in a building (e.g., roofs and walls) permit entry of birds, rodents, and other small animals, and dead spaces in walls permit their circulation among apartments in multiunit dwellings (Berg, McConnell, Milam, et al., 2008; Holt, Theall, & Rabito, 2012).

Waterborne Pathogens

Sanitation refers to measures to promote and establish favorable health conditions, especially those related to the community's water supply. People who live in substandard housing may not have safe drinking water, hot water for washing, or adequate methods of waste disposal. People in rural areas often depend on private wells, which may not be adequately maintained and tested for pathogens such as *Giardia lamblia*, *Cryptosporidium*, and *Escherichia coli*. These are primarily community health problems.

Pollution

Pollution is any harmful chemical or waste material discharged into the air, water, or soil. Examples of pollutants are gaseous fumes, asbestos, carbon monoxide, and cigarette smoke. Each year Americans generate millions of tons of waste in their homes and communities (U.S. Environmental Protection Agency [EPA], 2008).

Air Pollution Motor vehicle emissions are a major cause of *outdoor air pollution* in the United States. Other toxic air pollutants include asbestos; toluene; metals such as mercury, chromium, and lead compounds; and other emissions from factories and power plants. *Indoor pollutants* include radon; carbon monoxide; and allergens from dust mites, cockroaches, mold, rodents, and pets. Passive exposure to tobacco smoke is associated with respiratory disease and cancer; and environmental air pollution is linked to cardiovascular disease and respiratory viral infection (Kit, Simon, Brody, et al., 2013; National Cancer Institute, n.d.; Pope, Burnett, Turner, et al., 2012; U.S. Department of Health and Human Services [USDHHS], 2006).

Water Contamination Contamination in lakes, rivers, and streams ultimately affects both recreation and food production. Pollution occurs when inadequately treated or inappropriate quantities of human, industrial, or agricultural wastes are released into the water systems. If the pollution is severe enough, the water may become unsafe for human consumption.

Noise Substantial exposure to noise has been associated with a range of adverse health effects, including hearing loss, stress, elevated blood pressure, and loss of sleep. Noise is pervasive in our society—for example, from road traffic, jet planes, garbage trucks, construction equipment, lawn mowers, and loud music. People who live or work near major roads, bus depots, airports, and trucking routes are at greater risk, as are those in certain work environments (e.g., railroad workers).

Soil Improper waste disposal and excessive use of pesticides can contaminate soil. Agricultural, industrial, and manufacturing processes create solid and toxic waste. Animal, radioactive, and medical wastes pose special problems. Household products, such as paints, cleaners, oils, batteries, and pesticides, contain corrosive or toxic ingredients that contaminate the environment when disposed of improperly (e.g., in household trash or poured down the drain, on the ground, or into storm sewers).

Electrical Storms

According to the National Weather Service, deaths from lightning strikes lead all other categories of weather-related fatalities, exceeded in some years only by floods (Cooper & Kulkarni, 2011). Weather conditions play a major role in outdoor recreation programming. It is important for professionals, participants, and outdoor recreation providers to understand severe weather conditions, specifically thunderstorms and lightning, and the dangers associated with them.

KnowledgeCheck 24-3

- What are the major causes of injuries from MVAs (motor vehicle accidents)?
- List at least three tips for preventing food poisoning.
- List three sources of noise pollution.

 ThinkLike a Nurse 24-2

Identify an environmental problem in your neighborhood. What are some possible solutions?

SAFETY HAZARDS IN THE HEALTHCARE FACILITY

As many as 98,000 people die from medical injuries each year in U.S. hospitals (Pham, Aswani, Rosen, et al., 2012). Several characteristics of healthcare facilities pose safety hazards for residents and workers. We have discussed the hazard of infection in Chapter 23. Box 24-2 lists The Joint Commission's National Patient Safety Goals for 2013, which should give you an idea of the types of accidents that occur in healthcare agencies. If you would like to see a full explanation of the patient safety goals,

 Go to The Joint Commission Web site, at http://www.jointcommission.org/assets/1/6/2011_NPSGs_HAP.pdf

---

In its report *To Err Is Human: Building a Safer Health System*, the Institute of Medicine (IOM) estimated that as many as 98,000 hospitalized Americans die each year—not as a result of their illness or disease, but as a result of errors in their care (IOM, 2000). This figure does not reflect the many patients who survive but sustain serious injuries. Organizational factors contribute to errors and to safety problems in healthcare, including poor design, maintenance failures, unworkable procedures, shortfalls in training, less than adequate tools and equipment, and inadequate staffing. Disruptive behaviors, intimidation in the workplace, and a culture of disrespect among healthcare professionals have also been reported as significant barriers to patient safety.

Healthcare has traditionally had a hierarchical nature with the physician at the top. In addition, healthcare professionals have been taught to practice with autonomy. This combination of factors set the stage for a culture that does not respond well to questions about possible problems with patient care, particularly from subordinates. It is clear that such a culture needs to be repaired, and many healthcare organizations are working to address disrespectful behavior, staff reluctance to speak up about risks and errors, and blatant disregard of expressed concerns.

Key Point: *Since nurses are the healthcare professionals who spend the greatest amount of time with patients, research is beginning to document what physicians, patients, and nurses themselves have long known: How well clients are cared for by nurses affects their health and outcomes, and sometimes can be a matter of life or death.*

Studies have shown that greater numbers of patient deaths are associated with fewer nurses to provide care

(Aiken, Clarke, Sloane, et al., 2001), and less nursing time provided to patients is associated with higher rates of infection, gastrointestinal bleeding, pneumonia, cardiac arrest, and death from these and other causes (Kalisch, Tschannen, & Lee, 2012; Stimpfel & Aiken, 2013; Unruh & Zhang, 2012). In providing quality care to patients, nurses are indispensable to their safety.

What Are Never Events?

Never events can cause serious injury or death to a patient, and should *never* happen in a hospital. The list of never events has been expanded over time to mean events that are clearly identifiable and measurable, serious, and usually prevented. You can also gain insight into healthcare facility hazards by examining the following list of never events (Centers for Medicare & Medicaid Services, 2008; Watson, 2010):

- Foreign object (such as a sponge) left in patients after surgery
- Air embolism
- Administering the wrong type of blood
- Severe pressure ulcers
- Falls and trauma
- Injuries from burns, restraints, or bedrails
- Infections associated with urinary catheters
- Infections associated with intravenous catheters
- Symptoms resulting from poorly controlled blood sugar levels
- Surgical site infections following certain elective procedures (e.g., certain orthopedic surgeries, bariatric surgery for obesity)
- Deep vein thrombosis or pulmonary embolism following total knee and total hip replacement procedures.

The Institute for Healthcare Improvement (IHI), an independent, not-for-profit organization, launched the 100,000 Lives Campaign to recommend changes to reduce morbidity and death in American healthcare. At least three of the 100,000 Lives goals support the list of never events: Prevent adverse drug events, prevent central line infections, and prevent surgical site infections. To read the entire list of recommendations,

 Go to Chapter 24, **ESG Box 24-1, The 100,000 Lives Campaign,** on Davis*Plus*.

ThinkLike a Nurse 24-3

Many never events can be reduced by good nursing care. By preventing complications and maximizing reimbursement, nurses can prove their value to an organization and make the case for better staffing. Over which of the never events do you think nurses have the most control? Explain your thinking.

Understanding Errors in Healthcare— Root Cause Analysis

Root Cause Analysis (RCA) practice tries to solve problems by identifying and correcting the underlying cause(s) of events, as opposed to simply addressing their symptoms. By focusing correction on root causes, problem recurrence can be prevented. A **root cause** is typically a finding related to a process or system that has a potential for redesign to reduce risk, rather than an individual error. RCA provides an organized structure for analysis of errors and is designed to answer three basic questions:

1. What happened?
2. Why did it happen?
3. What can be done to prevent it from happening again?

The Joint Commission requires healthcare agencies to perform RCA for all unexpected occurrence involving death or serious physical or psychological injury, also known as **sentinel events**.

Example Problem: Falls

Although most falls occur in the home, they are a major concern in healthcare facilities as well. Falls are by far the most common incident reported in hospitals and long-term care facilities, occurring at one for every 2,000 patient stays (CDC, n.d.a; Centers for Medicare & Medicaid Services, 2011). Infants and older adults are especially at risk for injury from falls. Many patients have risk factors, such as poor vision, cognitive impairment, difficulty with walking or balance, orthostatic hypotension, weakness or dizziness from disease or therapy, and drowsiness from medications. Many cases involve falling from a bed, and falls occur more frequently on nights, weekends, and holidays. Most agencies have established procedures and safety features to prevent falls.

Equipment-Related Accidents

Equipment-related accidents usually occur when equipment malfunctions or is used improperly, for example when bed alarms fail to work or are set up incorrectly, when suction devices and infusion pumps are not working properly, oxygen cylinders are transported incorrectly, or wheelchairs and beds are not locked during transfer activities.

Fires and Electrical Hazards

Because most institutions promote a smoke-free environment, fire in a healthcare agency is more often related to anesthesia or improperly grounded or malfunctioning electrical equipment. Most healthcare agencies have policies for preventing electrical hazards. Nevertheless, patients and visitors do break the rules, so smoking cannot be discounted as a hazard.

When a fire occurs in a public building, an announcement is made over the communication system. Often words such as "Code Red" or "Code Yellow" are used in an effort to prevent panic among patients and visitors.

Depending on the situation, the announcement may ask visitors to leave the building. ✚ All personnel must know the fire escape route and follow hospital policy regarding fires. If you discover a fire, your first instinct may be to contain or put out the fire. Fight that instinct! Your first action is to rescue the patient—that is, move the patient(s) away from the area. Only then should you sound the alarm and attempt to confine the fire.

Restraints

A restraint is a device or method used for the purpose of restricting a patient's freedom of movement or access to his body, with or without his permission. The most obvious form of restraint is the use of physical force by another person. A restraint may also be (1) a mechanical device, material, or equipment, such as a cloth vest or siderails, or (2) a chemical restraint (medication) given to control disruptive behavior, such as sedatives and psychotropic agents.

- Devices such as casts and traction are not considered restraints (Centers for Medicare & Medicaid Services, 2008; The Joint Commission, 2009).
- Physical holding of a patient is not always considered restraint. Sometimes it is necessary to use devices or methods that involve the physical holding of a patient for routine physical examinations or tests.
- Restraints are classified according to the reason for their use: Medical-surgical restraints or restraints used for behavior management. Medicare has specific guidelines for each circumstance. Guidelines are more restrictive when restraints are used for behavior management.

As a safety measure, nurses traditionally restrained highly dependent older adults, patients with poor mobility, those with impaired cognitive status, and those they judged to be at risk for falls. However, it has been found that restraints make care more time consuming and do not reduce falls. Restraints are themselves a safety hazard, and actually increase the likelihood of injury. ✚ A restrained person has a natural tendency to struggle and try to remove the restraint, and as a result can become entangled and suffer nerve damage, circulatory impairment, and even suffocation. Restraint-imposed immobility can cause pressure ulcers, contractures, loss of strength, and other hazards of immobility. Emotionally, the person may suffer anger, fear, humiliation, and diminished self-esteem.

Avoid Restraints When Possible

Research indicates that less restraint use saves time and money, and reduces patient injuries (Chan, LeBel, & Webber, 2012; Tilly & Reed, 2008). The American Nurses Association along with other healthcare organizations have established evidence-based guidelines to show that a restraint-free environment is the standard of care (Said, A. & Kautz, D., 2013). For those reasons, healthcare facilities are trying to achieve that goal. When the decision is made to avoid restraints, it is essential to provide alternatives for keeping the patient safe. Multiple approaches are needed, including careful and ongoing assessment and surveillance, finding ways to communicate with the patient, and tailoring exercise programs, medication reviews, and environmental modifications to the needs of individual patients. **Key Point:** *Restraints never resolve the underlying problem; addressing the reason behind the patient's behavior is key to calming the patient* (Said, A. & Kautz, D., 2013).

To provide the safest possible care environment, The Joint Commission encourages healthcare facilities to:

- Promote a commitment to reduce the use of restraints and seclusion among all direct-care staff.
- Educate caregivers before they take part in any restraint-related activity.
- Document restraint episodes specifically, in detail.
- Maintain one-on-one viewing of patients in restraint and seclusion.
- Include staff members when deciding whether to explore new technology that is considered a safe alternative to traditional restraint devices.
- Budget for an adequate number of qualified staff to attend to patients.

Restraint Is Sometimes Necessary

Guidelines are slightly different depending on whether restraints are used to directly support medical healing or for a behavioral health reason (e.g., when a patient is irrational and pulling out his IV lines). Use restraints only as a last resort. As much as possible, use technology (such as bed alarms) and better anticipation of patient needs instead of restraints.

✚ If you must use restraints, Medicare, The Joint Commission, and other regulators require that restraints be medically prescribed and that you first try all less restrictive interventions.

Do Not Depend on Siderails

Based on the Centers for Medicare & Medicaid Services (CMS) standards siderails can be viewed as a restraint. A full-length siderail is a restraint when it is used to prevent the patient from getting out of bed regardless of whether he is able to do so safely. A half- or quarter-length upper siderail can be an aid to independence if it is used by the patient for the purpose of getting into and out of bed. Similarly, split rails are not considered restraints if a client requests them in order to feel more secure (Talerico & Capezuti, 2001).

Remember that older or cognitively impaired adults may regard siderails as a barrier rather than as a reminder that they need assistance. Several studies have shown that siderails may lead to serious falls and injuries. These findings have led healthcare providers to reevaluate the use of restraints and to recommend that siderails not be used routinely (Evans & Cotter, 2008; Sharkey, Van Leuven, & Radovich, 2012).

KnowledgeCheck 24-4

- What is a typical cause of fire in healthcare facilities?
- What measures should you take, and in what order, if a fire occurs in the hospital?

Mercury Exposure

Mercury is a heavy, odorless, silver-white liquid metal. Mercury is toxic in both acute and chronic exposure. It can be inhaled, ingested, or absorbed through the skin. It accumulates in muscle tissue and can cause renal and neurological disorders, especially in fetuses and neonates. Because of its shiny color and ability to form beads or balls, mercury is appealing to curious children. See Table 24-3 for potential health effects.

Products that may contain mercury include thermometers, thermostats, batteries, fluorescent light bulbs, blood pressure devices, and electrical equipment and switches. For more information about products and devices that may contain mercury,

 Go to Chapter 24, **Tables, Boxes, Figures; ESG Box 24-2, Products and Devices That May Contain Mercury,** on DavisPlus.

In 1998, the American Hospital Association (AHA) and the Environmental Protection Agency (EPA) launched a program to eliminate mercury-containing waste in the healthcare industry and prevent it from entering the environment via incinerators, landfills, and wastewater. Mercury thermometers are no longer being made in the United States. However, some people may still have them in their homes. Most, but not all, healthcare facilities have eliminated mercury thermometers and sphygmomanometers. You can help prevent mercury poisoning by taking an active role in eliminating mercury-containing items from your workplace. Some hospitals conduct thermometer exchanges, providing free or low-cost nonmercury thermometers to anyone who brings in a mercury thermometer.

Healthcare facilities must have policies and procedures for hazardous waste spills (e.g., mercury). These are required by The Joint Commission and federal agencies such as the EPA and the Occupational Safety and Health Administration (OSHA). You are not likely to encounter mercury exposure in acute care and ambulatory agencies.

Biological Hazards

As a nurse, you will place a high priority on the biological safety of patients. Institutionalized patients are at especially high risk from infectious microorganisms, some of which are highly resistant to antibiotics. To learn about or review healthcare-related infections, asepsis, and infection control, refer to Chapter 23.

Hazards to Healthcare Workers

Nursing is an active profession, and workplace injuries are all too common. Nurses sometimes hesitate to report they have been injured because they fear being labeled a complainer or troublemaker or being denied opportunities for promotion and other consequences. However, OSHA requires that employers show employees how to report a workplace injury and prohibits discrimination against employees who make such reports. You should always report an injury. By doing so, you help (1) pinpoint trends and areas of need in safety, and (2) ensure you will receive necessary treatment and follow-up. Common accidents include back injuries, needlestick injuries, radiation injury, and violence.

Table 24-3 ➤ Potential Health Effects of Mercury	
PRIMARY ROUTE	**POTENTIAL HEALTH EFFECTS**
Acute Effects	
Toxicity	Symptoms of chills, nausea, malaise, chest tightness and pain, dyspnea, coughing, stomatitis, gingivitis, excess salivation, and diarrhea. High levels can cause severe respiratory irritation, digestive disturbances, and severe renal damage.
Inhalation	Respiratory damage, wakefulness, muscle weakness, anorexia, headache, ringing in the ears, chest pain, inflammation of the mouth, and pneumonitis
Eye	Irritation and corrosion
Skin	Irritation and allergic dermatitis
Ingestion	Intestinal obstruction
Chronic Effects	
Primarily central nervous system	Numbness or tingling of the hands, lips, and feet; behavior and personality changes
Other	Fatigue, weakness, anorexia, weight loss, and gastrointestinal disturbances

Back Injury

Nursing personnel are consistently listed in the top 10 occupations for work-related musculoskeletal disorders (MSDs). Most often the MSD involves the shoulders and back (Bureau of Labor Statistics, 2012). The American Nurses Association (ANA) reports that 52% of nurses report chronic back pain (ANA, 2013), likely because many nursing tasks require bending and twisting of the torso, activities that can cause injury when the nurse does not use correct body mechanics. Among the most stressful activities are transferring patients (e.g., from toilet to chair), weighing patients, lifting a patient in bed, repositioning patients in beds or chairs, and changing bed linens.

Currently 10 states have laws requiring safe patient handling and the Veteran's Administration has guidelines that have been successful in decreasing work-related MSDs. However, healthcare facilities have not consistently implemented safe patient handling guidelines. In response, the ANA (2013) has developed national standards to guide healthcare facilities in this regard. The standards strive to create a culture of safety by requiring employers to develop a safe handling and moving program with policies, appropriate equipment, training, and accommodations for injured employees. Another critical element of the program is empowering nurses to (1) actively participate in creating and implementing safe handling measures and (2) promptly report hazards, incidents, and injuries in a "blame-free" environment.

Refer to Chapter 32 for information about body mechanics and how to safely lift and move patients. For more information about ANA's campaign to prevent musculoskeletal injuries,

 ANA's **Safe Patient Handling Web site,** at http://nursingworld.org/MainMenuCategories/WorkplaceSafety/SafePatient

or

 Go to Student Resources, Chapter 24, **Resources for Caregivers and Health Professionals,** on DavisPlus.

Needlestick Injury

Healthcare workers, mostly nurses and housekeeping staff, suffer up to 1 million injuries per year from needles and other "sharps," putting them at risk for infectious diseases such as hepatitis B and AIDS. The operating room is a high-risk area; surgeons experience about a quarter of all "sharps" injuries (Waljee, Sunitha, & Chung, 2013).

The federal Needlestick Safety and Prevention Act and OSHA standards required employers to maintain a log of sharps injuries and to purchase needleless systems and safer needle devices. Needlestick injury rates declined by more than 36% during the 3-year period following passage of that law. Nevertheless, a recent survey found that 26% of nurses still report having

had at least one injury from a sharp, usually a needle, contaminated with a patient's blood (Delahanty & Myers, 2007). The risk of needlestick injury increases for nurses who:

- Work in stressful environments
- Work varying or long shifts (longer than 12 consecutive hours)
- Have a low skill level, based on education level or experience.

Other risk factors include a lack of protective equipment, recapping needles and working in an area that requires higher than average use of needles. Although OSHA has fined hospitals for noncompliance, some employers still have not complied completely with the regulations. For suggestions about how you can prevent needlestick injuries,

 Go to Chapter 24, **Clinical Insight 24-1: Preventing Needlestick Injury,** in Volume 2.

For more discussion on how to handle needles safely,

 Go to Chapter 26, **Procedure 26-10B: Recapping Sterile Needles,** in Volume 2.

Radiation Injury

Radiation is the process of emitting radiant energy in the form of waves or particles. Ionizing radiation is used in computerized tomography (CT scans) in diagnostic radiology, linear accelerators in radiotherapy, and positron emission tomography (PET scans) in nuclear medicine. Patients are deliberately exposed to radiation during diagnostic tests and certain medical treatments. Healthcare workers who care for these patients are unavoidably exposed to small doses of radiation.

Take precautions to avoid excessive radiation exposure for the patient and yourself during x-ray procedures. **Key Point:** *Follow the principles of time, distance, and shielding when caring for a patient who is being treated with an internal radioactive implant:*

- *Time:* Organize nursing care to limit the amount of time with the patient.
- *Distance:* Perform near the patient only the nursing care that is absolutely necessary.
- *Shielding:* Wear protective shielding (e.g., a lead apron), if available, and wear a film badge if you deliver care that exposes you to radiation regularly. The film badge will indicate any radiation exposure.

Violence

The impact of violent acts on healthcare workers is widespread and includes injuries, higher-than-average staff turnover, increased requests for medical leaves, unusually high time-off and attendance issues, and stress-related illnesses (Papa & Venella, 2013). Hospital security may not be sufficient to protect you from injury if violence breaks out among patients, visitors, and/or staff. This is especially true in the emergency department (ED), which has 24-hour accessibility and may sometimes be crowded and chaotic. Under the stress of an acute illness, patients and family members alike may become anxious and angry and act out in ways that are unpredictable and atypical for them.

Violence typically begins with anxiety and escalates in stages through verbal aggression and then physical aggression. If you can relieve a patient's anxiety, you may be able to halt the progression to physical violence. Certain emotional and physical conditions increase the risk for patient aggression (refer to Assessing the Risk for Violence, in the following Practical Knowledge section).

Gang activity, which is widespread in U.S. cities, is another potential source of violence. As gangs spread, so does the likelihood that gang members will be treated in the ED or admitted to the hospital (Gillespie, Gates, & Berry, 2013; Taylor & Rew, 2011).

KnowledgeCheck 24-5

- What measures can healthcare workers use to reduce exposure to radiation?
- What safety measures help reduce equipment-related injuries in the healthcare facility?
- As a nurse, what can you do to help prevent injuring your back?

PracticalKnowledge
knowing **how**

This section provides focused assessments for certain safety risks; standardized nursing language for nursing diagnoses, patient outcomes, and general interventions for addressing patient safety; and specific nursing interventions for safety hazards discussed in the preceding Theoretical Knowledge section.

▓ ASSESSMENT

It is important to assess the client's immediate environment, developmental stage, and individual risk factors. The following will help you to perform focused assessments for falls risk, home safety, and risk for violence.

Assessing for Example Problem: Falls

Assess all inpatients for falls risk when they are admitted to the healthcare setting. For clients at risk for falls, repeat the risk assessment every 8 hours, and increase the frequency of monitoring. Also identify medications that increase the risk for falling (e.g., opioid analgesics, sedatives, and antihypertensives). Most institutions have policies and guidelines for assessing risk for falls. The following are some examples of methods you might use.

Morse Fall Scale

The Morse Fall Scale uses the following questions to assess a person's risk for falls:

1. Does the patient have a history of falling?
2. Does the person have more than one medical diagnosis?
3. Does the person use ambulatory aids, such as crutches or a walker?
4. Does the person have an IV line or a saline lock?
5. Is the person's gait normal or stooped or otherwise impaired?
6. What is the person's mental status (e.g., disoriented, forgetful)?

You can easily score, tally, and record those six variables on the patient's chart. The risk of falling varies greatly with different patient populations, different times of day, and different stages of the patient's illness. Age alone is not a predictor of falls, but the items scored by the scale are more common in older adults (Morse, 2001). Ideally, the Morse Fall Scale should be calibrated for each particular unit so that fall prevention strategies are targeted to those most at risk. Institutions implementing the Morse Scale should train personnel in the proper use of the scale (Morse, 2008, 2009). To see the complete Morse Fall Scale,

 Go to Chapter 24, **Tables, Boxes, Figures: ESG Figure 24-1,** on Davis*Plus*.

 Assessing Older Adults for Falls
For a flowchart summarizing falls assessment for older adults, refer to Figure 24-1.

Get Up and Go As a part of the routine assessment of all older adults, ask the patient (or caregivers) about falls. If they report a single fall or risk factors, conduct the Get Up and Go test to identify whether the patient is presently at risk for falls or needs further evaluation.

Timed Up & Go If the patient is seeking care because of a fall or if you observe any difficulty with ambulation, refer him to a practitioner with advanced skills and experience for a Timed Up & Go Test and a comprehensive fall evaluation. This is a version of the Get Up and Go test, in which the patient is asked to get up and walk 8 feet in 8.5 seconds or less. Primary care providers should annually perform a Timed Up & Go test for fall risk assessment for all patients over age 65 (American Academy of Neurology, 2008a, 2008b; Hendrich, 2007; Kenny, Rubenstein, Tinetti, et al., 2011; Podsiadlo & Richardson, 1991). To use the Get Up and Go test and the Timed Up & Go Test,

 Go to Chapter 24, **Assessment Guidelines and Tools, Get Up and Go Test** and the **Timed Up & Go Test,** in Volume 2.

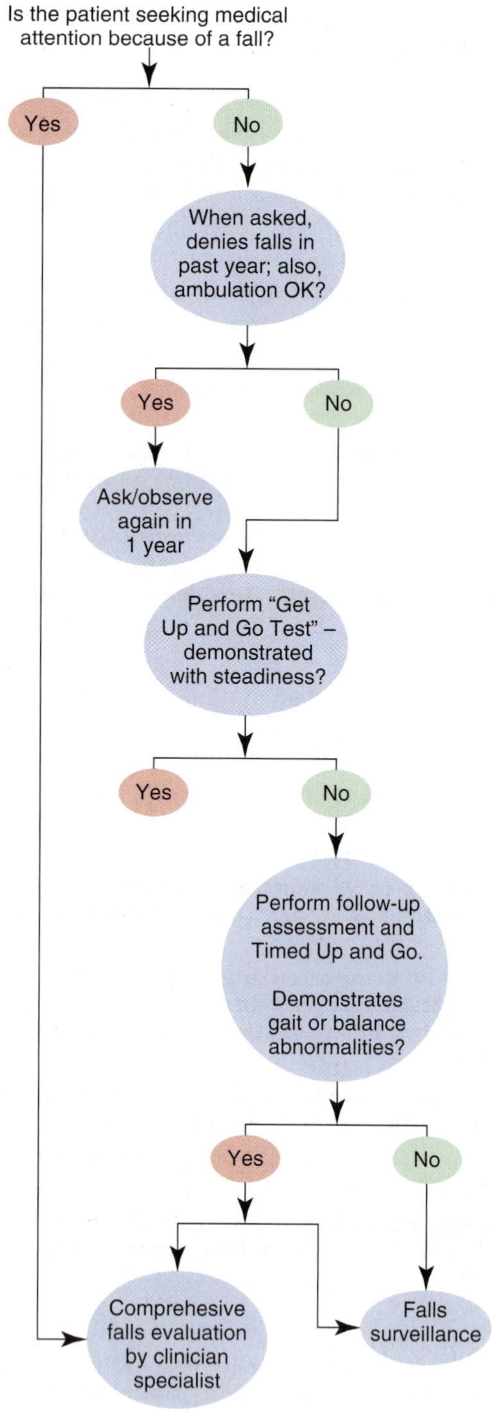
Is the patient seeking medical attention because of a fall?
Yes
No
When asked, denies falls in past year; also, ambulation OK?
Yes
No
Ask/observe again in 1 year
Perform "Get Up and Go Test" – demonstrated with steadiness?
Yes
No
Perform follow-up assessment and Timed Up and Go.
Demonstrates gait or balance abnormalities?
Yes
No
Comprehensive falls evaluation by clinician specialist
Falls surveillance

FIGURE 24-1 Falls assessment flowchart.

Assessing for Home Safety

As you know, many accidents occur in the home (e.g., fire, poisoning). Everyone should take a few minutes to check for environmental safety hazards.

- A **home safety checklist** is a convenient way for clients to identify potential hazards. For an extensive checklist you can print and use in a home assessment,

Go to Chapter Resources, Chapter 24, **ESG Figure 24-2, Home Safety Checklist,** on Davis*Plus*.

- **The safety assessment scale (SAS)** is an objective way to evaluate the dangers incurred by people with memory and cognitive deficits who live alone at home. You can use the short version of the SAS to assess the individual's risk status and decide whether she should have an in-depth evaluation. In addition to assessing for injury, this scale evaluates whether the cognitively impaired person is capable of cooking, taking medications independently, shopping, and performing other activities of daily living. To see this scale,

Go to **Assessment Guidelines and Tools, S.A.S. Safety Assessment Scale,** in Volume 2.

Assessing the Risk for Violence

You can be prepared to intervene and perhaps even prevent violence if you recognize risk factors and early warning signs (Flores, 2008; Woodrow & Guest, 2012).

1. Assess for factors that increase the risk for aggression:
   - Mental disorders, such as dementia, delirium, schizophrenia, and bipolar disorder
   - Being under the influence of alcohol or other drugs
   - Withdrawal from alcohol or other drugs
   - History of violence
   - Clinical conditions such as high fever, epilepsy, head trauma, and hypoglycemia
2. Assess for anxiety:
   - Agitation and restlessness
   - Pacing
   - Talking loudly, speaking rapidly
   - Gesturing widely
   - Be alert for verbal aggression, such as threats, sarcasm, and swearing.

KnowledgeCheck 24-6

- Which assessment tool would you use for a slightly confused home care client to assess her ability to safely live alone and perform activities of daily living?
- List the six risk factors that are assessed on the Morse Fall Scale.
- How should you screen older adults to see if they need a comprehensive falls evaluation?

ANALYSIS/NURSING DIAGNOSIS

How would your interventions differ for the following two diagnoses?

Risk for Falls related to poor vision secondary to cataracts

Risk for Falls related to muscle weakness, joint instability, and poor sense of balance

Etiologies The nursing diagnoses listed above illustrate that diagnosis etiologies are important because they affect your choice of interventions. Etiologies may include environmental hazards as well as the developmental and individual risk factors discussed in the preceding sections. Keep in mind that you must state *specific* etiologies for each individual—not just general ones such as "environmental hazards." For example:

Correct: Risk for Falls related to cluttered home environment and joint instability

Incorrect: Risk for Falls related to environmental and physical factors

NANDA-I Labels For NANDA-I labels to use in describing safety problems,

 Go to ESG, Chapter 24, **Standardized Language, NANDA-I Diagnoses and NOC Outcomes for Safety Problems,** on DavisPlus.

A few examples are: Risk for Contamination, Risk for Aspiration, and Risk for Poisoning. **Key Point:** *Use the diagnosis Risk for Injury only when the risk cannot be described by one of the more specific nursing diagnoses.*

PLANNING OUTCOMES/EVALUATION

The *NOC standardized outcomes* you use will depend on the nursing diagnosis. For some examples (e.g., Fall Prevention Behavior),

 Go to Chapter Resources, Chapter 24, **Standardized Language, NANDA-I Diagnoses and NOC Outcomes for Safety Problems,** on DavisPlus.

Individualized goals/outcome statements you might write for a client's safety diagnoses include the following:

- The child will be free of injury.
- (Client) will experience no physical injury due to environmental hazards.
- Falls will not occur.
- Family members will describe their planned escape routes in case of fire.

PLANNING INTERVENIONS/IMPLEMENTATION

NIC standardized interventions will be determined by the nursing diagnosis you use. To see the more than 50 interventions in the NIC domain (category) of Safety, and some interventions from other NIC domains that are applicable to safety needs,

 Go to Chapter 24, **Standardized Language, Examples of NIC Interventions Related to Safety,** on DavisPlus.

General Interventions Related to Safety

Specific nursing activities are designed to monitor and manipulate the physical environment to promote safety. The following are some general activities that provide

an overview of your role in patient safety in all types of settings and circumstances.

- Assess and continually monitor the safety needs of patients, based on their level of physical and cognitive function and past history of behavior.
- Assess and continually monitor safety hazards in the environment (i.e., physical, biological, and chemical).
- Remove hazards from the environment, when possible.
- Provide clients with emergency phone numbers.
- Modify the environment to minimize hazards and risk.
- Teach clients about specific safety measures.
- If an accident or injury occurs in the healthcare setting, file an incident report according to agency policy. See Chapter 18 for more information on this topic.
- Urge patients to be active members of the healthcare team (Box 24-3).

The QSEN Safety Competencies should also help you to understand your role in keeping patients safe. To review those competencies,

 Go to Chapter 24, **ESG Table 24-1, QSEN Safety Competency,** on DavisPlus.

BOX 24-3 ■ Speak Up

Speak up if you have questions or concerns, and if you don't understand, ask again. It's your body and you have a right to know.

Pay attention to the care you are receiving. Make sure you're getting the right treatments and medications by the right healthcare professionals. Don't assume anything.

Educate yourself about your diagnosis, the medical tests you are undergoing, and your treatment plan.

Ask a trusted family member or friend to be your advocate.

Know your medications and why you take them. Medication errors are the most common healthcare errors.

Use a hospital, clinic, surgery center, or other type of healthcare organization that has undergone a rigorous on-site evaluation against established state-of-the-art quality and safety standards, such as that provided by The Joint Commission.

Participate in all decisions about your treatment. You are the center of the healthcare team.

The Joint Commission encourages patients to become active, involved, and informed participants on the healthcare team, and for parents to do the same to help protect their children from medical errors. The preceding steps are based on research that shows that patients who take part in decisions about their healthcare are more likely to have better outcomes.

Source: Courtesy of Joint Commission on Accreditation of Healthcare Organizations. The complete Speak Up document is available at: http://www.jointcommission.org/multimedia/speak-up-know-your-rights/

Home Care Safety Interventions

Specific interventions follow for promoting safety related to particular hazards in home care. In this section, you will find boxes containing specific home safety interventions.

Prevent Poisoning in the Home

✚ In all cases of suspected poisoning, Call 911 or the local emergency number right away. Even if the person is having no symptoms, call the poison control center (PCC) as soon as possible. **The national PCC number is (800) 222-1222; they will connect you to a local PCC.**

Unintentional poisoning can affect people at all ages and from all walks of life. However, it may surprise you that middle-aged adults have the highest unintentional poisoning death rates.

For Children Nursing interventions focus on teaching parents how to childproof the home and what to do if someone ingests a poisonous substance. All homes should be equipped to handle an emergency if poisoning occurs. Teach parents to keep the telephone number for the nearest PCC easily accessible. If they suspect a child has ingested a poisonous substance, it is crucial to obtain help immediately so there is less time for the substance to enter the child's system.

For Adults Advise clients of the following:

■ Take only prescription medications prescribed by a healthcare professional.
■ Never take larger or more frequent doses of medications, particularly prescription pain medications, to try to get faster or more powerful effects.
■ Never share or sell your prescription drugs.
■ Be sure to follow directions on the label when taking medications, and read all warning labels.

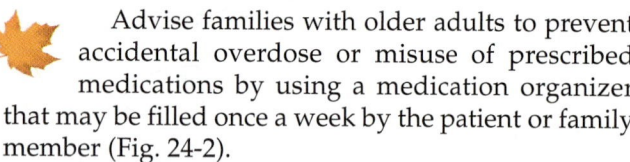
Advise families with older adults to prevent accidental overdose or misuse of prescribed medications by using a medication organizer that may be filled once a week by the patient or family member (Fig. 24-2).

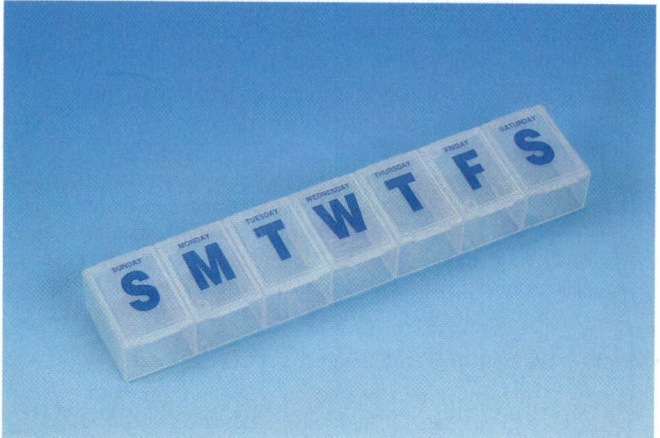

FIGURE 24-2 Medication organizer.

For steps to prevent poisoning, see Home Care: Preventing Poisoning in the Home. For actions to take if poisoning occurs at home,

 Go to Chapter 24, **Tables, Boxes, Figures; ESG Box 24-3, Home Care: If Poisoning Occurs at Home,** on Davis*Plus*.

Prevent Carbon Monoxide Poisoning

If CO intoxication is suspected, the person should be treated with 100% humidified oxygen. A simple blood test may be done to confirm CO levels in the blood. Nursing interventions include teaching prevention measures, such as the following:

■ Buy, install, and maintain a home CO detector.
■ Ensure that gas or wood-burning appliances are adequately vented to the outside.
■ Repair rust holes or defects in vehicles that could allow exhaust fumes to enter the passenger compartment.
■ Never use a kerosene heater, gas oven, or gas range to heat a house, even for a short time.
■ Never operate gasoline-powered engines, such as automobiles, generators, or lawn mowers, in confined spaces, such as garages or basements, or near open doors or windows.
■ Never burn charcoal inside a home, cabin, recreational vehicle, or tent—not even in a fireplace.

Prevent Home Fires

Nursing interventions include teaching families how to prevent fires and measures to take should a fire occur. Stress the following measures:

Have a Warning System Have working smoke alarms and change batteries every 6 months or more often. Keep a phone near the bed or chair for people who have limited mobility.

Have an Escape Plan Develop a home fire escape plan and practice it at least twice a year. Keep a rope or other type of ladder for escape from rooms above ground level. Have a fire extinguisher in the home, and know where it is located and how to use it. Check fire extinguishers regularly and replace them when they become outdated.

Have a Preventive Frame of Mind For example, when decorating Christmas trees and the exterior of your home, always use fire-safe lights. Do not leave old light sets hung on the outside of your home year after year. Always unplug Christmas tree lights before leaving home, and remove the Christmas tree from the home when it becomes dry. Other fire precautions include the following:

■ Never leave burning candles unattended. Do not use candles near curtains or other flammable materials.
■ With charcoal grills, use only charcoal starter fluids designed for barbecue grills.

Home Care

Preventing Poisoning in the Home

Young children will eat and drink almost anything. Most victims of accidental poisoning are children younger than the age of 5. Tips to prevent poisoning include the following:

Careful Words and Actions

➤ Never leave a small child unattended near household cleaning supplies or medicines, even for a moment. If you must answer the phone or doorbell, take the child with you.

➤ Children act fast; it takes only a moment for them to swallow something.

➤ Avoid taking medicines in front of children; children tend to imitate adults.

➤ Never call medicines or vitamins "candy." Instead, use the correct name ("cough medicine," and so on).

Careful Storage

➤ Store medicines or household chemicals on high shelves or in locked cabinets and drawers. Never leave them on kitchen or bathroom counters.

➤ Store all household chemicals away from food.

➤ Keep medicines and household chemicals in their original containers. Leave the original labels on. Do NOT store chemicals in containers that normally hold food.

➤ Use child-resistant packaging for medicines and household chemicals. Close the container securely after each use.

➤ Do not assume your child is safe around substances in child-resistant containers; research has shown that many toddlers and preschoolers can open them.

Careful Disposal

➤ Teach clients to take advantage of any community programs that take back unwanted medications for safe disposal (e.g., call the local trash service or a local pharmacy for options in your area).

➤ Teach clients how to safely dispose of outdated prescription medications:

Crush the medication or add water to dissolve it.

Mix the drugs with an undesirable substance such as kitty litter or used cooking grease to make it less desirable for pets and children to eat.

Place the mixture in an empty can or resealable bag and put it in the trash.

➤ Remove all identifying information from prescription labels before throwing containers in the trash or recycling them.

➤ It is not safe to dispose of drugs down the toilet or sink. Wastewater treatment plants are not fully designed to deal with medications, and small amounts have shown up in surface waters. Although there is no evidence of harm to humans or the environment, the long-term effects on people, animals, and the environment are unknown.

Careful Environment Checks

➤ Before purchasing a houseplant, verify that it is nontoxic.

➤ Examples of toxic plants are rhododendron, philodendron, English ivy, holly, mistletoe, and lily of the valley.

➤ Find out whether any plants growing in your yard are poisonous, and, if so, remove them.

➤ Teach children that they must never eat berries, wild mushrooms, or other edible-looking plants in yards, fields, and forests.

➤ A wide variety of plants can cause illness and even death in young children.

➤ Warn parents to keep children from chewing on windowsills, and so on, and to carefully clean up flakes of paint. Advocate for clients who need to have lead-based paint replaced in their homes.

➤ Lead-based paint can still be found in older homes, and some soil contains a high lead content. Young children often put dirt in their mouths and chew on furniture and window sills, especially when they are teething.

■ With gas grills, be sure that the hose connection is tight, and check hoses for leaks.
■ Store flammable materials (e.g., oil-soaked rags) in appropriate containers (e.g., metal container with a tight lid.
■ Do not smoke, especially in bed—and especially in a home where oxygen is in use.
■ Never use an open flame when oxygen is in use.

Promote Electrical Safety in the Home Make sure electrical outlets have covers. Routinely inspect electrical appliances for damaged cords; replace frayed cords. Do not place electrical cords under carpets, and make sure cords do not hang off of tables and countertops.

Know What to Do If a Fire Occurs The actions you take to extinguish a small fire depend on the source of the fire. For example, never pour water on a grease fire, and never discharge a fire extinguisher onto a pan fire. If there is an oven fire, turn off the heat and keep the door closed. If there is a microwave fire, keep the door closed, and unplug the microwave.

Key Point: *If the house is on fire, follow your escape plan. Crawl or stay low to the floor to avoid the smoke as much as possible.*

Prevent Scalds and Burns in the Home

Fire is not the only cause of thermal injuries. Teach clients how to avoid scalds and burns from other causes:

■ Turn pot handles toward the back of the stove so that children cannot tip them over.
■ Never wear loose-fitting clothing when cooking.

- **Key Point:** *Avoid warming infant formula and food in the microwave. Many parents ignore this advice, so also tell them to always check the temperature of formula and food carefully before giving it to the child.*
- Remove lids or other coverings from microwaved food carefully.
- Do not smoke, use matches, or drink hot liquids while holding an infant. Do not leave burning cigarettes unattended.
- Always check bath water temperature for children and older adults, and set water heater temperature low enough to prevent scalds.
- Place guardrails in front of radiators and fireplaces.
- Wear protective clothing and sunscreen when outside.

KnowledgeCheck 24-7

- Identify four safety measures that decrease the risk of scalds or burns in the child.
- What are some specific activities that reduce the possibility of fires in the home?

Example Problem Interventions: Prevent Falls at Home

Fall prevention may not seem like a lively topic, but it's important. Falls are a leading cause of injury among older adults. Nevertheless, fear of falling should not inhibit a person from living an active life. Instead, teach clients, especially older adults, measures for increasing the safety of their home environment (see the box, Home Care: Preventing Falls in the Home).

Teach clients, if they do fall at home, to take the following actions:

- Do not panic.
- Stay still for a few minutes to get over the shock.
- If you think you are okay, then slide over to a sturdy piece of furniture, get in a kneeling position, and push yourself up; then sit down until you recover.
- If you cannot move, try to cover yourself with something to keep warm until help arrives.

Prevent Firearm Injuries

Education is an essential intervention because of the frequency and severity of unintentional firearm injuries involving children. The American Academy of Pediatrics and other groups have mounted efforts to educate parents so that they will be able to make smart choices related to gun safety. You can help by teaching gun owners that it is important to store firearms unloaded and in a secure, locked container when not in use, and to store ammunition in a different location from the firearm. Suggest that they participate in gun safety courses and know the following rules for safe

gun handling (The National Rifle Association Headquarters, 2011):

- Always keep the gun pointed in a safe direction so that even if it were to go off it would not cause injury or damage.
- Never put your finger on the trigger until you are ready to shoot.
- Always keep the gun unloaded until ready to use it.
- Before cleaning a gun, make absolutely sure that it is unloaded. If you do not know how to open the gun and inspect the chamber(s), leave it alone and get help from someone who does.

Teaching Children Even if parents avoid having guns in their own home, it is possible that children will encounter them in other places. Urge parents to teach children safe behavior around firearms, and to be sure children know what to do if they see a gun (e.g., at a friend's house or in school) (The National Rifle Association Headquarters, n.d.):

1. Stop.
2. Don't touch it.
3. Leave the area.
4. Tell an adult.

Prevent Suffocation

Clients should recognize and teach children the universal sign for choking: grasping the neck between the thumb and index finger or clutching the neck with both hands (Fig. 24-3). It is also important to teach clients the following measures to prevent suffocation or asphyxiation:

- Inspect toys for small, removable parts.
- Do not attach pacifiers, rattles, or other infant toys to ribbons or strings.
- Do not use sweatshirts or jackets with neck tie strings.
- Position mobiles well above the crib, out of the infant's reach.
- Keep window blind cords out of the child's reach.
- Store plastic bags away from young children in a secure place.
- Ensure that the crib is designed to meet federal regulations: Crib slats must be less than $2\frac{3}{8}$ inches (6 cm) apart, and the mattress must fit snugly.
- When feeding children meat, cheese, or other firm foods, cut the food into very tiny pieces.
- Do not give a young child hard candy, chewing gum, nuts, popcorn, grapes, or marshmallows.
- Supervise children's balloon play, and dispose of burst balloons promptly.

Prevent Drowning

Drowning is a form of suffocation, but is discussed separately here for convenience. Teach clients the following water safety measures:

- Supervise activity when the child is near any source of water.

Home Care

Preventing Falls in the Home

Exercise Regularly

➤ Exercise at least 30 minutes every day. The amount of activity depends on age, physical condition, and the intensity of the exercise. Any activity is better than none (see Chapter 32 for more specific information). Tai chi, yoga, exercise classes, and weight training are helpful ways to improve balance, coordination, flexibility, and strength.

➤ Learn to use assistive devices, such as walkers and canes safely. Be sure rubber tips are not worn. Keep the walking aid by the bed at night.

Take Your Time

➤ You are more likely to fall when you are tired, sick, rushed, or emotionally upset.

➤ Walk and go up stairs carefully without hurrying; be careful not to be distracted while walking about.

➤ Do one thing at a time; complete it before going on to the next task.

➤ When getting out of bed or a chair, get up slowly and check your balance before standing or walking. Postural hypotension and dizziness on rising are a problem for some people taking medications for high blood pressure and other conditions.

Lighten Loads—Brighten Paths

➤ Carry things in several small loads instead of one very large load so you are able to see over them, especially on stairs.

➤ Use bags with handles instead of large boxes or laundry baskets to carry items.

➤ Make sure rooms are adequately lighted, use dim light (e.g., a night light) at night, and turn on the lights before entering a room.

➤ Have your eyes checked at least once a year.

➤ Clean eyeglasses frequently.

Don't Trip Yourself Up

➤ Ensure that shoes fit properly, and wear slippers with nonskid soles. Do not go barefoot.

➤ Avoid loose, trailing clothes. Keep hems of clothing at a length to prevent tripping.

➤ Older adults with leg or hip stiffness and pain may shuffle when walking; use of a cane or walker may help.

➤ Check tips of assistive devices, such as canes, walkers, and crutches, for the presence of intact nonskid covers.

➤ Use a ladder or step stool; do not stand on the top step of a stepladder; never climb on a chair.

Clear the Floor

➤ Tape or otherwise fasten phone and electrical equipment cords to the baseboard.

➤ Arrange furniture to provide wide walking areas.

➤ Keep clutter (e.g., toys, magazines, clothing) out of the walkways.

➤ Remove all scatter or throw rugs (or at least be sure they have nonskid padding under them).

➤ Wipe up all foods and fluids from the floor immediately.

➤ Apply an ice-melt product, salt, or sand to icy sidewalks, steps, and porches.

Use Caution on Stairs

➤ Keep stairs well lit.

➤ Keep stairs free of clutter.

➤ Install sturdy handrails and slip-resistant floor coverings on staircases. Fasten any stair coverings securely.

➤ For older adults and those with vision problems, paint the top and bottom steps white or put white stripes on the front edges of steps.

Minimize Bathroom Hazards

➤ Use shower chairs and raised toilet seats.

➤ Install grab bars and use a nonskid mat in the shower and tub.

➤ Install handheld shower attachments to make it easier to sit while showering and minimize the need to move and turn.

Childproof the Home

➤ Install window guards; never leave a window wide open.

➤ Use gates at the top and bottom of stairways for small children.

➤ Never leave a child alone on a changing table, even for a moment. Supervise young walkers to protect from falls.

➤ Remove chairs near counters or other areas where young children would be likely to climb. Push chairs all the way under dining table tops.

➤ Teach children to pick up their toys.

➤ Be sure that children wear helmets and other appropriate protective gear for bicycling, skateboarding, and other active sports.

 For Older Adults or Those With Limited Mobility:

➤ Use beds that are low to the floor.

➤ Keep a cordless phone in each room and by the bedside to make it easier to call for help if needed.

➤ Ask your doctor or pharmacist to review your medicines—both prescription and over-the-counter— to reduce side effects and interactions. This is especially important for psychotropic medications.

➤ Get treatment for postural hypotension and cardiovascular disorders, including dysrhythmias.

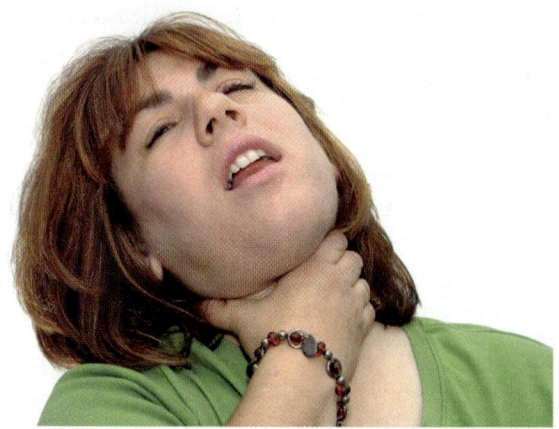

FIGURE 24-3 The universal sign for choking.

- Children up to age 4 are especially at risk for drowning and should never be left unattended in or near a bathtub, hot tub, swimming pool, or other source of water. Even wading pools, toilets, and mop buckets hold enough water to drown a small child.
- Do not allow children to run around a pool or to dive in shallow areas.
- If you have a pool, be sure it has a barrier (e.g., tall fence) to prevent children from gaining access.
- Insist that children use personal flotation devices (e.g., lifejackets, not float toys). (This is controversial. Some authorities regard flotation devices as toys that provide false security; others say anything that reduces a child's fear of the water is positive, because it is the fear reaction that leads to drowning.)

Choking Rescue

Teach adults the universal sign for choking (see Fig. 24-3) and basic first aid for choking, but explain that choking rescue is a skill that is best taught using supervised practice with a mannequin. Recommend that clients attend classes presented by organizations such as the Red Cross or the American Heart Association. The most important thing to remember when someone is choking is to have someone call 911 immediately.

The **choking rescue maneuver** is an emergency procedure for removing a foreign object lodged in the airway. It lifts the diaphragm and forces enough air from the lungs to create an artificial cough. The cough should move and expel the obstruction from the airway. The **Heimlich maneuver** makes use of abdominal thrusts only, whereas the American Red Cross (2008) alternates five back blows with five abdominal thrusts until the blockage is dislodged.

If you suspect airway obstruction in an adult, determine whether the victim is able to speak or cough forcefully (other signs include noisy breathing, loss of consciousness, and dusky skin, lips, and nail beds). Ask, "Are you choking?" If the person cannot speak or indicates he is choking, perform the Heimlich or choking rescue maneuver. Note that management of

choking is different for adults and children. Do not use the Heimlich maneuver for infants under 1 year of age.

For more detailed instructions about the choking rescue procedure,

 Go to Chapter 24, **Tables, Boxes, Figures; ESG Box 24-4, Rescue Maneuver for Choking: Infant Under 12 Months,** and **ESG Box 24-5, Rescue Maneuver for Choking: Adult or Child Over Age 12 Months,** on DavisPlus.

Prevent Take-Home Toxins

Most preventive measures apply to the workplace. However, you can teach clients who are at risk to remove work clothing and to shower, preferably in an open-air shower, before leaving work. If facilities for showering are not available, patient advocacy may be appropriate. (To learn about advocacy, see Chapter 42.) Before entering their homes, exposed workers who have not showered should remove their clothing, then shower immediately. When handling contaminated clothes or objects, they should wear gloves to reduce the risk of skin transmission. Laundering may not be effective in removing certain toxins from clothes.

ThinkLike a Nurse 24-4

You are having dinner in a restaurant and notice that the guest at the table beside you seems to be choking.

- What is the universal sign for choking?
- What is the first action you should take?

KnowledgeCheck 24-8

- List two things a person who works around workplace toxins can do to prevent bringing them into the home.
- What specific safety measures would you discuss with a mother to prevent choking in her 9-month-old child?

Intervention: Teaching for Safety Self-Care in the Community

In addition to teaching home safety to clients, you should also teach to promote safety self-care related to particular hazards in the community and environment. Some specific interventions follow for community hazards.

Motor Vehicle Safety

Anticipatory guidance and educational programs are important measures for improving motor vehicle safety for all age groups. You may also wish to become politically active on the issue of motor vehicle safety. For instance, you might petition your city council for a stop sign at a particularly dangerous intersection or a reduced speed limit on a highway in your area.

Also teach clients the following measures for avoiding motor vehicle injuries:

- Be cautious when walking or bicycling on the roadway, and observe the laws.

- Do not drink alcohol or take unprescribed or recreational drugs and drive. Have a designated driver.
- Do not engage in distracting activities while driving (e.g., using cell phones, texting, changing the music, applying cosmetics).
- Observe the speed limits.
- Always wear seat belts while driving, and periodically check belts to ensure safe operation.
- Make certain children are properly buckled in age-appropriate safety seats in the back seat of the car. If in doubt about the appropriateness or use of safety seats, ask the local police department to check the installation of your child safety seat. See Table 24-4 for types of car safety seats.

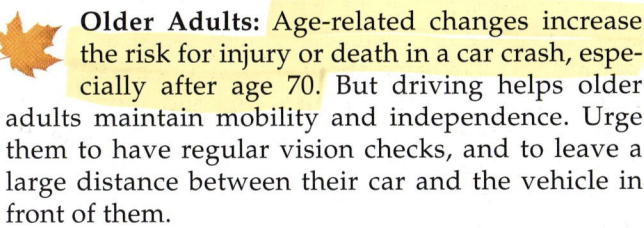 **Older Adults:** Age-related changes increase the risk for injury or death in a car crash, especially after age 70. But driving helps older adults maintain mobility and independence. Urge them to have regular vision checks, and to leave a large distance between their car and the vehicle in front of them.

Food Safety

Teach clients safe food handling and other preventive measures, such as the "4Cs of food safety": Clean, Cook, Combat cross-contamination, Chill. For further explanation of the 4Cs, refer to the Home Care box, Food Safety.

Fighting Vectorborne Pathogens

This section provides points you can use to teach clients about strategies to combat the vectors mosquitoes, ticks, and rodents (CDC, 2011c; EPA, 2007).

Mosquitoes Public strategies to control mosquitoes include spraying programs and digging ditches to promote drainage from stagnant areas. Individuals can help by taking the following actions.

- **Remove sources of stagnant water.** Empty standing water in old tires, buckets, toys, or other outdoor containers. Change water in birdbaths, fountains, wading pools, and potted plant trays at least once a week to destroy mosquito habitats. Keep rain gutters unclogged. Treat swimming pools with the proper chemicals and keep the water circulating.
- **Kill or repel mosquitoes.** Use EPA-registered mosquito repellents when necessary, and follow label directions carefully. All repellents and pesticides, whether used by an agency or the consumer, should have the name and amount of active ingredient on the label. No pesticide is 100% safe, so people must use them cautiously. Use "bug zappers" or citronella candles for evening outdoor activities.
- **Avoid mosquitoes, if you can.** Repair holes in window and door screens. Replace outdoor lights with yellow "bug" lights. They will attract fewer mosquitoes, but are not repellents. If you go into areas with high mosquito populations (e.g., salt marshes, deep woods), wear head nets, long sleeves, and long pants. If there is a mosquito-borne disease alert, stay indoors during the evening when mosquitoes are active.
- **Consult the experts.** Contact your local health department if you have questions about mosquitoes or about a spraying program.

Ticks When walking in tick-infested areas:

- Use DEET-containing insect repellant. Reapply it every few hours (or according to the label). DEET formulations as high as 50% are recommended for adults and children over 2 months of age. Use with caution for children. Wash off repellent at night before going to bed.
- When wearing sunscreen, apply sunscreen first and then repellent.
- Treat clothing with permethrin-containing or other insect repellents.
- Wear light-colored clothing. Ticks are attracted to dark colors; also, it is easier to see a tick on light-colored clothing.
- Wear long-sleeved shirts, tucked in. Pull socks up over pant legs.
- Check your body visually after walking in wooded areas, especially in the hair and skin folds. Use a mirror to view all parts of your body.
- Remove ticks right away. This can prevent some infections, such as Lyme disease or Rocky Mountain spotted fever. For instructions on how to remove attached ticks,

 Go to the CDC Web site in Chapter 24, **Resources for Caregivers and Health Professionals, Web Sites,** on Davis*Plus*.

Rodents and Other Animals To control rodents, raccoons, and other small animals, remove as many food and water sources as possible. Advise clients to:

- Cover food and clean up immediately after meals.
- Remove unwashed dishes from counters and in sinks.
- Keep garbage in closed containers that cannot be overturned.
- Repair holes and cracks in the exterior structure of the home, as well as interior walls, closets, attic, and around sinks and cabinets.
- Use commercial traps or hire professional exterminators.
- Participate in neighborhood cleanup projects.

➕ Keep in mind that rat and mice poisons and baits can be fatal and should not be used in areas accessible to children and pets.

Reducing Pollution

Teach families they can help to reduce pollution solid and hazardous wastes, as well as air and noise pollution of the environment. Refer to the following tips.

Table 24-4 ► TYPES OF CAR SAFETY SEATS

AGE	TYPE OF SEAT	GUIDELINES
Infants younger than 1 year old	"Infant-only" (These are small, may have carrying handles or be part of a stroller system.)	Use rear-facing seats until the infant is 1 year old and weighs at least 20 lb (Fig. 24-4).

FIGURE 24-4 Infant car seat with infant in rear-facing position in the middle of the back seat.

Toddlers and preschoolers	"Convertible" (can be used rear-facing, then converted to forward-facing) or "forward facing"	Rear-facing seats are safer for toddlers until they are age 2 yr. It is best to ride rear-facing as long as possible (until they reach the height and weight maximum specified by the seat manufacturer).
School-age children	Booster seats	After outgrowing their car safety seat, children should stay in a booster seat until the car seat belts fit properly (usually at about 4 ft 9 in. tall and between 8 and 12 years old). Booster seats are safer than a seat belt alone.
Older children	Car lap and shoulder belts	Children who have outgrown their booster seats should ride in the back seat until 13 years of age. Some experts recommend that anyone weighing <110 lb, regardless of age, ride in the back seat. Riding in the back seat is associated with a 40% reduction in the risk of fatal injury, and up to 46% in cars with airbags.

Note: These are guidelines, not legal requirements. Some states may also have laws governing types and use of car safety seats. You should be familiar with the laws in your area.

For in-depth information about child safety seats,

Go to the **American Academy of Pediatrics Web site** at http://www.aap.org/healthtopics/carseatsafety.cfm

Sources: American Academy of Pediatrics (AAP) (2011, updated 2013); CDC, National Center for Injury Prevention and Control (2006, updated 2013, and 2010d); NGC (2010); O'Keefe, L. (2009).

Self-Care

Food Safety

Clean

➤ Wash hands and surfaces often. Always wash your hands with soap and water before handling or preparing food and before eating.

➤ Don't be a source of foodborne illness yourself:

  ➤ Avoid preparing food for others if you have a diarrheal illness.

  ➤ Avoid changing a baby's diaper while preparing food.

➤ Wash produce. Rinse fresh fruits and vegetables in running tap water to remove visible dirt.

➤ Remove and discard the outermost leaves of a head of lettuce or cabbage.

➤ Never use a cutting board, knife, or other object that was used to prepare meat, poultry, or fish for any other purpose until it has been thoroughly washed in hot, soapy water.

➤ Be careful not to contaminate foods while slicing them up on the cutting board. Bacteria grow well on the cut surface of fruits or vegetables.

➤ Wash hands with soap after handling reptiles, birds, or baby chicks, and after contact with pet feces.

Cook

➤ Use a thermometer to measure the internal temperature of meat.

➤ Cook to temperatures sufficient to kill bacteria.

  Ground beef to an internal temperature of 160°F (71°C).

  Leftovers and casseroles, 165°F (74°C)

  Beef, lamb, and veal, 145°F (63°C)

  Pork and ground beef, 160°F (71°C)

  Whole poultry and thighs, 180°F (82°C)

  Poultry breasts, 170°F (77°C)

  Ground chicken or ground beef, 165°F (74°C)

  Stuffed fish, 165°F (74°C)

  Roast meats at an oven temperature of 300°F (149°C) or above

➤ Cook eggs until the yolk is firm. Do not eat raw or partially cooked eggs.

➤ Hold hot food above 140°F (60°C) and for no more than 2 hours.

Combat (Separate)

➤ Wash hands, utensils, and cutting boards after they have been in contact with raw meat or poultry and before they touch another food (to avoid cross-contamination).

➤ Put cooked meat on a clean platter, rather than back on one that held the raw meat.

Chill

➤ Refrigerate leftovers within 4 hours. Bacteria multiply quickly at room temperature.

➤ Avoid leaving cut produce (e.g., fruits, vegetables) at room temperature for a prolonged time.

➤ Chill cooked foods rapidly in a shallow (2-inch-deep) container. Large volumes of food will cool more quickly if they are divided into several shallow containers for refrigeration.

➤ Do not buy partially thawed items. Be sure they are frozen solid.

➤ Use a cooler to transport foods when the temperature is above 80°F (27°C).

➤ Store deli meat for only 1 or 2 days.

➤ Use thermometers in the refrigerator and freezer.

  Keep freezer temperature at 0°F (−18°C) or below.

  Keep refrigerator temperature at 40°F (4°C) or below.

➤ Thaw foods in the refrigerator or under cold running water. Use the microwave to thaw foods only if you are going to continue cooking them at that time.

➤ Pack lunches in insulated containers. You can refrigerate or freeze sandwiches before packing, to keep them cold.

Store

➤ Cover and date food.

➤ Store vegetables and fruit separately from uncooked meats.

➤ Do not store food in decorative containers unless they are labeled safe for food. Some crystal and pottery, for example, have high lead content.

➤ Store cleaning supplies away from food.

Report

Report suspected foodborne illnesses to your local health department. The local public health department is an important part of the food safety system. Often calls from concerned citizens are how outbreaks are first detected.

Other

➤ Never eat any food that has an odor or that might be spoiled.

➤ Be aware that some imported folk remedies, such as *greta* (which is used by some Hispanic patients for colic), may be contaminated with lead.

➤ Observe sanitation reports for selecting eating establishments in the community.

Sources: CDC (2005); FoodSafety.gov (n.d.); U.S. Food and Drug Administration (n.d.).

Hazardous Waste The following are tips for safe disposal:

- **Information.** Contact the local refuse disposal company for instructions about proper disposal of hazardous waste (e.g., paints, solvents, pesticides, cleaners, rechargeable batteries).
- **Products.** Use the least hazardous products available, and use only the amount necessary for a project. Share leftover materials with neighbors.
- **Motor oil.** Never dump motor oil into storm drains. For old oil and tires, call your local waste management company or a local quick-lube or tire dealer, for recommendations regarding disposal. You can also,

 Go to http://nextgen.valvoline.com/nextgen_why_recycle.html

- **Batteries.** Talk to an automotive dealer or repair service about recycling or trading in car and other batteries.

Solid Waste Proper disposal and recycling of solid wastes helps to prevent pollution. Remember the 4-Rs: Reduce, Reuse, Recycle, and Respond

*R*educe the amount of trash discarded (e.g., don't buy products that have unnecessary packaging).
*R*euse containers, bags, and products; sell or donate instead of throwing items out.
*R*ecycle. Use and buy recyclable and recycled products; compost yard trimmings.
*R*espond by educating others, expressing preferences for less waste (e.g., to manufacturers, merchants).

Also,

 Go to Chapter 24, **Supplemental Materials, The Consumer's Handbook for Reducing Solid Waste,** on Davis*Plus*, or go to http://www.epa.gov/waste/wycd/catbook/index.htm

Air Pollution To help reduce air pollution, pay attention to air quality warnings, and restrict time spent in high-traffic areas. You might also participate in car pools or use public transportation whenever possible.

Noise Pollution There are many interventions you can teach clients to help prevent irreversible hearing loss. Two specific interventions include avoiding exposure to continuous high noise levels and to wearing protective devices (e.g., ear plugs) in environments with a high noise level.

Electrical Storm Safety Measures

Another safety self-care intervention is to teach clients about safety in electrical storms. They should know that where there is thunder, there is also lightning. Advise clients to seek shelter when they are outside and hear thunder, in a large building if possible. Tell them to also stay away from open vehicles, including bicycles and motorcycles. If they cannot find shelter during a thunderstorm, they should stay away from tall objects, particularly a single tree in an open area; and crouch or sit in the lowest spot possible.

When inside during an electrical storm, stay away from plumbing outlets, and do not use corded telephones, computers, or other electrical equipment. As preventive measures, install ground fault interrupt switches and use surge protectors for electrical equipment.

Intervention: Promoting Safety in the Healthcare Facility

The following interventions will help you to prevent common accidents in the healthcare setting.

Interventions for Example Problem: Preventing Falls

Nursing interventions to prevent falls depend, of course, on the risk factors that were identified at the initial assessment.

Key Point: *Perhaps the single most important thing you can do to prevent falls is to identify those who are at risk for them.*

You will find other interventions in Box 24-4. For a care plan for Risk for Falls,

 Go to Chapter 24, **Care Plan: Risk for Falls,** on Davis*Plus*.

Reducing Electrical Hazards

Electrical hazards are a major cause of fires in healthcare agencies. The following interventions help reduce electrical hazards:

- Before use, have all electrically powered equipment and accessory equipment evaluated by facilities management.
- Participate in education and training programs for electrical safety are mandatory for all employees as established by The Joint Commission standards.
- If an electrical safety hazard is suspected, clearly label the malfunctioning equipment and send it for inspection.
- Use three-pronged electrical plugs whenever possible.
- Observe for breaks or frays in electrical cords.

Preventing and Responding to Fires

You must know your agency's procedures for responding to a fire, including how to evacuate patients from the building. Remember: **R-A-C-E.**

- **R**escue the patient—Remove the patient from immediate danger. Move patient(s) into the corridor, and close doors to the affected area.
- **A**ctivate the alarm—Report the location and kind of fire, and identify yourself. Activate the nearest alarm.
- **C**onfine the fire—Close all doors and windows. Turn off all oxygen valves after coordinating with the charge nurse.
- **E**xtinguish the fire—Use the proper extinguisher. Stay between the fire and the path to safety. Keep low.

BOX 24-4 ■ Preventing Falls in Healthcare Facilities

Provide a Safe Environment

- Determine the appropriate use of siderails based on the patient's cognitive and functional status. *Recent research performed in nursing homes suggests that removing or lowering siderails may help to prevent falls that occur when patients climb over them (Capezuti, Wagner, Brush, et al., 2007).*

- Keep the bed in a low position, except when giving care, with wheels locked (Fig. 24-5A).

- Make sure to lock wheels of wheelchairs, especially during transfer activities (Fig. 24-5B).

- Provide nonskid slippers (Fig. 24-5C).

- Keep water, urinal, bedpan, and tissues within easy reach of the patient.

- Place the call light within reach. Have the patient demonstrate the ability to call for the nurse.

- Provide a night light.

- Keep floors dry and free of clutter.

- For patients at risk for falls, place a warning sticker on the chart or door.

Assess, Teach, and Support

- Provide review and modification of medications, especially psychotropic medications.

- Provide gait training and advice on the use of assistive devices.

- Orient the person to surroundings (e.g., bathroom, chairs; you may need to label items).

- Offer to assist with toileting and transfer activities.

- Educate the patient and family regarding fall prevention strategies.

Policies, Procedures, Routines

- Consider instituting hourly rounds on your unit. *This has proven effective in reducing the number of falls.*

- Place disoriented patients in rooms near the nurses' station.

- Provide regular nursing surveillance of hospitalized older adults. *Research suggests that this can reduce their falls rate by about 50% (Shever, Titler, Kerr, et al., 2008)*

- Ask patients at risk for falling to wear red or brightly colored socks to alert caregivers.

- Communicate falls risk status during handover and transfer reports.

- Document changes in the patient's condition in the patient record.

Sources: Adapted from CDC, National Center for Injury Prevention and Control (2008); Kenny, R., Rubenstein, L. Tinetti, M., et al. (2011); Institute for Clinical Systems Improvement (ICSI) (2008); Joanna Briggs Institute (2010); National Guideline Clearinghouse (NGC) (2003, updated 2008); CDC, National Center for Injury Prevention and Control (2012); Stevens, J., & Sogolow, E. (2008).

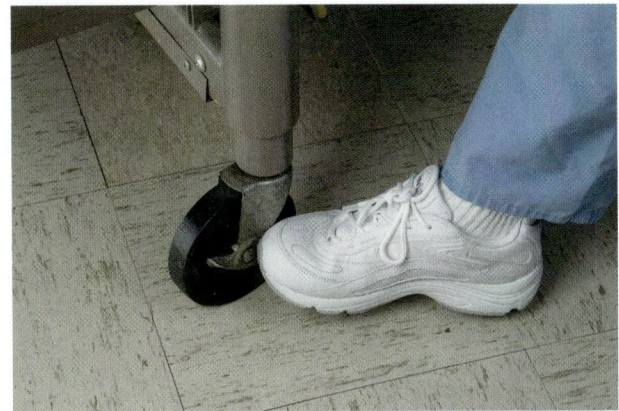

FIGURE 24-5 *A,* Locking the bed.

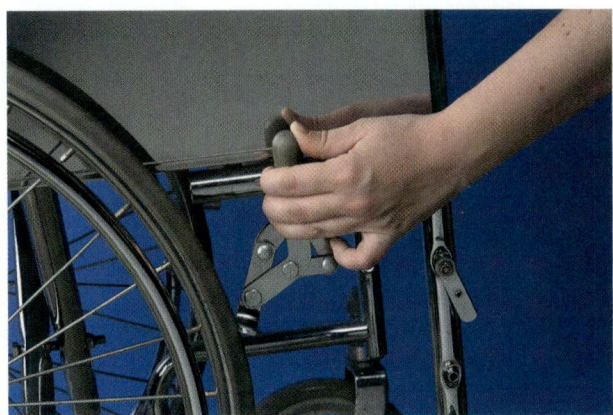

FIGURE 24-5 *B,* Safety locks on wheelchairs.

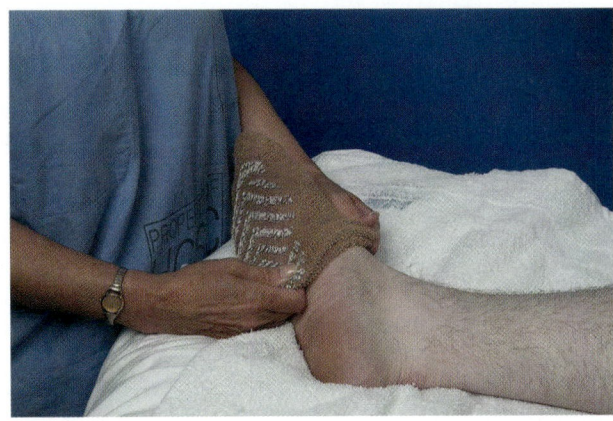

FIGURE 24-5 *C,* Applying nonskid slippers.

Toward Evidence-Based Practice

Compton, J., Copeland, K., Flanders, S., et al. (2012). **Implementing SBAR across a large multihospital health system.** *Joint Commission Journal on Quality and Patient Safety, 38(6),* 261–268.

Researchers assessed by survey (1) nurses' use of the SBAR (situation, background, assessment, and recommendations) standardized communication tool and (2) physician perception of communication quality after SBAR implementation. Findings indicated that more than half of nurses who participated in the study already used SBAR for critical communication. Findings indicated that:

- 72.6% of nurses demonstrated good or high proficiency with SBAR.
- Of 155 physicians, 78.1% said that the last report they received was adequate to make clinical decisions.
- Of the 27 physicians who indicated that the last report was not adequate, 25 had not received the report in SBAR format.
- Challenges included inconsistent use across facilities, lack of physician education about SBAR, and a tendency to view SBAR as a document rather than a verbal technique.

Vardaman, J., Cornell, P., Gondo, M., et al. (2012). **Beyond communication: The role of standardized protocols in a changing health care environment.** *Health Care Management Review, 37(1),* 88.

A qualitative case study of two hospitals collected data from 80 interviews with nurses, nurse managers, and physicians.

Results indicated that SBAR in addition to standardizing communication among nurses and physicians, SBAR may:

- Aid in rapid decision making by nurses, leading to better patient outcomes
- Provide a tool for less-tenured nurses to feel confident in communication
- Reinforce a move toward standardization in the nursing profession

Findings further suggest that standardized protocols may be a cost-effective method for hospital managers and administrators to accelerate the socialization of nurses, particularly new hires.

1. Identify a recent interaction you have had in which communication was difficult. What issues specific to the healthcare setting may encourage communication difficulties?

2. Communication problems among healthcare personnel can jeopardize patient safety. SBAR, a structured communication technique, has been adapted from aviation and the military as a strategy for clear communication based on a statement of the situation, background, assessment, and recommendations related to a clinical issue. Based on the findings from each of the studies, identify specific way that the use of SBAR can impact patient safety

 Go to Chapter 24, **Toward Evidence-Based Practice Suggested Responses,** on Davis*Plus.*

Key Point: *You should try to extinguish the fire only* **after** *you complete the R-A-C steps, and only a* **small** *fire that is contained to one area, such as a trash can. If the fire gets out of control, leave the area immediately.*

Extinguisher Classifications You should know where the extinguishers are located in your facility and know how to use them.

Most agencies use multipurpose (Class ABC) extinguishers.

Class A	Wood, paper, rubber, textiles, plastics
Class B	Flammable liquids, gases, oils, solvents, paints, or greases
Class C	Live electrical wires or equipment
Class D	Combustible metals (e.g., potassium, magnesium, titanium)
Class K	Kitchen fires involving cooking oils and fats

If you would like to read journal articles about evacuating patients,

 Go to Chapter 24, **Reading More About Safety,** on Davis*Plus.*

Preventing the Need for Restraints

Sometimes restraints are necessary: They may be needed to ensure the immediate physical safety of the patient or others, for instance. When that occurs, follow organization policies and always use the least restrictive restraint that ensures safety. To learn about applying and using restraints, see the Procedure Highlights box summary and

 Go to **Procedure 24-2, Using Restraints,** and **Clinical Insight 24-2, What You Should Know About Using Restraints,** in Volume 2.

Key Point: *Restraints are a last resort. The current standard of care is restraint-free.*

The following nursing interventions provide less restrictive alternatives to using restraints for patients who are confused or otherwise cognitively impaired.

Provide Consistency Keep the environment and the caregivers as consistent as possible. Family members may be able to interpret a patient's gestures or understand what is bothering him. To help relieve anxiety, encourage family and friends to remain with the patient around the clock for a few days after admission. Also encourage family and friends to help with care and to bring familiar objects from home.

Review the Patient's Medications Some may affect mental status or balance.

Provide Relaxation and Relieve Anxiety You may wish to try some of the following measures.

- Orient patients and families to their surroundings; reorient as often as necessary. This helps to relieve anxiety and prevent wandering.
- Have family and friends help with activities of daily living (ADLs). This also provides consistency.
- Use therapeutic touch and relaxation techniques, such as massage.
- Use the least invasive and most comfortable method to deliver care. For example, use a toileting schedule or provide a bedpan instead of inserting a urinary catheter; or encourage and provide oral fluids to avoid inserting an IV for hydration.
- Discontinue treatments that cause discomfort or agitation as soon as possible. For example, some patients become agitated and pull at or try to escape sensations from indwelling catheters, intravenous catheters, and nasogastric tubes.

Provide Frequent Assessment and Surveillance Use one-to-one supervision as needed—encourage family members and friends to stay or to hire sitters for clients who need supervision. Place patients with cognitive deficits or who need supervision for other reasons near the nursing station, and check on them frequently. Assess all patients regularly for cognitive changes.

Find Ways to Communicate It is important to communicate with patients who have cognitive deficits. Assess the patient's communication abilities to determine whether he can communicate what he needs and wants. You will need to be especially alert for body language, such as gestures, nods, and eye contact, as these may be the patient's only way of communicating. Speak clearly, calmly, and slowly. Smile, and face the patient. Ask the patient directly what she needs, for example, "Do you need the bathroom?" Word the question so the patient can answer with a yes or no.

Modify the Environment Some simple ways to prevent agitation and confusion are to reduce noise on the unit and provide adequate light. Music therapy is also calming to many patients. Use wedge cushions and body props for patients sitting in chairs to help them maintain good posture in the chair; these help keep them from slumping and falling out of the chair.

Use low beds for patients who are likely to fall or wander. In some situations it is best to remove bed rails. Keep doors to the unit locked if this is feasible and acceptable; in long-term care facilities, also lock outside doors. Have a staff member at main entrances and exits.

Ambularms and bed alarms are another alternative for restraints with patients who climb out of bed and are in danger of falling. The Ambularm is worn on the leg and signals when the leg is in a dependent position, such as over the siderail or on the floor. Another type of alarm is an integral bed alarm, which beeps if the patient's weight is off the mattress for more than a few seconds. For specific instructions about using alarms, see Procedure 24-1.

Anticipate Unmet Needs Often patients try to get out of bed because they have a need they cannot express. The best way to achieve restraint-free care is to individualize care to avoid the risky behavior. Look for the meaning of disruptive behaviors (e.g., wandering). Is the behavior a way of expressing an unmet need (e.g., is the patient thirsty or in pain)? The following are examples of actions to anticipate patient needs:

- Plan an elimination routine based on the patient's history. Patients often try to get out of bed because they need to go to the toilet.
- Provide pain relief and other comfort measures to decrease agitation.
- Provide diversional activities.

Sometimes restraints are necessary to ensure the immediate physical safety of the patient or others. When that occurs, follow organization policies and always use the least restrictive restraint that ensures safety. Also see Procedure 24-2 and Clinical Insight 24-2.

Responding to Mercury Spills

If a mercury spill is not properly cleaned, the mercury can remain in cracks and crevices for long periods of time and cause continuous exposure to mercury vapors. Large spills usually must be cleaned by a pollution control agency and can be very costly. It is especially difficult to remove mercury spills from carpets, so they usually have to be disposed of as hazardous waste. If you must clean mercury spills of 25 mL or less (e.g., from a broken, glass thermometer), consult Box 24-5.

Keeping Equipment Safe

The following interventions help ensure safe use of equipment:

- Seek advice if you are unsure how to operate the equipment.
- Make sure medical equipment has been properly inspected.
- Be alert to signs that the equipment is not functioning properly.
- Make sure that rooms are not cluttered with equipment.
- Follow agency policies regarding equipment brought from the patient's home (e.g., hair dryers, electric shavers, radios); usually these should be inspected for proper grounding and safe cords.

Coping With Violence

Some agencies have a "public safety room." Patients who have been arrested and brought to the hospital for

BOX 24-5 ■ What to Do If There Is a Mercury Spill

✚ Do not touch mercury droplets. Mercury vaporizes; the toxic vapors can be inhaled or absorbed through the skin.

In the Healthcare Agency

✚ If you are not trained in the procedure, do not attempt to clean up a mercury spill. Notify the environmental services department.

- Keep people and animals away from the area.
- Clean the spill promptly.
- If you are trained, use a commercially made mercury spill kit. All healthcare facilities should have them. Spill kits should contain gloves, protective glasses, mercury-absorbing powder, special mercury sponges, and a disposal bag. Some kits have filtered vacuum equipment.
- Follow agency guidelines and instructions in the kit.
- Clean beads off skin, clothing, and disposable items. Place cleaning materials and disposable items in the disposal bag and seal. Follow agency policy for laundering clothing.
- On hard surfaces, use a flashlight to search for beads.
- Change clothing that has been contaminated.
- Wash well. Shower and wash your hair as soon as possible so you do not unknowingly carry mercury home.

- Ventilate the area well to reduce the concentration of mercury vapors. Promote exhaust ventilation if possible.
- Complete an occurrence report.

In the Home and Community

- If you do not have a spill kit, wear rubber gloves and eye protection; use paper towels for cleanup and a plastic bag for disposal.
- Keep people and pets away from the area.
- Wipe beads off skin, clothing, and disposable items. Place disposable items in the plastic bag and seal with tape.
- On hard surfaces, use cardboard to scrape up the beads and pour them into a can or jar with a lid. Then wash the area.
- Shower or wash well.
- Keep the area well ventilated for several days.
- Do not use a broom or vacuum cleaner. These will just spread the mercury around and be contaminated by it.
- Do not flush mercury or cleaning materials down a toilet or drain.
- Do not wash and reuse contaminated materials.

---

blood and urine testing for alcohol and drug levels or any hostile patient who has risk factors for violence should receive care in the public safety room. The following are other interventions for preventing and protecting yourself from violence (Ackley & Ladwig, 2010; Bulechek, Butcher, Dochterman, et al., 2012; Doenges, Moorhouse, & Geissler-Murr, 2010; Flores, 2008; Wilkinson, 2013):

- Intervene to relieve anxiety. Anxiety often precedes violent behavior.
- Treat underlying medical conditions. For example, give medications or check blood glucose levels.
- Administer sedatives such as diazepam or lorazepam. There may be standing prescriptions for these.
- Use a calm, reassuring approach.
- Avoid using threatening, aggressive body language.
- Don't respond to anger with anger.
- Don't defend when the patient is verbally aggressive.
- Don't wear a stethoscope around your neck, dangling jewelry, or anything a patient might use to hurt you.
- If you know you will be receiving an angry patient, remove from the room objects that could be used as a weapon.
- Don't go into a room alone with an angry patient.
- Keep the room door open; do not let the patient get between you and the door.
- Remain at least an arm's length away from the angry patient.

- Do not turn your back on an angry patient.
- Do not touch the patient without permission, unless you intend to physically restrain him.
- Protect others in the environment. Follow the department's safety guidelines.
- As a last resort, use mechanical restraints if ordered and as necessary.
- Your priority must be your own safety and the safety of others in the area.

If you would like some guidelines for coping with the presence of gang members in the hospital,

 Go to Chapter 24, **Tables, Boxes, Figures; ESG Box 24-6, Guidelines for Coping With the Presence of Gang Members in the Hospital,** on Davis*Plus*.

Which Safety Interventions Can I Delegate?

As nurse manager on a clinical unit or as a primary care nurse, you may need to delegate safety promotion interventions to nursing assistive personnel (NAP). Which safety interventions would you delegate?

For all delegation decisions, refer to the discussion and guidelines in Chapter 7. One safety activity you might delegate is applying restraints. As in all delegation, you must first be sure that the NAP is competent to perform the skill. You may delegate the application of the restraints; however, you may *not* delegate the assessment of the patient's status nor the evaluation of the patient's response to the restraints. You may assign the NAP to (1) remove and reapply restraints to provide skin care and allow for supervised movement and (2) observe for skin excoriation under or around restraint location and report it to you.

You should be sure assistive personnel are aware of and follow all safety measures and institutional procedures. For example, you can expect the NAPs to remove clutter and spills in patient rooms, to provide patients with nonskid slippers, and to lock beds and wheelchairs.

For steps to follow in *all* procedures, refer to the Universal Steps for All Procedures found on the inside back cover of Volume 2. Go to the full procedures in Volume 2 to practice and learn the procedure steps. Use these procedure highlights later to help you review key points.

Procedure 24-1: Using a Bed Monitoring Device

➤ Select the correct type of alarm for your patient.

➤ Explain to the patient and family that the device alerts the staff when the patient tries to get out of the chair or bed.

➤ Apply or place the device; connect the control unit to the sensor pad.

➤ Connect the control unit to the nurse call system, if possible.

➤ Explain that the patient will need to call for assistance when she wants to get up.

➤ Disconnect or turn off the alarm before assisting the patient out of the bed or chair.

➤ Reactivate the alarm after assisting the patient back to the bed or chair.

➤ Understand that bed alarms do not prevent falls by themselves; they are used to improve the timeliness of staff response. Patients who are at risk for falls require increased observation and surveillance.

Procedure 24-2: Using Restraints

➤ Follow agency policy, state laws, and professional guidelines.

➤ Try alternative interventions, such as the following, first:

Bed/chair alarms

Patient sitters (nonprofessional staff hired to watch the patient)

➤ Use the least-invasive method among the various types of restraints:

Verbal restraints

Chemical restraints (e.g., antipsychotic or sedative medication)

Seclusion (safe containment to deescalate)

Physical restraints (4-point devices, tie-on, Velcro, leather)

➤ Use restraints only as a last resort to protect a patient and/or caregiver from injury; not for the convenience of the caregiver or as a punishment.

➤ Obtain the required consent form.

➤ Obtain a medical order before restraining, except in an emergency.

➤ Secure restraints in a way that allows for quick release.

➤ Ensure that restraints do not impair circulation or tissue integrity.

➤ Check restraints every 30 minutes.

➤ A prescriber must reassess and reorder the restraints every 24 hours.

➤ Release restraints and assess every 2 hours (more often for behavioral restraints).

Highlights of Procedures 24-1 and 24-2

To explore learning resources for this chapter,

For references cited in this chapter,

Go to Volume 2, **References Cited.**

Go to Davis*Plus* at **DavisPl.us/Wilkinson3.**

Chapter Resources for Chapter 24:

Response sheets for all learning activities

Resources for Caregivers and Health Professionals

Reading More About Promoting Safety (suggested readings)

Concept Map of chapter content

Interactive Case Studies

NCLEX-Style and Chapter Review Questions

Chapter Overview Podcasts

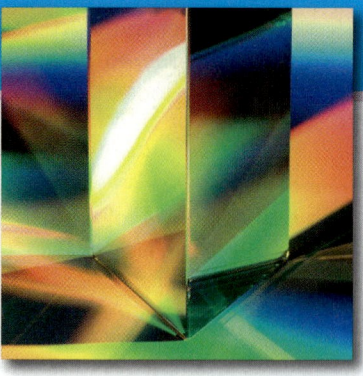

Facilitating Hygiene

Learning Outcomes

After completing this chapter, you should be able to:

➤ Explain how personal hygiene relates to health and well-being.

➤ Identify factors influencing personal hygiene practices.

➤ Discuss delegation of hygiene activities to nursing assistive personnel (NAP).

➤ Discuss the nurse's role in determining a client's self-care ability.

➤ Identify nursing diagnoses related to self-care ability and hygiene practices.

➤ Describe assessments to make when providing hygiene care of the skin, feet, nails, mouth, hair, eyes, ears, and nose.

➤ Describe the following types of baths: complete, assist, partial, towel, bag, shower, tub, and therapeutic.

➤ Apply the nursing process to common hygiene-related problems of the skin, feet, nails, mouth, hair, eyes, ears, and nose.

➤ Demonstrate nursing skills to promote patient hygiene (such as bathing, foot care, and bed making).

➤ Demonstrate care of the eyes, ears, and teeth, including glasses, contacts, hearing aids, and dentures.

➤ Discuss the relationship between a patient's overall well-being and the immediate environment.

Key Concepts

Activities of daily living
Hygiene
Self-care ability

Related Concepts

See the Concept Map on Davis*Plus*.

Meet Your Patients

You and a NAP (nursing assistive personnel) are to assist the following patients with their hygiene.

The first patient is Mrs. Williams, a 76-year-old woman of Indian heritage who was admitted yesterday after suffering a stroke that paralyzed her right side. Since the stroke, she has been unable to speak clearly and becomes frustrated as she attempts to communicate her needs. Her daughter says Mrs. Williams is a proud, independent, and tidy woman who has been living alone and caring for herself since her husband's death last year, even maintaining the yard and garden. She wears eyeglasses for reading and driving and has a hearing aid.

Your second patient is Mr. Gold, a 68-year-old Orthodox Jewish man admitted last week after a massive heart attack. Although his eyes are open, he does not respond to external stimuli. Because of Impaired Swallowing, Mr. Gold is unable to take food or fluid orally. A feeding tube was placed to ensure adequate nutrition and hydration. His oral mucous membranes and lips are dry and crusty. He is incontinent of urine and stool. Mr. Gold's son, Ira, tells you

that throughout his life Mr. Gold adhered to Orthodox Jewish law and requests that, in honor of his father, certain aspects of these laws be included in the care plan.

Think about the following questions now, then again after you have read the chapter. What immediate concerns come

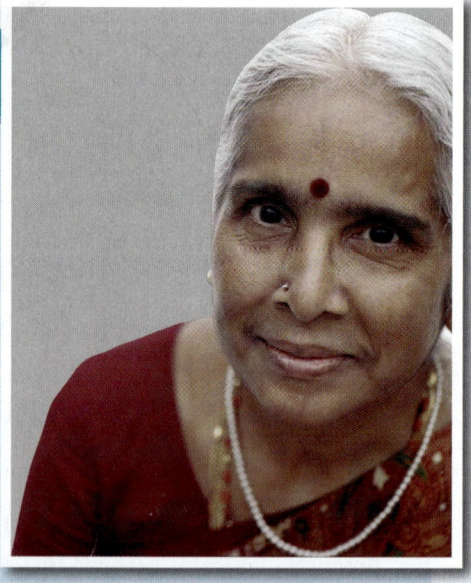

to your mind about each of these patients? How will you ensure that their hygiene needs are met? Are there any safety issues? Which parts of their hygiene care can you delegate, if any?

Theoretical Knowledge knowing **why**

This chapter provides the theoretical knowledge you need to answer the preceding questions, as well as others that will arise as you care for patients. It begins first with an explanation of the concepts of hygiene, activities of daily living, and self-care.

ABOUT THE KEY CONCEPTS

The concept of hygiene is the broadest of the key concepts because everything in the chapter is related to **hygiene**. However, the concepts of **activities of daily living** and **self-care ability** must also be considered key concepts because every aspect of hygiene must include consideration of these two ideas. That is, you need to know the patient's ability to perform an activity of daily living in order to know how to give appropriate hygiene care (e.g., can he wash his entire body, or just his hands and face?).

HYGIENE AND SELF-CARE

Hygiene describes activities involved in maintaining personal cleanliness and grooming. **Activities of daily living (ADLs)**, such as taking a bath or shower, washing hair, or brushing and flossing teeth promote comfort, improve self-image, and decrease infection and disease. Healthy people perform their own personal hygiene; however, some patients need assistance because of illness or injury. As a nurse, you are responsible for providing the necessary assistance and, at the same time, encouraging as much self-care as possible to promote activity, independence, and self-esteem.

What Factors Influence Hygiene Practices?

Every patient is unique, so as you would expect, personal hygiene practices vary greatly. To reflect caring, expand your understanding of the concept of hygiene to respect and accommodate each person's preferences and differences whenever possible.

Personal Preferences Some people prefer a shower, others a bath. One person may shower in the morning to wake up and feel clean for the day, whereas another bathes in the evening to relax before going to sleep. Choice of soaps and shampoos varies as well.

Culture and Religion or Spirituality Cultural and family values and beliefs about hygiene form the foundation for our beliefs as adults. Generally, people in North America consider daily bathing, use of deodorant, and brushing the teeth necessary to eliminate body odors. However, people in some cultures may find a weekly bath sufficient. Some religious or spiritual beliefs also influence hygiene practices. For example,

Orthodox Judaism prohibits receiving personal care from a member of the opposite sex.

Economic Status or Living Environment Inadequate bathing facilities or lack of money for hygiene supplies (e.g., lack of access to running water or soap) can influence how often a person bathes. People living in poverty must focus on meeting basic needs for food and shelter before they can spend money and energy on hygiene.

Developmental Level Parents and other caregivers perform hygiene care for infants and young children. Older children learn practices that become habits, such as brushing and flossing the teeth. As older children begin to perform their own hygiene independently, they are influenced by media and societal norms. For example, some preteens may avoid water and bathe only under parental duress, but teenagers, who are typically very self-conscious, may begin to take several showers a day. Many teenagers have oily skin and can tolerate frequent bathing, but as we age, the oil-producing sebaceous glands become less active. For adults, frequent bathing and the use of deodorant soap further dries the skin. Older adults may find it necessary to bathe only every 2 or 3 days, use less soap, and increase the use of skin moisturizers.

Knowledge and Cognitive Levels Not everyone has the knowledge needed to make appropriate decisions. For example, some people may not know the importance of flossing. Some women may not be aware of the importance of cleansing the perineum from front to back after using the toilet. Patient teaching is an important part of your hygiene care because most people will, eventually, be responsible for their own personal hygiene.

 Think**Like a Nurse** 25-1

Think about Mrs. Williams and Mr. Gold (Meet Your Patients). After reviewing each of the factors presented, determine the following for each patient:

- Which factor(s) will have the most influence on the hygiene practices of this patient?
- Why do you think so?
- How will this factor affect the individual plan of care?

How Does Health Status Affect Self-Care Ability?

Both physiological and emotional factors can interfere with a person's ability or willingness to perform hygiene measures.

Pain Pain severely limits the person's ability and motivation to perform ADLs. The pain itself, limited mobility caused by the pain, and drowsiness from analgesics used to manage the pain may all contribute to a self-care deficit.

Limited Mobility Limited mobility (e.g., from joint and muscle problems, injury, weakness, fatigue, surgery, prescribed bedrest, or pain) makes it difficult to perform hygiene activities. For example, a patient may be unable to bend over to wash her lower legs and feet, cut her toe-nails, or even raise her arms to wash and dry her hair. A patient who is weak or "lightheaded" may be afraid of falling and be reluctant to move about. Such a person needs help, especially getting into the bathtub or shower. Obstacles, such as IV lines, oxygen tubing, nasogastric tubes, indwelling urinary catheters, or casts, may also interfere with the patient's ability to perform self-care.

Sensory Deficits Sensory deficits diminish a person's ability to perform hygiene measures safely and independently. Safety is a priority for patients with sensory deficits. Consider these examples:

- A patient with macular degeneration (a visual deficit) is admitted to the hospital. Because he is unfamiliar with the new surroundings, he is unable to gather necessary supplies for grooming. You would need to provide direction, assistance, and understanding.
- A patient with a hearing loss is taking an anticoagulant (a medication to delay blood clotting). You may need to provide explicit written instructions about the importance of using an electric razor instead of his preferred double-edged razor.

Cognitive Impairment Cognitive impairment, such as is found in patients with dementia, delirium, psychoses, stroke, Alzheimer's disease, or traumatic brain injury, may make it impossible for the person to initiate his own grooming. The patient may be unable to determine the need for hygiene, much less know how to accomplish related tasks. For example, a patient with advanced Alzheimer's disease may actually forget how to care for himself and will need step-by-step direction. Because the person may also have difficulty interpreting stimuli in the environment, he may be fearful and resistant to hygiene measures performed by the nurse. Such cognitive deficits may require new or modified hygiene plans.

Emotional or Other Mental Health Disturbances These may diminish a person's ability to perform hygiene measures. Patients experiencing altered reality states, such as psychoses, delusions, or hallucinations, may dress inappropriately for the weather or the situation and have poor hygiene practices. Some are unable to make decisions about "what to do next" when bathing, dressing, and so on. A person who is depressed may neglect his grooming and hygiene because of a profound lack of energy or motivation.

KnowledgeCheck 25-1

- What are the benefits of personal hygiene?
- Why should you respect and accommodate your patients' hygiene preferences?
- Identify two economic or living environmental factors that may influence how frequently person bathes.
- Identify one example of a cognitive impairment that may make independent initiation of grooming impossible.
- Why may people experiencing depression neglect their grooming and hygiene?

PracticalKnowledge
knowing **how**

This section of the chapter will assist you to assess for and promote self-care abilities and to plan care for patients with Self-Care Deficits. Plan hygiene care around the patient's needs, not facility routines or staff convenience.

ASSESSMENT (SELF-CARE)

Assess your patient's functional status regularly. This enables you to identify the need to modify the care plan and set achievable goals for self-care. Focus on the patient's *ability* to perform hygiene measures and the need for assistance, not necessarily on the *quality* of these measures. For a focused hygiene assessment guide that includes assessment of self-care abilities, as well as the skin, feet, nails, oral cavity, hair, and eyes,

 Go to Chapter 25: **Assessment Guidelines and Tools,** **Assessment Guidelines: Hygiene,** in Volume 2.

For thorough assessment of those body systems, you can also refer to Volume 2 of Chapter 22, Health Assessment.

Assess Overall Self-Care Abilities

To describe a patient's self-care abilities, use a standardized functional status rating scale to assign a score to each response. Various scales are available, or you can create your own (see Box 25-1). Begin your assessment of self-care ability by conducting an initial interview with the patient and/or family, which includes the following:

Obtain a Health History Identify underlying illness, injury, or disease that might contribute to a self-care deficit or affect tolerance of hygiene procedures. *Cognitive impairment,* such as is found in patients with dementia, delirium, stroke, or traumatic brain injury, may make it impossible for the person to determine the need for hygiene, much less know how to accomplish related tasks. *Depression, psychoses,* or *delusions* may cause a profound lack of energy or motivation, causing patients to have poor hygiene and dress inappropriately for the *situation.*

BOX 25-1 ■ Functional Level Classification

1	Can do alone
2	Needs equipment or device; or someone to supervise
3	Needs hands on help; may also need an assistive device
4	Totally dependent; unable to assist

Assess Cognitive Ability and Physical Functioning

Determine overall grooming and cleanliness, level of consciousness, short- and long-term memory, ability to follow instructions, range of motion (ROM) and mobility, level of knowledge, and energy level.

Assess for Sensory Disturbances Assess for auditory, visual, tactile, or olfactory disturbances that interfere with the ability to perform hygiene care safely and independently. For example, a person who has decreased tactile sensation (sense of touch) may be at risk for burns because he is not able to determine the temperature of the bath water.

Assess Mobility Limited mobility (e.g., from IV lines, joint and muscle problems) makes it difficult to perform hygiene activities such as bathing.

Assess Pain Pain and analgesic side effects can severely limit the ability and motivation to perform ADLs.

Assess for Other Factors Identify other factors (e.g., cultural, religious) that may influence hygiene practices and preferences.

Determine Preferences and Practices Identify the patient's previous hygiene measures, normal routines, preferences, need for assistive devices, or any other existing problem areas.

 ### ThinkLike a Nurse 25-2

Answer the following questions for Mrs. Williams (Meet Your Patients):

- What factor(s) may interfere with Mrs. Williams's self-care ability?
- How can you ensure maximum independence with hygiene for her?
- How might you encourage her to strive toward optimal functioning?

ANALYSIS/NURSING DIAGNOSIS (SELF-CARE)

When a person is unable to perform one or more ADLs, a self-care deficit exists. NANDA International (2012) Self-Care diagnoses related to hygiene are Bathing, Dressing, Toileting, and Feeding, and sometimes Self-Neglect. Except for Feeding Self-Care Deficit, which is included in Chapter 27, you can find definitions and defining characteristics for each diagnosis if you

 Go to Chapter 25, **Standardized Language, NANDA-I Diagnoses to Describe Self-Care Abilities,** on DavisPlus.

Common Etiologies Common etiologies for Self-Care Deficit diagnoses include such factors as Activity Intolerance, Fatigue, decreased strength or endurance (e.g., as in emphysema, pneumonia, heart failure), and lack of motivation. Other etiologies were discussed in the Theoretical Knowledge section preceding (e.g., limited mobility; pain; developmental, knowledge and cognitive levels; and personal, cultural, and religious preferences).

The following are examples of nursing diagnoses:

Self-Care Deficit (Bathing, Dressing) related to Activity Intolerance secondary to heart failure

Self-Care Deficit (Bathing) related to cognitive and emotional effects of substance abuse

When writing self-care diagnoses, classify the patient's functional level if you have access to a standardized scale, such as the one found in Box 25-1. Otherwise, use descriptive terms such as *mild, moderate, severe,* and *total.* The following are examples of diagnostic statements you might write:

Using a scale: Bathing Self-Care Deficit **(2)** related to severe knee pain secondary to degenerative joint disease

Using descriptive words: Toileting Self-Care Deficit **(severe)** related to inability to walk to the bathroom secondary to muscle weakness

 ### ThinkLike a Nurse 25-3

- Which of the preceding NANDA-I self-care diagnoses apply to Mrs. Williams and Mr. Gold (Meet Your Patients)?
- Explain the reasoning for your choices.
- For each patient, what are the related factors for his or her Self-Care Deficit?
- Write a self-care diagnostic statement for Mrs. Williams and Mr. Gold.

PLANNING OUTCOMES/EVALUATION (SELF-CARE)

To see a bathing plan of care and care map,

 Go to Chapter 25, **Care Plan: Bathing Self-Care Deficit,** on DavisPlus.

The NOC standardized outcome Self-Care: Activities of Daily Living (ADLs) is appropriate for all of the Self-Care Deficit diagnoses. For outcomes for specific diagnoses,

 Go to Chapter 25, **Standardized Language, Selected Standardized Outcomes and Interventions for Self-Care Deficit Diagnoses,** on DavisPlus.

Individualized goals/outcome statements you might write for Self-Care Deficits include the following examples:

- Verbalizes satisfaction with body cleanliness and oral hygiene after a.m. care.
- Accepts assistance with ADLs or total care, if needed.

You will use the outcomes developed in the planning outcomes phase of the nursing process as the criteria for evaluating patient responses to self-care interventions.

PLANNING INTERVENTIONS/IMPLEMENTATION (SELF-CARE)

Although cleanliness can contribute to well-being, comfort, and health, it can also be stressful—for example, to critically ill patients, the frail elderly, and those with dementia. Adverse events may include decreased oxygenation or ventilation, hypertension, hypotension, intracranial hypertension, or even cardiorespiratory arrest (Robles, Corcoles, Torres, et al., 2002). This does not mean you should avoid hygiene care for such patients, but you may need to modify it and evaluate patient responses constantly as you work.

Even when a patient needs assistance with hygiene measures, the overall goal is to promote eventual self-care. Even if the patient is able to perform self-care, you might sometimes need to allow him to rest while you perform part of the care, for example, washing his feet and legs.

NIC standardized interventions for Self-Care Deficit diagnoses include Energy Management, Bathing, and Hair and Scalp Care. For other NIC interventions for self-care needs,

 Go to Chapter 25, **Standardized Language, Selected Standardized Outcomes and Interventions for Self-Care Deficit Diagnoses,** on Davis*Plus*.

Individualized interventions depend on the extent of the client's Self-Care Deficit, as well as the etiology of the problem. The following are some examples:

- Demonstrate the use of assistive devices (e.g., to help patient grasp and pull on socks).
- Use hook and loop (e.g., Velcro) fasteners instead of buttons and zippers.
- Allow sufficient time for all ADLs to prevent fatigue and frustration.
- Offer pain medication before ADLs.

You will find a thorough discussion of specific hygiene-care activities (e.g., care of the skin, oral hygiene) in the remainder of this chapter.

Types of Scheduled Hygiene Care

The following types of scheduled hygiene care are provided in most inpatient facilities (e.g., hospitals and long-term care settings). Although they are scheduled routinely, you should individualize these activities and involve the patient as much as possible.

Hourly Rounding (Comfort Rounds or Safety Rounds)

consists of seeing the patient every hour, on schedule. They are done to offer help with self-care needs such as pain relief, positioning, and toileting. Hourly rounding improves patient safety and greatly reduces call light use (Meade, Bursell, & Ketelson, 2007).

Early Morning Care is provided soon after the patient awakens. It includes preparing the patient for breakfast or other activities, such as diagnostic tests. As needed, assist with toileting, washing the face and hands, giving mouth care, and providing comfort measures.

A.M. (Morning) Care is hygiene care that occurs after breakfast. Depending on the patient's self-care ability, assist with toileting, bathing, oral hygiene, skin care,

hair care (including shaving if needed), dressing, and positioning or helping the patient transfer to a chair. You or the nursing assistive personnel (NAP) will also change or straighten bed linens, according to agency policy, and tidy the room.

P.M. (Afternoon) Care consists of preparing patients to receive visitors or afternoon rest. You may assist non-ambulatory patients with toileting, handwashing, and oral care; straighten bed linens; reposition the patient; and offer other comfort measures (e.g., pain medications).

H.S. (Hour of Sleep) Care is given before the patient goes to sleep. You should offer the same care as given in the afternoon, adding a back massage to help relax the patient. Also place within easy reach the call light, water glass, urinal, or anything else the patient may need during the night. Turn off lights and TV, and close the door before leaving the room (according to patient needs and preferences). For a back massage procedure,

 Go to Chapter 34, **Procedure 34-1,** in Volume 2.

Delegating Hygiene Care

In many institutions NAPs perform most of the hygiene care. However, you will need to carefully assess patients to ensure that it is safe to delegate their care. If the patient is unstable or the NAP is inexperienced or unfamiliar with the patient's limitations, you must assist or perform the care yourself. Read What Should I Know About Delegation and Supervision? in Chapter 7 for a review of making delegation decisions.

Before assigning a NAP to assist with a bath, shower, or toileting, give instructions about the following:

- Patient's limitations and restrictions, and the amount of assistance necessary
- Use of any assistive devices (e.g., cane, walker, or gait belt)
- Specific safety precautions to follow (e.g., use of gait belt or shower chair)
- Any obstacles present, such as drainage tubes, catheters, IV tubing, or bandages, and how to maintain them during bathing or toileting
- Observations to make during the procedure and why the observations are important (e.g., skin condition; presence of lesions; areas of special concern over bony prominences and under abdominal folds and breasts; presence, appearance, and amount of urine or stool; or the need to collect a specimen)

Remember, as the professional nurse, you are responsible for determining the meaning of the data reported to you by the NAP. Assisting with or supervising care (especially a bath) is an excellent opportunity for you to assess the patient's level of consciousness, short- and long-term memory, ability to follow instructions, ROM, skin condition, activity tolerance, and overall self-care ability.

ThinkLike a Nurse 25-4

Think of Mrs. Williams (Meet Your Patients). You have delegated her bathing and oral hygiene to a NAP.

- What information do you need to share with the NAP about this patient's needs, limitations, or preferences?
- What, if any, specific observations will you ask the NAP to make for Mrs. Williams?
- What, if any, specific observations will *you* need to make for Mrs. Williams?
- What action will you take if you determine that the patient's needs and preferences were not met by the NAP?

CARE OF THE SKIN

The preceding sections introduced you to the broad topic of hygiene and ADLs The rest of the chapter will deal with specific topics, such as care of the skin.

Quality and Safety Education for Nurses

Promoting Health and Safety Through Self-Care Management

Chapter Key Concept: *Hygiene, Self-Care Ability*

Competency: *Patient-Centered Care (Knowledge, Skills, Attitudes)**

Background. To promote patient health and safety requires patient-engagement and patient-provider partnership. An active partnership between the patient and healthcare provider establishes trust and encourages self-care management. Hand hygiene is considered the most significant action in breaking the chain of infection. Best practice regarding hand hygiene has primarily targeted healthcare workers without consideration of the role of the patient in the chain of infection (Landers, Abusalem, Coty, et al., 2012). Salcido (2012) reported an increase in hand hygiene compliance in healthcare workers (HCW) when engaging patients and having them ask the HCW, "Did you wash/sanitize your hands?" (p. 342).

Scenario: The student is caring for a patient with a surgical incision. A nurse enters the room and begins to remove the dressing without initiating hand hygiene.

Think about it: In this situation what are the implications for the student nurse in maintaining safe and effective care and prevention of infection?

➤ Identify specific strategies to engage the patient in self-care management to reduce the risk of infection.

➤ Debate the value of utilizing the patient-engagement strategy, "Did you wash/sanitize your hands?" as reported by Salcido (2012).

 Go to the QSEN Web site at **http://qsen.org/ competencies/pre-licensure-ksas/**

---

*The QSEN, KSA that is most pertinent is: *Engage patients or designated surrogates in active partnerships that promote health, safety and well-being, and self-care management.*

TheoreticalKnowledge knowing why

To assist patients with skin care, you must have theoretical knowledge about personal hygiene measures and the structure and function of the **integument** (skin).

Anatomy and Physiology of the Skin

The **integumentary system** consists of the skin, the subcutaneous layer directly under the skin, the hair, nails, and the sweat and sebaceous glands. The skin has two distinct layers, the epidermis and the dermis (see Fig. 35-1). The **epidermis** (the thicker, outer layer) consists of stratified squamous epithelial tissue composed of keratinized (dead) cells, which are fused to make the skin waterproof. The epidermis continually sheds (**desquamates**) and is completely replaced every 3 to 4 weeks. The epidermis contains melanin, a pigment that provides protection against the ultraviolet rays of the sun and that together with circulating blood gives skin its color. The **dermis** (the thinner, second layer) contains blood and lymphatic vessels, nerves, bases of hair follicles, and sebaceous and sweat glands.

Functions of the Skin

The skin has the following five main functions:

1. *Protection.* Intact skin is the body's first line of defense against bacteria and other microorganisms that can enter the body and cause infection. It also provides protection from thermal, chemical, and mechanical injury to underlying tissues. **Sebaceous glands** secrete an oily substance called *sebum*, which helps to waterproof and lubricate the skin and decrease bacterial growth.
2. *Sensation.* The skin contains sensory organs or receptors for heat, cold, pressure, touch, and pain.
3. *Regulation.* The skin helps maintain fluid and electrolyte balance by preventing the escape of excess water and electrolytes from the body. It helps to regulate body temperature through the processes of dilating and constricting blood vessels and activating or inactivating sweat glands. **Sweat glands,** concentrated in the axillae and external genitalia, excrete water in the form of perspiration; evaporation produces a cooling effect on the skin.
4. *Secretion/excretion.* The sweat glands secrete fatty acids and proteins and excrete nitrogenous wastes (*urea*), sodium chloride, and water in perspiration.
5. *Vitamin D formation.* The skin contains a form of cholesterol that is changed to vitamin D on exposure to ultraviolet light from the sun.

See Chapter 35 for more information about the structure and functions of the skin.

Factors Affecting the Skin

In addition to a person's hygiene practices, health status and developmental stage also affect skin condition.

Health Status

Anything that interferes with the hydration, circulation, and nutrition of the skin creates a risk to skin integrity. As you read each of the following factors, think whether it would be present for Mr. Gold (Meet Your Patients)?

- **Dampness.** Excessive perspiration (e.g., in fever and certain illnesses) and incontinence of urine or bowel cause the skin to become damp. The skin breaks down more easily when it is damp, especially in the skinfolds. This is called **maceration**.
- **Dehydration.** Fluid loss (e.g., from vomiting, diarrhea, or fever) and insufficient fluid intake can cause dehydration. This causes the skin to become dry and to crack easily.
- **Nutritional status.** People who are very thin or very obese are more likely to experience skin irritation and injury. *Morbid obesity* makes it physically difficult to reach all areas of the body, and can lead to development of odor and fungal conditions.
- **Insufficient circulation.** Immobility, vascular disease, and overall inadequate nutritional status may compromise circulation. This predisposes the patient to local tissue death and ulceration when skin cells do not receive enough oxygen.
- **Skin diseases.** Skin diseases such as impetigo (a bacterial infection of the skin) and *systemic diseases*, such as measles and chickenpox, cause lesions that create discomfort and require special hygiene care.
- **Jaundice.** A yellow discoloration of the skin can be caused by accumulation of bile pigments and is a symptom of certain diseases. Jaundice causes the skin to be itchy and dry.
- **Lifestyle and personal choices.** Some people damage their skin by exposure to ultraviolet rays because they want to be tan. Some use sunscreen; some do not. As another example, many people have skin tattoos or piercings, creating the risk for systemic and local infection and scarring.

Developmental Stage

Infants have fragile, easily injured skin. As a child matures, the skin becomes more resistant to injury and infection, but children need adults to provide or supervise the cleanliness of their skin. In adolescence, the sebaceous glands enlarge, and secretions increase. The skin becomes oily and susceptible to acne.

With aging, the skin changes in numerous visible ways, increasing the older adult's risk for skin problems, such as ulcers and reduced ability to heal. Refer to Table 25-1 for a description of normal skin changes in older adults.

KnowledgeCheck 25-2

- What are five functions of the skin?
- How does the skin help regulate body temperature?
- What changes take place in the skin as a person ages?

Table 25-1 ▶ Normal Skin Changes in Older Adults

STRUCTURE	CHANGE IN STRUCTURE AND ACTIVITY	CLINICAL EFFECTS
Epidermis	Thinner; decreased rate of cell turnover	Skin appears pale and somewhat translucent; slower healing.
Subcutaneous tissues	Thinner and more fragile, less fat	Decreased protection of bony prominences and thermoregulation
Collagen and elastin fibers in the dermis	Weaken and become less elastic	Skin becomes wrinkled.
Sebaceous and sweat glands	Activity decreases.	Skin becomes dry, scaly, and itchy. Temperature regulation in hot weather becomes more difficult.
Hormones (estrogen and progesterone)	Production decreases.	Contributes to drying and thinning of the skin.
Skin	Vascularity decreases.	Skin becomes cool and pale.
Hair follicles	Diminish in number and activity.	Hair becomes thin, grows more slowly.
Melanocytes (pigment cells)	Numbers decrease.	Hair turns gray or white; skin may become unevenly pigmented.
Nails	Thicken, become softer, growth rate diminishes.	Nails tear easily.
Skin growths	Become more common (e.g., warts, "liver spots," "age spots").	Most are caused by years of sun exposure; most are harmless (except for skin cancers, which are fairly common but not normal changes).

PracticalKnowledge
knowing **how**

ASSESSMENT (SKIN)

For a thorough discussion of skin assessment, including how to describe and document your observations, see Chapter 22. However, as you provide skin hygiene you should routinely assess the skin. For focused questions and observations,

 Go to **Assessment Guidelines and Tools, Focused Assessment: Guidelines for Assessing Hygiene** (section entitled Skin), in Volume 2.

Patients may be sensitive about skin problems or poor hygiene practices, so as you interview and examine the patient, do so in a nonjudgmental, respectful manner. Protect the patient's privacy by closing the curtain and exposing only the area being bathed or examined. Be mindful of the room temperature, and try to reduce drafts to avoid chilling the patient.

Subjective Data Ask the patient about his usual bathing and skin care practices and preferences, as well as the following:

- Past and current skin problems, including their effects on the patient's life
- Prescription and over-the-counter (OTC) or herbal remedies used to treat any skin problems
- Allergic skin reactions to food, medications, plants, skin care products, or other substances
- History of diseases or other factors that are known to cause skin problems, for example, decreased mobility, decreased circulation, incontinence, inadequate nutrition, or deficient knowledge

Objective Data Inspect each area of the skin in an orderly, head-to-toe manner, noting overall cleanliness, condition, color, texture, turgor, hydration, and temperature. Also look for rashes, lumps, lesions, and cracking. Look for drainage from wounds or around tubes. Observe for the following changes in skin color:

- **Pallor** in a light-skinned person may appear as pale skin without underlying pink tones. In a dark-skinned person, observe for an ashen gray or yellow color.
- **Erythema** is redness of the skin. It is related to vasodilation and inflammation. It is difficult to see in dark-skinned people, so you may discover it by palpating the skin for areas of increased warmth.
- **Jaundice**, a yellow discoloration of the skin, occurs in patients with impaired liver function. It is best seen in the sclerae of the eyes.
- **Cyanosis**, a bluish coloring of the skin, is caused by decreased peripheral circulation or decreased oxygenation of the blood. It may be related to cardiac, pulmonary, or peripheral vascular problems (e.g., arteriosclerosis). In dark-skinned patients, you can best see cyanosis by examining the conjunctivae, tongue, buccal mucosa, and palms and soles for a dull dark color.

KnowledgeCheck 25-3

- True or False: The professional nurse is responsible for making assessments.
- True or False: Assisting with the bath is an excellent time to assess the patient.
- To inspect for pallor in a dark-skinned person, which areas would you assess for an ashen gray or yellow color?
- What is the term that means "a bluish color of the skin"?
- Name two physiological causes of erythema.
- Where can you best see jaundice?

ANALYSIS/NURSING DIAGNOSIS (SKIN)

You should be familiar with the following common skin problems and observe for them as you provide skin care:

- **Pruritus** (itching) may lead to scratching and breaks in the skin and skin.
- **Dry skin** tends to crack, burn, or itch.
- **Maceration** is softening of the skin from prolonged moisture (e.g., urinary incontinence). It makes the epidermis more susceptible to injury.
- **Excoriation** is a loss of the superficial layers of the skin caused, for example, by scratching and by the digestive enzymes in feces.
- **Abrasion**, a rubbing away of the epidermal layer of the skin, especially over bony areas or prominences, is often caused by friction or shearing forces that occur when a patient moves or is moved in bed.
- **Pressure ulcers** are lesions caused by tissue compression and inadequate perfusion. See Chapter 35.
- **Acne** is an inflammation of the sebaceous glands that is common among adolescents and young adults.
- **Burns** are a type of traumatic injury caused by thermal, electrical, chemical, or radioactive agents.
  To see illustrations of most of those skin problems,

 Go to Chapter 22, **Procedure 22-2** and the **Abnormal Atlas** at the end of the chapter, in Volume 2.

Impaired Skin Integrity as the Problem

When you wish to focus on prevention or treatment of the *skin condition*, use the following NANDA-I (2012) diagnostic labels.

- **Risk for Impaired Skin Integrity.** *Definition:* At risk for alteration in epidermis and/or dermis.
  Risk factors: NANDA-I lists about 20 specific risk factors (e.g., radiation, extremes of age). It may be easier for you to remember the general conditions that affect the skin: dampness, dehydration, insufficient circulation, nutritional status (thin or obese), skin diseases, systemic diseases, and jaundice.
  Example: Risk for Impaired Skin Integrity related to immobility secondary to casts and traction
- **Impaired Skin Integrity.** *Definition:* Altered epidermis and/or dermis.
  Defining characteristics: Invasion of body structures, destruction of skin layers (dermis), disruption of skin surface (epidermis).
  Example: Impaired Skin Integrity related to decreased peripheral circulation secondary to arteriosclerosis

Impaired Skin Integrity as the Etiology

Impaired Skin Integrity may be the etiology of other nursing diagnoses. Certain skin problems place the patient at risk for infection by causing cracks or breaks in the skin. Others may contribute to discomfort and low self-esteem. The following are examples:

Risk for Infection related to skin lacerations and abrasions

Situational Low Self-Esteem related to appearance and self-consciousness about skin lesions secondary to severe eczema

 Think**Like a Nurse** 25-5

- Why are Mrs. Williams and Mr. Gold (Meet Your Patients) at risk for Impaired Skin Integrity?
- What are the specific kinds of skin integrity problems that pose an increased risk to both patients?

 PLANNING OUTCOMES/EVALUATION (SKIN)

For *NOC standardized outcomes* for problems of the skin, feet, nails, mouth, teeth, hair, eyes, ears, and nose,

 Go to Chapter 25, **Standardized Language, Selected Standardized Outcomes and Interventions for Hygiene Diagnoses,** on DavisPlus.

Two examples of NOC skin outcomes are Tissue Integrity: Skin and Mucous Membranes, and Self-Care: Hygiene.

Individualized goals/outcome statements you might write for a patient with skin problems include the following:

- Skin will remain intact and free of secretions.
- Skin will remain free of lesions.
- Patient will follow regimen to improve skin dryness.

 PLANNING INTERVENTIONS/IMPLEMENTATION (SKIN)

Some examples of *NIC standardized interventions* for skin integrity and skin care are Bathing, Perineal Care, and Wound Care. For others,

 Go to Chapter 25, **Standardized Language, Standardized Outcomes and Interventions for Hygiene Problems,** on DavisPlus.

Individualized nursing activities for patients with Impaired Skin Integrity include bathing and massage, which are presented in this section. You will usually delegate patient bathing to NAPs (Fig. 25-1). Therefore, your most important interventions may be to be certain that the patient actually gets a bath.

Bathing Bathing serves three purposes: health, social interaction, and pleasure or relaxation. Bathing removes perspiration and bacteria from the skin surface, helping to prevent body odor. The warmth from the warm water or bath wipes and the friction of bathing dilate the blood vessels near the surface of the skin,

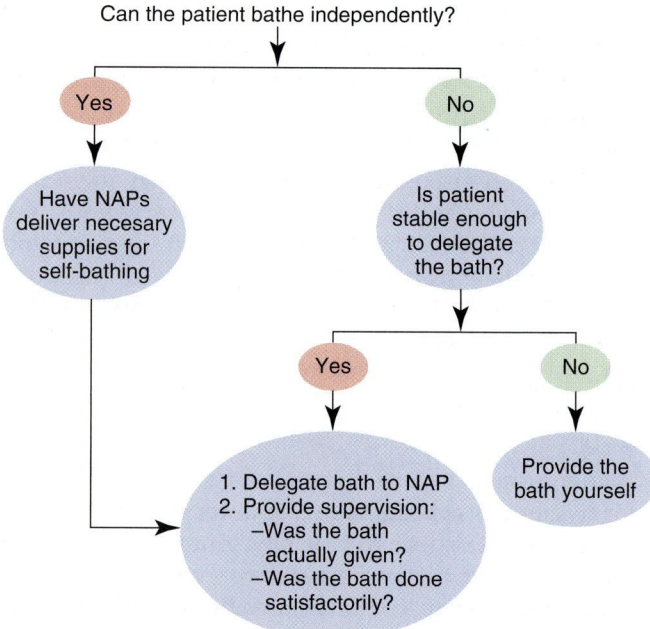

FIGURE 25-1 The RN should assess the patient, delegate bathing as appropriate, and provide supervision.

increasing the circulation. Bathing stimulates depth of respirations and provides sensory input. It can also be a time to strengthen the nurse–patient relationship, promote relaxation and comfort, enhance well-being, and improve self-image.

Back Massage Regardless of the type of bath used, when possible end the bath with a back massage to provide relaxation and stimulate circulation. As with all procedures, be sure there are no contraindications to massage (e.g., fractured ribs, burns, recent heart surgery). To learn a procedure for giving a back massage,

 Go to Chapter 34, **Procedure 34-1,** in Volume 2.

Choosing the Type of Bath to Meet Patient Needs

The type of bath you give depends on your nursing judgment; the patient's preference, self-care ability, and endurance; and the medical plan of care. **"Assist" bath** is a term commonly used to indicate that the nurse helps the patient with areas that may be difficult to reach, such as the back, feet, and legs. If a complete bath would be stressful to the patient, you may sometimes give a **partial bath**; that is, you will cleanse only the areas that may cause odor or discomfort, such as the axillae and perineum. A **complete bath** means you will wash the patient's entire body without assistance from the patient. For complete instructions,

 Go to **Procedure 25-1: Bathing: Providing a Complete Bed Bath Using a Prepackaged Bathing Product,** in Volume 2.

The following sections discuss other types of baths in detail.

Bed Baths and Modified Bed Baths

A **bed bath** is for patients who must remain in bed but who are able to bathe themselves. You will assist by placing the bath supplies on the bedside stand or overbed table.

Recent evidence supports the now widespread use of **prepackaged bathing products** (Clark & John, 2006). Prepackaged bathing products are a set of commercially prepared and packaged, premoistened, disposable washcloths that are warmed prior to use. Recent guidelines recommend the use of prepackaged bathing products. Studies suggest the following benefits:

- Helps assure consistency of bathing technique among caregivers
- Prevents inconsistent applications of emollients (moisturizers)
- Decreases the skin damage due to rough washcloths
- Decreases the potential for colonization of the skin and the spread of microorganisms with the use of tap water and basins. This is especially true of products containing chlorhexadine (Johnson, Lineweaver, & Maze, 2009; Ritz, Pashnik, Padula, et al., 2012; Rubin, Louthan, Wessels, et al., 2013; Sievert, Armola, & Halm, 2011).

Be certain the patient knows what the packaged bath is for and how to use it. Provide privacy, and place the call device within reach. If the patient cannot bathe all areas of his body, complete the bath for him.

The following are three modified types of bed bath:

- A **towel bath** is a type of bed bath in which you place a large towel and a bath blanket in a plastic bag, saturate them with a warmed, commercially prepared mixture, and use them to bathe the patient. Because the solution dries rapidly, there is no need to towel-dry the patient. Patients find towel baths satisfactory, and some agencies prefer towel baths because they take less time than a traditional bed bath. This is a preferred method for patients who have mild to moderate Impaired Skin Integrity or Activity Intolerance and for patients with dementia (e.g., Alzheimer's disease). See Procedure 25-2.
- A **bag bath** is a modification of the towel bath, in which you use 8 to 10 washcloths instead of a towel and bath blanket. They are moistened with water (preferably sterile, filtered, or distilled) or a pH-balanced no-rinse soap. They are then warmed and each part of the patient's body is cleansed with a fresh cloth.
- A **basin and water bath** is a type of bed bath, in which you use a disposable basin with water; washcloths; lotion; and a pH-balanced, no-rinse soap or a chlorhexidine-and-water solution. This may be done, for instance, if a patient refuses the prepackaged bath or if the patient is grossly soiled (i.e., large amounts of blood or feces). When you use a basin and water bath, you must be aware of the potential for healthcare-acquired infections (HAIs) related to (1) reusable basins and (2) the presence of biofilm in hospital waterlines and plumbing.

- Keep in mind that the potential exists for a bath basin to become a reservoir for microorganisms, leading to cross-contamination of the immediate environment and healthcare personnel. Therefore, if you must provide this type of bath, most recommendations are to use a disposable basin and not to re-use it.
- **Bath water.** Depending on the agency and the patient's condition, it may be safer to use of distilled, sterile, or filtered water in place of tap water to prevent skin contamination with bacteria biofilm. Some agencies have a serious problem with biofilm, whereas others do not; and some agencies have filtering systems that make the water safe to use. You must know the situation and the policy in your institution. When using tap water, it is a good idea to bathe the patient with a solution of chlorhexadine and water to combat any bacteria that may be present (Rubin, Louthan, Wessels, et al., 2013; Rutala, Weber, & HICPAC, 2008).

Key Point. *One size does not fit all! The more vulnerable the patient, the more caution you must exercise regarding basin and water bathing.*

Examples of patients who need special measures include the frail elderly, newborns, the critically ill, those who are immunocompromised, those having recent surgery or other loss of skin integrity, and patients requiring mechanical ventilation.

For the AACN guidelines for bathing adults, see Box 25-2.

Key Point: *Guidelines change frequently; be alert for practice changes.*

Shower

Most ambulatory patients prefer a shower. It is a time-saver and refreshing as well as cleansing. In a hospital or long-term care facility, some clients can manage a shower mostly on their own. You may need to prepare the client's bathing supplies, assist her to the shower, and help with areas of her body that she cannot reach. For complete information,

 Go to Chapter 25, **Clinical Insight 25-1: Assisting With a Shower or Tub Bath,** in Volume 2.

You will need to be sure the shower is clean and safe and that the water system is monitored as required by the healthcare agency. Primary prevention measures for nosocomial infections includes ensuring that the water system is designed and maintained in accordance with national standards, including the following:

- The hot water is maintained above 55°C (131°F).
- Routine sampling for bacteria is done.

Avoid showering and exposure to faucet water in patients who are immunocompromised or at high risk of infection. Use sponge baths instead.

Most hospitals and long-term care facilities have safety grab bars and handrails in the bathrooms, but these may need to be installed in the home.

BOX 25-2 ■ Guidelines for Bathing the Adult Patient

Bathing Frequency

For patients who are unable to provide self-care, assist with or provide a bath:

- daily or more frequently for comfort purposes (on patient request)
- to respond to diaphoresis
- to address a significant incontinence episode

Privacy and Timing of the Bath

Maintain patient privacy throughout the procedure.

Bath time should be determined based on:

- patient preference
- clinical stability
- patient's physiological tolerance to activity
- sleep pattern (uninterrupted sleep is essential to the healing process)

Bath Supplies and Products

Prepackaged bath products should be used in place of basin and tap water for regular bathing:

- Remove reusable basins from the environment to encourage use of prepackaged bathing products.
- If using a basin, use sterile or distilled water in place of tap water, unless the hospital has a filtering system that prevents biofilm in the waterlines.
- No-rinse pH-balanced cleansers with emollients help to protect the barrier function of the skin and reduce the risk of dry skin.
- Chlorhexidine gluconate (CHG) 2% prepackaged cloths are recommended to decrease the colonization of bacteria on the skin.
- Do not rinse; retain 2% CHG on the skin at all times.
- Do not use on mucous membranes (face or perineal area).

Adapted from: American Association of Critical-Care Nurses (AACN). (2013). AACN practice alert. Bathing the adult patient. Retrieved April 28, 2013, from http://www.aacn.org/wd/practice/content/practicealerts/bathing-adult-patient-practice-alert.pcms?menu=practice

Tub Bath

If a client is ambulatory but requires much assistance with bathing (e.g., because of pain and stiffness in the hands and arms) you may prefer a tub bath (see Clinical Insight 25-1 in Volume 2). It will be easier for you to wash and rinse the patient, and you will not get as wet as when you help with a shower. Immersion in the water also helps to soak areas that are crusty, scaly, or soiled and relaxes stiff, sore muscles and joints. Overall, tub baths are thought to be of greater benefit than a sponge or bed bath. Evidence suggests that hospital water supplies may serve as a reservoir for pathogens and play a role in their spread, so prevention of nosocomial infections related to the use of tubs should include a stringent maintenance and cleaning according to facility policy.

The tub should have handrails and a nonskid surface to prevent falls. Some patients need assistance getting into and out of a tub. Some kneel or squat first and then sit in the tub. For completely dependent patients, there are specially designed tubs that reduce the effort necessary to lift patients into and out of the tub. You can also use a hydraulic lift and a regular tub (Fig. 25-2).

Therapeutic Bath

The primary care provider may prescribe **therapeutic baths** for some patients. Given that current research suggests that hospital water supplies may serve as a reservoir for pathogens and play a role in HAIs, use of distilled, specially filtered, or sterile water would seem preferable, if in accord with provider prescription and facility policy. It is your responsibility to add the medically ordered substance, ensure appropriate temperature, and

assist the patient into the tub. Oatmeal or coal tar baths are examples of therapeutic baths used to treat specific skin conditions, such as chickenpox lesions or psoriasis. A warm sitz bath is another type of therapeutic bath; it helps to cleanse the perineum and soothe inflammation of perineal, vaginal, or rectal tissues. Use a disposable sitz tub if one is available. If a disposable tub is not available, clean the tub thoroughly at the end of the bath, preferably with a chlorhexidine-based product.

Perineal Care

The **perineum** (the area between the anus and vulva in a female, or the anus and scrotum in a male) is a dark, warm, moist area that supports bacterial growth. Perineal care promotes comfort and prevents odor, skin excoriation, and infection. You will usually give perineal care (including the external genitalia) along with a complete bed bath, but it may be needed at other times as well. Give perineal care more frequently if the patient is incontinent of urine or feces or has drainage from the area.

Because of personal, cultural, or religious beliefs, some patients may wish to have a same-sex caregiver provide the bath, or at least be present in the room. Whether you and the patient are of the same or opposite sex, perineal care may be embarrassing for you both. Perform care in a professional manner, and provide the patient with privacy (e.g., shut the door, pull bed curtains, drape properly). A matter-of-fact, sensitive approach puts most patients at ease. For information about providing perineal care refer to the Highlights of Procedures box and,

 Go to Chapter 25, **Procedure 25-4: Providing Perineal Care,** in Volume 2.

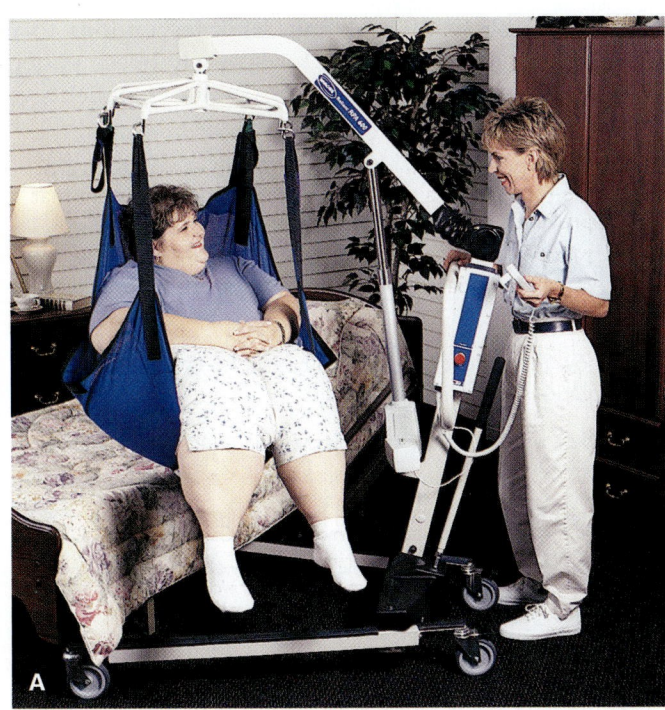
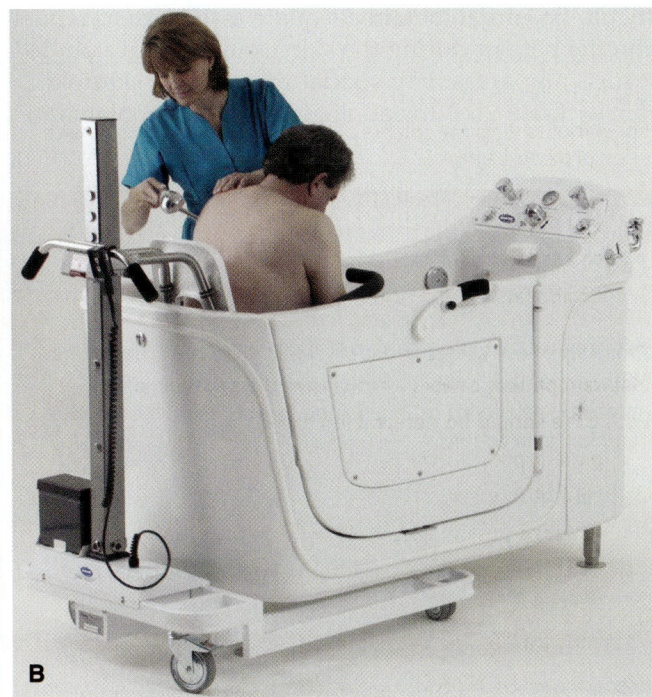

FIGURE 25-2 *A*, A hydraulic lift allows you to transport a patient to a bath or shower. *B*, A tub with a side-opening door enables patients to safely and easily enter the tub. (Courtesy of Carroll Health Care, London, Ontario, Canada.)

KnowledgeCheck 25-4

- What causes body odor?
- What is the best intervention to rid the skin of body odor?
- What is the rationale for providing perineal care?
- How can you protect patient privacy during perineal care?

 ## ThinkLike a Nurse 25-6

- Which of your patients (Meet Your Patients) will require nurse-assisted perineal care? Explain your reasoning.
- Which patient, if you are a woman, is most likely to be embarrassed by perineal care? Explain your reasoning.
- If you need more theoretical knowledge to answer these questions, what is it? Where could you find the information?

Bathing Patients With Dementia

Bathing should be a pleasant experience, not a stressful one. But patients with dementia tend to become agitated when told it is time to bathe, and often yell, scream, pinch, or hit their caregivers (Rasin & Barrick, 2004). The reason for the patients' agitation is usually that they experience pain, cold, fear, and loss of control. When the nurse meets patient comfort needs, (e.g., by maintaining the temperature of the prepackaged wipes or taking special care when washing arthritic joints), the patient becomes less agitated and aggressive behavior declines significantly. Nurses and NAPs sometimes focus, mistakenly, on the need to give a daily tub bath or shower. You can significantly reduce aggressive behaviors by giving a towel bath or bag bath instead (Konno, Stern, & Gibbs, 2013). Despite the common myths about bathing, keep in mind that:

- It does not take a large amount of water (e.g., a shower) to get a person clean. Prepackaged bathing products resulted in the use of significantly less product, a reduction in time to gather supplies and perform the bath, lower cost, and higher nurse satisfaction.
- The bath does not have to be performed at the same time every day, nor in the way "we have always done it here." You can educate families that a shower or tub bath is not the only ways to get clean.
- The patient will not be at more risk for skin problems or infections if a towel bath is used.
- It is not necessary to bathe a person who is resisting. You can adapt the approach, method, and time.
- Patients who are forced to bathe do not "just forget about it"; many stay upset and agitated for hours.

For more discussion of bathing myths and for instructions about providing a towel bath for a person with dementia,

Go to Chapter 25, **Clinical Insight 25-2, Bathing a Patient With Dementia,** in Volume 2.

 ## ThinkLike a Nurse 25-7

Suppose you have been providing towel baths to a patient who has mild dementia. One day a visiting family member says, "My father tells me he has not had a bath all week. What's going on here?" What would you do? How could you help to prevent this misunderstanding in the future?

Bathing Morbidly Obese Patients

Obesity is traditionally defined as a body mass index of 30 or higher (about 20% to 40% above one's ideal weight). Severe, or **morbid**, obesity exists when the body mass index (BMI) is 40 or higher (or body weight is 50% more than ideal weight). For the morbidly obese person, thorough skin assessment is essential, but it is difficult. Be sure to obtain adequate assistance to reposition the patient during the skin exam, so that you do not miss any areas. Pay special attention to skinfolds. Refer to Table 25-2 for etiologies of skin problems in morbidly obese clients, and for interventions to use when providing skin care for severely obese patients. Teach these interventions to NAPs and to patients who bathe independently.

Table 25-2 ► Skin Care for Morbidly Obese Clients

PROBLEM ETIOLOGY	INTERVENTIONS
Hygiene	
Morbidly obese clients find it physically difficult to reach all areas of the body. In addition, they may have limited mobility. Inability to maintain good hygiene may lead to odor and fungal infections.	Ask how the patient handles skin care at home. Use the same adaptations, if possible. Provide a trapeze to assist the patient to lift and reach difficult areas. Provide a handheld shower and long-handled brushes. Experts vary on the use of soap. Certainly the skin should be rinsed and dried well.
Moisture	
Skin in skinfolds stays damp because perspiration cannot evaporate. Moisture contributes to the development of fungal and other skin infections.	Use moisture barrier creams, particularly in skinfolds. Use fans, if permitted. Change linens often. Manage incontinence, including petrolatum barrier creams. If fungal infections occur, you may need a medical prescription for antifungal powders, sprays, cream, or ointment.
Pressure	
Pressure can be caused by limited mobility, by skin folds where skin rubs on skin, by tight clothing, catheters, and so on.	Reposition the patient frequently to redistribute the pressure of the skinfolds. Reposition catheters and tubes often; use tube holders to prevent rubbing. Separate the skin folds with towels.
Shear and Friction	
The patient is at risk for friction and shearing injury from pulling skin across the linens when moving in the bed and chair.	The ANA's (2013) position is that you should use specialized lifts and other equipment to move patients safely and avoid injury to yourself. If in an emergency you must move the patient, obtain sufficient help to avoid pulling the skin across the sheet or other surfaces. Do not use sheepskins. Use a waterproof and breathable mattress cover. Keep linens wrinkle-free. Provide a trapeze.
Nutrition	
Morbidly obese patients may have poor nutritional status because of lifestyle factors (e.g., fast-food intake and other poor dietary habits) and lack of exercise or mobility.	Recommend evaluation by a nutritionist. Monitor blood sugar. Encourage adequate protein intake.

Source: Beitz, J. M. (2014).

Bathing Older Adults

For older adults, especially the bed-bound and frail elderly, you must provide proper skin care and bathing techniques to prevent skin breakdown. At the same time, you should promote comfort and encourage independence in ADLs. Goals are to prevent drying of and injury to the skin. Bag baths adequately address the problems of skin dryness, itching, and irritation. They also improve skin integrity, and are far less distressing to frail older adults (White-Chu, & Reddy, 2011). Use a no-rinse pH-balanced cleanser to further protect the barrier function of the skin. Other interventions include avoiding use of soap, being sure to clean the skin immediately after soiling, and applying skin moisturizer. For further guidelines, see What If . . . Your Patient is an Older Adult, when you

Go to Chapter 25, **Procedure 25-1: Bathing: Providing a Complete Bed Bath Using a Prepackaged Bathing Product,** in Volume 2.

KnowledgeCheck 25-5

- A nurse has given a bath in which he washed a bedridden patient's entire body without assistance from the patient. What is the term for this bath?
- What are the advantages of a towel or bag bath?
- For which type of bath will you most likely have a medical prescription?

ThinkLike a Nurse 25-8

Which type of bath would be most appropriate for each of your patients (Meet Your Patients)? Provide rationales for your choices.

CARE OF THE FEET

Foot care is a necessary part of hygiene and essential at any age for tissue health, proper posture, and ambulation.

TheoreticalKnowledge
knowing why

When providing foot care, you will need theoretical knowledge about the structure of the feet, life span variations, and common foot problems. The feet provide support for the weight of the entire body and absorb a significant amount of shock during walking. Their musculoskeletal structure is complex, consisting of 26 bones and many muscles, tendons, and ligaments. The feet can be affected by congenital malformations, injuries, improper footwear, and medical conditions.

Developmental Variations

Foot problems tend to increase with aging. Because of diseases such as arteriosclerosis and peripheral vascular insufficiency, older adults often have decreased circulation to the lower extremities. This increases their risk for foot ulcers and infection. The incidence of diabetes is high among older adults, further

increasing the risk for infection secondary to delayed healing. In addition, the skin becomes dry, predisposing the older adult to cracking of the skin.

Common Foot Problems

In a recent survey in the United States, 83% of adults age 21 and older reported their foot health to be good to excellent. However, 78% reported that they had had at least one foot problem (e.g., pain, blisters, and athlete's foot) (Institute for Preventive Foot Health, 2012). Many foot problems are the result of improperly fitting shoes.

- A **corn** is a cone-shaped thickening of the epidermis caused by continuous pressure (e.g., from improperly fitting shoes) over bony prominences, such as the toe joints. Corns are often painful.
- **Calluses** are usually found over bony prominences in the weight-bearing part of the foot: the heels, soles, or plantar surfaces of the feet. They are similar to corns but cover a wider area and are not painful.
- **Tinea pedis**, or athlete's foot, is a fungal infection of the skin. It is aggravated by moisture accumulation in unventilated shoes. Symptoms include itching and burning skin with blisters, scaling, and cracking, especially between the toes. Athlete's foot may be contracted by walking barefoot in public showers.
- An **ingrown toenail** may result from improperly trimming the toenails and wearing poorly fitting shoes. The toenail grows inward into the soft tissues around it and the tissue at the nail border becomes swollen, inflamed, and painful. The nail may need to be surgically removed.
- **Foot odor** is produced when microorganisms growing on the feet interact with perspiration. The warm, moist environment created by shoes encourages both perspiration and bacterial growth.
- **Plantar warts** are painful growths caused by a virus. They may occur on any part of the sole of the foot but often develop under pressure points, such as the heel or ball of the foot.
- **Pressure ulcers** are lesions caused by unrelieved pressure that impairs the circulation, which usually occurs over a bony prominence. In patients who are immobile, the back of the heels, the ankles, and the great toes are common locations; but pressure ulcers do, of course, occur over other bony prominences.
- A **bunion** (hallux valgus) is a progressive disorder that begins at the enlargement of the first metatarsal joint at the base of the great toe and then progresses to leaning of the big toe, gradually changing the angle of the bones over time. A characteristic bump occurs slowly and continues to become increasingly prominent with aging. Tight-fitting shoes (particularly with high heels) are thought to be the cause of bunions in the large majority of patients. Genetics also play a role as do some diseases, such as arthritis. For illustrations and more information about bunions,

Go to the URL of the American College of Foot and Ankle Surgeons, at the link provided in **Resources for Caregivers and Health Professionals,** in Chapter 25 on DavisPlus.

Practical Knowledge
knowing **how**

The nursing focus for foot care is on prevention and early identification of problems. For associated *NOC standardized outcomes* and *NIC interventions* for patients with common foot problems,

 Go to Chapter 25, **Standardized Language, Selected NOC Outcomes and NIC Interventions for Hygiene Problems,** on *DavisPlus.*

ASSESSMENT (FEET)

Careful assessment of the feet allows for early detection of common foot problems. This chapter describes routine observations that you can make when giving foot care. For a thorough discussion of foot assessment, see Chapter 22 and,

 Go to Chapter 25, **Procedure 25-5, Pre-Procedure Assessments; and Assessment Guidelines and Tools, Guidelines for Assessing Hygiene,** in Volume 2.

The color and temperature of the feet provide data about circulation and oxygenation. For example, cold, dusky, or pale feet may indicate impaired circulation or tissue perfusion secondary to peripheral vascular disease.

ANALYSIS/NURSING DIAGNOSIS (FEET)

The following are examples of nursing diagnoses related to the feet:

- Impaired Skin (or Tissue) Integrity (feet) related to mechanical pressure from wearing shoes that do not fit properly
- Risk for Impaired Skin Integrity (feet) related to (1) decreased sensation secondary to diabetes mellitus and (2) decreased circulation to the feet secondary to arteriosclerosis
- Impaired Walking related to foot pain secondary to arthritis
- Risk for Injury (to feet) related to deficient knowledge of foot hygiene

PLANNING OUTCOMES/EVALUATION (FEET)

NOC outcomes for foot care are the same as for other areas of the body, as they relate to circulation, infection, tissue integrity, and wound healing. For example, Tissue Integrity: Skin and Mucous Membranes is useful for any area of the body.

Individualized goals/outcome statements you might write for a patient with foot problems include the following:

- Demonstrates proper cleansing, rinsing, and drying of the feet.
- Avoids trimming calluses.

- Wears shoes that fit properly.
- Inspects feet regularly.

PLANNING INTERVENTIONS/IMPLEMENTATION (FEET)

Examples of *NIC standardized interventions* include Foot Care, Skin Surveillance, and Circulatory Care: Arterial Insufficiency.

Individualized nursing activities related to care of the feet are those that prevent infection, odor, and trauma to the soft tissues of the feet. While performing foot care, teach the patient about self-care measures for care of the feet (see Self-Care: Teaching Your Client About Foot Care). To learn how to administer foot care,

 Go to Chapter 25, **Procedure 25-5: Providing Foot Care,** in Volume 2.

Diabetic Foot Care Because of impaired circulation and increased risk for infection, people who have diabetes are at high risk for problems with their feet. If they have neuropathy, they may not experience pain with a foot injury, so treatment may be delayed. If untreated, a seemingly minor foot lesion can progress to gangrene and require amputation. The instructions in the box Self-Care: Teaching Your Client About Foot Care are especially important for people with diabetes as well as for those with impaired peripheral circulation.

Knowledge Check 25-6

- What are some causes of ingrown toenails?
- What is the cause of foot odor?
- Why should you *not* apply lotion between the toes?

CARE OF THE NAILS

The nails are part of the integumentary system. They are composed of epithelial tissue. Healthy nailbeds are usually clean, pink, smooth, convex, and evenly curved. Present at birth, the nails change very little throughout life; however, as one ages, nails thicken, become ridged, and may yellow or become concave in shape.

Other changes are caused by certain pathological conditions. For example, trauma to the nail can lead to nail bruising or falling out; and inadequate diet or metabolic changes can cause the nails to become brittle. Also, patients with diabetes mellitus are much more prone to infection and must be vigilant about toenail care.

For NANDA-I diagnoses, *NOC standardized outcomes,* and *NIC interventions* for patients with common nail problems,

 Go to Chapter 25, **Standardized Language, Selected NOC Outcomes and NIC Interventions for Hygiene Problems,** on *DavisPlus.*

Self-Care

Teaching Your Client About Foot Care

Use the time during foot care to teach your client the following self-care activities. These measures are good advice for most people, but they are especially important for people who have diabetes or poor peripheral circulation.

Daily Foot Inspection

➤ Inspect the feet daily, using a mirror to view all surfaces. Check between the toes for cracks or redness. Look for calluses, blisters, wounds and lesions, or dry areas. If you cannot check your own feet, have someone else do it.

➤ If you have diabetes, have your feet checked regularly by a professional.

➤ Seek professional help for foot problems, such as poor circulation, corns, and ingrown toenails, and for trimming very thick nails—especially if you have diabetes.

Hygiene for Feet and Nails

➤ Wash, rinse, and dry the feet well.

➤ Avoid soaking the feet (if you are diabetic, or if there is decreased circulation to the feet).

➤ Apply a water-soluble lotion to feet, but do not use lotion between the toes, because it may cause maceration.

➤ Use an antifungal powder, if necessary, for athlete's foot.

➤ Do not cut or file callused areas.

➤ Cut and file toenails straight across. Do not use a razor blade on the nails or feet.

Shoes and Stockings

➤ Wear cotton or wool socks, which absorb perspiration.

➤ Wear well-fitted, sturdy shoes with nonskid soles and arch support. Natural materials, such as canvas and leather, are best because they allow air to circulate and perspiration to evaporate. Shoes should allow 1/2 to 3/4 inch of toe room.

➤ Avoid open-toed shoes, sandals, high heels, and flip flops. They do not protect the feet.

➤ Before putting on shoes, check for foreign objects; check that the inside of the shoe is smooth.

Protecting the Feet

➤ Avoid measures that impair circulation to the feet, such as wearing tight garters or knee stockings, or crossing the legs.

➤ Do not go barefoot, even when getting out of bed at night. Wear slippers.

➤ Do not put tape or over-the-counter corn medicines or pads or other medications (e.g., hydrogen peroxide) on the feet.

➤ Do not smoke. This further decreases circulation to the feet.

Seek Medical Attention for the Following:

➤ Pain in the feet or legs. This may be a sign of loss of circulation, serious infection, or nerve damage (neuropathy).

➤ Wounds or ulcers on the feet, especially if they don't seem to be healing

➤ A cut to the feet or lower legs that extends deep into the skin and bleeds significantly

➤ Generalized redness or red streaks surrounding a wound or ulcer on the feet or lower legs. This might be a sign of infection of the tissue (cellulitis).

➤ Fever greater than 101°F (38.5°C).

➤ Confusion. This can be a sign of that a wound infection has entered the bloodstream (septicemia). A change in mental status might indicate low blood sugar, which occurs with serious infection, or if the patient is diabetic.

➤ Foot problems, such as numbness or tingling, decreased sensation, cold skin temperature, corns, ingrown toenails, and for trimming very thick nails—especially if you have diabetes.

ASSESSMENT (NAILS)

When assessing the nails, you should obtain *subjective data* about the patient's usual nail care practices, any history of nail problems, and their treatments. To obtain *objective data*, inspect the nails for shape, contour, and cleanliness. Look for redness or swelling of the skin around the nails, and observe whether they are neatly manicured and trimmed appropriately, straight across. Unclean or rough fingernails may scratch or abrade the skin and create a risk for infection. Other nail changes may reflect an underlying disease process. In addition, the area under the nail can harbor direct and bacteria, which can be another source for transmitting microbes.

For more information about physical assessment of the nails, see Chapter 22, and

 Go to Chapter 25, **Assessment Guidelines and Tools, Guidelines for Assessing Hygiene,** in Volume 2.

ANALYSIS/NURSING DIAGNOSIS (NAILS)

There are no NANDA-I labels to describe nail problems. However, the following are examples of nursing diagnoses related to nail care:

■ Risk for Impaired Tissue Integrity related to ingrown nails secondary to trimming too close to the cuticle

■ Risk for Infection related to loss of skin integrity secondary to hangnails, cracked cuticles, or trauma from using sharp scissors or nail clippers

PLANNING OUTCOMES/EVALUATION (NAILS)

There are no *NOC outcomes* that relate especially to nail care, but you can use outcomes that relate more generally to circulation, infection, tissue integrity, wound healing.

Individualized goals/outcome statements you might write for a patient with problems related to the care of the nails may include the following:

- Demonstrates proper care of the nails.
- Trims fingernails with supervision.
- Seeks care of a **podiatrist** (physician who specializes in foot care) for toenail care.

PLANNING INTERVENTIONS/IMPLEMENTATION (NAILS)

Individualized nursing activities related to proper care of the nails include the following:

- Teaching for self-care (see the box Self-Care: Teaching Your Client About Nail Care)
- Providing nail care for dependent patients (the procedure for care of the fingernails is the same as for care of the toenails). Also,

 Go to Chapter 25, **Procedure 25-5: Providing Foot Care,** in Volume 2.

KnowledgeCheck 25-7

- True or False: Healthy nails are usually clean, smooth, and convexly curved.
- List at least three nail changes that occur with aging.
- List at least four things you should teach clients about self-care of their nails.

Teaching Your Client About Nail Care

Self-Care

➤ Inspect the nails daily.

➤ Trim nails with a nail clipper. (People with diabetes or circulatory problems should file only, because cutting poses a risk for injury to the tissues.)

➤ File the nails straight across, rounding the corners slightly to prevent scratching. Do not cut deeply into the lateral corners because this may cause ingrown nails.

➤ Remove hangnails by carefully removing them with cuticle clipper.

➤ Clean under the nails with an orangewood stick or other blunt instrument.

➤ Push back the cuticles gently.

➤ Use a moisturizing lotion to soften cuticles.

➤ Avoid biting nails.

➤ Consult a podiatrist for ingrown toenails or other nail problems.

➤ Recommend to patients with diabetes, circulatory insufficiency, or nail problems that they seek nail care from a podiatrist.

ORAL HYGIENE

To maintain the integrity of the mucous membranes, teeth, and gums, and to prevent tooth loss and gum disease, it is important to have (1) routine dental checkups, (2) adequate nutrition, and (3) daily mouth care (oral hygiene). Mouth care removes food particles and secretions. In addition, a clean mouth helps to promote a better appetite. It also reduces the incidence of healthcare-acquired pneumonia in older adults and critically ill patients in acute care settings.

Theoretical Knowledge
knowing **why**

Digestion of food begins in the mouth (oral cavity). The tongue and teeth begin digestion by breaking up food and mixing it with saliva. Front teeth, also called **incisors,** are for biting and tearing while the teeth in the back of the mouth, known as **molars,** are used for chewing. Saliva, produced by three pairs of salivary glands in the mouth, also acts as a mechanical cleaner of the mouth. The structures of the mouth pertinent to oral hygiene include the tongue, **gingiva** (gums), and teeth.

Developmental Variations

The first set of teeth (the **deciduous teeth**) erupts between 6 months and 2 years of age. By age 2, a child usually has 20 teeth (Fig. 25-3). Between the ages of 6 and 12 years, the deciduous teeth loosen, fall out, and are eventually replaced with 32 permanent teeth (Fig. 25-4). **Wisdom teeth** are the very back molars on either side of each jawbone.

 The tooth surface wears away with aging and the gums may begin to recede, resulting in bone and tooth loss and necessitating the use of dentures (false teeth). Other changes that may occur with aging are a brownish pigmentation of the gums and dryness of the oral mucosa, which is caused by decreased saliva production.

Risk Factors for Oral Problems

Oral health is influenced by heredity, nutrition, and oral hygiene. Therefore, any condition that prevents good oral hygiene can lead to oral problems. Such risk factors include the following:

- *History of periodontal disease*
- *Lack of money or insurance* for dental care
- *Pregnancy.* Increased estrogen during pregnancy increases the vascularity of the gingiva, so the gums may bleed easily and become puffy and tender. Good hygiene is needed to prevent infection.
- *Poor nutrition or eating habits.* Adequate intake of calcium, phosphorus, and vitamin D is essential for

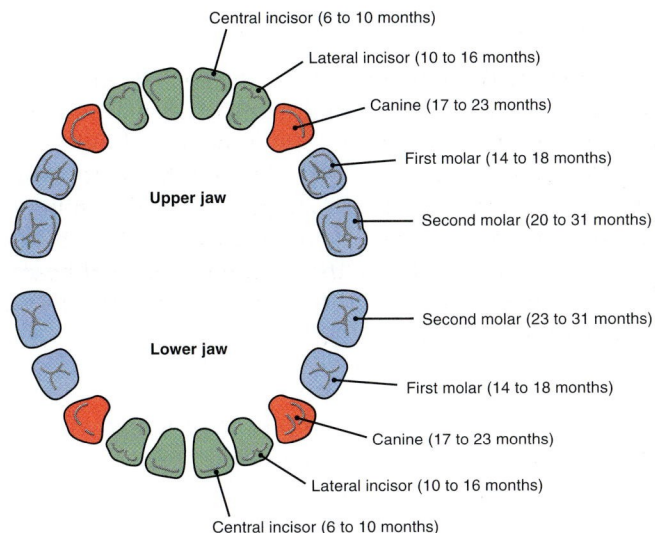

FIGURE 25-3 The 20 deciduous teeth. (Courtesy of P. Dillon (2007). *Nursing health assessment* (2nd ed.). Philadelphia: F. A. Davis.)

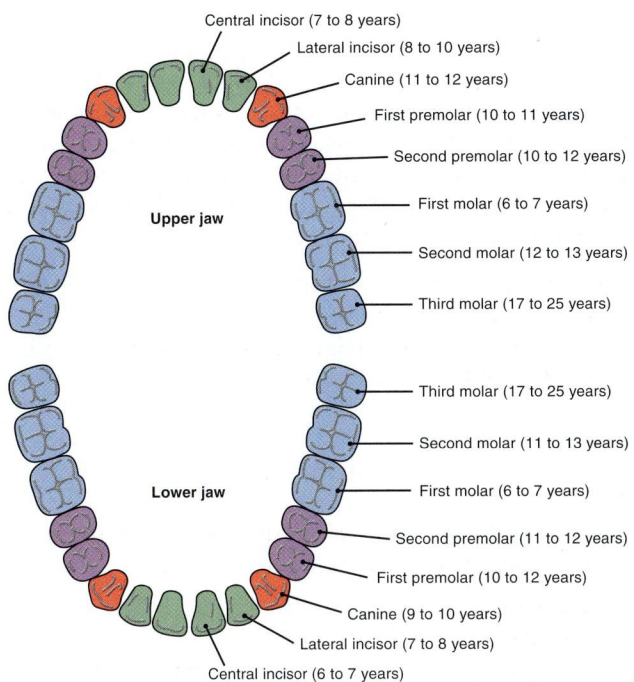

FIGURE 25-4 Most adults have 32 permanent teeth. (Courtesy of P. Dillon (2007). *Nursing health assessment* (2nd ed.). Philadelphia: F. A. Davis.)

healthy teeth and gums. Excessive intake of refined sugars leads to dental decay. One example of this is **baby-bottle tooth decay**, which occurs when parents put an infant or toddler to bed with a bottle or sippy cup of milk, fruit juice, or other sugary beverages. Carbohydrates in the fluid cause demineralization of the tooth enamel, leading to major decay of the upper and lower teeth.

■ *Medications.* The anticonvulsant phenytoin (Dilantin) causes gingival **hyperplasia** (excessive growth of cells). Other medications cause dryness of the mouth (e.g., diuretics, medications used to treat cancer, numerous calcium channel blocker agents [especially nifedipine], and tranquilizers such as chlorpromazine [Thorazine] and diazepam [Valium]).

■ *Medical treatments affecting the oral cavity include the following:*
Jaw surgery, which requires scrupulous oral hygiene to prevent infection
Radiation treatments of the head and neck, which can damage teeth and jaw structure and permanently damage the salivary glands.
Oxygen therapy, which dries the oral mucosa

■ *Any situation that causes dry mouth* predisposes to cracking of the mucosa, including heavy cigarette smoking, excessive alcohol use, inadequate fluid intake (e.g., being NPO), dehydration, and mouth breathing

■ Compromised self-care abilities may be caused by:
Decreased level of consciousness (e.g., a person who is comatose or heavily sedated), serious illness or injury, weakness, activity intolerance, or paralysis
Cognitive impairment (e.g., developmental delay, dementia)
Depression
Lack of knowledge or motivation to perform self-care

KnowledgeCheck 25-8

■ How do the teeth aid in digesting food?
■ How many deciduous teeth does a child usually have?
■ List at least three factors that cause dry mouth.
■ List at least two medications or medical treatments that can cause oral problems.
■ Name four situations that can compromise self-care ability for oral hygiene.

 ## ThinkLike a Nurse 25-9

■ For which of your patients, Mrs. Williams or Mr. Gold, does the Meet Your Patients scenario provide *actual data* to indicate that the patient is at risk for oral problems? What are the data?
■ Why is the patient's nursing diagnosis Risk for Impaired Oral Mucous Membrane instead of Impaired Oral Mucous Membrane?

Common Problems of the Mouth

Dental **caries** (cavities) and periodontal disease are the two most frequent problems affecting the teeth. They are discussed here along with other common mouth problems:

■ **Halitosis.** Also known as bad breath, halitosis results from poor oral hygiene, eating certain foods (e.g., garlic, onions), tobacco use, dental caries, infections, or even systemic diseases, such as uncontrolled diabetes or liver disease.

■ **Dental caries.** Failure to remove plaque is the primary cause of dental caries. **Plaque**, an invisible, destructive bacterial film that builds up on the teeth eventually leads to destruction of the tooth enamel. Untreated plaque can result in tooth loss. The plaque builds up with dead bacteria and forms hard deposits at the gumlines (**tartar**). The tartar causes deterioration of the supporting structures that hold the teeth in the gums and also attacks the bone tissue, causing the teeth to become loose. Other factors that contribute to the formation of cavities include excessive intake of refined sugars, a lack of brushing and flossing, and infrequent visits to the dentist.

- **Gingivitis** is inflammation of the gum tissue surrounding the teeth. If untreated, may progress to periodontal disease.
- **Periodontal disease (pyorrhea)** is the major cause of tooth loss in adults 35 years and older. It is an inflammation characterized by bleeding and receding gums and destruction of the surrounding bone structure. The patient experiences halitosis and complains of a bad taste in the mouth. When pyorrhea is advanced, the gums become infected, and the teeth loosen and may fall out or need to be removed.
- **Stomatitis**, an inflammation of the oral mucosa, has numerous causes, including bacteria, mechanical trauma, irritants, nutritional deficiencies, and systemic infection. Symptoms may include pain, halitosis, and increased salivation.
- **Glossitis**, an inflammation of the tongue, is caused by deficiencies of vitamin B_{12}, folic acid, and iron.
- **Cheilosis** is a cracking and/or ulceration of the lips, in the form of reddened fissures at the angles of the mouth. It is usually caused by vitamin B complex deficiencies.
- **Oral malignancies** must be detected as early as possible. Teach patients to see a dentist immediately if any of the following are present in the mouth: lumps, ulcers, white or red patches, bleeding, pain, persistent sores, or numbness.

KnowledgeCheck 25-9

- Identify and define several causes of halitosis.
- What are the two most common problems affecting the teeth?
- What is the end result of severe periodontal disease?

PracticalKnowledge
knowing **how**

You should assess the patient's oral cavity when performing or assisting with oral hygiene. This is particularly important for older adults because of the association between oral health and systemic disease. For *NANDA-I diagnoses, NOC standardized outcomes,* and *NIC interventions* for patients with problems of the mouth,

 Go to Chapter 25, **Standardized Language, Selected NOC Outcomes and NIC Interventions for Hygiene Problems,** on Davis*Plus.*

ASSESSMENT (ORAL CAVITY)

You might begin your subjective assessment by asking the patient about his usual hygiene practices. You should also interview the patient or examine his records for the risk factors for oral problems discussed in the preceding section (i.e., history of oral problems, nutritional status, access to dental care, medications such as anticonvulsants or diuretics, radiation therapy, oxygen therapy, NPO status, dehydration, and nasogastric tubes). Ask about tobacco and alcohol use.

As part of your objective assessment during hygiene care, inspect the lips, oral mucosa, gums, and tongue. Mucosa and gums should be pink and moist without lesions or bleeding. Look for loose, missing, or decaying teeth; tartar; stomatitis; and note any unusual odors or halitosis. Check to be sure the tongue is normal in color and without lesions.

 The Kayser–Jones Brief Oral Health Status Examination (BOHSE) is used to assess the oral cavity of older adults. It was specifically designed for nursing home residents who have either normal or impaired cognitive functioning, and can be used by a variety of nursing personnel. The tool assigns a numerical rating to findings for: the lymph nodes, lips, tongue, tissue inside the mouth, gums, saliva, condition of natural teeth, condition of artificial teeth, pairs of teeth in chewing position, and oral cleanliness.

For a copy of the BOHSE assessment,

 Go to Chapter 25, **ESG Table 25-2,** on Davis*Plus.*

To learn more about physical assessment of the oral cavity, refer to Chapter 22. Also,

 Go to Chapter 25, **Assessment Guidelines and Tools, Guidelines for Assessing Hygiene,** in Volume 2.

ANALYSIS/NURSING DIAGNOSIS (ORAL CAVITY)

In addition to Self-Care Deficit, discussed in the first part of the chapter, the following are examples of nursing diagnoses that may be useful in describing problems of the mouth:

- Risk for Infection related to mouth lesions
- Impaired Dentition (caries) related to inability to afford dental care
- Impaired Oral Mucous Membrane related to inability to manage mouth care secondary to impaired mobility

Oral and dental problems can be the etiology of other nursing diagnoses, for example:

- Deficient Knowledge related to lack of interest in learning about oral hygiene
- Imbalanced Nutrition related to lack of teeth for mastication
- Pain related to mouth lesions

PLANNING OUTCOMES/EVALUATION (ORAL CAVITY)

NOC standardized outcomes for oral problems include Oral Hygiene, Self-Care: Oral Hygiene, and Knowledge: Health Behavior.

Individualized goals/outcome statements you might write for mouth problems include the following:

- Oral mucous membranes will remain pink, moist, and intact.
- Demonstrates correct technique for brushing and flossing.
- Makes preventive dental visits every 6 months.

PLANNING INTERVENTIONS/IMPLEMENTATION (ORAL CAVITY)

For some clients, you may need only to provide the necessary supplies for mouth care. For others, you will need to assist or even completely provide care as often as necessary to keep the mouth clean and moist. Rinsing with mouthwash is not a substitute for a thorough cleaning of the teeth and mouth.

NIC standardized interventions for mouth care include Oral Health Maintenance, Self-Care Assistance, and Teaching: Individual.

Individualized nursing activities related to oral hygiene include (1) teaching for self-care (see the box Self-Care: Teaching Your Client About Oral Hygiene) and (2) assisting with and providing oral hygiene for dependent patients.

Denture Care

A patient may have a complete set of removable dentures or just an upper or lower plate. A **bridge**, or partial plate, consists of one or more artificial teeth. A bridge may be permanently fastened to other teeth, or it may be removable. Artificial teeth are fitted to the individual and should not be used by anyone else. If the person leaves the prosthesis out of his mouth for long periods, the shape of the gums will change, and it will no longer fit properly. Poorly fitted or loose dentures can lead to chewing difficulties and even nutritional deficiencies. The nurse's role is to ensure cleanliness by teaching for self-care (see the box Self-Care: Teaching Your Client About Oral Hygiene) or to provide denture care for dependent clients,

 Chapter 25, **Procedure 25-7: Providing Denture Care,** in Volume 2.

Oral Care for Critically Ill Patients

Patients in long-term care settings and critically ill patients in acute care settings are at high risk for healthcare-associated pneumonia. This is especially true for those dependent on a ventilator. Ventilator-associated pneumonia (VAP) is the most common hospital-acquired infection in critically ill patients. The teeth may be an

---

Teaching Your Client About Oral Hygiene

Measures to promote oral health and prevent periodontal disease and caries include the following:

Preventing Caries and Periodontal Disease

- Eliminate high sugar snacks between meals (ice cream, soft drinks, candy, gum, jams and jellies).
- Include in the diet cleansing, fibrous foods, such as raw fruits and vegetables.
- Include an adequate intake of calcium, phosphorus, and vitamins A, C, and D.
- Have regular dental checkups every 6 months.
- Brush teeth with a soft brush and toothpaste after each meal and at bedtime (some dentists say twice a day). Bacteria do the most damage to the teeth in the first 24 hours after eating.
- Floss between the teeth daily to remove food debris and stimulate the blood flow to the gingiva.
- Use a fluoride toothpaste to strengthen tooth enamel.
- You can make your own cleanser by combining one part baking soda with two parts salt.
- Follow the dentist's recommendations for topical applications of fluoride.

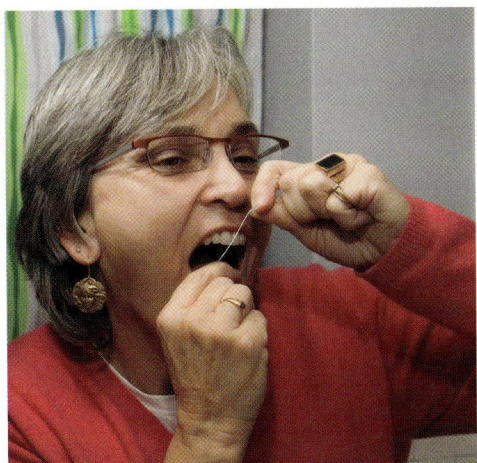

Flossing between the teeth is an essential part of oral hygiene.

Brushing and Flossing

- Make sure the brush is small enough to reach all teeth. If it is too firm, it can injure enamel and gum tissue.
- Electric toothbrushes are effective; however, you should consult your dentist about using waterspray units, because they can force debris into pockets of the gums.

Continued

➤ Brush at a 45° angle, from the gum to the tooth crown, using small circular or vibrating motions.

➤ When flossing: (1) Wrap one end of the floss around each of your middle fingers. (2) Hold about 1 to 2 inches of floss tightly between the fingers. (3) Insert floss between the teeth by gently moving it back and forth; do not force it. (4) Floss adjacent sides of both teeth to the gum tissue, but not into the gum, because you may injure the tissue. (5) Use a fresh section of floss when it becomes soiled or frayed. (6) Rinse your mouth well when you are finished. A variety of convenient flossing devices are available as an alternative to this method.

Oral Hygiene for Children

➤ Begin oral hygiene when the first tooth erupts. Use a washcloth, cotton ball, or gauze pad moistened with water.

➤ Do not put the child to bed with a bottle or sippy cup. Milk, juice, or any other liquid with sugar can lead to dental caries in the young child when the liquid sits on the teeth at night or for naps.

➤ Begin brushing the child's teeth with a soft toothbrush when she is about 18 months old. Start first using water only. Later, switch to a fluoride-containing toothpaste.

➤ Follow your dentist's instructions for giving a fluoride supplement.

➤ Schedule a visit to the dentist when all 20 deciduous teeth have erupted.

➤ See your dentist if you notice any problems, such as chipping, redness or swelling, caries, or misalignment.

➤ For school-age children, parents may need to supervise mouth care to be sure it is done adequately.

Care of Dentures

➤ If you have dentures or other removable prostheses ("bridges"), wear them. If you do not, the gums are likely to shrink, and you will have further gum loss.

➤ Clean dentures and bridges at least once a day, preferably after each meal.

➤ Remove dentures from the mouth to clean them.

➤ Use regular toothpaste or special denture-cleaning compounds.

➤ Do not use hot water on dentures; it may damage them.

➤ If the dentures have metal parts, do not soak them overnight in cleaning solutions.

➤ Store dentures in a denture cup, in distilled, sterile, or filtered water, to prevent drying. Do not wrap them in tissues because they may accidentally be thrown away.

➤ Clean dentures over a plastic pan or towel in the sink. They are fragile and may break if dropped.

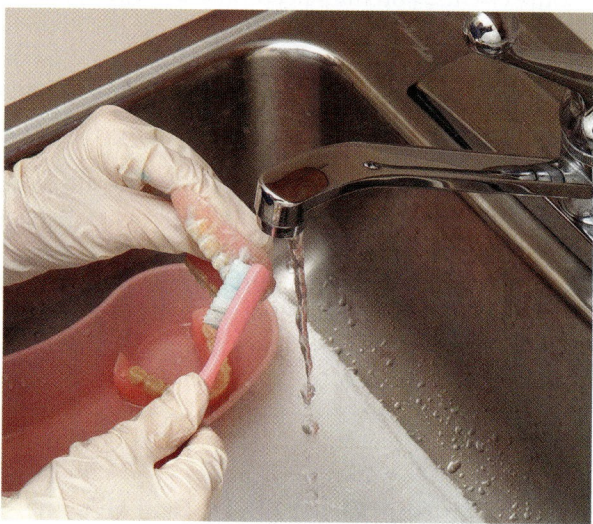

Dentures must be cleaned thoroughly as a part of daily oral hygiene.

important reservoir for bacteria that cause pneumonia. A simple and inexpensive way to reduce the risk of pneumonia for these patients is to keep their teeth clean, thus reducing the numbers of bacteria (AACN, 2007). The regimen includes the following:

- Brush the teeth twice a day.
- Use a soft toothbrush.
- Moisturize oral mucosa and lips every 2 to 4 hours.
- Use a chlorhexidine gluconate (0.12%) rinse twice a day during the perioperative period for patients who undergo cardiac surgery (adult patients).
- Use mouthwash inside the mouth twice a day for adult patients who are on a ventilator.

Oral Care for Unconscious Patients

Oral care for unconscious patients is particularly important because they often breathe through the mouth. If the patient is receiving oxygen per cannula or has a nasogastric or feeding tube inserted, the mucous membranes dry out even more.

✚ An unconscious patient often responds to oral stimulation by biting down, so use a padded tongue blade instead of your fingers to hold the mouth open. Also use a padded tongue blade when providing oral care for a patient with seizures to avoid the patient biting you.

Follow agency practices for the type and frequency of special mouth care. Some patients may need it every hour or two. You may use commercially packaged applicators or foam swabs to clean the mouth. Do not use lemon-glycerine swabs because they are drying to the mucosa and may cause changes in tooth enamel. Likewise, do not use hydrogen peroxide because it is irritating to oral mucosa and may alter the balance of normal flora of the mouth. To learn more about how to provide oral care for unconscious patients,

Toward Evidence-Based Practice

American Association of Critical-Care Nurses (AACN). (2007). AACN practice alert. Oral care in the critically ill. Retrieved April 20, 2013, from http://www.aacn.org/WD/Practice/Docs/PracticeAlerts/oral%20care%2004-2010%20final.pdf

This evidence report reviewed 14 references and graded the evidence for the conclusions they drew. They used a I to VI scale (Level VI = strongest support, Level I = weakest [manufacturer's recommendations only]). The following are two AACN recommendations for oral care in the critically ill:

- Use oral chlorhexidine gluconate (0.12%) rinse twice a day for adult patients undergoing cardiac surgery; not routinely for all patients. (Level V)
- Brush teeth, gums, and tongue at least twice a day. (Level II)

Yao, L.Y., Chang, C.K., Maa, S.H., et al. (2011). Brushing teeth with purified water to reduce ventilator-associated pneumonia. *Journal of Nursing Research, 19*(4), 289–297.

Researchers examined the effects of an oral care protocol on ventilator-associated pneumonia (VAP) rates on ventilator patients in an intensive care unit. The experimental group received a twice-daily oral care protocol of toothbrushing with purified water, elevating the head of the bed, and before-and-after hypopharyngeal suctioning. The control group received twice-daily mock oral care that was similar but did not include toothbrushing. After 7 days of toothbrushing with purified water, researchers found that cumulative VAP rates were significantly lower in the experimental group.

Lorente, L., Lecuona, M., Jiménez, A., et al. (2012). Ventilator-associated pneumonia with or without toothbrushing: A randomized controlled trial. *European Journal of Clinical Microbiology & Infectious Diseases, 31*(10), 2621–2629.

Patients in a medical-surgical intensive care unit (ICU) who were undergoing mechanical ventilation for more than 24 hours received regular oral care with 0.12% chlorhexidine digluconate. Patients were randomly assigned to receive toothbrushing in addition to regular oral care. Others did not receive toothbrushing. No statistically significant differences were found between the groups regarding the incidence of VAP with toothbrushing versus without toothbrushing. They concluded that adding manual toothbrushing to chlorhexidine oral care does not help to prevent VAP in critical care patients on mechanical ventilation.

1. Suppose you are a critical care nurse, using the AACN Practice Alert guidelines. For which of the two AACN recommendations would you most want to have further research evidence?

2. Which of the two studies above provides additional support for the AACN guideline? Explain your thinking.

3. How are the patients in the two studies alike or different from the patients for whom the AACN Practice Alert was designed?

 Go to Chapter 25, **Toward Evidence-Based Practice Suggested Responses,** on the Electronic Study Guide or *DavisPlus*.

 Go to Chapter 25, **Procedure 25-6: Brushing and Flossing the Teeth; Procedure 25-7: Providing Denture Care;** and **Procedure 25-8: Providing Oral Care for an Unconscious Patient,** in Volume 2.

Oral Care for Patients With Dementia

Poor oral health and dental pain affect general well-being and quality of life—specifically, on the ability to eat, type of diet, weight changes, speech, hydration, appearance, and social interactions. This is especially true for older adults with dementia, who have a high level of oral diseases and dental problems. Dental disease and pain may be the source of some of the behavior problems in this population. Because it is a challenge to provide oral hygiene for patients with dementia, staff sometimes neglect care. Residents may be uncooperative: refusing care, refusing to open the mouth, biting the toothbrush, and so on. Research is needed to identify the best interventions (Joanna Briggs Institute, 2004; Weening-Verbree, Huisman-de Waal, van Dusseldorp, et al., 2013). Meanwhile, for experts' suggestions for

ways to provide oral care to patients with dementia, see the What if . . . ? section,

 In Chapter 25, **Procedure 25-6: Brushing and Flossing the Teeth,** in Volume 2.

KnowledgeCheck 25-10

How would you position Mr. Gold (Meet Your Patients) to perform his oral hygiene?

CARE OF THE HAIR

Hair is an accessory structure of the skin. The hair helps to maintain body temperature, serves as a receptor for tactile sensation, and influences a person's self-image. Vellus hair is the short, fine hair present over much of the body. Terminal hair, which is coarser, darker, and longer, is found on the scalp, eyebrows, axillae, perineum, and legs. Sebaceous glands found at the base of the hair follicle secrete sebum, or oil, to lubricate hair and scalp. The condition of the hair is a measure of a person's overall health. See Chapter 22 for more information about changes in hair that occur through the life span and as a result of illness.

For *NOC standardized outcomes* and *NIC standardized interventions* for patients with problems related to care of the hair,

 Go to Chapter 25, **Standardized Language, Selected NOC Outcomes and NIC Interventions for Hygiene Problems,** on Davis*Plus*.

ASSESSMENT (HAIR)

For the purposes of hygiene, you will need information about the patient's history of hair problems or current conditions needing treatment (e.g., pediculosis), diseases or therapy that affect the hair (e.g., chemotherapy), and factors influencing the patient's ability to manage her hair and scalp care (e.g., Impaired Mobility). Ask the patient about special products she uses and about her preference for styling her hair. Inspect the condition and cleanliness of the hair, and inspect the scalp for dandruff, lesions, and so forth. For more complete information about assessing the hair, see Chapter 22. Also,

 Go to Chapter 25, **Assessment Guidelines: Hygiene,** in Volume 2.

ANALYSIS/NURSING DIAGNOSIS (HAIR)

Common problems associated with the hair and scalp include the following (also see Chapter 22):

- **Dandruff** is a condition in which there is excessive shedding of the epidermal layer of the scalp. Primary symptoms include itching and flaking of the scalp, which may be caused by fungal infection.
- **Pediculosis** is an infestation of head lice. Though frequently associated with poor hygiene practices, it knows no socioeconomic boundaries. Head lice spread through sharing of combs, brushes, hair ornaments, hats, and caps.
- **Alopecia,** or hair loss, can be very stressful and affect self-image. Abnormal hair loss, which may be gradual or sudden, can be caused by an autoimmune disorder, hormonal imbalance, thyroid disease, stress, fever, certain medications, or chemotherapy.

There are no NANDA-I labels that apply specifically to the hair. When the difficulty lies with self-care ability, you can, of course, use Dressing/Grooming Self-Care Deficit and Bathing/Hygiene Self-Care Deficit. Examples of other nursing diagnoses that may apply include the following:

- Risk for Impaired Skin Integrity related to secretions on the scalp
- Situational Low Self-Esteem related to alopecia secondary to chemotherapy

KnowledgeCheck 25-11

- List at least four assessments you should make of a patient's hair.
- What is pediculosis?
- What is alopecia?

PLANNING OUTCOMES/EVALUATION (HAIR)

As always, select outcomes based on the client's nursing diagnoses. *Individualized goals/outcome statements* you might write for a patient with problems related to the hair include the following:

- Scalp and hair are clean.
- By 9/18, brushes own hair.
- Hair and scalp are free from infestation, infection, irritation, or dryness.
- Verbalizes improved comfort and self-esteem.

PLANNING INTERVENTIONS/IMPLEMENTATION (HAIR)

Individualized nursing activities related to the care of the hair include daily brushing and combing of the hair, shampooing, and, for men, shaving and beard.

Providing Hair Care

Brush the hair daily to remove tangles, massage the scalp, stimulate the circulation, and distribute oil down the hair shaft. Use a stiff-bristled brush, but be sure the bristles are not sharp enough to injure the patient's scalp. Likewise, a comb with broken or uneven teeth or one that is too fine can break or snarl the hair or scrape the scalp. Comb tightly curled hair with a wide-toothed comb or pick. Encourage patients to brush and comb their own hair, if they are able to do so. Encouraging family members to assist with hair care will involve them in the patient's care and reduce feelings of helplessness. Do not cut a patient's hair unless he or she consents to the haircut. For a summary of a procedure for shampooing the hair, see the Highlights of Procedures box. For complete steps,

 Go to Chapter 25, **Procedure 25-9: Shampooing the Hair,** in Volume 2.

Shampooing the Hair Shampooing cleans the hair and scalp. It is soothing and relaxing to many patients. Hair can be shampooed while the person is in the shower, standing or sitting over a sink, or in bed. Protect the patient's eyes with a dry washcloth, and make sure the water temperature is appropriate for the patient. For patients who are unable to tolerate a standard shampoo procedure, you can use a dry shampoo as an alternative. However, it is not as effective as shampooing with water. Commercially prepared shampoo caps are available and have, in most institutions, replaced the dry shampoo method.

Hair Care for African Americans Hair care is equally important for all patients, so if a patient's hair requires special care, you must learn how to do it. The hair of African Americans varies in texture from some other ethnicities—it may be long or short, straight or kinky, thick or thin. Worn naturally, very curly hair can easily become entangled or matted, and it tends to be fragile and easily broken. The scalp also tends to be dry. The hair requires careful handling, especially if it has been chemically straightened, relaxed, or curled. Shampoo and groom the hair according to the person's preference, of course. In general, though, you should comb and brush the hair daily and apply a light oil to the scalp (e.g., mineral oil or a light moisturizing cream). Ask a family member to bring from home the product the patient prefers to use. Do not apply chemical relaxers to a patient's hair. Only a licensed beautician should do this.

Beard and Mustache Care

Beards and mustaches tend to collect food particles. They should be washed daily during a bath or shower and combed and trimmed as necessary. Do not shave a patient's mustache or beard without permission to do so. For details of beard and mustache care,

 Go to Chapter 25, **Procedure 25-10: Providing Beard and Mustache Care,** in Volume 2.

Shaving

Depending on the culture, shaving is an important part of grooming and helps patients feel better about their appearance. Many men shave their facial hair every day. Women may shave to remove axillary and leg hair. If the patient has a bleeding disorder or is taking anticoagulant medication, you should use an electric razor. For important points about shaving,

 Go to Chapter 25, **Procedure 25-11: Shaving a Patient,** in Volume 2.

Some dark-haired men (e.g., African Americans and Italians) have tightly curled facial hair, which curls back into the skin when shaved. An inflammatory reaction may occur, resulting in the formation of papules and pustules. In such cases, the man may wish to use a **depilatory** (hair-removing agent) instead of shaving. If you apply a depilatory, be sure to keep the chemical from contacting the patient's eyes, nose, mouth, and ears. Do not use a straight or safety razor to remove the depilatory, because it will irritate the skin. Some men with this condition prefer to grow a beard, especially when they are ill and unable to care for themselves.

CARE OF THE EYES

Usually you will not need to provide special hygiene care for the eyes. The eyelids and lashes keep dust and debris from entering the eyes, and tears continually cleanse and lubricate them. When necessary, you may gently cleanse the eyes, from the inner to the outer canthus, with a moistened washcloth (but with no soap). If there is

drainage or crusting, use a different cloth for each eye to prevent cross-contamination.

ASSESSMENT (EYES)

When performing hygiene care, inspect the eyes for redness, lesions, swelling, crusting, excessive tearing, or discharge. Also check the color of the conjunctivae. You should also ask the patient or check his records to see whether he wears glasses or contact lenses. If the patient wears glasses, ask when he uses them (e.g., for reading, for driving), and ask how well he sees without them. If the patient wears contact lenses, determine:

- The type of lens (hard, soft, long-wearing, disposable)
- How often he wears them (daily, occasionally) and for how long at a time
- Whether they are worn during sleep
- History of or current problems with lens usage (e.g., cleaning, removal)
- Usual practices for cleaning and storage
- History of or current problems with the eyes (e.g., redness, tearing, irritation, dryness, or "scratchy feeling")

These should be adequate data for hygiene care. However, it is not a complete eye assessment. For detailed information about assessing the eyes, see Chapter 22.

ANALYSIS/NURSING DIAGNOSIS (EYES)

Other than Bathing Self-Care Deficit, there is only one NANDA-I label specific to the eyes: Disturbed Sensory Perception: Visual. This label is of limited use for hygiene care. Other diagnoses that might occur include:

- Risk for Infection related to improper hand washing and improper lens cleaning
- Risk for Injury (to eyes) related to wearing lenses longer than recommended

PLANNING OUTCOMES/EVALUATION (EYES)

The only NOC standardized outcome specific to the eyes is Sensory Function: Vision. Its use is limited with regard to hygiene care; instead, you would use it if the client has a diagnosis of Disturbed Sensory Perception: Visual.

Individualized goals you might write for eye care include these examples:

- Demonstrates proper cleaning and storage of contact lenses.
- Eyes appear clean and without redness or drainage.

PLANNING INTERVENTIONS/IMPLEMENTATION (EYES)

For NIC standardized interventions related to eye care,

 Go to Chapter 25, **Standardized Language, Selected NOC Outcomes and NIC Interventions for Hygiene Problems,** on DavisPlus.

Individualized nursing activities related to the care of the eyes include providing eye care to unconscious clients, caring for eyeglasses and contact lenses, and caring for artificial eyes.

Eye Care for the Unconscious Patient

 Having lost the blink (corneal) reflex, comatose or critically ill patients need more frequent eye care (every 2 to 4 hours). Keep their eyes lubricated with saline or artificial tears to protect them from corneal abrasions and drying. You may also need to use a protective eye shield to keep the patient's eyes closed. Instill eye ointment or drops in the lower lids as ordered.

To review a procedure for administering eye medications,

Go to Chapter 26, **Procedure 26-2: Administering Ophthalmic Medications,** in Volume 2.

Caring for Eyeglasses and Contact Lenses

Eyeglasses need to be cleaned at least once a day. Using warm water and a soft cloth, clean gently to prevent scratching of the lens. Ask the patient whether the lenses require a special cleaning solution; some patients bring their own.

Key Point: *Label each patient's glasses, and store them in a safe place within the patient's reach, preferably in a glasses case in the drawer of the bedside table. They are expensive, so take care that they are not lost or damaged.*

An alternative to glasses, contact lenses are plastic discs worn on the cornea over the pupil. They float on the tears of the eye and stay in place because of surface tension. The cornea is nourished mainly by oxygen from the atmosphere and from tears, so in order to ensure an optimal supply of oxygen, contact lenses must be removed periodically. Wearing time varies from daily wear to up to around 30 days, depending on the type of lens. If you want more information about several different types of contact lenses:

Go to Chapter 25, **Supplemental Materials, Types of Contact Lenses,** on Davis*Plus.*

People usually care for their own contact lenses. Contact lens users must be careful to keep them free of microorganisms that could cause eye infections and to be careful to avoid eye irritation. Teach cleaning and disinfecting measures clients as needed (see the box Self-Care: Teaching Your Clients About Cleaning and Storing Contact Lenses), and follow those measures when you must care for a client's lenses.

If you need to remove a patient's lenses during an emergency, follow universal precautions and handle the lenses as you would any other valuable patient property.

 Never use your fingernails to remove a lens, as you may scratch the eye or damage the lens.

Self-Care

Teaching Your Clients About Cleaning and Storing Contact Lenses

➤ Cleaning and disinfecting procedures and solutions vary among manufacturers. Depending on the type of lens, use saline solutions or special rinsing and soaking solutions.

➤ Use a special container for the lenses, with a cup labeled for the left and right lens. Some lenses are stored in a solution; others are stored dry. Follow manufacturer's instructions.

➤ Always wash your hands before touching the eyes or the lenses.

➤ Be careful not to allow the lenses to come in contact with soaps, hair sprays, or cosmetics.

➤ Do not wear soft lenses while using eye drops or ointment (wait 1 hour after using drops and at least 4 hours for ointment).

➤ Be aware of the risk for eye irritation when in the presence of smoke or chemical vapors.

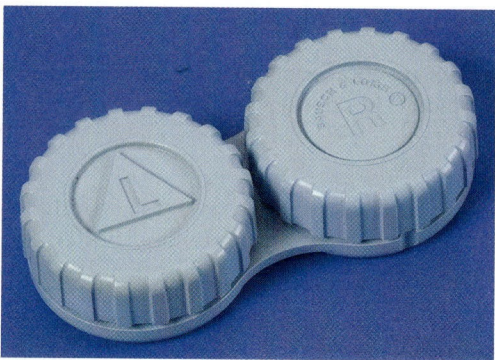

To avoid placing a contact lens in the wrong eye, lens cases are marked for the left and right eyes.

For more detailed instructions,

 Go to Chapter 25, **Procedure 25-12: Removing and Caring for Contact Lenses,** in Volume 2.

Caring for Artificial Eyes

An artificial eye is made to look like a natural eye. It can be made of glass or plastic. Some artificial eyes are permanently implanted in the socket, but others must be removed daily for cleaning of the prosthesis and the eye socket. If the patient is not able to perform his own eye care, ask about and follow his usual routines, when possible. To remove an artificial eye, wear procedure gloves. Using your dominant hand, raise the upper eyelid and depress the lower lid. Apply slight pressure below the eye to release the suction holding it in place (Fig. 22-5). Alternatively, you can use a small bulb syringe, place it directly on the eye, and squeeze to create suction and lift the eye from the socket. For details about removing, cleaning, and replacing an artificial eye, see the Procedures Highlights box and

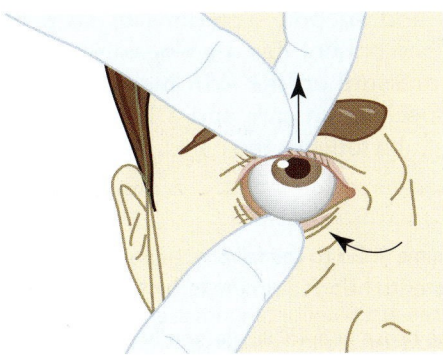

FIGURE 25-5 To remove a prosthetic eye, apply pressure just below the eye.

 Go to Chapter 25, **Procedure 25-15: Caring for Artificial Eyes,** in Volume 2.

KnowledgeCheck 25-12

- True or False: Eyes should be cleansed from the outer to the inner canthus.
- How can a contact lens wearer help prevent eye infections?
- After you have cleaned a prosthetic eye, should you dry it before reinserting it, or leave it wet? To answer this question, you may need to refer to Procedure 22-15, in the Highlights of Procedures box.

CARE OF THE EARS

Healthy ears require minimal care. However, you will need to help patients who have limited self-care abilities and teach others about self-care.

For example, **cerumen** (wax) impaction is a common cause of hearing loss, especially in older adults. People sometimes believe hearing loss is a normal part of aging and fail to seek treatment. Encourage them to see their primary care provider whenever hearing loss occurs.

Teach patients to avoid using rigid objects, such as bobby pins or toothpicks to clean their ears. Such instruments can traumatize the ear canal and may rupture the **tympanic membrane** (eardrum). Likewise, never use cotton-tipped applicators; they will push the cerumen further into the ear, causing a blockage.

For dependent patients, assess for drainage, excess cerumen, and hearing loss during the bath. Clean the auricle, and remove wax from the canal with the tip of the moistened washcloth. If cleansing with a washcloth does not effectively remove excess cerumen buildup, obtain a prescription for **cerumenolytic** drops and water irrigation. You can delegate ear cleaning and hearing aid care to the NAP if you are sure that the NAP knows how to perform these tasks. Describe what you want the NAP to observe and report to you. See Chapter 30 for information about ear irrigations.

Care of Hearing Aids A hearing aid is a battery-powered device that amplifies sound. Three types of

hearing aids are shown in Figure 25-6. Also, some patients wear a hearing aid in the temple pieces of their eyeglasses. People with severe hearing loss may wear a body hearing aid that clips onto the clothing or a harness-type carrier that connects by a cord to the earpiece. Digital hearing aids are rapidly replacing the analog models.

Hearing aids are expensive, so handle and store them properly. They require regular cleaning and replacement of batteries. Even with good care, they usually need to be replaced every 5 to 10 years, and earmolds usually need adjustment more often than that. Never place a hearing aid in water. For guidelines to remove, clean, and replace a hearing aid,

 Go to Chapter 25, **Procedure 25-16: Caring for Hearing Aids,** in Volume 2.

CARE OF THE NOSE

Usually the nose requires no special care. Have the patient remove excess secretions by gently blowing into a tissue with both nostrils open. Holding one nostril

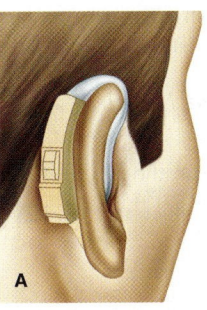
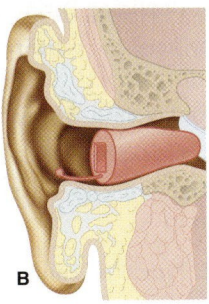
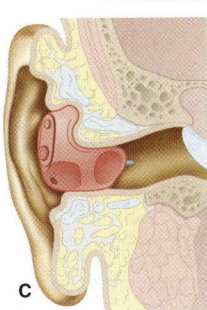

FIGURE 25-6 Hearing aids. *A,* The postaural (behind-the-ear) aid is the most widely used. A plastic tube connects it to an earmold. *B,* An in-the-canal aid is the least visible. *C,* The in-the-ear aid is made in one piece; all components are in the earmold.

shut can force secretions into the eustachian tubes. In debilitated or unconscious patients, dried secretions can interfere with respirations. Remove secretions by gently inserting a moistened cotton-tipped applicator into the nostrils. Occasionally you may need to instill saline into the nares and suction secretions to keep the airway patent. If the patient has a nasogastric (NG) tube, the constant pressure on the skin may cause breakdown. Provide special skin care and a lubricant at the point where the tube touches the nares.

For steps to follow in *all* procedures, refer to the inside back cover of Volume 2. Go to the full procedures in Volume 2 to practice and learn the procedure steps. Use these Procedure Highlights later to help you review key points.

Procedures 25-1, 25-2, and 25-3: Bathing: Providing a Complete Bed Bath Using a Prepackaged Bathing Product, Bathing: Providing a Towel Bath, and Bathing: Using a Basin and Water

➤ Use prepackaged bathing products.

➤ Check the temperature of the packaged bath wipes after microwaving.

➤ Avoid chilling or tiring the patient.

➤ Bathe the patient following the principles of "head to toe" and "clean to dirty."

➤ For extremities, cleanse from distal to proximal.

➤ Use a new wipe for cleansing the perineum and whenever the wipe becomes soiled.

➤ Perform hand hygiene when moving from a contaminated body part to cleanse a clean body part.

➤ If performing a basin and water bath, use a disposable basin and distilled, filtered, or sterile water, according to agency requirements. Use a CHG and water solution to bathe the patient and clean the pan. Store the basin upside down.

➤ Chlorhexidine gluconate (CHG) 2% prepackaged cloths decrease the colonization of bacteria on the skin and should not be rinsed.

Procedure 25-4: Providing Perineal Care

➤ Provide privacy; keep the patient covered as much as possible.

➤ Place waterproof underpad to protect the bed linens.

➤ Use warmed prepackaged wipes.

➤ Perform perineal care following the principle of "clean to dirty" (front to back).

Procedure 25-5: Providing Foot Care

➤ Inspect the feet thoroughly for skin integrity, circulation, and edema.

➤ Clean the feet with warmed prepackaged wipes; clean the toenails; rinse; and dry well.

➤ Trim the nails straight across, unless contraindicated. Check institutional policy; many institutions do not allow nurses to trim nails.

➤ File the nails with an emery board.

➤ Lightly apply lotion, except between the toes.

➤ Ensure that footwear or bedding is not irritating to the feet.

Procedure 25-6: Brushing and Flossing the Teeth

➤ Assess the teeth, mucous membranes, and swallowing ability.

➤ Position the patient to prevent aspiration (sitting or side-lying position).

➤ Hold the brush at a 45° angle, and brush the patient's teeth (or assist).

➤ Floss and rinse, using sterile, filtered, or distilled water according to agency policy.

➤ If the patient is at risk for choking, suction secretions as needed.

Procedure 25-7: Providing Denture Care

➤ Refer to Procedure 25-6, Brushing and Flossing the Teeth.

➤ Remove (and replace) the top denture before the lower denture.

➤ Tilt dentures slightly when removing and replacing.

➤ Handle dentures carefully, and place a towel in the sink to avoid breaking the dentures if you drop them.

➤ Use cool, agency-approved water and a stiff-bristled brush.

Procedure 25-8: Providing Oral Care for an Unconscious Patient

➤ Assess the condition of the teeth (or dentures), gums, and mucous membranes.

➤ Assess for the gag reflex.

➤ Position the patient to prevent aspiration.

➤ Brush and floss the patient's teeth.

➤ Suction secretions as needed

Procedure 25-9: Shampooing the Hair

➤ Determine the type of procedure needed. Assess the patient's ability to help and the condition of the hair and scalp.

➤ Identify hair care products needed for the procedure.

➤ Wash the hair with no-rinse shampoo or no-rinse shampoo cap.

➤ If basin and water are used, protect the bed from getting wet.

➤ Protect the patient's eyes and ears from soap and water.

➤ Towel-dry the hair.

➤ Take care not to burn the patient with the hair dryer, if one is used.

Procedure 25-10: Providing Beard and Mustache Care

➤ Assess the skin for redness, dry areas, or lesions.

➤ Trim the beard and mustache to the desired length with a comb and scissors or beard trimmer.

➤ Shampoo the beard and mustache.

➤ Apply conditioner, if desired.

➤ Towel-dry the beard and mustache, and comb and style as desired.

Procedure 25-11: Shaving a Patient

➤ Wear procedure gloves.

➤ Assess the skin for redness or dry areas.

➤ To soften the beard and moisten the skin:

  ➤ Apply a warm, damp towel to the face.

  ➤ Apply shaving cream or soap.

➤ To prevent skin irritation:

  ➤ Hold the skin taut, and shave the face and neck.

  ➤ If using a safety razor, hold the blade at a 45° angle to the skin.

  ➤ Apply after-shave product, if desired.

Procedure 25-12: Removing and Caring for Contact Lenses

➤ Instill one or two drops of wetting solution.

➤ Gently remove contact lenses; use your finger pads, not your fingernails.

➤ Clean and store contact lenses in sterile solution.

➤ Mark the containers "L" and "R" to identify the correct eye.

Procedure 25-13: Making an Unoccupied Bed

➤ Remove soiled linens without cross-contaminating other items in the room.

➤ Remake the bed with clean linens.

➤ Do not "shake" or "fan" linens.

➤ Work efficiently and safely.

➤ Ensure that there are no wrinkles in the bottom sheet or drawsheet.

Procedure 25-14: Making an Occupied Bed

➤ Maintain patient safety during the procedure.

➤ Assess the patient's ability to move and need for assistive equipment and patient-handling devices.

➤ Position the patient laterally near the far siderail, and roll soiled linens under him.

➤ Place clean linens on the side nearest you, and then tuck under the soiled linens.

➤ Roll the patient over the "hump," and position him on his other side, near you. Raise the near siderail.

➤ Move to the other side of the bed; pull soiled and clean linens through, and complete the linen change as in Procedure 25-13: Making an Unoccupied Bed.

➤ Place the bed in a low position, raise the siderails, and fasten the call light to the pillow.

Procedure 25-15: Caring for Artificial Eyes

➤ Have the patient lie down.

➤ Remove the artificial eye: Raise the upper eyelid; with dominant hand, depress the lower lid and apply slight pressure below the eye (or use a small bulb syringe).

➤ Clean the eye: Clean the eye with saline; store in saline or distilled, sterile or filtered water (per agency policy); label the container.

➤ Clean the edge of the eye socket with a moistened cotton ball.

➤ Reinsert the eye: Be sure the prosthesis is wet. Hold it with your dominant hand. Spread the patient's eyelids apart with nondominant hand, and guide prosthesis into the eye socket.

Procedure 25-16: Caring for Hearing Aids

➤ Keep hearing aids away from heat and moisture.

➤ Clean hearing aids with a damp cloth only.

➤ Avoid hairspray and other hair care products.

➤ Turn off hearing aids when not in use.

➤ Replace dead batteries immediately.

➤ Store hearing aids in a case with the battery compartment open.

➤ Keep hearing aids and batteries away from children and pets.

➤ To clean a hearing aid: Turn it off, remove it from the ear, cleanse the outer ear and the hearing aid, check the battery, reinsert it, turn it on, and check the volume with the patient.

THE CLIENT'S ENVIRONMENT

A comfortable environment contributes to the client's well-being. It is your responsibility, as a nurse, to see that the bedside unit and surroundings are clean, safe, and comfortable.

ASSESSMENT (SCANNING THE ENVIRONMENT)

Each time you enter a patient's room, you should scan the environment to see whether you need to make adjustments to ensure patient safety and comfort:

■ Is the room temperature comfortable?
■ Are the siderails up, when indicated?
■ Is the bed in low position, and the wheels locked?
■ Are bed linens clean and free of wrinkles?
■ Is the patient's call device within reach?
■ Is the overbed table clean and uncluttered?
■ Is there uncluttered walking space?
■ Are there unpleasant odors?

Each time you leave the room, ask, "What else can I do for you?" This ensures that you have not overlooked anything.

PLANNING INTERVENTIONS/IMPLEMENTATION (THE ENVIRONMENT)

Adequate ventilation; proper room temperature; low noise level; and neat, clean surroundings are important to ensure the patient's comfort.

Promoting Ventilation

Body secretions such as urine, feces, vomitus, or draining wounds cause odors in both inpatient facilities and the home. Odors can be offensive, and patients often feel embarrassed by them, so work quickly to free the environment of any sources of odors. Cleanliness is the best way to prevent odors. Other suggestions include the following:

- Provide good ventilation, if this is under your control. For example, open a window or use a fan.
- Empty and clean urinals, bedpans, or emesis basins promptly.
- Dispose of soiled dressings or other malodorous items in appropriate containers, and immediately remove them from the room.
- Unless contraindicated by the patient's illness, you can use a room deodorizer to help eliminate odors.
- Most institutions ban smoking in patient rooms, in part because of the odor.

Control Room Temperature

Although preferences may vary, a room temperature between 68°F and 74°F (20°C and 23°C) is usually comfortable for most patients. Those who are very ill, very young, or very old may need a higher than normal room temperature. If there is no thermostat in the room, you may need to provide blankets, open a window, provide a fan, and so on to adjust the room temperature.

Limit Noise

People who are ill are often sensitive to various environmental noises, such as an ice machine, suction equipment, paging systems, loud talking, and laughter. In addition, sleeping in a new and strange environment or in the presence of pain may be difficult. Make it a priority to control noise. Keep unnecessary conversations to a minimum, and speak quietly. Some hospitals have instituted a "quiet hour" to promote better rest. Others have installed decibel meters to help nurses be mindful of noise escalation during activity in the nurses' station.

Standard Bedside Equipment

In a hospital, standard bedside equipment usually includes a bed, bedside stand (end table), overbed table, and one or two chairs. The wall unit may consist of a call light, oxygen, suction and electrical outlets, and light fixtures and switches. The patient's personal items are usually kept in the bedside stand. Therefore, you should request permission from the patient before opening the stand. Personal hygiene items, bedpan, and urinal may also be kept in the lower cabinet of this stand.

Hospital Beds

Hospitalized patients spend a significant amount of time in bed. Hospital beds can be uncomfortable and may contribute to restlessness and poor sleep. Memory foam and moisture control mattresses are available and provide more comfort. However, they are expensive and not used routinely. Hospital beds are generally standard in size and higher and narrower than a home bed. This allows you to reach the patient more easily and safely.

Hospital beds are usually electronically controlled, so the patient and nurse can raise and lower the head and foot separately by the push of a button (see Fig. 25-7 for bed positions).

✚ Patient safety is your priority, so although you should raise the entire bed to a working level that is comfortable for you, be sure to place the bed in the lowest position before leaving the bedside. Long-term care settings usually have low beds to make it easier for ambulatory patients to transfer into and out of bed. As a part of the admission procedure, you will teach patients how to use the bed controls.

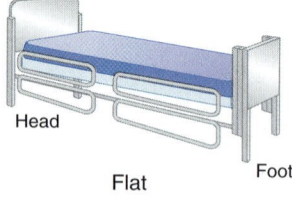

Head   Foot

Flat

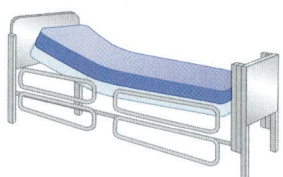

Semi-Fowler's position
(30° angle)

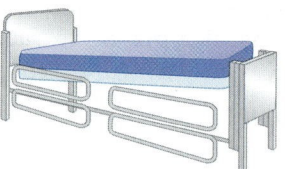

Trendelenburg's position

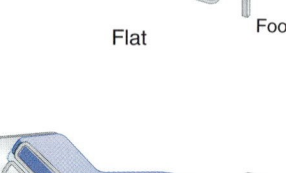

Fowler's position
(45° angle)

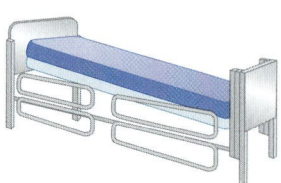

Reverse Trendelenburg's
position

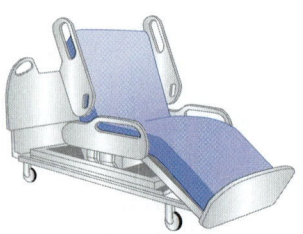

Sitting position
(special wound-care
beds; also adjust to
standing postion)

FIGURE 25-7 Hospital beds adjust to several positions.

Go to Chapter 11, **Procedure 11-1: Admitting a Patient to a Nursing Unit,** in Volume 2.

Patients may use siderails when moving into and out of bed. Siderails may help to prevent falls by patients with decreased consciousness. However, siderails are considered a passive restraint and may pose risk to a patient with a cognitive impairment. See Chapter 24 for additional information about the safe use of siderails and other equipment.

✚ Always lock the wheels on a hospital bed when it is stationary. For example, an unlocked bed could roll out from under an ambulatory patient who is moving from the bed to a chair. Ensure that the wheels are locked when you are helping the patient to a sitting position on the side of the bed or assisting with a transfer to a chair or stretcher.

Mattresses and Linens

Mattresses are usually firm and covered in a water-repellant material that resists staining and soiling and may be easily wiped down with a germicidal cleaner. A variety of special therapeutic mattresses are available to help reduce the effects of pressure over the bony prominences (e.g., sacrum, heels). See Chapter 35 for further discussion of special mattresses.

Using a mattress cover and/or pad promotes patient comfort and prevents soiling of the mattress. Plastic covers, however, do not allow moisture to escape, and contribute to skin maceration for patients who are incontinent or diaphoretic. Bed mattress covers, whether water-resistant, waterproof, or water-repellent, may lose their effectiveness over time, allowing moisture, blood, or bacteria to penetrate the mattress. Regularly check each medical bed mattress cover. If any visible signs of damage or wear such as cuts, tears, cracks, pinholes, snags, or stains are found, the cover should be immediately replaced to reduce the risk of infection (U.S. Food and Drug Administration, 2013).

Sheets may be fitted or flat. Other linens include drawsheets, washable incontinence pads, pillowcases, blankets, bedspreads, and gowns. If a plastic surface lies directly under the sheet, you should place a cloth or other absorbent pad between the patient and the sheet.

Bed Making

Clean, wrinkle-free bed linens help to promote comfort and a sense of well-being. In contrast, wrinkled and soiled linen can contribute to skin breakdown and pressure areas. Linens are generally changed daily after the bath and when soiled. If patients are up and about during the day, such as on a rehabilitation unit, beds are made daily, but bed linen may be changed weekly or only when soiled. If the patient is immobile or on bedrest, the bed is made while the patient occupies it. You or the NAP may make an unoccupied bed or an occupied bed. For more information about bed making,

 Go to Chapter 25, **Procedure 25-13: Making an Unoccupied Bed** and **Procedure 25-14: Making an Occupied Bed,** in Volume 2.

 Think**Like a Nurse** 25-10

For which of your patients (Meet Your Patients) will you most surely need to make an occupied bed? Why?

 ʇo explore learning resources for this chapter,

 Go to Davis*Plus* at DavisPl.us/Wilkinson3.

Chapter resources for Chapter 25:
   Response sheets for all learning activities
   Resources for Caregivers and Health Professionals
   Reading More About Facilitating Hygiene (suggested reading)
   Concept Map of chapter content
Interactive case studies
NCLEX-Style and Chapter Review Questions
Chapter Overview Podcasts

For references cited in this chapter,

 Go to Volume 2, **References Cited.**

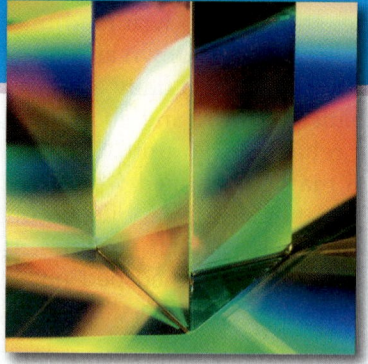

Administering Medications

Learning Outcomes

After completing this chapter, you should be able to:

▶ Name at least five sources of medication information.

▶ Distinguish among various nomenclature systems for naming and classifying drugs.

▶ Discuss the concepts and processes of pharmacokinetics, including drug absorption, distribution, metabolism, and excretion.

▶ Define onset, peak, and duration of drug action; therapeutic level, peak level, and trough level; and biological half-life.

▶ Compare and contrast primary, secondary, cumulative, and side effects; and adverse, toxic, allergic, anaphylactic, and idiosyncratic reactions.

▶ Define drug-drug interaction, antagonistic drug relationship, synergistic drug relationship, drug incompatibility, and medication contraindications.

▶ Correctly calculate drug dosages, including (1) conversion among the metric, apothecary, and household measurement systems and (2) working with units and milliequivalents (mEq).

▶ List the types of medication prescriptions, including the methods for communicating them.

▶ Discuss the agencies and legislation that help to ensure drug quality and safety.

▶ Describe nursing assessment before, during, and following the administration of a drug.

▶ Plan care for clients with problems of Risk for Injury and Noncompliance related to medications.

▶ Administer medications using the "three checks" and "rights of medication."

▶ Describe appropriate steps to take when communicating a medication error.

▶ Demonstrate the correct procedure for administering medications by the oral, enteral, inhalant, and parenteral routes.

▶ Demonstrate the intramuscular injection procedure at the following sites: ventrogluteal, deltoid, and vastus lateralis.

▶ Explain why the dorsogluteal site is no longer recommended for intramuscular injections.

▶ List five steps to incorporate in your practice to ensure safe medication administration and prevent a medication error.

Key Concepts

Medication administration
Medication safety
Pharmacology

Related Concepts

See the Concept Map on Davis*Plus*.

Meet Your Patients

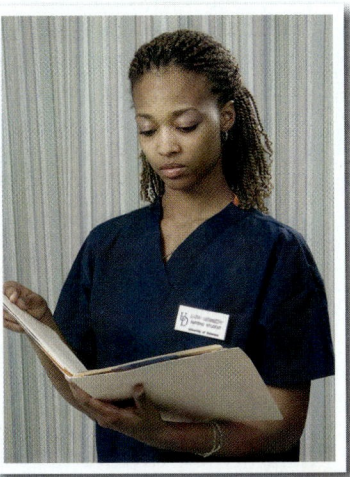

As a new nurse, you are scheduled to administer medications to five patients on the medical-surgical unit today for the first time. Your preceptor will be available as a resource. Your patients are:

- Margaret Marks, an 82-year-old woman who has a fractured hip and experiences periods of confusion.
- Cary Pearson, a 70-year-old man with feeding and swallowing difficulties who receives his medications through a gastrostomy tube.
- Cyndi Early, a 32-year-old woman with diabetes who is scheduled for surgery at 1000 today.
- James Bigler, a 44-year-old man who has had a repair of a compound fracture of the right arm and is receiving intravenous fluids and medications.
- Rebecca Jones, an 84-year-old woman with compression fractures of two lumbar vertebrae resulting from a fall.

You have reviewed your assignment but are unsure of where to begin. Should you visit your patients first and perform an assessment? Should you review the charts first? What should you do with the medication administration records (MARs)? There are so many questions running through your head, and you are a little nervous being on your own. Perhaps you could use the model of full-spectrum nursing (Chapter 2) to focus your thinking. In general, any time you give a medication, you will need to incorporate the following:

1. *Theoretical Knowledge:* Find out about the actions and expected effects of the medications you are to give.
2. *Patient Situation:* Assess the health status (e.g., disease process) of each patient as it relates to his medications.
3. *Critical Thinking:* Why is the drug being given? Is there anything about the patient's physiology that may alter his responses to the drug? Do you need to modify the administration procedure in any way?
4. *Practical Knowledge:* Be sure that you know the procedures for administering each medication safely.

By the time you complete this chapter, you will have the information you need to make those kinds of judgments. And remember that while you are a student, your instructor and the staff nurses will be there for support.

Theoretical Knowledge
knowing why

Pharmacology is the science of drug effects. It deals with all drugs used in society, legal and illegal, prescription and nonprescription, and "street" drugs. Because of their potential for harm as well as benefit, you should thoroughly understand the medications you administer.

ABOUT THE KEY CONCEPTS

The broadest concept identified in this chapter is **medication administration**. The concept of **medication safety** is intimately related to it. In order to administer medications without causing harm to patients, you will need theoretical knowledge of **pharmacology** (another key concept), as well as practical knowledge about safe procedures. You will identify many related concepts as you read this chapter (e.g., pharmacodynamics, pharmacokinetics). Try to understand how they relate to the three key concepts. If you can organize information this way in your mind, you are likely to remember it better.

HOW ARE DRUGS NAMED AND CLASSIFIED?

A **drug** is a chemical that interacts with a living organism and alters its activity. In healthcare, drugs are used in diagnosing, treating, or preventing a disease or other medical condition. The term *drug* is used interchangeably with *medication,* although some people think of the term *drug* as meaning an illegal substance.

Drug Names
A drug may have multiple names.

- **Chemical name** is the exact description of the drug's chemical composition and molecular structure. For example, *2-(p-isobutylphenyl) propionic acid* is the chemical name of the anti-inflammatory drug ibuprofen. The chemical name is rarely used in nursing practice.
- **Generic (nonproprietary) name** is assigned by the United States Adopted Name Council (USAN Council) when the developing manufacturer is ready to market the drug. This is usually similar to the chemical name, but in a simpler form.

- **Official name** is also the generic name that is listed in publications such as the *United States Pharmacopeia (USP)* and *National Formulary (NF)*. For example, *ibuprofen* is both a generic and an official name.
- **Brand (trade** or **proprietary) name** is what the drug is sold as in stores. The brand name is easily recognized because it begins with a capital letter and sometimes has a registration mark (®) at the upper right of the name. Different manufacturers of the same medication may give the medication different brand names. For example, Advil, Nuprin, and Motrin are all brand names for ibuprofen.

Prescription drugs require a written order from a healthcare provider (e.g., physician or advanced practice nurse) who is licensed by the state to prescribe or dispense drugs. **Nonprescription,** or **over-the-counter (OTC),** drugs may be purchased without a prescription and are assumed to be safe for the general population if consumers follow the manufacturer's directions. Some drugs are nonprescription at low doses but require a prescription for the consumer to purchase in a higher dose. For example, naproxen sodium 200 mg is sold over the counter as Aleve, whereas naproxen 500 mg is sold as Naprosyn and requires a prescription. Some drugs once available only by prescription may become OTC, such as with loratadine (Claritin).

Drug Classifications

It is not realistic to know everything about every drug, so "looking it up" must become second nature. If you learn the common characteristics for a drug classification, then when you encounter a new drug, you will be able to associate it with its classification and make inferences about its basic characteristics.

- By usage—why the drug is used
- By body system—where the drug works
- By chemical or pharmacological class—what the drug is made of

To see an explanation and examples of those classifications methods,

 Go to **ESG Table 26-1, Drug Classification System,** on *DavisPlus.*

A drug can be placed in more than one category in a classification system. Classified by usage, for example, ibuprofen (Motrin) can be an analgesic, anti-inflammatory, and an antipyretic agent. A drug can act on more than one body system, as well; in fact, most do. For example, diazepam (Valium) is used for its anti-anxiety effects, but it also decreases the activity of the intestinal system and other smooth muscles.

KnowledgeCheck 26-1

- Name three ways a drug may be classified.
- List at least four ways a drug could be named.

WHAT MECHANISMS PROMOTE DRUG QUALITY AND SAFETY?

Before the 20th century, the United States did not have mechanisms for publishing drug ingredients, regulations to govern the contents of drugs, or limitations regarding drug sales. People could buy medicines containing potent and dangerous ingredients, such as opium and alcohol. Now, reliable sources of drug information, state and federal regulations and standards controlling drug administration, and a variety of systems for storing and distributing medications in healthcare agencies all work together to protect consumers.

Drug Listings and Directories

Key Point: *When in doubt, look it up!* As a nurse, you are professionally, ethically, legally, and personally responsible for every dose of medication you administer. Always use current information when researching a medication. The following references have become the official standards for the healthcare industry:

Pharmacopoeia and Formularies The **United States Pharmacopoeia (USP)** is a directory of drugs approved by the Food and Drug Administration (FDA) that lists the physical and chemical composition of each drug. Any drug included in this book has met rigorous standards of quality, strength, and purity and the manufacturer is permitted to use the letters "USP" after the drug name. The **National Formulary (NF)** is another official resource for medication information in the United States. It identifies the therapeutic value of drugs as well as their formulas and prescriptions.

Nursing Drug Handbooks Available from textbook and other publishers, handbooks serve as a quick resource for dosage, side effects and nursing interventions associated with a drug.

Physician's Desk Reference (PDR) This book, commercially compiled by the pharmaceutical companies, lists manufacturers' prescribing information and is a standard resource for professionals prescribing and administering medication. The *PDR* does not include nursing interventions, but does contain information on dosing, routes of administration, and side effects.

Pharmacology Texts A textbook provides more information about physiology, pathophysiology, mechanism of action, and drug classifications than the drug formulary or a handbook. However, it may or may not have detailed information about the specific drug you are administering.

Electronic and Internet-Based Formularies The Internet, computer software, PDAs, and other handheld devices offer convenient access to formulary databases.

Pharmacist A clinical pharmacist can assist you with medication-related concerns (e.g., dosage calculations, compatibility).

Medication Package Inserts Most medications are packaged with an insert that provides information identical to that found in the drug formulary and specific for that particular drug.

Institutional Medication Policies and Procedures You should know the policies and protocols for medication administration for each institution in which you practice.

 Think**Like a Nurse** 26-1

Mr. Pearson (Meet Your Patients) has a medication, metoprolol (Lopressor), due at 0800. You are not familiar with this medication.

- What do you need to know before giving the drug?
- What resources might you use to learn about this medication?
- Which is the generic and which is the brand name of this medication?
- Select a nursing drug handbook and research this medication. What kinds of information are available to you in the book?
- Now look up the drug in a pharmacology text. How is that information similar to and different from the information in the handbook?

Legal Considerations

In the United States, drug administration is controlled by federal, state, and local laws. Standards of nursing care, state nurse practice acts, and organizational policies and procedures define your role and responsibilities in administering medications. You must be familiar with them to know what you can and cannot do. In addition, you must recognize the limits of your own experience, skills, and knowledge.

The Food and Drug Administration (FDA) of the U.S. Department of Health and Human Services regulates the testing, manufacture, and sale of all medications. This agency also monitors the safety and effectiveness of medications available to consumers. This process helps to ensure that ineffective or unsafe drugs are not marketed or are recalled, if later found unsafe. However, many medicinal products are *not* regulated by the FDA. For example, herbal remedies and some naturopathic supplements are considered "food products" and are not regulated, yet they are advertised as having health benefits.

Nurse Practice Acts

In most states, a nurse cannot prescribe or administer medications without an authorized provider's (e.g., advanced practice nurse, physician) order. The Board of Nursing also regulates the types and routes of medications that can be administered by the various levels of nurses. For example, a licensed practical nurse (LPN) in some states cannot administer intravenous medications, whereas other states requires additional education and experiences before LPNs can perform this skill. You should refer to your state's nurse practice act for your scope of practice. If you violate the state's nurse

practice act by giving medications without an order/prescription, your state's nursing board could revoke your license to practice nursing.

 Think**Like a Nurse** 26-2

Obtain a copy of your nurse practice act for the state in which you work. To find a copy,

 Go to the **National Council of State Boards of Nursing** Web site at https://www.ncsbn.org/contactbon.htm

What does your state's nurse practice act tell you about administering medications?

U.S. Drug Legislation

Various state and federal agencies regulate the manufacture and sale of medications. Each state must conform to federal regulations concerning medications. The states may, however, institute additional controls. Local governments may enact regulations for the use of alcohol and tobacco. For a historical list of U.S. laws regulating drug quality and safety,

 Go to Chapter 26, **ESG Table 26-2, U.S. Legislation for Drug Quality and Safety,** on Davis*Plus*.

For a history of additional activities to protect consumers and ensure drug safety,

 Chapter 26, Chapter Resources, **Resources for Caregivers & Professionals,** on Davis*Plus*.

Regulation of Controlled Substances

Controlled substances are drugs considered to have either limited medical use or high potential for abuse or addiction. Under the Controlled Substances Act (CSA) of the Comprehensive Drug Abuse Prevention and Control Act of 1970, it is illegal to possess a controlled substance without a valid prescription. For a summary of categories of controlled substances,

 Go to Chapter 26, **Tables, Boxes, Figures: ESG Table 26-3, Schedules for Controlled Substances,** on Davis*Plus*.

Controlled substances must be stored, handled, disposed of, and administered according to regulations established by the U.S. Drug Enforcement Agency (DEA). Only prescribers with a *national provider identification number* have the authority to prescribe controlled substances. Controlled substances must be stored in locked drawers within a second locked area. (This process is known as **double locking**.) The facility must also keep a record of every dose administered. A count of all controlled substances is performed at specified times, usually at change of shift. To facilitate counting and tracking inventory, drug manufacturers package many narcotics in sectioned containers, with each tablet separately and consecutively numbered (Fig. 26-1).

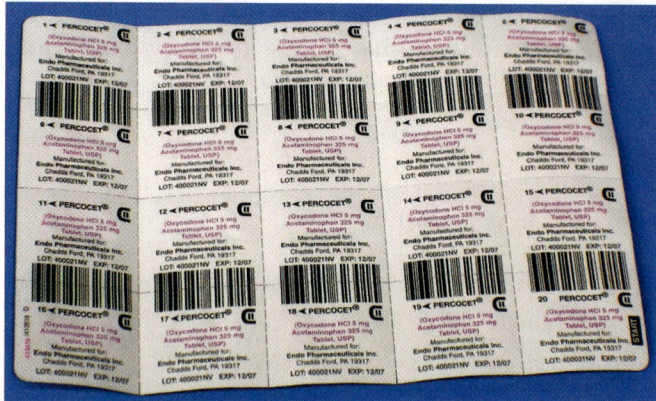

FIGURE 26-1 To facilitate counting, many narcotics are packaged in sectioned containers with each tablet numbered consecutively.

ThinkLike a Nurse 26-3

Locate the controlled substance area on your nursing unit.

- Is a double-locking system in place?
- Who is responsible for "carrying" the narcotics keys?
- What is done if there is a discrepancy between a narcotic sign-out sheet and the actual number of narcotic doses present?

Systems for Storing and Distributing Medications

Most inpatient healthcare facilities have specific areas designed for preparation of medications. Usually this is a central room ("medication room") or mobile cart. Some nursing units store drugs and supplies in a locked cabinet in or near patient rooms. Whatever the method, all drugs are secured in designated areas accessible only to nurses.

Stock Supply

Medications used most frequently may be kept in **stock supply** (bulk quantity), labeled, and in a central location. For example, acetaminophen elixir and cough syrups may be kept in large multidose bottles from which you measure doses for more than one patient. Stock supplies require you to measure the dose each time a patient needs it, so the potential for measurement error occurs more frequently. However, a bulk supply of medication is often very cost-effective.

Unit-Dose System

A locked, mobile cart is used, with drawers containing separate compartments for each patient's medications (Fig. 26-2). Extra drawers contain supplies, such as medication cups, syringes, and alcohol swabs. The pharmacy staff refills the drawers each shift or every 24 hours. Limited amounts of **prn** (give according to patient need) medications and stock medications are also kept in the mobile cart.

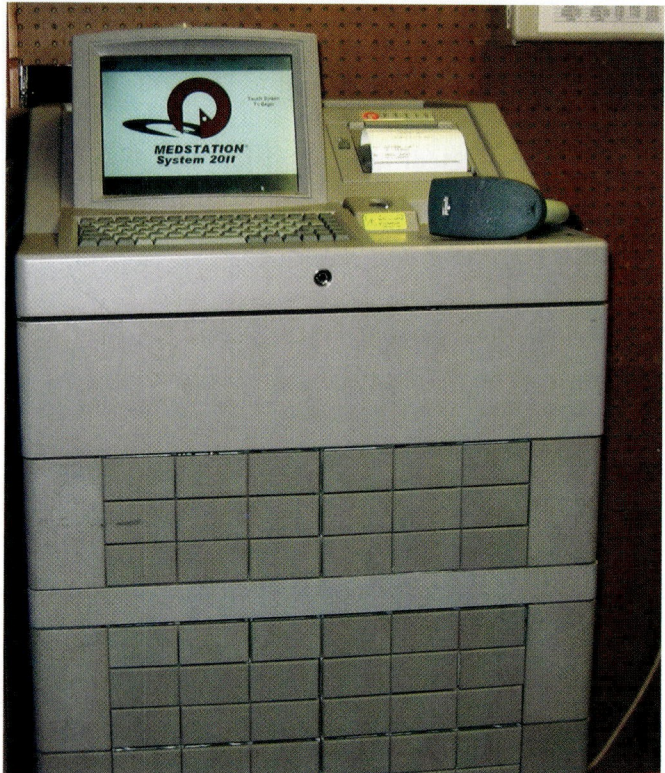

FIGURE 26-2 Medications may be kept in locked, mobile carts, with a drawer for each patient. Mobile (portable) medication carts are linked to the automated dispensing unit.

A **unit dose** is the prescribed amount of drug the patient receives at a single time. For example, if 800 mg of ibuprofen (Motrin) is prescribed to be given every 8 hours, the unit dose is 800 mg. Each unit dose (usually one tablet) is individually packaged and labeled with the drug name, dose, and expiration date. The pharmacist checks each unit dose before sending the drug to the nursing unit. You must recheck the drug and dose when preparing it for administration. The unit-dose system not only saves nursing time, but also is the safest method because of the double-check system.

Automated Dispensing System

An automated dispensing system is a computerized system similar to a unit-dose system. The locked cart contains all the medications frequently used on a particular nursing unit, and the computer database contains records and counts of the medications, as well as the medication prescriptions for each patient on the unit. Each nurse uses a password to access the machine and enters the data about the needed drug, after which the machine dispenses the medication. The medications are usually packaged in unit doses, but some bulk medications may also be kept on the cart. This method allows for immediate administration of newly prescribed medications, prn medications, controlled substances, and emergency medications because the nurse does not need to wait for the pharmacy to fill a prescription.

Self-Administration

At times while in the hospital, patients may self-administer medications. For example, sublingual nitroglycerin (used for chest pain) is self-administered in the outpatient setting, and some patients can continue self-administration of the drug while in the hospital. The drugs prescribed for self-administration are supplied in individual containers and stored at the bedside. Remind the patient to tell you when he takes a dose. This method promotes independence and allows you to evaluate the patient's ability to manage medications safely and accurately before she is discharged. Check the policy in your institution regarding self-administration of drugs.

KnowledgeCheck 26-2

- What legislation defines controlled substances in the United States?
- How is medication quality managed?

WHAT IS PHARMACOKINETICS?

Pharmacokinetics refers to the absorption, distribution, metabolism, and excretion of a drug (Fig. 26-3). These four processes determine the intensity and duration of a drug's actions. Each drug has unique pharmacokinetic characteristics. As you study these concepts, think how they relate to each other and to the key concepts pharmacology, medication administration, and medication safety.

What Factors Affect Drug Absorption?

Absorption refers to the movement of the drug from the administration site into the bloodstream. The rate of absorption determines when a drug can begin to exert its action; thus, absorption also influences metabolism and excretion. Absorption depends on the administration route, drug form, drug solubility, pH, blood flow to the area, and body surface area.

Route of Administration

Drugs are manufactured for a specific route of administration: oral, sublingual, buccal, inhalant, topical, enteral, and parenteral. They are absorbed at different rates for each route. Medications are available in a variety of forms.

Drugs are given for either local or systemic effect. The **local effects** of a drug occur at the site of application (e.g., certain topical applications of drugs to the skin), so no or limited absorption occurs. When given for a **systemic effect**, the drug must be absorbed into the bloodstream before it can be distributed to a distant location. A drug may enter the circulation either by injection into a vein or by absorption from other areas (e.g., muscle, stomach, mucous membranes).

Table 26-1 summarizes the preparations and the advantages and disadvantages of the various routes of administration. The choice of route is crucial in determining the suitability of the drug for a particular patient. For example, if your patient is vomiting, an

(Text continued on page 614)

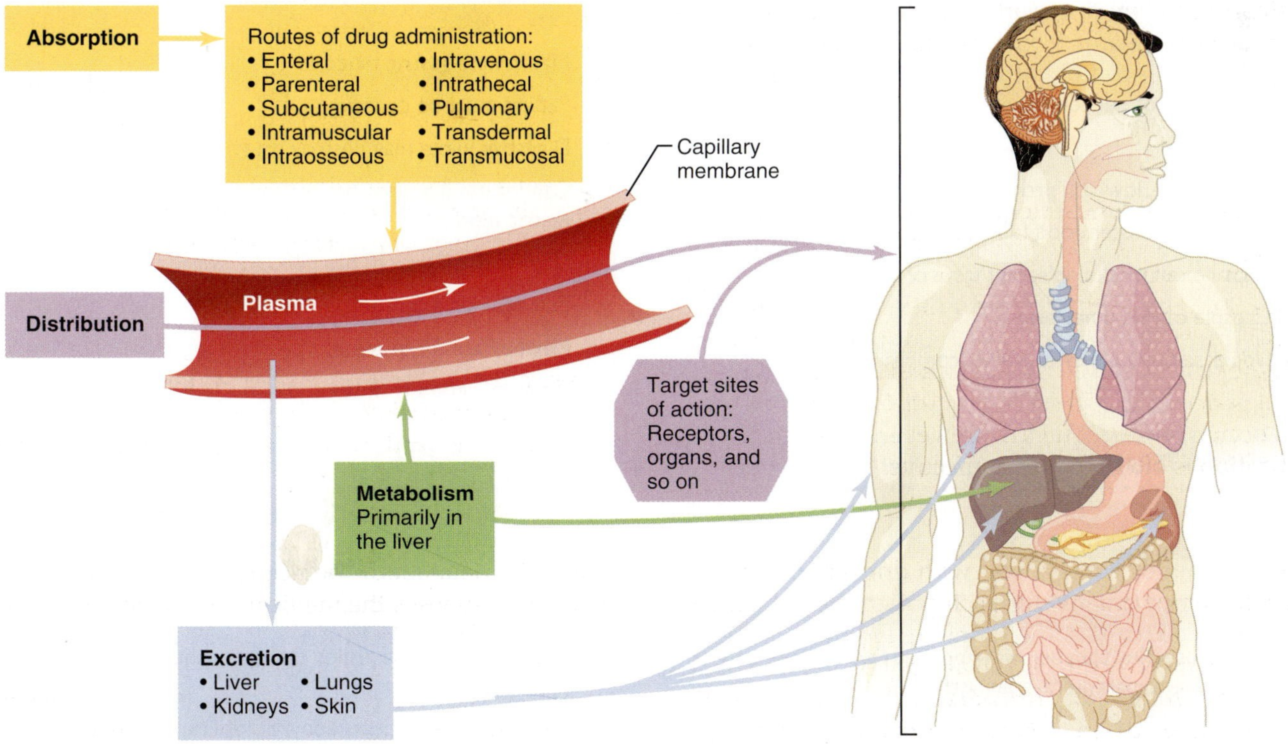

FIGURE 26-3 Pharmacokinetics is the study of drug absorption, distribution, metabolism, and excretion, which determine the intensity and duration of a drug's actions in the body.

Table 26-1 ➤ Advantages and Disadvantages of Routes of Administration

ROUTE: ORAL The drug is swallowed and absorbed from the stomach or small intestines.

Preparation types

- **Capsule**—A gelatinous container that holds the liquid, powder, or oil form of the drug. When swallowed, the gelatin container dissolves in the gastric juices.

- **Pill**—This term is rarely used now. *Tablet* is the preferred term.

- **Tablet**—A powdered drug is compressed into a hard, compact form (e.g., round, oval) that is easy to swallow and then breaks up into a fine powder in the stomach. The tablet is the most common oral preparation. *Enteric-coated tablets* have an acid-insoluble coating to keep them from dissolving in the stomach; they disintegrate in the alkaline secretions of the small intestine.

- **Time-released tablet or capsule**—A tablet or capsule formulated so that it does not dissolve all at once, but gradually releases medication over a few hours

- **Elixir**—A liquid containing water and about 25% alcohol that is sweetened with volatile oils (e.g., aromatic elixir); not as sticky or as sweet as syrups

- **Extract**—A very concentrated form of a drug made from animals or vegetables; may be a syrupy liquid or a powder

- **Fluid extract**—An alcohol-based solution of a drug from a vegetable source (e.g., belladonna); the most concentrated of the fluid preparations

- **Spirits**—A concentrated alcohol-based solution of a volatile (easily evaporated) substance or oil (e.g., ammonia, peppermint oil, orange oil); contains larger amounts of the substance than can be dissolved in water

- **Syrup**—An aqueous solution of sugar, used to disguise unpleasant taste of drugs

- **Tincture**—An alcohol or water-and-alcohol (with a high percentage of alcohol) solution made by extracting potent plants; may also be used externally (e.g., tincture of iodine)

- **Powder**—Finely ground drug(s), usually mixed with a liquid before ingesting; some are used internally, others externally. (Some are mixed with diluents for parenteral injection.)

- **Solution**—Drug(s) dissolved in a liquid carrier. *Aqueous solutions* are medications dissolved in water. (May be used orally, externally, and parenterally.)

- **Suspension**—Drug(s) that are suspended (not completely dissolved) in a liquid. *Aqueous suspensions* are suspended in water. *Never used for IV or intra-arterial routes*

Advantages	Disadvantages
■ Convenient	■ May irritate gastric mucosa.
■ Sterility is not needed for oral use.	■ Patient must be conscious.
■ Economical	■ Digestive juices may destroy drug.
■ Noninvasive, low-risk procedure	■ Cannot use if patient has nausea and vomiting or decreased gastric motility.
■ Easy to administer, good for self-administration	■ Cannot use if patient has difficulty swallowing.
■ Capsule can mask unpleasant taste of a drug.	■ Potential for aspiration
■ Capsule can be time-release	■ May be harmful to teeth.
■ Unpleasant taste may cause noncompliance.	■ Onset of action is slow.

ROUTE: ENTERAL The drug is given directly into the stomach or intestine (e.g., through a nasogastric (NG) or gastrostomy tube).

Preparation types

Same as for oral medications

Advantages	Disadvantages
■ Can be used for patients with Impaired Swallowing as an alternative to parenteral administration.	■ Not all tablets or capsules can be crushed; medications can clog the NG tube.
	■ NG tube itself presents some risk of aspiration.

Table 26-1 ➤ Advantages and Disadvantages of Routes of Administration—cont'd

ROUTE: SUBLINGUAL (a variation of transmucosal administration)—The drug is held under the tongue and absorbed across the sublingual mucous membrane.

Preparation types

Lipid-soluble lozenge (troche)—A flat, round preparation that dissolves when held in the mouth. May act locally or be absorbed through mucosa for systemic effect.

Tablet (See oral route.)

Advantages	Disadvantages
■ Used for local or systemic effects	■ May inadvertently be swallowed in the saliva.
■ Convenient	■ Not useful for drugs with unpleasant taste
■ Sterility not needed	■ May irritate the oral mucosa.
■ Quick delivery to general circulation	■ Patient must be conscious.
■ Bypasses stomach and intestines; absorbed directly into bloodstream	■ Useful only for highly lipid-soluble drugs
	■ Patient must hold the drug in place until it is dissolved, which may take a few minutes.
	■ Limited period of effectiveness, requiring frequent redosing

ROUTE: BUCCAL/TRANSMUCOSAL ADMINISTRATION Medication is held against the mucous membrane of cheek until it dissolves.

Preparation types

Lipid-soluble lozenge or tablet (See oral and sublingual routes.)

Spray—Can be dispersed to the nasal or pharyngeal mucosa for rapid absorption.

Advantages	Disadvantages
■ Same as sublingual	■ Same as sublingual
■ Rapid, convenient, portable	

ROUTE: TOPICAL (SKIN) The drug acts locally or is absorbed directly through skin (transdermal or percutaneous absorption).

Preparation types

Gel or jelly—A clear or translucent semisolid substance that liquefies when applied to the skin

Liniment—An oily liquid to rub into the skin

Lotion—An *emollient* (softening or soothing agent) for use on the skin; may be a clear solution, suspension, or emulsion

Ointment—A semisolid, fatty (usually petroleum jelly or lanolin based) substance for skin or mucous membranes; usually not water soluble

Paste—Similar to an ointment, but thicker and stiffer

Tincture (see oral route).

Transdermal patch—Releases constant, controlled amounts of medication, for systemic effect.

Aerosol spray or foam—A liquid or foam that is sprayed by air pressure onto the skin

Cream—A non-oily, semisolid substance applied to the skin

Advantages	Disadvantages
■ Continuous dosing	■ Effective only for lipid-soluble drugs and must be specially formulated.
■ Sterility is not needed.	■ May cause local irritation, especially if the patient is allergic to latex or tape.
■ For local or systemic effects	
■ Long-acting systemic effect	■ Discarded patches may pose danger of poisoning.
■ Useful if patient is unable to take oral medications	■ Leaves residue on skin.
■ Acceptable to most patients	■ Accurate doses can be difficult to obtain when the drug is in a tube or jar.

Continued

Table 26-1 ➤ Advantages and Disadvantages of Routes of Administration—cont'd

ROUTE: TOPICAL: INSTILLATIONS The drug is placed into a body cavity (e.g., urinary bladder, rectum, vagina, ears, nose, eye).

Preparation types

Solutions (for nose, ears, and eyes; enemas per rectum)—Drug(s) dissolved in a liquid carrier

Suppositories (for bladder, vagina, rectum)—Drug(s) mixed with a glycerin-gelatin or cocoa butter base and shaped for insertion into the body. They dissolve gradually at body temperature.

Jellies, creams (for vagina and rectum)—See skin route.

Advantages	Disadvantages
■ Continuous dosing	■ May be embarrassing for the patient.
■ Sterility is not needed	■ Absorption from the rectum is slow and if stool is present, there is local irritation, or if the patient defecates before the suppository melts.
■ Useful if patient is unable to take oral medications, when the oral drug has an unacceptable taste or odor.	■ Pain, if the patient has hemorrhoids.
■ Preferred when the patient is vomiting or unconscious.	■ As a rule, contraindicated when there is active rectal bleeding.
■ May be used for local or systemic effects	

ROUTE: TOPICAL: INHALATION A device (e.g., nebulizer, face mask) breaks the drug into finely dispersed particles, which are breathed into the respiratory passages. Some drugs are intended for local effects in the respiratory passages; others (e.g., anesthetic gases) are for systemic effects, especially in the brain.

Preparation types

Aerosols—Aerosols are liquids in very fine particles that can be inhaled into the lungs; they are sprayed under air pressure.

Gases—Gas is a basic form of matter (i.e., solid, liquid, and gas). A gas must be kept in a closed container; otherwise, the fast-moving molecules escape into the air. Examples are oxygen, nitrogen, carbon dioxide, and anesthetic gases.

Advantages	Disadvantages
■ Quick and efficient local and systemic route through the lungs	■ Requires special equipment.
■ May be given to unconscious patient.	■ May irritate lung mucosa.
■ Allows continuous dosing, and dosage can be easily modified.	■ Useful only for drugs that are gases at room temperature.
	■ May have unexpected systemic effect when only local effect is desired.

ROUTE: ALL PARENTERAL ROUTES Drug taken into the body other than through the digestive system.

Preparation types

Depends on route.

Advantages	Disadvantages
Patient may be conscious or unconscious.	■ Requires sterile procedures.
	■ Poses risk for infection because skin is broken.
	■ Requires skill.
	■ May cause some pain.
	■ Produces anxiety.
	■ More expensive than oral administration

ROUTE: PARENTERAL: INTRAVENOUS The drug is injected directly into the vein, either by bolus or slow infusion.

Preparation types

Aqueous solutions—Drug(s) dissolved in water

Table 26-1 ▸ Advantages and Disadvantages of Routes of Administration—cont'd

Advantages	Disadvantages
▪ Rapid effect because absorption is bypassed; therefore, good for emergency situations ▪ Patient needs only one needlestick, even for multiple doses.	▪ Poses risk of transient drug concentrations if drug is injected too rapidly. ▪ Limited to highly soluble medications. ▪ Poses risk for sepsis because pathogens may be introduced directly into the bloodstream. ▪ The patient must have usable veins. ▪ Cost of supplies and medications

ROUTE: PARENTERAL: INTRAMUSCULAR The drug is injected into the muscle mass.

Preparation types

Primarily aqueous solutions (see intravenous route), although some preparations (e.g., penicillin) are suspensions

Advantages	Disadvantages
▪ Rapid absorption, except for oily preparations or suspensions ▪ Allows use of drugs that are not stable in solution. ▪ Causes less pain (than do subcutaneous injections) from irritating drugs because they are deep in the muscle. ▪ Allows administration of a larger volume than does subcutaneous administration. ▪ Allows more rapid absorption than does subcutaneous or oral administration.	▪ May cause irritation and local reactions. ▪ Poses risk for tissue and nerve damage if site is improperly located. ▪ Cannot be used where tissue is damaged (e.g., bruised) or peripheral circulation is decreased.

ROUTE: PARENTERAL: SUBCUTANEOUS The drug is injected into the subcutaneous tissue under the skin

Preparation types

Primarily solutions—Drugs dissolved in a liquid carrier

Advantages	Disadvantages
▪ Allows faster action than does oral administration. ▪ Allows better absorption of lipid-soluble drugs than does intramuscular administration.	▪ Only very small amounts can be given. ▪ Absorption is relatively slow and often confined to the injected area.

ROUTE: PARENTERAL: INTRADERMAL The drug is injected under the skin, into the dermis. Most commonly used for diagnostic testing or screening or for injecting local anesthetic.

ROUTE: PARENTERAL: OTHER

Preparation types

Intraspinal—Injection of drug into the spinal canal

Intrathecal—Injection of drug into the subarachnoid space around the spinal cord

Epidural—Injection of drug between the vertebral spines into the extradural space.

Most commonly used for regional anesthesia and pain control.

Advantages	Disadvantages
Most rapid absorption Highly effective	Some patients may be anxious about administration method. Spinal route can produce hypotension, nausea, urinary retention, or headache.

oral drug will not be absorbed effectively in the stomach and would likely be expelled during vomiting. If the patient has diarrhea, rapid motility of the gastrointestinal (GI) tract would decrease absorption. If your patient Cary Pearson (Meet Your Patient) has a prescription for an oral medication, would you question the route? Why or why not?

Solubility of the Drug

Solubility refers to the ability of a medication to be transformed into a liquid form that can be absorbed into the bloodstream. Typically, absorption occurs more rapidly with highly soluble drugs. *Oral medications* must be water soluble and at least partially lipid soluble to be absorbed in the GI tract. Liquids (e.g., suspensions or solutions) are absorbed faster than tablets or capsules because the liquids are already dissolved.

- *Water-soluble drugs.* Drugs must be water soluble in order to dissolve in the *aqueous* (watery) contents of the GI tract. These drugs are more rapidly absorbed from the GI tract and take effect faster.
- *Lipid-soluble drugs.* Lipid solubility depends partly on the drug's chemical structure and partly on the environment at the site of absorption. Lipid-soluble drugs can penetrate lipid-rich cell membranes and enter the cells; whereas, water-soluble drugs (e.g., penicillin) cannot. That is why a highly fat-soluble drug (e.g., nitrous oxide) can easily pass through the blood brain barrier and effect sedation. Lipid-soluble drugs are preferred when a much longer acting effect is desired, since they are more slowly released into the circulatory system.

Solubility Factors Some drugs have been designed for delayed breakdown. **Enteric-coated** drugs cannot be broken down by gastric acids because the coating prevents the medication from being diluted before it reaches the intestines. In this way, the coating delays the action of the drug, which decreases the irritating effects on the stomach. **Timed-release (sustained-release)** medications are formulated to dissolve slowly, releasing small amounts for absorption over several hours.

✚ You should never crush or break enteric-coated and time-released medications; to do so would destroy their protective coatings.

Which of your patients (Meet Your Patient) is most likely to receive a water-soluble medication?

Effects of pH and Ionization

The **pH** (relative acidity or alkalinity) of the local environment also affects the absorption of a drug. The acid content of the stomach aids in transporting the medication across the mucous membranes, so *acidic* medications, such as aspirin, are more readily absorbed in the stomach than are *basic* (alkaline) medications, such as sodium bicarbonate, which are readily absorbed in the more alkaline small intestine. For best absorption, should Mr. Pearson's (Meet Your Patient) medications be acidic or alkaline preparations?

In solution, some of a drug's molecules are in **ionized** (electrically charged) form, and others in a **nonionized** (neutral or noncharged) form. The ionized molecules are lipid insoluble and thus cannot pass easily through the phospholipid layer of cell membranes. Drug molecules can be easily converted easily from one form to the other, depending primarily on the pH of the environment. For example, when aspirin is dissolved in the stomach acid, most of its molecules remain nonionized because of the low pH, so they easily pass through the membranes of the gastric mucosa and enter the bloodstream. If the person ingests an antacid before taking aspirin, the pH increases and the aspirin becomes more ionized, and will likely reduce the absorption and effects of the aspirin.

Blood Flow to the Area

Medications are absorbed rapidly in areas where blood flow to the tissue is greatest (e.g., oral mucous membranes). Areas with poor vascular supply (e.g., the skin, scarred areas) experience delayed absorption. Consider the following examples:

- Excessive exercise draws blood away from the stomach and intestines to the muscles. Which route would promote absorption for a person who has just exercised heavily: oral or intramuscular (IM)? Why?
- A person in shock has poor peripheral circulation. Which route would promote faster absorption: intramuscular or intravenous (IV)? Why?

For the first question, the IM route would be better for the person who has recently engaged in heavy activity. This is because medication injected deep into the muscle where there is a rich blood supply would be absorbed more readily, whereas medication administered orally must first dissolve and be absorbed in the GI tract. For the second question, the IV route would be more efficient for the person with poor circulation because drugs act more rapidly, even in healthy people, when they are injected directly into the bloodstream and do not have to be absorbed.

KnowledgeCheck 26-3

- Define *absorption.*
- How are drugs absorbed?
- What factors affect absorption?

How Are Drugs Distributed Throughout the Body?

Distribution is the transportation of a drug in body fluids (usually the bloodstream) to the various tissues and organs of the body. Because blood goes to all parts of the body, theoretically a drug can produce effects (intended or unintended) anywhere. The rate of distribution depends on adequate local blood flow in the **target area** (the site where the drug effects occur). It is also influenced by the permeability of capillaries to the drug's molecules as well as the protein-binding capacity of the drug. For a visual description,

 Go to Student Resources, **Pharmacokinetic Animation: Medication Absorption, Distribution, Metabolism, and Excretion,** on Davis*Plus*.

Local Blood Flow The blood supply of the target site affects distribution of a drug. For example, it is difficult to deliver a systemic medication to the skin and toes, where the blood vessels are very small. Factors that cause vasodilation in an area (e.g., application of warmth to an injection site, fever, and rest) increase circulation to area tissues. Factors that cause vasoconstriction (e.g., shock and chilling of the body) decrease circulation to the target tissue.

Membrane Permeability Drug molecules must leave the blood and cross capillary membranes to reach their sites of action. The capillary networks in some organs consist of tightly packed endothelial cells that prevent some drugs from crossing them. For example, the blood–brain barrier allows distribution into the brain and cerebrospinal fluid of only those drugs that are (1) lipid soluble (e.g., anesthetics and barbiturates) and (2) not tightly bound to plasma proteins. This barrier can be bypassed by injecting medications intrathecally (via the spinal canal) into the cerebrospinal fluid.

Protein-Binding Capacity For a given amount of a drug, some molecules bind to plasma proteins, and the remainder will be "free." Only free (unbound) drug molecules can produce pharmacological effects because only free molecules can be metabolized or excreted. For example, nearly all acetaminophen (Tylenol) molecules are free in the bloodstream and are therefore pharmacologically active. By contrast, about 99% of the anticoagulant warfarin (Coumadin) is bound in the blood; its effects are produced by only the 1% of warfarin molecules that are free. A drug's tendency to bind to plasma proteins depends mostly on its chemical structure. Some medical conditions also affect protein binding. For example, malnourishment and liver disease reduce the amount of protein (serum albumin) available for binding.

KnowledgeCheck 26-4

- Define *distribution*.
- What factors affect distribution of drugs in the body?

How Are Drugs Metabolized in the Body?
Metabolism (or **biotransformation**) is the chemical inactivation of a drug through its conversion into a more water-soluble compound or into metabolites that can be excreted from the body. Once a medication reaches its site of action, it is metabolized (changed into the inactive form) in preparation for excretion.

Metabolism takes place mainly in the liver, but medications can be detoxified also in the kidneys, blood plasma, intestinal mucosa, and lungs. If liver function is impaired (e.g., due to liver disease or aging), the drug will be eliminated more slowly, and toxic levels may accumulate. Disease states also affect drug metabolism. For example, patients with diabetes do not metabolize sugar effectively, so they should not take elixirs, which are high in sugar content.

Oral medications are absorbed from the GI tract and circulate through the liver before they reach the systemic circulation. Many oral medications can be almost completely inactivated in passing through the liver. This inactivation is known as the **first-pass effect**. For this reason, oral medications are formulated with a higher concentration of the drug than are parenteral medications. Alternatively, some medications can be given parenterally, allowing the drug to be distributed directly to target sites. For example, nitroglycerin undergoes this first-pass effect when taken orally; therefore, it is given sublingually or intravenously so that it bypasses the stomach and liver and reaches therapeutic levels in the blood.

KnowledgeCheck 26-5

- Define drug *metabolism*.
- Where are drugs metabolized?
- What factors affect drug metabolism?

How Are Drugs Excreted From the Body?
A drug continues to act in the body until it is excreted. For **excretion** to occur, drug molecules must be removed from their sites of action and eliminated from the body. Drugs may be metabolized completely, partially, or not at all when they are excreted. The following are common organs of excretion.

Kidneys The kidneys are the primary site of excretion. Adequate fluid intake facilitates renal excretion. If your patient has decreased renal function (e.g., as indicated by an elevated creatinine level), you should monitor for medication toxicity. Obtain a prescription for adjusted dosing if signs of toxicity are present.

Liver and GI Tract Some drugs broken down by the liver are excreted into the GI tract and eliminated in the feces. Others (e.g., fat-soluble agents) are reabsorbed by the bloodstream, distributed to the target site, and returned to the liver. This is called **enterohepatic recirculation**. The kidneys later excrete these compounds. Anything that increases peristalsis (e.g., diarrhea, laxatives, enemas, chronic bowel disease) accelerates drug excretion via feces. Inactivity, poor diet, and decreased peristalsis delay excretion, increasing the effects of a drug.

Lungs Most drugs removed by the lungs are not metabolized first. Gases and volatile liquids (e.g., general anesthetics) administered by inhalation usually are removed through exhalation. Other volatile substances, such as ethyl alcohol and paraldehyde, are highly soluble in blood and are excreted in limited amounts by the lungs. Strenuous exercise and deep breathing increase pulmonary blood flow and thereby promote excretion. By contrast, decreased cardiac output (as in shock) and hypoventilation (as can happen when a patient is in pain) prolong the period of time for drug elimination.

Exocrine Glands Drug excretion through the **exocrine** (sweat and salivary) **glands** is limited. The elimination of metabolites in sweat is frequently responsible for such side effects as dermatitis. Drugs excreted in the saliva are usually swallowed and absorbed as other orally administered agents.

 ThinkLike a Nurse 26-4

You are notified of a patient being transferred from the ICU to your unit. The patient is 79-year-old Hattie Banks, admitted 2 days ago to the ICU for digoxin toxicity.

- What theoretical knowledge do you have about the metabolism and excretion of digoxin (Lanoxin)?
- What assessments are important to make for Ms. Banks?

Concepts Relevant to Drug Effectiveness

In addition to the processes of absorption, distribution, metabolism, and excretion, you need to understand four other concepts related to a drug's effectiveness: (1) onset, peak, and duration of drug action; (2) therapeutic range; (3) bioavailability of the drug; and (4) concentration of the drug at target sites. As you read about them, try to relate these concepts to the key concepts of medication administration and medication safety.

Onset, Peak, and Duration of Action

Before reading on, think for a moment how the subconcepts *onset, peak,* and *duration* of action relate to the chapter key concept, *medication safety.* The **onset of action** is the time needed for drug concentration to reach a high enough blood level for its effects to appear. This is the **minimum effective concentration.** When the concentration of medication is highest in the blood, the medication has reached its **peak action.** The **duration of action** is that period of time in which the medication has a pharmacological effect (before it is metabolized and excreted) (Fig. 26-4). If the serum level of a medication falls below the minimum effective concentration, then the drug is not effective during that time. If the drug level exceeds the peak level, toxicity occurs.

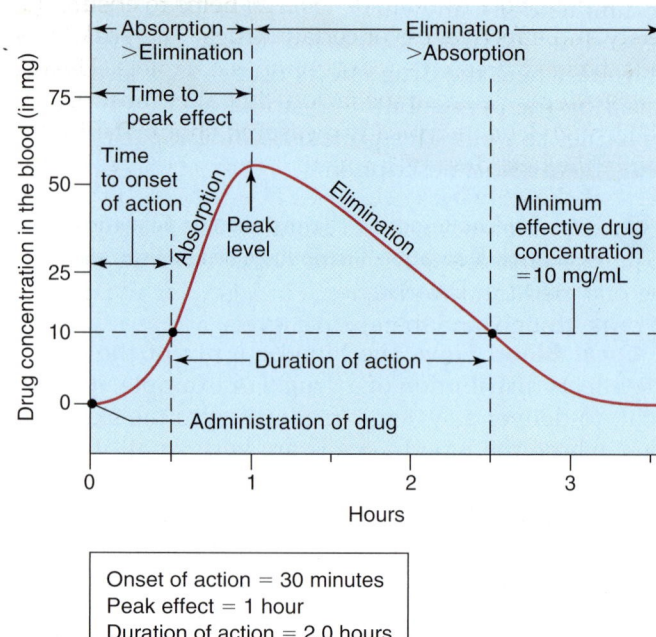

| Onset of action = 30 minutes |
| Peak effect = 1 hour |
| Duration of action = 2.0 hours |

FIGURE 26-4 Once the drug is administered and absorption begins, blood levels begin to rise. When the *minimum effective concentration* is reached, drug effects begin (*onset of action*). *Maximum effect* occurs at peak blood level.

 ThinkLike a Nurse 26-5

Refer to Table 26-1. James Bigler (Meet Your Patient) is having right arm pain and needs relief quickly.

- Would it be better to give him oral acetaminophen with codeine (Tylenol #3) or an IM injection of a similar-strength medication? Why?
- Do you have enough information to be completely sure your choice of route will bring the quickest onset of action? Explain.

Therapeutic Range

Even after absorption stops, distribution, metabolism, and excretion continue. When giving multidose medication (e.g., an antibiotic), the goal is to achieve a constant, therapeutic blood level. Because a fraction of the drug is constantly being excreted, repeated doses of the medication are given to achieve and maintain a constant therapeutic concentration.

Therapeutic range of a drug is a range of therapeutic concentrations. At onset of action, serum drug level is minimal.

Therapeutic level is the concentration of a drug in the blood serum that produces the desired effect without toxicity.

Peak level occurs when the drug is at its highest concentration (when the rate of absorption is equal to the rate of elimination). After that, metabolic and excretory processes begin to remove the drug from the tissues and blood.

Trough level occurs when the drug is at its lowest concentration, right before the next dose is due.

A test called a *peak and trough level* helps to ensure the safety and effectiveness of certain drugs. The peak level must be measured when absorption is complete. This, of course, depends on all the factors that affect absorption. The trough level is typically measured about 30 minutes before the next dose of the drug is due. The drug's half-life and the time between doses affect the trough level. You will sometimes need to monitor serum drug levels so the primary care provider can adjust the dose and timing of a medication as needed. For a graphic illustration of peak, trough, and therapeutic levels,

 Go to Chapter 26, **Tables, Boxes, Figures: ESG Figure 26-1, Peak and Trough,** on *DavisPlus*.

Biological Half-Life

A medication's **biological half-life** is the amount of time it takes for half of the drug to be eliminated. For example, tramadol (Ultram), a narcotic-like pain reliever, has a half-life of approximately 6 hours. This means if you take a 50-mg dose at 0800, by 1400 half of that dose (25 mg) will still be left in your body. In 12 hours, one-fourth of the initial dose (12.5 mg) will be left in your body. Liver and kidney disease, aging, absence of food, and slowed metabolic rate prolong half-life because of their effects on metabolism and excretion. Drug composition and distribution also affect half-life.

 ### Think**Like a Nurse** 26-6

Rebecca Jones (Meet Your Patients) received tramadol (Ultram) 50 mg for pain at 0800. The prescription allows the patient to have the drug every 6 hours. At 1400, you give her another 50 mg. Ultram is metabolized in the liver and excreted mainly in the urine.

- When this medication reaches onset of action, about how much tramadol does Ms. Jones now have in her body?
- If the normal half-life of tramadol is 6 hours, you would expect that Ms. Jones would still have about 25 mg of her first dose left in her body at the time of the second dose. Given her age, though, do you think she probably has more or less than 25 mg left at 6 hours? Why?

Concentration of Active Drug at Target Sites

The effectiveness of a medication depends ultimately on its concentration at the intended site. For example, a medication such as nitrofurantoin (Macrodantin) may be prescribed to treat a urinary tract infection. This drug is used because it is highly soluble in urine, and therefore tends to accumulate and concentrate in the bladder and kidneys, where the infection exists.

What Factors Affect Pharmacokinetics?

A drug's pharmacokinetics and therefore its effectiveness and safety are affected by the following factors:

- **Age.** Infants and young children need smaller doses because of their smaller body mass and immature body systems.

 Older adults may have declining liver and kidney function and are therefore at higher risk for drug toxicity.

Table 26-2 summarizes life span variations in pharmacokinetics.

- **Body Mass (Weight).** The final concentration of a drug in the body depends on the patient's body mass. The average adult dose is based on the drug quantity that will produce a particular effect in 50% of people 18 to 65 years of age and weighing 150 lb. Obviously, a person who is much larger or smaller than this "average" requires an adjusted dose.
- **Sex.** Men and women absorb drugs differently because women usually have lower muscle mass, a different hormone profile, and different fat and water distribution.
- **Pregnancy.** Most drugs are contraindicated during pregnancy because of their possible adverse effects on the embryo or fetus. Drugs known to cause developmental defects are called teratogenic drugs (e.g., alcohol; the anticonvulsant phenytoin [Dilantin]).
- **Environment.** Heat and cold affect peripheral circulation. A noisy environment may interfere with a person's response to anti-anxiety, sedative, or pain medications.
- **Route of Administration.** The route of administration influences the amount of a drug absorbed into the circulatory system and the distribution to the sites of action.
- **Timing of Administration.** The presence or absence of food in the GI tract affects an oral drug's pharmacokinetics. Biorhythms and cycles (e.g., drug-metabolizing enzyme rhythms, blood pressure cycles) also influence drug action.
- **Fluids.** Insufficient fluid intake affects the absorption of solid dosage forms.
- **Pathological States.** Intense pain decreases the effect of opioids; diseases causing circulatory, hepatic, or renal dysfunction interfere with pharmacokinetic processes.
- **Genetic Factors.** Abnormal susceptibility to certain chemicals is genetically determined. Enzyme deficiencies and altered metabolism change a patient's responses to a drug. For example, African Americans usually respond better to diuretics for blood pressure control than do other racial groups; and people of Asian descent metabolize some opioids at a slower rate. Use your critical thinking now. What important nursing intervention should you perform after you administer an opiate to an Asian patient?[1]
- **Psychological Factors.** Some patients have the same response to a placebo—a pharmacologically inactive substance—as they do to the active drug. If a person has faith that a drug will help him, a *placebo effect* similar to the effect of an active drug may occur. Emotional states, such as anxiety, may cause resistance

---

[1]How did you answer the question? If you said that you would need to observe closely for unexpected side effects, good thinking!

Table 26-2 ➤ Drug Therapy Across the Life Span

PHARMACOKINETIC PROCESS	CHILDREN	OLDER ADULTS
Absorption	■ Exaggerated in infants as a result of lack of gastric acidity and shorter intestines ■ More complete topical absorption results from a larger body surface and thinner epidermis. ■ Enteral route is unpredictable. ■ Decreased muscle tone makes absorption of parenteral drugs unpredictable. ■ Gastric pH is higher, so that medications absorbed in acid environments are absorbed much more slowly.	■ Delayed but more complete ■ Gastric pH is less acidic because of decreased acid production in the stomach. ■ Decreased gastric pH delays absorption of medications absorbed in acid environments. ■ Because of decreased intestinal motility, drugs remain in the system longer, allowing for more absorption.
Distribution	■ Protein binding may be a problem. ■ Greater chance of toxicity because of low albumin levels. ■ Water content in the child's body is higher than in adults, so water-soluble drugs are less concentrated in the child and fat-soluble drugs are more highly concentrated.	■ Low albumin level could create a problem with plasma protein binding. ■ Increased risk of toxicity owing to multiorgan slowdown. ■ Altered because of less lean mass ■ Less body water, greater body fat ■ Dehydration, poor nutrition, and electrolyte imbalances decrease absorption.
Metabolism	■ Metabolism may be altered because of immature liver. ■ Best to base dosage on body weight to avoid toxicity.	■ Presence of diseases may decrease metabolism of the drug. ■ Changes from age, higher blood concentration, and less excretion cause greater chances of toxicity. ■ Some drugs interfere with the liver's ability to metabolize another drug.
Excretion	■ Excretion is delayed as a result of immature kidneys. ■ Repeat dosing may cause problems.	■ Decreased glomerular filtration rate inhibits excretion from the kidneys. ■ Diminished renal function inhibits excretion, thereby increasing the risk of toxicity.

to tranquilizing drugs. Hostility toward or mistrust of medicine or health personnel can also interfere with a drug's effectiveness.

WHAT IS PHARMACODYNAMICS?

Pharmacodynamics, another subconcept of pharmacology, is the study of *how* medications achieve their effects at various sites in the body—how specific drug molecules interact with target cells and how biological responses occur. You will use knowledge of pharmacodynamics concepts to help you administer medications safely and to evaluate patient outcomes.

What Are Primary Effects?

Primary or **therapeutic effects** of medications are effects that are predicted, intended, and desired. The primary effects, in short, are the reason the drug was prescribed. All other consequences are **secondary effects** (unintended,

nontherapeutic). Both primary and secondary effects are dose related, so increasing the dose increases the effects. Medications are given for the following effects:

■ **Palliative effects** relieve the signs and symptoms of a disease but have no effect on the disease itself. For example, morphine sulfate may be given to a patient with cancer to manage pain, but it does not destroy cancer cells. The goal of palliative therapy is to make the patient as comfortable as possible when treatment options have been exhausted.

■ **Supportive effects** support the integrity of body functions until other medications or treatments can become effective. For a patient with a bacterial infection, you may give acetaminophen (Tylenol) to control fever until blood levels of the prescribed antibiotic are effective in combating the infection causing the fever.

■ **Substitutive effects** replace either body fluids or a chemical required by the body for improved functioning. You may, for example, administer insulin to a diabetic patient to replace the insulin no longer produced by the pancreas.

- **Chemotherapeutic effects** destroy disease-producing microorganisms or body cells. Two examples are (1) antibiotics, used to treat infections by killing or limiting the reproduction of certain bacteria and (2) antineoplastic drugs, used to treat cancer by limiting cell reproduction and destroying malignant cells.
- **Restorative effects** return the body to or maintain the body at optimal levels of health. For example, vitamin and mineral supplements are administered to many patients recovering from surgery.

KnowledgeCheck 26-6

- Name and define the four pharmacokinetic processes.
- How does absorption differ in children and older adults?
- What factors affect excretion?
- You are to administer the following drugs to Cyndi Early (Meet Your Patients): (1) insulin for her diabetes, administered subcutaneously, and (2) morphine to relieve her pain, administered intravenously. For which primary effect is each of these drugs being given?

What Are Secondary Effects?

All medications can cause secondary effects (e.g., side effects, adverse reactions, allergic reactions), which can either be harmless or cause injury and which can sometimes be predicted.

Side Effects

Side effects are unintended, often predictable, physiological effects of the medication to which patients usually adapt. They occur at the usual prescribed dose and may be immediate (e.g., dizziness) or delayed (e.g., constipation). For hospitalized patients, you will most often see side effects caused by analgesics, antibiotics, antipsychotics, and sedatives. The most common side effects are nausea, vomiting, diarrhea, dizziness, drowsiness, dry mouth, abdominal distention or distress, and constipation.

If side effects are significant, the medication may be discontinued. For example, digoxin (Lanoxin), which is given to regulate and strengthen the heartbeat, can cause cardiac irregularities, a side effect that can be life threatening. Persistent or undesired side effects may require symptom management with laxatives, antidiarrheals, and antiemetics. For example, levofloxacin (Levaquin), an antibiotic, may cause diarrhea, which is treated with antidiarrheal medication (e.g., loperamide [Imodium]).

Key Point: *As a primary nurse, your role includes teaching the patient what side effects to anticipate and how to manage them.*

Adverse Reactions

Adverse reactions are harmful, unintended, usually unpredicted reactions to a drug administered at the normal dosage. They are more severe than side effects and often require discontinuation of the drug.

- *Dose-related* adverse reactions result from the known pharmacological effects of the medication. For example, a diabetic patient treated with insulin may develop a very low blood sugar if too much insulin is administered.
- *Patient sensitivity* adverse reactions occur because the patient is unusually susceptible to the effects of the drug. Box 26-1 lists patients at high risk for adverse reactions.

The FDA defines **severe adverse reactions** as those that (1) are life threatening; (2) require intervention to prevent permanent impairment or death; or (3) lead to congenital anomaly, disability, hospitalization, or death. Health professionals must document serious adverse reactions according to agency policy and report them to the FDA MedWatch program. To make a report, contact the FDA by calling 1-800-332-1088, or

 Go to the **FDA Medwatch** Web site at http://www.fda.gov/medwatch/

You can also contact the Institute for Safe Medication Practices (ISMP) to report errors, close calls, or hazardous conditions. ISMP guarantees the confidentiality and security of the information received. For information on where and how to report errors,

 Chapter 26, Chapter Resources, **Resources for Caregivers and Health Professionals,** on Davis*Plus*.

BOX 26-1 ■ Risk Factors for Adverse Drug Reactions

Behavioral and Situational Factors

- History of allergies or previous adverse drug reactions
- Receiving treatment from two or more providers at the same time
- Taking multiple prescription drugs in addition to over-the-counter preparations and herbal remedies and supplements. This is also called polypharmacy.
- Taking a drug inconsistently
- Long-term use of a drug (may promote accumulation, leading to toxicity)

Physical Factors

- Concurrent illnesses (e.g., diabetes and renal failure)
- A change in the ability to absorb, metabolize, or excrete the drug (e.g., impaired hepatic or renal function)
- Confusion/cognitive impairment
- Very old or very young age
- Obesity or extreme thinness
- Dehydration or rapid change in hydration status

Toxic Reactions

Toxic reactions are dangerous, damaging effects to an organ or tissue. They are more severe than adverse reactions, sometimes even causing permanent damage or death. It may help to think of toxicity as poisoning. Antidotes are available for some medications; for example, naloxone (Narcan) is given for opiate toxicity. Toxicity may be caused by any of the following:

- *Overdosing* (administrating a dose that exceeds the prescribed amount). Examples are respiratory depression from excessive morphine and hypoglycemia from too much insulin.
- *Accumulation* of the drug in the tissues (related to long-term use or incomplete metabolism/excretion)
- *Abnormal sensitivity* or allergic response to the drug

Toxic reactions are usually localized, reversible, and immediate. However, they can be:

- Localized to a particular tissue or organ, or they can also affect several organ systems.
- Reversible (e.g., tinnitus caused by aspirin) or permanent (e.g., hearing loss caused by aminoglycoside antibiotics).
- Evident soon after administration; although, some toxic reactions take months or even years to develop (e.g., drug-induced cancers).

 ### ThinkLike a Nurse 26-7

- You have just looked up the antihypertensive drug lisinopril (Zestril) and found the following side effects:
  neutropenia, dizziness, headache, fatigue, depression, somnolence, paresthesia, hypotension, orthostasis, chest pain, nasal congestion, diarrhea, nausea, dyspepsia, impotence, rash, cough, muscle cramps, angioedema, lethargy, hypokalemia, decreased libido
  What strategy could you use to help you remember all the above side effects?
- You have checked the MAR for Margaret Marks (Meet Your Patients) and prepared her next dose of antibiotic for intravenous administration. The MAR also indicates that she is receiving morphine for pain and that her last dose was given 1 hour ago. When you enter the room, you find her apparently sleeping. You are not able to awaken her to verify her identity. What do you suspect is happening, and how should you respond? (If you need information about antibiotics and morphine, look it up in an appropriate reference.)

Allergic Reactions

In an **allergic reaction,** the immune system identifies a medication as a foreign substance that should be neutralized or destroyed. The patient experiences no problems with the first dose of the medication, but it acts as an antigen, activating the formation of antibodies against the drug. When the drug is again administered, the antigen–antibody binding complex prompts an allergic reaction.

Allergic reactions range from minor to serious; however, even a small amount of a medication can cause a severe reaction. Urticaria (hives), pruritus (itching), edema of soft tissue and mucosa, and rhinitis (inflammation of the nasal mucosa) usually occur within minutes to 2 weeks after exposure and are considered mild. Such reactions often disappear after the medication is discontinued and the blood level of the drug falls. Medications most frequently implicated in allergic reactions are antibiotics, biological agents, and diagnostic agents. For a list of specific drugs you can print and use,

 Go to Chapter 26, **Tables, Boxes, Figures: ESG Table 26-4, Medications Frequently Triggering Allergic Reactions,** on Davis*Plus.*

An **anaphylactic reaction** is a life-threatening allergic reaction that occurs immediately after administration. Anaphylaxis produces sudden constriction of bronchioles, edema of the larynx and pharynx, severe shortness of breath, wheezing, and severe hypotension (low blood pressure). Immediate treatment includes discontinuing the medication and giving epinephrine, IV fluids, steroids, and antihistamines. Respiratory support (e.g., oxygen, intubation, ventilation) may also be required.

➕ A patient who is allergic to one drug may also be allergic to other medications in the same class. For example, many patients who are allergic to penicillin are also allergic to cephalexin (Keflex), a synthetic penicillin.

Always explore the patient's allergy history and the patient's reaction to the medication. Remember to document allergies in the patient's chart, care plan, and MAR.

➕ People with severe allergic reactions should wear a Medic Alert bracelet (Fig. 26-5) that identifies the person and the allergen, and carry epinephrine for emergency injection.

 ### ThinkLike a Nurse 26-8

You are administering medications to your assigned patients (Meet Your Patients). What should you do in each of the following situations? Which patient should you attend to first? Explain your thinking.

- Ms. Jones has ibuprofen (Motrin) prescribed for back pain. She tells you she cannot take this medication because it makes her feel nauseated.
- Mr. Bigler had an open reduction internal fixation of his arm performed yesterday and is receiving an antibiotic, cefazolin (Ancef) 500 mg IV every 8 hours. He has already received three doses of this medication, and you initiated his 0800 dose about 10 minutes ago. He tells you that he thinks his throat is closing shut.

Idiosyncratic Reactions

An **idiosyncratic** reaction is an unexpected, abnormal, or peculiar response to a medication. Idiosyncratic reactions may take the form of extreme sensitivity to a medication, lack of response, or a paradoxical (opposite of

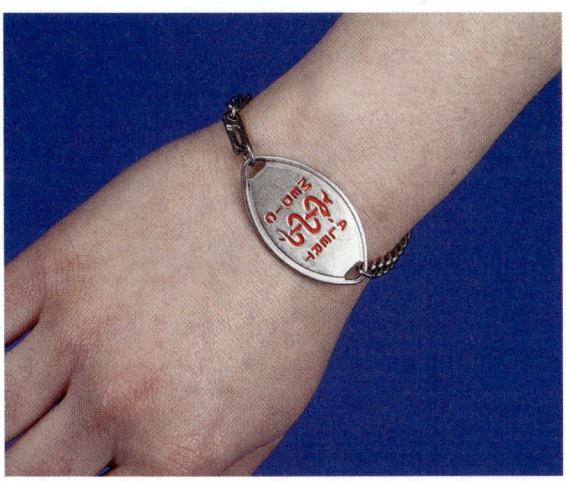

FIGURE 26-5 People with severe allergies to a medication should wear a Medic Alert bracelet.

expected) response, such as agitation in response to a sedative.

Cumulative Effect

A **cumulative effect** is the increased response to repeated doses of a drug that occurs when the rate of administration is greater than the rate of metabolism and excretion. This happens when (1) the body cannot metabolize a dose of the medication before the next dose is given, (2) excretion is slowed but absorption is normal or rapid, or (3) absorption is slowed. Unless the dose is changed, the medication accumulates in the system until a toxic level is reached. Opiates and barbiturates are known for their cumulative effects.

KnowledgeCheck 26-7

- Differentiate between primary and secondary effects of medications.
- List one adverse reaction for each of the following systems: blood, gastrointestinal, neurological, cardiovascular, hepatic, renal.
- What are some of the symptoms you will see in an anaphylactic reaction?
- What type of patient is most likely to experience an allergic reaction?

How Do Medications Interact?

When one drug alters or modifies the action of another, a **drug interaction** occurs. In an **antagonistic drug relationship**, one drug interferes with the actions of another and decreases the resultant drug effect—that is, the combined effect is less than that of one drug given alone. In a **synergistic drug relationship**, there is an additive effect; that is, the effect of both drugs together is greater than the individual effects. **Drug incompatibilities** occur when multiple drugs are mixed together, causing a chemical deterioration of one or both drugs. The result is an incompatible solution that should not be administered.

 You can usually recognize an incompatibility when the mixed solution takes on a changed appearance. However, you should always consult medication resources and compatibility charts *before* mixing medications. Then, after mixing, double-check the medication for changes in appearance.

As a nurse, you must know about drug interactions and monitor your patients for them. For a list of common drug-drug and drug-food interactions,

Go to Chapter 26, **Tables, Boxes, Figures: ESG Table 26-5, Drug-Drug and Food-Drug Interactions,** on DavisPlus.

The more drugs a patient takes, the higher will be the risk of a drug interaction. Other variables influence drug interactions: intestinal absorption, competition for protein binding, drug metabolism, renal excretion, and alteration of electrolyte imbalance. Drugs may also interact with certain foods. For example,

- High-fat foods and those low in fiber will delay stomach emptying and medication absorption by up to 2 hours.
- Acidic citrus fruits and juices enhance absorption of iron. Some citrus fruits, such as grapefruit, interact with medication in an antagonistic manner.
- Carbonated soft drinks can cause medications to dissolve faster, be neutralized, or experience a change in absorption rate in the stomach.
- Dairy products taken with an antibiotic such as tetracycline decrease the absorption of the drug in the stomach.
- Foods containing tyramine (e.g., aged, dried, or fermented products), when consumed while taking monoamine oxidase (MAO) inhibitors, may produce a hypertensive crisis.

To print and use a list of several medications that should be taken with food and those that should be taken on an empty stomach,

 Go to Chapter 26, **Tables, Boxes, Figures: ESG Box 26-1,** on DavisPlus.

KnowledgeCheck 26-8

- What type of interaction occurs when one drug interferes with the action of another?
- What interactions occur when one drug has an additive effect on another drug?
- What is drug incompatibility?

What Should I Know About Drug Abuse or Misuse?

You should be able to differentiate between the concepts that describe nontherapeutic use or effects of drugs.

- **Tolerance** is a decreasing response to repeated doses of a medication. The person then requires more of the drug to achieve the desired effect.

- **Dependence** is a person's reliance on, or need for the drug. Dependence leads to compulsive patterns of drug use wherein the user's lifestyle centers on procuring and taking the drug.
- **Drug misuse** is the nonspecific, indiscriminate, or improper use of drugs, including alcohol, over-the-counter (OTC), and prescription drugs. In performing self-care, people frequently misuse laxatives, aspirin, acetaminophen, ibuprofen, cough and cold remedies, and sleep-inducing drugs.

> Older adults are especially prone to misuse of laxatives in the self-treatment of constipation. Continued use of laxatives can led to dependence and other medical problems.

- **Drug abuse** is the inappropriate intake of a substance by amount, type, or situation, continuously or periodically. For example, consuming alcohol at work is considered abuse, but having a glass of wine with dinner is not. Drug abuse may or may not lead to drug dependence.
- **Illicit drugs**, also known as street drugs, are drugs sold illegally. Many are prescription drugs (e.g., hydrocodone [OxyContin or Vicodin]) sought for their mood-altering effects. Prescription drugs can be abused when taken for purposes other than medically intended.

HOW DO I MEASURE AND CALCULATE DOSAGE?

Medications are not always available in the exact dosage the patient needs. Therefore, you must be proficient in calculating drug dosages to be sure your patients receive the correct amount of medication.

Medication Measurement Systems

Medications are usually prescribed and measured using the metric system; however, a few are still dispensed using the apothecary and household systems. You will sometimes need to make conversions from one measurement system to another. To learn about how to convert medications doses within one system and between systems,

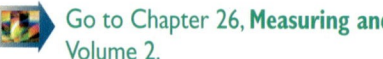 Go to Chapter 26, **Measuring and Calculating Dosage,** in Volume 2.

Metric System The metric system is the preferred system because it promotes accuracy by allowing for calculation of small drug dosages. A disadvantage of this system in the United States is that many people outside the healthcare system are not familiar with it.

Apothecary System The British apothecary system of measurement has been used in the United States since colonial times. Only a few medications (e.g., aspirin) are

measured using this system because it is less convenient and less precise. Apothecary measurements are usually written using Roman numerals, but you may also see them in Arabic numerals. For example, *5 grains* might be written as *grains V* or *gr V*.

✚ To avoid a dosage error, write out the intended unit of measurement (grains) so gr (grains) is not mistaken for gm (grams). (The Joint Commission, 2012)

Household System Because most people are familiar with the household system, it is easier to teach a patient about home medications using this system. However, nurses do not often use it because dosages measured in this system are less precise (e.g., teaspoons, ounces, cups) and can lead to medication dosing error.

Special Measurements: Units and Milliequivalents

Units Insulin, a drug used by diabetics to help control blood sugar, is measured in **units**, with 100 international units (U100) being the standard strength preparation. In this strength, 1 mL of the fluid medication contains 100 units of insulin. The following is a medication prescription using units: "NPH insulin 14 units subcutaneously every morning." Heparin, an anticoagulant, and penicillin are also prescribed in units.

✚ Not all units are the same. For example, 1 mL of heparin does *not* contain 100 units of heparin. You must always read the container label to know the number of units per milliliter.

Milliequivalents (mEq) indicate the strength of the ion concentration in a drug. A milliequivalent is the number of grams of a solid contained in 1 mL of a solution. Electrolytes, such as potassium chloride (KCl), are measured in mEq. The following is a prescription using mEq: "D_5W 1000 mL with KCl 40 mEq every 8 hours."

Key Point: *Note that units and mEq cannot be directly converted to the apothecary, metric, or household system.*

Calculating Dosages

You should be able to calculate accurately using several different methods and formulas. Inaccurate calculations result in incorrect dosages and could harm the patient. For expanded instructions on calculating dosages for adults and children,

 Go to Chapter 26, **Measuring and Calculating Dosage,** in Volume 2.

Several practice problems are available on Davis*Plus*. To use them,

 Go to Chapter Resources, Chapter 26, **Dosage Calculation Problems,** on Davis*Plus*.

WHAT MUST I KNOW ABOUT MEDICATION PRESCRIPTIONS?

Before administering any medication you must obtain a medication prescription from the care provider and verify that it is complete, correct, and legible.

- *For inpatients*, prescriptions for medications are either entered into an electronic health record for automated dispensing or printed in the medical orders section of the paper chart. This was traditionally referred to as an "order."
- *For outpatients* and for medications that will be filled by the patient (instead of the agency pharmacy). See Figure 26-6 for an example of a prescription that might be written and given to the patient or family. This is what was traditionally called a "prescription."

The term *prescription* is now used to refer to both the traditional inpatient *order* and the outpatient *prescription*. A written or printed outpatient medication prescription should contain the following essential elements:

- Patient's full name (some agencies and some states require the address of the patient)
- Name, address, and telephone number of the prescriber, including relevant credentials and legal registration number, such as the National Provider Identification (NPI) in the United States. Providers who are prescribing controlled substances must register with the federal Drug Enforcement Agency (DEA). The prescriber's DEA number must be included on the prescription. The NPI number is needed for Medicaid, Medicare, and durable medical equipment prescriptions.
- Date and time prescription was written
- Name of medication
- Dosage (including amount, frequency, and number of doses)
- Route of administration
- Signature of prescriber

Verifying Prescriptions

To verify a medication prescription, ask yourself the following questions:

- Is the prescription legible enough for me to read with certainty?
- Is the prescribed dose within the normally prescribed dosage range and comparable to any previously prescribed dose?
- Is the prescribed route appropriate?
- Is the drug appropriate for the patient? (For example, you would question an antihypertensive drug prescribed for a patient with hypotension.)
- Is the patient allergic to the prescribed medication?
- Are the administration times appropriate (for example, an antibiotic prescribed for every 6 hours, when the drug formulary indicates it should be taken every 24 hours)?

For outpatient prescriptions (to be obtained by the patient), ask yourself the following questions:

- What is the address and National Provider Identification (NPI) of the person prescribing?
- Is a DEA number included on prescriptions for controlled substances?
- How many doses are there before the prescription needs to be refilled?
- How many refills are prescribed?

KnowledgeCheck 26-9

- What are the essential parts of a medication prescription?
- How does an inpatient prescription (order) differ from an outpatient prescription?

What Abbreviations Are Used in Medication Prescriptions?

For a list of medication-related abbreviations you may see used when prescribing and documenting medications,

 Go to Chapter 26, **Tables, Common Medication-Related Abbreviations,** in Volume 2.

You should write out drug names in full. Abbreviations can be easily confused and many are not universally understood. However, you will see and use some abbreviations when administering and documenting medications (e.g., mL, mEq). Always do so carefully because some may be similar and confusing. Consult The

---

MICHELLE GRAVES, RN, FNP
NPI # GF 0110324
210 LINDEN STREET, SUITE 124
NEW YORK, NY 10032
(500) 443-7786 TEL.   (500) 443-7788 FAX

NAME _____   AGE _____

ADDRESS _____   DATE _mm/dd/yyyy_

Rx ILLEGAL IF NOT SAFTEY BLUE BACKGROUND

R

Lisinopril 20 mg i tablet PO qAM
sig #90

Refill X 3 times

DEA # AA3785000000

DO NOT SUBSTITUTE

To ensure brand name dispensing, check and initial box.

4RTE0045011

FIGURE 26-6 Example of a prescription.

Joint Commission's official Do Not Use list (Table 18-1) and know the acceptable abbreviations used in your facility. Also,

 Go to Chapter 26, **Tables, Institute for Safe Medication Practices (ISMP): List of Error-Prone Abbreviations, Symbols, and Dose Designations,** in Volume 2.

Types of Medication Prescriptions
Common types of medication prescriptions are based on the duration, frequency, and/or urgency of the prescription.

- **Standard written prescriptions** apply without a renewal date until the prescriber writes a prescription to alter or discontinue the medication or indicates on the original prescription a specific stop date. For example, "Give furosemide (Lasix) 20 mg IV-Push twice a day for 5 days." After 5 days, the prescription is discontinued, unless the provider renews it.
- **Automatic stop dates** are protocols that hospitals use for discontinuing medications after a certain length of time. Most narcotic prescriptions are in effect only for 7 days. If the medication is needed after the automatic stop date, the care provider must write another prescription.
- **STAT** prescription means that a single dose of medication is to be given immediately and only once. The word STAT or *now* should appear in the prescription, for example, "Give furosemide (Lasix) 20 mg IV push STAT," or "Give lorazepam (Activan) 1 mg IV push now."
- **Single** prescription, or *one-time prescription*, indicates that the medication is to be given only once at a specified time. Preoperative medications, given before surgery or diagnostic procedures or treatments, are an example of a single prescription. For example:
  Versed 25 mg intramuscularly on call for when surgical staff requests premedication to be administered
  Tetanus toxoid 0.5 mL intramuscularly before discharge
- **Standing orders.** When a unit has a standard population of patients—for example, coronary care patients or knee replacement patients—the primary care provider may develop a set of *standing orders*. These are officially accepted sets of prescriptions for this population of patient to be applied routinely by nurses for the care of patients. They establish guidelines for treating a particular disease or set of symptoms. For example:
  Coronary care or intensive care units (CCUs or ICUs) may have standing orders for the administration of nitroglycerin for chest pain (e.g., "Give nitroglycerin 0.4 mg sublingually q3–5 min for chest pain, to a maximum of 3 doses in 15 min").

  Many postoperative patients receive a prescribed number of injectable analgesic medications for pain relief. So, for all the postoperative patients on a unit, standing orders would include, "ketorolac (Toradol) 30 mg IV push q12hr for 2 days."

- **prn prescription.** The care provider may prescribe a medication to be given whenever the patient requires (prn), within the established parameters. A prn prescription requires the nurse to determine, in collaboration with the patient, when the medication is to be given. The prescription specifies (1) the condition for which the medication is to be given and (2) the minimum time intervals between doses.

Key Point: *The medication cannot be given more frequently than prescribed, even if symptoms persist.*

Pain medications, antiemetics (antinausea medications), and laxatives are usually given prn. For example:

Morphine 10 mg intramuscularly q3–4hr prn incisional pain.
Acetaminophen 650 mg PO q4hr prn for temp > 101°F.

How Are Medication Prescriptions Communicated?
Providers communicate medication prescriptions either in writing or verbally. The nursing implications are slightly different for each. The provider usually must cosign verbal and telephone prescriptions within 24 hours.

Written Prescriptions You will find **written prescriptions** either handwritten on a prescription form or preprinted standard medication orders and protocols. Some agencies accept medication orders or prescriptions transmitted electronically or via facsimile from the prescriber to the nurse, with the original copy provided later. To reduce the risk of errors with faxes and electronic transmission, always ensure that the content is legible.

Verbal Prescription A prescriber may sometimes give a **verbal prescription**, which is an oral order spoken to the nurse. When you receive a verbal prescription, you, as the RN, will write the prescription and sign it with the provider's name followed by your name and credentials. Medication names that sound the same can be confusing and lead to administering the wrong drug (Box 26-2). Repeat the prescription to the provider and spell the medication name to ensure accuracy—many drug names sound the same. Avoid taking verbal prescriptions, and use them only in urgent situations because they increase the risk for miscommunication and errors.

Telephone Prescription Prescribers may also give medication prescriptions via telephone. Usually this will be in response to a call you have placed to report a change in the patient's condition or the results of laboratory or other tests.

What Should I Do If I Think a Prescription Is Incorrect?
Key Point: *As a nurse, you are legally responsible for medications you administer.*

BOX 26-2 ■ Medications With Similar-Sounding Names

Alprazolam—lorazepam	NovoLog—Humalog
Baclofen—Bactroban	NovoLog—Novalin R
Cefzil, Keflin—Keflex	Ophthalgan—Auralgan
Celebrex—Celexa, Cerebyx	Percocet—Percodan
Cytoxan—Ciloxan	Phenergan—Phenaphen
Demerol—dicumarol	Procardia—Procardia XL
Digoxin—digitoxin	Quinine—quinidine
Glyburide—glipizide	Ranitidine—amantadine
Humalog—Humulin R	Serzone—Seroquel
Keflex—Kantrex	Taxotere—Taxol
Lamictal—Lamisil	Zantac—Xanax
Lodine—iodine	Zantac—Zyrtec
Morphine—meperidine	Zostrix—Zestril

If you believe a prescription is incorrect, do the following:

- Ask another nurse or physician to check the prescription.
- Look up the medication in a reliable resource (e.g., drug formulary) to verify spelling, usage, dosages, and routes.
- Contact the prescriber for clarifications, concerns, or questions.
- Do not assume you are correctly interpreting the prescription if you have any question at all.

Use your knowledge, common sense, and intuition when administering medications. To avoid errors, you must know and understand the procedures at your facility, be familiar with the medications you give, and always check the prescription. Each agency will have a policy specifying the procedure for checking medication prescriptions. For example, a unit secretary may copy the original prescription onto a MAR, but the nurse must check to be sure the transcription is correct.

 Most medication errors occur during the prescribing process; however, 50% are detected before these errors reach the patient (Mckay, 2012). Thus, this double check system is imperative.

▲ ThinkLike a Nurse 26-9

Find the errors in these medication prescriptions. Use a drug formulary or nursing drug handbook to check dosages, spelling, and so on.

- Ancef 10 g q6hr IV
- Capatril 25 mg orally twice a day
- Digoxin 0.125 mg daily
- Lasix 400 mg by mouth
- NTG gr 1/150 prn chest pain
- Tylenol orally prn fever

MEDICATION ERRORS

A **medication error** is any preventable event that may cause or lead to inappropriate medication use or harm to a patient. Medication errors occur with surprising frequency. They are among the most common adverse events that occur in hospitalized patients. The National Coordinating Council for Medication Error Reporting and Prevention (2012) estimates that 98,000 hospitalized patients die annually from medication errors.

The most common medication errors made by nurses are related to confusion caused by similar drug names, lack of knowledge of the drug (e.g., incorrect dosages, incorrect mixing), and lack of information about the patient (e.g., allergies, lab results, medical condition). Box 26-3 describes several causes of medication errors by nurses. For a list of drugs that can have devastating consequences when erroneously administered,

 Chapter Resources, Chapter 26, ISMP Web site, in **Resources for Caregivers and Health Professionals,** on DavisPlus.

How Can I Avoid Errors?

To ensure patient safety, begin by following the "three checks" and the six-plus "rights" found in the section Ensuring Safe Medication Administration for Inpatients, later in this chapter. You also must be familiar with and follow the variety of system-wide measures designed to prevent medication errors in your healthcare agency. For example, The Joint Commission recommends standardizing protocols for prescribing, administering, and documenting medication. Errors can be reduced in the home setting if the patient is prescribed the same dose at home as in the hospital.

Critical thinking may be your best way to avoid errors and improve patient care and safety. You need to learn from your mistakes and the mistakes of others, and you also need to think defensively. Ask "are we," "what if," and "why" questions: "Are we following standardized protocols for prescribing, administering, and documenting medication? What will happen if I don't do something or if I do something wrong? What assessments are required before and after I give this medication? Why am I hanging this IV or giving this medication?"

Error-Prevention Technology

Computers can decrease errors by improving access to information and communication among health professionals. Some healthcare agencies provide nurses with laptops and handheld mobile devices, putting at their fingertips detailed information about diseases, similar-sounding drugs, interactions, and side effects. A variety of error-prevention technologies can reduce the likelihood of medication errors.

BOX 26-3 ▪ Why Do Medication Errors Occur?

The following are several factors associated with medication errors:

Lack of Knowledge or Information

- Lack of knowledge of the drug (e.g., incorrect dosages, incorrect mixing, overly rapid infusion, drug interaction, adverse effects) is the most common factor contributing to medication errors.
- Lack of information about the patient (e.g., allergies, other medications, lab results, medical condition for which the medication is contraindicated). This is the second most frequent cause of errors.
- A drug is given by the wrong route.

Faulty Communication

- The written prescription is unclear, illegible, or transcribed incorrectly, resulting in administering the wrong drug or dosage (e.g., confusion between drugs with similar names).
- The telephone prescription is taken incorrectly.
- Protocol is not understood or is violated.
- A drug prescription is written on the wrong patient's chart.
- The wrong dosage is prescribed (e.g., by misplacing a zero or decimal point).
- Abbreviations are misunderstood.
- Poor, or no, documentation can result in error. For example, a nurse administers a medication yet fails to record it immediately afterward. A second nurse checking the patient's chart thinks the drug has not been given so administers a dose. The patient receives a double dose.

Equipment Errors

- Wrong equipment is used to administer the drug.
- Equipment malfunctions or is not used properly.

Calculation and Measurement Errors

- An error in calculating the dosage is made so the patient receives the wrong dose.
- There is confusion in the unit of measurement; for example, a drug is prescribed based on kilograms and dispensed or administered based on pounds (and vice versa).

Other

- Medication is improperly handled or stored.
- The patient's identity is not checked, and the wrong patient receives the medication.
- Lighting is inadequate.
- The nurse is fatigued, distracted, or interrupted.

Sources: Hayes, B., Klein-Schwartz, W., & Gonzales, L. (2009). Causes of therapeutic errors in older adults: Evaluation of national poison center data. *Journal of American Geriatrics Society, 57*(4), 653–658; The Joanna Briggs Institute. (2005). Strategies to reduce medication errors with reference to older adults. *Best Practice, 9*(4), 1–6; Pretorius, R., Gataric, G., Swedlund, S., et al. (2013). Reducing the risk of adverse events in older adults. *American Family Physician, 87*(5), 331–336; Roy, V., Gupta, P., & Srivastava, S. (2005). Medication errors: Causes & prevention. *Health Administrator, 19*(1), 60–64.

PICOT

Medication Safety

Situation: The student is preparing to administer medications to two clients in the subacute nursing setting. There are several medications to be administered to each client. The student has researched the medications, and knows that there are oral, subcutaneous, and intravenous medications to administer. Prior to preparing the medication the student reviews the medications, and calculates the doses to ensure accuracy.

PICOT Components:

P	Population/client	=	Nursing students
I	Intervention/indicator	=	Medication administration simulation
C	Comparator/control	=	Math testing only
O	Outcome	=	Safe medication administration skills
T	Time	=	Initial practice after graduation

Searchable Question: Do _____ (P) who receive _____ (I) demonstrate _____ (O) as compared to _____ (C) during _____ (T)

Example of Evidence: Medication errors have been identified as a cause of 6% of all sentinel events from 2004 through 2010 (The Joint Commission, 2010). Nursing students are often tested on medication calculation skills separately from the skill of administering medications. Shanks (2011) noted that psychomotor and cognitive skills needed to be integrated. Simulations that included calculating a pediatric dosage (mg/kg/day), administration of the medication, documentation, and evaluation of the efficacy allow the skills to be practiced in an environment that does not expose clients to harm. During the debriefing or reflection session that follows the simulation, the factors that contributed to an error or near miss can be identified, and further remediation can be utilized.

Practice Change. While this method may not be fail-safe, it allows students and new graduates to gain the knowledge and confidence to work through medication problems and arrive at accurate results (Shanks, 2011).

References: The Joint Commission (2010). *Summary data of sentinel events reviewed by The Joint Commission.* Oakbrook Terrace, IL: Author; Shanks, L. (2011). Medication calculation competency. *American Journal of Nursing, 111*(10), 67–69.

Technology cannot substitute for the need to adhere to all guidelines in medication administration. Rubin, Nash, and Safran (2012) present a case scenario that resulted in the death of a premature infant and a pretrial settlement of $8.25 million. The numerous systems in place failed to detect human error that caused the infant to receive an IV that contained 60 times the normal dose of sodium.

Computerized Prescriber Order Entry (CPOE)

CPOE helps prevent errors in reading and transcribing orders, particularly when handwritten orders are illegible. Electronic prescribing systems are safer when combined with decision-support tools that automatically alert prescribers to possible interactions, allergies, and other potential problems.

Barcoding Medications Barcode medication administration, especially when combined with CPOE, provides a highly effective system for identifying the right patient. It also transfers data electronically, eliminating the error-prone paper transcription process. When used correctly, barcoding at the unit-dose level prevents nurses from selecting an incorrect medication.

Smart Pumps IV infusion technologies, called smart pumps, used at the point of care can help you avoid programming the wrong dose into the pump and ensure the correct dose is delivered. Once they are programmed, the delivery rate does not change. An alarm will sound or the pump will stop if:

- A nurse attempts to program outside dosing limits.
- The flow is interrupted (e.g., a blocked line).

You must adhere to standard operating guidelines to use these pumps effectively to reduce errors (Cummings & McGowan, 2011). For more information on smart pump technologies, cases involving medication errors, and risk management strategies,

Chapter Resources, Chapter 26, the FDA Web site, in **Resources for Caregivers and Health Professionals,** on DavisPlus.

Automated Dispensing Cabinets (ADCs) Most healthcare institutions use ADCs. These systems are known to reduce medication errors when the built-in safety features are used, and the collaboration between pharmacy and nursing is ongoing (Mandrack, Cohen, Featherling, et al., 2012). ADCs in the pharmacy minimize human handling, which can also reduce error.

See the QSEN box for examples of errors that can occur when technologies for administering medication are misused.

Pediatric Considerations

Confusion between pounds and kilograms is a source of dosing error. You should weigh patients in kilograms

---

Quality and Safety Education for Nurses

Understanding the Limitations of Technologies for Medication Safety

Chapter Key Concept: Medication Safety

Competencies: Safety (Knowledge); Informatics (Knowledge, Skills, Attitudes)*

It is important to understand the limitations of safety enhancing technologies so that you can apply the technologies correctly (Informatics) and reduce the risk of patient harm (Safety).

Computerized physician order entry (CPOE). CPOE was hailed as the answer to prescribing errors and it has had many positive effects. However, several studies have reported mixed results: One documented 22 new types of errors, and one reported an *increase* in mortality after CPOE implementation. Factors contributing CPOE errors include:

➤ "Alert fatigue": the tendency for users to ignore frequent interruptions from warning messages

➤ Rigid programs that take users through multiple unnecessary screens or force unnecessary decisions. These encourage users to bypass decision points.

➤ False sense of security generated by the belief that automated systems prevent errors

Bar-code-assisted medication administration (BCMA). A high rate of false-positive alerts has led to practitioner overrides and work-around actions. Of particular concern is the practice of "back scanning" in which the patient's bar code is scanned *after* medication administration. This greatly increases the risk of error and constitutes negligence.

Smart pump problems. These include software limitations and practitioner misuse (e.g., turning off the pump's dose-checking feature and bypassing alerts). Such actions are ethically and legally indefensible, and do not meet standards of care.

Think about it. How does Informatics competency relate to the Safety competency? How can you avoid risky behaviors, contribute to the redesign of safety technologies, and put patient safety first when administering medications?

Sources: Amarasingham, R., Pantinga, L., Diener-West, M., et al. (2009); Elias, B. L., & Moss, J. A. (2011); Goedert, J. (2010); Han, Y. Y., Carcillo, J. A., Venkataraman, S. T., et al. (2005); Poon, E. G., Keohane, C. A., Yoon, C. S., et al. (2010); Sittig, D. F., & Singh, H. (2011); Trbovich, P. L., Pinkney, S., Cafazzo, J. A., et al. (2010).

* For specific Knowledge, Skills, and Attitudes,

 Go to the QSEN Web site **at http://qsen.org/ competencies/pre-licensure-ksas/**

---

when possible, because it is the standard measurement for pediatric prescriptions, medical records, and staff communication. Medication prescriptions should be written with the dose per kilogram of body weight so that the intended dosage can be easily double-checked by nurses and pharmacists. Pediatric-specific medication formulations and concentrations should be used when available, because they are safer than medications dispensed for adults.

What Should I Do If I Commit a Medication Error?

As a nurse, you have a duty to do no harm. With that said, if you make a medication error, even though you might be anxious about having put your patient at risk, embarrassed to admit that you made a mistake, or fear you could lose your job, you must immediately assess the patient's vital signs and physical status. Report your findings to the patient's primary care provider. Then follow the detailed guidelines about actions to take if you commit a medication error, which you will find when you,

 Go to **Clinical Insight 26-7: Taking Action After a Medication Error,** in Volume 2.

Follow your institution's policy regarding incident reports and other actions. Although an error does not actually occur until the patient has *taken* a medication, you may be required to file a report for an averted error or "near miss" (e.g., if you discover that the pharmacy has sent the wrong medication for a patient). **Near misses** are errors detected during the checking procedure before drug administration.

PracticalKnowledge
knowing how

Regardless of the type of medication or the route of administration, when administering a medication you should perform a medication-focused assessment, follow procedures for safe administration, and perform related interventions (e.g., explaining that a certain drug should be taken with food). The rest of this chapter explains these activities to you. Also be certain to become familiar with the guidelines, and

 Go to Chapter 26, **Medication Guidelines: Steps to Follow for All Medications (Regardless of Type or Route),** in Volume 2.

 Think**Like a Nurse** 26-10

Mr. Pearson (Meet Your Patients) refuses his 1400 dose of antibiotic, stating that he had just taken it. What actions do you take to ensure sound decision making and maintain patient safety?

ASSESSMENT

During your initial patient assessment, you will gather data needed to administer medications safely. The following are highlights of medication-related assessments.

Before Medicating Patients do the following:

- Measure vital signs
- Assess whether the patient's general condition is appropriate for the medication
- Evaluate your knowledge of the medication
- Identify biological factors that affect drug metabolism. Also,

 Go to Chapter 15, **Clinical Insight 15-1: Assessing for Biological Variations,** in Volume 2.

While Administering Medications assess the patient's:

- Mental status
- Coordination
- Ability to self-administer the drug
- Swallowing (for oral medications)

After Medicating Patients assess for:

- Effectiveness of the drug
- Side effects
- Signs of toxicity or adverse reactions

Medication History

When taking a medication history, explore the patient's allergy history. Allergic reactions occur with 5% to 10% of all prescriptions. You should also ask about the patient's history of illness, medications, attitudes toward medications, learning needs, and whether the patient (if a woman) is pregnant or breastfeeding. Also check relevant laboratory test results. For more discussion of the components to include in a medication history, and to print out a tool you can use for a full medication history and physical,

 Go to Chapter 26, **Supplemental Materials: Components of a Medication History,** on Davis*Plus*.

Physical Examination

The physical examination helps you to identify potential problems and the need for adapting medication administration procedures. For example, you will assess relevant body systems to confirm the need for the drug and to provide a baseline for evaluating the patient's responses. For oral medications, assess the patient's ability to swallow; for intramuscular medications, assess muscle mass. For more complete information about the physical examination related to medications,

 Go to Chapter 26, **Supplemental Materials: Physical Examination Related to Medications,** on Davis*Plus*.

ANALYSIS/NURSING DIAGNOSIS

The following are some examples of nursing diagnoses associated with patient medications:

Deficient Knowledge related to lack of motivation to learn about medications

Ineffective Family Therapeutic Regimen Management related to anxiety over child's health status
Risk for Aspiration related to Impaired Swallowing

For examples of other nursing diagnoses,

 Go to Chapter 26, **Standardized Language; Standardized Diagnoses, Outcomes, and Interventions Related to Medication Administration,** on DavisPlus.

A few nursing diagnoses represent medication side effects; however, because a wide range of adverse effects is possible, no attempt was made to include them all. The following sections discuss Risk for Injury and Noncompliance.

Risk for Injury

Risk for Injury may be related to polypharmacy, misuse, overuse, or underuse of medications.

Polypharmacy Many people self-prescribe or rely on OTC medications for relief of symptoms such as insomnia, headaches, joint pains, and indigestion. They may continue taking them in combination with prescribed medications. This practice is **polypharmacy**: the ingestion of numerous medications in an attempt to treat many conditions simultaneously. Polypharmacy increases the potential for adverse reactions and dangerous drug and food interactions.

Older adults are especially prone to polypharmacy. They typically take several medications prescribed for chronic diseases, and may self-medicate for symptoms related to the aging process (e.g., constipation). The likelihood of increased sensitivity to medications, drug interactions, and adverse drug effects increases as the number of medications taken by older adults increases (Perry, 2011). You should carefully assess the older adults' medication history to identify combinations that can be especially dangerous to them.

Misuse, Overuse, Underuse Some patients misuse, overuse, underuse, or use drugs inconsistently. They may even use them when contraindicated. For example, a person takes an antibiotic, "feels better" after a few days of the medication, and then stops taking it or takes it erratically as symptoms come and go. Such an inconsistent dosage schedule hinders the body's ability to achieve a blood level high enough to treat the infection or disease. Some drugs, for instance beta blockers, when taken inconsistently can be dangerous, even life threatening.

Noncompliance

Noncompliance (nonadherence) is failure to follow the treatment plan (e.g., not taking a prescribed medication, or skipping doses). You cannot assume that the reason a patient may be noncompliant is because he hasn't been taught the importance of following the treatment plan. Prescription medications are expensive. Faced with choosing between food and medicines, people on a limited budget or without health insurance often simply do not buy the more costly medications, or they may take only partial doses of maintenance medications (e.g., thyroid medications, oral hypoglycemics for diabetes). Some patients, particularly older adults, have visual and motor deficits that limit their ability to read labels and manipulate access (e.g., bottle caps, syringes). Other reasons for noncompliance include lack of symptoms, inability to tolerate side effects, lack of belief in the medication regimen, forgetfulness, and impaired mental capacity. Always investigate the patient's reasons for nonadherence so you can take the appropriate actions.

KnowledgeCheck 26-10

- What are the risks involved for patients who engage in polypharmacy?
- List at least three reasons for noncompliance with a medication regimen.

■ PLANNING OUTCOMES/EVALUATION

NOC standardized outcomes depend on the specific nursing diagnoses you choose. For NOC outcomes for selected nursing diagnoses,

 Go to Chapter 26, **Standardized Language; Standardized Diagnoses, Outcomes, and Interventions Related to Medication Administration,** on DavisPlus.

Individualized goals/outcome statements you might write should be stated so their achievement reflects resolution of the problem (NANDA-I label). The following are some examples:

After explanation, and within 1 week, describes the expected actions and side effects of his medications.
Self-administers his medications in the correct amounts and on the prescribed schedule.
After demonstration and practice, and within 1 week, correctly draws up and self-administers insulin.

■ PLANNING INTERVENTIONS/IMPLEMENTATION

NIC standardized interventions depend on the patient's nursing diagnoses, especially on the etiologies.

 Go to Chapter 26, **Standardized Language; Standardized Diagnoses, Outcomes, and Interventions Related to Medication Administration,** on DavisPlus.

Specific individualized nursing activities include preparing and administering medications and teaching clients to self-administer their medications. You will use specific, step-by-step procedures in Volume 2 for preparing and giving medications. Only the general principles are included in the Highlights of Procedures box in this volume. For specific, step-by-step procedures,

 Go to Chapter 26, **Procedures 26-1 through 26-18,** in Volume 2.

TEACHING PATIENTS ABOUT MEDICATION SELF-ADMINISTRATION

Teach the following information to patients to help them safely administer their own medications.

Know and Understand What You Are Taking You need to know and understand your drugs in order to take them safely and effectively.

- **When you are prescribed a new medication**, ask why you are taking it, how long you should take it, what side effects to expect, whether you should take it with food, and whether there are any special precautions.

  - **Ask what each drug is for and what it does.** This can prevent taking two medications that do the same thing, as can occur when you are seeing multiple providers (e.g., a podiatrist and an internist may both prescribe a medication to treat toenail fungus).

  - **Keep a list of your medications**, including doses and times taken. Take this list with you when you visit any healthcare provider or emergency department.

Take the Drug as Prescribed to achieve maximum safety and effectiveness.

- **Take the drug for the prescribed length of time** to make certain you receive its full benefit (e.g., some patients may take only part of an expensive antibiotic, hoping to "save it for later." However, if you do not take all of the medication, the infection may recur. Or antibiotic resistance may develop, leading to "super-infection," such as methicillin-resistant *Staphylococcus aureus* (MRSA).

  - **Older adults may forget to take their medications.** A simple plan you can follow at home, such as a written schedule or a meds calendar, might help, especially if the drugs are taken other than at mealtimes and bedtime.

  - **If you cannot see well**, ask a family member to write the schedule in large, black letters. Display it in a highly visible place.

  - **Some older adults may take the medication, only to forget shortly thereafter that they did so.** Use a divided pill container or a small glass filled with the medications for each dosage time during the day. If the a.m. container is empty, you will know you have taken the morning drugs and won't accidentally repeat them.

Communicate With Your Prescriber Notify your prescriber if you have side effects, adverse reactions, or questions. If you become pregnant, notify your primary care provider as soon as possible so your medications can be discontinued or adjusted.

Think About Safety Be aware of your safety and the safety of others.

- **Wear a Medic Alert bracelet** or necklace if you are a diabetic, take anticoagulants, or have allergies to any medication.

- **Do not take medications prescribed to others**, and do not share your medications with others.
- **If you take a variety of medications**, post a list of them in a prominent place that is easy to see in the event of an emergency.
- **Use childproof caps** if children have access to your medications. If no children are in the home, replace with simple closure cap for elderly patients who might have difficulty opening the containers.

 Families with young children visiting the homes of older adults need to be alert to the risk of accidental ingestion of medication.

- **Dispose of expired medications safely.** Do not place them in the trash within the reach of children. Disposing of drugs in the sink or toilet is not environmentally sound (e.g., they can appear in the community water supply). Your community may sponsor an "old medications discard day" or provide a place to discard drugs to avoid contamination. Some local pharmacies may offer medication disposal as a community service.

Administer Your Drugs Correctly, as follows:

- **Read the label carefully on the bottle each time** you take the medication so that you take the correct medication. Many pills look alike.
- **Take only the amount and dose prescribed.** If you have questions, call your prescriber.
- **To measure liquids, use kitchen measuring spoons** rather than tableware, which can vary in volume.

  - **If you have difficulty opening containers and administering your medications** because of pain or stiffness in the hands and fingers, ask family members and friends to help you. Ask the pharmacy and the primary care provider *not* to put childproof safety lids on containers for easier handling. Older adults are allowed to sign a release with their pharmacy to do this.

Store Your Drugs Safely Do not store a drug in a different container from the one it came in. The medication may lose its strength, or you may take the wrong medication. Store all your medications in a dry place out of the sunlight and away from the heat. If a medication requires a cold storage, be sure you return it to the refrigerator immediately after use.

Maintain Your Supply Your drugs need to be up to date and available when you need them.

- **Monitor your prescription amounts, and get refills before you run out.** If you get medications by mail, be sure you order them in plenty of time.
- **Check expiration dates**, and discard any **outdated** medications.
- **Do not take expired medications**; they may have lost their strength.

ENSURING SAFE MEDICATION ADMINISTRATION FOR INPATIENTS

Medication mistakes are the most common type of healthcare error. Errors include giving the dose at the wrong time, omitting doses, giving the wrong dose, and giving the dose without authorization. One safeguard is to develop a set routine for medication administration.

 Many errors occur as a result of interruption or distraction. It is best not to stop what you are doing when preparing or giving medication. One recommendation is to create a "sterile cockpit environment" (similar to takeoffs and landings in which the flight attendants are not disturbed) when preparing your medications (ISMP, 2008). You can do this by putting up "do not disturb" signs or wearing a bright yellow sash/apron to alert people not to disturb you when you are preparing or giving medication.

 Specifically, to help prevent errors when giving medications, perform "three checks" and "rights of medication" discussed following.

 Each time you administer a medication, be sure to follow the guidelines you will find,

In Chapter 26, **Medication Guidelines: Steps to Follow for All Medications (Regardless of Type or Route),** in Volume 2.

Three Checks

Check each medication three times:

1. *BEFORE you pour, mix, or draw up a medication,* check its label against the entry on the MAR. Be sure that the name, route, dose, and time match the MAR entry.
2. *AFTER you prepare the medication,* and before returning the container to the medication cart or discarding anything, check the label against the MAR entry again.
3. *AT THE BEDSIDE, check the medication again* before actually administering it.

Observing the "three checks" rule will help you to practice the "rights of medication."

Rights of Medication

Following the **rights of medication** means that you will give the (1) right medication to the (2) right patient in the (3) right dose using the (4) right route at the (5) right time with the (6) right documentation of the medication administration. This system helps you prevent medication errors.

Right Drug

Obviously, you must always administer the correct medication. That is one reason for reading each label

three times (see the "three checks"). Other ways to ensure giving the correct drug are to:

1. ***Think Critically.***
   - If you must take a verbal prescription, always repeat it back to the prescriber to be sure you have heard correctly. Spell the medication name. Many medication names sound the same when you hear them but are actually very different drugs (e.g., Isordil, Isuprel; see Box 26-2 for more examples).
   - Be familiar with the drugs you administer. If you don't know, look it up.
   - Always check the prescription to see whether there have been changes in the medication dosage, route, and so forth—especially after days off, after working a different shift, and after a break.
   - Ask yourself whether the medication prescription is suitable for the patient's condition. If not, question the prescriber.
   - Participate in daily patient rounds so you will be better informed about your patient's plan of care and why the medications are prescribed.

2. ***Be aware of the pitfalls in abbreviations, units of measurement, and handwriting.***
   - Double-check all prescriptions transcribed by hand to the MAR, especially when decimal points are involved.
   - Do not attempt to decipher illegible handwriting, confusing abbreviations, or units of measurement (e.g., mg and mL, or IU and IV). When in doubt, ask the prescriber to clarify.
   - Be alert for names that look very similar (e.g., Keflex and Keflin). It may be impossible to differentiate them when they are handwritten. Do not administer a drug prescribed by a nickname; be sure it is written out in full.

3. ***Perform the "three checks" of the label against the MAR.***
   - Read the label before and after you prepare the medication, and again at the bedside to verify that you selected the correct product name and strength.
   - Select the prescribed medication from the patient's drug drawer (unless it is a stock drug). Do not "borrow" from another patient's drawer.
   - Do not substitute one medication for another.
   - Even when using a unit dose, read the label. Avoid selecting medications based on size and color because many medications are the same size, shape, and color as others.
   - Be alert for similar-looking labels. If you are accustomed to withdrawing oxytocin (given IV to stimulate uterine contractions) from a small vial with a green label, you might be surprised to find that the small, green-label vial in your hand is actually hydroxyzine (Vistaril), which would harm the patient if given IV.
   - If a label is hard to read or comes off the container, return the container to the pharmacy. Never give a

medication from such a container. Also, do not transfer medications from one pharmacy container to another.

- **Heparin.** Physically separate the highly concentrated heparin sodium (10,000 units/mL in 1-mL vials) from the more diluted 1-mL vials for flushing heparin locks. There is a risk for fatal hemorrhage if the highly concentrated heparin solution is mistakenly used to flush an IV line. FDA-approved labeling now includes new color and design in order to distinguish various heparin concentrations in the vials. Be extremely careful when administering heparin to infants and children.

Right Dose

The right dose is the dose prescribed for the particular patient. Be sure the dose is within the recommended range for the patient's age, weight, and condition. The following are suggestions for avoiding dose errors:

- Perform the "three checks" of the container against the MAR. If the pharmacist has sent a dose different from the one prescribed, you may need to calculate how much of it to give. It is a good idea to have another nurse check your dosage calculations.
- For IV medications, use smart infusion pumps to help ensure the correct dose is delivered.
- How you prepare medications can affect the dose. When you must break a tablet, use a knife or a cutting device. If the tablet does not break evenly, discard and account for it. Also, when crushing a tablet to mix with liquid or food, clean the crushing device completely before and after using it to remove any pieces of a previously crushed drug.
- Read and write measurements carefully. It is easy to misread "mg" instead of "mL." There is a significant difference between 1 mg and 1 mL of IV morphine.
- Write out "international units" instead of abbreviating as "IU." IU can be confused with IV.
- Know how and when to use a zero. Always write a zero *before* a decimal point. It is easy to mistake .15 for 115 if the decimal point is written large or the 1 is written small (e.g., write "Lanoxin 0.125 mg," not "Lanoxin .125 mg"). Conversely, never write a decimal point and a zero *after* a whole number. The decimal point may be mistaken for a 1 (e.g., write "5 mg," not "5.0 mg").
- Question prescriptions for multiple tablets or vials as a single dose; most doses are one or two tablets or one single-dose vial.
- Question abrupt and excessive increases in dosage; most dosages increase gradually.
- Question prescriptions that are not consistent with the standard (protocol) dosage range for the patient's age, weight, and condition.
- Examine the standards of care and practice in your institution to see if they comply with the intent of The Joint Commission's National Patient Safety Goal related to safe dosing with anticoagulation therapy.

Right Time

- Check the prescription against the time to give the drug, and document the exact time of administration on the MAR.

> ✚ If the drug is not charted, never assume the patient received it as scheduled. If you do, the patient may not receive an essential medication; if you assume it has not been given and give it, the patient may receive an overdose.

- Medications are designed to be given at specific times to maintain constant therapeutic blood levels. However, you can give scheduled medications within a "window" of one-half hour before and one-half hour after the scheduled time, as a rule.
- Time oral medications in relation to meals. Give drugs that are irritating to the stomach (e.g., potassium, aspirin) with food; give drugs that absorb better on an empty stomach (e.g., tetracycline, iron supplement) before meals.
- Determine whether your patient is scheduled for any diagnostic procedures, surgery, or blood tests that require him to remain NPO. If so, you may need to hold oral or enteral medications, or have them changed to another route.
- If a drug has been delayed (e.g., for a diagnostic text), have the prescriber clarify when to administer the next dose in order to maintain constant therapeutic blood levels.

Right Route

Recall that drug absorption is highly dependent on the route of administration. The following are suggestions for ensuring the right route:

- Perform the "three checks," and be sure that the drug is in the proper form for the route prescribed, especially for time-released drugs.
- If the prescription does not specify a route, do not guess; clarify with the prescriber.
- Be sure the drug is in the proper form for the route prescribed. Many medications are available in multiple forms; others are made for one specific route. For example, cephalexin (Keflex), an antibiotic, comes in capsules, suspensions for oral use, and injectable forms for intramuscular and IV administration. By contrast, the antibiotic penicillin G procaine (Crysticillin) is prepared for IM injection and is *not* to be given intravenously.
- The right route also includes **right site**. If an intramuscular injection is prescribed, be sure the site is appropriate considering the age of the patient (child, adult, elderly) and the medical condition (e.g., if the site is traumatized or with compromised circulation, you would not use that site).

As an additional safety measure, draw up oral liquids only into an oral syringe to avoid inadvertent IV administration.

Right Patient

Just before giving the medication, always double-check the patient's identification (ID) bracelet. The Joint Commission's (2011) National Patient Safety Goals recommend using two methods of patient identification, so also ask the patient to state his name. It is best to say, "Please tell me your name," because patients with hearing impairment or confusion might respond "yes" incorrectly when asked, for example, "Are you Mary Smith?" Never skip this step, even if you are familiar with the patient. If you are busy and distracted, it is possible to enter the wrong room. Also, patients, especially when they are confused or emotionally disturbed, may move about. You may enter room 214 with a medication for Mr. Jones but discover an entirely different person in Mr. Jones's bed!

Do not leave medications at the bedside. Suppose you are taking an oral tablet to a patient's room. He is in the bathroom and says, "Just leave it; I'll take it when I come out." If you leave the tablet, how would you know whether he really took it? And what might happen if another, confused patient (or a visiting child) wandered into the room and took the tablet?

Be alert for patients with the same last name. It is common to have two patients with same or similar last names (e.g., Williamson, Wilkinson, Wilson, Wilkerson). Look for and place special alerts on charts and MARs to call attention to names that look or sound similar.

Computerized prescriber order entry (CPOE) and bar code medication administration transfer data electronically and provide a nearly foolproof system for identifying the right patient. However, you must still ensure order entry is made in the correct patient record.

Right Documentation

Most nurses consider documentation the sixth right. After administering a medication, document it immediately on the patient's MAR, as in Figure 26-7. To see an electronic MAR, go to Chapter 18. Be sure to document the following information:

- Name of medication given
- Dose of medication given
- Route of administration and injection site for parenteral medications
- Date and time administered
- Your name or initials as administering nurse

Most MARs are preprinted with the patient's name, name of the medication, dosage, and route administered

HOSPITAL MEDICATION ADMINISTRATION RECORD

Codes For Injection Sites

A - Left Anterior Thigh	H - Right Anterior Thigh
B - Left Deltoid	I - Right Deltoid
C - Left Gluteus Medius	J - Right Gluteus Medius
D - Left Lateral Thigh	K - Right Lateral Thigh
E - Left Ventral Gluteus	L - Right Ventral Gluteus
F - Left Lower Quadrant	M - Right Lower Quadrant
G - Left Upper Quadrant	N - Right Upper Quadrant

Mary Smith 086432

age 46 John Miller, M.D.

ALLERGIES: PCN, Sulfa

				mm/dd/yyyy	mm/dd/yyyy	mm/dd/yyyy
mm/dd/yyyy		Lanoxin 0.25mg po Q D	0900	09 JW		
mm/dd/yyyy		Rocephin ˙1 gm IV Q D	1200	1200 JW		
mm/dd/yyyy		Zinacef ˙1 gm IV Q 8 hr	0800 ⎫	08 JW		
			1600 ⎬			
			2400 ⎭			

SIGNATURE / SHIFT INDICATES	7-3	JW		
NURSE ADMINISTERING MEDICATIONS	3-11			
J Wilson, RN	11-7			

FIGURE 26-7 After administering a medication, immediately document the date, time, dose, route, and person administering the medication on the MAR.

(e.g., intramuscular, oral, or intravenous). If so, you need only to write the time you actually gave the medication, initial each medication, and sign the form one time. Write legibly in ink.

If for some reason (e.g., patient refusal, NPO for tests or procedures) you do not administer a prescribed medication, document that information on the MAR and write a nurse's note explaining why it was not given. For example:

06/20/15 0800—Pt NPO for surgery this a.m. 0800 meds held as prescribed. _____ Janet King, RN

When giving a PRN medication, in addition to recording on the MAR, write a nursing note describing your assessment and the time the drug was given. Then, after allowing time for the medication to be absorbed and take effect, evaluate and document the patient's responses. For example:

06/20/15 0800—Pt reports abdominal pain at incision site rated as a #6 on a scale of 1–10. Active bowel sounds auscultated. Resp 16 breaths/min, HR 88 beats/min, BP 130/84. Denies N/V. Morphine 10 mg given intramuscularly in right vastus lateralis. No injection-related complaints (see MAR). _____ Janet King, RN

06/20/15 0900-States pain relieved; "about 3" (scale of 1–10). Resp 14 breaths/min, HR 68 beats/min. BP 126/80. _____ J. King, RN

You are responsible for documenting the client's responses to all medications, including therapeutic effects, side effects, and unexpected or adverse reactions. Never document a drug before you give it; never document a medication given by someone else; and do not ask someone else to document medications you administer.

Other Rights

In addition to the six "rights" already discussed, patients also have the following rights about medications they receive:

- **Right Reason.** This includes the right to not receive unnecessary medications. For example, a tranquilizer or sleeping pill should be given because the patient is very anxious or cannot sleep, not for the convenience of caregivers who are weary of his incessant demands.
- **Right to Know.** This means that you tell the patient the name of the medication, why it is being given, its actions, and potential side effects.
- **Right to Refuse.** The patient has the right to refuse a medication regardless of her reasons and regardless of the consequences, except under certain circumstances (e.g., incompetency).

Some have advocated adding three additional rights: right form (of medication), right actions, and right response (Elliott & Liu, 2010).

ADMINISTERING ORAL MEDICATIONS

The oral route is the one most commonly used for medications. Recall what you already know about oral medications: Where are they absorbed? What are their advantages and disadvantages? What assessments should you make? If you cannot answer these questions, review Table 26-1 and the discussions of drug preparations and routes of administration. For an overview of administering various types of oral medications, see the Highlights of Procedures box. To see complete procedural steps,

 Go to Chapter 26, **Procedure 26-1: Administering Oral Medication,** in Volume 2.

Pouring Liquid Medications

Liquid medications are frequently used for children and older adults. They usually come in multidose bottles, so you will need to pour individual doses into a disposable, calibrated cup, as in Figure 26-8. When pouring, hold the bottle with the label inside your palm, so the liquid does not run over the label, making it difficult to read.

Buccal and Sublingual Medications

Buccal and sublingual medications, although placed in the mouth, are intended for absorption in the mucous membranes rather than in the GI tract. Some soluble forms of medications and enzyme preparations are

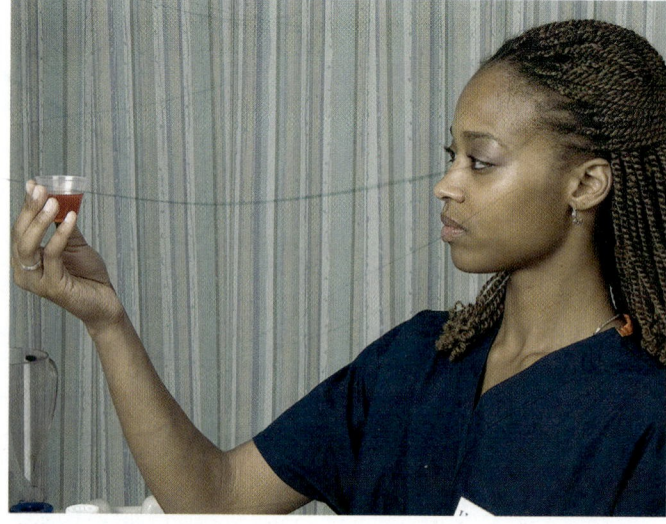

FIGURE 26-8 When pouring a liquid medication, measure the dose while holding the calibrated cup at eye level.

administered by this route and are rapidly absorbed, some within seconds. **Buccal medications** are held between the cheek and the gums; **sublingual medications** are held under the tongue.

Enteral (Nasogastric and Gastrostomy) Medications

For patients who cannot swallow or who have feeding tubes, you can give oral medications through nasogastric (NG), gastrostomy, or jejunal tubes. As with all routes of administration, check for drug interactions. Observe the following special considerations when administering enteral medications:

- *Hydrophilic medications,* such as psyllium (Metamucil)—Do not administer these through feeding tubes because they attract water and will solidify in the tube.
- *Crushing tablets*—Some tablets (e.g., enteric-coated or extended-release medications) should not be crushed, because crushing can change their action. Always check.
- *Continuous tube feedings*—Disconnect before giving medications.
- *Enteral tube suction*—Discontinue the suction for 30 minutes after administration and keep the tube clamped to allow time for the drug to be absorbed, if applicable.

For other procedures related to gastric and enteral tubes,

 Go to Chapter 27, **Procedure 27–2: Inserting Nasogastric and Nasoenteric Tubes, Procedure 27-3: Administering Feedings Through Gastric and Enteric Tubes, and Procedure 27-4: Removing a Nasogastric or Nasoenteric Tube,** in Volume 2.

Special Situations

Some oral medications can discolor or damage tooth enamel, have an objectionable taste, are difficult to swallow, or cause the patient to gag. Offer oral hygiene immediately after giving the medication. The following may also be helpful:

- **Medications that discolor the teeth.** Mix such drugs with liquid, have the patient drink the solution through a straw, and drink water afterward. Unless contraindicated, encourage the patient to drink a liberal amount of flavored liquid (e.g., juice) or water to dilute the medication.
- **Medications with an objectionable taste.**
  Have the patient suck on ice chips for several minutes before taking the medication. Ice numbs the taste buds.
  Store the medication in the refrigerator, unless contraindicated. The smell and taste are less objectionable when chilled, especially for oily liquids.

Use a syringe to place the medication on the back of the patient's tongue. There are fewer taste buds there.
Some medications can be constituted with flavored additive to make the elixir more appealing, particularly for children.

- **Contraindications to oral medications.** In the following situations, do not give the drug. Obtain a prescription for an alternative route or, if the patient is NPO, permission to give the medication with small sips of water. Patients who:
  Cannot swallow fluids. The risk for aspiration is too great.
  Have nausea or vomiting; the medication would be lost in the emesis.
  Are NPO.
  Are not coherent or are comatose.
- **Patients who have difficulty swallowing medications.** Some patients may gag, or the pills become "stuck" in their throat. It may help to crush soluble tablets and place them in liquids or in a small amount of applesauce or pudding. Remember that some forms (e.g., time-released tablets) should *not* be crushed, so check your drug reference sources to be certain. To learn more about which medication to take with or without food,

 Go to **ESG Box 26-1, Oral Medications Taken With or Without Food,** on Davis*Plus.*

KnowledgeCheck 26-12

- Describe two ways to ensure an accurate dosage when pouring liquid medications.
- What instructions should you give to a patient who is taking a sublingual medication?
- Explain the special steps required when administering enteral medications to a patient who is receiving continuous tube feedings.
- Describe three methods to use when administering objectionable-tasting drugs.
- For which patients are oral medications contraindicated?

Medicating Children Orally

Children are not motivated by logic. They do not grasp the cause and effect of "Take this, it will make you feel better." If they do not like the taste, they simply will not swallow it. Another challenge is that before the age of 5 years, a child may not be able to swallow tablets and capsules; therefore, most oral medications for children are prepared as sweetened and flavored liquids or chewable tablets. For very young children and infants, you must take care to prevent choking and aspiration. Parents can often suggest the best methods for getting their child to take medicines. For other parents, you may need to teach techniques for administering medications at home (see Self-Care: Teaching Parents About Medicating Children).

Self-Care

Teaching Parents About Medicating Children

1. Mark each bottle or syringe containing medication with a different color of tape or adhesive label. This makes each clearly distinguishable since many medication bottles look alike.

2. You can reuse syringes for oral medications until the markings or tape begins to wear off or the plunger becomes difficult to move. Wash syringes with warm, soapy water, rinse well, and allow to air dry.

3. Take your time when giving medication, and find a quiet environment. Don't rush the process. It can be frustrating to struggle with a young child who is resisting taking a medication, especially if your time is limited.

4. Give the medication at the same time each day so it becomes a matter of routine. It is easier to remember when a pattern is established.

5. If the child is old enough to understand, warn him when a medication has an unpleasant taste (e.g., "John, this doesn't taste very good, but you can have a big drink of juice as soon as you swallow it."). You may lose his trust if you surprise him with a bad taste.

6. Give the child a frozen fruit bar or frozen flavored ice pop just before the medication. This helps to numb the taste buds to weaken the taste of the medication.

7. To mask bad-tasting medicines, you can crush tablets or empty the contents of a capsule and mix with soft foods, such as applesauce, hot cereal, or pudding. This is helpful for children who might aspirate liquids, as well. (**Caution:** Check a drug reference book or with the prescriber before crushing a tablet or emptying a capsule. Some medications should not be crushed.)

8. Do not use essential foods in the child's diet (e.g., milk or orange juice) to mask the taste of medications. The child may later refuse a food he associates with the medicine.

9. ✚ To prevent choking or aspiration when giving liquids to infants and toddlers, hold the child in a sitting or semi-sitting position. Use a medicine dropper or syringe to place the medication between the gum and cheek. Instill the medication; avoid giving too much, too fast.

10. Always praise the child after she swallows the medication.

Medicating Older Adults Orally

Many interventions for older adults are the same as for patients of all ages (e.g., actions to facilitate swallowing, the content of the teaching). For those, review preceding section on Teaching Patients About Medication Self-Administration.

 In Chapter 26, **Procedure 26-1, Administering Oral Medication,** in Volume 2.

However, because of physiological changes associated with aging (see Table 26-2), certain problems occur more frequently in older adults. For example, older adults usually require smaller dosages of drugs, and physical responses to some medications are unpredictable. Therefore, interventions such as carefully observing for both therapeutic and undesired effects become even more important. The following interventions are for nurse-administered drugs (also see Box 26-4) and are not described in the self-administration discussion.

- **Address swallowing difficulties.** As the desire to drink decreases with age, the mouth often becomes drier, making it difficult to take large tablets. Crush tablets (if acceptable) or give drugs in liquid form. Try gently massaging the area just below the chin to initiate swallowing. For other strategies, collaborate with an occupational or speech therapist.

- **Accommodate slower reflexes and reasoning ability.** Allow more time to explain and administer medications. When teaching, keep instructions simple and repeat them often. Also reinforce the need to take the medication as prescribed. Some patients may think, "I don't feel any better when I take all this stuff." In the hospital, they may refuse to take

medications, or they may put the tablets in their mouths but spit them out when you leave the room. Stay with the patient until you see that he has swallowed the medications.

KnowledgeCheck 26-13

- What is the chief danger when administering oral medications to children?
- How can you help a person who has some difficulty swallowing oral medications?
- Keeping in mind that patients do have the right to refuse medications, how can you be sure that they are actually taking them and not spitting them out after you leave the room?

ADMINISTERING TOPICAL MEDICATIONS

Topical medications are applied directly to the skin or placed in body cavities by irrigation or instillation. Most must be applied two or three times per day for maximum effect. They have local or systemic effects, depending on how the drug is prepared, as in the following examples:

- *Local effects*—Zinc oxide ointment to protect the skin against irritation associated with bowel and bladder incontinence; corticosteroid creams for itching.
- *Systemic effects*—These are absorbed through the skin and mucous membrane (e.g., estrogen patches; also see Transdermal Medications, following).

Lotions, Creams, and Ointments

Before applying medications to the skin, assess for contraindications (e.g., skin irritation, open lesions, hypersensitivity). Use a cotton swab, tongue blade, or gloved

BOX 26-4 ■ Reducing Risk for Medication Errors for Older Adults

- **Be alert to unnecessary drug therapy.** It is not unusual for prescribers to be reluctant to stop a medication or simply forget to do so. The likelihood of a poor outcome increases as the number of drugs prescribed increases.

- **Request the indication for use** on all medication prescriptions.

- **Suggest primary care provider trials of nonpharmacological interventions** (such as warm massage and guided imagery) before prescribing medication for new symptoms.

- **Consider the "snowball effect."** This occurs when symptoms result as a side effect of prescribed medication, and the care provider then prescribes another drug to deal with the side effect. This results in yet another side effect, another drug, and so on. To interrupt this phenomenon, the prescriber can discontinue the medication, reduce the dose, or substitute one that the patient tolerates better.

- **Verify that a newly prescribed medication** does not have a documented drug-drug interaction. Check that the prescribed dosage is correct within the desired range.

- **When titrating drug doses, start low and go slow.** It's best to start with the lowest possible dose when starting a medication because adverse drug effects are dose related and older adults tend to be more sensitive.

- **Assess urinary status.** Many drugs are cleared through the renal system. Some have toxic effects on the kidneys, particularly for older adults.

- **Recommend safer drugs** if the prescriber initiates medication associated with adverse outcomes for older adults. The benefit must exceed the risk to the patient (Zwicker & Fulmer, 2008; Zwicker & Fulmer, updated 2012).

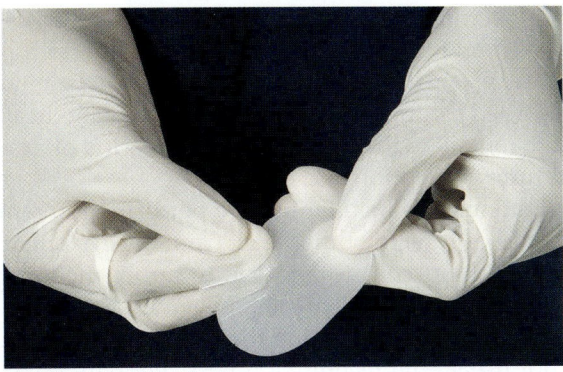

FIGURE 26-9 Patches allow constant, controlled amounts of medications to be released over a 24- to 72-hour period, giving a prolonged systemic effect. Wear gloves when removing and applying them.

Most patches are prepared with the correct dose already applied and should not be cut. Some gel patches can be cut and are self-adherent (e.g., lidocaine and diclofenac). Check the package insert or ask a pharmacist about proper handling, application, and disposal of patches. Wear gloves when applying, removing, and discarding transdermal patches (Fig. 26-9). See the Highlights of Procedures box and,

 Go to Chapter 26, **Procedure 26-7D: Applying Transdermal Medication,** in Volume 2.

PERFORMING IRRIGATIONS AND INSTILLATIONS

Washing out a body cavity with a steady stream of fluid or water is called **irrigation**. Sterile water, saline, or antiseptic solutions are flushed into the eyes, ears, throat,

finger to apply lotions, creams, and other ointments so that your skin does not absorb them. The Highlights of Procedures box summarizes key points for applying skin medications, including powders and aerosols. For the step-by-step procedure,

 Go to Chapter 26, **Procedure 26-7A: Applying Lotion, Cream, and Ointment,** in Volume 2.

Transdermal Medications

Designed to be absorbed through the skin, transdermal medications are prepared as patches made of a special membrane. Patches allow constant, controlled amounts of medications to be released over 24 hours or more, giving a prolonged systemic effect. Examples of drugs administered by patch include nitroglycerin (used to control angina or chest pain), scopolamine (used to treat motion sickness), nicotine (used to control smoking urges), and fentanyl (used to treat chronic pain).

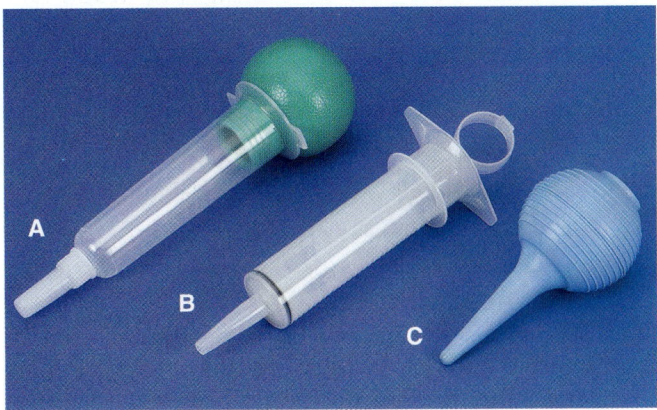

FIGURE 26-10 Syringes for administering enteral medications and performing irrigations and instillations. *A,* Asepto syringe: Plastic syringe with rubber bulb. *B,* Toomey (piston) syringe: Calibrated plastic syringe with removable tip that fits into the end of a tube (e.g., urinary catheter or enteral tube). For deep wound and bladder irrigations, and administration of enteral medications. *C,* Rubber bulb syringe, for ear irrigations.

vagina, rectum, or urinary tract to wash out the cavity. **Instillation** is the insertion of medication into a body cavity (e.g., eye drops) so the medication can be retained or absorbed through that body cavity. Some medications need to remain in the body cavity for a period of time for maximum absorption and effect.

Irrigations and instillations are performed to remove discharge or foreign bodies (e.g., from the eye or ear); to apply heat and cold to an area; to apply medications (e.g., antiseptics); and to prepare an area for surgery (e.g., an enema for cleansing the bowels). You will usually not use sterile technique unless there are breaks in the skin. Several types of syringes are used for irrigating and instilling medications and fluids. Each is calibrated to allow you to control the amount and speed of solution delivered into the cavity (Fig. 26-10).

Ophthalmic Medications

Ophthalmic ointments or solutions are used for their local effects, for example, to treat eye irritations, infections, and glaucoma or to lubricate the eye. During an eye examination, eye medications may be used to anesthetize the eye, dilate the pupil, or temporarily stain the cornea to identify abraded areas. Eye irrigation may be performed to remove foreign bodies, secretions, or harmful chemicals.

 Ophthalmic medications are packaged in small bottles or tubes with a label that states, "*For ophthalmic use only.*" Do not place any medication in the eye unless that statement appears on the container. Damage to the eye can result in permanent blindness.

The **cornea** (the transparent part of the sclera in front of the iris and pupil) is easily injured, so you should not place medications directly onto the eyeball. Take care to not touch the tip of the dropper or tube to the eye or conjunctiva; doing so may lead to bacterial growth on the container or damage the eye.

See Chapters 22 and 30 for information about the structure and function of the eyes. The Highlights of Procedures box summarizes key points in performing ophthalmic instillations. For the step-by-step procedure,

    Go to Chapter 26, **Procedure 26-2: Administering Ophthalmic Medication**, in Volume 2.

Otic Medications

Medications or solutions may be dropped into the ear to treat internal and external ear infections, to apply heat to the area, and to soften and remove earwax. Use solutions at body temperature because a solution that is too hot or too cold may cause vertigo, nausea, and pain. You will use clean technique when administering otic medications.

 To prevent infection, use sterile technique if the tympanic membrane (eardrum) has been ruptured or a surgical procedure has been done.

See Chapters 22 and 30 for information about the structure and function of the ear. The Highlights of Procedures box provides guidelines for performing otic instillations. For the complete procedure,

    Go to Chapter 26, **Procedure 26-3: Administering Otic Medication,** in Volume 2.

Nasal Medications

Clients usually self-administer nasal drops and sprays, many of which are available without a prescription. The most common nasal medications are used in the treatment of nasal congestion from colds, sinus infections, and so on. Nasal decongestants shrink swollen mucous membranes and allow for better airflow and drainage of mucus. Caution your patient that long-term use of decongestants may cause a **rebound effect**. This occurs when the medication is effective immediately after administration, but nasal congestion often recurs and even increases when the effects of the drug wear off. Thus, continual use of the drug becomes necessary to achieve nasal decongestion. Frequent use of or swallowing excess decongestant can also cause systemic side effects (e.g., increased heart rate, increased blood pressure). These effects can be serious in children; saline drops are safer for them.

See Chapters 22 and 30 for information about the structure and function of the nose. The Highlights of Procedures box provides guidelines for performing nasal instillations. For the complete procedure,

    Go to Chapter 26, **Procedure 26-4: Administering Nasal Medication,** in Volume 2.

Vaginal Medications

Vaginal medications come in various forms: foams, jellies, liquids (douches), creams, tablets, and suppositories. They may be used for contraception; to destroy bacteria in the vagina before gynecological surgery; to reduce vaginal dryness related to menopause; to treat vaginal itching or infection; or to induce labor. To keep suppositories firm enough to insert, store them in the refrigerator. After insertion, the body temperature causes the suppository to melt. Foams and jellies are inserted using an applicator or inserter. Apply a clean perineal pad if there is heavy drainage or if the woman is ambulatory (the medication may melt and drain from the vagina by gravity).

A **douche** is a vaginal irrigation using low pressure. Vaginal irrigations are used to administer antimicrobial solutions to prevent infection (e.g., before surgery), to remove irritating discharge, and to apply heat or cold (e.g., to reduce inflammation). In the acute care setting, you will usually use sterile supplies. However, this is not usually necessary when the irrigation is self-administered at home because people usually have some resistance to the microorganisms in their daily environment.

The Highlights of Procedures box provides guidelines for administering vaginal medications. For the complete procedure,

 Go to Chapter 26, **Procedure 26-5: Administering Vaginal Medication,** in Volume 2.

Rectal Medications

Rectal suppositories and liquid instillations (**enemas**) are used to encourage bowel movements or to treat systemic complaints. For example, antiemetic suppositories are often used to treat nausea. The rectal route may provide for higher blood levels of the medication than does the oral route because the venous blood from the rectum does not pass through the liver before entering the general circulation (review the discussion of the first-pass effect as needed). They can also be given in a colostomy stoma in certain patients. For advantages and disadvantages, see Table 26-1.

The Highlights of Procedures box provides guidelines for administering rectal medication. For the complete procedure,

 Go to Chapter 26, **Procedure 26-6: Inserting a Rectal Suppository, and Chapter 29, Procedure 29-3: Administering an Enema,** in Volume 2.

ADMINISTERING RESPIRATORY INHALATIONS

Nebulization is the production of a fine spray, fog, powder, or mist from a liquid drug. The patient inhales the medication mixture by breathing deeply through a mouthpiece attached to the nebulizer. Absorption is rapid because of the vascularity of the airways and alveoli.

Types of Nebulizers

The following are four types of devices for achieving nebulization:

- *Atomizers* disperse the medication in the form of large droplets.
- *Aerosol sprayers* suspend the droplets of medication in a gas (e.g., oxygen).
- *An ultrasonic (handheld) nebulizer* mixes a small volume of medication, usually less than 1 mL, with 3 mL of normal saline. The device forces air through the nebulizer and delivers medication and humidity as a fine mist. Because the particles are so small, the mist can be inhaled deep into the lungs.
- *A metered-dose inhaler (MDI)* (Fig. 26-11) is a type of nebulizer that delivers measured doses of a nebulized drug.

No matter which device is used, the smaller the droplets, the farther the medication can be inhaled into the respiratory tract.

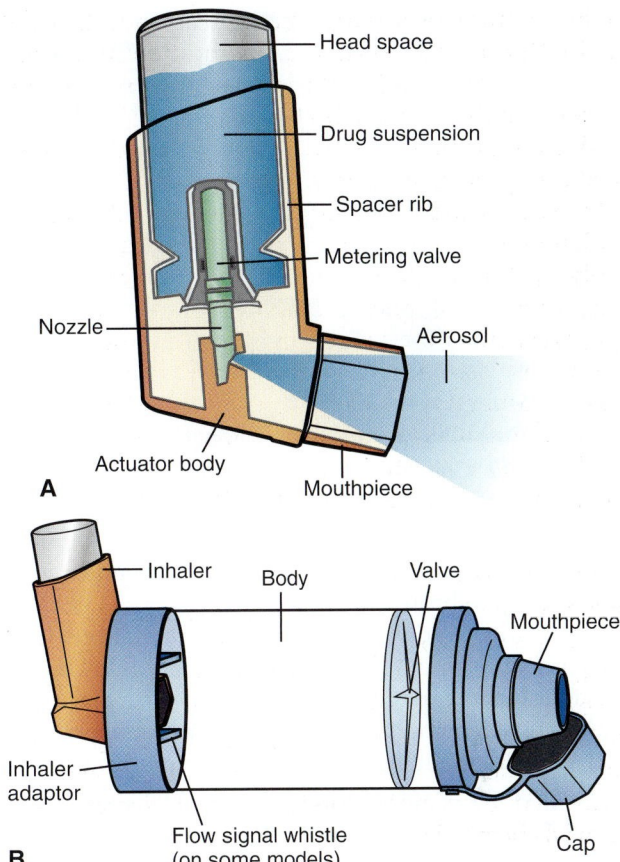

FIGURE 26-11 Inhalers. *A,* Metered-dose inhaler. *B,* Inhaler with a spacer.

Metered-Dose and Dry Powder Inhalers

A metered-dose inhaler (MDI) is a pressurized container prefilled with several doses of a drug and an eco-friendly substance, called hydrofluoroalkane, or HFA, for propelling the medication forward. The patient inhales while pushing the canister's pump to release a measured dose of medication through a mouthpiece (Fig. 26-11A). Sometimes an extender (spacer) is attached to the mouthpiece to enhance the delivery of medication into the respiratory tract (Fig. 26-11B). Medication is pumped into the extender instead of directly into the patient's mouth. The patient inhales the drug from the chamber.

A **dry powder inhaler (DPI)** is similar to an MDI. The medication is activated by a pump rather than by inhalation. Each powdered dose is in a blister pack that is activated according to the manufacturer's instructions. Once the dose is loaded, the patient simply takes a deep breath. DPIs are not designed to be used with a spacer.

The advantage of MDIs is that high doses of medication can be rapidly instilled in the lungs, producing local effects directly into the airway, while avoiding systemic side effects. Disadvantages are the need for manual dexterity, which is often compromised in older adults and young children; skill in coordinating the inhalation of the medication and the pushing of the canister to administer the dose; and the ability to inhale and exhale

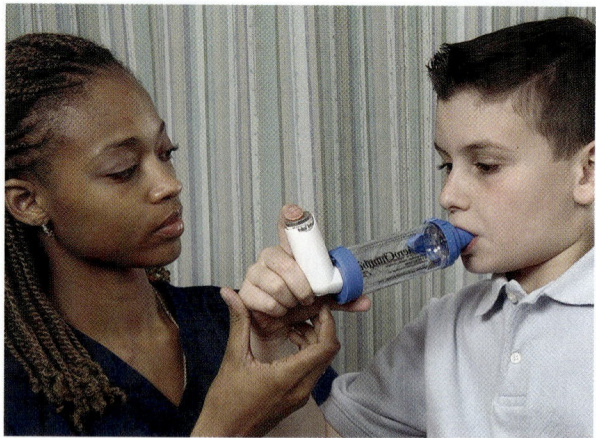

FIGURE 26-12 Child using a metered-dose inhaler with an extender.

deeply enough to allow penetration of the medication in the more distal bronchioles.

Patients frequently self-administer inhalations (most often bronchodilators or steroids) using an MDI. You may need to teach your patients how to use the device correctly (Fig. 26-12). Keeping track of how many puffs have been used is problematic for some users, which can lead to a canister being unexpectedly empty when needed. For this information, see the Highlights of Procedures box. Also,

 Go to Chapter 26, **Procedure 26-8: Administering Metered-Dose Inhaler (MDI) Medication,** in Volume 2.

KnowledgeCheck 26-14

- Why should you use a cotton swab, tongue blade, or gloved finger to apply corticosteroid creams and other topical medications?
- Most of the following routes are used for both local and systemic effects. Which one is used *only* for medications intended for systemic absorption (i.e., which one is not used for local effects): lotions, creams, ointments, transdermal patches, or irrigations?
- When administering eye drops, how can you prevent injury to the cornea?
- When should you use sterile technique when performing otic instillations?
- What are two of the undesired effects of self-administered nasal decongestants?
- What possible harm can result from vaginal douching?
- When is rectal instillation of a drug preferred over oral administration?
- When, as a rule, are rectal medications contraindicated?
- Define *nebulization.*
- What is the best way to determine if a metered-dose inhaler is empty?

ADMINISTERING PARENTERAL MEDICATIONS

Parenteral medications are those that are injected or infused into body tissues or into the bloodstream via various routes, including intradermal, subcutaneous,

intramuscular, or intravenous routes. Parenteral injections are absorbed faster and more completely than drugs given by other routes; therefore, the results are more predictable and the dosage can be measured more accurately. In addition, they can be used for patients who cannot take oral medications. However, tissue damage may result if the pH, osmotic pressure, or solubility of the medication is not appropriate to the tissue where the medication is given. For example, medications intended for injection into muscle may damage subcutaneous tissue. You must prepare and administer parenteral medications accurately, because the medications, once given, cannot be retrieved.

Equipment for Parenteral Medications

When administering injectable (parenteral) medications, you must know about various kinds of needles and syringes. You will also need to decide, based on each situation, what size and type of needle and syringe to use. For a summary of the sites and equipment used for parenteral administration,

 Go to Chapter 26, **Tables, Boxes, Figures: ESG Table 26-6, Parenteral Injections: Comparison of Sites and Equipment,** on Davis*Plus.*

Reusing Equipment at Home Many people (e.g., those who have diabetes) must give themselves repeated injections, perhaps several each day. Supplies for home use are expensive. Insurance may or may not cover the cost, or the person may not have insurance. Therefore, although health professionals and manufacturers recommend that disposable syringes and needles be used only once, some people find it practical to reuse them. If they do, you can help them to do it more safely by teaching them the content in

 Chapter 26, **Clinical Insight 26-1: Reusing Needles and Syringes: Home Care,** in Volume 2.

Needles

Needles are disposable, stainless steel sheaths that attach to a syringe. Figure 26-13 shows the parts of a needle. Needles are made in various lengths and gauges and with different bevel sizes.

Gauge refers to the inside diameter of the needle lumen. Needle gauges are numbered 14 through 30: the smaller the gauge, the larger the diameter (i.e., a 16-gauge needle has a larger diameter than a 20-gauge needle). Choose the gauge based on the patient's size and skin condition, the viscosity of medication used, and the speed of administration desired. Smaller needles (25- to 30-gauge) cause less pain and trauma to the tissue, so they are useful for patients who must have frequent or long-term injections (e.g., insulin and heparin). Larger needles, 14- to 18-gauge (or needleless systems), are used to infuse blood and more viscous medications or for rapid infusion of IV medications.

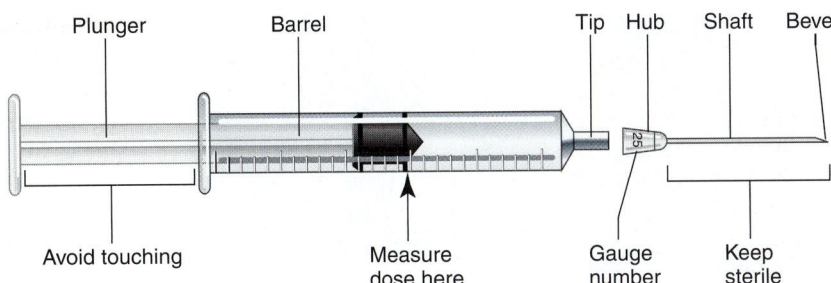

FIGURE 26-13 Parts of a needle and syringe.

Bevel is the slanted tip with a narrow slit. The slant of the tip creates an opening that will close quickly to prevent leakage of medication, blood, and serum. A long bevel tip is sharper and narrower and therefore causes less discomfort during injection. Long bevels are usually used for subcutaneous and intramuscular injections. Short bevels are used for intradermal or IV injections. For an illustration of a bevel,

 Go to **Procedure 26-11: Administering Intradermal Medication,** in Volume 2.

Needle Length is the distance from the tip to the hub (bottom) of the needle. Common needle lengths range from ⅜ inch to 3 inches. Choose the length according to the thickness of the patient's muscle and adipose tissue and the site in which the drug is to be injected. For example, use a longer needle for intramuscular injections, and a shorter one for intradermal injections. A 1½-inch needle is common for intramuscular injections, but you would use a shorter one for a child or a very thin person.

▲ ThinkLike a Nurse 26-11

- You are to give repeated intramuscular injections to a patient who is frail and has very little muscle mass (5 ft 5 in. tall and weighing 96 lb). You are to give 1 mL of a thin, watery medication. You have these needle sizes available: 16-gauge, 20-gauge, 25-gauge. Which would you use, and why?
- For the same patient, you have needles available in 1-inch and 1½-inch lengths. Which would you use, and why?

Filter Needles and Filter Straws are used to trap rubber or glass fragments when drawing up a medication from a vial or an ampule. You must replace the filter needle with a regular needle before injecting the medication into the patient or into the IV solution.

Safety Needles Many safety needle devices are available. Examples include a resheathing system with a sliding barrel that shields the needle, syringes with retractable needles, and needles with attached covers that reduce the risk of accidental puncture with contaminated needles (Fig. 26-14). Wing-tipped safety needles are also available for clinical use. To see some types of safety needles,

 Go to Student Resources, **Animations: Self-Resheathing Needle, Syringe With Retractable Needle, Winged Steel Needle, and "Add-On" Safety Feature for Needle,** on Davis*Plus.*

Syringes

A syringe consists of a barrel, plunger, and syringe tip (see Fig. 26-13). Because injections require strict sterile technique, you may touch the outside of the barrel and end of the plunger but not the inside of the barrel, hub, shaft of the plunger, or needle.

Syringes are usually made of plastic and are disposable. Some have the needle attached; others do not. The syringe tip, either **luer-lock** (twist on) or **non-luer-lock** (slip on), fits into the needle hub (Fig. 26-15). Syringes are made in various sizes, from 0.5 mL to 60 mL. The larger sizes are used for adding medications to IV solutions and for instillations and irrigations. You will usually use a 2-mL or 3-mL syringe for intramuscular injections. Three syringes are shown in Figure 26-16. For interactive exercises to familiarize yourself with syringe markings,

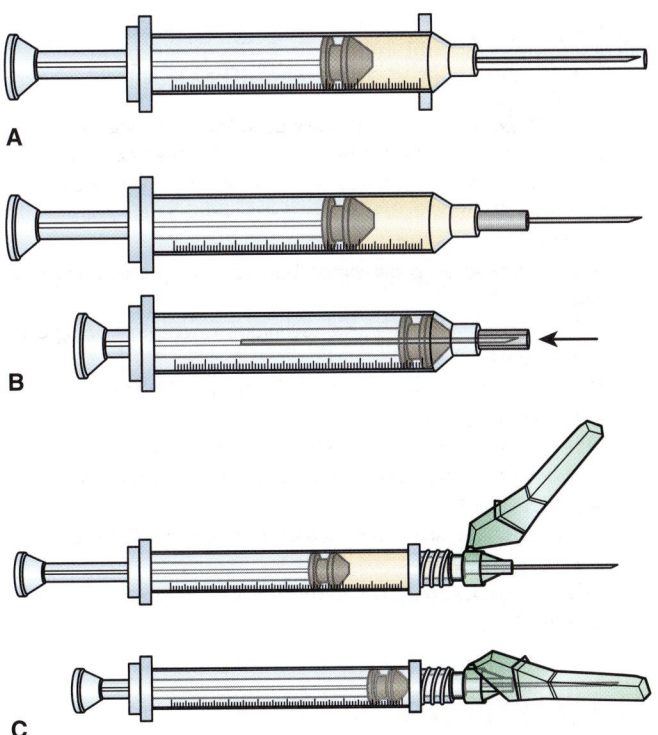

A

B

C

FIGURE 26-14 Needle safety features. *A,* Self-sheathing safety feature: Sliding needle shields attached to disposable syringes and vacuum tube holders. *B,* Syringe with retractable needle. *C,* Needles with covers.

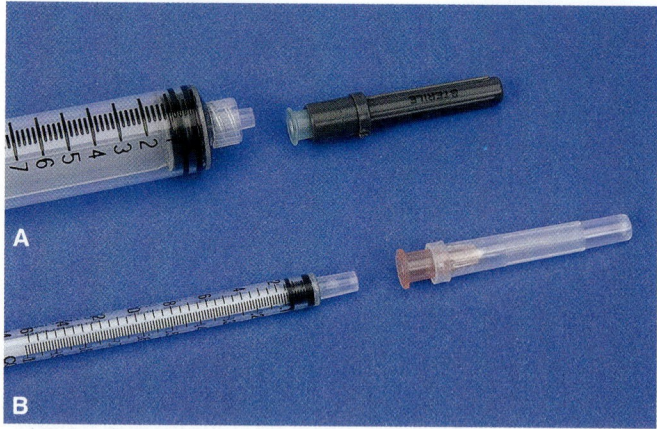

FIGURE 26-15 Syringe tips. *A,* Luer-lock (twist-on) tip. *B,* Non-luer-lock (slip-on) tip.

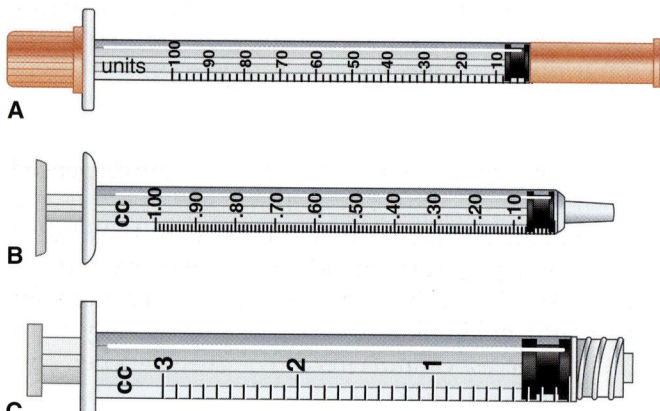

FIGURE 26-16 Syringe types. *A,* 100-unit insulin syringe marked in units. *B,* 1-mL tuberculin syringe marked in increments of 0.01 mL. *C,* 3-mL standard syringe marked in increments of 0.1 mL.

 Go to **Animations: Syringe Exercises,** on Davis*Plus.*

- **Standard syringes** are supplied in 3-, 5-, and 10-mL sizes. They are commonly supplied without needles or with 18-, 21-, 23-, or 25-gauge needles that are 0.5 to 3 inches long. They are calibrated and marked in 0.1-mL and 1- or 2-mL increments so that drugs can be measured accurately.
- **Tuberculin syringes** have a 1-mL capacity and are calibrated in 0.01-mL increments; they come with a small (usually 25- to 28-) gauge, short (½- to ⅝-in.) needle. Use tuberculin syringes to administer small, precise doses of medication (e.g., when medicating infants or children, for allergy tests, or when administering potentially dangerous medications, such as heparin).
- **Insulin syringes** are calibrated in units and are used to administer insulin. Insulin syringes are marked in 100 units per milliliter. They are made in 0.3-, 0.5-, or 1-mL sizes with very small-gauge needles (26- to 30-gauge).
- **Prefilled unit-dose systems** are reusable syringe holders that hold disposable, single-dose, prefilled

medication cartridges. No medication preparation is necessary, but you must check each cartridge and dose carefully because all of the cartridges look alike. You simply insert the cartridge into the holder and lock it in place. An auto-retractable needle on the syringe is intended to decrease the chance of needle stick. Pre-filled syringes for intravenous use have a luer-lock system or a blunt cannula to connect with the port. After administering the medication, dispose of the cartridge; keep the holder for reuse.

- **Disposable prefilled, self-contained systems** are available for hospitals, office practices, nursing homes, and self-administration. The injection plunger is attached to the medication barrel and twists in directly. This ready-to-use syringe reduces the risk of constituting or dosing errors. Because you do not need to remove the cartridge from the holder after using it, the risk of a needlestick injury is reduced (Fig. 26-17). To learn more about using prefilled systems,

 Go to Chapter 26, **Clinical Insight 26-2: Using Prefilled Unit-Dose Systems,** in Volume 2.

- **Safety syringes.** Many safety syringe devices are available. Examples include a resheathing system with a sliding barrel that shields the needle (Fig. 26-18), syringes with retractable needles that spring back into

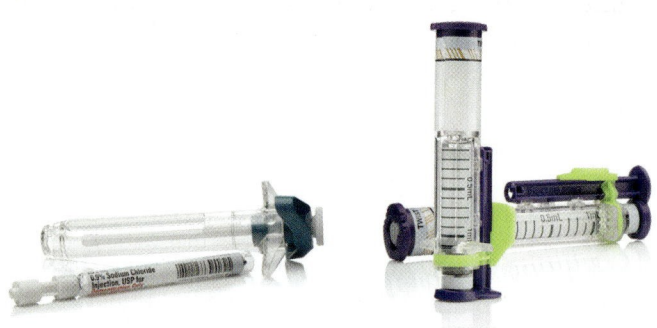

FIGURE 26-17 (*Left*) Prefilled unit-dose system. (*Right*) Disposable, prefilled, self-contained system.

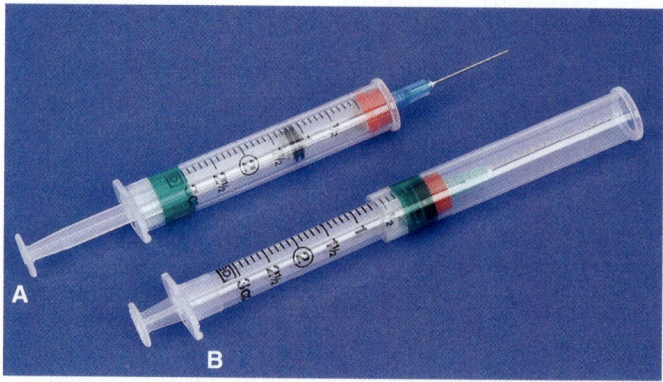

FIGURE 26-18 Special safety syringe. *A,* Needle guard position before injection. *B,* Needle guard position after injection.

the barrel of the syringe, and needles with attached covers that reduce the risk of accidental puncture with contaminated needles.

KnowledgeCheck 26-15

- What does the term *parenteral* mean?
- What are two disadvantages of the parenteral route?
- To maintain sterile technique, which part of a syringe must you *not* touch?
- You need to irrigate a wound. Which syringe size do you need: 0.5 mL, 3 mL, 5 mL, or 50 mL?
- Which syringe would you use for an intramuscular injection, as a rule: tuberculin, 50 mL, 5 mL, or 3 mL?

Drawing Up and Mixing Medications

Most injectable medications are packaged in single-dose or multidose ampules and vials. You will use slightly different techniques, depending on the container.

Drawing Up Medications From an Ampule

An **ampule** is a thin-walled, disposable glass container with a narrow neck that you must snap off to access the medication. To prevent injuries, use an ampule opener to snap the glass (Fig. 26-19). Each ampule holds a single dose of a liquid medication, usually 1 mL to 10 mL, although some hold 50 mL. Because glass fragments may be introduced into the medication, most agencies require you to use a filter needle or filter straw to draw up the medication. See the Highlights of Procedures box. Also,

 Go to Chapter 26, **Procedure 26-9A: Drawing Up Medication From Ampules,** in Volume 2.

Drawing Up Medications From a Vial

A **vial** is a single-dose or multidose plastic or glass container with a rubber stopper that reseals the top after each needle introduction. A plastic or metal cap covers the rubber stopper to protect it until it is used (Fig. 26-20). Because the vial is a closed system, you must inject air into it to withdraw the solution. Otherwise, a vacuum is created in the vial that makes withdrawal difficult. See the Highlights of Procedures box. Also,

 Go to Chapter 26, **Procedure 26-9B: Drawing Up Medication From Vials,** in Volume 2.

Nurses traditionally wipe the rubber stopper with alcohol after removing the cap, even on a single-dose vial; however, there is conflicting scientific justification for this practice as an infection control measure. The practice does remove dust and rubber particles from the top of the vial; however, using a filter needle or straw achieves that purpose as well. You will need to follow the policy of the institution in which you work.

Reconstituting Medications

Medications that are not stable in solution are dispensed as powders in vials. You must add a diluent or solvent to the powder to create a solution for injection. The diluent is usually sterile water or saline; however, each packaged vial includes the manufacturer's instructions for the amount and kind of solvent to add. For safety, use a plastic vial access cannula instead of a needle when possible. For guidelines,

 Go to Chapter 26, **Clinical Insight 26-3: Reconstituting Medication,** in Volume 2.

Mixing Medications in the Same Syringe

You can mix two medications in the same syringe (1) if they are compatible, (2) if the total dose is within accepted limits, and (3) if they are both to be given by the same route. This technique allows for efficient use of supplies and allows the patient to receive fewer injections.

Medications are *compatible* if they can be mixed without affecting their constituents or actions. Package inserts and medication references usually include compatibility information.

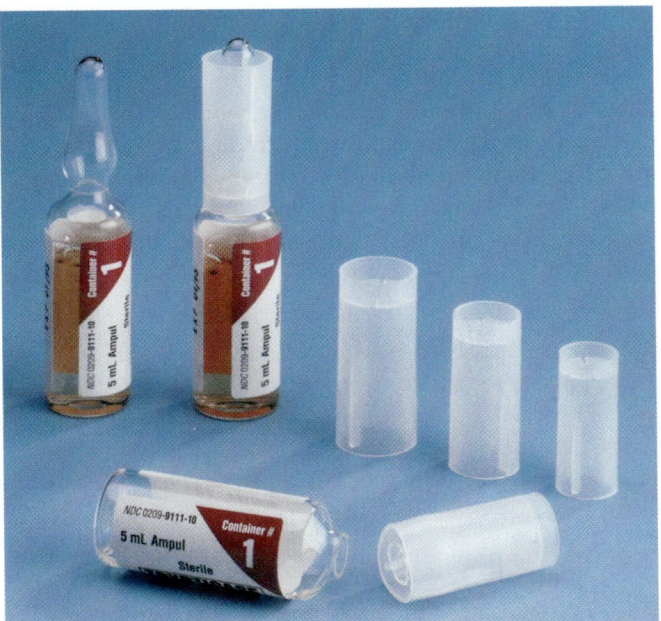

FIGURE 26-19 Safety device for opening glass ampules.
(Courtesy of Medi-Dose, Inc. EPS, Inc., Ivyland, PA.)

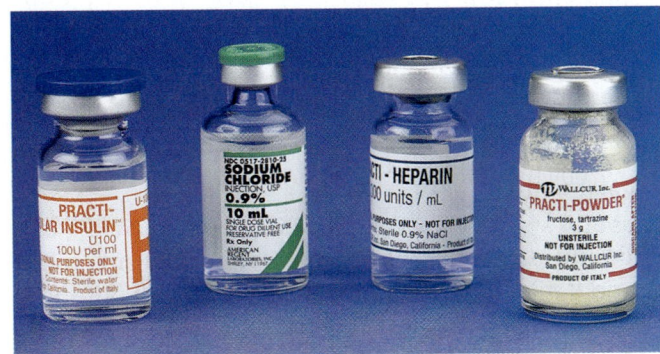

FIGURE 26-20 Vials containing medications.

Always check the compatibility before mixing medications together. If the contents of the syringe become discolored, there are visible particles in the solution, or there is a change in consistency, do not administer the medications.

When mixing medications in one syringe, you must follow these principles:

- Maintain sterile technique (as with all parenteral medications).
- Do not contaminate one container with medication from the other container. You must use a separate needle to withdraw from each vial (exceptions: when both are single-dose vials, and in the case of different types of insulin).
- Ensure the total, final dosage is correct by adding the volumes of the two medicines together and ensuring that this is the amount you have in the syringe.
- If you draw up too much of the second drug, or if your final measurement of the total for both drugs is incorrect, you cannot eject medication, because you cannot know how much of either drug you are ejecting. You must discard the syringe and medication and begin again.

 Never reuse a needle or syringe for drawing up a later dose of medication. A single-use vial contains only one dose of medication. Even if you do not administer the entire dose, the remaining amount must be discarded.

Key Point: *A single-dose vial should only be used one time for one patient, using a sterile needle and sterile syringe.*

See the Highlights of Procedures box for guidelines. For the complete steps,

 Go to Chapter 26, **Procedure 26-9C: Mixing Medication From Two Vials,** in Volume 2.

Accounting for Needle "Dead Space"

Some nurses believe a small amount of the patient's medication remains in the needle when an injection is given. Therefore, they recommended adding 0.2 mL of air to the syringe after measuring a medication for IM injection. Nurses are not in agreement regarding this practice and, unfortunately, there is scant research to provide evidenced-based guidance. Theoretically, on injection the air clears the needle of medication, ensuring that the patient receives the entire dose. However, because syringes are calibrated to account for medication left in the needle, and because the medication left in the needle after injection is the same amount as before the injection, many believe that air should not be added. We recommend that you add air only in the following situations:

1. *When the medication is irritating to subcutaneous tissues,* add 0.2 mL of air after measuring the proper dose. The air drives the medication deep into the subcutaneous tissue and creates an air lock above the medication, preventing it from tracking through subcutaneous tissue.

2. *When you change needles after drawing up the medication (e.g., replace a filter needle).* The new needle has air in it instead of medication. If you push the plunger until you see a drop of medication at the tip of the needle, you will see that you no longer have a complete dose in the syringe. Pulling in 0.2 mL air before changing the needle and then pushing the plunger until you see a drop of medication at the tip of the new needle will prevent the loss of medication with the needle change.

 Go to Chapter 26, **Clinical Insight 26-4: Measuring Dosage When Changing Needles,** in Volume 2.

Preventing Needlestick Injuries

Workplace injuries occur from needles and other "sharps," putting healthcare workers at risk for blood-borne diseases, such as hepatitis B, hepatitis C, and HIV (see Chapter 24). For this reason, special safety devices have been designed to reduce the risk of needlestick injuries through blunting, shielding, retracting needles, wing-tipped needles, and needles with attached covers as in Figure 26-14A, B, and C. Figure 26-18 is a photo of a safety syringe with a guard that pulls forward to cover the needle immediately after it is withdrawn from the skin to reduce the risk of accidental punctures with contaminated needles. You then dispose of both needle and sheath in a "sharps" container. Needles with attached covers reduce the risk of accidental punctures with contaminated needles.

The Centers for Disease Control and Prevention (CDC) and the Occupational Safety and Health Administration (OSHA) recommend the use of "needleless" systems. Most systems involve adapters that can be used with regular intravenous tubing and medication vials, permitting access through a valve system without a needle. Figure 26-21 shows three such devices.

Another needle-free system is the jet injection most often used for immunizations. The jet injectors drive liquid medication into the intradermal, subcutaneous, or intramuscular tissues by creating a narrow stream under high pressure that penetrates the skin. However, local reactions or injury, such as redness, bruising, and pain, occur more often with jet injectors than by use of a needle.

 Always dispose of needles, glass, and other "sharps" in clearly marked, usually red, puncture-proof containers (Fig. 26-22). Never force a needle into an already full container; you may be injured by sharps protruding from the top. Never put a needle or other sharp in a wastebasket, in your pocket, or leave it at the patient's bedside.

For tips to prevent needlestick injury,

 Go to Chapter 24, Promoting Safety, **Clinical Insight 24-2: Preventing Needlestick Injuries,** in Volume 2.

Recapping Contaminated Needles You should never recap a contaminated needle (e.g., after giving an

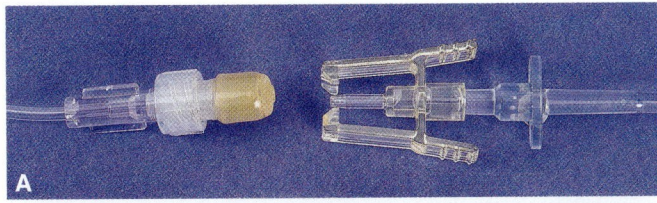

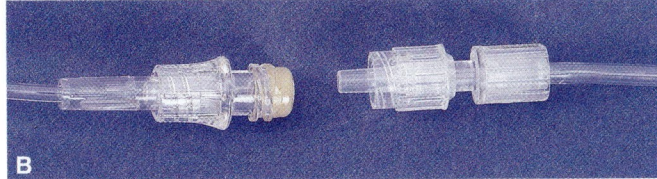

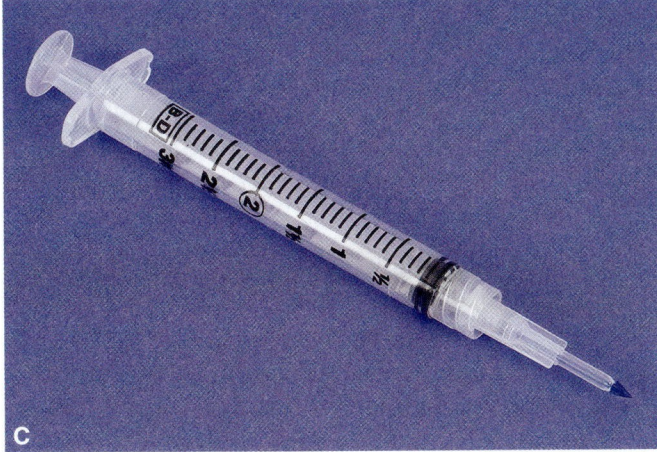

FIGURE 26-21 Needleless systems. *A,* Lever-lock cannula. *B,* Threaded lock cannula. *C,* Blunt-tipped syringe for drawing up medication.

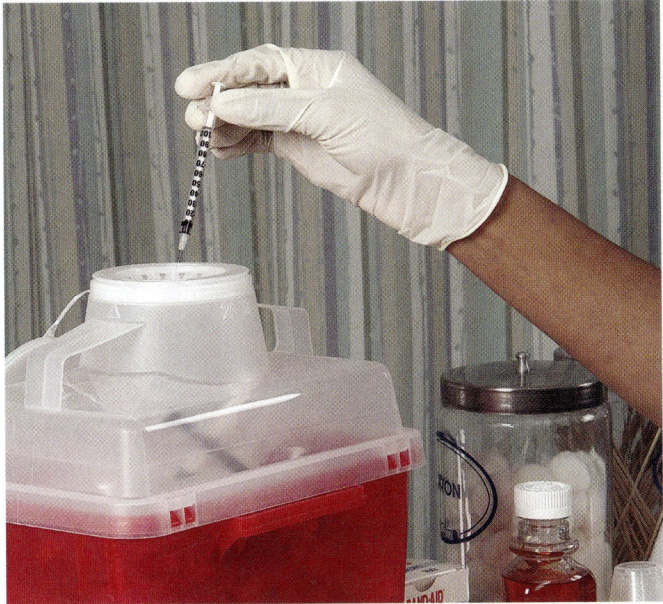

FIGURE 26-22 Disposal system for sharp objects, such as needles and glass. The container must be clearly marked, usually red, and puncture-proof.

injection); place it uncapped, needle pointing downward, directly into a sharps disposal container. However, you may occasionally find that you must recap a contaminated needle. The OSHA Fact Sheet (2012)

requires bending, recapping, or needle removal using a mechanical device or a one-handed technique. For step-by-step instructions,

 Go to Chapter 26, **Procedure 26-10: Recapping Needles Using a One-Handed Technique,** in Volume 2.

Recapping Sterile Needles OSHA and the National Institute of Occupational Safety and Health (NIOSH) (U.S. Department of Health and Human Services [USDHHS], NIOSH, 2012) do not advise against recapping sterile needles (e.g., after drawing up a medication), except to recommend needleless systems and safety systems. We suggest that you not use the one-handed "scoop" technique to recap a sterile needle because the risk of contaminating it is high. Consider one of the other methods described in Procedure 26-10.

Comfort and Safety Considerations

Parenteral techniques are invasive. They carry the potential for tissue trauma and provide a portal of entry for pathogens through the skin. You must, of course, maintain strict aseptic (sterile) technique to minimize the risk of infection. Moreover, your injection technique and choice of injection site are critical to patient comfort and safety. When choosing a site, consider the type, viscosity, and volume of the medication to be administered; the anatomical landmarks underlying injection sites; and the patient's situation (e.g., the condition of the tissues at the injection site, the accessibility of certain sites). The following are examples of judgment and technique errors and their consequences:

- Injecting a large volume of medication into a small muscle causes pain and may damage the tissues.
- Injecting into the wrong tissue (e.g., giving an intramuscular medication too shallowly into the subcutaneous tissue) may (1) accelerate or delay the rate of absorption and (2) cause tissue injury and pain.
- Incorrectly locating an injection site may result in bone or nerve injury when you insert the needle.
- An unsteady needle and syringe while injecting the drug could lead to pain and tissue trauma.
- Forgetting to aspirate before injecting risks administration of medication into an artery or vein instead of the muscle. This could result in an adverse, even fatal, effect.

Minimizing Discomfort

The discomfort associated with an injection comes from three sources: the prick of the needle, the pressure of the volume of the drug in the tissues, and chemical irritation caused by some drugs. Fear and anxiety magnify discomfort. Use the following techniques to reduce discomfort:

- Use the smallest needle suited for the site and medication.
- Use two needles when drawing up medications: one to withdraw the medication from the container, and the

second one for the injection. If the needle is not free of medication, it may irritate tissues as it is inserted.

- Do not administer too much solution into an injection site. If the total volume is more than the recommended amount, give it in two injections and at two sites.
- For intramuscular injections, help the patient assume a position that reduces muscle tension.
- For intramuscular injections, use the Z-track technique, discussed later in this chapter, to minimize pain and tissue irritation.
- Pull the skin taut, and insert the needle quickly to avoid pulling the tissues. Remove the needle quickly and at the same angle you inserted it.
- Steady the syringe with one hand while injecting the medication.
- Inject the medication slowly.
- Distract the patient from the procedure by talking to her.
- Apply gentle pressure (not massage) after injection unless contraindicated.
- Especially with children, acknowledge that they will feel some pain (e.g., "This may hurt a little bit."). If you deny or minimize the pain, the patient might lose trust in you and be even more anxious about future injections.
- After injecting a child, pat or hug him, speak softly to him, and perhaps play with him, so that he does not associate you only with pain.
- Other methods for decreasing pain can be cooling the skin (e.g., applying ice) or flicking or tapping over the injection area before injecting. Both send distracting signals to the brain so that when the needle comes, it can't process the stimulus as easily.

Developmental Stage

Because older adults may experience muscle atrophy or have decreased muscle mass, you may need to use a shorter needle.

Infants and children also require shorter, thinner needles. Also, you should ask a parent or another caregiver to immobilize an infant or young child to prevent injury during the injection.

The preferred intramuscular site for infants is the vastus lateralis muscle, because there are no major nerves

or blood vessels in the area and the gluteal muscles have not yet been developed by walking. For children who are walking, the site of choice is the ventrogluteal muscle because the muscle is more developed.

➕ Do not use the dorsogluteal site for patients of any age, including older children and adults, because of its location to major blood vessels and the sciatic nerve.

Intradermal Injections

Intradermal injections are given into the **dermis**, which is the layer of the skin located beneath the skin surface. The intradermal route is commonly used for allergy or tuberculosis (TB) testing. Most nurses use the patient's nondominant arm for TB screening and the dominant arm, chest, or upper back for all other tests (Fig. 26-23). Give only small amounts of medication by this route— about 0.1 mL. Use a 1-mL syringe and a short, small (26- to 28-gauge) needle, and insert at an angle of 5° to 15° (see Fig. 26-24).

➕ Do not apply pressure or massage the injection site, because the capillaries in the dermal tissue will quickly absorb the medication.

Refer to the Highlights of Procedures box for critical elements of intradermal injections. Also,

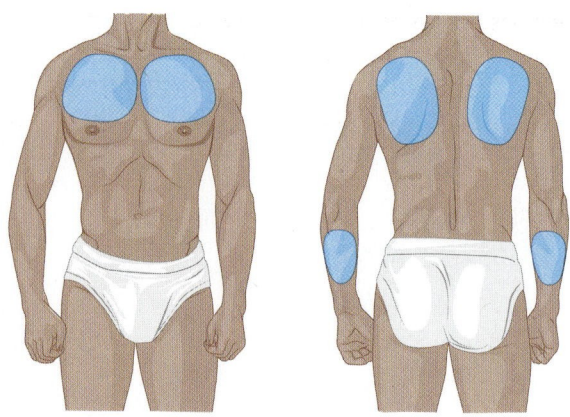

FIGURE 26-23 Sites commonly used for intradermal injection.

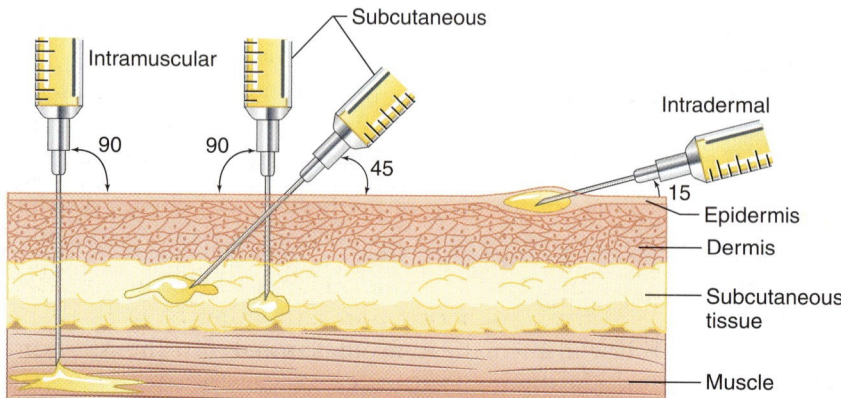

FIGURE 26-24 Standard angles of insertion for intramuscular, subcutaneous, and intradermal injections.

Toward Evidence-Based Practice

Agac, E., & Gunes, U. (2011). Effect on pain of changing the needle prior to administering medicine intramuscularly: A randomized controlled trial. *Journal of Advanced Nursing, 67*(3), 563–568.

One hundred patients rated the pain associated with two IM injections:

- One-needle technique—The same needle was used to both withdraw the medication and inject it.
- Two-needle technique—The needle was changed before administering the IM injection.

In both injections, air was pushed from the barrel after changing the needle, and the same investigator performed the actions. On a pain scale of 0 to 10, the overall pain score was 5.53 for the two-needle technique and 6.43 for the one-needle technique. Researchers recommended using a two-needle technique to promote patient comfort.

Zaybak, A., & Khorshid, L. (2008). A study on the effect of the duration of subcutaneous heparin injection on bruising and pain. *Journal of Clinical Nursing, 17*(3), 378–385.

Researchers studied the differences in bruising or pain when subcutaneous injections of heparin were given quickly or slowly in 50 patients who required treatment with heparin. Injections on the right abdomen were given over 10 seconds; on the left abdomen, over 30 seconds. Bruising occurred in 64% of patients who received the rapid injection and 42% of those receiving the slower injection. Pain intensity and pain duration were statistically significantly lower for the slower injection group, and the size of the bruising was smaller.

Ipp, M., Taddio, A., Sam, J., et al. (2007). Vaccine-related pain: Randomized controlled trial of two injection techniques. *Archives of Disease in Childhood, 92*(12), 1105–1108.

This study compared pain during a routine DPTaP-Hib immunization using a slow injection versus a rapid technique. Subjects were 113 healthy infants aged 4 to 6 months.

- Technique 1—One group received the IM dose using slow aspiration before injection, slow injection, and slow withdrawal.
- Technique 2—The other group's technique involved no aspiration, rapid injection, and rapid withdrawal.

Infants receiving the slower injection technique cried twice as often, cried longer, and took more time to have the vaccine injected. Researchers concluded that for the study participants, using a rapid injection technique is less painful than a slower technique and should be recommended for routine intramuscular immunization.

1. You are providing care to an older adult patient who is receiving heparin therapy via subcutaneous injection. Based on the Zaybak study, would you give subcutaneous doses over 10 seconds or 30 seconds?

2. You are working in a pediatric clinic. You want to administer IM medication and immunizations to children in as pain-free a way as possible. Would you give IM injection slowly or more rapidly? Why would you choose that technique?

3. Why do you think changing the needle after withdrawal of medication but prior to administration would be less painful?

 Go to Chapter 26, **Toward Evidence-Based Practice Suggested Responses,** on DavisPlus.

 Go to Chapter 26, **Procedure 26-11: Administering Intradermal Medication,** in Volume 2.

 Also go to Student Resources, **Animations: Angle of Injection,** on DavisPlus.

Subcutaneous Injections

Subcutaneous (subQ) injections are given into the subcutaneous tissue, the layer of fat located below the dermis and above the muscle tissue. Absorption is slower than it is through the intramuscular route because subcutaneous tissue does not have as rich a blood supply as muscle. However, speed of absorption varies with the subcutaneous site selected. Absorption is fastest in sites on the abdomen and arms; it is slower on the thigh and upper buttocks. Medication is absorbed more evenly from the abdomen than from the thighs and buttocks because it is affected less by activity.

You do not need to aspirate for blood return when giving a subcutaneous injection because of the shallow depth of the needle into the subcutaneous layer under the skin. The Highlights of Procedures box contains critical elements of the procedure. For the full procedure,

 Go to Chapter 26, **Procedure 26-12: Administering Subcutaneous Medication,** in Volume 2.

Choosing a Subcutaneous Site Avoid sites in which the subcutaneous tissue lies beneath burns, birthmarks, inflamed tissue, or scars. Do not use sites with lesions or sites over bony prominences, large underlying vessels, or nerves. When using the abdominal site, do not inject any closer than 5 cm (2 in. horizontally and vertically) from the umbilicus. For repeated injections, each injection should be at least an inch apart. It is important to rotate sites for repeated injections to minimize scarring and hardening of fatty tissue that will interfere with the absorption of medication. See Figure 26-25 for sites to use for subcutaneous injections.

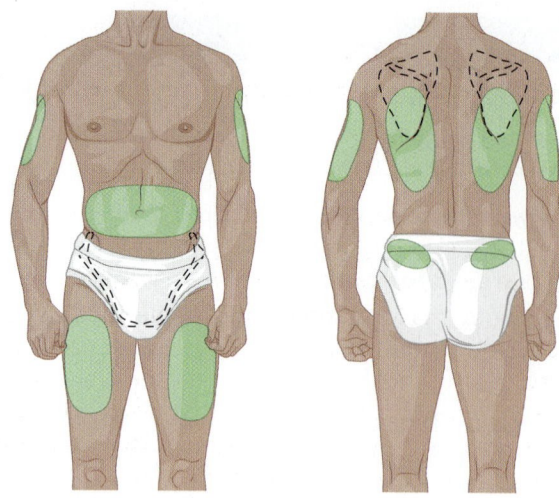

FIGURE 26-25 Sites used for subcutaneous injections.

Choosing a Subcutaneous Needle As a general rule, use a syringe with a small-gauge, short needle for subcutaneous injection—that is, long enough to penetrate beyond the skin into the fatty subcutaneous layer and yet not into the muscle. The needle length will vary depending on the amount of adipose the patient has and the type of injection that is needed (e.g., insulin, immunization, or other medication). For most subcutaneous injections, a ⅜- to ⅝-inch needle is preferred. However, shorter needles (e.g., ³⁄₁₆ to ⁵⁄₁₆ inch) are more comfortable for some insulin users.

The needle **gauge** for subcutaneous injection is typically 25- to 27-gauge; however, finer needles are preferred by many insulin users (e.g., 28- to 31-gauge). For children and persons with little or average subcutaneous fat, insert a standard length needle (⅝ in.) at a 45° angle; however, when using a shorter needle, inject at a 90° angle. Obese patients will need a longer needle (e.g., 1-inch) and a 90° angle for injection (Fig. 26-24), and the nurse needs to spread the skin taut rather than pinching.

✚ Inject only small amounts (0.5 to 1 mL) of water-soluble medication subcutaneously to avoid creating sterile abscesses (hardened, painful lumps under the skin).

Administering Insulin

Insulin must be administered subcutaneously or intravenously because it is a protein and would be destroyed in the gastrointestinal tract. Insulin is administered using a special insulin syringe. Insulin vials contain 100 units/mL. The prescriber will specify the number of units (**not** milliliters or milligrams) to administer. Insulin may be routinely prescribed in specific dosages at specific times or on a **sliding scale**, in which the amount of insulin prescribed is based on the patient's blood glucose level. However, some view the sliding scale as a reaction to hyperglycemia rather than

preventing its occurrence and a practice that may be dangerous (DeYoung, Bauer, Brady, et al., 2011). Others believe that when appropriately used, it is an effective type of correction insulin therapy (Magaji & Johnston, 2011). Sliding scale is used less now because basal insulin is available to stabilize blood sugar with fewer fluctuations, and because insulin pumps are in more common use. However, it can be useful when initiating insulin therapy and during times of physical stress (e.g., illness, surgery, trauma). Follow your institution's policy and the prescriber's guidance regarding the sliding scale.

People with diabetes usually administer their own insulin injections. Teach them to rotate injection sites to promote absorption and minimize tissue damage. Insulin is absorbed at different rates from different parts of the body. For hospitalized patients, you should document site rotation (usually on a diagram of the body) to prevent repeated use of the same site.

Categories of Insulin

To prevent errors and give insulin safely, you need to understand the categories of insulin and how they are used for blood sugar control.

- **Basal insulin** is given to cover the body's energy needs without taking the diet into account. Common basal insulins are NPH, insulin glargine (Lantus), and insulin detemir (Levemir).
- **Prandial** (mealtime) and **preprandial insulins**, such as regular insulin (e.g., Humulin R, Novolin R), are given to prevent high blood sugar after eating a meal. However, analogs with a more rapid acting onset than regular insulin (e.g., insulin lispro [Humalog], insulin aspart [NovoLog/NovoRapid], and insulin glulisine [Apidra]) are being added to the medication regime (Magaji & Johnston, 2011).
- **Correction insulin** is given to reduce an elevated blood sugar level that is not controlled by mealtime insulin. When a part of the patient's total daily dose requirements, this type of sliding scale blood sugar management may be effective. When used alone, it can create unpredictable glucose levels that may be dangerous.

Using two types of insulin can help keep blood sugar level in a target range. By mixing it in the same insulin syringe, your patient will need only one injection. For guidelines for mixing insulins,

 Go to Chapter 26, **Clinical Insight 26-5: Mixing Two Kinds of Insulin in One Syringe,** in Volume 2.

Appearance of Insulin

Regular (unmodified) insulin is rapid acting. It is a clear solution. If a vial of regular insulin is cloudy, you should discard it. Other types of insulin (e.g., modified, such as Lente, insulin glargine [Lantus], and neutral protamine Hagedorn [NPH]) are cloudy because of the addition of proteins, which slow the absorption of the drug, giving the insulin an intermediate to long duration of action. As a rule, remember "clear before cloudy"; that is, draw up the regular (clear) insulin first, and then draw up the modified (cloudy) insulin. In practice, though, you may rarely need to mix insulins because stable premixed insulins are available.

Storing Insulin

The length of time insulin can be stored depends on whether it is refrigerated or stored at room temperature. Discuss with your pharmacist or check the package insert to know how long the insulin will remain effective after the vial is opened. Also,

 Go to Chapter 26, **Supplemental Materials, Insulin Administration,** on Davis*Plus.*

Insulin Equipment

Insulin can be administered using a variety of tools. Regardless of the device, correct technique is essential for both nurses and patients who self-administer.

- **Disposable syringes** for subcutaneous injection are the most common.
- **Automatic injectors** are used by some patients for subcutaneous dosing. By pressing a button on the device, the injector releases the needle into the skin, releasing the insulin dose.
- **Insulin pumps** are becoming more common as a way to maintain glycemic control because of the benefit of fine-tuning the dosing. The pump consists of a tube with a needle on the end of it that is taped to the abdomen, and a computerized device that is worn at the waist. Insulin is received continuously from the pump. A button is pressed at mealtime to release an extra insulin dose.
- **Insulin pen devices** contain a cartridge and disposable needles to deliver certain doses with each injection. They are convenient and may help patients to avoid certain medication errors. However, the Institute for Safe Medication Practices (ISMP, 2013) strongly suggests that hospitals consider transitioning away from using them because of the risk of cross-contamination.
- **Nondisposable syringes** (glass syringe and metal needle) may be used repeatedly if they are sterilized after each use.
- **Spray injectors** forcefully spray the insulin dose into the skin. This involves a wider area of skin than would a regular injection.

KnowledgeCheck 26-16

- List three errors in technique that can occur when giving parenteral injections. State their possible consequences.
- Describe at least four ways to minimize the discomfort of an injection.
- Name two reasons for giving an intradermal injection.
- As a rule, what gauge and length of needle would you use for a subcutaneous injection?
- Why should people rotate injection sites when they must have repeated injections over a long time?

ThinkLike a Nurse 26-12

- What do intradermal and subcutaneous injections have in common?
- How are they different?

Administering Heparin

Heparin is a fast-acting medication that interrupts the blood-clotting process. It may be used for patients at risk for thrombus formation, for example, those who are immobile after major surgery, have undergone vascular surgery, or have problems related to blood clotting, such as cerebrovascular accident (stroke, brain attack) or myocardial infarction (heart attack). Because heparin is absorbed poorly from the gastrointestinal tract, it is given intravenously or subcutaneously. If mistakenly given intramuscularly, it will cause hematoma and pain.

 Heparin dosage is based on the patient's weight and results of blood coagulation studies, so always check laboratory values for coagulation studies before giving.

Give the injection deep into the subcutaneous tissue of the abdomen, at least 5 cm (2 in.) away from the umbilicus. Rotate sites. Because of the anticoagulant properties of heparin, you will need to modify your injection technique. For detailed guidelines,

 Go to Chapter 26, **Clinical Insight 26-6: Administering Anticoagulant Medication Subcutaneously,** in Volume 2.

Intramuscular Injections

Intramuscular (IM) injections (injections into muscle tissue) are absorbed faster than subcutaneous medications because of the rich blood supply in the muscles. Muscles can also tolerate more fluid—you can give as much as 3 or 4 mL of liquid in the large vastus lateralis and ventrogluteal muscles. The smaller the muscle, the less fluid it can tolerate. For example, you should usually give no more than 0.5 to 1 mL in the average deltoid muscle.

Conventional techniques require you to **aspirate** (pull back on the plunger of the syringe) before injecting medication intramuscularly to be sure the needle tip is not in a blood vessel. If there is no blood return, you are confident that the medication will not be injected into a blood vessel. However, there are insufficient evidence-based studies to support this conclusion. The CDC does not recommend aspiration before giving IM vaccines using the vastus lateralis and deltoid muscles *for vaccine administration* because there are no large blood vessels at these sites (CDC, n.d.). Others would limit the practice of aspiration to IM injections of large molecule medications such as penicillin (Crawford & Johnson, 2012). To promote better outcomes and less pain when administering IM injections to children, the practice of aspiration is not recommended (Walden & Vangilder, 2013). Since this has been a conventional practice and no evidence exists that aspirating for blood poses a risk to the patient, you should follow your institution's policies and procedures for IM injections.

Choosing an Intramuscular Site

When selecting an IM site, you should look for a site that is:

- A safe distance from nerves, large blood vessels, and bones
- Free from injury, abscesses, tenderness, necrosis, abrasion, or other pathology
- Large enough to accommodate the volume of medication to be given

Muscles commonly used are the vastus lateralis, ventrogluteal, and deltoid. Because of their proximity to major nerves and vessels, the rectus femoris and dorsogluteal are no longer recommended sites (Greenway, 2004; Walsh & Brophy, 2011). For a summary description of IM injection sites, refer to the Highlights of Procedures box. For the complete procedure,

 Go to Chapter 26, **Procedure 26-13: Locating Intramuscular Injection Sites,** in Volume 2.

Ventrogluteal Site—Site of Choice Whenever possible, use the ventrogluteal site for IM injections; it is the site of choice for adults and young children who are walking. The ventrogluteal site, located on the lateral hip, involves the gluteus medius and gluteus minimus muscles (Fig. 26-26). Because it is located away from major blood vessels and nerves, it is the safest and least painful site for IM injections. Be aware, though, that some medications and immunizations, such as those used to treat influenza/pneumonia, are normally given in the deltoid; be sure to check the package insert.

When learning to locate this site, many students notice that it feels "hard" when they palpate it. They worry the needle will hit the bone. In part, the muscle feels hard because there is little subcutaneous tissue over it.

To reassure yourself it is safe, examine a skeleton model with the muscles attached. Notice that the ilium is concave (curves in) and the muscle lies deep down in the "cup" it forms. If you are sure you have located the anterosuperior iliac spine and if you follow the procedure steps, you will not hit a bone. In fact, you are less likely to do so than were you to use other sites. For guidelines in locating the ventrogluteal site, refer to the Highlights of Procedures box and Procedure 26-13A (in Volume 2).

Dorsogluteal Site—Site to Avoid The dorsogluteal site consists of the gluteal muscles of the buttocks.

⊕ Avoid using the dorsogluteal site for IM injections because its close proximity to the sciatic nerve and superior gluteal artery increases the risk of (1) injection into a major blood vessel and (2) damage to the sciatic nerve. Furthermore, the site is difficult to identify accurately in older adults or in people with flabby skin.

Research found that nurses continue to use the dorsogluteal site, even though they are aware of its potential for complications, because of tradition, ease of mapping, and comfort level (Walsh & Brophy, 2010). **Key Point.** *Your avoidance of the dorsogluteal site gives you the opportunity to role model patient safety by demonstrating correct technique for locating the preferred site.*

Deltoid Site The deltoid site is located in the middle third of the upper arm (Fig. 26-27). The area has a small muscle mass with little subcutaneous tissue, so medications are absorbed rapidly. This muscle is easily accessible but is not well developed in many older adults. You should use it only for small amounts of up to 1 mL or when other sites are inaccessible. Avoid using the deltoid site in infants and assess children for adequate muscle mass before using it. However, the anterolateral thigh is preferred for children.

The deltoid muscle is small and lies close to the radial nerve and brachial artery. When locating this site, do not

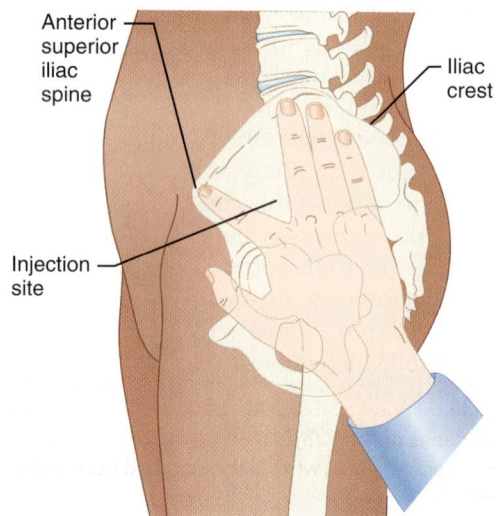

FIGURE 26-26 Locating the ventrogluteal site.

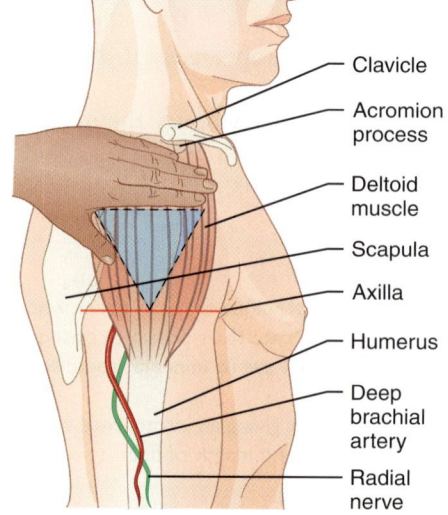

FIGURE 26-27 Locating the deltoid site.

merely roll up the sleeve; fully expose the entire upper arm and shoulder. Otherwise, you may miss the muscle mass and injure a nerve or blood vessel. For a guide to locating the deltoid site, see the Highlights of Procedures box and Procedure 26-13B (in Volume 2).

Vastus Lateralis Site The vastus lateralis muscle, located in the anterolateral thigh (Fig. 26-28), is the preferred site for young infants, particularly before walking age (Bartley, 2012; Jackson, Peterson, Nelson, et al., 2013) because it's usually the best developed and contains no large nerves or blood vessels, minimizing the risk for injury. Other advantages are that (1) drugs are rapidly absorbed from this area, (2) it can accommodate a larger volume of medication than can the deltoid, and (3) it is a convenient site for those who self-administer injections. A disadvantage is that the patient can see you administer the injection, and the psychological effect may create some discomfort. Also, because this muscle is used in walking, an ambulatory patient may notice more residual soreness than in another site.

To relax this muscle for injection, have the patient sit or lie flat with his knee slightly flexed. For children and adult patients with small muscle mass, you should grasp ("pinch up") the body of the muscle during injection to be sure that the medication reaches muscle tissue and the needle does not penetrate to the underlying bone. For a guide to locating the vastus lateralis site, refer to the Highlights of Procedures box and Procedure 26-13C (in Volume 2).

Rectus Femoris Site—For Adults Only The rectus femoris site, located in the anterior thigh, is no longer recommended for infants and children. In addition, you may rarely use it for adults, only when other sites are inaccessible or rapid absorption is needed. It is often used by patients who self-administer their IM injections because it is easy for them to reach. A disadvantage is that it is usually painful. Use a shorter needle when injecting

this site. For a guide to locating the rectus femoris site, refer to the Highlights of Procedures box and Procedure 26-13D (in Volume 2).

Choosing an Intramuscular Needle

Although a 1½-inch needle is considered "standard" for IM injections, you should choose the needle gauge and length based on the site, the size of the muscle, the amount of medication to be given, and the amount of adipose tissue over the muscle. In the deltoid muscle, for example, you might use a 23- or 25-gauge, 1-inch needle. But if the solution is viscous, you would need a larger-bore needle (e.g., 20-gauge). For a very thin person, you could use a 1-inch needle, even when injecting into the larger muscles. For an obese person, you might need a needle as long as 3 inches to penetrate adipose tissue and reach the muscle (long needles may not be available in many settings). As a rule, the angle of insertion for an IM injection is 90° (see Fig. 26-24). See Table 26-3 for needle length recommendations based on age and site for immunizations and vaccinations. The Highlights of Procedures box presents the key elements for IM injections. For the complete steps,

 Go to Chapter 26, **Procedure 26-14: Administering an Intramuscular Injection,** in Volume 2.

Z-Track Technique

The Z-track technique seals the needle track and prevents medication from leaking out of the muscle up through the needle track and into the subcutaneous tissues after the needle is withdrawn. The Z-track method is recommended for all IM injections, because it is less painful and helps to prevent irritation of subcutaneous tissues. It is particularly useful for irritating medications, such as iron preparations, that irritate or discolor subcutaneous tissue and for older adults who have reduced muscle mass. Procedure 26-14B, in Volume 2, describes the procedure for using the Z-track technique for intramuscular injections.

➕ For this technique, it is best to use the larger muscles: the ventrogluteal and vastus lateralis sites.

To see an animation of this method,

 Go to Student Resources, **Administering Animations, Z-track Injection,** on Davis*Plus.*

KnowledgeCheck 26-17

- Name three sites for giving IM injections.
- What is the preferred IM injection site for adults? Why?
- From which route is medication absorbed more rapidly: subcutaneous or IM? Why?
- For an "average" adult, what is the standard needle length for IM injections?
- Why is the dorsogluteal site *not* recommended?
- What are the disadvantages of the deltoid site?

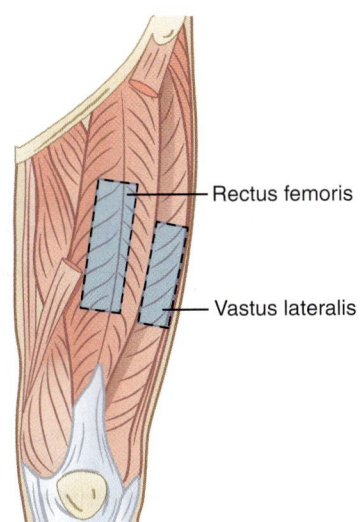

FIGURE 26-28 Locating the vastus lateralis.

Rectus femoris

Vastus lateralis

Table 26-3 ➤ Appropriate Needle Size Based on Age and Site for Vaccinations and Immunizations

AGE		NEEDLE LENGTH	SITE
Newborns (first 28 days)		⅝″*	Anterolateral thigh
Infants (1–12 months)		1″	Anterolateral thigh
Toddlers (1–2 years)		1–1 ¼″ ⅝–1″*	Anterolateral thigh Deltoid
Children and Teens (3–18 Years)		⅝–1″* 1–1 ¼″	Deltoid Anterolateral thigh
Adults (19 years and older)			
Male or Female	Less than 130 lb	⅝–1*″	Deltoid
Male	130–260 lb	1–1½″	Deltoid
Female	130–200 lb	1–1½″	Deltoid
Male	260+ lb	1½″	Deltoid
Female	200+ lb	1½″	Deltoid

*A ⅝″ needle may be used with the skin stretched tight and injection given at a 90° angle.

Source: Adapted from Centers for Disease Control and Prevention (2010a, updated 2012). Administering vaccines: Dose, route, site, and needle size. Retrieved June 23, 2013, from http://www.immunize.org/catg.d/p3085.pdf

- When using the vastus lateralis to give an IM medication to a person with small muscle mass, how can you ensure the medication reaches muscle tissue and the needle does not penetrate to the underlying bone?

Intravenous Medications

Intravenous (IV) medications are given through a catheter, or cannula, inserted into a vein. The onset of medication action takes place within seconds, so IV administration is especially useful in emergencies. However, because an IV drug begins to act immediately, there is no way for you to stop its action if an adverse reaction occurs (unless there is a known antidote). Review Table 26-1 for advantages and disadvantages of using the IV route. IV medications may be administered by a variety of programmable electronic pumps and infusers. These are discussed in Chapter 38.

Many IV push medications are irritating to vein walls and tissues around the vein. If the drug is accidentally injected into tissues, sloughing, pain, and abscesses may occur. To prevent complications, when administering IV medications, you should:

- Assess the patient before, during and after giving the medication.
- Determine whether the drug is compatible with the IV fluid that is infusing. Consult a pharmacist as needed.
- Determine whether the drug is compatible with the plastic IV bag and tubing. You may occasionally need to use a glass IV bottle and special tubing.
- Use sterile technique.

- Observe the insertion site often and check to be sure the cannula is in the vein before administering a medication. Figure 26-29 provides an example of damage that can occur when certain IV medications escape from the vein into surrounding tissues.
- Administer the medication slowly.
- Observe the patient carefully for signs of adverse reactions.
- Have an antidote on hand if the drug has potentially serious side effects. Be aware, though, that many drugs do not have an antidote.
- If your patient shows signs of serious allergic reaction, you will need to prepare to support the patient's airway, deliver oxygen, and administer medication to reduce the reaction.

The following sections explain how to administer IV medications by (1) adding medication to the large-volume primary or maintenance fluids, (2) IV push or bolus, (3) intermittent infusion (piggyback setup), (4) volume-control infusion sets, and (5) central venous access devices. You will find the procedures for initiating and maintaining intravenous fluids and using intermittent injection ports in Chapter 38.

Adding Medications to Large-Volume (Primary) Infusions

The safest way to administer a drug intravenously is to mix it into a bag of fluid that is already infusing (e.g., normal saline, lactated Ringer's solution, glucose). Vitamins, potassium chloride, oxytocin, and several blood pressure and cardiovascular drugs are commonly given

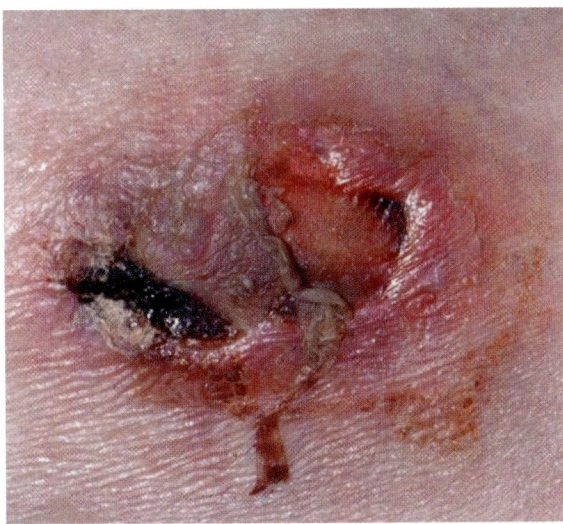

FIGURE 26-29 Tissue and skin injury after intravenous medication leaks into an infiltrated site. (Used by permission of the National Extravasation Information Service (UK). www.extravasation.org.uk)

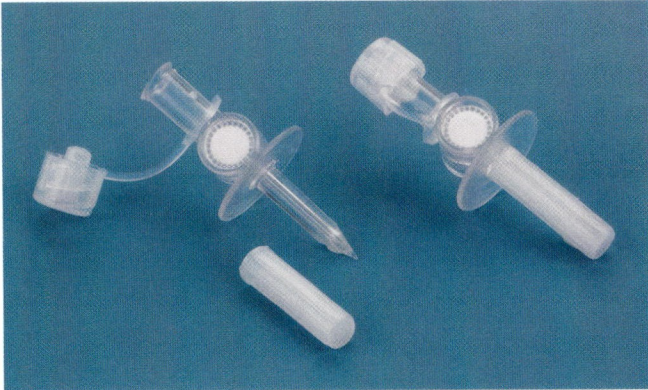

FIGURE 26-30 A reconstitution device is used to add medication from multidose IV vials while providing sterile air filtration. (Courtesy of Medi-Dose Inc./ EPS Inc., Ivyland, PA.)

this way. This method is useful when the drug can be infused continuously over a long period of time or when it must be given continuously to achieve the desired effect. The main disadvantage is the danger of infusing too much fluid, especially for children, older adults, and people with cardiac or renal disease. The drug may be premixed with the IV fluid in the pharmacy or you may occasionally need to add a drug to a bag of IV fluids.

 A safe method for mixing medication from multidose IV vials while providing sterile air filtration is to use a **reconstitution device**—designed with a sharp, thin, piercing spike to minimize coring and permit easy penetration of rubber top vials (Fig. 26-30). The luer-lock port maintains a secure closure between the device and the syringe. The hinged cap and the sheath over the spike help maintain sterility before use, minimize "touch" contamination, and ensure a closed system for disposal.

A safe method for adding medications to an IV container is to use a **transfer needle** or **cannula**—a blunted plastic needle with a double beveled tip (Fig. 26-31). One end is inserted into the powdered or liquid medication and the other end is inserted into a port of the IV bag. Solution is transferred from the IV bag into the medication vial, which you shake lightly to mix the medication. Then the medication is transferred back into the IV bag for administration.

Refer to the Highlights of Procedures box. Also,

 Go to Chapter 26, **Procedure 26-15: Adding Medications to IV Fluid,** in Volume 2.

IV Push Medications

IV push (bolus) medications are injected directly into a vein and enter systemic circulation immediately. IV push drugs are usually administered incrementally over a 1- to 10-minute time period. Read the package insert or ask the prescriber for specific guidelines on how fast the drug can be pushed. One minute can seem like a very

long time when you are pushing a medication, so don't guess—look at your watch!

 "IV push" does not mean the same thing as "give rapidly." If given too rapidly, IV drugs—particularly potassium—can be quite dangerous. Because you cannot retrieve the medication once it is injected, there is no margin for error.

To learn how to administer IV push drugs, refer to the Highlights of Procedures box, and

Go to Chapter 26, **Procedure 26-16: Administering IV Push Medication,** in Volume 2.

Intermittent Infusion

Many medications, such as antibiotics, are administered intravenously by intermittent infusion. Intermittent infusions may be given through the port of an infusing IV line or, if the patient does not need the additional fluids, through an intermittent injection port, also called a saline or heparin lock (Fig. 26-32).

Infusion Setup Most intermittent infusion medications are supplied in bags containing 50 to 250 mL of 5% dextrose in water (D_5W) or normal saline. The drug is given over a period of time, usually 30 to 60 minutes, and at regular intervals (e.g., every 6 hours). The small bag of diluted medication (the "secondary" bag) is attached to the primary IV infusion line for administration, usually

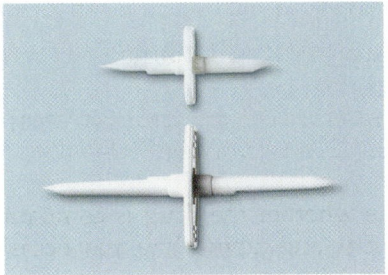

FIGURE 26-31 Transfer needles. (Courtesy of PFM Medical Ag.)

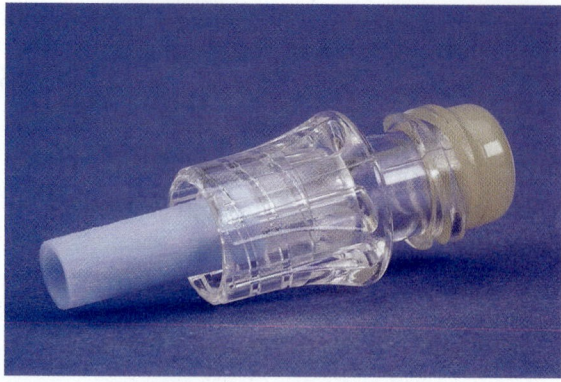

FIGURE 26-32 Intermittent injection port.

with a piggyback setup. With an **IV piggyback** setup, the smaller (secondary) container is connected to the primary (continuous) infusion line at the upper (primary) port (Fig. 26-33). This setup allows for intermittent use only and the infusion of one solution at a time.

A **tandem setup** allows for the simultaneous infusion of two IV bags, but is less commonly used than is a piggyback setup. For safety, most healthcare facilities require tandem infusions to be regulated via an IV pump.

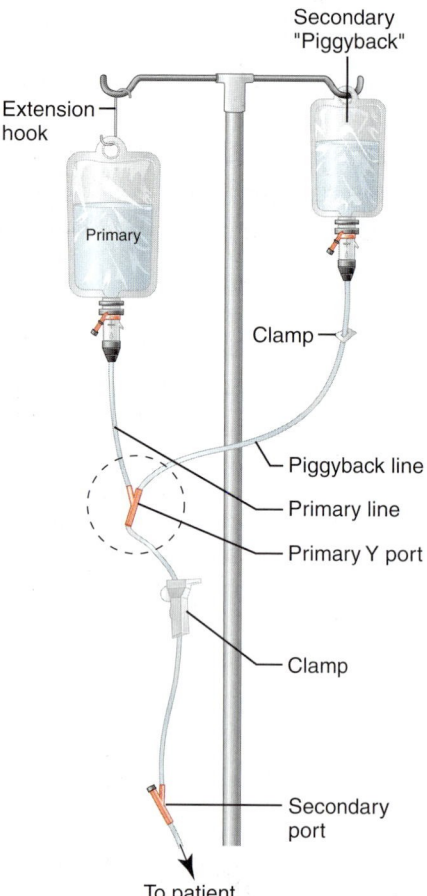

FIGURE 26-33 Piggyback setup is attached to the primary (continuous infusion) IV line at the upper port, allowing for intermittent infusion only.

Needleless Connections Traditionally, the secondary tubing was attached to the primary set tubing by inserting a needle into the port and taping it in place. However, most agencies now have needleless systems (see Fig. 26-21), which use a threaded or lever-type lock to make the connection. In addition to decreasing needle-stick injuries, a needleless system prevents contact contamination at the IV connection site.

Key Point: *You can help prevent catheter-related bloodstream infections by scrubbing the needleless IV connector for 15 seconds. Remember: "Scrub the Hub."*

When the secondary tubing is no longer needed, a disinfection cap containing either alcohol or chlorhexidine/alcohol solution is placed over the port (Fig. 26-34).

The Highlights of Procedures box provides guidelines for administering intermittent infusions. Also,

Go to Chapter 26, **Procedure 26-17B: Using a Piggyback Administration Set With a Gravity Infusion,** in Volume 2.

Volume-Control Infusion Sets

To effectively control the infusion of smaller amounts of solutions, particularly with pediatric patients, a volume-control infusion set (e.g., Buretrol, Soluset, Volutrol, or Pediatrol) may be used (Fig. 26-35). These are small fluid containers (100 to 150 mL) that are attached directly below the primary fluid container. The medication and the desired amount of IV fluid are added to the volume-control container and administered through the primary line. This system decreases the risk of overhydration because the amount of fluid that can infuse into the patient is limited to the amount that you place in the small container.

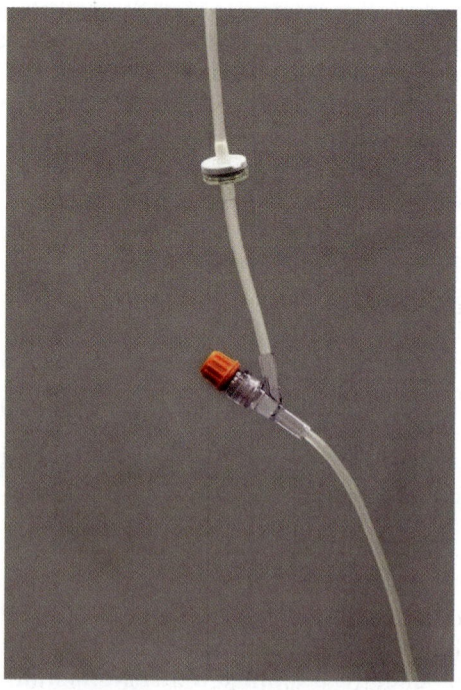

FIGURE 26-34 Disinfection cap for luer-lock needleless hubs. (Courtesy of Dr. Donna Clarren and Dr. Brian Oxhorn, Roseman College of Nursing.)

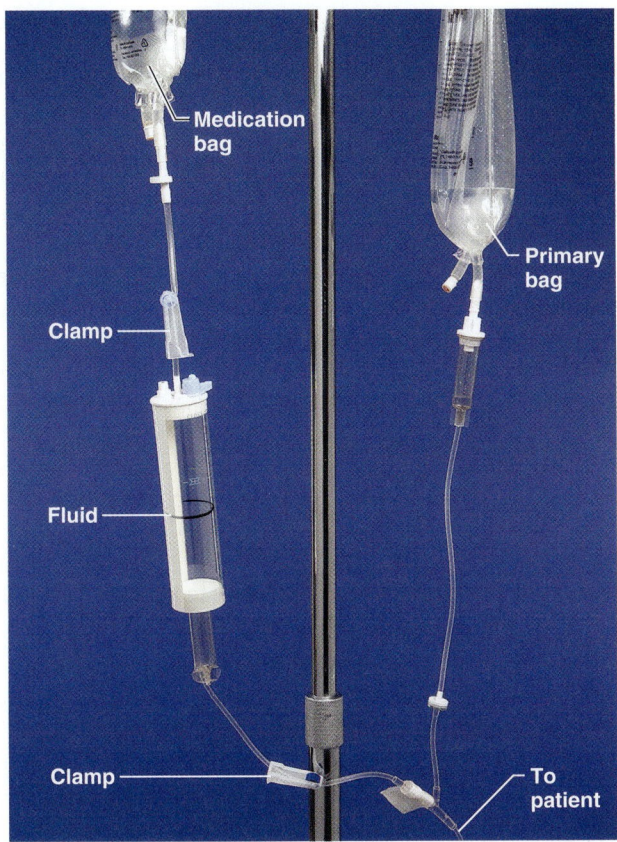

FIGURE 26-35 Volume-control infusion set for intermittent infusion administration; used when the fluid volume is critical and must be carefully monitored.

Central Venous Access Devices

Intravenous medication can be delivered through a central or peripheral vein. The most common reasons for a patient to have a **central venous access device (CVAD)** are to:

- Give long-term IV therapy
- Provide total parenteral nutrition when the patient cannot eat normally
- Have blood drawn without the trauma and complications of repeated venipuncture
- Provide vascular access when peripheral IV placement is difficult

External CVADs can be either tunneled or nontunneled. The *tunneled devices* are surgically implanted peripherally and tunneled to a central vein, typically the superior vena cava. *Nontunneled catheters* are inserted near the destination site. These catheters can be single- or multilumen. This category includes peripherally inserted central catheters (PICCs), which are inserted into the central circulation via a peripheral vein and can remain in place for months. For short-term use, the nontunneled central catheter can be inserted into the jugular, subclavian, or femoral veins.

An **internal**, or **implantable, port** is a CVAD that can remain in place and be functional for years. Access is

gained through the skin via a hollow port with a self-sealing silicone cap. These devices are inserted when long-term IV medication is needed or the medication is too irritating for a peripheral site. See Figure 26-36A for an example of a port for injecting medication into the subclavian vein.

Catheters for central venous delivery can be single- or multilumen (Fig. 26-36B). Although they are more convenient for administering different medications and fluid, some types of multilumen catheters have a higher infection rate than single-lumen catheters.

To learn how to administer medications through a CVAD, see the summary in the Highlights of Procedures box. Also,

Go to Chapter 26, **Procedure 26-18: Administering Medication Through a Central Venous Access Device,** in Volume 2.

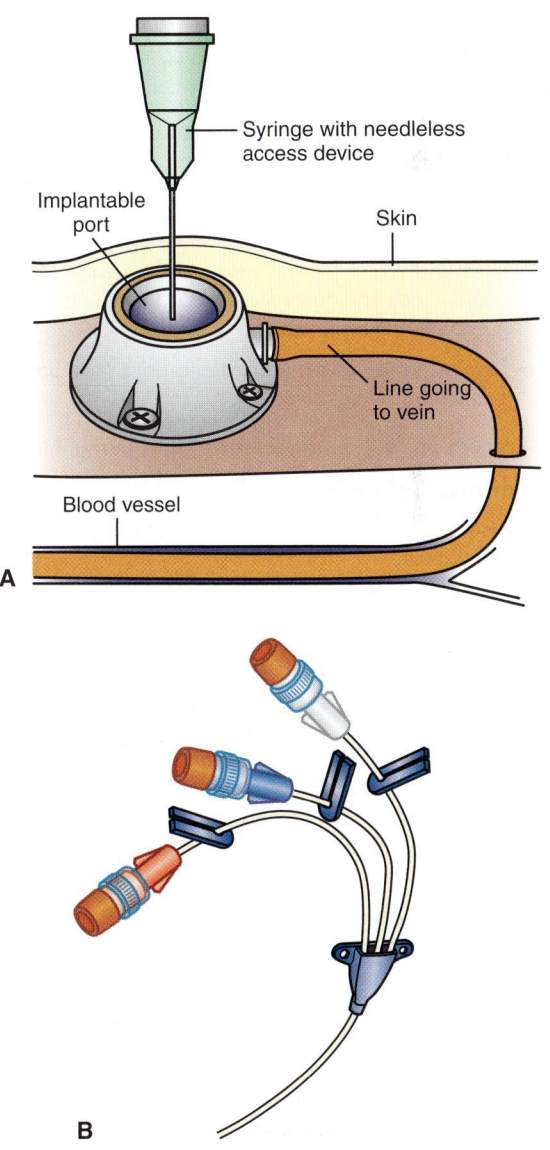

FIGURE 26-36 Central vascular access device: *A,* Implantable device. *B,* Multilumen catheter with blunt cannula, split septum, needleless access device.

For steps to follow in *all* procedures, refer to the Universal Steps for All Procedures found on the inside back cover of Volume 2. Go to the full procedures in Volume 2 to practice and learn the procedure steps. Use these procedure highlights later to help you review key points.

Procedure 26-1: Administering Oral Medication

➤ Observe the "three checks" and the "rights of medication": right patient, drug, dose, time, route, and documentation.

➤ *Tablets and capsules:* Pour the correct number into the medication cup.

➤ *Liquids:* Hold the plastic medication cup at eye level to measure the dose.

➤ Assist the patient to a high-Fowler's position, if possible.

➤ *Enterically administered medications:* Check for correct placement of the nasogastric or gastric tube.

➤ Correctly administer the medication.

　Powder: Mix with liquid, and give the mixture to the patient to drink.

　Lozenge: Instruct the patient not to chew or swallow it before dissolving it in his mouth.

　Tablet or capsule: Place the tablet or medication cup in the patient's hand or mouth, and instruct the patient to swallow with sips of liquid.

　Sublingual: Have the patient place the tablet under the tongue and hold it there until it is completely dissolved.

　Buccal: Instruct the patient to place the tablet between the cheek and gums and hold it there until it is completely dissolved.

➤ Stay with the patient until medications have been swallowed or dissolved.

Procedure 26-2: Administering Ophthalmic Medication

For instillations

➤ Use a high-Fowler's position, with the head slightly tilted back.

➤ Work from the inner to outer canthus when cleansing or instilling medication.

➤ Apply the medication into the conjunctival sac.

➤ Do not apply the medication to the cornea.

➤ Do not let the dropper or tube touch the eye.

➤ For eye drops, press gently against the same side of the nose for 1 to 2 minutes to close the lacrimal ducts. For an eye ointment, ask the patient to gently close his eyes for 2 to 3 minutes.

For irrigations

➤ Use a low-Fowler's position, with head tilted toward the affected eye, if possible.

➤ Check the pH in the conjunctival sac, if indicated.

➤ Use a Morgan lens or IV tubing to irrigate the eyes.

➤ For direct-flow irrigation, irrigate from the inner canthus to the outer canthus.

➤ Irrigate for 20 minutes or until the desired pH is reached.

Procedure 26-3: Administering Otic Medication

➤ Warm the solution to be instilled to body temperature.

➤ Assist the patient to a side-lying position, with the appropriate ear facing up.

➤ Straighten the ear canal. For an adult patient, pull the pinna up and back; for a child younger than 3 years, pull it down and back.

➤ Instill the prescribed number of drops into the ear canal.

➤ Do not force the solution into the ear or occlude the ear canal with the dropper.

➤ Instruct the patient to remain on his side for 5 to 10 minutes.

Procedure 26-4: Administering Nasal Medication

➤ Determine head position: Consider the indication for the medication and the patient's ability to assume the position.

➤ Explain to the patient that the medication may cause some burning, tingling, or unusual taste.

➤ Have the patient gently blow his nose and wash his hands afterward.

➤ Position the patient with the head down and forward for nasal sprays. Remember: "To spray your nose, look at your toes." For drops, assist the patient to a supine position with the head back.

➤ Place the tip of the sprayer into the right nostril, pointing the tip toward the outside of the nose (toward the outside corner of the right eye). Never point the tip toward the middle of the nose (the septum) or straight up (toward the sinus).

➤ Squirt the spray into the nose while patient inhales.

➤ Have the patient breath out through his mouth.

➤ Repeat for the other nostril.

➤ If the patient tastes the medicine, the head was not down or he did not inhale long enough. Advise him to put his head back down and sniff again without the medicine.

➤ If nose drops are used, ask the patient to stay in the same position for 1 to 5 minutes (depending on manufacturer's guidelines).

Procedure 26-5: Administering Vaginal Medication

For instillation

➤ Position the patient in a dorsal recumbent or Sims' position.

➤ Inspect and cleanse the vaginal area before administering the medication.

➤ Use a water-soluble lubricant.

➤ Insert the suppository or applicator along the posterior vaginal wall about 8 cm (3 in.).

➤ Instruct the patient to maintain the position for 5 to 15 minutes after the medication is inserted.

For irrigation (douche)

➤ Warm the irrigation solution to approximately 105°F (40.6°C).

➤ Hang the irrigation solution approximately 30 to 60 cm (1 to 2 ft) above the level of the patient's vagina.

➤ Position the patient in a dorsal recumbent position on a waterproof pad and bedpan.

➤ Lubricate the end of the irrigation nozzle.

➤ Insert the nozzle approximately 8 cm (3 in.) into the vagina, and start the flow of irrigation solution.

Procedure 26-6: Inserting a Rectal Suppository

➤ Before inserting the suppository, assess for contraindications, such as rectal surgery, rectal bleeding, or cardiac disease.

➤ Don gloves.

➤ Position the patient in the Sims' position.

➤ Lubricate the suppository.

➤ Insert the suppository past the internal sphincter about ½ to 1 inch in infants and 1 to 3 inches in adults. Never force the suppository during insertion.

➤ Instruct the patient to stay on his side for 5 to 10 minutes and retain (not expel) the suppository for about 30 minutes.

Procedure 26-7: Applying Medication to the Skin

➤ Wear gloves to avoid absorbing the medication through your own skin and to avoid cross-contamination.

➤ Before applying topical medication, cleanse the skin with soap and water.

➤ Do not apply medication to skin with open lesions, irritation, or known hypersensitivity.

➤ Avoid exposure to UV light/sunlight after applying medication.

➤ Assess for adverse skin reactions (e.g., hypersensitivity, redness, itching, or local irritation).

➤ Use gentle technique when applying topical medication to fragile skin, which is typical in older adults.

➤ Take care to not over-apply the medication.

➤ For transdermal patches, wear gloves when applying and removing; dispose of the patch in an appropriate receptacle, away from children and pets.

Procedure 26-8: Administering Metered-Dose Inhaler (MDI) Medication

➤ Identify the number of remaining inhalations in the canister. The "float method" is no longer recommended.

➤ Assist the patient to a seated position. Shake the inhaler. Remove the mouthpiece cap of the inhaler and insert the mouthpiece into the spacer while holding the canister upright.

➤ Remove the cap from the spacer.

➤ Ask the patient to breathe out slowly and completely.

➤ If a patient is unable to use the metered-dose inhaler independently, time the use of the device with the patient's own respirations.

➤ Place the spacer's mouthpiece into the patient's mouth and ask him to seal his lips around the mouthpiece. Press down on the inhaler canister to discharge one puff of medication into the spacer.

➤ Ask the patient to slowly inhale, and then hold his breath for as long as possible.

➤ If a second puff is needed, wait at least 1 minute and repeat.

Procedure 26-9: Preparing, Drawing Up, and Mixing Medication

➤ Maintain sterile technique.

➤ Recap the needle or vial access device (VAD) using a needle safety device or the one-handed method.

➤ Change the needle, if indicated.

Procedure 26-9A: Drawing Up Medication From Ampules

➤ Tap the ampule to remove medication trapped in the top of the ampule or shake it with a quick snap of the wrist.

➤ Use an ampule opener to break the ampule neck. Or wrap gauze or an alcohol swab in its wrapper around the neck of the ampule, and snap the ampule away from you.

➤ Use a filter needle or filter straw to withdraw the medication.

➤ Withdraw all of the medication from the ampule by inverting or tipping the ampule.

➤ Remove the filter needle and replace it with an appropriate size needle.

➤ Dispose of the broken ampule and filter needle in a sharps container.

Procedure 26-9B: Drawing Up Medication From Vials

➤ Scrub the rubber top of the vial with an alcohol prep pad or chlorhexadine gluconate (CHG)–alcohol product (for a multidose vial only).

➤ Draw air into the syringe equal to the amount of medication to be withdrawn.

➤ When inserting the needle or VAD through the rubber top of the vial, insert at a 45° to 60° angle, bevel up. Puncture the rubber top at that angle, but immediately raise to 90° as you insert the needle.

➤ Keeping the needle above the fluid line, inject air into the vial before inverting the vial and withdrawing the medication.

➤ Remove bubbles from the syringe, hold the vial at eye level, and check that the dose is correct before removing the needle.

Procedures 26-9C, D, and E: Mixing Medication From Two Vials, Mixing Medication From One Ampule and One Vial, and Using a Prefilled Cartridge and Single-Dose Vial—For Intravenous Administration

➤ Make sure the medications are compatible.

Continued

➤ Before beginning, determine the total volume of all medications to be put in the syringe and whether that volume is appropriate for the administration site.

➤ Maintain the sterility of the needles and medication.

➤ Avoid contaminating a multidose vial with a second medication.

➤ Carefully expel air bubbles.

➤ Withdraw the second medication very carefully because the medications are mixed as you pull back the plunger; therefore, you must withdraw the *exact* amount. If there is any excess, you must discard the contents of the syringe and start over.

➤ When opening ampules, protect yourself from injury.

➤ Use a filter needle or straw to withdraw medication from ampules; change to a needle of the proper length and gauge for administering the medication.

➤ When drawing up from a single-dose vial and ampule, draw up from the vial first.

➤ Do not use prefilled cartridges unless they have a safety needle; transfer the medication to a syringe with a safety device before administering.

➤ Always recap a sterile needle using a safety capping process or the one-handed scoop method.

Procedure 26-10: Recapping Needles Using One-Handed Technique

Procedure 26-10A: Recapping Contaminated Needles

➤ Recap a contaminated needle only if you cannot avoid it.

➤ Do not place your nondominant hand near the needle cap when recapping the needle or engaging the safety mechanism.

➤ If you are using a safety needle, engage the safety mechanism to cover the needle.

➤ Place the needle cap in a mechanical recapping device if one is available.

➤ If recapping devices are not available and you must recap the needle for your own and/or the patient's safety, use the one-handed scoop technique or one of the methods in Procedure 26-10B.

Procedure 26-10B: Recapping Sterile Needles

➤ Be sure to keep the needle and cap sterile.

➤ Do not place your nondominant hand near the needle cap when recapping the needle or engaging the safety mechanism.

➤ Use one of the following methods:

➤ Place the needle cap in a medication cup, and insert the needle into the cap.

➤ Place the cap on a clean surface so that the end of the needle cap protrudes over the edge of the counter or shelf, and scoop with the needle.

➤ Use a hard syringe cover: Stand it on end; insert the needle cap into the cover, and then insert the needle.

➤ Place the needle cap on a sterile surface, such as on open alcohol prep pad, and use the one-handed scoop technique. This is the least desirable method.

Procedure 26-11: Administering Intradermal Medication

➤ Have appropriate antidotes for certain injections readily available before beginning the procedure.

➤ Know the location of resuscitation equipment in case of a life-threatening adverse reaction.

➤ Maintain sterile technique and standard precautions.

➤ Use a 1-mL syringe and a 25- to 28-gauge, $\frac{1}{4}$- to $\frac{5}{8}$-inch needle with a short bevel.

➤ Be aware that an intradermal dose is small, usually about 0.01 to 0.1 mL.

➤ Administer the injection on the ventral surface of the forearm, upper back, or upper chest.

➤ Hold the syringe parallel to the skin at a 5° to 15° angle, with the bevel up.

➤ Stretch the skin taut to insert the needle.

➤ Do not aspirate.

➤ Inject slowly, and create a wheal or bleb.

➤ Do not wipe the site with alcohol, massage, or bandage the site.

Procedure 26-12: Administering Subcutaneous Medication

➤ Maintain sterile technique and standard precautions.

➤ Use a 1-mL syringe and a 25- to 27-gauge needle that is less than 1 inch long (usually $\frac{3}{8}$ to $\frac{5}{8}$ in.).

➤ A subcutaneous dose is typically no more than 1 mL.

➤ Most common injection sites: Use the outer aspects of the upper arms, abdomen, and anterior aspects of the thighs.

➤ Pinch the skin to inject, as a general rule.

➤ For an average-weight or thin patient, pinch up the skin and inject at a 45° angle. For an obese patient, inject at a 90° angle, if the adipose tissue pinches 2 inches or more, as a general rule. Use a longer needle and spread the skin taut instead of pinching.

➤ Do not aspirate when injecting heparin or insulin.

➤ Do not massage the site.

Procedure 26-13: Locating Intramuscular Injection Sites

➤ Always palpate the landmarks and the muscle mass to ensure correct placement.

Procedure 26-13A: Locating the Ventrogluteal Site

➤ On adults, a triangle is formed between your fingers when you place your palm on the head of the trochanter, index finger on the anterior superior iliac spine, and middle finger pointing toward or on the iliac crest. This is the preferred site for adults and children older than 7 to 12 months.

Procedure 26-13B: Locating the Deltoid Site

➤ The injection site is an inverted triangle on the upper arm. The base is the lower edge of the acromion process, and the tip is even with the top of the axilla. This is a good site in healthy adults for small-volume injection, especially when other sites aren't easily accessible because of drains or dressings.

Procedure 26-13C: Locating the Vastus Lateralis Site

➤ Midlateral thigh: On adults, one handbreadth below the head of the trochanter and one handbreadth above the knee. The site is the middle third of this area. This is the preferred site for infants who are not walking.

Procedure 26-13D: Locating the Rectus Femoris Site

➤ Middle third of the anterior thigh: Use this site only if no others are accessible. It is more painful than other sites.

Procedure 26-14: Administering an Intramuscular Injection

➤ Maintain sterile technique and standard precautions.

➤ Use a 1- to 5-mL syringe and a 21- to 25-gauge, 1-inch needle for deltoid site; 1½-inch needle for adults; 3-inch needle if the patient is obese.

➤ The usual volume is no more than 3 mL per injection. If the volume for injection is more than 3 to 5 mL, divide the dose into separate injections.

➤ Select an appropriate injection site, and identify the site using anatomical landmarks:

  ➤ The ventrogluteal site is preferred except in special circumstances (e.g., for many adult immunizations).

  ➤ The deltoid site is acceptable for IM doses of 1 mL or less.

➤ Inject at a 90° angle.

➤ Follow agency procedure regarding aspiration. If appropriate, aspirate before injecting. If blood appears, withdraw the needle, discard it, and start over.

➤ Press the plunger slowly to inject the medication (5 to 10 sec/mL).

➤ Z-track technique is recommended. Mnemonic:

Deliver	**D**isplace
All	**A**spirate
Injections	**I**nject (wait 5–10 seconds)
With	**W**ithdraw
Responsibility	**R**elease

Procedure 26-15: Adding Medications to IV Fluid

➤ Check the compatibility of the IV solution and medication.

➤ Refer to agency policy regarding maximum number of meds that can be added to one IV solution.

➤ Assess the patency of the IV site.

➤ Maintain the sterility of IV fluids and medication admixture.

➤ Affix the medication label to the bag, with the name and amount of medication, date and time administered, and your name or initials.

Procedure 26-16: Administering IV Push Medication

➤ Determine the type and amount of dilution needed for the medication.

➤ Determine the amount of time needed to administer the medication.

➤ Ensure the patency of the line before administration.

➤ Flush the line before and after administering the medication with normal saline. Flushing peripheral venous catheters with heparin 100 U/mL rather than with saline solution is recommended (Bertolino, Pitassi, Tinelli, et al., 2012).

➤ Maintain sterility.

Procedure 26-17: Administering Medications by Intermittent Infusion

➤ Ensure the compatibility of the IV solution and medication —both the solution in the primary IV system and in the secondary system.

➤ Assess the IV site and the patency of the line.

➤ Calculate the amount of medication to add to the solution.

➤ Use the correct amount and type of diluent solution.

➤ Use the correct rate of administration.

➤ Determine the correct primary line port in which to infuse the medication.

➤ Affix the correct label to the secondary bag identifying the infusate, patient name, start date and hour, discard date and hour, and your initials.

Procedure 26-18: Administering Medication Through a Central Venous Access Device

➤ First verify the medication can safely be administered through a central site.

➤ Scrub all surfaces of the catheter port, including the extension "tail," using an alcohol or CHG-alcohol combination product every time you enter the line.

➤ Flush the line before and after administering medication. Use saline, heparinized flush solution, or solution from the infusing IV line, according to agency policy.

➤ For multilumen catheters, flush all lumens.

➤ Clamp the line between the IV infusion set and the medication port. Open the clamp after medication is administered.

To explore learning resources for this chapter,

Go to Davis*Plus* at DavisPl.us/Wilkinson3.

Chapter Resources for Chapter 26:

Response sheets for all learning activities

Resources for Caregivers and Health Professionals

Reading More About Administering Medications (suggested readings)

Concept Map of chapter content

Interactive Case Studies

NCLEX-Style and Chapter Review Questions

Chapter Overview Podcasts

For references cited in this chapter,

Go to Volume 2, **References Cited.**

Supporting Physiological Functioning

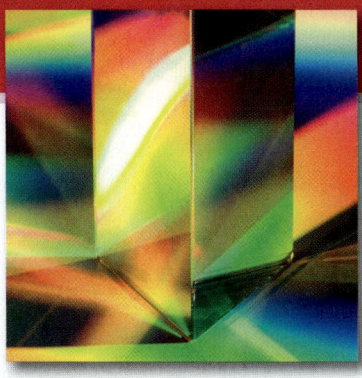

CHAPTER 27

Nutrition

Learning Outcomes

After completing this chapter, you should be able to:

- ➤ Identify the types, functions, metabolism, and major food sources of (1) the energy nutrients, (2) vitamins, (3) minerals, and (4) water.
- ➤ Differentiate among the various sources of nutritional information (e.g., USDA dietary guidelines, food guide ChooseMyPlate, DRIs, Nutrition Facts labels).
- ➤ Calculate a client's basal metabolic rate.
- ➤ Identify the primary nutritional considerations for various developmental stages.
- ➤ Discuss how each of the following affects and is affected by nutritional status: lifestyle choices, vegetarianism, dieting for weight loss, culture and religion, disease processes, functional limitations, and special diets.
- ➤ Describe tools and techniques for gathering subjective data about nutritional status.
- ➤ Compare the effectiveness of various anthropometric measurements.
- ➤ Calculate the body mass index for a client.

- ➤ Explain the significance of body mass index.
- ➤ List at least five physical assessment findings that indicate nutritional imbalance.
- ➤ Identify laboratory values that are indicators of nutritional status.
- ➤ Discuss the need for and advisability of vitamin and mineral supplementation.
- ➤ Describe nursing interventions for patients with special needs: Impaired Swallowing, NPO, older adults, and Nausea.
- ➤ Describe techniques for assisting patients with meals.
- ➤ Identify and discuss six nursing interventions for Imbalanced Nutrition: Less Than Body Requirements and six interventions for Imbalanced Nutrition: More Than Body Requirements.
- ➤ Safely provide enteral and parenteral nutrition for patients.

Key Concepts

Energy
Metabolism
Nutrition

Related Concepts

See the Concept Map on Davis*Plus*.

Example Problems

Overweight/Obesity
Underweight/Malnutrition

Meet Your Patients

As part of a class assignment, you are to assist a local business with its wellness program. You will be completing health risk appraisals and gathering the following data on each of the employees: height, weight, medical and nutritional history, and lifestyle practices. Today you will screen two employees, and then each will have blood drawn for a complete blood count (CBC), comprehensive metabolic panel, and lipid panel:

- **Isaac Schwartz**, a 65-year-old accountant, works long hours. He describes a sedentary lifestyle, no tobacco use, infrequent alcohol use, no medical problems, and a nutritional history of skipping meals and daily consumption of restaurant food. You measure his height as 69 in. and weight as 245 lb.
- **Sujing Lee**, a 29-year-old project manager, regularly works 65 hours per week. Sujing is 30 weeks pregnant. She does not smoke or drink and has never been hospitalized or had surgery. She has gained a total of 25 lb since becoming pregnant. Her diet consists mainly of

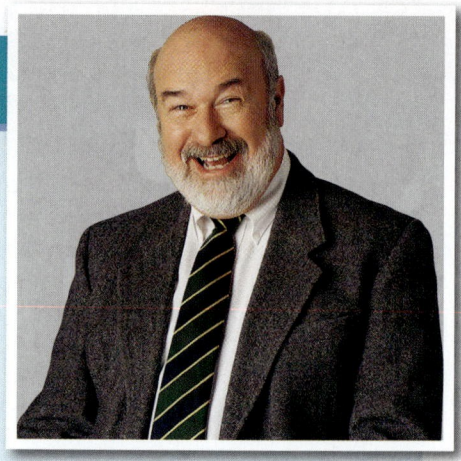

traditional Chinese food. She eats three meals a day and always brings lunch from home. Lately she has felt "tired all the time." At the screening, she weighs 126 lb and measures 63 in. tall.

At the end of your clinical day, you need to compile a report on the clients you have seen. How would you interpret the data on height, weight, and nutrition? What, if any, additional information do you need to help you evaluate their nutritional status? In this chapter, you will read about dietary recommendations, energy balance, and nutritional concerns across the life span. You will gain the theoretical knowledge to answer these questions, as well as practical knowledge about managing nutritional problems.

Theoretical Knowledge
knowing **why**

Organic, natural, low-fat, sugar-free, reduced-calorie, low-sodium, calcium-enriched . . . these are just a few of the hundreds of claims you find on packaged foods. Television and print ads hype nutritional supplements, weight-loss pills, and new diets, while the media carries conflicting reports on the benefits and dangers of phytochemicals, antioxidants, and *trans*-fatty acids. With so many options and different recommendations about what's healthy or not, it's no wonder that many people are confused about what to eat.

ABOUT THE KEY CONCEPTS

Nutrition is the study of food: how it affects the human body and influences health, and **metabolism**—specifically, how the body metabolizes food for **energy**. Good nutrition is essential to wellness, and poor nutrition contributes to disease, so clients need accurate, current, and appropriate nutritional information. Before you can give effective individualized advice, you need to know about the nutrients found in foods. In this chapter you will learn about concepts related to **energy**, for example, energy balance, nutrients, micronutrients, and factors that influence nutritional status.

WHAT ARE SOME RELIABLE SOURCES OF NUTRITION INFORMATION?

Standards and guides provide credible nutrition information. **Standards** are a reference for nutrient intake thought to meet the nutritional needs of most healthy population groups. They list nutrient amounts in measurements, such as grams and milligrams, and are not intended to indicate individual requirements or therapeutic needs. **Food guides** are more practical tools that you can use to educate patients and families. They specify the number of servings of foods needed daily so nonprofessionals can use them in making healthful meal choices. In general, standards and guides provide recommendations to healthy individuals but they are not sensitive to the needs of people experiencing metabolic or other medical problems.

Dietary Reference Intakes

The National Academy of Sciences, in a collaborative effort by the United States and Canada, has established standards, the **Dietary Reference Intakes (DRIs),** to promote the consumption of healthful nutrient levels. For carbohydrates and lipids, the *acceptable macronutrient distribution range (AMDR)* is used. To view the DRIs and AMDRs for males and females in various age groups,

Go to Chapter 27, **Supplemental Materials, Dietary Reference Intakes: Vitamins; Dietary Reference Intakes: Electrolytes** and **Water; Dietary Reference Intakes: Elements;** and **Dietary Reference Intakes: Macronutrients,** on Davis*Plus*.

The DRIs are a revision of the older Recommended Dietary Allowances (RDAs) for vitamins and minerals, protein, and total kcal that are thought to meet the needs of about 98% of individuals in a group. For vitamins and minerals, the DRI tables include RDAs and Adequate Intakes (AIs). AIs are the intakes adequate to meet the needs of all individuals in a group. For files you can download,

 Go to Browse by Subject, **U.S. Department of Agriculture, National Agricultural Library, Food and Nutrition Information Center,** a government Web site, at http://fnic.nal.usda.gov/

USDA Dietary Guidelines

In 1980, the U.S. Department of Agriculture (USDA) developed dietary guidelines for Americans. The guidelines are revised every 5 years. Box 27-1 presents the 2010 guidelines to help people evaluate their food habits and work toward general improvement in their diet. The guidelines do not specify daily amounts of food and nutrients.

The USDA intends this document to be a primary source of dietary health information for nutrition educators, policy makers, and healthcare providers. It is based on the latest scientific evidence and provides information about choosing a nutritious diet, maintaining healthy weight, achieving adequate exercise, and food safety to avoid food-borne illness. The dietary guidelines are updated every 5 years, so the new ones should be available after this book is published. To see the complete 2010 guidelines and the new guidelines when they are available,

 Go to the **USDA Dietary Guidelines** Web site, at http://www.cnpp.usda.gov/dietaryguidelines.htm

MyPlate

MyPlate is a colorful, four-part food guide for use as a dietary-teaching tool (Fig. 27-1) Based on USDA 2010 dietary guidelines, it visually illustrates a healthy meal—red for fruits, green for vegetables, orange for grains, and purple for protein with a separate blue section for dairy on the side.

MyPlate stresses the following concepts for healthy eating:

- Balancing calories by avoiding oversize portions.
- Eating more healthy food. That means making half the plate fruit and vegetables and making half of the grains whole grains.
- Eat less unhealthy food, for example, processed and high-sodium, high-sugar, and high-fat foods and snacks, and sugary and high-caffeine beverages.

BOX 27-1 ■ Dietary Guidelines for Americans 2010—Key Points

- Consume a variety of nutrient-rich foods and beverages daily.
- Adopt a balanced eating pattern (e.g., the USDA Food Guide) to meet recommended intakes.
- Limit the intake of saturated fats, *trans* fats, and cholesterol to less than 10% of calories. Replace them with mono- and polyunsaturated fats. Consume less than 300 mg of dietary cholesterol per day. Most fats should come from foods such as fish, nuts, and vegetable oils.
- Limit your intake of refined sugars, salt, and alcohol. Those aged 14 to 50 should limit their daily salt intake to 2,300 mg. However, those who are 51 and older; blacks; and people with hypertension, diabetes, or chronic kidney disease should reduce salt intake to 1,500 mg per day.
- Replace higher-fat protein foods with leaner meat, poultry, seafood, eggs, beans, unsalted nuts, and seeds.
- Increase the intake of fat-free or low-fat milk products, such as skim milk and cheese, cottage cheese, and yogurt.
- Achieve and maintain a healthy weight.
- Be physically active each day.
- Balance calorie intake with increase or decrease in activity.
- Choose a variety of fruits and vegetables each day, especially dark green, orange, red, and yellow vegetables and beans.

- Choose fiber-rich fruit, vegetables, and whole grains often. At least half the grains should come from whole grains.
- Women capable of becoming pregnant should consume iron-rich food and supplement with 400 micrograms (mcg) of folic acid.
- People 50 years and older should eat foods fortified with vitamin B_{12}.
- Cook, chill, and store foods to keep them safe from microorganisms.
- Clean hands, food contact surfaces, and fruits and vegetables. Do not wash or rinse meat and poultry. (Also see Chapter 24 for food safety.)

Source: Abstracted from U.S. Department of Agriculture and U.S. Department of Health and Human Services. (2011). Dietary guidelines for Americans 2010. Retrieved from http://www.cnpp.usda.gov/DGAs2010-PolicyDocument.htm; and CDC. (2009). Application of lower sodium intake recommendations to adults—United States, 1999–2006. *Morbidity and Mortality Weekly Report, 58*(11), 281–283. Retrieved from http://www.cdc.gov/mmwr/preview/mmwrhtml/mm5811a2.htm

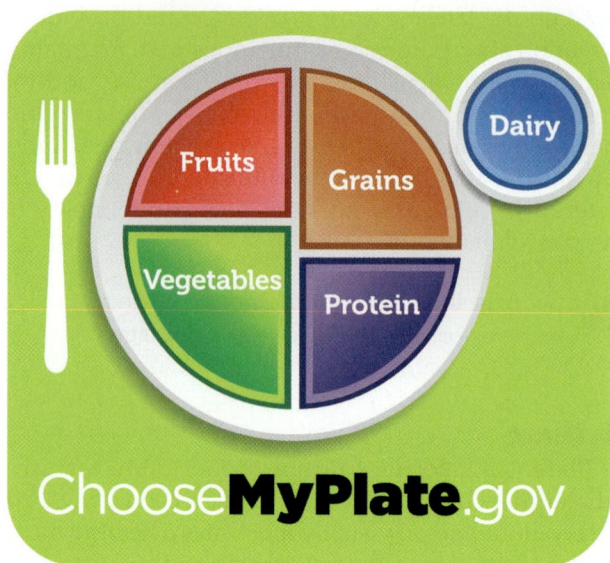

FIGURE 27-1 USDA Choose MyPlate. (From U.S. Department of Agriculture, www.choosemyplate.gov.)

MyPlate does not specify number of servings per day; it specifies measurable amounts, such as ounces and cups. For access to MyPlate,

 Go to the **MyPlate** Web site at http://www.Choose MyPlate.gov

MyPlate is also provided in Spanish, with the same foods as the English MyPlate. For the Spanish version,

 Go to http://www.choosemyplate.gov/en-espanol.html

MyPlate promotes healthy eating:

- *Activity.* MyPlate partners with Let'sMove to emphasize the importance of activity and exercise.
- *Choices.* MyPlate illustrates a meal that consists of 50% fruits and vegetable, as well as changing to fruit, vegetables, or unsalted nuts as snacks.
- *Personalization.* Eat the right amount of calories for you (one size does *not* fit all). To find the kinds and amounts of food you need to eat each day, based on personal factors, check the MyPlate Web site.
- *Proportionality.* Notice that the food group wedges are of slightly different sizes. The wedges are a general guide to how much food you should choose from each group. For example, the Vegetable group is a very large area, and the Protein area is slightly smaller. This gives you a general idea that you should eat many more servings of grains than of oils.
- *Variety.* Four different colors represent food groups. This illustrates the importance of variety in your diet; you need foods from all groups each day.
- *Tools for Success.* The SuperTracker, Daily food plans and sample menus are a few of the tools included on the site.

For information about serving sizes and nutrients provided by each food group when assisting patients with nutritional choices,

 Go to **Clinical Insight 27-1: 10 Tips for Building Healthy Meals,** in Volume 2,

or

 Go to Chapter 27, **Tables, Boxes, Figures: ESG Table 27-1, Serving Sizes for Daily Food Choices,** on Davis*Plus.*

For Asian, Latin American, Vegetarian, and Mediterranean diets, which include some of the traditional foods of those cultural groups,

 Go to the **Oldways Preservation and Exchange Trust** Web site at http://www.oldwayspt.org

For the Diabetes Food Plate,

 Go to the **American Diabetes Association** Web site at http://www.diabetes.org/food-and-fitness/food/planning-meals/create-your-plate/

The Diabetes Food Plate, unlike MyPlate, groups foods based on their carbohydrate and protein content. For example, you will find the plate divided into three sections, and the types of vegetables encouraged are non-starchy, such as spinach and green beans.

Food Guides for Older Adults

For an updated (2011) MyPlate for Older Adults,

 Go to the **Tufts University Friedman School of Nutrition Science and Policy** Web site at http://www.nutrition.tufts.edu/research/myplate-older-adults

The Tufts University MyPlate for Older Adults is consistent with the federal government's 2010 Dietary Guidelines for Americans, which recommend limiting foods high in *trans* and saturated fats, salt, and added sugars, and emphasize whole grains. The model also emphasizes whole fruits and vegetables in a range of colors. The MyPlate for Older Adults emphasizes nutrient-dense foods and stresses the importance of fluids by showing a circle representing glasses for fluids. It shows packaged fruits and vegetables in addition to fresh because they are easier to prepare and have a longer shelf life. This is important to consider when it is difficult for an older adult to make frequent trips to the grocery store. It also promotes physical activity with icons showing active adults.

Nutrition Facts Label

You are likely familiar with the **Nutrition Facts label** shown in Figure 27-2, because the U.S. Food and Drug Administration (FDA) requires this label on all packaged foods sold in the United States. The Nutrition Facts panel contains important information about serving

Toward Evidence-Based Practice

Scarmeas, N., Luchsinger, J., Mayeux, R., et al. (2007). Mediterranean diet and Alzheimer disease mortality. *Neurology, 69*, 1084–1093.

A Mediterranean diet (MeDi) consists of an average of nine servings of fruits and vegetables daily, whole grains, fish once or twice a week, and up to 5 ounces of red wine daily. It limits red meat and avoids *trans* fats and saturated fats, using instead olive oil for its antioxidant effect and canola oil and nuts to provide omega-3 fatty acids.

Researchers followed 192 community-based individuals diagnosed with Alzheimer's disease (AD) for 4.4 years. Eighty-five of the AD patients died during that period. Researchers concluded that adherence to the MeDi may reduce not only risk for AD but also subsequent disease course: Higher adherence to the MeDi is associated with lower mortality in AD.

Barberger-Gateau, P., Raffaitin, C., Letenneur, L., et al. (2007). Dietary patterns and risk of dementia. *Neurology, 69*, 191–193.

This study included 8,085 nondemented participants aged 65 and older in three cities in France. An independent committee validated 281 cases of dementia (including 183 AD). Daily consumption of fruits and vegetables was associated with a decreased risk of all-cause dementia; weekly consumption of fish was associated with a reduced risk of AD, but only among people carrying a high-risk AD gene; regular use of omega-3–rich oils was associated with a decreased risk for all-cause dementia. Researchers concluded that frequent consumption of fruits and vegetables, fish, and omega-3 rich oils may decrease the risk of dementia and AD, especially among those who do not carry the high-risk AD gene.

Vogiatzoglou, A., Refsum, H., Johnston, C., et al. (2008). Vitamin B_{12} status and rate of brain volume loss in community-dwelling elderly. *Neurology, 71*(11), 826–832.

This was a 5-year study of 107 community-dwelling elders aged 61 to 87 years with no cognitive impairment at the beginning of the study. They were assessed yearly by magnetic resonance imaging (MRI) scans, cognitive tests, and blood studies. The decrease in brain volume over the 5-year period was greater for those with lower vitamin B_{12} levels. Researchers concluded that low vitamin B_{12} status should be further researched as a cause of brain atrophy and likely cognitive impairment in the elderly.

1. Suppose you are a manager in a long-term care facility that specializes in treating residents with AD. You are planning nutritional interventions for these residents. Which of these three studies is best suited to your patients, and why?

2. How was the cognitive status of the subjects different in all three studies?

3. Based on the third study, vitamin B_{12} supplementation would most likely be of benefit to which of the following groups? Explain your thinking.
   a. People who have AD and want to extend their life expectancy
   b. Older adults who wish to prevent getting AD
   c. Older adults who want to avoid cognitive impairment from brain changes other than AD.

 Go to Chapter 27, **Toward Evidence-Based Practice Suggested Responses,** on Davis*Plus*

 Go to Chapter 27, **Resources for Caregivers and Health Professionals,** on Davis*Plus*

---

size, number of servings per package, total calories and calories from fat per serving, a list and amounts of the key nutrients in the food, and the *percent daily values* (% DV) for the nutrients listed on the panel. The % DV identifies the percentage that a serving of the food contributes to a consumer's overall intake of the nutrient listed. Updates to the label will reflect more typical serving sizes, listing added sugars when present, removing the "calories from fat" information, and proposed changes to the Daily Values.

Teaching your patients how to read these labels will help them to make wiser dietary choices. If you need a more thorough explanation of how to use Nutrition Facts labels,

 Go to the **USDA** Web site at http://www.fda.gov/downloads/Food/ResourcesForYou/Consumers/UCM079504.pdf

Knowledge Check 27-1
- What are the DRIs?
- List the current USDA dietary guidelines for Americans.

Think Like a Nurse 27-1
How might you use the various sources of nutritional information to evaluate the nutritional status of the clients introduced in the Meet Your Patients scenario?

WHAT ARE THE ENERGY NUTRIENTS?
The cells and tissues of the body depend for their functioning on building blocks called **nutrients**. Any one food may contain a variety of nutrients; for instance, cheese contains carbohydrates, protein, lipids, sodium, vitamins, and minerals. Some nutrients, called *macronutrients*, supply the body with energy (kilocalories),

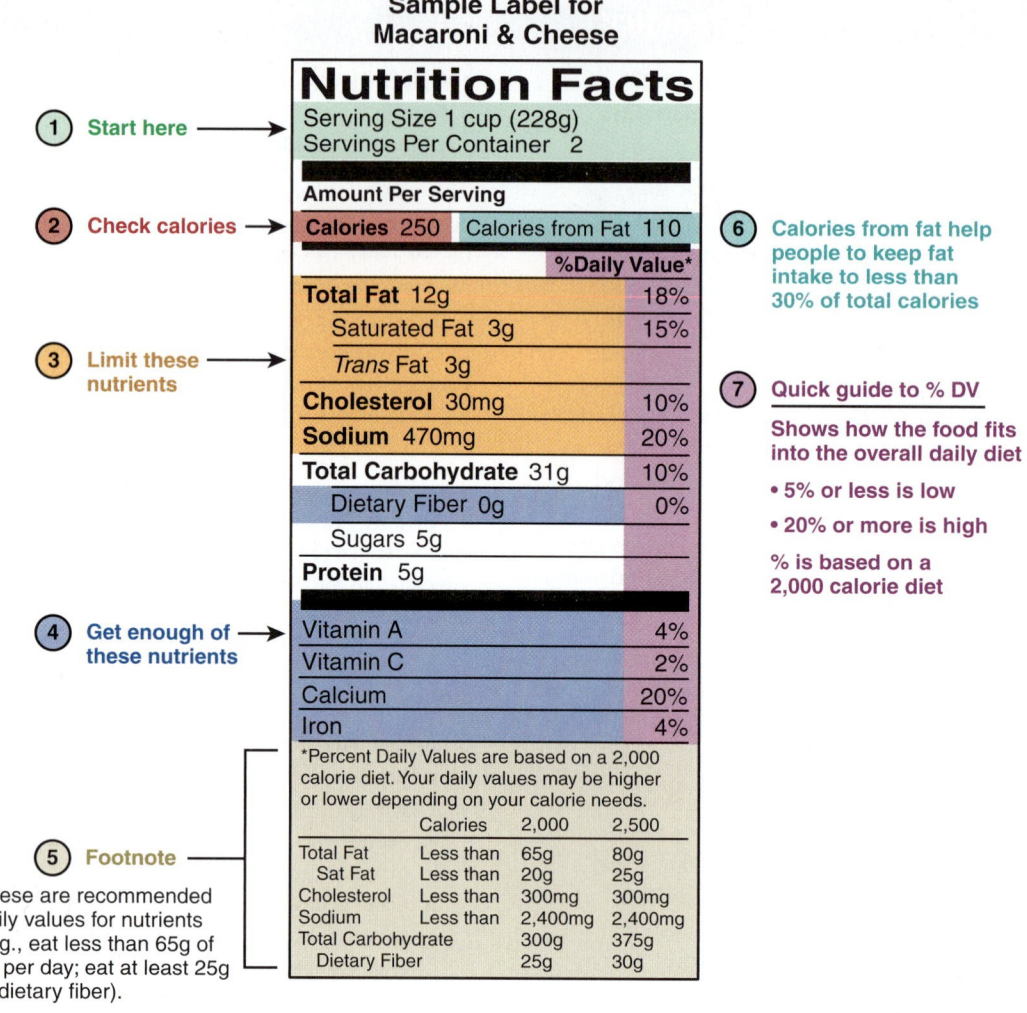

**Sample Label for
Macaroni & Cheese**

(1) Start here →

Nutrition Facts
Serving Size 1 cup (228g)
Servings Per Container 2

Amount Per Serving

(2) Check calories →

| Calories 250 | Calories from Fat 110 |

	%Daily Value*
Total Fat 12g	18%
Saturated Fat 3g	15%
Trans Fat 3g	
Cholesterol 30mg	10%
Sodium 470mg	20%
Total Carbohydrate 31g	10%
Dietary Fiber 0g	0%
Sugars 5g	
Protein 5g	

Vitamin A	4%
Vitamin C	2%
Calcium	20%
Iron	4%

(3) Limit these nutrients →

(4) Get enough of these nutrients →

*Percent Daily Values are based on a 2,000 calorie diet. Your daily values may be higher or lower depending on your calorie needs.

	Calories	2,000	2,500
Total Fat	Less than	65g	80g
Sat Fat	Less than	20g	25g
Cholesterol	Less than	300mg	300mg
Sodium	Less than	2,400mg	2,400mg
Total Carbohydrate		300g	375g
Dietary Fiber		25g	30g

(5) Footnote

These are recommended daily values for nutrients (e.g., eat less than 65g of fat per day; eat at least 25g of dietary fiber).

(6) Calories from fat help people to keep fat intake to less than 30% of total calories

(7) Quick guide to % DV

Shows how the food fits into the overall daily diet

• 5% or less is low

• 20% or more is high

% is based on a 2,000 calorie diet

FIGURE 27-2 A Nutrition Facts panel. (From U.S. Food and Drug Administration, 2007a).

whereas others, called *micronutrients,* help manufacture, repair, and maintain cells. In this section, we discuss the three classes of nutrients that provide the body with energy: carbohydrates, proteins, and lipids. Table 27-1 lists the sources of and requirements for macronutrients.

The body requires a constant supply of energy. Physiological mechanisms constantly convert stores of more complex forms of chemical energy into usable energy, which is then carried to individual cells. The term **metabolism** encompasses all the ways in which the body changes and uses nutrients. Two types of metabolic reaction, anabolism and catabolism, occur continually and are adjusted according to the needs of the body. **Anabolism** involves the formation of larger molecules from smaller ones. For example, if protein is needed for tissue repair, amino acids are recombined to form proteins. This process requires energy. **Catabolism** involves the breakdown of larger molecules into smaller components. One of the results of this separation is the release of energy. Most metabolic reactions, including metabolism of nutrients, are catalyzed by

enzymes; each is specific and catalyzes only one type of reaction.

Carbohydrates

Carbohydrates (CHOs) are the primary energy source for the body. **Simple carbohydrates,** commonly called *sugars,* are named according to the number of sugar (or *saccharide*) units making up their chemical structure. **Monosaccharides** (simple sugars) consist of a single unit; **disaccharides** are molecules made up of two saccharides. **Complex carbohydrates** consist of long chains of saccharides, called **polysaccharides. Dietary fiber,** a polysaccharide, is the indigestible "fibrous skeleton" of plant foods. Humans do not have the enzymes to digest fiber; thus, it provides no usable glucose. Carbohydrates perform several functions:

1. *Supply energy for muscle and organ function.* Carbohydrates, which are more easily and quickly digested than proteins and lipids, fuel strenuous short-term skeleton muscle activity and provide nearly all the energy for the brain. Humans store glucose in liver and skeletal muscle tissue as **glycogen.** Glycogen is

Table 27-1 ➤ Energy Nutrients

NUTRIENT	SOURCES	ENZYMES INVOLVED IN DIGESTION	REQUIREMENTS
Carbohydrates	*Simple sugars* occur mainly in corn syrup, honey, milk, table sugar, molasses, sugar cane, sugar beets, and fruits. *Complex carbohydrates* occur in vegetables, breads, cereals, pasta, grains, and legumes.	Salivary amylase (mouth) Ptyalin (mouth and stomach) Pancreatic amylopsin Intestinal: sucrase, lactase, maltase	There is debate about the amount of carbohydrate needed in the diet. Many popular diet plans alter carbohydrate intake: The Atkins diet is a low-carbohydrate plan, whereas the Pritikin and Ornish diets recommend high intake of complex carbohydrates. Body size and activity level affect the amount of carbohydrate used by the body. The 2002/2005 DRIs specify that adults should get 45%–65% of their calories from CHOs, or 130 grams per day (g/day).
Proteins	*Complete proteins* come mostly from animal sources: meat, poultry, fish, eggs, and milk products. *Incomplete proteins* are supplied by plant sources (e.g., grains, nuts, legumes, seeds, vegetables). They can be combined to make complete proteins.	Stomach: Pepsin Pancreas: Trypsin, chymotrypsin, carboxypeptidase Intestine: Aminopeptidase, dipeptidase	Protein needs depend on age, body size, and physical state. Needs are increased during growth periods, such as childhood and pregnancy. The average adult needs about 1 gram of protein per kilogram of body weight per day. The 2002/2005 DRIs specify that adults should get 10%–35% of their calories from protein, or 0.8 g/kg of body weight (46–56 g/day for an "average" person).
Lipids	*Saturated fats* occur in pork, beef, poultry, seafood, egg yolk, and dairy; coconut oil and palm oil. *Unsaturated fats (from plants)* occur in olives, olive oil, vegetable oils (peanut, soybean, cottonseed, corn, safflower), nuts, and avocados *Essential fatty acids (linoleic acid [omega-6] and alpha-linolenic acid [omega-3])* occur in polyunsaturated vegetable oils and in fatty fish (e.g., salmon). *Trans fats* occur in hydrogenated oils, some margarines, packaged baked goods, and many processed foods	Lingual: Lipase Gastric: Lipase, tributyrinase, bile salts Pancreatic lipase (steapsin)	There is debate about the appropriate amount of fat in the diet. The American Heart Association recommends that people obtain <30% of their calories from fat; <7% of calories should come from saturated fats, and <1% from *trans* fat. Clients with increased risk for heart disease may need stricter control. The 2002/2005 DRIs specify that adults should get 20%–35% of their calories from fat; children, 25%–40%.

Sources: Adapted from U.S. Department of Agriculture, Food and Nutrition Center (2002–2005). *Dietary guidance. DRI Tables. Dietary Reference Intakes: Macronutrients.* National Academy of Sciences. Institute of Medicine. Food and Nutrition Board. Retrieved from http://fnic.nal.usda.gov/dietary-guidance/dietary-reference-intakes/dri-tables; and American Heart Association (n.d.a) Fats 101. AHA recommendation. Retrieved from http://www.heart.org/HEARTORG/GettingHealthy/FatsAndOils/Fats101/Fats-101_UCM_304494_Article.jsp

converted back into glucose to meet energy needs. This process is called **glycogenolysis**. If carbohydrates are not available, proteins and lipids (fats) can also be used for energy.

2. *Spare protein.* If glycogen stores are low (for instance, in a person who is undernourished), physical activity causes the breakdown of body stores of protein (**gluconeogenesis**) and lipids (fats) to use for energy. But when proteins are used for energy, they are not available for their primary functions of tissue growth, maintenance, and repair. Fats are converted directly into an alternative fuel called **ketones**; ketones raise the acidity of the blood and can lead to acid–base imbalance. Fats are used for fuel in persons with diabetes, whose cells cannot use glucose for energy.

3. *Other physiological functions.* Carbohydrates enhance insulin secretion, increase satiety (feeling of fullness and satisfaction), and improve absorption of sodium and excretion of calcium. **Insulin** is a pancreatic hormone that promotes the movement of glucose into the cells for use.

To see the basic chemical structure of four types of carbohydrates,

 Go to Chapter 27, **Tables, Boxes, Figures: ESG Figure 27-1, Carbohydrates,** on Davis*Plus*.

Proteins

Proteins are complex molecules made up of *amino acids*. Every amino acid consists of a central carbon atom connected to a hydrogen atom, an acid, an *amine* (a region of the molecule containing nitrogen), and a side chain. Only the side chain varies from one amino acid to another. Just 20 different amino acids are the building blocks of most of the proteins in the human body (Table 27-2). The **essential amino acids** are significant in our diets because the body cannot manufacture them. They must be supplied by food or nutritional supplements. In contrast, the body can synthesize the 10 **nonessential amino acids,** so we do not need to obtain them from food. To see the basic structural formula for an amino acid and a polypeptide,

 Go to Chapter 27, **Tables, Boxes, Figures: ESG Figure 27-2, Amino Acids,** on Davis*Plus*.

For protein synthesis to occur, every amino acid necessary to build that protein must be available. **Complete protein** foods contain all of the essential amino acids necessary for protein synthesis. These usually come from animal sources. **Incomplete protein** foods (e.g., nuts, grains) do not provide all of the essential amino acids. However, by combining two incomplete proteins, a complete protein can be made. For instance, lentils (legumes) and rice (grain) with yellow peppers makes a healthy meal using complementary proteins; or almonds (nuts) with black beans (legumes) in a salad is another good choice. Yogurt (dairy) combined with sunflower and flax seeds (seeds) creates complementary proteins for a healthful vegetarian diet.

Protein Metabolism and Storage

Refer to Table 27-1: How many servings of protein did you eat yesterday? How many were complete proteins? How many were incomplete proteins? Do you think that protein foods accounted for more than 10% of your food intake yesterday?

Although protein digestion begins in the stomach, it occurs mostly in the small intestine, where enzymes break it down into amino acids. The body continually breaks down and resynthesizes protein into tissues, adjusting as needed to maintain overall protein balance. The body also maintains a balance between tissue protein and plasma protein. When amino acids are catabolized, the nitrogen-containing part is converted to ammonia (NH_3) and excreted in the urine as urea. Therefore, nitrogen balance reflects how well body tissues are being maintained.

Table 27-2 ➤ Amino Acids		
TYPE	**DESCRIPTION**	**EXAMPLES**
Essential	Must be obtained from the diet; cannot be made in the body.	Arginine,* histidine, isoleucine, leucine, lysine, methionine, phenylalanine, threonine, tryptophan, and valine
Nonessential	Easily synthesized by the body.	Alanine, asparagine, aspartic acid, cysteine,† glutamic acid, glutamine, glycine, proline, serine, and tyrosine**

*Considered by some to be "semiessential" because it cannot be synthesized at a rate that will support growth. Therefore, it is essential for children, but not for most adults.
†Considered conditionally essential. That is, essential in some situations (e.g., in immaturity, during severe stress).
Sources: American Heart Association (AHA). (n.d.a, updated 2011, June 29). Fats and oils: AHA recommendation. Retrieved March 4, 2014, from http://www.heart.org/HEARTORG/GettingHealthy/FatsAndOils/Fats101/Fats-and-Oils-AHA-Recommendation_UCM_316375_Article.jsp; Guyton, A. C., & Hall, J. E. (2011). *Textbook of medical physiology* (12th ed.), Philadelphia: W. B. Saunders; Lutz, C., & Przytulski, K. (2010). *Nutrition and diet therapy,* (5th ed.). Philadelphia, F.A. Davis; U.S. Department of Agriculture, Food and Nutrition Center (2002/2005). *Dietary Guidance. DRI Tables. Dietary Reference Intakes: Macronutrients.* National Academy of Sciences. Institute of Medicine. Food and Nutrition Board. Retrieved March 6, 2014, from http://fnic.nal.usda.gov/dietary-guidance/dietary-reference-intakes/dri-tables

Nitrogen balance occurs when intake and output of nitrogen are equal. A **positive nitrogen balance** exists when nitrogen intake exceeds output, making a pool of amino acids available for growth, pregnancy, and tissue maintenance and repair. **Negative nitrogen balance** exists when nitrogen intake is lower than nitrogen loss. This occurs in illness, injury (e.g., burns), and malnutrition.

Functions of Protein

Dietary proteins perform the following functions:

1. *Tissue building.* Protein is the structural material of every cell in the body. In fact, except for water, protein makes up the biggest part of the body. It is essential for growth, maintenance, and repair of body cells and tissues.
2. *Metabolism.* Proteins are essential for building body tissue. For example, proteins are precursors to digestive enzymes and hormones (e.g., thyroxine). **Enzymes** facilitate cellular reactions throughout the body. In addition, proteins combine with iron to form hemoglobin, the oxygen carrier in red blood cells.
3. *Immune system function.* **Lymphocytes** (specialized white blood cells) and antibodies (components of our immune system that defend against foreign invaders) are proteins.
4. *Fluid balance.* Because they attract water, proteins in cells and the bloodstream help regulate fluid balance.
5. *Acid–base balance.* Blood proteins function as buffers, helping to regulate acid–base balance.
6. *Secondary energy source.* As noted earlier, proteins can be broken down to provide energy when stores of the other energy nutrients are inadequate (Thompson & Manore, 2012).

Protein needs vary according to age, sex, weight, and health. Lean meat is nourishing and healthy as long as it is consumed in modest amounts and is not processed. Most North Americans eat more protein than they need, especially in the form of meat. There is no health benefit from eating more than the recommended amount of protein. In fact, there may be health risks in eating a diet that is high in animal protein. Animal proteins are high in saturated fat, which increases the risk for certain cancers and coronary artery disease, and which has been associated with kidney stones and calcium loss through the urinary system.

Lipids

Lipids are organic (carbon-containing) substances that are insoluble in water. They are made up of carbon, hydrogen, and oxygen—the same basic elements that make up carbohydrates. The term *lipid* comes from *lipos,* the Greek word for "fat." Lipids that are solid at room temperature are called *fats,* whereas those that are liquid at room temperature are called *oils.* For example, butter is a fat even when it is melted, because it would

be solid at room temperature. You will hear the terms *lipids* and *fats* used interchangeably.

People in developed countries typically eat a diet relatively high in fat. In the United States about 45% of our total kcal consumption comes from fat. Fat is an essential nutrient, but certain types when consumed in excess can also be a health hazard.

Lipid metabolism occurs in the small intestine, where bile and pancreatic enzymes begin splitting the fatty acids from their glycerol backbone. Lipids are stored as adipose tissue. Because lipids are insoluble in water, and because blood is primarily water, lipid absorption requires a solvent carrier.

Types and Sources of Lipids

The three types of lipids found in foods are glycerides, sterols, and phospholipids (Box 27-2). **Glycerides** (also called **true fats**) consist of one molecule of glycerol attached to one, two, or three fatty acid chains. *Glycerol* is an alcohol composed of three carbon atoms. *Fatty acids* are long chains of carbon and hydrogen atoms ending in an acid. Most glycerides found in foods are *triglycerides,* which are compounds consisting of a glycerol molecule attached to three fatty acids.

 Go to Chapter 27, **Tables, Boxes, Figures: ESG Figure 27-3, Lipids,** on DavisPlus.

Sterols are lipids, but they are not made of fatty acids. They consist of rings of carbon and hydrogen. The most important sterol in the body is **cholesterol**, a wax-like substance needed for the formation of cell membranes, vitamin D, estrogen, and testosterone. Cholesterol is synthesized in the liver, and it is also found in animal foods.

Phospholipids (which contain a phosphate group) are soluble in water. They are a key component of **lipoproteins**, which consist of phospholipids and a protein. Because they are water soluble, lipoproteins are the major transport vehicles for lipids in the bloodstream. By "wrapping" triglycerides with water-soluble phosphates and proteins, lipoproteins deliver these substances to body cells.

■ **Low-density lipoproteins (LDLs)** transport cholesterol to body cells. Diets high in saturated fats increase

BOX 27-2 ■ Types of Lipids

Glycerides	Fatty Acid Molecules	(bonded to)	Glycerol Molecules
Monoglycerides	1		1
Diglycerides	1		2
Triglycerides	1		3
Sterols	0		0
Phospholipids	1		2 + a phosphate group

LDLs circulating in the bloodstream and may result in fatty deposits on vessel walls, causing cardiovascular disease. As a result, LDL is often known as the "bad cholesterol."

- **High-density lipoproteins (HDLs)** remove cholesterol from the bloodstream, returning it to the liver, where it is used to produce bile; thus, a high blood level of HDL is considered protective against cardiovascular disease. It is often known as the "good cholesterol."

Saturated and Unsaturated Fatty Acids

Fatty acids are classified as saturated, unsaturated, or *trans* fats (Table 27-3). **Saturation** means that a substance is holding all that it is capable of holding (e.g., think of a wound dressing saturated with blood).

- An **unsaturated fatty acid** is one that is not completely filled with all the hydrogen it can hold. Therefore, it is lighter and less dense. Fats made up primarily of unsaturated fatty acids are called **unsaturated fats**.

Molecules of **monounsaturated fats** have one unfilled spot where hydrogen is not attached. **Polyunsaturated fatty acids** contain two or more unfilled spots for hydrogen. At the spot(s) where the molecule does not have hydrogen attached, it becomes kinked and does not pack together. This is why these fats are liquid at room temperature. Replacing saturated fats in the diet with mono- and polyunsaturated fats reduces the risk of heart disease and stroke. Dietary fat should mainly be polyunsaturated and unsaturated, from food sources, such as fish and nuts.

- **Saturated fatty acids** are those in which every carbon atom is fully bound to (or "saturated" with) hydrogen. The molecules pack tightly together at room temperature and are dense, solid, and heavy. A fat made up mostly of saturated fatty acids is called a **saturated fat**. Animal fats are the primary source of saturated fats in the North American diet; however, many processed foods contain saturated fats.

Table 27-3 ➤ Dietary Fats

TYPE OF FAT	SOURCES	EFFECT ON BLOOD CHOLESTEROL
Monounsaturated	Olives; olive oil, canola oil, peanut oil; cashews, almonds, peanuts, some legumes, and most other nuts; avocados	Lowers LDL and raises HDL.
Polyunsaturated	Corn, soybean, safflower, sesame, sunflower, and cottonseed oils; fish, nuts, and seeds	Lowers LDL and raises HDL.
Saturated	Whole milk, butter, cheese, and ice cream; lard; red meat; chocolate; coconuts, coconut milk, and coconut oil; palm oils; cocoa butter	Raises LDL and HDL.
Trans fats	Most margarines; vegetable shortening; partially hydrogenated vegetable oil; deep-fried chips; many fast foods (e.g., French fries, donuts); most commercial baked goods	Raises LDL.
Dietary Cholesterol	Foods from animals: meats, egg yolks, dairy products, organ meats (e.g., heart, liver), fish, and poultry	Raises cholesterol.

American Heart Association Recommendations

Limit foods high in saturated fat, *trans* fat, and/or cholesterol. Instead choose foods low in saturated fat, *trans* fat and cholesterol. Here are some helpful tips (AHA, n.d.a):

- Limit intake of whole-milk dairy products, fatty meats, tropical oils, partially hydrogenated vegetable oils, and egg yolks.
- Include a variety of fruits and vegetables in the diet: at least 4.5 cups/day
- Eat a variety of grain products; include whole grains: at least three 1-oz servings/day.
- Eat fish, particularly fatty fish, at least twice a week, 3.5-oz servings.
- Limit sodium intake to less than 1,500 mg/day.
- Include fat-free and low-fat milk products and legumes.
- Choose skinless poultry and lean meats.
- Choose fats and oils with 2 grams or less saturated fat per tablespoon (e.g., liquid and tub margarines, canola oil). Reduce saturated fat intake to less than 7% of total calories.
- Limit sugar-sweetened beverages to no more than 450 calories (36 oz) a week.
- Eat nuts, legumes, and seeds, at least four servings a week.

■ *Trans*-fatty acids are saturated fats created when food manufacturers add hydrogen to polyunsaturated plant oils, such as corn oil, to break the double carbon bonds and straighten out the molecules. This process solidifies the fat and extends the shelf life of the food. *Trans* fats are found in many margarines and other processed foods containing *hydrogenated vegetable oils.*

Saturated fats and *trans* fats are the main dietary factors in increasing blood cholesterol levels. They raise LDL cholesterol levels. The FDA mandates that *trans* fat content be listed on all food labels. Intake of saturated fats and *trans* fats should be limited.

Refer to Table 26-3: How many servings of fat did you eat yesterday? How many were saturated fats; how many were unsaturated?

Essential and Nonessential Fatty Acids

A fatty acid is considered **essential** if (1) the body cannot manufacture it and (2) its absence creates a deficiency disease. The essential fatty acids, **linoleic acid (omega-6)** and **alpha-linolenic acid (omega-3)**, help protect against heart disease. Omega-6 fatty acid is found mainly in polyunsaturated vegetable oils, nuts, and seeds. Omega-3 fatty acid can be obtained in adequate amounts by eating fatty fish (e.g., tuna, shellfish) twice a week (American Heart Association [AHA], last updated 2014).

Functions of Lipids

Lipids perform the following functions:

1. *Supply essential nutrients.* Food fats supply the essential fatty acids and aid in the absorption of fat-soluble vitamins.
2. *Energy source.* Although carbohydrates are the primary energy source during strenuous physical activity, our bodies burn fat for energy when we are engaging in sustained light activity, such as walking or mowing the lawn, and when we are at rest. The body also burns fat for energy when glycogen stores are exhausted.
3. *Flavor and satiety.* Lipids give food its creamy taste and texture and promote our sense of satiety (being "full"). Fats are digested more slowly than carbohydrates, so stomach emptying time is slower.
4. *Other functions of lipids.* Body fat provides insulation, protects vital organs, aids in thermoregulation, and enables accurate nerve-impulse transmission. In addition, lipids are a component of every cell membrane and are essential to cell metabolism.
5. *Cholesterol functions.* Cholesterol is a component of every cell in the body, where it lends suppleness and support. It is also an ingredient of bile, which helps digest fats, and serves as a precursor to all steroid hormones, including sex hormones. When lipid metabolism is "disordered," cholesterol contributes to atherosclerosis.

▲ ThinkLike a Nurse 27-2

Review the information you collected on the two employees (Meet Your Patients).

■ What conclusions, if any, can you make about their intake of carbohydrates, protein, and fats?

■ How might you gather additional data on their intake of the energy nutrients?

WHAT ARE THE MICRONUTRIENTS?

Vitamins and minerals are called **micronutrients** because they are required by the body in only very small amounts. Although they provide no energy, they are critical in regulating a variety of body functions.

Vitamins

Vitamins are organic substances that are necessary for metabolism or preventing a particular deficiency disease. Because the body cannot make vitamins, they must be supplied by the foods we eat. Vitamins are critical in building and maintaining body tissues, supporting our immune system so we can fight disease, and ensuring healthy vision. They also help our bodies to break down and use the energy found in carbohydrates, proteins, and lipids. Vitamins are especially critical during periods of rapid growth, pregnancy, lactation, and healing. Some evidence supports the claim that certain vitamins prevent chronic illness.

Table 27-4 summarizes information about vitamins, including specific functions and Dietary Reference Intakes (DRIs). Recommended Daily Allowances (RDAs) represent the daily dietary intake that is adequate to meet the needs of about 98% of all healthy individuals in a group, such as men, women, or infants. The American Academy of Pediatrics recommends that infants, children, and adolescents have a minimum daily intake of 400 international units (IU),* or 10 micrograms, of vitamin D (Wagner, Greer, & the Section on Breastfeeding and Committee on Nutrition, 2008). All breastfed, breast and bottlefed, and formula-fed infants who consume less than a liter of formula per day should receive oral vitamin D supplementation (American Academy of Pediatrics, 2008).

Fat-Soluble Vitamins The fat-soluble vitamins are A, D, E, and K. They are stored primarily in the liver and adipose tissues, although vitamin E is deposited in all body tissue. Because the body can store these vitamins, we do not need to consume them every day if we are consuming them in adequate amounts; however, diets extremely low in fat and disorders affecting fat digestion and absorption can lead to deficiency of fat-soluble vitamins. Because they are not readily excreted, excessive supplementation with the fat-soluble vitamins can lead to toxicity.

The USDA (2011g) now recommends 600 IU of vitamin D every day for most healthy adults age 70 and younger, and 800 IU for healthy people age 71 and older (Ross, Taylor, Yaktine, et al., 2011). This is sufficient for

---

*Although The Joint Commission includes the abbreviation *IU* on its "do not use" list, the abbreviation is used in other settings (e.g., on vitamin labels).

Table 27-4 ➤ Vitamins: Adult Dietary Reference Intakes (DRIs)*

VITAMIN	FUNCTION	RDA†	SOURCES	EFFECTS OF DEFICIENCY	SYMPTOMS OF EXCESS
Fat-Soluble Vitamins					
A	Night and color vision Cellular growth and maturity Maintaining healthy skin and mucous membranes Growth of skeletal and soft tissues Reproduction	Women: 700 mcg/day Men: 900 mcg/day	Fish liver oil, liver, butter, cream, egg yolk, yellow fruit, green leafy vegetables, fortified milk	Night blindness, xerosis, xerophthalmia, keratomalacia, skin lesions	GI upset, headache, blurred vision, poor muscle coordination, fetal defects
D‡	Regulates blood calcium levels. Regulates rate of deposit and resorption of calcium in bone.	15 mcg/day to age 70; then 20 mcg/day (AI), after age 71	Fish liver oil, fish, fortified milk, sunlight exposure	Bone and muscle pain, weakness, softening of bone, fractures, rickets	Fatigue, weakness, loss of appetite, headache, mental confusion, mental retardation in infants
E	Antioxidant Protects red blood cells and muscle tissue cells	15 mg/day, age 14+	Vegetable oils, nuts, milk, eggs, muscle meats, fish, wheat and rice germ, green leafy vegetables	Hyporeflexia, ataxia, hemolytic anemia, myopathy	Insufficient blood clotting, impaired immune system
K	Synthesis of clotting factors Bone development	Women age 19+: 90 mcg/day (AI) Men age 19+: 120 mcg/day (AI)	Green leafy vegetables, liver (Intestinal bacteria synthesize a form of vitamin K, so deficiency is unlikely.)	Increased bleeding	Jaundice and hemolytic anemia in infants
Water-Soluble Vitamins					
Thiamin	Cellular metabolism (producing energy from glucose and storing energy as fat) Nervous system function GI system function Cardiovascular system function	Women: 1.1 mg/day Men: 1.2 mg/day	Whole grains, enriched cereal, beef, pork, liver, peas, beans, nuts	Peripheral neuritis, loss of muscle strength, depression, memory loss, anorexia, constipation, dyspnea, decreased alertness and reflexes, fatigue, irritability, beriberi	Unlikely; readily excreted
Riboflavin	Cellular metabolism Antioxidant Tissue health and growth	Women: 1.1 mg/day Men: 1.3 mg/day	Milk, cheese, eggs, green vegetables, whole grains, enriched grains, bread, organ meats, poultry, fish	Tissue inflammation and breakdown: Sore throat, stomatitis, swollen tongue, facial dermatitis, anemia; poor wound healing	Unlikely; readily excreted

Table 27-4 ➤ Vitamins: Adult Dietary Reference Intakes (DRIs)*—cont'd

VITAMIN	FUNCTION	RDA†	SOURCES	EFFECTS OF DEFICIENCY	SYMPTOMS OF EXCESS
Niacin	Cellular metabolism to produce energy	Women: 14 mg/day Men: 16 mg/day	Enriched breads and cereals, chicken, tuna, liver, peanuts, dairy products	Weakness, poor appetite, indigestion, dermatitis, diarrhea, headache, dizziness, insomnia. Chronic: Central nervous system (CNS) damage (confusion, neuritis, dementia), pellagra	Facial flushing, itching, nausea, liver damage
B₆ (Pyridoxine)	Protein (and some carbohydrate) metabolism RBC production Neurotransmitter synthesis	Men and women through age 50: 1.3 mg/day Women 50+: 1.5 mg/day Men 50+: 1.7 mg/day	Meats, poultry, fish, beans, nuts, seeds, dairy products, enriched cereals	Rash, stomatitis, seizure, peripheral neuritis, depression	Irreversible nerve damage (i.e., extremity numbness, walking difficulties)
Pantothenic acid	Cell metabolism of fat and cholesterol Amino acid activation Heme formation	All adults: 5 mg/day (AI)	Occurs widely in most foods. Best sources: Meats, whole grain cereals, legumes	Deficiency is unknown.	Unlikely; readily excreted
Folacin (folate, folic acid)	Cellular metabolism Neurotransmitter synthesis Cell division DNA synthesis Hemoglobin formation	400 mcg/day (folic acid); 600 mcg/day when pregnant Women capable of becoming pregnant should take a daily supplement of 400–800 mcg	Green leafy vegetables, asparagus, liver, yeast, eggs, beans, fruits, enriched cereals	Megaloblastic anemia, neural tube defects	Increased seizure activity, hives, respiratory distress, itching, rash
B₁₂ (Cyanoco-balamin)	Metabolic reactions Maintain myelin sheath Hemoglobin synthesis	2.4 mcg/day	Dairy products, meat, poultry, fish, liver, milk, cheese, eggs	Classic triad of glossitis (inflamed tongue), weakness, and ascending paresthesia; pernicious anemia, irreversible nerve damage, memory loss, dementia	Unlikely; readily excreted

Continued

Table 27-4 ➤ Vitamins: Adult Dietary Reference Intakes (DRIs)*—cont'd

VITAMIN	FUNCTION	RDA†	SOURCES	EFFECTS OF DEFICIENCY	SYMPTOMS OF EXCESS
C	Collagen synthesis "Cementing" substance for capillary walls Antioxidant Iron absorption Immune function	Women: 75 mg/day Men (age 19+): 90 mg/day Additional 35 mg/day for those who smoke	Citrus fruits, tomatoes, potatoes, green vegetables, cauliflower	Anemia, tissue bleeding, easy bone fracture, gingivitis, petechiae, poor wound healing, joint pain, scurvy	Stomach inflammation, diarrhea, oxalate kidney stones

Note: 1 mcg = 40 International Units.

*Values in the table are RDAs unless marked (AI). Dietary Reference Intakes (DRIs) represent:

- Recommended Dietary Allowances (RDAs)—Intake set to meet the needs of 97%–98% of healthy individuals in a group.
- Adequate Intakes (AIs)—Believed to cover the needs of all individuals in the group.
- Upper Intake Levels (UIs)—The maximum daily intake likely to pose no risk of adverse effects.

†RDAs are usually less than adult values for infants and children, more for pregnant women, and highest for lactating women. RDAs for some vitamins (e.g., vitamin A) are higher for older adults and higher for men than for women.

‡The American Academy of Pediatrics recommends 10 mcg/day of vitamin D for infancy through adolescence (Wagner, Greer, & the Section on Breastfeeding and Committee on Nutrition, 2008). Other clinicians and researchers have suggested that the RDA for adults should be dramatically increased as well, to 20–25 mcg (800–1000 IU) for adults aged 50 and older (Jockers, 2007).

 Go to Chapter 27, **Supplemental Materials, Dietary Reference Intakes: Vitamins,** on Davis*Plus*.

Sources: Adapted from U.S. Department of Agriculture. (2011f) Dietary Reference Intakes (DRIs): Tolerable upper intake levels, vitamins. Food and Nutrition Board, Institute of Medicine, National Academies. Retrieved March 9, 2014, from http://iom.edu/Activities/Nutrition/SummaryDRIs/~/media/Files/Activity%20Files/Nutrition/DRIs/ULs%20for%20Vitamins%20and%20Elements.pdf; Complete reports are available at http://fnic.nal.usda.gov/dietary-guidance/dietary-reference-intakes/dri-tables; Lutz, C., & Przytulski, K. (2011). *Nutrition and diet therapy: Evidence-based applications* (5th ed.). Philadelphia: F.A. Davis.

most healthy adults; however, some adults may need more. These include those with very little sun exposure (or who consistently wear sun screen or protective clothing), dark skin, osteoporosis, impaired ability to absorb dietary fat, or who are taking medicines that interfere with vitamin D.

New research has revealed that women with very low levels of vitamin D are more likely to have cognitive impairment and higher risk of mental decline (Annweiler, Rolland, Schott, et al., 2012; Slinin, Paudel, Taylor, et al., 2012). Vitamin D is unique in that the body can synthesize it from a cholesterol compound in the skin when we receive adequate exposure to sunlight. However, adequate exposure is difficult in winter months for anyone living at a latitude of 40° or more north or south of the equator (e.g., in Canada and the northern United States). Newest recommendations are that adults age 50 years and older should receive 20 to 25 mcg (800 to 1,000 IU) of vitamin D per day.

Water-Soluble Vitamins The water-soluble vitamins include vitamin C and the B-complex vitamins: thiamine, riboflavin, niacin, pyridoxine (vitamin B_6), folic acid, pantothenic acid, biotin, and cyanocobalamin (vitamin B_{12}). Because these vitamins are soluble in water, excess amounts are regularly excreted by the kidneys in the urine. Thus, toxicity is rare except in people with renal disease. However, because excess amounts

are excreted, the body cannot store these vitamins; so they need to be consumed every day.

Minerals

Minerals are inorganic elements found in nature. They occur in foods either naturally or as additives, as well as in supplements. **Major minerals (macrominerals)** are minerals that the body needs in amounts of 100 mg/day or greater. **Trace minerals** are essential, but in a lower concentration. In the United States, calcium deficiency is one of the most common mineral deficiencies (Table 27-5).

Minerals assist in fluid regulation, nerve impulse transmission, and energy production; they are essential to the health of bones and blood and help rid the body of by-products of metabolism. Evidence also shows that minerals play key roles in disease prevention and treatment. For example:

1. Adequate *calcium* intake throughout the life span decreases the likelihood of osteoporosis (a condition marked by porous bones). The recommended daily intake of 1,200 mg for adults aged 50 years and older is difficult to achieve by diet alone (Food and Nutrition Board, Institute of Medicine, National Academies, 1997–2011; Lim, Hoeksema, Sherin, et al., 2009; National Guideline Clearinghouse [NGC], 2009; Ross, Taylor, Yaktine, et al., 2011).

Table 27-5 ➤ Minerals: Adult Dietary Reference Intakes*

MINERAL	FUNCTION	RDA†	SOURCES	EFFECTS OF DEFICIENCY	SYMPTOMS OF EXCESS
Macrominerals					
Calcium (Ca)	Bone and teeth formation, blood clotting, nerve conduction, muscle contraction, cellular metabolism, heart action	1,000 mg/day (AI), ages 19–50 1,200 mg/day (AI) ages 51+ 1,300 mg/day (AI), ages 9–18	Dairy products, sardines, green leafy vegetables, broccoli, whole grains, egg yolks, legumes, nuts, fortified products	Bone loss, tetany, rickets, osteoporosis	Kidney stones, constipation, intestinal gas
Magnesium (Mg)	Aids thyroid hormone secretion, maintains normal basal metabolic rate, activates enzymes for carbohydrate and protein metabolism, nerve and muscle function, cardiac function	*Men:* 400 mg/day (AI), ages 19–30; 420 mg/day, age 31+ *Women:* 310 mg/day (AI), age 19+	Whole grains, nuts, legumes, green leafy vegetables, lima beans, broccoli, squash, potatoes	Tremor, spasm, convulsions, weakness, muscle pain, poor cardiac function	Weakness, nausea, malaise
Phosphorus (P)	Bone and tooth strength, overall metabolism, formation of enzymes, acid–base balance	700 mg/day (AI), age 19+	Dairy products, beef, pork, beans, sardines, eggs, chicken, wheat bran, chocolate	Bone loss, poor growth	Tetany, convulsions
Potassium (K)	Intracellular fluid control, acid–base balance, nerve transmission, muscle contraction, glycogen formation, protein synthesis, energy metabolism, blood pressure regulation	4.7 g/day (AI)	Unprocessed foods, especially fruits, any vegetables, meats, potatoes, avocados, legumes, milk, molasses, shellfish, dates, figs	Muscle weakness (including weakness of heart and respiratory muscles), weak pulse, fatigue, abdominal distention. (Rarely occurs as a result of inadequate dietary intake. More likely due to losses from prolonged vomiting, diarrhea, or some diuretic drugs.)	Cardiac dysrhythmias, cardiac arrest, weakness, abdominal cramps, diarrhea, anxiety, paresthesia
Sodium (Na)	Water balance, acid–base balance, muscle action, nerve transmission, convulsions	1.5 g/day (AI), ages 19–50; 1.3 g/day, age 51–70; 1.2 g/day, age 70+	Table salt (NaCl), milk, meat, eggs, baking soda, baking powder, celery, spinach, carrots, beets	Dizziness, abdominal cramping, nausea, vomiting, diarrhea, tachycardia, convulsions, coma. (Rarely occurs except in heavy exercise and sweating.)	Thirst, fever, dry and sticky tongue and mucous membranes, restlessness, irritability, convulsion

Continued

Table 27-5 ➤ Minerals: Adult Dietary Reference Intakes*—cont'd

MINERAL	FUNCTION	RDA†	SOURCES	EFFECTS OF DEFICIENCY	SYMPTOMS OF EXCESS
Trace Minerals					
Copper	Aids in iron metabolism, works with many enzymes in protein metabolism and hormone synthesis	900 mcg/day (AI)	Liver, seafood, cocoa, legumes, nuts, whole grains	Rarely occurs: anemia, low WBC count, poor growth	Vomiting, nervous system disorders
Fluoride	Increases resistance to dental caries	*Women:* 3 mg/day (AI) *Men:* 4 mg/day (AI)	Fluorinated water, toothpaste, dental treatment, seaweed, fish, tea	Increased dental caries	Stomach upset, staining of teeth, bone pain
Iodine	Synthesis of the thyroid hormone, thyroxine	150 mcg/day	Iodized salt, salt water fish, dairy products, enriched white bread	Goiter, poor infancy growth, cretinism, hypothyroidism	Skin lesions, thyroid malfunction
Iron	Synthesis of hemoglobin, general metabolism (e.g., of glucose), antibody production, drug detoxification in the liver	*Women:* 18 mg/day, ages 19–50; 8 mg/day, age 50+ *Men age 19+:* 8 mg/day	Meats, eggs, spinach, seafood, broccoli, peas, bran, enriched breads, fortified cereals	Small, pale RBCs, anemia	Hemochromatosis
Zinc	Cofactor for many enzymes involved in growth, insulin storage immunity, alcohol metabolism, sexual development and reproduction	*Men:* 8 mg/day *Women:* 11 mg/day	Primarily meats and seafood; also legumes, peas, and whole grains	Skin rash, diarrhea, decreased appetite, hair loss, poor growth and development, poor wound healing	Reduced copper absorption, diarrhea, cramps, depressed immune function

*Dietary Reference Intakes (DRIs) represent:
- Recommended Dietary Allowances (RDAs)—Intake set to meet the needs of 97%–98% of individuals in a group.
- Adequate Intakes (AIs)—Believed to cover the needs of all individuals in the group.
- Upper Intake Levels (UIs)—The maximum daily intake likely to pose no risk of adverse effects.

Values in table are RDAs unless marked (AI).

†RDAs are usually less than adult values for infants and children, more for pregnant women, and highest for lactating women. RDAs for some minerals are higher for older adults and different for men and women.

 Go to Chapter 27, **Supplemental Materials, Dietary Reference Intakes: Elements; Electrolytes; and Elements,** on *DavisPlus*.

Sources: Adapted from National Institutes of Health, Office of Dietary Supplements, National Institutes of Health. (Last modified 2010). *Dietary Reference Intakes: Vitamins.* Retrieved March 9, 2014, from http://books.nap.edu/openbook.php?record_id=5776. Complete reports are available at http://fnic.nal.usda.gov/dietary-guidance/dietary-reference-intakes/dri-tables. Institute of Medicine of the National Academies, Food and Nutrition Board, Standing Committee on the Scientific Evaluation of Dietary Reference Intakes. (2010). DRIs for calcium, phosphorous, magnesium, vitamin D, and fluoride. Retrieved on March 9, 2014, from http://iom.edu/Activities/Nutrition/SummaryDRIs/~/media/Files/Activity%20Files/Nutrition/DRIs/ULs%20for%20Vitamins%20and%20Elements.pdf

2. *Iron* deficiency causes anemia, the most common nutritional problem worldwide.
3. *Magnesium* may decrease the risk of hypertension and coronary artery disease in women.
4. *Sodium,* consumed in high amounts (>2,500 mg/day), increases the risk for high blood pressure, heart attacks, and stroke.

Minerals are absorbed mostly in the small intestine. Salt and potassium are absorbed in the large intestine, however. If the body is deficient in a mineral, it absorbs more; if the body has enough, it absorbs less and excretes more in the feces. Minerals interact with other minerals, vitamins, and other substances to accomplish absorption and metabolism and perform their functions.

For example, iron absorption is enhanced in the presence of vitamin C, and vitamin D deficiency inhibits calcium absorption.

WHY IS WATER AN ESSENTIAL NUTRIENT?

Water is made up of hydrogen and oxygen. Water makes up about half of total body weight (55% to 65% in men and 50% to 55% in women). Men have greater muscle mass; muscle contains a relatively large amount of water. Water is distributed in two body compartments. **Intracellular fluid** is the water contained within each living cell. It makes up about 40% of the total body weight. **Extracellular fluid** is external to the cell membrane (e.g., in the fluid portion of blood and lymph and in the gastrointestinal [GI] tract); it accounts for 20% of body weight. Water is critical to the body because its functions are essential to life:

1. *Solvent.* Water is the basic solvent for the body's chemical processes.
2. *Transport.* Circulating as a component of blood, water serves as a medium for transporting oxygen, nutrients, and metabolic wastes.
3. *Body structure and form.* Water "fills in the spaces" in body tissues (e.g., in muscle).
4. *Temperature.* Water helps maintain body temperature. When body temperature rises, evaporation of sweat helps cool the body.

The amount of water a person requires varies according to the environmental humidity and temperature, activity level, age, and metabolic needs. The average AI for adult women is about 2.7 liters of water per day and 3.7 liters for men. Eighty percent of those amounts should come from fluids. We also obtain water in the foods we eat (Lutz & Przytulski, 2011). What foods can you think of that are high in water content?

Overall fluid balance is maintained when fluid intake in liquids, foods, and metabolic reactions matches fluid output through urine, feces, respiration, and sweat. Fluid and electrolyte balance is discussed in Chapter 38.

KnowledgeCheck 27-2

- What is the body's most usable energy source?
- Which nutrient's primary function is growth and repair of tissue?
- Identify five functions of adipose tissue (body fat).
- Which type of vitamin requires daily consumption to maintain appropriate levels?
- What distinguishes a major mineral from a trace mineral?
- Identify at least four functions of water.

WHAT MUST I KNOW ABOUT ENERGY BALANCE?

The energy in carbohydrates, proteins, and lipids is measured in terms of **calories**, or, more precisely, **kilocalories (kcal)**. A kcal is the amount of heat required to raise the temperature of 1 kg of water 1° centigrade. To maintain a stable weight, the number of kcal we consume must equal the number of kcal we burn. Any deviation results in weight loss or weight gain. Below is the amount of energy liberated from the metabolism of 1 gram of energy nutrients:

- Carbohydrates = 4 kcal/g
- Protein = 4 kcal/g
- Fat = 9 kcal/g

PICOT

Situation: The nurse is reviewing a client's intake and output (I&O) with him. The I&O are out of balance. The nurse begins to question the client further about other potential consequences of dehydration.

Searchable Question: Do _____ (P) who are _____ (I) demonstrate _____ (O) as compared to _____ (C) during _____ (T)

PICOT Components

P	Population/patient	= Elderly inpatients
I	Intervention/indicator	= Dehydration
C	Comparator/control	= Elderly community dwellers
O	Outcome	= Complications of dehydration
T	Time	= During hospitalization

Searching for the Evidence: Overall fluid balance is affected by diet, exercise, temperature, illness, and medication. Older people are also more susceptible to dehydration because of cognitive, sensory, motor impairments, which affect their activities of daily living (ADLs). They tend to take more medications and have more illness that can increase the risk for fluid imbalance. For example, the frail older person with exercise intolerance related to chronic pain may not be able to stay hydrated. If that person becomes ill, it is even more likely that the client will be unable to independently take in sufficient amounts of fluid. It is important to encourage all elderly people, inpatient and in the community, to consume small amounts of fluids throughout the day in order to maintain adequate fluid balance. Assessment questions that might point to a fluid imbalance would include those regarding intake, activity, and elimination patterns.

Source: Schold, J. M., De Groot, C., van de Cammen, T., et al. (2009). Preventing and treating dehydration in the elderly during periods of illness and warm weather. *Journal of Nutritional Health Aging, 13*(2), 150–157.

KnowledgeCheck 27-3

Imagine that you have just eaten a food consisting of 4 grams of protein, 18 grams of carbohydrate, and 1 gram of fat.

- What would your total kcal intake be?
- What percentage of your kcal is from carbohydrates? Protein? Fat?

A diet of too few kcal is likely also to lack essential nutrients. People who are undernourished may experience weakened immunity, stunted growth, and hormonal disruption. Too many kcal can cause obesity, which increases the risk for chronic diseases, such as diabetes, arteriosclerosis, hypertension, hyperlipidemia, and cancers. In determining total energy (kilocalorie) needs, consider two factors: the client's basal metabolic rate and the duration and intensity of daily physical activity.

What Is Basal Metabolic Rate?

The **basal metabolic rate (BMR)** is a measure of the energy used while at rest in a neutral temperature environment—the energy required for vital organs such as the heart, liver, and brain to function. *Direct measurement* of BMR requires use of a calorimeter: an insulated unit that measures temperature changes of water that are produced by exposure to a fasting individual at rest. Although it is very accurate, it is rarely used because most institutions do not have calorimeters and because the test requires a controlled environment and a 12-hour fast. Direct measurement of BMR is used primarily by researchers. *Indirect calculation* of BMR, sometimes called the resting energy expenditure (REE), includes the following:

- Measuring oxygen uptake per unit of time. This can be done in an exercise lab or with portable machines at the bedside. This is most often done for patients in intensive care units. Not all facilities have this capability.
- Serum thyroxine levels (a blood test).
- A formula for calculating BMR when precise measurement is not required (Box 27-3).

BOX 27-3 ■ Calculating Basal Metabolic Rate (BMR)

Women:	0.9 kcal/kg of body weight per hour
Men:	1.0 kcal/kg body weight per hour
Example:	Isaac Schwartz (Meet Your Patients) weighs 245 lb.

1 kilogram = 2.2 pounds.

Divide 245 by 2.2 to convert pounds to kilograms:

245 ÷ 2.2 = 111.3

Now complete the calculation:

1.0 × 111.3 × 24 hours = 2671.2

What Factors Affect Basal Metabolic Rate?

When interpreting test results, consider the following factors that influence BMR:

- *Body composition.* Lean body tissue has greater metabolic activity than do fat and bones. This explains why women, who have on average more adipose tissue than men, also have lower BMRs.
- *Growth periods.* BMR increases during periods of growth, such as the first 5 years of life, adolescence, pregnancy, and lactation.
- *Body temperature.* The BMR increases 7% for each 1°F (0.83°C) rise in body temperature.
- *Environmental temperature.* Cold weather, especially temperatures below freezing, causes a slight rise in the BMR to generate body heat and maintain normal body temperature.
- *Disease processes.* Diseases involving increased cellular activity, such as cancer, anemia, cardiac failure, hypertension, and asthma, result in BMR elevation. For the same reason, systemic injury (e.g., severe burns, traumatic injury) increases BMR.
- *Prolonged physical exertion.* Metabolic demands are also elevated during prolonged physical exertion (e.g., chopping wood, running).

How Do I Calculate a Client's Total Energy Needs?

The amount of energy required varies according to the intensity of the activity (Table 27-6). A person's total daily energy requirement is the number of kcal necessary to replace those used for basic metabolism plus those used in physical activities. The following are simple estimates based on activity level and age:

- Sedentary women and older adults need 1,600 kcal/day.
- Children, teenage girls, active women, and most men need 2,200 kcal/day.
- Teenage boys, active men, and very active women need 2,800 kcal/day.

However, these estimates have limited usefulness. For instance, is a woman who works a desk job but walks for 30 minutes a day sedentary, active, or somewhere in between? To calculate energy use more precisely, you need to know the person's age, weight, and physical activity, including the intensity and duration of the activity. See Table 27-7.

Heightened emotional states may also increase energy needs, not because they directly increase metabolic activity, but because they increase muscular activity in the form of muscle tension, restlessness, and agitated movements.

KnowledgeCheck 27-4

You have already calculated the expected BMR for Mr. Schwartz (Meet Your Patients) for a 24-hour period.

- If Mr. Schwartz describes himself as working at a desk 8 to 10 hours per day, lawn mowing manually every other week

Table 27-6 ➤ Levels of Physical Activity: Energy Expended and Examples*

INTENSITY LEVEL	LIGHT	LIGHT TO MODERATE	MODERATE	HIGH
Energy Expended	120–150 kcal/hr	150–300 kcal/hr	300–420 kcal/hr	420–700+ kcal/hr
Examples of Activities	Dressing Showering Shaving Rocking Writing Typing Standing	Housework (e.g., sweeping) Light gardening Mowing lawn (motorized) Painting Walking 2–3 mph Bicycling 5½ mph Canoeing 2–3 mph	Digging Mowing lawn (manually) Walking 3½–4 mph Ballet Ballroom dancing Golf (no cart) Tennis (doubles)	Shoveling snow Walking 5 mph Climbing Bicycling 15–25 mph Cross-country skiing Jogging 5 mph or 1 mile in 10 min Swimming Aerobic dancing

*Precise energy use varies with body weight. For example, an individual weighing 200 lb burns about 740 calories per hour during aerobic dance, whereas an individual weighing 125 lb burns about 470 during the same activity.

Table 27-7 ➤ Energy Needs Based on Weight and Activity

For *each pound of body weight*, a person needs the following per day:

ACTIVITY LEVEL	UNDERWEIGHT	NORMAL WEIGHT	OVERWEIGHT
Sedentary	13 kcal	13 kcal	9–11 kcal
Moderately active	18 kcal	16 kcal	13 kcal
Active	18–23 kcal	18 kcal	16 kcal

during the summer, and playing an occasional game of golf, how would you classify his general activity level?

- After interviewing Mr. Schwartz, you estimate his average caloric intake to be approximately 3,000 kcal per day. Determine whether his kcal intake is sufficient or insufficient to maintain his present activity level.

What Are Some Body Weight Standards?

Weight standards have been established to correlate weight with good health and longevity and to help determine a client's ideal body weight. The **general ideal weight guide** uses a formula to determine a reasonable weight based on height:

Men: 106 lb (47.7 kg) for the first 5 ft (150 cm), then add 6 lb/in. (2.7 kg/2.5 cm)
Women: 100 lb (45 kg) for the first 5 ft (150 cm), then add 5 lb/in. (2.25 kg/2.5 cm)
Add 10% for large body frame; subtract 10% for small body frame.

Various **height–weight tables** have been developed over the years (beginning as long ago as 1943).

Height–weight tables are based on statistical estimates and often include variations for age, sex, and body frame. Use standards and standardized tables with caution because they are based on limited samples and may create unrealistic expectations, especially at the low weight ranges. Consider the following example: You have two male clients; each weighs 200 lb. Mason is 72 in. tall, works out vigorously 5 days per week, and has 18% body fat. Travis is 72 in. tall, rarely exercises, and has 35% body fat. Which of these clients requires more kcal to maintain his present weight? Which of these clients is at lower risk for cardiovascular disease?

If you answered Mason, you are correct. Although both men have the same height and weight, Mason has more lean body mass. He will burn energy more rapidly and be able to eat more without gaining weight. Height–weight tables cannot replace a thorough assessment and analysis of body composition when attempting to determine a client's overall fitness.

To see the World Health Organization (WHO) (2006b) child growth standards (e.g., length and height-for-age, weight-for-age),

Go to http://www.who.int/childgrowth/standards/en/

Body composition analysis attempts to quantify lean body mass versus percentage body fat. Lean body mass includes muscle, bone, and connective tissue. Lean tissue weighs more than fat; thus, a person who engages in regular weight-bearing exercise and is physically fit may actually weigh more than an individual of similar appearance who is sedentary and unfit. Various methods to assess body composition, known as *anthropometric measurements,* are provided in the Assessment section later in the chapter.

ThinkLike a Nurse 27-3

Examine your dietary intake for the next 3 days to determine how balanced your diet is. Use the form on DavisPlus and record all intake.

- How does your diet compare to the USDA MyPlate or Canada's Food Guide in terms of:
  a. Servings of bread, cereal, rice, and pasta?
  b. Servings of vegetables?
  c. Servings of fruits?
  d. Servings of milk, yogurt, and cheese?
  e. Servings of meat, poultry, fish, dry beans, eggs, and nuts?
  f. Servings of fats, oils, and sweets?
- From what you have learned from this activity, what habits could you change in patterns of eating in order to achieve optimal nutrition?

WHAT FACTORS AFFECT NUTRITION?

Several factors influence nutritional needs and choices. Some can be modified; some cannot. The most influential factors are development, knowledge, lifestyle, culture, disease processes, and functional limitations. Parents and caregivers are the most important influences on the eating habits of children. For tips about how to be a role model for children and set good examples for healthy eating for life,

 Go to the **USDA** Web site at http://www.choosemyplate .gov/food-groups/downloads/TenTips/DGTipsheet12 BeAHealthyRoleModel.pdf

For more tips on how to encourage healthy eating in children,

 Go to Chapter 27, **Tables, Boxes, Figures: ESG Box 27-1, Healthy Eating for Children,** on Davis*Plus.*

Developmental Stage

At specific developmental stages, nutritional needs and eating patterns vary according to physiological growth, activity level, metabolic processes, disease prevention, and other factors.

Infants to One Year

Humans grow most rapidly during the first year of life. Birth weight doubles by 5 months of age and triples during the first year, with length increasing by 50%. A baby 20 inches long at birth grows to about 30 inches by age 1 year. Nutritional needs per unit of body weight are greater during this period than at any other time.

Calories and Protein The infant needs adequate protein for tissue building and enough carbohydrates to furnish energy and "spare" the protein. The period from conception into the second year of life is most critical to brain development. For maximum brain growth, the baby needs optimal nutrition. Severe protein-calorie deficiency in the last trimester of pregnancy or the first 6 months of life may decrease the number of brain cells by 20%.

Vitamins and Minerals Fetal iron stores are depleted at 4 to 6 months, so intake of iron becomes important. The infant needs calcium for bone growth and development of teeth, calcium and vitamin C for iron absorption, and vitamin D for calcium regulation.

Fluids Compared to adults, infants have a higher metabolic rate. They also have greater water loss through the skin, which makes up a greater proportion of the body. These factors, along with immature kidneys, mean that infants need proportionately more fluid than adults. To meet nutritional and fluid needs, the infant requires 1.5 to 2 ounces of breast milk or formula per pound of body weight per day.

Infant Feedings The only safe choices for meeting fluid and nutrient needs in the first months of life are breast milk and commercially prepared formulas. Breast milk is the ideal food for infants because it is matched to their nutritional requirements. It contains enzymes to digest fats, protein, and carbohydrates. In addition, it enhances maturation of the infant's immune system and provides passive immunity against a number of infections, including pneumonia, acute otitis media, and gastroenteritis. The American Academy of Pediatrics (AAP) supports the benefit of breastfeeding because of numerous other health benefits to infants, such as lower risk of sudden infant death syndrome (SIDS). Infants receiving breast milk in the first six months of life may also have less risk of developing diabetes mellitus later in life, obesity, asthma, and childhood leukemia (AAP, 2008; Ip, Chung, Raman, et al., 2007; Owen, Martin, Whincup, et al., 2007; Rosenbauer, Herzig, Kaiser, et al., 2007; Yamakawa, Yorifuji, Inoue, et al., 2013).

When breastfeeding is contraindicated or the mother chooses not to breastfeed, numerous commercial formulas are available. The most commonly used formula is modified cow's milk available in powder, liquid concentrate, or ready-to-use liquid. Other types include iron-fortified, soy, and hypoallergenic formulas.

➕ Infants younger than 1 year should not receive cow's milk because it may cause gastrointestinal bleeding and may place too much strain on the infant's kidneys. It also can contribute to iron-deficiency anemia.

➕ Honey and corn syrup should not be used as a source of carbohydrates in preparing infant formula. They are potential sources of botulism toxin, which can be fatal in children younger than 1 year old (Schlenker & Roth, 2010).

Boiling water prior to constituting infant formula depends on the water quality of the tap supply. When in doubt, consult the local health department. If unsure, the FAD recommends boiling rapidly for a minimum of 1 full minute and cooling completely before adding it to infant formula.*

At 4 to 6 months, infants may be started on solid foods, beginning with iron-fortified infant rice cereal. They progress to eating table food by 1 year of age. If solid foods are begun too early, they may trigger food allergies.

Healthy infants born at term have sufficient iron for their first 4 months. Iron supplements are usually given beginning at 4 to 6 months (depending on whether breast- or formula-fed), and they may continue after 12 months if iron needs are not being met (AAP, 2010). Fluoride might also be prescribed for infants without a fluoridated water supply.

Toddlers and Preschoolers

Toddlers grow more slowly in comparison to infants, and have fewer energy demands. Toddlers require about 900 to 1,800 kcal and 1,250 mL of fluid per day, depending on body weight. As the GI system matures, they are able to eat most foods and adjust to the adult pattern of three meals a day. By age 3, most children have all of their deciduous teeth and can chew adult food.

➕ Cut food into small pieces to avoid choking in toddlers who sometimes are "too busy" to chew food sufficiently. Sometimes young children "chipmunk" their food and can later choke on it. Do not give food when the child is in a car seat or bouncy chair, where choking is more likely and can occur without a parent noticing.

Toddlers Toddlers' diets are sometimes deficient in fat and meat. One- and 2-year-old children should drink reduced-fat (2%) milk or in some cases whole milk to provide adequate fat for the still-growing brain. Deficiencies in iron, calcium, and vitamins A and C are also common during this period. Parents need to offer a variety of foods to provide these essential nutrients. This can be a challenge, because toddlers assert their autonomy and manipulate their parents by refusing foods. They may take a long time to eat or refuse to eat at all.

Parents should not turn mealtime into a battle of wills or use foods to punish or reward; such reactions may affect the child's attitude toward food. To encourage the child to eat, you may offer parents the suggestions in the accompanying Home Care box.

Preschoolers Preschoolers' growth and nutritional needs are similar to those of toddlers; however, their eating patterns typically improve. They begin to form responses to specific foods, such as refusing all green vegetables or drinking less milk. They often refuse casseroles and foods with sauces, and they might also eat only one particular food for several days. Because they are active, preschoolers require nutritious between-meal snacks. Lifelong food habits are developed during this stage, so encourage families to widen the variety of foods offered to preschoolers and to investigate the diet provided by their child's day care or preschool. Between ages 2 and 5 fat should provide only about 30% of the child's intake.

School-Age Children

In the school-age period, growth and body changes occur gradually. Permanent teeth erupt, and the digestive system matures. School-age children need about 2,400 kcal and 1,750 mL of fluid per day. An adequate supply of vitamins and minerals is critical because the body is still growing and preparing for the demands of adolescence.

Parental control over food intake declines during these years. Peers and advertisers influence the child's food choices. The child eats away from home and may buy junk food with his lunch money or choose less nutritious foods in the school cafeteria. Even if the child brings lunch from home, he may trade his food or not eat lunch at all. Parents should encourage their children to eat breakfast to provide nutrients and energy to fuel problem-solving skills, memory, and sports and playground activities.

Home Care

Tips for Encouraging Toddlers to Eat

➤ Keep only nutritious foods in the house to avoid battles over nutrient-poor snacks.

➤ Serve foods in a "child-friendly" way; for example, arrange tortillas, cheese, tomato slices, and beans in a smiling face.

➤ Allow the child to "graze" throughout the day on healthful foods rather than insisting that she sit for formal meals at the table.

➤ Avoid "combined" foods, such as casseroles and stews.

➤ Limit consumption of sweets and snack foods.

➤ Do not use dessert as a reward for eating other foods (e.g., "You can't have cookies until you eat your meat").

➤ Offer healthy foods that are easy to eat (e.g., "finger foods" or those easily chewed)

---

*Water that is purified or bottled for use in infant formulas does not contain fluoride.

Poor eating habits may lead to obesity. Thirty-two percent of U.S. children are overweight: 18% of boys, and 15% of girls (Centers for Disease Control and Prevention [CDC], 2008). Leading causes of childhood obesity include the following:

- Routine consumption of high-fat, high-sugar fast foods, nutrient-poor foods, and high-calorie snacks and beverages
- Loss of family mealtime
- Eating in front of a TV, computer, or video game
- Lack of regular physical activity to burn the kcal consumed (Berkowitz & Borchard, 2009)

Adolescents

Adolescence is a time of dramatic growth and the development of the reproductive system. Boys experience an increase in muscle tissue and bone length and density. At menstruation, girls experience fat deposition. The needs of the adolescent body for energy, vitamins, and minerals approach those of the infant. In particular, adolescents need protein, calcium, iron, and B and D vitamins. Boys in particular seem to eat constantly. Adolescents have active lifestyles and snack often, preferring ready-to-eat, eat-on-the-run foods, such as chips, pizza, cookies, and fast foods. Unfortunately, most such foods have little nutrient value. Adolescents are responsible for their own food decisions, so the best approach for parents is to keep only healthful snack foods (e.g., cheese, fruit, raw vegetables) in the home.

For girls, the need for nutrients conflicts with intense social pressure to be slim. About half of all teenage girls report that they are either dieting or that they need to be. Eating disorders are a concern in adolescence. Most people with eating disorders exhibit their first symptoms before age 20, some as early as age 10. The majority of eating disorder sufferers are female (National Association of Anorexia Nervosa and Associated Disorders, n.d.). Underweight and undernutrition are discussed more in the Practical Knowledge Section.

Adults

Young adults continue to require adequate amounts of protein, vitamins, and minerals, but not at the same levels as in adolescence. If adults continue unhealthful behaviors developed in earlier stages, repercussions will begin to show up in adulthood. Calcium, vitamin D, folic acid, and iron continue to be critical, especially in women, for bone and reproductive health. U.S. Preventive Services Task Force (USPSTF) officials recommend that women capable of becoming pregnant should take a folic acid supplement of 400 to 800 mcg per day to lower the risk for neural tube defects in the fetus (Simmons, 2013; USPSTF, 2009).

The BMR of middle adults decreases, potentially causing weight gain if dietary intake and activity level are unchanged. Individuals may begin to experience chronic illnesses such as diabetes, hypertension, obesity,

and hyperlipidemia, often as a result of heredity or poor lifestyle choices. Dietary modification and exercise are essential to control these diseases. Overweight and obesity are discussed more fully in the Practical Knowledge section. For dietary strategies for preventing cancer,

 Go to Chapter 27, **Tables, Boxes, Figures: ESG Box 27-2, Dietary Strategies for Preventing Cancer,** on Davis*Plus*.

Pregnant and Lactating Women

Nutritional requirements increase dramatically during pregnancy as the mother provides for the nutritional needs of the fetus. Folic acid intake is critical in the first trimester of pregnancy (the first 13 weeks) to prevent neural tube defects; a daily supplement of 600 to 800 mcg is recommended during pregnancy. Adequate protein and calcium are important for growing muscle, brain, and bone tissues; iron is essential to maintain maternal and fetal blood supplies and stores during pregnancy. It is almost impossible to consume the recommended amount of dietary iron, so supplements are commonly prescribed, as are supplements of folic acid and calcium. Pregnant women need about 300 additional kcal/day in the second and third trimesters of pregnancy.

Pregnant women also need to be screened for gestational diabetes (GDM). Complication for the mother and the fetus/infant of uncontrolled GDM include increased childhood obesity, fetal macrosomia and primary cesarean section (Agency for Healthcare Research and Quality [AHRQ], 2012).

Women who are breastfeeding need 500 additional kcal per day. They continue to need additional protein and calcium, as well as increased fluid intake to make adequate amounts of breast milk. Needs vary based on the size of the baby and the frequency of breastfeeding. The quantity of the breast milk depends on an adequate supply of fluids and nutrients. However, the nutritional quality of the milk remains the same even if dietary intake is not adequate.

KnowledgeCheck 27-5

- Why is breast milk an ideal food source for infants?
- Why are an infant's nutritional needs per unit of body weight greater than at any other period of development?
- Why is it sometimes a challenge to meet the nutritional needs of toddlers?
- What is the challenge in meeting the nutritional needs of school-age children?
- Which age group experiences a growth spurt second only to that of infants?
- Why are energy (kcal) requirements less for older adults?

Older Adults

Nutritional needs of older adults vary only slightly from middle adulthood. Lean body mass, physical activity, and BMR decrease, so older adults tend to need fewer kcal; but they still need the same or higher levels of nutrients. However, it is not unusual for older adults to lose interest in eating and for the thirst sensation to decrease.

Older adults with chronic diseases may need to adjust to therapeutic diets low in salt, simple sugars, or fat. Unfortunately, the ability to taste and smell diminishes with age, and many clients find these diets unappealing. Other sensory changes, such as diminished vision or hearing, limit mobility and interaction, making it more difficult to purchase and prepare food. Tooth loss and gum disease limit chewing ability, forcing many older adults to eat only soft food. Arthritic hands may have difficulty preparing and eating food, and when they are no longer able to drive, many older adults must rely on local markets, where food choices may be limited and expensive. Other physical problems that may affect nutrition include gastroesophageal reflux, decreased gastric secretions, decreased intestinal peristalsis, and glucose intolerance.

See Table 27-8 for dietary requirements for adults older than 70 years. Notice the main difference is that older adults require smaller quantities of most foods. In general, they require slightly more of the milk/yogurt/cheese group and slightly less of all other groups, especially the breads/cereal group. Older adults need complex carbohydrates (i.e., fiber) to maintain bowel function. They should be sure to drink at least eight glasses of water or other fluids (e.g., soups) per day and choose primarily green leafy vegetables and brightly colored fruits to help prevent constipation and dehydration. All of this, of course, assumes their medical condition allows this type of diet.

Many older adults may need supplements of calcium, vitamin D, and vitamin B_{12}. For example: (1) As bone density decreases, calcium requirements increase, especially in women at risk for *osteoporosis*; and (2) low concentrations of vitamin B_{12} have been linked to cognitive decline in older adults (Clark, Birks, Nexo, et al., 2007; Orton, 2012; Ross, Taylor, Yaktine, et al., 2011).

With advancing age, older adults face many losses. As a result, depression and social isolation are common. Both negatively affect appetite. **Adult failure to thrive** is a complex disorder seen in many institutionalized older adults. It is characterized by weight loss, decreased activity and interaction, and increasing frailty.

ThinkLike a Nurse 27-4

Make a list of all the food products you have seen advertised on television and in magazines. What are the implications for the nutritional status of the public?

Lifestyle Choices

Nutrition-related lifestyle choices include the following:

Dietary Patterns The type of food consumed is as important as the amount of food to a person's overall health. Whole foods, such as fresh fruits and vegetables, whole grains, and legumes, promote health, whereas

FOOD GROUP	ADULTS ≥70 YEARS
Supplement of calcium, vitamin D, and vitamin B_{12}	As prescribed. Not everyone needs supplements. People should consult their healthcare providers.
Fats, oils, and sweets	Use sparingly
Milk, yogurt, and cheese group	3 servings
Meat, poultry, fish, dry beans, eggs, and nut group	2 or more servings
Vegetable group	3 or more servings
Fruit group	2 or more servings
Bread, fortified cereals, rice, and pasta group	6 or more servings
Water equivalents	8 or more servings

Table 27-8 ➤ Daily Food Requirements for Adults Older Than Age 70

Source: Tufts University Nutrition. (2011). MyPlate for Older Adults. Retrieved December 23, 2012, from http://www.nutrition.tufts.edu/research/myplate-older-adults

foods high in simple sugars, saturated and *trans* fats, and sodium increase the risk for health problems.

Work Environment Physically demanding work can cause fatigue and affect the quantity and quality of food consumed. When time pressure on the job makes it difficult to prepare and eat healthy food during a short lunch break, some workers may rely on convenience foods to save time.

Cooking Methods Up to one-half of the water-soluble vitamin content (vitamins B and C) is lost in the cooking water of boiled vegetables. Keeping foods hot longer than 2 hours results in even further loss.

Oral Contraceptive Use This method of family planning lowers the serum level of vitamin C and several B vitamins. Women with marginal nutrient intake may need vitamin supplements.

Using Food to Relieve Stress Food is commonly used to cope with stress, depression, loneliness, or boredom. For example, in highly stressful work environments some workers react by consuming high-calorie snacks beverages. Skipping meals, binge eating, or consuming too much of a single food (e.g., snack foods or chocolate) can result in poor nutrition, obesity, and low self-esteem.

Smoking Smokers use vitamin C faster than non-smokers. Vitamin C is also an antioxidant. The more a person smokes, the more vitamin is lost, and the more the body needs vitamin C to counteract the damage smoking causes to cells. Additionally, because vitamin C aids in absorption of iron, low levels of vitamin C also are linked to iron deficiency. If the person cannot quit smoking, a vitamin C supplement (2,000 mg/day) may help compensate.

Otherwise, there is some evidence suggesting folic acid found in leafy vegetables may protect against cancer in current and former smokers (National Institutes of Health, 2010).

Alcohol Alcohol contributes to obesity. A 12-oz beer contains 150 calories; a juice-based cocktail contains about 160 calories. This can add many unnecessary calories to the regular diet. In addition, alcohol significantly decreases the rate of fat metabolism. Excessive alcohol use interferes with adequate nutrition by (1) replacing the food in the person's diet, (2) suppressing the appetite, (3) decreasing the absorption of nutrients by its toxic effects on intestinal mucosa, and (4) impairing the storage of nutrients. People who use alcohol heavily need multivitamin supplements, especially B vitamins and folic acid.

Caffeine The most common sources of caffeine are coffee, soda, and energy drinks. Over the years, research reports have claimed a variety of dangers and health benefits for caffeine. Recently a privately funded group (Schardt, 2008) published an analysis of nine scientific reports in which they state that many of our accepted beliefs about coffee are myths. They report coffee does not create risk for dehydration, heart disease, or cancer, and has little or no role in hypertension. Caffeine may be associated with bone loss; however, its negative effect can be offset by as little as 2 tablespoons of milk. In high doses, caffeine can sometimes cause anxiety and stomach upset. On the positive side, caffeine can enhance mood and mental and physical performance. It aids the ability to burn fat for fuel instead of carbohydrates, and has been linked to a lower risk of Parkinson's disease, type 2 diabetes, stroke, and dementia (Schardt, 2008; van Dam, Willett, Manson, et al., 2006). So it appears that while the evidence is still mixed, caffeinated beverages in moderation are not the villains we once thought.

Vegetarianism

All vegetarian diets exclude red meat and poultry, but beyond this distinction is a wide spectrum of diets. **Semi-vegetarians** are the most inclusive, allowing fish, eggs, and dairy products as well as plant-based foods. **Ovo-lacto vegetarians** are somewhat more strict; they eat eggs and dairy products, but not fish. **Lacto-vegetarians** consume only dairy and plant-based foods. **Vegans** eat only foods of plant origin, and a **fruitarian** diet includes only fruits, nuts, honey, and vegetable oils. Soybeans, soy milk, tofu, and processed protein products can be used by all but fruitarians to enhance the nutritional value of the diet.

People choose vegetarian diets for a number of reasons. As noted in Chapter 16, some religions prohibit consumption of animal flesh or foods of animal origin. Ethical considerations related to humane treatment of animals also cause some people to adopt a vegetarian diet. However, many people adopt a vegetarian diet simply as a health choice, noting the abundant research indicating that vegetarianism reduces the risk of disease (e.g., ischemic heart disease) and promotes wellness by limiting fat intake.

Although ovo-lacto vegetarians have no higher rate of nutrient deficiencies than the meat-eating population, they must choose foods carefully to include enough of the following nutrients:

- *Vitamin B_{12}* is found only in animal products, such as eggs and milk. Vegans must eat foods fortified with B_{12} or take B_{12} supplements. Long-standing B_{12} deficiency can result in severe and irreversible neurological impairment.
- *Vitamin D* may be inadequately supplied by vegetarian diets, so vitamin D–fortified foods (e.g., soy and dairy milk are usually vitamin D fortified) should be included. Adequate sun exposure also helps to compensate for lack of dietary intake.
- *Calcium, iron, and zinc.* Vegans, fruitarians, and others who limit animal foods may need to supplement the diet with calcium, iron, and zinc. This is especially important for children and women who are pregnant or lactating.
  (a) *Iron:* The iron from plant foods is not absorbed as well as that from animal sources. However, it is easier to absorb dietary iron when it is eaten with foods containing vitamin C, so eating fruit or vegetables containing vitamin C with meals helps to compensate.
  (b) *Calcium:* Vegans, especially, may find it difficult to obtain enough dietary calcium. It is important to include fortified soy milk and calcium-rich vegetables (e.g., bok choy, broccoli, collards, Chinese cabbage, kale, mustard greens, okra, and fortified tomato juice). Calcium-fortified cereals are also available.
  (c) *Zinc:* A wide variety of foods contain zinc. Oysters contain more zinc than just about any other food. Meat and poultry also have a high zinc content. Although some grain and plant foods contain zinc, it is not as bioavailable from non-animal sources (National Institutes of Health, Office of Dietary Supplements, n.d.).
- *Protein* may be inadequate, especially in vegan children who do not care for the taste of soy milk, tofu, and other soy-based meat substitutes. For adults, a varied diet that meets normal nutrient and energy needs is also likely to supply adequate amounts of essential amino acids. Complementary proteins should be eaten throughout the day, but careful meal-by-meal balance of amino acids is usually not necessary. Review Table 27-1 and the discussion of complete and incomplete proteins earlier in the chapter.

- To ensure adequate nutrients it may be wise for vegetarians to consult a qualified nutrition professional, especially during periods of growth, breastfeeding, pregnancy, or recovery from illness. For recommended servings of vegetarian food groups, see MyVeganPlate (Fig. 27-3). This is presented in a similar manner to the ChooseMyPlate.org nutritional guidelines.

 Go to Chapter 27, **Tables, Boxes, Figures: ESG Table 27-2, Recommended Daily Servings for Vegetarian Meal Planning,** on Davis*Plus*.

As a vegetarian diet can be a healthy option, the USDA also has tips for vegetarian diet.

 Go to the **USDA** Web site at http://www.choosemyplate.gov/healthy-eating-tips/tips-for-vegetarian.html

Eating for Health and Athletic Performance

In recent decades the consumption of processed foods, grains, and beverages is cited as a cause of diseases, such as type 2 diabetes and obesity, heart disease, cancer, and many others. Consuming a diet high in meats and fish, fresh fruits and vegetables, nuts and seed, eggs, and other natural, whole foods is biologically healthier than the modern diet high in *trans* fats, preservatives, and chemical additives. Proponents of the paleo diet, named for the foods hunted and gathered by people of the Paleolithic era, advocate returning to a "caveman" diet for improved health and athletic performance. Foods to avoid are all processed foods, grains containing gluten, diary, refined sugar, legumes, potatoes, processed oils, and caffeine.

Dieting for Weight Loss

Many diets, including the *Dietary Approaches to Stop Hypertension* (DASH) diet, the American Heart Association diet, and others, are nutritionally sound, but many others are "fad diets," claiming to produce speedy, effortless, almost miraculous, weight loss. You can recognize fad diets by the following characteristics. They:

- Promise quick and dramatic weight loss, which is usually achieved only temporarily because it results from loss of body fluids.
- Limit the range of foods from which the dieter can select (e.g., only fruits and vegetables for the first week), leading to an imbalance in nutrients.
- Often recommend purchase of supplements and/or special packaged meals; in many cases, these are brands that they endorse or actually produce.
- Fail to include practical strategies that help dieters permanently change eating and activity patterns.

As soon as they achieve their weight-loss goal, fad dieters typically revert to former eating habits and regain the weight. In contrast, more moderate calorie-restriction diets, such as the American Heart Association diet:

- Describe food selection and preparation tips and other behavior modifications that can lead to slow, sustained weight loss.

- Promote a diet that includes a variety of food choices and a balance of nutrients.
- Encourage physical activity as a cornerstone of weight loss.
- Emphasize self-monitoring, cognitive strategies, and behavior modification.

 Go to the **USDA ChooseMyPlate.gov, Weight Management & Calories** Web site at http://www.choosemyplate.gov/weight-management-calories.html

Ethnic, Cultural, and Religious Practices

As described in Chapters 15 and 16, religion and culture can have a major impact on diet and lifestyle. The following are examples:

- Language barriers may make it difficult for a client to understand nutritional information. For those patients, simple visual aids may be useful.
- Ethnic/cultural food choices often reflect the foods that were plentiful in the region of origin (e.g., fish in coastal communities, coffee and cocoa beans in equatorial regions), as well as foods that were readily grown in the native soil (e.g., rice in warm wetlands, potatoes in colder climates).
- Other diet choices reflect a concern for food preservation: for instance, people from various geographic regions eat salted meats and dried fruits and cook with fiery spices to combat microbes.
- Certain religions may require fasting or abstaining from certain foods. For example, Roman Catholics fast on Ash Wednesday and Good Friday; kosher dietary laws prohibit eating pork and shellfish.
- The burden of childhood obesity is not spread equally across the U.S. population. For example, obesity has been increasing faster among lower socioeconomic groups and Mexican American and black children (U.S. Department of Health and Human Services, CDC, & National Center for Health Statistics, 2012).
- Cultural beliefs, perceptions, and attitudes about weight issues may often not match those of health providers. For example, some parents may perceive their children as cute and healthy, even though their BMI indicates they are obese. A slim body is not the ideal in all cultures.

Traditional diets of many cultures are healthful and should not be discouraged; in fact, contemporary adaptations made to these diets may compromise their nutritional quality.

Mediterranean Diet This diet is rich in olive oil, fish, fruits, vegetables, and nuts and low in dairy foods, processed foods and saturated fats, and red meat, and includes a glass of red wine. It has been linked to decreased risk of death from all causes, including deaths due to cancer and coronary artery disease in a U.S. population (Estruch, Ros, Salas-Salvado, et al., 2013; Mitrou, Kipnis, Thiébaut, et al., 2007).

Vegan
MY∧PLATE

Nutrition Tips:

*Choose mostly whole grains.
*Eat a variety of foods from each of the food groups.
*Adults age 70 and younger need 600 IU of vitamin D daily.
  Sources include fortified foods (such as some soymilks) or a vitamin D supplement.
*Sources of iodine include iodized salt (3/8 teaspoon daily) or
  an iodine supplement (150 micrograms).
*See www.vrg.org for recipes and more details.

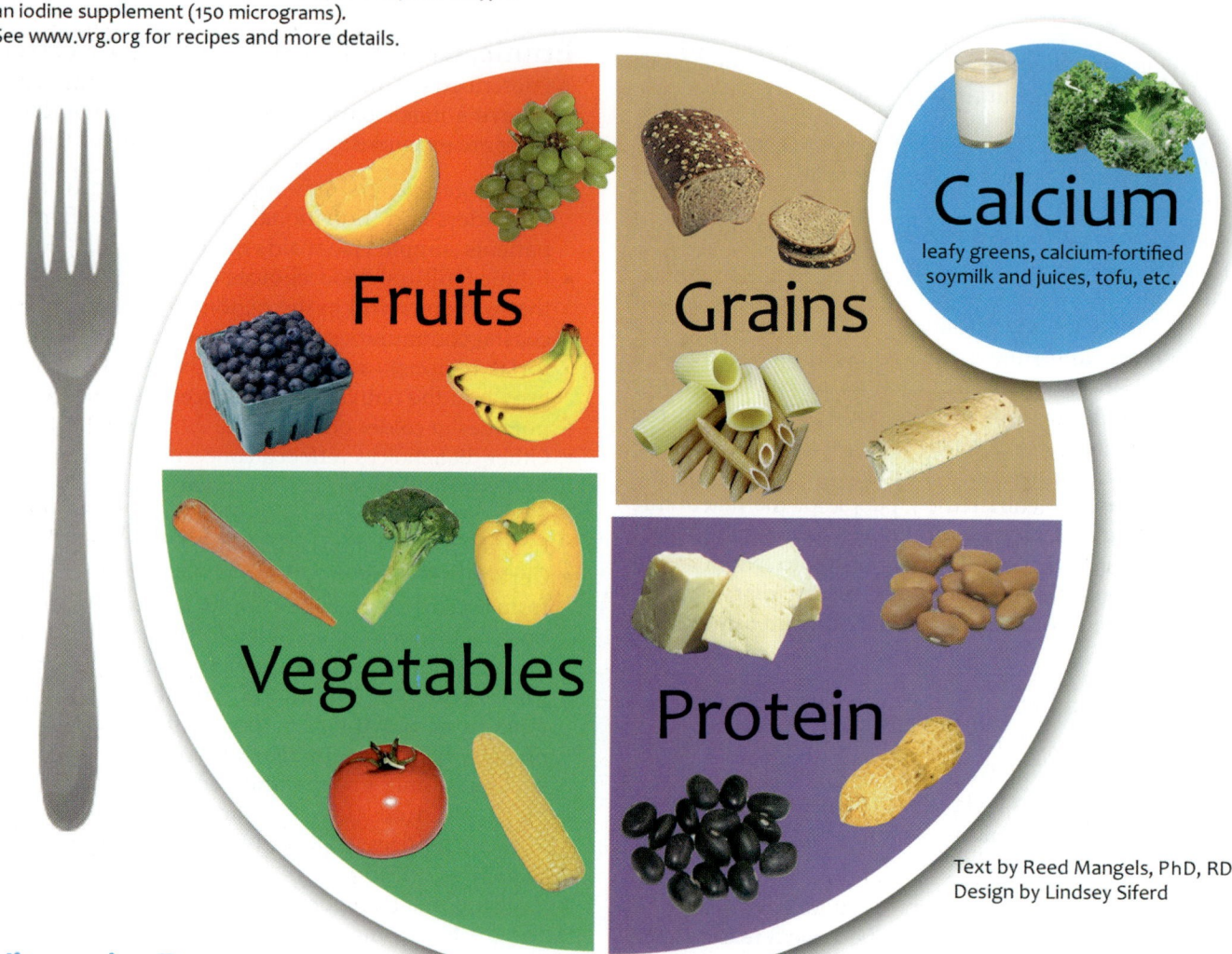

Fruits

Grains

Calcium
leafy greens, calcium-fortified
soymilk and juices, tofu, etc.

Vegetables

Protein

Text by Reed Mangels, PhD, RD
Design by Lindsey Siferd

Vitamin B12:

Vegans need a reliable source of vitamin B12. Eat daily a couple of servings of fortified foods
such as B12-fortified soymilk, breakfast cereal, meat analog, or Vegetarian Support Formula nutritional yeast.
Check the label for fortification. If fortified foods are not eaten daily,
you should take a vitamin B12 supplement (25 micrograms daily).

Note:

Like any food plan, this should only serve as a general guide for adults.
The plan can be modified according to your own personal needs. This is not personal
medical advice. Individuals with special health needs should consult a registered
dietitian or a medical doctor knowledgeable about vegan nutrition.

VRg. The Vegetarian
Resource Group P.O. Box 1463 Baltimore, MD 21203 www.vrg.org (410) 366-8343

FIGURE 27-3 MyVeganPlate. (Source: Vegan Resource Group. www.vrg.org)

Asian Diet The traditional Asian diet is a plant-based diet with a low amount of animal products. It consists of rice, fresh fruits, and vegetables, such as melons, bananas, tangerines, bok choy, cabbage, and other green leafy vegetables. Protein intake primarily consists of beans, nuts, and seeds, and occasional poultry, shellfish, and eggs. Health benefits of this diet include lower incidence of cardiovascular disease, diabetes, colon cancer, and obesity. Green and black teas contain antioxidants that may lower the risk of cancer.

Indian Diet The traditional Indian diet contains fresh, home-cooked foods containing a wide array of spices. The selection of meat is based on religious preference (e.g., Muslims don't eat pork; Hindus aren't permitted to eat beef; Buddhists are vegetarian). People who eat a traditional Indian diet that is high in fruits, vegetables, legumes, and nuts, and low in processed foods reap the benefit of low incidence of diabetes, heart disease, and other chronic diseases.

Hispanic Diet The Hispanic diet relies heavy on grains, especially rice, and legumes (e.g., beans), and corn-based products. Beans as a staple provide a diet rich in fiber, B vitamins, calcium, phosphorus, and iron; however, when prepared with lard, the health benefits diminish. The traditional Hispanic fare includes few fresh vegetables, except for tomatoes, which are rich in vitamins A and C, as well as potassium and iron. Diabetes type 2 is more prevalent among nonwhite Hispanics, due to a high rate of obesity. Sugary fruit beverages and soda are a common part of the contemporary Hispanic diet.

Disease Processes and Functional Limitations Affecting Nutrition

Chronic diseases (e.g., diabetes mellitus, GI disorders) can alter nutrient intake, digestion, absorption, use, and excretion. Any illness, especially when accompanied by fever, increases the need for protein, water, and calories to meet the demands of increased metabolic rate. Traumatic injury (e.g., burns, surgery) requires extra protein and vitamin C for wound healing and tissue rebuilding. People with long-term insufficient calorie intake (e.g., patients with cancer) also suffer from **protein-calorie malnutrition**, which is characterized by weight loss and muscle and fat wasting. A variety of other physical and psychological disorders and/or their treatments can adversely affect a client's nutrition:

Alcoholism Poor appetite is common in alcoholism, which results in decreased intake of food and therefore of nutrients. Alcohol can also interfere with the function of some vitamins.

Cognitive Function A person with a developmental delay, severe mental illness, confusion, or memory loss may be unable to remember what, when, or whether she has eaten.

Ability to Obtain and Prepare Food Paralysis or hemiplegia (e.g., from a stroke) can cause functional limitations that affect mobility and, hence, the ability to shop for food. Social factors also limit the ability to gather or procure food. People with limited income may be forced to choose between buying food, medication, or household utilities. Homeless people and others in extreme poverty are often reduced to eating from trashcans and dumpsters or consuming nonfoods, such as paper, grass, and clay.

Preparing food takes time and energy. A person with severe dyspnea from chronic obstructive pulmonary disease (COPD), for example, may not have the stamina to prepare a nutritious meal. Instead, she may eat prepared foods that are high in sodium content. Fatigue is also caused by advanced chronic disease, severe anemia, pregnancy, depression, or excess work.

Chewing and Swallowing Decayed or missing teeth and ill-fitting dentures make chewing difficult. The person often resorts to eating only soft foods, many of which lack fiber. Acute disorders affecting the throat, such as pharyngitis, make swallowing painful. Cancer of the larynx or esophageal strictures also makes swallowing painful or difficult, and frequently leads to avoiding food.

Stomach Function Heartburn, indigestion, and other stomach disorders are common. People may eat only bland foods or avoid certain foods to prevent the pain or burning that follow eating.

Peristalsis Peristalsis is the wave-like action that propels food through the intestinal tract. Bowel inflammation or infection, diverticula (outpouchings of the intestine), or tumors may increase peristalsis, thereby decreasing absorption of nutrients. In addition, high stress levels may either speed or slow transit time. If peristalsis is slow, the stomach may not empty properly (gastroparesis). This could lead to early satiety, nausea, or vomiting and affect nutrient intake. This is not unusual in patients with diabetes.

Intestinal Surface Area The amount of intestinal surface area may be diminished either by surgery or disease, thereby decreasing absorption of nutrients. This may result in malnutrition despite the fact that the patient is consuming adequate calories and protein.

Enzyme Secretion Liver, gallbladder, or pancreas problems affect the secretion of enzymes involved in digesting foods. Nearly 50 million Americans lack the enzyme (lactase) needed to digest milk. Up to 80% of blacks, 80% to 100% of Native Americans, and 90% to 100% of Asian Americans are lactose intolerant (National Digestive Diseases Information Clearinghouse, 2009, updated 2012).

Bariatric Surgery alters digestion to achieve rapid weight loss. The three types are restrictive, malabsorptive, and combined restrictive/malabsorptive. Restrictive procedures (sleeve gastrectomy, adjustable gastric banding). limit the stomach's capacity to hold food and reduce the passage through the GI tract. Malabsorption surgeries (intestinal bypass) are done to impair the uptake of food nutrients and fats. A combined approach uses stomach restriction and a partial bypass of the small intestine. Bariatric weight loss procedures increase the risk of nutrient deficiency, especially iron, copper, zinc, selenium, thiamine, folate, and vitamins B_{12}, and D. (Choban, Dickerson, Malone, et al., & the American Society for Parenteral and Enteral Nutrition, 2013).

Medications In addition to the direct effects of diseases and disorders, nutrition may be affected by the drugs and therapies used to treat them, as in the following examples:

- *Decreased appetite.* Some medications directly decrease appetite, for example, amphetamine and dextroamphetamine (Adderall), aspirin, diphenhydramine (e.g., Benadryl), and lithium carbonate (e.g., Lithobid).
- *Chemotherapy and radiation therapy.* These may cause oral ulcers, intestinal bleeding, or diarrhea—which interfere with eating and absorbing nutrients from food.
- *Altered metabolism.* Certain drugs alter nutrient metabolism; others increase or decrease nutrient excretion. Medication metabolism may also alter taste, changing the overall intake.
- *Effect on Specific Nutrients.* For example, acetylsalicylic acid (aspirin) decreases folate levels and increases excretion of vitamin C; laxatives may cause calcium and potassium depletion; and thiazide diuretics decrease the absorption of vitamin B_{12}.
- *Nausea and Vomiting.* Almost all oral medications have the potential to cause nausea or vomiting, thereby decreasing appetite. Examples include acetylsalicylic acid (aspirin), antibiotics, anticonvulsants, antidepressants, anti-inflammatory agents, antineoplastic agents (chemotherapy), asthma medications (especially theophylline), birth control pills, fluoride supplements, opioids, potassium chloride, and vitamin and mineral supplements.

KnowledgeCheck 27-6

- List at least three nutrients that may be more difficult to supply through a vegetarian diet.
- When selecting a program for weight loss, what factors should a person consider?
- Why should you encourage clients from various cultures to follow their traditional diets?
- Describe the effects on nutrition of (1) smoking and (2) heavy alcohol use.

Special Diets

Many people must follow a modified diet to assist in managing their illness. In addition, all inpatients at healthcare facilities must have a diet prescribed by their primary care provider. The following are the most commonly prescribed modified diets.

Regular Diet

A regular diet, also called the "house diet," is appropriate for clients without special nutritional needs. This diet is a balanced meal plan that supplies 2,000 kcal per day. Many facilities provide vegetarian and ethnic variations (Asian menu, kosher, and so on). Inpatients choose each meal from a list of menu choices.

Have you ever eaten "hospital food"? Or have you heard someone complain that hospital food is bland and unimaginative? There is some justification for that complaint. House diets must accommodate the varied tastes of all patients, so they are usually lightly seasoned. Selections are limited to avoid unpopular items (e.g., Brussels sprouts) and restrict fatty, fried, or gassy foods, which many patients tolerate poorly. However, you should refrain from making negative comments to patients about the food.

NPO

NPO means no food or fluid (including water) by mouth. This may be ordered before surgery or an invasive procedure to limit the risk of aspiration. Common examples are "NPO after midnight," or "NPO 8 hours prior to procedure." Most well-nourished, well-hydrated patients easily tolerate short-term NPO status. However, no one can tolerate prolonged periods of NPO. Intravenous fluids may be given to provide hydration, and clients who must remain NPO for a lengthy period need enteral (through a stomach tube) or parenteral (IV) nutrition to prevent malnutrition.

Diets Modified by Consistency

Patients undergoing surgery, bowel procedures, or acute illness may, for a short period of time, need a diet modified by consistency. Patients with chronic health concerns that affect their ability to chew or swallow (e.g., Impaired Dentition and Impaired Swallowing) may need long-term changes in the consistency of their diet (Table 27-9).

Diets Modified for Disease

Some health conditions require modification of dietary intake. The following are the most common diets:

- *Calorie-restricted.* For clients requiring weight reduction
- *Sodium-restricted.* For clients with blood pressure or fluid balance problems
- *Fat-restricted.* For clients with elevated cholesterol or triglyceride levels; may also be ordered for general weight loss
- *Diabetic.* To manage calories and carbohydrate intake for clients with diabetes mellitus
- *Renal diet.* To manage electrolytes and fluid for clients with renal insufficiency
- *Protein-controlled diet.* To manage liver and kidney disease

Table 27-9 ➤ Diets Modified by Consistency

DIET DESCRIPTION AND FOODS INCLUDED	COMMENTS
Clear Liquids. Provides fluids to prevent dehydration, and supplies some simple carbohydrates to help meet energy needs. *Foods Included:* Water, tea, coffee, broth, clear juice (usually apple, grape, or cranberry juice), Popsicles, carbonated beverages, and gelatin.	▪ Does not supply adequate calories, protein, and other nutrients, so timely progression to more nutritious diets is recommended. ▪ If clear liquids are required for more than 3 days, commercial clear liquid supplements are usually prescribed.
Full Liquids. Contains all the liquids included in the clear liquid diet plus any food items that are liquid at room temperature. *Foods Included:* Add to clear liquid diet: soups, milk, milk shakes, puddings, custards, juices, some hot cereals, and yogurt.	▪ Difficult to obtain a balanced diet on a full liquid plan; use for a short time only. ▪ If needed for a longer time, a professional dietitian should be involved in planning the diet. ▪ High-calorie, high-protein supplements are often added.
Mechanical Soft Diet. The diet of choice for people with chewing difficulties resulting from missing teeth, jaw problems, or extensive fatigue. *Foods Included:* Add to the full liquid diet: soft vegetables and fruits; chopped, ground, or shredded meat; and breads, pastries, eggs, and cheese.	▪ This diet can supply a full range of nutrients but is quite low in fiber. As a result, constipation is a risk. ▪ Many food items can be added to this diet by cooking them extensively or blending or grinding to alter their texture.
Pureed Diet. A pureed diet is a blended diet. It may have some or no foods excluded.	▪ Often liquids are added to the food to create a texture that may be scooped onto serving plates.

▪ *Antigen-avoidance diets.* For clients allergic to or intolerant of certain foods, such as a gluten-free diet for clients with celiac disease

▪ *Calorie-protein push.* Used when there is a need to heal wounds, maintain or increase weight, or promote growth. If the person cannot consume enough kcal by adding fats and proteins to his regular diet, high-calorie, high-protein supplements may be used.

ThinkLike a Nurse 27-5

Analyze the following diets. Which nutrients are missing or difficult to obtain from these diets?

▪ Clear liquid
▪ Full liquid

PracticalKnowledge
knowing **how**

Good nutrition not only is essential for health, but also is a key aspect of disease management. In the rest of this chapter, we look at assessing nutritional status and diagnosing and planning care for some nutrition problems. In addition, we discuss specifically the care of patients who are underweight/undernourished or overweight/obese.

Nutrition is a basic human need. But more than a physical necessity, it also has emotional associations. We eat when we are hungry, but we also eat for pleasure because the food tastes good! Food has become a part of most social events and activities. A certain food may symbolize one's cultural or religious affiliation or even be a political statement (e.g., refusal to eat lettuce in support of migrant workers). It is wise to keep in mind that food has different meanings to different people. Personal beliefs, habits, and preferences are as important as nutritional knowledge in determining what a person eats.

ASSESSMENT

There are two kinds of nutritional assessment: (1) screening assessments and (2) thorough, focused nutritional assessments. Usually you will perform a screening exam. If you identify nutritional risk factors, you then perform a focused nutritional assessment. For the components of a nutritional history,

 Go to Chapter 27, **Focused Nutritional Assessment,** the section entitled **Nutritional History, in Volume 2.**

SCREENING FOR NUTRITIONAL PROBLEMS

All hospitalized patients, especially those with obesity and patients at risk for nutritional deficit, should be receive a nutritional screening support plan within 48 hours of inpatient admission (Choban, Dickerson, Malone, et al., & the American Society for Parenteral and Enteral Nutrition, 2013). **Cursory screening** consists of evaluation of height, weight, and BMI coupled with a brief dietary history. Clients who are found to be at risk for nutritional problems should be further evaluated.

 It is especially important to assess nutritional status in elderly clients carefully to ensure that you detect marginal deficiencies before major problems occur.

- *The subjective global assessment.* This commonly used screening method makes use of information from the overall medical history and physical examination to evaluate a client's nutritional status.
- *The Nutrition Screening Initiative (NSI) (1991),* developed for older adults, identifies indicators of impaired nutritional status.
- *The Mini Nutritional Assessment (MNA),* also developed for older adults, can be used with clients of all ages (DiMaria-Ghalili & Guenter, 2008).

To learn more about those and other screening methods and for tools to use (e.g., to screen for dementia),

 Go to Chapter 27, **Screening for Nutritional Problems,** in Volume 2.

FOCUSED NUTRITIONAL ASSESSMENT

If screening reveals nutritional problems, perform a focused nutritional assessment to evaluate the client. The nutrition component of the complete physical assessment or any focused nutritional assessment includes both subjective (history) and objective (physical examination) data. To see and use a focused nutritional assessment,

 Go to Chapter 27, **Focused Nutritional Assessment,** in Volume 2.

Dietary History You can obtain a dietary history during any routine assessment. When you take a **dietary history**, whether you use a self-administered form or an interview, you collect general knowledge of the client's basic eating habits, food attitudes and preferences, cultural factors, and use of dietary supplements. A dietary history creates a picture of the client's food habits and eating behaviors.

24-Hour Recall A 24-hour recall requires the client to name all food eaten within a day. Simply ask questions such as, "Yesterday, what did you eat for breakfast/lunch/dinner/snacks?" A 24-hour recall is simple, requires no equipment, and can be used as often as required. However, accuracy of the data may be questionable, because some people have difficulty remembering everything they ate the previous day, and any single day may be atypical. Sometimes, a family member can help the client recall intake more accurately (Garibalia & Forster, 2008).

Food Frequency Questionnaire A food frequency questionnaire asks the client to identify the number of times per day, week, or month a particular food group is eaten (e.g., fruits, red meats). You can modify the questions according to the client's specific issues. Food frequency questionnaires provide a more global image of the client's nutritional intake than the 24-hour recall; however, accuracy is still a problem.

Food Record A food record is the most accurate food diary. It provides information on the quantity as well as the types of foods eaten. You ask the client in advance to keep a record of measured and weighed amounts of all foods he eats in a 3-day period. From the detailed information collected, you can analyze the total kilocalories and nutrient content for the recorded period. Although the food record provides meaningful results, it requires a high level of cognitive and psychomotor functioning that not all clients have. It also requires commitment to the process for 3 days, which may be difficult for some people. You may wish to remind some patients that there are Web sites that can help them with journaling their diet and tracking nutritional intake, goals, and energy expenditure. For examples,

 Go to Chapter Resources, Chapter 27, **Resources for Caregivers and Health Professionals,** on DavisPlus.

How Can I Assess Body Composition?

When assessing body composition (the proportion of fat in the body), you use **anthropometric measurements**. These are noninvasive physical examination techniques to determine body dimensions such as height and weight. Other examples are discussed in the following sections. Anthropometric measurements are used to assess growth rate in children; to indirectly assess adults' protein and fat stores; and to diagnose overweight, obesity, and underweight. To obtain accurate data, you must use standardized equipment and procedures and compare the data to existing reference standards for men and women.

Skinfold Measurements

Approximately half of body fat is located subcutaneously. Therefore, you will use measurement of skinfold thickness to estimate a person's body fat content. Skinfold thickness reveals information about current nutritional status as well as long-term changes in fat stores. Use a caliper to obtain the most accurate measurement. The most reliable location is the triceps for children and women and the subscapular area in men. The combined measurements of triceps skinfold and mid-upper arm circumference yield a better estimate of muscle and fat areas than a single measurement. For instructions on taking skinfold measurements,

 Go to Chapter 27, **Clinical Insight 27-2: Skinfold Measurement,** in Volume 2.

Circumferences

Another method of estimating the percentage of body fat is to use girth, or circumference measurements. Waist circumference is a complement to BMI for predicting obesity risk because BMI does not account for the difference between muscle and fat accumulation. *Mid-upper arm circumference* is routinely measured as part of screening. For people who are obese, *abdominal circumference* is the preferred measurement. *The waist-to-hip ratio (WHR)* evaluates obesity by assessing abdominal fat. A WHR of greater than 1 in men and greater than 0.8 in women indicates obesity. A high level of abdominal fat is associated with increased risk for hypertension, diabetes, hyperlipidemia, and cardiovascular disease. For specific instructions on measuring mid-upper arm circumference and WHR,

 Go to Chapter 27, **Clinical Insight 27-3: Measuring Circumferences to Evaluate Body Composition,** in Volume 2.

Body Mass Index

BMI can be precisely measured using scanning devices that measure *bioelectrical impedance*—the conduction of a harmless electrical charge through the client's body. Lean tissue readily conducts the charge, whereas adipose tissue does not. However, you will usually roughly estimate BMI by using the calculation formula in Box 27-4. You may also consult tables with precalculated values based on height and weight (National Heart, Lung and Blood Institute [NHLBI], n.d.). For an example of a height–weight BMI table,

 Go to Chapter 22, **Procedure 22-1: Performing the General Survey,** in Volume 2.

You can also find BMI calculators on the Web. Two reliable examples are at:

 Centers for Disease Control and Prevention, at http://www.cdc.gov/healthyweight/assessing/bmi/adult_bmi/english_bmi_calculator/bmi_calculator.html

and

 National Heart, Lung and Blood Institute, at http://www.nhlbi.nih.gov/guidelines/obesity/BMI/bmicalc.htm

The normal BMI for adults ranges from 18.5 to 24.9 (although this may vary slightly among professional organizations). The usefulness of BMI values is limited for athletes because of their highly developed muscle mass, and for pregnant and postpartal women because their increased weight is normal. In addition, BMI values have not been specifically calculated for people older than age 65. Despite these limitations, BMI is useful in identifying underweight and obese individuals.

KnowledgeCheck 27-7

- What is the most accurate type of food diary?
- Compare and contrast four nutritional screening approaches: cursory screening, subjective global assessment, Mini Nutritional Assessment, and Nutrition Screening Initiative.
- Identify three nutritional risk factors.

BOX 27-4 ■ Calculating Body Mass Index (BMI)

BMI = weight in kilograms ÷ (height in meters)^2
Example:

Robert weighs 165 lb. Convert his weight to kilograms:
$$165 ÷ 2.2 = 75 \text{ kg}$$

He is 71 inches tall. Convert his height to meters.
$$1 \text{ meter} = 39.37 \text{ inches.}$$

Divide 71 inches by 39.37 inches; he is 1.8 meters tall (rounded off)

His BMI is 75 kg ÷ (1.8)^2 = 23
The normal BMI for adults ranges from 18.5 to 24.9.

Classification of Body Mass Index Values

Classification	BMI (kg/m^2)
Severely underweight	<16
Moderately underweight	16–16.99
Mild underweight	17–18.49
Underweight	<18.5
Healthy weight	18.5–24.9
Pre-obese	25.0–29.9
Class I obesity	30.0–34.9
Class II obesity	35.0–39.9
Class III obesity	40.0 or higher

Source: Adapted from National Heart, Lung and Blood Institute (1998); and World Health Organization (2006a).

 ### ThinkLike a Nurse 27-6

1. Calculate your WHR.
2. Use Box 27-4 to calculate your BMI. Evaluate the result.
   - How useful are these data?
   - Do you feel you need to pursue a program of weight loss? Why or why not?

Imaging Techniques

Imaging techniques are not widely used to evaluate lean body mass because they are quite expensive to perform. Imaging methods include the following:

- *Dual-energy x-ray absorptiometry (DEXA)* is used to assess bone mineral content and density. Because lean tissue has different absorptive properties than does adipose tissue, this technique shows promise for wider use because it is quick and noninvasive.
- *Computed tomography (CT)* measures volume rather than actual body tissue composition. It can provide information about the quantity of adipose tissue, particularly in body cavities.
- *Magnetic resonance imaging* (MRI) is an excellent noninvasive method for directly assessing body composition. The cost and availability of the machinery, however, make it impractical for day-to-day evaluation of clients.

Underwater Weighing

Hydrodensitometry, or underwater weighing, is another method for determining body composition. It requires total submersion of the patient in a tank of water. Because fat readily floats, the person's buoyancy will vary depending on his percentage of body fat. This method is considered the gold standard for body composition measures. However, clinical use of this method is limited because it is impractical to use with children, the elderly, or individuals who are severely ill.

KnowledgeCheck 27-8

- What are the most reliable locations for skinfold measurement?
- What are the implications of an increased WHR?

What Physical Examination Findings Are Cues to Nutrient Imbalance?

To detect nutritional abnormalities, such as diabetes, you should assess physical findings, lifestyle, nutritional and medical history, dietary intake, anthropometric measurements, and laboratory testing (Box 27-5). Refer to Chapter 22 as needed for a review of physical examination techniques. For guidelines in performing a nutrition-focused physical examination,

 Go to Chapter 27, **Focused Nutritional Assessment,** in Volume 2.

BOX 27-5 ■ When to Assess for Diabetes

- Adults with BMI >25
- Physical inactivity
- High-risk ethnicity for obesity (e.g., American Indians, Alaskan Natives)
- First-degree relative with diabetes
- Women who have delivered a baby weighing more than 9 lb or diagnosed with gestational diabetes during pregnancy
- Hemoglobin A$_{1c}$ >5.7% (test for glucose control over a 2- to 3-month period)
- HDL cholesterol <35 mg/dL and/or triglyceride >250 mg/dL
- History of cardiovascular disease and/or hypertension
- Physical signs indicating low blood sugar (sweating, shakiness, anxiety, confusion, irritability, dizziness, difficulty speaking, lethargy, or loss of consciousness)
- Physical signs indicating high blood sugar (flushed skin confusion, weakness, labored breathing, sweet or fruity breath, nausea, loss of consciousness)
- Clinical conditions associated with insulin resistance (e.g., foot ulcers that are slow to heal)

If diabetes testing is normal, the American Diabetes Association (2011) recommends repeat evaluation every 3 years or more frequently, depending on risk factors.

KnowledgeCheck 27-9

- Identify at least 10 physical examination findings that would lead you to suspect nutritional problems.
- What factors would lead to poor wound healing?

What Laboratory Values Indicate Nutritional Status?

Various laboratory or biochemical indicators provide information about nutritional status. These include blood glucose, serum protein level and associated indices, total lymphocyte count, and hemoglobin. To see the norms for these lab tests,

 Go to Chapter 27, **Diagnostic Testing, Tests Reflecting Nutritional Status: Norms,** in Volume 2.

Blood Glucose

The blood glucose level indicates the amount of fuel available for cellular energy. Levels above the normal set point trigger the release of insulin, which causes the glucose to move into body cells and to be stored in the liver and muscles. A level below the normal set point triggers the release of glucagon, leading to the release of glucose from storage.

Hypoglycemia limits the fuel supply to the body, resulting in symptoms ranging from weakness to coma. Hypoglycemia is usually defined as blood glucose of less than 50 mg/dL, but some people may feel symptoms at higher levels. Often the cause is insufficient food intake, excessive physical exertion, or a disproportionate amount of hypoglycemic agents.

Hyperglycemia (blood glucose greater than 109 mg/dL fasting or greater than 127 mg/dL at random) may be a sign of diabetes mellitus, an endocrine problem, which may develop as a result of either insufficient insulin production or resistance to the existing supply of insulin. A high blood glucose level does not mean that there is more fuel available for cellular energy, though. A characteristic of diabetes is that although there is more than enough glucose in the blood, it cannot enter and be used by the cells. Repeated blood glucose measures are required before making a diagnosis of diabetes mellitus because glucose levels may be temporarily elevated as a result of excessive carbohydrate intake, growth, infection, or emotional and physical stressors.

A rise in blood sugar may produce weakness or fatigue. Prolonged elevations lead to weight loss, blurred vision, **polyphagia** (excessive hunger), **polydipsia** (excessive thirst), increased urination, **ketosis** (incomplete metabolism of fat due to inability to use carbohydrates as fuel), renal failure, and **peripheral neuropathy** (damage to nerves due to prolonged exposure to high glucose levels).

Patients with diabetes usually monitor their own blood sugar levels, but you may need to do it for some. Usually this is done by a fingerstick to obtain capillary blood for testing. Some devices can use blood from alternative sites such as upper arm, forearm, base of thumb, or thigh. Other types of monitors are available. For example, one kind uses a disposable sensor placed just under the skin. The sensor, worn like a watch, communicates with a receiver that reads the levels, and sounds if the blood sugar level is too high or too low. See the Highlights of Procedures box for a summary of the fingerstick procedure. For complete steps,

 Go to Chapter 27, **Procedure 27-1: Checking Fingerstick (Capillary) Blood Glucose Levels,** in Volume 2.

Serum Protein Levels and Indices

Protein molecules dissolve in blood to form plasma proteins. Tissue proteins are a combination of albumin and globulin, so serum protein levels are indicators of *protein stores*.

- **Albumin** is synthesized in the liver and constitutes 60% of total body protein. Low levels of albumin are associated with malnutrition, malabsorption, acute and chronic liver disease, and repeated loss of protein through burns, wounds, or other sources. The half-life of albumin is 18 to 21 days. As a result, there is a lag in detecting nutritional problems based on serum albumin. Albumin is also affected by fluid status and, therefore, is not an accurate measure in the patient with fluid imbalance. For example, a patient in positive fluid balance (taking in more than excreted) will have a falsely low albumin level.
- **Prealbumin** level fluctuates daily and is considered a better marker of acute change than albumin.
- **Transferrin** is a protein that binds with iron. Because it has a half-life of only 8 to 9 days, it allows for faster detection of protein depletion than does measuring albumin. Transferrin can be measured directly or indirectly (by a total iron-binding capacity test [TIBC]). It also reflects iron status. In a person with iron deficiency, the TIBC will be increased; in a person with anemia, the TIBC will be decreased.

Other markers are used to monitor *protein metabolism*:

- **Urea** is formed in the liver as an end product of protein metabolism and is excreted through the kidneys. As such, the serum blood urea nitrogen (BUN) level is an indicator of liver and kidney function. An elevated BUN level is seen with impaired kidney function, dehydration, excessive protein breakdown (often seen with diabetes mellitus, hyperthyroidism, or starvation) or excessive dietary protein intake. Low levels are seen with impaired liver function, fluid overload, and low protein intake.
- **Creatinine**, an end product of skeletal muscle metabolism, is excreted through the kidneys and is an excellent indicator of renal function. Increased levels may indicate impaired kidney function or loss of muscle mass.
- **Lymphocytes**, or white blood cells (WBC), are the body's first line of defense against microorganisms. For a detailed discussion of the role of WBCs in infection

control, as well as a discussion on the types of WBCs and their normal values, see Chapter 23. A decrease in total lymphocytes, known as **leukopenia**, is associated with malnutrition, protein deficiency, alcoholism, bone marrow depression, and anemia.
- **Hemoglobin** is composed of **heme**, an iron-rich compound, and **globulin**, a serum protein. Adequate iron intake is required to produce heme. Therefore, low hemoglobin levels may indicate inadequate iron intake or chronic blood loss. Globulin forms the backbone of hemoglobin as well as antibodies, glycoproteins, lipoproteins, clotting factors, and a variety of key enzymes. A decreased globulin level indicates insufficient protein intake or excessive protein loss.

May I Delegate Nutritional Assessments?

You may safely delegate to nursing assistive personnel (NAPs) the measurement of weight, height, and intake and output; (I&O) other nursing staff (e.g., licensed practical/vocational nurses) can collect a nutritional history. However, the registered nurse (RN) is responsible for reviewing and interpreting these findings. When delegating these tasks, you must also tell the NAP or licensed practical nurse (LPN) how often the measurements are to be made. Review Chapter 7 for making delegation decisions.

 KnowledgeCheck 27-10

- What are the likely causes of hyperglycemia?
- Why is it important to identify the serum albumin level?

 ThinkLike a Nurse 27-7

The Nutrition Screening Initiative (NSI) is completed for a 70-year-old.

- What major indicator on the NSI would indicate impaired nutritional status?
- What minor indicator would you likely see?
- What would malnourishment look like in the adult?
- What type of anthropometric findings would be typical of an older adult with poor nutrition patterns?
- What type of laboratory values would support impaired nutritional status?

ANALYSIS/NURSING DIAGNOSIS

For clients who have no symptoms of or risk factors for nutrition problems, use the diagnostic label Readiness for Enhanced Nutrition. NANDA-I defines this as "a pattern of nutrient intake that is sufficient for meeting metabolic needs and can be strengthened" (2012, p. 67).

Nutrition as the Problem

You can use the following NANDA-I labels to describe general nutrition problems:

- Adult Failure to Thrive
- Imbalanced Nutrition: Less Than Body Requirements
- Imbalanced Nutrition: More Than Body Requirements

- Risk for Imbalanced Nutrition: More Than Body Requirements
- Self-Care Deficit (Feeding)

As you have learned, nutrition problems have many causes. Etiologies for undernutrition include eating disorders, difficulties with chewing and swallowing, vomiting, alcoholism, food intolerances, metabolic disorders, digestive disorders, and absorption disorders. For overnutrition, etiologies include overeating, lack of exercise, and metabolic or endocrine disorders. The following nursing diagnoses may contribute to nutrition problems: Diarrhea, Health Behaviors (Nutrition), Impaired Swallowing, Nausea, Noncompliance (with prescribed diet), and Deficient Knowledge (nutrition).

The following is an example of a nutrition nursing diagnosis statement:

Imbalanced Nutrition: Less Than Body Requirements related to difficulty chewing and Impaired Swallowing

Nutrition as the Etiology

Nutritional problems can also be the etiology of problems in other functional areas, for example:

- Ineffective Breastfeeding r/t inadequate milk production 2° insufficient intake of calories and fluids
- Constipation r/t insufficient intake of fluids and fiber
- Diarrhea r/t excessive intake of alcohol and/or sugar
- Risk for Infection r/t inadequate intake of calories and protein
- Impaired (or Risk for Impaired) Skin Integrity r/t inadequate intake of protein and/or vitamin A
- Disturbed Sleep Pattern r/t excessive caffeine intake or to eating fatty and spicy foods near bedtime
- Impaired Social Interaction r/t low self-esteem 2° obesity

PLANNING OUTCOMES/EVALUATION

The overall *Healthy People 2020* nutrition goal for the United States population is to "promote health and reduce chronic disease associated with diet and weight" (U.S. Department of Health and Human Services [USDHHS], 2010, updated 2012). For specific objectives related to that goal,

 Go to Chapter 27, **Tables, Boxes, Figures: ESG Box 27-3, Nutrition and Weight Status Objectives From Healthy People 2020,** on Davis*Plus.*

 Also see the **Healthy People 2020** home page at www.healthypeople.gov

NOC standardized outcomes directly linked to nutritional problems include the following: Nutritional Status, Nutritional Status: Food and Fluid Intake, Nutritional Status: Nutrient Intake, and Weight Control.

You would choose other NOC outcomes based on the patient's nursing diagnosis. For example, for Situational

Low Self-Esteem related to obesity, you might use Self-Esteem; for Noncompliance (prescribed diet), you could use Adherence Behavior, Compliance Behavior, or Treatment Behavior: Illness/Injury.

Individualized goals/outcome statements you might write for a patient with nutrition-related problems include the following:

Loses 1 lb per week until ideal weight is attained.
Follows the prescribed modified diet that, at a minimum, meets the DRIs.
Eats a variety of foods that provide a balanced diet.

PLANNING INTERVENTIONS/IMPLEMENTATION

NIC standardized interventions directly linked to nutrition problems include the broad interventions of Nutrition Management, Nutrition Therapy, Nutritional Counseling, and Nutritional Monitoring. These interventions could probably be used for most nutrition problems, regardless of the etiologies. The other 13 interventions grouped under Nutritional Support address specific etiologies (e.g., Swallowing Therapy).

 Go to Chapter 27, **Standardized Language, NOC Outcomes and NIC Interventions Related to Nutrition,** on Davis*Plus.*

Individualized nursing actions are determined by the patient's nursing diagnosis. They may include, for example, counseling regarding vitamin and mineral supplementation, teaching clients on a limited budget how to buy nutritious foods, supporting special nutritional needs, and assisting clients with meals. These are discussed in the rest of this chapter.

Vitamin and Mineral Supplementation

Do you take a vitamin tablet every day? Do you know anyone who takes megadoses of vitamin C to prevent a cold? Or zinc to cure one? Noncredentialed nutrition "experts" recommend, and sell, megadoses of the entire alphabet of vitamin and mineral supplements to prevent cancer and heart attacks, improve your sex life, prevent aging, and work other miracles. However, conservative health professionals are often skeptical of high dose vitamin supplements, insisting that a nutritious diet supplies all the micronutrients you need. Somewhere in the middle, most likely, lies the truth. A growing body of research suggests that certain supplements provide health benefits, particularly calcium and vitamin D. Remember, too, that RDAs and AIs are for "average" needs. Individual needs for micronutrients vary. During periods of increased nutrient demands, it may be difficult to get enough nutrients from diet alone.

NIC Intervention—Nutritional Counseling

When teaching clients about supplements, keep the following principles in mind:

1. Dietary supplements may be appropriate for people whose diet does not provide the recommended

intake of specific vitamins. With a few exceptions, there is little evidence to suggest that people will be harmed by taking vitamin supplements in appropriate amounts (AHRQ, 2003).

2. Individual needs vary, and those needs should determine the specific nutrients and amounts used. For example:

   - Newborn infants are given a vitamin K injection to prevent hemorrhaging because they do not yet have bacterial flora in the gut to synthesize enough vitamin K.
   - Breastfed infants may need a vitamin D supplement (but not other vitamins) if the mother does not have an adequate diet or if the baby does not receive enough exposure to sunlight. Fetal iron stores are depleted at 4 to 6 months, so breastfed infants also need iron supplementation at that age.
   - Vegetarians who eat little or no animal products may need vitamin B_{12} or vitamin D supplementation.
   - Overweight children and those who have type 1 diabetes or hypertension, particularly Latino and African American children, are at risk for vitamin D deficiency.
   - Folic acid supplementation is recommended for people taking methotrexate (a drug used to treat certain types of cancer).
   - All women who are capable of becoming pregnant should take a daily folic acid supplement of 400 to 800 mcg in addition to the naturally occurring folate they eat in foods. Pregnant women need at least 600 mcg daily.
   - Most adults older than 50 years should obtain vitamin B_{12} from fortified foods or supplements.
   - Women age 50 and older should take calcium supplements to prevent osteoporosis; there is growing evidence that men may need to do so as well. Adults in the United States do not typically obtain adequate calcium from their diets.
   - Most calcium supplements come in combination with vitamin D to promote absorption of the calcium.
   - People who do not eat dairy products need supplemental calcium.

3. Food is the best source of nutrients. Supplements do not replace the need to eat a nutritious diet. Vitamins need carbohydrate, protein, and fat to do their work. Specific supplements for certain individual situations are more effective if the person also has an adequate diet.

4. Read supplement labels carefully. They provide information about toxicity levels, dosage, and side effects.

5. Encourage patients to ask their primary care provider's advice before taking vitamins.

6. Advise patients to follow the dosages recommended in the DRIs or RDAs.

7. Be certain that any health claims made for a supplement are based on sound research.

8. The long-term effects of most nutritional supplements have yet to be fully researched.

The same principles apply with regard to mineral supplementation. Supplements of specific minerals may be needed during growth periods (i.e., pregnancy, lactation, and adolescence), but as a rule healthy adults eating balanced diets do not need supplements. People who require mineral supplementation include those who refuse dairy products (and therefore lack calcium), and those with clinical problems such as iron-deficiency anemia, zinc deficiency (e.g., in alcoholism and long-term low-calorie diets), and treatment with certain diuretics (e.g., for hypertension).

Nutritious Foods on a Limited Budget

Hunger and malnutrition are not unusual among the poor in the United States. When your clients cannot afford to buy food, you should teach them about available assistance and make appropriate referrals to programs such as the following:

Supplemental Nutrition Assistance Program (SNAP) This is the new name for the federal Food Stamp Program. For low-income households, this program issues coupons that can be used to buy food to cover the household's needs.

Commodity Supplemental Food Program The federal government buys surplus food items to support certain agricultural products. These include both perishable and nonperishable commodities (e.g., peanut butter, cheese, green beans). The foods are made available to low-income pregnant and breastfeeding women, infants, children younger than 6 years old, and older adults at least 60 years old.

Women, Infants, and Children (WIC) This federal program provides free food to low-income women who are pregnant or breastfeeding and to children younger than age 5. Typical available foods are milk, eggs, cheese, cereals, juice, and infant formulas. They are intended to supplement the diet with protein, iron, and vitamins. They are not meant to supply all necessary food for the household.

National School Lunch and Breakfast Programs These federally assisted programs subsidize schools that provide free or reduced-rate breakfasts and/or lunches to low-income children. All students pay slightly less than the full cost of the meal. Lunches must supply about one-third of the child's DRIs for energy and nutrients.

NIC Intervention—Teaching: Individual

You can help your clients to use their food dollars creatively by teaching them to follow the suggestions in the Self-Care box.

Teaching Your Patients to Buy Nutritious Foods on a Limited Budget

Plan Ahead

➤ Look at the grocery advertisements in the paper or in their fliers, and plan meals around the sale items that are also the most nutrient dense.

➤ Make a list of the foods you need. This will help you to control impulse buying and extra trips to the store.

➤ Avoid eating at fast-food restaurants. Meals are more expensive and less nutritious than those you can prepare at home.

➤ If transportation is not a problem, buy fresh foods at farmers' markets, at consumer co-ops, and from neighbors who have gardens.

Buy Wisely

➤ Buy generic instead of more expensive and widely advertised brands.

➤ Watch for sales of nutrient-dense items. Stock up on and freeze them for future use if you do not need them right away.

➤ Buy in quantity—if it results in real savings and if you can use that amount of food before it spoils.

➤ Limit convenience foods (e.g., frozen dinners); they are expensive and often high in fat and sodium.

➤ Buy foods when they are in season; for example, fresh tomatoes are less expensive, and better tasting, in the summer than in the winter.

➤ Purchase oatmeal and cream of wheat instead of cold, sugared cereals. Buy in bulk rather than single-serving packages.

➤ Avoid shopping at convenience stores. Items are usually more expensive than in supermarkets.

➤ Buy inexpensive cuts of meat; avoid processed lunchmeats and hot dogs.

➤ Buy frozen concentrated fruit juices instead of juice in plastic jugs and cardboard boxes.

➤ Substitute dairy products, beans and lentils, and peanut butter for more expensive meat. Substitute powdered milk for whole milk.

➤ Read the Nutrition Facts panels on prepared foods to be sure you obtain the most nutrition for the money.

Supporting Special Nutritional Needs

Patients with impaired dietary intake and those who experience difficulty with swallowing, digestion, or elimination require specific nutritional interventions, such as the following.

Patients with Impaired Dietary Intake

Nutritional health is related to the type and amount of food patients consume. Physical illnesses that alter appetite, taste, and smell impair dietary intake. Medical restriction in intake, such as NPO, also affects nutritional status. Other factors leading to poor nutritional health include impaired ability to purchase and prepare nutritious food, and feed self.

Patients Who Have Nausea Nausea can cause vomiting and loss of appetite, leading to Impaired Nutrition. Nursing interventions include assessing for the cause of the nausea, and providing comfort and prevention measures. For other interventions,

 Go to **Clinical Insight 27-5: Interventions for Patients Who Have Nausea,** in Volume 2.

Loss of Appetite; Diminished Sense of Smell and Taste Refer to the section Stimulating the Patient's Appetite, later in this chapter.

NPO Patients who are to receive nothing by mouth (NPO) must receive glucose and electrolytes through either intravenous (IV) fluids (e.g., ½ NS, D5W, Lactated Ringers solutions), or total parenteral nutrition (TPN) and IV lipid infusion to meet the body's fluid and nutritional needs for prolonged periods of NPO.

✚ Remember, too, that remaining NPO for more than 3 days puts the patient at risk for malnutrition.

▪ Provide comfort measures for patients who cannot take food and fluids orally. Assist the patient with or provide oral hygiene. If allowed, provide ice chips, hard candy, chewing gum, or sips of water for rinsing the mouth.

▪ Advise family or visitors not to eat or drink around the patient, and try to schedule other activities for the patient at mealtimes.

   ▪ When older adults must be NPO for tests or procedures, schedule them early in the day to decrease the length of time the patient must be NPO. If testing must be late in the day, ask the primary care provider whether the patient can have an early breakfast.

Self-Care Deficit: Feeding You will find interventions in the section Assisting Patients With Meals.

Poor Selection of Nutritious Foods Advise clients to eat nutrient-dense foods and to eat essential foods first.

   Because the sense of taste is decreased, older adults may prefer concentrated sweets; and because they may also have a poor appetite, once they eat sweets they may not be hungry enough to eat other foods.

At least one study suggests that dementia, especially Alzheimer's disease, is less common among people who eat fruits and vegetables daily, eat fish once a week, and use fats rich in omega-3 fatty acids (e.g., walnut and soy oils) (Barberger-Gateau, Raffaitin, Letenneur, et al., 2007). Although this merely suggests there may be a connection, clients can benefit from this dietary advice.

Limited Ability to Purchase Nutritional Food Adults and children living in impoverished situations may qualify for government entitlement (e.g., Food Stamps, School Lunch Program) to supplement nutritional needs. Additionally, private, religious, and other charitable agencies (e.g., Harvesters) offer meals to those in need. Meals on Wheels are directed to the seniors living independently in their homes but who may have limited ability to buy and prepare nutritious meals. Refer to the Self-Care box Teaching Your Patients to Buy Nutritious Foods on a Limited Budget.

Patients with Impaired Swallowing, Digestion, or Elimination

Nutritional health is due in part to digestive function from **mastication** (chewing) all the way through passing stool. Dysfunction of the GI tract can reduce the transport, absorption, and elimination of food nutrients.

Dry Mouth This is typically an age-associated change. Advise clients to avoid caffeine; alcohol; tobacco; and dry, bulky, spicy, salty, or highly acidic foods. Offer sugarless hard candy or chewing gum to stimulate salivation (unless the patient has dementia). Use lip moisturizer and encourage frequent sips of water.

Impaired Swallowing The NANDA-I diagnosis Impaired Swallowing may be caused by mechanical obstruction (e.g., tumor), neuromuscular impairment (e.g., facial paralysis), stroke, cerebral palsy, or a host of other anatomical or physiological defects. Nutritional support for patients with Impaired Swallowing includes activities from the NIC intervention, Swallowing Therapy (Bulecheck, Butcher, Dochterman, et al., 2012, pp. 369–370). For a list of these activities,

 Go to **Clinical Insight 27-4: Interventions for Patients With Impaired Swallowing,** in Volume 2.

Gastroesophageal Reflux Advise clients not to eat just before bedtime and to elevate the head of the bed 30° to 40° to allow food to move out of the stomach before lying flat. It is also important to avoid overeating and bending over, and to take prescribed medications. They should also avoid fruit juices, fatty foods, chocolate, alcohol, and smoking; all of the stimulate reflux. If overweight, the client with reflux should lose weight.

Decreased Gastric Secretions To promote digestion for those with lessened gastric secretions, encourage regular meals, thorough chewing, and prescribed medication as needed. Food rich in vitamin D aids in calcium absorption.

Constipation To prevent problems with bowel elimination, advise patient to consume foods high in fiber. Soluble fiber allows more water to remain in the stool, which makes it softer and easier to pass. Insoluble fiber adds bulk to the stool for easier defecation. Patients should drink plenty of water—at least 64 ounces daily. Also, encourage exercise as physical activity aids GI motility needed to pass stool.

Glucose Intolerance Patients with glucose intolerance and insulin resistance should avoid concentrated, refined sugars, unless they have been told to use it to treat hypoglycemia. Complex carbohydrates (e.g., whole-grain cereals, vegetables) are better tolerated. Smaller, more frequent, nutritious meals may also be necessary.

Assisting Patients With Meals

Some patients are at risk for nutritional deficits as a result of a Self-Care Deficit (Feeding), which may be caused by loss of cognitive, musculoskeletal, or neuromuscular function; weakness; pain; or environmental barriers. Elderly patients, especially, are at risk for undernutrition or malnourishment in inpatient settings.

You should institute special nutrition interventions in patients who have one of the following:

- An involuntary weight loss of more than 5% in 30 days or 10% in 180 days.
- Leaving more than one-fourth of their food in the past 7 days or two-thirds of meals (based on a 2,000-kcal diet).
- A BMI of 19 or less.

NIC Interventions for this situation are Feeding and Self-Care Assistance: Feeding. Important nursing actions include assisting patients with meals. Other nursing activities include the following:

- Assess for functional deficits that contribute to Self-Care Deficit or Imbalanced Nutrition.
- Monitor intake for nutritional adequacy. Some patients may need liquid oral supplements of protein and calories.
- Collaborate with occupational and physical therapists in planning care.
- See that the patient has protein- and energy-enriched meals.
- Provide mid-afternoon snacks.
- Ensure the nutrition prescribed is actually implemented. Assign someone to be responsible for assisting the patient with meals as necessary. Include this in your instructions to NAPs and other assistive personnel.
- Refer the patient and family to an agency that can help them obtain a home health aide.

For guidelines more specific to assisting with meals, including care of patients with dementia,

 Go to Chapter 27, **Clinical Insight 27-6: Assisting Patients With Meals,** in Volume 2.

Example Problem: Overweight and Obesity

The BMI is commonly used to define weight status. A client with a BMI greater than 25 but less than 30 is considered **overweight** (or pre-obese). **Obesity** is a BMI of 30 or higher. The CDC data for 2009–2012 indicate more than one-third of adults over 20 years old are overweight (and not obese), while almost 36% are obese. Obesity rates did not differ between men and women. Almost 17% of youth were obese in 2009–2010. (UDHHS, CDC, National Center for Health Statistics, 2012).

Obesity and overweight together affect two-thirds of our adult population, and are associated with chronic diseases such as diabetes, hypertension, coronary artery disease and stroke, gallbladder disease, gout, and obstructive sleep apnea. A person who is 40% overweight is twice as likely to die prematurely as a normal-weight person (Ogden, Carroll, Kit, et al., 2012). Therefore, as a nurse you can assist your clients to achieve and maintain a healthy weight.

Obesity in Older Adults

The proportion of obese older adults has doubled in the past 30 years. Nevertheless, most older adults lead active and healthy lives and are not obese. Obesity is more prevalent in adults younger than age 70 and becomes less prevalent after that. Still, more than 15% of older adults are obese (Newman, 2009). However, according to the BMI thresholds set by the WHO, older people considered to be overweight are not at a greater mortality risk (Flicker, McCaul, Hankey, et al., 2010).

As we age we tend to be less active physically, but our eating patterns do not usually change. In addition, aging is associated with hormonal changes and slowing metabolism that cause accumulation of fat (e.g., decreased growth hormone and serum testosterone). Many of the chronic problems associated with aging are made worse by obesity (e.g., respiratory problems, arthritis, cardiovascular disease, cancer, and diabetes). For example, maintaining a BMI of less than 25 is particularly important in reducing diabetes risk, such as damage to the eyes, heart, kidneys, and other organs (National Diabetes Education Program, 2011).

Interventions are the same as for other groups: dietary modification, exercise, and use of community supports. Older adults may require more assistance in improving physical function so that they can exercise more. To avoid injuries, exercise should start at low intensity and progress gradually over several months.

ANALYSIS/NURSING DIAGNOSIS: OVERWEIGHT AND OBESITY

NANDA-I diagnoses define overweight and obesity in the following ways:

Imbalanced Nutrition: More Than Body Requirements is used when a person consumes nutrients in excess of metabolic needs. The defining characteristics are (1) triceps skinfold greater than 15 mm in men and 25 mm in women, or (2) weight 20% over ideal for height and frame.

Risk for Imbalanced Nutrition: More Than Body Requirements identifies the potential for an individual to experience intake of nutrients in excess of metabolic needs.

Etiologies Etiologies of the two preceding NANDA-I diagnoses include the following:

- Consuming more kcal than needed for activity, gender, height, and weight
- Reducing activity level without modifying food intake
- Genetic predisposition to obesity. For example, low BMR and excess adipose tissue distribution are common in certain ethnic groups.
- Ineffective coping mechanisms—for instance, the use of binge eating to reduce anxiety or relieve boredom
- Cultural influences—some cultural norms encourage excess weight, particularly as an indication of wealth.
- Decreased levels of thyroid hormone can lower BMR, causing weight gain.
- Ineffective Health Maintenance—for example, high-fat diet, inactivity, and avoidance of health assistance
- Impaired Physical Mobility, which limits physical activity and decreases energy expenditure

Obesity as Etiology of Other Problems Being overweight may lead to the development of other nursing diagnoses. Excess weight, and especially obesity, makes activity more difficult; therefore, over time, the person becomes more sedentary, and the body becomes deconditioned (weakened). The following are examples:

- Activity Intolerance r/t deconditioned state secondary to long-term sedentary lifestyle
- Decreased Cardiac Output r/t prolonged deconditioned state
- Constipation r/t inadequate physical activity
- Risk for Injury (and/or Risk for Falls) r/t deconditioned state and generalized weakness
- Social Isolation r/t poor self-image secondary to excess weight

PLANNING OUTCOMES/EVALUATION: OVERWEIGHT AND OBESITY

A part of your nursing role will be to work with clients to help achieve the Healthy People 2020 nutrition goals. To review them,

 Go to Chapter 27, **Tables, Boxes, Figures: ESG Box 27-3, Nutrition and Weight Status Objectives From Healthy People 2020,** on DavisPlus.

For *NOC standardized outcomes* for evaluating weight:

 Go to Chapter 27, **Standardized Language, NOC Outcomes, and NIC Interventions for Overweight/Obesity and Underweight/Malnutrition,** on DavisPlus.

Individualized goals/outcome statements include the following examples:

States pertinent factors contributing to weight gain.
Designs dietary modifications to meet individual long-term goal of weight control.

Accomplishes desired weight loss in a reasonable time frame (1 to 2 lb/week).

Incorporates appropriate physical activities requiring energy expenditure into daily life.

PLANNING INTERVENTIONS/IMPLEMENTATION: OVERWEIGHT AND OBESITY

For the *NIC standardized interventions* for overweight and obese clients,

 Go to Chapter 27, **Standardized Language, NOC Outcomes and NIC Interventions for Overweight/Obesity and Underweight/Malnutrition,** on Davis*Plus.*

Individualized nursing activities include the following:

- *Weigh the client weekly under the same conditions.* Weekly weighs allow the client to monitor his progress and can motivate him to follow the weight-loss regimen.
- *Suggest keeping a food diary for a number of days or weeks.* Research suggests that this can double diet weight loss. Analyzing the diary will provide valuable information on intake and circumstances that trigger eating. It may help to identify behavioral or coping issues. Keep in mind that many patients eat less than usual when they are keeping a food diary (Hollis, Gullion, Stevens, et al., 2008).
- *Educate the client about a healthy diet.* Lifestyle changes must be ongoing to maintain weight loss. For the client, the first step is to learn about a balanced diet and food quality.
- *Encourage the client to eat more fresh fruits and vegetables and fewer fatty foods and sugar-sweetened beverages.*
- *Discuss fat substitutes.* These are available to improve flavor and texture of low-fat foods while reducing total dietary fat. Recall that fats contain 9 kcal per gram, so reducing fat intake is an important part of most weight-loss diets. Fat substitutes are not absorbed; therefore, they contribute few kcal. The American Heart Association (n.d.b) states that fat substitutes, used appropriately, can provide flexibility in diet planning. Although the USDA (FDA) generally considers fat substitutes to be safe, long-term benefits and risks are not yet known. In addition, it is not unusual for people to experience diarrhea and stomach cramps when using fat substitutes.

- *Encourage the client to commit to regular exercise.* Increased physical activity will not only use up excess stores of fat but also increase the body's resting metabolic rate. Individuals should begin gradually with low-impact activities, such as walking for 20 minutes at least four times a week. The American College of Sports Medicine (ACSM) recommends 150 to 250 minutes of exercise per week to prevent weight gain. More than 250 minutes per week are needed to bring about significant weight loss—that is, 50 minutes on 5 days of the week or 40 minutes on 6 days of the week (Donnelly, Blair, Jakicic, et al., 2009; USDHHS, 2008). Although increased physical activity aids in weight control, advise your client to set realistic expectations for what exercise can achieve. A recent study concludes that overeating, more than a lack of exercise, is to blame for the American obesity epidemic (Swinburn, Sacks, Lo, et al., 2009).
- *Be encouraging and nonjudgmental.* Do so especially when there are setbacks.
- *Provide weight loss tips.* See the Self-Care box Teaching Weight Loss Tips.
- *For children, recommend the 5-2-1-0 program* (Marion County Children's Alliance, 2012). Children should have:
  5 – Servings of fruits and vegetables each day.
  2 – Hours or less of "screen" time per day.
  1 – Hour of physical activity per day.
  0 – Servings of sweetened beverages.

Self-Care

Teaching Weight Loss Tips

Getting Ready

Make a commitment.
➤ Promise yourself; promise others: "I will do this."

Set realistic goals.
➤ Aim to lose 1 to 2 lb/week. To do this you need to burn 500 to 1,000 calories more than you consume. Losing weight faster usually means losing water weight or muscle tissue rather than fat.

➤ Set "process" rather than "outcome" goals. For example, "I will exercise every day" instead of "I will lose 10 pounds this month." Changing your habits (your "processes") is the key to weight loss.

➤ Write your goals, your plan for achieving them, and your start date. This makes it reality, not just a thought.

➤ Review your goals each week. Readjust them as needed. If you are exercising more than you thought, adjust your goal upward, for example.

Plan for setbacks.
➤ Identify situations that might trigger eating or interfere with exercise; plan specific actions you will take to overcome them.

Continued

Beginning New Behaviors

Eat healthier foods.

➤ Eat more low glycemic fruits and high fiber vegetables.

➤ Limit fatty foods. Grill meats and vegetables rather than fry them. Substitute non-fat Greek yogurt for mayonnaise and sour cream. Try substituting applesauce in recipes that call for vegetable oil.

➤ Avoid sugar-sweetened beverages and high-sugar snacks. Consume foods with whole grains instead of those with bleached, processed flour. Sweeten food with agave or honey instead of refined sugar.

➤ Try using natural herbs and spices, extracts, and citrus to flavor food instead of adding salt and sugar.

➤ Be sure to add healthy foods to your diet, such as black beans, kale, walnuts and almonds, dark chocolate, pumpkin, quinoa, red wine, Brussels sprouts, eggplant, lentils, steel-cut oats, red beets, tuna, sweet potatoes, lean meat and fish, tomatoes, chia seeds, blueberries, spinach, flax seeds, and extra virgin olive oil.

➤ Don't be fooled by seemingly healthy foods. For example, light microwave popcorn contains high levels of sodium and the chemical diacetyl. Use a little extra virgin olive oil and balsamic vinegar instead of "light" salad dressings. Trail mix often contains chocolate chips or candies. Granola is high in sugar. Artichoke/spinach dip is high in fat. Flavored fat-free yogurt contains added sugar and artificial flavoring. Eat whole, natural foods without chemical additives and preservatives.

➤ Organic foods are healthier in that they reduce exposure to pesticide residues and antibiotic-resistant bacteria. But the published literature lacks strong evidence that organic foods are significantly more nutritious (Smith-Spangler, Brandeau, Hunter, et al., 2012).

Get active and stay active.

➤ If you have not been exercising, start slowly and build steadily, listening to your body's natural cues signaling injury.

➤ Work up to at least 250 minutes per week to lose weight and maintain the loss.

Get adequate sleep.

➤ For most people, this is 7 to 8 hours a night.

➤ New research suggests that sleep deprivation can affect levels of the appetite-regulating hormones leptin and ghrelin.

➤ Sleep loss can affect the type of food you crave. When you are tired you are less able to cope with stress and emotional triggers for eating, and more likely to crave comfort foods such as chocolate and ice cream.

"Sticking With It"

Keep a food diary.

➤ Recording what you eat can double your weight loss.

Decide what and when to eat.

➤ Decide what foods you will eat as well as when you will eat. For example, "I will eat only at the table, 3 meals and 2 snacks daily."

➤ Make a conscious effort to take small bites and eat slowly.

➤ Serve your food on small plates.

Shop wisely.

➤ Shop for food on a full stomach.

➤ Read food labels when purchasing food (for information about calorie and fat content).

Find ways to exercise.

➤ Lay out your exercise clothing ahead of time (e.g., at night if you exercise in the morning).

➤ Use the stairs instead of the elevator; park in the back of the parking lot, as far from the door as possible.

➤ Walk or bike to work when possible.

Get emotional support.

➤ Family members can help by not offering you desserts. Weight-loss support groups let you know you are not alone. An exercise partner can help keep you motivated.

Recognize lifestyle changes must be permanent.

Key Point: *Remember: Healthy eating, physical activity, and sleep are necessities, not luxuries!*

- *For children and adolescents,* weight loss is more effective when it involves the child, the parents, and the community in limiting soda (deRuyter, Olthof, Seidel, et al., 2012; Ebbeling, Feldman, Chomitz, et al., 2012) and junk food consumption and limiting hours spent watching television and playing video games. Children can be taught to make "best choices" regarding activities and the foods they eat (Speroni, Early, & Atherton, 2007). To learn more about obesity in adolescents and children,

 Go to Chapter 27, **Reading More About Nutrition,** on DavisPlus.

To see a sample care plan and care map for Imbalanced Nutrition: More than Body Requirements,

 Go to Student Resources, **Care Plan, Imbalanced Nutrition: More Than Body Requirements,** and **Care Map, Imbalanced Nutrition: More Than Body Requirements,** in Chapter 27, on DavisPlus.

Example Problem: Underweight and Undernutrition?

A BMI of less than 18.5 is considered underweight (see Box 27-4). For patients in long-term care settings, parameters include one of the following:

1. Involuntary weight loss of more than 5% in 30 days or 10% in 180 days
2. Leaving more than one-quarter of food in the past 7 days or two-thirds of meals based on a 2,000-kcal diet
3. A BMI of 19 or less

For hospitalized patients with serious illness, increased mortality is associated with a BMI of 21 or less (CDC, n.d., updated 2011).

A person becomes underweight when he consumes fewer kcal than needed based on his activity, sex, height, and weight. Consuming too few kcal may result in serious undernutrition; that is, insufficient intake of protein, fat, vitamins, and minerals. The causes of underweight status may be psychological, social, economic, or physiological (e.g., hospitalization, self-care deficits, illness, eating disorders). A person can also be malnourished with regard to specific nutrients without being underweight.

What Are the Signs of Severe Malnutrition?

Malnutrition is a condition of impaired development or function caused by a long-term deficiency, excess, or imbalance in energy and/or nutrient intake. Malnutrition caused by deficiency of protein in a diet that is primarily starches is called **kwashiorkor**. When protein sources in food are scarce and overall caloric intake is low, **marasmus** occurs, particularly in young children. Undernourished people are prone to infections. Symptoms of undernutrition resulting from insufficient food are reduced physical activity, weight loss, reduced height, abdominal enlargement, and hair loss. Other diseases develop as a result of specific vitamin and mineral deficiency, such as beriberi (neurological deficits), scurvy (delayed wound healing and poor bone growth), and pellagra (diarrhea and dementia). See Tables 27-4 and 27-5 for specific signs of vitamin and mineral excesses and deficits.

Malnutrition is most common in underdeveloped nations and among children, older adults, and people with chronic illnesses such as cancer, HIV, and COPD. Others at risk for malnutrition include those with the following:

- Serum albumin level 3.5 g/dL or less
- Nausea or vomiting lasting 3 days or more
- Clear liquid diet or NPO for 3 days or longer
- Increased nutritional requirements (e.g., wound healing, burns)
- Recent, unplanned loss of 10% or more of patient's usual weight

To assess for malnutrition in children, compare weight, height, and head circumference to the standards (norms) for the child's age. In cases of severe malnutrition, abdominal circumference can signal worsening disease. Other indicators in children include the presence of iron deficiency anemia and, in adolescents, a delay of stages of sexual maturation.

ANALYSIS/NURSING DIAGNOSIS: UNDERWEIGHT AND UNDERNUTRITION

Undernutrition as Problem When undernutrition is the focus of the patient's problem, the following NANDA-I labels may apply:

Adult Failure to Thrive
Imbalanced Nutrition: Less than Body Requirements

When the patient is at higher than normal risk for undernutrition, you can use *Risk for Imbalanced Nutrition: Less than Body Requirements*; however, this is not a NANDA-I diagnosis.

Undernutrition as Etiology Imbalanced Nutrition: Less Than Body Requirements may be the etiology of other nursing diagnoses. Compare the two following examples:

Imbalanced Nutrition: Less Than Body Requirements r/t Impaired Swallowing 2° pain with swallowing
Risk for Disproportionate Growth r/t Imbalanced Nutrition: Less Than Body Requirements 2° anorexia nervosa

For other etiologies and related diagnoses, and for help in choosing which to use for a patient,

 Go to Chapter 27, **Standardized Language, Nursing Diagnoses Associated with Undernutrition,** on DavisPlus.

Eating Disorders

Eating disorders stem from social pressures to be thin, fashion styled for slender body types, and even societal prejudices against people with obesity. Although all segments of society are affected, eating disorders are more common in women, and most report the onset of illness before the age of 20.

Anorexia Nervosa is a psychiatric disorder characterized by self-imposed, self-starvation. Some common physical signs include:

- Refusal to maintain body weight at or above minimally normal weight for age
- Intense preoccupation with weight and body shape
- Excessive facial or body hair (because of inadequate protein in the diet)
- Thinning, dry hair or hair loss
- Feeling cold and having a lower than normal body temperature
- Absent or irregular menstruation

Bulimia Nervosa refers to binge eating (eating an excessive amount of food in a short period of time) followed by self-induced vomiting or laxative abuse to purge food. People with bulimia people also have many of the same physical signs as anorexia as well as tooth decay or erosion of enamel resulting from repeated vomiting. Salivary glands are swollen. People with bulimia lack energy, feel bloated, and have low levels of potassium and other serum electrolytes. Feelings of guilt, anxiety, or depression are common.

Serious medical complications for anorexia and bulimia nervosa include osteoporosis and increased risk for fractures; brain damage; decreased resistance to infection; cardiac, renal, liver, and metabolic disorders; and even death. You will need to recognize the warning signs of eating disorders, such as the behavior changes described in Box 27-6.

PLANNING OUTCOMES/EVALUATION: UNDERWEIGHT AND UNDERNUTRITION

The NOC standardized outcome for assessing weight is Weight: Body Mass. If it becomes necessary to monitor nutritional status, you could use the labels of Nutritional Status: Food and Fluid Intake and Nutritional Status: Nutrient Intake.

Individualized goals/outcome statements include the following:

Progressively gains weight toward desired goal.
Verbalizes willingness to follow diet.
Body mass and weight are within normal limits.
Laboratory values (e.g., albumin, CBC) are within normal limits.
Recognizes factors contributing to underweight.

PLANNING INTERVENTIONS/IMPLEMENTATION: UNDERWEIGHT AND UNDERNUTRITION

NIC standardized interventions for undernutrition include Appetite, Nutritional Status, and Weight: Body Mass. For others,

---

BOX 27-6 ■ Warning Signs of an Eating Disorder

Food Behaviors
- Deliberate self-starvation with weight loss.
- Continuous dieting.
- Skips meals.
- Takes only tiny portions.
- Will not eat in front of others.
- Always has an excuse not to eat.
- Usually has a diet soda or coffee in hand.
- Eats only food that is low in fat.

Appearance and Body Image Behaviors
- Wears baggy clothes.
- Complains of being fat.
- Obsesses about clothing size.
- Spends lots of time looking in the mirror.

Exercise Behaviors
- Exercises excessively and compulsively.
- May tire easily.
- Pushes self beyond normal expectations.

Social Behaviors
- Tries to please everyone and withdraws if unsuccessful.
- Tries to care for everyone but self.
- Tries to control what and where family eats.
- Relationships tend to be superficial or dependent.

Emotional Behaviors
- Intense fear of gaining weight

 Go to Chapter 27, **Standardized Language, NOC Outcomes and NIC Interventions for Adult Failure to Thrive, Overweight/Obesity and Underweight/Malnutrition,** on *DavisPlus.*

Individualized nursing activities for clients who are underweight or undernourished include the following:

- **Assess for recent changes in physiological status as underlying cause of weight loss or undernourishment** (e.g., pain, fatigue, illness, and immobility).
- **Offer high-calorie and high-protein (nutrient-dense) foods.** Serve these foods when the person is most likely to be hungry. Avoid food with little nutritional value; when intake is limited, it is essential that it not be wasted on empty calories.
- **Consult with a dietitian.** Discuss strategies to increase the nutritional content of foods.
- **Weigh the client regularly under the same conditions.** Weigh the client one to two times per week if nutritional status is severely jeopardized to assess the effectiveness of the therapeutic plan.

- **Offer high-protein supplements.** Offer nutritious high-protein supplements between meals to increase intake of protein and kcal. It may be easier for the client to drink a small amount of a supplement than to eat enough food to supply the equivalent nutrients.
- **Suggest community resources** (e.g., Meals on Wheels for clients with Adult Failure to Thrive). Additional assistance may be needed to improve access to food.
- **For eating disorders, see that the client is referred for appropriate counseling** (e.g., dietitian, mental health professional).

The following sections discuss more fully nursing interventions for improving the appetite, as well as alternative feeding methods.

Stimulating the Patient's Appetite

Illness, with its accompanying pain, anxiety, and medications, often causes appetite loss. This is especially true for institutionalized patients, who have little control over food choices and preparation. You will need to make an effort to see that hospitalized patients eat the food that is served. It is not enough merely to order meals and deliver the trays. The following measures may help improve appetite and intake and, subsequently, nutritional status:

- **Offer frequent, small meals.** This helps prevent gastric distention and improves appetite by keeping the patient from being overwhelmed with a large amount of food.
- **Suggest smokers refrain for 1 hour before a meal.**
- **Restrict liquid intake with meals** to prevent gastric distention or feeling full before the patient consumes sufficient nutrients.
- **Keep the patient's environment neat and clean** and free of unpleasant sights, odors, and medical equipment. These often trigger loss of appetite. For example, remove bedpans, urinals, and the emesis basin from the room before mealtimes.
- **Order a late food tray or warm the food** if the patient is not in his room during mealtime.
- Provide or assist with **frequent oral hygiene.**
- **Provide a pleasant eating environment.**
- **Serve foods attractively**; vary textures, colors, and flavors; arrange the tray so the person can easily reach the food.
- **Position the person comfortably** for mealtime.
- **Find out what the person likes to eat**, and encourage family and friends to bring foods from home.
- **Control pain around the clock**, and avoid painful treatments before meals.
- **If the patient receives a nutritional supplement, delay the meal for at least an hour afterward.**
- **Encourage meals with friends** for those who live alone, or meals at a senior center.
- **Provide nutrient-dense foods** (e.g., add ice cream to appropriate beverages and foods).

- **Arrange for a home health aide** to shop and prepare meals for those who are unable to leave home for groceries, or arrange for Meals-on-Wheels.

Providing Enteral Nutrition

If a patient cannot meet his nutritional needs through an enhanced diet and measures to stimulate the appetite, you may need to use an alternative feeding method. Feeding can occur through the intestinal tract as enteral nutrition, or intravenously as parenteral nutrition. **Enteral nutrition** (tube feeding) refers to the delivery of liquid nutrition into the upper intestinal tract via a tube. Tube feeding may be used in addition to or instead of oral intake. It is the preferred method of feeding for a patient who has a functioning intestinal tract but needs nutritional support (e.g., patients with high metabolic needs, such as those with trauma, burns, or severe malnutrition; neurological disorders that affect swallowing; anorexia nervosa; prematurity; failure to thrive; or specific bowel diseases). Tube feeding may be a short- or long-term therapy.

Enteral feedings are preferred to parenteral (i.e., intravenous) nutrition because they maintain peristalsis and have a lower incidence of infections (Marik & Zaloga, 2004). However, there are a number of risks associated with enteral feedings. If enteral formula is aspirated into the lungs, it can lead to infection, pneumonia, abscess formation, adult respiratory distress syndrome (ARDS), and in some cases death. The high glucose content of enteral formulas provides a medium for bacterial growth. Other complications include diarrhea, nausea and vomiting, nasopharyngeal trauma, alterations in drug absorption and metabolism, and various metabolic disturbances.

There have been some instances where enteral feedings have been mistakenly connected to intravascular (IV) lines and feeding solutions have been infused into veins. These events, termed "tubing misconnections," are potentially fatal to the patient (The Joint Commission, 2006, 2007; Millin & Brooks, 2012; U.S. Food and Drug Administration, 2005). An enteral device manufacturer and a professional organization dedicated to improving patient care by advancing the science and practice of nutrition support therapy have cooperated to develop the "BE A. L. E. R. T." safety campaign to increase the safety of patients on enteral nutrition (see Box 27-7). To reduce feeding misconnections, only use an enteral-only fitting at the proximal end of the feeding administration set. This safety device can be distinguished from a traditional Leur connector so it cannot be attached to an intravenous line or syringe (Institute for Safe Medication Practice, 2014).

Administer feedings at room temperature, and be sure to check the expiration date of any feedings before starting an infusion. In this volume, the Highlights of Procedures box summarizes a procedure for enteral feedings. For complete instructions,

 Go to Chapter 27, **Procedure 27-3: Administering Feedings Through Gastric and Enteric Tubes,** in Volume 2.

Quality and Safety Education for Nurses

Safe Use of Parenteral Nutrition

Chapter Key Concept: *Nutrition*

Competency: *Quality Improvement (Knowledge, Skill, Attitudes); Evidenced-Based Practice (Skills, Attitudes); Safety (Knowledge, Skills, and Attitudes)**

Clinicians at Scripps Memorial Hospital (SMH) in La Jolla, California, theorized that their poor processes and variation in methods in the use of parenteral nutrition (PN) were producing inconsistent patient outcomes, thus increasing patient risk. The following is a description of how they set out to correct this by identifying the root causes of the problems and standardizing care.

Problems Identified: Clinicians first organized a multidisciplinary team to collect and analyze data,

develop better practices, and evaluate outcomes. They found several problems: inappropriate use of PN, poor glycemic control in patients on PN, inconsistent and confusing ordering practices, insufficient calorie replacement, and insufficient laboratory monitoring.

Corrective Interventions: Implementing the American Society for Parenteral and Enteral Nutrition's (A.S.P.E.N.) guideline for PN, revising the PN order form, educating physicians and other clinicians, and establishing twice weekly PN rounds. The group measured specific quality indicators before and after implementing the new procedures. The following table shows the top four measures:

Safety Measure	Pre-Intervention (2007)	Post-Intervention (2009)
Compliance with 10 Mandatory Components of a PN Order Form (A.S.P.E.N. guideline)	20%	100%
Appropriate use of parenteral nutrition	60%	97%
Baseline labs ordered before PN starts	30%	80%
Kcal delivered are within 10% of estimated need	54%	85%

Results/Conclusions: In addition to improving compliance, the new procedures resulted in significant costs savings.

Think About It: Parenteral nutrition is a high-risk treatment associated with serious complications, including death. (1) Do the above measures mean that patient outcomes are

improved? (2) In what specific ways does this QI project demonstrate the QSEN competencies of Quality Improvement, Safety, and Evidenced-Based and Practice? (3) Which specific knowledge, skills, and attitudes does it address?

Source: Boitano, Bojak, McCloskey, McCaul, et al. (2010).

*To learn about specific Knowledge, Skills, and Attitudes,

 Go to the QSEN Web site at http://qsen.org/competencies/pre-licensure-ksas/

BOX 27-7 ■ Be A.L.E.R.T

To reduce errors and help ensure safe enteral nutrition, use the following mnemonic:

A   **Aseptic** technique------------------------------------- When preparing and delivering enteral formula, practice good hand hygiene; wear gloves when handling feeding tube; avoid touching can tops, container openings, spike, and spike port.

L   **Label** enteral equipment------------------------------ with patient name and room number, formula name and rate, date and time of initiation, and nurse initials.

E   **Elevate** the head of the bed------------------------- a minimum of 30° for feedings whenever clinically possible; may mitigate risk of reflux and aspiration of gastric content.

R   **Right** patient, **Right** formula, **Right** tube---------- Match formula to patient's feeding order; verify **enteral** tubing set connects formula container to feeding tube.

T   **Trace** all lines and tubing back to patient----------- Avoid misconnections—trace all lines from origin to patient; only enteral-to-enteral connections.

Sources: © 2009 Nestlé HealthCare Nutrition, Inc. The BE A. L. E. R. T. poster is a joint effort of the American Society for Parenteral and Enteral Nutrition (A.S.P.E.N.) and Nestlé HealthCare Nutrition, Inc. Retrieved from http://www.nutritioncare.org/Professional_Resources/Patient_Safety/Patient_Safety/; A.S.P.E.N. (2009). Special report: Enteral nutrition practice recommendations. *Journal of Parenteral and Enteral Nutrition,* Retrieved from http://www.nutritioncare.org/wcontent.aspx?id=2078

Patients may receive enteral or parenteral nutrition in the home as well as in inpatient settings. The box Home Care: Home Nutritional Support reviews teaching related to alternative feeding methods in the home. You should review these topics with the patient or caregiver.

Types of Enteric Tubes

Enteric tubes are available in various materials, lengths, diameters, and types. Choose the type of tube you need based on the intended use and the length of time you anticipate it will be left in place. This chapter focuses on the use of enteral tubes as a route for feeding; however, they are inserted for other reasons, as well:

- To lavage the stomach (e.g., when there is disease, surgery, or bleeding in the GI tract, and in cases of poisoning or medication overdose)
- To collect a specimen of stomach contents for laboratory tests
- To prevent nausea, vomiting, and gastric distention postoperatively.

These are complicated therapies to manage at home, so patients typically go home with a referral for a home care nurse to assist in the transition from hospital to home and follow-up with nutritional support service.

When a nasogastric (or orogastric) tube is placed so the stomach can be emptied (lavage), larger bore, tubes made of polyvinyl chloride (PVC), are used. These are called **Salem sump tubes** (Fig. 27-4). A Salem sump tube has a lumen for drainage and one to allow air to enter the stomach. The air port (pigtail) is usually blue. A **Levin tube**, also used for drainage, has a single lumen, with holes in the tip and along the sides.

Selecting a Feeding Tube

Short-term (<6 weeks) enteral feedings are usually delivered through a nasogastric (NG) or a nasoenteric (NE) tube. As a nurse, you may be asked to place a small-bore, **nasogastric** or a **nasojenunal (NJ) feeding tube**. The tube is inserted through one naris, passed through the nasopharynx into the esophagus, and finally into the stomach. Placing the tube through the mouth is an option (oropharyngeal), but this method is more likely to trigger gagging or unconscious chewing on the tube. The Highlights of Procedures box in this volume provides a summary of a procedure for inserting nasogastric and nasoenteric tubes. For the entire procedure,

Go to Chapter 27, **Procedure 27-2: Inserting Nasogastric and Nasoenteric Tubes,** in Volume 2.

A **nasoenteric (NE) tube** is longer than an NG tube, extending through the nose down into the duodenum or jejunum (if it extends into the jejunum, it is called an NJ tube). A small, flexible tube is preferred for feeding (Fig. 27-5). An NE tube may be used instead of an NG tube for patients at risk for aspiration. This includes patients who have a decreased level of consciousness, absent or diminished gag reflex, or severe gastroesophageal reflux.

Home Care | Home Nutritional Support

Clients frequently administer enteral and parenteral nutrition at home. To assist the client or caregiver with the management of home nutritional therapy, teach the following aspects:

- *Formula.* Review the type of formula the patient should receive. Enteral or IV solutions are clearly marked with their contents. Emphasize that the caregiver double-check that the correct solution is being used and that the expiration date and time have not been reached before administering any feeding.

- *Administration.* Carefully review how to administer the feeding. Emphasize the need for handwashing before hanging the infusion. After a period of time, the client may be able to tolerate delivering 1 to 3 L of enteral feeding at night. The rate must be increased at the beginning and decreased when ending the delivery. If parenteral nutrition is administered at home, be sure that the client or caregiver is aware of proper technique.

- *Access device.* Review the care required for the access device, including site care, dressing changes, and flushing.

- *Storage.* Stored enteral and parenteral nutrition must be refrigerated to prevent bacterial contamination.

- *Monitoring.* Instruct the client or caregiver to report a rise in temperature, weight loss, change in bowel movements, decrease in urine output, or change in condition.

- *Follow-up.* Arrange for the client to be weighed and assessed regularly to monitor the adequacy of the feedings. Often clients weigh at home and report to the primary care provider's office or the nutrition support team for ongoing monitoring of progress and review of lab work.

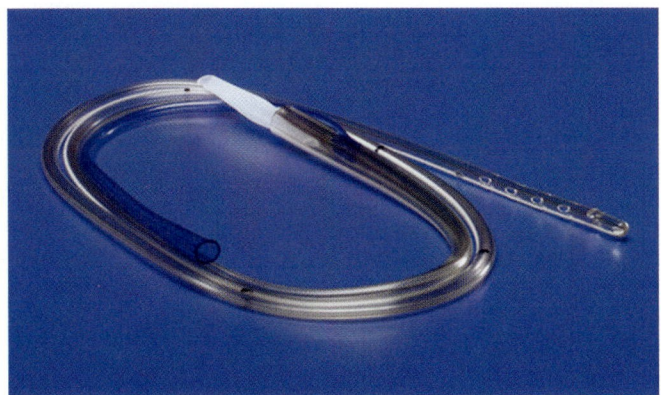

FIGURE 27-4 A large-bore, polyvinyl-chloride (PVC) Salem sump tube used for gastric lavage.

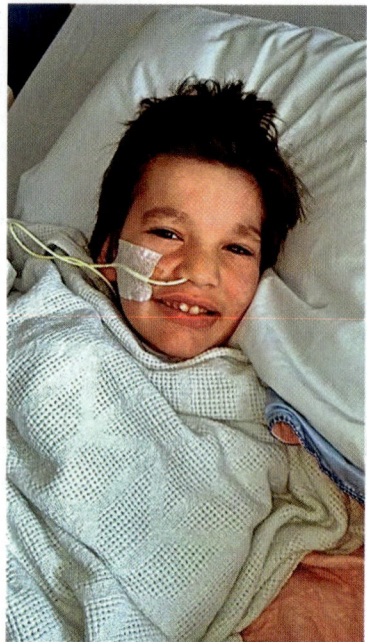

FIGURE 27-5 A small lumen, flexible nasoenteric feeding tube provides continuous nutrition to patients with impaired swallowing.

The **lumen** (inside diameter) of a feeding tube is measured using the **French (Fr) scale**: the larger the lumen, the larger the diameter. Most feeding tubes for adults are measured in French units (each Fr unit is

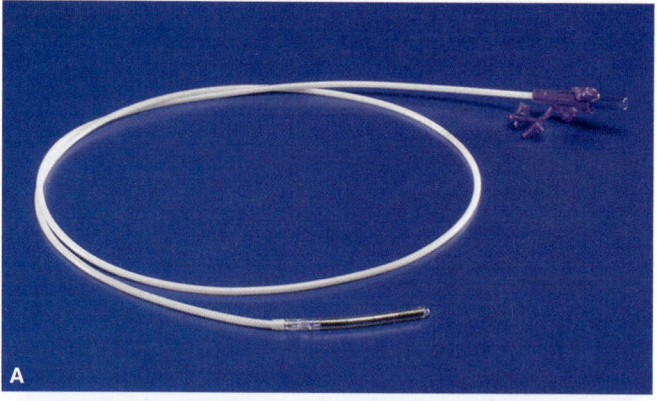

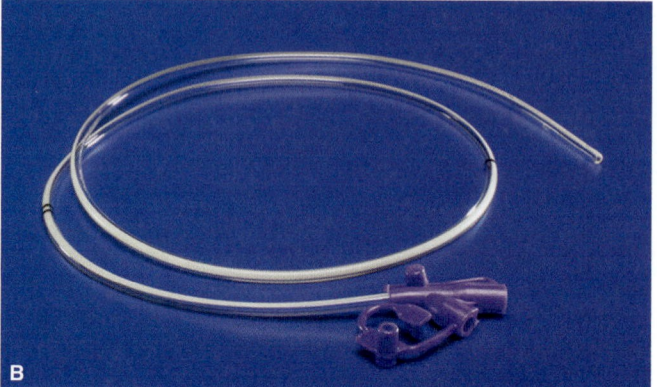

FIGURE 27-6 *A,* A double-lumen, weighted (Dobhoff) feeding tube. *B,* A nonweighted (kangaroo) feeding tube.

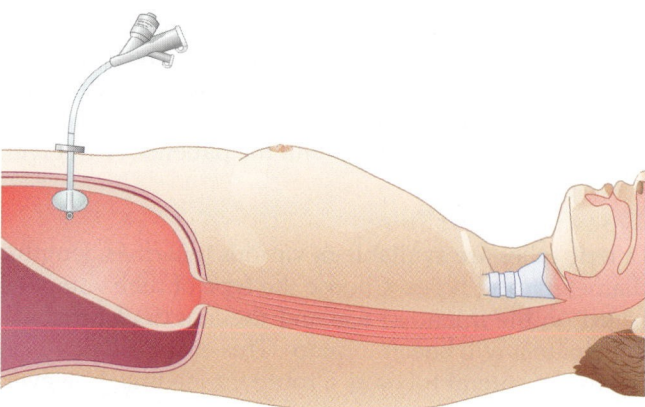

FIGURE 27-7 A percutaneous gastrostomy (PEG) tube for feeding.

about 0.33 mm), and designated as either small bore (5-12 Fr) or large bore (14 Fr or larger) tubes. Large-bore NG tubes, such as the Salem sump (Fig. 27-4), are occasionally used for feeding, but are converted to a smaller tube within the first 2 days. Smaller tubes are less flexible, less comfortable, and are more commonly used if it is necessary to empty (lavage) the stomach. Figure 27-6 shows two types of feeding tubes.

For long-term feedings, a **gastrostomy tube (G-tube), percutaneous endoscopic gastrostomy tube (PEG)** (Figs. 27-7 and 27-8), **jejunostomy tube (J-tube, PEJ),** or **gastrostomy button (G-button)** (Fig. 27-9), is preferred. These are placed surgically or laparoscopically through the skin and the abdominal wall into the stomach or jejunum. They can also be placed endoscopically. The surgical incision is sometimes sutured tightly around the tube to hold it in place and prevent leakage. You must use surgical asepsis to care for a new incision.

A gastrostomy tube can be converted to a **G-button** once healing has taken place. Historically, a PEG or PEJ was reserved for clients needing long-term nutritional support. However, that trend is changing. Patient comfort

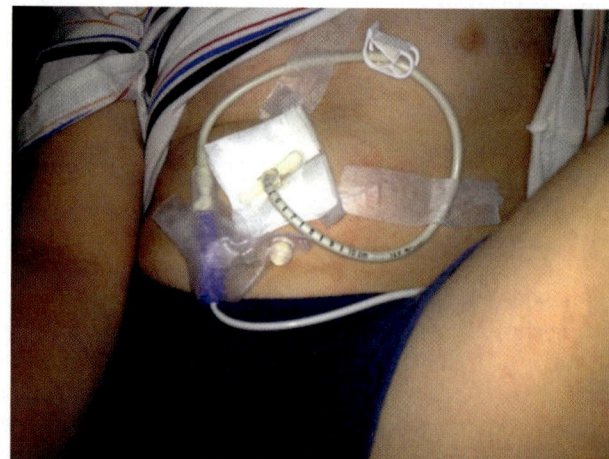

FIGURE 27-8 A PEG feeding tube is more convenient and comfortable than a nasogastric tube.

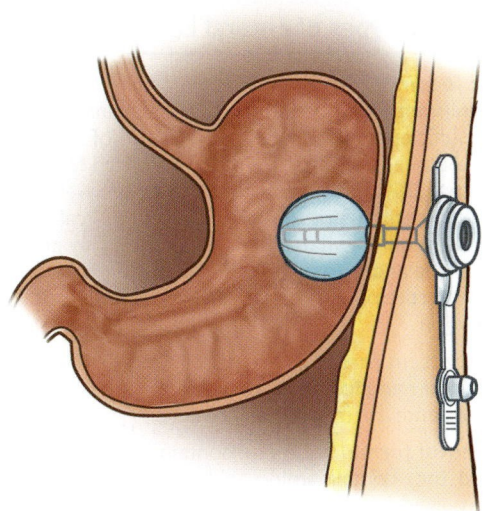

FIGURE 27-9 A gastrostomy button (G-button) in place for feeding.

and improved technology leading to ease of insertion have made PEG or PEJ an option even for short-term use. The G-tubes and G-buttons, which can be capped off flush with the abdominal wall when not in use, are the most comfortable of all for long-term use.

Checking Feeding Tube Placement

NG and NE feeding tubes are placed without direct visualization. As a result, there is risk of placing the tube into the respiratory tract. Therefore, you must check the location of the tip of the feeding tube before each enteral feeding or once per shift for continuous feedings. Failure to verify placement could be disastrous because it may result in infusion of formula into the lungs.

Radiographic Verification

Radiographic verification is the most reliable method for confirming tube placement, and must be performed before the first feeding is administered. All feeding tubes contain markings that can be detected by radiographic films. Reliable bedside assessment is necessary because even when the tube is initially placed correctly in the stomach (or intestine), it may later move upward. No other method alone reliably verifies tube placement.

Bedside Methods

No bedside method alone is reliable. Feeding tube placement can be checked by testing the pH of the aspirate in combination with other methods for bedside verification (see Clinical Insight 27-7). If in doubt, obtain a radiograph to determine tube location.

Bedside methods include the following:

- **Measuring the pH (acidity) of the aspirate and inspecting color, character, and volume.** Gastric fluid is typically clear, odorless, and green with a pH of 5.0 or less. If the tube has migrated into the lungs, the aspirate would be pale yellow and cloudy with a pH of 7.0 or higher. Testing the acidity of the gastric aspirate is currently the most reliable bedside method of checking that the tube is in the stomach. However, the following conditions can affect the accuracy of pH testing:

  If blood is present, either from epistaxis or gastric bleeding, the pH will resemble the pH of blood (7.35).

  If the patient is receiving medications to control stomach acidity (e.g., antacids, H2 blockers, or proton pump inhibitors), the gastric pH may be as high as 6.

  Because of the frequency of such situations, even the pH method should be used in combination with other verification methods (American Society for Parenteral and Enteral Nutrition [A.S.P.E.N.], 2009b).

- **Measuring the residual volume of the aspirate** and observing for unexpected changes in the volume. A dramatic increase in the residual volume may indicate that a small bowel tube has moved into the stomach. Large gastric residual volume (GRV) might also mean the patient is not digesting the feeding and may need a promotility agent (e. g., metoclopramide) to improve bowel function. The patient with large GRV is at greater risk for aspiration. Check GRV every 4 hours during the first 48 of gastric enteral feeding. After that, GRV checks can be done every 6 to 8 hours in stable patients.

- **Injecting air into the feeding tube** (the "whoosh test"). If the tube is in the stomach, injecting 5 to 30 mL of air produces a gurgling sound audible by listening with a stethoscope over the stomach. This is the least reliable method for checking placement of an NG or NE tube. Because the lungs and stomach lie close together, the sounds created by sending air through the tube can easily be transmitted to nearby areas of the body, causing you to err in determining tube placement.

- **Measuring the tube that extends outside of the body.** At the time it is placed, the feeding tube should be marked where it exits the body (e.g., the abdominal wall, the naris). If there is a change in the length of the external portion of the tube, it may have moved out of the original placement site. A consistent measurement may help to verify tube placement (Peter & Gill, 2009).

- **Capnometry** tests for carbon dioxide (CO_2). The presence of CO_2 with the placement of an NG or NE tube would indicate that the tube has been placed in the respiratory tract. This method is not yet in wide use, and is best used only at the time the tube is placed. Figure 27-10 is a CO_2 detector.

- **Measuring bilirubin, trypsin, and pepsin in the aspirate** provides a positive determination that the tube is placed in the stomach. Test devices for these three gastric components are not yet commercially available (Elpern, Killeen, Talla, et al., 2007; Peter & Gill, 2009).

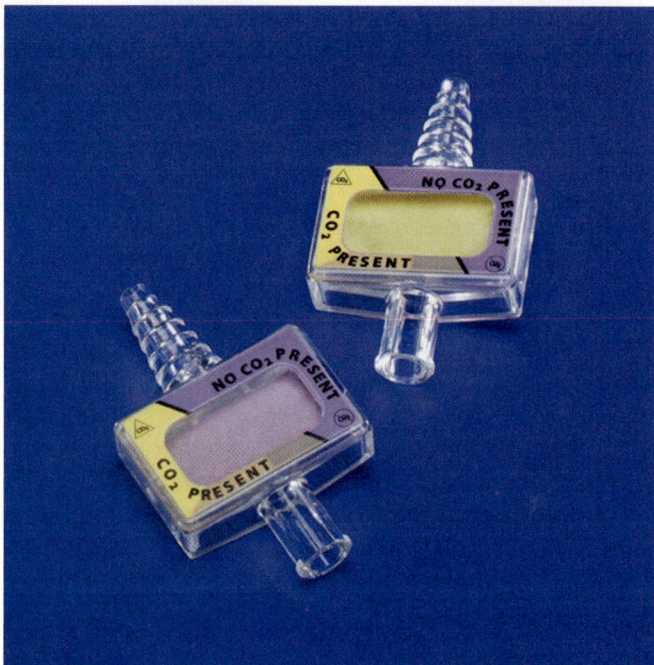

FIGURE 27-10 A carbon dioxide detector for checking feeding tube placement.

 No longer recommended: Adding dye to enteral feedings as a method for identifying aspiration of gastric contents is not recommended because it has been associated with several adverse effects, including gastric bacterial colonization, diarrhea, systemic dye absorption, and death (AACCN, 2005b, revise 2009).

Remember, you should not rely on any one of these methods alone. Always use them in combination. For more information and guidelines for checking enteral tube placement,

Go to Chapter 27, **Clinical Insight 27-7: Checking Feeding Tube Placement,** in Volume 2.

Knowledge Check 27-11
- When is enteral nutrition the preferred alternative feeding?
- Identify and describe the types of enteral nutrition tubes.
- List four tube placement verification techniques.

Administering Enteral Feedings
In a few institutions, enteral feeding formulas are blended in the kitchen, but most use one of the many commercially prepared products. The type of product selected depends on the patient's health condition. Products vary in nutritional components and caloric concentration (Box 27-8).

Feeding Schedules
Feedings may be delivered on a continuous, cyclic, or intermittent schedule. **Continuous feedings** provide a constant flow of formula and an even distribution of nutrition throughout the day. For example, an infusion of 50 mL/hr for 24 hours of a 1 kcal/mL formula provides

---

BOX 27-8 ■ Types of Enteral Feeding Solutions

- **Basic feeding formulas** are used for clients who have no significant nutritional deficits but are unable to eat or drink sufficiently. They provide 1 kcal/mL of solution, and meet the needs of most clients. A standard formula contains 12%–20% of kcal from protein, 45%–60% of kcal from carbohydrates, and 30%–40% of kcal from fats. They also contain vitamins and minerals. They are usually lactose free and contain complex forms of carbohydrates, fats, and proteins. Therefore, they require digestion and absorption.

- **High-protein formulas** are for clients who have a substantial need for protein, such as those with burns, open wounds, or malnutrition.

- **Elemental formulas** do not contain complex proteins; instead, they contain amino acids or peptides. They are reserved for patients with severe small bowel absorptive dysfunction. These formulas are fiber free and highly osmotic. Their use is controversial.

- **Diabetic formulas** are for clients who require tube feedings to meet nutritional needs but have type 1 or type 2 diabetes mellitus. These formulas control carbohydrate intake.

- **Renal formulas** are for clients who require tube feedings to meet nutritional needs but have renal failure or renal insufficiency as comorbidity. These formulas limit potassium, sodium, and nitrogen intake.

- **Pulmonary formulas** provide 55% of the calories as fat so that less CO_2 is produced per unit of oxygen consumed. They are used, for example, for patients with lung disease.

- **Fiber-containing formulas.** Because fiber has a potential protective effect for multiple disease states, including diverticulosis, colon cancer, diabetes, and heart disease, fiber-containing formulas may be used for patients in long-term care facilities or patients who require enteral feedings for a prolonged period of time.

1,200 kcal per day. Continuous infusions are usually administered via small-bore NG, NJ, PEG, or PEJ tubes, or G-buttons, to patients in debilitated states who require intensive nutritional support. Feedings may be interrupted for periodic instillation of medications or flushing with water.

- **Pump-controlled infusions** are recommended for jejunal feedings and for gastrostomy feedings given by continuous infusion to decrease gastroesophageal reflux. A feeding pump ensures a steady flow rate.
- **Gravity feedings** can also be used, but the rate of delivery is not precise, and they increase the risk of gastroesophageal reflux, diarrhea, and aspiration. You regulate the drip rate by adjusting a clamp on the tubing, much the same as adjusting an IV rate.

Cyclic feedings are administered regularly; however, the infusion time is less than 24 hours per day. Nocturnal feedings are a form of cyclic feedings. The patient is able to eat meals and participate in activities throughout the day but receives an infusion of enteral formula at night while at rest. Another variant is a 20-hour infusion. A 4-hour break allows time for the feeding pump to be disconnected for hygiene and other activities.

Intermittent feedings are given to supplement oral intake or for patients who want greater mobility to take part in activities, such as physical therapy. Feedings are given on a regular or periodic basis several times a day, usually over 30 to 60 minutes. An example of a prescription for a *regular feeding* is, "Give 250 to 500 mL of enteral nutrition every 4 to 6 hours." *Periodic feedings* are often based on oral intake and are considered to be more physiologically similar to normal eating patterns. Consider the following periodic feeding prescription:

If the client consumes 90% to 100% of the ordered diet, give no additional feeding.
>75% but <90%, give 100 mL of formula after each meal.
>50% but <75%, give 200 mL of formula after each meal.
>25% but <50%, give 300 mL of formula after each meal.
0 to 25% of the ordered diet, give 400 mL of formula.

Intermittent feedings are sometimes given by **bolus**, if the patient can tolerate this method. In this method, you use a syringe to deliver 300 to 400 mL of formula through the tube over a 5- to 10-minute period. This is the easiest method to teach family members for home care, and it frees the patient from mechanical devices that limit activity. But because the fluid is given more rapidly by this method, it increases the risk for respiratory aspiration and for stomach distention. You can use it only with gastric tubes, never with intestinal tubes.

Open and Closed Feeding Systems

An **open system** is exposed to the environment. One example is to open cans of formula and use a syringe to inject the formula into the tube; alternatively, you can pour it into a reservoir (e.g., a plastic bag). You should flush and clean the system after each delivery. Most agencies require that an open-system feeding not hang for more than 4 hours.

A **closed system** is a prefilled system (e.g., a bag or a bottle) that functions much like IV fluid. The nurse spikes the container with tubing that is attached to the feeding pump or run through a manually controlled drip chamber. Closed systems decrease the risk of contamination. A prefilled closed-system container can safely hang for 24 to 48 hours if you use sterile technique. You can measure out the specified amount in the drip chamber, allowing the remainder of the container to be used later in the day.

Monitoring Patients Receiving Enteral Nutrition

For patients receiving enteral nutrition, you will need to monitor tube placement, skin condition, laboratory values (especially blood glucose, BUN, and electrolytes), feeding residual, and GI status. This will allow you to detect complications that affect metabolism or fluid and electrolyte balance and to assess responses to enteral feeding. Feedings may need to be increased or decreased depending on the patient's changing clinical condition. In addition, enteral feeding solutions provide an ideal medium for bacterial growth. For guidelines,

 Go to Chapter 27, **Clinical Insight 27-8: Monitoring Patients Receiving Enteral Nutrition,** in Volume 2.

Also,

 Go to Chapter 27, **Clinical Insight 27-9: Preventing Infection in Patients Receiving Enteral Feedings,** in Volume 2.

Removing Feeding Tubes

When a patient's condition has stabilized and she no longer requires enteral nutrition, the feeding tube may be removed. A PEG tube is usually clamped if feedings are no longer required. The Highlights of Procedures box summarizes a procedure for removing a feeding tube. For a complete set of steps to follow,

 Go to Chapter 27, **Procedure 27-4: Removing a Nasogastric or Nasoenteric Tube,** in Volume 2.

 ## Think**Like a Nurse** 27-8

Your client has dementia and is frequently agitated. She has been progressively losing weight. An interdisciplinary team recommended enteral nutrition due to poor oral intake; however, the client has repeatedly pulled out her NG tube and had an episode of aspiration pneumonia last month. What recommendations might you consider at the next meeting?

Providing Parenteral Nutrition

Parenteral nutrition (PN) is the delivery of nutrition intravenously into a large, central vein. This is the preferred method of feeding for clients who cannot be nourished through the GI tract. Some clients (e.g., those with shortened small bowel secondary to injury or disease) who are able to meet some of their nutritional needs may use PN in addition to some oral intake to meet caloric and nutrient needs. Others, such as clients who are severely malnourished, have extensive burns or trauma, or have conditions that require resting the GI system, are nourished entirely by PN.

PN solutions usually contain a 10% to 70% concentration of dextrose in water (but usually not more than 20%) along with amino acids, and can provide 20 to 30 kcal per kilogram per day, depending on the patient's calculated energy need. Note, though, that the most common concentrations of glucose provide only 200 kcal per liter. PN also contains vitamins, minerals, and trace elements. Standard PN formulas are available at many healthcare facilities; however, PN can be modified to meet individual needs.

The type of venous access device used to administer PN will depend on the components of the PN and the anticipated duration of PN. Because PN solutions

For steps to follow in *all* procedures, refer to the Universal Steps for All Procedures found on the inside back cover of Volume 2. Go to the full procedures in Volume 2 to practice and learn the procedure steps. Use these procedure highlights later to help you review key points.

Procedure 27-1: Checking Fingerstick (Capillary) Blood Glucose Levels

➤ Have the patient wash hands with warm soap and water. Dry well with a clean towel.

➤ Don procedure gloves.

➤ Cleanse the patient's finger with soap and water and let it dry thoroughly.

➤ Prepare the lancet and meter and obtain a clean test strip that is correct for the meter.

➤ Stick the side of the fingertip.

➤ Place the drop of blood on the test strip.

➤ At the indicated time, read the glucose level on the digital display. (Follow the manufacturer's instructions.)

Procedure 27-2: Inserting Nasogastric and Nasoenteric Tubes

➤ Place the patient in a sitting or high-Fowler's position.

➤ Measure the length of the tube:

NG tubes: Measure from the tip of the nose to earlobe and from earlobe to the xiphoid process.

Nasoenteric tubes: Add 8 to 10 cm (3 to 4 in.) to the NG measurement, as directed.

➤ Lubricate the tube with a water-soluble lubricant.

➤ Ask the patient to hyperextend the neck and breathe through the mouth.

➤ Insert the tube gently through the nostril; advance the tube as the patient swallows.

➤ Instruct the patient to tilt the head forward, drink water, and swallow.

➤ Withdraw the tube immediately if respiratory distress occurs during or immediately after insertion.

➤ Confirm tube placement initially by x-ray. Always reconfirm tube placement with a combination of bedside methods before giving feedings or medicine.

➤ Secure the tube to the nose and to the patient's gown.

Procedure 27-3: Administering Feedings Through Gastric and Enteric Tubes

➤ Check the medical prescription for the type of formula, rate, route, and frequency of feeding.

➤ Confirm that an x-ray of tube placement was performed.

➤ Confirm tube placement at the bedside before administering the feeding.

➤ Elevate the head of the bed at least 30° to 45° during the feedings and for an hour after administration.

➤ For intermittent feedings, check gastric residual volume before feeding.

For continuous feeding: Check at least once every shift. If the residual is not within normal limits, hold the feeding and recheck in 1 hour. If still not within normal limits, notify the physician.

For gastrostomy and PEG tubes and gastrostomy buttons (G-buttons): Check residual volume every 4 hours.

For jejunostomy tubes: Residual volumes are not checked.

➤ Flush tubing with 30 mL of water before and after feeding (every 4 hours for continuous feedings), and before and after medication administration.

➤ Change the tube feeding administration set and other supplies a minimum of every 24 hours.

➤ Continuous feedings should be infused by pump.

Procedure 27-4: Removing a Nasogastric or Nasoenteric Tube

➤ Verify the primary provider's prescription for removal of the tube.

➤ Assist the patient to a sitting or high-Fowler's position.

➤ Inject 10 mL of air through the main lumen to clear the tube of secretions.

➤ Ask the patient to hold his breath, and gently, but quickly, withdraw the tube.

➤ Discard the equipment.

➤ Provide or assist with care of nose and mouth.

Procedure 27-5: Administering Parenteral Nutrition

➤ Perform pre-procedure assessments: Check patient record (e.g., to confirm CVC tip placement), check blood glucose, and assess patency of the line.

➤ Position the patient supine.

➤ Examine the PN solution for leaks, cloudiness, and particles. If the solution contains lipids, also look for a brown layer, oil droplets, or oil on the surface. Have a coworker verify.

➤ Identify the patient, using two identifiers; have a coworker verify.

➤ Compare the bag with the patient's ID band and with the original prescription.

➤ Observe meticulous sterile technique in the appropriate steps of the procedure. During all steps, observe careful aseptic (clean) technique. Or follow agency policy.

➤ Use a filter.

➤ Attach the new administration set to the new bag.

➤ Prime the tubing (either now or after placing in the pump).

Highlights of Procedures 27-1 through 27-6

➤ Place the tubing in the infusion pump; set the rate.

➤ Clamp the catheter and the old administration set.

➤ Remove gloves, perform hand hygiene, and don clean gloves.

➤ Observe meticulous sterile technique in the appropriate steps of the procedure. During all steps, observe careful aseptic (clean) technique.

➤ Scrub all surfaces of the needleless connector and luer-locking threads with an antiseptic pad.

➤ Determine patency of the IV line.

➤ Trace the tubing back to the patient, attach the new infusion tubing to the designated PN lumen (usually the largest one), and secure the luer-lock connection.

➤ Start the infusion.

➤ Label tubing.

Procedure 27-6: Administering Lipids

➤ Lipids require a special administration set.

➤ Position the patient supine.

➤ Be certain lipids are not cold.

➤ Examine the bottle for a layer of froth or separation into fat globules or layers.

➤ Complete the infusion within 20 hours.

➤ Use new tubing for each bottle of lipids.

➤ If infusing simultaneously with PN, use a separate port below the PN filter.

➤ Take vital signs before infusing, then every 10 minutes for 30 minutes, and observe for side effects.

➤ Begin the infusion slowly. If no reactions occur after 30 minutes, adjust to the prescribed rate.

are hypertonic, they should be administered in a large, high-flow vein through a central venous access catheter. The subclavian vein has been the site of choice; however, the jugular vein is preferred for tunneled catheters and implanted ports. Peripherally inserted central catheter (PICC) lines are also used for PN.

➕ All PN catheters must have chest x-ray confirmation that the tip is in the lower portion of the superior vena cava adjacent to the right atrium (see Fig. 27-11) before beginning the first infusion. High blood flow through the superior vena cava causes rapid dilution of the concentrated PN and thereby prevents vessel damage. Some types of PN solutions may be infused via a peripheral vein, but this is not usual.

Lipid emulsions contain essential fatty acids, triglycerides, and supplemental kcal. They are administered weekly for patients who rely on PN to prevent essential fatty acid deficiency. They also add calories to the PN mixture so that lower glucose concentrations can be used, thus reducing the risk of glucose fluctuations. Most IV fats are supplied by safflower or soybean oil. They provide 1.1 to 3 kcal/mL.

You may administer lipids at the same time as the PN, through a peripheral line or by Y-connector tubing through a central line. Lipids are also sometimes added to the PN solution (this is called a 3-in-1 admixture), and administered over a 24-hour period. The Highlights of Procedures box summarizes procedures for administering parenteral nutrition and lipid emulsions. For the complete procedures,

 Go to Chapter 27, **Procedure 27-5: Administering Parenteral Nutrition** and **Procedure 27-6: Administering Lipids,** in Volume 2.

To learn about monitoring and maintenance of patients receiving parenteral nutrition,

 Go to Chapter 27, **Clinical Insight 27-10: Monitoring and Maintaining Patients Receiving Parenteral Nutrition,** in Volume 2.

 To explore learning resources for this chapter,

 Go to DavisPlus at DavisPl.us/Wilkinson3.

Chapter Resources for Chapter 27:
 Response sheets for all learning activities
 Resources for Caregivers and Health Professionals
 Reading More About Nutrition (suggested readings)
 Concept Map of chapter content
Interactive Case Studies
NCLEX-Style and Chapter Review Questions
Chapter Overview Podcasts

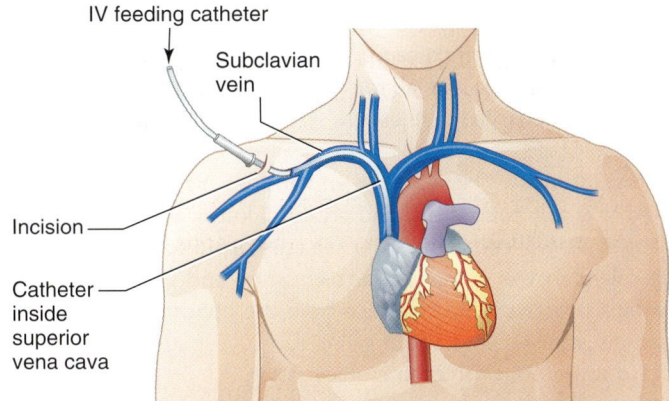

FIGURE 27-11 The subclavian vein is the site of choice for parenteral nutrition.

For references cited,

 Go to Volume 2, **References Cited.**

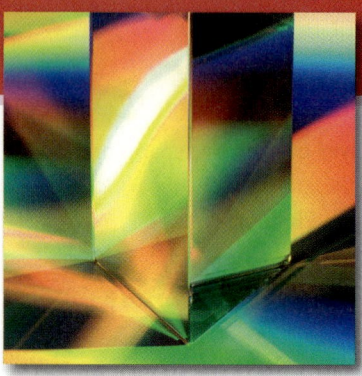

CHAPTER 28

Urinary Elimination

Learning Outcomes

After completing this chapter, you should be able to:

➤ Describe the normal structure and function of the organs in the urinary system.

➤ Describe the processes of urine formation and elimination.

➤ Discuss factors that affect urinary elimination.

➤ Describe the contents of a nursing assessment and physical examination focused on urinary elimination.

➤ Accurately measure urine output.

➤ Describe procedures for collecting various types of urine specimens.

➤ Describe diagnostic tests used in identification of urinary elimination problems.

➤ Discuss common elimination problems: urinary tract infection, urinary retention, and urinary incontinence.

➤ Identify nursing diagnoses associated with altered urinary elimination.

➤ Describe nursing interventions that promote normal urination.

➤ Provide care for clients experiencing urinary problems.

➤ Perform urinary catheterizations following accepted procedures.

➤ Discuss nursing care appropriate for clients who have a urinary diversion.

Key Concepts

Urinary elimination

Related Concepts

See the Concept Map on Davis*Plus*.

Example Problems

Urinary incontinence

Urinary retention

Urinary tract infections

Meet Your Patient

During your assigned clinical experience at University Hospital, the registered nurse (RN) asks you to complete the admission process for Marlena, a 55-year-old woman who is complaining of frequent, painful urination. As you interview her, Marlena becomes embarrassed. "I really don't enjoy talking about this," she admits. When she asks to use the bathroom, you ask her to give you a midstream clean-catch urine sample. She returns with a small specimen of pink-colored, strong-smelling urine. "I have a strong urge to go and then I hardly have any urine. It burns like crazy during my stream," she reports.

You close the door and interview Marlena in private about her usual urination pattern and current symptoms. Your calm approach and straightforward manner put her at ease. She confides that she is sexually active and that her symptoms began after spending the weekend with her new partner. You take her vital signs: oral temperature,

99.4°F (37.4°C); radial pulse, 88 beats/min; respiratory rate, 20 breaths/min; and blood pressure, 108/72 mm Hg.

The emergency department (ED) physician asks you to perform a dipstick urinalysis on the urine sample and to send the urine sample to the lab for culture and sensitivity. He says: "Well, what do you think we need to do next?" How would you answer his question?

As you gain theoretical and practical knowledge in this chapter, we will return to this case study to discuss how you might answer the physician's question and support Marlena's recovery. You will also have the opportunity to examine your feelings about giving care that patients may regard as personal or even embarrassing.

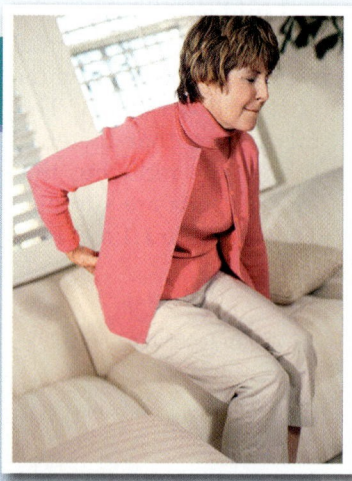

ABOUT THE KEY CONCEPTS

The key concept of **urinary elimination** is important because many of your nursing activities focus on promoting normal elimination. Your understanding of urine formation and elimination will help you will help you to choose and provide the best independent and collaborative interventions for patients with urinary elimination problems.

Theoretical Knowledge
knowing **why**

A variety of factors, including personal hygiene, age, nutrition, stress, sexual activity, and medications, play a role in urinary health. That's why it is vitally important that you take a holistic approach to patients who have altered urinary elimination patterns.

HOW DOES THE URINARY SYSTEM WORK?

The body removes from food and fluids the nutrients necessary for essential bodily functions, such as physical activity, self-repair, and mental operations. Waste products are left in the blood and in the bowel. The organs of the urinary system that help to excrete wastes and maintain a balance of chemicals and water in the body include the kidneys, ureters, bladder, and urethra (Fig. 28-1).

The Kidneys Filter and Regulate

The kidneys filter metabolic wastes, toxins, excess ions, and water from the bloodstream and excrete them as urine. If kidney function is impaired, these substances reach toxic levels and damage body cells. The kidneys also help to regulate blood volume, blood pressure, electrolyte levels, and acid–base balance by selectively reabsorbing water and other substances. Secondary functions of the kidneys are to produce erythropoietin, secrete the enzyme renin, and activate vitamin D_3 (calcitriol). The kidneys are located against the posterior abdominal wall behind the peritoneum (they are **retroperitoneal**). The average kidney weighs about 5 ounces and is the shape of a kidney bean (see Fig. 28-1).

The outer layer, or **cortex**, of the kidney is composed of millions of microscopic functional units, called *nephrons* (Fig. 28-2). The inner layer, or **medulla**, consists of 8 to 10 wedge-shaped cones, called the *renal pyramids*. The renal pyramids are made up of bundles of collecting tubules. The innermost area is the **renal pelvis**. Funnel-shaped extensions known as **calyces** (singular: **calyx**) enclose the central portion of each renal pyramid and direct urine into the renal pelvis.

The Nephrons Form Urine

The **nephron** is the basic structural and functional unit of the kidney (see Fig. 28-2). There are about 1 million nephrons in each kidney. Each nephron consists of:

- A double-walled hollow capsule, the **Bowman's capsule**, enclosing a **glomerulus**, a knotty ball of capillaries
- A series of filtrating tubules
- A collecting duct

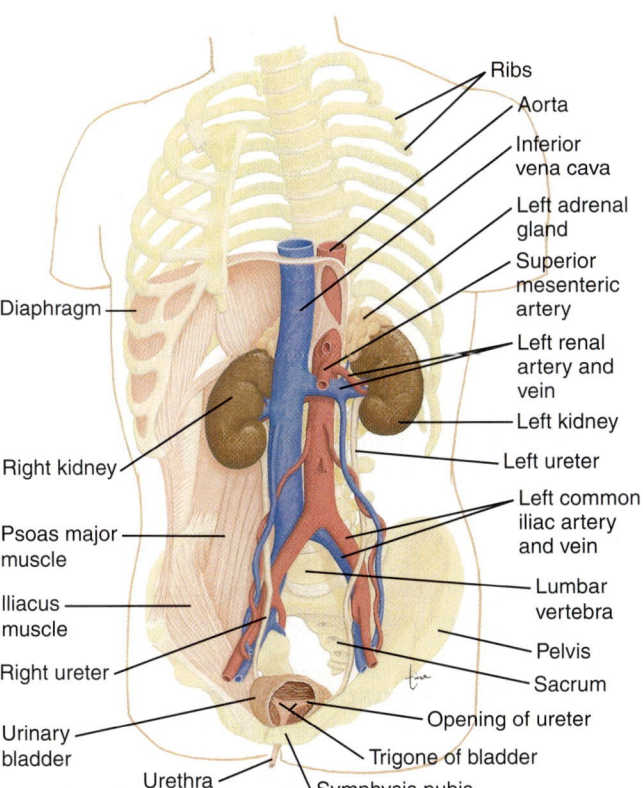

FIGURE 28-1 The organs of the urinary system include the kidneys, ureters, bladder, and urethra.

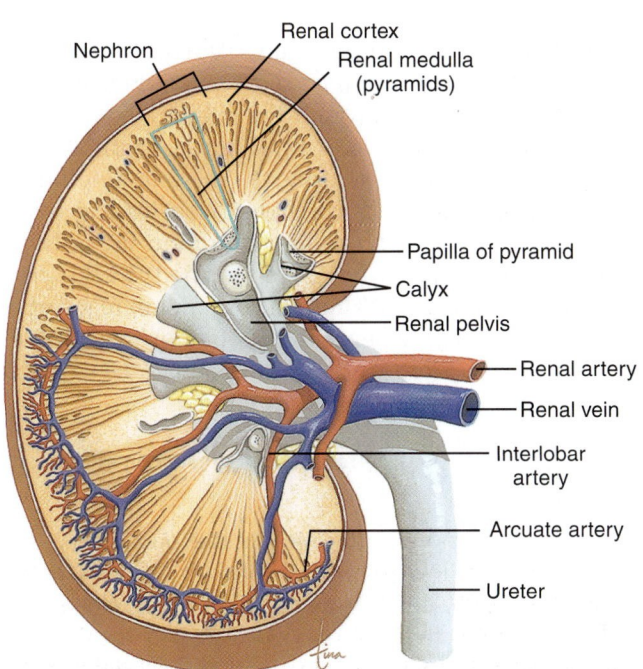

FIGURE 28-2 A cross section of the kidney, showing the renal cortex, medulla, pyramids, and calyces.

Together, these structures act as a microscopic filter, controlling the excretion and retention of fluids and solutes according to the body's moment-by-moment needs. Urine is formed by filtration, reabsorption, and secretion, as discussed next.

For a detailed view of a nephron,

 Go to Chapter 28, **Tables, Boxes, Figures: ESG Figure 28-1,** on Davis*Plus.*

Glomerular Filtration

Figure 28-3 summarizes the process of urine formation. The first step, **filtration**, occurs in the glomeruli. The renal arteries bring blood to the kidneys and into the glomeruli. Blood pressure forces plasma, dissolved substances, and small proteins out of the porous glomeruli into Bowman's capsule to form a liquid called **filtrate**. The **glomerular filtration rate** is the amount of filtrate formed by the kidneys per minute. Unless the glomerular capillaries are inflamed or damaged, large molecules, such as blood cells and blood proteins, are too large to filter across their walls. Glomerular filtrate resembles blood plasma, except that it contains much less protein and no blood cells.

Renal blood flow progressively decreases with aging, primarily because of changes to the micro blood vessels to the kidney. This decline in glomerular filtration is the most important functional deficit caused by aging (Besdine, 2013).

To see an animated explanation of the processes of osmosis, diffusion, filtration, and active transport,

 Go to **Animations: Osmosis, Diffusion, Filtration, and Active Transport,** on Davis*Plus.*

Tubular Reabsorption

The filtrate moves from Bowman's capsule into a highly twisted tubule (*proximal convoluted tubule,* Fig. 28-3). As the filtrate journeys through the tubule, 99% is reabsorbed into the peritubular capillaries. Approximately 1% of filtrate returns, as urine, to the *collecting tubule,* which transports it into the ureters. Wastes and toxins that remain in the blood after filtration are actively transported into the filtrate (reabsorbed) in the *distal* and *collecting tubules.* Water and sodium are reabsorbed in these structures when antidiuretic hormone (ADH) and aldosterone are secreted. For an animated explanation of urine formation and elimination,

 Go to **Animations: Formation and Elimination of Urine,** on Davis*Plus.*

When the amount of fluid in the body decreases (e.g., because of low intake or blood loss), the posterior pituitary gland secretes more ADH. This causes the distal and collecting tubules to reabsorb more water into the blood. At the same time, the adrenal cortex secretes more aldosterone, which increases the reabsorption of sodium, and water follows sodium back

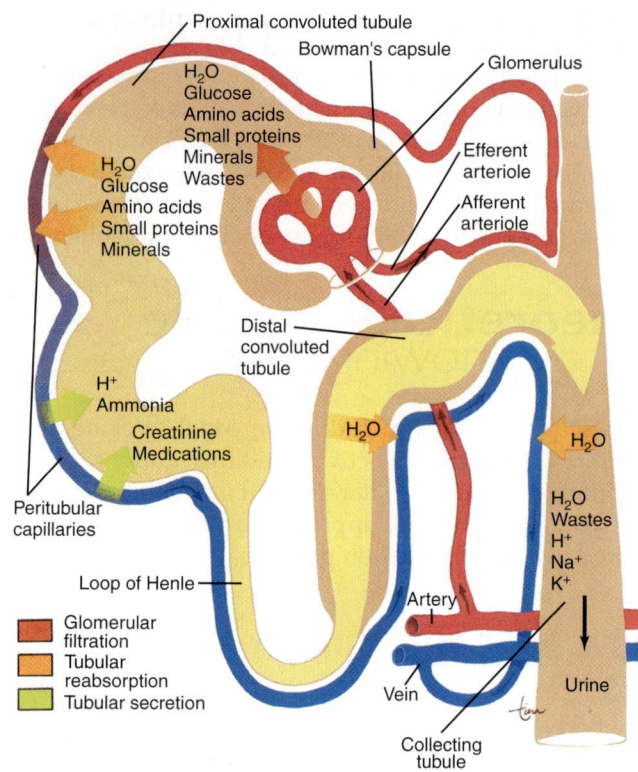

FIGURE 28-3 A schematic representation of the formation of urine.

into the blood. ADH and aldosterone thus have the effect of maintaining normal blood volume and blood pressure.

When the amount of water in the body increases (e.g., as in ingestion of excessive fluids), ADH is suppressed and the opposite effect occurs. Urine becomes dilute and water continues to be eliminated until its concentration returns to normal (Scanlon & Sanders, 2011).

Tubular Secretion

Some substances are actively secreted from the blood in the peritubular capillaries into the renal filtrate. For example, metabolic waste products, such as ammonia and creatinine, and some medications are secreted into the filtrate and then eliminated in urine. In addition, the kidneys help maintain the normal pH of blood by secreting hydrogen ions (H^+).

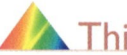 Think**Like a Nurse** 28-1

If a client is suffering from impaired kidney function, what signs and symptoms might you expect to see?

The Ureters Transport Urine

The remaining organs of the urinary system transport or store the urine once it is formed. From the collecting tubules, urine travels into the renal pelvis and enters the ureter. Each kidney has one ureter, approximately 26 to 30 cm (10 to 12 in.) long and 1.25 cm (0.5 in.) in diameter (see Fig. 28-1). The ureters contract in peristaltic waves to move urine toward the bladder. At the opening between the ureter and the bladder is a flap of mucous membrane that acts as a one-way valve, allowing urine to enter the bladder but preventing backflow (**reflux**) into the ureter.

The Urinary Bladder Stores Urine

The urinary bladder (see Fig. 28-1) is a sac-like organ that receives urine from the ureters and stores it until discharged from the body. The wall of the bladder consists of four layers:

- An innermost mucous membrane seals off the remaining layers from exposure to urine.
- A layer of connective tissue supports the mucous membrane.
- Three layers of longitudinal and circular smooth muscle fibers are collectively called the **detrusor muscle**.
- An outermost layer of fibrous connective tissue covers the detrusor layer.

When the bladder is empty, it shrivels and its elastic wall becomes heavily folded. As it receives newly formed urine, it expands and the wall becomes smooth. An average, normal bladder can store 500 mL (1 pint) of urine, but it may distend when needed to a capacity twice that amount. You cannot palpate an empty bladder, but a full or distended bladder extends upward to form a pear shape that you can feel in the suprapubic region.

The Urethra Transports Urine

The urethra transports urine from the bladder to the body's exterior. In women, the urethra is about 3 to 4 cm (1.5 in.) long and is anchored to the anterior wall of the vagina by connective tissue; it opens at the **urinary meatus** between the clitoris and vaginal opening. Because the female urethra is so short, women are especially prone to urinary tract infection from microorganisms residing in the vagina and rectum. In men, the urethra extends about 20 cm (8 in.) from the bladder to the urinary meatus at the distal end of the penis. As it leaves the bladder, the male urethra passes through a surrounding gland known as the **prostate**. In addition to urine, the male urethra also carries semen.

The mucous membrane of the urethra (in both men and women) is continuous with the bladder and the ureters. Therefore, infection in the urethra can easily spread through the bladder and up into the kidneys.

KnowledgeCheck 28-1

- Identify the major structures of the urinary system.
- What are the functions of the kidneys?
- Briefly describe how urine is formed.
- What role do the ureters, bladder, and urethra play in urinary elimination?

HOW DOES URINARY ELIMINATION OCCUR?

Where the bladder connects to the urethra is a thickening of smooth muscle, called the **internal urethral sphincter**. When closed, the internal sphincter keeps urine in the bladder from entering the urethra. When the bladder contains 200 to 450 mL of urine (50 to 200 mL in children), the distention activates stretch receptors in the bladder wall. The stretch receptors send sensory impulses to the *voiding reflex center* in the spinal cord, triggering motor impulses that cause the detrusor muscle to contract and the internal sphincter to relax. The internal urethral sphincter is not under voluntary control.

Voiding (also called **urination** or **micturition**) occurs when contraction of the detrusor muscle pushes stored urine through the relaxed internal urethral sphincter into the urethra. This triggers the conscious urge to void. However, voiding may be voluntarily delayed by inhibiting release of a second, **external urethral sphincter**. When the person is ready to urinate, the brain signals the external sphincter to relax, and urine flows through the urethra. Further contraction of the detrusor muscle normally forces out any urine remaining in the bladder. After the detrusor muscle relaxes, the bladder begins to fill with urine again.

As you can see, voiding and control of urination require that, in addition to normal functioning of the bladder and urethra, the brain, spinal cord, and nerves supplying the bladder and urethra be intact. The person must be aware of the need to urinate and able to respond by either inhibiting the reflex or by emptying the bladder.

Normal Urination Patterns

The kidneys produce urine at a rate of about 50 to 60 mL per hour, or 1,500 mL per day. However, output may fluctuate by 1,000 mL to 2,000 mL depending on various factors discussed in the next section. Most people void about five or six times per day, even eight times is normal—typically after awakening, after each meal, and just before bedtime. When fluid intake is increased, urination will be more frequent. Sometimes frequent urination is a sign of other medical problems, such as diabetes or urinary tract infection.

Characteristics of Normal Urine

Specific gravity is a measure of dissolved solutes in a solution. As the concentration of the urine solutes increases, specific gravity increases. The specific gravity of distilled water is 1.000 because there are no dissolved solutes. The normal specific gravity range for urine is 1.002 to 1.030. A very low specific gravity (e.g., 1.001) may indicate the kidney is ineffective in concentrating urine; a high specific gravity (e.g., 1.029) means the person is dehydrated. As fluid intake increases, urine becomes dilute and lighter in color to almost clear as it approaches a specific gravity of 1.000. In contrast, if fluid intake is low or there have been fluid losses, as with diarrhea or vomiting, the urine darkens as the specific gravity rises. Characteristics of urine are discussed in depth later in this chapter. Also,

 Go to Chapter 28, **Procedure 28-3B: Measuring Specific Gravity of Urine**, in Volume 2.

 Think**Like a Nurse** 28-2

- How does Marlena's (Meet Your Patient) urinary elimination pattern differ from normal?
- What would you expect to find if you measured her specific gravity?
- Marlena's symptoms suggest a urinary tract infection. How might this be related to the fact that she is sexually active?

WHAT FACTORS AFFECT URINARY ELIMINATION?

Given the complex structure and physiology of the urinary organs, it isn't surprising that many of the following variables affect their function.

Developmental Factors: Infants and Children

A newborn's kidneys produce 15 to 60 mL of urine per kilogram of body weight per day. Newborns do not concentrate urine well and, therefore, may void up to 25 times during the first 24 hours of life. The normal specific gravity of their urine is 1.008. Over the first weeks of life, the urine gradually becomes more concentrated, and the well-hydrated infant produces eight to ten wet diapers a day. Infants do not have voluntary control of voiding because neuromuscular functioning is immature.

The timing of toilet training is highly variable and is influenced by family and culture (e.g., the presence of older children who can act as role models). In the United States, most parents begin toilet training when their child is between 18 and 36 months of age. This timing can vary widely. Before toilet training can occur, toddlers must be able to control the external urethral sphincter, sense the urge to void, communicate their need to use the toilet, and remove their clothing. Toddlers usually stay dry in the daytime before they can go without a diaper all night. Occasional wetting (**enuresis**) is entirely normal in children, even in the early school years, especially when the child is intensely involved in a game, test, or other absorbing activity. Such events should be accepted calmly and not punished.

Nocturnal enuresis, or nighttime bedwetting, occurs in approximately 5% to 10% of 5-year-old children, 1.5% to 5% of 9- and 10-year-olds, and 1% of those aged 15 years and older. Males have higher prevalence rates than females at all age points (Brown, Pope, & Brown, 2011).

Primary nocturnal enuresis is bedwetting in a child who has not achieved consistent dryness at night. **Secondary enuresis** occurs in a child who has had at least 6 months of nighttime dryness.

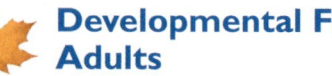
Developmental Factors: Older Adults

The size and functioning of the kidneys begin to decrease at about age 50, and by age 80 only about two-thirds of the functioning nephrons remain. This results in a decline in filtration rate, which affects the ability to dilute and concentrate urine, but does not normally create problems unless an illness alters fluid balance. For example, when older adults lose fluids and electrolytes through vomiting and diarrhea, it is difficult for their kidneys to maintain acid–base and electrolyte balances. Chronic diseases such as arteriosclerosis, common in older adults, can reduce blood flow and impair renal function. Decreased kidney function places older adults at risk for drug toxicity, as well.

The potential volume of the bladder decreases because of a loss of elasticity in the bladder wall; thus, older adults need to urinate more frequently, especially during the night (**nocturnal frequency**). Loss of elasticity and muscle tone also decreases the ability of the bladder to empty completely. Retention of urine after voiding then increases the risk for bladder infections. In women, childbearing may have weakened the pelvic muscles, which can lead to leakage of urine. In older men, the prostate gland may be enlarged, causing urinary frequency and hesitancy. Most older men have some degree of difficulty starting urination or reduced force of the urinary stream, and may experience dribbling.

Personal, Sociocultural, and Environmental Factors

Many people put off voiding while they are working, watching TV, or busy with other tasks. Delaying urination promotes urinary stasis and can lead to bladder infections. Other situations can inhibit voiding, as well, such as the following:

- *Anxiety*. A person who is anxious and tense cannot relax the abdominal and perineal muscles and the external urethral sphincter. It is then difficult to void.
- *Lack of Time*. Most people find it difficult to void when they feel rushed; therefore, when helping patients to void, make sure you have scheduled enough time for them to relax fully.
- *Lack of Privacy*. Many people require privacy for voiding and if they are in a restaurant or other unfamiliar environment, they may be embarrassed even to ask for directions to a bathroom. Some hospitalized clients may also avoid asking for assistance to the bathroom.

- *Loss of Dignity.* In Chapter 11, we talked about the loss of dignity that hospitalized patients experience. Patients who need assistance with toileting may be especially vulnerable to such feelings, especially if they require catheterization or a bedpan. It is important, therefore, to acknowledge such feelings and encourage the patient to participate in other aspects of self-care, such as bathing and dressing.
- *Cultural Influences.* Some patients will state personal, cultural, or religious requirements for toileting assistance to be provided by a person of the same gender, or they will wait until a visit from a family member before acknowledging their need for help with voiding.

Nutrition, Hydration, and Activity Level

Substances that contain caffeine, such as coffee, tea, cola, and chocolate, act as diuretics and increase urine production. Consuming large amounts of alcohol impairs the release of ADH, resulting in increased production of urine. In contrast, a diet high in salt causes water retention and decreases urine production.

The kidneys also conserve water when a person is dehydrated, such as after heavy exercise or when fluid intake is inadequate. This causes the urine to be concentrated and low in volume. During prolonged periods of physical activity, especially in hot weather, the body loses sodium and other electrolytes rapidly through sweat; for this reason, electrolyte replacement beverages may be more beneficial than plain water in helping to prevent dehydration for prolonged or vigorous-intensity activity (Thompson & Manore, 2012). For most adults, pale to clear urine indicates adequate hydration.

KnowledgeCheck 28-2

- What quantity of urine in the bladder will stimulate the urge to void?
- Identify at least three methods for determining whether hydration is adequate and urine output is within normal limits.

Medications

Various medications affect urination. Phenazopyridine hydrochloride (Pyridium), a bladder analgesic, turns the urine a deep orange-red color. *Diuretics,* sometimes called "water pills," treat blood pressure, fluid retention, and edema by increasing elimination of urine. Diuretics are classified as thiazide, potassium-sparing, or loop-acting diuretics (Box 28-1). In contrast, a number of medications have a side effect of urinary retention. They inhibit the free flow of urine because of *anticholinergic effects* (e.g., medications relax smooth muscle). See Box 28-2 for a listing of the most common medications associated with urinary retention.

Still other medications are **nephrotoxic** (damaging to the kidneys). These include some antibiotics, such as gentamicin (Garamycin) and amphotericin B (Amphotec, a fungicide), and high doses or long-term use of aspirin and ibuprofen.

BOX 28-1 ■ Common Diuretic Classes

Thiazide diuretics are used to treat high blood pressure by reducing the amount of sodium and water in the body. They also dilate blood vessels, thereby lowering blood pressure.

Potassium-sparing diuretics reduce the amount of water in the body. Unlike other diuretic medicines, these medicines do not cause potassium loss.

Loop-acting diuretics cause the kidneys to excrete more urine by reabsorbing less water. This reduces the amount of water in the body and lowers blood pressure.

Medications that have significant interactions with diuretics include digoxin, antihypertensives, lithium, certain antidepressants (especially when taking thiazide or loop-acting diuretics), and the immunosuppressant cyclosporine, especially when the patient is taking a potassium-sparing diuretic.

Common side effects of diuretics include weakness, muscle cramps, skin rash, increased sensitivity to sunlight (with thiazide diuretics), dizziness, lightheadedness, joint pain.

The following medications are sometimes used to treat various bladder conditions.

- **Anticholinergics** inhibit involuntary contractions of the bladder, increase capacity of the bladder, and delay the urge to void for people with urge incontinence. They may be given orally or transdermally. Transdermal medications are used to treat urge incontinence caused by overactive bladder. The patch relieves symptoms up to 4 days.
- **Antidepressants** (e.g., duloxetine or imipramine) can reduce stress incontinence by causing bladder muscles to relax. Some drugs work by stimulating the nerve that controls the urethral sphincter.
- **Antispasmodics** help to relax the bladder and prevent urge incontinence. For example, propantheline bromide (Pro-Banthine) is prescribed to stop bladder muscle contractions (overactive bladder).
- **Muscarinic receptor antagonists** (e.g., tolterodine tartrate) block nerve receptors in the smooth muscle of the bladder. These medications control bladder contraction and reduce urinary frequency for people suffering from overactive bladder and urge incontinence.
- **Estrogen** is used to improve the blood flow to the urethral tissues and increase thickness of mucosal and urethral tissues. Estrogen is not FDA-approved for treatment of stress incontinence, although may be prescribed for other reasons.
- **Botulinum toxin** injections control spasms of overactive bladder by relaxing the muscles. It has FDA approval for use in overactive bladder related to nerve damage, such as with spinal cord injury or multiple sclerosis.

Surgery and Anesthesia

Reproductive and Urinary Tract Surgeries can affect urine solutes, urine characteristics, and the ability to pass urine normally. Manipulation of the urinary tract frequently leads to trauma, bleeding, or the introduction of bacteria into a normally sterile tract. Swelling after diagnostic or invasive procedures and childbirth may cause urinary retention.

Surgery in the Pubic Area, Vagina, or Rectum is associated with a high incidence of trauma to the urinary organs, lower abdominal swelling, loss of pelvic muscle control, and increased pressure on the kidneys, ureters, or bladder. Surgery on the reproductive organs, such as hysterectomy in women or transurethral resection of the prostate in men, usually requires the use of an indwelling catheter (tube) for draining the bladder postoperatively. The urine may be red or pink-tinged after any invasive urinary tract surgery or procedure.

Anesthetic Agents can decrease blood pressure and glomerular filtration, thus decreasing urine formation. Spinal anesthesia decreases the patient's awareness of the need to void, which may lead to bladder distention.

Pathological Conditions

Disorders of the urinary system that affect urinary elimination include the following:

- *Infection or inflammation* of the bladder, ureters, or kidneys
- **Renal calculi** (kidney stones) or tumors, which obstruct the normal flow of urine
- In older men, **hypertrophy** (excessive growth) of the prostate gland due to benign or cancerous lesions, which interferes with flow of urine from the bladder into the urethra

Diseases involving other systems can indirectly affect urinary function. For example:

- *Cardiovascular and metabolic disorders* decrease blood flow through the glomeruli and thus impair filtration and urine production.
- *Nervous system* conditions that affect control of the urinary system organs will impair urinary elimination. After a stroke or spinal cord injury, for example, some patients may lose bladder control. *Neurogenic bladder* occurs as a result of impaired neurological function. The person cannot perceive bladder fullness or control the urinary sphincters. The bladder becomes flaccid or spastic, causing frequent involuntary loss of urine.
- *Systemic infection*, especially when accompanied by a high fever, causes the kidneys to reabsorb and retain water.
- *Immobility and impaired communication* may interfere with the ability to get to the bathroom in time or to communicate the need for assistance. This may result in urination in inappropriate settings or at inappropriate times.

- *Cognitive changes* that alter perception of the urge to void or severe psychiatric conditions involving altered perception or ability to manage activities of daily living may lead to **incontinence**, which is involuntary loss of urine.

KnowledgeCheck 28-3

- What common medications increase the amount of urine voided?
- What types of medications are associated with urinary retention?
- What types of conditions or surgeries are associated with a high incidence of altered urination?

Example Problem: Urinary Tract Infections

Normally urine is free of bacteria, viruses, and fungi. A urinary tract infection (UTI) occurs when microorganisms, usually *Escherichia coli*, which usually live harmlessly in the colon, enter the urethra and begin to multiply, overwhelming the normal flora. An infection limited to the urethra is called **urethritis**. **Cystitis** occurs when bacteria travel up the urethra into the bladder, causing a bladder infection. If not treated promptly, the infection may progress superiorly (upward) to the ureters or kidneys (**pyelonephritis**).

Several biological safeguards are in place in the urinary system to prevent UTIs. One-way valves at the junction of the ureters and bladder help prevent urine from backing up toward the kidneys. In addition, the flow of urine during urination helps wash bacteria out of the body. In men, the prostate gland produces secretions that slow bacterial growth. But despite these safeguards, infections still occur.

Risk Factors for Urinary Tract Infection

People who are more prone to UTIs include the following:

- *Sexually active women.* During sexual activity, perineal pathogens may enter the urethra. Because a woman's urethra is short, pathogens, particularly *E. coli*, can gain rapid access to the bladder.
- *Women who use spermicidal contraceptive gel.* Spermicides reduce normal flora in the vagina, allowing pathogens to multiply unrestricted.
- *Pregnant women.* Some pregnant women are more prone to UTI because of hormonal changes and because of pressure of the uterus on the bladder.

  - *Older women.* The loss of estrogen associated with menopause leads to drying of the mucosa in the vagina and urethra and a decrease in protective normal flora.
- *Men with an enlarged prostate.* An enlarged prostate may develop as a result of aging or cancerous changes. Pressure from the prostate creates difficulty emptying the bladder, resulting in stagnant urine, which provides an excellent medium for the growth of bacteria.

- *People with kidney stones.* Kidney stones (*renal calculi*) obstruct the flow of urine, creating stagnation, and irritate the urinary tract as they are passed.
- *Anyone who has an indwelling catheter.* Indwelling catheters pose several risks:

  Failing to maintain a closed drainage system increases the risk for infection by allowing bacteria to enter the catheter; the catheter provides a pathway for bacteria to migrate up into the urinary system (Chenoweth, Gould, & Saint, 2014; Gould, Umscheid, Agarwal, et al., 2009; Wald, Fink, Makic, et al., 2012).

  The catheter irritates the mucosal lining of the urethra, which then creates a portal of entry for microbes. The longer the catheter is indwelling, the higher is the risk of developing UTI (Bernard, Hunter, & Moore, 2012).

  The urine collection bag is a reservoir for microorganisms.

- *People who have diabetes mellitus.* Glucose in the urine provides nutrients for bacteria to multiply.
- *Immunocompromised patients.* Susceptible hosts (e.g., neonates, elderly, those receiving immunosuppressive drugs, people with weakened immune systems) are less able to maintain a healthy balance of microbes in the urinary tract.
- *People who have a history of UTIs.* Anyone with a previous UTI is more likely to experience a recurrence. This may be related to the absence of certain antigens against bacteria that attach to the lining of the urethra (National Kidney and Urologic Diseases Information Clearinghouse, 2011).

Recognizing and Treating Urinary Tract Infections

The presence of bacteria in a symptomatic patient is used in the medical diagnosis of UTI. To assist in the diagnosis of UTI, assess for the signs and symptoms.

Back pain	Foul-smelling urine
Bladder spasms	Hematuria
Chills	Nausea and vomiting
Dysuria	Pyuria
Edema	Urgency
Fever	Urinary frequency

Key Point: *The classic signs of UTI are urinary WBCs, pyuria, dysuria, urgency, and frequency.*

Signs of fever, bacteriuria, and abnormal blood values do not predict catheter-associated urinary tract infections (CAUTI) (Madigan & Neff, 2003) and UTIs in older adults (Rowe & Juthani-Mehta, 2014). Catheter-associated UTIs are generally assumed to be benign. Such infection in otherwise healthy patients is often asymptomatic and is likely to resolve spontaneously with the removal of the catheter (Hooton, Bradley, Cardenas, et al., 2010). Occasionally, infection persists and leads to such complications as prostatitis, epididymitis, cystitis, pyelonephritis, and gram-negative bacteremia, particularly in high risk

patients (Grabe, Bjerklund-Johansen, Botto, et al., 2013; Parker, Callan, Harwood, et al., 2009a, 2009b).

Antibiotics are used to treat UTI. The length and type of treatment depends on the location and severity of infection. In general, a bladder infection may be treated with oral antibiotics for 1 to 5 days.

 Elderly people and those with chronic underlying illness, such as diabetes, are often prescribed a longer course of treatment, sometimes up to 14 days.

In contrast, pyelonephritis (kidney infection) may require IV antibiotics for several days followed by a course of oral antibiotics. Preventive antibiotic treatment is not recommended for people requiring long-term urinary catheterization (Hooton, Bradley, Cardenas, et al., 2010; Grabe, Bjerklund-Johansen, Botto, et al., 2013; Lo, Nicolle, Classen, et al., 2008; Wound, Ostomy, and Continence Nurses Society [WOCN], 2008). Drug resistance develops easily; therefore, antibiotics are reserved for symptomatic infections (Muzzi-Bjornson & Macera, 2011).

Think**Like a Nurse** 28-3

As you may have concluded, Marlena (Meet Your Patient) has a UTI. What additional history questions would you like to ask Marlena?

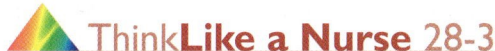

Example Problem: Urinary Retention

Urinary retention is an inability to empty the bladder completely. Etiologies include obstruction, inflammation and swelling, neurological problems, medications, and anxiety.

Obstruction Among men, an enlarged prostate is the most common cause of obstruction in the lower urinary tract. Other obstructions include stones lodged in the urethra, strictures or scars from previous injury, tumors or blood clots in the urinary system, and fecal impaction. Impacted stool distends the rectum and causes forward pressure on the urethra, interfering with the flow of urine out of the bladder.

Inflammation and Swelling Obstruction may also occur as a result of inflammation and swelling, for example, from infection or surgery in the pelvic region. Swelling narrows the diameter of the urethra so that urine cannot flow freely.

Neurological Problems Recall that voiding requires that the brain, spinal cord, and nerves supplying the bladder and urethra must be intact. Conditions that affect innervation of the bladder include spinal cord tumors or injury, herniated disk, and viral infections involving perineal nerves (e.g., genital herpes).

Medications Anesthesia and other medications can also cause temporary problems with urination. Box 28-2 provides examples of medications with anticholinergic or alpha-adrenergic effects that may impede urine flow.

BOX 28-2 ■ Medications Associated With Urinary Retention

Class	Use	Medication
Antihistamine	Treat allergy symptoms	fexofenadine (Allegra)
		diphenhydramine (Benadryl)
		chlorpheniramine (Chlor-Trimeton)
		cetirizine (Zyrtec)
Anticholinergics/antispasmodics	Treat stomach cramps, muscle spasms, and urinary incontinence	hyoscyamine (Levbid, Cystospaz, Gastrosed)
		oxybutynin (Ditropan, Oxytrol)
		tolterodine (Detrol)
		propantheline (Pro-Banthine)
Tricyclic antidepressants	Treat anxiety and depression	imipramine (Tofranil)
		amitriptyline (Elavil)
		nortriptyline (Aventyl)

Source: National Kidney and Urologic Diseases Information Clearinghouse. (2007, updated June 29, 2012). *Retention.* NIH Publication No. 08-6089. Retrieved December 10, 2013, from http://kidney.niddk.nih.gov/kudiseases/pubs/UrinaryRetention/

Anxiety Painful urination may produce anxiety and lead to voluntary withholding of urination.

Example Problem Urinary Incontinence

Urinary incontinence (UI) is a lack of voluntary control over urination. Urinary incontinence will affect at least 1 in 4 women and 1 in 9 men at some point in their lives.

Incidence rises with age, with as many as 30% to 50% of elderly women being affected (Rainsbury, Fabricius, & McLarty, 2011). Incontinence is associated with skin impairment, obesity, UTIs, self-rated poor health, reduced mobility, depression, social isolation, and increased caregiver burden (Dowling-Castronovo, 2013).

The total number of people affected by incontinence is presumed to be greater than current estimates because healthcare providers often fail to ask specific questions about it or people are embarrassed to admit to experiencing leakage of urine. Incontinence affects people of all ages and social and economic levels. It affects both sexes, but women are twice as likely as men to have this condition. Risk factors for incontinence also include older age, neurological disease (e.g., stroke), obesity, sedentary lifestyle, depression, and diabetes.

Although incontinence is common, it is not a normal change that occurs with aging. This myth is pervasive and often leads older adults to avoid seeking treatment. Many people do not mention leakage of urine to healthcare providers because they are embarrassed, believe nothing can be done, or believe it is an inevitable condition of older age. These views may lead to restriction of activities and ultimately to loneliness, depression, and isolation (Dowling-Castronovo & Bradway, 2012).

In men, UI is most often related to benign prostatic hyperplasia (enlarged prostate) or to prostatectomy. In women, it is often related to childbirth, specifically to vaginal delivery. Incidence is even higher among those who required episiotomy or forceps- or vacuum-assisted birth. Other risk factors for UI are perimenopausal status, high body mass index (BMI), diabetes, and current cigarette smoking.

Types of Urinary Incontinence

The two major types of urinary incontinence are transient and established. **Transient incontinence**, also called acute or reversible, is characterized by a sudden onset of usually reversible signs and symptoms. Causes include urinary tract infection and medications, especially diuretics. **Established urinary incontinence** is also known as chronic or persistent incontinence (Dowling-Castronovo & Bradway, 2012).

The Agency for Healthcare Research and Quality guidelines identified the following types of UI:

- **Urge incontinence** is the involuntary loss of larger amounts of urine accompanied by a strong urge to void. It is often referred to as **overactive bladder**.
- **Stress incontinence** is an involuntary loss of small amounts of urine with activities that increase intra-abdominal pressure. Etiological factors include pregnancy, childbirth, obesity, chronic constipation, and straining at stool. Activities that produce leakage of urine also include exercise, laughing, sneezing, coughing, and lifting.
- **Mixed incontinence** is a combination of urge and stress incontinence.
- **Overflow incontinence** is the loss of urine in combination with a distended bladder. Causes of overflow incontinence include fecal impaction, neurological disorders, and enlarged prostate (NANDA-I, 2012).

- **Functional incontinence** is the untimely loss of urine when no urinary or neurological cause is involved. NANDA-I (2012) defines functional incontinence as the "inability of a usually continent person to reach the toilet in time to avoid unintentional loss of urine" (p. 193). This type of incontinence occurs because of physical disability, immobility, pain, external obstacles, or problems in thinking or communicating that prevent a person from reaching a toilet.
- **Reflex incontinence** is loss of urine when the person does not realize the bladder is full and has no urge to void. Central nervous system disorders and multisystem problems are common causes. NANDA-I (2012) defines reflex urinary incontinence as the "involuntary loss of urine at somewhat predictable intervals when a specific bladder volume is reached" (p. 195). Tissue damage from radiation, cystitis, bladder inflammation, or radical pelvic surgery can also trigger reflex incontinence.

The following are other types of incontinence.

- **Enuresis**, which tends to be familial, is involuntary urination after about 5 to 6 years of age, when control is usually established. Enuresis is *primary* if bladder training was never achieved and *secondary* if control was established and then lost. Enuresis has been associated with stress (e.g., marital discord), UTI, allergies, abnormal electroencephalographic patterns, sleep disorders, hearty laughing, and small bladder capacity; however, the cause is not always apparent.
- **Nocturnal enuresis** (bedwetting) can persist until age 10 or later. If one parent had nighttime bedwetting as a child, there is a high chance the child will also experience it. Most often children outgrow the condition. Only a small percentage of the secondary type is caused by a medical condition, such as UTI, urinary obstruction, diabetes, pressure on the bladder from extreme constipation, or neurological disorders of the spinal cord.

Practical Knowledge
knowing **how**

As a nurse, you will monitor and assist clients with urinary elimination, teach them about body functions, and work collaboratively with the healthcare team to facilitate normal urinary function. In the remainder of the chapter, we discuss these activities. Also see the Nursing Care Plan and the Care Map.

ASSESSMENT

To assess urinary elimination, you will use data from the nursing history, physical examination, and diagnostic and laboratory reports.

Nursing History

Because urination patterns vary among individuals, you will need a nursing history to determine what is normal for a particular person. As you interview the client, pay attention to her reaction to your questions. Many people are embarrassed about discussing urination. Tailor your assessment to the client's needs, and use language that makes her comfortable. For a set of interview questions,

 Go to Chapter 28, **Assessment Guidelines and Tools, Urinary Elimination History Questions,** in Volume 2.

 Think**Like a Nurse** 28-4

In the Meet Your Patient scenario, some assessment findings were given for Marlena. What additional physical assessments might you perform to complete this urinary tract assessment?

Physical Assessment

Physical assessment for urinary elimination includes examination of the kidneys, bladder, urethra, and skin surrounding the genitals, as appropriate. For a complete discussion of physical examination of the genitourinary system,

 Go to Chapter 22, **Procedure 22-17: Assessing the Male Genitourinary System,** and **Procedure 22-18: Assessing the Female Genitourinary System,** in Volume 2.

Knowledge Check 28-4

- What should you discuss with your client when performing a nursing history focused on urinary elimination?
- What are the key elements of a physical assessment for a client with urination problems?

 Think**Like a Nurse** 28-5

After gathering a focused nursing history pertaining to urinary elimination, you check your patient's vital signs: oral temperature, 99.4°F (37.4°C); radial pulse, 88 beats/min; respiratory rate, 20 breaths/min; and blood pressure, 108/72 mm Hg. What other physical assessment findings might you expect?

Assessing the Urine

In addition to observations already mentioned, assessment of the urine includes measuring urine output and conducting a variety of bedside tests.

Measuring Intake and Output

Measuring urine output is part of a comprehensive plan to monitor a client's fluid status. Recall that the kidneys produce urine at a rate of approximately 50 to 60 mL per hour, or 1,500 mL per day. However, urinary output fluctuates depending on the quantity of fluids the patient drinks and on other factors, such as the ability of the heart to circulate the blood, adequate kidney functioning, and the ability of the patient to void the urine.

Urine output might be low if the person is sweating excessively or has significant vomiting and diarrhea. High fever can contribute to reduced urine output.

You must know both the intake and the output (I&O) as well as relevant physical condition to interpret the meaning of the patient data. For example, if urine output is low, you cannot assume the patient's kidneys are not working properly. If his intake is also low, he may be dehydrated. But what does it mean if his intake is high and his output low? Yes, this could mean his kidneys are not working well. However, it could also mean that his kidneys are producing urine but that he has urinary retention because of something that is obstructing flow.

To measure fluid intake, record all fluids the patient drinks or receives intravenously. Include the following items as fluid intake: oral fluids, semiliquid foods, ice chips, IV fluids, tube feedings, and irrigations instilled and not withdrawn immediately. Fluid output includes the following items: urine output, gastrointestinal fluid loss (e.g., emesis), liquid feces, and drainage (e.g., from suction devices or wounds). Explain to the client, family members, and all caregivers that I&O are being monitored. Posting a sign at the bedside or on the door to the room is a helpful reminder. When possible, have the client assist you with monitoring.

You will usually total the I&O at the end of each shift, as well as for each 24-hour period. In intensive care units, you may measure I&O hourly. Most healthcare facilities have standardized I&O forms. I&O may be recorded on a separate form or be part of a flowsheet. To see examples, see Figure 18-2.

 Go to Chapter 18, **Forms: Nursing Assessment Flow Sheet,** in Volume 2.

For more discussion of intake and output, go to Chapters 18 and 38.

Observe standard precautions when handling urine to prevent exposure to body fluids. Always wear disposable procedure gloves, and avoid splashing the urine and contaminating your uniform. The method you use to measure urine is dictated in part by the amount of help the client needs with urination.

Voided Urine

Many ambulatory clients need no assistance with urination. Be sure to inform them you are monitoring their I&O, and explain how they can help. Place a specimen "hat" (collection container) under the toilet seat to collect urine, or have male clients void into a urinal. Periodically measure the output and empty the urine into the toilet. For clients who can assist with recording the I&O, provide a bedside clipboard.

For the client with mobility problems, use a bedpan or urinal to collect urine output. Use a fracture pan for clients with a fracture of the pelvis, lower back, or legs or for clients who have casts, splints, or braces on their legs. Male clients may void into a urinal while remaining in bed.

 Go to Chapter 29, **Procedure 29-2: Placing and Removing a Bedpan,** in Volume 2.

For complete instructions for measuring urine output from a bedpan or urinal,

 Go to Chapter 28, **Procedure 28-1A: Measuring Urine Output From a Bedpan or Urinal,** in Volume 2.

Urine From a Catheter

An **indwelling urinary catheter**, also known as a Foley or a retention catheter, is a flexible tube that is inserted through the urethra into the bladder. It is held in place by a balloon that is inflated in the bladder above the detrusor muscle. Catheter insertion and ongoing care are discussed in the Planning Interventions/Implementation section of this chapter.

You will usually measure urine output from the indwelling catheter at the end of each shift unless otherwise prescribed. Clients who require close monitoring of I&O will have a special collection bag with a measuring chamber. Often this is used to assess hourly urine output.

For complete instructions for measuring urine from a catheter,

 Go to Chapter 28, **Procedure 28-1B: Measuring Urine From an Indwelling Catheter,** in Volume 2.

Obtaining Samples for Urine Studies

Many disorders of the urinary system can be assessed by examining urine. You will perform some of these tests at the bedside. For others, you will collect a specimen that is analyzed in the lab. The various types of urine samples are discussed in the text that follows.

Freshly Voided Specimen

To collect a freshly voided sample, collect the urine in the same manner as when you are measuring intake and output. Pour the urine into a specimen container labeled with the patient's name, the date, and the time of collection. Many facilities require packaging the container in a moisture-proof specimen-handling bag. Follow agency policy on additional packaging. Transport the specimen to the lab as soon as possible (according to agency policies). If there is a delay in getting the specimen to the lab, most agencies recommend refrigeration.

 Go to Chapter 28, **Procedures 28-1: Measuring Urine** and **28-2: Obtaining a Urine Specimen for Testing,** in Volume 2.

Clean-Catch Specimen

Many diagnostic tests require a clean-catch urine specimen. The client must cleanse the genitalia before voiding and collect the sample in midstream because the initial flow of urine may contain organisms from the urethral meatus, distal urethra, and perineum. A midstream sample is free of these contaminants. The Highlights of Procedures box in this chapter summarizes key steps in collecting a clean-catch sample. For the complete procedure,

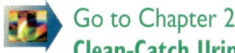 Go to Chapter 28, **Procedure 28-2A: Collecting a Clean-Catch Urine Specimen,** in Volume 2.

Sterile Urine Specimen

A sterile urine specimen aids in determining the presence of a urinary tract infection. You can obtain a sterile urine specimen by inserting a catheter into the bladder or by withdrawing a sample from an indwelling catheter. Do not take the specimen from the collection bag because that urine may be several hours old.

 Never disconnect the catheter from the drainage tube to obtain a sample. Interrupting the system creates a portal of entry for pathogens, thereby increasing the risk of contamination.

For a description of the steps involved in obtaining a sterile specimen from an indwelling catheter, see the Highlights of Procedures box and also

 Go to Chapter 28, **Procedure 28-2B: Obtaining a Sterile Urine Specimen From a Catheter,** in Volume 2.

24-Hour Urine Collection

A 24-hour urine collection, may be prescribed to evaluate some renal disorders by showing kidney function at different times of the day and night. You will need to use a large container and preserve all the urine voided in the 24-hour time period. For details about how to collect this type of specimen, see the Highlights of Procedures box, and also

 Go to Chapter 28, **Procedure 28-2C: Collecting a 24-Hour Urine Specimen,** in Volume 2.

Routine Urinalysis

A routine urinalysis (UA) is one of the most commonly prescribed laboratory tests. It is used as an overall screening test as well as an aid to diagnosing renal, hepatic, and other diseases. Urinalysis requires a freshly voided sample.

Urinalysis techniques include "dipstick" testing and/ or microscopic analysis. Dipstick testing is commonly performed at the bedside; microscopic examination is done in the lab. Box 28-3 contains several terms used to describe urine characteristics and quantity. For the expected findings and common variants of urinalysis,

 Go to Chapter 28, **Diagnostic Testing, Urinalysis,** in Volume 2.

Bedside Testing (Dipstick)

Dipstick testing can determine pH and specific gravity and the presence of protein, glucose, ketones, and occult blood in the urine. Commercially prepared kits contain a reagent designed to detect a specific substance (e.g., glucose). The reagent may be a paper test strip, a fluid, or a tablet. When contacted by the urine, a chemical reaction causes a color change that you compare to a color chart (Fig. 28-4). You will need good lighting to evaluate the test strip results. Read the kit label to be certain that you

are using the correct reagent and that the kit is not past the expiration date. Follow the manufacturer's directions regarding the amount of urine needed and the time needed for the reagent to develop. For guidelines for dipstick testing and delegation,

Go to Chapter 28, **Procedure 28-3A: Dipstick Testing of Urine,** in Volume 2.

BOX 28-3 ■ Terms Associated With Urination

Acute renal failure (ARF): An acute rise in the serum creatinine level of 25% or more. May be caused by inadequate blood flow to the kidney, injury to the kidney glomeruli or tubules, or obstruction of kidney outflow.

Anuria: The absence of urine, often associated with kidney failure or congestive heart failure. This term is used when urine output is less than 100 mL in 24 hours.

Dysuria: Painful or difficult urination. May be associated with infection or partial obstruction of the urinary tract as well as medications that trigger urinary retention.

End-stage renal disease (ESRD): A chronic rise in serum creatinine levels associated with loss of kidney function that must be treated with dialysis or transplantation. Also known as chronic renal failure (CRF).

Enuresis: Involuntary loss of urine

Frequency: The need to urinate at short intervals

Hematuria: Blood in the urine. May be due to trauma, kidney stones, infection, or menstruation.

Micturition: To start the stream of urine; to urinate; release urine from the bladder

Nephropathy: A broad term meaning disease of the kidney

Nephrotoxic: A substance that damages kidney tissue. Some antibiotics (gentamicin, tobramycin, and amikacin), nonsteroidal anti-inflammatory drugs (NSAIDs), lead, and contrast media have the potential to be nephrotoxic.

Nocturia: Frequent urination after going to bed. May be caused by excessive fluid intake as well as a variety of urinary tract and cardiovascular problems.

Nocturnal enuresis: Involuntary loss of urine while asleep

Oliguria: Urine output of less than 400 mL in 24 hours. For pediatric patients, oliguria is <0.5–1.0 mL/kg per hour.

Pessary: An incontinence device that is inserted into the vagina to reduce organ prolapse or pressure on the bladder

Polyuria: Excessive urination. May be caused by excessive hydration, diabetes mellitus, diabetes insipidus, or kidney disease.

Proteinuria: The presence of protein in the urine. May be a sign of infection or kidney disease.

Pyuria: Pus in the urine. May be caused by lesions or infection in the urinary tract.

Urgency: A sudden, almost uncontrollable need to urinate.

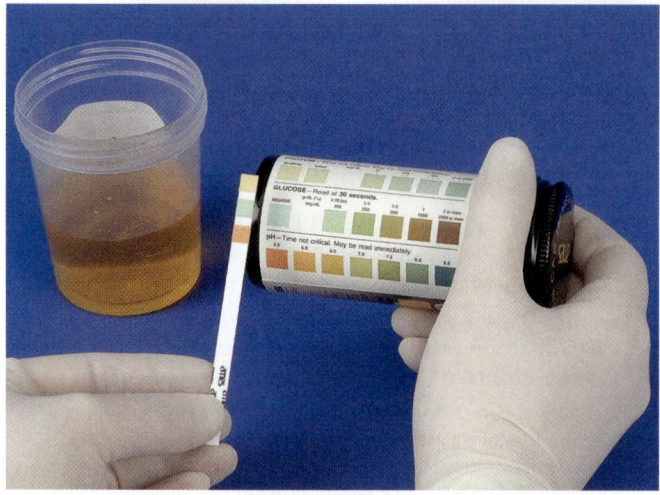

FIGURE 28-4 Commercial testing kits contain a reagent for a specific substance. A chemical reaction with the urine causes a color change that you interpret using a color chart.

Specific Gravity

Specific gravity, an indicator of urine concentration, can be measured with a reagent strip. However, when you need to be precise and accurate, you should use a refractometer. Specific gravity is usually tested in the laboratory, but it is a nursing responsibility in some settings. For guidelines when testing urine specific gravity,

 Go to Chapter 28, **Procedure 28-3B: Measuring Specific Gravity of Urine,** in Volume 2.

A **refractometer** (Fig. 28-5) measures the extent to which a beam of light changes direction when it passes through the urine (the *refractive index*). If the concentration

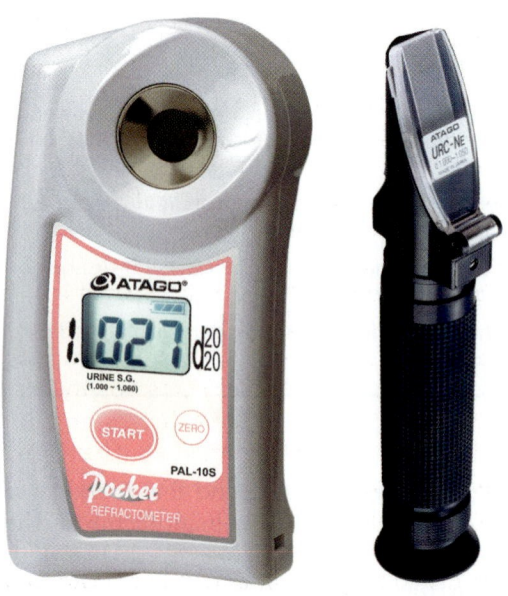

FIGURE 28-5 A refractometer indicates urine concentration by measuring the extent to which a beam of light is refracted ("bent") when passed through the urine.
(Courtesy of Atago USA, Inc.)

of solids is high, the light is refracted more. The method is quick and easy to perform and requires only a few drops of urine. A refractometer is more precise, requires a much smaller specimen, is more compact, and poses less risk of spills and exposure to body fluids than does a urinometer, which for the most part is no longer used.

KnowledgeCheck 28-5

- Explain how to collect a clean-catch urine specimen.
- You are caring for a patient on a hospital unit from 0700 to 1200. Based on the following information, calculate the I&O and comment on your findings.
  Receiving IV fluid at 125 mL/hr
  0800 breakfast—4 oz juice, toast, scrambled eggs, 8 oz coffee
  0930—3 oz water
  0700 to 1200—wound drainage: 360 mL
  0700 to 1200—urine output per indwelling catheter: 180 mL

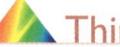 ThinkLike a Nurse 28-6

- Why do you think the first voided urine is discarded at the start of a 24-hour urine collection?
- Below are the dipstick findings you obtained on the clean-catch specimen from Marlena (Meet Your Patient).

Urinalysis	Result
pH	8.0
Specific gravity	1.030
Protein	Negative
Glucose	Negative
RBCs	Trace
Nitrite	+1
WBCs	+2
Bilirubin	Negative
Ketones	Negative
Urobilinogen	Negative

  a. Identify the abnormal findings.
  b. What would you expect the findings of her urine culture and sensitivity to demonstrate?

Blood Studies

Blood urea nitrogen (BUN) and creatinine levels are commonly measured to assess renal function and hydration. For normal ranges,

 Go to Chapter 28, **Diagnostic Testing, Blood Studies: BUN and Creatinine,** in Volume 2.

Common Diagnostic Procedures

A variety of diagnostic procedures may be performed on the urinary tract. These procedures are conducted in the operating room, procedure suite, or radiology department. Typically nurses are responsible for preparing the client for the procedure, assisting with specimen collection, delivering aftercare, and sometimes assisting the physician. For a discussion of urinary system studies and the nursing responsibilities associated with them,

 Go to Chapter 28, **Diagnostic Testing, Studies of the Urinary System,** in Volume 2.

ANALYSIS/NURSING DIAGNOSIS

Urinary elimination problems are described by several nursing and medical diagnoses. NANDA-I diagnoses specific to urinary elimination include the following:

Functional Urinary Incontinence
Impaired Urinary Elimination
Reflex Urinary Incontinence
Risk for Urge Urinary Incontinence
Stress Urinary Incontinence
Urge Urinary Incontinence
Urinary Retention
Overflow Urinary Incontinence
Readiness for Enhanced Urinary Elimination
Risk for Infection (Urinary Tract)
Risk for Ineffective Renal Perfusion

Urinary problems may also be the etiology of other nursing diagnoses, such as the following:

Anxiety related to urinary urgency and recent episode of incontinence
Disturbed Body Image secondary to new urostomy
Acute Pain related to bladder spasms and urinary tract infection
Social Isolation related to frequent periods of incontinence

PLANNING OUTCOMES/EVALUATION

The general goal related to urinary elimination is that patients will comfortably void approximately 1,500 mL of light yellow urine in 24 hours. Because normal urine elimination patterns vary, the frequency and amount of urine are based on the individual's pattern, food and fluid intake, medications, and other factors.

NOC standardized outcomes for urinary problems, regardless of the specific problem, are the following: Kidney Function, Urinary Continence, Urinary Elimination, Self-Care: Toileting, and Tissue Integrity: Skin & Mucous Membranes (because urinary elimination problems often place the patient at Risk for Impaired Skin Integrity).

Individualized goals/outcome statements you might use to evaluate the effectiveness of interventions for urinary problems include the following:

- Will resume his normal urination pattern by (date).
- Will discuss feelings about his urostomy.
- Will have no visible blood in urine after 2 days on antibiotics.
- Responds to the urge to void in a timely manner.
- After voiding, states he feels he has emptied his bladder completely.
- Postvoiding residual volume is <150 mL.

PLANNING INTERVENTIONS/IMPLEMENTATION

For *NIC standardized interventions* for patients with urinary elimination nursing diagnoses,

 Go to Chapter 28, **Standardized Language, NIC Interventions for Urinary Problems,** on Davis*Plus.*

You should select nursing activities to meet individual needs and address problem etiologies. *Specific nursing activities* for patients with elimination problems fall into the following categories: promoting normal urination, preventing urinary tract infection, managing urinary retention, managing urinary incontinence, and caring for patients who have urinary diversions. The rest of this chapter discusses those activities.

Promoting Normal Urination

As a nurse, you should have a repertoire of independent nursing activities for promoting normal urination. These include providing privacy, positioning, scheduling elimination, providing and monitoring fluid and nutrition, and assisting with hygiene.

Provide Privacy

Although urination is a normal physiological process, most people consider it a private matter. Taking a matter-of-fact approach confirms to patients that you are comfortable with this aspect of care. Provide privacy when discussing or providing care related to urination. Excuse visitors from the room, draw the dividing curtains in shared rooms, and close the door to the room. Whenever possible, give the patient time alone to void. Do not, for example, hover outside the bathroom door asking, "Are you okay?" or "Are you finished?" However, if the client is weak and frail, you may need to remain with him.

Assist With Positioning

Most men stand to void and may have difficulty voiding in other positions. Whenever possible, assist the patient to the bathroom to use the toilet and allow him to assume his preferred position. Alternatively, provide a bedside commode or urinal for the patient to use. To place a urinal, position the patient in a semi-Fowler's position with the legs slightly spread. Place the urinal on the bed between the patient's legs, and insert his penis into the urinal.

Women generally find an upright seated or squatting position to be the most comfortable position for voiding. If a female patient must remain in bed, provide a bedpan. Place her in a semi-Fowler's position to urinate unless contraindicated. Raise the siderails or provide an overhead trapeze so that the patient will have grip holds to maneuver herself onto and off the bedpan. If the patient is very weak, you may need an assistant to help you position her on the bedpan, and you may need to stay with her to help her maintain her position. For the steps involved,

 Go to Chapter 28, **Procedure 29-2: Placing and Removing a Bedpan,** in Volume 2.

Quality and Safety Education for Nurses

Managing Urinary Incontinence

Chapter Key Concept: *Urinary Incontinence*

Competency: *Patient-Centered Care (Knowledge, Skills, Attitudes); Evidenced-Based Practice (Knowledge, Skills, Attitudes)**

Scenario: Dashondra Simms, RN, lives in a rural area and works in a urology practice. After participating in a radio interview to provide information about urinary incontinence, many women call the urology practice to ask for help. Dashondra asks each woman how she manages her incontinence, where she obtains information, if the condition has changed her quality of life, and if she would be willing to participate in an incontinence support group. Dashondra's notes reveal a population with unmet healthcare needs. To address this, she decides to develop a patient-centered, evidence-based program to increase participants' knowledge and confidence about managing their incontinence.

First, Dashondra accesses the National Guideline Clearinghouse Web site to obtain evidence-based guidelines for different incontinence management techniques. She searches databases such as MEDLINE and CINAHL for peer-reviewed studies that identify the psychosocial needs of patients, cultural or ethnic differences in managing incontinence. She also consults colleagues for their opinions.

Dashondra organizes a planning meeting with the women and asks them about the emotional impact of living with incontinence. The women talk about their feelings of self-worth, dignity, and confidence being affected. Self-image, sexuality, and their sense of freedom also emerged as specific psychosocial issues. The women identified that the following would be of value to them in an incontinence self-management program: education about new treatments, a monthly support group meeting, an online forum for members, and telephone or e-mail access to the nurse as desirable components of the program.

Think about it:

➤ How did Dashondra establish an evidence base for educating group members?

➤ How did she make the intervention patient centered?

➤ In what ways did Dashondra use information technology to help her design the program?

_____

Source: Hayder, D., & Schnepp, W. (2010); Schröder, A., Abrams, P., Andersson, K. E., et al. (2009); Wilson (2004).

*For specific Knowledge, Skills, and Attitudes,

 Go to the QSEN Web site at http://qsen.org/ competencies/pre-licensure-ksas/

Facilitate Toileting Routines

Most patients void on awakening, after meals or drinking a large volume of fluid, before bedtime, or during the night for some. Identify your patient's pattern, and stick to it as much as possible. If you anticipate a change in the pattern for elimination, inform the patient. For example, if the patient is to receive a diuretic, explain that he will need to urinate more often. Similarly, if the patient is scheduled for a diagnostic procedure or activity, inform him ahead of time so that he may void before the activity begins.

Provide assistance to all patients who have mobility problems and those who use the bedpan. Discuss with all NAP the need to offer assistance so that patients experience minimal delays.

Promote Adequate Fluids and Nutrition

Adequate hydration promotes urinary tract function and flushes the system of waste products. Unfortunately, many people do not drink an adequate amount of fluid. Water is the preferred fluid because soda, coffee, and tea often contain caffeine or additives that may cause diuresis. However, the amount of fluid is more important than the type. If the patient will not or cannot drink water, provide the fluid he prefers. Most people should drink at least 8 to 10 eight-ounce glasses of fluid daily (also known as the 8-by-8 rule) unless health problems limit the fluid. See Box 28-4 for strategies to increase your patient's fluid intake.

BOX 28-4 ■ Strategies to Increase Patients' Fluid Intake

- For patients with limited mobility, keep water or other liquids in easy reach.
- You may need to remind young children or patients with cognitive or psychiatric disorders to drink fluids.
- For patients who have increased fluid needs, provide goals for intake, and frequently remind them to drink.
- Many foods have a high fluid content. If the patient requires additional fluid for hydration, consider adding soup and watery foods, such as watermelon, to the diet. In contrast, if the patient requires fluid restriction, you will have to account for these foods into the fluid balance.
- Try offering liquids with a straw. Patients tend to drink more this way.
- Chilled drinks might be more appealing, particularly if the patient's mouth is dry. Offer beverages with ice if they are to be served cold.
- Provide good mouth care. Patients will often drink more readily if their mouth feels fresh.

Assist With Hygiene

Urine is irritating to the skin. Therefore, perineal cleansing is an integral part of toileting hygiene. Many ill patients are unable to do this for themselves, so you may need to provide perineal care. If the patient can ambulate to the bathroom, you merely need to assist with her usual cleansing routines. You may assist the patient by pouring warm periwash over the genitals while she is seated on the toilet, the bedside commode, or on the bedpan. Be sure to rinse with warm water because soap may be drying to the genital mucosa. Also offer a moist washcloth or towelette for washing hands after toileting. For further information,

 Go to Chapter 25, **Procedure 25-4: Providing Perineal Care,** in Volume 2.

KnowledgeCheck 28-6

- Identify activities that promote normal urination patterns.
- Write at least two nursing diagnostic statements that would be appropriate for Marlena in the Meet Your Patient scenario.

Interventions for Example Problem: Urinary Tract Infections

An important part of UTI treatment is prevention of future UTIs. The accompanying Self-Care box presents the

teaching points that you should include in your sessions with patients at risk for or recovering from a UTI.

Interventions for Example Problem: Urinary Retention

Clients with a mechanical obstruction to urine flow are treated by surgical removal or repair of the obstruction (e.g., resection of the prostate gland, removal of bladder calculi). For clients who have loss of bladder tone, collaboratively you may:

- Administer cholinergic medications, such as bethanechol chloride (Urecholine), which promote bladder emptying by stimulating contraction of the detrusor muscle.
- Administer alpha-adrenergic antagonists, such as tamsulosin (Flomax), which reduce urethral resistance and improve bladder emptying.
- Use **Credé's maneuver** (apply manual pressure over the bladder to promote emptying).
- Perform urinary catheterization.

Independent nursing interventions for patients with urinary retention include the following:

- Monitor I&O.
- Assess for risk factors for urinary retention (e.g., prostatic hypertrophy; pelvic surgery; and medications with anticholinergic side effects, such as diazepam [Valium], some antidepressants, and diphenhydramine [Benadryl]).
- Inspect and palpate for bladder distention.
- Apply heat to the lower abdomen to relax the muscles near where the bladder lies.
- Run water nearby, or place the patient's hands in warm water. Hearing running water can stimulate the urge to urinate.
- Pour distilled water over the perineum, or assist the patient to take a warm sitz bath.
- Measure the urine that remains in the bladder immediately after the patient voids. This is known as **post-void residual urine (PVR).** PVR can be measured with a portable noninvasive bladder ultrasound device (bladder scanner) or by insertion of a straight catheter.

 Go to Chapter 28, **Procedure 28-1C: Measuring Post-Void Residual Urine Volume (PVR) With a Portable Bladder Scanner,** in Volume 2.

- Advise the patient to contact a medical professional:
  If not previously evaluated for urinary hesitancy, dribbling, or weak urine stream
  For fever, vomiting, side or back pain, shaking chills, or passing little urine for 1 to 2 days
  For blood in the urine, cloudy urine, frequent or urgent need to urinate, or a discharge from the penis or vagina

---

Self-Care

Teaching Your Client About Preventing UTI

➤ **Drink at least 8 to 10 eight-ounce glasses of water per day** to keep urine dilute and to flush bacteria from the urinary tract. The Institute of Medicine (2006) recommends even more, particularly with heat exposure or prolonged exercise. Water is best. Some reports claim a benefit to drinking cranberry juice because cranberries contain a substance that keeps bacteria from sticking on the walls of the bladder (Jepson, Williams, & Craig, 2012). However, this practice is controversial (Guay, 2009).

➤ **Urinate when you first feel the urge.** Do not make a habit of postponing urination because bacteria can multiply in stagnant urine.

➤ **Always wipe from front to back** after urination or defecation.

➤ **Wear cotton underwear** because nylon or other synthetic fabrics prevent evaporation of moisture. Also avoid tight-fitting clothing in the groin area. Bacteria and other microorganisms grow well in a warm, moist environment.

➤ **Urinate after having intercourse** to flush away bacteria that might have entered the urethra.

➤ **If you have a history of UTI,** avoid using a diaphragm, spermicidal contraceptive gel, or unlubricated or spermicidal condoms.

➤ **Avoid bubble baths** and baking-soda baths if you have a history of UTI.

➤ **Promptly report any symptoms of UTI** to your healthcare provider.

Self-Catheterization Patients with spinal cord injuries or neurological disorders use intermittent catheterization to drain the bladder and limit the risk of infection. Many actually perform **intermittent self-catheterization**, although caregivers may assist. Although you will use sterile technique for catheterization, most patients who self-catheterize use clean technique. In spite of this difference, intermittent catheterization carries a lower risk of infection than does an indwelling catheter (Hooton, Bradley, Cardenas, et al., 2010). The goals of intermittent self-catheterization are to (1) completely empty the bladder and (2) prevent urinary tract infections. To teach patients the procedure for self-catheterization,

 Go to Chapter 28, **Clinical Insight 28-4: Teaching Clients About Clean, Intermittent Self-Catheterization,** in Volume 2.

Urinary Catheterization

Catheterization is the introduction of a pliable tube (catheter) into the bladder to allow drainage of urine. Urinary catheterization is performed to:

- Obtain a sterile urine specimen.
- Drain the bladder for surgical or diagnostic purposes or when emptying is incomplete after urination.
- Prevent or treat bladder overdistention and urinary retention (e.g., after surgery) when other measures fail.
- Measure PVR if a portable bladder ultrasound device is unavailable or if the results are inconclusive.
- Protect excoriated skin from contact with urine.
- Reduce the need for unnecessary movement of patients who are near death.

Indwelling urinary catheterization is associated with the complications of bacteriuria and UTI. A catheter provides a connection between the external environment and a normally sterile system. In addition, when the patient has an indwelling catheter, microorganisms are no longer flushed from the urethra through voiding.

✚ In fact, an indwelling urinary catheter is the most common cause of nosocomial infections. To reduce the risk of bacterial contamination, asepsis and maintain a closed system is critical when inserting and caring for a urinary catheter (Gould, Umscheid, Agarwal, et al., 2009). Catheterization can injure the urethra if the catheter is too large, is not well lubricated, is forced through strictures, or is inserted at an incorrect angle.

Types of Urinary Catheters

There are a variety of catheter types and materials to choose from, depending on whether the patient requires catheterization for long-term or short-term use, has product sensitivity, or is at increased risk for infection.

- **Silver-alloy** coated catheters may reduce the risk of catheter-associated urinary tract infections for up to 14 days (WOCN, 2009; Schumm & Lam, 2010).

Silver-coated catheters are not, however, routinely used for short-term catheterization because they are more costly than standard catheters.

- **Silicone elastomer or Teflon-bonded** are coated latex catheters. The coating reduces friction and tissue irritation during insertion and while the catheter remains in place. These catheters must not be used in patients with latex sensitivity (WOCN, 2009).
- **Polyvinyl chloride (PVC)** catheters are inexpensive and commonly used for intermittent catheterization. They are more rigid and therefore less comfortable for indwelling use (WOCN, 2009).
- **100% silicone catheters** are used primarily for long-term catheterization. They cause less tissue irritation and prevent encrustation. They are safe for patients with latex sensitivity.
- **Hydrogel coated** catheters can be made of either latex or silicone. They cause less urethral trauma during insertion, resist encrustation, and can remain in place up to 12 weeks (Turner & Dickens, 2011). This type of *lubricant and/or antimicrobial coating* helps prevent infection.

✚ Always check for latex or Teflon and iodine allergies before performing a catheterization.

Straight Catheter A **straight catheter** is a single-lumen tube that is inserted for immediate drainage of the bladder (e.g., to obtain a sterile urine specimen, to measure postvoid residual volume (PVR), or to relieve temporary bladder distention). After the bladder is empty or the sample obtained, the catheter is removed and the patient resumes voiding independently.

Indwelling Catheter An **indwelling catheter**, also known as a *Foley* or *retention catheter*, is used for continuous bladder drainage (e.g., when the bladder must be kept empty or when continuous urine measurement is needed). It is usually a double-lumen tube: one lumen is used for urine drainage, and the second lumen is used to inflate a balloon near the tip of the catheter. A triple-lumen indwelling catheter is used when the patient requires intermittent or continuous bladder irrigation. Men usually need a larger lumen (e.g., 18 Fr) than do women.

The inflated balloon holds the catheter in place at the neck of the bladder. The balloon is sized according to the volume of fluid used to inflate it. For most patients you will use a 5-mL balloon; for children 3-mL; and for achieving hemostasis after a prostatectomy, a 30-mL balloon.

Figure 28-6 illustrates the different types of catheters.

Suprapubic Catheter A **suprapubic catheter** is used for continuous urine drainage when the urethra must be bypassed (e.g., after gynecological surgery or where there is prostatic obstruction). A suprapubic catheter is inserted through an incision above the symphysis pubis (Fig. 28-7). It may be sutured in place initially. Once the stoma tract has healed, a standard indwelling catheter

Toward Evidence-Based Practice

Buchko, B. L., & Robinson, L. E. (2012). An evidence-based approach to decrease early post-operative urinary retention following urogynecologic surgery, _Urologic Nursing_, 32(5), 260–264, 283.

The purpose of this project was to identify evidence and develop a protocol to prevent postoperative urinary retention in women undergoing urogynecologic surgery. The goals were to decrease the incidence of urinary retention, reduce the frequency of intermittent catheterization, and reduce the duration of indwelling catheterization in these patients. An algorithm was developed that defined when and how to assess the patient for urinary retention using a portable bladder scanner. Treatment protocols related to intermittent catheterization, indwelling catheterization, or continued monitoring were then added. An educational program was also developed to teach nurses how to use the algorithm. Research is ongoing to measure patient outcomes and determine the effectiveness of this program.

Bernard, M. S., Hunter, K. F., & Moore, K. N. (2012). A review of strategies to decrease the duration of indwelling urethral catheters and potentially reduce the incidence of catheter-associated urinary tract infections. _Urologic Nursing_, 32(1), 29–37.

The authors evaluated current literature for research-based strategies to reduce the length of time of urinary catheter placement and the effect of these strategies on the incidence of catheter-associated urinary tract infections (CAUTI). The length of time an indwelling catheter is in place is the greatest risk factor for development of a CAUTI, yet assessment of the continuing need for the catheter is often overlooked. Both nurse-led and informatics-led interventions demonstrated a significant reduction in duration of catheterization. In both interventions, nurses played a critical role and impacted the development of CAUTI in their patients.

1. What are the benefits in reducing the duration of indwelling catheterization in postoperative patients?

2. Assessment of urinary retention has traditionally been done with either bladder palpation or straight catheterization. What are the advantages of utilizing a portable bladder scanner in assessing urinary retention?

3. In addition to reducing the likelihood of CAUTI, what other benefits may occur with early removal of an indwelling catheter?

Go to Chapter 28, **Toward Evidence-Based Practice Suggested Responses,** on Davis*Plus*.

---

is usually used and is held in place by inflation of the balloon.

Catheter Sizing Catheters are sized by the *diameter* of the lumen; the larger the number, the larger the lumen. For example, 8- and 10-Fr catheters are used for children; they are smaller in diameter than the 14- and 16-Fr catheters typically used for adults. Catheters also come in different *lengths*: A 22-cm catheter is appropriate for women, whereas for men you will need a 40-cm catheter.

Supplies for Urinary Catheterization

The supplies used for inserting an indwelling catheter are usually prepackaged. Included in the kit are sterile gloves, swabs or cotton balls, a solution for cleansing the urethral meatus, sterile lubricant, a sterile indwelling

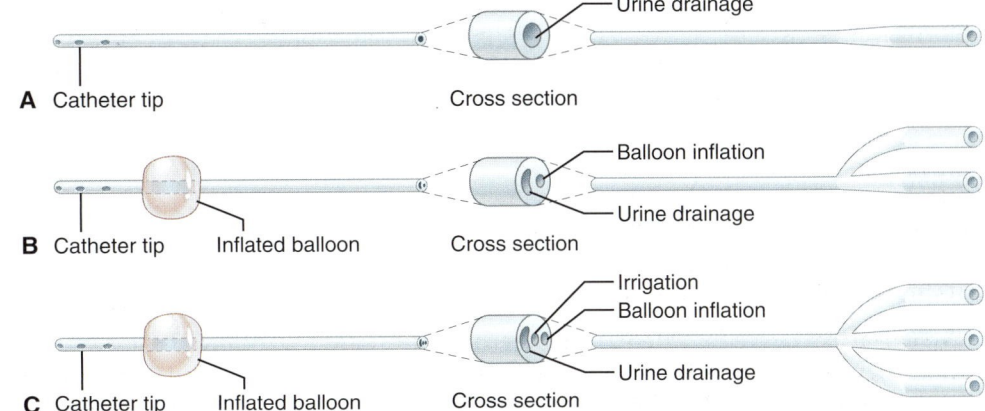

FIGURE 28-6 Types of catheters. *A,* A single-lumen catheter is used to obtain a urine sample or immediately drain the bladder. *B,* A double-lumen catheter is the most commonly used indwelling catheter. *C,* A triple-lumen catheter is inserted when the patient requires irrigation of the bladder.

A Catheter tip — Urine drainage — Cross section

B Catheter tip — Inflated balloon — Balloon inflation — Urine drainage — Cross section

C Catheter tip — Inflated balloon — Irrigation — Balloon inflation — Urine drainage — Cross section

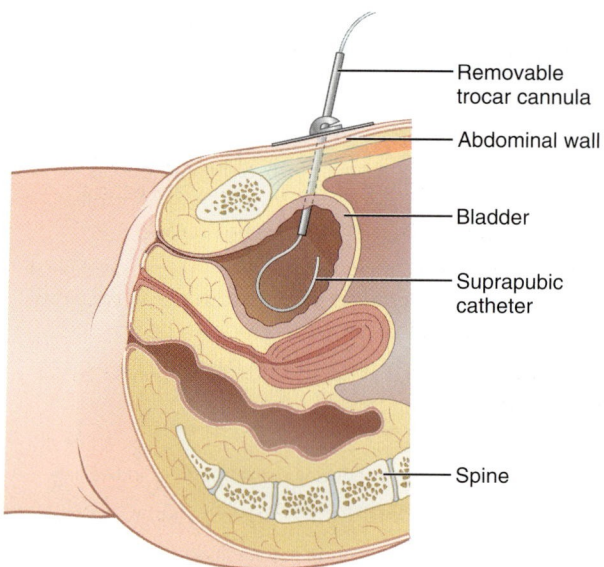

Removable
trocar cannula

Abdominal wall

Bladder

Suprapubic
catheter

Spine

FIGURE 28-7 A suprapubic catheter drains urine from a surgically created opening into the bladder, bypassing the urethra.

catheter, a syringe filled with sterile water to inflate the retention balloon, drainage tubing, and a drainage collection bag. Kits contain the most common catheter sizes, usually 12, 14, or 16 Fr. Pediatric kits contain 8- or 10-Fr catheters. The smallest diameter catheter possible that provides proper drainage is recommended to minimize urethral trauma (Lo, Nicholle, Classen, et al., 2008).

KnowledgeCheck 28-7

- Describe the difference between a catheter used for straight catheterization and one used for ongoing drainage.
- Why is intermittent catheterization preferred for patients who must be catheterized over lengthy periods of time?

Urinary Catheter Insertion

To insert a urinary catheter, you will need to gather the appropriate supplies and prepare the patient. Explain to the patient the reason for the catheter insertion, the expected length of time the catheter will be needed, and the sensations he is likely to have. Most patients experience a sensation of pressure and some discomfort (but not pain) when a catheter is inserted. Explain that when the catheter is inserted it may feel as though he is voiding, but the urine is going into the tube, not onto the bed. If there is swelling or bleeding in the urinary tract, insertion may be painful.

Many patients feel embarrassed during this procedure. A professional approach, along with good draping and other privacy measures, helps relieve discomfort or distress. As you are draping the patient, offer to answer any further questions he may have.

Use a dorsal recumbent position for women and a supine position for men. For female patients, make

sure to lower the section of the bed called the knee gatch, so that you can easily visualize the urinary meatus. You may need to place a firm cushion under the patient's buttocks to prevent her sinking into a soft mattress and obscuring visibility of the meatus. For women who are unable to assume a dorsal recumbent position, consider Sims' or a lateral position (Fig. 28-8). Cleaning around the meatus and perineum is mandatory prior to insertion of the catheter. For a brief summary, see the Highlights of Procedures box; for the complete procedure,

Go to Chapter 28, **Procedure 28-4: Inserting a Urinary Catheter,** in Volume 2.

Caring for the Patient With an Indwelling Catheter

The best practice care is always to remove a urinary catheter that is not necessary (Institute for Healthcare Improvement, 2011).

Key Point. *Remember above all, when providing care for a patient with an indwelling catheter, keep it closed, keep it flowing, and keep it clean.*

Prevent Urinary Tract Infection UTIs are the most common healthcare-associated infection. Approximately 80% of all UTIs are associated with indwelling urinary catheters (Moola & Konno, 2010). An indwelling catheter is connected to a drainage tube and collection bag, which

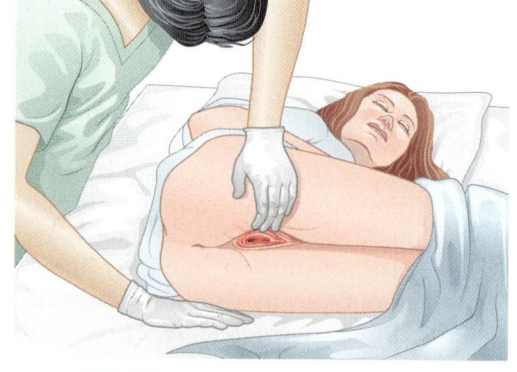

A

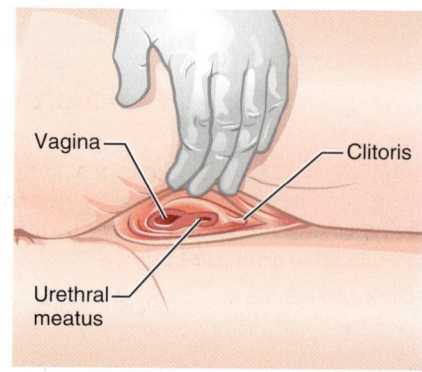

Vagina

Clitoris

Urethral
meatus

B

FIGURE 28-8 *A, B,* For women who cannot assume a dorsal recumbent position, you can use the side-lying position and lift the superior buttock to expose the urethral meatus.

For steps to follow in *all* procedures, refer to the Universal Steps for All Procedures found on the inside back cover of Volume 2. Go to the full procedures in Volume 2 to practice and learn the procedure steps. Use these procedure highlights later to help you review key points.

Procedure 28-1: Measuring Urine

➤ Don clean procedure gloves.

➤ Record the amount of urine on the input and output (I&O) flow sheets.

Procedure 28-1A: Measuring Urine Output From a Bedpan or Urinal

➤ Place the bedpan or urinal in the proper position and encourage your patient to begin voiding. Remain close by or instruct the patient to press the call light button when finished.

➤ Pour the urine from the bedpan or urinal into a graduated measuring device. Place on a flat, even surface and read the amount at eye level.

Procedure 28-1B: Measuring Urine From an Indwelling Catheter

➤ Open the drainage spout and allow urine to drain into the measuring device, being careful to avoid touching the spout to the inside of the container. Place the measuring device on a flat even surface and read the amount at eye level.

Procedure 28-1C: Measuring Post-Void Residual Urine Volume (PVR) With a Portable Bladder Scanner

➤ Assist the patient to a supine position. Uncover only the patient's lower abdomen and suprapubic area.

➤ Select the patient's gender.

➤ Palpate the symphysis pubis and apply ultrasound gel midline on the abdomen above the symphysis pubis.

➤ Position the scanner head in the gel and aim it towards the bladder and slightly downward.

➤ Press and release the SCAN button. Hold the scanner steady until the scan is finished.

➤ Read the bladder volume measurement.

➤ Repeat the scan several times to ensure accuracy.

➤ Press "DONE" when finished. Print the results by pressing PRINT.

Obtaining a Urine Specimen for Testing

Procedure 28-2: Obtaining a Urine Specimen for Testing

➤ Don clean procedure gloves

Procedure 28-2A: Collecting a Clean-Catch Urine Specimen

➤ Wash the perineum or the end of the penis first with antiseptic solution, then with an antiseptic solution. (For women, wash from front to back; for men, use a circular motion from the urethra outward.)

➤ Ask the patient to begin voiding. After the stream begins, collect a 30- to 60-mL specimen.

➤ Maintain sterility: Do not touch the inside of the container or the container lid. Avoid getting toilet paper, feces, pubic hair, or anything else in the urine sample.

➤ Place the lid on the container; label the container with the patient's name, the date, and the time of collection.

➤ Follow agency policy on additional packaging.

➤ Transport the specimen to the lab as soon as possible. If there is a delay in getting the specimen to the lab, most facilities recommend refrigeration.

Procedure 28-2B: Obtaining a Sterile Urine Specimen From a Catheter

➤ Wearing procedure gloves, empty the drainage tube of urine.

➤ Don clean gloves, and swab the specimen port with an antiseptic swab.

➤ Insert the needleless access device with a 10-mL syringe into the specimen port, and aspirate the amount of urine you need.

➤ Transfer the specimen into a sterile specimen container.

➤ Maintain sterility: Do not touch the needleless access device, the inside of the container, or the container lid.

➤ Label the specimen container with the correct patient identification and transport it to the lab in a timely manner.

Procedure 28-2C: Collecting a 24-Hour Urine Specimen

➤ Ask the patient to void. Record the time. Discard this first voiding.

➤ Collect all urine voided during the next 24 hours.

➤ Label the storage container with the patient's name, date, and time the test ended. Transport it to the lab after the collection is complete. Otherwise, place the urine in a refrigerator designated for specimen storage per agency policy.

Procedure 28-3: Testing Urine at the Bedside

➤ Follow the manufacturer's directions carefully regarding the amount of urine needed.

Procedure 28-3A: Dipstick Testing of Urine

➤ Read the kit label to be certain that you are using the correct reagent and that the kit has not passed the expiration date.

➤ Read the reagent strip at the exact time indicated on the label. You will need adequate lighting to evaluate the results.

➤ Dipstick testing is considered a preliminary test for screening.

Procedure 28-3B: Measuring Specific Gravity of Urine

➤ Before use, be sure the equipment is calibrated to 1.000 according to the manufacturer's instructions.

➤ Use fresh urine. If you cannot perform the test within 1 hour, refrigerate the specimen.

➤ Place a drop of urine on the glass plate and close the flap.

Continued

➤ Hold the refractometer up to the light when looking through the eyepiece.

➤ Read the specific gravity by looking for the point where the contrast line between the dark and light fields crosses the scale.

➤ Clean the instrument when finished.

Procedure 28-4: Urinary Catheterization

➤ Allow adequate time for catheterization: Experienced nurses need at least 15 minutes. You will need more time if problems arise—and even more if you are a novice.

➤ Take an extra pair of sterile gloves and an extra sterile catheter into the room.

➤ Be sure that you have good lighting.

➤ Work on the right side of the bed if you are right-handed and on the left side if you are left-handed.

➤ Drape the patient for privacy.

➤ Perform perineal care before the procedure; wash your hands; open the kit.

➤ Don sterile gloves and maintain sterile technique while manipulating the supplies in the kit and performing the procedure.

➤ For indwelling urinary catheterization, do not pretest the balloon by inflating it before insertion, especially with silicone catheters. The practice can cause the balloon to form cuffs, and arm the patient's urethra.

➤ Generously lubricate the catheter before insertion.

➤ Once you have touched the patient with your nondominant hand, do not remove that hand from the patient.

➤ Insert the catheter 5 to 7.5 cm (2 to 3 in.) for women, 17 to 22.5 cm (7 to 9 in.) for men, until urine flows.

➤ Drain the bladder; collect needed samples; measure urine; and then remove the catheter if it is intermittent. If the catheter is indwelling, inflate the balloon and connect the drainage bag.

Procedure 28-5: Applying an External (Condom) Catheter

➤ Application of a condom (external) catheter is a clean procedure.

➤ Clean and dry the penis before catheter application.

➤ When applying the condom, stabilize the penis with your nondominant hand.

➤ Leave a gap of 2.5 to 5 cm (1 to 2 in.) between the condom and the tip of the penis to prevent skin irritation.

➤ Use only the tape supplied in the application kit to secure the catheter.

➤ For condom catheters that contain adhesive material on the inside of the condom, grasp the penis and gently compress the condom onto the shaft.

➤ Be certain that the tubing from the end of the catheter to the drainage bag is free from kinks.

Procedure 28-6: Removing an Indwelling Catheter

➤ Use clean technique. Wash hands before and after removing the catheter. Wear clean procedure gloves.

➤ Be sure to remove the stabilization device or tape securing the catheter to the patient.

➤ Obtain a sterile specimen if needed.

➤ Connect a syringe to the balloon port and allow the balloon to self-deflate or withdraw the fluid slowly. Follow manufacturer's instructions. Check the balloon size on the valve port to verify that all fluid has been removed.

➤ If the balloon does not empty completely do not pull on the catheter. Report to the charge nurse or the primary care provider before continuing.

➤ Observe the first few voidings after the catheter is removed.

Procedure 28-7: Irrigating the Bladder or Catheter

Procedure 28-7A: Intermittent Bladder or Catheter Irrigation

➤ Drape the patient, exposing only the specimen removal port or the irrigation port on a three-way catheter.

➤ Because of the risk of infection, never disconnect the drainage tubing from the catheter.

➤ Use a sterile irrigation solution, warmed to room temperature.

➤ Instill the irrigation solution slowly.

➤ Repeat the process as necessary.

Procedure 28-7B: Continuous Bladder Irrigation

➤ Drape the patient, exposing only the irrigation port of the catheter.

➤ Using aseptic technique, attach the connecting tubing to the irrigation solution container.

➤ Prime the tubing.

➤ Don clean procedure gloves.

➤ Pinch the irrigation port of the catheter and connect the irrigation tubing to the port.

➤ Regulate the flow of the irrigant.

➤ Monitor urine output.

constitute a closed system. To minimize the chance for catheter-associated urinary tract infection, the system cannot be opened at any point. Meticulous hand hygiene and cleanliness of all ports using disinfectants is imperative for preventing the spread of infection (CDC, 2013)

Maintain Free Flow of Urine Free flow of urine prevents backflow of urine into the bladder, which can cause bladder distention and injury. Adequate urine production flushes pathogens out of the bladder, provides natural irrigation of the tubing, and prevents stasis of urine. Stasis of urine also provides a medium for growth of microorganisms.

Maintain Skin and Mucosal Integrity To maintain skin and mucosal integrity, secure the tubing to the leg. This prevents traction of the tubing and irritation to the urinary tract. Hygiene and perineal cleansing also reduces irritation from the encrustation of urine and feces along the tubing.

For a comprehensive list of nursing activities to help you meet the preceding goals,

 Go to Chapter 28, **Clinical Insight 28-1: Caring for a Patient With an Indwelling Catheter,** in Volume 2.

Bladder Irrigation

You may perform an irrigation to maintain patency of a urinary catheter, to wash out the bladder (e.g., remove blood clots in the bladder after surgery), or to instill medications into the bladder. An intermittent irrigation is most commonly used for medication instillation, whereas a continuous irrigation is used to maintain patency when blood, clots, or debris is anticipated. Routine intermittent irrigations (e.g., every shift, every week) are sometimes prescribed to ensure patency; however, these have not shown any benefit in preventing catheter blockage and should be avoided (WOCN, 2009).

A client requiring a continuous irrigation should have a triple-lumen catheter in place: one lumen for injecting water into the balloon when the catheter is inserted, another for the irrigating solution to flow into the bladder, and a third for the solution and urine to flow out of the bladder.

✚ A double-lumen catheter system may need to be opened for irrigation and therefore creates a high risk for infection. Although "open" irrigation was used in the past, it is no longer recommended.

The Highlights of Procedures box provides overviews of bladder irrigation. For complete procedures,

 Go to Chapter 28, **Procedure 28-7A: Intermittent Bladder or Catheter Irrigation,** and **Procedure 28-7B: Continuous Bladder Irrigation,** in Volume 2.

Removing an Indwelling Catheter

Removing a urinary catheter is a simple task, but you must monitor patients carefully afterward. Gather the necessary supplies, and tell the patient what you are about to do, what she will feel, and that you will need to monitor her urination after removal. Explain that this procedure is usually painless.

Cleaning around the meatus and perineum is mandatory prior to removing the indwelling urinary catheter. After removing the catheter, ask the patient to notify you the first time she voids. Note and record the time and amount of the first voiding and the appearance of the urine. Compare the patient's intake to output for the next 8 to 12 hours, and palpate the bladder for distention. A portable bladder scanner may also be used to quantify the amount of any retained urine. The catheter may have caused some edema of the urethra, which can interfere with voiding at first. Therefore, you must assess regularly for bladder distention until normal voiding is reestablished. The same is true for patients who have had rectal, perineal, or lower abdominal surgery, which may also create perineal edema.

If a catheter is in place for several weeks and the urine has been draining continuously, the bladder does not stretch and contract as it does in normal voiding. Therefore, the muscle loses tone and the patient may require bladder retraining. Agencies have differing procedures for this. One method is to begin clamping the catheter for certain periods of time (e.g., 1 to 4 hours) to allow the bladder to fill, and then releasing the clamp to allow urine to drain from the bladder. This should stimulate the bladder muscle and improve tone. However, there is limited evidence to support a practice guideline for clamping the catheter before discontinuing it (Hadwen, 2011).

For hospitalized patients who have had a urinary catheter for a short time, it may be a good idea to time catheter removal for late at night instead of in the morning. A review of research found that when this was done, patients (on average) held urine in the bladder for a longer period of time before voiding in the morning. This led to a larger volume for the first void after the catheter was discontinued. Patients with late-night catheter removal were discharged sooner and without needing to have the urinary catheter reinserted for urine retention (Griffiths & Fernandez, 2009).

For guidelines to follow when removing a retention catheter,

 Go to Chapter 28, **Procedure 28-6: Removing an Indwelling Catheter,** in Volume 2.

KnowledgeCheck 28-8

- What actions should you take before inserting a catheter?
- When caring for a client with an indwelling catheter, you notice sandy particles around the urethral meatus. What should you do?
- How often should the urine collection bag be emptied?

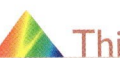 ThinkLike a Nurse 28-7

- You are caring for a patient who had an indwelling catheter removed 12 hours ago. The patient has not voided. What action should you take?

Interventions for Example Problem: Urinary Incontinence

Because urinary incontinence is so prevalent, you are likely to be called on to deal with this problem in your practice. Most incontinence is managed with skin care and behavioral interventions, but medications are sometimes used.

Perineal Skin Care

Normal urine is acidic. When it remains in contact with the skin, it becomes alkaline, causing dermatitis and skin excoriation. It is essential to keep the skin, clothing, and bedding clean and dry, especially after any leakage of urine. Commercially prepared perineal cleansers contain a surfactant that loosens soiling on the skin. This reduces the need for more aggressive cleansing with washcloths and tap water. Many of these preparations also do not require rinsing. Barrier creams may be used for irritated skin; antifungals may be prescribed (e.g., nystatin [Mycostatin]) to prevent or eliminate fungus growth. You may use absorbent products as an adjunct to other control measures, especially for those with intractable UI.

Behavioral Interventions

Nurses have taken the lead in investigating incontinence and treatment options. Aggressive nursing intervention can help to improve patients' quality of life, capacity for physical activity, and self-esteem. It can also help to reduce healthcare costs for the patient.

There are five categories of nonpharmacological treatment options nurses commonly provide independently: lifestyle modification, bladder training, pelvic floor muscle rehabilitation, anti-incontinence devices, and supportive interventions (Schröder, Abrams, Andersson, et al., 2009). These therapies have been proven to be effective for most patients.

Lifestyle Modification

Changes in lifestyle that can reduce incontinence. Some patients find improvement when limiting consumption of caffeine, cigarette, alcohol, and spicy and citrus foods that irritate the bladder. Timing prescribed diuretics in the morning, engaging in low impact exercise (not high impact), and avoiding constipation also improves urinary control. People with a BMI greater than 30 who suffer urinary incontinence may consider losing weight to control symptoms.

Bladder Training

The goal of bladder training is to enable the patient to hold increasingly greater volumes of urine in the bladder and to increase the interval between voidings. This involves patient teaching, scheduled voiding, and self-monitoring using a voiding diary. In addition to teaching the mechanisms of urination, teach distraction and relaxation strategies to help inhibit the urge to void. Other techniques include deep breathing and guided imagery.

Scheduled Voiding

This is a form of bladder training involving timed voiding and habit retraining. The client must be mentally and physically capable of self-toileting. Initially the patient may be scheduled to attempt voiding every 2 hours or even more often. As a pattern develops and the person gains greater control, the length of time between voiding may be increased. Scheduled voiding is usually combined with other techniques, including lifestyle adjustments and pelvic muscle exercises.

For detailed instructions for improving urinary control (e.g., bladder training, scheduled voiding, and pelvic floor muscle rehabilitation),

 Go to **Clinical Insight 28-2: Caring for Patients With Urinary Incontinence,** in Volume 2.

Pelvic Floor Muscle Rehabilitation

Pelvic floor muscle exercises (PFMEs), also known as Kegel exercises, are a mainstay of UI treatment for women. PFMEs strengthen perineal muscles and help to prevent and treat stress, urge, and mixed UI. PFMEs are the most commonly used method for preventing and reversing incontinence in women for the first year after giving birth. This approach may also prevent or reduce urinary incontinence in older women and in men undergoing prostate surgery. To be successful, the patient must do the exercises correctly and practice them daily. PFMEs should include 10–15 contractions three times a day. A period of 2 to 3 months may be required before treatment is effective (Herbruck, 2008; Price, Dawood, & Jackson, 2010).

Vaginal Weight Training

Vaginal weight training may be used as an adjunct to PFMEs. A small, weighted cone is placed in the vagina and the patient is instructed to attempt to retain the weight for 15 minutes while ambulatory. This method, however, has not shown better outcomes than performing standard PFMEs (Gameiro, Moreira, Gameiro, et al., 2010).

Biofeedback

Biofeedback has been advocated by some women as an adjunct to PFMEs. Electrodes attached to the skin on the perineum provide feedback to the patient about the perineal contraction.

Supportive Interventions

Supportive interventions focus on helping the patient reach the toilet, urinate independently, and perform toileting self-care. When continence cannot be achieved, absorbent products with waterproof coverings are available. Under no circumstances should you refer to these as "diapers." To do so is disrespectful of the patient's dignity.

Key Point: *Reassure the patient that urinary incontinence is not inevitable or shameful and that it can usually be treated effectively.*

ThinkLike a Nurse 28-8

How do you feel about instructing patients about pelvic floor muscle exercises? Do you think a woman should always provide this instruction? Explain your thinking.

Anti-incontinence Devices

Anti-incontinence devices are designed to reduce the incidence of UI or provide a pathway for urine flow. When anti-incontinence devices are used, it is important to observe for vaginal or urinary tract infection, blood in the urine, and vaginal erosion. The devices include the following:

- **An intravaginal support device** or **pessary** is a removable device inserted into the vagina. It is designed to relieve pressure of the pelvic organs on the urethra and is an effective treatment for stress incontinence. When used long term, monitor for vaginal infection and ulceration.
- **An external occlusive device** is removed before voiding. For women, a urethral meatus covering is used. For men, a penis clamp is a reusable, soft spongy rubber device used to control stress incontinence or dribbling urine, common with an enlarged prostate.
- **An internal urethral meatus plug** is a disposable, single-use device, typically used for activities that cause stress incontinence. It may be used by men and women.
- A **valved catheter** allows urine to be drained on a schedule.
- An **indwelling urethral catheter** is used as a last resort to control the flow of urine and protect the perineal skin. **Self-intermittent catheterization** can be used to drain the bladder and prevent leakage of urine, especially for those with overflow incontinence.
- A **bed alarm** can be used to wake the patient if incontinence occurs.
- An **external collection device** may also be used. Condom catheters, also known as urosheaths, are most commonly used for men who have adequate bladder emptying and intact genital skin. To learn how to apply a condom catheter, see the Highlights of Procedures box for a summary of the procedure. Also,

 Go to Chapter 28, **Procedure 28-5: Applying an External (Condom) Catheter,** in Volume 2.

Complementary Alternative Methods

There are no alternative methods that have been proven to cure urinary incontinence; although some treatments show promise in reducing the symptoms (e.g., acupuncture and biofeedback). Several small-scale studies have indicated that acupuncture may be effective in relieving symptoms in urge and mixed incontinence (Engberg, Cohen, & Sereika, 2009; O'Dell & McGee, 2006). A *sacral nerve stimulator* is an electronic device used for patients who do not respond to behavioral treatment or medication for urge incontinence. The lead wire is placed near

the sacral nerve and acts like a bladder pacemaker for better urinary control.

Managing Enuresis

Occasional wetting (called *enuresis*) is entirely normal in children even in the early school years, especially when the child is intensely involved in a game, test, or another absorbing activity, or when restricted from using the toilet. Parents should accept such events calmly and not punish the child (see Home Care: Managing Enuresis in Children).

Children, especially older ones, can be embarrassed by *nocturnal enuresis,* or bedwetting, not to mention the inconvenience it poses. Young children may feel anxious about using the bathroom in a clinic, hospital, or any unfamiliar environment. They may be especially anxious about using a bedpan. Also, be aware that the stress of an illness or hospitalization may cause a child to regress in his ability to toilet independently. You may need to schedule regular trips to the bathroom and to watch for nonverbal cues that the child needs to void.

ThinkLike a Nurse 28-9

What treatment options for incontinence have you seen used in your clinical experience? What options do you believe should be used more frequently? Less frequently? Explain your thinking.

Treatments for Urinary Incontinence

Behavioral interventions, such as timed voiding and pelvic floor muscle training, also known as Kegel exercises, are the first-line management options for urinary incontinence. Pelvic floor muscle exercises

---

Home Care

Managing Enuresis in Children

➤ Reassure parents that in most cases loving acceptance and passage of time provide the cure.

➤ Cover the mattress with plastic.

➤ Limit fluid intake in the evening.

➤ Wake the child to urinate just before the parents go to sleep.

➤ Use a bed alarm that wakens the child when wetting occurs. Over time, this conditioning may be effective; however, once the alarm is removed, the child may relapse into enuresis.

➤ If bedwetting persists into the school-age years, the child should receive a thorough medical evaluation to rule out underlying disease processes.

➤ Parents should plan to bathe the child in the morning rather than at bedtime to minimize urine odor.

➤ Medication can be effective for managing nocturnal enuresis in some children. Medication is helpful when the child is not sleeping at home.

(PFME) should be continued for at least 3 months before moving to more aggressive treatment. The following medical and surgical treatments may be used to manage UI:

- *Medications.* Although not the treatment of choice, some forms of incontinence may respond to pharmacological treatment (e.g., drugs to improve urethral sphincter muscle functioning or to relax the detrusor muscle and increase bladder capacity). Medications include topical estrogen for women who have UI associated with urogenital atrophy, and anticholinergic drugs such as oxybutynin (Ditropan) and tolterodine (Detrol), which inhibit involuntary bladder contractions.
- *Devices.* Indwelling intravaginal devices, such as pessaries, may be useful for some women with pelvic organ prolapse in reducing urinary incontinence (Herbruck, 2008). Intraurethral devices to manage incontinence are not used routinely, but instead reserved to prevent occasional leakage, for example, during exercise.
- *Sacral nerve stimulation* might be recommended for the treatment of urge incontinence in women who have not responded to conservative treatment.
- *Surgical treatment,* such as a creating a sling of muscle and tissue that holds the bladder and uterus and other pelvic organs in place to relieve the pressure that can cause discomfort and incontinence. Other surgical options include enlarging the bladder size and improving the muscular capacity for bladder emptying. However, this surgery is reserved for those who do not respond to other bladder therapies, medication, or self-catheterization.

Key Point: *Do not use absorbent products, handheld urinals, and other toileting aids to routinely manage urinary incontinence, unless used to supplement other therapy.*

For more information about helping patients to manage urinary incontinence,

 Go to Chapter 28, **Clinical Insight 28-2: Caring for Patients With Urinary Incontinence,** in Volume 2.

Caring for Patients With a Urinary Diversion

A **urinary diversion**, or **urostomy**, is a surgically created opening for elimination of urine, required when the bladder must be removed or bypassed. Diversion surgeries are used to treat patients who have conditions such as birth defects, cancer, trauma, or disease of the urinary system. Risks associated with urinary diversions are primarily infection and permanent kidney damage, which can occur from *hydronephrosis* (distention of the kidneys with urine, which results from obstruction of the ureter).

What Are the Types of Urinary Diversions?

There are four major diversion options, following:

- **Cutaneous ureterostomy.** This surgery reroutes the ureter(s) directly to the surface of the abdomen, forming a small stoma. It may be unilateral or bilateral. The procedure has limited use because it provides a pathway for pathogens on the skin to directly enter the kidney. The stomas are small and difficult to fit with a collection appliance.
- **Conventional urostomy (ileal conduit, Bricker's loop, ileal loop).** This is the most common type of urinary diversion (Fig. 28-9). A small piece of ileum is removed with blood and nerve supply intact. The remainder of the ileum is reconnected to prevent disruption of flow through the bowel. The free segment of ileum is sutured closed at one end, and the other end is brought out to the abdominal wall to create a stoma. The result is a small pouch into which the ureters are implanted. Urine, along with mucus from the ileum, drains continuously from the stoma and is collected in a pouch that the patient wears.
- **Continent Urinary Reservoir (ileal reservoir, Indiana pouch).** A continent urinary reservoir (Fig. 28-10) is a variation of the ileal conduit. Urine drains from the ureters into a surgically created ileal pouch. The stoma created on the abdomen contains a nipple valve to keep urine from leaking. Rather than having urine flow constantly, the patient inserts a catheter into the stoma to drain urine through the valve. A second valve prevents reflux of urine back into the kidneys.
- **Neobladder.** A neobladder mimics the function of a urinary bladder. A portion of intestine is made into a pouch or reservoir that is connected to the urethra. Urine is then passed through the urethra, similar to the normal passage of urine. The patient will need to void by bearing down or applying manual pressure over the bladder (Credé's maneuver), but may also need to perform intermittent self-catheterization to fully empty the bladder.

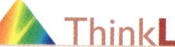 Think**Like a Nurse** 28-10

What types of challenges or problems do you think a patient with a urinary diversion might experience?

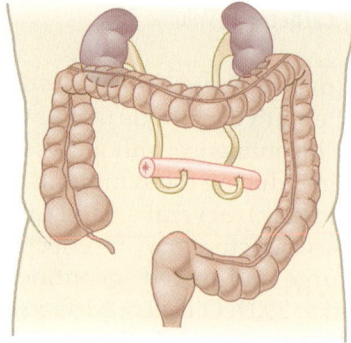

FIGURE 28-9 An ileal conduit is the most common urinary diversion.

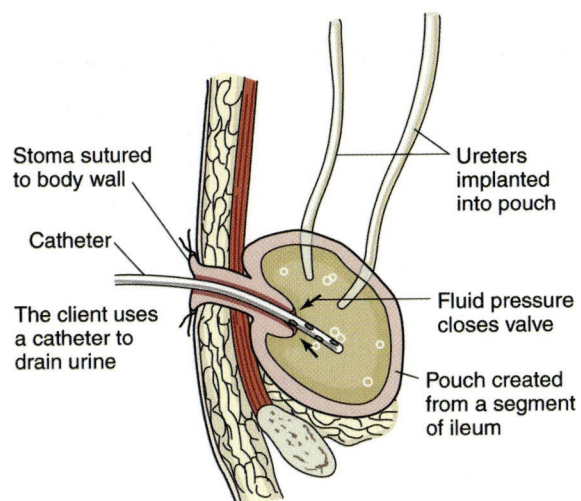

FIGURE 28-10 A continent urostomy allows the client to manage urine without the need to wear an ostomy appliance.

Interventions for Patients With Urinary Diversions

A patient with a urinary diversion requires physical and psychological care. Initially you may need to assist the patient with all aspects of his care. However, the goal is for the patient to become comfortable with his changed body and to assume self-care.

Patients with a stoma experience a variety of reactions. Patients with continent urinary reservoirs are usually more comfortable with their stoma because of the control it offers while avoiding the embarrassment, odor, and inconvenience of a conventional urostomy. Your attitude and willingness to discuss the body changes associated with an ostomy will help your patient begin his adjustment. In many communities, the local ostomy association has counselors available to visit patients, discuss the psychological changes associated with a urinary diversion, and help them with physical care of the stoma. Most counselors are adept because they too have ostomies. They are able to share practical and personal information with patients based on their own experience with similar challenges.

For guidelines specifically for caring for a patient with a urinary diversion,

 Go to Chapter 28, **Clinical Insight 28-3: Caring for Patients With Urinary Diversions; Clinical Insight 28-4: Teaching Clients About Clean, Intermittent Self-Catheterization; and Procedure 29-6: Changing an Ostomy Appliance,** in Volume 2.

Patients With Neobladder or Continent Urinary Reservoir Continent urinary reservoir patients will also need instruction in inserting a catheter through the stoma to release the urine. Patients with a neobladder will need to learn to void by bearing down or applying manual pressure over the bladder, but may also need to learn clean intermittent self-catheterization.

 To explore learning resources for this chapter,

 Go to DavisPlus at DavisPl.us/Wilkinson3.

Chapter Resources for Chapter 28:
  Response sheets for all learning activities
  Resources for Caregivers and Health Professionals
  Reading More About Urinary Elimination (suggested readings)
  Concept Map of chapter content
Interactive Case Studies
NCLEX-Style and Chapter Review Questions
Chapter Overview Podcasts

For references cited in this chapter,

 Go to Volume 2, **References Cited.**

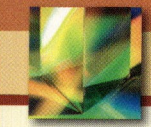

Nursing Care Plan

Client Data

Desmond Washington, a 69-year-old man, comes to the clinic 4 weeks after having a prostatectomy for prostate cancer. He was discharged from the hospital on postoperative day 4 and went home with an indwelling urinary catheter. The catheter was removed at his last visit, 9 days after surgery.

Mr. Washington is meticulously groomed. He is friendly, greeting other patients in the clinic and chatting with the clinic personnel. When his nurse brings him to an exam room and asks how he feels, he says, "I saw the sun come up today. I appreciate that more now. The good Lord has given me a new lease on life, and I intend to use it!" His nurse continues, "That's great, Mr. Washington. How have you been doing since the catheter was removed?" Mr. Washington's smile fades. He lowers his voice and says, "You know, I think that's the worst part of this whole thing. I hate wearing these diapers—they make me feel, well, like an old man. I'm certainly not ready for this."

The nurse continues, "Do you have *any* control of your urine?" Mr. Washington explains, "I may go for hours and stay dry, and then it seems for no reason, I wet myself. Take yesterday, for example. I was sitting on the sofa watching the ball game when someone came to the door. I got up to answer the door, and all of a sudden, I felt wet. I didn't even have anything to drink so I could make it through the afternoon and stay dry. And if I cough? Forget it. Can something be done so I can hold my urine again?"

Nursing Diagnosis

Stress Urinary Incontinence related to disruption of the urinary sphincter and related pelvic muscles by surgery as evidenced by client report of involuntary loss of urine with increased intra-abdominal pressure.

NOC Outcomes	Individualized Goals/Expected Outcomes
Urinary Continence (0502) Urinary Elimination (0503)	*By the next visit, Mr. Washington will:* 1. Describe three things he can do that will help regain urinary continence. 2. Explain three interventions to cope with leaked urine. 3. Report that he is drinking adequate amounts of fluids during the day.

Nursing Interventions and Activities	Rationale

NIC Interventions
Urinary Elimination Management (0590)
Urinary Incontinence Care (0610)

Nursing Activities	
1. Obtain midstream voided urine specimen for urinalysis.	Urinary tract infection can cause or worsen incontinence (Goode, Burgio, Richter, et al., 2010; Joseph, 2006).
2. Identify factors that contribute to Mr. Washington's incontinence by using an incontinence diary.	Identifying activities or other factors that cause loss of urine control can guide specific interventions. A diary facilitates monitoring over time and can identify patterns that could otherwise be missed (Rainsbury, Fabricius, & McLarty, 2011; Robinson, 2006; Shultz, 2012).

Nursing Care Plan (continued)

Nursing Interventions and Activities	Rationale
3. Teach pelvic floor muscle exercises (PFMEs).	PFMEs strengthen pelvic muscles and enhance sphincter control. They have been shown in some studies to increase urinary continence without side effects in men who have undergone prostatectomy (Glazener, Boachie, Buckley, et al., 2011; Rainsbury Fabricius, & McLarty, 2011; Sighinolfi, Rivalta, Mofferdin, et al., 2009; Van Kampen, De Weerdt, Van Poppel, et al., 2000; Vaughan, Goode, Burgio, et al., 2011).
4. Use biofeedback when needed in conjunction with PFME training to help Mr. Washington isolate pelvic floor muscles.	Biofeedback allows clients to receive auditory or visual (or both) cues when the proper muscles are contracted, so they learn what the proper muscle contraction feels like. Biofeedback also allows the nurse or therapist to objectively measure strength of contractions (Campbell, Glazener, Hunter, et al., 2012; Herderschee, Hay-Smith, Herbison, et al., 2011; Robinson, 2006).
5. Teach timed voiding. Have Mr. Washington void on a schedule of every 2 hours.	Voiding on a schedule of every 2 hours can reduce the amount of urine in the bladder, thus reducing the likelihood of leakage with activities of daily living (Shultz, 2012).
6. Explain the need to drink adequate fluids and *not* limit fluids in an effort to prevent incontinence. Help Mr. Washington identify ways to drink a minimum of 1,500–2,000 mL/day.	Adequate fluid intake is important to maintain dilute urine, which is less irritating to the bladder; to maintain systemic hydration; and to reduce the risk for constipation, which can contribute to urinary incontinence (Rainsbury, Fabricius, & McLarty, 2011; Robinson, 2006).
7. Assist the client in selecting appropriate absorbent products that collect urine strictly for temporary management while continence management is ongoing.	Proper absorbent garments and pads can collect and trap urine, keep skin clean and dry, reduce odor, and minimize the risk of soiling accidents (National Institute for Health and Clinical Excellence, 2013; Robinson, 2006).
8. Help the client develop a personal hygiene routine that will maintain skin integrity.	Proper hygiene will reduce the risk of skin irritation and infection. Use warm (not hot) water, and pat (don't scrub) the perineal area. A barrier cream will repel fluid and protect the skin from urine.
9. Offer referral to a support group.	Support groups provide a sense of community and enhance problem-solving skills of members. Mr. Washington may feel less embarrassment when he discovers that others share his problems (Robinson, 2006).
10. Explain that urinary incontinence is common after prostatectomy, but that it may be only temporary.	Urinary incontinence can be a troubling complication of prostatectomy for many men. Fortunately, it often resolves within 6 to 12 months after surgery (Yu Ko & Sawatzky, 2008).

There are other treatment recommendations that are supported by research or have been identified anecdotally to be useful for some clients (WOCN, 2003). These include reducing caffeine consumption; eliminating bladder irritants, such as artificial sweeteners, spicy foods, and citrus from the diet; losing weight; and quitting smoking. In addition, it is important for nurses to understand the pathophysiology of urinary incontinence differs between men and women and that interventions that are successful in women may or may not be equally successful in men.

(continued)

Nursing Care Plan (continued)

Evaluation

At the end of the visit, Mr. Washington said, "I didn't know there were things I could do about the leaking urine. Before surgery, all I cared about was getting rid of the cancer. I don't need a support group for me but maybe I'll lead one!" Mr. Washington had been placing folded paper towels in his underwear to collect urine because he thought absorbent products were too expensive, but with guidance from his nurse he identified products he could afford. He liked that they would not be visible through his clothing.

At Mr. Washington's next visit, the nurse will review the initial collaborative goals and stated outcomes and perform a client assessment to determine whether the goals were reached in the stated time frame.

Mr. Washington currently has a positive attitude and is focused on "beating" his cancer first and on managing complications of surgery second. As time passes, incontinence may persist and may become more frustrating for him once he is fully recovered from surgery. Mr. Washington initially declined referral to a support group, but he may be more interested in joining one in the future for help dealing with long-term consequences of prostatectomy.

References

Campbell, S. E., Glazener, C. M. A., Hunter, K. F., et al. (2012). Conservative management for postprostatectomy urinary incontinence. *Cochrane Database Systematic Reviews, 1,* CD001843. DOI: 10.1002/14651858.CD001843.pub4

Glazener, C., Boachie, C., Buckley, B., et al. (2011). Urinary incontinence in men after formal one-to-one pelvic-floor muscle training following radical prostatectomy or transurethral resection of the prostate (MAPS): Two parallel randomised controlled trials. *Lancet, 378*(9788), 328–337. http://dx.doi.org/10.1016/S0140-6736(11)60751-4

Goode, P. S., Burgio, K. L., Richter, H. E., et al. (2010). Incontinence in older women. *Journal of the American Medical Association, 303*(21), 2172–2181. http://dx.doi.org/10.1001/jama.2010.749

Herderschee, R., Hay-Smith, E. C., Herbison, G. P., et al. (2011). Feedback or biofeedback to augment pelvic floor muscle training for urinary incontinence in women. *Cochrane Database Systematic Review 7,* CD009252. DOI: 10.1002/14651858.CD009252.

Joseph, A. C. (2006). Noninvasive therapies for treating post-prostatectomy urinary incontinence. *Urologic Nursing, 26*(4), 281–285, 269.

National Institute for Health and Clinical Excellence. (2013, March 1 corrected). *Urinary incontinence in women: The management of urinary incontinence in women* [Full guideline draft] (National Collaborating Centre for Women's and Children's Health, Author). Retrieved March 17, 2014, from http://www.nice.org.uk/nicemedia/live/13019/62658/62658.pdf

Rainsbury, P. G., Fabricius, M., & McLarty, E. (2011). Management of urinary incontinence in primary care. *InnovAiT, 4*(1), 23–30. http://dx.doi.org/10.1093/innovait/inq041

Robinson, J. P. (2006). Pathology and management of postprostatectomy incontinence. In D. B. Doughty (Ed.), *Urinary & fecal incontinence: Current management concepts* (3rd ed., pp. 255–265). St. Louis, MO: Mosby Elsevier.

Shultz, J. M. (2012). Rethink urinary incontinence. *Nursing 2012, 42*(11), 32–40.

Sighinolfi, M. C., Rivalta, M., Mofferdin, A., et al. (2009). Potential effectiveness of pelvic floor rehabilitation treatment for postradical prostatectomy incontinence, climacturia, and erectile dysfunction: A case series. *Journal of Sexual Medicine, 6*(12), 3496–3499. http://dx.doi.org/10.1111/j.1743-6109.2009.01493.x

Van Kampen, M., De Weerdt, W., Van Poppel, H., et al. (2000). Effect of pelvic-floor re-education on duration and degree of incontinence after radical prostatectomy: A randomised controlled trial. *Lancet, 355*(9198), 98–102.

Vaughan, C. P., Goode, P. S., Burgio, K. L., et al. (2011). Urinary incontinence in older adults. *Mount Sinai Journal of Medicine, 78*(4), 558–570. http://dx.doi.org/10.1002/msj.20286

Wound, Ostomy, and Continence Nurses Society (WOCN). (2003). Identifying and treating reversible causes of urinary incontinence. *Ostomy/Wound Management, 49*(12), 28–33.

Yu Ko, W. F., & Sawatzky, J. V. (2008). Understanding urinary incontinence after radical prostatectomy: A nursing framework. *Clinical Journal of Oncology Nursing, 12*(4), 647–654. http://dx.doi.org/10.1188/08.CJON.647-654

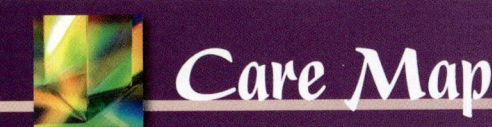

Care Map

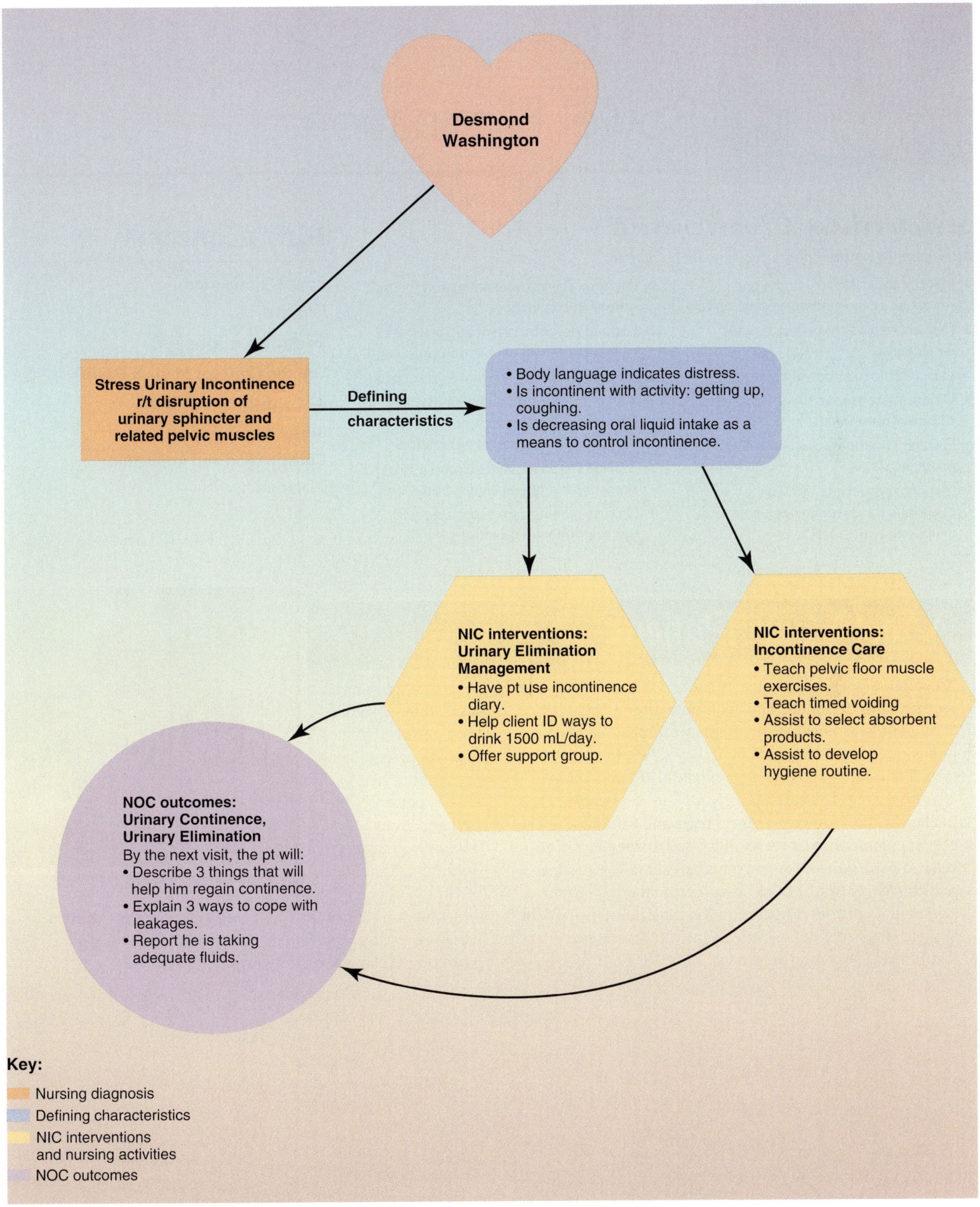

Desmond Washington

Stress Urinary Incontinence r/t disruption of urinary sphincter and related pelvic muscles

Defining characteristics

- Body language indicates distress.
- Is incontinent with activity: getting up, coughing.
- Is decreasing oral liquid intake as a means to control incontinence.

NIC interventions: Urinary Elimination Management
- Have pt use incontinence diary.
- Help client ID ways to drink 1500 mL/day.
- Offer support group.

NIC interventions: Incontinence Care
- Teach pelvic floor muscle exercises.
- Teach timed voiding
- Assist to select absorbent products.
- Assist to develop hygiene routine.

NOC outcomes: Urinary Continence, Urinary Elimination
By the next visit, the pt will:
- Describe 3 things that will help him regain continence.
- Explain 3 ways to cope with leakages.
- Report he is taking adequate fluids.

Key:
- Nursing diagnosis
- Defining characteristics
- NIC interventions and nursing activities
- NOC outcomes

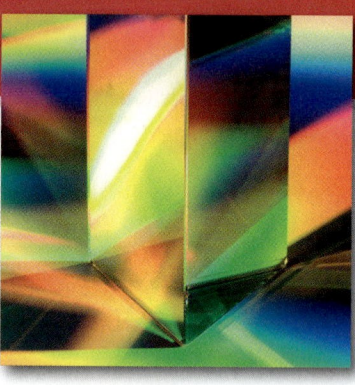

CHAPTER 29

Bowel Elimination

Learning Outcomes

After completing this chapter, you should be able to:

➤ Identify the basic structures and functions of the gastrointestinal system.

➤ Discuss factors that affect bowel elimination.

➤ Describe normal bowel elimination.

➤ Differentiate among the various types of bowel diversions.

➤ Discuss common bowel elimination problems.

➤ Identify appropriate nursing history questions to assess bowel elimination problems.

➤ Perform a physical examination focused on bowel elimination.

➤ List and describe diagnostic tests used to identify bowel elimination problems.

➤ Formulate nursing diagnoses associated with altered bowel elimination.

➤ Describe nursing interventions that promote normal bowel elimination.

➤ Provide care for clients experiencing alterations in bowel elimination.

➤ Discuss nursing care associated with the use of bowel diversions.

Key Concepts

Bowel elimination
Motility

Related Concepts

See the Concept Map on *DavisPlus*.

Example Problems

Bowel incontinence
Constipation and impaction
Diarrhea

Meet Your Patient

You are assigned to care for Mrs. Zeno, a frail 96-year-old woman who broke her hip last month after a fall at home. Mrs. Zeno was hospitalized for surgical repair of her hip and is now in a skilled nursing facility (SNF) for rehabilitation. The nursing assistive personnel (NAP) informs you that Mrs. Zeno has eaten poorly for the past week, only picking at the food on her meal trays and refusing the protein supplements that were added to her diet. Mrs. Zeno tells you she would like to go home: "I have my routine and the foods I like. I think I'd be better there." As you review the chart in preparation for clinical, you note that she has not had a bowel movement (BM) for 3 days. Her last BM was small and very hard.

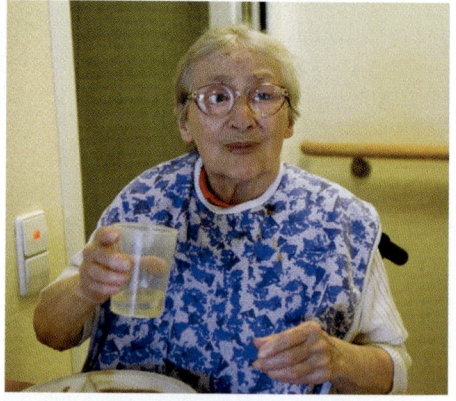

What additional assessments should you perform? What, if anything, is of concern about her bowel pattern? What actions should you take with Mrs. Zeno?

In this chapter, you will gain theoretical and practical knowledge to help you answer those questions and provide care for clients with bowel elimination concerns.

744

TheoreticalKnowledge
knowing **why**

Bowel elimination is a normal process by which we eliminate waste products from our bodies. In this chapter you will come to understand concepts underlying the function of the gastrointestinal tract as well as factors that affect bowel elimination.

ABOUT THE KEY CONCEPTS

Bowel elimination is one of the overarching concepts in this chapter—the "hook" on which you hang your theoretical knowledge. The other key concept, **motility**, helps you to understand how normal elimination occurs and what changes take place in problems such as constipation and diarrhea. Other, more specific, concepts will flesh out your understanding of bowel elimination. For example, when you grasp the concept of bowel diversion, you will how it relates to various bowel elimination problems. As you study the chapter, identify the concepts and try to understand how they are connected. This will help you to care for clients with any medical diagnosis affecting bowel elimination.

WHAT ARE THE ANATOMICAL STRUCTURES OF THE GASTROINTESTINAL TRACT?

The gastrointestinal (GI) tract is a smooth-muscle tube approximately 10 m (30 ft) long, running through the body from the mouth to the anus. Its major functions are to digest and absorb the nutrients present in food and to eliminate food waste products as feces. The structures of the GI tract are the mouth, pharynx, esophagus, stomach, small intestine, large intestine, rectum, and anus (Fig. 29-1).

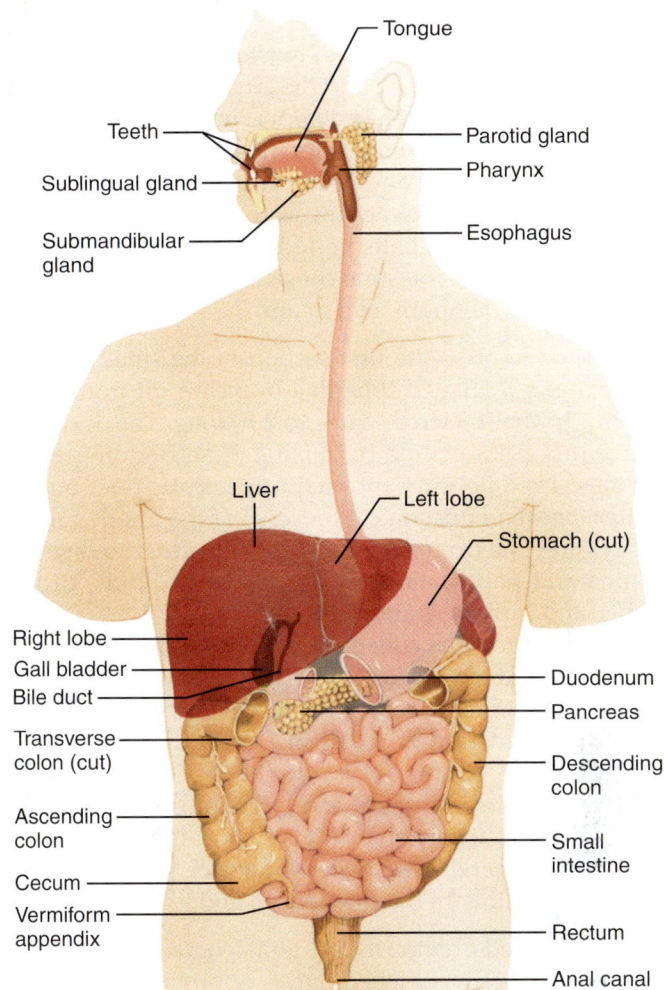

FIGURE 29-1 The gastrointestinal tract extends from the mouth to the anus. The major functions of the GI system are to digest and absorb the nutrients in food and to eliminate food waste products as feces. (*Source:* Scanlon, V., & Sanders, T. (2010). *Essentials of anatomy and physiology* (6th ed., p. 371). Philadelphia: F. A. Davis. Used with permission.)

The Upper Gastrointestinal Tract

The upper part of the GI tract consists of the mouth, pharynx, esophagus, and stomach.

Mouth Mechanical digestion begins in the mouth with **mastication**, or chewing. Food is torn into small pieces, mashed, moistened with saliva, formed into a bolus, and then swallowed into the esophagus. Glands in the mouth secrete enzymes, such as ptyalin and salivary amylase, which begin the digestion of carbohydrates.

Pharynx The pharynx is the back part of the throat where food and air pass after chewing. To prevent choking and aspiration, a flap of connective tissue, called the **epiglottis**, closes over the trachea when food is swallowed.

Esophagus The esophagus is a tube of smooth muscle, which alternately contracts and relaxes in waves of **peristalsis** to push the bolus toward the stomach. The bolus travels the length of the esophagus (about 25 cm, or 10 in.) in about 15 seconds. The *cardiac sphincter* (also called the *gastroesophageal sphincter*) relaxes to allow food to pass into the stomach. When the cardiac sphincter constricts, it prevents acidic stomach contents from flowing back into the esophagus.

The Stomach The stomach is a distensible sac that extends from the esophagus to the small intestine. The stomach stores food while it churns and mixes it, providing further mechanical breakdown. Chemical digestion continues in the stomach, which secretes hydrochloric acid (HCl), a protein-digesting enzyme called *pepsin;* and *gastric lipase,* an enzyme that begins the digestion of lipids. The stomach lining also secretes a mucous coating that protects the stomach from being corroded by HCl. Food remains in the stomach an average of 4 hours. It leaves the stomach and enters the small intestine as a liquid, called **chyme**.

The Small Intestine

The small intestine is a folded, twisted, and coiled tube that connects the stomach and the large intestine. About 2.5 cm (1 in.) in diameter and approximately 6 m (20 ft) long if fully extended, it occupies most of the abdominal cavity. Most digestion and absorption of food occurs in the small intestine. Chyme travels through it slowly, by peristalsis; peristalsis halts periodically to allow for absorption. The small intestine consists of three segments: the duodenum, jejunum, and ileum.

- The **duodenum** is the first section of the small intestine. It is a C-shaped tube that branches off from the stomach, about 30 to 60 cm (1 to 2 ft) long. The duodenum processes chyme by mixing it and adding enzymes. The bile duct and main pancreatic duct both enter the small intestine at the level of the duodenum, providing bile from the liver and gallbladder to digest lipids and pancreatic enzymes to digest lipids, proteins, and carbohydrates.
- The **jejunum** is the coiled midsection of the small intestine. It is about 1.8 to 2.4 m (6 to 8 ft) long and forms the connection between the duodenum and ileum. Its major function is to absorb carbohydrates and proteins.
- The **ileum** joins the small and large intestine. It is responsible for absorption of fats; bile salts; and some vitamins, minerals, and water. However, nutrients are absorbed mainly in the duodenum and jejunum.

As mentioned previously, the total length of the small intestine, if it were stretched out, is approximately 6 m (20 ft), but in the body it is much shorter because it is folded to provide a vast surface area for absorption. The inner wall of the small intestine is covered by millions of tiny finger-like projections called **villi** (Fig. 29-2). The villi are covered with even tinier projections, called **microvilli**. The combination of folds, villi, and microvilli increases the surface area of the small intestine greatly, facilitating absorption of nutrients.

The Large Intestine

The **large intestine**, also known as the **colon**, is larger in diameter than the small intestine (6.3 cm, or 2.5 in.) but shorter in length—about 1.5 to 1.8 m (5 to 6 ft). It extends from the ileum of the small intestine to the anus. It contains seven segments: the cecum, ascending colon, transverse colon, descending colon, sigmoid colon, rectum, and anus (Fig. 29-3).

Undigested food entering the first portion of the large intestine, the **cecum**, consists mostly of cellulose and water. The connection of the ileum to the cecum is controlled by the **ileocecal valve**. Under most conditions, the valve prevents backflow of chyme from the colon into the small intestine. The **appendix** is a small, finger-like appendage off the cecum. It is believed to be a **vestigial organ**—one whose significance has diminished over time—however, it is lined with lymphatic tissue and may play a role in immune function.

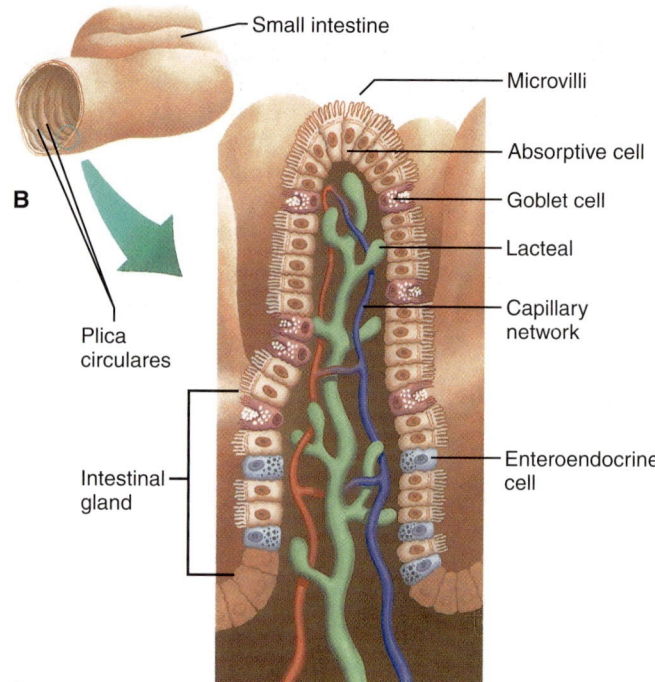

FIGURE 29-2 The small intestine is highly folded, providing a vast surface area for absorption of nutrients. The microvilli form a brush border, which is the site of most nutrient absorption. A, Section through the small intestine showing the plica circulares (circular folds) of the mucosa and submucosa. B, Microscopic view of a villus showing the internal structure. (*Source: Scanlon, V., & Sanders, T. (2010). Essentials of anatomy and physiology* (6th ed., p. 383). Philadelphia: F. A. Davis. Used with permission.)

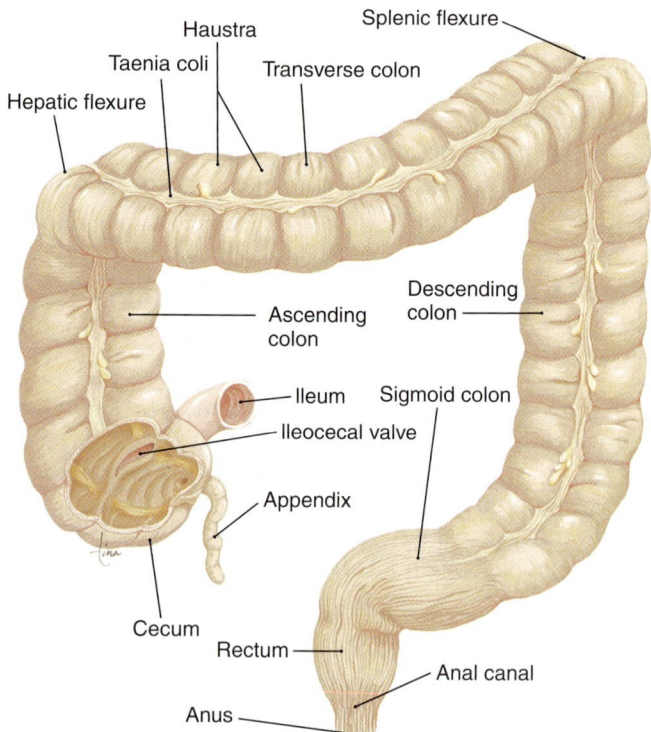

FIGURE 29-3 The large intestine shown in anterior view. The term *flexure* means a turn or bend. (*Source: Scanlon, V., & Sanders, T. (2010). Essentials of anatomy and physiology* (6th ed., p. 385). Philadelphia: F. A. Davis. Used with permission.)

The next three segments, the **ascending**, **transverse**, and **descending colon**, ring the small intestine. The **sigmoid colon** is a final, small segment of bowel that twists medially and downward to connect with the rectum and anus.

The colon secretes mucus, which facilitates smooth passage of stool, and absorbs water, some vitamins, and minerals. Approximately 80% of the fluid that enters the colon is reabsorbed along its passage. Normal flora in the colon aid in the digestive process. These bacteria are responsible for producing vitamin K and several of the B vitamins.

The large intestine has two sets of muscles that give it a puckered appearance. Longitudinal muscles, known as **taenia coli**, run lengthwise along the colon surface. Tension in these muscles gathers up the colon into pouched segments known as **haustra** all along its length (see Fig. 29-3). In addition, the colon wall contains circular muscles that, together with the taenia coli, cause the colon to expand and contract in length and width to achieve haustral churning, peristalsis, and mass peristalsis.

- **Haustral churning** moves digestive contents around within each haustra. This action promotes reabsorption of water.
- **Peristalsis** continues throughout the length of the large intestine, where it propels intestinal contents toward the rectum and anus.
- **Mass peristalsis** is a powerful contraction along a lengthy segment of bowel. It is facilitated by the **gastrocolic reflex**, which is triggered by food entering the stomach and small intestine. Mass movements usually occur only one to three times each day, and they are responsible for most of the propulsion of the contents in the transverse and sigmoid colon.

The Rectum and Anus

The **rectum** is approximately 15 cm (6 in.) long and is continuous with the **anus**, the last 2.5 cm (1 in.) of the colon. A highly vascular folded tube, the rectum is free of waste products until just before defecation.

The anus has two ring-like muscles that function as sphincters. The **internal sphincter** involuntarily relaxes and opens when stool is present in the rectum. The **external sphincter** is under voluntary control. Voluntary relaxation of the external sphincter allows stool to be expelled from the body (Fig. 29-4). The anus is highly vascular. Chronic pressure on the veins within the anal canal, as with prolonged sitting or retained feces, can cause **hemorrhoids** (distended blood vessels within or protruding from the anus).

KnowledgeCheck 29-1

- What are the major functions of the small intestine and large intestine?
- How do the rectum and anus control elimination of feces from the body?

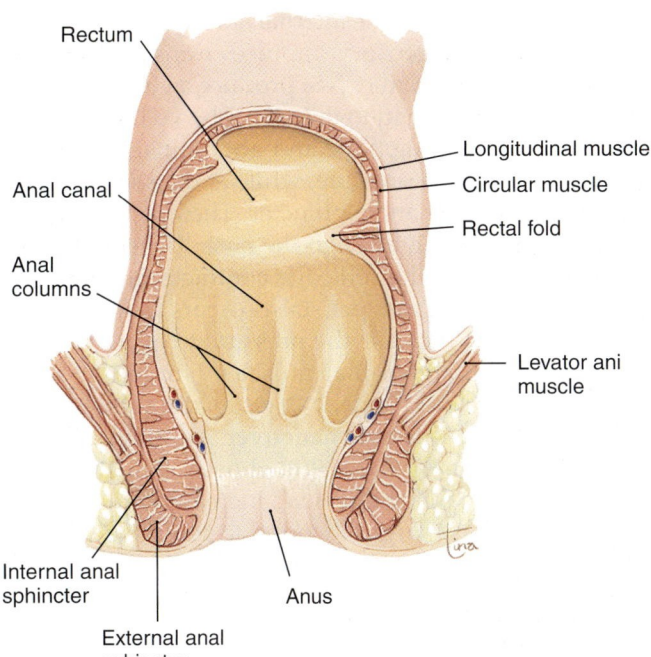

FIGURE 29-4 Internal and external anal sphincters shown in a frontal section through the lower rectum and anal canal. (*Source:* From Scanlon, V., & Sanders, T. (2010). *Essentials of anatomy and physiology* (6th ed., p. 387). Philadelphia: F. A. Davis. Used with permission.)

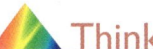 ThinkLike a Nurse 29-1

Based on your knowledge that hemorrhoids are dilated blood vessels in the anal canal, what symptoms would you expect a patient with hemorrhoids to exhibit?

HOW DOES THE BOWEL ELIMINATE WASTE?

As you have learned, reabsorption of water from chyme in the large intestine results in a semisolid mass known as **feces**. Feces are a mixture of fiber and undigested food, shed epithelial cells, inorganic material (e.g., calcium and phosphates), bacteria, and water. Small amounts of fat may be present. Feces are usually brown because **bile salts**, which aid in the digestion of fat, are excreted in the feces. Bile is normally golden yellow, but the action of bacteria in the GI tract changes the color to brown. Bacteria are also responsible for the odor of feces.

Flatus, or gas, is formed in the digestive process. Some is swallowed air that accompanies the intake of food. A small portion diffuses from blood into the GI tract. However, most of the gas is created by bacterial fermentation in the colon.

The Process of Defecation

The process by which the bowel eliminates waste is called **defecation**. When fecal material reaches the rectum and causes it to distend, (a) stretch receptors are stimulated to start contraction of the sigmoid colon and rectal muscles, and (b) the internal anal sphincter relaxes. At the same time, sensory impulses transmitted to the central nervous system (CNS) produce a conscious urge to defecate. We respond to this signal by voluntarily contracting our diaphragmatic and abdominal muscles to increase downward pressure, while at the same time relaxing the external anal sphincter. These actions allow feces to be propelled through the anus. If we ignore the signal to defecate, the reflexive contractions ease for a few minutes, until mass peristalsis occurs again.

A person can increase the pressure to expel feces by contracting the abdominal muscles (straining) while maintaining a closed airway (e.g., holding the breath). This is called the **Valsalva maneuver**. Although it assists with the passage of stool, you should caution clients with heart disease, glaucoma, increased intracranial pressure, or a new surgical wound to avoid the Valsalva maneuver because it increases pressure within the abdominal cavity, raises blood pressure, and is associated with an increased risk for cardiac arrhythmias.

Normal Defecation Patterns

The sheer volume of over-the-counter (OTC) products to treat "irregularity" suggests that bowel function problems are common. Nevertheless, many people avoid the topic of bowel elimination—it is not typically something they chat about with their neighbors. As a result, many patients have unanswered questions about their bowel function and may turn to you for information.

Part of the confusion about bowel function is that there is a wide range of "normal." The frequency of BMs may range from several times per day to once a week. As long as the person passes stools without excessive urgency (needing to rush to the toilet), with minimal effort and no straining, without blood loss, and without the use of laxatives, you can regard bowel function as normal.

Normally stool is approximately 75% water and 25% solid when expelled. This combination yields a soft, formed semisolid. If passage through the colon is slowed, more water is reabsorbed from the feces. The stool becomes dry and hard, requiring more effort to pass. If transit time through the colon is faster than normal, less water is reabsorbed, and stools are watery.

🌈 Think**Like a Nurse** 29-2

- Based on your knowledge of normal bowel function, how would you describe Mrs. Zeno's (Meet Your Patient) bowel function? Is it normal or abnormal?
- What additional information, if any, do you need to know to answer this question?

WHAT FACTORS AFFECT BOWEL ELIMINATION?

Each person develops an elimination pattern that is based on several factors, discussed in the sections immediately following.

Developmental Stage

Bowel elimination patterns change throughout the life span.

Infant During the first few days of life, the term newborn passes meconium through the anus. **Meconium** is green-black, tarry, sticky and odorless. It is formed by swallowed mucus, hair, and amniotic fluid. Stools transition to a yellow-green color over the next few days. After that, the appearance of the feces depends largely on the type of feeding the infant receives. Breastfed babies pass golden yellow stools, whereas formula-fed babies pass tan stools. Initially babies defecate frequently, usually after each feeding—especially when they are breastfeeding. The stools tend to be watery while the large intestine is still immature. Gradually normal flora develop in the colon, and stools become firmer and less frequent.

Children The ability to control defecation typically develops at about 2 to 3 years of age. Toilet training requires neural and muscular control as well as conscious effort. The child must be aware of the urge to defecate, be able to maintain closure of the external anal sphincter while getting to the toilet, and be able to remove clothing. When toddlers become engrossed in play, they sometimes ignore the need to move their bowels, and soiling is common. As children mature, they gradually learn to gain more control. In fact, school-age children and adolescents often delay defecation until they have come home or have completed an activity.

Adults The bowel pattern set in childhood normally continues into late adulthood if the client consumes adequate fiber and fluid and engages in regular physical activity.

 However, peristalsis, intestinal smooth muscle tone, perineal muscle tone, and sphincter control normally decrease with aging. These physiological processes can contribute to bowel elimination problems among older adults, especially if they decrease their activity and fiber intake.

Personal and Sociocultural Factors

Privacy is important to most people, as is sufficient time to have a bowel movement without feeling the need to hurry. Clients working in fast-paced jobs may have difficulty even consciously recognizing the need to defecate, and some habitually ignore the need, promoting bowel dysfunction. Parents and caregivers of infants and toddlers may postpone their own toileting needs because of fear of leaving the children alone. Some clients are embarrassed by the thought that anyone might realize they are having a bowel movement and will wait until they are entirely alone before even entering the bathroom.

Have you ever heard the following phrase: "He puts his stress in his gut"? Stress does have a major influence on motility of the GI tract. It may cause diarrhea or constipation, and it is a primary risk factor in the development of *irritable bowel syndrome,* a disorder associated with bloating, pain, and altered bowel function.

Nutrition, Hydration, and Activity Level

Foods and Fiber Regular intake of food promotes peristalsis. People who eat on a regular schedule are likely to develop a regular pattern of defecation, whereas irregular eating creates irregular bowel elimination. Adequate intake of high-fiber promotes peristalsis and defecation. Bulky foods absorb fluids and increase stool mass. The increased mass stretches bowel walls, initiating peristalsis and the defecation reflex. Most people should have at least five servings of high-fiber foods each day.

Some foods have specific effects in the bowel. For example, the active bacteria in yogurt stimulate peristalsis, while at the same time promoting healing of intestinal infections. Low-fiber foods, such as pasta and other simple carbohydrates and lean meats, slow peristalsis. Foods like broccoli, onions, and beans lead to excess gas in many people. Spicy foods may also cause gas, as well as more frequent bowel movements.

Dietary Supplements Dietary supplements can also affect bowel function. For example, calcium supplements may cause constipation, whereas magnesium loosens stools. Supplemental vitamin C softens stools and, in high doses, may cause diarrhea in sensitive clients.

Fluids A minimum of six to eight 8-ounce glasses (1,500 to 2,000 mL) of fluid per day is required to promote healthful bowel function. Inadequate fluid intake or excessive fluid loss, as in diarrhea or vomiting, slows peristalsis and leads to dry, hard stools that are difficult to pass (Fritz & Pitlick, 2012). Excessive fluid intake (especially beverages with high sugar content) may lead to rapid passage through the colon and soft or watery stools. Different types of fluids have varying effects on sensitive individuals. For instance, consuming large amounts of milk may cause constipation in some people. Coffee promotes peristalsis in many clients and may even cause loose stools in sensitive clients.

Activity Physical activity seems to stimulate peristalsis and bowel elimination. In addition, sedentary people are likely to have weaker abdominal muscles. Clients with health concerns that limit activity (e.g., shortness of breath, pain, or required bedrest) often experience constipation.

Medications

Many medications may affect peristalsis. All oral medicines have the potential to affect the function of the GI tract. Examples include the following:

- *Antacids,* often used for heartburn, neutralize stomach acid but may slow peristalsis.
- *Aspirin and other nonsteroidal anti-inflammatory drugs (NSAIDs),* such as naproxen and ibuprofen, irritate the stomach. Repeated use can lead to ulceration of the stomach or duodenum.
- *Antibiotics* given to combat infection decrease the normal flora in the colon. The result is often diarrhea. Bacterial populations can be maintained with supplements of probiotics (e.g., acidophilus) or daily consumption of yogurt (Salfi & Holt, 2012).
- *Iron,* a common mineral supplement, is available as an over-the-counter (OTC) medication and is often prescribed for the treatment of anemia. Iron has an astringent effect on the bowel and is notorious for causing constipation and changing stool color to black. It also causes nausea if taken when there is no food in the stomach.
- *Pain medications,* particularly opioids (narcotics), slow peristalsis and are associated with a high incidence of constipation.
- *Antimotility drugs,* such as diphenoxylate (Lomotil), may be used to treat diarrhea. They work by slowing peristalsis.
- *Laxatives* are used to treat constipation. In general, laxatives work by stimulating peristalsis (see Box 29-1). They are frequently abused by people who self-medicate with OTC drugs, who may become dependent on them, requiring ever-increasing dosages until the intestine fails to work properly.

BOX 29-1 ■ Types of Laxatives

- **Stool softeners** enable moisture and fat to penetrate the stool, thereby softening it and making it easier to pass. Example: docusate sodium. Effectiveness of stool softeners in relieving chronic constipation is being questioned, but they are still in use.

- **Osmotic laxatives** work by drawing water into the bowel from surrounding tissue, resulting in bowel distention. Examples: polyethylene glycol, lactulose.

- **Lubricant laxatives** coat the stool and the GI tract with a thin waterproof layer. Example: mineral oil. Because the lubricant coats the entire GI tract, it may interfere with the absorption of nutrients. Mineral oil is potentially dangerous in debilitated patients. Inhaled droplets can lead to a form of pneumonia.

- **Stimulant laxatives** are bowel irritants. They irritate the intestinal wall, stimulating intense peristalsis. Examples: senna, bisacodyl, castor oil.

- **Bulking agents** are high in fiber. They must be combined with sufficient fluid intake to be effective. The fiber attracts fluid into the colon, and the increased bulk of the stool stimulates the urge to evacuate. These are considered the safest form of laxative, but may interfere with absorption of some medicines. They are the drug of choice for chronic constipation. Examples: Metamucil, Citrucel, psyllium, FiberCon.

- **Chloride channel activators** increase intestinal fluid and motility to help stool pass.

- **Combination laxatives** are laxatives that contain more than one type of laxative ingredient. The most common type is a combination stimulant laxative and stool softener.

Surgery and Procedures

Clients undergoing anesthesia and surgery often experience sluggish bowel elimination. The delay in bowel elimination may be caused by a variety of circumstances:

Anesthesia General anesthesia (which renders the patient unconscious) and analgesics (administered pre-operatively and postoperatively for pain) slow bowel motility. Spinal anesthesia and epidural anesthesia are less likely to cause this effect.

Stress Regardless of the type of anesthesia, most clients find surgery a stressful event. As you may recall from Chapter 12, if stress activates the general adaptation syndrome (GAS), autonomic nervous system and endocrine responses ensue. Among those responses is a slowing of peristalsis.

Manipulation of the Bowel During Surgery Abdominal or pelvic surgery in which the bowel is manipulated may result in a **paralytic ileus**, a cessation of bowel peristalsis. Although peristalsis halts, the bowel continues to produce secretions. Without peristalsis, secretions remain stagnant, causing distention and discomfort. To decrease the complications of paralytic ileus, patients who have had bowel surgery typically have a nasogastric (NG) tube with low constant or intermittent suction. The NG tube removes secretions until peristalsis returns. To review insertion of an NG tube or management of a patient with an NG tube,

 Go to Chapter 27, **Procedure 27-2: Inserting Nasogastric and Nasoenteric Tubes,** in Volume 2.

Decreased Mobility After surgery, patients often experience discomfort that affects mobility. This further hinders GI motility and increases the risk for constipation.

Perineal Surgery Patients who have had surgical interventions involving the perineal region (e.g., an episiotomy after childbirth) may fear pain or that their sutures will "tear" or "break" during bowel elimination, and therefore they resist the urge to evacuate their bowel.

Anal Sphincter Surgery Patients who have had surgery that disrupts the anal sphincter may experience uncontrolled rectal drainage after surgery.

Pregnancy

In early pregnancy, many women experience fluid loss due to "morning sickness"—periods of nausea and vomiting. As the pregnancy progresses, the growing uterus crowds and displaces the intestines, and the increased level of progesterone slows intestinal motility. As a result, pregnant women often experience constipation, decreased appetite, and irregular food intake. In addition, the increasing pressure of the uterus and the increased blood volume of normal pregnancy increase the woman's risk for hemorrhoids.

PICOT

Constipation in Pregnancy

Situation: The nurse is interviewing a 27-year-old pregnant client with a history of constipation, gas, and general abdominal discomfort after eating. The client reports increasing her dietary intake of fluid and fiber, but with limited results. Focused assessment reveals hypoactive bowel sounds and a firm abdomen. She is anxious about taking medication during pregnancy. The nurse wants to learn more about nonpharmacological interventions for constipation.

PICOT Components

P Population/client   = Pregnant women

I Intervention/indicator = Increased physical activity

C Comparator/control   = Fiber and liquids only

O Outcome   = Relief from constipation

T Time   = During pregnancy

Searchable Question: Do _____ (P) who receive _____ (I), as compared to _____ (C) demonstrate _____ (O) during _____ (T)?

Example of Evidence: The effect of hormones on the bowel, as well as the increased iron intake in prenatal vitamins often causes early pregnancy constipation. The increasing size of the uterus, and decreased maternal activity can further contribute to constipation. Many clients find relief with increased fiber and fluid intake. A commitment to daily exercise will also increase peristalsis, promoting fecal movement. The client on bedrest can also benefit with thigh strengthening and ROM exercises.

Application to Practice: The nurse discusses with the client ways in which she can incorporate increased physical activity into her lifestyle during pregnancy.

Reference: Trottier, M., Erebara, A., & Bozzo, P. (2012). Treating constipation during pregnancy. *Canadian Family Physician, 58*(8), 836–838.

ThinkLike a Nurse 29-3

- Review the case of Mrs. Zeno (Meet Your Patient). What factors may be affecting her bowel elimination?
- What additional information do you need?

Pathological Conditions

Several disorders affect bowel function. Among them are neurological disorders that affect innervation of the lower GI tract, cognitive conditions that limit the ability to sense the urge to defecate, pain or immobility that leads to sluggish peristalsis, and pathological conditions of the GI tract. Constipation and diarrhea are discussed in the Nursing Diagnosis section of the chapter. Other common disorders are food allergies, food intolerances, and diverticulosis.

Food Allergies The National Institute of Allergy and Infectious Diseases (NIAID) characterizes a **food allergy**

as an adverse health effect arising from an immune response that occurs reproducibly on exposure to a given food (NIAID, 2011, updated 2013). Some common food allergens include dairy products, egg whites, shellfish, gluten, peanuts and other nuts, citrus fruits, and soy. Immune responses to foods manifest as a variety of symptoms ranging from a mild rash to anaphylactic shock. Common GI symptoms suggesting food allergy include constipation, diarrhea, a red, blistering rash around the anus, abdominal discomfort, bloating, excessive gas, and intestinal bleeding (Boyce, Assa'ad, Burks, et al., 2010).

Food Intolerances In contrast to a food allergy, a **food intolerance** is specifically linked to the GI system. It produces such symptoms as GI discomfort, pain, gas, bloating, diarrhea, or constipation after the person consumes the food. An example is *lactose intolerance*, a deficiency of the enzyme lactase, which is responsible for the breakdown of milk sugar (lactose). Such symptoms can mimic those of a food allergy, but food intolerances are not caused by immune responses.

Diverticulosis When the colon must repeatedly move highly compacted fecal material, over time the longitudinal and circular muscles enlarge. This increases force on the mucosal tissues, causing them to "balloon" out between the muscles and to form pouches in which fecal matter becomes trapped. The development of these saclike outpouchings of mucosa through the muscle layers of the colon wall is a condition called **diverticulosis**. In some cases, the pouches become infected, a condition called **diverticulitis**, and antibiotics or surgery is required. People whose diets are low in fiber or consist mainly of refined foods are especially at risk for diverticulosis. Obesity and red meat intake are also risk factors (Humes, 2012).

KnowledgeCheck 29-2

- What is a normal defecation pattern?
- Identify the factors that affect bowel elimination.

WHAT IS A BOWEL DIVERSION?

As you know, various pathologies affect the GI tract—causing motility changes, inflammation, and so on. Many can be treated with medication (e.g., laxatives, anti-inflammatory drugs). However, some conditions require surgical intervention, such as bowel diversions.

A **bowel diversion** is a surgically created opening for elimination of digestive waste products. The procedure is performed for clients with a variety of conditions, including cancer, ulcerations, trauma, or inadequate blood supply. A client with a bowel diversion does not eliminate via the anus. Instead, the **effluent** (output, fecal material) is expelled through a surgically created opening in the abdominal wall, called a **stoma** or **ostomy**. The effluent ranges from liquid to solid, depending on the part of the bowel that is being diverted.

Bowel diversions may be temporary or permanent. *Temporary bowel diversions* are common after surgical

interventions for benign conditions of the bowel. They allow healing of the distal portion of the bowel. Once adequate healing has occurred, surgical **reanastomosis** (reconnection) of the bowel is performed, and the patient once again has BMs from the anus. *Permanent bowel diversions* are performed if the bowel is necrotic (dead) or cannot be salvaged because of severe disease or trauma.

Ileostomy

An **ileostomy** brings a portion of the ileum through a surgical opening in the abdomen, bypassing the large intestine entirely. Recall that most of the water is absorbed from the feces in the large intestine. Therefore, drainage at this level is liquid and continuous. The patient must wear an ostomy appliance at all times to collect the drainage. Some variations of an ileostomy are designed to control drainage more effectively and to cause less body image disturbance. However, many clients are not candidates for these procedures because of their underlying disease.

- A **Kock pouch**, or **continent ileostomy**, creates an internal pouch, or reservoir, to collect ileal drainage (Fig. 29-5A). To drain the pouch, the patient inserts a tube through the external stoma into the pouch several times per day. This alternative avoids continuous drainage and allows the patient to be free of an ostomy appliance.
- A **total colectomy with ileoanal reservoir** is a surgical procedure in which the colon is removed, a pouch is created from the ileum, and the ileum is connected to the rectum (Fig. 29-5B). The patient evacuates the bowel on

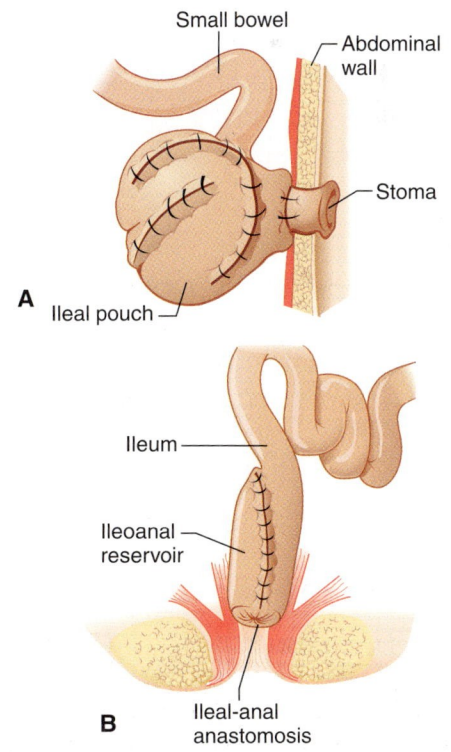

FIGURE 29-5 Ileostomy variations. A, Continent ileostomy (Kock pouch). B, Ileoanal reservoir.

the commode in the usual manner. Although this procedure should result in continence of bowel elimination, the feces will still be liquid.

Colostomy

A **colostomy** is a surgical procedure that brings a portion of the colon through a surgical opening in the abdomen. The location of the colostomy determines the consistency of the feces eliminated, as well as the need to wear an ostomy appliance (Fig. 29-6). The closer the colostomy is to the ascending colon and the ileocecal valve (between the small and large intestine) (Fig. 29-3), the more liquid and continuous the drainage will be. In contrast, a colostomy close to the sigmoid colon will produce solid feces. Colostomies near the rectum, such as sigmoid colostomies, can often be controlled by diet and irrigation. As a result, the client may not need to wear an ostomy appliance to collect drainage.

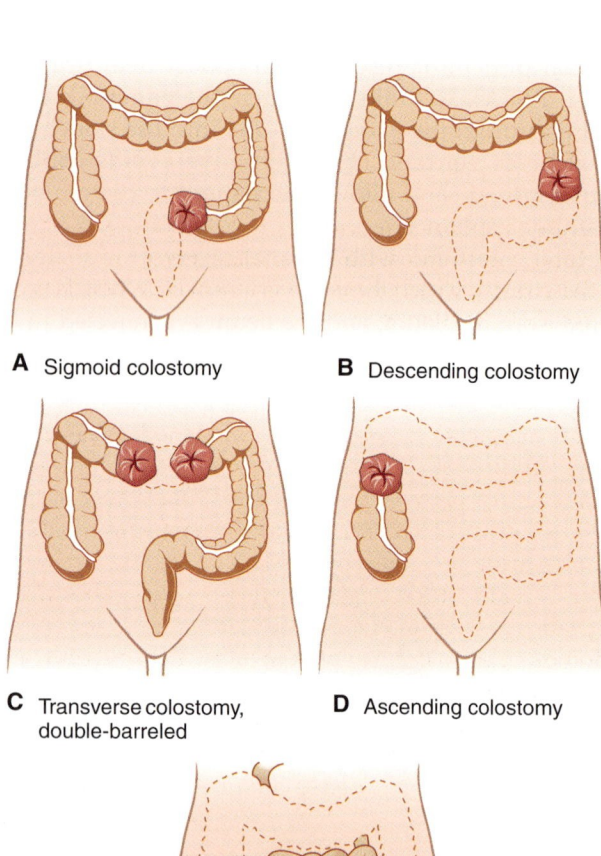

A Sigmoid colostomy   **B** Descending colostomy

C Transverse colostomy, double-barreled   **D** Ascending colostomy

E Ileostomy

FIGURE 29-6 *A–E,* Location of various bowel diversion ostomies. Shaded areas indicate sections of the bowel that are removed or being "rested." The closer the colostomy is to the ascending colon ("higher"), the more liquid and continuous the drainage will be.

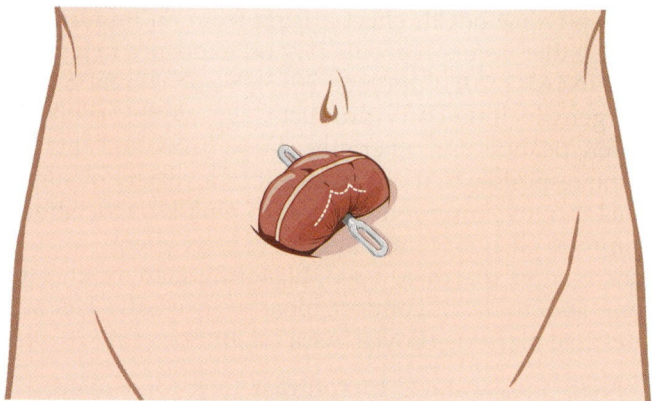

FIGURE 29-7 A loop colostomy.

A colostomy created in the transverse colon is usually temporary and may be either a double-barreled or loop colostomy.

- A **double-barreled colostomy** (see Fig. 29-6C) has two separate stomas that externalize the bowel on both sides of the portion that has been removed. The proximal stoma is the functioning end that drains fecal material. The distal stoma may drain mucus and is sometimes called a mucous fistula.
- A **loop colostomy** (Fig. 29-7) consists of a segment of bowel brought out to the abdominal wall. The posterior wall of the bowel remains intact, but a plastic rod is wedged under the bowel to keep it from slipping back into the abdomen. The anterior wall is incised, and the mucosal surface is left visible and open to air. It, too, has a functioning proximal end and limited drainage from the distal end.

You may also be interested in seeing an animation about colostomies at

 Go to **Animations: Colostomy,** on *DavisPlus.*

KnowledgeCheck 29-3

- What changes in bowel elimination are associated with constipation? With diarrhea?
- Why are bowel diversions performed?
- What determines the nature of the effluent from a bowel diversion?

PracticalKnowledge
knowing **how**

As a nurse, you will monitor and assist clients with bowel elimination, teach about bowel function, and work collaboratively with the healthcare team to facilitate normal bowel function in well and ill clients. In the remainder of the chapter, we discuss these activities.

ASSESSMENT

To assess bowel elimination, you must obtain a focused nursing history, perform a physical examination focused on elimination, and review diagnostic and laboratory data. For guidelines for physical examination and for a list of questions to use in a focused bowel assessment,

 Go to Chapter 29, **Assessment Guidelines and Tools, Focused Assessment: Bowel Elimination,** in Volume 2.

Focused Nursing History

Because bowel patterns vary, you will need a nursing history to determine what is normal for each client. As you interview clients, pay attention to their reactions to your questions. Many people are embarrassed by discussion about bowel function. Tailor your assessment to the client's needs, and use language that makes the client comfortable. Remember to ask the client about her medications because many have the potential to cause constipation (e.g., antacids, antidiarrheals, calcium and iron supplements) (Box 29-2). For clients with a bowel diversion, you will also gather data on the client's usual care of the stoma, use of appliances, and adjustment to the ostomy.

Focused Physical Assessment

Physical assessment for bowel elimination includes examination of the abdomen, rectum, and anus, as well as characteristics of normal and abnormal stool (Table 29-1). Observe the size, shape, and contour of the abdomen, and listen to bowel sounds. You might also palpate the anus

---

---

and rectum for the presence of stool or masses. When auscultated:

- *Normal bowel sounds* are high-pitched, with approximately 5 to 15 gurgles every minute.
- *Hyperactive bowel sounds* are very high-pitched and more frequent than normal. They may occur with small bowel obstruction and inflammatory disorders and may produce diarrhea.
- *Hypoactive bowel sounds* are low-pitched, infrequent, and quiet. A decrease in bowel sounds indicates decreased peristalsis, which can result in constipation.
- *Absent bowel sounds.* If after listening for 3 to 5 minutes you hear no bowel sounds, you can describe them as *absent*. Absent bowel sounds indicate a lack of intestinal activity, which may occur after abdominal surgery and indicate a paralytic ileus.

For complete details about a focused assessment of bowel function,

 Go to Chapter 22, **Procedure 22-14: Assessment of the Abdomen** and **Procedure 22-19: Assessing the Rectum and Anus,** in Volume 2.

KnowledgeCheck 29-4

- What should you discuss with your client when performing a nursing history focused on bowel elimination?
- Describe the physical assessment you would perform for a client with constipation.

Diagnostic Tests

Several diagnostic tests may be performed to assess for bowel elimination problems (e.g., to screen for colorectal cancer, to diagnose diverticulosis). They may be classified as indirect or direct visualization studies. **Indirect visualization studies** are radiographic views of the lower GI tract. The simplest of the tests is an abdominal flat plate, an anterior to posterior (AP) x-ray view of the abdomen used to detect gallstones, fecal impaction, and distended bowel.

Direct visualization studies are used for diagnostic and treatment purposes. They are invasive procedures and are conducted by a gastroenterologist, who inserts various instruments (e.g., *endoscopes*) to examine the interior of the GI tract. The nurse's role during these studies is to prepare the patient for the test, function as an assistant, and provide aftercare. You might need to assist the patient to the appropriate position, monitor the patient's tolerance of the procedure, provide pain medication or sedation to keep the patient comfortable during the exam, and provide reassurance to the patient as the test proceeds. For a description of the most common visualization tests,

 Go to Chapter 29, **Diagnostic Testing, Direct Visualization Studies of the Gastrointestinal Tract** and **Indirect Visualization Studies of the Gastrointestinal Tract,** in Volume 2.

Table 29-1 ➤ Normal Characteristics of Feces and Variations

STOOL CHARACTERISTIC	CONDITION	AGE GROUP	DESCRIPTION
Frequency	Normal	Infants*	Bottlefed—1 to 3 stools/day; Breastfed—4 to 6 stools/day
		Adults	Daily; 2 to 3 BMs/week
	Variations (Hypermotility)	Infants*	>6 stools/day
		Adults	>3 stools/day
	Variations (Hypomotility)	Infants*	Bottle fed—<1 stool every day or 2 Breastfed—<1 stool/week
		Adults	<1 stool/week
Color	Normal	Infants*	Dark green (1st week); then yellow
		Adults	Brown
	Variations		*Bile* pigment gives feces a brown color. Infant stools are yellow because of their rapid passage.
			White or clay-colored stool may indicate absence of bile (e.g., as in bile duct obstruction) or use of some antacids.
			Light brown stool may indicate diet high in milk products and low in meat.
			Pale, fatty stool may indicate malabsorption of fat.
			Black, tarry stool (melena) may indicate use of iron medications or upper GI bleeding; eating large quantities of red meat, spinach, and dark green vegetables may cause feces to be almost black.
			Red stool may indicate bleeding in lower intestinal tract or hemorrhoids.
			Stool darkens the longer it is left standing after defecation.
Quantity	Normal	Adults	Approximately 150 g/day
	Variations		Quantity varies with amount of food eaten, from 100 to 400 g per day.
Shape	Normal		Approximately the diameter of the rectum: about 2.5 cm (1 in.) in diameter
	Variations		Narrow, pencil-shaped stool may indicate intestinal obstruction or constriction, or rapid peristalsis. Small, marble-shaped stool may indicate slow peristalsis, with longer time in the large intestine.
Consistency	Normal		Formed, soft, moist
	Variations		Consistency is related to gastric motility and is affected by food and fluid intake.
			Hard stool indicates constipation. The more time spent in the large intestine, the more water is reabsorbed, and the harder the stool. May also indicate dehydration.
			Liquid stool may indicate diarrhea; rapid peristalsis (e.g., from infection).
Odor	Normal		Pungent; affected by foods eaten
	Variations		Normal odor is created by putrefaction and fermentation in the lower GI tract. Odor is also influenced by the pH of the stool, which is normally neutral or slightly alkaline.
			Strong, foul odors may indicate blood in the stool, especially in the upper GI tract, or infection.

*All information about infant stool patterns applies after passage of meconium.

For nursing care before, during, and after each of these tests,

 Go to Chapter 29, **Tables, Boxes, Figures: ESG Box 29-1, Direct Visualization Studies of the Gastrointestinal Tract,** and **ESG Box 29-2, Indirect Visualization Studies of the Gastrointestinal Tract,** on *DavisPlus*.

 Think**Like a Nurse** 29-4

A client asks you why he must perform a bowel prep with a strong laxative before having a colonoscopy. How might you reply?

Laboratory Studies of Stool

Stool specimens may be analyzed to detect blood, infection, or parasitic infestation. The client must void first and then defecate into a clean, dry bedpan, bedside commode, or a special container (half hat) placed under the toilet seat. A small sample is obtained and sent to the laboratory for analysis or analyzed at the bedside. To obtain a specimen from an infant or young child, you will collect freshly passed feces from a diaper.

Handling Stool Specimens

✚ Wear clean gloves when you handle the container or manipulate stool specimens. Use tongue blades to transfer the stool specimen to the container provided by the lab. Do not contaminate the outside of the specimen container.

In most cases you will need approximately 2.5 cm (1 in.) of formed stool or 20 to 30 mL of liquid stool. If blood, mucus, or purulent material is present, be sure to include this with the sample. Transport the specimen to the laboratory as soon as possible. If that is not possible, consult the laboratory for appropriate storage. Usually you will need to refrigerate the specimen until it can be received in the lab.

Testing for Fecal Occult Blood

Blood from the GI tract may be visible to the eye or **occult** (hidden), especially when passed through the stool from higher up in the intestine. You can perform the test for occult blood at the bedside, although some institutions require that it be done in the laboratory. The test is called a *guaiac test* or *fecal occult blood test*. It requires use of a special reagent that detects the presence of **peroxidase**, an enzyme present in hemoglobin. Only a small smear of stool is required. For home testing, remind patients to wash their hands before and after collecting stool. The Highlights of Procedures box in this chapter summarizes the skill. For the complete procedure, including medications and foods to avoid before the test,

 Go to Chapter 29, **Procedure 29-1: Testing Stool for Occult Blood,** in Volume 2.

Colorectal cancer is the third most common cancer in both women and men, with African Americans having the highest incidence of colorectal cancer compared with other races (American Cancer Society, 2013). Screening can detect colorectal polyps so they can be removed before becoming cancerous. Annual guaiac-based fecal occult blood testing is recommended for all patients 50 to 75 years of age and older as one method of screening for colorectal cancer (some guidelines suggest every 2 years). The recommended age for annual testing drops to the age of 40 years for high risk adults or 10 years younger than the age at which the youngest affected relative was diagnosed with colorectal cancer (National Guideline Clearinghouse [NGC], 2012). Some suggest the cutoff age to stop screening should be age 75, or an expected remaining life span of less than 10 years. Based on 2011 data, a little more than half of adults aged 50 and older were screened for cancer at the recommended intervals (American Cancer Society, 2013).

Assessing for Pinworms

Pinworms (an intestinal parasite) are small, white, thread-like worms that spread through human-to-human transmission, by ingesting (swallowing) infectious pinworm eggs and/or by entry through the anus (e.g., when eggs attach to a person's fingers and are transferred to the anal area by scratching or touching the anus). Once present, the pinworms live in the cecum. They come to the anal area to deposit eggs during the night and migrate back up through the rectum during the day. In assessing a child, you can spread the buttocks while the child is sleeping and examine the anus to see whether any pinworms are visible to the naked eye. You can also test for the presence of the eggs with tape. In the morning, as soon as the patient awakens, press clear cellophane tape against the anal opening. Remove the tape immediately, and place it adhesive side down on a slide. Alternatively, or in addition, insert a cotton-tipped swab gently into the rectum for not more than 2.5 cm (1 in.). Smear the specimen on a slide for microscopic inspection for parasites and eggs. You may also check at night by using a flashlight. The test may need to be repeated on consecutive days.

 Think**Like a Nurse** 29-5

You are reviewing a client's chart and note that the client was tested for fecal occult blood. The results are as follows:

3/10/16 negative for occult blood
3/11/16 no BM
3/12/16 no BM
3/13/16 no BM
3/14/16 positive for occult blood
3/15/16 negative for occult blood
3/16/16 negative for occult blood

What can you conclude? What questions do these findings raise?

■ ANALYSIS/NURSING DIAGNOSIS

Common nursing diagnoses related to bowel elimination include the following:

- *Bowel Incontinence* is a change in normal bowel habits characterized by involuntary passage of stool. It is more common among women and older adults. Other risk factors include neurological diseases, stroke, sphincter damage, and inflammatory bowel disease.
- *Constipation.* Because frequency of bowel elimination varies, constipation is usually defined as a decrease in the frequency of bowel movements resulting in the passage of hard, dry stool. Constipation can be a temporary problem wherein symptoms resolve in a short time. Nearly everyone experiences constipation at some point. *Chronic constipation* typically lasts 3 months or longer and may persist for years. Unrelieved constipation may eventually result in a **fecal impaction**, in which dry, hard stools lodged in the rectum cannot be passed.
- *Risk for Constipation* is an appropriate diagnosis for clients at increased risk because of bedrest, medications such as opioids, or surgery. You might use this diagnosis for a client with a condition or taking medications known to decrease peristalsis.
- *Perceived Constipation* is an appropriate diagnosis for a client who makes a self-diagnosis of constipation and uses laxatives, suppositories, or enemas to ensure a daily bowel movement.
- *Diarrhea* is the passage of loose, unformed, or watery stools.
- *Dysfunctional Gastrointestinal Motility* is a broad label that encompasses increased, decreased, ineffective, or absent peristaltic activity within the GI system. If you use this label, you need to specify whether the GI motility is increased, decreased.
- *Toileting Self-Care Deficit* is impaired ability to perform or complete own toileting activities.

For definitions and defining characteristics of these diagnoses, consult a nursing diagnosis handbook or

 Go to Chapter 29, **Standardized Language, Nursing Diagnoses Associated With Bowel Elimination,** on *DavisPlus.*

Bowel elimination problems may also form the etiology of other nursing diagnoses and collaborative problems. Examples include the following:

- Social isolation r/t embarrassment secondary to bowel incontinence
- Potential Complication: Electrolyte imbalance secondary to diarrhea. Older adults, very young children, and infants are at especially high risk.
- Impaired Skin Integrity r/t irritating effects of feces secondary to diarrhea
- Anxiety r/t perceived need for a daily bowel movement
- Disturbed Body Image r/t bowel diversion

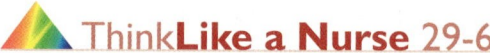 **ThinkLike a Nurse 29-6**

- What data do you have about Mrs. Zeno's (Meet Your Patient) bowel function?
- What else would you like to know about her bowel function? What other symptoms often accompany these cues?
- Which NANDA-I nursing diagnosis best describes this cue cluster?
- In addition to this nursing diagnosis, what other data in the scenario might also be contributing to her infrequent BMs?
- From the scenario data, how would you describe the etiology of Mrs. Zeno's problem?
- What questions do you still have about the etiology?

■ PLANNING OUTCOMES/EVALUATION

The general bowel elimination goal is that the patient will have soft, formed bowel movements regularly.

For *associated NOC standardized outcomes* for bowel elimination diagnoses,

 Go to Chapter 29, **Standardized Language, Selected Standardized Outcomes and Interventions for Bowel Elimination Diagnoses,** on *DavisPlus.*

When bowel elimination is the etiology, choose outcomes linked to the problem side of the diagnosis. For example, for Impaired Skin Integrity r/t irritating effects of diarrhea stool, the NOC outcomes might fall within Tissue Integrity: Skin and Mucous Membranes.

Individualized goals/outcome statements depend on the nursing diagnosis. Because normal bowel elimination patterns are individualized, regularity is based on the individual's pattern. Examples include the following:

Will resume his normal bowel pattern by (date).
Will discuss his feelings about his colostomy.

■ PLANNING INTERVENTIONS/IMPLEMENTATION

Bowel elimination is a normal physiological function. It is important for you to convey an attitude of acceptance and display professionalism when providing care for patients with bowel elimination problems.

A few examples of *NIC standardized interventions and activities* for patients with bowel elimination problems include: Bowel Incontinence Care, Constipation/Impaction Management, Diarrhea Management, Bowel Management, and Teaching: Individual. For a more comprehensive list of NIC interventions for various nursing diagnoses,

 Go to Chapter 29, **Standardized Language, Selected Standardized Outcomes and Interventions for Bowel Elimination Diagnoses,** on *DavisPlus.*

Specific nursing activities to promote normal bowel function and relieve elimination problems are found in the following sections. Both independent and dependent interventions are discussed.

Promoting Normal or Regular Defecation

Promoting regular defecation entails a number of independent nursing activities. These include providing privacy, positioning, timing, providing hydration and nutrition, promoting exercise, and teaching clients when they should seek medical assistance.

Provide Privacy

Try this exercise. Imagine that your class assignment for today is to stand in front of the classroom and describe to the class your normal pattern of defecation, including frequency, appearance, and other characteristics of the stool. How would you feel about that? Would you do it?

Although defecation is a normal physiological function, most patients consider it a very private matter. Taking a matter-of-fact approach confirms to patients that you are comfortable with this aspect of care. Provide privacy for your patient when discussing or providing care related to bowel elimination. For example, excuse visitors from the room, draw the dividing curtains in shared rooms, and close the door. Many patients are embarrassed by the odor of bowel movements and therefore may ignore the urge to defecate. Using an aromatic spray or other odor-reducing product may help to reduce embarrassment.

Assist With Positioning

An upright seated or squatting position is the most comfortable for defecation and decreases the need to strain. When possible, assist the patient to the bathroom to use the toilet. An alternative is to place a bedside commode next to the bed for patients who are unable to ambulate to the bathroom. A patient who must remain in bed should assume a semi-Fowler's position to use the bedpan. Patients who are unable to assume this position because of surgery, trauma, or other medical conditions must use supine or side-lying positions. These positions are unnatural for bowel elimination and place the patient at risk for constipation.

Raise the siderails or provide an overhead trapeze so that the patient can grip them to maneuver on and off the bedpan. If the patient is very weak, you may need an assistant to help you position him on the bedpan. In addition, you may need to stay with the person while he uses the bedpan to help him maintain his position. The Highlights of Procedures box in this chapter provides a summary of this skill. For the complete procedure,

 Go to Chapter 29, **Procedure 29-2: Placing and Removing a Bedpan,** in Volume 2.

Consider the Timing of Defecation

Recall that food entering the duodenum triggers mass peristalsis. As a result, the urge to defecate often occurs after meals. Advise patients not to ignore this urge, because doing so may lead to constipation. For patients who are ambulatory, allow some free time after meals to use the restroom. Assist those who cannot toilet independently to ambulate to the bathroom or use the bedpan. Discuss with NAPs the need to offer help without waiting to be asked so that patients experience minimal delays.

Support Healthful Intake of Food and Fluids

Teach clients the importance of a balanced diet in promoting soft, formed, regular bowel movements. Encourage a daily intake of 25 to 30 grams of fiber to provide bulk, attract water into the stool, and promote peristalsis. The diet should be rich in fresh fruits, dried fruits, vegetables (especially raw), whole-grain foods, flaxseed, popcorn, dried beans, peas, and legumes.

Without adequate fluid intake, a high-fiber diet can actually cause constipation. Recommend a minimum intake of 1,500 mL of fluid per day to keep stool soft and aid in production of mucus to lubricate the colon. Ideally, a person should drink eight to ten 8-ounce glasses of fluid daily (2,000 to 2,400 mL). Water is the preferred fluid because soda, coffee, and tea often contain caffeine or additives that promote diuresis. However, because the diuretic effect of these fluids is minimal, they are acceptable for clients who simply will not drink enough plain water.

Key Point: *Adding fiber does not help to relieve opioid-induced constipation unless the patient's current intake is deficient.* In fact, excessive fiber might put the patient at risk for bowel obstruction due to the opioid-induced decreased peristalsis, delayed gastric emptying, and prolonged intestinal transit time of the feces (Pitlick & Fritz, 2013).

Encourage Exercise

Physical activity increases peristalsis and promotes defecation. Encourage patients to exercise three to five times per week and to engage in daily walking or light activity. Assist hospitalized or institutionalized patients to ambulate as soon as their condition permits. Even limited activity, such as getting out of bed or walking 10 feet, decreases the risk for constipation.

Provide range-of-motion (ROM) exercises for patients who must remain on bedrest. Even passive ROM (the joints are moved through ROM by the nurse) promotes peristalsis. Chapter 32 provides additional information about activity and ROM exercises, if you need it.

For clients who can assist with exercise, the following exercises promote abdominal and perineal strength:

- *Thigh strengthening.* Have the client slowly bring one knee up to his chest, briefly hold it, then lower the leg to the bed. Repeat this pattern alternating legs. Encourage the client to perform this exercise several times per hour while he is awake.
- *Abdominal tightening.* Have the client tighten and hold the abdominal muscles for a count of five and then relax. This core exercise works the abdominal muscles used during defecation.

Managing Flatulence

Recall that flatus is a natural by-product of digestion. When gas is excessive or leads to complaints of abdominal distention, cramping, or discomfort, it is known as **flatulence**. Some people develop flatulence after eating gas-producing foods, such as beans, cabbage, cauliflower, onions, or highly spiced foods. For others, flatulence occurs when fiber intake is increased. Clients with irritable bowel syndrome experience a cluster of symptoms that include flatulence. Constipation is often accompanied by flatulence because digestive by-products undergo prolonged fermentation in the colon. Use the following interventions to help clients manage flatulence:

- Teach clients to be aware of and avoid foods that trigger flatulence.
- Teach clients to follow self-care strategies (identified earlier) for maintaining regular bowel movements.
- Encourage patients who have had surgery with gaseous anesthesia to ambulate and perform bed exercises to stimulate peristalsis and the passage of gas.
- In severe cases, you may need to insert a rectal tube to aid in the elimination of flatus. For a summary, see the Highlights of Procedures box. To learn the entire procedure,

 Go to Chapter 29, **Procedure 29-5: Inserting a Rectal Tube,** in Volume 2.

Teach Clients When to See a Primary Care Provider

Obviously many GI symptoms are normal and do not require treatment. For example, everyone has excessive flatus and abdominal distention at some time—perhaps as a result of a high-fat, high-sugar meal. And it is common for bowel movements to occasionally become a little irregular. However, clients need to know when a symptom may be signaling a more serious condition.

Teach clients to see their primary care provider for the following if a symptom lasts longer than 3 weeks or is disabling:

- Blood in the stool (unless they have hemorrhoids and this is not an unusual occurrence for them)
- Severe stomach pain
- Change in bowel habits
- Unintended weight loss
- Constipation is not relieved after trying fiber, fluids, and exercise

KnowledgeCheck 29-5

Identify at least five independent nursing actions that you can take to encourage regular elimination in a well client.

 ThinkLike a Nurse 29-7

How could you facilitate regular bowel elimination for Mrs. Zeno (Meet Your Patient)? What information do you need?

Interventions for Example Problem: Diarrhea

Diarrhea may occur as a result of contaminated food, a viral infection, or dietary change, or as a side effect of a medication. Patients with diarrhea are at risk for fluid and electrolyte imbalance, particularly potassium. Ideally, oral liquids replace the lost fluid and potassium. Infants, young children, and the frail elderly are most vulnerable and may require hospitalization and intravenous fluid replacement therapy. Ideally, oral liquids replace the lost fluid and potassium.

Nursing interventions focus on treating the diarrhea itself, as well as its associated problems (cramping, fluid and electrolyte imbalances, and Impaired Skin Integrity):

Preventive Interventions

Diarrhea can be prevented in the following ways:

- **Teach hand hygiene.** Teach patients to wash their hands often. This helps prevent diarrhea caused by viruses and other pathogens.
- **Provide information about foods that can cause diarrhea.** Highly spiced foods, high-fat foods, greasy snacks, or large quantities of raw fruits and vegetables may cause diarrhea in some patients. Tell patients to keep track of foods that trigger diarrhea and to eat them in moderation.

Monitoring Interventions

During the diarrhea episode, assess and monitor the following:

- **Monitor stools.** Assess frequency, amount, color, and consistency of stools to determine the severity of the diarrhea.
- **Monitor fluid balance.** Monitor intake and output, body weight, and vital signs to assess hydration. Also assess skin turgor and moistness of mucous membranes.
- **Monitor serum electrolyte levels.**
- **Monitor skin integrity.** Assess the perineal area for alterations in skin integrity. Clients with diarrhea may experience perianal irritation and excoriation.

Treatment Interventions

Treatments include medications, diet modification, and attention to fluid balance and skin integrity.

Medications Opiates (e.g., paregoric) and opiate derivatives (e.g., loperamide) are the primary antidiarrheal drugs prescribed. Although they slow peristalsis and inhibit diarrhea, they may cause drowsiness; advise patients, especially older adults, to use them with caution. Pepto-Bismol (bismuth subsalicylate) is a readily available OTC medication that is useful for traveler's diarrhea because it has antimicrobial and antisecretory properties.

Antidiarrheal medications are not recommended for acute diarrhea. In many cases, diarrhea is a response to infection or unusual foods and serves as a mechanism to rid the body of the pathogens or troublesome food. Although antidiarrheal medications are available without a prescription, caution patients to avoid using them unless instructed by their healthcare provider. Medication is usually reserved for use with chronic diarrhea—diarrhea that has persisted for more than 1 month.

Diet and Fluids During the acute episode, the patient may need to modify his diet to control the diarrhea.

- **Teach the patient about, or provide, a clear liquid diet**, including electrolyte replacement fluids (e.g., Pedialyte or sports drinks that have been diluted by 50% or more). Clear broth and gelatin are also good choices.
- **Encourage your patient to sip liquids** or take ice chips or Popsicles often to replace the losses.
- **Reduce the amount of fiber** in your client's diet by cutting back servings of whole grain bread and fresh fruits and vegetables.
- **Limit foods containing caffeine**, such as coffee, strong tea, and colas.
- **Avoid a sudden large intake of fluid or food** when resuming a normal diet, because this may trigger mass peristalsis.
- **Plain yogurt and other probiotic foods** consumed daily may help to prevent the diarrhea caused by antibiotics. Other medications may also cause diarrhea. A change in medications may be required.
- **Continue breast milk** for breastfed infants with acute diarrhea. There should be no need for interruption. In fact, breastfeeding has a well-known protective effect against the development of enteritis, promotes faster recovery, and provides improved nutrition.
- **Advise a BRAT diet** if a child with diarrhea has an appetite. A BRAT diet consists of bananas, (white) rice, applesauce, and toast. These are easy to digest, provide calories for energy without gastric irritation, and help offset potassium loss. Although developed for pediatric use, the BRAT diet is sometimes used for adults.

Interventions for Example Problem: Constipation

Many of the nursing strategies to prevent and treat constipation are identical to the activities that promote regular bowel elimination.

Short-Term Constipation

Short-Term Constipation is usually caused by the person's lifestyle. Clients most likely to experience constipation are those who (1) have decreased activity or are on bedrest, (2) are receiving opioids or other medications that slow peristalsis, and (3) have decreased fluid and fiber intake. The following are some interventions:

- **Increase the intake of high-fiber foods** if intake is inadequate (normal adult Recommended Dietary Allowances (RDA) and Adequate Intakes (AI) is 25 to 38 grams, depending on age and sex).

- **Increase fluid intake.**
- **Increase physical activity.**
- **Provide privacy for using the toilet.**
- **Assist the patient to a seated or squatting position** whenever possible. A semi-Fowler's position is preferred for a client on bedrest.
- **Allow the patient uninterrupted time to use the toilet**, especially after meals, when mass peristalsis occurs.
- **Encourage the patient not to ignore the urge to defecate.**
- **Assess for complications** such as impaction and hemorrhoids.

Chronic Constipation

Chronic constipation may be associated with physiological factors such as dysfunctional intestinal motility, nervous system problems, and dysfunctional anorectal musculature. Chronic constipation causes significant psychological distress and decreased quality of life for many clients, and it may result in complications, which include intestinal impaction, anal fissures, hemorrhoids, volvulus (twisted loop of the intestine), intestinal obstruction, rectal ulcers, fecal seepage, and bowel perforation.

Many laxatives are readily available without prescription and are used by clients to treat actual or perceived constipation. However, lifestyle changes and nonprescription medications do not usually prevent or adequately treat chronic constipation. Therefore, laxatives may be prescribed (Box 29-1). *Bulking agents* are the preferred medications for treating constipation. They are actually fiber in a nonfood source. Habitual laxative use, except for bulking agents, may cause reliance on medications for bowel elimination and, ironically, may lead to further constipation. See Self-Care: Teaching Your Patient About Laxative Use for key points to discuss with patients about managing constipation.

Older Adults

Screen older adults for risk factors, including a history of polypharmacy and taking laxatives. Other risk factors include impaired cognitive status, inadequate fluid intake, inadequate dietary fiber, reduced mobility, lack of privacy for toileting, and reliance on others for assistance. These are the same as risk factors for all ages, but they are more likely for older adults. Prevention measures are the same for all ages. However, for those unable to walk or who are restricted to bed, exercises such as trunk rotation, pelvic tilt, and leg lifts may be helpful. For older adults, osmotic laxatives (e.g., PEG and lactulose, bulking agents) have been found to be beneficial (The Joanna Briggs Institute, 2008).

Fecal Impaction

Fecal impaction is the presence of a hardened fecal mass in the rectum. The impaction often blocks the passage of normal stool and sets up a vicious cycle of furthering

Teaching Your Patient About Laxative Use

Discuss the following topics with clients who have concerns about the frequency of their bowel movements or ask about laxatives.

1. The frequency of BMs may range from several times per day to once per week. As long as stools are passed without excessive urgency, with minimal effort and no straining, and without the use of laxatives, bowel function may be regarded as normal.

2. To maintain normal bowel function:

   ➤ Eat a well-balanced diet that includes five servings of whole grains, fresh fruits, and vegetables.

   ➤ Drink eight to ten glasses of fluid per day.

   ➤ Engage in daily exercise to stimulate peristalsis.

   ➤ Set aside uninterrupted time after breakfast or dinner for using the toilet.

   ➤ Do not ignore the urge to defecate.

   ➤ Whenever there is a significant or prolonged change in bowel habits, report this to your healthcare provider.

3. If you are experiencing constipation, choose bulking agents, such as Metamucil or psyllium, to treat the problem rather than other OTC laxatives. Be sure to drink plenty of water when using bulking agents.

---

hardening. Liquid stool may leak, seeping around the hardend mass, and the patient may report feelings of fullness, bloating, constipation, diminished appetite, and a change in bowel habits. You can detect fecal impaction by digital examination of the rectum. To treat a fecal impaction, you will use enemas or digital removal of stool. Once the impaction has been removed, establish a bowel regimen to prevent recurrence of impactions.

Administering Enemas

An **enema** is the introduction of solution into the rectum to soften feces, distend the colon, and stimulate peristalsis and evacuation of feces. Some enema solutions are chosen because they irritate the mucosa of the rectum and sigmoid colon and assist with forceful evacuation of stool.

Before administering a prescribed enema, explain the purpose of the enema and what the patient can expect. For example, the patient will probably experience some cramping with a large-volume enema. Reassure the patient that you will be immediately available to help her to the restroom or onto the bedpan.

Responses to an enema are governed by the height of the solution container, the speed of flow, the concentration of the solution, and the resistance of the rectum. Hypotonic and isotonic solutions are easier to retain. Muscle tone and history of constipation or other bowel disorders determine the resistance of the rectum. A client with a long history of constipation is more likely to be able to tolerate a large-volume enema, because the rectum and colon have become distended over time.

Enemas may be classified as cleansing, retention, or return-flow. The primary care provider generally prescribes the specific type to administer to a patient. The Highlights of Procedures box summarizes the steps for administering an enema. To learn the full procedure for various types of enemas,

 Go to Chapter 29, **Procedure 29-3: Administering an Enema,** in Volume 2.

Cleansing Enemas

Cleansing enemas promote removal of feces from the colon. They may be used to:

- Treat severe constipation or impaction.
- Clear the colon in preparation for visualization procedures, such as colonoscopy.
- Empty the colon when starting a bowel training program.
- Clear the colon for surgeries of the lower GI tract and for some pelvic surgeries.

A cleansing enema may be given "high" or "low." A "low" enema is given by standard procedure. A "high" enema attempts to clear as much of the large intestine as possible. With a "high" enema, the client receives initial instillation of the fluid in the left lateral position. The client then moves to the dorsal recumbent position and then the right lateral position for the remainder of the instillation. This turning process allows the fluid to follow the shape of the large intestine.

Cleansing enema solutions include hypotonic solutions and hypertonic solutions.

- **Hypotonic solutions** (saline, tap water, and soap). With hypotonic solutions, you introduce a large volume (500 to 1,000 mL for adults, 100 to 250 mL for infants) of fluid into the rectum. The volume distends the intestine and leads to rapid evacuation of stool.

  ✚ Large-volume solutions may be contraindicated in patients who have weakened intestinal walls.

- **Hypertonic solutions**, in contrast, are usually smaller in volume (70 to 120 mL, or 2.5 to 4 oz, for adults). The hypertonic solution attracts water into the colon, causing distention and stimulating peristalsis and defecation (Table 29-2).

  ✚ Hypertonic solutions may be contraindicated for patients who tend to retain sodium or water (e.g., those with renal failure and congestive heart failure).

Retention Enemas

Retention enemas introduce a solution into the colon that is meant to be retained for a prolonged period. Consequently the volume is small, usually 90 to 120 mL (3 to 4 oz). The following are the most common forms of retention enemas.

Table 29-2 ▶ Solutions Commonly Used in Enemas

SOLUTION	EXAMPLES	ACTION	TIME UNTIL BM	ADVERSE EFFECTS
Hypotonic	500–1,000 mL of tap water	Large volume distends the colon, thereby stimulating peristalsis; water also softens stool.	15 minutes	Fluid and electrolyte imbalance, especially water intoxication, is possible if enema is not expelled.
Isotonic	500–1,000 mL of normal saline (0.9% NaCl solution)	Large volume distends the colon, thereby stimulating peristalsis; some softening of stool also occurs.	15 minutes	Fluid and electrolyte imbalance, especially sodium retention
Hypertonic	120–180 mL of sodium phosphate (e.g., Fleet); available as a commercially prepared solution	Attracts water into the colon, thereby causing distention.	Rapid acting: 5–10 minutes	Sodium retention
Oil	90–120 mL of mineral oil, cottonseed oil, or olive oil; available as a commercially prepared solution	Softens the feces, lubricates the rectum.	Varies widely. An oil-retention enema is often given 1–3 hours before a cleansing enema is administered.	
Soapsuds	Pure Castile soap is added to tap water or saline.	Intestinal irritation stimulates peristalsis.	Varies	Only pure Castile soap is safe. Other soaps and detergents can cause bowel inflammation.
Carminative	For example 1:2:3 "MGW" solution (e.g., 30 mL magnesium, 60 mL glycerin, and 90 mL water)	Provides relief from abdominal distention caused by flatus.		

- **Oil-retention enemas** instill 90 to 120 mL of oil into the rectum to soften stool and lubricate the rectum. This type of enema may be used to assist a client to pass hard stool or before digital removal of stool. It may also be used in conjunction with a cleansing enema—at least 1 hour before the cleansing enema.
- **Carminative enema** is a procedure in which 60 to 180 mL (2 to 6 oz) of solution are instilled into the rectum to help expel flatus and relieve bloating and distention. This procedure is used after abdominal or pelvic surgery when peristalsis is slow to return and the client experiences pressure from gas. Solutions may be commercially prepared or prepared on the unit. A common carminative enema is the "MGW" enema; a mixture of magnesium sulfate, glycerin, and water in a ratio of 1:2:3 (e.g., 15 mL of magnesium sulfate, 30 mL of glycerin, and 45 mL of water).
- **Medicated enemas** may be used to instill antibiotics to treat infections in the rectum or anus or to introduce anthelminthic agents for treatment of intestinal worms and parasites.
- **Nutritive enemas** administer fluid and nutrition through the rectum for patients who are dehydrated and frail. They are most commonly used in hospice care as a means to provide hydration for dying patients.

Return-Flow Enemas

A return-flow enema, known as a *Harris flush*, may be ordered to help a patient expel flatus and relieve abdominal distention. For adults, approximately 100 to 200 mL (3 to 7 oz) of tap water or saline is instilled into the rectum. The rectal tube and solution container are then lowered below the level of the rectum to encourage return flow of the solution. This process is repeated several times, or until distention is relieved. If the solution becomes thick, discard it and begin again with new solution.

Digital Removal of Stool

If fecal impaction does not respond to use of stool softeners and enemas, you will need to digitally remove feces from the rectum. Digital removal is accomplished by breaking up the hardened mass into pieces and manually extracting the pieces. You may administer an oil-retention enema at least 30 minutes before digital removal to soften the stool and decrease the patient's discomfort during the procedure.

Aside from discomfort, the pressure generated in the rectum may stimulate the vagus nerve, slowing the heart rate. For that reason, you must have a prescription from the primary care provider.

For a summary of this procedure, see the Highlights of Procedures box. For complete steps,

 Go to Chapter 29, **Procedure 29-4: Removing Stool Digitally,** in Volume 2.

KnowledgeCheck 29-6

Identify the types of enemas available for use.

- How do hypotonic and isotonic enemas differ from hypertonic enemas?
- What actions can you take to make the patient more comfortable when he receives an enema?

ThinkLike a Nurse 29-8

Mrs. Zeno (Meet Your Patient) begins to pass liquid stool. What actions should you take? Explain your reasoning.

Interventions for Example Problem: Bowel Incontinence

Bowel incontinence (or *fecal incontinence*) is the inability to control the discharge of feces and flatulence. One study suggests that 17% of Medicare patients report fecal incontinence (FI), and that patients with FI had a greater chance of institutionalization (Shah, Chokhavatia, & Rose, 2012). Physiological conditions causing bowel incontinence include conditions that affect innervation of the rectum and anus, uncontrolled diarrhea, impaction resulting in leakage of stool, and cognitive or emotional changes that alter perception of the urge to defecate. Bowel incontinence is also created by functional limitations—for example, when a client recognizes the need to have a BM but cannot get to the toilet independently or in time to defecate in the toilet.

Clients with persistent bowel incontinence require special nursing care to prevent Impaired Skin Integrity because of the moisture and the activity of enzymes in the stool. In addition, bowel incontinence may be embarrassing. As clients worry about future episodes, anxiety escalates. Refer to the Nursing Care Plan and Care Map for a patient with fecal incontinence near the end of this chapter. In general, nursing interventions include the following:

- Monitor the pattern of BMs.
- Provide a bedpan or assist the patient to the bathroom at regular intervals and at times BMs are most likely to occur.
- Change clothing and/or bed linens as soon as possible to prevent skin irritation and embarrassment.
- Provide prompt hygiene care after any episodes of incontinence.
- Monitor skin for evidence of breakdown. Use moisture-barrier cream if redness or irritation is noted.
- Review diet, fluid intake, activity, and medicines. Work with the primary care provider to alter the above factors to encourage regular bowel movements.

- Consider a bowel training program (discussed in a following section).
- Consider using containment or indwelling methods to prevent fecal drainage from soiling clothing. Research on patient outcomes of most of these methods is limited.

Absorbent Products

You may use absorbent products to prevent fecal drainage from soiling clothing and linens. For small quantities of stool, a long, rectangular pad or a belted absorbent shield can be placed inside clothing. For larger quantities, adult incontinence garments are used. They may pull on like underwear or fasten like a diaper. Moisture-resistant pads placed under the patient help to protect bed linens. When using absorbent products, remember these important points:

Key Point: *Never refer to incontinence pads as "diapers" when caring for adults or children who have been toilet trained. This inappropriate reference may cause embarrassment and lower the patient's self-esteem.*

 Never place the plastic side of the pad next to the patient's body. This holds moisture next to the skin, which leads to irritation and breakdown.

- Use state-of-the-art skin protection products, such as perineal cleansers and skin barrier products.
- Change the pad as soon as possible after defecation. Keep the skin scrupulously clean.

External Fecal Collection Devices

You may apply an external fecal incontinence pouch to protect perianal skin or to collect large fecal samples. The pouch collects fecal drainage, keeping feces away from the skin. This is a common approach for clients with uncontrolled diarrhea. Pouch systems vary widely. Most often, a moisture-proof barrier is applied around the anus, and a plastic pouch is secured to the barrier (Fig. 29-8). The equipment may be the same as that used for patients with an ostomy, which is discussed later in the chapter.

External collection systems can prevent skin breakdown, minimize odor, track output accurately, and enhance patient comfort. However, they are not typically used for patients who are ambulatory, agitated, or active in bed because the device may be dislodged, causing skin breakdown. **Key Point:** *External systems cannot be used effectively when the patient has Impaired Skin Integrity because they will not seal tightly.*

- Assess the system regularly to ensure that it has not become dislodged and that no leaks have occurred.
- Change the fecal pouch at least every 72 hours (per protocol) and whenever there is evidence of leakage.
- Empty the fecal pouch when it is one-third to one-half full to prevent it from getting too heavy.
- Pay close attention to the perianal skin as you perform your assessment. You may need to use moisture-barrier cream on the surrounding skin.

The Highlights of Procedures box summarizes the procedures for placing both external fecal drainage devices. To learn the procedures,

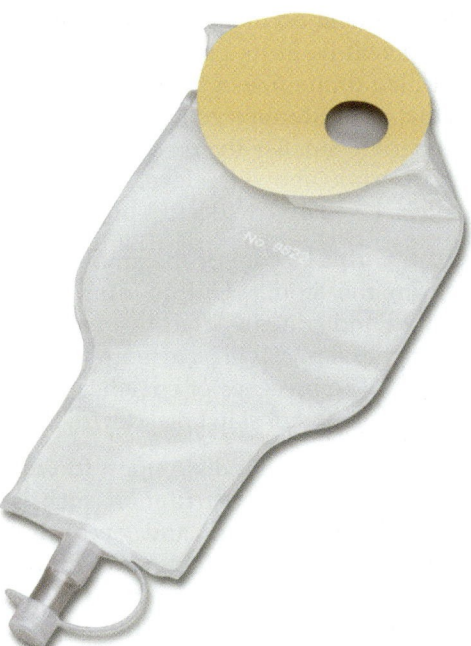

FIGURE 29-8 A fecal incontinence pouch. A skin barrier is applied around the anus and a plastic pouch is secured to the barrier. (Courtesy of Hollister Incorporated, Libertyville, IL.)

 Go to Chapter 29, **Procedure 29-8: Placing Fecal Drainage Devices,** in Volume 2.

Indwelling Fecal Drainage Devices

Indwelling fecal drainage devices are used to collect liquid stool from bedbound, immobilized ill patients. They consist of a soft, latex-free catheter and a collection bag (Fig. 29-9). The tube is inserted and a balloon on the end is filled with saline or water. Internal devices protect perianal skin, protect caregivers from potentially infectious stool, and are thought to decrease urinary tract infections. They are FDA approved, but only for 29 consecutive days, and not for pediatric patients. Other contraindications include patients who have severe hemorrhoids; recent bowel, rectal, or anal surgery or injury; rectal or anal tumors; or stricture or stenosis.

You must follow the manufacturer's recommendations carefully for insertion and maintenance. When the bag is filled, empty or replace it, depending on the type. You must also monitor to confirm placement and may need to irrigate the device. To learn more about placing and caring for a patient with an indwelling fecal drainage device, see the Highlights of Procedures box and,

 Go to Chapter 29, **Procedure 29-8B: Inserting an Indwelling Fecal Drainage Device, and Clinical Insight 29-1: Caring for a Patient With an Indwelling Fecal Drainage Device,** in Volume 2.

Bowel Training

A bowel training program assists the patient to have regular, soft, formed stools. It is appropriate for clients who have chronic constipation, impaction, or bowel

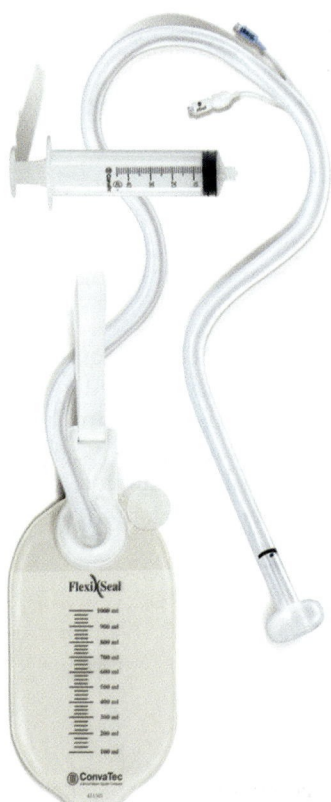

FIGURE 29-9 An indwelling fecal drainage device. (Courtesy of ConvaTec Inc., Skillman, NJ.)

incontinence. Elements of a bowel training program include the following:

- Plan the program with the patient and caregiver.
- Gradually increase fiber in the diet while monitoring consistency of the stool.
- Increase fluid intake to at least eight glasses of water per day, if not contraindicated.
- Initiate a designated uninterrupted time for defecation: usually after meals, especially in the morning.
- Provide privacy for the patient during the designated time.
- Develop a staged treatment plan if constipation develops. Usually additional fiber is added as a first measure. A stool softener is next, followed by a suppository such as bisacodyl (Dulcolax).
- Regularly modify the plan based on the patient's response.

KnowledgeCheck 29-7

- What are the major patient care concerns associated with bowel incontinence?
- What are the elements of a bowel training program?

Caring for Patients With Bowel Diversions

Patients experience a variety of reactions to a bowel diversion, and each person has unique physical and psychological needs. Initially you will care for the ostomy, but the goal is for the patient to assume self-care. For a full description of the care of an ostomy appliance, including changing and emptying,

 Go to Chapter 29, **Clinical Insight 29-2: Guidelines for Ostomy Care;** also see **Procedure 29-6: Changing an Ostomy Appliance,** in Volume 2.

Ongoing Assessments

Always begin care with a thorough assessment of the stoma, the stool, and the skin.

Assess the Stoma A healthy stoma (Fig. 29-10) ranges in color from deep pink to brick red, regardless of the patient's skin color, and is shiny and moist. Pallor or a dusky blue color indicates ischemia, and a brown-black color indicates necrosis. Immediately after surgery the stoma will be swollen and enlarged. As the inflammation

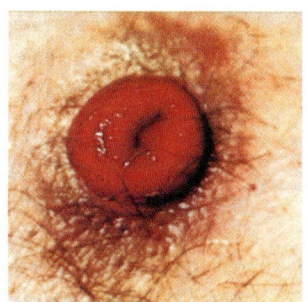

FIGURE 29-10 A healthy stoma is deep pink to brick red and is shiny and moist.

subsides and healing occurs, the stoma will shrink. By 6 to 8 weeks, it will be at its permanent size. Stoma size varies according to the size of the person and the part of the bowel that was externalized (Fig. 29-6). An ileostomy stoma is generally smaller than a colostomy stoma. The stoma will protrude above the level of the abdomen by approximately 1.3 to 2.5 cm (0.5 to 1 in.).

Assess the Output Monitor the amount and type of drainage from the stoma. Output from an ileostomy stoma is liquid and contains digestive enzymes. An ostomy lower in the GI tract will have more solid output and fewer enzymes. The presence of enzymes in the effluent increases the likelihood of skin breakdown.

Assess the Skin Pay close attention to the skin surrounding a stoma for signs of irritation, such as redness, tenderness, skin breakdown, and/or drainage. Skin breakdown may lead to infection, pain, and leakage.

Helping Patients Adapt to the Diversion

Patients experience a variety of reactions to a bowel diversion, and each person has unique needs. Initially you will care for the ostomy, but the goal is to have the patient assume self-care and a normal life. The first step in that direction is for the patient to adjust to the presence of an ostomy. If the patient has been sick before the surgery and the ostomy leads to less pain or discomfort, the transition may be easier. Similarly, patients with continent ostomies may adapt more easily to their stoma.

Toward Evidence-Based Practice

Li, C. C., Rew, L., & Hwang, S. L. (2012). The relationship between spiritual well-being and psychosocial adjustment in Taiwanese patients with colorectal cancer and a colostomy. *Journal of Wound Ostomy & Continence Nursing, 39*(2), 161–169.

Participants were 45 Taiwanese patients, aged 42 to 83 years, who were diagnosed with colorectal cancer and underwent colostomy surgery. They completed a questionnaire that examined relationships among demographic and clinical characteristics, spiritual well-being, and psychosocial adjustment to the colostomy. Participants reported strong family relationships but poor adjustment in sexual relationships. Spiritual well-being was significantly associated with psychosocial adjustment and was found to play an important role for patients when faced with psychosocial adjustment related to a colostomy.

Poletto, D., & Silva, D. M. (2013). Living with intestinal stoma: The construction of autonomy for care. *Revista Latino-Americana de Enfermagem, 21*(2), 531–538.

Ten people who received a stoma, and their family members, participated in two semi-structured interviews to investigate which care provided in the postoperative period played the largest role in promoting autonomy. The study identified common factors that influence the development of autonomy, including (1) the need to carry out stoma care; (2) receiving health support and care after discharge from hospital; (3) the family's support in developing autonomy; and (4) returning to daily activities and social reinsertion. The authors suggested that health professionals are fundamental to the process of developing autonomy by working as educators, supporting the achievement, and encouraging the care and the return to activities.

1. Based on these studies, write three nursing interventions you would use to help a patient accept and adapt to a stoma.

2. Suppose you wanted to know whether those interventions would be effective for patients with other medical conditions. For example, would the interventions that help clients adapt to a stoma help other clients to adapt to a different issue? Think of at least two health conditions for which you might want to perform the two studies just described. Explain your thinking.

 Go to Chapter 29, **Toward Evidence-Based Practice Suggested Responses,** on DavisPlus.

Ostomy patients no longer have sphincter control, so they may need to modify their diet. You can promote adaptation by teaching the client about diet modifications. Box 29-3 discusses the effects of some foods on a patient with an ostomy.

With the exception of a temporary double-barreled colostomy, ostomy care is a lifelong task. Patients must learn about appliances, stoma care, and ongoing management of the ostomy. In many hospitals and large communities, you can find an enterostomal therapy nurse to assist patients with their ongoing care and to provide consultation on ostomy appliances. For more interventions to promote physical and psychological adaptation,

 Go to Chapter 29, **Clinical Insight 29-2: Guidelines for Ostomy Care,** in Volume 2.

Colostomy Irrigation

Colostomy Irrigation may be indicated as an occasional intervention for constipation or in a select population of patients. Consult with the ostomy nurse and/or physician to see if colostomy irrigation is appropriate for your patient. A stoma above the descending colon

usually has liquid output that cannot be controlled. Therefore, it is not irrigated. Patients with an ostomy in the descending or sigmoid colon may use colostomy irrigation as a means to control bowel evacuation and possibly eliminate the need to wear an ostomy pouch.

Colostomy irrigation is similar to an enema. The nurse or patient inserts a flexible tube into the stoma and instills a traditional enema solution. The patient may use a special plastic sleeve over the stoma or an ostomy appliance to direct the output into the toilet. After evacuation of the bowel, the client may wear a small covering over the stoma instead of a pouch. See the Highlights of Procedures box for a summary. For the complete procedure,

 Go to Chapter 29, **Procedure 29-7: Irrigating a Colostomy,** in Volume 2.

KnowledgeCheck 29-8

- How can you help a patient adapt psychologically to living with a bowel diversion?
- What does a healthy stoma look like?
- Why is skin care around a stoma so important?

BOX 29-3 ■ Dietary Changes Associated With an Ostomy

Note: These are only suggestions. Each person must, by trial and error, discover what works best for him.

General Guidelines for Patients

- Initially you may be asked to follow a bland, low-residue or soft diet for a month or two to prevent obstructions and GI upsets. Advance the diet by adding one new food at a time.
- Eat three or more meals daily at regular times.
- People with ostomies may require additional fluid to compensate for the loss of the large intestine.
- Avoid chewing gum, as it may cause you to swallow air, causing a noisy stoma.
- Avoid foods that cause gas, odor, blockage, or loose stools. Eventually introduce them into your diet one at a time and be aware of their effects.
- Chew your food well to avoid blockage of the stoma.
- Avoid excessive weight gain.

Foods That May Cause Gas or Odor

Alcohol, beer, carbonated beverages

Asparagus, beans, broccoli, Brussels sprouts, cabbage, cauliflower, cucumbers, garlic, onions

Dairy, eggs

Fish, cod liver oil, nuts, peanut butter

Foods That May Help Control Gas or Odor

Buttermilk, yogurt

Cranberry juice

Parsley

High-Fiber Foods That May Cause Blockage

You can eat some of these foods (e.g., mushrooms, shrimp) if you cut them into small pieces and chew them very thoroughly.

As long as blockage does not occur, these foods should not necessarily be avoided, but used carefully.

- Foods with seeds (e.g., raspberries)
- Foods with tough skins (e.g., corn, dried fruits, pears, tomatoes)
- Mushrooms
- Nuts, popcorn
- Raw or minimally cooked fruits and vegetables (e.g., coleslaw, Chinese stir-fried vegetables, oranges, apple skins)
- Shrimp, lobster
- Stringy foods (e.g., celery, coconut, spinach, bean sprouts, green beans, orange pulp)

Foods That May Cause Loose Stools

Alcohol, beer, caffeine, chocolate, licorice

Milk

Baked beans, cooked cabbage, onions

Bran cereal, whole grains

Prunes, raisins

Note: Never restrict fluids in an effort to control diarrhea.

Foods That May Alleviate Diarrhea

Bananas **R**ice (white) **A**pplesauce **T**oast (BRAT diet) and other starchy foods (e.g., rice, bread, potatoes)

Cheese and creamy peanut butter

Sources: Lutz, C., & Przytulski, K. (2010). Nutrition and diet therapy: Evidence-based applications (5th ed.). Philadelphia: F.A. Davis; United Ostomy Associations of America (2005, updated 2011). Ostomates food reference chart. In Diet & nutrition guide. http://www.uoaa.org/ostomy_info/pubs/uoa_diet_nutrition_en.pdf

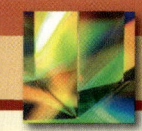

Nursing Care Plan

Client Data

Olivia Grimaldi, 59 years old, is admitted to the orthopedic unit after having a total knee replacement. She is receiving intravenous opioid analgesics for pain. Mrs. Grimaldi's nurse sits down to talk and complete the nursing admission assessment. The conversation turns to a discussion of bowel habits.

Nurse: Mrs. Grimaldi, we pay special attention to bowel elimination because many people on this unit have problems. How often do you have a bowel movement?

Mrs. G: Not as often as I'd like. I used to be very regular, but lately everything is all mixed up.

Nurse: What has changed? Tell me what's going on.

Mrs. G: Oh, it's so embarrassing. I haven't told anyone about this.

Nurse: When did this problem start?

Mrs. G: Everything started going bad when I fell and landed on this knee a few months ago. Nothing was broken, but the pain has been just awful. I knew I had arthritis, but I never felt anything like this. I couldn't sleep, the pain was so bad. The doctor put me on some pain pills—narcotics—and they helped, but I got so constipated. I started using laxatives to go to the bathroom, but I kept needing to use more and more. Sometimes I would take a laxative and then I would have to get to the bathroom quickly. I had a couple of accidents because I couldn't get to the toilet quickly enough.

Nurse: I think this is something we'll be able to help you with, Mrs. Grimaldi.

The nurse discovers that Mrs. Grimaldi drinks about 32 to 40 ounces of fluid each day and has used several stimulant laxatives and enemas to relieve her constipation. Her mobility has been significantly impaired for the past 2 months.

Nursing Diagnosis

Bowel Incontinence related to overdistention of the rectum secondary to chronic constipation, as evidenced by client report of constipation when taking opioids and subsequent fecal incontinence with the use of laxatives.

NOC Outcomes	Individualized Goals/Expected Outcomes
Bowel Continence (0500) Bowel Elimination (0501)	*By discharge, Mrs. Grimaldi will:* 1. Be free from fecal impaction. 2. Begin to establish a regular pattern of stool evacuation. 3. Describe four actions she can take to reduce the risk of constipation. *Within 1 month, Mrs. Grimaldi will:* 1. *Control stool passage without any episodes of fecal incontinence.*

NIC Interventions

Bowel Management (0430)
Bowel Training (0440)

Nursing Activities	Rationale
1. Conduct a comprehensive assessment of all factors related to fecal incontinence and impaired bowel elimination.	Fecal incontinence has multiple possible causes. The best nursing interventions are those based on client assessment (Bliss & Norton, 2010). Constipation is attributed to immobility, weak straining ability, use of constipating drugs, neurological disorders, lack of dietary fiber, and poor fluid intake (Fritz & Pitlick, 2012).

Nursing Care Plan (continued)

Nursing Activities	Rationale
2. During physical examination, inspect the perianal skin for possible causes of fecal incontinence or skin irritation resulting from exposure to liquid stool.	Congenital abnormalities and hemorrhoids can lead to incontinence. Skin tags can make cleansing difficult and lead to minor soiling that is difficult to distinguish from actual fecal incontinence (Bliss & Norton, 2010).
3. Inquire about Mrs. Grimaldi's access to the bathroom and toileting facilities at home and work. Provide regular toileting assistance as long as the client needs it during her hospitalization.	A lack of convenient access to the toilet can precipitate fecal incontinence (Song, 2012).
4. Work with Mrs. Grimaldi to establish a bowel reeducation program, starting with bowel cleansing.	Cleansing is indicated for rectal impaction or palpable stool in the descending or sigmoid colon. Cleansing with manual disimpaction, laxatives, and/or enema removes any potential blockages to stool elimination (Jamshed, Lee, & Olden, 2011; Rao & Go, 2010).
5. Ensure that Mrs. Grimaldi drinks 30 mL/kg of fluids per day and gradually increase dietary fiber with bran or with bulking agents. Mrs. Grimaldi is drinking only about 1,200 mL of fluid per day. If she weighs 125 lb (56.7 kg), she would need to drink at least 1,700 mL of fluid per day.	Increasing fluid intake may help to normalize stool consistency in clients with constipation who do not have adequate fluid intake (Leung & Rao, 2011; Linari, Schofield, & Horrom, 2011). Increasing dietary fiber improves stool consistency and reduces fecal incontinence (Leung & Rao, 2011; Shakil, Church, & Rao, 2008); however, unless the diet is deficient in fiber, adding fiber does not necessarily alleviate constipation. Bulk should be added to the diet slowly to reduce the risk of bloating, gas, or diarrhea. Dosing of bulking agents can be increased weekly until desired results are achieved; the results are more important than the amount of fiber ingested.
6. Teach Mrs. Grimaldi about how her body works to produce stool; ways to gently signal the body to defecate; the importance of responding to the urge to defecate; and how immobility, medications, and dehydration can cause constipation.	Gaining knowledge about bodily functions allows clients to be active participants in their care. Addressing causes of constipation can reduce the risk of recurrence (Fritz & Pitlick, 2012; Rao & Go, 2010).

Evaluation

Review initial outcomes and goals. Reassess daily progress toward stated discharge goals.

The day before Mrs. Grimaldi's discharge she had no palpable stool on physical exam, and she no longer needed the intravenous analgesics; her patient-controlled analgesia (PCA) pump was discontinued. She was drinking approximately 20 mL/kg per day of fluids, she had begun taking 2 tablespoons of psyllium dissolved in water every morning, and she had a bowel movement each of the previous 2 days with stool of normal consistency for the first time in more than a month. She was able to state the actions she would take at home: Continue the bulk supplements, try to increase her fluid intake to 30 mL/kg per day, use nonconstipating analgesics, and increase her mobility each day. The nurse charted that the goals were met.

References

Bliss, D. Z., & Norton, C. (2010); Bulechek, F., Butcher, H., & Dochterman, J. (2012); Fritz, D., & Pitlick, M. (2012); Gallagher, P., O'Mahony, D., & Quigley, E. (2008); Jamshed, N., Lee, Z. E., & Olden, K. W. (2011); Leung, F. W., & Rao, S. S. (2011); Linari, L. R., Schofield, L. C., & Horrom, K. A. (2011); Moorhead, S., Johnson, M., Maas, M., et al. (Eds.). (2012); Rao, S. S., & Go, J. T. (2010); Rohwer, K., Bliss, D. Z., & Savik, K. (2013); Shakil, A., Church, R., & Rao, S. (2008); Song, H. J. (2012).

Care Map

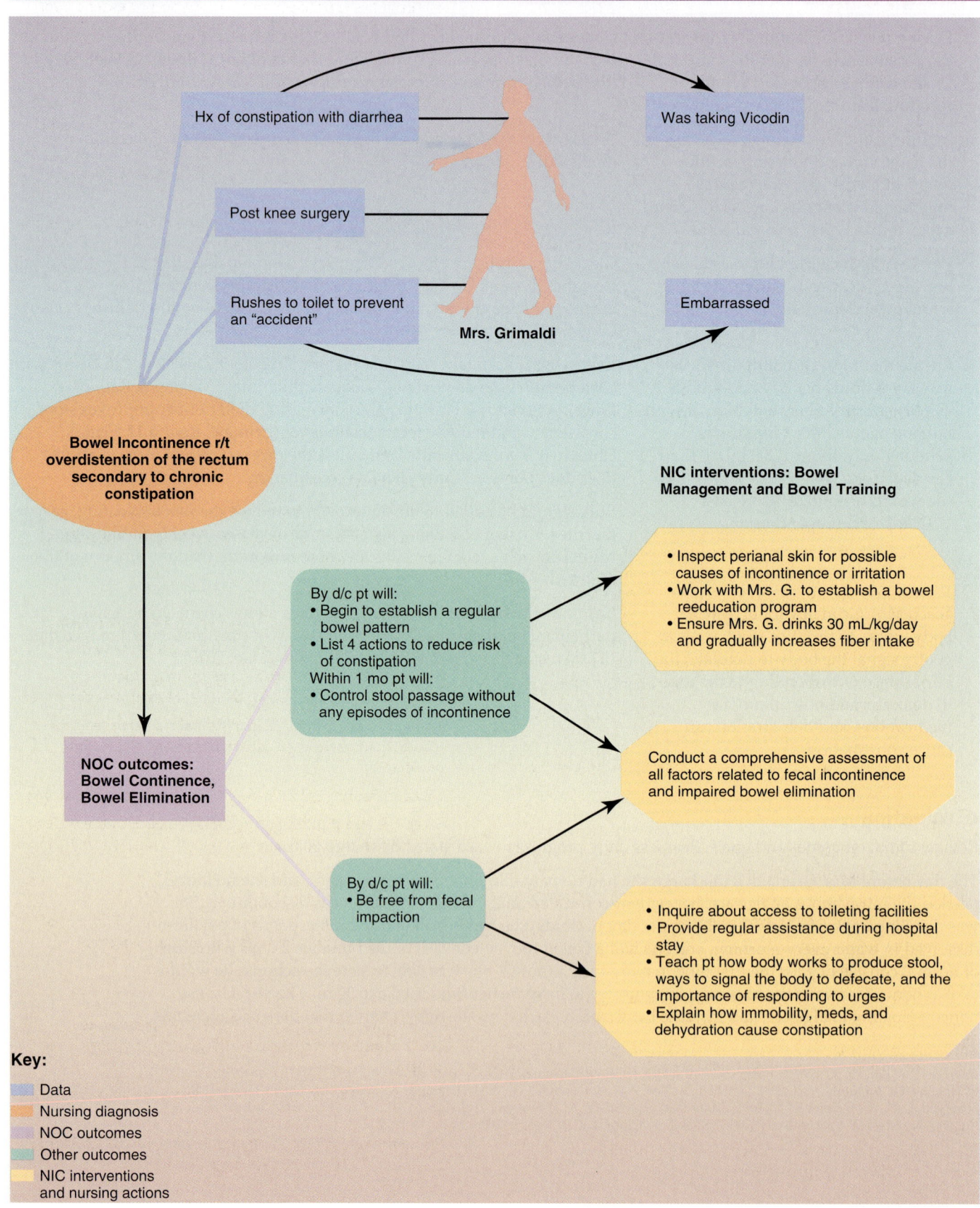

Hx of constipation with diarrhea

Was taking Vicodin

Post knee surgery

Rushes to toilet to prevent an "accident"

Mrs. Grimaldi

Embarrassed

Bowel Incontinence r/t overdistention of the rectum secondary to chronic constipation

NIC interventions: Bowel Management and Bowel Training

By d/c pt will:
- Begin to establish a regular bowel pattern
- List 4 actions to reduce risk of constipation
Within 1 mo pt will:
- Control stool passage without any episodes of incontinence

- Inspect perianal skin for possible causes of incontinence or irritation
- Work with Mrs. G. to establish a bowel reeducation program
- Ensure Mrs. G. drinks 30 mL/kg/day and gradually increases fiber intake

NOC outcomes: Bowel Continence, Bowel Elimination

Conduct a comprehensive assessment of all factors related to fecal incontinence and impaired bowel elimination

By d/c pt will:
- Be free from fecal impaction

- Inquire about access to toileting facilities
- Provide regular assistance during hospital stay
- Teach pt how body works to produce stool, ways to signal the body to defecate, and the importance of responding to urges
- Explain how immobility, meds, and dehydration cause constipation

Key:
- Data
- Nursing diagnosis
- NOC outcomes
- Other outcomes
- NIC interventions and nursing actions

For steps to follow in *all* procedures, refer to the Universal Steps for All Procedures found on the inside back cover of Volume 2. Go to the full procedures in Volume 2 to practice and learn the procedure steps. Use these procedure highlights later to help you review key points.

Highlights of Procedures 29-1 Through 29-8

Procedure 29-1: Testing Stool for Occult Blood

➤ Persons age 50 or older should be screened every 1 to 2 years for occult (hidden) blood in the stool. Some guidelines suggest annual screening. High-risk groups require initial screening at a younger age.

➤ Patients should avoid foods that may alter the accuracy of the test for 3 days before collecting the stool specimen.

➤ Review the patient's medications. If the patient is taking salicylates, NSAIDs, iron, anticoagulants, or colchicines, consult with the physician.

➤ Take care that the sample is not contaminated by urine or menstrual blood.

➤ Test two small stool samples from separate areas of the large sample.

➤ Following the manufacturer's directions, place the correct number and size of drops of developer solution into the "windows" of the opposite side on the Hemoccult slide.

➤ Record a positive result if the slide windows turn blue.

Procedure 29-2: Placing and Removing a Bedpan

➤ Determine whether the patient will need to use a regular bedpan or a fracture pan.

➤ Don clean procedure gloves.

➤ Help the patient to achieve a position on the bedpan that will be most helpful in facilitating elimination. Use a semi-Fowler's position whenever possible. Modify the position based on the patient's condition.

➤ Provide toilet tissue, clean washcloths, and towels for the patient to perform personal hygiene when elimination is complete. Assist if the patient cannot perform these tasks independently.

Procedure 29-3: Administering an Enema

➤ Generously lubricate and gently insert the rectal tube.

➤ Instill warm solution at a slow rate.

➤ For best results:

  ➤ Be sure patient is properly positioned (left lateral with knee flexed, if possible).

  ➤ Instruct her to retain the solution for 3 to 15 minutes, depending on the type of enema.

  ➤ Assist the patient in a sitting or squatting position to promote defecation.

➤ Before leaving the bedside, implement fall prevention measures that are appropriate for your patient.

➤ Use nursing judgment to modify the procedure based on the patient's mobility and ability to follow your instructions.

Procedure 29-4: Removing Stool Digitally

➤ Be aware that this procedure is both painful and embarrassing to your patient.

➤ Trim and file your fingernails so they do not extend over the ends of your fingertips.

➤ Obtain baseline vital signs, and determine whether the patient has a history of cardiac problems or other contraindications.

➤ Determine whether the procedure will be accompanied by suppository insertion or enema administration.

➤ Use only one or two gloved fingers, and remove stool in small pieces.

➤ Allow the patient periods of rest, and monitor for signs of vagal nerve stimulation.

➤ Teach the patient lifestyle changes necessary to prevent stool retention.

Procedure 29-5: Inserting a Rectal Tube

➤ A rectal tube may be used to facilitate the passage of gas for clients experiencing intestinal distention.

➤ Position the patient on his left side.

➤ Lubricate the tip of the tube; insert 10 to 12.5 cm (4 to 5 in.).

➤ Attach the collecting device to the end of the tube.

➤ Leave the tube in place for 15 to 20 minutes.

➤ Assist the patient to move about in bed; the knee-chest position is ideal if tolerated.

Procedure 29-6: Changing an Ostomy Appliance

➤ Change the pouch every 3 to 5 days, as a general rule.

➤ Empty the old pouch before removing it, if possible.

➤ Remove the wafer or pouch, pulling down from the top with one hand while holding counter-tension with the other.

➤ Assess the stoma and the peristomal skin area (e.g., for discoloration, swelling, redness, irritation, excoriation, bleeding).

➤ Use a measuring guide to determine the size of the stoma.

➤ Trace the size of the opening onto the back of the wafer, and cut the wafer opening about 2 to 3 mm ($\frac{1}{16}$ to $\frac{1}{8}$ in.) larger.

➤ Apply the new wafer with gentle pressure.

Note: Some pouches come with the wafer attached, some without. These instructions assume that the wafer is attached.

Procedure 29-7: Irrigating a Colostomy

➤ Consult with the ostomy nurse and/or physician to see if colostomy irrigation is appropriate for your patient.

➤ Determine the patient's normal bowel pattern before surgery.

➤ Prime the tubing before irrigation, using 500 to 1,000 mL, preferably 1,000 mL, of warm tap water.

Continued

Highlights of Procedures 29-1 Through 29-8—cont'd

➤ Position the patient in front of or on the toilet or bedside commode. If the patient is immobile, place her in left side-lying (Sims') position, and use a bedpan.

➤ Prepare the new appliance before removing the existing one.

➤ Examine the stoma and peristomal skin.

➤ Lubricate the cone at the end of the tubing and insert it gently.

➤ Allow approximately 30 minutes for evacuation.

➤ Remove the sleeve, and rinse, dry, and store it.

Procedure 29-8: Placing Fecal Drainage Devices

Procedure 29-8A: Applying an External Fecal Collection System

➤ Select the fecal management system appropriate for the patient.

➤ Obtain assistance as needed.

➤ Place the patient side-lying.

➤ Cleanse and dry the perineal area; clip hair as needed.

➤ Spread the buttocks and apply the device; avoid gaps and creases.

➤ Hang the drainage bag lower than the patient.

Procedure 29-8B: Inserting an Indwelling Fecal Drainage Device

➤ Select the fecal management system appropriate for the patient.

➤ Obtain assistance as needed.

➤ Place the patient left side-lying.

➤ Remove any indwelling device.

➤ Cleanse and dry the perineal area;

➤ Prepare the device according to instructions (e.g., remove residual air from the balloon).

➤ Lubricate the balloon generously with water-soluble lubricant.

➤ Spread the buttocks and gently insert the balloon end of the catheter.

➤ Inflate the device with water or saline.

➤ Remove the syringe from the inflation port; gently tug the catheter.

➤ Position the tubing, avoiding kinks; position the collection bag lower than the patient.

To explore learning resources for this chapter,

Go to DavisPlus at DavisPl.us/Wilkinson3.

Chapter Resources for Chapter 29:

    Response sheets for all learning activities

    Resources for Caregivers and Health Professionals

    Reading More About Bowel Elimination (suggested readings)

    Concept Map of chapter content

Interactive Case Studies

NCLEX-Style and Chapter Review Questions

Chapter Overview Podcasts

For references cited in this chapter,

Go to Volume 2, **References Cited.**

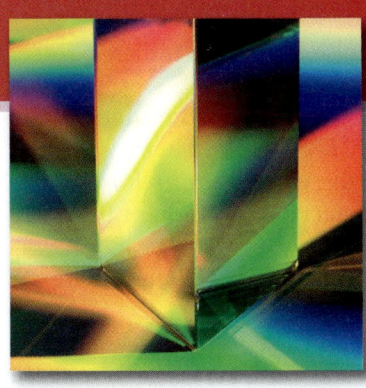

CHAPTER 30

Sensation, Perception, & Cognition

Learning Outcomes

After completing this chapter, you should be able to:

➤ Identify the components of the sensory experience.

➤ Compare and contrast sensory deprivation and sensory overload.

➤ List factors placing clients at risk for altered sensory perception.

➤ Discuss the hazards of sensory deficits in vision, hearing, taste, smell, touch, and proprioception.

➤ Identify factors that affect sensory stimulation.

➤ Assess clients for signs and symptoms of altered sensory perception.

➤ State nursing diagnoses and outcomes appropriate for clients with problems of sensory perception.

➤ Describe nursing interventions to prevent sensory deprivation and sensory overload.

➤ Describe nursing interventions for clients with sensory deficits.

➤ Discuss strategies to enhance communication with clients with sensory deficits.

Meet Your Patients

■ Joshua is a 28-year-old patient in the intensive care unit (ICU). He had a car accident 3 weeks ago and has had several surgeries to repair a fractured femur, ruptured spleen, and intracranial bleeding. He was ventilated mechanically for 10 days and has had numerous invasive procedures. The nurses report that he is very confused and has been hallucinating.

■ Richard is a 90-year-old man who has been a resident at a skilled nursing facility for 10 years. He has no visitors, never leaves his room, has no television or radio in the room, and no longer speaks. He does not respond to verbal or tactile stimulation. He lies in bed in a fetal position. When staff members try to move him, he moans and howls.

Consider how these patients are similar and how their care might overlap. It seems hard to imagine that these patients could have much in common. What similarities can you see? What differences? As you read this chapter, follow these cases and other examples illustrating the effects of altered sensory or perceptual function.

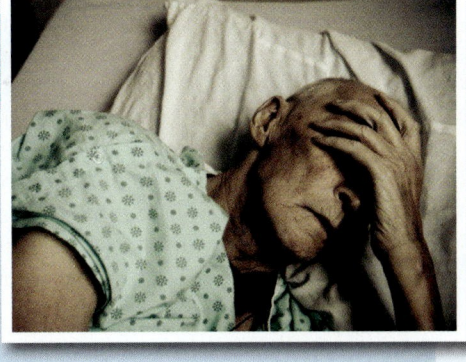

Theoretical Knowledge
knowing why

We experience the world through our senses. Vision, hearing, smell, taste, touch, and our sense of our body in space all help us to interpret and interact with our environment in a meaningful way. To grow, develop, and function, we must be able to sense and respond to sensory input.

Many patients who are being treated for one condition also have a preexisting sensory deficit (e.g., a diabetic client whom you are teaching self-injection may also be blind). Others develop alterations in sensory function as a result of their illness or of medications they are taking. The Joint Commission (2010) requires that you address the communication needs of patients with vision, speech, hearing, language, and cognitive impairments. This chapter will help you provide care for such patients.

ABOUT THE KEY CONCEPTS

Throughout your nursing career, you will care for patients with altered sensory function. To best meet their patient care needs, you will need to understand how the concepts of **sensation, reception**, and **perception** influence their sensory experience. In this section you will also learn about related concepts, including those needed to care for patients who experience sensory deprivation, overload, or deficits.

COMPONENTS OF THE SENSORY EXPERIENCE

Our senses give us information about the environment inside and outside of our bodies. The purpose of sensation is to allow the body to respond to changing situations and maintain homeostasis. A sensory experience involves four components in the nervous system: stimulus, reception, perception, and an arousal mechanism. A **stimulus** may be a sight, sound, taste, touch, pain, or anything that stimulates a nerve receptor. The brain must receive and process it to make it meaningful.

Reception

Reception is the process of receiving stimuli from nerve endings in the skin and inside the body. A receptor converts a stimulus to a nerve impulse and transmits the impulse along sensory neurons to the central nervous system (CNS). Some receptors remain activated for as long as the stimulus is applied. However, most receptors *adapt* to stimuli; that is, their response declines with time. Adaptation explains why, over time, you become unaware of an unpleasant smell or the persistent hum of an air conditioner.

Receptors usually respond to only one type of stimulus. For example, taste buds in the mouth detect sweet, sour, salty, or bitter, whereas receptors in the retina

detect light rays. The following are examples of the many types of sensory receptors in the body:

- *Mechanoreceptors* in the skin and hair follicles detect touch, pressure, and vibration.
- *Hair cells* are receptors for hearing. Located in the cochlea of the ear, they detect sound waves. In the vestibular apparatus of the ear, receptors for equilibrium and balance also detect acceleration of the body and position of the head.
- *Thermoreceptors* in the skin detect variations in temperature.
- *Proprioceptors* in the skin, muscles, tendons, ligaments, and joint capsules coordinate input to enable us to sense the position of our body in space (proprioception).
- *Photoreceptors* located in the retina of the eyes detect visible light.
- *Chemoreceptors* for taste are located in our taste buds. *Olfactory receptors* (chemoreceptors for smell) are located in the epithelium of the nasal cavity.

Perception

Perception is the ability to interpret the impulses transmitted from the receptors and give meaning to the stimuli. After the receptors generate nerve impulses, the impulses travel along neural pathways to the spinal cord and brain. They are then relayed to specialized locations in the brain where perception of the stimuli occurs (Fig. 30-1). For example, vision is perceived in the occipital lobes, hearing in the temporal lobes, and touch in the somatosensory area. Perception requires functioning of the sensory receptors, the reticular activating system, neural pathways, and brain.

Perception occurs when the person becomes aware of the stimulus and receives the information. It would not be possible to process all the stimuli that constantly bombard us. The brain discards about 99% of all sensory information as irrelevant and unimportant. For example, you are usually unaware of your clothing touching your body. However, if you focus on it, you can feel it. Perception of a stimulus is affected by several factors:

- *Location* of the receptors and pathway activated
- *Number* of receptors activated
- *Frequency* of action potentials generated (which varies according to the intensity of the stimulus)
- *Changes* in location, number, and frequency

Past experiences, knowledge, and attitude also influence perception.

Arousal Mechanism

For the central nervous system to perceive, interpret, and react to incoming stimuli, it must be active. The **reticular activating system (RAS)**, located in the brainstem, controls consciousness and alertness. The neurons of the RAS make connections between the spinal cord, cerebellum, thalamus, and cerebral cortex, relaying visual, auditory,

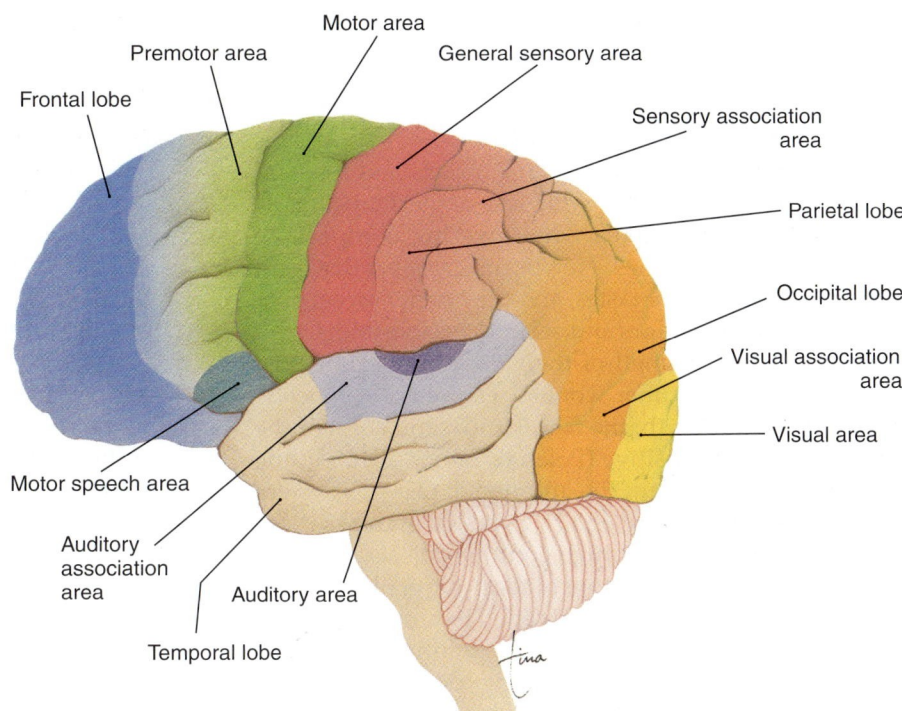

FIGURE 30-1 Special sensory areas of the brain receive and interpret stimuli from the sensory receptors. (*Source*: Scanlon, V., & Sanders, T. (2014). *Essentials of anatomy and physiology* (7th ed.). Philadelphia: F. A. Davis. Used with permission.)

and other stimuli that help keep us awake, attentive, and observant. Without such stimuli, the CNS becomes lethargic, and the person may lose consciousness. Anesthesia, sedatives, opioids, and some other drugs depress the RAS, as does a darkened, quiet environment. Not surprisingly, as you will learn in Chapter 34, sleep is regulated by the RAS.

The level of stimuli needed to maintain arousal varies: Some people feel optimally alert in bright, noisy, fast-paced environments, whereas others prefer much lower levels of stimulation. As discussed earlier, the brain adapts to constant stimuli, such as a ticking clock. Thus, to maintain arousal, some variation in stimuli is required, such as different pieces of music or an ever-changing view.

Responding to Sensations

Once a stimulus is perceived, the brain either discards it, stores it in memory, or sends impulses along motor pathways to various parts of the body (e.g., the muscles, the heart, and so on), bringing about a response. Humans respond to sensations when they are alert and receptive to stimulation. For example, a fatigued new mother may wake up to the soft cry of her infant yet sleep through the persistent ringing of the doorbell. The response to a stimulus is based on the following factors:

Intensity An intense stimulus excites more receptors, leading to a greater response. For example, a bright, glaring light can cause you to respond by squinting and shielding your eyes, whereas a dim light may cause little reaction.

Contrast Contrast is also stimulating. Imagine being outside in cold, windy weather. If you enter an unheated garage, you instantly feel warmer because the building blocks the wind. If you then go inside a room with a blazing fireplace, you will need to take off layers of clothing rapidly because the contrast in temperature will make you feel hot.

Adaptation Often we take stimuli for granted. Recall your first clinical experience. Did you notice the noise and activity on the unit? Nurses become accustomed to the noise, lights, activity, and even alarms and are able to "tune them out." These stimuli are new to many patients, so they notice them and may have difficulty resting.

Previous Experience Prior experience with a stimulus affects ongoing responses to the same stimulus. Have you ever seen a patient scrunch her eyes, grit her teeth, or turn away from an injection before you are even ready to give it? This may mean that she has memory of a prior negative experience with injections.

KnowledgeCheck 30-1

- What is the difference between reception and perception?
- What are the four components of a sensory experience?
- What is the role of the reticular activating system in the sensory experience?

FACTORS AFFECTING SENSORY FUNCTION

Among the many factors affecting sensory function are developmental stage, culture, health status, medications, stress level, personality, and lifestyle.

Developmental Variations

People have differing sensory perceptual abilities at different stages of life. In addition, the need for and use of sensory stimulation differs throughout life.

Newborns Newborns can track objects and respond to light, but their vision is far less acute than that of older children and adults. Their hearing is especially acute at low frequencies. Newborns can also discriminate between different tastes, and they prefer sweet over sour. They react to odors and seem to be able to discriminate between the smell of their own mother's breast milk and that of another woman. The sense of touch is keenly present at birth; the face, hands, and soles of the feet are the most sensitive (Polan & Taylor, 2010). In the first months of life until the autonomic nervous system matures, newborns are easily overstimulated by the loud noises, bright light, high contrast objects, and sensitive areas (back and bottom of feet), particularly when more than one sense is involved. They defend themselves from sensory overload by exhibiting avoidance behaviors, such as crying, mottling, poor feeding and sleeping, and even yawning.

Infants Infants require sensory stimulation to grow and develop normally. Tactile stimulation through cuddling, feeding, and soothing creates a bond between infant and caregivers, provides comfort and pleasure, and teaches the infant about the external environment. Exposure to voices, music, and ambient noise develops the auditory nervous system. By 1 year of age, the child can discriminate between different sounds and often recognizes the source. Lights, colors, and contrast allow the infant to observe the world in which she lives.

Children and Adolescents In early childhood, visual acuity improves; full depth perception is achieved during the preschool period. Hearing is usually fully developed in young children; however, they may experience reversible hearing loss as a result of frequent ear infections and cerumen impaction. In contrast to toddlers, who often lose their balance when walking, older children are sure and steady on their feet. During the school-age years and adolescence, children are developmentally driven toward peers, and the increased social interaction provides a wealth of sensory stimulation.

Adults and Older Adults By early adulthood, senses are at their peak, unless they are affected by illness or injury. As the adult ages, all of the senses are affected. Table 30-1 describes sensory changes associated with aging.

Table 30-1 ➤ Sensory Function Changes With Aging	
SENSE	**CHANGES ASSOCIATED WITH AGING**
Vision	The vitreous humor becomes thinner, and "floaters" appear in the visual field.
	The lens becomes discolored and opaque; the pupil becomes smaller. Therefore, less light reaches the retina, limiting vision.
	The lens becomes less flexible and less able to focus on near objects.
	The ciliary body contracts and the lens thickens, bringing loss of visual acuity, decreased ability to accommodate to distance and sudden changes in illumination, and decreased night vision.
	Peripheral vision decreases.
	Tear production decreases.
Hearing	Cerumen is drier and more solid, creating hearing loss.
	Scarring occurs (e.g., from previous inflammation over the life span).
	Hearing changes commonly include presbycusis (hearing loss of high-frequency tones) and decreased speech discrimination.
Taste	Taste buds atrophy and decrease in number, so there is less ability to perceive tastes, especially sweetness. Dry mouth may alter the sense of taste.
Smell	Atrophy and loss of olfactory neurons decreases the ability to perceive smell (which may also alter the sense of taste).
Touch	Loss of sensory nerve fibers and changes in the cerebral cortex decrease the ability to perceive light touch, pain, and temperature variations.
Kinesthesia	Kinesthetic changes include a decrease in muscle fibers and diminished conduction speed of nerve fibers, resulting in slowed reaction time, decreased speed and power of muscle contractions, and impaired balance. These place older adults at increased risk for falling.

Older adults experience a generalized decrease in the number of nerve conduction fibers, resulting in slower reflexes and delayed response to stimuli. Structural changes also occur in the aging eye and ear. Sensory decline with aging may cause withdrawal, depression, social isolation, and hallucinations. Keep in mind that aging is not the only cause of sensory deficits in older adults.

Culture

Culture affects the nature, type, and amount of interaction and stimulation that people feel comfortable with. People of different cultural backgrounds tend to prefer differing amounts of eye contact, personal space, and physical touch. Compare the day-to-day experience of an older adult living in a remote farming community to someone living in an extended family home in the center of a large city. The amount of stimulation perceived as normal would be very different for each of these people. You may think your hospitalized patient needs quiet time alone to rest. However, if he is accustomed to being surrounded by a large family, he may actually rest better in the midst of what seems like chaos to you. Also, use touch advisedly. For some people it is comforting; for others, it may be offensive.

Illness and Medications

Neurological disorders, such as multiple sclerosis, slow the transmission of nerve impulses. Diseases that affect circulation (e.g., atherosclerosis) may impair function of the sensory receptors and the brain, thereby altering perception and response. Reduced or lack of oxygen (anoxia) harms and even destroys cells, causing widespread damage to the neurologic system.

Some conditions affect specific sensory organs. For example, diabetic retinopathy is the leading cause of blindness among adults ages 20 to 74. Hypertension, too, can damage the retina of the eyes.

Physiologic injury to the brain may occur from trauma, as follows:

- *Closed head injury* (e.g., acute concussion) occurs when brain tissue is compressed from bleeding, bruising, fluid, or increased pressure inside the skull, for example after a fall.
- *Penetrating injury* occurs when a foreign object enters into the brain, resulting in damage to the brain tissue or structure.

Medications that cross the blood brain barrier affect neurologic or sensory function by damaging or killing brain cells. For example, aspirin and furosemide (Lasix) become ototoxic if taken for a long period of time and impair function of the auditory nerve. CNS depressants, such as opioid analgesics and sedatives, blunt reception and perception of stimuli.

Stress

Have you ever been under a great deal of stress? How did it feel? When you are under stress, do you find yourself looking for or avoiding stimuli? Obviously, stress provides added stimulation. As a result, a person who is bored may add stress. By setting a goal, such as running a marathon, the person undertakes a series of activities to reach that goal. In that regard, stress provides sensory stimulation at a time when the person may have been experiencing deprivation.

However, stress can cause too much stimulation. Physical illness, pain, hospitalization, tests, and surgery are all stressors that can lead to sensory overload—more stimuli than the person can handle. Jason (Meet Your Patients) has been under tremendous physical and emotional stress as a result of his injuries and surgeries. His situation is one in which you might want to limit unnecessary stimuli (e.g., noise, lights, too many visitors).

Personality and Lifestyle

Are you the kind of person who likes to have people around all the time? Do you thrive on noise and action? Or are you the kind of person who loves to curl up with a book and a cup of tea? Clients, too, vary in their personalities and lifestyles. Some people, by nature, like excitement, change, and stimulation; others prefer a more predictable and quiet life. Clients are at risk for sensory alterations if their previous level of stimuli does not match their current level. Health problems, a change of environment, or loss of a partner can each create changes in stimuli.

KnowledgeCheck 30-2

- List five major factors that affect sensory function.
- Compare and contrast the sensory changes in childhood with those in older adulthood.

SENSORY ALTERATIONS

Humans are constantly striving to achieve **sensoristasis**, a state of optimal arousal. Sensory alterations occur when the body experiences meaningless or limited stimulation (sensory deprivation), excessive stimulation (sensory overload), or sensory deficits.

Example Problem: Sensory Deprivation

Sensory deprivation is a state of RAS depression caused by a lack of meaningful stimuli. When environmental stimuli are deficient, the remaining stimuli, such as distant noises, minor pain, and cold extremities, can become overly noticeable or distorted, filling in the "sensory gap" and causing the patient a level of distress that is out of proportion to the intensity of the stimulus. Clinical manifestations include problems with perception, cognition, and emotion (Box 30-1).

PICOT

Sensory Overload in the ICU

Situation: The nurse is caring for a client with an impulse control disorder who is admitted to the ICU after sustaining traumatic injuries from motorcycle accident. The client has a history of violent outbursts; the nursing team is meeting with a psychiatric social worker to develop an appropriate plan of care.

PICOT Components

P	Population/patient	=	Hospitalized patients with impulse control disorder
I	Intervention/indicator	=	Sensory overload in ICU
C	Comparator/control	=	Patients without a psychiatric history
0	Outcome	=	Violent behavior
T	Time	=	During hospitalization

Searchable Question: Do _____ (P) who are _____ (I) demonstrate _____ (O) as compared to _____ (C) during _____ (T)

Example of Evidence: Clients with a psychiatric history who are admitted to the acute medical facility pose special challenges for the nursing staff. Priorities include ensuring safety for this client and others, including healthcare staff. Initial assessment should focus on patterns and types of violent behavior, frequency, and characteristics of targeted victims. The nurse would also assess for possible triggers to agitation. In addition to collecting the client's psychiatric and medication history, the nurse would also be alert to potential high stress situations during hospitalization, such as sensory overload, that precipitate negative behaviors.

Practice Change: Healthcare staff will modify the environment to avoid exposing clients to excess sensory stimulation.

Reference: Flannery, R. B., Jr. (2005). Precipitants to psychiatric patient assaults on staff: Review of empirical findings, 1990–2003, and risk management implications. *Psychiatric Quarterly, 76*(4), 317–326. doi:10.1007/s11126-005-4965-y

The following situations increase the risk for sensory deprivation:

- Impaired sensory reception (e.g., neurological injury, dementia, depression, sleep deprivation, sensory losses, and CNS depressant medications)
- Inability to transmit or process stimuli (e.g., nerve or brain injury)
- Restricted mobility
- Sensory deficits (e.g., vision, hearing)
- A nonstimulating, monotonous environment. Examples include children in orphanages; people in prison; homebound disabled and older people; patients in nursing homes and other institutions; and hospitalized patients in isolation, seclusion, or private rooms.
- Being from a different culture and unable to interpret received cues

Example Problem: Sensory Overload

Sensory overload develops when either environmental or internal stimuli—or a combination of both—exceed a higher level than the patient's sensory system can effectively process. This sometimes occurs in patients who, because of neurological or psychiatric disorders, are unable to adapt to continuing, nonmeaningful stimuli. Some clinical manifestations of sensory overload are similar to those of sensory deprivation (see Box 30-1).

Hospitalized patients often experience sensory overload due to a combination of physical discomfort, anxiety, separation from loved ones, and the experience of being in the unfamiliar hospital environment. Medications that stimulate the CNS may also contribute to overload, as will substances, such as caffeine. In

BOX 30-1 ■ Signs of Sensory Deprivation and Sensory Overload

Sensory Deprivation	Sensory Overload
Irritability	Irritability
Confusion	Confusion
Reduced attention span	Reduced attention span
Decreased problem-solving ability	Decreased problem-solving ability
Drowsiness	Drowsiness (due to insomnia)
Depression	Muscle tension
Preoccupation with somatic complaints (e.g., heart palpitations)	Anxiety
Delusions (misinterpretations of external stimuli)	Inability to concentrate
Hallucinations (seeing, hearing, feeling, tasting, or smelling something that is not there)	Decreased ability to perform tasks
	Restlessness
	Disorientation

addition, physical conditions that activate the CNS (e.g., hyperthyroidism, acute brain injury) contribute to sensory overload. Some mental health conditions (e.g., psychosis, sensory integration disorder, attention deficit hyperactivity disorder) are exacerbated by high intensity noise and light in the environment.

KnowledgeCheck 30-3

- How does sensory deprivation occur?
- Identify five signs of sensory deprivation.
- How does sensory overload occur?
- Identify five signs of sensory overload.

 ## ThinkLike a Nurse 30-1

Review the stories of Joshua and Richard (Meet Your Patients). How are these patients similar? What factors may have contributed to each patient's current concerns?

Example Problem: Sensory Deficits

Sensory deficits may stem from impaired reception, perception, or both. Of the six basic sensory deficits discussed here, impaired vision and hearing are the ones you are most likely to encounter in nursing practice. Drawing on your personal experience, think how many people you know who wear glasses or contact lenses or who wear a hearing aid. How many do you know whose vision or hearing is not completely corrected by such aids? You can see that sensory deficits are common.

A sudden onset of a deficit is unnerving and may lead to disorientation and anxiety. Gradual changes allow the person to adapt, often without even realizing the extent of it. The patient who has progressively lost hearing may, over time, keep turning up the sound on his radio and telephone and not realize that others find the sound blaring. When there is a deficit in one sense, the other senses may become sharper to compensate (e.g., a person who is blind may develop more acute hearing). Six sensory deficits are discussed in the following sections.

Sensory Deficit: Impaired Vision

Vision occurs when light rays that focus on the retina trigger a nerve impulse that is transmitted to the visual area of the brain in the occipital region. Visual deficits may result from trauma or disease of the eye, microvascular problems, or CNS disorders. Common causes of visual deficits include age-related changes, refractive errors, orbital trauma, cataracts, glaucoma, diabetic or hypertensive retinopathy, macular degeneration, or loss of visual fields after a stroke (Box 30-2). Changes in vision affect all aspects of daily living and may severely limit mobility and interaction.

Sensory Deficit: Impaired Hearing

Hearing occurs when sound waves entering the ear canal are converted to vibrations and transferred from

BOX 30-2 ■ Common Visual Deficits

- **Myopia**, or nearsightedness, means that the patient is able to see close objects well but not distant objects. For example, a person with 20/200 vision can see an object from 20 feet away that a person with normal sight could see from a distance of 200 feet.

- **Hyperopia**, or farsightedness, implies that the eye sees distant objects well. A person with hyperopia may have 20/10 vision—he can see an object from 20 feet that a normal eye can see from 10 feet; however, near vision is impaired.

- **Presbyopia** is a change in vision associated with aging. The lens becomes less elastic and less able to accommodate to near objects. If you're older than 40 years of age, there's a good chance you may be experiencing this problem.

- **Astigmatism** is caused by an irregular curvature of the cornea or lens that scatters light rays and blurs the image on the retina. The person has blurred vision with distortion.

- **Cataracts** are a clouding of the lens, resulting in blurred vision, sensitivity to glare, and image distortion.

- **Glaucoma** is a type of vision loss caused by increased pressure in the anterior cavity of the eyeball that distorts the shape of the cornea and shifts the position of the lens, resulting in loss of peripheral vision. It can eventually lead to blindness.

- **Macular degeneration** is the loss of central vision due to damage to the *macula lutea*, the central portion of the retina. The leading cause of visual impairment in U.S. residents older than age 50, it is characterized by slow, progressive loss of central and near vision. It is usually present in both eyes.

- **Strabismus** (crossed eyes), in which one eye deviates from a fixed image, can cause permanent vision loss.

the middle ear to the inner ear. Vibrations cause the hair cells in the cochlea to bend, generating impulses that are carried by cranial nerve VIII to the brain. The auditory area in the brain is located in the temporal lobes. The auditory area interprets the sound and allows you to determine the direction from which the noise is coming. See Chapter 22, Figure 22-5, for an illustration of the structures of the ear.

Hearing deficits may result from injury or disease in structures of the ear, the nerves, or the brain (Box 30-3). Inability to hear decreases the ability to communicate and thus hampers social interaction. It may interfere with a patient's ability to understand instructions from healthcare professionals and create a safety hazard due to inability to hear warnings.

Sensory Deficit: Impaired Taste

Taste imparts flavor and interest to food. Taste deficits may decrease the pleasure associated with eating; weight loss and malnutrition may result. Taste depends on the functioning of the taste buds on the tongue and, to a lesser extent, on the soft palate. Four types of taste

BOX 30-3 ■ Common Hearing Deficits

- **Conduction deafness** results when one of the structures that transmits vibrations is affected. It may be a temporary or permanent condition caused by infection of the middle ear, a punctured tympanic membrane, or arthritis of the auditory bones. A hearing aid may be helpful for conduction deafness.

- **Nerve deafness** occurs when there is damage to cranial nerve VIII or the receptors in the cochlea. It may result from ototoxic medications (e.g., gentamicin) or viral infections that affect cranial nerve VIII. Chronic exposure to loud noise may also lead to nerve and receptor impairment.

- **Presbycusis** is a progressive sensorineural loss associated with aging. It results from deterioration of the hair cells in the cochlea. Presbycusis leads to diminished ability to hear high-pitched sounds and to distinguish sounds in a noisy environment. Hearing aids may be of no value in sensorineural hearing loss.

- **Central deafness** results from damage to the auditory areas in the temporal lobes. Tumor, trauma, meningitis, or CVA (cerebrovascular accident, i.e., stroke) in the temporal lobe may cause this.

- **Tinnitus** is a term used to describe ringing in the ears. Most tinnitus comes from damage to the microscopic endings of the nerve in the inner ear, for example, trauma, turbulent blood flow, hypertension, ear infection, medications, otosclerosis, or arthritic changes of the bones of the ear.

- **Impacted cerumen** is a condition in which earwax becomes tightly packed in the ear canal, blocking the canal. Patients with impacted cerumen may experience a feeling of fullness or pain, decreased hearing, or tinnitus.

- **Otosclerosis** is a hardening of the bones of the middle ear, especially the stapes. The stapes becomes fixed, leading to poor sound transmission to the inner ear. The cause of this disorder is unknown.

- **Otitis media** is a middle ear infection. It is a common childhood illness that may be caused by viruses or bacteria.

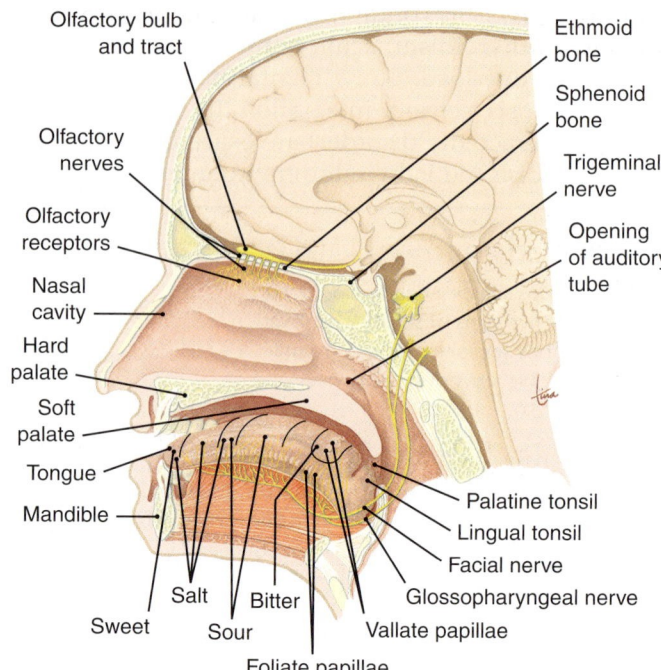

FIGURE 30-2 Structures concerned with the sense of smell and taste. (*Source:* Scanlon, V., & Sanders, T. (2014). *Essentials of anatomy and physiology* (7th ed.). Philadelphia: F. A. Davis. Used with permission.)

BOX 30-4 ■ Medications That Cause Tast Disturbance

Numerous medications can cause a foul or metallic taste. This unpleasant side effect can result from medication taken orally, IM, or IV.

- Antibiotics (metronidazole, rifampin, clarithromycin, tetracycline)
- Anticonvulsants (phenytoin and carbamazepine)
- Antihistamines and decongestants
- Antihypertensive (captopril) and cardiac medications (ACE inhibitors)
- Antiretroviral drugs (indinavir)
- Antithyroid medication
- Carbon anhydrase inhibitors, used to treat glaucoma (acetazolamide, methazolamide)
- Chemotherapy agents (procarbazine, vinblastine, vincristine, dacarbazine)
- Lithium carbonate
- Antipsychotics
- Antidepressants
- Statins
- Muscle relaxants (methocarbamol)

buds exist: sweet, sour, salty, and bitter. A proposed fifth taste bud, glutamate, can detect savory flavors. The buds for sweet and salty tastes are primarily on the tip of the tongue; for sour taste, on the two lateral sides of the tongue; and for bitter taste, primarily on the posterior tongue and the soft palate (Fig. 30-2). When stimulated, taste buds generate nerve impulses that travel along the facial and glossopharyngeal nerves (cranial nerves VII and IX, respectively) to the taste area in the parietal–temporal cortex. Foods stimulate different combinations of taste buds. That stimulation, together with the sense of smell, produces the vast number of tastes we can perceive.

Impaired taste most commonly results from **xerostomia** (excessively dry mouth), which may be caused by medications (Box 30-4), decreased saliva production, inadequate fluid intake, poor nutrition, or poor oral hygiene. Other causes of taste deficits include the common cold; infections of the nose, sinuses, mouth, or salivary glands; smoking; vitamin B_{12} or zinc deficiency; dental fillings and inlays; dementia; and injury to the mouth, nose, or head. A metallic taste in the mouth can occur during pregnancy due to hormonal fluctuations or from more serious causes such as cancer, peptic ulcer, and kidney disease.

Sensory Deficit: Impaired Smell

The sense of smell is triggered when chemoreceptors in the upper nasal cavities detect vaporized chemicals. Chemoreceptors generate impulses carried by the olfactory nerve (cranial nerve I) into the olfactory area in the temporal lobes (see Fig. 30-2). Vaporized molecules can be detected from a distance, so the sense of smell can serve as an early warning system for detection of smoke and noxious chemicals.

The sense of smell is vital to the sense of taste. Recall the last time you had a cold or nasal congestion. When the sense of smell is lost (**anosmia**), food does not taste the same. Patients who are unable to smell food lose their appetite, and nutritional deficits may result. Permanent anosmia may develop after cranial nerve damage, a tumor, or atherosclerosis. It may also be inherited and nonpathological. Zinc deficiency, heavy smoking, cocaine use, rhinitis, and sinusitis can cause reversible anosmia.

Nurses may make therapeutic use of a patient's sense of smell. **Aromatherapy**, the use of odors for therapeutic effect, has become one of the most widely practiced complementary therapies among nurses in the United States. Olfaction has been shown to play a role in memory, mood, and safety. See the box Complementary & Alternative Modalities (CAM): Essential Oils. Refer also to Chapter 42 for more information about aromatherapy.

Sensory Deficit: Impaired Tactile Perception

Touch is crucial to growth and development. It provides pleasure, warns us of injury, and transmits information about the external environment. The dermis of the skin contains receptors for the cutaneous sensations of light touch, pressure, heat, cold, and pain. Information from these receptors is transmitted to the sensory areas in the parietal lobes. The number of cutaneous receptors determines the sensitivity of an area and the amount of space devoted to that region in the sensory cortex area. The hands and face have the most receptors and therefore the largest area in the sensory cortex.

A person's ability to perceive touch is often measured in terms of *two-point discrimination*, that is, the ability to perceive as distinct two close but separate points pressed against the skin. On the lips and fingertips, a person can normally distinguish between points less than 4 mm apart, whereas on the torso, normal two-point discrimination is greater than 2 cm.

Loss of tactile sensitivity can be caused by a cerebrovascular accident (stroke), brain or spinal tumor or injury, or peripheral nerve damage caused by diabetes, Guillain-Barré syndrome, or chronic alcoholism.

Complementary & Alternative Modalities (CAM)

Essential Oils

Aromatherapy is the use of naturally extracted aromatic essences from plants to balance, harmonize, and promote the health of body, mind, and spirit. It is a natural, noninvasive treatment system designed to affect the whole person, not just the symptom or disease. Essential oils are thought to work by promoting the body's natural ability to balance, regulate, heal, and maintain itself. Some oils may be used topically in certain situations (e.g., minor burns). Beginning research supports the following; however, the evidence base is not strong.

➤ **Eucalyptus, *Eucalyptus globulus* or *Eucalyptus radiata*.** Helpful in treating respiratory problems, such as coughs, colds, and asthma. Used to treat burns, wounds, and insect bites. Also helps to boost the immune system and relieve muscle tension.

➤ **Ylang-Ylang, *Cananga odorata*.** Helps one to relax, and can reduce muscle tension. Good antidepressant. Used for anxiety, hypertension, and stress.

➤ **Geranium, *Pelargonium graveolens*.** Helps to balance hormones in women, good for balancing the skin. Can be both relaxing and uplifting, as well as antidepressant. Used for acne and oily skin.

➤ **Peppermint, *Mentha piperita*.** Used in treating headaches; sinusitis; vertigo; muscle aches; asthma; and digestive disorders such as slow digestion, indigestion, nausea, and flatulence.

➤ **Lavender, *Lavandula angustifolia*.** Relaxing, and also useful in treating wounds and burns, and for skin care. Also used for asthma, itching, labor pains, colic, and dysmenorrhea.

➤ **Lemon, *Citrus limonum*.** Uplifting, yet relaxing. Helpful in treating wounds and infections, and for house cleaning and deodorizing. Sometimes used for athlete's foot, colds, and warts.

➤ **Clary sage, *Salvia sclarea*.** Natural pain killer, helpful in treating amenorrhea and muscular aches and pains. Relaxing, and can help with insomnia. Also helpful in balancing hormones. Used to treat sore throat, stress, and exhaustion.

➤ **Tea tree, *Melaleuca alternifolia*.** A natural antifungal oil, good for treating all sorts of fungal infections including vaginal yeast infections, "jock itch," athlete's foot, and ringworm. Used for insect bites, itching, and migraine. Also helps to boost the immune system.

➤ **Roman chamomile, *Anthemis nobilis*.** Relaxing, and can help with sleeplessness and anxiety. Also good for muscle aches, arthritis, and tension. Useful in treating wounds and infection. Used for insomnia, nausea, PMS, and earache.

➤ **Rosemary, *Rosmarinus officinalis*.** Uplifting and promotes mental stimulation. Also stimulating to the immune, circulatory, and digestive systems. Good for muscle aches and tension.

ThinkLike a Nurse 30-2

- Why do you think a person with impaired tactile perception is at risk for injury?
- Speculate as to the possible nature of injuries that might occur.

Sensory Deficit: Impaired Kinesthetic Sense

Kinesthesia, or muscle sense, is a complex process involving **proprioceptors** that detect stretch in muscles to create a mental picture of how the body is positioned. Conscious muscle sense is perceived in the parietal lobes. Unconscious muscle sense occurs in the cerebellum, which coordinates movement.

Problems of the inner ear commonly impair kinesthesia. The vestibular apparatus of the inner ear has hair cells that detect rotation or acceleration of the body. Because the vestibular cell nuclei also receive input from neurons involved in vision, a mismatch between the position or acceleration of the head and the visual field can result in motion sickness. This is why it is not advisable to read a book while riding in a car traveling on a winding road.

Parkinson's disease, other neurological disorders, tumors, cerebrovascular accident, and even certain medications can impair kinesthesia. Kinesthetic deficits place the patient at risk for balance and coordination problems and falls. For activities that enhance proprioception, see the Home Care box Sensory Deficits—Safety and Health Measures, later in this chapter.

Seizures

A **seizure** is the abrupt onset of disturbance in electrical activity in the brain—a group of neurons fires abnormally. This results in motor symptoms, such as rhythmic jerking of the limbs. Symptoms and the duration of the seizure vary, depending on the area of the brain affected. In addition to motor symptoms, the person may have a decreased level of consciousness or a loss of consciousness. This places the patient at high risk for injury from falls. Half of the people newly diagnosed with a seizure disorder will have generalized seizures.

Seizures are not uncommon. Incidence is highest for those younger than age 10 or older than age 65. Males are more likely to have seizures than females, especially children. Three-quarters of children with seizures outgrow the events (Epilepsy Foundation of America, n.d.). Most seizures last less than 3 or 4 minutes.

In 7 out of 10 people with seizures, no identifiable cause can be found. Among adults, the most common cause is a tumor or head trauma. The most common reason for seizures in a person with epilepsy is failure to take prescribed antiseizure medication. Other common triggers are ingesting mood altering substances, sleep deprivation, stress, illness, fever, and hormone fluctuations. Additionally, high contrast patterns and flashing or flickering lights (e.g., video games, strobe lights) can provoke seizure activity.

 Go to Chapter 30, **Clinical Insight 30-1: Seizure Precautions**, in Volume 2.

KnowledgeCheck 30-4

- Discuss the difference between myopia and hyperopia.
- What is the difference between conduction deafness and nerve deafness?
- Identify three factors that may impair the sense of taste.
- How is the sense of smell triggered?
- What areas of the body have the greatest number of tactile receptors?
- What type of health concerns may be generated by kinesthetic deficits?

ThinkLike a Nurse 30-3

Imagine that you are experiencing sensory deficits. Which deficits would you find most challenging?

PracticalKnowledge
knowing **how**

As a nurse, you should always consider your client's sensory perceptual status. Sensory deficits, excess, and overload influence a person's safety and quality of life and may be especially troublesome for those in inpatient facilities.

 ASSESSMENT

Assessment of sensory perception includes a history and physical exam to gather data about the following (see Chapter 22):

- Factors affecting sensory perception
- Mental status, including mood, affect, cognition, and memory
- Level of consciousness
- Recent changes in sensory stimulation
- Use of sensory aids
- The client's environment
- The support network
- Focused examination of vision, hearing, taste, smell, touch, balance, ability to respond to stimulation, muscle tone, coordination

Nursing Interview In your nursing interview, you will assess the client's usual and current state of sensory function, as well as gather a history of sensory problems and use of sensory aids. In addition to interviewing the client and family, assess the environment and client situation for factors that may alter sensory function. The rest of the Assessment section provides a brief overview of each of those items.

Physical Assessment Physical assessment of sensory function requires assessment of the six senses. For guidelines,

Go to Chapter 22, **Procedure 22-16: Assessing the Sensory Neurological System, Procedure 22-6: Assessing the Eyes,** and **Procedure 22-7: Assessing the Ears and Hearing,** in Volume 2. Also refer to Chapter 30, **Assessment Guidelines and Tools, Hearing Screening in Older Adults,** in Volume 2.

For a guide to bedside physical assessment of sensory function,

 Go to Chapter 30, **Assessment Guidelines and Tools, Bedside Assessment of Sensory Function,** in Volume 2.

Assess Changes in Sensory Function

To assess changes in sensory function, you will need to obtain a history of the client's usual sensory function as well as information about the client's current status. For a list of questions you can use for this purpose,

 Go to Chapter 30, **Assessment Guidelines and Tools, Nursing History: Sensory Perceptual Status,** in Volume 2.

Assess Risk Factors for Impaired Sensory Perception

You should perform a comprehensive assessment for any patient at increased risk for sensory alterations:

- Older adults
- People who are bedbound or homebound
- Patients in intensive care units
- Those with acute or chronic brain injury, limited mobility, or known sensory deficits, especially if the change has been acute.

Routinely assess developmental level, health status, medications, stress and coping mechanisms, personality, history of head trauma, and lifestyle related to sensory alterations.

Assess Mental Status

Sensory alterations may trigger changes in mental status, and altered mental status can interfere with sensory perception. A check of mental status includes assessment of behavior, appearance, response to stimuli, speech, memory, and judgment. Normal findings include an ability to express and explain realistic thoughts with clear speech, follow directions, listen, answer questions, and recall significant past events.

You can assess many of those factors as you interact with the client. For example, if you have asked the client the questions covered in your nursing interview, you have already formed an impression about his appearance, speech, ability to express himself, and other facets of mental status. In addition, you must specifically assess the client's level of orientation. Chapter 22 presents additional discussion of mental status screening and orientation.

Assess Level of Consciousness

Level of consciousness (LOC) is one indicator of cerebral function. It includes arousal (from alert to deeply comatose) and orientation (to time, place, person, and situation). An alert client will respond to auditory stimuli. If the client does not respond, progress to tactile and then painful stimuli. Remember, however, that if your client does not speak your language he may not respond to questions or commands. The Glasgow Coma Scale is commonly used to assess LOC. It assesses eye, motor, and verbal responses. The FOUR (Full Outline of Un-Responsiveness) Scale adds brainstem reflexes and respirations. To use the Glasgow Coma Scale or the FOUR Scale for assessing level of consciousness,

 Go to Chapter 22, **Procedure 22-16: Assessing the Sensory Neurological System,** in Volume 2.

If you are not using a coma scale, document your findings specifically and objectively in your nursing notes. Be sure to assess whether the patient is alert, confused, lethargic, obtunded, stuporous, or comatose. For explanations of those states and observations to make,

 Go to Chapter 30, **Assessment Guidelines and Tools, Nursing History: Sensory Perceptual Status (section, Assess Mental Status),** in Volume 2.

Assess Use of Sensory Aids

Sensory aids are devices that assist with sensory function. They include glasses, contact lenses, hearing aids, canes, and walkers. For sample interview questions,

 Go to Chapter 30, **Assessment Guidelines and Tools, Nursing History: Sensory Perceptual Status,** in Volume 2.

Assess the Environment

The environment is an important source of stimulation. Consider how different the environment is for Joshua and Richard (Meet Your Patients). Joshua is in a crowded space with lights and noise 24 hours per day. He has had a number of invasive procedures and is most likely receiving pain medication. In contrast, Richard is in a quiet room with little exposure to light, noise, or touch. As Joshua's and Richard's situations demonstrate, a healthcare environment can have too many or too few stimuli. As part of your assessment, observe how the client is responding to the conditions of the environment.

Compare Patient's Personality and Lifestyle With the Current Environmental Situation In healthcare facilities, patients are subjected to lights, noises, and odors that cause them anxiety. They may hear others who are crying out in pain. A patient from a small family and a quiet environment may develop sensory overload by the stimulation in a hospital setting. Even someone used to a rapid-paced lifestyle may experience overload, particularly when experiencing pain, nausea, dizziness, or other symptoms of illness. In contrast, a person used to an active lifestyle may find the hospital setting intolerable (boring).

Assess the Effect of the Environment on Sensory Deficits For a patient with age-related hearing changes, the noise of the healthcare environment may make it difficult to decipher voices. A patient with visual deficits or impaired balance will often modify his home environment to improve function in the home; however, when the patient is hospitalized or moved to a long-term care facility, these aids may no longer be feasible. To assist the patient, you must determine which environmental conditions worsen sensory deficits and which help to compensate.

Assess the Support Network

For a client with a sensory deficit, his support network may serve as a buffer or a hindrance. For example, an older adult with macular degeneration has progressive loss of vision. If he lives alone, the effect of the visual loss will be quite different than if he lived with an extended family. Support persons may help the client to adapt to deficits by assuming chores that the client can no longer perform or by providing comfort to the client so he is less distressed by the sensory losses.

A support network can also be influential when clients are experiencing sensory deprivation or overload. Recall that Richard (Meet Your Patients) has no visitors. What influence do you think frequent visits by family members would have on Richard? If you say that Richard would receive more stimulation and may have less sensory deprivation, you are correct. Family members can also help clients who are confused from sensory alterations by reorienting and calming the client.

KnowledgeCheck 30-5

- Identify six areas you should assess for a client with known or suspected sensory alterations.
- What factors must be evaluated when it is known that a client uses a sensory aid?
- Identify at least two ways that you can assess vision and hearing deficits at the bedside.

 ThinkLike a Nurse 30-4

How would you assess Joshua and Richard (Meet Your Patients) for sensory alterations? You may need to review the Meet Your Patients scenario at the beginning of this chapter to answer this question.

ANALYSIS/NURSING DIAGNOSIS

NANDA International (2012) identifies the following diagnostic labels for use with sensory-perceptual problems. For definitions of the following labels,

 Go to Chapter 30, **Standardized Language, Selected NOC Outcomes and NIC Interventions for Sensory Perceptual Nursing Diagnoses,** on DavisPlus.

Acute Confusion
Chronic Confusion

Impaired Environmental Interpretation Syndrome
Impaired Memory
Risk for Peripheral Neurovascular Dysfunction
Unilateral Neglect

Disturbances and deficits in sensory perception may also be the etiology of other nursing diagnoses. Examples include the following:

Risk for Falls r/t visual impairment
Risk for Injury r/t reduced tactile sensation
Bathing Self-Care Deficit r/t kinesthetic impairment
Feeding Self-Care Deficit r/t visual impairment
Deficient Diversional Activity r/t reluctance to be in social situations because of hearing impairment
Imbalanced Nutrition: Less Than Body Requirements r/t loss of appetite secondary to impaired taste
Social isolation r/t embarrassment about Impaired Memory

PLANNING OUTCOMES/EVALUATION

For *NOC standardized outcomes* associated with sensory perception diagnoses,

 Go to Chapter 30, **Standardized Language, Selected NOC Outcomes and NIC Interventions for Sensory Perceptual Nursing Diagnoses,** in the Student Resources on DavisPlus.

Individualized goals/outcomes statements you might write for a client with Disturbed Sensory Perception include the following:

- Compensates for visual impairment by maximizing the use of touch and hearing.
- Verbalizes the importance of eating nutritious foods, despite the fact they "taste funny."
- Demonstrates proper use of her hearing aid.
- Participates in at least one unit activity daily.

As always, use the goals and outcomes you write to evaluate the client's responses to nursing interventions. The outcomes focus your data collection; comparing the new data against the outcomes allows you to determine patient progress.

PLANNING INTERVENTIONS/IMPLEMENTATION

For *NIC standardized interventions* associated with sensory perception nursing diagnoses,

 Go to Chapter 30, **Standardized Language, Selected NOC Outcomes and NIC Interventions for Sensory Perceptual Nursing Diagnoses,** on DavisPlus.

Specific nursing activities to address sensory perception problems are based on the nursing diagnosis chosen, especially on its etiology. Common nursing activities are discussed in the following sections.

Self-Care

Teaching Your Client About Sensory Perceptual Health

Vision

➤ Have regular eye examinations.

Infants and preschoolers—Screen at their routine office visits.

Young adults—Complete eye exam at least three times between the ages of 20 and 39.

At age 40—Have a baseline screening, and based on that information, the ophthalmologist will determine how frequently your eyes need to be re-examined.

 Age 65 and older—Complete eye exam every 1 to 2 years to check for cataracts and other eye conditions (American Academy of Ophthalmology, 2009).

➤ If you are at risk for eye disease, have more frequent eye exams, regardless of your age. For example, if you: (1) take steroids; (2) are of African ancestry; (3) have a family history of eye disease, diabetes, or high blood pressure; (4) or have any symptoms. Your ophthalmologist will recommend how often you should have an exam.

➤ Call your healthcare provider for prompt examination if you have eye pain, discharge, a change in vision, or bleeding.

➤ Have your prescriptions for glasses or contact lenses reviewed at each screening and updated if needed.

➤ Be sure that visual screening is done at your child's elementary school. If not, consult your pediatrician or other care provider.

➤ Work with your primary healthcare provider to control conditions such as hypertension and diabetes.

➤ If you are pregnant, obtain early and adequate prenatal care to prevent the danger of premature birth and exposure of the newborn to high-volume oxygen.

➤ Keep sharp or pointed tools (e.g., scissors) out of reach of infants, toddlers, and preschoolers.

➤ Teach children to walk carefully, tool point downward, when carrying pointed tools or other objects.

➤ Teach children to stay away from projectile activities, such as lawn mowing.

➤ Keep the child away from firearms and fireworks.

➤ Insist that your child use eye protection when playing sports such as tennis or baseball.

➤ Insist that children wear helmets when skating or riding bicycles and that teenagers wear helmets when riding motorcycles.

➤ For children who wear glasses, be sure the lenses are made of shatterproof safety glass.

Hearing

➤ Auditory screening is often performed in elementary school; however, most adults do not have their hearing screened regularly. If you work in an area with a high noise level, you should have your hearing checked regularly. Early detection may prevent hearing loss.

➤ If you are pregnant:

Obtain early prenatal care.

Avoid ototoxic drugs.

Be sure you are tested for syphilis and rubella (German measles).

Avoid anyone you suspect may have rubella.

➤ Children with frequent ear infections require evaluation to determine whether hearing loss has occurred.

 Middle and older adults may begin to experience difficulty distinguishing voices in a crowd or hearing the television or radio. These are indications of hearing loss and should be evaluated; you may need a hearing aid.

➤ Hearing loss is not a "natural part of aging."

Taste

Dental health is an important aspect of maintaining taste. Decayed teeth, gum disease, and other disorders of the mouth may affect the ability to taste. Have your teeth cleaned and examined at least yearly. You may need additional dental work to promote oral health.

Promoting Optimal Sensory Function

Optimal sensory function requires periodic health screening along with early identification and treatment of health problems. Comprehensive healthcare is the ideal approach, because sensory problems are often related to other health disorders. For example, to protect his vision, a client with hypertension needs to have periodic eye examinations and to control his blood pressure. See the Self-Care box for information to teach your clients about self-care to promote their vision and hearing. For additional information on health promotion and health screening, see Chapter 43.

Interventions for Example Problem: Sensory Deprivation

If your assessment indicates the client is at risk for sensory deprivation, include specific strategies for prevention in the nursing care plan. Be sure to communicate this information to nursing assistive personnel (NAPs) so they can participate in this aspect of care. Interventions will include (a) providing stimulation and (b) supporting the patient's ability to perceive and interpret stimuli. Ideally you will use the following as preventive actions.

Visual Stimulation For visual stimulation, help the patient with glasses to apply them whenever she is not sleeping. Make sure eyeglasses are clean and in good repair. This will allow the patient to receive available stimuli. Put artwork on the walls, furnish colorful pajamas and robes, and place pictures or flowers where the patient can see them. Unless the patient objects, open curtains during the daytime to allow sunlight to enter the room. Avoid keeping the patient in a dark room, except to promote sleep.

Auditory Stimulation To stimulate hearing, help the patient with a hearing aid to apply it whenever she is not sleeping. Check that the hearing aid has working batteries and the sound is set at the appropriate level. When possible, move the patient to a quiet area to avoid background noise when communicating.

Olfactory Stimulation Stimulate the sense of smell with fruits and flowers, or even aromatherapy. Pleasant smells may also stimulate appetite.

Tactile Stimulation Use touch carefully in your patient care activities. You may want to hold a patient's hand while talking or provide a back rub with morning and bedtime care. Gentle hand massage is sometimes effective in calming agitated patients. Another form of touch, called healing touch, using the patient's energy fields has the potential to aid in pain control and facilitate self-healing (Harwick, Pulido, & Adelson, 2012). However, people do respond differently to being touched, so adjust the amount of touch you provide according to the patient's reaction.

Audiovisual Media A television or radio in the room may provide meaningful stimulation. Teach NAPs to choose appropriate music and programs for the patient. Inappropriate choices (e.g., cartoons with laugh tracks) offer meaningless stimulation and may lead to sensory deprivation.

Social Interaction Social interaction is a type of stimulus. The following are some social interaction measures:

- Make regular contact with the patient. Introduce yourself, and address the patient by name.
- Provide continuity of care by assigning the same personnel whenever possible.
- Encourage patients to have some form of social interaction. For example, urge long-term care patients to take part in scheduled activities. Assist acute care patients out of bed for meals or visits from family and friends. Advise staff members to visit at intervals or encourage patients to leave their rooms. Children may play video games with others online.
- Avoid isolating the patient when at all possible. Ensure that any patient in isolation receives adequate stimulation from nurses, family members, or assistive personnel.

Minimizing Anxiety and Confusion Minimize anxiety and confusion so the patient can accurately perceive stimuli. For example:

- Explain all procedures and care. This will decrease anxiety and help orient confused clients.

- Hang a calendar in the room, along with a schedule of activities.
- A large clock on the wall is also helpful.
- Encourage family members to bring in familiar objects from home.
- If the patient is disoriented, provide information at each visit. For example, "Good morning, Mr. Booker. My name is Elsa. I am the nurse taking care of you this morning. It is a few minutes after 8 in the morning. I'm going to take your blood pressure and get you ready for breakfast."

Communication Develop alternative methods of communication when interacting with clients with aphasia, or who speak another language, or who have difficulty hearing. Communication boards, a magic slate, pictures, or writing may be helpful. You might also hang a message board in the room and ask family members to post photos, cards, or notes. Computers are useful if the patient has one; and texting might also be used.

Pet Therapy Consider using pet therapy. Many facilities have resident pets or can arrange to have pets visit. A singing bird may delight a resident who cannot be out of bed. In long-term care facilities, resident cats often favor bedbound clients for their frequent naps. Pet therapy can increase socialization, lower blood pressure, and decrease loneliness and pain (Braun, Stangler, Narveson, et al., 2009).

Collaboration Collaborate with other healthcare team members in caring for clients with sensory deprivation. Music therapy, activities, physical therapy, speech therapy, nutritional therapy, and occupational therapy may all be valuable in the care of the client. Carefully monitor the use of sedating medications that may contribute to sensory deprivation.

Self-Stimulation Finally, when they are able, teach patients to provide their own stimulation by counting, singing, reading, playing video games, social networking, or reciting poetry.

 Think Like a Nurse 30-5

Which of the strategies to treat sensory deprivation would be most appropriate for Richard (Meet Your Patients)?

Interventions for Example Problem: Sensory Overload

Sensory overload is sometimes an unfortunate outcome of hospitalization. To prevent or treat sensory overload, consider the following strategies. Oddly, some of the interventions are the same as those for preventing sensory deprivation.

- **Control visual stimuli.** Minimize unnecessary light. Instruct NAPs to be aware of appropriate light levels, especially at night. Use a flashlight instead of turning on room lights, for example.

■ **Control auditory stimuli.** Minimize unnecessary noise. Instruct NAPs to be aware of appropriate noise and light levels, especially at night. Speak in a moderate tone of voice, using a calm and confident manner. Do not speak about the client to others in his presence, even when he seems unresponsive. Consider the use of earplugs for the client.

■ **Control olfactory stimuli.** Reduce noxious odors by promptly emptying commodes and bedpans, removing meal trays, using deodorant sprays, and keeping wounds covered.

■ **Control tactile stimuli.** Some patients are overly sensitive to touch, though. In those instances, you must minimize irritating stimuli.

■ **Use radio and TV appropriately.** Choose programs to meet the client's interests. Do not leave the TV or radio on 24 hours a day.

■ **Minimize stress.** Stressors create internal stimuli such as anxiety. Observe for the client's reaction to environmental stimuli. Remove annoying or bothersome stimuli if possible.

Introduce yourself when meeting the client and address him by name.

Provide a calm presence; for example, do not hurry with care or speak rapidly.

If possible, provide a private room and limit visitors. Reduce unessential tasks by other health team members.

Control pain and nausea with ordered medications.

Teach clients about stress reduction techniques.

Provide relaxing music that promotes visualization and deep-breathing techniques.

■ **Promote adequate sleep and rest.** Establish a schedule for care that allows for uninterrupted periods of sleep and rest. Besides preventing interruptions during rest periods, a schedule will provide the client with advance notice of what to expect during the day. Instruct NAPs and family members on the importance of allowing the client adequate rest and the need to avoid interruptions.

 Think**Like a Nurse** 30-6

Review the scenario of Joshua, the young ICU patient with sensory overload (Meet Your Patients).

■ Which strategies to prevent sensory overload would be most appropriate for an ICU patient?

■ Which would be least likely to be successful or not feasible based on the setting?

Provide rationale for your choices. You may need to visit an ICU or talk with classmates who have been to an ICU to answer this question.

Interventions for Example Problem: Sensory Deficits

Recall that in addition to sensory deprivation and sensory overload, many clients have sensory deficits. The Joint Commission (2010) requires that you address the communication needs of patients with vision, speech, hearing, language, and cognitive impairments. Regardless of the primary medical diagnosis, you may need to modify your approach to the client or alter the environment. Describe the sensory deficits on the nursing care plan, along with strategies to deal with them. For example, if the patient recovering from an abdominal surgery has no vision in his left eye, nursing orders should specify to approach the patient from the right.

Interventions for Visual Deficits

Visual deficits range from minor problems requiring corrective lenses to complete blindness. Surgical procedures of the eye may cause temporary visual problems. Problems that limit movement of the head may limit peripheral vision but have no effect on central vision. To provide care for the client with visual deficits, you will need to describe fully the scope of the deficit on the care plan. For the client with sight, your interventions focus on enhancing vision.

■ Make sure eyeglasses are clean, in good repair, and of the proper prescription. Place them within easy reach or help the client put them on if necessary.

■ Offer a magnifying lens or large-print books and magazines for clients with presbyopia.

■ Provide enough light, but avoid glare: (1) Use soft, diffuse lighting; (2) provide sunglasses, visors, or hats with brims when the client is outdoors.

■ For information on caring for contact lenses, see Chapter 25, and

 Go to Chapter 25, **Procedure 25-12: Removing and Caring for Contact Lenses,** in Volume 2.

For clients with severely limited vision:

■ Be sure that all staff are aware of the client's limited vision.

■ Provide an uncluttered environment, and do not rearrange furniture.

■ Place the call bell, phone, and self-care items within easy reach.

■ Consider books on tape or Braille for the client.

■ Keep the bed in a low position.

■ When helping the client walk, ask which side she prefers to have you on. Offer her your arm and allow her to grasp it.

■ For safety measures, see Home Care: Sensory Deficits—Safety and Health Measures.

■ If a visually impaired client uses a guide dog, do not distract the dog. A guide dog in a harness is working and should be approached only with the owner's permission.

To learn about communicating with visually impaired clients,

 Go to Chapter 30, **Clinical Insight 30-2: Communicating With Visually Impaired Clients,** in Volume 2.

Interventions for Hearing Deficits

A hearing impairment can limit communication and place the client at risk for social isolation. In addition, clients with impaired hearing are unable to receive warnings. This places them at risk for injury (e.g., they may not hear a fire alarm). Your interventions should focus on supporting auditory function, improving communication, and creating a safer environment.

Support Auditory Function If the client has a hearing aid, check to make sure that it is working, the batteries are functional, and the sound is adjusted to a comfortable level. Encourage your client to wear her hearing aid as much as possible. A significant number of people with hearing impairment do not wear hearing aids. To review care of a hearing aid,

 Go to Chapter 25, **Procedure 25-16: Caring for Hearing Aids,** in Volume 2.

Inspect ear canals for cerumen impaction, a common cause of conduction hearing loss. For key information about otic irrigation, see the Highlights of Procedure 30-1 box and,

 Go to Chapter 30, **Procedure 30-1: Performing Otic Irrigation,** in Volume 2.

Other support measures include closed-caption television, which allows the client to read the dialogue and continue to enjoy his favorite shows or stay current with the news. For telephones, the client might want to consider sound amplification or conversion to text-telephone service. Finally, some clients may also be candidates for hearing aid dog service.

Adapt and Improve Communication For a client with hearing impairment, provide written instructions to ensure that she understands the teaching and instructions.

For additional suggestions for communicating with hearing-impaired persons,

 Go to Chapter 30, **Clinical Insight 30-3: Communicating With Hearing-Impaired Clients,** in Volume 2.

Promote Safety ✚ Suggest that your client modify the home environment. For example, install blinking lights that alert the person to an incoming phone call or the ring of a doorbell. Blinking alarm clocks, burglar alarms, and smoke detectors are also available. Also refer to the accompanying Home Care box Sensory Deficits—Safety and Health Measures. For institutionalized patients, keep background noise to a minimum, and keep a call bell within easy reach of the patient.

KnowledgeCheck 30-6

- Identify three safety measures that may be used with clients with visual impairment.
- Identify three safety measures that may be used with clients with hearing impairment.

Interventions for Olfactory Deficits

An impaired sense of smell diminishes taste and denies the client the pleasure of enjoying food. This often leads to weight loss. Home safety issues are also a concern for the client who cannot smell. Measures to protect the client with olfactory impairment are found in the Home Care box Sensory Deficits—Safety and Health Measures.

Interventions for Gustatory Deficits

Many people find great pleasure from the different tastes of food. Without the gustatory sense, a client may eat less and be at risk for nutritional deficits and weight loss. If the client has lost weight, be sure to check the fit of any dentures or dental appliances. Weight changes may affect their fit and make it even harder to eat.

For hospitalized clients, provide frequent oral hygiene. Assess for sores or open areas in the mouth. These require prompt treatment because they may become infected and further damage the sense of taste. Teach clients to eat foods separately or drink water between bites to distinguish the taste of the food more readily. Seasonings, salt substitutes, spices, or lemon may improve the taste of foods and encourage the client's appetite (see the Home Care box Sensory Deficits—Safety and Health Measures).

Interventions for Tactile Deficits

Patients with peripheral vascular disease, spinal cord injury, diabetes, cerebrovascular accident, trauma, or fractures are at risk for diminished tactile sensation. They may not notice a cut or wound in an area with limited sensation. For institutionalized patients, inspect the affected area daily and teach the patient to continue this practice at home. Look for open areas, cuts, abrasions, or areas of erythema. Any of these findings requires care.

Highlights of Procedure 30-1

Procedure 30-1: Otic Irrigation

➤ Warm the irrigating solution to body temperature.

➤ Assist the patient into a sitting or lying position, with the head tilted slightly toward the affected ear.

➤ Straighten the ear canal by pulling up and back on the pinna. For a young child, pull down and back to straighten the canal.

➤ Instruct the patient to notify you if he experiences any pain or dizziness during the irrigation.

➤ Place the tip of the nozzle (or syringe) into the entrance of the ear canal, and direct the stream of irrigating solution gently along the top of the ear canal toward the back of the client's head.

➤ Continue irrigating until the canal is clean.

➤ Perform an otoscopic examination.

➤ Place a cotton ball loosely in the outer ear.

Home Care

Sensory Deficits—Safety and Health Measures

To promote safety and health, instruct clients on the following points:

Visual Deficits

➤ Do not use throw or area rugs on any floors.

➤ Keep spaces uncluttered.

➤ Orient the client to new surroundings, for example, "The couch is directly ahead 3 feet. There is a table next to it."

➤ Do not rearrange furniture.

➤ Keep the bed in a low position.

➤ Clients with significant visual impairment should be evaluated for the ability to drive. Many people resist giving up driving privileges, because this severely limits their lifestyle. However, poor vision places the driver, passengers, pedestrians, and other drivers at risk for harm.

Hearing Deficits

➤ Install blinking lights that alert the person to an incoming call or the ring of a doorbell.

➤ Install blinking alarm clocks, burglar alarms, and smoke detectors.

Olfactory Deficits

➤ Have gas appliances regularly inspected and maintained to prevent gas leaks.

➤ Check smoke detectors and replace batteries regularly.

➤ If you cannot detect food spoilage by smell or taste, date foods and inspect them for any evidence of spoilage. Spoilage usually causes changes in the color and consistency of canned, fresh, or leftover foods.

Gustatory Deficits

➤ Perform frequent oral hygiene to encourage appetite and enhance the sense of taste.

➤ Enhance the meal experience by concentrating on the visual appeal of the meal, the plates, and the dinner table.

➤ Avoid bland, overcooked food. Use spices liberally unless they are contraindicated.

➤ Vary food texture, color, and temperature to provide more interest.

Tactile Deficits

➤ Use a bath thermometer to monitor water temperature and prevent burns.

➤ Change position frequently to relieve pressure on bony prominences.

➤ Use properly fitting shoes and socks.

➤ Immediately report any signs of circulatory impairment (e.g., declining motor function, cool temperature, gray-blue coloration).

➤ Inspect daily for open areas, cuts, abrasions, or areas of redness.

Kinesthetic Deficits

Kinesthesia, or muscle sense, is enhanced by activities that tone muscles and increase coordination. These activities are helpful for individuals of any age. Examples include the following:

➤ Rhythmic movement (e.g., t'ai chi, dance, yoga)

➤ Aerobic activities, such as walking, running, or bicycling

➤ Strength training, such as weight-bearing exercise or use of light weights

➤ Flexibility activities, such as stretching

➤ Balance conditioning with eyes open and closed (e.g., standing on one foot)

➤ Putting joints through full range of motion, especially rotational movements

---

Also see the Home Care box Sensory Deficits—Safety and Health Measures.

If the patient consents, you can stimulate the sense of touch by brushing his hair, giving a back rub, or touching him when giving care. You may need to use firm pressure for him to feel the touch. Frequent turning and positioning may also help. Use a bed cradle, and keep bed linens loose to keep them off the skin as much as possible.

Although traditionally we have thought of touch as a caring and healing intervention, there is actually not a lot of empirical evidence that supports its use as a nursing intervention. Furthermore, there are wide differences in how touch is perceived among both patients and nurses. Use touch carefully, considering personal and cultural preferences, observing the patient's reaction, until research evidence provides clear guidelines for practice (Gleeson & Higgins, 2009; Gleeson & Timmins, 2005).

Interventions for Confused Clients

Confusion interferes with the ability to interpret stimuli accurately. It can be temporary or permanent. Confusion is an aspect of both delirium and dementia. **Delirium** is an acute, reversible state of confusion caused by medications and a variety of physiological processes, such as hypoxia, metabolic disturbances, infection, or sensory alterations. It may be accompanied by changes in the level of consciousness. In contrast, **dementia** is a chronic and progressive deterioration in mental function caused by physical changes in the brain and is not associated with changing levels of consciousness.

To promote patient orientation, use simple communication, decrease anxiety, keep the patient safe, and provide continuity of care. Notice that some of the following interventions are the same as for preventing sensory deficit.

Toward Evidence-Based Practice

Iwamoto, Y., & Hoshiyama, M. (2012, September). Time orientation during the day in the elderly with dementia. *Physical & Occupational Therapy in Geriatrics,* 30(3), 202–13. doi:10.3109/02703181.2012.713453

Researchers were interested to find out what time of day elderly patients with dementia were most lucid. Using the Mini-Mental State Examination (MMSE) and a time estimation test, they learned that time orientation was affected more in the morning than in the afternoon. Meals did not have an effect on orientation to time.

O'Keeffe, E., Mukhtar, O., & O'Keeffe, S. (2010). Orientation to time as a guide to the presence and severity of cognitive impairment in older hospital patients. *Journal of Neurology and Neurosurgical Psychiatry,* 82, 500–504. doi:10.1136/jnnp.2010.214817

Assessing orientation to time is an important part of the mental status exam. Researchers assessed a sample of 262 patients with dementia or delirium to learn what part of the time orientation is most indicative of cognitive functioning. Failure to correctly identify either the year or month was a highly sensitive measure for detecting cognitive impairment. The severity of disorientation to time was strongly associated with the severity of dementia.

1. According to the Iwamoto and Hoshiyama study about time orientation in elderly with dementia, what would the best of time of the day be for performing nursing care that requires cooperation?

2. What would the best of time of the day be for providing orientation to an elderly client with dementia?

3. Suppose you are working in a skilled nursing facility and do not know the residents yet. If you have only a brief opportunity to interact with an elderly patient, what questions might you ask to get a sense of the severity of dementia or delirium prior to planning care?

4. Other than orientation to time, what other questions might you ask the resident to assess cognitive functioning?

Go to Chapter Resources: Chapter 30; **Toward Evidence-Based Practice Suggested Responses,** on Davis*Plus.*

Promote Orientation Introduce yourself and state the client's name each time you meet with him. Wear a readable (large, plain type) nametag to reinforce your introduction. Also identify the day, date, and time as you interact. Provide visual clues to time, such as opening the drapes during the day and closing them at night, and placing calendars and clocks where they are easy to see. Also place personal objects, photos, and mementos in the immediate environment, and discuss them with the client. Encourage the patient to participate in familiar activities, such as bathing.

Simplify Your Communications The patient cannot interpret stimuli accurately and may not understand what you say. Speak slowly and allow adequate time for the client to answer any questions you raise. Face the client and speak calmly, simply, and directly. Provide simple explanations for all care and treatments. Use short sentences with few words: "It's bath time," rather than, "Let's go have a bath and get you all nice and clean for visitors." Do not offer too many choices because this further confuses the already confused patient.

Relieve Anxiety People with dementia (a common cause of confusion) are often anxious, worried, and fearful. Find ways to make the person feel more secure and comfortable before you focus on the content of your conversations.

- Gently hold or pat the patient's hand, but use touch cautiously.
- Realize that the person is probably distressed and is doing the best he can. Be affectionate, reassuring, and calm, even when things make no sense.

- Try to respond to the person's feelings instead of the content of his words. This helps to reassure her. For example, if a woman is constantly searching for her husband, don't say, "Your husband is not here." Rather, say, "You must miss your husband," or "Tell me about your husband."
- If the person has difficulty finding the right word, supply it for him unless it upsets him. This helps control his frustration.
- If you do not understand what the patient is trying to say, ask him to point to it or describe it (e.g., "What does a zishmer look like?").
- Consider using alternative therapy, such as music therapy.

Provide for Safety Recognize that the client's decision making may be poor. Maintain a safe environment. For example, store medications away from the patient's reach, keep doors and windows closed securely, and use bed or chair monitors to prevent wandering.

Provide Continuity of Care When Possible It helps to establish a routine for care and assign the same caregivers each day.

Knowledge Check 30-7

- What are the major concerns associated with loss of smell and taste?
- What safety measures should be taught to a client with tactile impairment?
- How can you best assist a client who is confused?

Interventions for Unconscious Patients

The unconscious patient requires reality orientation even though he is unable to interact with you. In addition to some of the preceding suggestions, you should include the patient's support persons in the care. Teach them the necessary strategies. You can also usually incorporate more touch into the plan of care.

 Safety measures are a priority for unconscious patients. Keep the bed in low position when you are not at the bedside, and keep the siderails up. If the patient's blink reflex is absent or her eyes do not close totally, you may need to give frequent eye care to keep secretions from collecting along the lid margins. The eyes may be patched to prevent corneal drying, and lubricating eye drops may be necessary. Oral care is also important because the unconscious patient does not take fluids by mouth.

Interventions for Patients at Risk for Seizures

 You need to take measures to protect patients who are at risk for seizures. Pad the head, foot, and siderails of the bed and place oral suction at the bedside. If a seizure occurs, you may need to perform suctioning after the episode to prevent aspiration of oral secretions. Do not attempt to open the mouth and insert a padded tongue depressor. This can result in airway obstruction by pushing the tongue back into the pharynx. When anxious, the first responder also could break teeth trying to insert the depressor.

For a more comprehensive discussion of nursing care for patients with a seizure disorder,

 Go to Chapter 30, **Clinical Insight 30-1: Seizure Precautions,** in Volume 2.

 ThinkLike a Nurse 30-7

 What types of interventions would be most appropriate for Joshua and Richard (Meet Your Patients)—that is, interventions for sensory deficits, sensory deprivation, sensory overload, or confusion?

 To explore learning resources for this chapter,

 Go to Davis*Plus* at **DavisPl.us/Wilkinson3.**

Chapter Resources for Chapter 30:
  Response sheets for all learning activities
  Resources for Caregivers and Health Professionals
  Reading More About Sensation, Perception, & Cognition (suggested readings)
  Concept Map of chapter content
Interactive Case Studies
NCLEX-Style and Chapter Review Questions
Chapter Overview Podcasts

For references cited in this chapter,

 Go to Volume 2, **References Cited.**

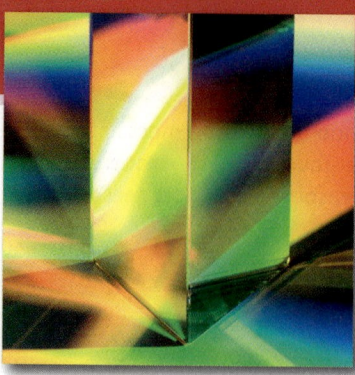

CHAPTER 31

Pain

Learning Outcomes

After completing this chapter, you should be able to:

- Define *pain*.
- Classify pain according to origin, cause, duration, and quality.
- Describe the physiological changes that occur with pain.
- Discuss two physiological mechanisms involved in pain modulation.
- Discuss factors that influence pain.
- Identify the effect of unrelieved pain on each of the body systems.
- Discuss nonpharmacological pain relief measures.
- Describe pharmacological measures, including nonopioid analgesics, opioid analgesics, and adjuvant analgesics.
- Describe chemical and surgical pain relief measures.
- Explain why pain should be considered the fifth vital sign.
- Identify the steps involved in creating a pain management program for a client.
- Individualize goals and interventions for clients with a nursing diagnosis of Acute Pain.
- Individualize goals and interventions for clients with a nursing diagnosis of Chronic Pain.
- Explain how to use a patient-controlled analgesia (PCA) system.
- Describe a method for evaluating a pain management program.

Key Concepts

Pain
Pain management

Related Concepts

See the Concept Map on Davis*Plus*.

Meet Your Patient

As a special experience, your instructor has arranged for you to spend a half-day in the intensive care unit (ICU). As you enter the ICU, you are a little apprehensive. Your patient today is a 23-year-old Asian woman who was in an automobile accident yesterday and sustained chest and abdominal injuries. You walk into the room with your clinical instructor to meet your patient, Ms. Eunice Chu Ling. She was taken to the operating room during the night to have her spleen removed. She is intubated (meaning she has an endotracheal tube in her airway that is connected to a ventilator), has an intravenous line running, and a chest tube on the left side that is draining bloody fluid. Her parents and siblings are in the room sitting rigidly in the chairs, smiling at you. Ms. Chu Ling is awake and grimacing. You want to ask her if is she is in pain, but she cannot speak.

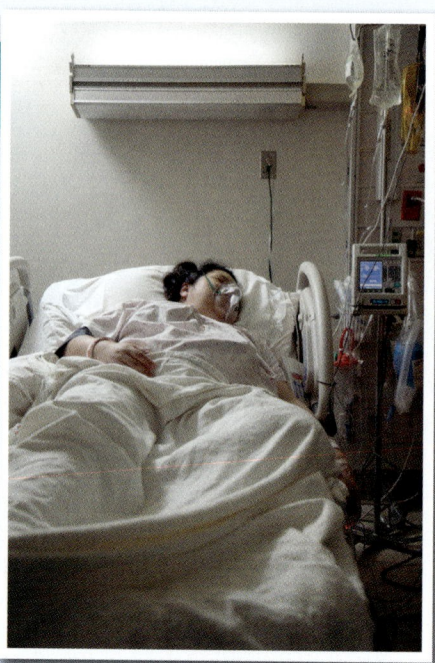

ABOUT THE KEY CONCEPTS

In this chapter, you will begin to understand the key concept of pain. Related concepts, such as transduction, transmission, perception, and modulation will help you to know what pain is and why it occurs; how to better assess it; and how to manage patients' experience of acute and chronic pain (acute and chronic pain are also related concepts you will learn in the chapter).

Theoretical Knowledge
knowing **why**

Pain is one of the most distressing symptoms nurses deal with, and it is the most frequent reason people seek medical attention (American Academy of Pain Management, 2005, updated 2011). Most of the top 10 causes of death, such as heart disease, cancer, and chronic lower respiratory diseases, are associated with pain. As more people age and experience these chronic illnesses, you are likely to encounter more patients in pain. The following are some facts about the incidence of pain:

- More than 1 in 4 American adults experience pain lasting more than 24 hours.
- About 100 million American adults—more than the total affected by heart disease, cancer and diabetes combined—are affected by chronic pain (Institute of Medicine, 2011)
   - About one-fourth to half of community-dwelling older adults report pain that interferes with normal functioning.
- An estimated 1 in 5 adults experiences pain or physical discomfort that disrupts sleep a few nights a week or more.
- In spite of measures to relieve pain, 50 percent to 75 percent of hospitalized patients die in moderate to severe pain.
- Non-Hispanic white adults reported pain more often than adults of other races. Women and men reported pain at about the same frequency.
- The most commonly reported types of pain are headaches, facial aches, joint pain, and lower back, neck pain.

WHAT IS PAIN?

The International Association for the Study of Pain (IASP) and the American Pain Society (APS) define pain as "an unpleasant sensory and emotional experience association with actual or potential tissue damage, or described in terms of such damage" (APS, 1994, p. 16; Merskey & Bogduk, 1994, p. 971). Pain is the most common reason people seek medical care in the United States. The pain experience can significantly interfere with a person's quality of life, affecting nearly every aspect of life. For instance, severe back pain can affect a patient's job performance, engagement in social activities, sexual intimacy, sleep and rest, ability to exercise, and ability to perform activities of daily living. These factors, in turn, can affect the intensity of the patient's pain, as well as his response to pain.

Margo McCaffery, a nursing expert on pain, describes pain as "whatever the person says it is, and existing whenever the person says it does" (1968, p. 95). In other words, pain is a subjective experience. Unlike a pulse or blood pressure, you cannot measure pain objectively. In addition, your expectations of your patients' pain will be influenced by your own values, ideals, and life experiences. As McCaffery's definition indicates, you will need to put aside your personal beliefs about pain and focus on the *patient's* experience.

Pain can cause sleep loss, irritability, cognitive impairment, functional impairment, and immobility, and thus it can be destructive to the patient and family. Although we usually think of pain in this negative context, pain is also protective, warning us of potential injury to the body. Recall the last time you touched a hot object with your bare hand. Undoubtedly, you quickly pulled your hand away when you felt discomfort. Without the ability to sense pain, you might have been burned. Pain can also prompt us to change our actions: After you have been sitting at the computer for a while, muscle pain may prompt you to get up and stretch or go out for a walk; or the gastrointestinal discomfort we experience after overeating may remind us to eat more moderately in the future.

You will be able to manage pain more effectively if you can recognize the type of pain the patient is experiencing. But remember that patients often experience more than one kind of pain. Pain can be classified by the origin of pain, cause, duration, and quality of pain.

Origin of Pain

The origin of pain refers to the site where pain is felt, and not necessarily the source of pain.

Cutaneous or **superficial pain** arises in the skin or the subcutaneous tissue. If you have ever touched a hot object or received a paper cut, you have experienced superficial pain. Although the injury is superficial, it may cause significant short-term pain.

Visceral pain is caused by the stimulation of deep internal pain receptors. It is most often experienced in the abdominal cavity, cranium, or thorax. Visceral pain is not well localized and can be described as tight, pressure, or crampy pain. The description of the quality and extent of the pain often serves as a strong clue to the cause. Menstrual cramps, labor pain, gastrointestinal infections, bowel disorders, and organ cancers all produce visceral pain.

Deep somatic pain originates in the ligaments, tendons, nerves, blood vessels, and bones. Deep somatic pain is localized and can be described as achy or tender. A fracture or sprain, arthritis, and bone cancer can cause deep somatic pain.

Radiating pain starts at the origin but extends to other locations. For instance, the pain of a severe sore throat may extend to the ears and head. Or the pain of an episode of gastroesophageal reflux ("heartburn") may radiate outward from the sternum to involve the entire upper thorax.

Referred pain occurs in an area that is distant from the original site. For example, the pain from a heart attack may be experienced down the left arm, through the back, or into the jaw. See Figure 31-1 for other examples of referred pain.

Phantom pain is pain that is perceived to originate from an area that has been surgically removed. Patients with amputated limbs may still perceive that the limb exists and experience burning, itching, and deep pain in that area.

Psychogenic pain refers to pain that is believed to arise from the mind. The patient perceives the pain despite the fact that no physical cause can be identified. Psychogenic pain can be just as severe as pain from a physical cause. See the discussion of somatoform pain disorder in Chapter 12, if you would like more information.

Cause of Pain

Physical pain is either nociceptive or neuropathic. These two types of pain differ in the way they affect the patient as well as in how they are treated.

Nociceptive pain is the most common type of pain experienced. It occurs when pain receptors, which are called **nociceptors**, respond to stimuli that are potentially damaging, for example, as a result of noxious thermal, chemical, or mechanical stimuli. Nociceptive pain may occur as a result of trauma, surgery, or inflammation. It is most commonly described as aching. Two types of nociceptive pain are:

- Visceral pain (i.e., pain originating from internal organs)
- Somatic pain (i.e., pain originating from the skin, muscles, bones, or connective tissue)

Neuropathic pain is a complex and often chronic pain that arises when injury to one or more nerves results in repeated transmission of pain signals even in the absence of painful stimuli. The nerve injury may originate from any of a variety of conditions, such as poorly controlled diabetes, a stroke, a tumor, alcoholism, amputation, or a viral infection (e.g., shingles or HIV/AIDS). Some medications, such as chemotherapeutic agents, can trigger nerve injuries that may cause neuropathic pain even after the medication is discontinued. Neuropathic pain is described as burning, numbness, itching, and "pins and needles" prickling pain.

Duration of Pain

Acute pain has a short duration and is generally rapid in onset. It varies in intensity and may last up to 6 months (American Pain Society, 2006). This type of pain is most frequently associated with injury or surgery. It is protective in that it indicates potential or actual tissue damage. Although acute pain may absorb a patient's physical and emotional energy for a short time, it is helpful for the patient to know that it will generally disappear as the tissues heal.

Chronic pain is pain that has lasted 6 months or longer and often interferes with daily activities. It can be related to a progressive disorder, or it can occur when there is no current tissue injury, as in neuropathic pain. Patients with chronic pain may experience periods of remission and exacerbation. Unlike acute pain, chronic pain is often viewed as insignificant and may lead to withdrawal, depression, anger, frustration, and dependence. Next to incurability, chronic pain is the most feared aspect of contracting cancer or other progressive diseases.

Intractable pain is both chronic and highly resistant to relief. This type of pain is especially frustrating for the patient and care provider. It should be approached with multiple methods of pain relief.

Quality of Pain

The words patients use to describe the quality of their pain help care providers to determine the probable cause and most effective treatment. Patients may describe pain quality with a variety of adjectives, such as *sharp* or *dull, aching, throbbing, stabbing, burning, ripping, searing,* or *tingling*. They may refer to its periodicity as *episodic, intermittent,* or *constant*. Patients also use a variety of terms to convey the intensity of their pain, such as *mild, distracting, moderate, severe,* or *intolerable*.

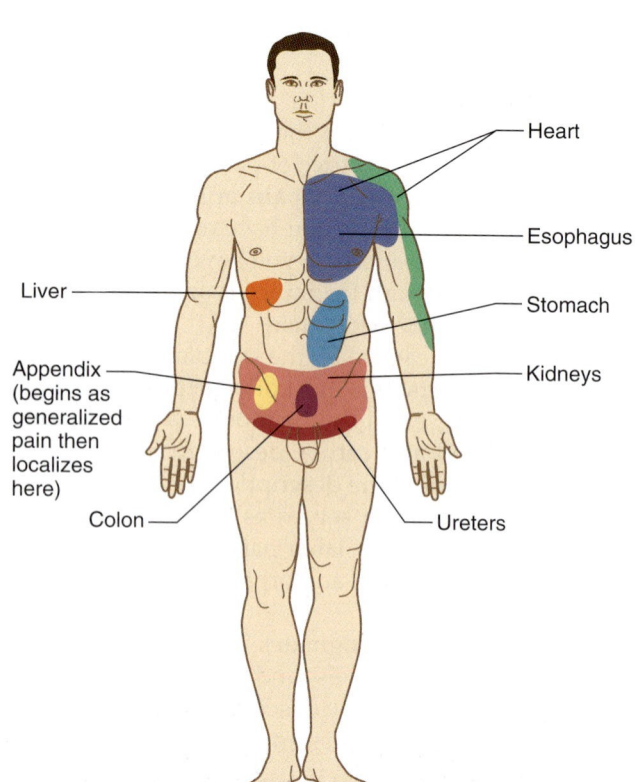

Heart

Esophagus

Liver

Stomach

Appendix (begins as generalized pain then localizes here)

Kidneys

Colon

Ureters

FIGURE 31-1 Most common areas of referred pain.

KnowledgeCheck 31-1

How would you classify the pain that the following patients are experiencing?

- A patient with metastatic cancer
- A patient with back pain that was the result of an automobile injury a year ago
- A patient who had bowel surgery yesterday
- A patient with a fractured leg
- A patient who just had his leg amputated but feels as though the leg is still there
- A patient who just received a paper cut while turning the pages of a book.

ThinkLike a Nurse 31-1

How would you expect a patient with neuropathic pain to appear?

WHAT HAPPENS WHEN SOMEONE HAS PAIN?

Review the story of Eunice Chu Ling in the Meet Your Patient scenario. Eunice had been in an auto accident that caused severe injuries. She has had surgery and requires monitoring and invasive devices, such as a ventilator and IV line. She is awake but cannot speak. However, through the maze of equipment you can see that she is grimacing. Consider these aspects of Eunice's experience as we explore the physiology of pain.

Transduction

Pain-sensitive nociceptors are found in the skin, subcutaneous tissue, joints, walls of the arteries, and most internal organs. The skin has the highest density of nociceptors, and the internal organs the least. Eunice's injuries, surgery, and procedures have stimulated nociceptors throughout her body. In a process called **transduction**, nociceptors become activated by the perception of potentially damaging mechanical, thermal, and chemical stimuli.

Mechanical Stimuli **Mechanical stimuli** are external forces that result in pressure or friction against the body. Eunice's injuries are predominantly of this type. They involve stretching of tissue in joints and body cavities related to bleeding and swelling, and compression of body tissues caused by the force of the accident. Other types of mechanical stimuli are surgical incisions, friction or skin shearing that occurs from sliding down in bed, or pressure from a mechanical device, such as a cast or brace.

Thermal Stimuli **Thermal stimuli** result from exposure to extreme heat or cold. If you've ever touched a hot object and rapidly pulled away or suffered an earache when outdoors on a cold day without a hat, you have experienced pain from thermal stimuli.

Chemical Stimuli **Chemical stimuli** can be internal or external. Lemon juice or any acidic substance on an open area in the skin causes sharp, sudden pain. This is an example of pain from *external* chemical stimuli. In contrast, the chest pain experienced during a myocardial infarction (heart attack) is caused by *internal* chemical stimuli; specifically, the chemical changes that result from tissue ischemia. Another example of a chemical source is ingestion of lead-based paint chipping from a deteriorating residence built before the 1940s. The lead poisoning (also called plumbism) produces neurological damage, headache, and other multisystem effects.

In the Meet Your Patient scenario, the physical cues that Eunice may be in pain include bruising, swelling, surgical incisions, and her tubes and IV. However, you will not always see physical, external cues when tissue injuries are present. This is especially true of injuries caused by internal chemical stimuli. This is one reason you need to believe the patient's report of pain.

Tissue damage prompts the release of substances such as bradykinin, histamine, and prostaglandins, which activate nociceptors in the surrounding tissues. Bradykinin is also a powerful vasodilator that triggers a release of inflammatory chemicals that cause the injured area to become red, swollen, and tender. Inflammation is the most frequent cause of pain.

Transmission

Peripheral nerves carry the pain message to the dorsal horn of the spinal cord in a process known as **transmission** (Fig. 31-2). Pain messages are conducted to the spinal cord along either of two types of fibers:

- **A-delta fibers** are large-diameter myelinated fibers that transmit impulses at 6 to 31 meters per second.

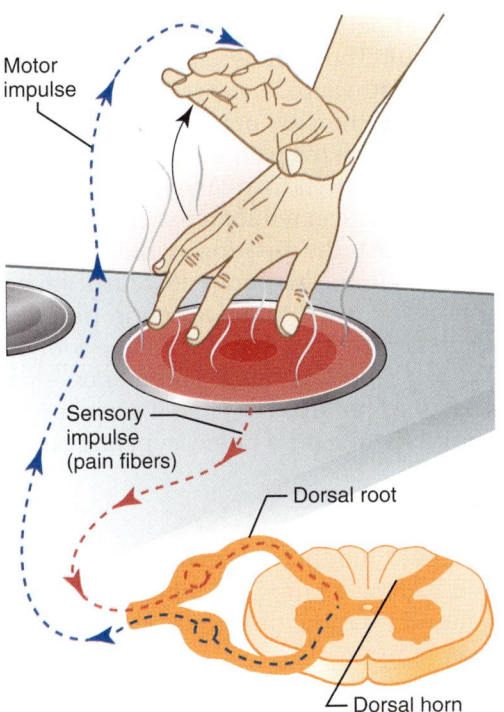

FIGURE 31-2 After nociceptors are activated, pain is transmitted along A-delta fibers or C fibers to the dorsal horn of the spinal cord. From there, the pain message is sent to the brain for perception.

These fibers transmit *fast pain impulses* from acute, focused mechanical and thermal stimuli. For instance, when you bump your knee, the initial sharp pain is carried by A-delta fibers. Pleasurable stimuli to skin receptors, such as from massage, also stimulate A-delta fibers.

- **C fibers** are smaller unmyelinated fibers that transmit *slow pain impulses*, that is, dull, diffuse pain impulses that travel at a slow rate. C fibers conduct pain from mechanical, thermal, and chemical stimuli. If you bump your knee, the lingering ache in the tissue will be carried by C fibers.

At the dorsal horn of the spinal cord, the impulses ascend through via spinothalamic tracts to the brain stem and the thalamus. This process requires chemicals called neurotransmitters (e.g., *substance P*). Most pain impulses are sent to the thalamus of the brain, which acts as an integrating center to direct the impulses to three regions of the brain: (1) the somatosensory cortex perceives and interprets physical sensations; (2) the limbic system is involved in emotional reactions to stimuli; and (3) the frontal cortex is involved in thought and reason. The person now perceives pain.

To see how the pain is transmitted along different nerve routes,

 Go to **Animations: Pain Pathway** on Davis*Plus.*

Pain Perception

Perception involves the recognition and definition of pain in the frontal cortex. The point at which the brain recognizes and defines a stimulus as pain is called the **pain threshold**. The number and intensity of stimuli necessary to produce pain, as well as the duration and characteristics of the pain produced, vary from patient to patient. Although the pain threshold usually remains fairly constant for an individual over time, repeated experience with pain can reduce a patient's threshold.

Pain tolerance is the duration or intensity of pain that a person can endure. This varies not only from person to person but also for the same person in different situations. For example, a mother donating a kidney to her child may not report as much postoperative pain as if she had a kidney removed because it was cancerous. Extreme sensitivity to pain is called **hyperalgesia**.

Pain Modulation

A process called **modulation** changes the perception of pain by either facilitating or inhibiting pain signals through the endogenous analgesia system and the gate-control mechanism.

The Endogenous Analgesia System

In the **endogenous analgesia system,** neurons in the brain stem activate descending nerve fibers that conduct impulses back to the spinal cord. These impulses trigger the release of endogenous opioids and other substances to block the continuing pain impulses and provide pain relief. **Endogenous opioids** are naturally occurring analgesic neurotransmitters (enkephalins, dynorphins, and beta endorphins) that inhibit the transmission of pain impulses and the release of substance P. Endogenous opioids bind to opiate receptor sites in the central and peripheral nervous systems at four receptor sites, designated as mu (∞), kappa (∞), delta (∞), and sigma (∞). These sites are also involved in reception when patients take pain medicines. Each of the receptor sites has a different affinity for various medications. Nonpharmacological measures, such as exercise, meditation, visualization, and music therapy, can also prompt the release of endogenous opioids.

The Gate-Control Theory

Pain impulses can also be modulated at the spinal level. The **gate control theory of pain modulation** describes the mechanism of pain sensation, based on the idea that the perception of pain does not occur by direct stimulation of only nociceptors (pain-producing fiber). Instead, pain is perceived by the interplay between two different kinds of fibers—those that produce pain and those that inhibit pain.

As slow-pain impulses travel along C (small) fibers from the periphery to the brain, they encounter a "gate" that either allows or blocks the transmission of pain sensation to the brain. If the source of stimulation is non-painful, the gate would be blocked to feeling pain. Likewise, noxious stimulation keeps the gate open to pain. Imagine that you've just hit your arm against a hard surface. Almost without thinking, you reach down and rub the area. Your massage stimulates skin receptors. These send sensory impulses along fast A-delta (large) fibers, which quickly excite inhibitory neurons at the "gate." These neurons in turn block some of the pain signals being carried along the slower C fibers (Fig. 31-3). Another application of the gate control theory is use of a Sitz bath after childbirth to produce relief from pain at the perineum. The warm water and gentle pressure block the gate to the perception of pain in the brain. The gate control theory is the basis for development and use of the transcutaneous electrical nerve stimulation (TENS) to relieve pain. (See Nonpharmacological Pain Relief Measures later in this chapter.)

Descending impulses from the brain, including impulses related to mood or emotion, are also thought to open or close the gate. For this reason, medications for depression are sometimes used for patients with chronic pain. Nonpharmacological therapies, such as meditation, exercise, relaxation techniques, and laughter, may also compete with C fiber impulses and block the gate. These strategies are discussed later in this chapter.

On a purely physiological basis, pain is simply transduction, transmission, perception, and modulation. However, as we discuss next, our experience of pain involves far more than these four processes.

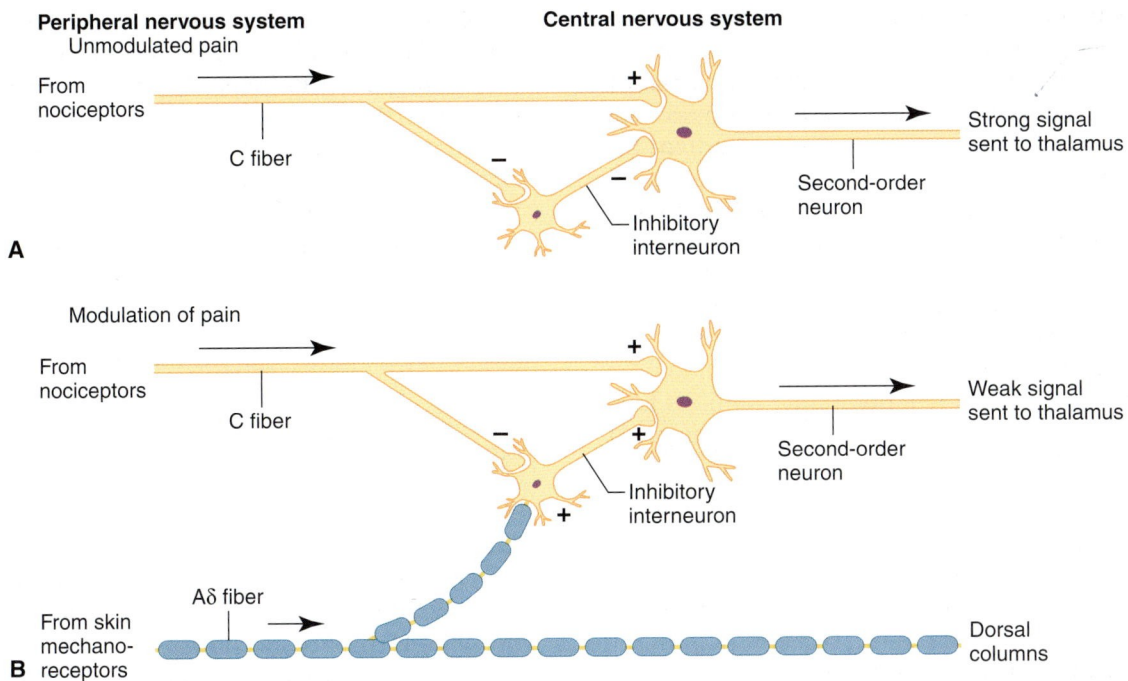

FIGURE 31-3 The gate-control theory of pain modulation. *A,* Normally, C fibers carrying slow-pain signals block inhibitory interneurons and transmit their signals across the synapse unimpeded. *B,* A-delta fibers carrying pleasurable signals (e.g., from touch) excite inhibitory interneurons, which then block the transmission of slow-pain signals (+ equals transmission, − equals no transmission).

 KnowledgeCheck 31-2

- What must occur to generate pain?
- What are the four physiological steps involved in the pain process?

ThinkLike a Nurse 31-2

Based on what you have learned about pain modulation, what nursing interventions might help Eunice (Meet Your Patient) be more comfortable?

WHAT FACTORS INFLUENCE PAIN?

Think back to the last time you experienced significant pain. Was it obvious to others that you were in pain? Were you demonstrative? Quiet? Withdrawn? Did you moan or cry out? Now recall Eunice Chu Ling's reaction. What accounts for these different responses to pain?

Pain is universal, yet each person experiences and responds to pain differently. This uniqueness gives you a hint about its nature: Pain is a complex phenomenon that influences and is influenced by emotions, age, sociocultural factors, and communication and cognitive impairments.

Emotions

The most common emotions associated with pain are fear, guilt, anger, helplessness, and loneliness. In Meet Your Patient, imagine how Eunice Chu Ling must be feeling. How might her feelings affect and be affected by her pain?

Fear Some patients (e.g., Eunice) fear that their pain means their illness or injury is life threatening. Others fear their pain will eventually become intolerable. Many fear that if they ask for pain relief, they will be judged as weak or that they will become addicted to pain medications. When such fears remain unresolved, can prolong or increase the patient's pain.

Confusion and Helplessness In addition to fear, Eunice is also probably experiencing confusion and helplessness. Depending on her role in the accident, she may also feel angry or guilty. Fortunately, family members have come to visit, but when they leave and she is by herself, Eunice may experience loneliness or even a sense of abandonment.

Anxiety and Depression As you learned in Chapter 13, anxiety and depression are common in people who are ill or hospitalized. Anxiety is most often associated with acute pain, but the anticipation of pain may also trigger anxiety. Waiting for surgery or a procedure that you know will be painful offers plenty of time to think about the unpleasantness and to become anxious. In contrast, depression is most often linked with chronic pain, especially intractable pain.

Previous Pain Experience Emotional responses to pain are affected by previous pain experiences. Often patients who have had numerous painful experiences are more anxious about the prospect of experiencing pain and are more sensitive to pain. This is especially troublesome for children and adults who require a series of surgeries or painful treatments for their medical conditions. Conversely, patients who have had effective pain relief in the past are usually less anxious and are more confident they will achieve satisfactory pain relief.

From your own pain experiences, you can see that people in pain do not experience one single emotional reaction to the experience. Instead, a flood of feelings may overwhelm them, and these emotions in turn may escalate their pain. Often patients get in a vicious cycle: Illness and pain trigger emotional reactions, and the emotional reactions exacerbate the pain.

Rarely is pain purely physical or emotional. Instead, it is usually a combination of both. Interventions to relieve pain may relieve feelings of fear and helplessness, and interventions addressing these emotions, such as reflective listening and gentle touch, often aid in pain relief.

 ThinkLike a Nurse 31-3

Imagine being in a situation similar to that of Eunice Chu Ling. What emotions might you experience?

Developmental Stage

The behavior people exhibit when they have pain is strongly influenced by their stage of development.

Infants and Children.

Newborns have the same sensitivity to pain as older infants and children; preterm infants may have a greater sensitivity (McCaffery & Pasero, 1999). The most common kind of pain that children experience is acute pain resulting from injury, illness, or necessary medical procedures. Infants and small children usually respond to pain by crying loudly. However, in premature and term newborns, the experience of pain does not always evoke detectable behavioral response. Indicators of pain in neonates might be as subtle as skin mottling, grimacing, twitching, crying, poor feeding, increased or decreased activity, averting gaze, temperature fluctuation, elevated blood pressure, and decreased oxygen saturation. As a result, even though an infant has a low pain score based on behavioral assessment tools, he may not be pain free (American Academy of Pediatrics et al., 2001b; Slater, Cantarella, Franck, et al., 2008).

Older Adults

Pain occurs in approximately ½ to ¾ of the geriatric population. Estimates are that as many as 45% to 80% of nursing home residents have significant undertreated pain (Takai, Yamamoto-Mitani, Okamoto, et al., 2010). Some older adults may be unable to report pain because of cognitive impairment. Often their discomfort is evident only in nonverbal cues, such as grimacing, rapid blinking, withdrawal, labored breathing, altered gait, or decreased activity. Some older patients respond to pain in atypical ways, such as mental confusion or collapse

(American Geriatrics Society [AGS], Panel on Persistent Pain in Older Persons, 2009; Flaherty, 2007, revised 2012). Undertreated pain often leads to other problems that diminish the quality of life, such as social isolation, depression, sleep disturbances, and mobility-related problems.

Sociocultural Factors

We learn our responses to pain through interaction with family and social support groups. Beliefs about the value of expressing pain or minimizing it are often tied to culture. As you care for clients of various backgrounds, you may notice patterns of behavior. Some patients may gain comfort from crying or moaning when they are in pain, whereas some cultures may value silence and brave endurance of pain. Be careful, however, not to assume that patients will react in the same as others of the same ethnic or cultural group. Each patient is unique. For example, do you respond to pain in exactly the same way as your parents and siblings?

The family and friends of patients in pain also have culturally determined responses to the experience. From the Meet Your Patient scenario, recall how Eunice Chu Ling's family is responding. Although you may think it odd that they are smiling, they may be doing so because they want to make a favorable connection with you, the nurse, because you are responsible for providing care to Eunice. As a nurse, you will be caring for many people in pain and will see a wide variety of responses. Avoid reaching hasty conclusions about the meaning of those responses.

Nurses, too, are affected by their culture. Most nurses respond compassionately to those in pain. However, if you fail to recognize that pain is a unique multidimensional experience, you may misjudge a patient's reaction to injury, surgery, or other discomforts. Disparities exist in the treatment of chronic pain among people of different racial backgrounds. Clinicians should strive to provide culturally competent care and adequate pain control to every patient.

Communication and Cognitive Impairments

One of your greatest challenges as a nurse will be caring for patients in pain who have impaired cognition or communication (e.g., patients who have suffered stroke or dementia, who are intubated, or who have limited command of the local language). Although people with dementia might not appear to be experiencing pain, there is no evidence they have less pain than do other older adults. Cognitively impaired adults are not less sensitive to pain but may rather fail to interpret sensations as painful. Or they might not be able to effectively communicate their pain to others. Although they may not be able to recall their pain, they nonetheless still experience it (Horgas, Yoon, & Grall, 2012; McAuliffe, Brown, & Fetherstonhaugh, 2012). These patients are at risk for underassessment of pain and inadequate pain relief (Baldridge & Andrasik, 2010; Horgas, 2007). You will need to consider their behavioral cues as a form of self-report.

Common nonverbal cues of pain include decreased activity, grimacing, frowning, crying, moaning, and irritability. Less obvious indicators you may see in cognitively impaired patients include the following:

- Facial expressions (e.g., a sad or frightened expression, rapid eye blinking)
- Vocalizations (e.g., noisy breathing, profanity, verbally abusive language)
- Changes in physical activity (e.g., fidgeting, increased pacing or rocking, disruptive behavior)
- Changes in routines (e.g., refusing food, difficulty sleeping)
- Mental status changes (e.g., increased confusion)
- Physiological cues include elevated blood pressure, respiration, and pulse. Be aware, however, that the absence of these cues does not automatically mean that pain is absent.

KnowledgeCheck 31-3

- What are the most common emotional responses to pain?
- What factors influence behavioral responses to pain?

 ## ThinkLike a Nurse 31-4

Eunice Chu Ling is unable to communicate verbally because of her intubation. She is grimacing in pain. After you medicate her for pain, how would you determine whether her pain has been relieved?

HOW DOES THE BODY REACT TO PAIN?

Bodily reactions to pain are influenced by the stage of the pain experience, as well as the intensity, duration, and quality of the pain. Pain triggers a variety of changes in the body. The onset of acute pain activates the sympathetic nervous system. As discussed in Chapter 12, this fight-or-flight (stress) response is protective. It minimizes blood loss, maintains perfusion to vital organs, prevents and fights infections, and promotes healing.

If the pain continues, the body adapts, and the parasympathetic nervous system takes over. However, the pain receptors continue to transmit the pain message so that the person remains aware of the tissue damage. Again, this is largely protective; for example, the pain you feel for several days after you sprain your ankle reminds you to stay off it until it is fully healed.

The severity and duration of the pain significantly affect how the person continues to respond to it. Often the person is able to ignore mild pain, but pain that is severe and unrelieved can consume thoughts and change daily living patterns. Box 31-1 identifies common pain responses.

BOX 31-1 ■ Common Pain Responsese

Physiological (Involuntary) Responses

Sympathetic Responses (Acute Pain)

Dilated blood vessels to the brain, increased alertness

Dilated pupils

Impaired GI motility

Increased heart rate and force of contraction

Increased respiratory rate, shallow breathing

Increased systolic blood pressure

Pallor

Parasympathetic Responses (Deep or Prolonged Pain)

Changeable breathing patterns

Constricted pupils

Decreased pulse rate

Decreased systolic blood pressure, feeling faint, possible syncope

Withdrawal

Behavioral Responses (Voluntary)

Agitation, striking out, fidgeting

Grimacing, frowning, fearful facial expression, grinding teeth

Guarding, bracing, or rubbing the painful area

Moaning, groaning, crying, sighing, crying

Rapid speech (acute pain); slow, monotonous speech (chronic pain)

Withdrawing from painful stimuli, resisting certain movements with care

Eating and sleeping poorly

Reduced energy, reduced interest in others, reduced activity level and mobility

Change in gait

Psychological (Affective) Responses

Anger

Anxiety

Depression

Exhaustion

Fear

Hopelessness

Irritability

Unrelieved Pain

Unrelieved pain can produce harmful effects in various body systems.

Endocrine System Ongoing pain triggers excessive release of hormones, including adrenocorticotropic hormone (ACTH), cortisol, antidiuretic hormone (ADH), growth hormone (GH), catecholamines, and glucagon. Insulin and testosterone levels decrease. These hormone shifts activate carbohydrate, protein, and fat catabolism (breakdown), hyperglycemia, and poor glucose use. The inflammatory process, combined with these endocrine and metabolic changes, can result in weight loss, tachycardia, fever, increased respiratory rate, and even death.

Cardiovascular System   Unrelieved pain leads to hypercoagulation and an increase in heart rate, blood pressure, cardiac workload, and oxygen demand. The combination of hypercoagulation and increased cardiac workload may lead to unstable angina (chest pain), intracoronary thrombosis (clot formation in the vessels that supply the heart), and myocardial ischemia and infarction (heart attack).

Musculoskeletal System   Unrelieved pain causes impaired muscle function, fatigue, and immobility. Poorly controlled pain can prevent the patient from performing activities of daily living and engaging in physical therapy.

Respiratory System   Patients in pain tend to breathe shallowly—to limit thoracic and abdominal movement in an effort to reduce pain. This is called **splinting**. Splinting reduces tidal volume (air exchanged with each breath) and increases inspiratory and expiratory pressures. These changes can lead to pneumonia and atelectasis as well as underventilation (retained carbon dioxide, also called hypercarbia) and respiratory acidosis.

Genitourinary System   Unrelieved pain causes release of excessive amounts of catecholamines, aldosterone, ADH, cortisol, angiotensin II, and prostaglandins. These hormones lead to decreased urinary output, urinary retention, fluid overload, hypokalemia, hypertension, and increased cardiac output.

Gastrointestinal (GI) System   In response to pain, intestinal secretions and smooth muscle tone increase, and gastric emptying and motility decrease.

KnowledgeCheck 31-4

- What are the effects of untreated pain on each of the body systems?
- How might untreated pain affect the progress of a patient recovering from major illness?

PracticalKnowledge
knowing **how**

As we discussed earlier, a person's *pain threshold* is the point at which that person perceives a stimulus as painful, whereas *pain tolerance* is the amount of pain a person is able to endure. Both differ greatly from person to person. Increases in pain may indicate change in condition or a need for more aggressive pain management. Practical knowledge includes knowing how to assess for and manage patients' pain.

ASSESSMENT

A comprehensive pain assessment includes pain location and quality, intensity, aggravating and alleviating factors, timing and duration, and goals for pain relief. Additionally, you need to ask questions that reveal the patient's functional ability and goals, and psychological/social factors, such as depression or substance abuse (ICSI, 2005, updated 2011). To treat pain effectively, you must first understand the patient's perception of pain. To do this, begin with a pain history. Each agency will have different assessment forms for this history. For a list of questions that are typically asked,

   Go to Chapter 31, **Assessment Guidelines and Tools, Focused Assessment: Pain Assessment,** in Volume 2.

You should also make ongoing assessments regularly and, of course, accept the patient's report of pain.

Patient Self-Report   This is the most reliable indicator of pain, even for those with mild cognitive impairment (American Association of Critical Care Nurses, 2013; Herr, Bjoro, & Decker, 2006). Self-report is especially important for patients with chronic pain. When pain is ongoing, the autonomic nervous system eventually adapts, so physiological and behavioral signs become less evident (Schneider, 2006–2007).

Patient Satisfaction   Patient satisfaction with healthcare can be directly related to how well pain is managed. To ensure patient comfort and satisfaction, teach patients about pain management options and expected outcomes as you assess their responses to pain interventions. This helps involve them in their care and allows for making rapid adjustments to their regimen (Bozimowski, 2012).

Pain, the Fifth Vital Sign

The American Pain Society recommends assessing for pain as the fifth vital sign. This means that you should ask patients to rate their pain intensity whenever you take a full set of vital signs (Berdine, 2002; Molony, Kobayashi, Holleran, et al., 2005; Pasero, 1997). By simply raising the question with each vital signs check, you will prompt your clients to report pain more often. Also, teach nursing assistive personnel (NAP) to ask patients about their pain when taking vital signs and to report their findings to you. Box 31-2 provides the clinical approach to pain assessment recommended by the Agency for Health Care Policy and Research (AHCPR). Perform pain assessments routinely, but not limited to:

- On admission to a healthcare facility
- Before and after each potentially painful procedure or treatment
- When the patient is at rest, as well as when involved in a nursing activity

BOX 31-2 ■ Recommended Clinical Approach to Pain Assessment—Agency for Healthcare Policy and Research

Ask about pain regularly. **A**ssess pain systematically.

Believe the patient and family in their reports of pain and what relieves it.

Choose pain control options appropriate for the patient, family, and setting.

Deliver interventions in a timely, logical, coordinated fashion.

Empower patients and their families.

Enable patients to control their course to the greatest extent possible.

Source: Agency for Healthcare Policy and Research (AHPR), Public Health Service, U.S. Department of Health and Human Services (USDHHS). (1994). *The clinical practice guideline for the management of cancer pain.* AHCPR Publication no. 94-0592. Rockville, MD: Author.

■ Before you implement a pain management intervention, such as administering an analgesic drug, and 30 minutes after the intervention
■ With each check of vital signs, if the pain is an actual or potential problem
■ When the patient complains of pain

Assessing Pain in Children

You can assess pain in children through self-report, behavioral observation, or physiological measures. Be sure to consult the parents about the child's stress signals and reaction to pain. With children, use art and play as a way to assess the child's understanding of pain and the pain management plan. Choose age-appropriate toys to engage the child in acting out feelings. Sometimes this indirect method is more effective than directly asking the child. Remember, most children are fearful about injections and may deny pain if they think that describing their pain will lead to an injection. You can also use a pain-rating scale consisting of simple illustrations of faces. For an example,

 Go to Chapter 31, **Assessment Guidelines and Tools, Using Pain Scales,** in Volume 2.

Culturally Competent Assessments

Three words—*pain, hurt,* and *ache*—seem to be used across many cultures to describe pain (Pasero & McCaffery, 2011). You might also use descriptions of *burning, itching,* and *cramping* when asking patients about their pain experience. For this reason, many pain assessment tools can be successfully translated into various languages. If you work in an area where there are many non-English-speaking patients, you may benefit from pain assessment tools that have been translated into the languages

you are most likely to encounter. To see pain translated into common languages,

 Go to Chapter 31, **Tables, Boxes, Figures: ESG Box 31-1, Pain in a Sample of Languages,** on Davis*Plus.*

Difficult-to-Assess Patients

Patients who are under anesthesia or those receiving sedation are difficult to assess for pain. Those with a brain injury may mimic pain-like behavior. Patients with Alzheimer's disease with severe cognitive and expressive deficits are also a challenge for assessing the extent of pain. It may not be possible to elicit a reliable self-report for pain, and their behavioral cues might not be reflective of the pain experience either.

When using a pain scale for cognitively impaired patients, you must allow sufficient time for the patient to respond. There are many pain assessment tools. The Pain Assessment in Advanced Dementia (PAINAD) Scale is a five-item, observational tool, specifically geared to older adults with dementia. The areas for rating include breathing, negative vocalization, facial expression, body language, and consolability. Lower scores indicate less pain. To see this tool,

 Go to Chapter 31, **Tables, Boxes, Figures: ESG Table 31-1, Pain Assessment in Advanced Dementia (PAINAD) Scale,** on Davis*Plus.*

You need to judge the intensity and quality of pain based on patient history and current environment. Does the patient have an underlying painful condition? What is the likely source of pain? Are there physical signs that indicate the patient has increased pain with movement, turning, or other motions? Nonverbal signs of pain become important cues for such patients.

Nonverbal Signs of Pain

In addition to the patient's verbal report of pain, you must recognize other responses that may signal pain (see Box 31-1). Pay attention to the patient's physical signs and symptoms. Is the blood pressure or pulse elevated? Does the client appear ashen? These are signs of sympathetic nervous system stimulation. You will see these signs if the pain is acute. If the pain is unresolved or chronic, the blood pressure and pulse may be lower than normal, and the patient may report feeling faint. These are signs of parasympathetic nervous system stimulation.

Key Point: *However, there can be underlying physiological conditions, medications, or hemodynamic changes that cause changes in vital signs. And, likewise, an absence of vital sign changes doesn't necessarily indicate an absence of pain.*

For guidelines to help you assess for nonverbal signs of pain,

 Go to Chapter 31, **Clinical Insight 31-2: Guidelines for Assessing Pain,** in Volume 2.

Quality and Safety Education for Nurses

Assessing and Treating Pain in Cognitively Impaired Patients

Competency: *Patient-Centered Care (Knowledge, Skills, Attitudes)**

Scenario: Mr. Fagin, who has dementia, has been hospitalized for prostate cancer that has metastasized to his pelvis, femur, and ribs. Mr. Fagin seems confused and is loudly singing hymns and banging his hands against his table in rhythm. The RN goes to Mr. Fagin's room, observes him carefully, and speaks with him. When asked if his bones hurt, he nods his head "yes." She also asks Mrs. Fagin about her husband's usual responses to pain. Mrs. Fagin states that her husband has always been very religious and often sings hymns when upset. She also says that he never complained about aches and pains in the past and that she believes he is now having "quite a bit of pain." She says, "I can't stand to see him suffer." The nurse checks the medication administration record (MAR) and obtains the prescribed prn opioid analgesic. While Mrs. Fagin speaks gently to her husband, the nurse administers the opioid analgesic. She documents the medication in the MAR, noting Mr. Fagin's behaviors prior to being medicated. Thirty minutes later the nurse observes Mr. Fagin eating dinner with his wife. His body and facial expression are relaxed, and he has stopped singing. Before leaving, the nurse asks Mr. and Mrs. Fagin whether they would like a visit from the hospital chaplain.

Think about it: A central nursing duty in the patient-centered care competency is alleviating pain and suffering. (1) How is

Mr. Fagan's situation is different from that of a patient with normal cognitive function? (2) What knowledge, skills, and attitudes did the nurse apply that demonstrate competency in pain management (and, therefore, in patient-centered care), particularly for the patient with dementia? As you think about it, consider the following:

➤ Why was it important to ask Mrs. Fagin about her husband's usual behavior?

➤ Was it appropriate to ask the Fagins whether they wanted a visit from the chaplain?

➤ How did the nurse show respect for Mr. and Mrs. Fagin's preferences, values, and needs?

➤ Singing loudly doesn't seem like to be an obvious indication of pain; what other factors let the nurse know Mr. Fagin was in pain?

➤ How is pain assessment modified for cognitively impaired patients?

➤ Do you see how the nurse recognized Mr. Fagin and his wife as full partners in care?

For specific Knowledge, Skills, and Attitudes,

 Go to the QSEN Web site at **http:www.qsen.org.ksas_ prelicensure.php**

Using Pain Scales

To help you assess the intensity of the pain as well as any changes in the pain, you can choose from among a variety of pain scales. Select a pain scale by considering the patient's age, level of education, language skills, eyesight, and developmental level. Keep in mind that when using a simple pain intensity scale, children can communicate the quality of pain before they are developmentally capable of indicating the intensity (O'Rourke, 2004). Once you choose a particular pain scale for a patient, use it consistently to prevent confusion and allow for comparison. To see some pain scales you might use,

 Go to Chapter 31, **Assessment Guidelines and Tools, Using Pain Scales,** in Volume 2.

KnowledgeCheck 31-5

- How often should you assess the patient for pain, if pain is a potential problem for the patient?
- What are some of the common pain scales used?
- Who should determine if the patient is in pain?

ThinkLike a Nurse 31-5

What pain rating scale would you use to assess Eunice (Meet Your Patient)? Why?

ANALYSIS/NURSING DIAGNOSIS

For nursing diagnoses, NOC outcomes, and NIC interventions associated with Pain,

 Go to Chapter 31, **Standardized Language, NANDA-I Diagnoses, NOC Outcomes, and NIC Interventions Associated With Pain,** on DavisPlus.

The following NANDA-I labels are commonly used when pain is the focus of the problem:

- *Acute Pain.* Pain with an anticipated or actual duration of <6 months.
- *Chronic Pain.* Pain with an anticipated or actual duration of >6 months.

Notice that NANDA-I uses only duration, not speed of onset or severity, to differentiate between Acute Pain and Chronic Pain.

Pain affects many areas of functioning. Therefore, it is often the etiology of other nursing diagnoses, such as the following:

> *Ineffective Sexuality Pattern* related to pain in joints
> *Sleep Deprivation* related to chronic back pain of more than a year's duration

When writing a pain nursing diagnosis, specify the location of the pain and any etiological or precipitating factors that you are aware of. For example:

> Acute Pain (headache) related to changes of position and secondary to increased intracranial pressure.

Also identify any knowledge deficits, fear of addiction, or any other fears or beliefs that may interfere with effective pain management. Focusing on the specific nature of pain enables you to choose the most useful interventions.

PLANNING OUTCOMES

The overall objective when working with a client in pain is to prevent pain whenever possible or, if it is present, to reduce or eliminate pain.

NOC standardized outcomes for pain include these examples: Physical Comfort Status, Pain Control, Pain Level, and Pain: Disruptive Effects.

Individualized goals/outcome statements you might write for a client with pain include the following:

- By day 2 post-op, will require only oral analgesics.
- Within 15 minutes of PCA injection, reports pain is <3 on a 0–10 scale.
- Reports that chronic pain does not prevent her from performing activities of daily living.
- Pain Control: Uses pain relief diary (4: Often demonstrated) (NOC)

Use the goals set in the planning outcomes phase to evaluate the pain relief obtained from nursing and medical interventions.

PLANNING INTERVENTIONS/IMPLEMENTATION

When planning care, remember that each situation is unique. For example, one terminally ill patient may request complete relief of pain even if this leads to heavy sedation. Another may prefer that the pain be decreased to a just manageable level so he can interact with his family or complete any unfinished business. The patient and family must be part of the pain management program. Generally, the most effective and least invasive method of pain control is preferable. Remember to include nonpharmacological interventions.

Although overall care of the patient depends on the cause of the pain, whether pain is acute or chronic, and on the patient's unique situation, there are nursing interventions and activities that address pain, regardless of its cause.

NIC standardized interventions for pain include Analgesic Administration, Sedation Management, Pain Management, Behavior Modification, and several others (see the Standardized Language table on DavisPlus).

Individualized nursing activities (including focused assessments) for clients with Acute Pain and Chronic Pain include the following:

- Actively listen to the patient's reports of pain.
- Support the patient in maintaining an active role in treatment by including her as part of the pain management team.
- Provide prescribed analgesics promptly.
- Assess for response to analgesics and nonpharmacological measures, including level of sedation. Make assessments approximately 30 to 60 minutes after

the administration of an oral medicine. Injectable medications work more quickly, so adjust the assessment time accordingly.

- Alter the treatment if the pain is not adequately relieved.
- Provide interventions to manage the side effects of medications.
- Reduce anxiety and fear by offering explanations about care and medications, by allowing the patient to be in control of his pain management, and by providing positive encouragement.
- Consult with the healthcare team about complex pain management issues.
- Delegate appropriate pain management strategies to a NAP.

See Box 31-3 for a list of strategies that may be delegated to NAPs.

Nonpharmacological Pain Relief Measures

Integrating complementary therapies into a pain management plan can help ease chronic pain and reduce the need for drug therapy (Bishop, Yardley, & Lewith, 2008; Ernst, 2008; Hart, 2008). According to the 2007 National Health Interview Survey (NHIS), 38% of adults used some form of complementary and alternative medicine (CAM) when confronted with pain or stress (Barnes, Bloom, & Nahin, 2008).

Nonpharmacological measures, such as exercise, meditation, visualization, and music therapy, can prompt the release of endogenous opioids. They offer an alternative for people with mild pain who do not wish to take potent drugs for pain relief. For many patients, they are satisfying and empowering. However, they should be used as an adjunct to pharmacological therapies for patients with moderate to severe pain.

BOX 31-3 ■ Pain Management Tasks That May Be Delegated to Nursing Assistive Personnel

Nursing assistive personnel (NAP) may assist you in caring for patients with pain. However, you may never delegate the responsibility to assess the patient's pain, monitor the patient's response to pain management strategies, or evaluate the pain management plan. The following tasks may be delegated:

- Repositioning, using pillows for support
- Back rub or massage
- Providing darkness and quiet in the room for sleep
- Straightening sheets
- Mouth care
- Soft music of the patient's preference
- Using distraction (talking or setting up a favorite game for the patient)

Cutaneous Stimulation

Cutaneous stimulation (stimulation of the skin) is a method of pain relief based on the gate-control theory of pain. As we discussed earlier, skin stimulation sends impulses along the large sensory fibers, which in turn excite inhibitory interneurons in the spinal cord to "close the gate." This process diminishes the patient's perception of pain. Cutaneous stimulation works best on pain that is localized and not diffuse.

TENS Units A **transcutaneous electrical nerve stimulator (TENS)** is a battery-powered device about the size of a pager that is worn externally. TENS units consist of electrode pads, connecting wire, and the stimulator. The pads are directly applied to the painful area. Once activated, the unit stimulates A-delta sensory fibers. A TENS unit can be worn intermittently or for long periods of time, depending on the patient's pain.

PENS Units **Percutaneous electrical stimulation (PENS)** combines a TENS unit with percutaneously placed (through the skin) needle probes to stimulate peripheral sensory nerves. PENS is effective in short-term management of acute and chronic pain. PENS therapy in some patients promotes physical activity, increases the sense of well-being, reduces the use of nonopioid medication, and improves sleep.

Spinal Cord Stimulator Chronic neurological pain may be treated by a surgically implanted **spinal cord stimulator (SCS)**. The SCS produces a tingly sensation that interferes with the perception of pain.

Acupuncture Application of extremely fine needles to specific sites in the body to relieve pain is called **acupuncture**. It is believed to stimulate the endogenous analgesia system. Acupuncture is well documented to provide relief from low back pain (Lee, Choi, Lee, et al., 2013). It is used to relieve dental pain and has been used extensively after surgery and chemotherapy to treat nausea. Of all the complementary therapeutic approaches, acupuncture enjoys the most credibility in the medical community (Hart, 2008). There have been some reports in which acupuncture has led to light-headedness, which may be a concern for patients who are at risk for falls.

Acupressure Similar to the ancient art of acupuncture, from which it evolved, **acupressure** stimulates specific sites in the body. However, instead of needles, fingertips provide firm, gentle pressure over the various pressure points. This process may have a calming effect through the release of endorphins. Patients can be readily taught key points to stimulate so that they can self-administer acupressure at any time.

Massage Massage has been shown to be effective in reducing pain (Cassileth, Trevissan, & Jyothirmai, 2007). By providing cutaneous stimulation and relaxing the muscles, **massage** helps to reduce pain. **Effleurage**, or the use of slow, long, guiding strokes, is used for obstetrical

patients during labor and as back rubs for postsurgical patients. Massage requires little effort from the patient and may improve sleep. For most patients, superficial massage is soothing and relaxing, both mentally and physically. However, some patients do not like to be touched, and you should always obtain verbal permission for a massage.

Application of Heat and Cold The application of cold causes vasoconstriction and can help prevent swelling and bleeding. Cold can be especially effective in reducing the amount of pain that occurs during procedures. Apply a cold pack to the site before and after a procedure to reduce pain. Heat promotes circulation, which speeds healing. Use caution with these methods, however, because the skin may be injured by extremes of either hot or cold. Also, because the addition of moisture to heat or cold amplifies the intensity of the treatment, take extra precautions when applying moist heat or cold.

✚ To safely use heat and cold:

- Avoid direct contact with the heating or cooling device. Cover the hot or cold pack with a washcloth, towel, or fitted sleeve.
- Apply heat or cold intermittently, for no more than 15 minutes at a time, to avoid tissue injury.
- Check the skin frequently for extreme redness, blistering, cyanosis (blue color), or blanching (white color).
- If any of these occur, discontinue the treatment immediately and notify the provider.

Contralateral Stimulation Why does a patient experiencing pain in the right arm experience some relief when lotion is applied and rubbed into the left arm? The principle involved is called **contralateral stimulation**—stimulating the skin in an area opposite to the painful site. Stimulation may be in the form of scratching, rubbing, or applying heat or cold. This intervention is especially helpful if the affected area is painful to touch, under bandages, or in a cast. It has provided some relief to patients who have phantom pain after an amputation.

Immobilization

Immobilizing a painful body part (e.g., with splints) may offer some relief. It is particularly helpful with arthritic joints. You must remember to remove the splints at regular intervals so that the patient can exercise the area to strengthen the site and prevent further injury. Patients in severe pain have the tendency to immobilize a painful area by limiting its use.

Cognitive–Behavioral Interventions

Cognitive–behavioral therapy attempts to alter patterns of negative thoughts and to encourage more adaptive thoughts, emotions, and actions. It is used to decrease depression and anxiety, both of which play a role in pain. Cognitive therapy helps patients to deal with their pain by fostering a sense of control over their illness and decreasing feelings of helplessness. Be sure to obtain the patient's permission before using these methods, because psychological or spiritual distress may occur if she considers them inconsistent with her belief system. Because they are complementary therapies, several of these interventions are discussed in more detail in Chapter 46. If you wish to read more about them,

 Go to Chapter 46, **Holistic Healing**, on Davis*Plus*.

Distraction

Distraction is a method of drawing the patient's attention away from the pain and focusing on something other than the pain. It is based on the belief that the brain can process only so much information at one time. When distraction works, the patient has only a peripheral awareness of pain. You may have responded to this strategy in the past. Have you ever had a headache or muscle pain go away when you became busy with other activities? Although distraction can be used for severe pain, it is most effective for mild to moderate pain and for brief periods of time (e.g., for a short procedure such as an injection or infusion). Some patients experience an increase in pain and may become fatigued and irritable when they are no longer distracted. Distraction is useful with all ages, but it should not be used in place of analgesics.

Distraction can be visual, tactile, intellectual, or auditory. The usefulness of the different methods varies among patients.

- *Visual* tactics, such as watching a football game on TV, serve as effective distraction for some patients.
- *Tactile* distraction such as massage, hugging a favorite toy, holding a loved one, or stroking a pet is effective for still other patients.
- *Intellectual* distraction includes becoming engrossed in a crossword puzzle or playing a challenging game.
- *Auditory* distraction in the form of music therapy has been shown to reduce anxiety during childbirth and appears to improve mood and pain tolerance. Music therapy has also been shown to improve patients' perceived effectiveness of pain. Patients' self-reports show pain is reduced and relaxation is achieved more easily. Physiological measures, such as respirations, heart rate, blood pressure, and muscle tension, indicate a less intense pain experience (American Music Therapy Association, n.d.). Music should not be limited to adults; it can be used for infants and children as well.

Relaxation Techniques

Relaxation techniques reduce pain in a variety of medical conditions, especially in chronic pain. In **sequential muscle relaxation (SMR)**, or progressive relaxation, the person sits comfortably and tenses a group of muscles for 15 seconds and then relaxes the muscle while breathing out. After a brief rest, this sequence is repeated using another set of muscles. Patients often start at the facial muscles and work downward to the feet.

Guided Imagery

Guided imagery uses auditory and imaginary processes to affect emotions and help calm, divert, and relax (Hooten, Timming, Belgrade, et al., 2013). Acute and chronic pain, physical and psychological, may respond to guided imagery; however, it is more effective for chronic pain. Audio media featuring guided imagery can help patients use their imagination to create images of temporary escape that will elicit a sense of well-being (Lewandowski, Good, & Draucker, 2005). For a script for a guided imagery session,

 Go to Chapter 12, **Supplemental Materials**, on Davis*Plus*.

Diaphragmatic Breathing

Diaphragmatic breathing is an effective measure to invoke relaxation and improve tissue oxygenation for pain management. The goal is to train patients to intentionally take slow, even breaths using the diaphragm to inhale and exhale at the same rate for five to eight breaths per minute.

Hypnosis

Hypnosis involves the induction of a deeply relaxed state. Once the person is in this state, the hypnotist offers therapeutic suggestions to provide relief of symptoms. For example, the hypnotist may suggest to a patient with arthritis that the pain can be turned down, like the volume of a radio. Special training in hypnotherapy is required.

Therapeutic Touch

Therapeutic touch (TT) was developed by nurses and derived from the ancient practice of laying on of hands. Despite its name, therapeutic touch does not require physical contact. It focuses on the use of the hands to direct energy fields surrounding the body. Although research studies on its effect are not consistent, some patients become relaxed and require less pain medication after a session of therapeutic touch.

Humor

Humor has positive effects on a patient's physical and emotional health. For most people, laughter is positive and indicates mental well-being. Humor may boost the immune system as well. It is especially helpful when used before a painful procedure because it lessens anxiety and serves as a form of distraction. Some institutions have humor carts and even humor rooms containing humorous videos, books, and playful items, such as bubbles, fingerpaints, and puppets. Humor is helpful for both children and adults, but it must always be in good taste and age-appropriate. Involve the patient in choosing the humor material, because what one person considers very funny another person may not.

Expressive Writing

Expressive writing can help reduce chronic pain. Some recommend structured writing sessions in which the patient describes stressful events for a specified period of time over consecutive days. This type of therapy is best when done in conjunction with a knowledgeable practitioner to provide direction and support (Hart, 2008). Others benefit from frequent journaling in an informal way, expressing feelings, fears, or what comes to mind.

 ThinkLike a Nurse 31-6

What has been your experience with using nonpharmacological pain relief measures to manage your own pain? How would you incorporate these methods into your nursing practice?

Pharmacological Pain Relief Measures

Analgesics are classified into three groups: nonopioids, opioids, and adjuvants. Many health practitioners use the World Health Organization's (WHO) three-step ladder to assist in the selection and titration of an analgesic (Fig. 31-4). Each step on the ladder represents severity of pain, by which the analgesic selection is determined. Choice of treatment is based on the level of pain the patient is experiencing. Patients in severe pain should start at the third step. Titration is accomplished according to the patient's response. Monitoring should be regular and continuous. If the patient's pain is not controlled, adjust by moving up the pain ladder. To apply the ladder correctly, you need to know the interactions and side effects of all the drugs recommended on each step.

Base decisions about the use of analgesics on a thorough pain assessment using valid and reliable pain assessment tools, as well as knowledge of the drug to be administered (see Assessment). Prior to first dose, verify the patient's drug allergy status.

Dosing Administer analgesics at regular times throughout the day if the patient has pain that lasts throughout the day. First, determine the dosage that relieves pain at the patient's desired level, then observe how long the first dose lasts. Administer the next dose before the last dose wears off. Around-the-clock (ATC) dosing prevents the patient from experiencing severe pain several times a day and is believed to be better than prn (as needed) dosing for pain. Explain to the patient

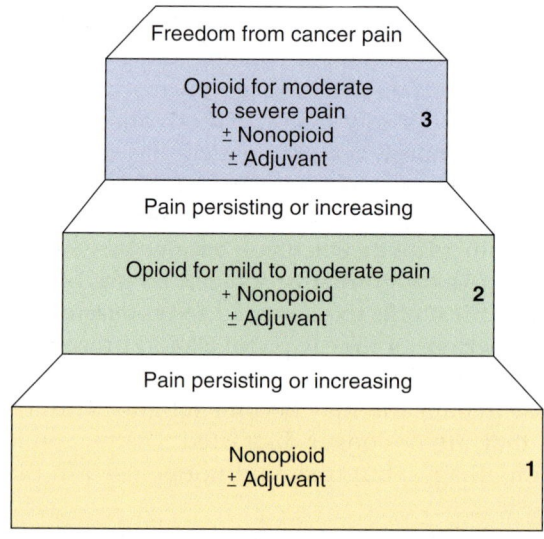

FIGURE 31-4 The WHO three-step analgesic ladder. (World Health Organization (WHO). (1990). Cancer pain relief and palliative care: Report of a WHO expert committee. WHO Technical Report series, No. 804. Geneva, Switzerland: Author. Used with permission.)

Toward Evidence-Based Practice

Cole, L. C., & Lobiondo-Wood, G. (2012). Music as an adjuvant therapy in control of pain and symptoms in hospitalized adults: A systematic review. *Pain Management Nursing.* Advance online publication. pii:S1524-9042(12)00144-0. doi:10.1016/j.pmn.2012.08.010.

Seventeen randomized controlled trials were reviewed in a search for the terms *music, music therapy, pain, adults, inpatients,* and *hospitalized* from January 2005 to March 2011. These included surgical, medical, medical-surgical, intensive care, and pregnant patients. These studies supported the use of music as an adjuvant approach to pain management in hospitalized adults.

Topcu, S. Y., & Findik, U. Y., (2012). Effect of relaxation exercises on controlling postoperative pain. *Pain Management Nursing,* 13(1), 11–17.

Sixty patients undergoing upper abdominal surgery were studied. Pain levels were assessed before and after relaxation exercises using the verbal pain scale. Pain levels were reduced after relaxation exercises.

1. For patients using alternative or integrative therapies, such as guided imagery, music, and relaxation to manage pain in various situations, why do you think these techniques might be effective?

2. When teaching alternative or integrative therapies for managing pain, how might you best prepare the setting in order to maximize the effectiveness of the technique?

3. Can you think of reasons patients might resist trying alternative or integrative methods for managing chronic pain? What would you do to encourage patients who seem to oppose the idea of practicing nonpharmacological pain management?

 Go to Chapter 31, **Toward Evidence-Based Practice Suggested Responses,** on DavisPlus.

that ATC dosing will keep pain at an acceptable level throughout the day and allow her to function at an optimal level. For optimal pain management, avoid administering small, frequent, ineffective, partial doses within a range; this results in underdosing.

Studies show higher nonsteroidal anti-inflammatory drug doses give longer duration of action rather than greater pain relief in the short term (McQuay, Derry, Eccleston, et al., 2012).

Nonopioid Analgesics

Nonopioid analgesics include a variety of medications that relieve mild to moderate pain. Many also reduce inflammation and fever. Several of these medications, including acetaminophen (Tylenol), aspirin, ibuprofen (Advil, Motrin), and naproxen (Aleve), are available over the counter. All may be used for acute and chronic pain. Most have an onset of action within 1 hour. Box 31-4 features a number of commonly used nonopioid analgesics.

The analgesic properties of acetaminophen and aspirin are often underestimated. Research indicates that 650 mg of aspirin or acetaminophen may relieve as much pain as 50 mg of oral meperidine or 3 to 5 mg of oxycodone, both of which are opioid analgesics. Nevertheless, nonopioid analgesics are often compounded with opioids. This allows for a lower dose of opioid to be administered and reduces the incidence of side effects.

Nonsteroidal Anti-Inflammatory Drugs

The largest group of nonopioid analgesics is made up of nonsteroidal anti-inflammatory drugs (NSAIDs). These include aspirin, ibuprofen, and several others. NSAIDs act primarily in the peripheral tissues by interfering with the production of prostaglandins. Prostaglandins sensitize pain receptors and are involved with inflammation.

One of the most common side effects of NSAIDs is gastric irritation and bleeding. Because of the risk of GI bleeding, the long-term use of nonselective NSAIDs, such as naproxen, oxaprozin, and piroxicam, is generally not recommended in older adults. Additionally, they can lead renal failure, high blood pressure, and heart failure in geriatric patients (American Medical Directors Association [AMDA], 2012).

Taking the medication with food, lowering the dose, or using enteric-coated pills can reduce the incidence of this side effect. Some of the newer NSAIDs are less irritating to the GI so they markedly decrease gastric irritation and bleeding. However, they are expensive and available only by prescription. Combining two nonsteroidal anti-inflammatory drugs (NSAIDs) is not often recommended because it increases the risks of side effects and may not be more effective.

Aspirin is a unique NSAID. In addition to reducing inflammation, fever, and pain, it can inhibit platelet aggregation (clumping), the first step in clot formation. For that reason, NSAIDs should be used with caution in patients with impaired blood clotting, renal disease, and gastrointestinal bleeding or ulcers.

Myocardial infarction, stroke, and thrombophlebitis (a clot in the peripheral veins) are all associated with platelet aggregation. Because of this property, low-dose aspirin (usually 81 mg) is prescribed to decrease risk of these disorders. Regular use of aspirin prolongs clotting time, so teach patients who use aspirin that they will bruise easily and will bleed more if cut. Taking a small daily dose of aspirin to prevent myocardial infarction does not seem to increase the side effects for patients taking other NSAIDs.

Acetaminophen

Unlike most nonopioid analgesics, acetaminophen has very little anti-inflammatory effect. Instead it has analgesic and fever-reducing properties. It has fewer side effects and is probably the safest of the nonopioids. It does not affect platelet function, rarely causes gastrointestinal problems, and can be used in patients who are allergic to aspirin or other NSAIDs. However, even in recommended doses (up to a maximum of 4,000 mg daily), it can cause severe hepatotoxicity (liver toxicity) in patients who take excessive quantities, or who consume alcohol or have liver disease.

KnowledgeCheck 31-6

- How do NSAIDs induce pain relief?
- What is the main side effect of NSAIDs?
- In which patients are NSAIDs contraindicated?

Adjuvant Analgesics

Adjuvant analgesics reduce the amount of opioid the patient requires. They may be used as a primary therapy for mild pain or in conjunction with opioids for moderate to severe pain. They are especially useful if the patient experiences significant side effects from escalating doses of opioids. Adjuvant analgesics are frequently used in managing neuropathic pain, in which they may be the primary treatment or may be used in conjunction with opioids. Drugs in this category include anticonvulsants,

---

BOX 31-4 ■ Commonly Used Nonopioid Analgesics

Chemical Name	Brand Name
Acetaminophen	Tylenol
Acetylsalicylic acid (aspirin)	Excedrin, Bayer, others
Celecoxib	Celebrex
Diclofenac	Voltaren, Cataflam
Etodolac	Lodine
Ibuprofen	Motrin, Advil, others
Indomethacin	Indocin
Ketoprofen	Oruvail
Nabumetone	Relafen
Naproxen	Naprosyn, Aleve, Anaprox

antidepressants, local anesthetics, topical agents, psychostimulants, muscle relaxants, neuroleptics, corticosteroids, and others.

Opioid Analgesics

Opioids are natural and synthetic compounds that relieve pain, although they vary in potency. To some degree, opioids work by finding pain receptor sites to bind with and block the pain impulse. Keep in mind that the process of achieving analgesia is more complex than this. Opiate receptors include mu, delta, kappa, and sigma receptors; however, mu receptors are most effective in relieving pain.

- **Mu agonists** stimulate mu receptors and are used for acute, chronic, and cancer pain. They include codeine, hydrocodone (Vicodin), morphine, hydromorphone (Dilaudid), fentanyl, methadone, and oxycodone. These are excellent medications for **breakthrough pain**—pain that "breaks through" relief provided by long-acting analgesics. Breakthrough analgesia refers to a rescue or extra dose. Drugs used for breakthrough pain should have a rapid onset and short duration. There is no maximum daily dose limit and no "ceiling" to the level of analgesia from mu agonists. You can steadily increase the dose to relieve pain.
- **Agonist-antagonists** are another group of opioids. They stimulate some opioid receptors but block others. Agonist-antagonists are rarely used, but are appropriate for moderate to severe acute pain. This group of drugs includes mixed agonist-antagonists, such as pentazocine (Talwin) and nalbuphine (Nubain), and partial agonists, such as buprenorphine (Buprenex). Agonist-antagonists should not be given to patients taking mu agonists (e.g., morphine) because they may act as antagonists at the mu receptor sites and reduce or reverse the analgesia from the mu agonist.

Opioid Effectiveness

The effectiveness of opioids for pain relief can vary depending on individual differences in metabolism. Some patients metabolize opioids poorly; others very rapidly. Body mass alone is not the sole factor for appropriate opioid dosing (D'Arcy, 2008b; Patanwala, Edwards, Stolz, et al., 2012), even though existing opioid regimens tend to be based on lean body mass.

Chronic pain is relatively resistant to effective long-term, opioid analgesia. Although opioids are shown to be effective for certain types of pain, their usefulness is not appreciable in improving physical function with the activities of daily living. Additionally, chronic use of opioids can invoke other hazards, including overdose, physical dependence, and sedation/cognitive impairment (Hooten, Timming, Belgrade, et al., 2013).

Patient Misconceptions About Opioids

Some people may be concerned about using opioids because they fear respiratory depression, drug tolerance, drug dependence, and addiction. Respiratory depression can be treated with naloxone (Narcan), an opioid antagonist.

- **Tolerance** to opioids can occur, but increasing the dose or changing the route of administration can correct that problem. There is no ceiling on the analgesic effects of opioids. Because of the problem of cross-tolerance, opioid rotation and new opioid compounds are used to produce better pain relief (D'Arcy, 2008b).
- **Physical dependence** leads to withdrawal symptoms when the medication is stopped abruptly; it can be prevented by decreasing the dose slowly over time.
- **Key Point:** Psychological dependence, *commonly called* addiction, *occurs in very few patients even after long-term prescribed use of opioids for pain.*

Thus, fear of addiction should not prevent patients from receiving opioids for appropriate pain relief (Pasero, Manworren, & McCaffery, 2008; Patterson, 2008).

Screening for Abuse Potential

Be aware that patients with chronic pain *can* become addicted to or abuse medications. But the addiction is not necessarily *just* because they're taking opioids for pain, but because of their tendencies toward abuse. Considering the prevalence of substance abuse in the general population, assessing the risk for abuse is important for all patients with chronic pain.

Healthcare professionals often fail to recognize substance abuse unless they actively screen for it. Although you may be uncomfortable asking questions about alcohol and illicit drug use, gathering a reliable substance use history is important to provide a foundation for good pain management. This history should include information on the pattern and amount of alcohol intake because patients whose tolerance for alcohol is high may require a higher dose of opioids. Screening should be an integral part of chronic pain management using a validated risk assessment tools, such as the following:

- The **Opioid Risk Tool (ORT).** This is a five-question, yes/no self-report designed to predict a patient's tendency for aberrant behaviors when prescribed opioid analgesia.
- The **Screener and Opioid Assessment for Patients With Pain (SOAPP).** This is a longer, highly reliable tool that may be more appropriate for high-risk populations or when the clinician has time for a thorough assessment.

You can't rely on the normalcy of behavior to indicate opioid abuse. Random drug screening will show opioid use even when aberrant behavior is not evident (Schneider, 2006–2007). To use the Opioid Risk Tool,

 Go to Chapter 31, **Tables, Boxes, Figures: ESG Table 31-2, Using the Opioid Risk Tool,** on Davis*Plus.*

Side Effects of Opioids

Most opioids share the same general side effects, but there are some differences among the specific drugs. You should know, or look up, the side effects of the specific opioid you are to administer.

The most common side effects are nausea, vomiting, constipation, and drowsiness. Other side effects of opioids include difficulty with urination, dry mouth, sweating, tachycardia, palpitations, constipation, bradycardia, rashes, urticaria (hives), or pruritus (itching). Some side effects, such as drowsiness and nausea, improve after a few doses. Large doses may lead to respiratory depression and hypotension.

Most patients experience some degree of sedation at the beginning of opioid therapy or when the dose is increased.

✚ Always assess the patient for level of alertness and respiratory status before you administer an opioid. Excessive sedation will precede respiratory depression. Monitor postoperative patients who receive opioids for sedation and respiratory depression every 1 to 2 hours during the first 12 to 24 hours after surgery.

Be aware that some patients may have a **paradoxical reaction** to opioids. That is, their pain may actually increase despite receiving increasing doses of opioids (Hooten, Timming, Belgrade, et al., 2013).

For an example of an agitation sedation rating scale,

 Go to Chapter 31, **Assessment Guidelines and Tools, Focused Assessment: Richmond Agitation-Sedation Scale,** in Volume 2.

See Box 31-5 for strategies to prevent common side effects.

KnowledgeCheck 31-7

- What are the most common side effects of opioids?
- Identify at least three things that you should monitor when administering opioids.
- What is the risk of addiction to opioids for patients with acute pain?

Equianalgesia

Equianalgesia refers to the approximately equal analgesia that a variety of opioids will provide. Equianalgesic

---

BOX 31-5 ■ Preventing and Treating Side Effects From Opioids

Before deciding to add another medication to treat a side effect, consider changing the dose or frequency of the current opioid or changing to another opioid.

Side Effect: Constipation

- Add more fruits, vegetables, and fiber to the diet. Keep in mind, though, this does not help relieve opioid-induced constipation unless the patient's current fiber intake is deficient. Excessive fiber might even put the patient at risk for bowel obstruction due to the opioid-induced decreased peristalsis (refer to Chapter 29, as needed).
- Increase exercise routine. Even walking short distances will help.
- Increase oral fluid intake to eight 8-ounce glasses of water per day.
- If needed, administer stool softeners.
- If the above are not effective, administer a mild laxative.
- If constipation continues, soften stool with glycerin suppository and follow up with a soapsuds enema.

Side Effect: Nausea and Vomiting

- Reduce opioid dose by combining nonpioid or adjuvant drugs.
- Teach patients that nausea will usually subside after several doses.
- Premedicate or medicate consecutively with an antiemetic. Be aware this may increase sedation, depending on the antiemetic chosen.
- Teach relaxation techniques.

Side Effect: Pruritus

- Reduce opioid dose by combining with nonpioid or adjuvant drugs.
- Use cool packs, lotion, or topical anesthetics.

- Administer antihistamines, such as diphenhydramine (Benadryl). Be aware that this may increase sedation.
- Teach the patient that he can generally expect to develop a tolerance to pruritus.
- Use distraction techniques, which frequently work well.

Side Effect: Respiratory Depression

- Assess the patient's respiratory status *before* administering the opioid and frequently afterward.
- Reduce the opioid dose by combining with nonpioid or adjuvant drugs.
- Reduce the opioid dose by 25% when you observe signs of oversedation.
- If the patient is not responsive or is only minimally responsive, stop the opioid and administer an antagonist, such as naloxone (Narcan), diluted and very slowly. After dosing with a narcotic antidote, reassess the patient for respiratory depression. Naloxone is metabolized more quickly than opioids and therefore repeat dosing might be needed.

Side Effect: Drowsiness

- Assess the patient to ensure that the drowsiness is due to opioid administration and not from another cause.
- Teach the patient that drowsiness will generally subside after a few days as she develops tolerance.
- If analgesia is adequate, reduce the opioid by 25%.
- Discontinue all other nonessential CNS depressant medications.
- During the daytime, offer simple stimulants, such as caffeine.
- Offer a lower dose more frequently to decrease peak concentration.
- Consider another opioid or route of administration.

dose calculations provide a starting point when changing from one opioid to another or from one route of administration to another. For example, a parenteral dose of 5 mg of morphine is equivalent to 60 mg of parenteral codeine or 100 mg of oral codeine in terms of the analgesic effect it produces. As another example, 5 mg of parenteral morphine is the equivalent of 15 mg of oral morphine. These doses are approximate and vary according to the number of doses, the variety of opioids the patient has received, and the needs of the patient. To see a table of equianalgesic dosages among opioids,

 Go to Chapter 31, **Tables, Boxes, Figures: ESG Table 31-3, Equianalgesic Doses of Commonly Used Opioid Analgesics,** on Davis*Plus.*

Routes of Administration for Opioid Analgesics

Use the safest and least invasive route to relieve pain using opioids.

Oral The oral route is convenient, safe, and generally produces steady analgesic levels. It is the preferred route of administration unless rapid onset of analgesia is desired. Use the oral route to provide relief for mild to severe pain. Oral patient-controlled analgesia (oral PCA) is being used in some hospitals to eliminate the delay between the patient's request for medication and the nurse's administration of it.

Nasal A rich supply of blood in the intranasal area provides the drug easy access to systemic circulation. The mixed agonist–antagonist opioid butorphanol and the mu agonist sufentanil can be administered intranasally. One drawback to this route is that it may cause burning or stinging.

Transdermal The transdermal route delivers a continuous release of drug for up to 72 hours. It is a convenient alternative for a patient who requires constant opioid treatment for pain, however it does not provide immediate relief. Fentanyl (Duragesic) is commonly given as a transdermal patch.

Key Point: *Use with care on patients who are febrile (increased body temperature increases absorption of the drug). Inform the patient and family about safe storage and proper disposal of transdermal patches. Proper dating and removing patches after the dose is complete can prevent confusion and dosing errors.*

Rectal Suppositories are an excellent alternative to the oral route, especially in infants and young children and when the patient is vomiting, has a gastrointestinal obstruction, or is at risk for aspiration. The rectal route may be contraindicated in patients with neutropenia or thrombocytopenia because of the potential to cause rectal bleeding while inserting the suppository.

Subcutaneous The subcutaneous route may be used for intermittent injections and continuous administration of opioids. Continuous subcutaneous infusion (CSCI) is appropriate for people who cannot tolerate oral opioids or who have dose-limiting side effects from oral administration (e.g., nausea) and who also have limited venous access. Frequently, CSCI of opioids is used for chronic cancer pain and in palliative care. Hydromorphone and morphine are the drugs most commonly used. Absorption and distribution vary based on the placement site chosen. It is better absorbed, is safer, and provides more continuous relief than the intramuscular (IM) route. Small portable medication pumps allow the patient to be mobile. However, some patients find this method painful and time consuming.

Key Point: *Teach patients and their families how to use the pumps, needles, syringes, and other equipment. Because of the small volume of drug (2 to 3 mL per hour) that can be absorbed, two sites may be needed if higher doses are required.*

Intramuscular (IM) IM injections are painful, the onset of action is slow, and absorption is unreliable. With repeated administration, sterile abscesses and fibrotic tissue can result. The IM route should be avoided in all patients, but especially in children because they often refuse pain medication to avoid having an injection.

Intravenous (IV) The IV route produces immediate pain relief and is desirable for acute or escalating pain. It is most commonly used for short-term therapy and for hospitalized patients who can be monitored. It is, however, also used in the home care setting for patients with cancer and other pain who are unable to tolerate oral opioids. Methods of IV delivery include continuous infusions, bolus, and PCA. Patients on a continuous infusion can deliver a bolus for breakthrough pain or procedures such as wound care. Drawbacks to this route include the need for venous access and the need to maintain a patent line. Patients who previously used oral opioids may find the IV equipment cumbersome but they typically report less pain and fewer side effects than with the oral route.

Intra-articular A pain pump is implanted into a joint during arthroscopic surgery as a measure to control postsurgical pain. A pain pump provides relief to patients by delivering continuous infusion of local anesthetic directly to the surgical site.

Intraspinal and Epidural Analgesics Intraspinal analgesia requires placement of a catheter in the subarachnoid space (for intrathecal analgesia) or the epidural space by an anesthesiologist or a certified registered nurse anesthetist (CRNA). The epidural space is generally preferred because it poses less risk of complications although they can occur, such as dural puncture, infection, hematoma, and nerve damage (see Fig. 31-5). Placement of the catheter, as well as the type and concentration of medication, determines the area affected by the medication. Higher doses are needed for epidural than for intrathecal administration.

The most commonly used opioids for epidural administration are morphine sulfate (Duramorph), fentanyl citrate (Sublimaze), and hydromorphone (Dilaudid). Local

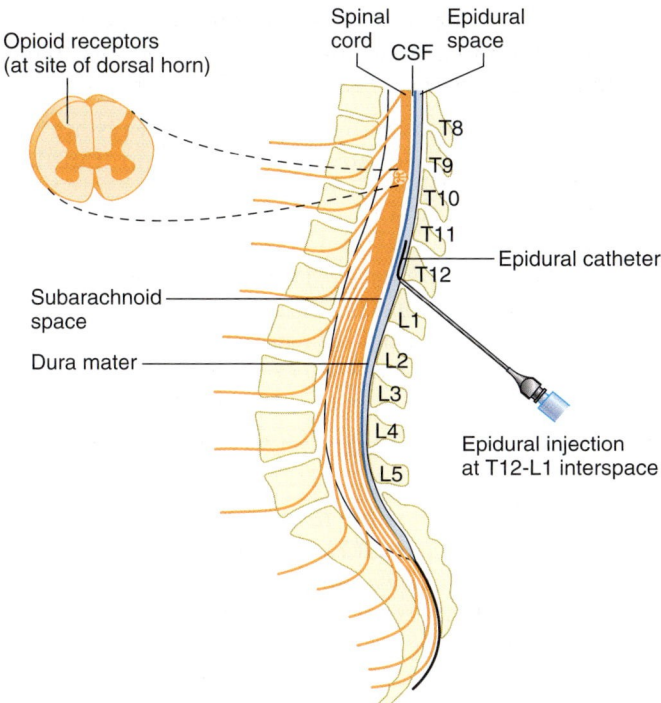

Opioid receptors
(at site of dorsal horn)

Spinal cord

CSF

Epidural space

T8
T9
T10
T11
T12

Epidural catheter

Subarachnoid space

Dura mater

L1
L2
L3
L4
L5

Epidural injection
at T12-L1 interspace

FIGURE 31-5 Placement of an epidural needle and catheter.

anesthetics are frequently combined with the opioids to reduce the total amount of drug necessary to produce analgesia. For nursing care activities associated with caring for a client with an epidural catheter for pain management,

 Go to Chapter 31, **Clinical Insight 31-1: Caring for a Patient With an Epidural Catheter,** in Volume 2.

Peripheral Nerve Catheter Pain Management Therapy
Infusion of regional anesthesia directly to nerves through a catheter provides pain relief during and for the first few days after certain surgeries (e.g., knee, shoulder, ankle).

Patient-Controlled Analgesia (PCA)
PCA pumps are an effective and safe way to deliver opioids by IV, epidural, or subcutaneous routes. They provide excellent pain relief and give the patient a sense of control over the pain. The system consists of a programmable infusion pump, a syringe (or bag), IV tubing, and a button that the patient presses to self-administer a dose. The success of the pump depends on programming a dose that can be administered frequently enough to manage the patient's pain effectively. Rarely, providers order a low continuous rate of infusion (basal rate) that can be supplemented with patient-demand doses.

Most PCA pumps can be programmed with 1- or 4-hour maximum lockout interval to prevent overdosing. If the patient reaches the set limit, the pump will automatically trigger a "lockout" even if the patient keeps pressing the button. You will need to educated patients about this lockout feature, as some might avoid activating the pump in fear of overdosing.

If you are teaching the patient about use of the PCA pump in the postoperative period, make sure he is alert enough to understand the directions and has been given

a hearing aid or glasses, if needed, before you offer your explanation. Encourage patients to administer a dose before potentially painful activities, such as walking or physical therapy. PCA pumps are contraindicated in patients who have limited ability to understand direction.

Because of the potential to overdose the patient, only nurses who are trained in PCAs should set up the pump and the program.

 As a safeguard, another nurse should do an independent double-check of the setup before patient use.

The accompanying Highlights of Procedures box summarizes the key points involved in use of the PCA. For detailed instruction on use of a PCA pump,

 Go to Chapter 31, **Procedure 31-1: Setting Up and Managing a Patient-Controlled Analgesia by Pump,** in Volume 2.

▲ Think**Like a Nurse** 31-7
- What routes of opioid administration have you seen in your clinical rotation?
- What types of pain relief and side effects have you observed?
- What routes of administration would you like to see? Why?

Highlights of Procedure 31-1

For steps to follow in *all* procedures, refer to the Universal Steps for All Procedures found on the inside back cover of Volume 2. Go to the full procedure in Volume 2 to practice and learn the procedure steps. Use these procedure highlights later to help you review key points.

Procedure 31-1: Setting Up and Managing Patient-Controlled Analgesia by Pump

➤ Determine the patient's baseline vital signs, cognitive status, physical mobility, and pain level.

➤ Review the physician prescription for PCA, including the demand dose, the lockout interval between each dose, initial bolus (loading) dose, the basal rate (if prescribed), and the 1-hour or 4-hour lockout dose limit.

➤ Determine whether the patient has an allergy to prescribed medication.

➤ Verify PCA with two nurses before initiating PCA, after any change in pump settings, change of shift, any transfer in care, and when wasting the remainder of medication.

➤ Insert the medication cartridge/syringe into the pump, prime the connecting tubing, and lock the pump.

➤ Set the pump for the demand dose, the lockout interval, loading dose (if prescribed), basal rate (if prescribed), and the 1-hour or 4-hour lockout dose limit.

➤ Connect the tubing into the patient's maintenance IV line.

➤ Start the pump.

➤ Place the button that controls dosing within reach of the patient.

➤ Change tubing per facility protocol.

Chemical Pain Relief Measures

Nerve blocks and **epidural injection** are types of regional anesthesia. An anesthetic agent is injected into or around the nerve that supplies sensation to a specific part of the body. Most nerve blocks affect a network of nerves called a *plexus.* Nerve blocks may be used for short-term pain relief after surgical procedures or for long-term management of chronic pain.

Local anesthesia is the injection of local anesthetics into body tissues. Short-acting agents, such as lidocaine, and long-acting agents, such as marcaine, may be used. Local anesthetics are injected into subcutaneous tissue for minor surgical procedures. They may also be injected into joints and muscle for pain relief. Pumps are commonly used to administer local anesthetics at surgical sites for postoperative pain relief.

Topical anesthesia involves applying an agent that contains cocaine, lidocaine, or benzocaine directly to the skin, mucous membranes, wounds, or burns. Topical anesthesia is quickly absorbed and provides pain relief for mild to moderate pain. Many topical anesthetic agents are available over the counter. Sunburn relief agents, gel products for tooth and gum pain, and first aid sprays are forms of topical anesthetics.

Radiofrequency Ablation Therapy

Radiofrequency ablation therapy uses electromagnetic waves that travel at the speed of light to target nerves that carry pain impulses. This procedure is used to provide longer term pain relief than that provided by injections of steroids or pain relievers and nerve blocks.

Surgical Interruption of Pain Conduction Pathways

Surgical interruption of pain conduction pathways results in permanent destruction of nerve pathways and is used as a last resort for intractable pain. The various options depend on the type and location of pain.

- **Cordotomy** interrupts pain and temperature sensation below the tract that is severed. This is most frequently done for leg and trunk pain.
- **Rhizotomy** interrupts the anterior or posterior nerve route that is located between the ganglion and the cord. Anterior interruption is generally used to stop spastic movements that accompany paraplegia, and posterior interruption eliminates pain in the area innervated. This procedure may be safely performed at any level along the spine but is most often used for head and neck pain produced by cancer.
- **Neurectomy** is used to eliminate intractable localized pain. The pathways of peripheral or cranial nerves are interrupted to block pain transmission.
- **Sympathectomy** severs the paths to the sympathetic division of the autonomic nervous system. The outcomes of this procedure are improvement in vascular blood supply and the elimination of vasospasm. It is used to treat the pain from vascular disorders, such as Raynaud's disease.

Surgical therapies disrupting pain pathways are not widely used because of advances in oral and transdermal opioid therapies.

KnowledgeCheck 31-8

- Identify three types of chemical pain relief measures.
- What type of patient might be suitable for surgical interruption of a pain pathway?

Misconceptions That Interfere With Pain Management

Key Point: *Pain is invisible to others but it exists when the patient says it does. It exists even when there are no sure signs of pain or an apparent cause.*

Patients, caregivers, and clinicians sometimes have beliefs about pain or pain management strategies that interfere with the treatment plan. For instance, one older patient may fear that severe pain is a sign of weakness and try to endure it. Others might perceive pain as a part of the normal physical declines that accompany aging instead of an acute situation that requires treatment. An athlete might believe "no pain, no gain," although actually pain can signal a problem. Or a family member may worry that pain medication may make the patient nonfunctional. Others might fear addiction to pain medication even though non-narcotic analgesics are not addictive.

The beliefs of healthcare providers can also interfere with pain management. For example, nurses and other caregivers sometimes doubt the patient's report of pain because:

- Most people don't have pain from that particular illness or procedure.
- There is no obvious, physical cause for the pain.
- They are concerned about drug-seeking behavior and patient addiction.

As you care for patients in pain, remain open to the patient's description of pain, and work with the patient and caregivers to provide pain control. Table 31-1 highlights some of the most common misconceptions about pain.

Managing Pain in Older Patients

Pain, particularly persistent pain, is common among older adults, especially those suffering from degenerative spine conditions, arthritis, nightly leg pain, or pain as a result of cancer. Pain management among older patients is especially complex. Most older adults have at least one chronic condition and take multiple medications. Adding analgesics to a complex medication regimen increases the likelihood of drug interactions. In addition, drug distribution is altered in older patients because of changes in blood

Table 31-1 ➤ Common Misconceptions Among Patients and Caregivers About Pain

FALLACY	TRUTH
The caregiver is more objective than the patient about the amount of pain experienced.	The patient's report is the "gold standard," and the patient is the authority.
You should wait until the pain is severe before taking medication.	You should take pain medication early and on a scheduled basis even if pain is not severe.
There is a significant danger of addiction to pain medications.	Patients in pain rarely become addicted to their pain medications.
Pain is a normal component of aging.	Pain is a symptom that something is wrong and should be treated.
Complaining of pain will label the person as a "bad patient."	The patient should report pain so that it can be treated.
Patients should have severe pain only if they have major surgery.	Even minor surgery and injury can produce severe pain.
Patients will have visible physical or behavioral signs if they are really in pain.	Even when patients are in severe pain, they may not exhibit physical or behavioral signs.

flow to the organs, protein binding, and the difference in body composition. Older adults are at great risk for undertreatment of pain because they and their caregivers may be reluctant to administer analgesics for fear of producing confusion, excessive sedation, drug interactions, and respiratory depression (AGS, Panel on Persistent Pain in Older Persons, 2009).

Another problem for sufficiently treating pain in older adults is that pain is often unrecognized because of dementia, coexisting medical conditions, sensory impairment, or inability to verbally communicate the quality or intensity of pain. Poor pain management can result in falls, poor sleep, delayed healing, reduced activity, prolonged hospitalization, anxiety, and poor quality of life (Horgas, 2007). At the same time, there is a risk of overtreatment due to the higher peak effect and longer duration of pain relief that they experience as a result of changes associated with aging (AGS, Panel on Persistent Pain in Older Persons, 2009; Christo, 2009).

Persistent pain is not a normal part of aging and should not be ignored. For updated recommendations, see the American Geriatrics Society (AGS) Panel on Pharmacological Management of Persistent Pain in Older Persons,

 Go to Chapter 31, **Tables, Boxes, Figures: ESG Table 31-4, AGS Panel on Pharmacological Management of Persistent Pain in Older Persons**, on DavisPlus.

The AGS guidelines for managing persistent pain in older adults no longer recommend that seniors use over-the-counter (OTC) or prescription NSAIDs, such as aspirin or ibuprofen, before being prescribed an opioid medication. In light of increased cardiovascular risk and gastrointestinal toxicity in this population, the AGS Panel recommends the following:

- Consider opioid therapy for all patients with moderate to severe pain or diminished quality of life due to pain.

- Consider acetaminophen for treatment of persistent pain, particularly musculoskeletal pain, in light of its effectiveness and safety.
- Consult the guidelines about the use of adjuvant therapy for older persons with recurring pain.

ThinkLike a Nurse 31-8

- Which groups of patients are most at risk for inadequate pain management?
- What can you do to assist each group?
- How do past pain experiences affect present pain experience?

Managing Pain in Patients With Substance Abuse or Active Addiction

It is important to differentiate between physical dependence, which is expected and treatable, and addiction. **Addiction** is a state of psychological dependence in which a person uses a drug compulsively and will engage in self-destructive behavior to obtain the drug. Many studies have shown that the properly managed, short-term medical use of opioid analgesic drugs is safe and rarely causes addiction with the exception of those with a personal or family history of drug abuse or mental illness (National Institutes of Health [NIH], National Institute on Drug Abuse, 2001, revised 2011).

Nevertheless, substance abuse is a common problem within our society and is a problem among individuals from all backgrounds. Behaviors that may indicate substance abuse or addiction include the following:

- Repeated requests for injections of an opioid or atypical high dosing when pain should normally be diminishing with recovery from an injury or surgery
- Refusal to try oral medication for pain relief
- "Doctor shopping"—moving from provider to provider in an effort to obtain multiple prescriptions for the drug(s) they abuse
- "Pharmacy shopping"—using multiple pharmacies to dispense controlled substances

If you observe these signs, assess the patient carefully because the signs may also indicate untreated withdrawal or increased pain due to complications. When dealing with clients with active addiction, try to assume a nonjudgmental approach.

Although it is important to recognize opioid addiction, you must be careful not to undertreat pain in patients whom you know or suspect to abuse substances. As a nurse, you will be in a position to help maintain the balance between providing adequate pain relief and protecting against inappropriate drug use.

 ## ThinkLike a Nurse 31-9

You are preparing to give your patient a bath. When you remove his bath equipment from under the bedside table, you find illicit drugs mixed in with the bath equipment. What would you do?

Pain Relief From Placebos

A **placebo** is defined as "any medication or procedure, including surgery, that produces an effect in a patient because of its implicit or explicit intent, not because of its specific physical or chemical properties" (McCaffery & Pasero, 1999, p. 36). Placebos contain inactive substances that do not chemically provide analgesia. Clearly, placebos can relieve pain for some patients. How they do so is not well understood. Theories include operant conditioning, faith, anxiety reduction, and endorphin release. Although use of placebos may be appropriate in clinical trials, they are not suitable for pain management for the following reasons:

- If the patient responds to a placebo, it does not mean that the patient did not have pain. In classic studies done in the 1950s, 36% of patients demonstrated adequate pain relief from a placebo injection the day after abdominal surgery (Evans, 1974). However, there is no way to determine in advance which patients will experience pain relief; therefore, you risk inadequately treating the patient.
- Even in the same patient, placebos may relieve pain at one time and not at another.
- Ethically, the most important reason for not using placebos is that their use involves deceit. If discovered, and it frequently is, the patient's trust in healthcare professionals will be diminished, if not destroyed.

Teaching the Patient and Family About Pain

Patients and caregivers tend to cope more effectively when they are well informed. Because pain can interfere with a patient's learning, be sure to include the patient's family in your teaching. If the patient is discharged from the facility with a prescription for opioids, teach the family how to monitor for excessive sedation and to call the healthcare provider if pain relief is not adequate.

You should discuss the following topics with the patient and family:

- The cause of the pain, if it is known
- The normal duration of the pain, if known (e.g., postoperative pain generally decreases every day as tissues heal)
- How to use the selected pain scale; ask for a demonstration of use
- The overall pain management plan
- Information about the analgesic prescribed—dose, interval, and route of administration
- If opioids are prescribed, explanation that the risk of addiction is extremely low
- Nonpharmacological ways to treat pain
- Side effects to observe for
- The need to alter the treatment plan if relief is not achieved
- How to contact the healthcare team regarding side effects, missed doses, change in condition, or ineffective pain management

Documentation

Thoroughly document the pain management plan and the patient's responses. Documentation may be narrative, in either nursing or interdisciplinary notes, or recorded on a pain management flowsheet. Although documentation varies from facility to facility, it typically reflects the entire spectrum of the nursing process:

- The expected outcome for pain management
- The patient's pain level at the present time
- The patient's response to any intervention for pain
- Any adverse reactions that may have resulted from the analgesic
- Planned interventions to improve the pain relief if needed

Typically, pain management flowsheets contain a column for time, pain ratings, and analgesic used, including dose and route, vital signs, and side effects. They are tailored to the patient population, the type of pain being monitored, and the clinical setting. For example, the pain flowsheet for a patient on an IV PCA pump will be more complex than a pain flowsheet for a patient on oral medications at home. Documentation is important because typically pain recall is poor and patients often underestimate their pain after the fact. If pain is not adequately documented, there is no way to prove that it was accurately assessed. For an example of a pain flow sheet,

 Go to Chapter 31, **Tables, Boxes, Figures: ESG Figure 31-3, Pain Flow Sheet,** on Davis*Plus*.

■ EVALUATION

Evaluation is critical to a pain management program. Compare your findings with the expected outcomes to determine whether the pain management strategy is effective. Questions to ask include the following:

- Are the patient's pain scores consistently at or better than the desired level? Are they improving?
- Is the patient's behavior, mobility, range of motion, mood, and affect consistent with pain relief?
- What is the quality of the patient's life, according to the patient's standards?

In addition to evaluating the extent to which the pain was relieved, you need to determine which interventions were or were not effective, as well as any adverse reactions to these interventions. Close examination of the patient's pain relief diary should provide most of the data you need for evaluation. For a sample of a client diary,

 Go to Chapter 31, **Assessment Guidelines and Tools, Focused Assessment: Pain Relief Diary,** in Volume 2.

It is important to reassess the patient's pain regularly. An increase in pain may be a sign of inadequate pain management, but it may also be a sign of developing complications. Before implementing a change in the treatment plan, you should determine whether the pain management plan was carried out correctly. If the decision of the healthcare team is to make a change, remember to evaluate again the effect of this change. Do not assume your intervention will provide adequate pain relief.

NURSING PROCESS IN ACTION

Mary Jean Thompson, 30 years old, was admitted to the hospital with severe abdominal pain and underwent an appendectomy yesterday. The surgeon has prescribed hydromorphone (Dilaudid) 2 mg tablet PO q4 hr prn for pain. Ms. Thompson doesn't like the idea of taking pain medication and waits until she rates her pain a 9 or 10 on a scale of 0 to 10 before requesting medication. Even after the medication, her pain never drops below a 7 on a scale of 0 to 10 and she is unwilling to turn or ambulate because of the pain.

When you perform your assessment, she tells you she does not want to be sedated. "I hate that groggy, drugged feeling. I'm willing to have some pain to avoid that." After you discuss the importance of pain management to aid in healing and ability to participate in activities and therapy, Ms. Thompson states that she would like to have a pain score of 3 to 4 today. See the accompanying plan for her pain management.

Pain Management: Nursing Care

Nursing Diagnosis: Acute Pain (surgical incision) related to possible inadequate analgesia (drug and dosing) because of reluctance to take pain medication, as manifested by not requesting medication until her pain is at a score of 9

EXPECTED OUTCOMES	NURSING INTERVENTIONS	RATIONALE
On a scale of 0–10, the patient will verbalize pain relief at a score of 3 or below while in bed and 4 or below while ambulating at all times.	Assess and document the patient's verbal and nonverbal expressions of pain relief with each check of vital signs, with every procedure and ambulation, and when the patient is at rest.	Assessment is necessary to determine the effectiveness of the prescribed medications. Assessment and documentation are legal responsibilities for the nurse as well.
	Discuss with the prescriber the need to modify medication dose or type if pain relief measures are ineffective. Recommend PCA.	Ineffective pain management will cause the patient increased stress and can lead to further complications because the patient will be unwilling to move.
	When you obtain new pain orders for a PCA morphine pump, educate the patient about the pump.	A patient using PCA requires instruction about safe use of the pump.
	Provide nonpharmacological interventions, such as a back rub or other techniques described in this chapter, before rest or sleep, with any exacerbation of pain, and after painful procedures such as ambulation.	Nonpharmacological interventions are synergistic and enhance the relief the opioid gives (Shin & Kolanowski, 2010).
The patient will demonstrate pain relief by participating in ambulation and turning within 24 hours.	Teach the patient to press the self-administered pain medication using the PCA before activities.	Peak blood levels enable the patient to ambulate, cough and deep-breathe, and perform activities of daily living.

To explore learning resources for this chapter,

Go to DavisPlus at DavisPl.us/Wilkinson3.

Chapter Resources for Chapter 31:
    Response sheets for all learning activities
    Resources for Caregivers and Health Professionals
    Reading More About Pain (suggested readings)
    Concept Map of chapter content
Interactive Case Studies
NCLEX-Style and Chapter Review Questions
Chapter Overview Podcasts

For references cited in this chapter,

Go to Volume 2, **References Cited.**

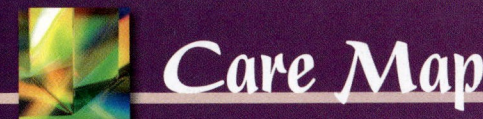

Care Map

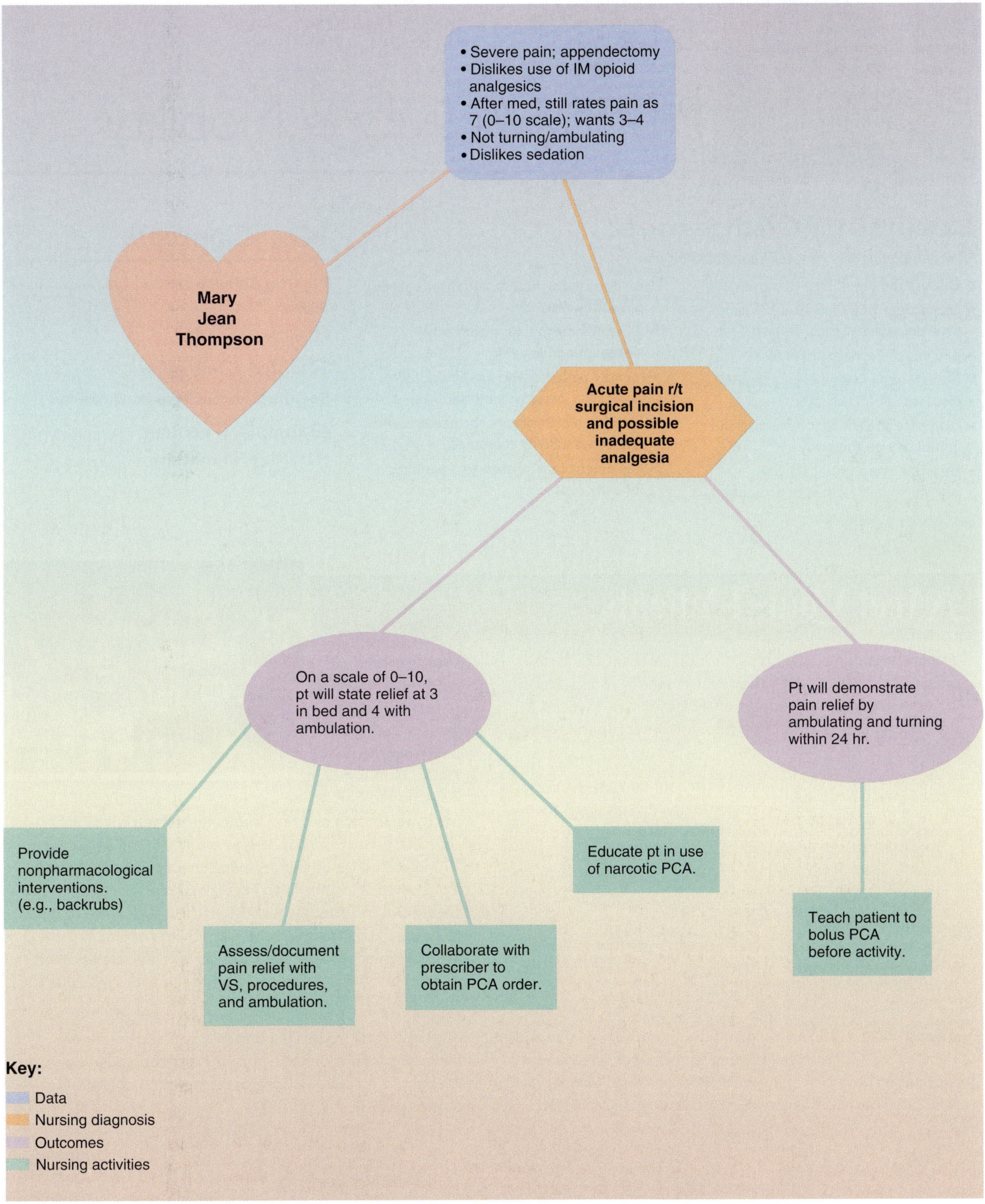

- Severe pain; appendectomy
- Dislikes use of IM opioid analgesics
- After med, still rates pain as 7 (0–10 scale); wants 3–4
- Not turning/ambulating
- Dislikes sedation

Mary Jean Thompson

Acute pain r/t surgical incision and possible inadequate analgesia

On a scale of 0–10, pt will state relief at 3 in bed and 4 with ambulation.

Pt will demonstrate pain relief by ambulating and turning within 24 hr.

Provide nonpharmacological interventions. (e.g., backrubs)

Assess/document pain relief with VS, procedures, and ambulation.

Collaborate with prescriber to obtain PCA order.

Educate pt in use of narcotic PCA.

Teach patient to bolus PCA before activity.

Key:

Data
Nursing diagnosis
Outcomes
Nursing activities

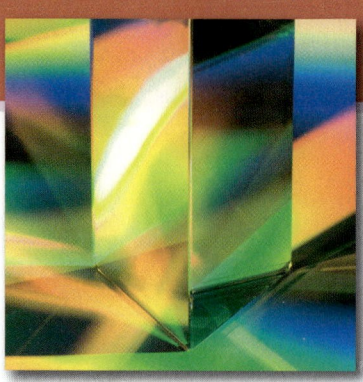

CHAPTER 32

Physical Activity & Mobility

Learning Outcomes

After completing this chapter, you should be able to:

> Discuss the physiology of movement.
> Use proper body mechanics when providing patient care.
> Discuss the concept of fitness.
> Describe the five types of exercise discussed in this chapter.
> Compare the effects of exercise and immobility on the body.
> Describe the physical activity recommended for health promotion,
> cardiovascular fitness, and maintenance of healthy weight.
> Discuss factors that affect body alignment and activity.
> Identify patients who are at risk for immobility or activity intolerance.
> Develop a plan of care for patients with decreased activity tolerance.
> Implement care related to a patient's mobility problems.

Key Concepts

Physical Activity
Fitness
Mobility

Related Concepts

See the Concept Map on DavisPlus.

Example Problem

Hazards of immobility

Meet Your Patients

You are attending a health promotion series at the local hospital in order to fulfill the requirement in your state for continuing nursing education. For the next 4 weeks, the topic is exercise. In the group, you meet the following people:

- Phillip Flanders is a 40-year-old accountant. He works long hours in an office setting doing work that is sedentary and requires concentration. Although he is not physically active, he often feels tired. He does not exercise regularly. Many of his friends have suggested that he begin some kind of exercise program to improve his energy and health. Phillip would like to learn how to get started with an overall fitness program that works with his work and family life. Before getting started, he makes an appointment with his primary care provider for a thorough health evaluation.
- Peter Phan is 28 years old and is a marathon runner and triathlete. On average, he runs 35 miles per week and cycles at least twice per week. Peter has had plantar fasciitis in the past that was painful and caused him to

miss exercise. Peter would like to learn what he can do to prevent other injuries.

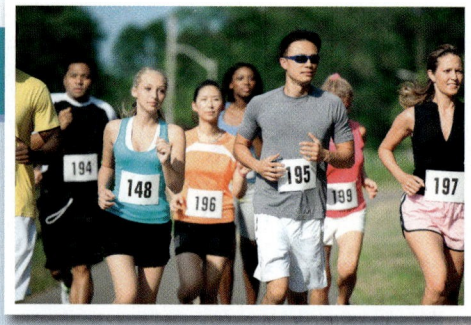

- Helen Jillian is 72 years old. She has hypertension and high cholesterol levels for which she takes four medications. She is 5 ft 1 in. tall and weighs 290 lb. Recently she began having chest pain when starting a brisk walk. Her physician prescribed nitroglycerin for the chest pain, and after a thorough cardiac evaluation told her to enroll in this class and the CardioFit program at the hospital. She does not understand why she is being asked to do these things because activity seems to trigger her chest pain.

In this chapter, you will find answers to each of these patient questions about activity and exercise. In addition, you will learn more about assisting patients with mobility problems.

Theoretical Knowledge
knowing **why**

Primitive nomadic people were active just meeting their daily needs. Tribes commonly journeyed to hunt for game; women were on foot gathering roots, fruits, and other edible plants. Survival depended on physical activity, such as changing locations to find food or escape a dangerous situation. Later, the shift to an agricultural society reduced the need for most people to hunt and gather food. However, even farming was hard work and people were physically active most of the year.

Today, with modern grocery distribution systems, we expend little to no energy to obtain food. In addition, there are many occupations in which people spend hours at a desk or in front of a computer screen. Many of today's leisure activities, (e.g., watching television, playing video games) are also sedentary. Even though fitness equipment and health clubs are popular, the overall level of fitness in the United States is declining. Nearly half of adolescents do not engage in regular, moderate to vigorous activity. And, more than two-thirds of adults do not achieve the recommended amount of physical activity needed for health and fitness. Regular exercise, one study found, does not reduce the risk of an otherwise sedentary lifestyle (e.g., greater risk of diabetes, cardiovascular disease, obesity, and premature death) (Gray, 2012). To get enough exercise, most people need to make a conscious effort to build exercise and activity into their lives. This chapter will help you to understand why that is important.

ABOUT THE KEY CONCEPTS

Two concepts are widely used to describe human movement: physical activity and fitness. Physical **activity** is bodily movement produced by the contraction of skeletal muscle that increases energy expenditure above a baseline level (U.S. Department of Health and Human Services [USDHHS], 2008). **Exercise** is a subconcept of physical activity. It is planned, structured, and repetitive and purposeful for improving or maintaining physical fitness, physical performance, or health (Caspersen, Powell, & Christenson, 1985). **Fitness** (or physical fitness) is the ability to carry out activities of daily living with vigor and alertness, without undue fatigue, and with enough energy for leisure pursuits and to respond to emergencies (USDHHS, 2008).

As you read this chapter, you will learn how the key concepts of activity, fitness, and mobility are related, and how they relate to subconcepts, such as exercise and body mechanics. Once you have a grasp of these concepts, you should be able to apply them to any patient, regardless of their particular health problem or medical diagnosis.

PHYSIOLOGY OF MOVEMENT

Activity and exercise require body movement (**mobility**). Mobility depends on the successful interaction among the skeleton, the muscles, and the nervous system.

Skeletal System

The skeletal system includes bones, cartilage, ligaments, and tendons. The skeleton forms the framework of the body, protects the internal organs, produces blood cells, and stores mineral salts (e.g., calcium) and fat.

Bones consist of a hard outer shell with a spongy interior (Fig. 32-1). There are 206 bones in the human body. Some bones are long (such as the femur and humerus), some short (phalanges and metacarpals), some flat (sternum and cranial bones), and some are irregularly shaped (vertebrae and tarsal bones). The short, flat, and irregular bones contain red bone marrow that produces red blood cells.

Bones feel strong and tough, so it is easy to forget that they are composed of living tissue that is constantly building and remodeling. **Osteoclasts** are specialized cells that function as housekeepers in the bone by breaking down old or damaged tissue. **Osteoblasts** repair damaged bone and build new bone to keep the skeleton strong. A delicate balance exists between the actions of the osteoblasts and the osteoclasts.

When two bones come close together (**articulate**), a joint is formed. Body movement occurs at the joints. Joints are classified based on the amount of movement they permit:

- **Synarthroses** are immovable joints (e.g., the sutures between the cranial bones). In youth, these joints have some flexibility to allow growth, but they gradually become rigid.

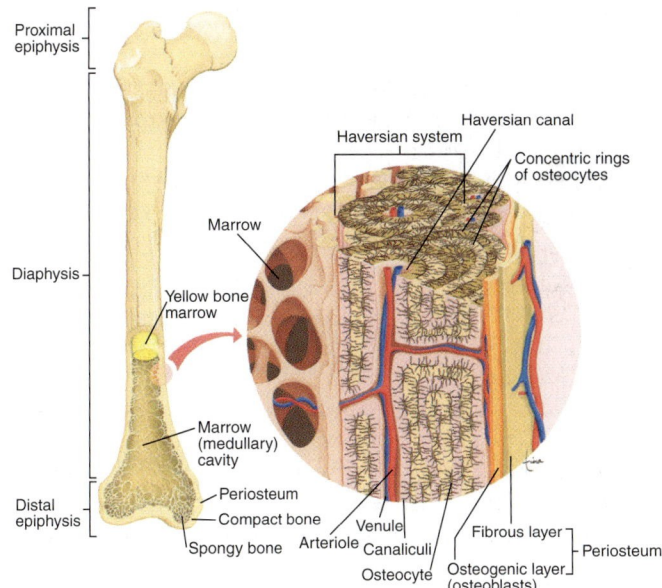

FIGURE 32-1 Bone is complex living tissue.

- **Amphiarthroses** allow for limited movement. Examples are the joints between the vertebrae and pubic bones.
- **Diarthroses,** or **synovial joints,** are freely movable because of the amount of space between the articulating bones. Synovial joints are filled with **synovial fluid,** and the joint surfaces of the articulating bones are covered with smooth **articular cartilage** (connective tissue found in the joints and skeleton). The synovial fluid and articular cartilage prevent friction as the bones move. Table 32-1 identifies the types of movable joints in the body.

Cartilage, ligaments, and tendons serve as the interface between the skeleton and the muscles. Ligaments are fibrous tissues that connect most movable joints. Ligaments are flexible to allow freedom of movement, but strong and tough so they do not yield under force of movement. Tendons are fibrous connective tissues that attach muscles to the bone. Muscles span a joint and attach by tendons to two different bones.

Muscles

Muscles make up 40% to 50% of body weight. When they contract, they cause movement. The type of movement depends on the type of muscle: skeletal, smooth, or cardiac.

- **Skeletal muscle** moves bones and joints.
- **Smooth muscle,** occurring in the digestive tract and other hollow structures, such as the bladder and blood vessels, produces movement of food through the digestive tract, urine through the urinary tract, and blood through the circulatory system.
- **Cardiac muscle** is a unique form of muscle that has the ability to contract spontaneously. It is responsible for the beating of the heart.

Muscles attach to bone at two points: (1) at the *point of origin*, to the more stationary bone, and (2) at the *point of insertion*, to the more movable bone. The "belly" (thickest part) of the muscle lies between these two points. When a skeletal muscle contracts, it shortens, thus causing one bone to move at the joint. Muscles work in pairs. For example, the biceps brachii contracts to flex the forearm (bend the elbow joint). When the biceps contracts, the opposing muscle, the triceps brachii, relaxes. Similarly, contraction of the triceps is associated with relaxation of the biceps (Fig. 32-2).

Nervous System

The nervous system controls the movement of the musculoskeletal system. Motor nerves are either autonomic or somatic. The **autonomic nervous system** consists of the sympathetic and parasympathetic nervous systems, which innervate involuntary muscles, such as the heart, blood vessels, and glands. The **somatic nervous system** innervates the voluntary skeletal muscles.

When you make a conscious decision to bend your elbow, the thought originates in the motor area of your cerebral cortex. The upper motor efferent nerves communicate with the lower motor neurons that conduct impulses to the muscles. When the muscle receives sufficient stimuli, it contracts the biceps as the triceps relaxes and moves the elbow. Movement also occurs through reflex mechanisms. Common reflexes include the knee-jerk reflex and corneal reflex. Reflexes are discussed at length in Chapter 22.

A muscle contraction, whether conscious or reflexive, stimulates afferent nerves that convey information to the cerebral cortex and the cerebellum. This information helps control and coordinate movements.

Table 32-1 ➤ Types of Synovial Joints		
TYPE	**DESCRIPTION**	**EXAMPLES**
Ball-and-socket	A rounded head (ball) fits into a cup-like structure (socket) to allow movement in all planes in addition to rotation.	Shoulder and hip joints
Condyloid	An oval-shaped bone fits into an elliptical cavity to allow movement in two planes at right angles to each other.	Wrist
Gliding	Two flat plane surfaces move past each other.	Intervertebral joints
Hinge	A convex surface fits into a cavity, allowing flexion and extension.	Knee and elbow
Pivot	The joint is formed by a ring-like object that turns on a pivot. Motion is limited to rotation.	The atlas and axis of the first vertebrae and base of the skull
Saddle	One bone surface is concave in one direction and convex in the other. The other surface has the opposite construction so that the bones fit together. Movement is possible in two planes at right angles to each other.	Carpal–metacarpal joint of the thumb

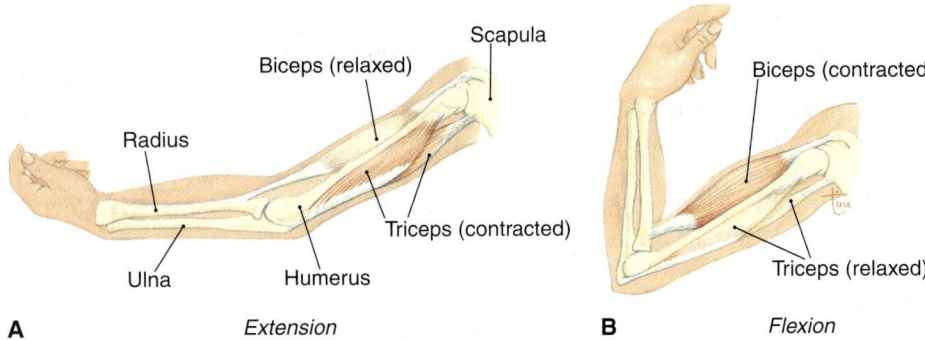

FIGURE 32-2 Antagonistic muscles. *A,* Extension of the forearm. *B,* Flexion of the forearm.

KnowledgeCheck 32-1

- Name three purposes of the skeletal system.
- Define the following movements: abduction, adduction, flexion, extension, circumduction, internal rotation, supination, and pronation.
- Identify three types of muscle.
- How do the muscles and the nerves interact?

BODY MECHANICS

Body mechanics is a term used to describe the way we move our bodies. It includes four components: body alignment, balance, coordination, and joint mobility. You should always use good body mechanics and teach them to patients for back safety and injury prevention. In addition to discussing those components, this chapter also presents some guidelines to use when teaching your patients about safe movement and lifting.

The following are concepts used to describe problems with muscle mass, strength, or mobility.

Body Alignment

Body alignment, or posture, is an important aspect of body mechanics. Proper posture places the spine in a neutral (resting) position. There are four natural curves to the spine (Fig. 32-3). Proper posture maintains these natural curves because it allows movement to occur with less stress and fatigue; the bones are aligned, and the muscles, joints, and ligaments can work at peak efficiency. Good posture contributes to the normal functioning of the nervous system and improves feelings of well-being (see the Self-Care box Tips to Maintain Proper Posture). Most posture problems result from a combination of the following:

Accidents, injuries, and falls
Careless sitting, standing, or sleeping habits
Excessive weight
Foot problems or improper shoes
Negative self-image
Occupational stress
Poor sleep support (mattress)
Poorly designed workspace
Visual difficulties
Weak muscles or muscle imbalance
Skeletal misalignment or malformation (e.g., scoliosis, kyphosis)

Self-Care

Tips to Maintain Proper Posture

➤ Avoid standing in one position for a lengthy period. If you cannot change positions, elevate one foot on a stool or box, and alternate foot placement frequently.

➤ Do not lock your knees when standing upright.

➤ Keep your stomach muscles tight to support your back.

➤ Do not bend forward at the waist or neck when you are working in a low position.

➤ When you are seated at your desk, work at a comfortable height.

➤ Do not wear high-heeled or platform shoes for long periods of time.

➤ Do not slump when you sit.

➤ Sit close to your work.

➤ Use a chair that supports your back in a slightly arched position.

➤ Sit with your feet flat on the floor and your knees below your hips.

➤ Sleep on a mattress that is firm but not extremely hard.

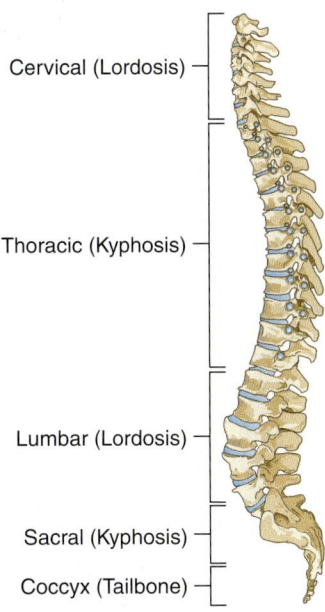

Lateral (side) spinal column

Cervical (Lordosis)

Thoracic (Kyphosis)

Lumbar (Lordosis)

Sacral (Kyphosis)

Coccyx (Tailbone)

FIGURE 32-3 There are four natural curves to the spine.

Balance

The body achieves balance when it is in alignment. For your body to be balanced, your line of gravity must pass through your center of gravity, and your center of gravity must be close to your base of support. The **line of gravity** is an imaginary vertical line drawn from the top of the head through the center of gravity. The **center of gravity** is the point around which mass is distributed. In the human body, the center of gravity is below the umbilicus at the top of the pelvis. The **base of support** is what holds the body up. The feet provide the base of support.

To avoid injury when moving objects, place your center of gravity closest to your base of support and stand with your head erect, buttocks pulled in, abdominal muscles tight, chest high, shoulders pulled back, and feet wide (Fig. 32-4). Use a wide stance, with feet apart and one foot forward when standing for a long period of time. The broader the base of support, the lower the center of gravity, and the easier it is to maintain balance.

Coordination

Smooth movement requires coordination between the nervous system and the musculoskeletal system. Voluntary movement is initiated in the cerebral cortex. However, the cerebellum coordinates movements. As you may recall, *proprioception*—the awareness of posture, movement, and position sense—is largely controlled by the cerebellum. The basal ganglia, located deep in the cerebrum, assist with coordination of movement. Damage to the motor cortex, cerebellum, or basal ganglia affects coordination of movement. For example, a stroke affecting the motor cortex alters gait and changes posture.

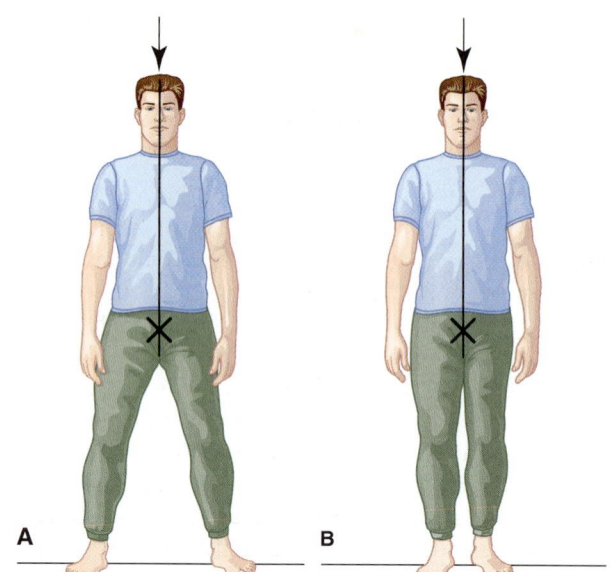

FIGURE 32-4 *A*, With a wide stance, the center of gravity (x) is closer to the base of support. *B*, With a narrow stance, the body is less stable.

Joint Mobility

The key concept **mobility** refers to a person's ability to move within the environment (*Taber's Cyclopedic Medical Dictionary*, 22nd ed.). Joint movement allows us to sit, stand, bend, walk, and perform other activities. **Range of motion (ROM)** is the maximum movement possible at a joint. **Active range of motion** (AROM) is movement of the joint performed by the individual without assistance. The patient independently moves his joints through flexion, extension, abduction, adduction, and circular rotation. AROM involves strength and flexibility; and is part of being physically fit. For that reason, stretching exercises are included in a comprehensive exercise program. **Passive ROM** (PROM) involves moving joints through their ROM when the patient is unable to do so for himself. For other terms describing body movement,

 Go to Chapter 32, **Tables, Range of Motion at the Joints,** in Volume 2.

To see animations of joints and range of motion,

 Go to **Animations: Range of Motion Animations,** on Davis*Plus*.

Body Mechanics Guidelines

Principles of body mechanics are the rules that allow you to move your body while reducing your risk for injury. Historically, nurses have used body mechanics guidelines as the cornerstone of safe practice for moving and lifting patients. However, because of patient characteristics and condition (e.g., obesity), as well as the patient care environment, you cannot rely on body mechanics alone to prevent injury. Think about it. A patient's weight is not evenly distributed or may be positioned awkwardly. He might be combative or simply a moving target (Howard, 2010; Waters, Nelson, Hughes, et al., 2009). There is no reason to "prove yourself" by transferring without the use of an assistive device (e.g., lift, transfer board, or other staff). The American Nurses Association (ANA) launched the national campaign *Handle With Care* to reduce the risk of back and musculoskeletal injuries among nurses. This campaign emphasizes the use of assistive devices to decrease the risk of injury and recommends virtually no manual lifting (ANA, n.d.). For guidelines to help you assess patients' transfer abilities and use good body mechanics,

 Go to Chapter 32, **Clinical Insight 32-1: Applying Principles of Body Mechanics,** in Volume 2.

KnowledgeCheck 32-2

- Identify the four components of body mechanics.
- Give at least five guidelines for good body mechanics.

ThinkLike a Nurse 32-1

While you are attending the health promotion class, Helen Jillian (Meet Your Patients) develops chest pain and must be assisted to a wheelchair for transport to the emergency department.

- Based on what you know about body mechanics, how would you be able to assist Ms. Jillian?
- What additional information do you need to know?

PHYSICAL ACTIVITY AND EXERCISE

Physical activity refers to bodily movement and energy expenditure involving contraction of the skeletal muscles above basal level. Bodily movement can be grouped into two basic categories:

- **Baseline activity** refers to the light-intensity activities of daily living, such as standing, walking slowly, and lifting lightweight objects.
- **Exercise (health-enhancing physical activity)** is more than baseline to produce health-enhancing benefits. People who are physically fit are able to perform activities of daily living with vigor and alertness and with enough energy to enjoy work and leisure activities. (USDHHS, 2008)

Types of Exercise

Health-enhancing physical activity (exercise) may be classified according to the type of muscle contraction it involves and according to whether it uses oxygen for energy.

Isometric exercises involve muscle contraction without motion. They are usually performed against an immovable surface or object, for example, pressing the hand against a wall. The muscles of the arm contract, but the wall does not move. Each position is held for 6 to 8 seconds and repeated 5 to 10 times. Isometric training is effective for developing total strength of a particular muscle or group of muscles. It is often used for rehabilitation because the exact area of muscle weakness can be isolated and strengthening can be administered at the proper joint angle. This kind of training requires no special equipment, and there is little chance of injury. Patients who are bed-bound can use this form of exercise to maintain or regain muscle strength.

Isotonic exercise involves movement of the joint during the muscle contraction. A classic example of an isotonic exercise is weight training with free weights. As the weight is moved throughout the ROM, the muscle shortens and lengthens. Calisthenics, such as chin-ups, push-ups, and sit-ups, all of which use body weight as the resistance force, are also isotonic exercises.

Isokinetic exercise is performed with specialized apparatuses that provide variable resistance to movement. Isokinetic exercise combines the best features of both isometrics and weight training by providing resistance at a constant, preset speed while the muscle moves through the full ROM. Specialized machines available at health and fitness facilities and physical therapy departments are used for this form of exercise.

Aerobic exercise acquires energy from metabolic pathways that use oxygen—the amount of oxygen taken into the body meets or exceeds the amount of oxygen required to perform the activity. Aerobic exercise uses large muscle groups, can be maintained continuously, and is rhythmic in nature. It increases the heart and respiratory rates, thereby providing exercise for the cardiovascular system while simultaneously exercising the skeletal muscles. Jogging, brisk walking, and cycling are common forms of aerobic exercise.

Anaerobic exercise occurs when the amount of oxygen taken into the body does not meet the amount of oxygen required to perform the activity. Therefore, the muscles must obtain energy from metabolic pathways that do not use oxygen. Rapid, intense exercises such as lifting heavy objects and sprinting are examples of anaerobic exercise.

Planning and Evaluating a Fitness Program

A well-rounded fitness program focuses on flexibility, resistance training, and aerobic conditioning. The **mode** of exercise is the type of activity. Aerobic (endurance) and muscle-strengthening (resistance) physical activities both promote better health. Factors when designing or evaluating an exercise program include the following:

Flexibility Training Stretching before exercise helps warm up the muscles and prevents injury during exercise. Stretching after exercise cools the muscles and limits post-exercise stiffness.

 As we get older, joints and muscles become stiffer. A regular flexibility program helps maintain mobility as aging occurs.

Resistance Training Movement against resistance increases muscular strength and endurance. Perhaps the most common type of resistance training is weight lifting. When a person is exercising for strength, the goal is to increase the amount of resistance with each exercise (i.e., lift more weight). When a person is exercising for endurance, the goal is to increase the number of repetitions with each exercise (i.e., lift the weight more times).

Aerobic Conditioning Fitness and body composition are improved by aerobic conditioning. Components of aerobic conditioning include intensity, duration, frequency, and mode. Intensity is how hard one is exercising. Box 32-1 describes three common tests used to evaluate exercise intensity.

Amount of Physical Activity Duration is the amount of time one is exercising. To achieve and maintain healthy level of fitness, the USDHHS recommends 150 minutes/week or more of moderate-intensity physical activity (e.g., brisk walking) coupled with increasing the activity every day (USDHHS, 2008). The **frequency** of exercise should be 3 to 5 days per week, although the more often and the longer the duration, as tolerated, the better.

Older adults at risk for falls should engage in balance exercises at least 3 days per week. Muscle strengthening should be performed for all major muscles but not on consecutive days. Walking is an excellent form of physical activity for those who can walk safely.

See Box 32-2.

BOX 32-1 ■ Tests for Determining Exercise Intensity

Target Heart Rate Method

In the target heart rate method, the target heart rate (THR) is calculated from an estimate of maximum heart rate. The estimated maximum heart rate is calculated using the following formula:

$$\text{Maximum heart rate} = 220 - \text{age}$$

The THR is calculated as a percentage of the maximum heart rate. Most persons can exercise at 60% to 80% of the maximum heart rate.

For example, consider a 50-year-old woman. Her maximum heart rate is 170 beats/min. To exercise at 75% intensity, her target heart rate is 128 beats/min.

$$\text{Maximum heart rate} = 220 - 50 = 170$$

$$\text{Target heart rate} = 0.75 \times 170 = 128$$

The person's heart rate during exercise should be 128 beats/min, excluding warm-up and cool-down.

Talk Test

The talk test evaluates exercise intensity based on the person's ability to talk while exercising. Short phrases interspersed with breaths or feeling like you can "just respond" is considered an appropriate level of exercise. If you are too short of breath to answer, the level of intensity is too high. An ability to carry on a conversation indicates that you are not exercising hard enough.

Borg Rate of Perceived Exertion Scale®

The Rate of Perceived Exertion (RPE) scale is easy to use. The person who is exercising selects the rating based on how difficult the exercise feels at that time. The exerciser selects one of eight categories that best describes the intensity of activity. RPE ratings range from *No Exertion at All* to *Extremely Hard*. *Extremely Hard* is associated with exercise that corresponds to almost 100% of maximum heart rate. *Somewhat Hard* corresponds with 75% of maximum heart rate; this is the level you should encourage for most individuals.

Sources: Borg, G. (1998). *Borg's perceived exertion and pain scales.* Stockholm, Sweden: Human Kinetics; Foster, C. (2004). "Talk test" measures exercise intensity. *Medicine & Science in Sports & Exercise, 36*(9), 1632–1636.

BOX 32-2 ■ U.S. Department of Health and Human Services 2008 Physical Activity Guidelines for Americans

Children and Adolescents

- Engage in at least 1 hour of physical activity daily.
- Physical activity should be enjoyable. A variety of activities will improve adherence.
- Most activity should be aerobic, either moderate or vigorous intensity.
- At least 3 days/week, children and teens should participate in vigorous-intensity exercise as well as muscle- and bone-strengthening physical activity.

Adults and Older Adults

- To gain substantial health benefits, get at least 150 minutes per week of moderate-intensity or 75 minutes a week of vigorous-intensity aerobic physical activity, or an equivalent combination of moderate- and vigorous-intensity aerobic activity. More frequent exercise (i.e., 300 minutes/week) is even more beneficial.
- Engage in aerobic activity throughout the week in episodes of at least 10 min. Longer periods of time provide additional benefits.
- For additional health benefits, perform moderate or high-intensity muscle and bone-strengthening activities on 2 or more days per week.

Specific to Older Adults

- Older adults unable to perform 150 minutes of moderate-intensity aerobic activity per week should be as physically active as abilities and conditions allow.
- Include exercises that maintain or improve balance, tone, and muscle strength.

Adults, Children, and Adolescents With Disabilities

- Be as physically active as abilities allow with guidance from their healthcare provider.

Healthy Pregnant and Postpartum Women

- Consult with the healthcare provider regarding activity level throughout pregnancy. If the pregnancy or postpartum recovery is uncomplicated, then those who regularly engage in vigorous-intensity aerobic activity or in high amounts of activity can continue with this regimen.
- If not already engaged in vigorous-intensity physical activity, get at least 150 minutes of moderate-intensity aerobic activity per week, preferably spread throughout the week after consulting with healthcare provider.

Source: Adapted from U.S. Department of Health and Human Services (USDHHS). (2008). *2008 physical activity guidelines for Americans.* Retrieved from www.health.gov/paguidelines

Many people become discouraged because they don't see immediate results from their efforts. However, subtle changes occur long before the person sees changes in weight or shape. Not only can instructional fitness videos, trainers and group exercise make participation more engaging, but they also help to improve form and safety through demonstration of proper technique. Tips to help develop an exercise program are included in the Self-Care box Teaching Clients How to Set Up a Fitness Program.

Key Point: *Anyone with a chronic condition or symptoms of a new health issue should be under the care of a healthcare provider.*

Benefits of Regular Exercise

Regular physical activity each week, sustained for months and years, can produce long-term health benefits. Strong evidence links regular physical activity with a lower risk for early death, heart disease, stroke, type 2

Teaching Clients How to Set Up a Fitness Program

If you are older than 40, smoke or drink, are sedentary, are overweight, or have a chronic health condition, have a medical evaluation before starting an exercise program.

Getting Started

➤ Choose a variety of exercises that you enjoy and feel comfortable doing, such as walking, biking, dancing, or a team sport.

➤ Find allies. Exercising with someone else can make it more fun. If you choose to exercise by yourself, pick a friend with whom you can discuss your exercise progress.

➤ Vary your routine. You may be less likely to get bored or injured.

➤ Choose a comfortable time of day.

➤ Don't get discouraged. It can take weeks or months before you notice some of the changes from exercise.

➤ Forget "no pain, no gain." Although a little soreness is normal after you first start exercising, pain isn't. Stop if you hurt.

➤ Make exercise fun. Find fun things to do, such as taking a walk through the park or watching your favorite show while riding a stationary bike.

➤ Sign a contract committing yourself to exercise.

➤ Find an accountability partner. A fitness program is not only more enjoyable when shared with someone else but also is more successful with others for whom you are accountable.

➤ Keep a daily log of your activities.

➤ Think about joining a health club. The cost gives some people an incentive to exercise regularly.

Exercise Tips

➤ Warm up your muscles for 5 to 10 minutes before your main session of aerobic exercise.

➤ Maintain your exercise intensity for 30 to 45 minutes.

➤ Gradually decrease the intensity of your workout (cool down) and then stretch for 5 to 10 minutes at the end of your workout.

➤ Accumulate physical activity throughout the day. For example:

   Take the stairs instead of the elevator.

   Go for a walk during your coffee break or lunch.

   Walk all or part of the way to work.

   Park your car at the far end of the parking lot.

➤ Wear good, shock-absorbing footwear. Shoes that do not support your feet will cause stress on leg bones and the back and, over time, lead to injury.

➤ Alternate easy and hard exercise days, or alternate modes of exercise (e.g., alternate running, swimming, and biking).

➤ Take a day off periodically. The body needs a chance to rest and allow bones, joints, and muscles to rest and repair.

➤ To avoid becoming dehydrated, drink at least 8 ounces of fluid before the exercise, and then pause regularly during the exercise for more. If you are thirsty after the exercise session, drink until you feel satiated. Water is still the best liquid to drink during and after exercise. However, you can't rely on feeling thirsty as a reminder to replace fluid lost through sweating; one of nature's dirty tricks is that exercise suppresses thirst.

---

diabetes, hypertension, hyperlipidemia, metabolic syndrome, colon and breast cancers, and depression.

For those who have been inactive, walking is a good form of exercise. And for older adults, the risk of injury to joints is lower than other forms of physical activity. Even brisk walking for as little as 30 minutes a day, when done consistently, promotes weight loss and maintenance of normal weight when combined with diet; lowers the risk of disability; and promotes better heart and lung function and muscular fitness. Moderate-intensity walking helps older adults to improve strength, balance, and muscle tone, which helps to prevent falls and to improve overall physical stamina. Otherwise, moderate intensity exercise enhances psychological well-being, reduces depressive symptoms, and improves memory and mental clarity in older adults (Jitramontree, 2010).

Weight-bearing exercise reduces loss of bone density in adults and older adults (USDHHS, 2008). Resistance training does not lead to weight loss; instead, it may increase loss of fat mass and improve muscle tone and strength (Donnelly, Blair, Jakicic, et al., 2009). Exercise is associated with an overall decrease in mortality in men and women of all ages and an overall improvement in quality of life for people in all ethnic groups and across the life span. People with disabilities also benefit from physical activity (USDHHS, 2008). Box 32-3 presents numerous other benefits of regular exercise.

Risks Associated With Exercise

Armed with theoretical knowledge, you should be able to teach your clients realistically about the risks associated with exercise and thereby help them to exercise safely. Risks include cardiac injury, musculoskeletal injury, dehydration, hypoglycemia, and temperature regulation problems. Keep in mind that the benefits of exercise far outweigh the risks. Advise clients to follow the tips in the Self-Care box Teaching Your Patient How to Prevent Back Injury to exercise safely and help prevent injury.

Cardiac Injury Fear of triggering a cardiac event prevents some people from exercising. However, exercise

BOX 32-3 ■ Benefits of Regular Exercise

Cardiovascular System

- Improves pumping action of the heart.
- Decreases heart rate, heart rate variability, and blood pressure.
- Improves circulation by increasing the number of capillaries.
- Improves venous return to the heart.
- Increases blood volume and hematocrit.
- Increases high-density lipoprotein (HDL).
- Decreases low-density lipoprotein (LDL) and total cholesterol.
- Decreases risk of thrombophlebitis.

Respiratory System

- Improves pulmonary circulation.
- Improves gas exchange at the alveolar–capillary membrane, and overal aerobic capacity.
- Dilates bronchioles to increase ventilation.

Musculoskeletal System

- Improves skeletal development in children.
- Increases muscle mass, strength, power, and endurance.
- Improves flexibility.
- Increases coordination.
- Helps maintain joint structure and function; reduces risk of osteoarthritis.
- Improves bone mass and mineral density.
- Improves gait speed, stability, and balance.

  - Improves bone mass with aging; reduces risk of osteoporosis.
  - Reduces risk of falls and helps older adults maintain an independent lifestyle.

Nervous System

- Speeds nerve impulse transmission.
- Reduces sympathetic response to exercise.
- Improves reaction time.

Endocrine System

- Increases sensitivity to insulin at the receptor sites.
- Increases efficiency of metabolic processes.
- Improves temperature regulation.

- Facilitates weight management.
- Decreases adipose surrounding organs.

Gastrointestinal System

- Improves appetite.
- Improves abdominal muscle tone.
- Decreases risk of colon cancer.

Urinary System

- Increases efficiency of kidney function.

Integumentary System

- Improves skin tone as a result of improved circulation.

Immune System

- Reduces susceptibility to minor viral illnesses.
- Reduces systemic inflammation.

Mental Health

- Boosts energy level.
- Release endorphins, which assist with pain control and stress management.
- Improves self-esteem and body image.
- Provides a nonpharmacological way to relieve symptoms of anxiety and depression.
- Leads to positive outlook and sense of optimism.

  - Promotes clearer thinking and improved memory in older adults.

- Enhances feelings of well being and diminishes depressive symptoms.
- Relieves some stress.
- Can be a source of social interaction.

Overall Health

- Burns calories to achieve and maintain healthy body weight.
- Leads to reduced abdominal obesity.
- Improves overall stamina.
- Reduces fatigue.
- Increases sleep time and improves sleep quality.

Source: Adapted from President's Council on Sports, Fitness, and Health. (2010, June). Exercise comes of age: Medicine for older adults. *Research Digest, 10*(3), 1–3. Retrieved from https://www.presidentschallenge.org/informed/digest/docs/june2010digest.pdf

itself is rarely life threatening, especially when compared with the alternative (*not* exercising). Before starting an exercise program or significantly increasing the intensity of normal workouts, seasoned athletes as well as rank beginners should be screened for underlying health problems, such as high blood pressure, thickened heart muscle (cardiac hypertrophy), electrical abnormalities, and blood vessel abnormalities. In people without underlying heart disease, recreational drug use

is an important cause of sudden cardiac arrest, whether during exercise or at rest.

Musculoskeletal Injury High-impact exercises, such as running or aerobic dance, may pose a risk for injuries to bones, joints, and muscles. However, you can prevent most such injuries by gradually increasing the activity level or varying activities. Walking is an exercise that most people can do without injury. Injury can also occur from lifting weights. Free weights can cause injury if the

Teaching Your Older Adult Patient About Increasing Physical Activity and Exercise

What Are the Benefits of Physical Activity for an Older Adult?

➤ Improves and maintains strength so you can stay as independent as possible.

➤ Maintains balance and prevents falls.

➤ Gives you more energy to do the things you want to do.

➤ Helps you to sleep better and feel more rested.

➤ Perks up your mood and helps reduce depression.

➤ Prevents or delays some diseases like diabetes, heart disease, and cancer.

What Kind of Physical Activity Should I Do?

➤ Get at least 30 minutes of *endurance* activity almost every day. Exercise that makes you breathe hard builds strength and staying power.

➤ Wear a step counter to monitor your level of *endurance* activity. Set goals and monitor your progress. If you are taking 10,000 or more steps per day, you are probably getting an adequate amount of physical activity.

➤ Incorporate *resistance* into your exercise; use some kind of weight or isometric activity to build strength. Remember that you can do more and are less likely to fall when your muscles are strong.

➤ Do things to work on your *balance* (e.g., standing on one foot). This can help to prevent falls.

➤ Daily stretching will help you be more *flexible* and prevent injury.

Who Should Exercise?

Almost anyone can do some type of physical activity, but before starting a new exercise program check with your healthcare provider if you experience:

➤ Any change in your health in the past 6 months

➤ Shortness of breath or dizziness

➤ Chest pain or pressure, or fluttering heart

➤ Joint pain or swelling

➤ Unexplained weight loss

➤ An infection with fever

➤ Eye problems

➤ Blood clot

➤ Hernia

➤ Recent hip surgery or joint injury

Source: Adapted from the National Institutes of Health, National Institute on Aging. (2011, updated 2013). *Exercise and physical activity: Your everyday guide from the National Institute on Aging.* Retrieved from http://www.nia.nih.gov/HealthInformation/Publications/exercise.htm

Teaching Your Patient How to Prevent Back Injury

➤ Poor posture is one of the main causes of back pain. Make a conscious effort to maintain good posture at all times.

➤ Use a firm mattress that provides adequate support.

➤ Sit with your knees slightly lower than your hips.

➤ If you must stand for a long period of time, flex your hip and raise one foot on a stool or object 6 to 8 inches off the ground. Periodically switch legs.

➤ Wear comfortable, low-heeled shoes. Avoid high heels as much as possible.

➤ Avoid restrictive clothing that inhibits your ability to use good body mechanics.

➤ Follow principles of body mechanics at all times (e.g., use wide base of support, and do not lift with your back) but keep in mind manual lifting techniques are based on loads that weigh far less than typical patients.

➤ Manual lifting techniques are based on the assumption that the load is stable and held close to the body.

➤ Exercise regularly to maintain your optimal weight and strengthen the muscles of your body.

➤ Include abdominal exercises in your routine. Strong abdominal muscles help support the back.

➤ Avoid lifting excessive weight.

➤ Avoid exercises or movements that cause spinal flexion (e.g., toe-touches, sit-ups with knees extended), excessive flexion of the neck (e.g., abdominal crunches with neck curved to chest), or spinal rotation (twisting).

person lifts too much weight or uses poor body mechanics when lifting. Working with a fitness trainer to learn correct form and what are appropriate weights markedly decreases the risk of injury. In addition, exercise machines provide some degree of control and are less likely to cause injury.

Dehydration It is possible to become dehydrated with prolonged exercise, with warm temperatures, or as a result of health problems or medications. During an intense exercise period, the body can lose 2 liters of fluid for every hour of exercise. It is important to drink water before, during, and after the exercise period. Water is still the best choice during and after exercise. Some sports drinks include glucose and electrolytes for replacement and quick energy and can be used for endurance activities or prolonged, intense activity.

Temperature Regulation Problems Hyperthermia can occur when the person exercises in a hot climate. Hyperthermia is often accompanied by dehydration. **Heat exhaustion** is a potentially life-threatening event. Signs of heat exhaustion include light-headedness, nausea, headache, fatigue, hyperventilation, loss of concentration, and abdominal cramps. Body temperature rises, but the skin is clammy and cold. In contrast, **hypothermia** can occur when the person does not wear proper clothing or is exposed to cool water for an extended period of time. Hypothermia is characterized by fatigue, confusion, and lack of coordination.

KnowledgeCheck 32-3

- Identify and describe four types of exercise.
- State the components of an exercise program

ThinkLike a Nurse 32-2

- How would you address Helen Jillian's (Meet Your Patients) concerns about the risks associated with engaging in an exercise program?
- Peter Phan (Meet Your Patients) has experienced a number of injuries as a result of his exercise. Based on your knowledge of exercise, what questions would you like to ask Peter about his exercise program?

FACTORS AFFECTING MOBILITY AND ACTIVITY

Recall that physical activity is bodily movement produced by the contraction of skeletal muscles. **Mobility** refers to a person's capacity for bodily movement, or how well the person is able to move about in the environment. Factors influencing activity and mobility include developmental stage, nutrition, lifestyle, attitudes, external factors, diseases, and physical abnormalities. These factors are discussed in the next sections.

Developmental Stage

Neuromuscular development is related to age. A newborn can move his extremities and turn his head from side to side, but he is unable to get from place to place. As the child matures, motor skills and coordination develop. In spite of that, children in the United States are becoming more sedentary, contributing to the continuing rise of obesity among children, adolescents, and adults. The Centers for Disease Control and Prevention (CDC) reports the following:

- More than one-third of adults and almost 18% of youths were obese in 2012. Obesity rates did not differ between men and women. Older adults were more likely to be obese than younger adults (USDHHS, 2012).
- Obesity rates for children have more than doubled, while quadrupling in adolescents in the last three decades. Among children, aged 6 to 11, nearly 18% are obese, compared to 7% in 1980; and now 21% of those ages 12 to 19 are, compared to 5% at that time (Ogden, Carroll, Kit, et al., 2014).
- Only 36% of young adults get regular physical activity in their spare time.

- Only 26% of young adults were doing strength training at least twice per week, which is a minimum recommendation for adults of all ages (CDC, updated 2014).

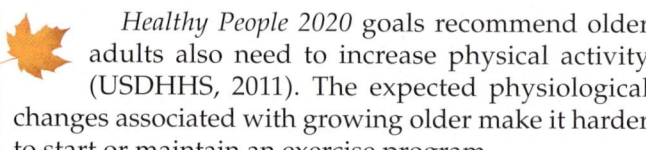

Healthy People 2020 goals recommend older adults also need to increase physical activity (USDHHS, 2011). The expected physiological changes associated with growing older make it harder to start or maintain an exercise program.

The result is increased risk for chronic health problems. For a discussion of neuromuscular development across the life span and associated nursing considerations as it affects activity and exercise,

 Go to Chapter 32, **Tables, Boxes, Figures: ESG Table 32-1, The Influence of Developmental Stage on Activity and Exercise,** on *DavisPlus*.

Nutrition

In the United States, obesity is a major health problem. Centers for Disease Control and Prevention report more than one-third of adults in the United States are obese (Ogden, Carrol, Kit, et al., 2014). Obesity often leads to health problems, which indirectly reduces activity and can in turn contribute to further obesity. For example, joint injuries and osteoarthritis are more prevalent with obesity, which in turn reduces a person's physical activity. Unhealthy eating patterns, such as large portions, consumption of convenience foods, and a diet high in saturated fat and simple carbohydrates, play a major role in the obesity problem. Although the obese person has plenty of calories available to expend on exercise, movement becomes more difficult as body size increases.

In contrast, people with chronic disease may be in negative nitrogen balance—that is, they do not have adequate protein stores available to maintain or repair body tissue. They experience muscle wasting and fatigue, which lead to reduced activity levels.

Lifestyle

Over the last century, manual labor has declined and work environments have become increasingly sedentary. As a result, individuals need to look toward leisure time for exercise and fitness activities. This requires making time for exercise. Personal values about exercise and fitness determine when, or whether, exercise becomes part of a person's routine.

Some people enjoy exercise. Others see it as pure drudgery or as "something I have to do." A person's culture and support system define what exercise the person is likely to accept. For example, swimming requires wearing a bathing suit. People raised in a culture that values modesty may not choose swimming as a form of exercise. Walking, which allows the person to dress in modest clothing, would be a preferred form of exercise.

Stress

How is your stress level? A high stress level can produce fatigue. Although you may view exercise as one more thing you don't have time for, exercise is energizing and can be used to relieve stress. For example, taking a brisk 20-minute walk during a study break may allow you to continue working for several more hours. You can also use this technique when caring for patients. Hospitalized patients and family members often experience a great deal of stress. Helping the patient take a walk to the courtyard, or instructing family members how to handle the wheelchair so they can take a walk around the block, often will help lessen some of the strain.

Environmental Factors

Environmental factors affecting exercise include weather, pollution, neighborhood conditions, finances, and support systems. Weather has a strong influence on activity level. Cold, damp weather encourages people to stay inside, whereas warm, sunny weather makes it fun to go outside and exercise. Encourage patients to choose a variety of activities that they enjoy so they can exercise regardless of the weather. When air quality is poor, suggest indoor activities in order to reduce exposure to allergens and pollutants.

Neighborhood conditions, such as crime or lack of parks, influence attitudes about outside activities. Mall walking is an example of a successful way to incorporate exercise into daily patterns when neighborhood conditions do not encourage activity. Joining a gym or engaging in sports might be practical for some budgets. However, many activities, such as walking or playing basketball or tennis in the community park, are inexpensive.

The support system is perhaps the most influential external factor. Family and friends who are active are likely to promote and support your efforts to exercise. Those who are sedentary may not encourage you to be more active or lose weight.

Diseases and Abnormalities

Diseases and abnormalities in various body systems can negatively influence body alignment, balance, coordination, and joint mobility. In the next sections, we describe some disorders that affect activity and exercise.

Congenital Abnormalities of the Musculoskeletal System

The following are common congenital abnormalities that affect appearance, motor function, and mobility:

- **Syndactylism** is the fusion of two or more fingers or toes. Most cases involving the hands are treated surgically at an early age to limit the effect on fine motor development.
- **Developmental dysplasia of the hip (DDH)** is a congenital abnormality of the development of the femur, acetabulum, or both that shows as hip dislocation.

- **Foot deformities**, such as clubfoot (talipes equinovarus), occur in about 4% of all newborns. Serial casts or surgery may be used to correct the defect and preserve function.
- **Scoliosis** is a lateral curvature of the spine. Scoliosis can result from congenital bone disorders, neuromuscular impairment, or trauma, but approximately two-thirds of cases have no known cause and are termed idiopathic scoliosis. Idiopathic scoliosis is classified as infantile, juvenile, or adolescent depending on the age at onset.

Diseases Related to Bone Formation or Metabolism

Bone formation abnormalities may be congenital, related to dietary deficiencies, or the result of bone disease.

- **Osteogenesis imperfecta (OI)** is a congenital disorder of bone and connective tissue that is characterized by brittle bones that fracture easily. Infants with OI are often born with fractures and continue to fracture with minimal trauma or even spontaneously. Prompt recognition and treatment of fractures helps prevent deformities.
- **Achondroplasia**, or dwarfism, occurs when the bones ossify (harden) prematurely.
- **Paget's disease** is a metabolic bone disease in which increased bone loss results in pain, pathological fractures, and deformities. This disorder usually affects the skull, vertebrae, femur, and pelvis.
- **Vitamin D and calcium** are needed to form and maintain bone. Deficiencies lead to porous bones. In children, prolonged deficiencies can cause the long bones of the legs to become bowed, retard growth, and lead to frequent fractures.

Diseases Affecting Joint Mobility

Diseases of the joints may be degenerative or inflammatory. The most prevalent type of degenerative joint disease is **osteoarthritis (OA)**. OA involves a loss of articular cartilage in the joint, with pain and stiffness as the primary symptoms. Patients may also have decreased ROM and **crepitus**, a creaking or grating sound, with joint motion. Symptoms are aggravated by weight-bearing and joint use and are relieved by resting the affected joints. OA is more common in women, older adults, and people who are overweight.

Rheumatoid arthritis (RA) is a systemic autoimmune disease involving chronic inflammation of the joints and surrounding connective tissue, frequently resulting in difficulty in performing activities of daily living (ADLs). RA causes joint pain, deformity, and loss of function; patients may also experience fever, fatigue, weakness, and weight loss. RA occurs most frequently in the fingers, wrists, elbows, ankles, and knees. It occurs in 1% to 2% of the population, with a greater incidence in women. The illness usually begins in mid-life, but persons in any age group can be affected. Those in the 30- to 50-year-old range are the most frequently affected age group (Swann, 2007). Unlike OA, RA does not improve with rest. Pain is most intense when the person arises from bed. Pain and joint deformities may so severely affect mobility that patients cannot care for themselves.

Ankylosing spondylitis is a chronic inflammatory joint disease characterized by stiffening and fusion of the spine and sacroiliac joints. The inflammation occurs where the ligaments, tendons, and joint capsule insert into the bone. The disease usually develops in young adults, equally in men and women. Signs and symptoms include low back pain and stiffness and decreased ROM of the spine. The convex lumbar curve is lost, and the upper spine curve increases, causing kyphosis (see Chapter 22 for review).

Gout is an inflammatory response to high levels of uric acid. Crystals form in the synovial fluid, and small white nodules, or *tophi*, form in the subcutaneous tissues. Gout produces painful joints and severely limits activity during acute flare-ups.

Problems Affecting Bone Integrity

Osteoporosis is a decrease in total bone density, which occurs when osteoclast activity outpaces that of the osteoblasts. The internal structure of the bone diminishes, and the bone collapses in on itself. Normally bone mass continues to increase up to the third decade of life. After age 30, bone loss begins. Women experience a rapid decline in bone mass at menopause. In men, a gradual loss continues. As bones become porous, they become weak, leading to vertebral collapse or fractures of the long bones of the arms and legs. Fractures may occur spontaneously or with very slight trauma.

Genetics, body frame, menopausal status, chronic disease and lifestyle choices also play a role. The most common risk factors for osteoporotic fracture are advanced age, low bone mineral density, and previous fracture as an adult. Smoking, low calcium and vitamin D intake, excess alcohol use, and sedentary lifestyle also increase the risk (National Institutes of Health, National Institute on Aging, 2012).

The best treatment for osteoporosis is prevention. Teach adolescents and adults to eat a balanced diet high in calcium, fluoride, and other minerals, and to start an exercise program they can continue throughout their lives.

 Advise older women that weight-bearing exercise can help decrease the rate of bone loss, and advise them to ask their provider about medications to reduce bone mineral loss (National Osteoporosis Foundation, n.d., a)

The National Osteoporosis Foundation (n. d., b) recommends calcium intake for adults age 50 and older to be 1,200 mg/day and vitamin D 800 to 1,000 IU daily to prevent bone loss. Phosphorus is another important bone mineral. But if there is a disproportionate amount of phosphorus compared to the amount of calcium in the diet, bone loss can occur.

They urge people of all ages, but particularly postmenopausal women, to avoid smoking because tobacco reduces the absorption of calcium in the intestine. In addition, more than two drinks of alcohol per day decreases the matrix of the bone and reduces the body's ability to absorb calcium. Other pharmacological options for postmenopausal women include estrogen, parathyroid hormone, and calcitonin.

Osteomyelitis (infection of the bone) may develop after bone injury or surgery. It can be difficult and expensive to treat and can leave the patient with permanent disability. Bone contains microscopic channels that are impermeable to most of the natural defenses of the body. Once bacteria enter these channels, they multiply rapidly.

Bone tumors may also affect form and function. Tumors in the bone cause considerable pain and severely limit activity.

Trauma

Trauma can affect the entire musculoskeletal system. One of the most significant forms of trauma is a **fracture**, or a break in the bone (see Fig. 32-5). Signs and symptoms of a fracture include tenderness at the site, loss of function, deformity of the area, and swelling of the surrounding tissues. However, x-ray is required for definitive diagnosis. Fractures are classified according to the extent of damage. The type and severity of fracture determine whether casting, traction, or surgical repair is necessary. For a classification and description of several types of fractures,

Go to Chapter 32, **Supplemental Materials: Fractures,** and to **Tables, Boxes, Figures: ESG Figure 32-1, Types of Fractures,** on Davis*Plus*.

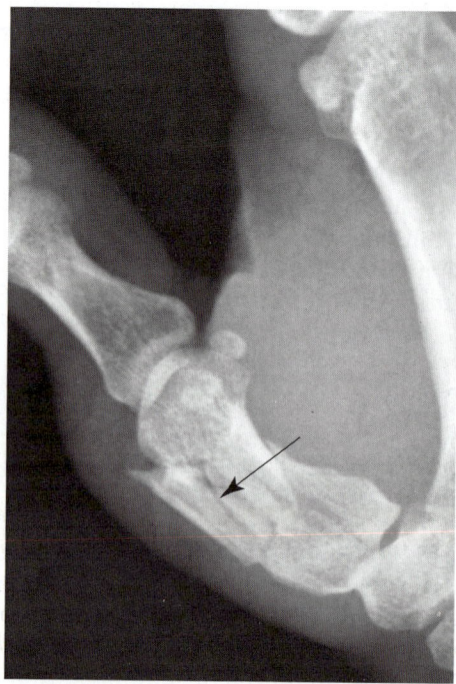

FIGURE 32-5 Fracture in hand occurring after traumatic injury.

To learn about caring for a cast in the home, refer to the Home Care box Teaching Care of a Cast at Home.

Sprains and strains are more common than fractures. A **sprain** is a stretch injury of a ligament that causes the ligament to tear. A partial tear can usually heal with rest, but a complete tear often requires surgery to stabilize the joint. A **strain** is an injury to muscle caused by excessive stress on the muscle. Both strains and sprains cause pain at the site of injury, swelling, and loss of function. As you can see, the signs and symptoms are the same as those of a fracture. As a result, x-ray studies are used to distinguish these injuries. Initial treatment of fractures, sprains, and strains include rest, ice, compression, and elevation.

Stretching and tearing injuries to the meniscus (knee cap), lateral knee ligaments, and Achilles tendon are also fairly common. Magnetic resonance imaging (MRI) studies are done to determine the extent of injury. Rest and ice are necessary, but often surgical repair is needed to achieve full healing.

Disorders of the Central Nervous System

Any disorder that affects the motor centers of the brain or the transmission of nerve impulses will affect mobility. Cerebrovascular accident (stroke), head or spinal cord injury, multiple sclerosis (a disorder affecting nerve transmission), and myasthenia gravis (a disease caused by antibodies to the acetylcholine receptors at the neuromuscular junction) are examples. Progressive degenerative disorders of the neurological system also affect mobility and coordination. For example, Parkinson's disease is a progressive degeneration of the basal ganglia. It produces tremor, rigidity, and difficulty coordinating movement.

Diseases of Other Body Systems

Diseases affecting other body systems may affect mobility and activity tolerance, as in the following examples:

- ■ *Respiratory disorders.* Any disorder that affects oxygenation limits exercise tolerance. Chronic obstructive

---

Home Care

Teaching Care of a Cast at Home

➤ Always keep the cast clean and dry.

➤ Before bathing, cover the cast with a plastic bag and tape the opening shut or use a commercial cast cover with Velcro straps. Do not place the cast into water unless it is made of water-repellent material. Keep in mind that waterproof casts are not for all types of fractures. They can't be used for recently manipulated fractures or when skin pins are used.

➤ If the cast gets wet enough that the skin gets wet under the cast, it may break down and infection may occur. Dry it immediately with a blow dryer on the cool setting. Be careful—skin can be burned using the hot setting. If you have any trouble getting the cast dry, the cast may need to be replaced. Call the healthcare provider if the cast doesn't dry properly.

➤ Sweating under the cast enough to make it damp may cause mold or mildew to develop. Call the healthcare provider if you notice odor coming from the cast.

➤ ✚ Never put anything inside the cast. Do not try to scratch the skin under the cast with any sharp objects, such as a hanger or pencil. This may break the skin under the cast and cause it to become infected. Do not use powders, ointments, or lotions inside the cast.

➤ Sometimes when swelling goes down, the cast can become loose and rub on the skin. If this is the case, advise your patient to call the primary provider to look at the cast.

➤ Check the circulation by gently squeezing a finger or toe below the cast. It should blanch (turn lighter) and quickly return to a pink color. The fingers and toes should be warm to the touch, able to move freely, and not tingling or numb.

➤ Do not trim the cast or break off any rough edges. This may weaken or break the cast. If a fiberglass cast has a rough edge, use a metal file to smooth it or call the healthcare provider.

➤ A sling may be needed for support if the cast is on the hand, wrist, arm, or elbow. It is helpful to wrap soft sheepskin or padding behind the neck to protect the skin and make it feel more comfortable.

➤ If the cast is on the foot or leg, do not walk on or put any weight on the injured leg, unless the doctor allows it.

➤ If the primary provider allows walking on the cast, be sure to wear the cast boot. The boot is to reduce wear and tear on the bottom and has a tread to prevent slipping and falling.

➤ Crutches may be needed to walk if a cast is on the foot, ankle, or leg. Make sure the crutches are adjusted properly before leaving the hospital or the doctor's office.

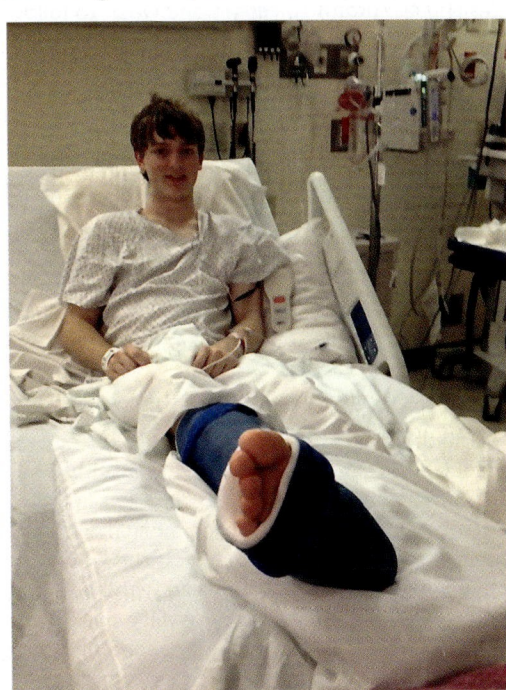

pulmonary disease, asthma, and pneumonia are associated with shortness of breath, which becomes worse with increased activity.

- *Circulatory disorders.* Impaired arterial circulation limits oxygen delivery to the tissue. As activity increases, skeletal muscle pain develops. Impaired venous circulation causes leg swelling and discomfort, which are relieved by elevating the legs. As a result, patients may become relatively sedentary to relieve the pain and discomfort.
- *Fatigue.* Acute illnesses, such as influenza, produce fatigue and limit activity for short periods of time. Disorders that produce long-standing fatigue include anemia, anorexia nervosa, cancer, depression, and grief.
- *Bedrest* is part of the treatment for a variety of disorders. For example, a woman with a high-risk pregnancy may be placed on bedrest. You will learn more about bedrest and the effects of immobility in the following section.

KnowledgeCheck 32-4

- In which age groups are you more likely to see health concerns that affect mobility?
- What types of disorders limit activity or mobility?

- What are the signs and symptoms of a fracture?
- What is the difference between a strain and a sprain?

 ThinkLike a Nurse 32-3

- Your teenage daughter complains when you ask her to take a calcium supplement and encourage her to exercise. What information should you provide so she understands why these measures are important?
- Phillip Flanders (Meet Your Patients) has never been involved in a regular exercise program. Phil works as an accountant, and most of his friends are work associates. Phil's siblings are overweight and do not exercise. Both of his parents died of heart disease. Many of Phil's friends have suggested that he begin exercising to improve his energy and health. What recommendations can you make to Phil to make it more likely that he will start and continue an exercise routine?

Example Problem: Hazards of Immobility

Most people take their mobility for granted until illness, disease, or trauma affects their ability to move. Even short periods of immobility may be difficult. If you've ever had the flu or an illness that sent you to bed, you know that it can take several days to return to your pre-illness state, especially for older adults and people with

---

Quality and Safety Education for Nurses

Effects of Teamwork and Collaboration on Outcomes

Chapter Key Concept: Mobility

Competency: Teamwork and Collaboration (Knowledge, Skills, Attitudes); Patient-Centered Care (Knowledge, Skills, Attitudes)*

Situation: Mr. Lee underwent surgery to repair a ruptured quadriceps tendon in his left leg. His discharge instructions did not include information specific to quadriceps tendon repair but provided general guidelines about wound care, signs and symptoms to report, and when to follow up with the physician.

At his 2-week post-op visit, Mr. Lee was making good progress. The surgeon gave him a prescription to start physical therapy, telling him that the therapists at a nearby location knew his protocols. He also told Mr. Lee that he could drive and return to work, but that he should "listen to his body" and rest when he was tired or in pain. Mrs. Lee mentioned that the drive to work was 1 hour each way and wondered if that was too much. After the surgeon left, the nurse removed the staples from the incision and talked to Mr. and Mrs. Lee about potential complications and how to perform wound care.

The next day, Mr. and Mrs. Lee met with Bernadette, a physical therapist at the location the doctor suggested. She scheduled Mr. Lee for therapy on Mondays, Wednesdays, and Thursdays, which fit her schedule. During the first visit Mrs. Lee could hear her husband moaning with pain. On the second visit, Mrs. Lee remarked that the knee was very swollen but the therapist disagreed with her, noting that other patients had much more swelling than Mr. Lee. One week later Mr. Lee went to the surgeon's office afraid that something was wrong. He was experiencing severe pain and

a fever of 101°F. The surgeon concluded that the knee was not damaged or infected, but that it was very inflamed. He told Mr. Lee he should not have scheduled back-to-back therapy sessions and that he was "overdoing" it. It took 2 weeks before the pain, swelling, and fever subsided.

Think about it: Patient-centered care, teamwork, and collaboration are considered integral to patient safety and quality care. (1) Were Mr. Lee's outcomes affected by the team's communication pattern? Identify the problems. (2) Did Mr. Lee's care reflect patient-centeredness? While developing your answers, consider the following questions and concepts:

➤ How would you describe this team's functioning?

➤ What barriers to team functioning do you think might exist in this scenario?

➤ What could the office nurse have done to improve collaboration?

➤ How did teamwork and communication affect safety?

➤ What system changes would you make to improve communication?

➤ Did the team value Mrs. Lee's input? How might outcomes have been different if Mrs. Lee had been recognized as a full partner in planning or providing care? Do you think quality, safety, costs, and patient satisfaction were affected?

To learn about specific Knowledge, Skills, and Attitudes,

 Go to the QSEN Web site at http://qsen.org/ competencies/pre-licensure-ksas/

underlying chronic illness. Severe illness associated with prolonged immobilization causes physiological changes in almost every body system, along with psychological changes. Some changes are reversible, but others are not. These changes are discussed below.

Effect of Immobility on Muscles and Bones

Even a couple of days in bed can leave you feeling tired and weak, because the musculoskeletal system is one of the first systems affected by immobility. Inactivity causes significant wasting of the gastrocnemius, soleus, and leg muscles that control flexion and extension of the hip, knee, and ankle. Confinement to bed leads to 7% to 10% loss of muscle strength (atrophy) per week. Immobility also causes the joints to become stiff. The strongest muscles, usually the flexors, pull the joints in their direction, leading to **contractures**, or joint **ankylosis** (fusion of the joints).

Immobility affects parathyroid function, calcium metabolism, and therefore bone formation. The result of these changes is osteoporosis, calcium depletion in the joints, and **renal calculi** (kidney stones) due to increased excretion of calcium. These changes place the patient at risk for pathological fractures with minimal trauma.

Effects of Immobility on the Lungs

Immobility decreases the strength of all muscles, including those involved in chest wall expansion, which also affects ventilation. When a patient is in bed, the depth of respirations decreases, and secretions pool in the airways. The strength to effectively cough and expectorate secretions diminishes as muscle tone of the abdomen and chest decrease. As a result, pooled secretions block air passages and alveoli, decrease oxygen and carbon dioxide exchange, and often lead to atelectasis (collapse of air sacs), or pneumonia. Even a sedentary lifestyle affects the capacity to increase ventilation in response to exercise (see Chapter 36 if you want more information about ventilation).

Effect of Immobility on the Heart and Vessels

Immobility increases the workload of the heart and promotes venous stasis. When you are active, the skeletal muscles of the legs help pump blood back to the heart. Recall that the veins are thin-walled vessels with valves. Muscle activity propels blood toward the right side of the heart, and the valves prevent backflow of blood. To compensate for immobility, heart rate and stroke volume increase to maintain blood pressure. But with immobility, cardiac reserves are lessened, which means the heart is less able to respond to demands above baseline. Without muscle activity, the force of gravity causes blood to pool in the periphery, which leads to edema. Fluid in the tissue (e.g., heels or sacrum) is more prone to pressure injury.

In addition to venous pooling, immobility leads to compression and injury of the small vessels in the legs and decreased clearance of coagulation factors, causing blood to clot faster. These three changes—stasis, activation of clotting, and vessel injury—make up what is known as **Virchow's triad**, a trilogy of symptoms associated with a greater chance of thrombus formation, such as deep vein thrombosis (DVT).

An immobile person is also more prone to **orthostatic hypotension**. Prolonged bedrest inactivates the baroreceptors involved with constriction and dilation of the blood vessels. As a result, when a person who has been immobilized changes position, he is less able to maintain his blood pressure. The patient complains of feeling dizzy and light-headed and may be unable to support his own weight.

Effects of Immobility on Metabolism

Inactivity increases the level of serum lactic acid and decreases adenosine triphosphate (ATP) concentrations. As ATP concentrations decrease, so do the body's energy reserves. In response, metabolic rate drops, protein and glycogen synthesis decrease, and fat stores increase. Together, these effects cause glucose intolerance and reduced muscle mass. Immobility also triggers the release of epinephrine, norepinephrine, thyroid hormones, adrenocorticotropic hormone (ACTH) from the pituitary gland, and aldosterone from the kidneys. These changes in hormones are the same as occur in the stress response; so, as you can see, immobility can be a stressor in itself.

Effects of Immobility on the Integument

External pressure from lying in one position compresses capillaries in the skin, obstructing skin circulation. Lack of circulation causes tissue ischemia and possible necrosis (death). Nursing interventions include frequent turning and skin care to prevent wounds, known as pressure ulcers, from forming (see Chapter 35 as needed).

Effects of Immobility on the Gastrointestinal System

Immobility slows peristalsis, which leads to constipation, gas, and difficulty evacuating stool from the rectum. In extreme circumstances, a **paralytic ileus** (cessation of peristalsis) may occur. When peristalsis slows, appetite diminishes and food also is digested slowly. The net effect is usually decreased calorie intake and inability to meet the protein demands of the body. Body muscle is broken down as a fuel source, causing further wasting.

Effects of Immobility on the Genitourinary System

Being supine inhibits drainage of urine from the renal pelves and bladder. Urine becomes stagnant, which creates an ideal environment for infection and kidney stone formation. Immobility triggers a rise in calcium levels,

BOX 32-4 ■ Preventing Complications of Bedrest

- Position the patient to allow for lung expansion and prevent atelectasis and pneumonia.
- Provide a healthy diet to prevent loss of muscle mass.
- Prevent orthostatic hypotension by having the patient sit on edge of bed before the first time out of bed.
- Turn the patient every 2 hours to prevent pressure on the skin and minimize edema.

which also contributes to stone formation. Diminished muscle tone leads to a decrease in bladder tone, and many patients have difficulty voiding in a bedpan or urinal.

Psychological Effects of Immobility

Prolonged immobility, whether in the hospital or at home, leads to isolation and mood changes. In the 1960s, the effects of immobility were studied among astronauts. Along with the many physical effects of immobility, these healthy men showed signs of depression, anxiety, hostility, sleep disturbances, and changes in their ability to perform self-care activities. Patients who are in bed for long periods of time can suffer all these problems, as well as disorientation, apathy, and altered body concept. Other notable psychological effects of immobility/bedrest included a diminished ability to concentrate, recall sequential events, problem-solve, and perform self-care.

For tips on preventing complications of bedrest, see Box 32-4.

KnowledgeCheck 32-5

- Identify the effects of immobility on the cardiovascular, musculoskeletal, and integumentary systems.
- Why might immobility be referred to as a stressor?
- What are three effects of immobility on the GI system?
- What changes in mood might be seen with immobility?

PracticalKnowledge
knowing **how**

As you have seen in the preceding sections, immobility can result in serious health consequences. In the remainder of the chapter, we discuss nursing activities to promote activity and exercise and eliminate the hazards of immobility.

■ ASSESSMENT

Perform an assessment focused on mobility and exercise for any patient who has musculoskeletal concerns, is obese, has limited mobility, or is confined to bed or home. As always, you will validate the nursing history data with physical examination. Box 32-5 defines a variety of terms used to describe problems with muscle mass,

strength, or mobility. For a comprehensive focused assessment tool,

Go to Chapter 32, **Assessment Guidelines and Tools, Focused Assessment: Assessing Activity and Exercise,** in Volume 2.

To help you with focused mobility assessments in the home, see the Home Care box Home Assessment for a Patient With Mobility Concerns.

Focused Nursing History

A nursing history focused on activity and exercise addresses usual activity, fitness goals, mobility problems, underlying health problems, lifestyle, and external

Home Care

Home Assessment for a Patient With Mobility Concerns

Assess the Environment

- Are there stairs or other obstacles that the patient must negotiate?
- What aspects of the home environment assist with patient care?
- What aspects of the home environment hinder patient care?
- What is the patient's history of falls or other mobility concerns?
- Would the patient benefit from assistive equipment (e.g., hospital bed, walker)?
- Can the patient negotiate the distance between the bedroom, bathroom, and kitchen?

Assess the Family's or Caregivers' Abilities and Needs

- Who is providing care?
- Is the available care sufficient to meet the patient's needs?
- Are additional support persons available to assist with care?
- Can the caregiver safely move the patient in bed or assist the patient out of bed?
- What are the health concerns or physical limitations of the caregivers?
- What is the backup plan if the family or caregiver can no longer meet the patient's needs?

Assess Resources

- What community resources are available to the patient or caregiver (e.g., Meals on Wheels, physical therapy, Visiting Nurses Association)?
- Are the patient and caregiver willing to use community resources?
- What services are provided by the patient's insurance?
- Can the patient or family afford private services? If so, what services are they interested in?

BOX 32-5 ■ Terms Used to Describe Problems with Muscle Mass, Strength, or Mobility

Atrophy is a decrease in the size of muscle tissue due to lack of use or loss of innervation.

Clonus is spasmodic contraction of opposing muscles resulting in tremorous movement.

Flaccidity is a decrease or absence of muscle tone.

Hemiplegia is paralysis of one side of the body.

Hypertrophy is an increase in the size or bulk of a muscle or organ.

Paraplegia is paralysis of the lower portion of the trunk and both legs.

Paresis is partial or incomplete paralysis.

Paresthesia is numbness, tingling, or burning due to injury of the nerve(s) innervating the affected area.

Quadriplegia is paralysis of all four extremities.

Spasticity is a motor disorder characterized by increased muscle tone, exaggerated tendon jerks, and clonus.

Tremor is involuntary quivering movement of a body part.

---

factors. When caring for patients with very limited activity, assessing the ability to perform ADLs or instrumental activities of daily living (IADLs) may be more appropriate. Recall that ADLs focus on hygiene, feeding, toileting, and transfer out of bed. In contrast, IADLs focus on tasks that are instrumental in helping a patient maintain independent living status. Assessment tools for ADLs and IADLs were presented in Chapter 3.

Focused Physical Assessment

Important data to include in a physical assessment related to activity and exercise include vital signs, height, weight, body mass index, body alignment, joint function, gait, muscle strength, and activity tolerance. This section summarizes a few of these components.

Before beginning the exam, be fully aware of the patient's mobility status and any restrictions in movement, pain, injury, or otherwise. As you move through the exam, observe for pain, inflammation, and mobility limitations in all areas. For a thorough discussion of physical assessment of the musculoskeletal system, see Chapter 22. For an illustration of joint ROM,

 Go to Chapter 32, **Tables, Range of Motion at the Joints,** in Volume 2.

For guidelines when performing ROM exercises,

 Go to Chapter 32, **Clinical Insight 32-3: Tips for Performing Passive Range-of-Motion Exercises,** in Volume 2.

The Functional Independence Measure

Also known as the FIM Scale, the functional independence measure is used to assess the severity of patient disability and how much assistance is required for the person to carry out ADLs. The dimensions on the assessment include eating, bathing, grooming, upper body dressing, lower body dressing, shower transfer, toilet transfer, bladder and bowel management, mobility, safe use of stairs, problem-solving, expression, social interaction, cognitive comprehension, and memory. On admission, patients are scored for baseline and then serially until discharge and later in the outpatient or home setting to monitor improvement.

Gait

The way a person moves communicates a great deal about his general state of health, mood, and risk for falls. You might want to assess abnormal gaits in patients with injury, neurological issues, or with the following characteristics:

- **Antalgic gait**—limp to avoid pain when bearing weight on the affected side
- **Propulsive gait**—a stooped, rigid posture, with the head and neck bent forward; movement forward is by small, shuffling steps with involuntary acceleration; also known as festinating gait; common in Parkinson's disease
- **Scissors gait**—legs flexed slightly at the hips and knees with the thighs crossing in a scissors-like movement; common with cerebral palsy, stroke, or spinal tumor
- **Spastic gait**—a stiff, foot-dragging walk caused by one-sided, long-term, muscle contraction; seen with cerebral palsy, head trauma, or brain tumor
- **Steppage gait**—an exaggerated motion of lifting the leg to avoid scraping the toes of a foot with footdrop (foot appears floppy with the toes pointing down); seen with Guillain-Barré syndrome
- **Waddling gait**—a distinctive rolling motion in which the opposite hip drops; seen in patients with muscular dystrophy or developmental dysplasia of the hip; characteristic gait in late pregnancy.

 Go to Chapter 22, **Volume 2, Abnormal Atlas: Abnormal Gaits,** on Davis*Plus.*

Activity Tolerance

To promote the benefits of physical activity, people need to pace themselves during exercise, especially those who have been inactive. Health professionals can teach people to rate the perceived level of exertion and monitor target heart rate. Target heart rate requires a pulse check during exercises and staying within 50% to 85% of the maximum heart rate. To figure this out, take 220, subtract the person's age, and then multiply times 0.5 for a target heart rate for low intensity exercise; or multiply times 0.85 for maximum heart rate during high intensity exercise.

For more information about optimal target heart rates during exercise, see Box 32-1 or

 Go to the American Heart Association Web site. **Target Heart Rates** are available at http://www.heart.org/ HEARTORG/GettingHealthy/PhysicalActivity/Target-Heart-Rates_UCM_434341_Article.jsp

KnowledgeCheck 32-6

- Describe a focused assessment for a patient experiencing mobility concerns.
- Identify the assessment methods (inspection, palpation, percussion, and auscultation) used when performing a physical examination focused on mobility concerns.

ThinkLike a Nurse 32-4

Review the Meet Your Patients scenario. Which, if any, of the class participants requires a physical examination focused on mobility concerns? Explain your reasoning.

ANALYSIS/NURSING DIAGNOSIS

Nursing diagnoses that specifically describe activity and exercise problems include the following:

- *Activity Intolerance* is a state in which a patient has insufficient physical or psychological energy to carry out daily activities.
- *Impaired Physical Mobility* is limitation of independent purposeful movement of the body. Impaired Physical Mobility is a broad, general diagnosis. Use the following, more descriptive diagnoses when the patient has specific deficits: Impaired Bed Mobility, Impaired Walking, Impaired Wheelchair Mobility, and Impaired Transfer Ability.
- *Risk for Disuse Syndrome* exists when a patient's prescribed or unavoidable inactivity creates the risk for deterioration of other body systems.
- *Sedentary Lifestyle* is a habit of life that is characterized by a low physical activity level.

Mobility problems may also be the etiology of other diagnoses. The following are examples:

- Acute Pain r/t musculoskeletal injury.
- Ineffective Health Maintenance r/t prescribed bedrest.
- Risk for Injury r/t unsteady gait.

Keep in mind that Immobility, especially bedrest, can be the etiology of problems in all body systems, as well as psychosocially. For more examples and for further information about mobility diagnoses,

 Go to Chapter 32, **Standardized Language, NANDA-I Diagnoses for Activity and Exercise Problems,** on DavisPlus.

To see a nursing care plan and care map for the diagnosis Impaired Physical Mobility,

 Go to Chapter 32, **Nursing Care Plan, Impaired Physical Mobility and Care Map,** on DavisPlus.

PLANNING OUTCOMES/EVALUATION

For *associated NOC standardized outcomes* for mobility diagnoses,

 Go to Chapter 32, **Standardized Language, Selected NOC Outcomes for Energy Maintenance and Mobility,** on DavisPlus.

Individualized goals/outcome statements depend on the nursing diagnosis used. Because activity and exercise abilities are individualized, goals must consider the patient's current condition, expected condition changes, lifestyle, and values. Examples:

Will independently transfer to the wheelchair by [date].

Will discuss his feelings about his activity restrictions by [date].

PLANNING INTERVENTIONS/IMPLEMENTATION

Because attitudes about fitness and activity vary widely, mobility is often a difficult topic. Some people are devastated by activity limitations caused by disease or treatment. Others are able to accept these changes. For these reasons, it is important for you to convey an attitude of acceptance about the patient's current activity level and provide care that helps the patient achieve his optimal level of function.

For *NIC standardized interventions and activities* for patients with mobility problems,

 Go to Chapter 32, **Standardized Language, Selected NIC Interventions for Activity and Exercise Management and Immobility Management,** on DavisPlus.

Individualized nursing activities to promote exercise and mobility include promoting exercise, preventing injury from exercise, positioning patients, moving patients in bed, transferring patients out of bed, performing ROM exercises, and assisting with ambulation. The rest of this chapter will explain those interventions.

In addition, when caring for patients with specific diseases and abnormalities, you will need to add the following interventions:

- **For congenital anomalies**—Nursing responsibilities include early detection and referral for additional treatment, and parent counseling.
- **For bone formation abnormalities**—Nursing responsibilities include collaborative treatments, providing comfort, and patient education to promote mobility. Also teach patients to consume a balanced diet that meets the minimum recommendations for vitamins and minerals.
- **For joint mobility problems**—Nursing activities focus on providing comfort and teaching about medications. If mobility is severely restricted, you will also assist patients with ADLs.
- **For osteomyelitis or bone tumors**—Nursing activities include collaborative treatments, patient education about the treatment plan, and providing comfort.

Promoting Exercise

Nurses are in a perfect role to encourage and educate people of all ages to be active for healthy living. Here are some common steps to help people attain and maintain fitness. Also see the Self-Care box Teaching Clients to Set Up a Fitness Program.

- *Personalize the benefits of regular physical activity.* In other words, find out what motivates your patient. For instance, your patient might want to lose weight and improve his physical appearance. Yet another patient might be interested in improving the quality of sleep or overcoming periods of low energy during the day.
- *Set personal goals for physical activity.* Simple, realistic goals tend to be best. Be sure to define them so they are specific and measurable.
- *Include a variety of activities to keep the patient from feeling bored.*
- *Remind your patient to recognize and appreciate success.*
- *Suggest strategies to achieve the patient's goals.* For instance, you might suggest a fitness program that is fun and entertaining. You can also inform your patient about ways to avoid joint injury or falls.
- *Provide encouragement.* Sometimes just the right approach is a positive, enthusiastic one. You might offer praise for taking steps toward health and fitness. Support from spouse, family members, friends, and coworkers can improve compliance and consistency.

- *Promote physical exercise as an enjoyable activity.*
- *Discuss barriers to regular activity and elicit ways to overcome those obstacles.*

People give various reasons for failing to develop a regular exercise program. See Box 32-6 for suggestions on dealing with such objections.

Preventing Injury From Exercise

As previously discussed, the benefits of exercise outweigh any associated risks. Advise clients to follow the tips in the Self-Care boxes Teaching Clients How to Set Up a Fitness Program and Teaching Your Patient How to Prevent Back Injury. Also re-read the theoretical knowledge in the section Risks Associated With Exercise if you need a review.

Positioning Patients

Healthy people regularly shift position to maintain comfort. However, many patients are unable to move without assistance. They require a change of position at least every 2 hours to prevent skin breakdown, muscle discomfort, damage to superficial nerves and

---

BOX 32-6 ■ Suggestions for Overcoming Objections to Exercise

Objection	Suggestion
"I hate to exercise."	Pick activities that you enjoy.
"I burn out on exercise."	Plan ahead and build in rest days and varied activities.
"I am self-conscious about going to the gym and don't have the motivation to exercise by myself."	Find a friend to exercise with, or develop a reward system for yourself if you continue to exercise. An exercise "buddy" can help increase motivation and consistency in the weekly routine.
"I am too busy with work or family."	Develop a routine that you can do at lunchtime, or exercise with your family.
"I find exercise boring."	Change your routine frequently.
"I can't afford to join a health club, hire a fitness trainer, or buy expensive equipment."	Just get active doing things you enjoy. Go for a brisk walk, or play with your grandkids. Some of the best core exercises require no equipment at all (e.g., push-ups, planks). You can also use a chair, jump rope, or many things around the house to build into your fitness routine.
"I'm too tired to exercise."	The hardest part is getting started, but after a few minutes or so, you'll feel better and have more energy after you finish.
"Exercise hurts."	Make sure to exercise at your target heart rate, and plan a rest day after every weight-lifting session.
"I don't have time."	Schedule your exercise time. If need be, schedule several short 10- to 15-minute sessions throughout the day, and do more as time allows. It all adds up and will benefit you.
"I have pain about all the time."	Take pain medication an hour or so before starting physical activity. If fatigue is the problem, try to arrange schedule to keep a balance of rest and activity as well as avoid stimulants (e.g., caffeine or nicotine) that might interfere with the quality of sleep.
"I have difficulty getting around sometimes."	Stretch adequately before starting exercise, but not to overstretch joints. Also, you will need to walk on smooth, even surfaces.
"I am diabetic and have trouble with my feet. My vision is not very good, either."	Be sure shoes fit properly and the area is well-lit.
"I'm too old to exercise."	It's never to late to get active, and any physical activity you do is better than none. Exercises that build strength, stamina, flexibilty and balance improve the quality of life and reduce the risk for falls.

blood vessels, and contractures. Immobile people are more prone to pressure injury as a result of reduced circulation, impaired oxygen exchange to the tissues, and edema.

A firm mattress provides support to the patient's body and makes it easier to turn the patient (because he does not sink down into the mattress). Most hospital mattresses are firm. However, when you provide home care, you will find mattresses of various types and conditions. To provide additional support, you can place a piece of plywood under a sagging mattress.

A clean, dry bed also makes it easier to turn the patient and decreases the risk of skin maceration or pressure ulcer formation. Bedding should provide coverage and warmth but not be tucked in so tightly as to restrict movement.

Protecting the Nurse's Back

According to the U.S. Bureau of Labor Statitics (2013), healthcare workers providing direct patient care rank fifth in the number of work-related musculoskeletal injuries. Nurses are at risk for back and shoulder injury as a result of manual moving and repositioning of patients, residents, or clients. Rising obesity rates in the United States, aging of the workforce, and the shortage of nurses impact the physical demands on caregivers (CDC, n.d., updated 2014).

To protect yourself from back injury as you move patients, avoid manual lifting as much as possible. Some lifts and patient care tasks require multiple staff members to accomplish safely, and, because low staffing makes this teamwork difficult, nurses often attempt these tasks alone (Waters, Nelson, Hughes, et al., 2009). Use assistive equipment and devices, as recommended by the ANA (2013), and always make sure you have adequate help. The amount of help you need depends on the size of the patient, the level of assistance the patient can offer, your size and strength, and the equipment or lines attached to the patient.

Other measures to reduce the risk for injury for nurses include the following:

- Avoid slippery or wet surfaces during ambulation or moving patients.
- Remove physical obstructions (e.g., cabinets, toilets) when moving or transferring patients.
- Arrange a clutter-free environment that allows for free movement of equipment and personnel.
- Watch out for uneven floor surfaces or movable rugs.
- Lock wheels of furniture and equipment before moving patients.
- Avoid moving patients through too small a width to the entrance way.

Positioning Devices

Devices used to maintain body alignment, prevent contractures, and promote comfort are briefly discussed in the next sections. Positioning devices are commonly used to help minimize the risk for the example problem, Hazards of Immobility. For guidelines for using common positioning devices, including hip abduction pillows,

 Go to Chapter 32, **Clinical Insight 32-2: Using Common Positioning Devices,** in Volume 2.

Adjustable Beds

An adjustable bed, often referred to as a hospital bed, assumes a variety of positions. You can elevate or lower the head of the bed, and elevate the foot of the bed. Often the bed breaks, or "gatches," at the knee to keep the patient from sliding down when the head is elevated. You can also adjust the height of the bed. You should raise the bed to waist height when providing care so that you can use proper body mechanics; place the bed in its lowest position before helping a patient get out of bed or if the patient is at risk for falling.

Several types of specialized beds are used in treating and preventing pressure ulcers. These include alternating, low air loss, immersion (air-fluidized), and oscillating beds. The mattresses may be composed of air, water, or gel. Special beds are discussed further in Chapter 35. A circular bed and Stryker frame are used in the care of patients with severe mobility restrictions. Both can rotate a patient from supine to prone. With the advent of low-pressure specialized beds, these latter two types of beds are now in limited use.

Pillows

Pillows are the most common devices used to assist with positioning, provide support, and elevate body parts. They help position a patient by molding to the body and expanding the weight-bearing area. You will need a variety of sizes to position patients who are unconscious, paralyzed, frail, or who have had surgery. To obtain the right size or type (e.g., abductor pillows), or if pillows are not available, you can use folded blankets or towels. Foam wedge pillows are useful for elevating the upper body when an adjustable bed is not available and for abducting the hips after hip surgery.

Siderails

Most hospital beds are equipped with siderails. The rails may run the full length of each side of the bed or consist of an upper or lower rail on each side.

Siderails are designed to ensure patient safety. They serve as a reminder that the patient should call for assistance before getting out of bed and provide a grip for the patient who is able to reposition himself in bed. Although siderails are designed to protect patients, they can be a source of injury. Patients can get tangled in the railing or fall between the bed and rail, and confused patients may injure themselves trying to climb over the rails.

Siderails may also be considered a form of restraint, so follow your agency's policy for use and be sure to discuss their purpose with patients and family. See Chapter 24 if you need to review restraint use.

Trapeze Bar

A trapeze bar is a triangular-shaped device that is attached to an overhead bed frame (see Clinical Insight

32-2). The patient can use the base of the triangle as a grip bar to move up in bed, turn, and pull up in preparation for getting out of bed or getting on and off the bedpan. Patients can use the trapeze to move about in bed and to exercise their upper extremities. Frail patients may not be able to use a trapeze bar because of the amount of effort it requires.

Footboard

When a person is supine, the toes tend to point downward toward the bed (**footdrop**), and the feet are in plantar flexion. Able-bodied persons usually shift position throughout the night, so the foot and leg muscles are periodically contracted and relaxed. In contrast, the patient who is unable to move independently will experience a shortening of the gastrocnemius muscle and may have difficulty walking again if prolonged plantar flexion occurs. A footboard is a device placed at the end of the bed to prevent footdrop and outward hip rotation, but it does not relieve heel pressure (Fig. 32-6). For the footboard to be effective, the heels must be touching it. Each time you turn the patient, you may need to reposition the footboard to ensure proper position.

Other Positioning Devices

The following are other positioning devices used in the clinical setting:

- **Trochanter rolls** are made from tightly rolled towels, bath blankets, or foam pads. They are placed snugly adjacent to the hips and thighs to prevent external rotation of the hips. To learn how to make them,

 Go to Chapter 32, **Clinical Insight 32-2: Using Common Positioning Devices,** in Volume 2.

- **Hand and wrist splints** may be manufactured or fashioned from rolled washcloths. Often splints are custom made for patients. The purpose of splints is to hold the wrist and hand in natural position and prevent claw-hand deformities.

- **Hand rolls** prevent hand contractures. Some are commercially made. Otherwise, you can make a hand roll from a tightly rolled washcloth.

- **Hip abduction pillows** prevent internal hip rotation and hip adduction when the patient is in a supine position. These wedge-shaped pieces of spongy material are used after femoral fracture, hip fracture, or surgery. Lateral indentations and straps that wrap around the patient's thighs hold the patient in the correct position.

- **Boots** made of spongy rubber with heel cutouts and ankle cushioning prevent footdrop, skin breakdown, and external hip rotation ✚ If any part of the boot is made of a latex product, be sure the patient does not have a latex allergy before applying.

- **Foot cradles** are metal or plastic devices that are secured at the foot of the bed to hold bedding up off the toes and feet, allowing for free movement.

- **High-top sneakers** may be used to prevent heel drop, but they do not reduce heel pressure. They do help in positioning hips and pelvis to prevent hip rotation.

- **Sandbags** are small fabric bags filled with sand. They are used in the same manner as pillows and trochanter rolls; however, they provide firmer support.

Positioning Techniques

In the next section we briefly describe the various ways to position patients. Table 32-2 illustrates these positions; identifies potential problems associated with them; and offers solutions to prevent the problems. The positions are also described and illustrated in Chapter 22, Table 22-1.

Fowler's Positions

Fowler's position is a semisitting position, in which the head of the bed is elevated 45° to 60°. This position promotes respiratory function by lowering the diaphragm and allowing the greatest chest expansion. It is also an ideal position for some patients with cardiac dysfunction. Common variations include **semi-Fowler's position,** in which the head of the bed is elevated only 30°, and **high-Fowler's position,** in which the head is elevated 90°.

In the **orthopneic position,** the head of the bed is elevated 90° and an overbed table with a pillow on top is positioned in front of the patient (Fig. 32-7). Have the patient lean forward, resting his arms and head on the pillow. This position is helpful for a patient with shortness of breath.

Lateral Positions

The **lateral position** is a side-lying position with the top hip and knee flexed and placed in front of the rest of the body. The lateral position creates pressure on the lower scapula, ilium, and trochanter but relieves pressure from the heels and sacrum. The **lateral recumbent position** is side-lying with legs in a straight line (see

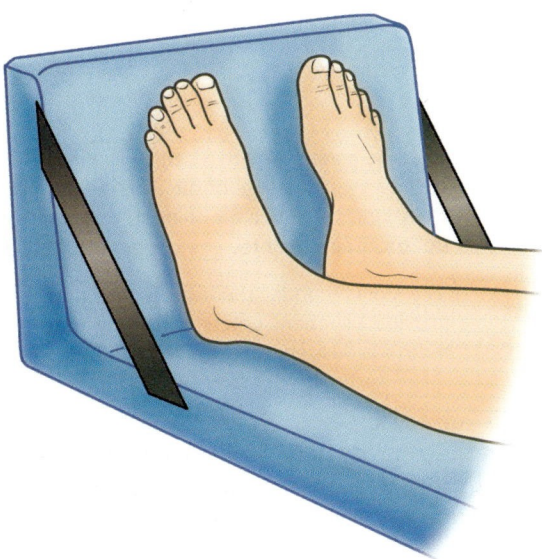

FIGURE 32-6 A footboard is placed at the end of the bed to prevent footdrop.

Table 32-2 ➤ Positioning a Bed-Bound Patient

POSITION	POTENTIAL PROBLEM	SOLUTIONS
Fowler's	Hyperextension of the neck	Use a small pillow under the head and neck.
	Posterior flexion of the lumbar curvature	Use a firm mattress.
		Position the patient so that the angle of elevation begins at the hip.
	Dislocation of the shoulders	Position a pillow under the forearms to prevent pull on the shoulders.
	Flexion contracture of the wrist and edema of the hands	Support the hands on pillows in alignment with the forearms.
	Flexion contracture of the fingers and abduction of the thumbs	Use hand splints if appropriate, or provide a large roll in the palm of the hand.
	External rotation of the legs	Place sandbags or rolls alongside the trochanters and upper thighs.
	Hyperextension of the knees	Place a small pillow under the lower legs from the ankles to below the knees. Do this for short periods only; avoid pressure on the popliteal area.
	Footdrop	Use a footboard or high-top sneakers to hold the feet in dorsiflexion.
Lateral	Lateral flexion of the neck	Place a pillow under the head and neck to provide alignment.
	Internal rotation and adduction of the upper shoulder and limited respirations	Place a pillow under the upper arm, and comfortably flex the lower arm.
	Internal rotation and adduction of the femur	Support the upper leg from groin to foot with pillows.
	Twisting of the spine	Align the shoulders with the hips.
	Flexion of the cervical spine	Place a pillow under the head and neck to provide alignment, unless drainage from the mouth is desired.
Prone	Hyperextension of the lumbar curvature, pressure on the breasts in women or genitals in men, impaired respirations	Place a small pillow under the abdomen.
	Footdrop	Move the patient down in bed so the feet extend over the edge of the mattress, or place a small pillow under the shins so that the toes do not touch the bed.
	Lateral flexion of the neck	Place a pillow under the head and neck to provide alignment, unless drainage from the mouth is desired.

Table 32-2 ➤ Positioning a Bed-Bound Patient—cont'd

POSITION	POTENTIAL PROBLEM	SOLUTIONS
Sims'	Internal rotation and adduction of the upper shoulder and limited respirations	Place a pillow under the upper arm, and comfortably flex the arm at the elbow.
	Pressure on the shoulder and axilla of the inferior arm	Position the lower arm behind and away from the back.
	Internal rotation and adduction of the femur	Support the upper leg from groin to foot with pillows.
	Twisting of the spine	Align the shoulders with the hips.
	Footdrop	Support the feet in dorsiflexion with sandbags.
	Hyperextension of the neck	Place a pillow under the head and neck to provide alignment.
Supine	Internal rotation of the shoulders and extension of the elbows	Position the upper arms next to the body. Place pillows under the forearms, and position the wrists in slight pronation.
	Flexion of fingers and abduction of the thumbs	Use hand splints if appropriate, or provide a large roll in the palm of the hand.
	Flexion of the lumbar curvature and hips	Provide a firm mattress, or place a small pillow under the lumbar curvature.
	External rotation of the legs	Place sandbags or rolls alongside the trochanters and upper thighs.
	Hyperextension of the knees	Place a small pillow under the lower legs from the ankles to below the knees.
	Footdrop	Use a footboard or high-top sneakers to hold the feet in dorsiflexion.

Table 22-1). The **oblique position** is an alternative to the lateral position that places less pressure on the trochanter. The patient turns on the side with the top hip and knee flexed; however, the top leg is placed behind the body (Fig. 32-8).

Prone Position

In the **prone position**, the patient lies on his abdomen with his head turned to one side. This is the only position that allows full extension of the hips and knees. It also allows secretions to drain freely from the mouth and thus is helpful for an unconscious patient. However, this is the most difficult position to move an unconscious or frail patient into, because it requires the greatest amount of manipulation to position the patient appropriately. The prone position creates a significant lordosis (inward curving of the spine in the lower back)

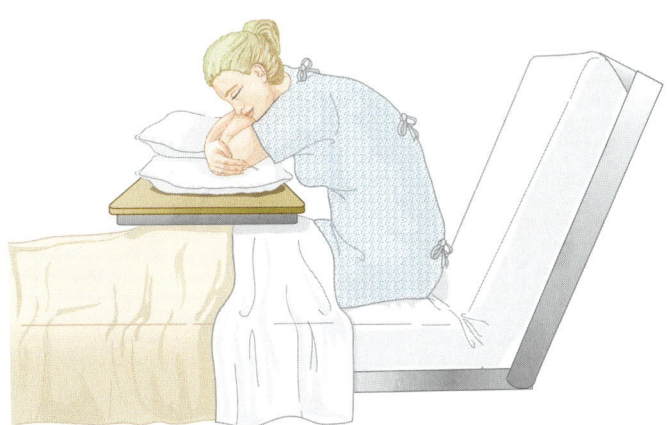

FIGURE 32-7 The orthopneic position is ideal for a patient with shortness of breath.

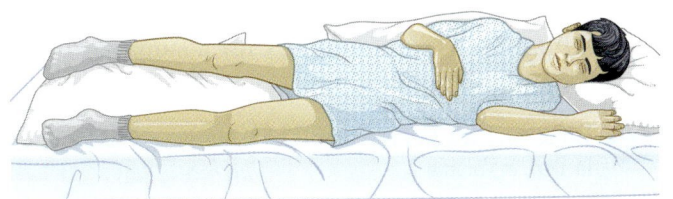

FIGURE 32-8 The oblique position is a modified lateral position that places less pressure on the trochanter.

and rotation of the neck. Therefore, it should not be used for patients with cervical or lumbar spine problems. You should not use the prone position for patients with cardiac or respiratory difficulty because it inhibits chest wall expansion and, therefore, oxygenation. As a rule, you can use this position only for short periods of time.

Sims' Position

Sims' position is a semiprone position. The lower arm is positioned behind the patient, and the upper arm is flexed. The upper leg is more flexed than the lower leg. Sims' position facilitates drainage from the mouth and limits pressure on the trochanter and sacrum. This is an ideal position for administering an enema or a perineal procedure.

Supine Position

In the **supine position**, also known as the **dorsal recumbent position**, the patient lies on his back with head and shoulders elevated on a small pillow. The spine is aligned and the arms and hands comfortably rest at the side.

KnowledgeCheck 32-7

- Describe the following positions: Fowler's, lateral, prone, Sims', and supine.
- What is the advantage of the oblique position versus the lateral position?
- Identify and describe six positioning devices.
- What are three uses for siderails?

ThinkLike a Nurse 32-5

You are providing care for a young man who is recovering from Guillain-Barré syndrome, which produces a reversible paralysis after viral illness. He has been healthy until this present illness. How would you position this patient? Explain your reasoning.

Moving Patients in Bed

To position patients, you must be adept at moving and lifting them in bed. This involves positioning the patient in the length of the bed, as well as turning with as little friction and shearing on the skin as possible. Moving patients in bed is a common intervention to help minimize the risk for the example problem, Hazards of Immobility.

Moving Up in Bed Frail patients tend to slide down in bed because of gravity and their inability to correct their position. Elevating the head of the bed accentuates the slide and places the patient in an awkward position. If the patient is light in weight or able to provide assistance, you will be able to move her independently (see the Highlights of Procedures box for a summary). For complete instructions,

 Go to Chapter 32, **Procedure 32-1A: Moving a Patient Up in Bed,** in Volume 2.

Turning in Bed Turn patients at least every 2 hours to protect their skin and prevent other complications of immobility. For efficient use of time, try to time turning to coincide with moving the patient up in bed. Use pillows and other positioning devices to help the patient maintain the new position (see the Highlights of Procedures box for a summary). For a complete description,

 Go to Chapter 32, **Procedure 32-1B: Turning a Patient in Bed,** in Volume 2.

Logrolling Logrolling is a special turning technique used when the patient's spine must be kept in straight alignment. You will need at least two nurses for this procedure, more if the patient is large. Logrolling moves the patient's body as a unit. One nurse is positioned at the level of the patient's head. The other staff members are distributed along the length of the patient. All must move the patient in unison (see the Highlights of Procedures box for a summary). For a complete description,

 Go to Chapter 32, **Procedure 32-1C: Logrolling a Patient,** in Volume 2.

Friction-Reducing Devices You can use one of a variety of friction-reducing devices when moving a patient in bed. Transfer roller sheets are thin, low-friction fabric sheets that may be placed beneath the drawsheet to facilitate moving the patient in bed (Fig. 32-9). A scoot sheet is also a thin, low-friction fabric sheet that is often positioned under the drawsheet of the patient, but it is attached to a mechanical crank (Fig. 32-10). By turning the crank, a single person can move a patient up in bed. Transfer roller sheets are relatively inexpensive and are widely available on clinical units. If one is not available, you can improvise by placing a large, clean, unused plastic bag under the drawsheet to help you move the

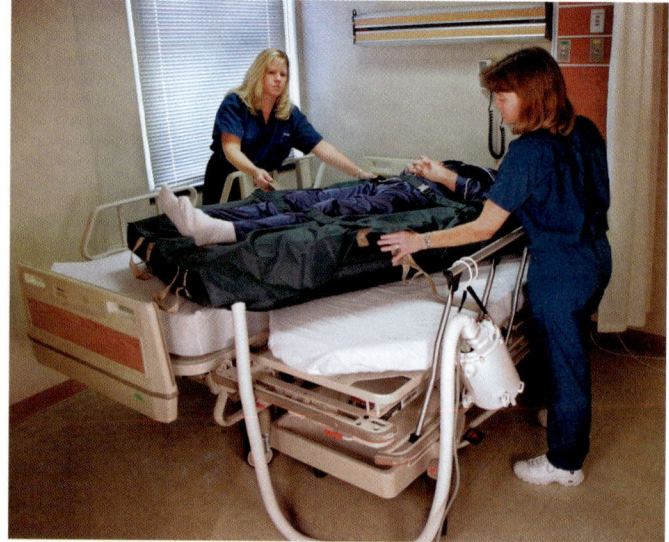

FIGURE 32-9 A transfer roller sheet reduces friction and facilitates movement.

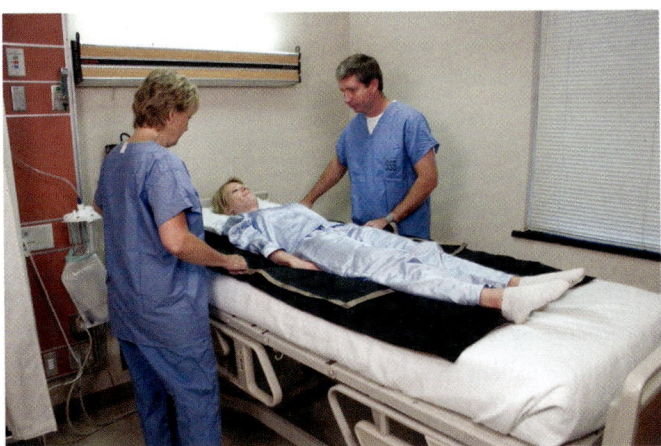

FIGURE 32-10 A scoot sheet allows one or two nurses to easily move a patient up in bed.

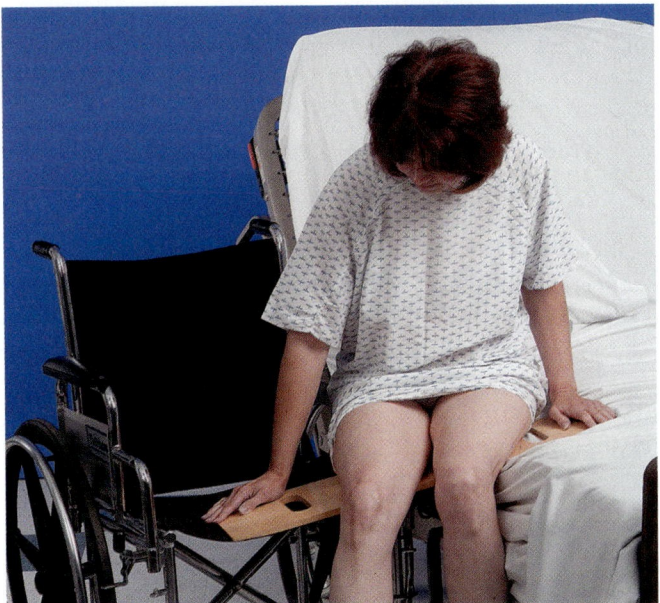

FIGURE 32-11 Transfer boards are used by patients with chronic mobility problems to increase their independence.

patient. The plastic bag reduces drag and facilitates movement. However, unlike the thin fabric of transfer sheets, plastic allows moisture to pool under the patient. Consequently, you should not leave a bag in place under the drawsheet.

Transferring Patients Out of Bed

Stretchers and wheelchairs are used to transport patients between units and to tests or procedures. A stretcher is usually reserved for the patient who is weak, sedated, or has a condition that does not permit transfer by wheelchair. A wheelchair may be used for transport or as part of an activity program. In addition, you may transfer patients to a stationary chair to increase their general activity level (see the Hightlights of Procedures box for a summary). For complete procedural steps,

 Go to Chapter 32, **Procedure 32-2A: Transferring a Patient From Bed to Stretcher, Procedure 32-2B: Dangling a Patient at the Side of the Bed,** and **Procedure 32-2C: Transferring a Patient From Bed to Chair,** in Volume 2.

To know what type of assistive device is appropriate for patient safety and to prevent back injury to the nurse,

 Go to Chapter 32, **Clinical Insight 32-1, Applying Principles of Body Mechanics,** in Volume 2.

Transfer Board

A **transfer board** is a wood or plastic device designed to assist with moving patients. Using a transfer board reduces your risk of injury and promotes a smooth transfer. Place the board under the patient on the side to which he will be moved. It is best to use a drawsheet to slide the patient across the board (Fig. 32-11). Transfer boards are also used by patients with long-standing mobility problems to increase their independence.

Mechanical Lift

A **mechanical lift** is a hydraulic device used to transfer patients. Place a fabric sling under the patient, and attach chains or straps from the sling to the lifting device (Fig. 32-12). A mechanical lift is especially useful when providing care for obese and immobile patients. Lifts are often used in home care because they allow one person to transfer the patient safely. Most lifts position patients in a seated position and thus are ideal for assisting the patient into a chair. Others suspend the patient in a supine position; they may be used to transfer the patient from bed to stretcher or to suspend the patient while the bed is made. Many such lifts include scales that weigh the patient while he is suspended in the sling. Some mechanical lifts are mounted on the ceiling to reduce caregiver back injuries and increase patient safety (see Fig. 32-13).

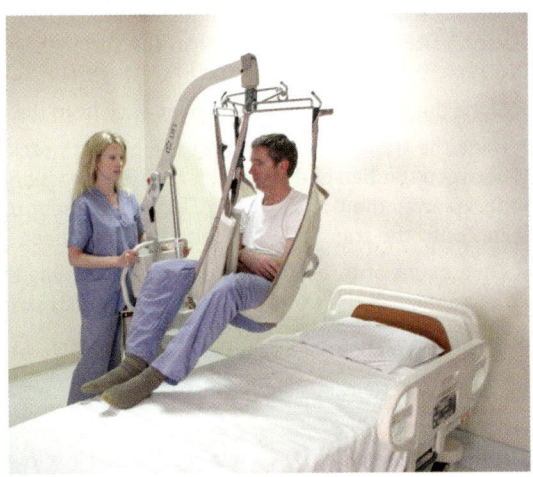

FIGURE 32-12 A mechanical lift is useful when providing care to patients with impaired mobility.

For steps to follow in *all* procedures, refer to the Universal Steps for All Procedures found on the inside back cover of Volume 2. Go to the full procedures in Volume 2 to practice and learn the procedure steps. Use these procedure highlights later to help you review key points.

Procedure 32-1A: Moving a Patient Up in Bed

➤ Use a friction-reducing device to move the patient if the patient can assist with movement. Use a full body sling if the patient cannot assist.

➤ Remove the pillow. Have the patient flex her neck, fold her arms across her chest, and place her feet flat on the bed.

➤ Position a nurse on either side of the patient.

➤ Use a wide base of support.

➤ Have the patient, on the count of 3, push off with his heels as you shift your weight forward.

Procedure 32-1B: Turning a Patient in Bed

➤ Use a friction-reducing device and drawsheet to move the patient. Position at least one nurse on each side of the bed.

➤ Place the patient's near leg and arm (e.g., the left arm and leg when turning to the right) across his body, and abduct and externally rotate the far shoulder.

➤ Each nurse places one arm at the level of the patient's shoulders and the other at the level of the patient's hips. Each nurse shifts her weight as both simultaneously roll the patient in the intended direction.

Procedure 32-1C: Logrolling a Patient

➤ Move the patient as a unit to the opposite side of the bed; raise the siderail on that side.

➤ Move to the side of the bed that the patient will be turning toward; lower the siderail.

➤ Each staff member evenly distributes his arms across the patient's length. One nurse is responsible for moving the head and neck as a unit.

➤ Shift your weight backward as you roll the patient toward you.

Procedure 32-2A: Transferring a Patient From Bed to Stretcher

➤ Move the patient to the side of the bed where the stretcher will be placed.

➤ Position the stretcher next to the bed, and lock it in place.

➤ Keep the destination device (i.e., bed to stretcher or vice versa) situated a little lower than the surface the patient is on.

➤ Using the drawsheet, roll the patient away from the stretcher.

➤ Place the transfer board against the patient's back halfway between the bed and stretcher. Position a friction-reducing device over the transfer board. Turn the patient to his back and onto the transfer board with the drawsheet.

➤ On a count of three, use the drawsheet to slide the patient across the transfer board onto the stretcher.

Procedure 32-2B: Dangling a Patient at the Side of the Bed

➤ Place the patient in a supine position, and raise the head of the bed to 90°.

➤ Apply a gait transfer belt, and place the bed in a low position.

➤ Stand facing the patient with a wide base of support. Place your foot closest to the head of the bed forward of the other foot.

➤ Position your hands on each side of the gait transfer belt.

➤ Rock onto your back foot as you move the patient into a sitting position, and pivot to bring the patient's legs over the side of the bed.

➤ Stay with the patient as he dangles.

Procedure 32-2C: Transferring a Patient From Bed to Chair

➤ Ask the patient to wear nonskid footwear.

➤ Place the bed in the low position, and lock the wheels.

➤ Assist the patient to dangle at the side of the bed (see Procedure 32-2B).

➤ Brace your feet and knees against the patient. Bend your hips at the knees, and hold on to the transfer belt.

➤ If two nurses are available to assist with the transfer, one nurse should be on each side of the patient.

➤ Instruct the patient to place her arms around you between your shoulders and waist. Ask the patient to stand as you move to an upright position by straightening your legs and hips.

➤ Instruct the patient to pivot and turn with you toward the chair.

➤ Ask the patient to flex her hips and knees as she lowers herself to the chair. Guide her motion while maintaining a firm hold on her.

➤ If the chair is a wheelchair, lock the wheels.

Procedure 32-3: Assisting With Ambulation

➤ Ask the patient to wear nonskid footwear.

➤ Place the bed in low position, and lock the wheels.

➤ Assist the patient to dangle at the side of the bed (see Procedure 32-2B).

➤ If two nurses are available, each nurse should stand facing the patient on opposite sides of the patient.

➤ Brace your feet and knees against the patient. Bend your hips at the knees, and hold onto the transfer belt. Pay attention to any known weakness.

➤ Instruct the patient to place her arms around you between your shoulders and waist (the location depends on the height of the patient and the nurses). Ask the patient to stand as you move to an upright position by straightening your legs and hips.

➤ Allow the patient to steady herself for a moment.

➤ One nurse: Stand at the patient's side, placing both hands on the transfer belt. If the patient has weakness on one side, position yourself on the weaker side.

➤ Two nurses: One nurse stands on each of the patient's sides, grasping hold of the transfer belt.

➤ Slowly guide the patient forward. Observe for signs of fatigue or dizziness.

➤ If the patient must transport an IV pole, allow the patient to hold onto the pole on the side where you are standing. Assist the patient to advance the pole as you ambulate together.

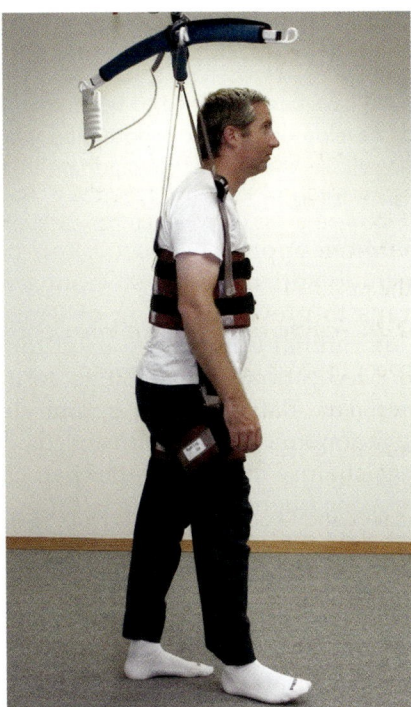

FIGURE 32-13 A ceiling mounted mechanical lift is used to support patients in the standing position.

Standing assist devices are mechanical lifts that help the patient move from a sitting to a standing position or support a patient in the standing position. A sling is positioned around the back and under the arms of the patient (Fig. 32-14). Specialized chairs and wheelchairs are also available. Each has a mechanical lift in the seat that rises to assist the patient to a standing position. Mechanical lift devices reduce the risk of back and musculoskeletal injury.

Transfer Belt
A **transfer belt** is a heavy belt several inches wide that is used to facilitate transfer or provide a secure

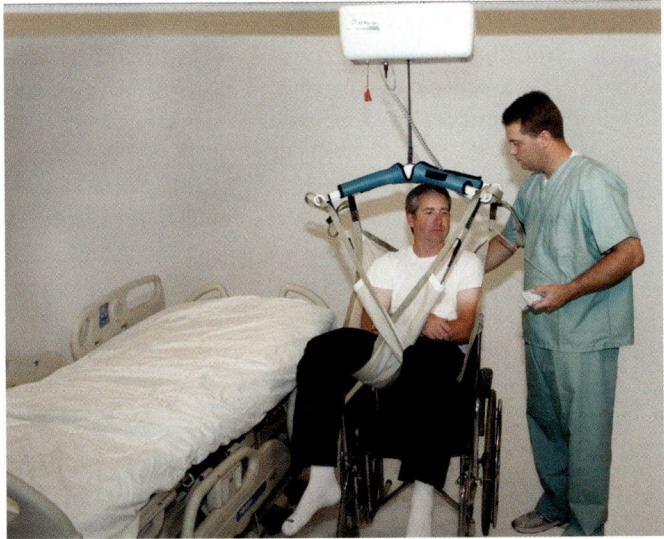

FIGURE 32-14 A mechanical lift with a sling chair is used to safely transfer an immobile patient into a wheelchair.

mechanism to hold the patient when ambulating. Apply the belt around the patient's abdomen, close to the patient's center of gravity. The belt may have external grip holds, or you may grip the entire belt with your hand (Fig. 32-15).

➕ The fit should not be overly tight or cause the patient discomfort. You should be able to easily place your hand under the belt. Do not place it over the rib cage, as this could compromise breathing. Do not use a transfer belt around the patient's hip. This could cause unsteadiness and lead to a patient fall. You would not use a transfer belt after abdominal surgery or with other abdominal wound, colostomy, or internal organ contusion or other injury.

KnowledgeCheck 32-8

- What criteria determine whether your patient should be logrolled when he is repositioned?
- How often should you turn and reposition a patient?
- Identify the most appropriate device for the following activities:
  Transferring an obese patient from a bed to a stretcher
  Assisting an immobile patient to a recliner chair
  Helping a weak patient from bed to chair

Performing Range-of-Motion Exercises
Patients with limited mobility are at risk for developing complications of disuse, such as muscle atrophy, joint stiffness, and contractures. To limit the complications of

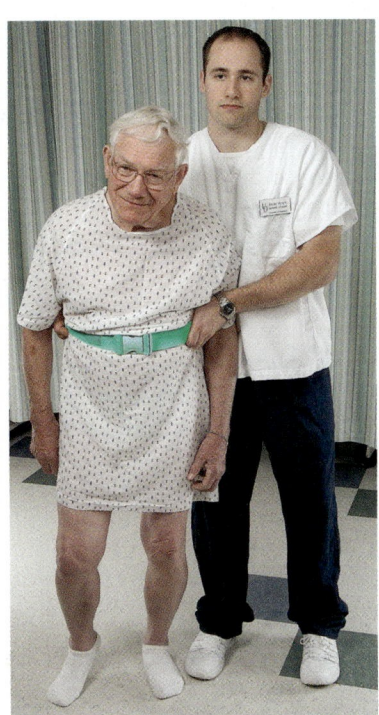

FIGURE 32-15 A transfer belt is placed close to the patient's center of gravity. It may have external grip holds to facilitate transfer or provide a secure mechanism to hold the patient when ambulating.

immobility, patients recovering from illness, injury, or surgery often perform AROM as a rehabilitation procedure. Additionally, movement with ADLs improves joint mobility, circulation, muscular strength,

Passive range of motion (PROM) is movement of the joints through their range of motion by another person. Both AROM and PROM improve joint mobility, increase circulation to the area exercised, and help maintain function. However, AROM also improves and respiratory and cardiac function. For an explanation of how to perform PROM,

 Go to Chapter 32, **Clinical Insight 32-3: Tips for Performing Passive Range-of-Motion Exercises,** in Volume 2.

Continuous passive motion, also called CPM, is a device that repetitively but gently flexes and extends the knee joint. The CPM machine is often used after knee replacement or other knee procedures to allow the joint to improve range of motion, eliminate the problem of stiffness, and prevent the development of adhesions, which can limit motion further.

Assisting With Ambulation

Prolonged bedrest is no longer the standard of care. However, as a nurse, you will provide care to patients whose illnesses and injuries curtail their ability to walk and be active. Assisting patients with ambulation includes physical conditioning to prepare the patient for ambulation, as well as assisting the patient to walk.

Physical Conditioning

Patients who have been confined to bed for more than a week or who have sustained major injury require conditioning before they are able to resume walking. The following conditioning exercises are summarized here; they are explained in detail,

 Go to Chapter 32, **Clinical Insight 32-4: Assisting With Physical Conditioning Exercises to Prepare for Ambulation,** in Volume 2.

Quadriceps and Gluteal Drills The quadriceps muscle group and the gluteal muscles are the largest muscles of the body. Patients who are confined to bed can perform isometric exercises to prepare them for walking.

Arm Exercises Patients use the biceps and triceps muscles when getting out of bed and for crutch walking. Exercises to help prepare the patient for ambulation include using a trapeze bar, and doing "push-ups" off the mattress or a chair.

✚ Be mindful of any cardiac or musculoskeletal precautions that restrict arm movement, weight-bearing on the hands and wrists, or other upper body injury. If lymphedema is present in the upper extremities, do not encourage arm exercises or use of the trapeze, unless directed by the primary care provider.

Dangling Use this position to prepare the patient to get up in a chair, to stand, or to ambulate.

✚ Patients who have been confined to bed frequently become light-headed or develop orthostatic hypotension when first getting up. Dangling allows the patient to experience being upright with limited risk of falling.

Some common approaches used for orthostatic problems include antiembolism stockings with compression wraps to prevent pooling of venous blood. Sometimes abdominal binders are used for this purpose as well. Medication is available to control orthostatic hypotension. Patients with spinal cord injury experiencing autonomic dysfunctions need a high-back reclining wheelchair so the back of the chair can be lowered (and someone might even have to lift up their legs for a few minutes) until blood pressure stabilizes. Tilt-table therapies are also used.

Daily Activities Moving around in bed and performing ADLs (e.g., brushing one's hair) exercise many of the muscle groups needed for ambulation. Getting up into a chair accustoms the patient to an upright posture and is an important predictor of success with ambulation.

Assisting the Patient to Walk

Before getting the patient out of bed, assess his readiness to walk. Also obtain the appropriate equipment and assistance. Move floor rugs and loose objects from the path of the patient and caregiver. Be sure the floor is not slippery. When possible, use a transfer belt. Have a chair or additional assistance available on the first few attempts at ambulation.

✚ If the patient becomes faint or begins to fall, do not attempt to hold him up by yourself. Instead, protect the patient as you guide him to a seated or lying position. Create a wide base of support, and project forward the hip closest to the patient. Help the patient slide down your leg as you call for help (Fig. 32-16). Protect the patient's head as his body descends.

The Hightlights of Procedures box summarizes ambulation with one-nurse assist and with two-nurse assist. For the complete procedures,

 Go to Chapter 32, **Procedure 32-3A: Assisting With Ambulation (One Nurse),** and **Procedure 32-3B: Assisting with Ambulation (Two Nurses),** in Volume 2.

🍁 **Assisting Older Adults** When assisting older adults to ambulate, find out how much assistance, if any, the patient typically requires and modify support as needed. Consider the following nursing interventions.

■ Observe constantly during ambulation for weakness and fatigue. Plan for periods of rest during ambulation, if needed. The older adult might become

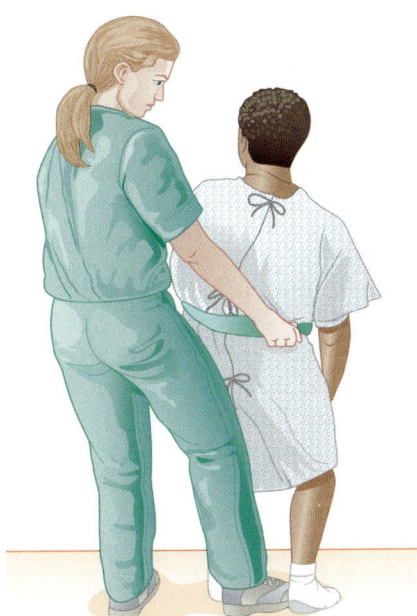

FIGURE 32-16 If the patient begins to fall, the nurse guides the patient gently to the floor or to a chair.

fatigued more quickly and recover more slowly from the physical demands of walking, especially if a heart or lung condition is present.

- ✚ Move the patient gradually to a sitting position and allow him to dangle at the bedside before coming to a standing position. Observe for dizziness or light-headedness.

- ✚ Assess for falls risk factors. For example, some medications cause dizziness or lethargy; and patients with neurological or cognitive disorders, such as Parkinson's or Alzheimer's disease, have a greater potential for falls. For more information about assessing a patient's risk for a fall see Chapter 24.

- ✚ To reduce the risk for falling in the home, recommend family place nonskid strips on stairs or other smooth flooring.

- ✚ Assistive devices, such as walkers, canes, and transfer belts, can be useful for older adults or others who require additional support.

- ✚ Be cautious when using a transfer belt for the patient with osteoporosis or back pain. Too much pressure from the belt can cause injury or pain.

KnowledgeCheck 32-9

- Identify four principles to be followed when performing PROM.
- Describe activities that can promote a patient's readiness for ambulation.
- What action should you take if a patient begins to fall when ambulating?

Mechanical Aids for Walking

A variety of aids is available to promote stability and independence when walking. Some aids are intended for short-term use; others will be incorporated into the patient's lifestyle. Some patients consider the use of aids a sign of weakness or inconvenience. As a result, they avoid using the aid and increase their risk of falls. However, most people dread loss of independence, so you can promote the use of walking aids by stressing their importance in helping the person maintain independence.

 Go to Chapter 32, **Clinical Insight 32-6: Teaching Patients to Use Canes, Walkers, and Crutches,** in Volume 2.

Canes

The following are three basic types of canes used (Fig. 32-17):

- *Single-ended cane with a half-circle handle.* This is ideal for the patient who needs minimal support and is able to negotiate stairs.
- *Single-ended cane with a straight handle.* This is ideal for the patient with hand weakness who has good balance.
- *Multiprong canes.* A multiprong cane usually has three or four prongs, and all types have a straight handle. These canes provide a wide base of support and are useful for patients with balance problems.

Walkers

A walker is a lightweight metal frame device with four legs that provides a wide base of support as a patient ambulates. Various forms of walkers are available. Some models have wheels that allow the walker to be rolled forward; others have a seat that allows the patient to rest periodically (Fig. 32-18). These walkers are best for patients whose mobility problems are related to fatigue or shortness of breath rather than gait instability.

Braces

Braces support joints and muscles that cannot independently support the body's weight. They are most commonly used in the lower extremities. Physical

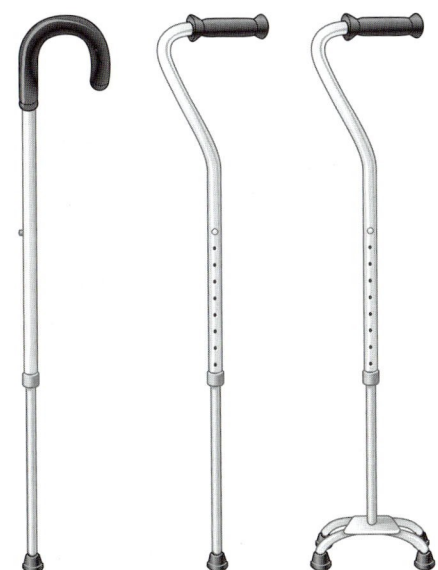

FIGURE 32-17 Three types of canes.

medicine specialists usually fit the brace. Nursing responsibilities include assisting the patient into and out of the brace and monitoring the condition of the skin under the brace.

Crutches

Crutches are commonly used for rehabilitation of an injured lower extremity. The purpose of using crutches is to limit or eliminate weight-bearing on the leg(s) by forcing the user to rely on strength in the arms and shoulders for support. Two forms of crutches are available.

The *forearm support crutch* is more likely to be used by a patient with permanent limitations. It is usually constructed of lightweight aluminum with a hand hold and a forearm support (Fig. 32-19A).

Axillary crutches are for both short- and long-term use (Fig. 32-19B). Properly fitted axillary crutches support the body weight in the hands and arms, not the axilla. For guidelines on how to measure a patient for an axillary crutch,

 Go to Chapter 32, **Clinical Insight 32-5: Sizing Walking Aids,** in Volume 2.

Crutch walking taxes the arms and hands and may cause discomfort to the axillae, arms, and palms where the patient is bearing weight. There are five crutch gaits: two-point gait, three-point gait, four-point gait, swing-to gait, and swing-through gait. Two-point and four-point gait are used for partial weight-bearing, whereas three-point gait is used when weight-bearing must be avoided. Swing-to and swing-through are used when weight-bearing is permitted.

For basic gaits and guidelines for teaching patients to use crutches,

 Go to Chapter 32, **Clinical Insight 32-6: Teaching Clients to Use Canes, Walkers, and Crutches,** in Volume 2.

To see animations of crutch gaits,

 Go to **Animations: 5 Types of Crutch Gaits,** on Davis*Plus.*

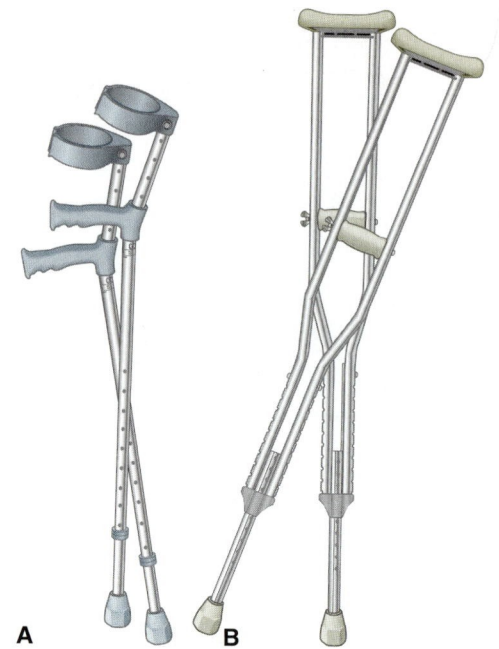

FIGURE 32-19 Crutches. *A,* Forearm support crutches. *B,* Axillary crutches.

KnowledgeCheck 32-10

- What type of cane should a patient with significant balance problems use?
- When are forearm support crutches used?
- Identify five crutch gaits.

 ### ThinkLike a Nurse 32-6

Discuss crutch walking with your peers and family. What instruction would facilitate the best understanding of proper crutch-walking technique?

 To explore learning resources for this chapter,

 Go to Davis*Plus* at DavisPl.us/Wilkinson3.

Chapter Resources for Chapter 32:

Response sheets for all learning activities

Resources for Caregivers and Health Professionals

Reading More About Physical Activity & Mobility (suggested readings)

Concept Map of chapter content

Interactive Case Studies

NCLEX-Style and Chapter Review Questions

Chapter Overview Podcasts

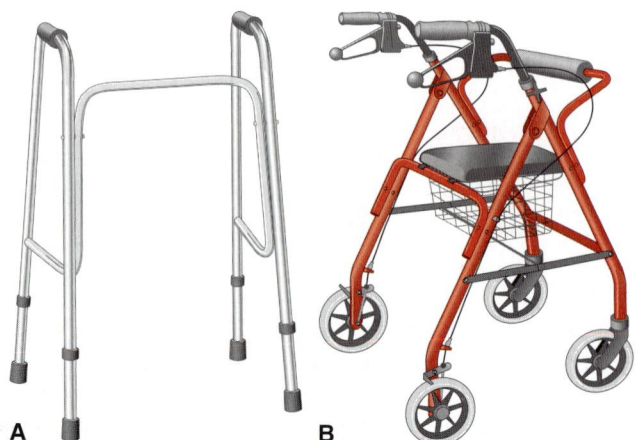

FIGURE 32-18 Walkers. *A,* The basic walker is picked up and advanced as the patient steps ahead. *B,* Some walkers have wheels and seats that allow the patient to rest periodically.

For references cited in this chapter,

 Go to Volume 2, **References Cited.**

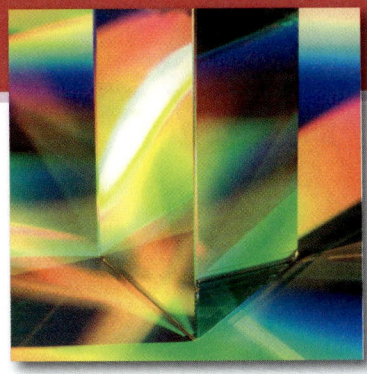

CHAPTER 33

Sexual Health

Learning Outcomes

After completing this chapter, you should be able to:

➤ Identify the female and male reproductive organs.

➤ Describe the physical, emotional, social, and spiritual aspects of human sexuality.

➤ Explain how gender, gender identity, and sexual orientation contribute to expression of sexuality throughout the life cycle.

➤ Differentiate between typical and atypical forms of sexual expression.

➤ Explore physical and psychological issues that affect sexuality and sexual functioning.

➤ Complete a sexual history as part of a comprehensive nursing assessment.

➤ State nursing diagnoses to describe sexuality problems.

➤ Explain how sexual health is challenged by high-risk sexual behaviors, sexually transmitted infections (STIs), menstrual problems, infertility, negative intimate relationships, sexual harassment, rape, and disorders of the sexual response cycle.

➤ Provide nursing interventions that enhance sexual well-being.

➤ Discuss strategies to increase your personal comfort and confidence in providing holistic nursing care.

➤ Describe approaches for dealing with inappropriate sexual behavior from patients or in the work environment.

Key Concepts

Sexual dysfunction

Sexual health

Sexuality

Related Concepts

See the Concept Map on Davis*Plus*.

Meet Your Patients

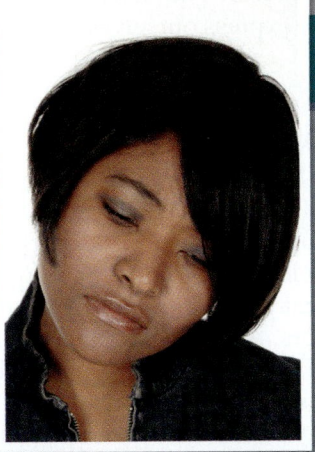
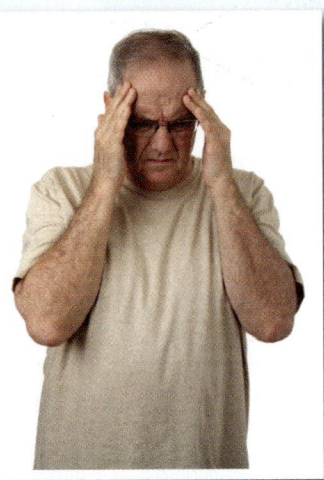

■ Two days after undergoing a fine-needle aspiration to evaluate a small breast mass, Jocelyn Carter's surgeon informed her that the mass was malignant. He recommended a mastectomy (removal of the breast). Today, she arrives alone at the surgery registration area. You ask how she is feeling, and she tells you that the past week has been a whirlwind of activity. "I had to arrange childcare, cancel a business trip, and organize the house so that I could take a few days off to have the surgery. My husband is working overseas this fall, so he couldn't be here to help me. Honestly, I don't know how I'm feeling. I haven't had time to think about it." A few minutes later, as she waits in the surgery holding area, she begins to cry. You hold her hand and ask whether she would like to talk. She asks you, "Do you think my husband will still want me? I'm afraid he will be turned off when he looks at me."

■ Gabriel Thomas comes to the outpatient clinic complaining of a throbbing headache for the past 3 days. He explains that he has tried several over-the-counter (OTC) medicines and has had no relief. You check his blood pressure, and measure the reading at 240/130 mm Hg. When

Meet Your Patients (continued)

you ask whether he has ever been treated for high blood pressure, he replies, "Are you another one of these people trying to get me to take drugs that will ruin my sex life?"

- Frank Thanee, who has heart disease, had a mitral valve replacement 3 days ago. He has been transferred to the cardiology floor for an additional day of hospitalization. His partner, Greg, has spent the past 3 days at the hospital and has just left to check on the apartment and feed their cat. Frank confides that he is worried about his parents' expected visit. "I've never been able to tell them about Greg. They wouldn't be able to understand it, never mind approve. I don't know how to handle this. What do you think I should do?"

Although each of these clients has a different medical diagnosis, all are experiencing a concern related to

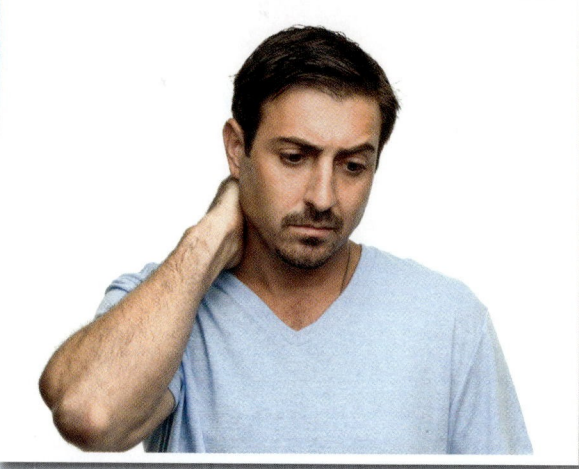

sexuality. In this chapter, we explore the relationship between health and sexuality, and the nurse's role in promoting sexual health.

Theoretical Knowledge
knowing **why**

When a baby is born, the first question the parents ask is, "Is it a boy or a girl?" In fact, many parents want to know the gender of their baby early in the pregnancy at the first sonogram. Hopes and dreams of future parent–child relationships (e.g., mother–daughter) often begin to form even during the first months of pregnancy. As you will learn, sexuality encompasses much more than gender. It includes how we perceive ourselves, how we relate to others, and how we express ourselves as sexual beings.

ABOUT THE KEY CONCEPTS

Like many people, you may have been socialized to avoid talking openly about sexuality. As a nurse, though, you will find that you must discuss a variety of issues pertaining to sexuality that are vital for clients' optimal wellness. Some of these discussions may include sexual dysfunctions, infections, or behaviors. As you learn about concepts related to sexuality and sexual function, you will be challenged to confront and set aside your own biases to comfortably and competently address your clients' sexual health needs.

SEXUAL AND REPRODUCTIVE ANATOMY AND PHYSIOLOGY

The role of the reproductive system in human life extends far beyond its basic function of producing children. It influences body image, sexual desire, and sense

of sexual identity. The first step in exploring human sexuality is to understand the basics of reproductive anatomy and physiology.

Female Reproductive Organs

The female reproductive system consists of a pair of ovaries and fallopian tubes, the uterus, vagina, and external genital tissues (Fig. 33-1). **Ova** (eggs) are produced in the ovaries and travel through the fallopian tubes to the uterus. If fertilization occurs, the embryo embeds in the wall of the uterus for further development.

The **vagina** is a muscular tube that receives sperm during sexual intercourse, allows the exit of menstrual flow if fertilization does not occur, and serves as a birth canal at the end of pregnancy.

The external genitalia and the mons pubis are a source of pleasurable sensations. The **mons pubis** is a pad of fatty tissue over the symphysis pubis. It is covered with coarse hair and contains sensitive nerve endings. The external genitalia, or **vulva**, consist of the clitoris, labia majora, labia minora, Bartholin's glands, urinary meatus, and vaginal introitus. The **clitoris** contains erectile tissue, blood vessels, and nerves. It is extremely sensitive and reacts to pleasurable stimuli. The **labia minora** also engorge and become sensitive during sexual stimulation. External genital organs, such as the clitoris, are protected by the **labia majora**.

The breasts are important to female sexual arousal; in fact, some women can be brought to orgasm solely by caressing the breasts and nipples. The mammary glands, enclosed within the breasts, are also part of the reproductive system. Their function is to produce milk to provide nourishment for an infant after birth.

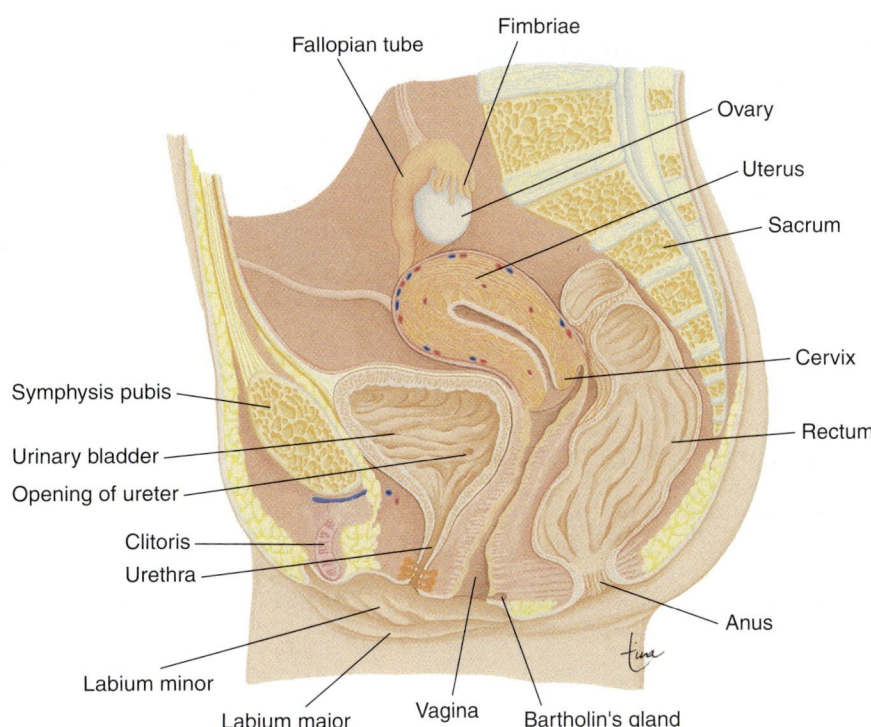

FIGURE 33-1 The female reproductive system.

The Menstrual Cycle

Menstruation begins with puberty and involves hormone changes that prepare the body for pregnancy. The phases of the menstrual cycle are triggered by hormonal changes (Fig. 33-2).

Menstrual Phase Menstruation usually lasts 3 to 7 days, averaging 5 days. During this phase, the uterus sheds the endometrial lining and several ovarian follicles develop. Follicle-stimulating hormone (FSH) from the anterior pituitary gland begins to increase during this phase, leading to a rise in estrogen levels.

Follicular Phase This phase begins on the first day of menstrual bleeding and is associated with growth of ovarian follicles and regrowth of the endometrium of the uterus. This phase ends with **ovulation**, or release of the ovum from the mature follicle, around day 13 or 14 of the menstrual cycle. Luteinizing hormone (LH) levels from the anterior pituitary gland rise, as does the estrogen level.

Ovulatory Phase A surge in LH and FSH occurs, lasting about 16 to 36 hours. The follicle then ruptures and the egg is released for fertilization. Estrogen peaks and progesterone rises, which stimulates growth of the endometrium.

Luteal Phase If fertilization occurs, the endometrium thickens to support an embryo. The pregnancy hormone, called chorionic gonadotropin, is produced. Pregnancy tests are based on detecting levels of this hormone. If fertilization does not occur, progesterone levels drop, and menses begins.

Male Reproductive Organs

The male reproductive system consists of the testes and a series of ducts and glands that transport sperm. Sperm are produced in the testes and transported through the epididymis, ductus deferens, ejaculatory duct, and urethra (Fig. 33-3). Along the path, the reproductive glands (seminal vesicles, prostate, and bulbourethral glands) add secretions that mix with the sperm to produce semen.

The penis functions in the urinary system to transport urine from the bladder to the outside of the body. It also has important functions in the reproductive system. Within the penis are three sections of erectile tissue: the corpus cavernosum and sections of corpus spongiosum above and below the urethra. During sexual arousal these erectile tissues fill with blood, making the penis erect. **Ejaculation** (the expulsion of semen) is brought about by peristalsis of the reproductive ducts and contraction of the prostate and muscles of the pelvic floor. With each ejaculation, approximately 100 million sperm cells are expelled in 2 to 4 mL of semen.

KnowledgeCheck 33-1

- Identify the major structures of the female reproductive system.
- Summarize the phases of the menstrual cycle.
- Identify the major structures of the male reproductive system.

SEXUALITY

What do you think of when you see the term *sexuality*? What images come to mind? The World Health Organization (WHO) notes that "sexuality is experienced and

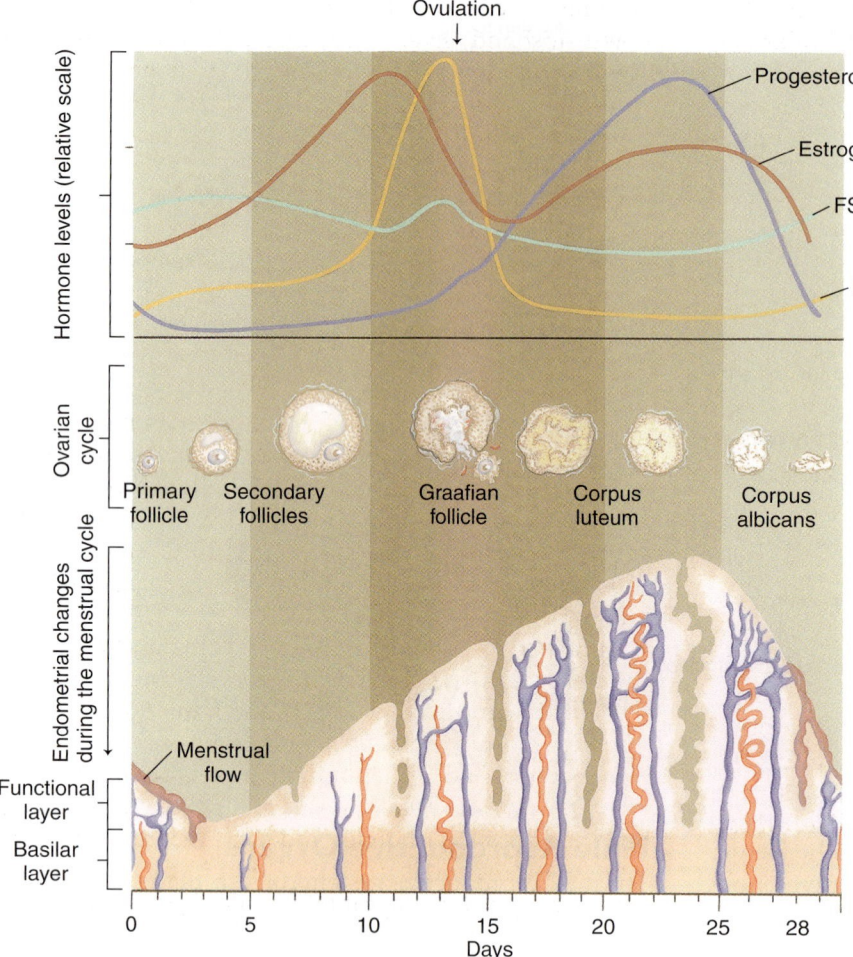

FIGURE 33-2 The menstrual cycle. Hormone levels and endometrial thickness throughout the cycle are shown.

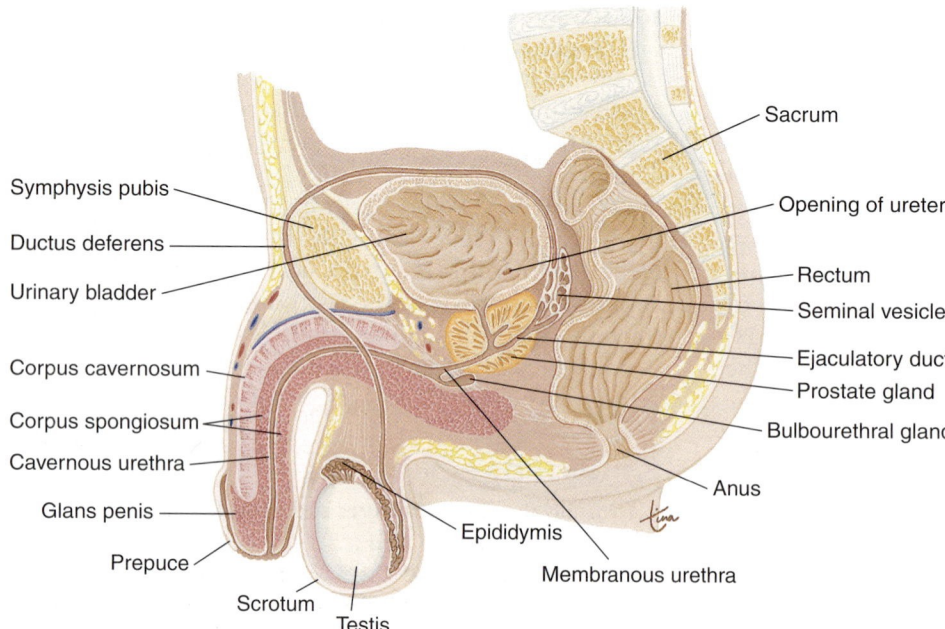

FIGURE 33-3 The male reproductive system.

expressed in thoughts, fantasies, desires, beliefs, attitudes, values, behaviors, practices, roles and relationships." **Sexuality** is recognized as a "central aspect of being human throughout life and encompasses sex, gender identities and roles, sexual orientation, eroticism, pleasure, intimacy and reproduction" (WHO, 2006, updated 2010). **Sexual identity** is a person's perception of his or her gender, gender identity, gender role, and sexual orientation. All of these are also a part of the person's overall self-concept (see Chapter 13 to review self-concept).

What Is Gender?

People often think of *sexuality* as a synonym for *sex*. This is inaccurate. In fact, even the word *sex* has multiple meanings. For example, *sex* is used to describe intimate pleasurable activity (e.g., "We had sex yesterday") or to indicate whether an individual is male or female (e.g., "What sex is your baby?"). In this chapter, we use the term **gender** to indicate biological sex status (male or female) and follow the World Health Organization's definition of sexuality.

Gender is determined at the moment of conception, when an ovum is fertilized by a sperm. The ovum always provides an X chromosome, whereas the sperm may contribute either a second X chromosome, which results in a female offspring, or a Y chromosome, resulting in a male offspring (Fig. 33-4).

Gender Roles

Gender roles are the societal norms for gender-appropriate behavior. During the 1950s, the media portrayed the father in a suit who went off to work to support his family. Mother, in her apron, spent the day cooking, cleaning, and caring for her perfect children and devoted husband. Even then, many Americans did not identify with this stereotype, and today it may seem unreal. But many of these values remain embedded at some level within our contemporary culture (Fulcher & Coyle, 2011).

Historically in Western culture, people expected men to be strong and control their feelings, and women to be gentle and express their feelings. Boys received positive reinforcement for "masculine" behaviors, such as competitiveness, and ridicule or teasing for showing emotions or being passive. In girls, "feminine" behaviors, such as passivity and cooperation were reinforced, whereas assertiveness was often labeled as unacceptable aggression. In the past 50 years, expectations regarding gender roles have changed and expanded. Women now perform jobs formerly thought to be "for men only" (e.g., physician, police officer) and men are active in professions once dominated by females (e.g., teaching, nursing).

Today, many parents encourage some **androgyny** in their children. The word *androgyny* is a combination of the Greek words for male, *andro*, and female, *gyn*. By one of its definitions, *androgyny* refers to a blending of traditional masculine and feminine roles. It means that everyone has some skills, traits, and behaviors that may be classified as "masculine" and some that may be "feminine." Androgyny is a positive trait in that it gives an individual greater adaptability in life situations.

▲ ThinkLike a Nurse 33-1

- Provide at least three examples of nonconformity to traditional gender role expectations.
- As a parent, how might you encourage androgyny in your children, if you wished to do so?

Gender Identity

Gender identity, one component of sexual identity, is the image we have about ourselves as a man or woman. It is an internal experience: whether we "feel like" a woman or a man. However, when a person forms a gender identity that is not the same as their biological gender, he or she is considered **transgendered** (or "differently gendered"). The *Diagnostic and Statistical Manual of Mental Disorders* (DSM-5) replaced the concept of gender identity disorder with gender dysphoria and emphasizes that gender nonconformity is not a mental disorder (American Psychiatric Association [APA], 2013a).

Key Point: *You should understand the numerous and different terms associated with the concept of "transgender" to provide nonjudgmental and appropriate care (e.g., transsexual, intersexed, transvestite, heterosexual, homosexual, or bisexual) (Dickinson, Cook, Playle, et al., 2012; Walsh, Barnsteiner, De Leon Siantz, et al., 2012).*

- **Transsexuals** are people who identify with the opposite gender from their biology—for example, a person with the physical appearance and reproductive organs

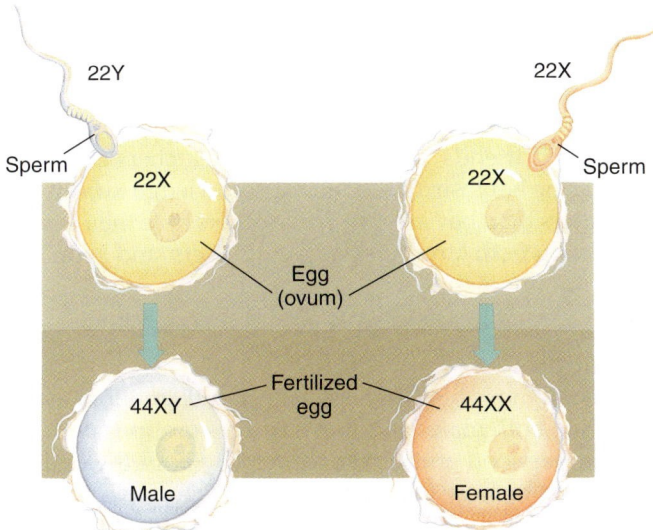

FIGURE 33-4 The woman provides the X chromosome, and the man may contribute either a second X chromosome, which results in a female offspring, or a Y chromosome, resulting in a male offspring.

of a woman who "feels" and perceives herself to be a man. It is common for transsexuals to express dissatisfaction with their gender at an early age. They may insist that they will grow up to be the opposite gender. Their preference for dress and play is typically those of the other gender.

■ **Preoperative transsexuals** are adults who alter their physical appearance through dress, makeup, and/or the use of hormones so that their external appearance corresponds to their gender identity. After extensive counseling and successfully living in the opposite gender role for a period of time, they may decide to undergo surgery to reconstruct their external genitalia and remove the reproductive organs of the biological birth gender. After sex reassignment surgery, the **postoperative transsexual individual** legally changes gender. In an inpatient facility, during the perioperative period, assignment to a single room is more appropriate.

■ **Intersexed** people (formerly referred to as **hermaphrodites**) are born with ambiguous sexual organs. For example, the person may have female internal organs (ovaries, a uterus), but enlarged clitoral tissue resembling a penis. Initially, a developing embryo is in an **undifferentiated sexual state**—neither male nor female until about the seventh week of pregnancy when the gonads form into either testes or ovaries. A mutation of any of the genes involved in sexual differentiation or an alteration in hormonal secretion may result in altered genitalia. Parents must decide whether to have the child undergo surgery to make the assigned sex consistent with the physical appearance or to delay assignment and allow the child to choose at a later time.

■ A **transvestite** (or **cross-dresser**) is a person (male or female) who occasionally or frequently wears the clothing characteristic of the opposite sex, particularly the under-garments, as a form of sexual expression. The person often carries out this behavior in secret. Cross-dressers may be heterosexual, homosexual, or bisexual (see the next section, What Is Sexual Orientation?).

KnowledgeCheck 33-2

■ How is gender determined?
■ Distinguish gender, gender role, and gender identity.
■ What is androgyny?

 ThinkLike a Nurse 33-2

Do you believe that androgyny is a positive attribute? Explain your thinking.

What Is Sexual Orientation?

Sexual orientation refers to the general tendency of a person to feel sexually attracted to people of a certain gender. Because most people in Western culture are thought to be **heterosexual** (sexually attracted to members of the opposite sex), heterosexuality is the predominant cultural expectation. However, in the mid-20th century, the research of Alfred C. Kinsey indicated that a population's sexual orientation falls on a bell curve, with the majority of people experiencing at least some attraction to people of the same gender (Kinsey 1948, reprinted 1998). Kinsey theorized that society influences people to sublimate homosexual feelings and choose exclusively heterosexual relationships.

Klein, Sepekoff, and Wolf (1985) described sexual orientation as an ongoing dynamic process, with people's gender-based inclinations changing over time. In truth, we do not fully understand what makes up sexual orientation or how it develops. With increasing research on the biological aspects of sexual orientation, more professionals are concluding that people come to "recognize" the object of their sexual desire rather than "choose" or "prefer" it. Therefore, "sexual orientation" is probably a more accurate term than "sexual preference."

Heterosexuality

Heterosexuals are people who are sexually and emotionally attracted to members of the opposite sex. In informal conversation, people may refer to this segment of the population as *straight*. Many major religious traditions reinforce heterosexual behaviors and gender roles. Although some heterosexuals have had same-gender sexual thoughts or limited experiences during childhood, adolescence, or adulthood, they still consider themselves heterosexual and have relationships with people of the opposite gender.

Homosexuality

The focus of sexual attraction for **homosexuals** is a person of the same gender. Homosexuals may be referred to as *gay* men and *lesbian* women. Accurate prevalence statistics are difficult to obtain because most of the studies rely on self-report data. Homosexuality is not an aspect of the dominant culture and is prohibited by some religions. As a result, there has been significant discrimination against homosexuals. It can be difficult for gays and lesbians to share this aspect of their lives with employers, colleagues, family, and friends, as well as with researchers and pollsters. Some homosexuals openly acknowledge to both self and others that they are gay, while others hide their sexual orientation from family, friends, employers, and people in their communities.

Bisexuality

A person who is **bisexual** is sexually and emotionally attracted to both males and females. This group is perhaps least understood and least accepted by both the heterosexual and homosexual communities. They are less likely to be found in long-term monogamous relationships and often experience feelings of isolation. However, some bisexuals maintain stable and satisfying marriages because of their sustained sexual attraction to and amiable relationship with their spouse and the importance they place on parenting. Compatibility within the marriage depends on the partner's acceptance of the bisexual spouse's sexual orientation and sexual relationships outside the marriage, if any.

KnowledgeCheck 33-3

- What are the majority and minority sexual orientations in our culture?
- What is meant by *transgender*?

ThinkLike a Nurse 33-3

- What sexual orientations are you comfortable working with?
- Would you have difficulty working with a transsexual or other transgendered client?

How Does Sexuality Develop?

We are sexual beings from birth to death. Expression of our sexuality evolves through the life span. If you require additional discussion on sexuality and developmental stages,

Go to Chapters 9 and 10, **Expanded Discussion,** on *DavisPlus.*

Birth Through Preschool

Beginning at birth, parents, caregivers, and others respond to the infant with preconceived thoughts of what that gender role entails. The first 2 years of life can be highly sensual; as infants are nursed, stroked, bathed, and massaged, they develop their first attachment experience through bonding with the parent or caregiver (Fig. 33-5). It is not unusual for children in this age group to touch their genitals and enjoy being nude. This behavior is part of their exploration of their bodies and is a normal part of child development. By age 3, most children recognize gender differences and know the names of body parts. Toddlers are interested in their bodies and curious to see the genitals of others.

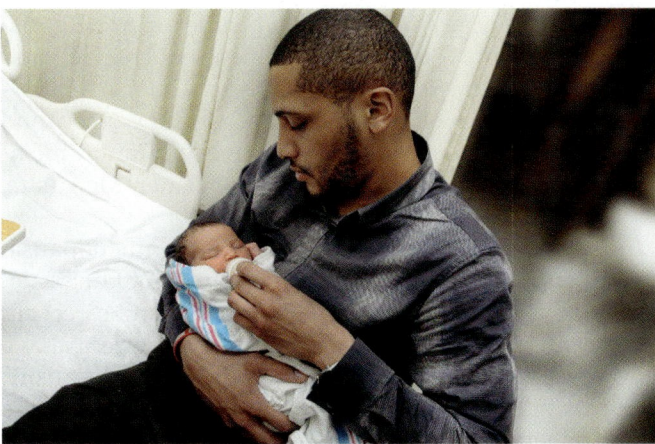

FIGURE 33-5 Parent–infant attachment occurs through daily contact and care through activities such as feeding, bathing, and holding.

By age 5, children mimic adults by holding hands or hugging. Adults, who find these actions amusing or endearing, frequently reinforce such behaviors. Young children also may practice getting married, playing house, or playing doctor. It is not unusual for preschool children to masturbate and ask questions about "where babies come from." Parents should give factual answers without offering explanations beyond what the child asks.

School Age Through Puberty

The school-age child strongly identifies with the same-sex parent and has mostly same-sex friends. Through interaction at home, school, and other activities, children gain awareness of gender roles and emerging gender identity.

From age 8 to 12, the child is in transition between childhood and puberty. Secondary sex characteristics become apparent. In females, breast buds form, and pubic hair appears. For a significant number of girls, **menarche** (beginning of menstruation) occurs. Boys become more muscular, the voice deepens, hair in facial and axillae develop, and the genitals begin to increase in size. The first attraction, either heterosexual or homosexual, may occur during this stage, and the child may begin to masturbate more frequently, but privately. For information on the Tanner stages of sexual development in boys and girls,

Go to Chapter 22, **Procedures 22-17** and **22-18,** in Volume 2.

Many school-age children are curious and may ask explicit questions about sexual activity, reproduction, and sex roles. Parents and nurses should answer with facts and follow up with age-appropriate printed material. When children reach age 10 to 12, parents should begin teaching them basic information about approaching body changes, menstruation, sexual intercourse, and reproduction.

Adolescents

Adolescence is a time of heightened sexual interest and activity. There are two reasons for this: (1) the hormonal changes accompanying puberty and (2) the culture's emphasis on sex. Masturbation is common. It is a safe and comforting sexual activity that has neither interpersonal nor disease risks. However, some adolescents may encounter parental, cultural, or religious disapproval of masturbation.

Sexual exploration usually begins with kissing, moves on to fondling, and can lead to genital contact. This progression may occur over a period of years, or there may be an early initiation of oral, vaginal, or anal intercourse. In 2011, 47% of teenagers in U.S. high school students surveyed had engaged in sexual intercourse (Centers for Disease Control and Prevention [CDC], 2012a). However, the birth rate for adolescents and teenagers reached a record low in 2011 (CDC, updated 2013a). The incidence of oral sex is increasing in U.S.

youth. Two-thirds of youths between the ages of 15 and 25 have engaged in oral sex (Copen, Chandra, & Martinez, 2012). Many teens believe that this behavior allows them to maintain their virginity and incorrectly assume that it carries no health risks. Sexuality education in the home and school dispels myths and prepares teens for adult roles. To make informed choices as they move toward adulthood, adolescents need information about body changes, interpersonal relationships, **contraception** (birth control), and preventing **sexually transmitted infections (STIs)**.

To review physical changes of adolescence, see Chapters 9 and 22.

Young Adults

Not so many years ago it was generally assumed that young adults would abstain from sexual intercourse until marriage. The husband and wife would then become sexually active and start a family. Today, the age of first marriage is higher than in previous decades and young adults engage more openly in sexual activity outside of marriage. Many young adults practice **serial monogamy**, in which the partners are mutually faithful but make no lifelong commitment. When the relationship ends, each partner usually enters another monogamous relationship.

During early adulthood, people define their sexual identity and resolve issues related to their sexual orientation and self-concept. As a part of sexual maturity, they develop an intimate relationship in which there is both communication and respect. Many people find a life partner during this period and make long-term plans, which often include parenting. However, some adults continue to struggle with their sexual identity, sexual orientation, or ability to form or commit to intimate relationships.

Young adults often wonder whether their sexual behaviors and responses are normal (e.g., "How often do most people have intercourse?" "Do other women have an orgasm every time they have sex?"). Many still need information about birth control, prevention of STIs, and relationship and communication issues.

Middle Adults

Adults in the middle years experience life changes that may enhance physical and emotional intimacy. For many parents, their children are now young adults who no longer rely on parental support, and they have more privacy and time to spend together. However, new stressors may arise. In times of economic downturn, for example, middle-aged adults are also one of the groups most seriously affected. In addition, this may also be a time when physical changes and chronic diseases emerge that could affect sexual patterns.

Female Transitions Women transition through **menopause** (cessation of menstruation), a process that varies widely. Some are relieved that the prospect of childbearing has ended, while others may mourn the loss of the ability to give birth. Normal physiological changes include decreased vaginal secretions and vaginal wall thinning that result from decreased levels of estrogen and progesterone. These changes may result in painful intercourse and decrease a woman's desire for sexual activity. Some women also experience hot flashes, sleep disturbances, and mood changes.

Male Transitions As a result of the aging process or health conditions (e.g., type 2 diabetes or hypertension), men may experience erectile difficulty. They may perceive this problem as a threat to their masculinity and sexual attractiveness, and their self-image may suffer. Men also experience a decrease in the sex hormone testosterone. Many men remain fertile into old age, although sexual desire and the ability to achieve and maintain erection decrease gradually with aging.

It may be a challenge for you to view middle adults as individuals who engage in and enjoy sexual relations. Patients of this age may remind you of your parents and thus it may be difficult for you to see them as persons who have sexual relationships. Holistic nursing care requires you to assess and formulate strategies to address their sexual concerns.

Aging Adults

Most older adults are sexually active and regard sexuality as an important part of life. Little evidence exists to support the premise that age-related changes result in decreased sexual relationships (Delamater, 2010). A substantial number of men and women engage in vaginal intercourse, oral sex, and masturbation even in their 80s and 90s (Delamater, 2010; Lindau, Schuman, Laumann, et al., 2007; Taylor & Gosney, 2011). You should recognize that older adults have sexual needs (e.g., reassurance from a sexual partner or sexual stimulation) and sexual problems (e.g., lack of closeness).

Sexual problems are more likely to result from failing physical health and medication side effects than from age alone. For example, as noted earlier, men with diabetes are more likely to have difficulty achieving and maintaining an erection. Other obstacles for sexual expression are lack of a partner (especially for women) and lack of privacy (e.g., for those who live with family members or in a long-term care facility) (Bauer, McAuliffe, Nay, et al., 2013).

As a result of age-related changes, postmenopausal women report less sexual stimulation and reduced desire, so they tend to need more foreplay and direct clitoral stimulation for sexual enjoyment. They may have fewer orgasms or orgasms that are weaker in intensity. Nevertheless, some women "rediscover" sexual desire after menopause.

Older women may complain of loss of vaginal lubrication and experience pain during intercourse, caused by vaginal thinning and dryness. You can help your patients by suggesting water-soluble lubricants to counteract vaginal dryness and enhance pleasurable sensations during sexual activity.

Some men report erectile difficulty and need more time and more direct genital stimulation to achieve erection. It may take longer to ejaculate, and the orgasmic contractions may be less intense. When penetration is not possible (e.g., because of male erectile dysfunction), many couples find satisfaction with alternate forms of sexual stimulation and expression.

In the past, many healthcare providers have hesitated to offer sexual counseling out of fear that such intimate discussion might offend their patients. Older adults may also hesitate to discuss their sexual problem with healthcare providers unless encouraged to do so. You should address the topic as you would any other area (e.g., "We have discussed your medical needs and your dietary needs; let's now discuss your sexual needs"). Once you introduce the subject and people feel comfortable, they are usually eager for advice and solutions (American Geriatric Society Foundation, updated 2012).

You can help aging clients to understand that sexual feelings do not necessarily disappear with age, and sexual expression need not stop (Fig. 33-6). For example, sexual expression may include hugging, caressing, oral sex, and mutual manual stimulation. In addition, you may suggest ways to adapt coital positions to accommodate bodily changes, for example, when a partner is obese or has joint immobility.

KnowledgeCheck 33-4

- Why is it important to consider sexuality throughout the life cycle?
- What are the two major contributing factors to adolescents' heightened sexual interest and activity?
- What aspects of human sexuality are associated with young and middle adulthood?
- What challenges to sexuality may be found in the aging adult?

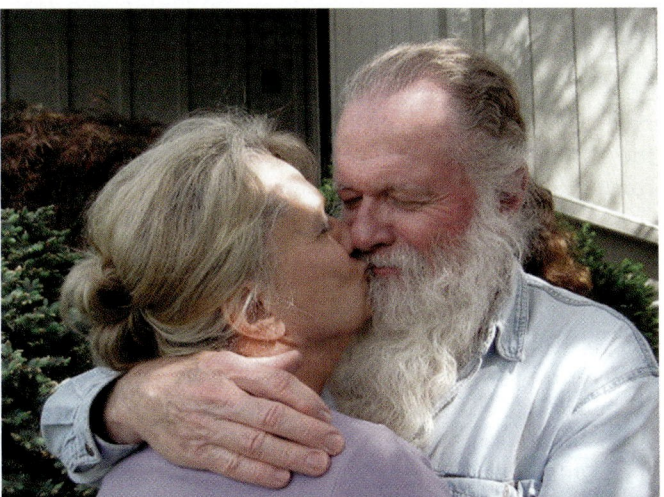

FIGURE 33-6 Healthy older adults maintain sexual intimacy.

What Factors Affect Sexuality?

Culture, religion, lifestyle, sexual knowledge, and physical health all influence our attitudes toward sexuality, sexual behaviors, and intimate relationships. This section will help you begin to broaden your understanding of the key concepts of sexuality and sexual health to provide nonjudgmental, holistic care to people who have a wide range of values, lifestyles, and states of well-being.

Culture

Culture influences our ideas about gender role, gender identity, marriage, sexual expression, and social responsibilities. However, it is not unusual for people to be **ethnocentric**—that is, to see their own culture and sexual behaviors as the norm for all. Because the United States is a multicultural country, beliefs and practices related to human sexuality vary widely. Consider the following examples of cultural influences:

- Puritan and Victorian-era legacies have influenced many European Americans, some of whom consider sex to be "not nice," particularly if engaging in certain sexual activities or positions.
- African Americans are influenced by the dominant Anglo-Saxon culture, their African heritage, history in America, and current economic and social situation. Marriage rates for blacks are lower than for other ethnic groups, in part because of economics, an unequal gender ratio (84 males per 100 females), and cultural acceptance of single parenting (Hummer & Hamilton, 2010; Hyde & DeLamater, 2010).
- Many Latinos have strong ties to the Roman Catholic Church and a tradition of rigidly defined gender roles. The norm in Hispanic culture is for the male to be given more freedom as a child, but he is expected to be a virile, responsible provider for his family as an adult. In contrast, the female is typically raised to be more passive and obedient throughout her life.
- Asian Americans and Muslim Americans tend to be the most sexually conservative of the major U.S. cultural groups.

Culture determines what is acceptable and what is not. In some societies, **polygamy** (marriage to more than one partner) may be acceptable. Another culture may permit or prohibit sexual play among children. Many cultures have special rites of passage at puberty, such as the Jewish bar mitzvah for boys and bat mitzvah for girls, or the Native American vision quest.

Generally, you should honor cultural practices unless they are harmful. An example of a harmful practice is female genital mutilation (formerly known as **female circumcision**), which is illegal in most countries but is still performed among certain tribes. In this procedure, the labia majora, labia minora, and clitoris are excised, and/or the vagina is sutured closed (**infibulation**). Infibulation may be done to ensure that the girl remains a virgin, whereas clitoral excision is meant to reduce sexual desire and ensure that the woman remains faithful to her husband. In addition to its psychosocial consequences, the procedure carries a high risk of infection and can cause the development of scar tissue that makes vaginal birth impossible. The U.S. Congress passed a law in 1996 making female genital mutilation for girls younger than 18 a federal offense. The World Health Organization in 1997 and again in 2010, with the support of the United Nations, issued statements to abolish the practice of female genital mutilation (WHO, 2010, updated 2013).

Religion

Religion also has a powerful influence on sexuality. Religious practices restricting premarital sex, birth control, homosexuality, abortion, extramarital relationships, and masturbation are common. Some religions restrict opposite gender healthcare providers and have rules about body coverings and modesty. Even education about the structure and function of the human body is governed by some religions. The "sexual revolution" that began in the 1960s has led to permissive sexual values in the broader Western culture. When these values conflict with a person's traditional religious values, anxiety and sexual dysfunction may result. To review the influence of religion on health, see Chapter 16.

 ThinkLike a Nurse 33-4

How have religion and culture influenced your views on sexuality?

Lifestyle

Life experiences encompass our interactions with others and the environment. Family, socioeconomic status, employment factors, and interpersonal relationships shape our lifestyle, although they do not fully determine it. Consider the following examples:

- Having a beloved brother reveal to you that he is gay might alter your perception of homosexuality. Similarly, being raised by a same-sex couple might affect your view of gender roles.
- Growing up in a low-income neighborhood in which prostitution is a visible and accepted part of the environment might influence your views on acceptable sexual behavior.
- Dedication to a high-stress job or family demands might leave you too exhausted to desire sex with your spouse.
- Being in an abusive relationship would affect how you feel about yourself and might cause you to avoid intimacy in the future.

Lessons learned through day-to-day experience create powerful impressions on our views and often modify cultural and religious influences.

Sexual Knowledge

Although sexuality and family life are part of the curriculum in many public schools, you cannot assume that young adults have adequate sexual knowledge. Community values play a large role in determining how sexuality is viewed and taught. Thus, even if a state mandates sex education, a particular school may limit discussion on reproduction, STIs, birth control, intimacy, exploitive relationships, domestic abuse, or rape, believing that these topics are best addressed by the family or church. In addition, many children are home-schooled or taught in private or church-affiliated schools that do not allocate any class time to sex education. Even in schools with a comprehensive curriculum, parents have the right to exclude their child from sex education classes. Do not let your clients' age, level of education, or life experiences lead you to make assumptions about their knowledge of sexuality. For example:

- A married person may not be sexually active.
- A woman with several children may not know what is involved in a pelvic exam or how conception occurs.
- A highly educated person may be uninformed regarding his body structure and function.

It is difficult for most people to admit to a professional that they lack knowledge. Therefore, you must assess each client's knowledge and understanding of sexual terms. At times you may need to use the vernacular or "street" terminology to be understood. You can then introduce medically specific terminology.

KnowledgeCheck 33-5

- What sexual knowledge would you expect an adult male with children to have?
- What sexual knowledge would you expect a nursing student to have?

Health and Illness

Sexuality involves body, mind, and spirit so it is not surprising that health status affects sexuality. For example, healthful nutrition and physical exercise are commonly reported to increase satisfaction in sexual relationships, whereas obesity and inactivity can undermine one's own feelings of attractiveness or one's attraction for one's partner. The importance of sexuality is readily apparent in the clinical setting. For example, the clients in the Meet Your Patients scenarios all expressed concerns related to their sexuality.

Physical Illness

Diseases, injuries, and medical treatments may demand lifestyle changes in multiple areas, including sexual functioning.

- **Heart disease or respiratory disease** may cause people to restrict sexual activity because of fatigue, dyspnea, or fear of overstressing the heart.
- **Diabetes mellitus** leads to neurological changes that may cause male erectile dysfunction; women may experience vaginal dryness and loss of orgasmic

ability. In addition, vaginal yeast infections are common with diabetes, causing itching and painful intercourse.

- **Cancer** may be accompanied by body image changes, fatigue, treatments that create nausea, and fear of death—all of which may lead to feeling unattractive, with a reduced desire for sexual activity.
- **Spinal cord injury** may make it impossible for the person to feel physical stimulation. Depending on the level of the injury, the person may or may not experience psychogenic or reflexogenic genital arousal. Some men may be able to achieve erection and ejaculation and are fertile; others may have no genital response.

Surgeries

Surgery may alter a person's body image. At the least, surgery leaves a physical scar. At worst, it removes a body part or creates other disfigurement. When the surgery involves body parts important to sexual functioning (e.g., a breast, a testicle), the effect is even more likely to be negative. Some people may avoid sex because of sexual esteem issues (e.g., feeling unattractive, concern about partner's reaction). This may be especially true after a hysterectomy, mastectomy, orchiectomy, prostatectomy, or colostomy (or other ostomy).

- **Hysterectomy** (surgical removal of a uterus) may enhance the sexual experience if it relieves pain and bleeding that were present before surgery. In contrast, some women report difficulty becoming aroused or having less intense orgasm after hysterectomy. These problems may be related to trauma to nerves in the pelvic area, to the absence of uterine contractions during orgasm, or to anxiety because the woman's gender identity is tied to childbearing.
- **Mastectomy** (surgical removal of a breast) can have a significant influence on a woman's self-esteem and negatively impact sexuality. Research found that among sexually active women, body image problems were related to breast reconstruction, fertility, hair loss from chemotherapy, weight gain or loss, and a partner's difficulty understanding one's feelings (Katz, 2011).
- **Prostatectomy** (removal of the prostate gland, usually to treat prostate cancer) may be accompanied by erectile and other sexual dysfunction.
- **Orchiectomy** (removal of the testicle) is usually performed for testicular cancer. Males can experience infertility, which is associated with loss of self-concept, sexual identity, and intimacy (Bradford, 2012).
- A **colostomy** is a surgical procedure that brings a portion of the colon through a surgical opening in the abdomen (see Chapter 29 for review). The patient must usually wear a pouch, in which to expel feces. Ostomy surgery profoundly impacts sexuality. Patients with ostomies often experience body image difficulties; loss of desire for intercourse; fears about leakage, noise from flatulence, and pain; and concern about how their partners will react (Schuler, 2013).

If a person becomes disabled while in a marriage or other committed relationship, the strain can threaten the relationship. In contrast, a person who is single or has a lifelong disability may experience difficulty establishing an intimate relationship because of physical limitations, social isolation, poor self-image, or discrimination. A need for intimacy still exists even when people lose interest in sexual activities. Communication about sexual needs and desires may be difficult for couples, but as a nurse, you can support and facilitate discussions of your patients' concerns. Holistic rehabilitation programs may offer comprehensive services and promote discussions regarding sexuality and relationship issues.

Mental Health Disorders

Psychiatric disorders can lead to interpersonal disruptions and difficulty with sexual expression.

- A depressed person experiences significant loss of interest in activities that previously brought pleasure. Thus it is common for people with depression to avoid engaging in interpersonal activities, including sex.
- Conversely, a person with hypomania or mania may be preoccupied with pleasurable activities and increased sexual activity, as well as verbalization and acting out. Both extremes are disruptive to a relationship.
- For a person with psychosis, interpersonal relationships and sexual patterns are disrupted by lack of contact with reality or frank delusions.

Counseling for the couple is important when symptoms are controlled. During times of acute illness, it is vital that the partner have medical and psychological support.

Medications

Many medications used to treat health problems have unwelcome sexual side effects. Gabriel Thomas (Meet Your Patients) clearly illustrates the concern some clients have about commonly prescribed medications. Table 33-1 lists a number of drugs and their effects on sexual function.

Medications may be prescribed to enhance sexual function, particularly for men experiencing erectile dysfunction (ED), for example, those with diabetes mellitus or who are taking beta-adrenergic blocking agents to treat high blood pressure. Three oral drugs are available for impotence: sildenafil, vardenafil, and tadalafil. These drugs generally work within 1 hour of administration, but have no effect without sexual stimulation. They increase blood flow to the corpus cavernosum of the penis.

➕ Medications used to treat ED should be used with caution in patients with cardiovascular disease because of its vasodilation effects and is contraindicated in patients receiving nitrate drugs. You should conduct a careful medication history and conduct the appropriate patient teaching.

Table 33-1 ➤ Effects of Drugs on Sexual Function

MEDICATION	POSSIBLE EFFECT
Alcohol	In limited quantities, alcohol may enhance desire and function. However, heavy or chronic use may lead to decreased libido, orgasmic dysfunction, and erectile dysfunction.
Anti-anxiety agents	Decreased libido, delayed ejaculation
Anticonvulsants	Decreased libido, prolonged painful erections, difficulty achieving orgasm
Antidepressants	Decreased libido, difficulty achieving orgasm Bupropion (Wellbutrin) and trazodone (Desyrel) are least likely to cause sexual side effects.
Antihistamines	Decreased libido, decreased vaginal lubrication
Antihypertensives	Decreased libido, erectile dysfunction, delayed ejaculation Calcium channel blockers are least likely to cause sexual difficulties.
Chemotherapy	Fatigue, decreased libido
Opioids	Decreased libido, erectile dysfunction
Stimulants (cocaine, methamphetamines)	Initially stimulants cause increased intensity of the sexual encounter; however, with continued use, sexual dysfunction develops.

KnowledgeCheck 33-6

- Identify four factors associated with physical illness that may affect sexuality or sexual functioning.
- What determines our sexual attitudes?

SEXUAL HEALTH

The World Health Organization defines **sexual health** as "a state of physical, emotional, mental, and social well-being related to sexuality; it is not merely the absence of disease, dysfunction, or infirmity. Sexual health requires a positive and respectful approach to sexuality and sexual relationships, as well as the openness and opportunity to have pleasurable and safe sexual experiences, free of coercion, discrimination, and violence. For sexual health to be attained and maintained, the sexual rights of all persons must be respected, protected, and fulfilled" (WHO, 2006, updated 2010). To promote sexual health effectively, you will need theoretical knowledge about sexual responses, modes of sexual expression, and problems affecting sexuality.

 ThinkLike a Nurse 33-5

Examine your own beliefs about sexuality. Identify areas of concern you have regarding sexuality. How do you think this will affect your ability to assist patients with sexual health concerns?

What Is the Sexual Response Cycle?

The **sexual response cycle** is the sequence of physiological events that occur when a person becomes sexually aroused. Based on research conducted in the 1950s, Masters and Johnson (1966) identified a four-stage

sexual response: excitement, plateau, orgasm, and resolution (Fig. 33-7). Some scholars have suggested that the stage of desire be added to the original Masters and Johnson model. In some people, desire can either precede or follow excitement (Basson, 2001, 2008).

Although it is most intense in the genitals, sexual response is a total body response, involving many physiological changes (e.g., increased heart rate, flushing). The emotional and mental aspects of sexual activity are equally important to the person's satisfaction. The body has many **erogenous zones** (areas that cause sexual arousal when stimulated): the genitals, the skin, lips, ears, breasts, buttocks, and thighs. Box 33-1 shows normal physiological changes in sexual response that occur with aging.

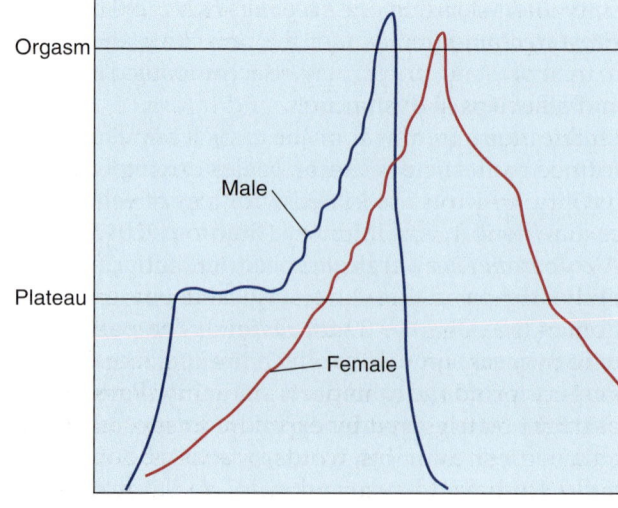

FIGURE 33-7 The sexual response cycle.

BOX 33-1 ■ Normal Physiological Changes in Sexual Response That Occur With Aging

Sexual Response Stage	Changes in Women	Changes in Men
Desire	Decreased libido	Decreased libido
Excitement and plateau	Delayed nipple erection	Delayed nipple erection
	Reduced labial separation and swelling	Delayed and less-firm erection
	Reduced vaginal expansion	Longer excitement stage
	Reduced lubrication	Decreased pre-ejaculatory emissions
	Decreased elevation of the uterus	Reduced muscle tension
	Reduced muscle tension	Reduced lifting of the scrotum and testes
	Reduced vaginal tone (in those who have had multiple vaginal deliveries); results in less stimulation during intercourse	Shorter phase of impending orgasm
		May require more direct stimulation to achieve and maintain an erection
Orgasm	Reduced spread of sexual flush	Shorter ejaculation time
		Fewer ejaculatory contractions
		Reduced volume of ejaculate
Resolution	No cervical dilation	More rapid loss of erection
		Longer refractory period
		Nipple erection lasts longer after orgasm

Sources: Ginsberg, T. (2010). Male sexuality. *Clinics in Geriatric Medicine, 26*(2), 185–195; Kennedy-Malone, L., Fletcher, K., & Plank, L. (2004). *Management guidelines for nurse practitioners working with older adults.* Philadelphia: F.A. Davis; Running, A., & Berndt, A. (2003). *Management guidelines for nurse practitioners working in family practice.* Philadelphia: F.A. Davis; Stanley, M., Blaire, K.A., & Beare, P.G. (2005). *Gerontological nursing: Promoting successful aging with older adults* (3rd ed.). Philadelphia: F.A. Davis; Tsitouras, P. (2011). Male menopause: Just the facts. *Clinical Geriatrics, 19*(8), 28–32; University of California, Santa Barbara. (2012). Aging and the sexual response cycle. SexInfo, Online. Retrieved from http://www.soc.ucsb.edu/sexinfo/article/aging-and-sexual-response-cycle-0; Yee, L. (2010). Aging and sexuality. *Australian Family Physician, 39*(10), 718–721.

Desire

Desire is a stage of varying length characterized by an interest in sexual intimacy. Desire occurs in the mind and is communicated either verbally or through body language. This communication may be subtle and easily misread. In different cultures, behaviors meant to communicate desire may vary along gender lines. **Libido** is an individual's typical level of desire. Desire increases in proportion to the level of the sex hormones (e.g., a man with low testosterone is not as interested in sex). For women, desire reaches a peak each month near the time of ovulation, when estrogen levels are high.

In many people, desire is readily aroused by erotic stimuli, such as sights, sounds, and fantasies. However, research indicates that a majority of women and a minority of men do not experience desire until after they have become aroused; in these people, physical excitement prompts the desire for sex (Basson, 2001, 2008).

What is considered "sexual" or "attractive" can vary greatly, because societal, cultural, and personal values influence the range of stimuli that provoke sexual desire. Desire may last only moments or be ongoing for years. Transient sexual thoughts are fleeting moments of desire that might be triggered by exposure to sexually explicit media or erotic thoughts, words, or actions. Love and desire do not have to occur within a sexual relationship; this kind of example of desire can last for years.

Excitement

Excitement is the body's physical response to desire. During excitement the following bodily changes occur: Heart rate, blood pressure, and respiratory rate increase; muscles tense (**myotonia**); nipples become erect; and genital and pelvic blood supply increases (**vasocongestion**). In women, vasocongestion leads to vaginal lubrication, swelling of the breasts, rise of the uterus, and swelling of the labia and clitoris. In men, erection begins as the penis increases in length and diameter. The testes rise closer to the body, and the scrotum thickens.

Excitement may lead to further sexual activity, but this is not inevitable. For both sexes, the person may lose and regain initial physical excitement many times without advancing to the next stage. Excitement may be communicated verbally or through body language.

Plateau

If stimulation continues, the person reaches the **plateau** phase. Plateau is associated with continued increases in pulse, respiratory rate, blood pressure, and muscle tension. Some people flush around the face, neck, and chest in this phase. In women, the areolae become firmer, the clitoris retracts into the clitoral hood, Bartholin's glands lubricate, and the lower vagina swells and narrows. With a male partner, the vagina tightens around the man's penis, increasing his sexual stimulation. In men,

Toward Evidence-Based Practice

The sexual behaviors of older adults and the relationship between quality of life and sexuality in older adults is the subject of ongoing research.

▌ **Penhollow, T. M., Young, M., & Denny, G. (2009). Predictors of quality of life, sexual intercourse, and sexual satisfaction in older adults.** *American Journal of Health Education, 40(1), 13–22.*

This study attempted to identify aspects of sexuality that have the greatest influence on sexual intercourse, sexual satisfaction, and overall quality of life of residents in a retirement community. Sexual self-confidence was found to be the single most important predictor of sexual intercourse and sexual satisfaction and (for women) quality of life. Cultural (sexual acceptance, sexual priority), psychological (sexual desire, sexual self-confidence, and control), and social factors (satisfaction in relationship and social life) help to explain sexual satisfaction beyond the physical health.

▌ **Syme, M., Klonoff, E., Macera, C., et al. (2013). Predicting sexual decline and dissatisfaction among older adults: The role of partnered and individual physical and mental health factors.** *Journals of Gerontology Series B: Psychological Sciences and Social Sciences, 68(3), 323–332.*

Researchers measured the concept of sexual unwellness in adults 63 to 68 years of ages. The majority of adults (64.2%) were sexually active at least once a month to once a day or more. Fatigue symptoms, history of diabetes, and poor spousal health were associated with a lack of sexual satisfaction and inability to maintain the sexual relationship. Gender differences revealed that women were more likely to report a lack of sexual satisfaction, which was usually partner related. For males, spousal support and good spousal health decreased the risk of unsatisfactory sexual relations.

▌ **Doll, G. (2013). Sexuality in nursing homes: Practice and policy.** *Journal of Gerontological Nursing, 39(7), 30–37.*

Administrators or social workers in 91 nursing homes responded to a survey regarding sexual expressions of residents in nursing homes and residential care facilities. Results revealed that residents engaged in sexual talk (85%) (e.g., sexually explicit language, verbal propositioning); demonstrated sexual acts (85%) (e.g., masturbation, fondling, intercourse); formed romantic relationships (66%); and showed implied sexual acts (60%) (e.g., reading pornography). The reactions of the nursing staff varied, from informing the supervisor (68.9%), trying to respectfully help the resident (51.1%), following the facility's policy (41%), ignoring the issue (27.8%) to panic (20%).

1. What trend in the research about sexuality in older adults do you see?

2. In the Penhollow study, what was the single most important factor influencing sexual satisfaction and quality of life, other than physical health? What additional factor was identified in the Syme study? What do you think nurses can do to promote it?

3. Based on these studies, how do you think nurses can affect the quality of sexuality in older adults?

 Go to Chapter 33, **Toward Evidence-Based Practice Suggested Responses,** on Davis*Plus*.

---

the ridge of the glans penis becomes more prominent, pre-ejaculate (two or three drops of fluid) is emitted, and the testes rise closer to the body. The person may achieve, lose, and regain the plateau phase several times without experiencing orgasm.

Orgasm

Orgasm occurs at the peak of the plateau phase. At the moment of orgasm, the sexual tension that has been building is released. The heart rate, respiratory rate, and blood pressure reach their peak, and there is loss of voluntary muscle tone.

- *In women,* spinal cord reflexes cause powerful rhythmic contractions of the vagina, uterus, anus, and pelvic floor muscles; feelings of warmth spread through the pelvic area. The cervical canal dilates, allowing easy transport of the sperm to the uterus. Orgasm may last for a few seconds or up to nearly a minute.
- *In men,* spinal cord reflexes cause the urethra, anus, and pelvic floor muscles to contract followed by **ejaculation** (the expelling of semen through the urethra). For men, orgasm usually lasts no more than 30 seconds.

The intensity of orgasm varies among individuals and in each individual from one sexual experience to another. Orgasm may involve intense spasm associated with intense focus on the sexual pleasure, or it may be signaled by as little as a sigh or subtle relaxation.

Resolution

Resolution is the period of time following orgasm. The muscles relax, and the body returns to its pre-excitement state. Immediately after orgasm, men experience a **refractory period**, during which they cannot achieve an erection. The duration of this period varies among individuals and increases with age. Women experience no refractory period—they can either enter the resolution stage or return to the excitement or plateau stage immediately following orgasm.

Identify the phase of the sexual response cycle described.

- This phase is reached if there is ongoing stimulation. This stage may be achieved, lost, and regained several times without the occurrence of orgasm.
- This stage occurs in the mind and may be communicated between potential sexual partners either verbally or through body language.
- This phase is associated with the release of sexual tension.

 ## ThinkLike a Nurse 33-6

Critique the theory of Masters and Johnson, as represented in the preceding discussion of the sexual response cycle. How would you respond to the statement that the theory does not adequately address variation among individuals and even within an individual's sexual response?

What Are Some Forms of Sexual Expression?

People express their sexuality and gain sexual satisfaction in different ways. Although opinions vary, a range of behaviors is socially acceptable and therefore considered "normal" by most people in our society. These behaviors are discussed in the next few sections.

Developing Intimate Relationships

Developing intimate relationships involves a willingness to take risks and offer trust. Intimacy involves openness, mutual respect, caring, commitment, protection, honesty, and devotion. Although we often think of intimate relationships as sexual, they are not necessarily so. Furthermore, in our society, many sexual relationships occur without intimacy.

Fantasies and Erotic Dreams

Most men and women have sexual fantasies. They may be related to past experiences, dreams, or desires; or stories heard, seen, or read. Sexual fantasies serve to increase self-esteem and sexual arousal and serve as an outlet to explore sexual desires. People in long-term monogamous relationships may fantasize to bring variety and excitement into a routine sexual encounter. Erotic dreams are also common among both men and women. Nocturnal orgasm may or may not occur with the dream.

Masturbation

Masturbation is self-stimulation of the genitals. Although there are many techniques, men typically hold and stroke the shaft of the penis, and women typically stimulate the clitoris manually. Young children touch their genitals as a part of body exploration, but they quickly learn either that touching certain areas is not acceptable or that it should be done in private. Adolescents, particularly males, may masturbate frequently. Adults may masturbate for sexual release when a partner is not available or for variety in a partnered relationship. Sex

therapists often recommend masturbation as a means to resolve orgasm difficulties in women and ejaculatory problems in men.

Religious and social taboos discouraging masturbation are common. Some people mistakenly believe that masturbation is harmful, causing acne, warts, blindness, or insanity. More commonly masturbation is considered a "dirty," shameful, or perverted act. For example, former U.S. Surgeon General Joycelyn Elders retired after receiving some criticism for advocating masturbation as a method of safe sex.

Shared Touching

Mutual masturbation, or shared touching, may be an alternative to sexual intercourse. This is particularly appealing to individuals who seek to maintain their virginity, decrease the risk of STIs, or for those who have mobility or other physical problems that make intercourse difficult. Mutual masturbation is recognized as a form of safer sex because body fluids are not likely to be exchanged. This behavior can be satisfying because it allows for a significant level of sexual intimacy and for participants to experience orgasm.

Sexual Intercourse

Sexual intercourse and **coitus** are terms used to describe penile penetration of the vagina. People use a variety of positions for intercourse, depending on preference, mobility, cultural and religious influences, the relationship, and other personal beliefs. For some women, manual stimulation of the clitoris is also necessary to achieve orgasm. Partners typically do not reach orgasm at the same time, despite the romantic preoccupation with this phenomenon.

Unprotected coitus may lead to conception, so the couple should use some method of contraception if they want to avoid pregnancy. Because it involves exchange of body fluids, sexual intercourse may also lead to the transmission of infections. Using a lubricated condom decreases this risk, but it is not a foolproof measure to prevent STIs.

Oral–Genital Stimulation

Both heterosexual and homosexual couples practice oral–genital stimulation (oral sex). Couples in committed relationships may engage in it for sexual variety or as foreplay. Oral sex provides intimacy, without an unplanned pregnancy, and many believe that it does not affect their virginity status. For the latter reasons, oral sex has become prevalent among adolescents. Oral–genital contact may, however, lead to STIs.

Cunnilingus is the oral stimulation of a woman's genitals. **Fellatio** is stimulation of the male genitals by a partner's mouth. Although swallowing semen is not a health issue, it may be a matter of personal preference as to whether the recipient ejaculates in the partner's mouth. Dental dams, plastic wrap, or latex condoms can be used to prevent the transmission of STIs.

Anal Stimulation or Anal Intercourse

Both homosexual and heterosexual couples engage in oral–anal stimulation (called **anilingus**). Objects for sexual stimulation, or the partner's finger, tongue, and mouth, may be used to stimulate the anus. **Anal intercourse** (also termed *sodomy*) is the insertion of the penis into the partner's rectum. When a couple engages in anal intercourse, lubrication is essential to lessen the chance of tiny tears to the rectal mucosa or damage to the anal sphincter. A lubricated condom can be used to lessen the chance of STIs. The condom must be changed before vaginal penetration to avoid the transfer of *Escherichia coli* bacteria from the rectum to the vagina. Couples should follow the same precaution when using objects for sexual pleasure.

Celibacy

Celibacy, or abstinence, is a state in which an individual refrains from sexual activity. Traditionally, a celibate is a person who remains unmarried, often for religious reasons, and sublimates sexual desire through prayer, meditation, and service. There are numerous reasons a person may remain celibate:

- Fear of or lack of desire for intimate relationships
- Childhood sexual trauma
- A developmental or physical disability that limits opportunities for meeting prospective partners, limits privacy, or interferes with the ability to communicate or act on desires
- The desire to focus energies elsewhere because of a low libido.
- The need to regain balance after the loss of a relationship, whether through separation, divorce, or death.

Married couples may also be celibate and have a happy stable relationship. Others might be celibate after the loss of a relationship, whether through separation, divorce, or death, often feeling a considerable void.

Alternative Forms of Sexual Expression

The *DSM-5* (APA, 2013a) describes eight categories of sexual deviation or **paraphilias**: exhibitionism disorder, fetishism disorder, frotteurism disorder, pedophilia disorder, sexual masochism disorder, sexual sadism disorder, transvestic disorder, and voyeurism disorder. Some people may experience guilt, shame, and depression about their paraphilia, while others are distressed only by societal disapproval, restrictions, and possible criminal charges associated with their mode of expression. If you need more information about paraphilias,

 Go to Chapter 33, **Supplemental Materials: Alternative Forms of Sexual Expression,** on Davis*Plus*.

Important things you can teach parents and other caregivers to do to reduce children's risk of sexual violence, predators, or other unhealthy exposure are contained in the Self-Care box Teaching Children About Predators.

Self-Care

Teaching Children About Predators

Set the Stage for Open Discussion

➤ Talk openly and directly with your child about her own development and sexuality. This establishes trust and makes it easier for the child to come to you when she has questions.

➤ Be open to your child's questions. Acting embarrassed discourages further conversation.

➤ Assure your child that she won't get in trouble for "tattling" on someone who asks her to keep a secret about sexual or touching encounters.

➤ Make discussion a natural part of growing up—don't save it "for later."

Know What's Going On

➤ Be involved in your child's everyday life and ask questions—that is, where he is, who he's with, what he's doing, what his closest friends are doing.

➤ Know the other adults your child is around. Go to your child's activities and get to know the adults involved.

➤ Know what he watches on TV, the iPod or iPad, the computer, or media games.

➤ Locate computers in a central area in the home where you can monitor Internet use.

➤ Install a parental control to limit access to and monitor Web sites that would expose your child to sexual content or predators.

➤ Know if sexual predators live near you. Check out the sexual predators registry in your area.

➤ Establish curfew times and contingency communications if curfew is breached. Teach your child to use a code word that communicates he is in trouble.

Just Say No

➤ Teach your child about body parts that are private and should not be touched or seen by others—except for medical reasons.

➤ Teach your child to firmly say no and get away if someone tries to touch or look at her in a way that makes her feel uncomfortable.

➤ Urge your child to tell you or another trusted adult if someone tries to touch or look at private areas or if the person tries to show the child his or her own private body parts.

➤ Teach your child never to get in the car with strangers and never go near a stranger's car for any reason.

➤ Always use a buddy system to prevent the child from being alone.

➤ Teach your child to yell, "Help! Stranger!" if anyone tries to follow her, walking or in a car.

➤ Place limits on Internet use.

➤ Teach children not to disclose personal information in public settings or on the Internet, even social networking sites.

- What are aspects of an intimate relationship?
- Identify solitary types of sexual expression and those that may be conducted with a partner.

What Problems Affect Sexuality?

Sexual well-being is a complex mesh of physical, emotional, cognitive, social, and spiritual components. Therefore, it is not surprising that many people experience challenges to their sexual health. Difficulties can arise in loving, healthy and in dysfunctional relationships. Sexual dysfunction may be temporary and situational, or it may be long standing.

Sexually Transmitted Infections

An STI may be caused by bacteria, virus, fungi or parasites. STIs are spread through direct sexual contact with an open wound or with body fluids, such as semen, vaginal secretions, or blood that contains pathogens. Contrary to many myths, STIs are not transmitted by casual touching, coughing, or other indirect means.

STIs are among the most common infectious diseases in the United States today. More than 20 different STIs have been identified and affect millions of men and women each year. **Reportable** (or **notifiable**) **diseases** have a significant effect on public health. When healthcare providers diagnose a reportable disease, mandatory reporting laws require it to be reported to the local public health department or the Centers for Disease Control and Prevention (CDC). Examples include the following:

- *Chlamydia trachomatis.* The most common transmitted infection in the U.S. is also known as the "silent infection" because the infected person may not have symptoms. Chlamydia can cause serious damage to a female's reproductive system if untreated. About 1 in 15 sexually active persons will become infected. In 2011, an estimated 2.8 million cases occurred, although 1.4 million cases were diagnosed and treated (CDC, 2012b, updated 2013).
- *Gonorrhea.* This infectious disease is caused by a bacterium and is a common STI among sexually active teenagers and young adults. An estimated 820,000 new cases occur each year, although in 2011, 321,849 cases were reported to the CDC (2012c, updated 2013).
- *Syphilis.* Although 46,042 new cases were reported in 2011, the actual number of cases is higher. This STI is caused by a bacterium that is transmitted from person to person by direct contact with the syphilis sore, which can occur on the external genitalia, vagina, lips, mouth, anus, and in the rectum. If left untreated, long-term neurological complications and even death may occur (CDC, 2012d, updated 2013).
- *Genital Human Papillomavirus.* Also called HPV, this STI can infect the genital areas, mouth, and throat of males and females. It can also cause genital warts and certain types of cancers (e.g., cervical, genital, oropharyngeal). Many people with HPV do not know they

are infected, and in many instances the STI will go away without intervention. There are more than 40 types of HPV and it is possible for a person to get more than one type. The HPV vaccine is recommended to minimize the chance of contracting HPV (CDC, 2013b).

Nearly two-thirds of all STIs occur in people younger than 25 years. Because many STIs have few or no initial symptoms, an infected person can transmit the infection without knowing it. For example, up to 90% of women infected with gonorrhea or chlamydia have no symptoms. To find out whether a patient has an STI, you must obtain a culture, that is, a swab of secretions from the genitals. In a man, the swab is put into the urethral opening. In a woman, the swab is obtained from secretions near the cervix. A culture of the throat or rectum is obtained if the person has had oral or anal sex.

Many STIs can be treated fairly easily with antibiotics; however, if left untreated, they may cause serious problems. In women, the pathogens can travel up through the uterus into the fallopian tubes and cause pelvic inflammatory disease (PID). Untreated PID may cause sterility.

The best ways to prevent STIs are to practice abstinence or to participate only in a committed, mutually monogamous sexual relationship with someone who has never had an STI and is at low risk for one. Risk for an STI increases if a person has unprotected sex or sex with more than one partner. Other risk factors include alcohol and drug use, sharing needles, and noncompliance with the STI treatment regimen.

To read about various STIs, their symptoms, treatment, and effect on sexual functioning, fertility, and childbearing,

 Go to Chapter 33, **Tables, Boxes, Figures: ESG Table 33-1, Common Sexually Transmitted Infections (STIs),** on Davis*Plus*.

Dysmenorrhea

Dysmenorrhea is painful menstruation caused by strong uterine contractions that cause ischemia of the uterus. The patient may experience cramping, lower abdominal pain, back and upper thigh pain, headache, vomiting, and diarrhea. Treatments include bedrest, application of heat to the back and abdomen, and analgesics such as aspirin and other nonsteroidal anti-inflammatory drugs (NSAIDs), for example, ibuprofen or naproxen.

Premenstrual Syndrome

Premenstrual syndrome (PMS) is characterized by physical and emotional changes occurring 3 to 14 days before the onset of the woman's menstrual period. Physical symptoms include headaches, constipation, breast tenderness, and weight gain associated with bloating, abdominal swelling, or swelling of the hands and feet. Some women feel as though they are on an emotional roller coaster, with periods of depression, anxiety, irritability, tension, and an inability to concentrate. Some women have difficulty maintaining social interactions at work or school because of severe emotional symptoms. Client teaching for PMS is discussed later in this chapter.

Women experiencing more severe forms of menstrual cycle dysfunction (**premenstrual dysphoric disorder [PMDD]**) become seriously depressed for a week or more before their periods. In contrast, PMS is shorter, usually milder, and involves more physical symptoms. A woman can suffer from both PMS and PMDD at the same time, or may have one and not the other.

KnowledgeCheck 33-9

- Identify three methods to decrease the transmission of STIs.
- What are physical and emotional symptoms of premenstrual syndrome (PMS)?

Negative Intimate Relationships

Many couples are happy, and their sexual relationship becomes even more satisfying as they mature. However, some intimate relationships are not mutually satisfying, even when they do not involve neglect, or physical or emotional abuse. Couples may be involved in a celibate or loveless union for financial security, social status, for "the sake of the children," or because of cultural or religious restrictions regarding divorce. In reality, many relationships fall in between—sometimes satisfying and other times less so—depending on a wide variety of factors, such as stress, physical and mental illness, hormones, fatigue, distractions, low self-esteem, and financial pressure. The most negative relationships involve *domestic violence* (also called *intimate partner violence*), which may include physical and/or emotional intimidation, assault, and rape.

Although either gender partner may be a victim of domestic violence, most often a man is the perpetrator. The anger, domination, and physical violence of the partner lead to fear, intimidation, and submission in the victim. Often victims come to believe they deserve the abuse and may hesitate to admit the cause of their injuries, even in hospital settings. Many abused women are either emotionally or financially dependent on their partner and believe staying in the relationship is their only option. If you wish to learn more about abuse and violence, see Chapters 9 and 10.

Sexual Harassment

Sexual harassment occurs when a person in power makes unwanted sexual advances that implicitly or explicitly relate to the victim's employment, academic status, or success. "Advances" can take the form of sexual comments or behaviors (such as touching). Because of the power imbalance, the victim may keep silent and suffer physically and psychologically. **Sexual assault** includes contact with or without penetration, sexual touching of intimate parts, and any unwanted sexual activity in situations of intoxication, coercion, or misconception.

PICOT

Sexuality, Dementia, and Competency

Situation: The adult children of a widow with early onset Alzheimer's disease are concerned about their mother's sexual advances directed at another resident at the assisted living facility. Although the residents are, legally, consenting adults, the children are concerned about their mother's judgment and sexual appropriateness.

PICOT Components:

P	Population/client	=	Adults with early onset Alzheimer's disease
I	Intervention/indicator	=	Nonpharmacological behavior modification
C	Comparator/control	=	No sexual relationships
O	Outcome	=	Appropriate, consensual sexual relationships
T	Time	=	Late adulthood

Searchable Question: Do _____ (P) who receive/are exposed to _____ (I) demonstrate _____ (O) as compared to _____ (C) during _____ (T)?

Example of Evidence: All people have needs for intimacy, companionship, and touch. Clients with dementia pose a particularly difficult situation for both family and professionals, who may consider sexual behavior to be inappropriate, based on the elderly client's age, setting, situation, or health issues. The central question for you to answer is whether the client is competent. The family and staff need to carefully and sensitively assess the following areas: Is the client's mental status suited to engaging in a consensual, sexual relationship? Who is initiating sexual contact? Is the client able to consent to sexual intimacy? Is the client aware of emotional and physical potential risks, such as the relationship ending? Is the sexual activity consistent with behavior the client exhibited prior to the onset of the dementia? Although there are no established treatment guidelines, various nonpharmacological plans may help to assure appropriate expression of sexuality.

Practice Change: After obtaining a thorough sexual assessment, the nurse may plan nonpharmacological behavior modification for the client to demonstrate appropriate sexual behaviors and meet the client's intimacy needs.

Joller, P., Gupta, N., Seitz, D. P., et al. (2013). Approach to inappropriate sexual behaviour in people with dementia. *Canadian Family Physician, 59*(3), 255–260.

Sexual harassment may take two forms: (1) In *quid pro quo,* the employer makes the employee feel that she must engage in unwelcome sexual advances to maintain employment. (2) In *hostile environment* situations, the sexual advances are more subtle, but persistent, and create an intimidating environment.

Rape

Although rape is actually a crime of violence rather than of sex, we discuss it here because it often involves the sexual organs and usually has negative effects on the victim's sexuality. **Rape** is nonconsensual vaginal, anal, or oral penetration. It occurs through force, by the threat of bodily harm, or when the victim is incapable of giving consent. All states consider rape, even within a marriage, to be a crime.

Victims of rape range from infants to older adults and may be either gender, although females are more likely to be victims. One in 6 women and 1 in 33 males are victims of attempted or completed rape (National Institute of Justice, 2010). Forced oral assault, multiple assailants, and weapons are more likely involved with male victims. In two-thirds of cases, the victim knows or is related to the assailant, especially when the victim is a young child (National Institute of Justice, 2010; Rennison & Rand, 2008). People with developmental disabilities, especially mental retardation, are at double the risk for sexual assault than the general population.

- **Group (gang) rape** occurs when more than one person sexually assaults a victim. Group rape usually occurs when drugs and alcohol are involved.
- **Statutory rape** is sexual activity between an adult and a person under the "age of consent" (this ranges from 14 to 18 years of age, depending on state regulations). This charge may be filed even when the sex is consensual.
- **Date rape** is rape by an acquaintance when the assault occurs during an agreed-on social encounter or date. Although date rape is not a lesser violation, our society tends to blame the woman when date rape occurs.

Many rapes go unreported. Rape is an assault that involves significant psychological and physical injury; however, the police often become involved because the victim requires medical attention. After a rape or other forms of sexual assault, care may be delayed, particularly for teens, if alcohol or drugs are involved. Other reasons for not reporting rape include fear of the assailant, fear of consequences to the assailant, knowledge of the low conviction rate for rapists, the desire to avoid a trial, shame and embarrassment, past sexual history, self-blame, wanting to "move on," and the wish to deny the event and its possible consequences.

In addition to psychological and physiological trauma, the rape victim is at risk for STIs and pregnancy. Three-quarters or more of sexually assaulted teens experience post-traumatic stress disorder. Referral to a local sexual assault support group is critical. A *sexual assault nurse examiner (SANE)* is a registered nurse who has received special training in the immediate care of sexual assault victims. To learn about providing care to sexual assault victims,

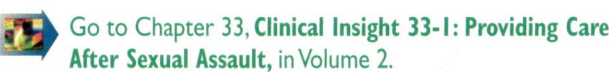 Go to Chapter 33, **Clinical Insight 33-1: Providing Care After Sexual Assault,** in Volume 2.

Sexual Response Cycle Disorders

Disorders in various stages of the sexual response cycle may affect desire, arousal, excitement, and orgasm.

Low Libido

Low libido (hypoactive sexual desire) manifests as a significant decrease in or absence of both sexual fantasies and sexual activity. Low libido may affect both men and women. It can be transient or long term. The person may experience low libido only with one particular partner, or the lack of desire can extend to all sexual activity. Persons with low libido may reluctantly engage in sexual encounters or avoid all sexual contact. However, once sexual activity has been initiated, the person is usually able to achieve orgasm.

Factors contributing to hypoactive sexual desire include sexual trauma, a negative attitude toward sex, negative relationships, and biological factors (e.g., hormone deficiencies, perimenopause, side effects of various medications). Low sexual desire, in both men and women, may respond positively to testosterone administration.

Arousal Disorders

In women, arousal disorders manifest as minimal or absent pelvic congestion and vaginal lubrication even though desire may be present.

- **Dyspareunia**, or painful intercourse, further decreases sexual desire. Dyspareunia is often caused by vaginal dryness resulting from hormonal changes, the aging process, tampons, and medications, including antihistamines. A water-based lubricant or saliva helps to resolve vaginal dryness. Other causes of female dyspareunia include vaginal or urinary tract infections, pelvic inflammatory disease, and endometriosis.

  Dyspareunia in men most commonly results from urinary tract infection or **phimosis**, a condition in which the foreskin of the penis is too tight. **Balanitis**, inflammation of the penis, is another cause of dyspareunia in men.
- **Vaginismus** is a rare disorder affecting desire and arousal. It is characterized by intense involuntary contractions of the perineal muscles, which close the vaginal opening and prevent penile penetration. Vaginismus may be associated with psychological disorders (e.g., negative attitudes toward sex, history of sexual abuse or trauma) or physiological disorders (e.g., trauma during childbirth).
- **Erectile dysfunction (ED)**, formerly known as *impotence* is a sexual arousal disorders in men. Men with ED have persistent or recurring inability either to achieve or to maintain an erection sufficient for satisfactory sexual performance. The most common cause of ED is diseases of the blood vessels (e.g., hypertension, high cholesterol, or diabetes). ED may also result from underlying neurological (e.g., spinal cord injury, Parkinson's disease, stroke) or endocrine problems (diabetes). Common psychological problems that contribute to ED include performance anxiety, childhood sexual abuse, relationship

issues, or mental illness. Some medications can also cause ED, such as antihistamines, antidepressants, antipsychotics, and antihypertensives. While testosterone plays a major role in libido (desire), it has only a minor role in erectile function.

Orgasmic Disorders

Orgasmic disorder is a delay in or absence of orgasm after a normal sexual excitement phase. Once a woman has had orgasms, it is uncommon for her to lose that ability unless there has been a sexual trauma, poor sexual communication, a conflicted sexual relationship, a mood disorder, a medical condition, or direct physiological effects from a drug. Orgasmic disorder is more prevalent in younger women who have not had adequate sexual experience to learn how to reach orgasm. It is not unusual for a woman to require manual clitoral stimulation to reach orgasm because not all women can achieve orgasm through intercourse alone.

Men, too, can experience orgasmic disorders. Some cannot achieve orgasm during intercourse, but are able to reach orgasm through masturbation or manual or oral stimulation by their partner.

Premature ejaculation occurs when the male reaches orgasm and ejaculates before, at the time of, or shortly after penetration. The disappointment of both partners may lead to issues with self-esteem, sexual avoidance, and ED. There are sexual techniques as well as medications that can help to delay ejaculation.

Retrograde ejaculation occurs when the semen empties into the bladder instead of being ejaculated through the urethra. Normally this cannot occur because the internal bladder sphincter closes in the orgasmic phase. However, some medications, prostate surgery, and spinal cord injuries may lead to retrograde ejaculation, resulting in sterility.

KnowledgeCheck 33-10

- Identify three forms of sexual victimization.
- In which phases of the sexual response cycle can sexual dysfunction occur?

PracticalKnowledge
knowing **how**

Although you understand the importance of comprehensive client assessment, you may find it difficult to gather information related to sexuality. Students, and some nurses, may be shy, or may be concerned that the client will be embarrassed to talk about sexual topics since these matters are personal and private, and can threaten a person's self-esteem. Including sexuality as a routine part of your nursing assessment reinforces the concept that sexuality is an integral part of life and provides an opportunity for much-needed patient teaching. Many patients will not raise the topic of sexuality, so to meet patient needs, you must include this topic in your assessment.

ASSESSMENT

The extent to which you will assess a client's sexual health status varies. For example, for a woman with a suspected STI, you would perform a comprehensive health assessment and a focused sexual health assessment. Similarly, clients with illnesses that affect their sexual functioning should receive a full assessment. Jocelyn Carter (Meet Your Patients) is an example. Recall that chronic illness can have a profound effect on sexual functioning (e.g., Frank Thanee and Gabriel Thomas in the Meet Your Patients scenario). A focused sexual health assessment is needed in the following situations:

Pregnancy, infertility workup, request for birth control
Menstrual cycle irregularities or problems
Annual health visit
Unusual discharge from or change in genital organs
Urination problems
As part of a comprehensive physical examination
A known sexual problem (e.g., dyspareunia)
Illness or surgeries that may affect sexual function (e.g., arthritis, colostomy)
Medications

Sexual History

Most healthcare facilities use a standard nursing assessment form. Some address sexuality in a comprehensive manner, but most have only a few superficial questions or nothing at all. You will need to be sensitive to your client's verbal and nonverbal cues to identify and explore relevant issues that are not on the form. For topics to include in a sexual history and for suggestions for questions to ask,

Go to Chapter 33, **Assessment Guidelines and Tools, Focused Assessment: Guidelines and Questions for Taking a Sexual History,** in Volume 2.

Tips for Taking a Sexual History   When you are asking personal questions, always provide privacy. It is one thing to discuss blood pressure in the presence of family, but quite another to discuss sexual health issues, which may threaten the very core of a relationship. For example, a wife is not likely to discuss domestic violence with her abusing husband at her side, and an 18-year-old man will probably not admit to having sex with another man when his father is present. For other suggestions,

Go to Chapter 33, **Clinical Insight 33-2: Guidelines for Taking a Sexual History,** in Volume 2.

Focused Physical Examination

Sexual health assessment includes a physical examination focused on the reproductive system. For detailed instructions about performing these examinations,

Go to Chapter 22, **Procedure 22-17: Assessing the Male Genitourinary System,** and **Procedure 22-18: Assessing the Female Genitourinary System,** in Volume 2.

If there is reason to suspect that a client has an STI, you should obtain cultures of any discharge or lesions. Other laboratory tests may also be ordered.

KnowledgeCheck 33-11

What techniques can you use to increase comfort and communication during a sexual history assessment?

ThinkLike a Nurse 33-7

Review the three case scenarios in the Meet Your Patients discussion. Consider the following questions for each patient:

- Would you be comfortable caring for and responding to each of these patients?
- What topics, if any, that have been raised by these patients would be difficult for you to handle?
- How would you answer each of the patients' questions?

ANALYSIS/NURSING DIAGNOSIS

NANDA-I has two nursing diagnoses for describing sexual problems. The following discussion should help you differentiate between them.

Ineffective Sexuality Patterns Use this diagnosis when the patient expresses concerns about his sexuality. Examples of such concerns might include conflict about sexual orientation, value conflicts, fear of acquiring an STI, lack of knowledge about how to adapt sexual techniques to altered body function, lack of privacy, not having a partner, or impaired relationship with the partner.

Sexual Dysfunction This diagnosis applies when there is an actual change in sexual function during the phases of desire, excitation, or orgasm that the patient views as unsatisfying, unrewarding, or inadequate. This includes sexual response cycle disorders, such as low libido, arousal disorders, orgasmic disorders, vaginismus, premature ejaculation, and erectile dysfunction. If these defining characteristics for Sexual Dysfunction do not seem to "fit" the patient, then use the more general diagnosis, Ineffective Sexuality Patterns.

There is much overlap between these two NANDA-I diagnoses. The only defining characteristic of Ineffective Sexuality Pattern is that the patient reports difficulties, limitations, or changes in sexual behaviors or activities; Jocelyn Carter (Meet Your Patients), for example, is not actually experiencing problems with sexual satisfaction or performance. She is expressing a broader concern about her sexuality—about her future desirability as a sex partner. Therefore, the better diagnosis for her is Ineffective Sexuality Patterns. The same is true for Gabriel Thomas, who is expressing fear that he may have sexual problems in the future.

Sexual Dysfunction is the more specific diagnosis for physiological problems and for concerns about sexual performance. Thus, it is best to use Sexual Dysfunction when the patient has one or more of the following defining characteristics:

Changes in achieving sexual satisfaction
Change of interest in self or others
Inability to achieve sexual satisfaction
Verbalization of a sexual problem
Actual or perceived limitations imposed by disease or therapy
Changes in ability to achieve perceived sex role
Seeking confirmation of desirability

Etiologies of Sexuality Diagnoses

Several other nursing diagnoses may be the cause of sexuality problems. The following are the more common ones:

- *Activity Intolerance* and *Fatigue* (e.g., from cardiac or respiratory disease) may cause the person to alter her lifestyle, including sexual activity, to conserve energy. Lack of energy may decrease the person's interest in sex, or it may require a change in the mode of sexual expression.
- *Impaired Physical Mobility* (e.g., as occurs with arthritis, spinal cord injuries) may affect a person's ability to interact, meet potential partners, and perform sexually (e.g., assume certain positions, make certain movements).
- *Fear* that sexual activity may be dangerous can inhibit desire and the ability to perform (e.g., after heart surgery). This diagnosis may also apply to the client's partner, who may afraid that sexual activity will hurt the client after surgery, or hurt a pregnant partner or the baby.
- *Chronic Pain* may directly affect interpersonal relationships, interest in sex, or comfort during sexual intimacy. It may cause fatigue, indirectly affecting sexuality.
- *Chronic Low Self-Esteem* may result from chronic health problems and their consequences (e.g., loss of employment, inability to perform parenting roles). Sexual expression may also become a challenge, yet the intimacy and reassurance that accompanies sexual encounters can be vital to self-esteem and a sense of wholeness.
- *Self-Care Deficits.* For clients who need assistance with activities of daily living (ADLs), for example with toileting, family or caretakers often find it difficult to accept and facilitate sexual relationships. When a person with a physical disability lives in a residential facility, lack of opportunity and privacy may interfere with sexual expression (Fig. 33-8).
- *Delayed Development.* Relationship challenges also exist for people who are developmentally disabled. Those with very low cognitive functioning are unable to seek out or understand sexual relationships. Unfortunately, this makes them vulnerable to sexual abuse. Sex education is vital for these individuals to help them understand body structure and function, relationship issues, and ways to avoid exploitation and abuse.

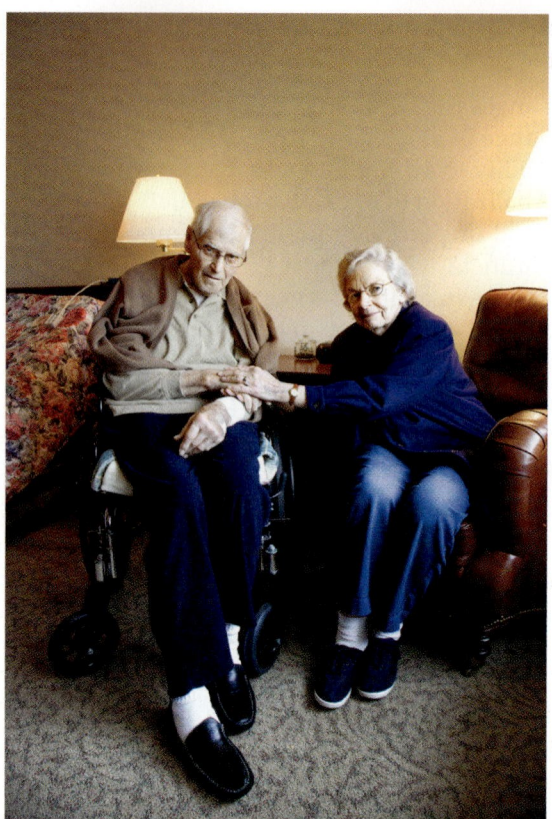

FIGURE 33-8 Adults with physical restrictions or those living within group settings, such as skilled nursing care, can maintain sexual relationships.

Sexuality Problems as Etiologies of Other Diagnoses

Sexuality problems can be the etiology of other nursing diagnoses, for example:

- *Disturbed Body Image* related to change in appearance secondary to orchiectomy (removal of a testicle)
- *Pain (during coitus)* related to inadequate vaginal lubrication secondary to aging
- *Fear* related to sexual abuse by father
- *Rape-Trauma Syndrome* (Note that you do not need an etiology for this nursing diagnosis. It is self-explanatory, as are most syndrome diagnoses.)

ThinkLike a Nurse 33-8

Give a specific example (patient situation) for each of the defining characteristics of Sexual Dysfunction listed in the preceding section.

▮ PLANNING OUTCOMES/EVALUATION

For *NOC standardized outcomes* associated with Ineffective Sexuality Patterns and Sexual Dysfunction,

 Go to Chapter 33, **Standardized Language, Examples of NOC Outcomes for Sexuality Problems,** on Davis*Plus.*

Individualized client outcomes and goals, as always, depend on the nursing diagnosis you identify. For Sexual Dysfunction and Ineffective Sexuality Patterns, you might write the following desired outcomes:

- Expresses comfort with sexual orientation.
- Describes plans for resolving values conflicts about extramarital sex (e.g., will talk to his minister).
- Describes techniques for preventing STIs.
- Reports using a condom for all sexual activities involving exchange of body fluids.

The following are examples of outcomes that apply specifically to Sexual Dysfunction:

- Communicates sexual needs and preferences to partner.
- Maintains penile erection through orgasm.
- Describes ways to adapt positions for intercourse to accommodate painful knee joints.

PLANNING INTERVENTIONS/IMPLEMENTATION

For *NIC standardized interventions* and selected nursing activities for sexuality,

 Go to Chapter 33, **Standardized Language, Examples of NIC Interventions and Nursing Activities for Sexuality Problems,** on Davis*Plus.*

Specific nursing activities for sexuality problems depend on the etiology of the problem and on the goals selected. Broadly speaking, nursing interventions involve teaching about sexual health and self-care, counseling for altered sexual functioning, and dealing with inappropriate sexual behavior. Those interventions are discussed in the following sections.

You will also find a nursing care plan and care map for Ineffective Sexuality Problems on the following pages.

Teaching About Sexual Health

Before you begin teaching, take the time to get to know your client and find out what she already knows about sexuality. The time you take putting the client at ease is well spent. When you develop rapport and trust, the client will be more likely to speak openly with you about sensitive or embarrassing topics, to retain what you teach, and to feel free to ask questions. Offer to include the partner in the discussion if the client wishes. See Chapter 19 for a review of teaching and learning.

As part of teaching focused on sexuality, you should discuss prevention of STIs with all clients and discuss contraception with clients who are heterosexual or bisexual. Other common topics are presented in the next sections.

Body Function and Reproduction

A person's age, experience, and educational level do not ensure knowledge of sexual functioning. Before you begin any teaching, explore your client's knowledge base by asking open-ended questions such as "What questions do you have about sex?"

Visual aids (e.g., a diagram of reproductive system anatomy) are helpful. For example, for pregnant clients you could use drawings and charts illustrating fetal development. Most agencies provide handouts and brochures so that clients can review information at home.

As part of your general discussion on sexuality and bodily function, you may wish to discuss common myths and misconceptions about sex. Below are several statements about sex that provide a good starting point for discussion. **Key point: *The statements are all false.***

- You can't get pregnant the first time you have sex.
- You can't get pregnant if you're using a condom.
- You can tell the size of a man's penis by the size of his feet.
- You always have symptoms if you have an STI.
- People over 70 don't have sex.
- A vaginal orgasm is better than a clitoral orgasm.
- If the relationship is good, the man and woman will achieve simultaneous orgasm.
- It is not healthful to have intercourse during menstruation.
- The only normal position for intercourse is face-to-face. Anything else is deviant or at least "not nice."
- Only "dirty" people have STIs. You will not get an STI if your partner has good hygiene habits.
- If a woman does not have an orgasm, she does not really love her partner. The same is true for a man.

Douching

Teach women that douching is unnecessary and is associated with significant risks. It can wash away the lactobacilli that clean the vagina and protect it from infection. Women who douche are at increased risk for some STIs and for PID (Gollub, Cyrus-Cameron, Armstrong, et al., 2013; Rew, 2009). Furthermore, douching is essentially useless as a method of contraception. Some women douche because they notice an odor. Reassure them that this is normal during certain times of their menstrual cycle. If the odor doesn't disappear after washing, they should see their healthcare provider.

Menstruation

Many women require information about self-care to dispel myths about menstruation. For example, it is not dangerous to engage in sexual activity during menstruation. The bloody fluid is from the uterus, not the vagina, so intercourse will not harm the vagina. Actually, some women and men enjoy sex more during menstruation because the increased vascularity, warmth, and lubrication in the pelvic region increase their pleasurable sensations, and orgasm may relieve women's menstrual cramps. If the flow is very heavy, the woman can place protective padding under her buttocks to protect the bed linens. Some women use a diaphragm to keep the flow from entering the vagina during sexual activity.

To prevent odor, the woman should use good perineal hygiene, bathe or shower every day, and change pads or tampons frequently. Advise women to follow the manufacturer's directions for tampons to reduce the risk for toxic shock syndrome. Deodorized pads and tampons are not very effective and can cause irritation to the vulva and vagina.

For mild cramping occurring before or during menses, aspirin and other NSAIDs, such as ibuprofen or naproxen, are effective and can be taken unless contraindicated for other reasons. These drugs inhibit uterine contractions and have analgesic properties. A warm bath or heating pad may be comforting; lying supine also keeps the abdomen warm.

Premenstrual Syndrome

For women with PMS, you may suggest a variety of nonpharmacological treatments: getting adequate sleep; eating small, frequent meals; reducing dietary intake of sugar, caffeine, alcohol, and salt; taking vitamin and mineral supplements; and exercising. Selective serotonin reuptake-inhibiting drugs (SSRIs) such as fluoxetine (Prozac) and sertraline (Zoloft) are increasingly being used as a front-line therapy for managing symptoms of PMS.

Menopause

Hormone replacement therapy (HRT) (estrogen-only, progestin-only, or combination) remains the most effective treatment to relieve symptoms of menopause, such as itching, dryness, discomfort with intercourse, hot flashes, sleep disturbances, and other symptoms. HRT can either increase or decrease risk of heart disease, depending on when hormone therapy is started; how long women remain on it; and individual differences. HRT can help prevent loss of bone density in menopausal women, which leads to fewer hip fractures among users. Also beneficial is the reduced risk of colorectal cancer.

The risks associated with long-term use in a small number of women include heart disease, blood clots, breast and ovarian cancer, and dementia. Therefore, consumers, healthcare providers, and third-party payors have become more conservative in using HRT or reserving treatment for short-term use. Counsel women to discuss the risks and benefits of HRT with their primary care provider, and inform them that there are some natural remedies and bioidentical therapies that may provide symptom relief (see the related CAM box).

Self-Examination

Breast self-examination and testicular self-examination are vital aspects of sexual health. For more information and for details about these assessments, see Chapters 9, 22, and 42.

Breast Exam Any change in how the breasts normally look and feel should be immediately provided to the healthcare provider. The American Cancer Society (ACS) (2012, updated 2013) recommends that women in their 20s and 30s should have a clinical breast exam at

CAM for Perimenopausal Symptoms

Help, including hormone therapy, is available for perimenopause symptoms. In addition to finding a primary care provider with whom to discuss their symptoms, you might advise women to try the following:

➤ Eat a balanced diet, low in fat and rich in calcium.

➤ Use supplemental vitamins, if necessary.

➤ Get adequate sleep.

➤ Exercise daily.

➤ Avoid tobacco use.

➤ Limit alcohol and caffeine.

➤ Drink plenty of water to counteract the drying effect of low estrogen levels.

➤ Use soy products (e.g., soy milk, tofu, and soy flour), which are rich in phytoestrogens that are converted during digestion to very weak estrogens.

➤ Try the herbal remedies red clover and black cohosh.

➤ Use natural progesterone cream, which is made from a yam root. Women usually apply a small amount of the cream for 12 days out of each month.

least every 3 years, be educated on the benefits and limitations of breast self-exam (BSE), and taught how to conduct a BSE. Women should have yearly mammograms to screen for breast cancer after age 40. Although some researchers and professional groups have contrary recommendations (e.g., mammograms every 2 years for women ages 50 to 74), these guidelines represent an extensive review of the health literature and input from an expert advisory group.

Testicular Exam   The ACS (2012) advises men to be aware that a lump in the testicle could be a sign of testicular cancer. However, because the benefit of testicular self-exams has not been studied enough to show they reduce the death rate from this cancer, the ACS does not make a recommendation about monthly self-exams. However, after puberty checking for lumps is a good idea, especially if the man had undescended testicle or family history of testicular cancer.

Preventing Sexually Transmitted Infections

STIs are a worldwide health concern, and education is a key component of prevention. The only absolutely safe sex is total avoidance of sexual activity with a partner. However, most adults do not choose abstinence. The next safest sex occurs within a long-term, mutually monogamous relationship. Other safer sex practices involve the consistent, correct use of a condom and limiting the number of sexual partners. For information about the use of male and female condoms,

Go to Chapter 33, **Clinical Insight 33-3: Teaching Your Patient to Use a Condom,** in Volume 2.

Teach your clients the proper use of condoms and encourage them to discuss sexual feelings, activity, and safety with their partners. If people are not comfortable talking about birth control, STIs, and safer sex with a potential partner, they need to consider whether it is wise to begin a sexual relationship. Planned Parenthood advocates the following behaviors for safer sex:

- Be honest about current sexual practices and sexual history, as well as sexual health concerns.
- Avoid the exchange of body fluids, including semen, blood, and vaginal secretions, by correctly and consistently using latex barriers.
- Avoid contact with genital sores or growths.
- Have routine checkups for infection.
- Consult a healthcare provider for diagnosis and treatment of symptoms such as abnormal discharge from the vagina, penis, or rectum; a burning sensation with urination; sores in the genital area; or painful intercourse.
- Accept responsibility for your actions.

Also advise clients to choose a healthcare provider with whom they can comfortably discuss these issues. Freedom to speak frankly and openly about their sexual health concerns is important to their health. Assure them that testing, examination, and treatment for STIs are always confidential.

Contraception

For clients who are heterosexual or bisexual, your sexual health teaching may include methods for preventing unwanted pregnancies. Several fertility control and family planning strategies are available, each with advantages and disadvantages. For information on several fertility control methods,

Go to Chapter 33, **Tables, Fertility Control Methods,** in Volume 2.

Counseling for Sexual Problems

The PLISSIT model was developed as a guideline for counseling for sexual problems (Annon, 1976). Basic nursing education does not prepare you to provide sex therapy. However, the first three PLISSIT steps have been successfully adapted to address sexual knowledge deficits, which you are qualified to treat. The acronym PLISSIT represents the following:

*P*ermission. Permission means that you communicate an open, accepting attitude so that the client feels free to ask open-ended questions and express concerns and feelings and to engage in sexual behaviors with a consenting partner. For example, you might state, "Many women experience decreased vaginal lubrication after menopause. Tell me how well you have been lubricating."

*L*imited Information. Supplying limited information may include teaching about normal sexual functioning, expected changes in sexual functioning, medication side effects, and medical and surgical impacts on sexuality. For example, you might say, "Some women experience decreased vaginal lubrication because of decreased levels of certain hormones."

Specific Suggestions. You might make specific suggestions for self-care, as presented in this chapter. For example, you might say, "Some women have found that using a water-soluble lubricant is helpful."

Intensive Therapy. If these interventions do not relieve the client's concerns, you should refer the client to someone with specialized knowledge of sexual health. For example: "You might consider discussing this with your gynecologist."

Dealing With Inappropriate Sexual Behavior

Nursing involves intimate contact. We see people disrobed, literally touch bodies, and discuss private topics. In most cases, patients recognize this as professional behavior associated with providing healthcare. Occasionally they may respond inappropriately. For example, a client may make sexually suggestive comments, request sexually related care that is not required (e.g., ask you to bathe his genitalia when he can do it adequately himself), disrobe or expose body parts that are not involved in the care delivered, or touch or grab you as you provide care. The following are the most common reasons for sexually inappropriate behaviors:

- Confusion
- Neurological disorders, especially those involving the frontal lobe
- Mental illnesses
- Poor impulse control
- Misinterpretation of nursing care
- Need to have power or control over others, especially when the client feels powerless in other aspects of his life
- Worries about sexual functioning
- Unrealistic view of nursing based on sexual stereotypes

If you believe a client is demonstrating inappropriate sexual behaviors, immediately tell the client that the behavior is inappropriate. Do not express anger, but use clear statements, such as, "I don't like your comments. They are inappropriate and make me feel uncomfortable. Please stop." Next, let the client know what behavior you expect. Be direct with your comments. If the client is exposing himself, let him know what you expect him to wear ("I expect you to keep your pajama bottoms on"). If the client is attempting to touch you, tell him, "Don't touch me." Refocus the client's attention to the care you are delivering ("Hold still now, while I tape your IV"). If you are extremely uncomfortable or the client persists in the comments or actions, leave the room and report the incident to your instructor or the nurse assigned to the client. Your instructor may need to change your assignment. You

may also wish to consider discussing the situation with the client while another person is in the room.

Sexual harassment is a unique form of inappropriate sexual behavior (refer to Sexual Harassment in the Theoretical Knowledge section). If you believe you are being sexually harassed, you should confront your harasser and clearly state your concerns. If you feel unable to confront your harasser (e.g., if the harasser is a teacher or supervisor), keep a written record of the events, and report your concerns to the worksite or school official in charge of personnel. By law, all worksites and educational environments must have a written procedure for handling cases of sexual harassment. It will tell you how to file a grievance, what forms you need to use, to whom to report the incident, and details of the procedure for a hearing and resolution. For further information, see Chapter 45.

PUTTING IT ALL TOGETHER

Consider the three patients discussed in the Meet Your Patients scenario. Each situation illustrates how important sexual identity is to the sense of self. Each of the patients is concerned about how their medical problem might affect their sexuality:

- Jocelyn Carter is worried about how surgery will affect her relationship with her husband.
- Gabriel Thomas is concerned that blood pressure medications will impair his sexual abilities.
- Frank Thanee, recovering from open-heart surgery, is focused on explaining his long-term same-sex relationship to his family.

To help patients identify and resolve sexual health concerns, you will need to examine your own beliefs and values. The self-knowledge gained from examining your own views on sexuality will help you to be open to your patients' sexual concerns. The full-spectrum nursing model can help you to find the best approach when dealing with sexual health. Following, we use the three patients from Meet Your Patients to illustrate how this works.

Thinking

Theoretical Knowledge A sound knowledge base enables you to teach and respond sensitively to all your clients. Many myths and taboos surround the subject of sexuality, so it is important that you remain objective and current regarding these topics. You will need theoretical knowledge about sexuality, the effect of health concerns on sexual function and expression, and treatment of sexual health problems. What knowledge do you already have that would enable you to address Gabriel Thomas's concerns? What knowledge do you still need?

Critical Thinking To help Gabriel Thomas, you will need to focus on what he is experiencing and critically examine his concerns in light of what is known about

(text continued on page 877)

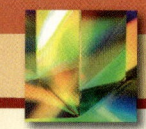 Nursing Care Plan

Client Data

Emilio Juarez is a 50-year-old man hospitalized for cardiac monitoring after an acute myocardial infarction (MI, heart attack). He has no history of diabetes or hypertension. Mr. Juarez owns a computer software company and is active in the community (president of the Chamber of Commerce).

After dinner, Mr. Juarez's nurse sits down to teach Emilio and his wife, Luz, about the medications he will be taking. She also begins to talk to them about a cardiac rehabilitation program. Mr. Juarez asks, "What do you mean by 'activity restriction'? Do I have to stop doing all the things I did before?" The nurse asks, "What things are you thinking about?" Mr. Juarez hesitates, then says, "Oh, like working in the yard, going up the stairs, and, you know, personal things." Mrs. Juarez immediately says, "There is no need to talk about that now. The most important thing is for my Emilio to feel better and get home—there is plenty of time for other things later." The nurse tells the Juarezes that many couples are anxious about resuming sexual activity after a heart attack and says, "I'd like to give you some information about that and answer any questions you might have."

Nursing Diagnosis

Ineffective Sexuality Patterns related to lack of knowledge about post-MI sexual activity and reluctance to ask questions, as evidenced by Mrs. Juarez's comment, "There is no need to talk about that now."

NOC Outcomes	Individualized Goals / Expected Outcomes
Sexual Identity (1207) Sexual Functioning (0119) Body Image (1200)	*By discharge, Mr. Juarez will:* 1. Be able to identify two resources he can use to learn more about sexual activity after myocardial infarction. 2. Commit to attending the cardiac rehabilitation classes offered at the hospital. *During and by the end of the cardiac rehabilitation program, Mr. Juarez will:* 1. Identify stressors in his life related to sexual activity. 2. Report a desire to resume sexual activity to pre-MI levels. 3. Resume previous sexual activity. 4. Discuss any problems encountered.

Nursing Care Plan (continued)

NIC Interventions/Activities	Rationale

NIC Interventions

Sexual counseling (5248)
Body image enhancement (5220)
Anxiety reduction (5820)

Nursing Activities

1. Initiate discussions about sexual activity after MI, beginning with general, nonthreatening statements.

Clients and significant others are often too embarrassed to ask about sexual matters. The client's perception of his sexuality impacts personal and social behavior outside the bedroom (Steinke, 2002; Svedberg, Johansson, Persson, et al., 2012). Patients should be reassured that after recovery from an MI, sexual activity presents no great risk of another MI ("Sex After Heart Attack," Mayo Clinic, 2013).

2. Allow Mr. Juarez to control the discussion of sexual matters.

The subject of sexual activity should be raised with patients within the context of cardiac rehabilitation (Cooper, Skinner, Nherera, et al., 2007; Paull, Arndt, Petkovski, et al., 2011). This shows respect for the client's privacy and his sexual being. Controlling what issues are discussed and when enhances self-esteem (Steinke, 2000; Paull, Arndt, Petkovski, et al., 2011).

3. Listen carefully to Mr. Juarez's verbal and nonverbal expression of concerns.

Anxiety interferes with patients' return to sexual activity after an acute cardiovascular event (Moser, 2007). Some men may overtly express uninterest in discussing sexual matters; others avoid the topic by joking, avoiding eye contact, or brushing off concerns as not pressing. Men commonly avoid verbalizing feelings in this area because of the personal nature and threats to masculine identity. Although depressive symptoms are more common in women after an MI and contribute to higher rates of rehospitalization, men also show depression (Moser, 2007; Parashar, Rumsfeld, Reid, et al., 2008).

4. Seek consultation from other members of the healthcare team as needed.

When nurses are uncomfortable talking about sexual matters and do not initiate the conversation, the client may think sexual activity is prohibited after MI. It is imperative that healthcare professionals incorporate sexuality into the plan of care to effectively meet the care needs of their clients (Parker & Yau, 2011; Paull, Arndt, Petkovski, et al., 2011).

5. Include Mrs. Juarez in counseling as much as possible, with Mr. Juarez's consent.

Marriage and close interpersonal relationships allow each member to support the other and alleviate negative effects of stress. The client and spouse may have different perceptions of recovery, anticipated needs, sexuality, and other uncertainties that must be addressed to minimize stress (Baird & Eliasziw, 2011).

(continued on next page)

Nursing Care Plan (continued)

NIC Interventions/Activities	Rationale

Nursing Activities

6. Be clear about exploring Mr. and Mrs. Juarez's specific concerns, and correct any misinformation.

Anxiety about sexual activity after MI often arises from misconceptions. Fewer than 1% of MIs occur during sexual activity ("Sex After Heart Attack," Mayo Clinic, 2013). There is no evidence suggesting that sexual activity poses a risk for sudden death ("Sex After Heart Attack," Harvard Health Letter, 2013). Regular exercise, such as in a cardiac rehab program, reduces the risk of MI from sexual activity (DeBusk, Drory, Goldstein, et al., 2000; Muller, 2000). For some cardiac patients, sexual problems begin before a heart attack. Erectile dysfunction, the consistent inability to sustain an erection, affects more than 50% of men older than 60 and is a recognized symptom of cardiovascular disease. The typical period of maximum risk (which is still very low) is within 4 weeks of the MI (DeBusk, Drory, Goldstein, et al., 2000). Exercise training after acute MI improves cardiovascular efficiency and reduces myocardial oxygen demand during customary activities, including sexual activity (Miner, 2006). Erectogenic drugs, when used correctly, do not increase overall cardiovascular risk in patients after an MI (Cooper, Skinner, Nherera, et al., 2007).

7. Discuss the risks of using drugs for erectile dysfunction together with nitrates.

An unsafe drop in blood pressure can occur when erectile dysfunction medication is taken with nitrates (Cooper, Skinner, Nherera, et al., 2007). Men should be taught to contact their prescribers if they experience an erection lasting more than 4 hours or if a change in vision occurs.

Nursing Care Plan (continued)

Evaluation

After Mrs. Juarez left for the evening, the nurse returned to bring Mr. Juarez a medication. He said, "Thanks for bringing that up and for leaving the booklet. I love my wife, and I was worried. I sure didn't want to have another heart attack. She was embarrassed to let on that it is important to her, but we will be sure to make use of the rehab program." The nurse followed up later by giving the Juarezes a DVD that discusses sexual issues, which they can take home and watch in privacy and comfort when they are ready to do so.

References

Baird, D., & Eliasziw, M. (2011). Disparity in perceived illness intrusiveness and illness severity between cardiac patients and their spouses. *Journal of Cardiovascular Nursing, 26*(6), 481–486.

Cooper, A., Skinner, J., Nherera, L., et al. (2007). *Clinical guidelines and evidence review for post myocardial infarction: Secondary prevention in primary care and secondary care for patients following a myocardial infarction (full NICE guideline)*. National Collaborating Centre for Primary Care and Royal College of General Practitioners. Retrieved from http://www.nice.org.uk/cg48

DeBusk, R., Drory, Y., Goldstein, I., et al. (2000). Management of sexual dysfunction in patients with cardiovascular disease: Recommendations of the Princeton Consensus Panel. *American Journal of Cardiology, 86*(2), 175–181.

Miner, M. M. (2006). Sexual activity after myocardial infarction: When to resume the use of erectogenic drugs. *Current Sexual Health Reports, 3*(1), 30–34.

Moser, D. K. (2007). The rust of life: Impact of anxiety on cardiac patients. *American Journal of Critical Care, 16*(4), 361–369.

Muller, J. E. (2000). Triggering of cardiac events by sexual activity: Findings from a case-crossover analysis. *American Journal of Cardiology, 86*(Suppl. 2A), 14F–18F.

Parashar, S., Rumsfeld, J. S., Reid, K. J., et al. (2008). Impact of depression on sex differences in outcome after myocardial infarction. *Circulation: Cardiovascular Quality and Outcomes, 2*, 33–40.

Parker, M., & Yau, M. (2011). Sexuality in women with spinal cord injury. Occupational Therapy Australia, 24th National Conference and Exhibition, 29 June–1 July 2011 (#35501). *Australian Occupational Therapy Journal, 58*(Supp. 127).

Paull, G., Arndt, P., Petkovski, D., et al. (2011). Sexuality and chronic cardiovascular disease—a neglected area of practice: The role of the occupational therapist in a cardiac rehabilitation setting. Occupational Therapy Australia, 24th National Conference and Exhibition, 29 June–1 July 2011 (#35503). *Australian Occupational Therapy Journal, 58*(Supp. 127).

Sex after heart attack. (2013). *Harvard Health Letter, 37*(8), 5.

Sex after heart attack. (2013) *Mayo Health Clinic Letter, 31*(4), 7.

Steinke, E. E. (2000). Sexual counseling after myocardial infarction. *American Journal of Nursing, 100*(12), 38–43.

Steinke, E. E. (2002). A videotape intervention for sexual counseling after myocardial infarction. *Heart & Lung, 31*(5), 348–354.

Svedberg, P., Johansson, I., Persson, S., et al. (2012). Psychometric evaluation of the 25-Item Sex After MI Knowledge Test in a Swedish context. *Scandinavian Journal of Caring Science, 26*(1), 203–208.

Care Map

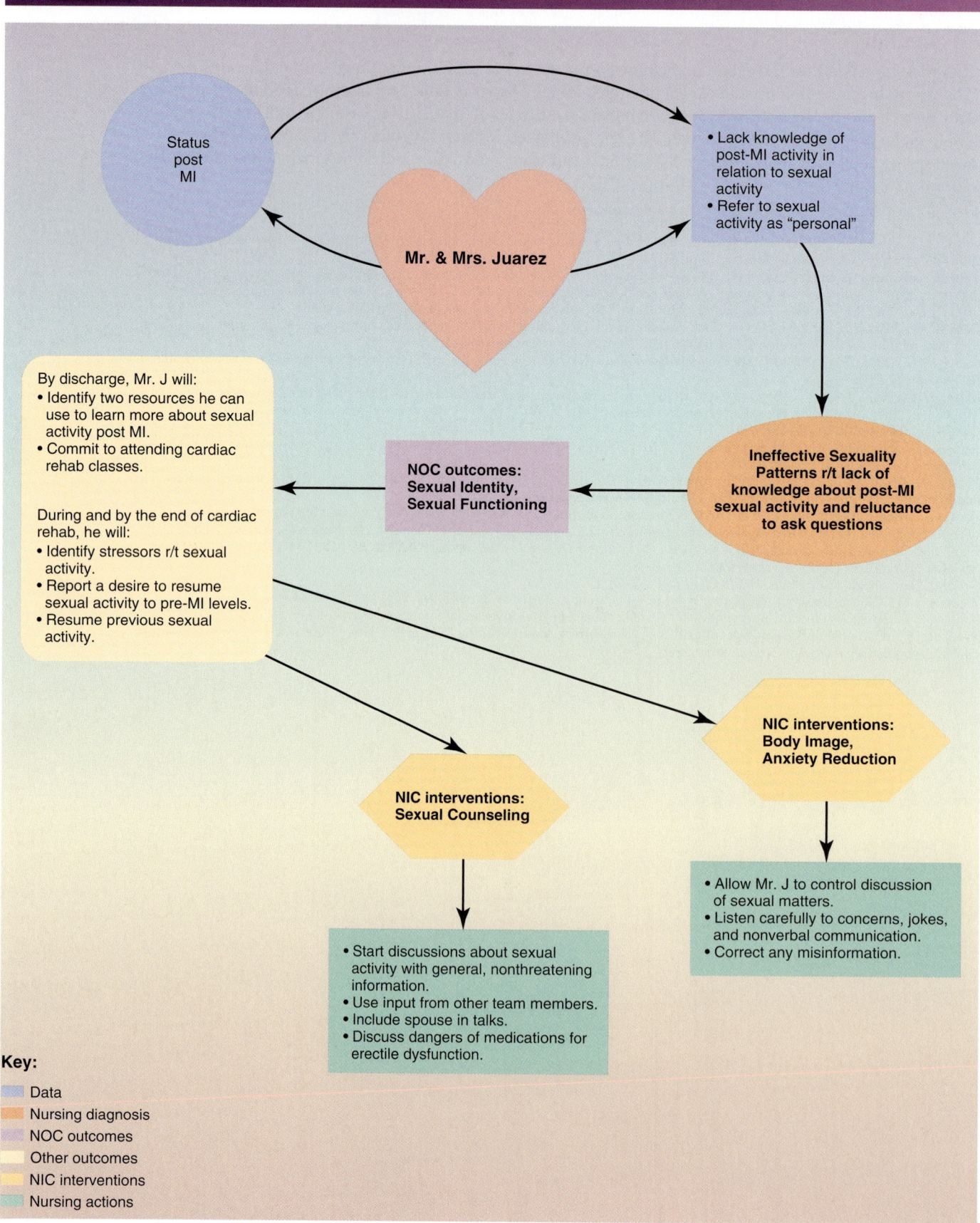

Status post MI

Mr. & Mrs. Juarez

- Lack knowledge of post-MI activity in relation to sexual activity
- Refer to sexual activity as "personal"

By discharge, Mr. J will:
- Identify two resources he can use to learn more about sexual activity post MI.
- Commit to attending cardiac rehab classes.

During and by the end of cardiac rehab, he will:
- Identify stressors r/t sexual activity.
- Report a desire to resume sexual activity to pre-MI levels.
- Resume previous sexual activity.

NOC outcomes:
Sexual Identity,
Sexual Functioning

Ineffective Sexuality Patterns r/t lack of knowledge about post-MI sexual activity and reluctance to ask questions

NIC interventions:
Body Image,
Anxiety Reduction

NIC interventions:
Sexual Counseling

- Allow Mr. J to control discussion of sexual matters.
- Listen carefully to concerns, jokes, and nonverbal communication.
- Correct any misinformation.

- Start discussions about sexual activity with general, nonthreatening information.
- Use input from other team members.
- Include spouse in talks.
- Discuss dangers of medications for erectile dysfunction.

Key:
- Data
- Nursing diagnosis
- NOC outcomes
- Other outcomes
- NIC interventions
- Nursing actions

hypertension and its treatment. You will need to prioritize your concerns about Mr. Thomas, balancing the need to control his blood pressure with his sexual requirements. Help him consider the consequences of various approaches, for example, by discussing alternative forms of sexual expression.

Doing

Practical Knowledge When dealing with sexuality, communication skills are essential practical knowledge. Your verbal and nonverbal skills demonstrate to patients your comfort with sensitive topics. Consider the situation of Jocelyn Carter. Suppose you responded to Jocelyn's question by telling her, "That's the least of your worries." How do you think she would feel? Now consider what might happen if you responded, "You must be worried about your sexual relationship. Tell me a little more about what you're feeling."

Nursing Process To help Mr. Thomas, you will need to assess his knowledge and concerns, clearly identify his problems (elevated blood pressure and Ineffective Sexuality Pattern), and use the nursing process to develop a plan of care that is acceptable to him. When working with patients with sexual health concerns, tailor your approach to each individual's needs, just as you do in all areas of health.

Caring

Self-Knowledge To help patients identify and resolve sexual health concerns, you will need to examine your own beliefs and values. The self-knowledge gained from examining your own views on sexuality will help you to be open to your patients' sexual concerns. What are your beliefs about sex and sexuality? Are you uncomfortable around people whose sexual orientation is different from yours? Imagine how you would feel if Frank Thanee asked you for help with his family relationships.

 To explore learning resources for this chapter,

Go to DavisPlus at DavisPl.us/Wilkinson3.

Chapter Resources for Chapter 33:
  Response sheets for all learning activities
  Resources for Caregivers and Health Professionals
  Reading More About Sexual Health (suggested readings)
  Concept Map of chapter content
Interactive Case Studies
NCLEX-Style and Chapter Review Questions
Chapter Overview Podcasts

For references cited in this chapter,

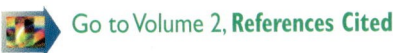 Go to Volume 2, **References Cited.**

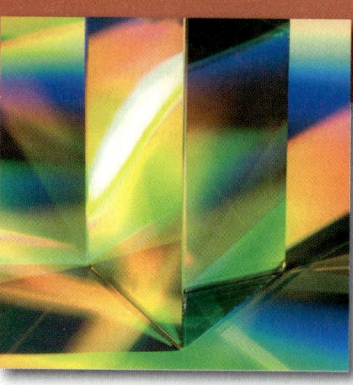

CHAPTER 34

Sleep & Rest

Learning Outcomes

After completing this chapter, you should be able to:

➤ Explain why rest and sleep are important.
➤ Describe the functions and physiology of sleep.
➤ Explain circadian rhythms and how they relate to sleep.
➤ Identify factors that influence rest and sleep.
➤ Discuss how sleep impacts physical, mental, and spiritual well-being.
➤ Describe nursing implications for age-related differences in the sleep cycle.
➤ Identify at least five common sleep disorders.

➤ Perform a comprehensive sleep assessment using appropriate interview questions, a sleep diary, and a sleep history.
➤ Formulate nursing diagnoses that identify sleep problems that may be treated through specific nursing interventions.
➤ Plan, implement, and evaluate nursing care related to specific nursing diagnoses addressing sleep problems.

Meet Your Patients

You are a nurse working on a surgical unit. Today you are meeting with Anne for preoperative teaching. She is scheduled for a complete hysterectomy next Monday. She has a secondary diagnosis of fibromyalgia, a chronic disorder characterized by widespread muscle pain and nonrestorative sleep.

Anne is a 49-year-old married woman with three children. She works full-time and manages the family with her husband. She says, "I'm a little nervous about the surgery, but I know I need it. But I haven't been sleeping well because of thinking about it." Anne tells you that she has actually had trouble sleeping for the last 20 years. "I take an Ambien pill, 10 mg, every night to help me sleep. Will I be able to get that in the hospital? I really can't sleep at all without it," explains Anne.

As you continue the interview, Anne explains that she suffered from physical and emotional abuse as a young woman and has had sleep problems ever since. She has been to counseling, but that did not improve her sleep. In

addition to her upcoming surgery, she has been coping with the recent death of her father. You realize that sleep-promoting measures will be an important part of her nursing care.

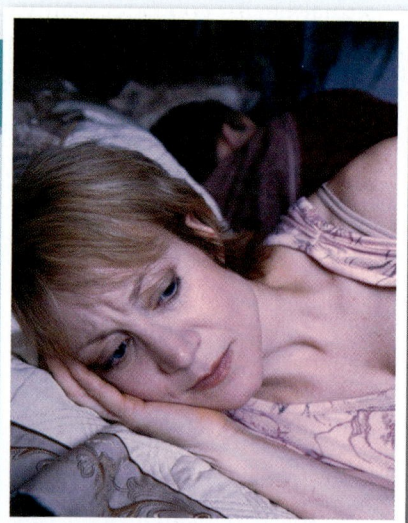

What clues would cause you to suspect that Ann will have difficulty sleeping while in the hospital? What characteristics of the hospital environment might interfere with Anne's sleep? You may not have enough theoretical knowledge and experience to feel confident about your answers to these questions, but use your present knowledge and your life experiences to think about them.

Theoretical Knowledge
knowing **why**

Have you felt tired after waking up from a night's sleep? Have you ever been tired, but not sleepy, and, after relaxing a while, felt your normal energy return? How do you think sleep and rest are different? How are they alike? This chapter will help you to make those distinctions.

ABOUT THE KEY CONCEPTS

In this chapter we will examine the concepts of rest and sleep, along with related concepts (e.g., stages of sleep, sleep disorders).

Rest is a condition in which the body is inactive or engaging in mild activity, after which the person feels refreshed. A person at rest is calm, at ease, relaxed, and free of anxiety and stress (Fig. 34-1). People rest by doing things that they find calming and relaxing.

Sleep is a cyclically occurring state of decreased motor activity and perception (Fig. 34-2). Body functions slow, and metabolism falls by 20% to 30%, so the body conserves energy. Sleep is characterized by altered consciousness: A sleeping person is unaware of the environment and responds selectively to external stimuli. For example, an alarm clock, bright light, or other meaningful stimuli usually awaken a sleeper, but everyday background noises and soft light do not.

Although necessary and beneficial, rest without sleep is inadequate. At rest, the body is disturbed by all exterior stimuli, whereas in sleep it is screened from them by altered consciousness. Thus, sleep restores the body; rest alone cannot do this.

WHY DO WE NEED TO SLEEP?

We spend more time sleeping than in any other single activity: about 8 hours a day, or 2,688 hours a year—nearly one-third of our lives! So why is sleep so important?

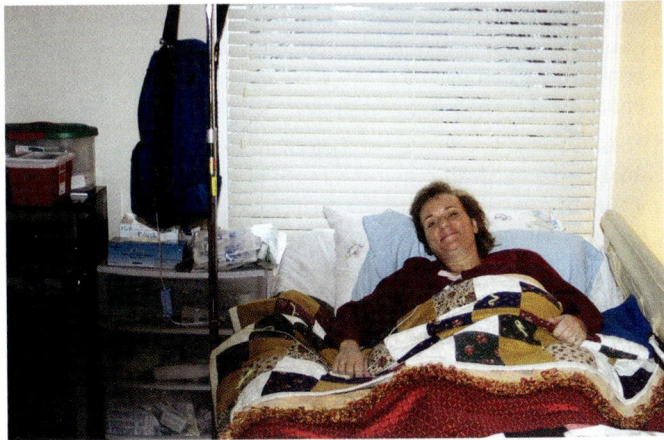

FIGURE 34-1 Woman receiving hospice care resting comfortably.

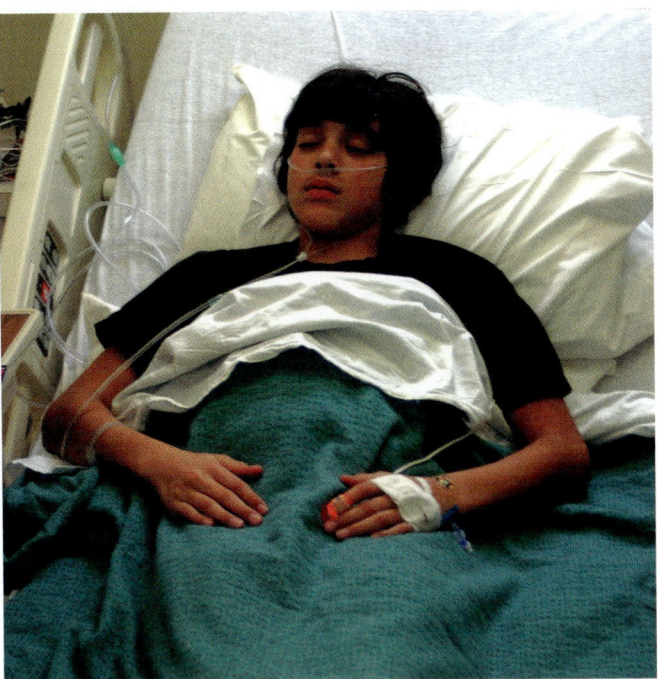

FIGURE 34-2 Boy sleeping in hospital setting.

Before you try to answer, think back to the last time you slept poorly. Remember the mental fogginess, the physical fatigue, the feeling of slight nausea? Poor quality or insufficient length of sleep for even one night can reduce mental performance, and long periods of sleep deprivation can result in stress-related illnesses (e.g., cardiac events) and injuries (e.g., from an automobile accident). The reason is that sleep and rest are essential for physical, mental, and spiritual well-being.

Sleep affects almost every tissue in our bodies. Sleep isn't essential just for the brain; it also affects growth and stress hormones, and even hormones that affect appetite and control body weight. Research also indicates that sleep strengthens the immune system (Cohen, Doyle, Alper, et al., 2009; Ranjbaran, Keefer, Stepanski, et al., 2007) and helps the body to fight infection. Lack of sleep increases the risk heart disease, stroke, infections (National Institutes of Health, 2013), and possibly even cancer (Hakin, Wang, Zhang, et. al., 2014).

Sleep is an important regulator of energy metabolism. Despite the fact that some regions of the brain are more active during sleep than when we are awake, total energy output is reduced during sleep, giving the body time for restoration and repair. Without sleep, the body is less able to tolerate glucose and yet responds with insulin resistance. Sleep restriction is also linked to increased appetite through changes in the appetite control hormones, leptin and ghrelin. Additionally, not enough sleep leads to reduced energy expenditure, all of which can lead to obesity and type 2 diabetes. (Broussard, Ehrmann, van Cauter, et al., 2012).

Sleep may also improve learning and adaptation. It gives the individual a chance to mentally repeat and rehearse facts and situations before they are encountered in wakeful life. Some evidence suggests that sleep and dreaming may facilitate the storage of long-term memory, perhaps by assisting the brain in reorganizing and storing information (National Institutes of Health, 2010, reviewed 2012).

 Older adults have an even greater need for sleep to protect against the natural decline in cognitive function that comes with aging (Mander, Tao, Lu, et al., 2013).

Sleep also appears to reduce stress and anxiety, improving our ability to cope and concentrate on activities of daily living. More sleep also reduces the body's sensitivity to pain (Roehrs, Harris, Randall, et al., 2012).

 Similarly, nonrestorative sleep contributes to widespread pain, which is common in older adults (McBeth, J., Lacey, R. J., & Wilkie, R., 2014).

Sleep/rest and illness are interrelated (Fig. 34-3). Illness and injury increase the need to sleep and at the same time make it difficult to sleep. In turn, lack of sleep increases the susceptibility to illness by compromising the immune system. People who are ill or injured need more sleep to restore energy needed for tissue repair and healing. However, they often have difficulty resting because of pain and other symptoms of their illness.

For further discussion of sleep theories,

 Go to Chapter 34, **Supplemental Materials: Theories of Sleep,** on Davis*Plus*.

KnowledgeCheck 34-1

- Compare and contrast sleep and rest. How are they different? Alike?
- Why is promoting sleep an important nursing intervention?

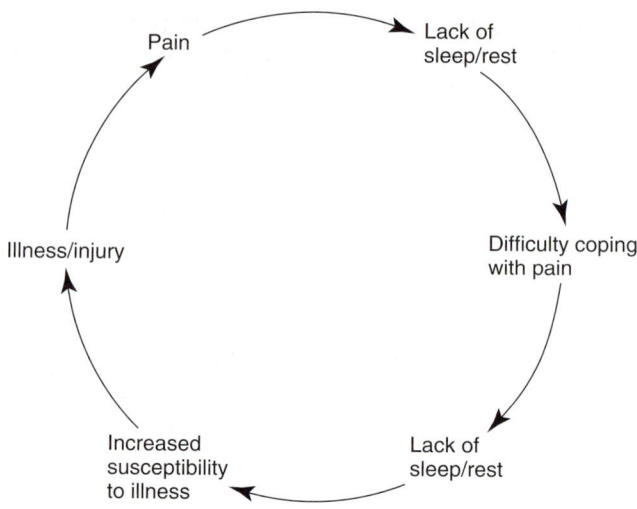

FIGURE 34-3 Relationship between sleep/rest and illness. Lack of sleep and rest increases susceptibility to illness. Likewise, the pain and stress of illness disturb sleep.

ThinkLike a Nurse 34-1

What effect do you think surgery will have on Anne's sleep (Meet Your Patient)? Why?

HOW MUCH SLEEP DO WE NEED?

Key Point: *Sleep needs vary widely among individuals. Even though the accepted standard has been 8 hours per night for adults, there is really no amount or pattern of sleep that is best suited for all people.*

PICOT

Acupuncture for Neuropathic Pain

Situation: The nurse is caring for a client with peripheral neuropathy secondary to uncontrolled diabetes. The client is showing signs of daytime drowsiness, irritability, and restlessness. He states he has trouble sleeping, but does not want to take medication for pain. He is willing to try alternative therapies.

PICOT Components

P	Population/client	= Sleep-deprived adults with chronic pain
I	Intervention/indicator	= Acupuncture
C	Comparator/control	= No acupuncture
O	Outcome	= Decreased pain and increased sleep
T	Time	= (none needed)

Searchable Question: Do _____ (P) who receive/are exposed to _____ (I) demonstrate _____ (O) as compared to _____ (C)?

Example of Evidence: Persistent neuropathic pain can interfere with quality of life and impair sleep. It has been associated with depression, anxiety, and loss of sleep. Acupuncture has been helpful in decreasing neuropathic pain. In one study, 77% of clients reported pain relief after six courses of acupuncture. Therefore, the client with neuropathic pain might use acupuncture to rest more comfortably and minimize the sleep disturbances that were impairing the sleep and rest cycle.

Application to Practice: The client who reports unsatisfactory sleep requires a more in-depth sleep history, including questions about the quality of sleep, sleep hygiene, napping, and bedtime routines. A complete medication and pain history should be obtained. As sleep disturbance may increase a patient's pain, the nurse may decide to explore with the healthcare team the possibility of suggesting acupuncture to a patient who is dealing with chronic pain.

Vinik, A. I., & Casellini, C. M. (2013). Guidelines in the management of diabetic nerve pain: Clinical utility of pregabalin. *Diabetes, Metabolic Syndrome, and Obesity. 6*, 57–78. doi:10.2147/DMSO.S24825

Some people are refreshed after napping for 15 or 20 minutes; others feel groggy after napping; others cannot nap at all. Many people routinely awaken several times a night and do not report being tired, whereas others report fatigue and loss of mental clarity if their sleep is even minimally interrupted. In spite of individual variations, however, different sleep patterns are characteristic of different age groups.

Infants and Children Infants have an overall greater total sleep time than any other age group. Newborns sleep as much as 16 to 18 hours a day, in periods ranging from one to several hours. Sleep time gradually decreases over the next few months, but throughout the first year of life, a minimum of 14 hours of sleep per day is recommended (Centers for Disease Control and Prevention, 2013b). Most infants sleep several hours during one overnight period, with a morning and afternoon nap each day.

The U.S. Centers for Disease Control and Prevention (CDC) (2013a) recommends that toddlers get 12 to 14 hours of sleep; preschoolers, 11 to 13 hours; and adolescents aged 10 to 17, 8.5 to 9.5 hours. There has been concern that U.S. children are getting too little sleep. As a result, children with insufficient sleep experience problems with behavior, coping, and school performance, as well as health risks.

Adults After the first year of life, sleep duration gradually lessens (Table 34-1). In most adults, sleep of 7 to 8 hours is fully restorative; however, there are wide individual variations. In some cultures, total sleep time is divided into an overnight sleep period and a midafternoon nap.

Older Adults
Older adults spend significantly less time sleeping but need more rest than younger adults. Usually older adults rest or nap during the day, go to bed early, and get up early. They take

longer to fall asleep, and their arousal periods during sleep are longer and more frequent. Frequent waking is commonly due to physical discomfort, anxiety, and nocturia (Polan & Taylor, 2010). If sleep is interrupted, the person needs to increase the total time in bed in order to get adequate sleep. Otherwise, she may experience fatigue, irritability, and impaired cognition.

 ThinkLike a Nurse 34-2

- How much sleep might Anne (Meet Your Patient) need in a normal night?
- How will a good night of sleep benefit Anne while she is in the hospital?
- If you were preparing for an important test, would it be better to stay up all night studying, or should you try to get a good night of sleep?
- How many hours of sleep do *you* need to feel rested and function well the next day? Compare notes with family members, friends, and classmates. Do they all need the same amount of sleep as you?

PHYSIOLOGY OF SLEEP

Our environment plays a role in the physiology of our sleep, so let's begin with an exploration of circadian rhythms, by which the body maintains synchronicity with nature. **Synchrony** occurs when something happens at the same time or works or develops on the same time scale as something else.

How Do Circadian Rhythms Influence Sleep?

Biorhythms are "biological clocks" that are controlled within the body and synchronized with environmental factors (e.g., gravity, electromagnetic forces, light, and darkness). Biorhythms influence many physical and mental functions. For example, body temperature is typically lowest when the person wakes up in the morning, and female menstruation follows an approximately 28-day cycle, like the lunar cycle on which our calendar months are based.

A **circadian rhythm** is a biorhythm based on the day–night pattern in a 24-hour cycle. The term comes from the Latin words *circa*, meaning "about," and *dies*, meaning "day"—once a day. A person's circadian rhythm is regulated by a cluster of cells in the hypothalamus of the brainstem that respond to changing levels of light. Circadian rhythm affects our overall level of functioning; for example, most people have a higher energy level in the daytime and less energy at night. However, some people are more alert and active in the morning, and others function at a higher level in the afternoon or evening.

Do you feel sleepy at about the same time each night? Do you often awaken before the alarm clock goes off? If so, that's because the timing of sleep and waking is also influenced by your circadian biorhythm. Sleep quality is best when your sleep and wake times

Table 34-1 ➤ Average Sleep Requirements	
AGE GROUP	**HOURS/DAY**
Newborns (birth–4 weeks)	16–20
Infants (4 weeks–1 year)	14–16
Toddlers (1–3 years)	12–14
Preschoolers (3–6 years)	11–13
Middle and late childhood (6–12 years)	10–11
Adolescents (12–18 years)	8.5–9.5
Young adults (18–40 years)	7–8
Middle-age adults (40–65 years)	7
Older adults (65 years and older)	5–7

are in synchrony with your circadian rhythm. For this reason, people who work evening and night shifts (e.g., healthcare workers, police officers) can suffer significant sleep deprivation until their bodies adjust to the new pattern. Changing time zones can also disrupt sleep–wake cycles and can thus be troublesome for people who travel frequently. Hospitalization can also interfere with a patient's circadian rhythm. Noises, lights, waking the patient for vital signs or medications, altered normal bedtime rituals, absence or presence of family members, homesickness, recent losses, worry, fear of the unknown, and pain may compromise the patient's quality of sleep and the ability to fall and stay asleep (Meltzer, Davis, & Mindell, 2012).

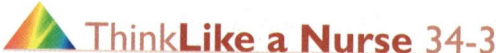

ThinkLike a Nurse 34-3

What may upset Anne's circadian rhythm?

How Is Sleep Regulated?

What makes us fall asleep? What happens in the brain during sleep? The mechanisms of sleep are complex and poorly understood, but we know that sleep is controlled by centers in the lower part of the brain that produce sleep by actively inhibiting wakefulness. As just noted, a major factor in regulating sleep is the amount of light received through the eyes. The increasing light of a dawning sky signals the hypothalamus (Fig. 34-4) to induce gradual arousal from sleep. Another collection of nerve cell bodies within the brainstem, called the **reticular formation**, is responsible for maintaining wakefulness. The reticular formation is activated by stimuli from the cerebral cortex. Together, these reticular and cortical neurons are called the **reticular activating system (RAS)**. Neurotransmitters associated with excitatory and inhibitory sleep mechanisms include catecholamines, acetylcholine, serotonin, histamine, and prostaglandins.

An **electroencephalogram (EEG)** is used to record the electrical activity of the neurons in the brain. Electrical impulses are transmitted from the brain through electrodes attached to the scalp. These impulses create five different wave patterns, or *brain waves*. Figure 34-5 shows examples of different types of brain waves during sleep:

- **Alpha waves** are high-frequency, medium-amplitude, irregular waves. These occur in the drowsy stage.
- **Beta waves** are high-frequency, low-amplitude, irregular waves. These occur during periods of wakefulness.

Fatigue and Sleep Deprivation Among Healthcare Workers

Self-Care

Extended work hours and rotating shift work significantly increase fatigue and impair on-the-job performance and safety.

Impact of Fatigue

➤ Lapses in attention and memory; poor concentration

➤ Irritability

➤ Reduced motivation, apathy, and indifference

➤ Diminished reaction time

➤ Impaired judgment and decision making

➤ Altered communication

➤ More errors, needlestick and sharps injuries, and adverse events to patients

Fight Sleepiness on the Job

➤ Be honest with yourself about how you tolerate rotating shifts, night shift, and longer shifts (e.g., 12 hours), and schedule accordingly. Plan rest days in between consecutive work days.

➤ Engage in conversation with others, not just listen and nod.

➤ Do something that requires physical action periodically, even if it means just geting up and moving around.

➤ Take frequent breaks (e.g., every 1 to 2 hours) during the night shift, if possible.

➤ Be smart about your caffeine use; that is, don't take caffeine when you don't need it to stay awake, and avoid caffeine at the end of your shift before sleep.

➤ Practice good sleep hygiene measures during your off hours. See the Self-Care box Teaching Your Patients About Sleep Hygiene.

Source: Adapted from The Joint Commission. (2011). Health care worker fatigue and patient safety. *The Joint Commission Sentinel Event Alert, 48,*1–4. Retrieved from http://www.jointcommission.org/assets/1/18/sea_48.pdf

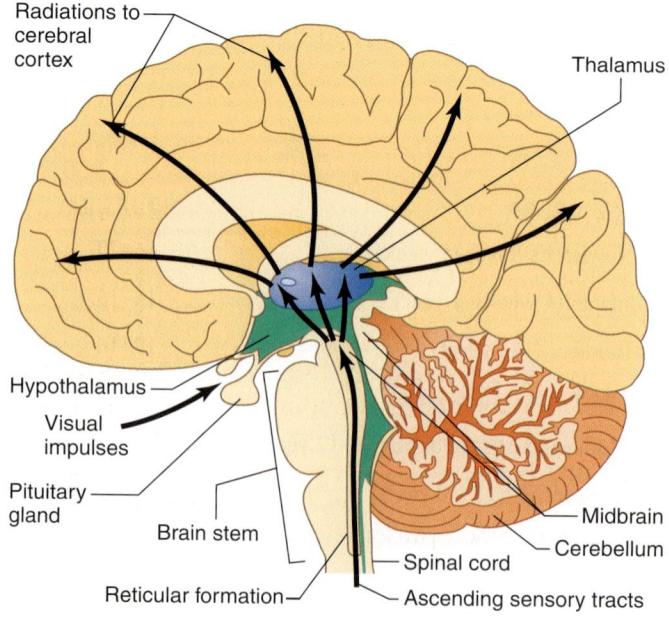

FIGURE 34-4 The reticular activating system works to regulate sleep and wakefulness.

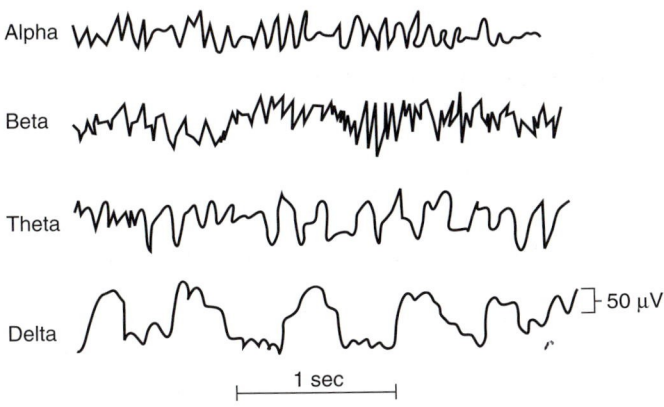

FIGURE 34-5 Four different types of brain waves.

- **Spindles** or **K-complexes** are peaked, irregular wave-forms that occur in the earlier phases of NREM sleep.
- **Theta waves** are high-amplitude waves that are common in children but rare in adults. These occur with delta waves when transitioning to a deeper sleep stage.
- **Delta waves** are low-frequency, high-amplitude, regular waves common in deep sleep.

The EEG of a waking person differs greatly from that of a sleeping person. In general, the greater the brain activity is, the more rapid will be the brain waves on the EEG. While the person is awake, brain waves are very rapid, irregular, and low in amplitude, mostly alpha and beta waves. Many neurons are firing at different intervals, at different times, and with different strengths. When a person is relaxed without intense stimulation of the senses, the EEG records mostly alpha activity. During sleep, alpha waves disappear. They are replaced by slower, higher amplitude delta waves.

What Are the Stages of Sleep?

There are two distinct types of sleep, NREM and REM. The body moves back and forth between them during the sleep cycle.

NREM Sleep

NREM (non–rapid eye movement) sleep is generally the restful phase of sleep in which physiological function is slow. NREM sleep is also called slow-wave sleep (SWS) because it is characterized by the presence of delta waves. NREM is divided into three stages, each deeper than the one preceding it. The parasympathetic branch of the autonomic nervous system becomes progressively more dominant during each stage of NREM sleep. During this phase, muscles relax; body temperature lowers; and heart rate, respirations, and blood pressure decrease.

REM Sleep

During **REM** (rapid eye movement) sleep the brain becomes highly active and the brain waves resemble those of a person who is fully awake. Rapid eye movements occur, which can often be detected even though the sleeper's eyelids are closed. More spontaneous awakenings occur during this stage than any other.

REM sleep is essential for mental and emotional restoration. Loss of REM sleep impairs memory and learning. A person who is deprived of REM sleep for several nights will usually experience *REM rebound*; that is, the person will spend a greater amount of time in REM sleep on successive nights, keeping the total amount of REM sleep constant over time.

Sleep Cycles

Cycling between REM and NREM sleep produces restorative rest. The American Association of Sleep Medicine (2007) identifies four stages of sleep (three NREM stages and the REM stage) have been identified, based on brain activity and other physiological characteristics (Table 34-2). The NREM/REM sleep cycle repeats four to six times throughout the night, depending on the total amount of time spent sleeping (Fig. 34-6). Each cycle lasts about 90 to 100 minutes. The first REM period may last only about 20 minutes, but with each cycle, the REM period lengthens until, in the last cycle of a typical 8-hour sleep period, REM may last as long as 60 minutes. The amount of time spent in each sleep stage varies over the life span.

KnowledgeCheck 34-2

- List the stages of sleep.
- Describe the progression of a typical sleep cycle for a young adult.
- Describe the physiological activity characteristic of each stage of sleep.
- What is the stage that must be "made up" if not enough time is spent in it?

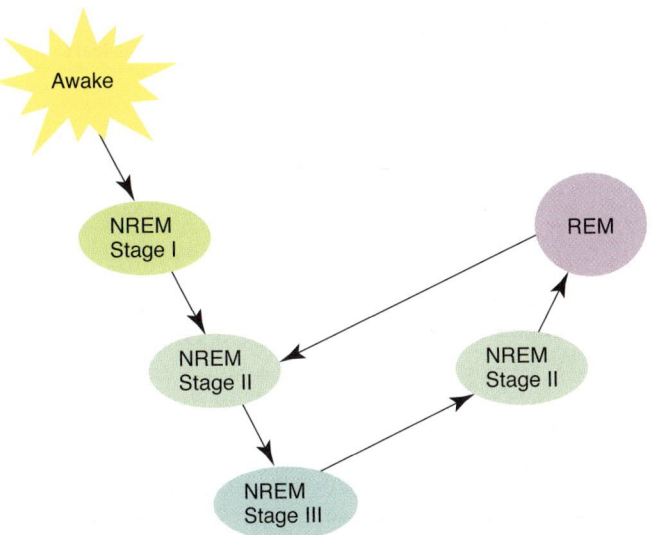

FIGURE 34-6 The normal adult sleep cycle. All but NREM stage I are repeated four or more times a night.

Table 34-2 ➤ Characteristics of Stages of Sleep

STAGE	TYPICAL BRAIN WAVE TYPE	CHARACTERISTICS
W (Wakefulness)	Beta waves with some alpha waves	Ranges from full alertness to the early stages of drowsiness.
		Reading eye movements
		Eye blinks with eyes open or closed
NI (NREM)	Alpha waves with occasional low frequency theta waves	Transition between wakefulness and sleep
		Slow eye movements
		Light sleep; can be awakened easily
		Relaxed but aware of surroundings
		Groggy, heavy lidded
		Regular, deep breathing; eyelids open and close slowly.
		Accounts for about 5% of total sleep.
		Dreams are usually not remembered.
NII (NREM)	Theta waves, K-complexes and sleep spindles	Light sleep
		Easily roused
		Temperature, heart rate, and blood pressure decrease slightly.
		Accounts for about 50% of total sleep.
NIII (NREM)	Delta waves; sawtooth waves	Deep sleep
		Difficult to rouse; if awakened in this stage, may be confused.
		Parasympathetic nervous system predominates: temperature, pulse, respirations, and blood pressure slow even more.
		Skeletal muscles are very relaxed.
		Snoring may occur.
		Some dreaming may occur, but dreams are less vivid than those that occur in REM sleep. This sleep stage is especially important for restorative processes such as healing, growth, and tissue renewal.
		Makes up 20-25% of total sleep time.
REM	5–30 minutes (usually at least 20–30)	Highly active sleep with spontaneous awakenings
		Less restful than NREM sleep
		Eyes move rapidly and small muscles twitch.
		Essential for mental and emotional restoration
		Metabolism, temperature, pulse, and blood pressure increase.
		Pulse may be rapid and irregular.
		Apnea may occur.
		Gastric secretions increase.
		Deep-tendon reflexes are depressed.
		Dreaming occurs.
		If awakened, person will react normally.
		Accounts for about 25% of total sleep.

WHAT FACTORS AFFECT SLEEP QUALITY AND DURATION?

People vary not only in the amount of sleep they need, but also in their sleep patterns. **Sleep quality** has both subjective and objective components. It is related to (1) the total amount of sleep, (2) how well the person slept, and (3) whether the person obtained the needed amounts of NREM and REM. Several factors affect the amount and quality of sleep.

Age

Age is an important factor affecting the duration of sleep (see Table 34-1). But sleep *patterns* are also affected by age. For example, newborns and young children experience prolonged REM sleep periods; young adults spend about 25% of their sleep in REM sleep; and

 older adults typically enter REM sleep quicker and spend more time in this active phase of sleep.

Children and Adolescents

A survey by the National Sleep Foundation found that 2 out of 3 young children experience sleep-related problems a few times a week. The problems included trouble falling asleep, frequent awakenings, nightmares, and heavy snoring (CDC, 2013a, 2013b). Environmental stimuli, such as the sounds and lights of other family members' activities, may make it difficult for a young child to sleep, or the child may have difficulty "winding down" after hectic activities in the late afternoon and early evening hours.

- *Toddlers and preschoolers* may be frightened to go to bed because of imaginary figures or intruders, or they may waken frequently at night because of bad dreams, the need to use the bathroom, illness, heavy snoring, tossing off the bedclothes, or falling out of bed. Some have difficulty self-calming enough to achieve a restful state before falling asleep.
- *School-age children* may suffer significant sleep disturbances because of anxiety or depression. Others might have more temporary sleep difficulty related to isolated situations, stress, excitement, or social concerns, such as anticipating a school event or sports competition.
- *In adolescence,* the growth spurt that occurs increases the need for sleep (Polan & Taylor, 2010), yet only 31% of high school students report getting at least 8 hours of

sleep on an average school night (CDC, 2010). At the same time, teenagers may not sleep well because of increased demands at school; staying up late to study, watch television, text or social network; dating or staying out late with friends; or using alcohol or drugs. Some teens consume large amounts of caffeinated colas and other beverages that can delay or disturb sleep.

Young Adults

College students may pull "all-nighters" to cram for exams or experience difficulty falling asleep or staying asleep because of worries about grades or future career choices. Young adults may drive themselves too hard to succeed, prompting late nights at work or sleep loss due to hectic travel schedules or work-related stress. Others might not obtain enough sleep because of social and personal entertainment choices during the night. Others might work evening or night shifts.

Sleep for parents of young children is often interrupted. Breastfeeding mothers typically need to feed their infants one or more times each night until the infant begins solid foods. Parents of toddlers often wake to care for a child who is having a nightmare, is ill, or needs to use the bathroom. The National Sleep Foundation (2008) survey found that some parents lose as many as 200 hours of sleep a year because of their children's poor sleeping patterns.

Middle-Aged and Older Adults

Middle-aged adults may experience sleep difficulties because of the depression, anxiety, and tension that result from the stress and competing demands on time, such as work or career, the need to care for a parent, marital discord, worry about teenaged children, or financial problems. The lack of sleep compounds the problem, leading to reduced ability to cope, and again to lack of sleep. Sleep interruptions are common due to access to technology, such as text messaging and social networking. As a physiological example, menopausal women may be awakened by hormonal fluctuations. Obstructive sleep apnea (OSA) also plays a role in insufficient sleep.

Older adults may suffer sleep disturbances because of nocturia, the side effects of medications, underlying illnesses, depression, discomfort, or pain. In addition, the levels of melatonin, the natural hormone that controls sleep, decline in the latter decades of life.

Lifestyle Factors

Lifestyle factors influencing sleep include work, exercise, nutrition, and use of medications and drugs. As noted earlier, a person who changes work shifts frequently may find it difficult to sleep at the right time or for long enough to feel rested and restored. Moreover, people who cross time zones frequently because of travel may experience difficulty falling asleep, early wakening, or daytime fatigue.

Physical Activity If it occurs at least 2 hours before bedtime, exercise promotes sleep. Fatigue from a normal physically active day is thought to promote a restful night's sleep. However, the more tired a person is, the shorter the first period of REM sleep will be. Additionally, sedentary lifestyle is a factor for sleep disorder.

Diet Foods can either promote or interfere with sleep. A meal high in saturated fat near bedtime may interfere with sleep. Dietary L-tryptophan and adenosine are essential amino acids (meaning the body does not produce its own), found in milk, cheese, and animal products, that may help to induce sleep by converting into serotonin.

Carbohydrates seem to promote relaxation through their effects on brain serotonin levels. In general, satiation induces sleep, whereas many people, especially infants and children, have difficulty falling asleep when they are hungry.

Nicotine and Caffeine Central nervous system stimulants, such as nicotine and caffeine, interfere with sleep. Smokers tend to have more difficulty falling asleep and are more easily roused than nonsmokers. People who stop smoking often experience temporary sleep disturbances during the withdrawal period. Caffeine blocks adenosine and thereby inhibits sleep. However, individuals vary greatly in their sensitivity to caffeine. Some people can consume coffee throughout the day and evening and suffer no loss of sleep, whereas others cannot consume even small amounts of caffeine early in the day without suffering sleep difficulty later.

Alcohol Consumption of alcohol, especially if heavy, may hasten the onset of sleep; however, it disrupts REM and slow wave sleep and may cause spontaneous awakenings with difficulty returning to sleep. In addition, in some people heavy alcohol consumption can prompt vivid dreams during REM sleep. Because alcohol is a diuretic, it can interrupt sleep by inducing nocturia.

Medications Many of the medications people take cause either sleeplessness or excessive grogginess and sedation. Medications to induce sleep (i.e., hypnotics) tend to increase the amount of sleep while decreasing the quality. Zolpidem tartrate (Ambien) promotes normal REM sleep and appears to influence sleep quality less than do other hypnotics. Amphetamines, tranquilizers, and antidepressants reduce the amount of REM sleep; barbiturates, in addition, interfere with NREM sleep. Opioids, such as morphine, suppress REM sleep and cause frequent awakening. Beta blockers are reported to cause sleep disorders and nightmares.

Illness

Illness increases the need for sleep and rest. At the same time, its associated mental and physical distress can cause sleep problems. Fear of the unknown outcome of an illness and role changes associated with hospitalization can cause anxiety. Disease symptoms, such as fever, pain, nausea, and respiratory conditions (e.g., shortness of breath,

dyspnea, sinus congestion), can also interfere with sleep. Specific disease conditions altering the quality of sleep include allergies, hyperthyroidism, and Parkinson's disease.

Anxiety increases gastric secretions, intestinal motility, heart rate, and respirations, all of which contribute to a restless night. Anxiety also stimulates the sympathetic nervous system, increasing the level of norepinephrine. This decreases stage III and REM sleep and leads to more awakenings. Depression may be associated either with too much sleep or with difficulty sleeping.

Environmental Factors

Environmental factors can promote or inhibit sleep. Some people need a cool room, whereas others need warmth. Some prefer heavy blankets, and others like to sleep with just a light sheet. Noise can also inhibit sleep, but a person can become habituated to noise over time and be less affected by it. Some people routinely fall asleep to music or while listening to a radio or television. Often loud noises are needed to awaken a person in NREM stages III and REM sleep.

Any change in the usual environmental stimuli can affect sleep. For example, a patient used to falling asleep next to his wife may have trouble sleeping alone in a hospital bed. Equipment noise, the muffled sounds of a busy medical-surgical unit, or the labored breathing or snoring of a roommate also can interfere with the patient's ability to sleep.

When people who are accustomed to sleeping in a dark room are hospitalized, they may have trouble falling asleep because of light outside their window or filtering into the room from the hallway. However, light can be therapeutic for some patients suffering from sleep problems. Exposure to bright light can alter circadian rhythms in some adults.

 Light therapy has not been shown to be effective in older adults with dementia living in skilled nursing facilities (Haesler, 2004).

KnowledgeCheck 34-3

- For each of the following patients, propose at least two factors that might affect sleep:
  A newborn in the neonatal intensive care unit
  A preschooler being treated for pneumonia
  An adolescent with cancer
  A breastfeeding mother of a newborn
  An older man who has fractured his hip
- Identify at least three types of environmental stimuli that can disturb sleep.

WHAT ARE SOME COMMON SLEEP DISORDERS?

Sleep disorders are classified by their signs and symptoms. The more common disorders fall into two groups:

- **Dyssomnias**—Sleep disorders characterized by insomnia or excessive sleepiness. They include insomnia, sleep–wake schedule (circadian) disorders, sleep apnea, restless leg syndrome, hypersomnia, and narcolepsy.

- **Parasomnias**—Patterns of waking behavior that appear during sleep (e.g., sleepwalking)

Insomnia

Insomnia as defined by the Diagnostic and Statistical Manual, 5th edition (DSM-5), is the predominant complaint of dissatisfaction with sleep quantity, associated with the inability to fall asleep, remain asleep, or go back to sleep. The sleep disturbance causes significant distress or impairments in social, occupational, academic, behavioral, and other important areas of functioning. True insomnia occurs at least 3 nights per week, and is present for 3 months or longer, even when there is ample opportunity for sleep (American Psychological Association, 2013).

Sleep difficulty may be *transient/short term* (less than a month) or *chronic* (longer than a month). People with sleep difficulty usually report an insufficient quantity and quality of sleep and wake without feeling refreshed, even though they are often observed to sleep more than they perceive that they do.

Insomnia is the most common sleep disorder. Two out of three people say they have trouble sleeping at least once a week (National Sleep Foundation, 2011), but 10 to 20% of the general population meet the DSM-5 diagnostic criteria for insomnia disorder (American Psychological Association, 2013). It is more prevalent in women and in adults older than 60 years; those who suffer from chronic illness (e.g., hypertension, obesity, cancer, thyroid disorders) (Institute of Medicine, 2006; Budhiraja, Roth, Hudgel, et al., 2011); and shift workers (Budhiraja, Roth, Hudgel, et al., 2011).

Daytime consequences of insomnia, which include symptoms of excessive daytime sleepiness, poor concentration, fatigue, lethargy, and irritability. Insomnia can also create an increased risk for depression, anxiety, and possibly cardiovascular disorders (Wilson, Nutt, Alford, et al., 2010). Or it may be the presenting symptom of other primary sleep disorders, such as restless leg syndrome.

Recent evidence suggests a link between abnormal hypothalamic–pituitary–adrenal gland activity and insomnia and mood disorders (Roth, Roehrs, & Pies, 2007). Insomnia may occur as a result of illness, depression, anxiety disorders, acute stress, substance abuse, side effects of medications (e.g., steroids, central adrenergic blockers, bronchodilating agents), or inadequate sleep hygiene (e.g., watching TV in bed, drinking caffeine-containing beverages before bedtime).

Primary care providers can diagnose and manage most cases of insomnia. Once underlying medical or psychiatric conditions have been identified and treated, a combination of behavioral and pharmacological therapy may be effective. The use of medication to induce sleep is controversial because some types can become habit forming, become less effective when taken continuously, and

can have serious side effects. However, sedative–hypnotic treatment is justified in short-term insomnia to avoid the negative effects of insomnia on mood and performance. Short-term aggressive treatment may prevent the development of chronic insomnia.

Sleep–Wake Schedule (Circadian) Disorders

Abnormalities in sleep–wake schedules may be caused by rapid time-zone changes (jet lag), shift work, or a change in total sleep time from day to day. Symptoms include decreased vigilance, decreased ability to perform psychomotor tasks, and short sleep episodes *(microsleeps)* that the person is not aware of. People suffering jet lag need several days to adjust their sleep–wake schedule.

Restless Leg Syndrome (RLS)

Restless leg syndrome (RLS) is a disorder of the central nervous system characterized by an uncontrollable movement of the legs while resting or before sleep onset. It tends to run in families. It affects 5% to 15% of Americans (U.S. Deptartment of Health and Human Services, et al., 2005, revised 2011). Children and young adults experience 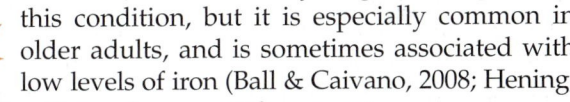 this condition, but it is especially common in older adults, and is sometimes associated with low levels of iron (Ball & Caivano, 2008; Hening, 2007) and use of some antidepressants.

It tends to be familial, more often occurring in women than in men. Symptoms include unpleasant creeping, crawling, itching, or tingling sensations in the legs. Symptoms are relieved only by moving the legs, which prevents the person from relaxing and falling asleep.

If RLS is severe, treatment may include **neuroleptic** agents and medication used to treat Parkinson's disease (Birath & Martin, 2009). People with RLS should avoid stimulants (e.g., caffeine). Other self-care measures include walking, massaging, stretching, heat or cold compresses, medication, vibration, and acupressure. Some people with severe symptoms might require anticonvulsant medication to control the creeping and crawling sensation in the legs (National Sleep Foundation, n.d.).

Sleep Deprivation

Sleep Deprivation is a NANDA-I nursing diagnosis. It is not actually a sleep disorder, but rather a result of prolonged sleep disturbances (e.g., insomnia and parasomnias), resulting from NREM or REM deprivation, or both. According to the CDC (2013b), nearly 30% of adults reported an average of less than 6 hours of sleep per day. Persons experiencing sleep deprivation are likely to feel drowsy during the day or a general feeling of malaise. They have difficulty performing daily tasks, impaired cognitive processing, problem-solving, and decision making; restlessness, perceptual disorders, slowed reaction time, irritability; and somatic (body) complaints (e.g., hand tremors).

Toward Evidence-Based Practice

Broussard, J. L., Ehrmann, D. A., Van Cauter, E., et al. (2012). **Impaired insulin signaling in human adipocytes after experimental sleep restriction: A randomized, crossover study.** *Annals of Internal Medicine, 157*(8), 549–557.

Sleep may be an important regulator of energy metabolism. The investigators found that in people who were sleep deprived, the body's fat cells' response to insulin reduced by 30%, thereby increasing the risk for insulin resistance, type 2 diabetes, and obesity.

Roehrs, T. A., Harris, E., Randall, S., et al. (2012). **Pain sensitivity and recovery from mild chronic sleep loss.** *Sleep, 35*(12), 1667–1673.

With a small sample of healthy adults, investigators found that increased sleep time lessens daytime sleepiness and reduces pain sensitivity.

Ong, J. C., Stepanski, E. J., & Gramling, S. E. (2009, February 15). **Pain coping strategies for tension-type headache: Possible implications for insomnia.** *Journal of Clinical Sleep Medicine, 5*(1), 52–56.

Study participants reported both stress and sleep problems as a trigger of headaches, and going to sleep as a strategy for dealing with pain. Study findings suggest that too much or too little sleep can lead to headaches; people with headaches often take naps to deal with headache pain. Chronic insomnia can occur from napping during the day.

Ruiter, M. (2012, June 11). **Top risk of stroke for normal-weight adults: Getting under 6 hours of sleep.** Presented at Sleep 2012, the annual meeting of the Associated Professional Sleep Societies. Abstract #0829.

The 3-year study of 5,666 adults ages 45 and older found that stroke risk was four times higher with less than 6 hours of sleep a night versus 7 to 8. Enrollees in the *Reasons for Geographic and Racial Differences in Stroke (REGARDS)* study were of normal weight and at low risk for sleep apnea. They had no history of stroke, no symptoms, and were not at high risk for sleep apnea. Chronic sleep deprivation (<6 hours of sleep per night) is thought to increase the risk of stroke as a result of changes in the autonomic functions of the body, including blood pressure, heart rate, inflammation, and glucose levels.

1. Sleep deprivation produces detrimental effects for many people, even those of normal weight and at low risk for sleep apnea. In what other ways do you think sleep deprivation creates problems for the body?

2. Considering the findings of the REGARDS study, what else would you want to know if your patient has been getting less than 6 hours of sleep per night?

3. On one hand, sleep can be a way for people with headaches to deal with the pain. On the other hand, too much sleep, such as daytime naps, can wreak havoc in getting a good, restful sleep at night. How would you use the Ong study to guide patients who are dealing with the pain of a migraine?

 Go to Chapter 34, **Toward Evidence-Based Practice Suggested Responses,** on Davis*Plus.*

Insomnia is a major contributor to injuries caused by motor vehicle accidents and other unintentional fatal injuries (American Academy of Sleep Medicine, 2014).

Functional imaging studies contrasting sleep-deprived and well-rested brains reveal the importance of adequate sleep for memory and learning (Chee & Chuah, 2008; Walker, 2009). If sleep deprivation is severe and prolonged, delusions, paranoia, and other psychotic behavior may occur. Studies of sleep-deprived adults revealed changes in the levels of certain immunoglobulins and other markers of the immune system (Hui, Hua, Diandong, et al., 2007; Ranjbaran, Keefer, & Stepanski, 2007), which means going without sleep can weaken the body's protection against infection.

Illness and hospital care are common causes of sleep deprivation, especially for patients in critical care units (CCUs). In this environment, lights are on most of the time, and equipment noise, frequent treatments, and assessments all combine with the client's fragile physical condition to create sleep deprivation. Likewise, health-care providers who work long and late hours or rotating day–night shifts experience serious fatigue that can lead to medical error, increased risk of occupational injury, and patient injury or death (The Joint Commission, 2011).

Hypersomnia

Hypersomnia is excessive sleeping, especially in the day-time. People with excessive daytime sleepiness doze, nap, or fall asleep at times and in situations when they need or wish to be awake and alert. The sleep disorders that commonly cause hypersomnia are obstructive sleep apnea and narcolepsy. Hypersomnia may also be caused by disorders of the central nervous system, kidney, or liver or by metabolic disorders (e.g., diabetic acidosis and hypothyroidism). It can also be a symptom of depression.

Sleep Apnea

Sleep apnea is a periodic interruption in breathing during sleep—an absence of air flow through the nose or mouth during sleep. Typically the soft tissue of the pharynx and soft palate collapse and obstruct the airway. Episodes may occur several or a hundred times a night and may last up to 1 minute or longer. During periods of apnea, the oxygen level in the blood drops, and the carbon dioxide level rises, causing the person to wake up. This may result in cardiac dysrhythmias (irregularities) and increases in pulse and blood pressure. Many people with sleep apnea complain of unrefreshed sleep, fatigue and morning headache, and easily falling asleep during sedentary activity; however, some may experience mild sleep apnea without any symptoms (Epstein, Kristo, Strollo, et al., 2009).

OSA is diagnosed clinically by reports of at least five witnessed breathing interruptions or awakenings due to gasping or choking events per hour (Epstein, Kristo, Strollo, et al., 2009). To definitively diagnose sleep apnea, a sleep study consisting of an EEG, monitoring of arterial oxygen saturation, and an electrocardiogram (ECG) is recommended. Treatment depends on the type of apnea involved. Untreated sleep apnea is associated with polycythemia, hypertension, angina, coronary artery disease, right-sided heart failure, stroke, impotence, depression, personality changes, and mood swings. The two main types of sleep apnea (obstructive and central) have different etiologies. **Mixed apnea** is a combination of the two main types.

Obstructive Sleep Apnea Obstructive sleep apnea (OSA) is caused by airway occlusion (usually by the tongue or palate) during sleep, but the person continues to try to breathe. Sleeping partners often report that the person snores, snorts, grunts, or thrashes about during sleep. Airway occlusion may also be due to a collapse of the hypopharynx or from other structural abnormalities (e.g., enlarged tonsils, adenoids, a deviated nasal septum, or thyroid enlargement). Although most often males over age 40, particularly if overweight, are affected by sleep apnea, the condition occurs in females of any age and weight. Treatment of OSA might involve surgery to remove any obstruction within the airway or applying CPAP (continuous positive airway pressure) treatment. This is a device that delivers oxygen using forced air pressure and keeps the airways open when apnea occurs. Patients with OSA should avoid alcohol and smoking and lose excess weight (Epstein, Kristo, Strollo, et al., 2009). ✚ Caution patients with sleep apnea about driving if drowsy. They are 5 to 7 times more likely to have a motor vehicle accident than those without apnea (Laugsand, Strand, Vatten, et al., 2014).

Central Sleep Apnea Central sleep apnea (CSA) is a complete suspension of breathing resulting from a dysfunction in central respiratory control. Only about 10% of sleep apnea is central in origin. People with CSA tend to awaken during sleep and, therefore, experience daytime sleepiness.

Snoring

Snoring is a hallmark sign of OSA, but it does not necessarily indicate OSA. Even so, snoring can significantly reduce the quality of sleep for the bed partner. Snoring results when the muscles at the back of the mouth relax during sleep, obstruct the airway, and vibrate with each breath. Obstruction is usually more pronounced when the person sleeps on his back. Many treatments have been invented to open the air passages, such as nose tapes or even surgery. Saline sprays, nose drops, and cortisone sprays are also used—all with mixed success.

Narcolepsy

Narcolepsy is a chronic disorder caused by the brain's inability to regulate sleep–wake cycles normally. The distinction between being asleep and being awake are blurred. At various times, the person with narcolepsy experiences a sudden, uncontrollable urge to sleep lasting from seconds to minutes, even though the person sleeps well at night. The person cannot avoid the sleep episodes but awakens easily.

Narcolepsy is characterized by sleepiness, slurred speech, slackening of the facial muscles, a feeling of impending weakness of the knees, paralysis, and hallucinations. Performance is impaired during these micro-sleep episodes. Sleep episodes can come on suddenly, even while the person is having a conversation. If they occur while the person is driving, working, or operating machinery, they can be dangerous. People with narcolepsy awaken from episodes of unavoidable sleep feeling refreshed (National Institute of Neurological Disorders and Stroke, 2009, updated 2011). Some have other symptoms, such as **cataplexy**, a sudden loss of muscle tone usually triggered by an emotional event (e.g., laughter, surprise, or anger), but most only have hypersomnia.

Narcolepsy affects up to 1 in every 2,000 Americans, males about as often as females (National Institute of Neurological Disorders and Stroke, 2009, updated 2011). It can develop at any age, but symptoms typically first appear during adolescence and early adulthood. Each micro-sleep episode begins in the REM stage instead of progressing through the NREM stages first. People with narcolepsy do not tolerate irregular sleep–wake patterns, such as shift work, and have difficulty staying awake with passive activity, such as watching television. The condition is controlled by central nervous system stimulants, such as methylphenidate (Ritalin), with little evidence of tolerance, dependence, or abuse.

Other individuals might suffer **pseudo-narcolepsy**, which is characterized by involuntary episodes of sleep but are related to acute or chronic sleep deprivation. When the person is well rested, the episodes resolve.

KnowledgeCheck 34-4

- What is the most common dyssomnia?
- What factors in the hospital may contribute to sleep deprivation in patients?
- What are the clinical signs of sleep deprivation?
- Why are sleeping pills not recommended for chronic insomnia?
- Why is snoring significant?

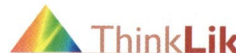

ThinkLike a Nurse 34-5

Compare and contrast insomnia and hypersomnia. How are they different? How are they alike?

Parasomnias

The parasomnias include sleepwalking, sleeptalking, bruxism, night terrors, REM sleep behavior disorders, and nocturnal enuresis.

Sleepwalking Sleepwalking (somnambulism) occurs during stage III of NREM sleep, usually 1 to 2 hours after the person falls asleep. The sleeper leaves the bed and walks about, with little awareness of surroundings. He may perform what appear to be conscious motor activities (e.g., brush his teeth, make coffee), but he does not wake up. The person is not aware of sleepwalking and has no memory of the event on awakening. The event may last 3 to 4 minutes or longer. Children sleepwalk more than adults do. If the child does not outgrow the condition or serious safety risks exist, medication may be given to suppress the deepest stage III sleep. Stress, fatigue, and some drugs can trigger sleepwalking.

Sleeptalking Sleeptalking occurs during NREM sleep, just before the REM stage. It does not usually interfere with the person's rest but may be disturbing to a bed partner.

Bruxism Bruxism grinding and clenching of the teeth, usually occurs during stage II NREM sleep. It can eventually erode tooth enamel and loosen the teeth. The noise can also disturb the bed partner's sleep.

Night Terrors Night terrors are sudden arousals in which the person (often a child) is physically active, often hallucinatory, and expresses a strong emotion such as terror. Children experiencing night terrors typically cry or scream in fear, thrash about, and resist all attempts by their parents or other caregivers to hold or console them. The child appears to be fully awake, but she is not; in fact, children in the midst of night terrors are extremely difficult to awaken. Episodes may last from 10 to 30 minutes. However, the child typically returns to sleep without awakening, and in the morning has no memory of the event. Unlike *nightmares* (unpleasant, frightening dreams), which occur during REM sleep, night terrors occur during stage III (deep NREM) sleep.

REM Sleep Behavior Disorders REM sleep behavior disorders are associated with REM (or dreaming period) sleep, in which the sleeper violently acts out the dream. People have actually injured themselves or others without waking.

Nocturnal Enuresis Nocturnal enuresis (bedwetting) is nighttime incontinence past the stage at which toilet training has been well established (Polan & Taylor, 2010). It has incorrectly been associated with dreaming; however, most incidents occur during NREM sleep, during the first third of the night when the child is difficult to arouse. It may be distressing to the child and family because of the importance society places on continence, the inconvenience of keeping bed linens clean, and the misconception that the child is bedwetting to act out against parents. Because the great majority of children outgrow enuresis, the best strategy is patience (McCance & Huether, 2009). If the problem persists, the child should have a full medical evaluation.

Secondary Sleep Disorders

Secondary sleep disorders occur when a disease causes alterations in sleep stages or in quantity and quality of sleep. The following are the most common causes:

- **Depression.** Depressed people may spend a great deal of time in bed. However, in general, they have difficulty falling asleep, experience less slow-wave (deep) sleep, spend less time in REM sleep, awaken early, and have less total sleep time.
- **Hyperthyroidism or hypothyroidism.** An increase in thyroid secretion causes an increase in stage III sleep; hypothyroidism causes a decrease in those stages. Hyperthyroidism increases metabolic rate, making it difficult for the person to fall asleep.
- **Pain.** Both acute and chronic pain interfere with sleep. Chronic pain affects both the quality and quantity of sleep. It inhibits sleep, increases arousals during sleep, and causes longer waking intervals during the night.
- **Airway passage obstruction or CNS dysfunction.** These conditions were discussed under Sleep Apnea.

Disorders That Are Provoked by Sleep

Sleep-provoked disorders are those that occur when signs and symptoms of the disease appear or become worse during sleep. Diseases affected by sleep include the following (McCance & Huether, 2009):

- **Coronary artery disease**. During REM sleep, dreams may increase heart rate and provoke angina and ECG changes.
- **Asthma**. People with asthma may experience bronchospasm during REM sleep. In adults, asthma attacks frequently occur during the night as the esophageal sphincter relaxes and reflux results. In children, they occur mostly during the final two-thirds of the night, when there is less stage III sleep.
- **Chronic obstructive pulmonary disease (COPD).** Persons with COPD experience lowered oxygen tension and increased carbon dioxide retention during sleep, especially during REM sleep, when neuromuscular control is normally depressed. This can result in pulmonary spasm and transient pulmonary hypertension.
- **Diabetes.** Blood glucose levels vary during sleep. When diabetes is uncontrolled, it may profoundly affect the blood sugar level during sleep, when the person is not alert enough to deal with it. Therefore, patients with uncontrolled diabetes may need to have blood glucose levels monitored during sleep.

- **Gastric and intestinal ulcers.** During REM sleep, people with duodenal ulcers secrete up to 20 times more gastric acid than do people who do not have duodenal ulcers. Peptic ulcers also contribute to increased acid, often producing nocturnal epigastric pain and sleep loss.
- **Epilepsy.** Seizures are sensitive to sleep patterns. Sleep deprivation can trigger seizures, increase their intensity, or cause seizures to last longer. Some forms of epilepsy are especially reactive to sleep cyles or transitions between sleep states (Schachter, Shafer, & Sirven, 2013).

KnowledgeCheck 34-5

- List and define at least three parasomnias.
- Describe ways in which depression can affect sleep.
- List two sleep-provoked disorders, and explain how the sleep stage affects the disease.

PracticalKnowledge
knowing **how**

Because sleep enhances wellness and speeds recovery from illness, promoting sleep is an important independent nursing intervention. In this section, you will learn how to assess for signs of sleep disturbance, as well as specific interventions to facilitate sleep for each client.

ASSESSMENT

It is important to assess usual sleep patterns and rituals for all patients who are being admitted to the hospital or seeking help for a sleep problem. A brief assessment for all patients should include questions about the following:

- Usual sleeping pattern
- Sleeping environment
- Bedtime routines/rituals
- Sleep aids
- Sleep changes or problems

Key Point: *The nurse would conduct a more in-depth sleep assessment for patients who wake up at least three times a night; those who take more than 30 minutes to fall asleep; and if the difficulty falling or staying asleep has been going on for more than 30 days.*

For a list of additional questions you can use to obtain this information,

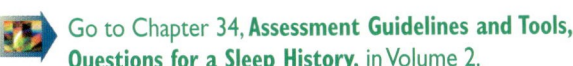 Go to Chapter 34, **Assessment Guidelines and Tools, Questions for a Sleep History,** in Volume 2.

If the person reports experiencing satisfactory sleep, that is an adequate assessment, and you merely need to support her usual sleep patterns and rituals. When you suspect a sleep problem, you will perform a more in-depth assessment, such as a detailed sleep history or sleep diary.

A **sleep history** (self-report) includes in-depth questions about the person's usual times for sleep, any

preparation, preferences and routines, quality of sleep, napping habits (if any), and whether she wakes early and cannot return to sleep.

A **sleep diary** provides very specific information on your patient's patterns of sleep. This allows you to identify trends in sleep/wakefulness and associate behaviors interfering with sleep. You will usually tell the patient to keep the diary for 14 days; remind him that it is important to be diligent in maintaining it.

For examples of a sleep history and a sleep diary,

 Go to Chapter 34, **Assessment Guidelines and Tools, Questions for a Sleep History** and **Sleep Diary,** in Volume 2.

To find the National Sleep Foundation Sleepiness Diary online,

 Go to Chapter 34, **Resources for Caregivers and Healthcare Professionals,** on DavisPlus.

An **actigraph** is a device worn on the wrist or may be an application on a mobile device that estimates a person's sleep and wake patterns, including time spent in various sleep stages. A **sleep study** is most useful in detecting sleep apnea and other sleep disorders, such as narcolepsy, night terrors, and periodic limb movement disorder. One of the most common sleep studies performed in a sleep lab is **polysomnography,** which records brain wave activity, eye movement, oxygen and carbon dioxide levels, vital signs, and body movements during the sleep phases.

ANALYSIS/NURSING DIAGNOSIS

It is important to determine whether lack of sleep is a problem, is a symptom of a problem, or is contributing to (etiology of) a different problem. For health promotion applications, use the NANDA-I diagnosis Readiness for Enhanced Sleep when a client has no particular sleep problem but wishes to move to a higher level of functioning in the area of sleep.

Sleep as the Problem

When you wish to focus on interventions to promote sleep, use the following NANDA-I labels on the problem side of the nursing diagnosis.

Use *Insomnia* for patients who have a disruption in the amount of quality of sleep to the extent that it impairs functioning.

Use *Sleep Deprivation* as the nursing diagnosis when the patient's amount, consistency, or quality of sleep is decreased over prolonged periods of time. Defining characteristics of Sleep Deprivation are more severe than those for Disturbed Sleep Pattern, so nursing activities may focus as much on relieving symptoms (e.g., confusion, paranoia) as on sleep promotion.

Use *Disturbed Sleep Pattern* as the diagnosis when assessment data points to a time-limited sleep problem due to external factors (e.g., inability to sleep in the unfamiliar hospital environment). The problem should be one that can be treated by nursing therapy. Add modifying words to specify the type of sleep problem, as in the examples. This will help you to focus goals appropriately.

- Disturbed Sleep Pattern (difficulty falling asleep) related to worries about family
- Disturbed Sleep Pattern (difficulty falling and remaining asleep) related to noise of hospital environment and need for scheduled treatments
- Disturbed Sleep Pattern (premature awakening) related to sleeping aid dependence and lack of knowledge of nonpharmacological aids for insomnia
- Disturbed Sleep Pattern (excessive daytime sleeping) related to effects of biological aging and depression
- Disturbed Sleep Pattern (altered sleep–wake patterns) related to frequent rotations of shift and overtime

Carefully describe the etiologies for sleep problems, because they determine your interventions.

 ## ThinkLike a Nurse 34-6

In the following nursing diagnoses, how do you think your interventions would be different for each diagnosis? Disturbed Sleep Pattern related to:

- Changes in bedtime routines
- Exercising within 2 hours before sleep
- Drinking caffeinated beverages, eating chocolate, and drinking alcohol
- Emotional or physical pain
- Drug dependence or withdrawal
- Physical illness

Sleep Pattern as an Etiology

Disturbed Sleep Pattern and Sleep Deprivation affect many areas of functioning, so they often are the etiology of other nursing diagnoses, as in these examples:

- Risk for Injury or Falls related to sleepwalking (or REM sleep behavior disorder or narcolepsy)
- Fatigue (or Activity Intolerance) related to chronic insufficient quality or quantity of sleep (e.g., secondary to insomnia)
- Ineffective Coping related to decreased cognitive functioning and awareness, secondary to lack of sleep
- Disturbed Thought Processes related to decreased cognitive functioning, secondary to lack of sleep
- Anxiety (or Fear) related to fear of death from sleep apnea

Sleep Pattern as a Symptom

Difficulty sleeping may be one of the symptoms of another problem. For example, a client may have Spiritual Distress related to challenges to belief system *as manifested by nightmares, sleep disturbances, and verbalization of inner conflict about beliefs.* In this instance, you would focus on interventions for Spiritual Distress, assuming that the sleep pattern would improve as the Spiritual Distress is resolved. Other nursing diagnoses that may cause sleep loss include Anxiety, Chronic Sorrow, Death Anxiety, Decisional Conflict, Complicated Grieving, Diarrhea, Impaired Gas Exchange, Nausea, Pain, and Relocation Stress Syndrome.

KnowledgeCheck 34-6

- For a chronic, long-term sleep problem, would you use a diagnosis of Sleep Pattern Disturbance, Sleep Deprivation, or Readiness for Enhanced Sleep?
- Name at least two nursing diagnoses that might have a sleep problem as the etiology.
- Name at least one nursing diagnosis that might have a sleep problem as the defining characteristic.

■ PLANNING OUTCOMES/EVALUATION

NOC standardized outcomes linked to the NANDA-I sleep labels are as follows:

- For Disturbed Sleep Pattern: Rest, Sleep, and Personal Well-Being
- For Sleep Deprivation: Rest, Sleep, and Symptom Severity
- For Insomnia: Concentration, Endurance, Fatigue Level, Mood Equilibrium, Personal Health Status, Personal Well-Being, Quality of Life, Rest, and Sleep

When sleep disturbances are the etiology of another nursing diagnosis, you will need to use the NOC outcomes associated with that diagnosis. For example:

Nursing diagnosis: Anxiety related to Sleep Deprivation
NOC outcomes for Anxiety: Anxiety Control, Coping

Individualized goals/outcome statements you might use to evaluate the success of interventions to promote sleep include the following:

- Verbalizes feeling rested or feeling less fatigue.
- Falls asleep within 30 minutes; sleeps 6 hours without awakening.
- Maintains a sleep–wake pattern that provides sufficient energy for the day's tasks.
- Demonstrates self-care behaviors that provide a healthy balance between rest and activity.
- Identifies stress-relieving rituals that enable falling asleep more easily.
- Demonstrates decreased signs of sleep deprivation.
- Verbalizes feeling less fatigued and more in control of life activities.

■ PLANNING INTERVENTIONS/IMPLEMENTATION

NIC standardized interventions for Sleep Deprivation and Sleep Pattern Disturbance include the following: Coping Enhancement, Energy Management, Environmental Management: Comfort, Relaxation Therapy, and Sleep Enhancement. Linkages have not yet been established for Insomnia.

Specific nursing activities for clients with sleep problems are described in the next sections.

For a care plan and care map for Sleep Pattern Disturbance,

 Go to Chapter 34, **Care Plan** and **Care Map,** on or *DavisPlus.*

Schedule Nursing Care to Avoid Interrupting Sleep

Use nursing judgment to decide when a procedure must be done and when it is more important for your patient to sleep. Healthcare routines usually allow time for rest periods. In addition, you may consider the following:

- Some patients need to rest after a procedure or after meals.
- If the person looks sleepy, give a prescribed sleeping pill early to avoid waking him later in the evening.
- You can often alter routines; for example, you can allow the patient to sleep as long as he can in the morning and bring his breakfast later. Or if the care provider has prescribed a sleeping pill, give it early in the evening if he seems sleepy.
- Cluster care to avoid unnecessary interruptions in sleep. Unless the patient is critically ill, do not wake him for morning vital signs if he is sleeping.
- Keep the noise level to a minimum. Be aware that activities, conversation, and equipment, even outside the patient's room, can disrupt sleep (Meltzer, Davis, & Mindell, 2012).

For examples of NOC outcomes and NIC interventions for sleep diagnoses,

 Go to Chapter 34, **Standardized Language: Selected NOC Outcomes and NIC Interventions for Sleep Diagnosis,** on *DavisPlus.*

Create a Restful Environment

Many people find it difficult to sleep in a strange bed, even a comfortable one. Hospital beds are not noted for their luxury, but you can help make them more comfortable.

- Be sure the bed linens are tight on the bottom and loose on top to allow movement.
- Keep linens clean, dry, and free of irritants. Perspiration on the hospital gown or linens can lead to chill.
- Good body alignment also facilitates relaxation. Use extra pillows, a blanket from home, or any other item that may help the patient rest.
- Keep the room dark and quiet, unless the patient prefers a light.
- As much as possible, control the temperature of the room and provide good ventilation.

 For steps to follow in *all* procedures, refer to the Universal Steps for All Procedures found on the inside back cover of Volume 2. Go to the full procedures in Volume 2 to practice and learn the procedure steps. Use these procedure highlights later to help you review key points.

Highlights of Procedure 34-1

Procedure 34-1: Giving a Back Massage

➤ Warm the lotion.

➤ Raise the bed to working height.

➤ Position the patient comfortably on her side or prone.

➤ Place lotion on your hands.

➤ Rub down the length and then up the sides of the back.

➤ Never rub directly over the spine.

➤ Apply gentle thumb pressure on either side of the spine at the midback, pushing outward for about 2.5 cm (1 in.) along the trapezius muscle.

➤ Always apply pressure away from the spine, not toward it.

➤ Go to the spots that felt the tightest or that the patient states are tight. Work in small circles, using gentle thumb pressure.

➤ Gently shake the scapula.

➤ Apply horizontal strokes across the scapula, using your thumb.

➤ Apply pressure in circles using the heels of your hands down both sides of the spine.

➤ Apply horizontal strokes using the heels of your hands across the latissimus dorsi muscle.

➤ Gently rub your hands up either side of the spine from the base of the back to the base of the neck, and then down the sides of the back.

Promote Comfort

Pain, itching, and nausea may all be deterrents to rest and sleep in an ill person. Be sure to offer pain medications at their scheduled times, and before the patient's sleep time. Other comfort measures include providing a restful environment (see the preceding intervention) and offering fluids, cool cloths, or a massage or back rub. For detailed instructions for back massage,

 Go to Chapter 34, **Procedure 34-1: Giving a Back Massage,** in Volume 2.

Also see the accompanying Highlights of Procedure 34-1 box.

Support Bedtime Rituals and Routines

Most people have some kind of a routine before bed, be it reading, watching TV, drinking warm milk, or praying or meditating, to allow them to prepare for sleep. For children, a favorite doll, blanket, bedtime story, as well as brushing their teeth and hair, may enhance sleepiness. Be sure to include any routines or rituals in the nursing plan of care to ensure continuity. Advise patients who smoke not to smoke after the evening meal.

Offer Appropriate Bedtime Snacks or Beverages

Complex carbohydrates (e.g., bread, cereal) seem to help most people sleep. A small amount of protein (e.g., milk, cheese) with the snack reduces the sugar boost and keeps blood glucose more stable. The dietary amino acid L-tryptophan promotes sleep. Advise the client to avoid alcohol, especially in the evening. Although it may induce sleepiness at first, alcohol interferes with the deep sleep cycle. The client should also avoid taking caffeine-containing foods and beverages (e.g., tea, coffee, energy drinks, chocolate, colas) after the evening meal. Advise the client to drink plenty of fluids during the day but to restrict fluids close to bedtime. Nicotine is a stimulant and should be avoided.

Promote Relaxation

You will base your choice of relaxation strategies on your repertoire of techniques and on patient preference. Relaxation strategies may include a massage, a warm bath, or one of the following:

- *Guided imagery* can be used to help your patient move in his mind to a safe place, where relaxation is possible. You may ask the patient what type of place will soothe him and "guide" him there through visualization. See Chapter 12 if you need to review.
- *Progressive muscle relaxation,* relaxing each muscle independently and progressing from head to toe, may help to promote sleep.
- *Music therapy* has been shown to be effective in promoting relaxation. Some patients respond well and can put away their troubles while listening to music, whereas others may find music irritating. Slow, quiet music or a recording of forest or ocean sounds may be soothing.

You may wish to refer to Chapter 46 for more details about relaxation strategies.

Maintain Patient Safety

A person who sleepwalks needs protection from injury because the risk of falling is great (e.g., stairs). Intravenous infusions, catheters, and nasogastric tubes can produce injury if they are pulled out of the body when the person gets out of bed. Guide sleepwalkers back to bed, and remember that they startle easily, so be gentle and quiet.

Safe Sleep for Infants

✚ Infant suffocation is a common cause of death in infants, and is often associated by infant position and the sleep environment, such as use of blankets, pillows, and infant positioners. The safest position for infants under 3 months of age is supine position (not on the side) on a firm sleep surface, and sharing a room but not a bed. Commercial positioning devices are not recommended to keep infants on their backs unless prescribed (American Academy of Pediatrics Task Force on Sudden Infant Death Syndrome & Moon, 2011; CDC, 2012).

Teach About Sleep Hygiene

Most people with sleep problems manage them at home by creating a restful environment, relaxing, avoiding distractions, and trying various sleep strategies without using sleep-inducing medication. Refer to the Self-Care box (Teaching Your Client About Sleep Hygiene) when teaching clients self-care for sleep.

Administer and Teach About Sleep Medications

When considering sleep medications, it is important for the patient to understand the options, be aware of potential side effects, and know what questions to ask. Some medications are habit forming; others may have unpleasant side effects. When patients first start taking prescription sleep aids, they should use caution during morning activities until they are sure how the drug affects them. Long-term effects of these medications are not known. As a general rule, they are not recommended for long-term use. Some natural or homeopathic aids can lead to rest and sleep.

Prescription Sleep Medications

You should be familiar with the various prescription and nonprescription sleep medications your patients may be taking.

Nonbenzodiazepines   These sedative/hypnotics have a short half-life, which means that they are eliminated from the body quickly and do not cause daytime sleepiness. They are also selective, meaning that they target specific receptors that are thought to be associated with sleep rather than depressing the entire central nervous system. Examples are zolpidem tartrate (e.g., Ambien) and zaleplon (e.g., Sonata). The newest type of sedative/hypnotic, although not technically a nonbenzodiazepine, is ramelteon (e.g., Rozerem). It is the first sleep drug not designated as a controlled substance. It works by targeting melatonin receptors.

General side effects of nonbenzodiazepines include drowsiness, dizziness, fatigue, headache, and unpleasant taste. Long-term effects of these medications are not yet known, although an increased risk of fatal overdose has been reported.

Benzodiazepines   This class of sedative/hypnotics is the first-line treatment for insomnia, and includes both long-acting and short-acting drugs. Long-acting medications linger in the body and potentially cause daytime drowsiness. Many benzodiazepines were originally

Teaching Your Client About Sleep Hygiene

Self-Care

➤ Follow a regular routine for bedtime and morning awakenings.

➤ Go to bed each night at the same time, even on days you are off work.

➤ If you cannot fall asleep in 30 minutes, get up and do something nonstimulating, but avoid using the computer. The wavelengths of blue light emitted from the screen arouse the brain into a wakeful state. When you feel sleepy, go back to bed.

➤ Use relaxation methods to promote sleep; read a book, pray, or meditate.

➤ Avoid going to bed angry; and stay clear of emotional discussions before going to sleep.

➤ Don't depend on sleeping aids; be aware of the potential dangers of sleeping medications.

➤ Use your bedroom only for sleep; do not turn your bedroom into the family room.

➤ Avoid caffeine, alcohol, tobacco products, and heavy meals before going to sleep. Remember that some beverages and foods, such as black tea, chocolate, and cola, contain caffeine. Alcohol interferes with the transition to deeper phases of sleep. Heavy alcohol consumption can contribute to breathing impairment during the night.

➤ Avoid eating carbohydrates (e.g., crackers, cereal, or bread) before bed; they boost blood glucose levels, so a few hours later, the rapid drop in sugar will wake you.

➤ Use aromatherapy to relax.

➤ If you take prescription drugs, ask your prescriber or pharmacist about the side effects.

➤ Use earplugs to block out noise.

➤ Walk or exercise in the early evening at least 1 hour before going to sleep; doing so will raise your body temperature and tire your muscles. Even 15 minutes a day of exercise will give your body the activity and oxygen it needs to help you relax more and sleep better.

➤ Take a warm bath just before going to sleep. This will raise your body temperature and relax you to help you fall asleep more easily.

 ➤ Avoid naps during the day, unless you are an older adult who takes short "power naps." Daytime napping can lead to nighttime insomnia.

➤ Don't try to "catch up" on sleep. Rise at your regular time, even if you went to bed later than usual.

➤ Try to keep your bedroom as dark as possible. Even an illuminated bedroom clock is a source of light that can be distracting when trying to fall asleep. Either replace the clock or block the light with something.

➤ Close your eyes and visualize something peaceful when trying to fall asleep. Imaging your favorite, relaxing place where you find comfort or familiarity can relax you and help you get to sleep.

➤ Try progressive relaxation to fall asleep. Follow recorded instructions directing you in a sequence of relaxing certain muscle groups.

---

formulated to treat anxiety. Examples are diazepam (e.g., Valium), alprazolam (e.g., Xanax), flurazepam (e.g., Dalmane), lorazepam (e.g., Ativan), and triazolam (e.g., Halcion). The risk for rebound insomnia and dependency and tolerance, especially in older adults, is greater with this class of sleep-inducing drugs. They are potentially dangerous when combined with alcohol and some medications.

Barbiturates These sedative/hypnotics and anticonvulsants are rarely prescribed for insomnia because of the risk of addiction, abuse, and overdose. Examples are amobarbital (e.g., Amytal), pentobarbital (e.g., Nembutal), and secobarbital (e.g., Seconal).

Tricyclic Antidepressants At times, primary care providers prescribe antidepressants to promote sleep. Although none of these medicines is specifically FDA approved for this purpose they have shown clinical benefit for some people with insomnia who also suffer with depression. Examples are amitriptyline (e.g., Elavil), doxepin (e.g., Sinequan), imipramine (e.g., Tofranil), and nortriptyline (e.g., Aventyl, Pamelor). Older adults are particularly at risk for daytime sleepiness and dizziness.

Nonprescription Sleep Medications

Nonprescription sleep medications usually contain an antihistamine, which may induce drowsiness that lasts into the next day. It is important to check the ingredient label of any over-the-counter (OTC) medication to see whether it contains an antihistamine. Advise clients that OTC sleep medications can interact with other medicines they may be taking, so they should consult their prescriber or pharmacist before using them. An example is diphenhydramine hydrochloride (Benadryl). Other nonprescription sleep aids include the following:

■ *Melatonin*. Melatonin is a natural hormone produced by the pineal gland to modulate sleep. Commercial products containing melatonin are widely sold as sleep aids; however, the effectiveness remains controversial. Although approved by the Food and Drug Administration (FDA) and generally safe for short-term use, melatonin is unregulated and varies in strength and purity across manufacturers and may pose a risk for people taking blood thinners, such as warfarin. There also is increased risk of seizure in children with brain disorders.

■ *Herbal sleep aids*. Herbal remedies for sleep problems include chamomile tea, valerian root, hops, lavender, and passionflower. These herbal remedies have not undergone extensive testing for benefits and safety and have not been proved to be effective sleep aids.

KnowledgeCheck 34-7

- What is the classification of zolpidem (Ambien)? Why is it an especially desirable medication for sleep?
- What are two other classes of medications that are sometimes prescribed for sleep?
- Describe three independent nursing interventions to promote sleep.
- Why should people contact their prescriber before taking nonprescription sleep aids?

PUTTING IT ALL TOGETHER

Anne (Meet Your Patient) has arrived back on the surgical unit after her surgery. She has a urinary catheter, oxygen mask, IV line, and morphine by patient controlled analgesia (PCA) for pain control. She is nauseated from the anesthesia and moaning in pain. Her husband, Eric, and their three children are there to greet her, and they are worried. Anne looks dreadful! "With all this equipment, and her moaning, is she going to be okay?" Eric asks. He tells you that Anne didn't sleep at all the night before surgery. "She was nervous and didn't want to take a sleeping pill because we were supposed to be at the hospital by 5:30 a.m.," he explains.

You perform an initial assessment. Anne's vital signs are as follows: BP, 118/74 mm Hg; pulse, 88 beats/min and regular; respirations, 26 breaths/min; and T, 99.48°F. Her lungs are clear, the dressing is dry and intact, and the urinary catheter shows a small amount of light yellow urine draining from the bladder. The oxygen mask is partially off. You check Anne's oxygen saturation. It is 99%. The notes from the operating and recovery rooms indicate that Anne has not received anything for pain in more than 90 minutes. The PCA is connected, but the pump supplies analgesia only when the patient triggers the device. Anne has been groggy and does not understand or remember that she must push the button to obtain pain medication. You trigger a bolus of morphine and show Anne and the family how the PCA works. You realize that she is sedated and may not remember what you have taught her, but Eric assures you that they will be staying for the day and will reinforce your instruction.

Several minutes later Anne is calm. Her respirations have slowed to 20 breaths/min, and she is lightly snoring. Eric sighs in relief. "I guess she'll sleep for a while now," he says. You explain that she will sleep with the pain medication, but it will not be as restful as good-quality sleep.

"With the morphine she will wake frequently and not get much REM sleep—that's a type of sleep we all require for health," you explain.

You were able to gather data preoperatively from Anne about her sleep habits and routines. You are also aware that Anne has had chronic sleep problems. In the nursing care plan, you have written the diagnosis Disturbed Sleep Pattern related to pain (secondary to fibromyalgia), dependence on Ambien, anxiety, grief, stresses of surgery, and unfamiliar environment. You tell Eric that you would like him to bring from home Anne's pillow, toothbrush, and face cream because she has indicated that these are all part of her usual bedtime ritual. When Eric volunteers that Anne sometimes listens to music before bedtime, you suggest that he also bring her favorite music.

At dinnertime, Eric and the kids go home and gather Anne's belongings. When they return, she is more alert and comfortable. She tells them she feels exhausted, but not in pain. When you make your rounds, you explain that you would like to keep her usual bedtime routine and that she will be getting Ambien this evening. She is visibly relieved by your comments.

This scenario demonstrates full-spectrum nursing and shows how a nurse can make a difference for patients and their families by recognizing the need for sleep and providing appropriate interventions.

To explore learning resources for this chapter,

Go to Davis*Plus* at **DavisPl.us/Wilkinson3.**

Chapter Resources for Chapter 34:
    Response sheets for all learning activities
    Resources for Caregivers and Health Professionals
    Reading More About Sleep & Rest (suggested readings)
    Concept Map of chapter content
Interactive Case Studies
NCLEX-Style and Chapter Review Questions
Chapter Overview Podcasts

For references cited in this chapter,

Go to Volume 2, **References Cited.**

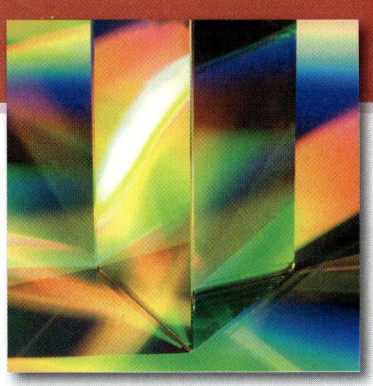

CHAPTER 35

Skin Integrity & Wound Healing

Learning Outcomes

After completing this chapter, you should be able to:

➤ Discuss the factors that affect skin integrity.

➤ Identify wounds based on accepted classification schemes.

➤ Describe the three phases of wound healing.

➤ Distinguish primary intention healing, secondary intention healing, and tertiary intention healing.

➤ Describe three types of wound drainage.

➤ Review the major complications of wound healing.

➤ Explain the factors involved in the development of pressure ulcers.

➤ Use the Braden scale to assess risk for pressure ulcers.

➤ Assess and categorize pressure ulcers based on the pressure ulcer staging system.

➤ Provide nursing care that limits the risk of pressure ulcer development.

➤ Differentiate the kinds of chronic wounds.

➤ Accurately chart assessment of a wound.

➤ Demonstrate appropriate techniques for irrigating a wound.

➤ Describe care of a wound with a drain.

➤ Differentiate the five forms of wound debridement.

➤ Discuss the different kinds of tissue found in wounds.

➤ Discuss when and how to use absorbent, alginate, collagen, gauze dressings, transparent films, hydrocolloids, hydrogels, and foam and antimicrobial dressings.

➤ Describe guidelines to follow when applying heat or cold therapy.

➤ Demonstrate bandage and binder application.

Key Concepts

Skin integrity
Wound
Wound healing

Related Concepts
See the Concept Map on Davis*Plus*.

Example Problem
Pressure ulcers

Meet Your Patient

William Harmon is a 78-year-old man who fell 3 days ago. His fall resulted in a fractured left hip. He was admitted to the hospital and underwent an open reduction and internal fixation (ORIF) of the left hip. Today is his second postoperative day. He is still bed bound and is unable to roll or pull himself up in bed.

Mr. Harmon's weight on admission was 140 lb (63.64 kg). His height is 73 in. His family reports that he has been steadily losing weight. He expresses little interest in eating and says he has been depressed since his wife died last year.

While performing your assessment of Mr. Harmon, you notice that a large dressing covers the left hip incision. You loosen the dressing and see the staples are intact at the incision site and there is a minimal amount of serosanguineous

drainage on the bandage. As you turn him in bed, you see a 10 cm by 6 cm reddened area on his coccyx and a 2 cm by 3 cm purple bruise-like area on his left heel. Mr. Harmon now has three wounds, an intentional surgical wound and two pressure ulcers

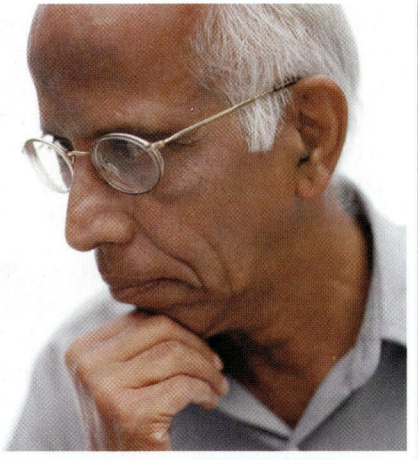

that have resulted from his impaired mobility. How will you care for each of these wounds? What factors contributed to each of the wounds, and how will you promote healing?

Theoretical Knowledge
knowing why

The integumentary system consists of the skin, hair, nails, sweat glands, and the subcutaneous tissue below the skin. The skin is the largest organ of the body. The major functions of the skin include protection of the internal organs, unique identification of an individual, thermoregulation, metabolism of nutrients and metabolic waste products, and sensation.

ABOUT THE KEY CONCEPTS

For optimal function, **skin integrity** must be preserved—that is, all layers of the skin must be intact. A **wound** is a disruption in the normal skin integrity. It is easy to see how the concepts of skin integrity and wound are related; they are opposites. You will use your knowledge of both these concepts as you protect your patients' skin and promote the physiological process of **wound healing**.

WHAT FACTORS AFFECT SKIN INTEGRITY?

To understand skin integrity, you need to understand the structure of the skin (Fig. 35-1).

Epidermis The **epidermis** is the outer portion of the skin. The epidermis is made up of four or five layers, of which the most important are the inner and outer layers.

- The **stratum corneum**, the outermost layer, is composed of numerous thicknesses of dead cells. Functioning as a barrier, it restricts water loss and prevents fluids, pathogens, and chemicals from entering the body.
- The **stratum germinativum**, the innermost layer of the epidermis, continually produces new cells, pushing the older cells toward the skin surface. In the dermal layer, the **keratinocytes** are protein-containing cells that give the skin strength and elasticity. Deeper in the epidermis are **melanocytes**, which produce melanin, a pigment that gives skin its color and provides protection from ultraviolet light. **Langerhans cells** are mobile. Their function is to phagocytize (engulf) foreign material and trigger an immune response.

Dermis The **dermis** lies below the epidermis and above the subcutaneous tissue. It is made of irregular fibrous connective tissue that provides strength and elasticity to the skin and is generously supplied with blood vessels. Within the dermis are sweat glands, sebaceous (oil) glands, ceruminous (wax) glands, hair and nail follicles, sensory receptors, elastin, and collagen.

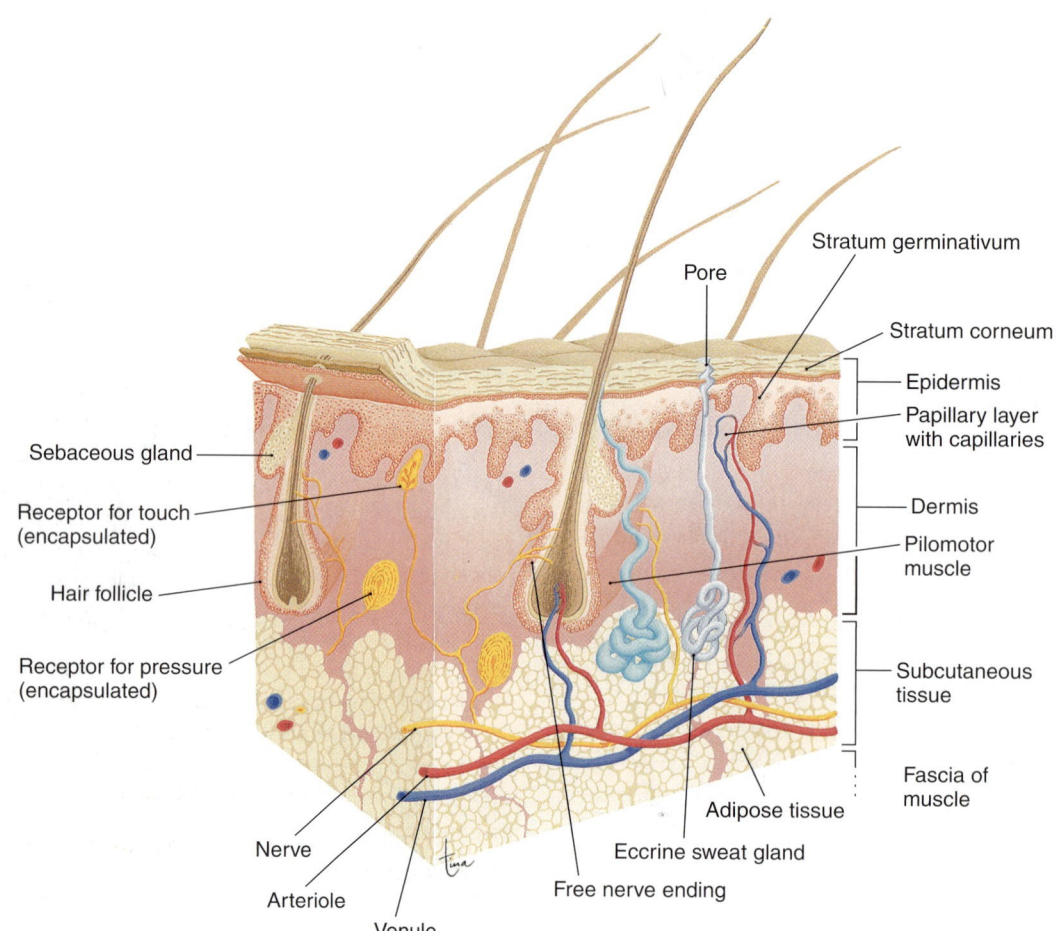

FIGURE 35-1 The structure of the skin.

Subcutaneous Tissue The subcutaneous layer is composed primarily of connective and adipose tissue. It provides insulation, protection, and a reserve of calories in the event of severe malnutrition. This layer varies in thickness in different body sites. Sex hormones, genetics, age, and nutrition also influence the distribution of subcutaneous tissue.

For optimal function, all layers of the skin must be intact. Breaks in the skin (e.g., surgical incisions, injuries) increase the risk of infection. In the following sections you will learn about factors that influence the ability to maintain intact skin and heal wounds (e.g., age).

Age-Related Variations

Age affects the condition and structure of the skin. Infants, for example, are born with varying amounts of *vernix caseosa*, a creamy substance that protects their skin. Their skin is thinner and more permeable than that of adults, which predisposes infants to skin breakdown (e.g., diaper rash). The subcutaneous layer (brown fat) and sweat glands are not fully developed, especially for preterm infants. As a result, in the first few weeks of life thermoregulation is inadequate, and the infant must be swaddled to maintain body heat.

The skin of infants and young children feels smooth, but as they are exposed to sun and other environmental elements, skin texture becomes coarser. Sex hormones released during puberty increase sebaceous and sweat gland activity, which leads to perspiration odor and sometimes acne. In women, high estrogen levels may contribute to the softening of connective tissue and cause striae and darkening of the skin, particularly on the face, areolae, nipples, vulva, and umbilicus, particularly in people with dark skin.

As adults age, the activity of the sebaceous and sweat glands diminishes, resulting in drier skin. **Xerosis** (itchy, red, dry, scaly, cracked, or fissured skin) is a problem for up to 85% of older adults and can be a threat to the integrity of their skin. Along with loss of lean body mass, the subcutaneous tissue layer thins, giving the individual a sharp, angular appearance. Excess weight can offset this change of appearance, though. The strong bond between the epidermal and dermal layer decreases as the dermal layer loses elasticity as a result of changes in its collagen fibers. These changes make the skin prone to breakdown and prolong wound-healing time. Regeneration of healthy skin takes at least twice as long in an 80-year-old as in a 30-year-old. In addition, many older adults have chronic diseases that interfere with healing. Diabetes, for instance, predisposes to infection, and liver dysfunction interferes with synthesis of blood-clotting factors.

Impaired Mobility

A healthy person moves and shifts position unconsciously when he senses pressure or discomfort. However, for people who are unable to move independently, the weight of the body on the bed or chair causes an increase in pressure leading to skin breakdown. Impaired mobility is caused by conditions that require complete bedrest or that seriously limit activity (e.g., paralysis, extreme fatigue, high-risk pregnancy, sedation, casts, traction, and altered sensory perception).

KnowledgeCheck 35-1

- Identify the major functions of the skin.
- What is the function of the stratum corneum, the outermost layer of the skin?
- What is the function of the subcutaneous layer?
- What effect does aging have on skin?
- What effect does immobility have on skin?

Nutrition and Hydration

Skin condition reflects overall nutritional status, and at the same time nutritional intake affects the skin. Adequate intake of protein, cholesterol, calories, fluid, vitamin C, and minerals is essential to maintaining skin integrity.

Protein Healthy skin depends on adequate protein levels to maintain the skin, repair minor defects, and preserve intravascular volume. As protein levels decline from excess loss or inadequate intake, minor defects cannot be repaired, fluid leaks from the vascular compartment of dependent areas, and edema (excess fluid in the tissues) develops. Edema decreases skin elasticity and interferes with the diffusion of oxygen to the cells. Therefore, the skin becomes prone to breakdown.

Cholesterol Low cholesterol levels predispose patients to skin breakdown and inhibit wound healing. Patients on low-fat tube feedings may experience deficiencies in cholesterol, fatty acids, and linoleic acid. Together, these fats aid in providing fuel for wound healing and maintain a waterproof barrier in the stratum corneum.

Calorie Intake If calorie intake is inadequate, the body uses proteins for energy (catabolism); they are then unavailable for building and maintenance functions (anabolism) (see Chapter 27 as needed). When undernutrition is prolonged, the person experiences weight loss, loss of subcutaneous tissue, and muscle atrophy. As a result, padding between the skin and the bones decreases, predisposing the skin to pressure ulcers.

Ascorbic Acid, Zinc, and Copper Vitamin C, or ascorbic acid, is involved in the formation and maintenance of collagen, so a deficiency can delay wound healing. Zinc and copper are also involved in collagen formation, and deficiencies of either may impair healing.

Hydration Skin turgor depends on hydration. Poor skin turgor may occur as a result of dehydration, whereas edema may result from overhydration. Both dry, dehydrated, as well as edematous, overhydrated, skin are prone to injury, especially when exposed to pressure, shearing, friction, and moisture. For further discussion on fluid requirements, see Chapter 38.

Diminished Sensation or Cognition

Clients with peripheral vascular disease, spinal cord injury, diabetes, cerebrovascular accident, trauma, or fractures often have diminished tactile sense. They are therefore more prone to skin breakdown. If you've ever touched a hot surface and quickly pulled back your hand, you know the importance of tactile sensation.

Clients with diminished sensation are less able to sense a hot surface and would likely suffer a burn. A cut or wound in an area with limited sensation may go unnoticed and therefore untreated. They are also unable to feel pressure in an affected area. As a result, they may not shift position to relieve pressure over bony prominences or be aware that shoes or clothing are constricting.

PICOT

Pressure Ulcers and the Malnourished Older Adult

Situation: While caring for an emaciated patient after surgery, the nurse notes two new wounds on the patient's bony prominences. Pressure ulcers have developed secondary to the patient's immobility, friction, shear, and postoperative drainage.

PICOT Components:

P Population/patient = Malnourished adults

I Intervention/indicator = Nutritional supplements

C Comparator/control = Diet without supplements

O Outcome = Improved (or faster) healing time

T Time =

Searchable Question: Do _____ (P) who receive/are exposed to _____ (I) demonstrate _____ (O) as compared to _____ (C) during _____ (T)?

Example of Evidence: Protein intake has been associated with improved wound healing. To prevent pressure wounds, many acute care facilities recommend that patients' diets have increased protein content, as do many long-term care facilities. To examine the effect of nutritional intervention in pressure ulcer care, researchers reviewed six clinical trials using oral nutritional supplementation (ONS) enriched with arginine, vitamin C, and zinc for pressure ulcer care. Results showed pressure ulcer healing and reduced risk of developing pressure ulcers.

Practice Change: The nurse caring for patients at risk for pressure wounds needs to address the patient's nutritional needs, including a diet high in protein.

Schols, J. M., Heyman, H., & Meijer, E. W. (2009). Nutritional support in the treatment and prevention of pressure ulcers: An overview of studies with an arginine enriched oral nutritional supplement. *Journal of Tissue Viability, 18*(3), 72–79.

Clients with impaired cognition (i.e., Alzheimer's disease, dementia, altered level of consciousness) are at higher risk to have skin breakdown because they are not aware of the need to reposition. Cognitive impairment can be subtle and difficult to recognize. Talk to your patient's family or caregiver and review past medical records so that the plan of care can be adjusted.

Impaired Circulation

The vascular system brings oxygen-rich blood to the tissues and removes metabolic waste products. Circulatory impairment interferes with tissue metabolism. *Impaired arterial circulation* restricts activity, produces pain, and leads to muscle atrophy and thin tissue that can lead to ischemia and necrosis. *Impaired venous circulation* results in engorged tissues containing high levels of metabolic waste products that make the tissue susceptible to edema, ulceration, and breakdown. Both forms of circulatory impairment delay wound healing. Circulatory impairment is one of the main causes of chronic wounds.

Medications

Side effects and idiosyncratic reactions to medications can affect skin integrity and wound healing. Any medication that causes pruritus (itching), dermatoses (rashes), photosensitivity, alopecia, or pigmentation changes can result in changes that impair skin integrity or delay healing (Fig. 35-2). The following are examples:

- *Blood pressure medications* decrease the amount of pressure required to occlude blood flow to an area, creating a risk for ischemia.
- *Anti-inflammatory medications*, such as over-the-counter (OTC) nonsteroidal anti-inflammatory drugs (NSAIDs, e.g., ibuprofen) and steroids (e.g., prednisone), inhibit wound healing.
- *Anticoagulants* (e.g., heparin, warfarin [Coumadin]) can lead to extravasation of blood into subcutaneous tissue. As a result, even minimal pressure or injury can cause a hematoma.
- *Chemotherapeutic agents* delay wound healing because of their cellular toxicity.
- *Certain antibiotics, psychotherapeutic drugs,* and *chemotherapy agents* for cancer increase sensitivity to sunlight, increasing the risk for sunburn.
- *Several herbal products*, such as those containing lavender and tea tree oil, cleanse the skin but also have a drying effect.

Moisture on the Skin

Excessive exposure to moisture leads to **maceration** (softening of the skin) and increases the likelihood of skin breakdown. Incontinence and fever are the most common sources of moisture. Bowel incontinence is particularly troublesome because feces contain digestive enzymes and microorganisms that can readily lead

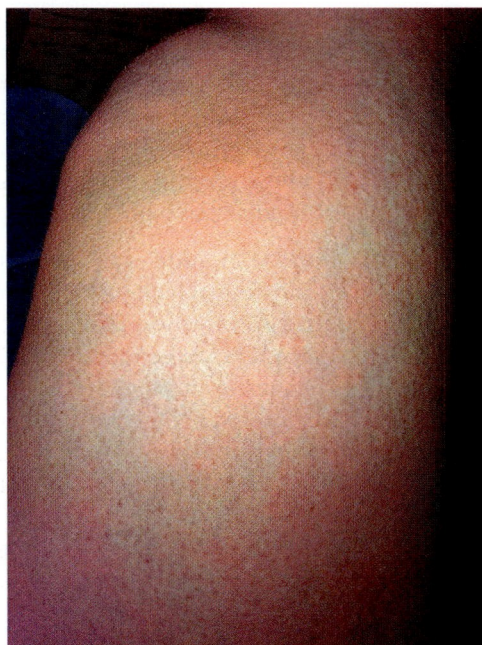

FIGURE 35-2 Skin reaction to medication.

to **excoriation** (denuding) of superficial skin layers. This can lead to **moisture-associated skin damage (MASD)**, **dermatitis** (inflammation of the skin), pressure ulcers, and infection.

Fever

Fever is a risk factor for skin breakdown for two reasons. First, it leads to sweating, which can cause maceration. Second, it increases the metabolic rate, thereby raising the tissue demand for oxygen. An increased demand for oxygen is difficult to meet if there is any circulatory impairment or tissue compression secondary to pressure.

Contamination or Infection

Contamination of a wound refers to the presence of microorganisms in the wound. All chronic wounds are considered contaminated. As bacteria begin to increase in number, a wound is said to be **colonized**, though the microorganisms are causing no harm. Wounds are colonized from the surrounding skin and local skin organisms, the external environment, and internal sources, usually from the mucous membranes of the gastrointestinal system. The acid nature of the skin keeps bacteria attached to the skin (Zulkowski, 2013). A wound becomes **critically colonized** when the bacteria begin to overwhelm the body's defenses. Critical colonization may be detected by subtle signs, such as an increase in drainage, or by more pronounced signs, such as a new foul odor, a change in color of the wound bed, new tunneling of the wound, or absent or friable granulation tissue.

An **infection** implies the microorganisms are causing harm by releasing toxins, invading body tissues,

and increasing the metabolic demand of the tissue. Infection of the skin makes it more vulnerable to breakdown and impedes healing of open wounds. If not stopped, bacteria can then gain access to the systemic circulation.

Lifestyle

Some lifestyle habits affect skin integrity:

- *Tanning* exposes the skin to ultraviolet radiation, thereby increasing the risk for skin cancer as well as drying the skin.
- *Hygiene habits* that involve either excessive or insufficient skin hygiene are not healthy for skin integrity. Frequent bathing and use of soap remove skin oils and may lead to drying, which jeopardizes the skin's barrier function. Infrequent cleansing of the skin contributes to excessive oiliness, clogged sebaceous glands, and inadequate removal of microbes on the skin, which can then infect a wound or lesion.
- *Regular exercise* improves circulation, which is necessary for skin integrity and wound healing.
- A *nutritious diet* provides the nutrients needed to maintain skin integrity, as already discussed.
- *Smoking* compromises the oxygen supply to the tissues, making skin more prone to breakdown and delaying wound healing. It also interferes with vitamin C absorption, which is needed for collagen formation.
- *Body piercings and tattoos* present a risk for infection and scarring. Complications, which occur in about 20% of piercings, include local infections, sepsis, endocarditis, hepatitis, and toxic shock syndrome. Intraoral and perioral piercings can result in gingivitis, damage to teeth and gums, and choking. Advise patients to become informed about the procedure and about aftercare and to find reputable piercers.

KnowledgeCheck 35-2

- Identify the factors that affect skin integrity.
- What nutritional components are essential to maintain skin?

ThinkLike a Nurse 35-1

- Review the case of William Harmon (Meet Your Patient). What risks, if any, does Mr. Harmon have for skin breakdown or delayed healing?
- What additional information do you need to know to fully evaluate his risk?
- What risks do you have for impaired skin integrity? What actions can you take to protect your skin?

WOUNDS

Wounds are a disruption in the normal integrity of the skin. Wounds may be intentional, such as a surgical wound, or unintentional, such as a cut or a pressure ulcer.

Types of Wounds

Wounds are classified according to length of time the wound has existed, as well as the condition of the wound (e.g., contamination, severity).

Skin Integrity The simplest wound classification system is based on the integrity of the skin. If there are no breaks in the skin, the wound is described as **closed**. Contusions (bruises) or tissue swelling from fractures are common closed wounds. A wound is considered **open** if there is a break in the skin or mucous membranes. Open wounds include abrasions, lacerations, puncture wounds, and surgical incisions. A compound fracture may also lead to an open wound caused by the projection of bone through the skin. Several open and closed wounds are described in Table 35-1.

Length of Time for Healing The length of time for wound healing varies according to the skin integrity and the factors affecting it, discussed in the previous section. **Acute wounds** are expected to be of short duration. In a healthy person, these wounds heal spontaneously without complications through the three phases of wound healing (inflammation, proliferation, and maturation). Wounds that exceed the expected length of recovery are classified as **chronic wounds**. The natural healing progression has been interrupted or stalled because of infection, continued trauma, ischemia, or edema. Chronic wounds include pressure, arterial, venous, and diabetic ulcers. These wounds are frequently colonized with several types of bacteria, and healing is slow because of the underlying disease process. Unless the type of wound is properly diagnosed and the underlying disease process treated, a chronic wound may linger for months or years (Table 35-2).

Level of Contamination **Clean wounds** are uninfected wounds with minimal inflammation. They may be open or closed and do not involve the gastrointestinal, respiratory, or genitourinary tracts (these systems frequently harbor bacteria). There is very little risk of infection for a clean wound. **Clean-contaminated wounds** are surgical incisions that enter the gastrointestinal, respiratory, or genitourinary tracts. There is an increased risk of infection for these wounds, but there is no obvious infection.

Contaminated wounds include open, traumatic wounds or surgical incisions in which a major break in asepsis occurred. The risk of infection is high for these wounds. Wounds are considered **infected** when bacteria counts in the wound tissues are above 100,000 organisms per gram of tissue. However, the presence of *beta-hemolytic streptococci*, in any number, is considered an infection. Signs of wound infection include erythema and swelling around the wound, fever, foul odor, severe or increasing pain, large amount of drainage, or warmth of the surrounding soft tissue.

Depth of the Wound **Superficial wounds** involve only the epidermal layer of the skin. The injury is usually the result of friction, shearing, or burning. **Partial-thickness wounds** extend through the epidermis but not through the dermis. **Full-thickness wounds** extend into the subcutaneous tissue and beyond. The descriptor **penetrating** is sometimes added to indicate that the wound involves internal organs. Wound depth is a major determinant of healing time: The deeper the wound, the longer the healing time.

KnowledgeCheck 35-3

- Explain the difference between an acute and a chronic wound.
- Describe the wound categorization system based on the level of contamination.
- How does wound depth affect healing?

Table 35-1 ▶ Types of Wounds	
TYPE	**DESCRIPTION**
Abrasion	A scrape of the superficial layers of the skin; usually unintentional but may be performed intentionally for cosmetic purposes to smooth skin surfaces
Abscess	A localized collection of pus resulting from invasion from a pyogenic bacterium or other pathogen; must be opened and drained to heal
Contusion	A closed wound caused by blunt trauma. May be referred to as a bruise or ecchymotic area.
Crushing	A wound caused by force leading to compression or disruption of tissues. Often associated with fracture. Usually there is minimal or no break in the skin.
Incision	An open, intentional wound caused by a sharp instrument
Laceration	The skin or mucous membranes are torn open, resulting in a wound with jagged margins.
Penetrating	An open wound in which the agent causing the wound lodges in body tissue.
Puncture	An open wound caused by a sharp object. Often there is collapse of tissue around the entry point, making this wound prone to infection.
Tunnel	A wound with an entrance and exit site

Table 35-2 ➤ Chronic Wounds

TYPE	ETIOLOGY	CHARACTERISTICS
Pressure Ulcers	Caused by pressure, resulting in tissue ischemia and injury	Appearance depends on the stage or tissue layers involved. Pressure ulcers tend to be located over bony prominences. Can cause serious tissue damage.
Arterial Ulcers	Caused by inadequate circulation of oxygenated blood to the tissue, which leads to tissue ischemia and damage	Ulcer appears "punched out," small and round with smooth borders. The wound base is usually pale with or without necrotic tissue. They tend to occur over the distal part of the leg, especially the ankles, toes, side of the foot, and shin. The surrounding skin appears shiny, thin, and dry and is cool to touch. Often there is loss of hair in the surrounding area. The area has delayed capillary refill time, and patients may complain of pain that worsens with increased activity. Arterial ulcers are most common in lower extremities but can occur anywhere. This type of ulcer can lead to serious injury and even death.
Venous Stasis Ulcers	Caused by incompetent venous valves, deep vein obstruction, or inadequate calf muscle function, resulting in venous pooling, edema, and impaired microcirculation of the skin	Usually located around the inner ankle, or in the lower part of the calf. Surrounding skin is reddened or brown and edematous. Wounds are usually shallow, with irregular wound margins. The wound bed appears "ruddy" or "beefy" red and granular. Drainage may be moderate to heavy depending on amount of edema. Pain usually occurs with leg dependence and dressing changes.

Wound Healing Process

All wounds heal through a physiological process in which epithelial, endothelial, and inflammatory cells, platelets, and fibroblasts migrate into the wound to bring about tissue repair and regeneration. The process is essentially the same regardless of the type of injury or the type of tissues involved.

Types of Healing

Wounds may heal by regeneration or by primary, secondary, or tertiary intention.

Regenerative/Epithelial Healing When a wound affects only the epidermis and dermis, **regenerative/epithelial healing** takes place. No scar forms and the new (regenerated) epithelial and dermal cells form new skin that cannot be distinguished from the intact skin. Partial-thickness wounds heal by regeneration.

Primary Intention Healing When a wound involves minimal or no tissue loss and has edges that are well approximated (closed), **primary (first) intention** healing takes place (Fig. 35-3A). Little scarring is expected. A clean surgical incision heals by this method.

Secondary Intention Healing Healing by **secondary (second) intention** occurs when a wound (1) involves extensive tissue loss, which prevents wound edges from approximating, or (2) should not be closed (e.g., because it is infected). Because the wound is left open, it heals from the inner layer to the surface by filling in with beefy red **granulation tissue** (a form of connective tissue with an abundant blood supply) (Fig. 35-3B). Epithelial tissue may appear in the wound as small pink or pearl-like areas. **Key Point:** *Do not mistake this as a sign of infection. Wounds that heal by secondary intention heal more slowly, are more prone to infection, and develop more scar tissue. Pressure ulcers (discussed later) and infected wounds are examples.*

Tertiary Intention Healing A wound heals by **tertiary (third) healing,** also called *delayed primary closure,* when two surfaces of granulation tissue are brought together (Fig. 35-3C). This technique may be used when the wound is clean-contaminated or contaminated. Initially the wound is allowed to heal by secondary intention. When there is no evidence of edema, infection, or foreign matter, the wound edges are closed by bringing together the granulating tissue and suturing the surface. Such wounds require strict aseptic technique during all dressing changes because they are prone to infection. Tertiary intention healing creates less scarring than does secondary, but more than primary intention healing.

Phases of Healing

Wound healing occurs in three stages: inflammatory, proliferative, and maturation (Fig. 35-4).

Inflammatory Phase—Cleansing The inflammatory (cleansing) phase lasts from 1 to 5 days and consists of two major processes: hemostasis and inflammation.

- *Hemostasis.* At the time of injury, tissue and capillaries are destroyed, causing blood and plasma to leak into the wound. Area vessels constrict to limit blood

Primary intention

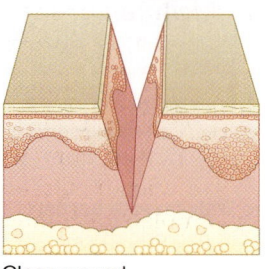 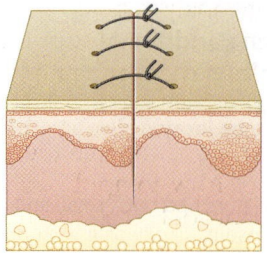 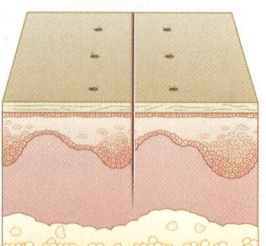

A Clean wound   Sutured early   Results in hairline scar

Secondary intention

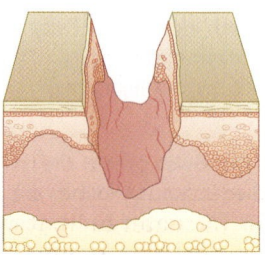 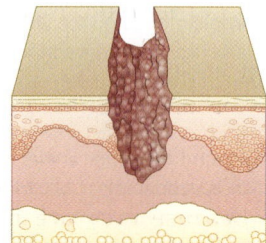 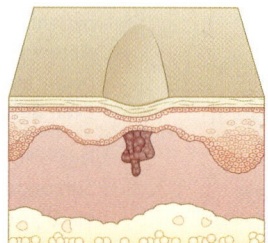

B Wound gaping and irregular   Granulation occurring   Epithelium fills in scar

Tertiary intention

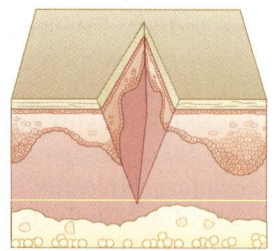 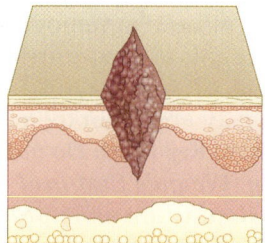 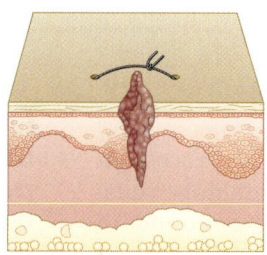

C Wound not sutured   Granulation partially fills   Granulating tissue sutured
                                       in wound   together

FIGURE 35-3 *A,* In a wound with minimal tissue loss, the edges may be sutured together, resulting in rapid healing and minimal scarring. *B,* A wound that heals by secondary intention heals from the inner layer to the surface. Healing takes longer, and there is scarring. *C,* A wound that heals by tertiary intention is initially healed by secondary intention and later sutured.

loss. Platelets aggregate (clump together) to slow bleeding. At the same time, the clotting mechanism is activated to form a blood clot.

- *Inflammation.* The inflammatory reaction is characterized by edema, erythema, pain, temperature elevation, and migration of white blood cells into the wound tissues. Within 24 hours, macrophages begin engulfing bacteria (**phagocytosis**) and clearing debris. Along with plasma proteins and fibrin, they form a scab on the wound surface, which seals the wound and helps prevent microbial invasion.

Proliferative Phase—Granulation The proliferative phase is also called regeneration or healing. It occurs from days 5 to 21. Cells develop to fill the wound defect and resurface the skin. **Fibroblasts** (connective tissue cells) migrate to the wound where they form **collagen**, a protein substance that adds strength to the healing wound. New blood and lymph vessels sprout from the existing capillaries at the edge of the wound. The result is the formation of granulation tissue, a beefy red tissue that bleeds readily and is easily damaged. As the clot or scab is dissolved, epithelial cells begin to grow into the

wound from surrounding healthy tissue and seal over the wound (**epithelialization**).

Maturation Phase—Epithelialization The maturation phase (or remodeling) is the final phase of the healing process. It begins in the second or third week and continues even after the wound has closed. Over the next 3 to 6 months, the initial collagen fibers that were laid in the wound bed during the proliferative phase are broken down and remodeled into an organized structure (e.g., scar tissue), increasing the tensile strength of the wound. A wound that has healed by primary intention leaves little scarring. Even so, a scar is only 80% as strong as the original tissue.

KnowledgeCheck 35-4

Identify the type of wound healing (primary, secondary, or tertiary intention):

- A wound that heals from inner layer to the surface
- A wound with approximated edges
- A wound that heals by approximating two surfaces of granulation tissue
- A wound that is sutured and has minimal or no tissue loss

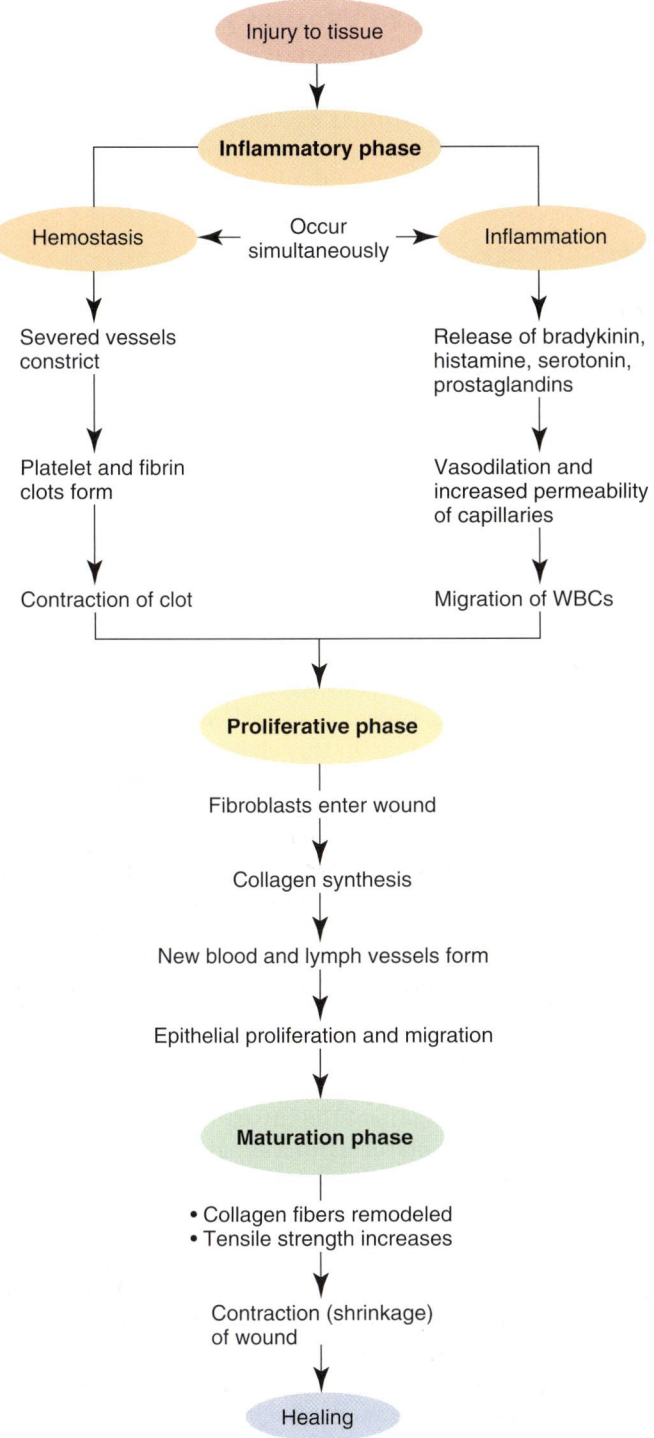

Injury to tissue

↓

Inflammatory phase

Hemostasis ← Occur simultaneously → Inflammation

Severed vessels constrict

Release of bradykinin, histamine, serotonin, prostaglandins

Platelet and fibrin clots form

Vasodilation and increased permeability of capillaries

Contraction of clot

Migration of WBCs

↓

Proliferative phase

Fibroblasts enter wound

↓

Collagen synthesis

↓

New blood and lymph vessels form

↓

Epithelial proliferation and migration

↓

Maturation phase

• Collagen fibers remodeled
• Tensile strength increases

↓

Contraction (shrinkage) of wound

↓

Healing

FIGURE 35-4 Stages in the wound healing process.

Wound Closures

Wounds that heal by primary and tertiary intention may be closed in several ways. Adhesive strips, sutures, staples, surgical glue, negative-pressure closure, and compression are the current choices.

Adhesive Strips In the following situations, adhesive strips (e.g., Steri-Strips) are used:

■ Closing superficial low-tension wounds, such as skin tears or lacerations

■ Closing the skin on a wound that has been closed subcutaneously to aid in healing and reduce scarring
■ Giving additional support to a wound after sutures or staples have been removed

Adhesive strips are often kept in place until they begin to separate from the skin on their own. For a summary of how to apply adhesive skin closures, see the Highlights of Procedures box. For complete instructions,

 Go to Chapter 35, **Procedure 35-10: Placing Skin Closures,** in Volume 2.

Sutures The traditional wound closures are sutures ("stitches"). Suturing leads to small puncture wounds along the track of the laceration or incision. Several types of suture materials are available.

■ *Absorbent sutures* are used deep in the tissues, for example, to close an organ or **anastomose** (connect) tissue. Because they are made of material that will gradually dissolve, there is no need to remove absorbent sutures.
■ *Nonabsorbent sutures* are placed in superficial tissues and require removal, usually by the nurse. For a summary of how to remove sutures and staples, see the Highlights of Procedures box. For complete steps,

 Go to Chapter 35, **Procedure 35-12: Removing Sutures and Staples,** in Volume 2.

Surgical Staples Made of lightweight titanium, surgical staples provide a fast, easy way to close an incision (Fig. 35-5). They are also associated with a lower risk of infection and tissue reaction than are sutures. The downside of staples is that some wound edges are more difficult to align. The most common sites for wound stapling

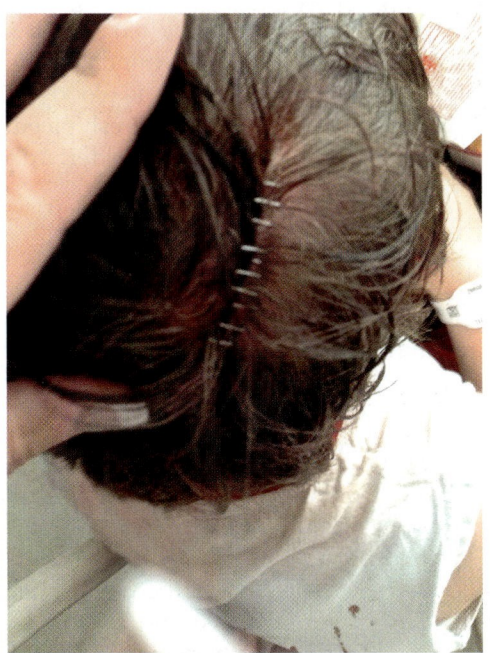

FIGURE 35-5 Surgical stables in the scalp.

are arms, legs, abdomen, back, scalp, or bowel. Wounds on the hands, feet, neck, or face should not be stapled.

Surgical Glue This is a relatively new method for wound closure. It is safe for use in clean, low-tension wounds. It is an ideal wound closure method for skin tears.

Advanced Wound Treatments

Collaborative treatments are necessary for wounds that will not heal despite aggressive care. Such treatments include the following:

- **Surgical options**, such as extensive debridement, skin grafts, secondary closure of the wound, and flap techniques (partially detached tissue placed over a wound) are used for complicated wounds.
- **Hyperbaric oxygen therapy (HBOT)** is the administration of 100% oxygen under pressure to a wound site. HBOT increases oxygen concentration in the tissue, stimulates the growth of new blood vessels, and enhances white blood cell (WBC) action.
- **Platelet-derived growth factor** augments the inflammatory phase of wound healing and accelerates collagen formation in the wound.

Types of Wound Drainage

Drainage is the flow of fluids from a wound or cavity. It is often referred to as exudate and is fluid that oozes as a result of inflammation. Exudate may take several forms.

- **Serous Exudate.** Clean wounds typically drain serous exudate. It is watery in consistency and contains very little cellular matter. Serous exudate consists of *serum*, the straw-colored fluid that separates out of blood when a clot is formed.
- **Sanguineous Exudate.** You will often see sanguineous exudate with deep wounds or wounds in highly vascular areas. Sanguineous exudate is bloody drainage. It indicates damage to capillaries. Fresh bleeding produces bright red drainage, whereas older, dried blood is a darker, red-brown color.
- **Serosanguineous Drainage.** In new wounds, you will most commonly see serosanguineous drainage, a combination of bloody and serous drainage.
- **Purulent Exudate.** The thick, often malodorous, drainage that is seen in infected wounds is called purulent exudate. It contains pus, a protein-rich fluid filled with WBCs, bacteria, and cellular debris. It is commonly caused by infection from **pyogenic** (pus-forming) bacteria, such as streptococci or staphylococci. Normally, pus is yellow in color, although it may take on a blue-green color if the bacterium *Pseudomonas aeruginosa* is present.
- **Purosanguineous Exudate.** Red-tinged pus is called purosanguineous exudate. It indicates that small vessels in the wound area have ruptured.

Complications of Wound Healing

Recall that wounds heal by moving through the phases of inflammation, proliferation, and maturation. At times, this process is interrupted by complications. The most common complications are hemorrhage, infection, dehiscence, evisceration, and fistulas.

Hemorrhage

Whenever a capillary network is interrupted or a blood vessel is severed, bleeding occurs. **Hemostasis** (cessation of bleeding) usually occurs within minutes of the injury. Hemostasis is delayed, however, when large vessels are injured, a clotting disorder exists, or the client is on anticoagulant therapy. If bleeding begins again after initial hemostasis, something is probably wrong. Possible causes include a slipped suture, erosion of a blood vessel, a dislodged clot, or infection. The risk of hemorrhage is greatest in the first 24 to 48 hours following surgery or injury. Bleeding may be internal or external.

Internal Bleeding Swelling of the affected body part, pain, and changes in vital signs (i.e., decreased blood pressure, elevated pulse) may indicate internal bleeding. By *internal bleeding,* in this chapter, we are referring to a **hematoma**, a red-blue collection of blood under the skin, which forms as a result of bleeding that cannot escape to the surface. A large hematoma causes pressure on surrounding tissues. If the hematoma is located near a major artery or vein, it may impede blood flow.

External Hemorrhage External hemorrhage is relatively easy to recognize. You will see bloody drainage on the dressings and in the wound drainage devices. When there is a brisk hemorrhage, blood often pools underneath the client as the dressings become saturated. To be sure that you are aware of the full extent of the bleeding, remember to look underneath the patient.

Infection

Microorganisms can be introduced to a wound during an injury, during surgery, or after surgery. Suspect infection if a wound fails to heal. Localized swelling, redness, heat, pain, fever (temperatures higher than 38°C [100.4°F]), foul-smelling or purulent drainage, or a change in the color of the drainage may also indicate infection. The symptoms are likely to occur in a contaminated or traumatic wound within 2 to 3 days. In a clean surgical wound, you will usually not see signs and symptoms of an infection until the fourth or fifth postoperative day. Incisions that begin draining within 5 to 7 days of surgery are at risk for dehiscing.

Dehiscence

Rupture (separation) of one or more layers of a wound is called **dehiscence** (Fig. 35-6). Wound dehiscence is most likely to occur in the inflammatory phase of healing, before large amounts of collagen have been deposited in the wound to strengthen it. The most common causes of

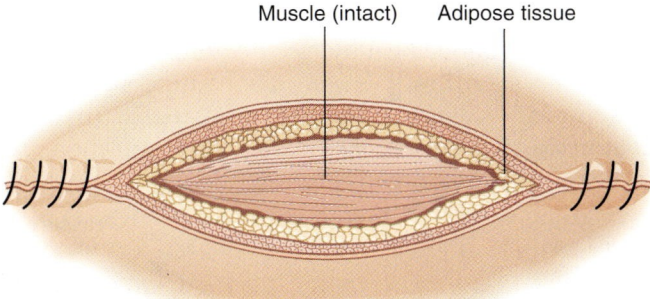

FIGURE 35-6 Dehiscence is separation of one or more layers of a wound. It is most common in the inflammatory phase of healing.

dehiscence are poor nutritional status, inadequate closure of the muscles, wound infection, or increased tension on the suture line (coughing, lifting an object). Obese clients are also more likely to experience dehiscence because fatty tissue does not heal readily and the patient's mass increases the strain on the suture line.

Dehiscence is usually associated with abdominal wounds. Patients often report feeling a "pop" or tear, especially with sudden straining from coughing, vomiting, or changing positions in bed. Usually there is an immediate increase in serosanguineous drainage. Nursing interventions include maintaining bedrest with the head of the bed elevated at 20° and the knees flexed. To prevent *evisceration*, a binder may be applied. The provider should be notified of the dehiscence to examine the wound.

Evisceration

Evisceration is total separation of the layers of a wound with internal viscera protruding through the incision (Fig. 35-7). This rare complication is a surgical emergency. Immediately cover the wound with sterile towels or dressings soaked in sterile saline solution to prevent the organs from drying out and becoming contaminated with environmental bacteria. Have the patient stay in bed with knees bent to minimize strain on the incision. Do not put a binder on the patient. Notify the surgeon

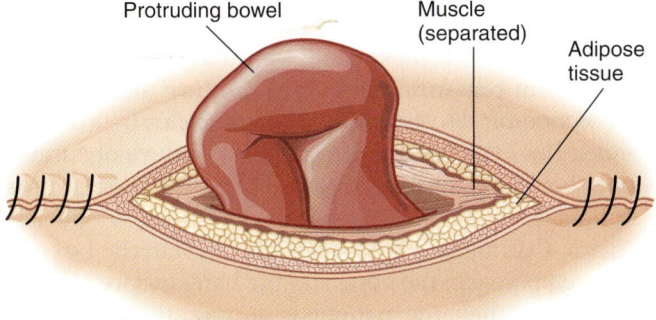

FIGURE 35-7 Evisceration is total separation of the layers of a wound with internal viscera protruding through the incision.

and ready the patient for surgery (see Chapter 39 for perioperative care).

Fistulas

A **fistula** is an abnormal passage connecting two body cavities or a cavity and the skin. Fistulas often result from infection or debris left in the wound. An abscess forms, which breaks down surrounding tissue and creates the abnormal passageway. Chronic drainage from the fistula may lead to skin breakdown and delayed wound healing. The most common sites of fistula formation are the gastrointestinal and genitourinary tracts. Figure 35-8 illustrates a fistula between the rectum and vagina.

KnowledgeCheck 35-5

- Describe four types of wound closures.
- Identify five types of wound complications.
- Describe three signs of internal hemorrhage.
- Differentiate between dehiscence and evisceration.

ThinkLike a Nurse 35-2

Recall the case of Mr. Harmon (Meet Your Patient). What form of wound healing (primary, secondary, or tertiary) is he undergoing? How long would you expect it to take before his wounds heal?

CHRONIC WOUNDS

A chronic wound is one that has not healed within the expected time frame. It has not moved through the repair process in an orderly fashion (inflammation, proliferation, maturation). Wounds that do not heal within 2 to 4 weeks may be considered chronic. Pressure ulcers are a type of chronic wound.

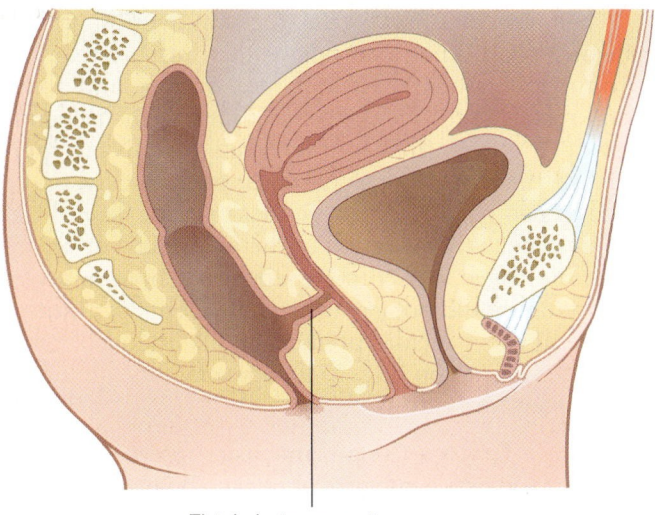

Fistula between rectum and vagina (enterovaginal)

FIGURE 35-8 A fistula is an abnormal passage connecting two body cavities or a cavity and the skin. Fistulas are most common in the gastrointestinal and genitourinary tracts.

Pressure Ulcers

Pressure ulcers (formerly called *decubitus ulcers*, *pressure sores*, and *bedsores*) are localized areas of injury to the skin, and possibly the underlying tissue, usually over a bony prominence. We discuss them separately because vigilant nursing care can prevent most pressure ulcers; if they do form, nurses play a major role in their treatment. In fact, a higher rate of pressure ulcers may signal overall poor care. Additionally, patients who develop pressure injuries have generally longer hospital lengths of stay, are more likely to be readmitted within 30 days after discharge, and may even be more likely to die during the hospital stay than those without this complication (Lyder, Wang, Metersky, et al., 2012). Unless the pressure injury is present on admission (POA), in most circumstances Medicare will decline payment for treatment for that ulcer.

How Do Pressure Ulcers Develop?

Patients at risk for developing pressure ulcers are those with immobility, friction and shear, moisture, incontinence, poor nutrition, perfusion, age, skin condition, and altered level of consciousness (Stechmiller, Cowan, Whitney, et al., 2008). Pressure ulcers are caused by unrelieved pressure, or pressure in combination with shearing forces. These compromise blood flow to an area, resulting in *ischemia* (inadequate blood supply) in the underlying tissue. Tissue ischemia leads to tissue anoxia (lack of oxygen) and cell death.

Key Point: *The key variables in ischemia are time and pressure. Small amounts of pressure over an extended period of time or a large amount of pressure for a short period of time results in tissue ischemia. Pressure ulcers can occur in as little time as 2 hours, though they may take as long as 5 days for the full extent of tissue damage to be known.*

When ischemia first occurs, the skin over the area is pale and cool. When you relieve the pressure (e.g., by turning the patient), vasodilation occurs, and extra blood rushes to the area to compensate for the ischemic period. The area flushes bright red (**reactive hyperemia**). If the redness does not disappear quickly, tissue damage has occurred. The redness should last about half as long as the duration of the ischemia. For example, if the tissue was compressed for an hour, reactive hyperemia should not last more than about 30 minutes.

Several other factors predict the likelihood of pressure ulcer formation (Fig. 35-9). Some factors are intrinsic and some are extrinsic.

Intrinsic Factors Certain intrinsic (internal) factors alter skin and tissue integrity or oxygen delivery capabilities, decreasing the amount of force required to create a pressure ulcer. Examples include immobility and impaired sensation, as occur with spinal cord injuries, stroke, or coma; poor nutrition; edema; aging; low arteriolar pressure; and fever. Septicemia is one of the most

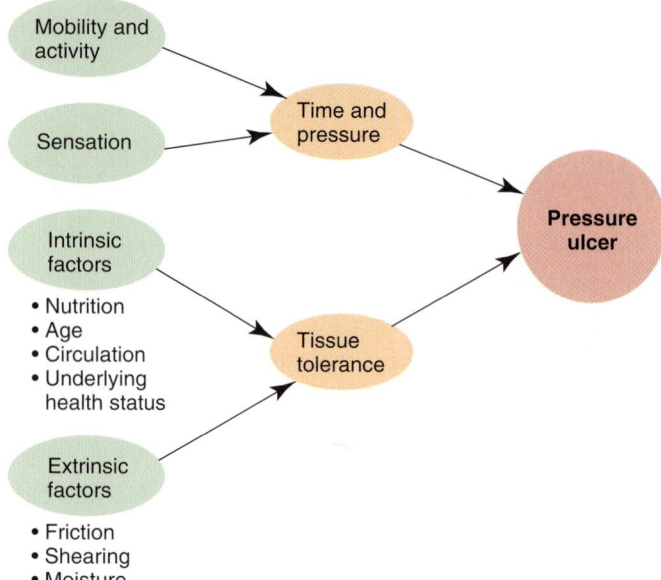

FIGURE 35-9 Several factors contribute to the development of pressure ulcers.

common principal reasons for hospitalization among patients with secondary pressure ulcers (Russo, Steiner, & Spector, 2008). The previous section, "What Factors Affect Skin Integrity?," discussed a variety of intrinsic factors.

Poor nutrition or dehydration can weaken the skin and lead to pressure ulcers. Adequate intake of calories, protein, vitamin C, and zinc is necessary to prevent pressure ulcers and promote healing of injured tissue (Institute for Clinical Systems Improvement [ICSI], 2012).

Extrinsic Factors The following extrinsic (external) factors contribute to the development of pressure ulcers:

- *Friction* damages the outer protective epidermal layer, decreasing the amount of pressure needed to develop skin lesions (Black, Baharestani, Cuddigan, et al., 2007).
- *Shearing* occurs when the epidermal layer slides over the dermis, causing damage to the vascular bed. It most commonly occurs when the head of the bed is elevated and the patient slides downward, causing shear in the sacral area. When shearing occurs, the amount of pressure needed to occlude circulation is cut in half.
- *Moisture*, especially in the form of urine, feces, or perspiration, macerates the skin and decreases the amount of pressure required to produce ulceration.
- *Compression* can also cause pressure ulcers by reducing blood flow to a body area. This most commonly occurs over bony prominences, but can also occur under casts, splints, endotracheal tubes, and other assistive devices (Black, Cuddigan, Walko, et al., 2010). Skin can be compressed between the bone and the hard surface of a bed or chair. When the patient is supine, these pressure points are the occiput, scapulae, elbows, sacrum, and heels. Figure 35-9A–D illustrates the pressure points in the supine, lateral, prone, and sitting positions.

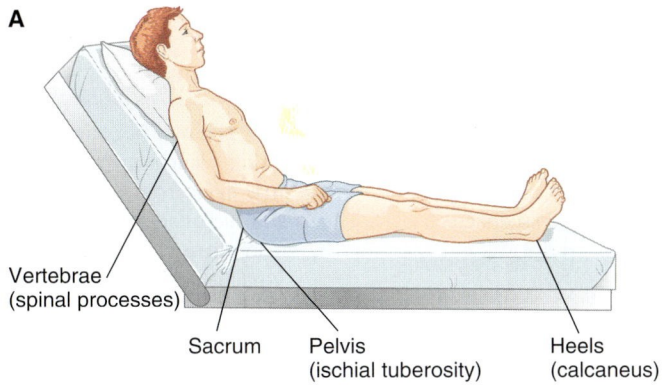

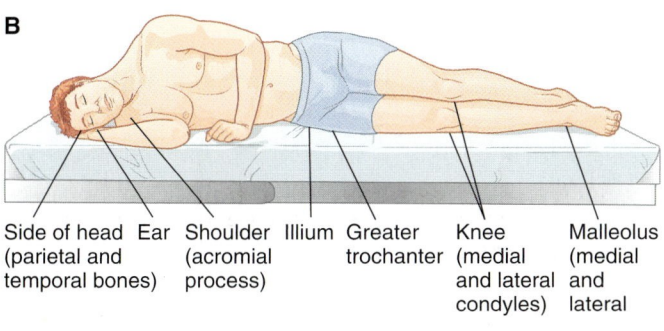

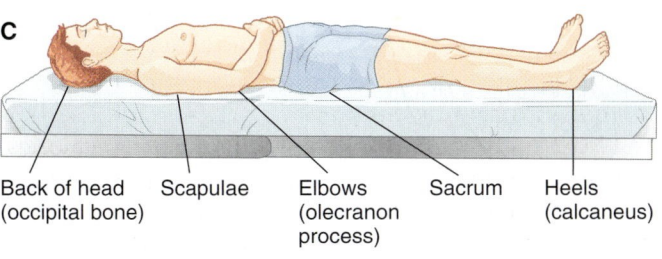

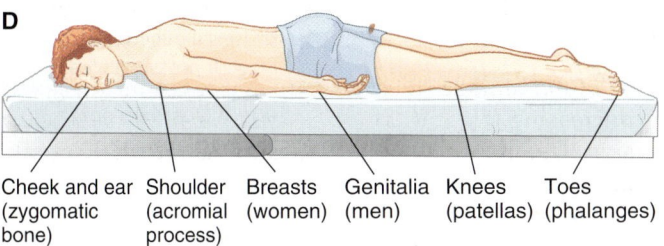

FIGURE 35-10 *A–D,* Most commonly, pressure ulcers develop over the bony prominences. *A,* Sitting. *B,* Lateral. *C,* Supine. *D,* Prone. (Adapted from AHRQ Clinical Practice Guidelines.)

How Are Pressure Ulcers Staged?

Pressure ulcers are classified by the degree of tissue involvement (Table 35-3). The National Pressure Ulcer Advisory Panel (NPUAP) developed a standardized staging system. Only wounds caused by pressure are staged. Other classification systems exist to describe other chronic wounds, such as diabetic foot ulcers and venous stasis ulcers.

Key Point: *Healing ulcers are not "reverse" staged. The healing process cannot cause a stage IV pressure ulcer to become a stage III. Pressure ulcers become progressively shallower by filling in with granulation*

tissue, but lost muscle, subcutaneous fat, and dermis are not replaced. Therefore, reverse staging does not accurately characterize what is physiologically occurring in the ulcer (NPUAP, n.d.). Instead, pressure ulcers maintain their original staging classification throughout the healing process, but they are described as healing (e.g., "stage IV ulcer: healing" or "stage I ulcer: healing").

Other Types of Ulcers

This chapter focuses primarily on pressure ulcers. However, not all lower extremity ulcers are related to pressure.

Venous Stasis Ulcers are irregularly shaped lesions caused by venous congestion, often from damage to valves in the veins (e.g., from deep vein thrombosis). They occur usually between the inside ankle and the knee, not necessarily over a bony prominence, and are typically red in color, shiny and taught, and may even feel warm or hot. Fluid drainage can be significant.

Diabetic Foot Ulcers occur when diabetes causes the narrowing of arteries, decreasing oxygenation to the feet that results in delayed healing and tissue necrosis. Because people with diabetes lose protective sensation, they may walk on sores, continuously damaging the tissues. Diabetic foot ulcers, often painless, occur mainly on the plantar surface of the foot, the ball of the foot, or top and bottom of the toes. Patients with diabetic foot ulcers are highly susceptible to wound infection because of the poor sensation, circulation, and immune protection (Woo, Santos, & Gamba, 2013).

Arterial Ulcers occur when there is a non-pressure-related blockage of arterial blood to an area (e.g., by a clot or stenosis of the arterioles), causing ischemia and tissue necrosis. This type of wound usually occurs over the lower leg, ankle, or bony areas of the foot. The wound bed tends to be dry and pale, with little drainage. Arterial ulcers are usually very painful, especially at night.

For more detailed information about these three types of ulcers,

 Go to Chapter 35, **Supplemental Materials,** on Davis*Plus.*

KnowledgeCheck 35-6

- What stage pressure ulcer does Mr. Harmon (Meet Your Patient) have?
- What factors have contributed to its development?

 Think**Like a Nurse** 35-3

Based on your knowledge of the factors that have contributed to Mr. Harmon's pressure ulcer development, what actions may lead to healing of the pressure ulcer? *Note:* To answer this question, you do not need to know about wound care (e.g., irrigation) for a pressure ulcer.

Table 35-3 ➤ Staging Pressure Ulcers

STAGE	CLINICAL FINDINGS	DISCUSSION
Stage I Pressure Ulcer — Epidermis — Dermis — Fat — Muscle — Bone NPUAP.org | Copyright © 2011 Gordian Medical, Inc. dba American Medical Technologies	Localized area of intact skin with nonblanchable redness, usually over a bony prominence. The area may be painful, firm, soft, or warmer or cooler as compared with adjacent tissue. Discoloration will remain for >30 minutes after pressure is relieved.	Dark skin may not have visible blanching; its color may differ from that of the surrounding area. Therefore, stage I may be difficult to detect.
Stage II Pressure Ulcer NPUAP.org | Copyright © 2011 Gordian Medical, Inc. dba American Medical Technologies	Involves partial-thickness loss of dermis. Stage II pressure ulcers are open but shallow and with a red pink wound bed. There is no slough. May also be an intact or open/ruptured serum-filled blister; or a shiny or dry shallow ulcer without slough or bruising.	Do not use this stage to describe skin tears, tape burns, perineal dermatitis, maceration, or excoriation. Do not mistake moisture-associated skin damage or fungal infections for Stage II pressure ulcer. Stage II ulcers do not involve sloughing or bruising.

Table 35-3 ➤ Staging Pressure Ulcers—cont'd

STAGE	CLINICAL FINDINGS	DISCUSSION
Stage III Pressure Ulcer 	A deep crater characterized by full-thickness skin loss with damage or necrosis of subcutaneous tissue. May extend down to, but not through, underlying fascia. Undermining (deeper-level damage under boggy superficial layers) of adjacent tissue may be present. Bone/tendon is not visible or directly palpable.	Some stage III pressure ulcers can be extremely deep when located in an area with significant adipose layers.
Stage IV Pressure Ulcer 	Involves full-thickness skin loss with extensive destruction, tissue necrosis, or damage to muscle, bone, or support structures. Exposed bone/tendon is visible or directly palpable. Slough or eschar may be present. Undermining and sinus tracts (blind tracts underneath the epidermis) are common.	The depth of a stage IV pressure ulcer varies by location. They can be shallow on the bridge of the nose, ear, occiput, and malleolus because these areas do not have subcutaneous tissue. Stage IV ulcers can extend into muscle and supporting structures (e.g., fascia, tendon, or joint capsule). Often require a full year to heal. Even once healed, the site remains at risk for future injury because the scar is not as strong as the original tissue.

Continued

Table 35-3 ➤ Staging Pressure Ulcers—cont'd

STAGE	CLINICAL FINDINGS	DISCUSSION
Suspected Deep Tissue Injury 	An area of skin that is intact but discolored. It might be purplish or deep red, painful, boggy, or have a blister.	Occurs owing to damage of underlying soft tissue from pressure or shear. Findings can be subtle enough that often DTI is not recognized until after severe tissue damage has occurred. May heal or evolve further and become covered by thin eschar, rapidly exposing additional layers of tissue even with optimal treatment. In darker pigmented individuals, discoloration might go undetected.
Unstageable Pressure Ulcer	Involves full-thickness skin loss. The base of the wound is obscured by *slough* (tan, yellow, gray, green, or brown necrotic tissue) or *eschar* (tan, black, or brown leathery necrotic tissue).	Until enough slough and/or eschar is removed to expose the base of the wound, the true depth, and therefore stage, cannot be determined. *Stable eschar* is dry, adherent, and intact without erythema or fluctuance. Do not remove stable eschar, as it serves as "the body's natural cover."

Reprinted with permission. Wound, Ostomy and Continence Nurses Society (WOCNS). (2007, revised 2014). *Position statement: Pressure ulcer staging* (p. 52). Mount Laurel, NJ: Author. Retrieved from http://npuap.org/pr2.htm

PracticalKnowledge
knowing**how**

As a nurse, you will care for many patients who have wounds or who are at risk for skin breakdown. In the remainder of the chapter, we will discuss how to maintain skin integrity, prevent pressure ulcers, and treat wounds.

▬ ASSESSMENT

The National Pressure Ulcer Advisory Panel (NPUAP) recommends nurses perform a comprehensive wound assessment while identifying other health problems and their impact on wound healing. Existing wounds require additional assessment. A thorough skin assessment includes a nursing history, physical examination, and diagnostic testing. For a list of competencies for nurses treating pressure ulcers (NPUAP, 2010),

Go to Chapter 35, **Tables, Boxes, Figures: ESG Box 35-1, Competencies for Registered Nurses Treating Pressure Ulcers,** on DavisPlus.

Focused Nursing History

To assess wound healing ability and the risk for skin breakdown, you will need to gather data on factors that affect skin integrity (discussed previously): age, mobility, nutrition, hydration, sensation, circulation, medications, moisture, lifestyle, underlying health and disease status, and the presence of microorganisms. Also consider the psychosocial issues related to coping with chronic wounds (Woo, 2011). For instance, you will need to assess with care and compassion how the patient copes with the pain of a chronic wound, handles the loss of control and independence, is adapting to changes in body image, deals with the financial burden of caring for complex wounds, and adjusts to the social isolation that comes with impaired mobility and chronic illness. For history questions to help you assess these factors,

 Go to Chapter 35, **Assessment Guidelines and Tools, History Questions for Skin and Wound Assessment,** in Volume 2.

For example, patients with poor circulation, such as those with diabetes, atherosclerosis, or low blood pressure, are at risk for tissue injury. Patients who use tobacco or are anemic have reduced oxygen supply in the blood, predisposing them to pressure ulcers. Those with limited mobility or reduced sensation because of nerve damage, head injury, stroke, spinal cord injury, or diabetes, experience a loss of protective sensations to reposition themselves (ICSI, 2012).

Pressure Ulcer Risk Assessment Measures

Patients may have multiple risk factors for skin problems. A comprehensive risk assessment tool enables you to evaluate the cumulative risk. Among the most commonly used tools are the Braden and Norton scales. To see these scales,

 Go to Chapter 35, **Assessment Guidelines and Tools, The Braden Scale for Predicting Pressure Sore Risk,** and **The Norton Scale for Assessing Risk of Pressure Ulcers,** in Volume 2.

The Braden Scale is used to identify persons at risk for developing pressure ulcers. The Braden scale evaluates six major risk factors: sensory perception, moisture, activity, mobility, nutrition, and friction and sheer. The final score reflects the patient's risk; the lower the score, the more likely the patient will develop a pressure ulcer. A score of 18 or less for hospitalized patients indicates risk. Interventions should be based on individual risk factors, as well as the total score. You should use this scale to assess the patient on admission to the facility and again in 48 to 72 hours or per facility policy. Studies have shown the second score to be more predictive, probably related to an increased awareness of the patient's status. The Braden Q is a modified scale used in children.

The Norton Scale assesses risk based on the patient's physical condition, mental state, activity, mobility, and incontinence. A low score indicates a high risk. Some have suggested that the Norton scale should be modified by adding categories for skin appearance, medication, and nutrition.

 ## ThinkLike a Nurse 35-4

Review the Braden scale. Apply this risk assessment scale to Mr. Harmon (Meet Your Patient).

- What additional information, if any, do you need to complete these assessments?
- Calculate a Braden score based on Mr. Harmon's risk factors if he had also been incontinent of urine twice that day.

Focused Physical Examination

Physical assessment of skin integrity focuses on the two following areas:

Inspecting the Skin Inspect all areas of the body routinely. Evaluate the skin for color, integrity, temperature, texture, turgor, mobility, moisture, lesions, and hair distribution. Check pressure points for erythema, tenderness, or edema. Assess all bony prominences of individuals "at risk" for skin breakdown routinely. Include skin under special garments, such as shoes, heel elevators, and antiembolism stockings. Also assess vulnerable pressure points for bed- or chair-bound patients. See Chapter 22 if you need more details on skin assessment.

Assessing Mobility and Activity Level Patients who are have some degree of immobility are at a higher risk for developing pressure ulcers, and should be closely monitored to detect early signs of the formation of pressure-related wounds (Wound, Ostomy and Continence Nurses Society [WOCNS], 2010). See Chapter 32 if you need additional information about activity and mobility.

Assessing Treated Wounds

All wounds require a focused assessment. Assessment frequency depends on the condition of the wound, the work setting, the patient's overall condition and underlying disease process, the type of wound, and the type of treatment used for the wound. If you are providing wound care, you will assess the wound with every treatment. Assessment parameters include the following. Also, for a wound assessment summary,

 Go to Chapter 35, **Assessment Guidelines and Tools, Physical Examination: Wound Assessment,** in Volume 2.

Location Describe the wound location in anatomical terms. For example, describe an incision from cardiac surgery as a midsternal incision extending from the manubrium to the xiphoid process. An accurate description of the location is important because:

- *Location influences the rate of healing.* Wounds in highly vascular regions, such as the scalp or hands, heal more rapidly than wounds in less vascular regions, such as the abdomen or a heel.

- *Location affects movement.* Wounds that can be readily stabilized heal more rapidly than those in areas that are affected by the constant stress of movement.
- *Location can give you clues to the wound etiology.* A wound over a bony prominence could be related to pressure, whereas one on the bottom of the foot could be a diabetic foot ulcer.

Type of Wound Is it an acute wound? If the wound is sutured, examine the closure. Are the wound edges approximated (together)? Is there tension on any aspect of the wound? Are the stitches intact? Or is this a chronic wound?

Size Measure the length and width of the wound in centimeters. It is important that nurses use a ruler and measure a wound the same way. The NPUAP recommends using a head-to-toe orientation, the longest length head to toe, and the widest width side to side, perpendicular (90° angle) to length, encompassing the entire wound. Use serial photographs with grids showing the wound's dimensions, especially if the wound has an irregular border, to document the baseline and wound healing (European Pressure Ulcer Advisory Panel [EPUAP] and NPUAP, 2009). To measure wound depth, gently insert a sterile cotton-tip applicator into the deepest part of the wound. Measure the applicator from the tip in the wound bed to the skin level.

Undermining or Tunneling Assess the wound edges for any undermining or tunneling. Pay close attention to any tissue that appears to have a separation either in tissue type or plane, as frequently tunnels may be found. Measure the depth and location of any undermining or tunneling using the face of a clock as a guide. If the top of the wound is 12:00 and the bottom of the wound is 6:00, for example, record "2 cm of undermining is present from 1:00 to 4:00" or "6 cm tunnel exists at the center of the wound tracking in the 3:00 direction."

Periwound Examine the skin surrounding the wound. Skin discoloration may indicate a hematoma or additional injury to the surrounding tissue. Look for maceration, undermining, crepitus, blistering, erythema, and epiboly, slough, and eschar.

- **Maceration** is caused by excessive moisture from pooled drainage on intact skin for periods of time or when a moist dressing is inappropriately applied, left on too long, or overlaps onto healthy skin. The skin may appear as pale and wrinkled or "pruned," and may flake and peel.
- **Undermining** will produce a boggy feel around the wound.
- **Crepitus** is gas trapped under the skin. If you palpate the surrounding skin and feel a crackling sensation, this is crepitus. Crepitus may be due to air leaking from the lung in a chest wound or may indicate the presence of gas-producing bacteria.
- **Erythema**, **swelling**, or other signs of irritation indicate that the surrounding tissue is in jeopardy.

Quality and Safety Education for Nurses

Improving Wound Care With Information Technology

Competency: *Informatics (Knowledge); Quality Improvement (Knowledge); Evidenced-Based Practice (Attitudes)**

Situation: Information technology (IT) can have a significant impact on wound care management—from reducing documentation time to tracking outcomes. Extensive documentation of wound care is required for both clinical and reimbursement reasons. Electronic documentation systems eliminate duplication. They save time by using data entered once and adding it in all the other fields where it is required. This allows for more time to spend in patient care.

In addition to reducing paperwork, wound management software incorporates best practices into care management algorithms, decision supports, and alerts based on the type and stage of each wound. Changes in wound characteristics or new patient information initiates computer prompts that request more information or suggest treatment changes. For example, if the patient begins a new medication that can delay wound healing, a prompt may ask whether another medication may be used instead, or the prompt might suggest more frequent monitoring of wound characteristics.

When you upload photographs and multiple measurements of the patient's wound(s), they become part of the electronic care plan and pop up in chronological order so that you can visualize how the wound is healing. Clinicians can also set reminders for initiating future steps or referrals, eliminating the need to rely on memory and reducing errors.

Think about it: Informatics is the use of information and technology to communicate, manage knowledge, mitigate error, and support decision making. Can you think of how other patient conditions can benefit from specific management software? What might the information technology software look like for patients with high blood pressure or obesity?

➤ What data would be collected?

➤ What information might be generated from the data?

➤ What errors might be prevented?

For specific Knowledge, Skills, and Attitudes,

 Go to the QSEN Web site at **http://qsen.org/ competencies/pre-licensure-ksas/**

Source: DeGaspari, J. (2013). Not skin deep: Lower costs and better outcomes in wound care. *Healthcare Informatics.* Retrieved from http://www.healthcare-informatics.com/article/not-skin-deep-lower-costs-and-better-outcomes-wound-care

Epiboly is closed or rolled wound edges. Examine wound edges for epithelial tissue and contraction. Epiboly may indicate that epithelial cells have moved down and rolled under the wound edges. Once the cells reach the wound bed, they will stall wound healing.

Slough is usually soft, stringy, and pale yellow or gray.

Eschar, also known as an *unstageable pressure ulcer*, is thick, hard, and black or brown.

Extent and Type of Tissue in Wound Base Assessment of the types of tissue and their amounts can give you an idea of the severity of the wound, treatment options, and/or healing of the wound. Table 35-4 outlines different types of tissue you might see in a wound bed. Viable (living) tissue must be distinguished from nonviable tissue. Many wounds may have different types of tissue at the same time. Describe each type with percentages. For example, "80% of the wound bed contains granulation tissue, and 20% remains necrotic." Granulation tissue is evidence of healing. A pale color or dry texture may indicate a delay in healing. Necrotic tissue of any type will delay wound healing and should be removed. The exception is stable eschar on a heel that is firmly attached to the healthy wound edges without signs of infection.

Drainage Determine whether exudate is present. If so, describe the amount, color, consistency, and odor. Compare changes in the exudate to the patient's previous status.

- *Amount.* Describe the amount as none, light, moderate, or heavy. Drainage amounts vary according to the type of wound (i.e., venous stasis ulcers usually produce more drainage than arterial ulcers).

- *Drains.* If a drain is present, measure the amount of fluid in the collection container.
- *Color.* Describe the color or consistency as serous or clear, serosanguineous, sanguineous, purulent, or seropurulent (composed of serum and pus).
- *Odor.* Describe odor as absent, faint, moderate, or strong. Clean the wound of all exudate or foreign material before assessing for odor because odor characteristics vary depending on the wound moisture, organisms, amount of nonviable tissue, or types of dressings used. Odor may indicate fistula formation or bacterial contamination. For example, if a patient has an abdominal wound that was odorless but begins to smell of bile or feces, you should carefully assess for presence of a fistula.

Wound and Tissue Pain Routinely ask your patients about pain or discomfort related to the wound or wound care (EPUAP and NPUAP, 2009). You will need to develop a pain management plan if the patient is uncomfortable. Always take seriously the patient's complaint of pain, especially if there is a sudden increase. Pain is often an early symptom of infection. In the immunocompromised patient, pain may be the only symptom of infection.

Nutritional Status Screen and assess the nutritional status of each patient admitted with a pressure ulcer; and whenever there is a change in the patient's condition (WOCNS, 2010). A referral to the dietitian for early assessment and intervention may be necessary if nutritional problems are present. Sufficient calories are needed for wound healing. This may involve adding oral supplemental meals, or even enteral or parenteral nutrition (Association for the Advancement of Wound Care, 2005, revised 2010).

Table 35-4 ▶ Types of Tissue in the Wound Bed

TYPE OF TISSUE	DESCRIPTION	NURSING GOAL
Slough	Soft, moist, devitalized (necrotic) tissue; may be white, yellow, tan; may be stringy, loose, or adherent to bed.	Debride the wound.
Eschar	Necrotic tissue; dry, thick, leathery; may be black, brown, or gray depending on moisture level.	Debride the wound.
Granulation Tissue	Pink to red moist tissue; made of new blood vessels, connective tissue, and fibroblasts; surface is granular or pebble-like.	Cleanse, protect. Promote epithelialization.
Clean, Nongranulating	Absence of granulation tissue, but bed is pink, shiny, and smooth.	Cleanse, protect. Promote growth of healthy tissue.
Epithelial	Regenerating epidermis; may appear pink or pearly white as it crosses the wound bed; may begin as a ring around the wound or from epithelial cells lining hair follicles.	Cleanse, protect.

Assessing Untreated Wounds

For an untreated wound, make the same assessments as for a treated wound. Also, make additional assessments that allow you to determine the immediate treatment needed. For example, assess for bleeding. If bleeding is profuse, apply direct pressure to the site. If bleeding continues after you apply pressure for 5 minutes or if blood is spurting from the wound, call the provider immediately. Severe pain, numbness, or loss of movement below the wound also requires immediate, comprehensive evaluation. For a description of focused assessment for an untreated wound,

 Go to Chapter 35, **Assessment Guidelines and Tools, Physical Examination: Wound Assessment,** in Volume 2.

Also determine whether the patient needs a tetanus immunization. Tetanus-prone wounds include compound fractures, gunshot wounds, crush injuries, burns, punctures, foreign object injuries, wounds contaminated with soil, and wounds neglected for more than 24 hours. An immunization should be given if:

- The last immunization was 10 years ago or longer (Immunization Action Coalition, U.S. Department of Health and Human Services, Centers for Disease Control and Prevention [CDC], 2012).
- The wound is contaminated with dirt or debris or is a burn, and the most recent tetanus immunization was given more than 5 years ago.
- It is uncertain when the patient last received an immunization.

Evaluating Pressure Ulcer Healing

In addition to the Braden and Norton risk assessments previously described, the Agency for Healthcare Research and Quality (AHRQ) and NPUAP recommend use of the *PUSH tool* to evaluate pressure ulcers (NPUAP, 1998). The tool provides a comprehensive means of reporting the progression of a pressure ulcer. Surface area, exudate, and type of wound tissue are scored and totaled. As the ulcer heals, the total score falls. To see the PUSH tool,

 Go to Chapter 35, **Assessment Guidelines and Tools, The PUSH Tool for Evaluation of Pressure Ulcers,** in Volume 2.

Laboratory Data

You should integrate laboratory data with your history and physical assessment findings. The most common laboratory assessments related to skin integrity are protein levels, complete blood count, erythrocyte sedimentation rate, glucose, thyroid and iron levels, coagulation studies, and wound cultures. To learn more about these tests and see the normal ranges,

 Go to Chapter 35, **Diagnostic Testing: Tests for Assessing Wounds,** in Volume 2.

Wound cultures may be ordered to determine the types of bacteria present. Local or systemic signs of infection, suddenly elevated glucose levels, pain in a neuropathic extremity, or lack of healing after 2 weeks in a clean wound may indicate the need for a wound culture. Cultures may be obtained by swab, aspiration, or tissue biopsy.

Swabbing The most common and most noninvasive method to obtain a culture is with a swab. Swab specimens have been shown to be acceptably accurate in representing bacteria counts biopsied from a wound (Mutluoglu, Uzun, Turhan, et al., 2012). The WOCNS (2007, revised 2011) recommends using swab cultures as a reasonable alternative to biopsy in the clinical setting. However, other recent studies refute this, claiming deep tissue biopsies are the most accurate way to detect infection (Aggarwal, Higuera, Deimemgian, et al., 2013).

The Highlights of Procedures box summarizes swabbing. For the full procedure,

 Go to Chapter 35, **Procedure 35-1: Obtaining a Wound Culture by Swab,** in Volume 2.

Needle Aspiration Specifically trained providers (e.g., physicians, advanced practice nurses) may perform needle aspiration of a wound. This involves insertion of a needle into the tissue to aspirate tissue fluid. Organisms present in the tissue fluid can then be detected. Needle aspiration is an invasive procedure, with the risk of inadvertent needle damage to tissue and underlying structures.

Tissue Biopsy The most accurate method for culturing a chronic wound is *tissue biopsy.* It has long been considered the "gold standard." Tissue is removed from the wound edge by a specially trained provider. However, many facilities do not have the equipment needed to process tissue samples. This is an invasive procedure. It creates a risk of sepsis, causes pain, and disrupts the wound bed, sometimes delaying healing.

KnowledgeCheck 35-7

- What should be included in a wound assessment?
- What is the preferred method of wound culture that may be performed by a registered nurse (RN)?
- Identify three types of laboratory data that may be associated with a delay in wound healing.

What Assessments Can I Delegate?

Initial assessment of a wound, as well as ongoing evaluation of a wound that requires treatment, must be done by the RN. You may delegate to nursing assistive personnel (NAP) inspection of the skin for evidence of skin breakdown. Instruct the NAP to notify you of redness, tissue warmth, or drainage that they observe during their care of the patient. You may also delegate turning and position changes to the NAP. You must provide them with the times for the turning and how they should position the patient at each turn. A turning chart at the bedside is helpful. Turning and movement prevent tissue damage from ischemia, thereby preventing pressure ulcers.

ANALYSIS/NURSING DIAGNOSIS

The following nursing diagnoses are appropriate for patients who are at risk for skin breakdown or for patients who have wounds.

- *Risk for Impaired Skin Integrity* is appropriate for patients who have one or more risk factors for skin breakdown (e.g., immobility, incontinence, extremes of age, impaired circulation, impaired sensation, undernutrition, emaciation). NANDA International (2009) recommends that you use a risk assessment tool (e.g., Norton or Braden scale) to identify these patients.
- *Impaired Skin Integrity* is appropriate for patients who have experienced damage to the epidermis or dermis, for example, patients who have superficial wounds or stage I or II pressure ulcers.
- *Impaired Tissue Integrity* is appropriate for patients with wounds that extend into the subcutaneous tissue, muscle, or bone. Use this diagnosis for patients with deep wounds or stage III or IV pressure ulcers.
- *Risk for Impaired Tissue Integrity* is appropriate for clients with Impaired Skin Integrity who are at risk for delayed healing. For example, Mr. Harmon (Meet Your Patient) has a stage I pressure ulcer but is at risk for further progression of the ulcer because of his age, nutritional state, and the presence of another wound. Note that this is not a NANDA-I diagnosis; however, it is useful in the situation described.

Skin problems and wounds can be the etiology for other nursing diagnoses as well, for example:

- *Risk for Infection* is an appropriate diagnosis if the patient has a traumatic wound or is immunosuppressed, undernourished, or immobile.
- *Pain* is a diagnosis that may be used for patients who are experiencing discomfort from the wound or from the treatments required to heal the wound.
- *Disturbed Body Image* should be used if the patient is experiencing distress about the wound. Consider this diagnosis even if the patient is expected to make a complete recovery. Some patients experience extreme distress about wounds. You will certainly want to consider this diagnosis if the patient experiences an injury that is expected to result in disfigurement.

PLANNING OUTCOMES/EVALUATION

For associated NOC standardized outcomes for skin and tissue integrity diagnoses,

 Go to Chapter 35, **Standardized Language, Selected Standardized Outcomes and Interventions for Skin and Wound Diagnoses,** in Volume 2.

Individualized goals/outcome statements should address the need to maintain intact skin or heal the wound. For patients who have a diagnosis of Risk for Impaired Skin Integrity, you might write a goal such as the following:

Maintains intact skin throughout treatment, as evidenced by good skin turgor with no erythema, edema, or breaks in the skin.

For patients who have a wound (actual Impaired Skin Integrity or Impaired Tissue Integrity), you might write a goal such as the following:

Wound will heal by May 1, as evidenced by a progressive decrease in the size of the wound, a decrease in drainage from the wound, improvement in the condition of the surrounding skin, and no evidence of infection (erythema, purulent drainage, or odor).

PLANNING INTERVENTIONS/IMPLEMENTATION

For NIC standardized interventions for skin and tissue integrity problems,

 Go to Chapter 35, **Standardized Language, Selected Standardized Outcomes and Interventions for Skin and Wound Diagnoses,** in Volume 2.

Specific nursing activities directed at maintaining skin integrity or healing wounds focus on preventing and treating pressure ulcers and other chronic wounds, providing wound care, and applying heat and cold therapies. In the next section, we discuss these nursing therapeutic measures.

Interventions for Example Problem: Pressure Ulcers?

Pressure ulcers are extremely difficult and time-consuming to treat. As a result, prevention is the most important nursing intervention. Healthy People 2020 proposed two public health objectives focused on pressure-related skin injury: 1) to reduce the proportion of nursing home residents with a current diagnosis of pressure ulcers, and 2) to reduce the rate of pressure ulcer-related hospitalizations among older adults (U.S. Department of Health and Human Services, 2010, updated 2013). The ICSI (2012) has made preventing pressure ulcers one of 12 goals in its 5 Million Lives Campaign. Institute for Healthcare Improvement (IHI) recommended the six crucial elements in preventing pressure ulcers discussed in the following sections (IHI, 2011).

Conduct a Pressure Ulcer Admission Assessment for All Patients

Most agencies use a standardized risk assessment, such as the Braden and Norton scales, to assess the risk of pressure ulcers (see the previous section, Assessment).

You should use these scales to assess every patient on admission to any type of facility (hospital, nursing home, or with home health care). Risk factors found in addition those on the scales will place your patient at even higher risk. Examples include age, fever, incontinence, immobility, hypotension, and poor dietary intake, edema.

Reassess Risk for All Patients Daily

✚ Reassess your hospitalized patient for risk daily because his condition can change frequently and rapidly. Any time your patient's condition changes or he is transferred to another unit, reassess his risk. Monitor a nursing home resident weekly for the first 4 weeks, then quarterly or whenever the patient's condition changes or deteriorates. Reassess home patients at every visit (WOCNS, 2007, revised 2011).

Once a patient is identified as being at risk for developing pressure ulcers, prevention strategies can be implemented. Inform all members of the healthcare team (i.e., physical therapists, transporters, physicians, dietitians) of at-risk patients. Using visual cues, such as stickers on charts or dots on ID bands, can help remind staff.

Inspect Skin Daily

Skin care begins with regular inspection of the skin—at least daily for patients at risk—and usually every 8 to 12 hours for institutionalized patients. You must have adequate light to detect subtle, early skin changes. Use a penlight to inspect bony prominences if direct sunlight is not available. Be sure to check pressure points for erythema, tenderness, or edema. Instruct family members and caregivers about the importance of early detection of skin problems. In obese patients, skin damage can occur under breasts, under abdominal folds, between thighs, or anywhere skin is in contact with skin.

Manage Moisture

Excess moisture creates a risk for skin breakdown. Use the following nursing actions to help you manage moisture:

Incontinence Care Check the patient at regular intervals (e.g., when turned) and provide skin care as soon as possible after each incontinent episode. Apply incontinence or moisture barrier creams to protect perineal skin from urine and stool (WOCNS, 2010). Wipes and spray skin protectant products are comparable in preventing moisture-related skin breakdown. Wipes are more cost effective during hospitalization; however, the spray product preserves skin integrity over a longer period of time, beyond average hospitalization duration (Brunner, Droegemueller, Rivers, et al., 2012). Use undergarments or products that wick moisture away from the skin. For persistent bowel incontinence, consider using a pouching system or fecal containment device to contain protect the skin from the effluent

(National Guideline Clearinghouse [NGC], 2006, revised 2014).

Bathing Soaps and bathing techniques can contribute to skin breakdown, so be careful to keep the skin clean and intact. Diaphoretic (sweaty) patients may need frequent bathing, as sweat can be irritating to sensitive or injury-prone skin. Older adults most likely will not need daily bathing because they experience decreased oil and sweat production. Use warm, distilled or filtered water—not hot. Hot water dries the skin, especially for older adults. Gently bathe fragile skin, using a minimum of force and friction; washcloths can be abrasive. Use a mild, emollient cleansing soap only if needed and not routinely. Be sure to rinse thoroughly and gently pat the skin dry. Soaps are drying to the skin because they remove skin oils and may interfere with the ability of the skin to hold water (Ayello & Sibbald, 2012, updated; Joanna Briggs Institute, 2007).

Lotion and Massage If the patient's skin is dry, apply a moisturizing lotion using a gentle massaging motion to promote circulation and wound healing.

✚ Do not massage over bony prominences, as this can irritate the area and lead to tissue injury (NPUAP, 2007; National Guideline Clearinghouse [NGC], 2006, revised 2014).

Linens Keep the linens soft, clean, dry, and free from wrinkles by changing or straightening them frequently. Moisture and wrinkles in the sheets can damage skin integrity.

Optimize Nutrition and Hydration

Nutrition is vital to skin integrity. Patients with rapid weight loss, high metabolic demands, limited intake, or decreased serum albumin levels are particularly at risk for pressure ulcer development. Monitor hydration status and offer water (if appropriate) whenever you reposition the patient. Patients at risk and those with pressure ulcers should take 1 mL of fluid with every kcal consumed per day (National Guideline Clearinghouse [NGC], 2006, revised 2014).

Carefully review the diet ordered for at-risk patients, and assess what the patient is eating. The diet may need to be modified to achieve adequate calorie and protein intake. Protein requirements are 1.25 to 1.5 grams per kilogram of body weight per day (National Guideline Clearinghouse [NGC], 2006, revised 2014) or may be as high as 2 g/kg/day for deeper pressure ulcers or multiple wound sites, so high-protein supplements are often prescribed (Collins & Schnitzer, 2013). Individuals with nutritional and pressure ulcer risks require 30 to 35 kcal per kilogram of body weight per day (NGC, 2006, revised 2011).

Consider the consistency of the diet as well. A soft diet may be helpful for a patient who is frail or is missing teeth. Tube feeding or parenteral nutrition may be prescribed to supplement oral intake if the patient is unable to consume adequate quantities of calories and protein. You may need to make a dietary referral.

Minimize Pressure

Most patients who are at risk for pressure ulcers have mobility problems. As a result, you must provide frequent position changes. This is one of the most important interventions for preventing pressure ulcers. You may delegate turning and position changes to the NAP. Turning and movement prevent tissue damage from ischemia, thereby preventing pressure ulcers (Joanna Briggs Institute, 2008a, 2008b).

Turning and Repositioning Reposition the patient at least every 2 hours (Armstrong, Ayello, Capitulo, et al., 2008; Bergstrom, Bennett, Carlson, et al., 1994; NPUAP, 2007; WOCNS, 2010). However, patients with very fragile skin or little subcutaneous tissue might need to be repositioned more frequently. At-risk individuals who are chair bound should be repositioned every hour or taught to shift their weight every 15 minutes. Place a turning schedule at the bedside so that all caregivers can participate in the prevention strategy. For an example of a patient turning schedule,

 Go to Chapter 35, **Tables, Boxes, Figures: ESG Box 35-2, Scheduled Position Changes,** on Davis*Plus*.

Use the Rule of 30 to guide your positioning: Elevate the head of the bed 30° or less, and when the patient is on her side, position the patient at a 30° angle to avoid direct pressure on the trochanter. If the head of the bed is elevated more than 30°, limit the time in this position to minimize pressure and shear (NPUAP, 2007).

To protect skin during turning or repositioning, use lift devices or draw sheets, heel and elbow protectors, or sleeves and stockings. Never drag a patient when pulling her up in bed. Use a minimum of two people when moving patients in bed National Guideline Clearinghouse [NGC], 2006, revised 2014).

Support Surfaces Various support surfaces are available for preventing and treating pressure ulcers. They do so by redistributing pressure and controlling moisture to prevent bacterial growth on the skin (microclimate between the skin and the surface of the bed). Support surfaces for redistributing pressure include specialty mattresses, and alternating and dynamic bed systems. These products may consist of static air, alternating air, gel, foam, or fluid, and are available in several sizes and shapes for beds, chairs, exam tables, and operating room tables (Fig. 35-10). Limit the number of linen layers between the treatment support surface and patient (ICSI, 2012).

Any patient at risk should be placed on a pressure-redistributing device. People lying on ordinary foam mattresses are more likely to get pressure ulcers than those lying on a higher-specification foam mattress (McInnes, Jammali-Blasi, Bell-Sye, et al., 2011). Support surfaces alone will not prevent skin breakdown but should be coupled with effective turning and positioning schedules (NPUAP, EPUAP, 2009).

Protect heels by using products that completely raise the heels off the bed (ICSI, 2012). Pillows may not be enough to redistribute the weight of your patient's foot. Pressure redistributing devices are also made for chairs and wheelchairs. Donut-type devices, bunny boots, rigid splint, IV bags, rolled towels or sheet, and sheepskin should not be used (NPUAP, 2007; WOCNS, 2010; National Guideline Clearinghouse [NGC], 2006, revised 2014).

To see a decision-making tree developed by the AHRQ to guide selection of appropriate support surfaces,

 Go to Chapter 35, **Tables, Boxes, Figures: ESG Figure 35-2: Decision Tree Guiding Selection of Appropriate Support Surfaces,** on Davis*Plus*.

What Are Adjunctive Wound Care Therapies?

The use of adjunctive therapies is the fastest growing area in pressure-related wound management. Nurses apply adjunctive therapies that include negative pressure wound therapy, electrical stimulation, hyperbaric oxygen, radiant heat, tissue growth factors, ultrasound, bioengineered skin equivalents, and surgical options.

- **Negative Pressure Wound Therapy.** Negative pressure wound therapy (NPWT) promotes healing by secondary and tertiary intention. Using a specialized pump, negative pressure is placed on a wound packed with foam or gauze dressings to create a vacuum. The subatmospheric pressure improves wound healing by reducing the edema in swollen tissues; promoting granulation tissue formation; and removing exudate and infectious material. Negative pressure promotes granulation tissue formation by "stretching" cells and stimulating blood vessel growth and wound perfusion. The Highlights of Procedures box summarizes this procedure. For complete guidelines,

 Go to Chapter 35, **Procedure 35-6: Applying a Negative Pressure Wound Therapy (NPWT) Device,** in Volume 2.

- **Silver Dressing.** Silver-coated dressings or silver-based cream may act as a barrier to bacterial penetration in the wound bed. Silver may eradicate biofilms of colonized bacteria.

Go to Chapter 35, **Tables, Boxes, Figures: ESG Table 35-1: Silver Dressings Used in Chronic Wound Management,** on Davis*Plus*.

- **Electrical Stimulation.** Electrical currents are transferred across tissues to aid in chronic wound healing.

Electrodes are placed around the wound bed and connected to a machine that produces an electrical impulse. This therapy stimulates cellular growth through development of fibroblasts, new collagen, and increased blood flow and tissue oxygenation.

- **Hyperbaric Oxygen Therapy.** Hyperbaric oxygen therapy (HBOT) is the administration of 100% oxygen under pressure. HBOT increases oxygen concentration in the tissue, stimulates the growth of new blood vessels, and enhances white blood cell (WBC) action.

- **Tissue Growth Factors.** Tissue growth factors are proteins that occur naturally in the body and cause specific cells to grow and replicate. Platelet-derived growth factor has been used in chronic wound healing. It is indicated for diabetic and other nonhealing wounds that are free of necrotic tissue and have good vascularity.

- **Ultrasound.** Another adjunctive therapy used in chronic wound healing is ultrasound. Sound waves are emitted by a control unit and handheld sound head or transducer. Vibrations from the transducer create sound waves that pass into the tissue, causing it to vibrate and heat up. This stimulates movement of fluid within and between cells and aids in debridement and increased cell metabolism.

- **Bioengineered Skin Substitutes.** This is a group of substances that aids in the temporary or permanent closure of wounds. Substitutes may be actual human epidermis or dermis from organ donation, animal cells, or synthetic material. They can be used to treat partial- and full-thickness wounds.

- **Surgical Options.** Complicated wounds require the use of surgical options, such as extensive debridement, skin grafts, secondary closure of the wound, and **flap techniques** (partially detached and rotated tissue placed over a wound to fill in the deficit).

KnowledgeCheck 35-8

- Identify the major interventions for preventing pressure ulcers.
- What nursing diagnosis is most appropriate for a patient at risk for pressure ulcer development?

What Patient and Family Teaching Do I Need to Do?

Teaching the at-risk patient and family about pressure ulcer prevention is a key prevention strategy. Include the following topics in your teaching:

- Characteristics of healthy skin
- Appearance of skin that has experienced unrelieved pressure
- Skin care and hygiene
- Protection of the skin and prevention of pressure ulcers
- Importance of adequate nutrition
- Techniques for turning and positioning
- Importance of frequent position changes
- Use of pressure-redistributing devices

- Skin changes that should be reported to healthcare professionals

The following are some simple tips for taking care of wounds at home that you can teach families (ICSI, 2012). If the wound is:

Wet → dry it
Open → cover it
Unclean → clean it
Necrotic → don't scrub it
Dry → moisten it

What Wound Care Competencies Do I Need?

Care planning to meet the complex, individualized needs of a patient with a chronic wound involves the entire multidisciplinary team (e.g., physical therapists, dietitians, infection control specialist, wound specialist). Your wound assessment will guide your choice of interventions, which depend on the nature of the wound. Consider these two examples:

- A patient with a diabetic foot ulcer must have all the pressure taken off that area because every step traumatizes healing tissues. The appropriate dressing must be selected; in addition, this patient will need to wear a special shoe that is specially made for patients with neuropathy.

- Patients with a venous stasis ulcer commonly wear compression garments (e.g., elastic hose, stocking, or multilayer compression wrap). These provide continuous pressure to the veins, which improves venous return and helps the ulcer to heal (O'Meara, Cullum, Nelson, et al., 2012). Before applying elastic compression, be sure the limb is not increasing in edema. Lower extremity arterial disease must be ruled out before applying compression as it can compromise arterial circulation. Avoid thigh-high elastic stockings because they tend to roll and cause a tourniquet effect (ICSI, 2012). See Chapter 32 if you need more information about compression stockings.

Wound care is more than placing a dressing into a wound. It incorporates all of the strategies for preventing that wound, as well as treating it. ESG Box 35-1 lists RN competencies for treating pressure ulcers (NPUAP, 2010). These interventions can also be used in treating other types of acute and chronic wounds.

Go to Chapter 35, **Tables, Boxes, Figures: ESG Box 35-1, Competencies of Registered Nurses for Treating Pressure Ulcers,** on Davis*Plus.*

Cleansing Wounds

Cleansing removes exudate, slough, foreign materials, and microorganisms from the wound. This helps promote healthy tissue healing. Always clean a wound initially and with each dressing change. To cleanse a wound, gently pat the surface with gauze soaked with saline or other prescribed wound cleanser. If there is granulation tissue, be careful not to disrupt it.

Historically, antiseptic solutions, such as Dakin's, acetic acid, hydrogen peroxide, povidone-iodine, chlorhexidine, and alcohol, were used to cleanse all types of wounds. However, antiseptic solutions can damage granulating tissue and should not be used on healing tissue (AHRQ, 2005, updated 2010). Recent clinical evidence suggests that polyhexanide/betaine may be nontoxic and effective in enhancing wound healing (Wilkins & Unverdorben, 2013). Antiseptic solutions should be reserved for new wounds, those that won't heal, or wounds in which the bacterial burden is more harmful than the solution itself.

Because normal saline is physiological, it is safe and it will not harm injured or healing tissue. It will adequately cleanse most wounds if a sufficient amount is used to thoroughly flush the wound. Drinkable tap water can also be used to cleanse wounds (WOCNS, 2010) and is as effective as saline (Fernandez & Griffith, 2008, 2012). However, the decision to use tap water should be based on the nature and complexity of the wound and the patient's general condition, including the presence of comorbid conditions (e.g., diabetes) and immunological status (Watret & McLean, 2013). Additionally, there is some concern over biofilm in hospital water delivery systems (Christina, Spagnola, Casini, et al., 2014). To reduce this risk of microbial contamination, purified water instead of tap should be used for cleansing wounds.

Liquid or foam skin cleansers that are pH balanced may be used to cleanse periwound skin or incontinence effluent. They are not for use in wounds. **Key Point:** *The most important thing to remember is to use universal precautions to minimize the risk of cross-contamination when cleansing periwound or other non-wound skin.*

Irrigating Wounds

Nurses commonly use irrigation (**lavage**) to cleanse wounds by flushing. To remove debris from a wound, introduce the irrigation solution with a gentle amount of force. Ideal irrigation pressures range from 4 pounds per square inch (psi) to 15 psi. To remove material adhering to the wound bed use a 35-mL syringe attached to a 19-gauge angiocatheter to deliver the solution at approximately 8 psi (ICSI, 2012). Pressures above 15 psi increase the risk of driving bacteria into the tissues, as well as causing mechanical damage.

Some agencies use a piston syringe for irrigation. Do not use a bulb syringe as it increases the risk of aspirating the drainage. Commercial irrigation systems are also available, such as whirlpool agitators, whirlpool hose sprayers, pressurized canisters, and pulsed lavages. Closely evaluate the amount of pressure they deliver before you use these devices. High-pressure irrigation systems (35–70 psi) may dislodge healing granulation tissue, especially in chronic wounds. High pressure can cause pain and also drive bacteria deeper into the wound compartment, leading to increased risk of infection (Gabriel & Schraga, 2013, updated).

There is a risk of splattering when irrigating, so you need to use gowns, masks, and goggles. Sterile technique is used for acute surgical wounds, wounds that have recently undergone sharp debridement, or when prescribed by the provider. The majority of wound irrigations use clean technique. The Highlights of Procedures box provides a summary of the procedure. For the complete steps,

Go to Chapter 35, **Procedure 35-2: Performing a Sterile Wound Irrigation,** in Volume 2.

Caring for Wounds With Drainage Devices

A variety of drains may be inserted into wounds to allow fluid and exudate to exit. Drains prevent excessive pressure from building up in the tissues. Drains are usually

Toward Evidence-Based Practice

Fernandez, R., & Griffiths, R. (2012). The effects of water compared with other solutions for wound cleansing. *Cochrane Database of Systematic Reviews*, 2; Art. No.: CD003861. doi:10.1002/14651858.CD003861.pub3. Retrieved from http://summaries.cochrane.org/CD003861/the-effects-of-water-compared-with-other-solutions-for-wound-cleansing

Use of saline versus tap water for cleansing wounds is debated. Normal saline is traditionally preferred because it cleanses without interfering with the normal healing process. However, tap water is used commonly in the community for cleaning wounds and for care of chronic wounds because it is generally free of pathogens, while easily accessible and inexpensive. Analysis of findings from 24 clinical studies showed no differences in the rates of infections among

acute and chronic wounds in adults and children cleansed with tap water compared with those washed with saline.

1. What trend in the research about cleansing wounds do you see compared with previous times?

2. If study findings indicate little difference in wound infection when tap water is used for cleansing, then what would you recommend to those using tap water in the community?

3. What implications does using tap water for cleaning wounds have when sending patients home after surgery?

 Go to Chapter 35, **Toward Evidence-Based Practice Suggested Responses,** on Davis*Plus*.

placed during a surgical procedure. Some are sutured into place, whereas others are simply placed into the cavity.

Types of Drains

A *Penrose drain* is a flexible, flat latex tube that is placed in the wound bed but usually not sutured into place. A clip or pin may be attached to the drain at the insertion site to keep it from slipping into the wound. You may be asked to advance the drain by gradually removing it from the wound bed. For example, the surgeon may prescribe, "Advance the Penrose drain 6 mm (1/4 in.) per day." Each day you will pull the drain out of the wound 6 mm (1/4 in.) until the drain is finally removed. The Highlights of Procedures box summarizes this procedure. For complete guidelines,

 Go to Chapter 35, **Procedure 35-13: Shortening a Wound Drain,** in Volume 2.

Some drains are attached to a collection device. Examples include Hemovac and Jackson-Pratt and drains (Fig. 35-11). The provider may order a device to be "placed to suction." This means you will compress the device to create suction and facilitate removal of drainage (Fig. 35-12). The Highlights of Procedures box summarizes this procedure. For complete guidelines,

 Go to Chapter 35, **Procedure 35-14: Emptying a Closed-Wound Drainage System,** in Volume 2.

If a specific pressure is to be applied, some drains can be connected to wall suction. The provider will prescribe the amount of suction. For example: "Place Hemovac to 20 mm Hg suction at all times."

Nursing Activities for Maintaining Drains

As a nurse you are responsible for monitoring wound drains. The provider will describe the number and type of drains present. Describe drain placement according to the position on the clock face. Consider the patient's head to be at the 12 o'clock position. Some patients have more than

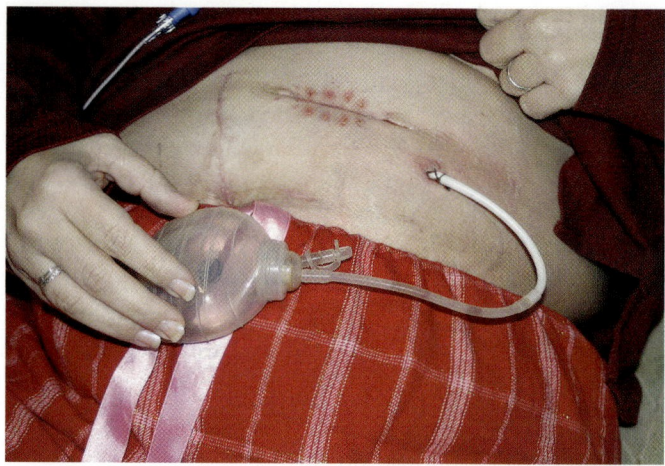

FIGURE 35-12 Compress the bulb of the Jackson-Pratt drain to create suction and remove wound drainage.

one drainage device in a wound. Label the drains numerically with a marker or by placing tape on the collection apparatus so that each caregiver provides consistent care.

When removing dressings or irrigating wounds, be very careful to avoid dislodging the drain. Remember, many drains are not sutured in place. Monitor the amount and character of the drainage and record this information in your nursing notes as well as on the intake and output (I&O) record.

Report to the provider any significant change in the amount or character of the drainage. If you suspect a drain is occluded, check the drain line from the insertion site to the collection device. Remove any kinks in the tubing. If this does not correct the problem, notify the provider of the blockage.

You need to empty the collection apparatus at a designated volume to maintain suction. As the device fills, suction pressure decreases. If there is significant drainage, you may need to empty the device several times during your shift.

KnowledgeCheck 35-9

- Identify goals for wound care before applying a dressing to a wound.
- What solutions are used to cleanse a wound?
- How can you control the amount of force applied for wound irrigation?
- Identify three nursing responsibilities when caring for a client with a wound drain.

ThinkLike a Nurse 35-5

- Describe the percentage and type of tissue found in Mr. Harmon's (Meet Your Patient) wounds.
- What are the goals of treatment for each of Mr. Harmon's wounds?

Debriding a Wound

Debridement is the removal of devitalized tissue or foreign material from a wound. It also helps remove cells that are alive but not functioning (**senescent**) from the

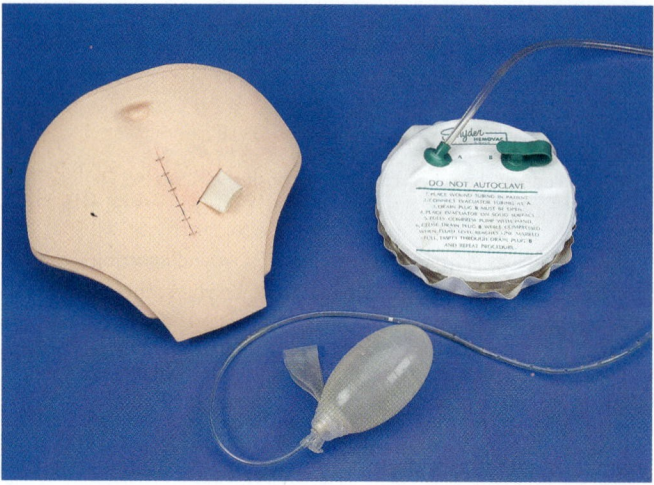

FIGURE 35-11 *Left,* Penrose drain. *Center,* Jackson-Pratt device. *Right,* Hemovac drainage system.

wound bed and edges. Removal of necrotic tissue, exudate, and infective material helps stimulate wound healing and prepare the wound bed for advanced therapies or biological agents. There are five types of debridement: sharp or surgical, mechanical, enzymatic, autolytic, and biotherapy or maggot therapy.

Sharp Debridement

Sharp debridement is the use of a sharp instrument, such as scalpel or scissors, to remove devitalized tissue. This method provides an immediate improvement of the wound bed and preserves granulation tissue. A physician, nurse, or physical therapist may perform this procedure at the bedside if they have received specialized training. If a wound requires extensive debridement, it may be performed in the operating room. Many stage IV ulcers extend into the bone, so a bone biopsy is often performed at the same time. The biopsy will detect **osteomyelitis**, extension of the infection into the bone.

Mechanical Debridement

Mechanical debridement may be performed via lavage (discussed in a preceding section), the use of wet-to-dry dressings, or hydrotherapy (whirlpool).

- **Wet-to-Dry Dressings.** Coarse gauze moistened with normal saline is packed into the wound, allowed to dry, and then removed, perhaps several times a day. This form of debridement was common once, but has declined in use because it causes pain and provides only **nonselective debridement.** That is, it removes not only debris but also granulation tissue. If you must use this method, medicate the patient beforehand with opioid analgesics. Rewetting the gauze aids in its removal and decreases the pain, but it may eliminate the debriding action of the dressing change.

- **Hydrotherapy or Whirlpool Treatments.** Hydrotherapy or whirlpool treatments also provide nonselective debridement. This is a vigorous form of debridement reserved for wounds with a large amount of nonviable tissue, such as burns. Hydrotherapy is usually performed in the physical therapy department once or twice per day. The wound is placed in a whirlpool containing tepid water for a prescribed amount of time (perhaps 5 to 15 minutes). Do not expose the wound directly to the water jets.

  Whirlpool treatments increase the risk for periwound maceration, contamination by waterborne infections, and cross-contamination. Therefore, strict adherence to infection control measures is essential. Use hydrotherapy with caution in patients with venous stasis ulcers because it leads to vasodilation, which may increase edema and congestion. Persons with diabetic neuropathies are at increased risk for burns because of a decrease in sensory abilities.

Enzymatic Debridement

Enzymatic debridement uses proteolytic agents to break down necrotic tissue without affecting viable tissue in the wound. To use an enzymatic product, clean the wound with normal saline, apply a thin layer of the cream, and cover with a moisture-retaining dressing. This may be done once or twice daily, depending on the product. Apply the product only to devitalized tissue because it might cause some local irritation.

Autolysis

Autolysis is the use of an occlusive, moisture-retaining dressing and the body's own enzymes and defense mechanisms to break down necrotic tissue. This process takes more time than the other techniques, but it is tolerated better. The procedure involves applying the dressing and observing the fluid that collects under it (wound fluid may be tan in color). The dressing is normally changed every 72 hours, or sooner if drainage breakthrough occurs. At that time, the wound is cleansed before a new dressing is applied. Observe the wound closely and regularly for signs of infection, such as an increase in pain or a foul odor. Autolysis is contraindicated in the presence of infection or immunosuppression.

Biotherapy or Maggot Debridement Therapy

Maggot debridement therapy is the use of medical-grade larvae of the greenbottle fly to dissolve dead and infected tissue from wounds. The larvae secrete enzymes that liquefy dead tissue and create an alkaline environment. The enzymes are neutralized when they come in contact with normal tissue, so healthy tissue is unharmed. The larvae also digest bacteria from the wound. This therapy is effective and simple to use, though containing the larvae within the dressing can be problematic (Opletalova, Blaizot, Mourgeon, et al., 2012). Larvae are usually changed every 48 to 72 hours and disposed of as biohazardous medical waste. The use of maggots can be emotionally disturbing to both patients and nurses, so take this into consideration and discuss it with the patient.

Providing Moist Wound Healing

A physiological wound environment is one that maintains the right amount of moisture for cells to flourish. More than 65% of the human body is composed of water. The skin maintains this level of moisture by allowing water vapor to escape into the air around us in small amounts. With damage to the skin, body cells can dehydrate and die, so wound dressings must function as a barrier to water vapor loss.

Primary **dressings** are ones that are placed in the wound bed and actually touch the wound. A **secondary dressing** is one that covers or holds a primary dressing in place. Many dressings can act as both, touching the wound bed and securing themselves to the wound with some type of adhesive. Figure 35-13 shows various sizes of gauze dressings.

The type of dressing used on a wound depends on the characteristics of the wound and the goals of treatment. The dressing of choice should:

- Prevent drying of the wound bed.
- Absorb drainage.
- Keep the surrounding tissue dry and intact.

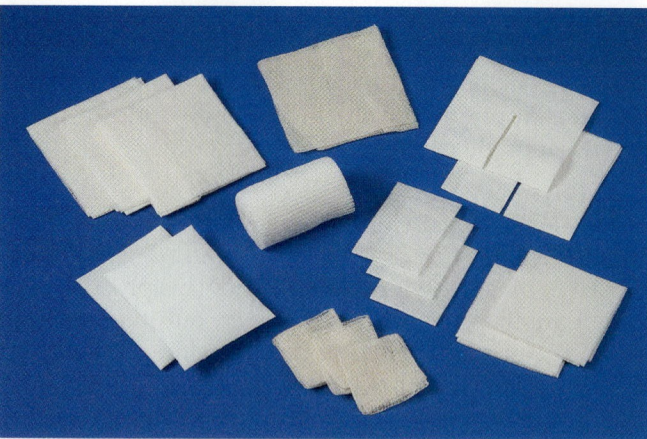

FIGURE 35-13 Gauze dressings are available in a variety of shapes and forms.

- Protect from contamination and infection.
- Aid in hemostasis.
- Debride the wound.
- Eliminate dead space.
- Prevent heat loss.
- Splint the wound site.
- Provide comfort to the patient.
- Control odor.
- Minimize scarring.

Choosing the Dressing

When choosing a dressing, ask yourself whether it will achieve the purposes listed above. Also consider how long the dressing should stay in place, how often it needs to be changed, and whether it can it be removed without damaging fragile skin or the wound itself (Table 35-5).

Ideally, the dressing will facilitate the goals of moist wound healing (preceding). There is no single "recipe" for healing a wound. Each wound must be treated and dressed individually based on the patient history and assessment. Many wound materials are available, and new products are continually introduced. The "newest" dressing is not necessarily the best for the wound. Many products carry hefty price tags, so it must be determined that the benefit achieved is worth the extra cost. Choose the dressing based on what the wound needs and not the manufacturer's brand name. Perform ongoing reassessment of your dressing choice every time you assess the wound, modifying dressings and treatments as the wound evolves.

The Highlights of Procedures box summarizes procedures for applying dry, wet-to-damp (moist-to-moist), transparent film, and hydrocolloid dressings. For complete steps,

 Go to Chapter 35, **Procedure 35-4: Removing and Applying Dry Dressings; Procedure 35-5: Removing and Applying Wet-to-Damp Dressings; Procedure 35-7: Applying and Removing a Transparent Film Dressing,** and **Procedure 35-8: Applying a Hydrating Dressing (Hydrocolloid or Hydrogel),** respectively, in Volume 2.

KnowledgeCheck 35-10

- What should you consider when choosing a dressing?
- Describe the five types of wound debridement.
- Identify the purposes of a wound dressing.
- Differentiate among the different categories of dressings.
- What types of dressings may be used for wounds with a large amount of exudate?
- What form of dressing is appropriate for a wound with an eschar that needs to be eliminated?

Securing Dressings

What you will use to secure a dressing depends on wound size, location, amount of drainage, frequency of dressing changes, patient's activity level, and type of dressings used. Tape, ties, bandages, secondary dressings, and binders are among the choices. Tape is most commonly used. It is available in several forms:

- **Adhesive tape** provides stability to a dressing. It is tough and durable and can be used if you need to apply pressure to a wound. It leaves a residue on the skin and can cause trauma to surrounding intact skin when it is removed. However, commercial adhesive removers are available to remove the residue and can be used to loosen tape as it is removed.
- **Foam tape** readily molds to the contours of the body and is ideal for dressings over joints.
- **Nonallergenic tape and paper tape** are best for sensitive skin. Ask patients whether they have any history of tape allergies or irritation, and use a tape that the patient has tolerated well in the past.

To tape a dressing, place strips of tape at the ends of the dressing, and space them evenly over the remainder of the dressing. The Highlights of Procedures box summarizes a procedure for taping dressings. To see the complete procedure,

 Go to Chapter 35, **Procedure 35-3: Taping a Dressing,** in Volume 2.

If a dressing requires frequent changes, you can use **Montgomery straps** with ties to secure the dressing (Fig. 35-15). Montgomery straps decrease the amount of pulling and irritation of skin around a wound. Apply the adhesive part of the straps to the skin at the ends of the dressing and at evenly spaced intervals. Lace the cloth ties between the straps to secure the dressing. Change the ties whenever they become soiled. Keep the straps in place until they begin to loosen from the skin.

Consider using thin hydrocolloids, low-adhesion foam dressings, or skin sealants under tape to also help prevent skin tears. For the fragile skin of older adults or infants, use porous tapes and avoid unnecessary tape use.

Controlling Infection

A wound provides a portal of entry or exit for microorganisms. When caring for patients with closed wounds, follow CDC Standard Precautions. For patients with

(text continued on page 928)

Table 35-5 ▶ Types of Wound Dressings

DRESSING TYPE AND DESCRIPTION	USE	CAUTIONS	WOUND SIZE
Absorbent dressings ■ Made from highly absorptive layers of fibers such as cellulose, cotton, or rayon ■ May or may not have an adhesive border. Procedure 35-4: Removing and Applying Dry Dressings Procedure 35-5: Removing and Applying Wet-to-Damp Dressings	■ Can be used as a primary or secondary dressing to manage drainage from partial- or full-thickness wounds. ■ Highly absorptive. Used for wounds with moderate to large amounts of drainage.	■ Do not use to pack undermining wounds. ■ Do not use if the wound is not draining. This can dry out the wound bed and damage tissue.	Moderate to large
Alginates ■ Fibers derived from brown seaweed and kelp. ■ Available in pad or rope form.	■ Very high absorbency (20 to 40 times their weight). ■ Promote a moist environment. ■ Facilitate autolytic debridement. ■ Ideal for wounds that have depth, tracts, tunneling, or undermining.	■ Will adhere to the wound bed if there is no drainage. ■ When the alginate comes in contact with exudate, a nonadhesive gel is created. Must irrigate this gel from the wound before placing the next dressing. ■ Allergy to antibiotic components, or to seaweed or kelp.	Large
Antimicrobials (Antibiotic & Antifungal) ■ Available as ointments, impregnated gauzes, pads, gels, foams, hydrocolloids, and alginates. ■ Commonly contain silver and cadexomer iodine.	■ Reduce exudate and prevent infection by reducing bacteria in the wound. ■ Promote collagen deposition. ■ Can be used on partial- or full-thickness wounds, malodorous wounds with little to large amounts of drainage, or highly contaminated or infected wounds.	■ Allergy to iodine or silver	Large
Collagens ■ Made from bovine (cow) or porcine (pig) sources and made into sheets, pads, powders, and gels.	■ Use with partial- and full-thickness and contaminated or infected wounds. ■ Absorb exudate. ■ Promote a moist wound bed for healing. ■ Stimulate wounds to produce collagen fibers and granulation tissue in the wound bed. ■ Do not stick to the wound bed and are easy to apply and remove.	**Key Point:** *If using porcine dressings, check that your patient has no religious practices that would forbid this use. In particular, check with your Jewish and Muslim patients.*	Minimal to large

Continued

Table 35-5 ▶ Types of Wound Dressings—cont'd

DRESSING TYPE AND DESCRIPTION	USE	CAUTIONS	WOUND SIZE
Foams ■ Made from semipermeable hydrophilic foam that forms an impermeable barrier over the wound. ■ Made into wafers, rolls, and pillows; have film coverings; and are adhesive or nonadhesive.	■ Absorbent; for wounds with moderate to heavy exudates. ■ Thermal insulation ■ Promote a moist environment. ■ Do not stick to wound bed. ■ Used under compression. ■ Protect friable periwound skin. ■ Can be shaped around body contours. ■ May be used in combination with alginates or films.	■ Do not use with wounds that have tunneling or tracts. ■ Not recommended for dry, desiccated wounds. ■ May macerate periwound skin, if dressing becomes oversaturated.	Minimal to large
Gauze ■ Simplest and most widely used dressings. ■ Made of woven and nonwoven fibers of cotton, rayon, polyester, or a combination of these. ■ Some are impregnated with antimicrobial agents, medications, or moisture, and others contain petrolatum to keep the wound moist.	■ Cleansing ■ Protection ■ Used for packing large wounds, cavities, or tracts, deep or dirty wounds, or heavily draining wounds. ■ Used in combination with amorphous hydrogels, saline, or medications. ■ May be packed as sterile or nonsterile, in bulk or in smaller packages.	■ Labor intensive ■ Can stick to wound tissue and damage new, regenerated cells with gauze removal. ■ Does not ensure a moist wound environment, as they allow for fluid evaporation. ■ May be applied incorrectly, as it must be fluffed to avoid pressure or overpacking of a wound. ■ Dressing change interval is dependent on the amount of fluid saturation of the gauze. Frequent dressing changes disrupt the wound bed and cause the wound to become hypothermic (cold), which physiologically impairs cell growth for healing.	Large
Hydrocolloids ■ Wafers, pastes, or powders that contain hydrophilic (water-loving) particles. 🏠 Procedure 35-8: Applying a Hydrating Dressing (Hydrocolloid or Hydrogel)	■ Hydrophilic particles interact with water to form a gel that keeps the wound moist. ■ Provide a protective layer against friction/caustic agents and bacteria. Also reduce pain. ■ Ideal for wounds with minimal exudates (e.g., partial thickness wounds, stage II pressure ulcers). ■ Promote autolysis.	■ Not the dressing of choice for wounds that require frequent dressing changes. ■ Opaque. Do not allow the wound to be visualized. ■ Not recommended for wounds surrounded by friable or sensitive skin (difficult to remove). ■ Should not be used on infected wounds because they are impermeable to oxygen, moisture, and bacteria.	Light to moderate

Table 35-5 ▷ Types of Wound Dressings—cont'd

DRESSING TYPE AND DESCRIPTION	USE	CAUTIONS	WOUND SIZE
	■ Used under compression. ■ Mold to the shape of the body, making them useful for difficult areas, such as heels or between buttocks. ■ Use around stomas to create an even surface on which to place the ostomy appliance. ■ Do not require a secondary dressing.	■ When an exudate comes in contact with the hydrocolloid material, it can produce an odor that might be confused with a malodorous wound. Clean the wound bed first before determining if it is malodorous. ■ May facilitate the growth of anaerobic bacteria. ■ Should not be used on wounds with tunneling or tracts because these wounds must be packed and allowed to drain. Wound should be shallow enough that the hydrocolloid touches the wound bed.	
Hydrogels ■ Sheets, granules, or gels with a high water content, creating a jelly-like consistency that does not adhere to the wound bed. Procedure 35-8: Applying a Hydrating Dressing (Hydrocolloid or Hydrogel)	■ Enhance epithelialization to promote a moist environment. ■ Rehydrate the wound bed. ■ Promote autolysis. ■ Soft, cooling texture promotes comfort. ■ Soften slough or eschar in necrotic wounds.	■ Have limited absorptive capabilities (not practical for wounds with significant exudate). Require a secondary dressing. ■ Easily macerate periwound skin due to high moisture content.	Minimal
Skin sealants and moisture barriers ■ Skin sealants—made from liquid transparent copolymer. ■ Moisture barrier ointments—petrolatum, dimethicone, or zinc-based products that can be applied to skin to protect it from exudate, moisture, urine, and feces.	■ Simple and fast to use, and if needed, should be used with each dressing change. ■ Can be wiped or sprayed on skin to protect it from wound exudate and moisture, friction, and skin stripping from adhesives. ■ Provide a barrier of protection over vulnerable skin from the effects of moisture and mechanical and chemical skin injury.	■ Ointments impair the adhesion of wound dressings or tapes.	Any
Transparent films **(See Fig. 35-14)** ■ Clear and semipermeable. Procedure 35-7: Applying and Removing a Transparent Film Dressing	■ Promote a moist environment. ■ Occlusive with oxygen permeability. ■ Promote autolysis. ■ Often used to dress IV sites. ■ Prevent external bacterial contamination. ■ Allow wound assessment without removing or disturbing the dressing. ■ Can be placed over joints without inhibiting movement.	■ If used over wounds that are draining, the tissues will become macerated. ■ Adhere to the skin, so do not use them on friable skin.	Minimal to none

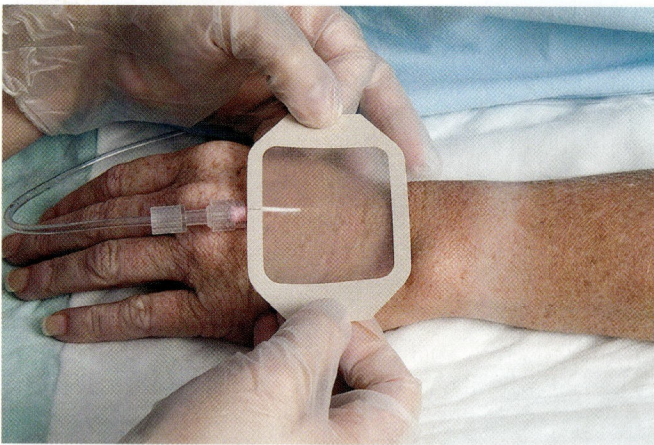

FIGURE 35-14 IV sites are commonly dressed with transparent film dressings.

open or draining wounds, follow CDC Tier Two: Contact Level Precautions in addition to Standard Precautions. See Chapter 23, and also,

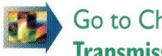 Go to Chapter 23, **Clinical Insight 23-4: Following Transmission-Based Precautions**, in Volume 2.

The following nursing activities will also aid in preventing and controlling wound infections:

Asepsis Measures

If the patient has an infection, place her in a private room or in a room with a patient who has an active infection caused by the same organism and no other infections. Follow any additional specific precautions for the microorganism identified. Most important, wash your hands frequently.

Use clean gloves when caring for the patient with a wound. Remove gloves and wash your hands before coming in contact with another patient. Change your gloves after removing a soiled dressing and before applying a clean dressing.

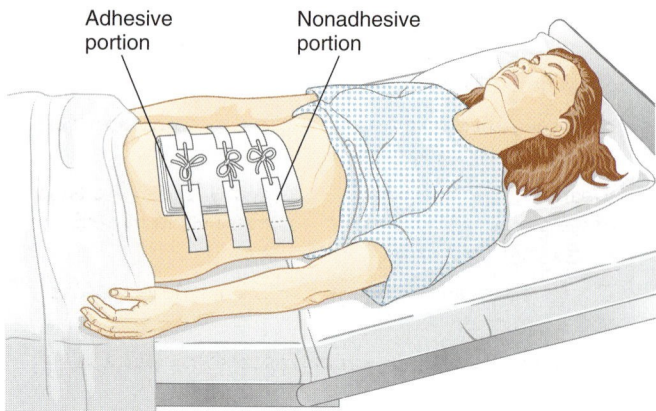

Adhesive portion   Nonadhesive portion

FIGURE 35-15 Montgomery straps with ties may be used to secure a dressing that requires frequent changing.

If a patient has multiple wounds, treat the least contaminated wound first, then progress to the most contaminated. Wash your hands and change gloves between each wound.

Sharp Debridement Use sterile instruments for sharp debridement. Monitor the patient for signs and symptoms of sepsis (fever, tachycardia, hypotension, altered level of consciousness) after sharp debridement. Remember, only specially trained providers can do sharp debridement. **Key Point:** *Keep in mind there are reasons not to debride a wound. It is imperative not to remove eschar if the wound has poor circulation at the ulcer site. You would also leave alone a stable heel eschar. Additionally, debridement would not benefit the patient who is critically unstable or with a grave prognosis (Association for the Advancement of Wound Care [AAWC], 2005, revised 2010).*

Dressings and Supplies Acute wounds may require sterile dressings. Use clean dressings for chronic wounds. However, even a chronic wound may require sterile dressings if the patient is immunocompromised. Carefully dispose of contaminated dressings in biohazard waste receptacles. Discard unused dressings if they become contaminated.

Store patient dressing supplies in a clean and dry area. Do not share supplies among patients. Access only the number of supplies you need for the dressing change. Do not touch the supply of dressings with gloves that have come in contact with the wound. Discard unused dressings if they have become contaminated.

 ### Think**Like a Nurse** 35-6
What would be the best method to secure dressings for Mr. Harmon (Meet Your Patient)?

Supporting and Immobilizing Wounds
Binders and bandages are used to hold a dressing in place, apply pressure to a wound to impede hemorrhage, and support and immobilize an injured area, thereby promoting healing and comfort. Before applying a bandage or binder, determine the purpose of the application and assess the part being bandaged.

Binders
Binders may be used to keep a wound closed when there is danger of dehiscence, or to immobilize a body part to aid in the healing process. They are typically used on large areas of the body and are designed for a specific body part. They may be made of cloth or elasticized material and fasten with straps, pins, or Velcro. The most common binders are the following:

- *A triangular arm binder or sling* is used to support the upper extremities. Because commercial slings are readily available, you will rarely use a triangular sling.

- *A T-binder* is used to secure dressings or pads in the perineal area.
- *An abdominal binder* is used to provide support to the abdomen, for example, when there is an abdominal incision or an open abdominal wound healing by secondary intention. The binder decreases the risk of dehiscence.

To learn a procedure for applying binders, see the Highlights of Procedures box, and

 Go to Chapter 35, **Procedure 35-10: Applying Binders,** in Volume 2.

Bandages

A bandage is a cloth, gauze, or elastic covering that is wrapped in place. With the exception of a sling, most bandages come in rolls and in various widths, commonly 1.5 to 7.5 cm (0.5 to 3 in.). Use a narrow width on small body parts, such as a finger, and wider bandages on arms and legs.

- **Cloth bandages** are most commonly used as slings to immobilize an upper extremity or to hold large abdominal dressings in place.
- **Gauze** is the most frequently used type of bandage. It is available in many sizes and forms and readily

(text continued on page 931)

Highlights of Procedures 35-1 Through 35-15

 For steps to follow in *all* procedures, refer to the Universal Steps for All Procedures found on the inside back cover of Volume 2. Go to the full procedures in Volume 2 to practice and learn the procedure steps. Use these procedure highlights later to help you review key points.

Procedure 35-1: Obtaining a Wound Culture by Swab

➤ Position the patient for easy access to the wound and in a manner that will allow the irrigation solution to flow freely from the wound with the assistance of gravity.

➤ Don clean nonsterile gloves.

➤ Remove the soiled dressing, and dispose of gloves and dressing.

➤ Don clean gloves and fill a 35-mL syringe with an attached 19-gauge angiocatheter, with 0.9% (normal) saline solution; open the culturette package.

➤ Holding the angiocatheter tip 2 cm from the wound bed, gently irrigate the wound (superior to inferior).

➤ If using Levine's technique, press the culture swab against an area of red granulating tissue, and rotate.

➤ Or if using the Z-stroke technique, swab the wound from margin to margin in a 10-point, zigzag pattern, avoiding contact with the wound edge.

➤ Reinsert the swab into the culturette tube (aerobic or anaerobic culture, depending on the type of wound and type of organism); label the tube; and have the specimen transported to the lab.

Procedure 35-2: Performing a Sterile Wound Irrigation

➤ Administer pain medication 30 minutes before the procedure, if necessary.

➤ Position the patient for easy access to the wound and in a manner that will allow the irrigation solution to flow freely from the wound with the assistance of gravity.

➤ Don protective equipment: gown, face shield, and clean gloves.

➤ Remove the soiled dressing, and dispose of gloves.

➤ Set up a sterile field with a sterile irrigation kit or a 35-mL syringe and a 19-gauge angiocatheter with needle removed, dressing supplies, and irrigation solution.

➤ Wearing sterile gloves, fill either the syringe and angiocatheter or the piston-tip syringe with irrigation solution.

➤ Holding the syringe 2 cm (¾ to 1 in.) from the wound bed, gently irrigate the wound with a back-and-forth motion, moving from the superior aspect to the inferior aspect.

➤ Dry the tissue surrounding the wound with sterile gauze.

➤ Apply a new dressing. Consider applying a waterproof skin protectant if the wound drainage is heavy.

➤ Dispose of used equipment and soiled dressings in a biohazard container.

➤ Reposition the patient and change any linens that got wet.

Procedure 35-3: Taping a Dressing

➤ Place the patient in a comfortable position that provides easy access to the wound.

➤ Ensure the skin surrounding the dressing is clean and dry.

➤ Choose a tape that is appropriate for the dressing.

➤ Place the tape parallel to the incision.

➤ Tear strips that extend 1–1½ inches beyond the dressing edge.

➤ Apply tape without pulling or stretching.

➤ Smooth tape with your fingertips.

Procedure 35-4: Removing and Applying Dry Dressings

➤ Administer pain medication 30 minutes before the procedure, if necessary.

➤ Place the patient in a comfortable position that provides easy access to the wound.

➤ Wearing clean (nonsterile) gloves, gently loosen the edges of the tape to remove the soiled dressing and discard it in a biohazard receptacle.

➤ Change gloves and cleanse the wound gently with saline-moistened gauze.

➤ Assess the wound for location, appearance, odor, and drainage.

➤ Apply a dry dressing.

➤ Secure the dressing with tape.

Continued

Procedure 35-5: Removing and Applying Wet-to-Damp Dressings

➤ Assess for pain, and medicate 30 minutes before the procedure, if necessary taping dressing wound

➤ Place the patient in a comfortable position that provides easy access to the wound.

➤ Wearing clean nonsterile gloves, gently loosen the edges of the tape to remove the soiled dressing and discard in a biohazard receptacle.

➤ Change gloves and cleanse the wound gently with saline-moistened gauze.

➤ Assess the wound for location, appearance, odor, and drainage.

➤ Don clean nonsterile gloves and apply a single fluffed layer of moist, fine-mesh gauze to the wound. Be sure to place gauze in all depressions of the wound.

➤ Apply a second moist, fluffed layer over the first layer. Repeat this process until the wound is filled with moistened sterile gauze.

➤ Cover the moistened gauze with an absorbent, surgical pad.

➤ Secure the dressing with tape or Montgomery straps. Perform hand hygiene and date and time the dressing.

Procedure 35-6: Applying a Negative Pressure Wound Therapy (NPWT) Device

➤ Administer an analgesic if needed.

➤ Select an appropriate dressing, per NPWT unit directions, to fill the entire wound cavity.

➤ Obtain and set up the NPWT unit.

➤ Don clean gloves and remove the old dressing and discard in biohazard receptacle.

➤ Prepare a sterile field for supplies.

➤ Don sterile gloves for new surgical wounds; or clean gloves for chronic wounds.

➤ Irrigate/cleanse the wound.

➤ Apply appropriate dressing per NPWT unit protocol.

Procedure 35-6A: Open Pore Reticulated Polyurethane Foam (i.e., Vacuum Assisted Closure Therapy [V.A.C.])

➤ Cut the foam to fill the wound cavity.

➤ Do not place foam into blind/unexplored tunnels.

➤ Do not allow the foam dressing to overlap onto healthy skin.

Procedure 35-6B: Gauze Dressing Application (i.e., Chariker–Jeter Method)

➤ Measure the length of the drain.

➤ Moisten the gauze.

➤ "Sandwich" the drain in the moistened gauze and place in the wound base.

➤ Tuck the gauze into any undermining areas to ensure contact with the wound bed.

➤ Apply a strip or dollop of ostomy paste 1 cm from wound edge and secure the drain as needed.

For Both Types of Dressing

➤ Connect tubing attached to the dressing to the evacuation tubing going to the collection system.

➤ Position the tubing and connector away from bony prominences and skin creases.

➤ Ensure the clamps are open on all tubing.

➤ Turn on the pump and set to prescribed settings.

➤ Listen for audible leaks and observe for dressing collapse.

➤ Change the canister once a week or sooner if it fills.

Procedure 35-7: Applying and Removing a Transparent Film Dressing

➤ Place the patient in a comfortable position that provides easy access to the wound.

➤ Remove the soiled dressing, if necessary.

➤ Cleanse the surrounding skin and wound.

➤ Assess the condition of the wound.

➤ Apply the transparent film dressing to the wound by removing the center backing and holding the dressing firmly by the edges.

➤ Place over the wound and press out wrinkles and air.

Procedure 35-8: Applying a Hydrating Dressing (Hydrocolloid or Hydrogel)

➤ Place the patient in a comfortable position.

➤ Remove the soiled dressing, if necessary.

➤ Cleanse the wound, if necessary.

➤ Assess the wound, or other area where the hydrocolloid dressing will be applied, for size, location, appearance, exudate, odor, and signs and symptoms of infection.

➤ Apply the hydrating dressing.

Procedure 35-9: Placing Skin Closures

➤ Place the patient in a comfortable position that provides easy access to the wound.

➤ Cleanse the surrounding skin and wound.

➤ Assess the wound and determine the size and type of skin closure needed.

➤ Peel the skin closure from the card at a 90° angle.

➤ Place closures across the wound without tension starting at the middle of the wound.

➤ Place closures $1/8$ in. (3 mm) apart along the entire wound.

Procedure 35-10: Applying Binders

➤ Choose a binder of the correct type and size for the intended purpose.

➤ Make sure the binder is positioned properly to provide support but not compromise circulation or impair breathing.

➤ Pad any pressure areas or skin abrasions.

➤ *Abdominal binder:* Assess the patient every 2 to 3 hours to assure that the binder has not slipped up or down or is creating pain. Fasten from the bottom up.

> *Triangular strap binder:* Position the patient's arm across the chest with elbow flexed slightly. Place one end of the triangle over the shoulder of the uninjured arm, and allow the triangle to fall open so that the elbow of the injured arm is at the apex of the triangle.

> *T-binders:* They come in two basic types—those for females have a perineal strap; those for males have a split in the perineal strap.

Procedure 35-11: Applying Bandages

> Bandage the body part in its natural position.

> Work from distal to proximal position.

> Choose a bandage of the proper width.

> Clean the wound (if present).

> Apply primary dressing as prescribed.

> Apply the bandage as needed to secure the primary dressing.

Procedure 35-12: Removing Sutures and Staples

Procedure 35-12A: Removing Sutures

> Place the patient in a comfortable position that provides easy access to the wound.

> Use the forceps to pick up one end of the suture. Slide the small scissors around the suture, and cut near the skin.

> With the forceps, gently pull the suture in the direction of the knotted side to remove it.

Procedure 35-12B: Removing Staples

> Position the staple remover so that the lower jaw is on the bottom.

> Place both tips of the lower jaw of the staple remover underneath the staple.

> Lift slightly on the staple, ensuring that it stays perpendicular to the skin.

> Gently squeeze the handles together and lift the staple straight up.

> Place the removed staples on a piece of gauze.

> Dispose of the removed staples in the sharps container.

> Apply dressing or Steri-Strips if needed.

Procedure 35-13: Shortening a Wound Drain

> Before shortening a wound drain, make sure it is secured tightly.

> Firmly grasp the full width of the drain at the level of the skin and pull it out by the prescribed amount (e.g., 5 mm, [1 in.]).

> Insert a sterile safety pin through the drain at the level of the skin.

> Hold the drain tightly, and insert another pin above your fingers.

> Using sterile scissors, cut the drain a little above the safety pin closest to the skin.

Procedure 35-14: Emptying a Closed-Wound Drainage System

> Don personal protective equipment as needed, including nonsterile procedure gloves, gown, and eyewear.

> Properly dispose of contaminated items into designated biohazard waste receptacles.

> Measure drainage.

> Document on I&O sheet.

> Report excess volume to the primary healthcare provider.

---

conforms to the shape of the body. It may also be impregnated with medications for application to the skin or with plaster of Paris, which, when dried, hardens to form a cast.

- **Elastic** bandages are used to apply pressure and give support (e.g., to improve venous circulation in the legs). Ace bandages are the most common form of elasticized bandage.

- **A rolled bandage** is a continuous strip of material (gauze, stretchable gauze, or elastic webbing) that you unroll as you apply it to a body part. To apply a roller bandage, hold the free end in place with one hand, and use the other hand to pass the roll around the body part. Start at the distal end and move toward the body. This will prevent the bandage from trapping blood in the distal end. Exert equal tension on each pass (or turn).

Go to Chapter 35, **Procedure 35-11: Applying Bandages**, in Volume 2.

Using Heat and Cold Therapy

Local application of heat or cold has been used for therapeutic purposes for centuries. Temperature-sensitive nerve endings respond readily to temperatures between 59°F and 113°F (15°C and 45°C). Response to heat or cold depends on the area being treated, the nature of the injury, duration of the treatment, patient age, physical condition, and the condition of the skin.

Monitor the patient especially carefully in the following situations:

- **Extremes of Age.** The very young and the very old are the least tolerant of heat and cold therapies.
- **Sensory Impairment.** Patients with sensory impairment are at increased risk for injury related to use of heat and cold therapy because they may not perceive temperature changes, burns, or ischemia.
- **Highly Vascular Areas.** Highly vascular areas, such as the fingers, hand, face, and perineum, are very sensitive to

temperature changes and thus are at high risk for injury from heat and cold.

- **Application to a Large Area.** Application of cold or heat to a large body surface area decreases the patient's tolerance of the treatment. Application to a small area is best tolerated.
- **Injured Skin or Wounds.** Intact skin tolerates heat and cold therapy better than skin that has been injured or has open wounds.

Safety Measures

 For patient safety, observe the following precautions when applying heat and cold:

- Avoid direct contact with the heating or cooling device. Cover the hot or cold pack with a washcloth, towel, or fitted sleeve.
- Apply hot or cold intermittently, leaving it on for no more than 15 minutes at a time in any one area. This precaution helps prevent tissue injury (e.g., burns, impaired circulation). It also makes the therapy more effective by preventing *rebound phenomenon*: At the time the heat or cold reaches maximum therapeutic effect, the opposite effect begins.
- Check the skin frequently for extreme redness, blistering, cyanosis (blueness), or blanching. When heat or cold is first applied, the thermal receptors react strongly, and the person feels the temperature intensely. Over about 15 minutes, the receptors adapt to the new temperature, and the person notices it less. Caution clients not to change the temperature when this occurs because doing so can cause tissue injury.

Applying Heat Therapy

Local application of heat is used to relieve stiffness and discomfort associated with musculoskeletal problems. It may also be used for patients with wounds. Heat increases blood flow to an area through the mechanisms of vasodilatation, increased capillary permeability, and reduced blood viscosity. Increased blood flow brings oxygen and white blood cells to the wound and aids in the healing process. Heat promotes the delivery of nutrients and removal of waste products from the tissue, promotes relaxation, and decreases stiffness and muscle tension.

When heat is applied to a large area of the body, vasodilatation may cause a drop in blood pressure and a feeling of faintness. Warn patients to be alert for this effect if they will be administering heat at home.

Moist Heat Adding moisture to heat amplifies the intensity of the treatment. Moist heat can be applied in several forms, depending on the skin condition.

- *Washcloth or towel.* If heat is being applied for relaxation and the skin is intact, you can soak a washcloth or towel in warm water and wring out the excess moisture before applying to the skin.
- *Gauze compress.* If there are any open areas, you will need to use a sterile gauze compress.
- *Soaks and baths* also provide moist heat. A **soak** involves immersion of the affected area. Soaking helps

cleanse a wound and remove encrusted material. A **bath** is a modification of a soak in which a special tub or chair may be used. The most commonly used bath is a sitz bath (Fig. 35-16). A **sitz bath** soaks the patient's perineal area. Disposable sitz baths are often used to help prevent infection.

Dry Heat Dry heat may be applied with electric heating pads, disposable hot packs, or hot water bags. Caution patients to place the heating pad or device over the body area and never to lie on it. The pad or bag should be covered with its own cover or a towel.

- *Electric heating pad*s have the advantage of providing a constant temperature, but the risk of burns is high.
- *Aquathermia pads* (Fig. 35-17) may also be used for dry heat application. Aquapads are plastic or vinyl pads that circulate water in the interior of the pad to create a constant temperature.
- *Disposable hot packs and hot water bags or bottles* are also available. Hot water bags are common in home use, but not in healthcare agencies because of the danger of burns from improper use.

For guidelines (including water temperatures) for applying moist and dry heat,

Go to Chapter 35, **Clinical Insight 35-1: Applying Local Heat Therapy,** in Volume 2.

Applying Cold Therapy

The application of moist or dry cold causes vasoconstriction and decreases capillary permeability. It produces local anesthesia, reduces cell metabolism, increases blood viscosity, and decreases muscle tension. It also slows bacterial growth. Applications of cold are used to prevent or limit edema and reduce inflammation, pain, oxygen requirements, and bleeding. Cold therapy is often used to treat fevers and sports injuries (e.g., sprains, strains, fractures, and contusions), and to

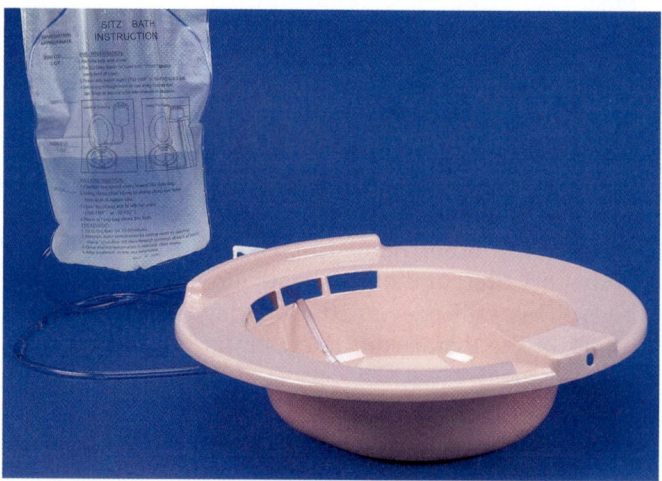

FIGURE 35-16 A Sitz bath soaks the patient's perineal area.

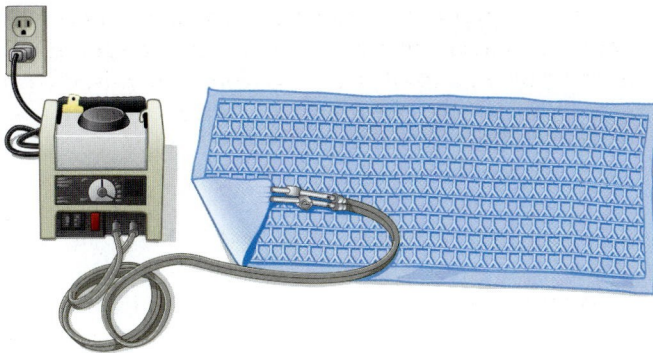

FIGURE 35-17 Aquapads circulate water in the interior of the pad to create a constant temperature.

prevent swelling after surgery (e.g., an ice bag may be applied to the perineum after childbirth; an ice collar may be applied to the throat after a tonsillectomy). Cold applications have the following side effects:

- *Elevated blood pressure.* Because cold causes vasoconstriction, it may increase the patient's blood pressure.
- *Shivering.* Prolonged cold may cause shivering, a normal response as the body attempts to produce heat.
- *Tissue damage.* Prolonged exposure to cold may cause tissue damage from impaired circulation.
  For guidelines in applying cold therapy,

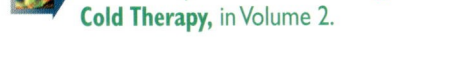 Go to Chapter 35, **Clinical Insight 35-2: Applying Local Cold Therapy,** in Volume 2.

KnowledgeCheck 35-11

- What is the effect of adding moisture to heat or cold treatments?
- How long should heat or cold be applied to an area?
- What precautions should you take before using heat or cold therapy?

CarePlanning & Mapping

For a care plan and care map for Impaired Skin Integrity,

 Go to Chapter 35, Student Resources, **Care Plan** and **Care Map,** on DavisPlus.

 To explore learning resources for this chapter,

 Go to DavisPlus a **DavisPl.us/Wilkinson3.**

Chapter Resources for Chapter 35:
  Response sheets for all learning activities
  Resources for Caregivers and Health Professionals
  Reading More About Skin Integrity & Wound Healing (suggested readings)
  Concept Map of chapter content
Interactive Case Studies
NCLEX-Style and Chapter Review Questions
Chapter Overview Podcasts

For references cited in this chapter,

 Go to Volume 2, **References Cited.**

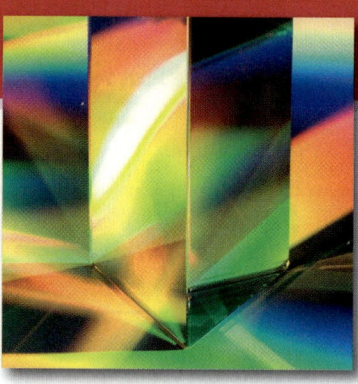

CHAPTER 36

Oxygenation

Learning Outcomes

After completing this chapter, you should be able to:

- ➤ Describe the structure and function of the respiratory systems.
- ➤ Identify individual, environmental, and pathological factors that influence oxygenation.
- ➤ Assess oxygenation, breathing, and gas exchange.
- ➤ Interpret diagnostic testing related to oxygenation, breathing, and gas exchange.
- ➤ Develop nursing diagnoses related to oxygenation, breathing, and gas exchange.
- ➤ Plan outcomes and interventions for maintaining and improving oxygenation.
- ➤ Safely and correctly perform common nursing procedures related to oxygenation, breathing, and gas exchange.
- ➤ Evaluate adequacy of oxygenation, breathing, and gas exchange, and modify nursing activities appropriately based on outcomes.

- ➤ Describe a procedure for safe oxygen administration.
- ➤ Describe measures for mobilizing airway secretions.
- ➤ Implement measures for promoting optimal respiratory function (e.g., positioning).
- ➤ Explain how to suction the upper and lower airways.
- ➤ Provide care for patients requiring artificial airways.
- ➤ Provide care for patients requiring mechanical ventilation.
- ➤ Provide care for patients requiring chest tubes.
- ➤ Provide measures to promote oxygenation.
- ➤ Recognize medications used to enhance pulmonary function.
- ➤ Use identified outcomes to evaluate care for patients with oxygenation problems.

Key Concepts

Oxygenation
Respiration
Ventilation

Related Concepts

See the Concept Map on Davis*Plus*.

Example Problem

Upper respiratory infections
Influenza
Pneumonia

Meet Your Patients

In a pulmonary clinic, your student assignment is to (1) perform a focused assessment related to breathing and oxygenation, (2) perform common therapeutic interventions related to breathing and oxygenation, (3) identify desired outcomes and evaluate achievement of those outcomes, and (4) plan for follow-up and home care needs. In the course of your clinical day, you care for the following clients:

- Mary is a 4-year-old girl with a history of asthma. Her mother, Ms. Green, has brought her in because of an "asthma attack." Mary is sitting on her mother's lap and

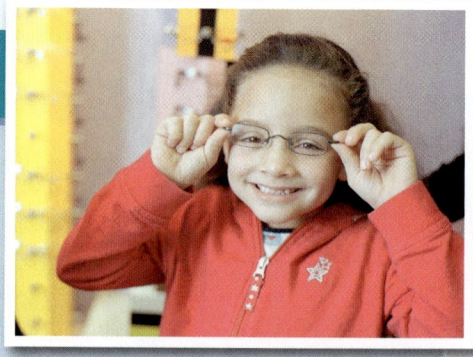

breathing rapidly through an open mouth. Her cough sounds congested and wheezy. The nurse practitioner has prescribed a nebulized treatment containing albuterol (Proventil) and ipratropium bromide (Atrovent).
- Mr. Chu is a 78-year-old man complaining of cough, sore throat, fatigue, and weakness. His temperature is

Meet Your Patients (continued)

100.4°F (38°C), pulse is 90 beats/min, respirations are 26 breaths/min, and blood pressure (BP) is 166/82 mm Hg.

■ William is a 19-year-old male who has had a sudden onset of right-sided chest pain and shortness of breath. His chest x-ray revealed a right pneumothorax, and he is currently receiving 35% oxygen by face mask while

waiting for an ambulance to transport him to the hospital for further evaluation.

Each of these patients is experiencing an oxygenation problem. In this chapter you will learn a variety of assessment techniques and interventions to support breathing, oxygenation, and gas exchange for patients such as these.

Theoretical Knowledge
knowing why

The pulmonary, cardiovascular, musculoskeletal, and neurological systems work together to achieve oxygenation. The musculoskeletal and neurological systems regulate the movement of air into and out of the lungs. The lungs oxygenate the blood, and the heart circulates the blood throughout the body and back to the lungs. In this chapter, we focus on the pulmonary system; Chapter 37 presents the cardiovascular system. Remember, however, that the two systems work together. Changes in one system create changes in the other.

ABOUT THE KEY CONCEPTS

The concept **oxygenation** refers to how well the cells, tissues, and organs of the body are supplied with oxygen. The concepts of **respiration** and **ventilation** are the two major processes that occur in the pulmonary system to oxygenate the blood. All of the problems and interventions in this chapter relate in some way to oxygenation, respiration, or ventilation. Knowledge of these concepts will help you to understand the rationale for interventions such as airway suctioning, oxygen, mechanical ventilation, and chest tubes.

THE PULMONARY SYSTEM

The pulmonary system has two major components: the *airway* and the *lungs*. The following presents a brief review of the anatomy and physiology of the pulmonary system and explains how breathing is controlled. For more in-depth information, consult anatomy and physiology texts, or

 Go to Chapter 36, **Supplemental Materials: Structures of the Pulmonary System,** on Davis*Plus.*

The Airway

The airway consists of the nasal passages, mouth, pharynx, larynx, trachea, bronchi, and bronchioles (Fig. 36-1). Air flows through these structures into and

out of the lungs. In addition, the airway structures do the following:

■ *Moisten the air*—A moist mucous membrane lining adds water to inhaled air.
■ *Warm the air*—Blood flowing through the vascular airway walls transfers body heat to the inhaled air.
■ *Filter the air*—(1) Specialized cells in the lining of the airways secrete sticky mucus to trap foreign particles. (2) **Cilia,** tiny hair-like projections from the walls of the airways, move rhythmically to sweep trapped debris up and out of the airway.

Upper Airway Located above the larynx, the upper airway includes the nasal passages, mouth, and pharynx. The *pharynx* (throat) contains the openings to the esophagus and trachea. The *trachea* lies just in front of the esophagus. The *epiglottis,* a small flap of tissue superior to the larynx, closes off the trachea during swallowing so that food and fluids do not enter the lower airway. The epiglottis opens during breathing to allow air to move through the airway.

Lower Airway Located below the larynx, the lower airway includes the trachea, bronchi, and bronchioles. The lower airway is considered sterile. The **trachea,** sometimes called the "windpipe," extends from the larynx to the point at which it divides to form the right and left mainstem bronchi. As the airways branch and become smaller, they have progressively thinner and less cartilage, until it disappears completely in the smaller bronchioles. The walls of the bronchi and bronchioles contain layers of smooth muscles. Spasm of these muscles (**bronchospasm**) narrows the airway and obstructs airflow.

The Lungs

The *lungs* are soft, spongy, cone-shaped organs. They are separated by the **mediastinum,** which contains the heart and great vessels. The right lung has three lobes; the left lung has two lobes. The upper portion of each lung, the *apex,* extends upward above the clavicle. The lower portion of each lung, the *base,* rests on the diaphragm. Knowing the location of lung tissue beneath the chest wall helps you to perform a complete and accurate assessment of the lungs.

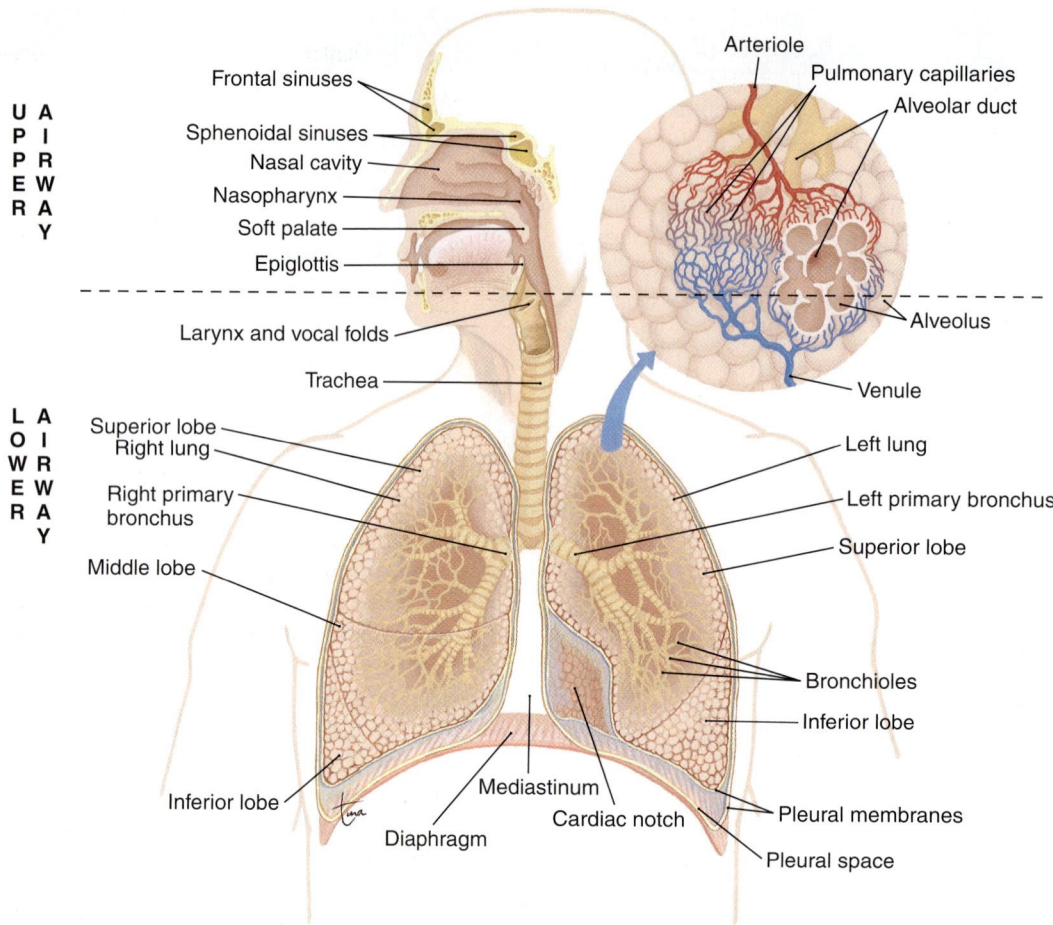

FIGURE 36-1 An anterior view of the respiratory system. The upper airway lies above the larynx. The lower airway, located below the larynx, is considered sterile.

The lungs are composed of millions of **alveoli**—tiny air sacs with thin walls surrounded by a fine network of capillaries. Gases (oxygen and carbon dioxide) easily pass back and forth between the alveoli and capillaries. Alveoli are composed of two types of cells (Fig. 36-2).

- *Type I alveolar cells* are the gas exchange cells.
- *Type II alveolar cells* produce **surfactant**, a lipoprotein that lowers the surface tension within alveoli to allow them to inflate during breathing.

KnowledgeCheck 36-1

- What happens to inhaled air in the airways? How does this occur?
- In which structures of the lung does gas exchange take place?
- What does surfactant do for alveoli?

 ### ThinkLike a Nurse 36-1

You are assigned to care for an adult patient who has a medical condition with which you are not familiar. You look it up and find that the condition causes a dramatic loss of surfactant. Based on your knowledge of the function of surfactant, what problems is this patient at high risk for developing?

WHAT ARE THE FUNCTIONS OF THE PULMONARY SYSTEM?

Two of the key concepts in this chapter are major processes that occur in the pulmonary system: ventilation and respiration. **Ventilation** is the movement of air into and out of the lungs through the act of breathing. **Respiration** is the exchange of the gases oxygen and carbon dioxide in the lungs.

Pulmonary Ventilation

Oxygenation of the blood, and ultimately of organs and tissues, depends on adequate ventilation. Ventilation must move enough air through the lungs to make adequate oxygen available to the alveoli. Ventilation is accomplished through cycles of inhalation and exhalation. To see an animated demonstration of the physiology of ventilation,

 Go to **Cardiovascular/Pulmonary Animations: Pulmonary Ventilation,** on DavisPlus.

Inhalation Expansion of the chest cavity and lungs creates negative pressure inside the lungs, causing air to

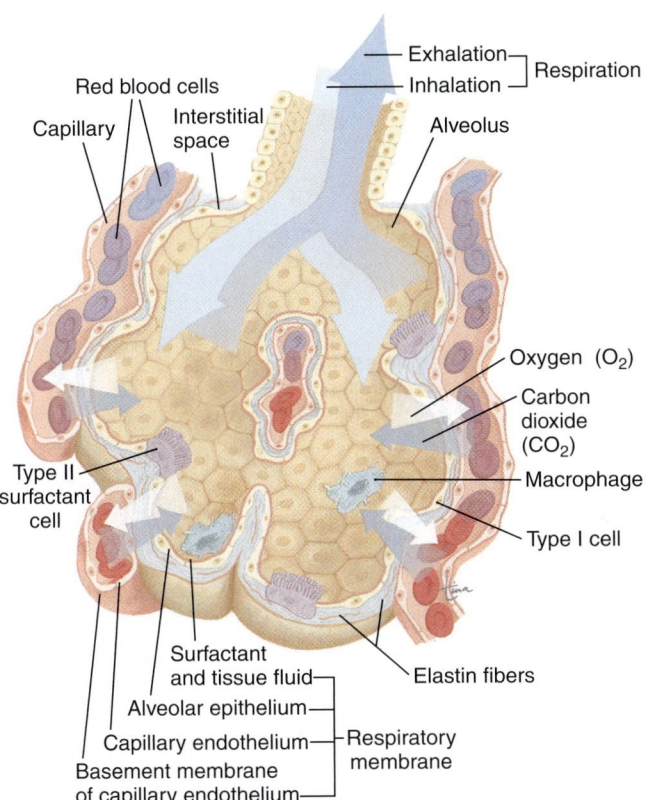

FIGURE 36-2 Alveolar structure showing type I and type II cells. Type I alveolar cells are the gas exchange cells. Type II alveolar cells produce surfactant.

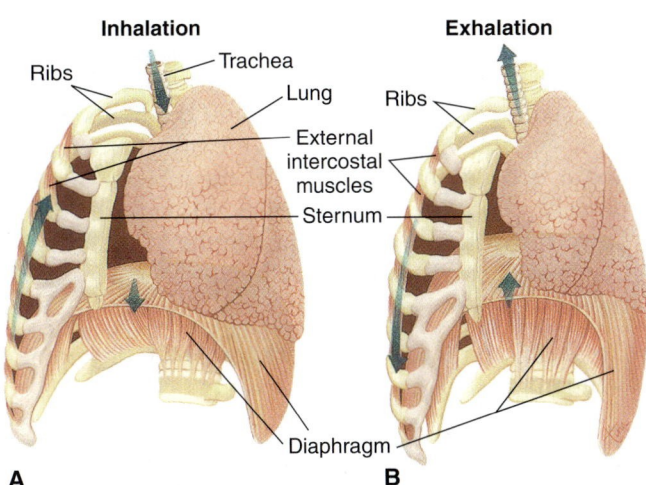

FIGURE 36-3 *A,* During inhalation, the diaphragm contracts, pulling the chest cavity and lung bases downward; the intercostal muscles pull the rib cage up and outward. *B,* In exhalation, the diaphragm relaxes, the lung bases move upward, and the ribs and intercostal muscles move down and in, resulting in lung compression.

be drawn in through the nose or mouth and airways. This is **inhalation**. The *diaphragm* is the major muscle of breathing. When it contracts with each inhalation, the chest cavity is pulled downward, pulling the lung bases downward with it. *Intercostal muscles*, the small muscles around the ribs, also contract on inhalation and pull the ribs outward, slightly expanding the chest cavity and lungs. The pleural membrane covering the lungs adheres ("sticks") to the pleural membrane lining the chest cavity, so the lungs expand. Lung expansion creates negative pressure and draws air in through the only opening to the outside, the trachea (Fig. 36-3A).

Exhalation When the diaphragm and intercostal muscles relax, **exhalation** allows the chest and lungs to return to their normal resting size (Fig. 36-3B). The reduction in size causes the pressure inside the chest and lungs to rise above atmospheric pressure, so air flows out of the lungs. Exhalation requires no energy or effort.

What Factors Affect Ventilation?

The adequacy of ventilation is affected by the rate and depth of respirations, lung compliance and elasticity, and airway resistance.

- **Respiratory rate and depth** are almost self-explanatory. **Rate** is how fast you breathe, and **depth** is how much

your lungs expand to take in air. These processes affect oxygen and carbon dioxide levels in the blood.
- **Hyperventilation** occurs when a person breathes fast and deeply to move a large amount of air through the lungs, causing too much carbon dioxide to be removed by the alveoli. Mild hyperventilation can occur in response to **hypoxemia** (a low level of oxygen in the blood). When blood oxygen is low, ventilation increases to draw additional air (and oxygen) into the lungs. However, as ventilation increases, carbon dioxide levels fall. Severe hyperventilation is usually triggered by medication, central nervous system abnormalities, high altitude, heat, exercise, panic, fear, or anxiety.
- **Hypoventilation** occurs when a decreased rate or shallow breathing moves only a small amount of air into and out of the lungs. Hypoventilation can lead to hypoxemia because less air (carrying oxygen) reaches the alveoli. The concern is that hypoxemia will progress to **hypoxia** (an oxygen deficiency in the body tissues).
- **Lung elasticity** (or elastic recoil) refers to the tendency of the elastin fibers to return to their original position away from the chest wall after being stretched (think of stretching a rubber band, then letting go of it). Alveoli that have been overstretched, as with emphysema, lose their elastic recoil over time. This loss of elasticity allows the lungs to inflate easily but inhibits deflation, leaving stale air trapped in the alveoli.
- **Lung compliance** refers to the ease of lung inflation. Normally the lungs inflate easily. Lung compliance is reduced by increased lung water (edema), loss of surfactant, or conditions that cause elastin fibers in the lungs to be replaced with scar tissue (collagen).

- **Airway resistance** is the resistance to airflow within the airways. The larger the diameter of the airway, the more easily air moves through it. Normally, airway resistance is very low, so it takes little effort to move large volumes of air into and out of the lungs. However, even small decreases in airway diameter (as might occur with secretions in the airway or mild bronchospasm) markedly increase airway resistance. Mary, the little girl with asthma in the Meet Your Patients scenario, is undoubtedly experiencing airway resistance.

To see an animated demonstration of the physiology of ventilation,

 Go to **Animations: Cardiovascular/Pulmonary Animations: Physiology of Ventilation,** on DavisPlus.

KnowledgeCheck 36-2

- What is the difference between ventilation and respiration?
- Describe how the diaphragm, accessory muscles, and pressure changes within the lungs create inhalation and exhalation.
- How does hypoventilation affect risk for hypoxemia and hypoxia?

Respiration (Gas Exchange)

Respiration refers to gas exchange, that is, the oxygenation of blood and elimination of carbon dioxide in the lungs. Although nurses commonly use the term *respirations* to mean "breaths" in an assessment of vital signs, strictly speaking this is not accurate: You cannot measure gas exchange by counting breaths per minute. Gas exchange occurs at two equally essential levels: external (in the lungs) or internal (in other body tissues).

External Respiration Alveolar–capillary gas exchange (or **external respiration**) occurs in the alveoli of the lungs. Oxygen (O_2) diffuses across the alveolar–capillary membrane into the blood of the pulmonary capillaries; carbon dioxide (CO_2) diffuses out of the blood and into the alveoli to be exhaled (Fig. 36-4). The rate of diffusion depends on the thickness of the membrane and the total surface of lung tissue available for gas exchange. Examples of conditions that slow diffusion are pleural effusion (fluid around the lungs), pneumothorax (lung collapse), and asthma (bronchospasms). If blood is not adequately oxygenated in the alveoli, hypoxemia (low blood-oxygen levels) occurs. Getting oxygen into the blood as it flows through the lungs is only the first step in oxygenation.

Internal Respiration Capillary–tissue gas exchange (or **internal respiration**) occurs in body organs and tissues. Oxygen diffuses from the blood through the capillary–cellular membrane into the tissue cells, where it is used for metabolism. From the cells, CO_2, a waste product of cellular metabolism, diffuses through the capillary–cellular membrane into the blood, and then is transported to the lungs and exhaled. Tissue oxygenation requires both adequate external respiration and adequate

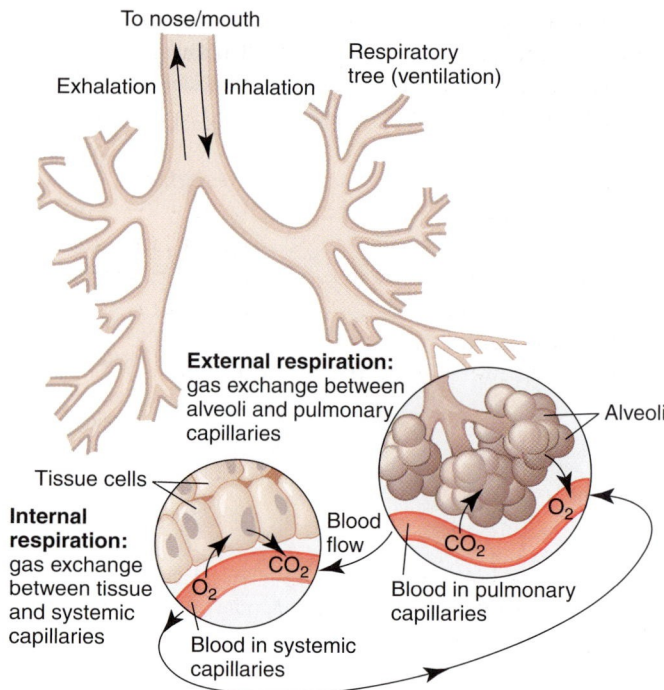

FIGURE 36-4 External respiration occurs at the alveolar–capillary membrane. Internal respiration occurs at the tissue–capillary membrane.

peripheral circulation. Limitations in either function may lead to hypoxia (oxygen deficiency in body tissues). In addition, if tissue cells are using more oxygen for metabolism than normal (e.g., during a high fever), hypoxia will occur unless more oxygen is made available to the tissues.

 Think**Like a Nurse** 36-2

William (Meet Your Patients) has a right pneumothorax. Which of the two factors affecting the rate of gas diffusion is causing William to be hypoxemic? If you do not know what a pneumothorax is, look it up.

How Is Breathing Controlled?

The respiratory centers in the brainstem control breathing using feedback from chemoreceptors and lung receptors. Voluntary control from the **motor cortex** can override the involuntary respiratory centers, but only temporarily. This allows a person to continue breathing while doing activities such as talking, singing, swallowing, whistling, and blowing.

- **Chemoreceptors**, located in the medulla of the brainstem, the carotid arteries, and the aorta, detect changes in blood pH, O_2, and CO_2 levels and send messages back to the central respiratory center in the brainstem. In response, the respiratory center increases or decreases ventilation to maintain normal blood levels of pH, O_2 (PO_2), and CO_2 (PCO_2). Normally the blood CO_2 level provides the primary stimulus to breathe. High CO_2 levels stimulate breathing to eliminate the excess CO_2. A secondary, though important, drive to breathe is hypoxemia. Low blood O_2 levels stimulate breathing to get more oxygen into the lungs.

- **Lung receptors**, located in the lung and chest wall, are sensitive to breathing patterns, lung expansion, lung compliance, airway resistance, and respiratory irritants. The respiratory center uses feedback from the lung receptors to adjust ventilation. For example, if the lung receptors sense respiratory irritants such as dust, cold air, or tobacco smoke, the respiratory center triggers airway constriction and a more rapid, shallow pattern of breathing.

For a brief overview of the nervous system,

 Go to Chapter 36, **Supplemental Materials: The Nervous System,** on Davis*Plus*.

KnowledgeCheck 36-3

- Describe two ways in which breathing is controlled.
- The level of which gas (oxygen or carbon dioxide) is the primary stimulant for breathing?

 ThinkLike a Nurse 36-3

A patient has adequate blood oxygen levels based on a pulse oximeter reading of 98%. Can you conclude that organ and tissue oxygenations are adequate? Explain your thinking.

WHAT FACTORS INFLUENCE PULMONARY FUNCTION?

Factors that influence pulmonary function include developmental stage, the environment, individual and lifestyle factors, medications, and pathophysiological states.

Developmental Stage

Normal development influences lung, heart, and circulatory function, all of which affect oxygenation. Developmental factors have less effect on function in young and middle adults than in older adults.

Infants

Premature infants (less than 35 weeks' gestation) do not have a fully developed alveolar surfactant system. Surfactant is the substance that keeps air sacs inflated for effective respiration. Therefore, premature infants are at high risk for **respiratory distress syndrome (RDS).** RDS is characterized by widespread **atelectasis** (collapse of alveoli). The premature infant also has immature pulmonary circulation. Together with hypoventilation, this leads to hypercarbia (high CO_2 blood levels) and hypoxemia.

Infants born at term are also at risk for oxygenation problems (e.g., infection and airway obstruction) for the following reasons:

- Because the newborn's lower airway structures are immature and small, an infectious agent can spread rapidly.

- The infant's airways are quite narrow in diameter and, therefore, easily obstructed by edema, mucus, or a foreign body, such as meconium passed at birth.
- The central nervous system for preterm, and even some term, infants is immature, leading to periodic breathing patterns and apnea.
- The immune system of infants in the first few months of life is immature. Although at birth infants enjoy the benefit of some maternal immunoglobulin circulating in their system, this protection is limited and not sufficient for fighting certain infections.
- By age 6 months, infants can grasp small objects and put them in their mouth. This new skill, combined with small airway diameter, puts them at risk for choking on small objects.

Toddlers

As the toddler's respiratory and immune systems mature, the risk for frequent and serious infections diminishes. However, *upper respiratory infections* (URIs) remain common because (1) the tonsils and adenoids are relatively large, predisposing to tonsillitis, and (2) many children are exposed to new infectious agents in preschool and day care. Most children recover from URIs without difficulty.

Toddlers actively explore the environment and often put objects in their mouth, which puts them at risk for other respiratory problems, for example:

- *Acquiring and transmitting infections* through toys and other objects
- *Airway obstruction* from aspiration of small objects (e.g., candy, buttons, coins, peanuts, grapes, and so on). The toddler's airway is still relatively short and small and may be easily obstructed.
- *Drowning* in very small amounts of water around the home (e.g., in a bucket of water or toilet bowl)

Preschool and School-Age Children

Preschool and school-age children have developed mature lungs, heart, and circulatory system that can adapt to moderate stress and change. Healthy children typically have bouts of tonsillitis or URIs, which usually resolve without difficulty. Viral infections, such as croup and pneumonia, are common, especially in preschoolers and younger school-age children. Exercise-induced (and other) asthma is also a problem. Unfortunately, as early as middle school children may begin social habits such as tobacco use that can have long-term adverse effects on oxygenation in both the pulmonary and cardiovascular systems.

Adolescents

In adolescence, the lungs develop adult characteristics. The average adolescent is developmentally at little risk for lung diseases. Some may, however, be developing behaviors and habits, such as tobacco use, that can create risk throughout life.

- As do adults, young people often begin smoking for social reasons (e.g., peer pressure, advertising, desire to feel cool), but nicotine addiction perpetuates the habit.
- The use of e-cigarettes is becoming more common. Recent studies indicate that they do not deter smoking and actually contribute to nicotine addiction.
- Adolescents make fewer routine healthcare visits than do younger children, and as a result may not receive the recommended influenza vaccines.
- And finally, exercise-induced asthma is still a problem in this age group.

Young, Middle, and Older Adults

Unhealthy practices (e.g., smoking and a lack of aerobic exercise) of adolescence often continue into adulthood. About 1 in 5 U.S. adults is a cigarette smoker (*Vital Signs*, 2011). Half the adults who smoke were regular smokers by their 18th birthday (American Lung Association, 2011; Schiller, Lucas, & Peregoy, 2012).

Changes in the respiratory system that begin in middle age and increase in older adulthood may become significant when the person experiences stressors such as infection, surgery, anesthesia, and emotional problems. The number of cells and the efficiency of the organs decline in a subtle and progressive way as a person ages. Keep in mind, though, that endurance training and regular exercise minimize the rate of these changes. In fact, an older person who is physically conditioned by regular exercise may have better lung function than will a younger adult who is not well conditioned.

 Older adults tend to experience the following changes:

- *Reduced lung expansion and less alveolar inflation,* especially in the bases of the lungs. This is because (1) costal cartilage begins to calcify, reducing chest wall movement during breathing; (2) the lungs have less recoil ability; and (3) the alveoli lose elasticity.
- *Difficulty expelling mucus or foreign material* due to a less effective cough reflex, drier mucus, and fewer cilia in the airways.
- *Diminished ability to increase ventilation* when oxygenation demands increase (e.g., with exercise). As diaphragm strength decreases, vital capacity is reduced; therefore, exhalation becomes less efficient, causing progressive air-trapping.
- *Declining immune response,* especially cell-mediated immunity, T-cell activity, and the inflammatory response
- *Gastroesophageal reflux disease* is more common in older adults, creating a risk for aspirating stomach contents into the lungs. This may result in an inflammatory response.
- *Chemoreceptors* that control breathing respond more slowly to increased O_2 demand or rising levels of

CO_2, making hypoxemia more likely when respiratory problems occur.

All of these changes put older adults at risk for respiratory infections. URIs that would be mild and short lived in a younger person may quickly lead to pneumonia in an older adult.

Environment

Environmental factors, such as the following (stress, allergic reactions, air quality, altitude, and temperature and humidity), affect oxygenation.

Stress

The stress response stimulates the release of catecholamines from the sympathetic nervous system resulting, which (1) increases the tendency of blood to clot (e.g., as in pulmonary embolus), and (2) suppresses the immune system and inflammatory response. A chronically suppressed immune and inflammatory response increases the risk for all infections, including respiratory. For additional information on the effects of stress, see Chapter 12.

Allergic Reactions

An **allergy** is a hypersensitivity, or overresponse, to an antigen. Pulmonary allergens include such things as dust, dust mites, cockroach particles, pollen, molds, newsprint, tobacco smoke, animal dander, and sometimes foods.

Hay Fever Hay fever is an allergic reaction affecting the eyes, nose, and/or sinuses. It causes the release of *histamine*, which is largely responsible for accumulation of nasal fluid, swollen nasal membranes, nasal congestion, and itchy, swollen, watery eyes. Antihistamines are effective in combating hay fever.

Asthma Asthma is an allergic reaction occurring in the bronchioles of the lungs. *Slow-reacting substance of anaphylaxis* (SRS-A) is released, which causes bronchoconstriction and lower airway edema and spasms, making breathing difficult and ineffective. Because histamine is not a major factor in causing the asthmatic reaction, antihistamines have little effect in the treatment of asthma. Asthma is the most common serious chronic disease of childhood, and it can be life threatening. In adults, a significant amount of asthma is caused or made worse by their workplace environment, especially among adults ages 45 to 64 years, African Americans, and other minorities (Centers for Disease Control and Prevention [CDC], 2012a).

Air Quality

Air pollution triggers respiratory problems (e.g., lung cancer, carbon monoxide poisoning) that interfere with oxygenation. Even healthy people may experience headache, coughing, and other symptoms when exposed to air pollution. People with existing respiratory disease may become unable to function. Some sources of air pollution are natural (e.g., forest fires), but the most common and damaging sources result from human activities (e.g., automobile exhaust emissions). Indoor air pollutants include carbon monoxide, nitrogen oxides, radon, and suspended particles (e.g., dust, mold spores, aerosols, and tobacco smoke). Pollutants are most harmful to infants, toddlers, older adults, and people with heart or lung disease. For more information about air quality,

 Go to Chapter 36, **Supplemental Materials: Air Quality Affects Oxygenation,** on Davis*Plus.*

Altitude

Atmospheric pressure falls from 760 mm Hg at sea level to 523 mm Hg at 10,000 feet. Oxygen pressure falls proportionally, leading to decreased oxygen diffusion from alveoli into capillaries (impaired gas exchange). Low oxygen levels at high altitudes can cause hypoxemia and hypoxia. If a person is suddenly exposed to low oxygen levels, arterial chemoreceptors stimulate ventilation, making more oxygen available in the alveoli and at the tissue level. Over the long term, people who live at high altitudes undergo physiological changes that facilitate oxygenation, including an increase in the following:

- Ventilation, which brings more oxygen into the lungs
- Production of red blood cells (RBCs), which aids in the transport of oxygen to organs and tissues
- Lung volume and pulmonary vasculature, which results in increased surface area for alveolar–capillary gas exchange
- Vascularity of body tissues, which allows for improved oxygen delivery to the tissues
- Production of hemoglobin, which readily binds with oxygen so that the tissue cells can use oxygen even when oxygen pressure is low in the environment.

Temperature and Humidity

When it is very hot or very cold, the body must expend additional energy to main a constant body temperature (e.g., 98.6˚F). The additional energy increases the amount of oxygen the body is using. Breathing hot or cold air can also dry and irritate the airway, causing bronchospasm. This decreases the size of the airway and makes it more difficult to move air in and out of the lungs, causing shortness of breath, especially in those with respiratory conditions such as asthma or chronic obstructive pulmonary disease (COPD). High humidity also contributes to shortness of breath.

Lifestyle

Lifestyle factors that affect oxygenation include pregnancy, occupational exposure to hazards, nutrition, obesity, exercise, smoking, and substance abuse.

Pregnancy During pregnancy, oxygen demand increases dramatically. Maternal metabolism increases by approximately 15% during the last half of pregnancy,

increasing the demand for O_2. At the same time, the enlarging uterus pushes upward against the diaphragm, limiting its downward movement. In response, the maternal respiratory rate increases in order to increase *minute ventilation* (amount of air moved into and out of the lungs in 1 minute) (Hall, 2011).

Occupational Hazards Occupational hazards may affect pulmonary function by irritating airways or causing cancer. Toxic agents may be categorized as follows:

- *Chemicals and their fumes* irritate the sensitive membranous lining of the lungs and airways and may lead to lung cancer or leukemia. Even common household cleaners can emit toxic fumes.
- *Products of combustion* (e.g., carbon monoxide) are known causes of lung cancer and chronic lung disease.
- *Microorganisms,* such as viruses, fungi, and mold, may lead to infections and precipitate asthma.
- *Fine particles* (e.g., coal dust and asbestos) suspended in the air can be inhaled into the smallest airways, causing irritation and toxic reactions, including cancer.

Nutrition The body needs an appropriate balance of proteins, carbohydrates, fats, and other nutrients for proper immune function. A healthy diet builds resistance to disease and infection, promotes normal cellular function and tissue repair, and maintains a healthy weight. Poor nutrition, especially in those with pulmonary disorders, can lead to loss of ventilatory muscle strength, making breathing more difficult.

Obesity is defined as a body mass index (BMI) above 30. Obesity causes multiple health problems, many of which affect pulmonary function. The following are two examples:

- *Respiratory infections.* Excess abdominal fat presses upward on the diaphragm, preventing full chest expansion, leading to hypoventilation and dyspnea on exertion. The risk for respiratory infection then increases because lower lung lobes are poorly ventilated and secretions not removed effectively.
- *Sleep apnea.* When the person lies down, chest expansion is limited even more. Excess neck girth and fat deposits in the upper airway often lead to obstructive sleep apnea, a condition characterized by daytime sleepiness, loud snoring, and periods of apnea lasting 10 to 120 seconds (Porth & Matfin, 2010).

Exercise Exercise increases metabolic demands. The body responds by increasing the heart rate and the rate and depth of breathing. Lack of exercise has the opposite effect. A sedentary lifestyle reduces the capacity to increase ventilation in response to exercise.

Substance Abuse People abuse various kinds of substances, including prescription medications. Excess use or overdose of respiratory depressants such as opioids, sedatives, anti-anxiety agents, and hypnotics can cause hypoventilation, apnea, and respiratory failure, in some instances resulting in death. Over-the-counter (OTC) medications and other legally available products, such as alcohol, caffeine, glue, and aerosols and other inhalants, also have abuse potential and can be lethal. A large amount of alcohol, for example, depresses respiratory and vasomotor centers of the brain. Illicit drugs, including stimulants (e.g., amphetamines, cocaine), hallucinogens (e.g., LSD, PCP), marijuana, and in some states "bath salts," also have adverse effects on the respiratory system. And of course, an overdose of these substances can depress respirations and increase the risk for aspiration.

Smoking

Tobacco smoke contains tiny particles of tar and approximately 200 known toxic chemicals, more than 60 of which are known to cause cancer. Tobacco smoke constricts bronchioles, increases fluid secretion into the airways, causes inflammation and swelling of the bronchial lining, and paralyzes cilia. These effects lead to reduced airflow and increased production of secretions that are not easily removed from the airways. Lung inflammation stimulates the release of enzymes that break down elastin and other alveolar wall components. Continued smoking leads to chronic bronchitis, obstruction of bronchioles and alveolar walls, and emphysema. Cigarette smoking is estimated to be the cause of more than 80% of cases of lung cancer. The longer a person smokes and the more cigarettes he smokes, the greater the risk for cancer and other chronic lung diseases (American Lung Association, 2010; MedlinePlus, n.d., last updated 2009).

Roughly 1 in every 5 American adults smokes. However, once a person stops smoking, the body begins to repair the damage. In the first few days, the person will cough more as the cilia begin to clear the airways. Then the coughing subsides, and breathing becomes easier. Even long-time smokers can benefit from smoking cessation (Box 36-1).

BOX 36-1 ■ Benefits of Smoking Cessation

- Life expectancy increases.
- Blood pressure and heart rate decrease.
- Circulation to the extremities improves within 2 hours.
- Carbon dioxide levels in the blood begin to drop within 4 hours.
- Oxygen levels in the blood begin to improve within 8 hours.
- Digestion improves.
- Coughing, congestion, and shortness of breath decrease.
- Overall energy increases.
- Lungs increase ability to clean themselves, thereby reducing the risk of infection.
- Risk of heart attack decreases and returns to that of a nonsmoker in 1 year.
- Risk of lung and other cancers, stroke, and chronic obstructive lung disease decreases.

Secondhand Smoke Also known as **environmental tobacco smoke** (ETS), **second-hand smoke** is a general term for any smoke that non-smokers are exposed to. There are two types of second-hand smoke:

- **Mainstream smoke** refers to the smoke that a smoker inhales and then exhales.
- **Side-stream smoke** refers to the smoke released from the end of a lit cigarette, cigar, or pipe. Side-stream smoke accounts for 85% of the ETS in a smoky room, so although it is no worse for you than mainstream smoke, it makes up the bulk of smoke that non-smokers may encounter.

The Environmental Protection Agency (EPA) classifies secondhand smoke as a Group A carcinogen, meaning it is a substance known to cause cancer in humans. There is no safe level of exposure to secondhand smoke. Even short exposure can make blood platelets stickier, causing damage to blood vessel lining and disturbing the heart rate. Secondhand smoke is the third leading cause of preventable death in the United States (EPA, 2011). Children younger than 18 months are especially vulnerable to lower respiratory tract infections related to secondhand smoke (American Lung Association, n.d.).

The Healthy People 2020 (Healthypeople.gov, 2010) identified the goal of reducing illness, disability, and death related to tobacco use and secondhand smoke exposure by establishing policies to reduce exposure to secondhand smoke, increase the cost of tobacco, restrict tobacco advertising, and reduce illegal sales to minors.

KnowledgeCheck 36-4

- What are the major risks to oxygenation related to developmental factors?
- What environmental and lifestyle factors that influence ventilation can be avoided or minimized?

ThinkLike a Nurse 36-4

Review the Meet Your Patients scenario at the beginning of this chapter.

- Which patient(s) may be experiencing developmental, environmental, or lifestyle-related problems with oxygenation?
- Identify any additional information you need to know to answer this question.

Medications

Many drugs can interfere with pulmonary function by depressing respirations. Respiratory depressants generally act by depressing central nervous system (CNS) control of breathing or by weakening the muscles of breathing. They include general anesthetics, opioids (e.g., morphine), anti-anxiety drugs (e.g., diazepam [Valium]), sedative-hypnotics (e.g., barbiturates), neuromuscular blocking agents, and magnesium sulfate. Drugs that block beta-2 adrenergic receptors (e.g., used to lower the blood pressure) have little effect on healthy lungs but can lead to serious bronchiole constriction in people with asthma.

Medications are also used to improve respiratory function. A few examples include bronchodilators, anti-inflammatory agents such as corticosteroids, cough suppressants, expectorants, and decongestants.

For a more extensive discussion of individual medications that either interfere with or improve respiratory function,

 Go to Chapter 36, **Supplemental Materials: Medications That Can Interfere With Oxygenation** and **Medications Used to Improve Oxygenation,** on Davis*Plus*.

Pathophysiological Conditions

Poor exchange of oxygen and carbon dioxide at the alveolar–capillary membrane or the tissue level alters the levels of O_2 and CO_2 in the blood. Unchecked, it affects oxygenation in tissues and organs and can be life threatening. Box 36-2 describes some alterations in gas exchange.

Alterations in gas exchange are caused by a number of disorders that affect the structure, function, and regulation of the pulmonary and cardiovascular systems. Because it is difficult to separate pulmonary and cardiovascular causes and effects, both are included in the discussion of pulmonary disorders that follows. For a thorough description of these diseases and pathological conditions, consult a medical-surgical nursing text, or

 Go to Chapter 36, **Supplemental Materials: Pathophysiological Conditions That Influence Gas Exchange,** on Davis*Plus*.

KnowledgeCheck 36-5

- What are some indirect indicators of tissue oxygenation?
- How are hyperventilation and hypoventilation related to carbon dioxide levels?
- What are the effects of carbon dioxide levels on the nervous system?

 ## ThinkLike a Nurse 36-5

You are assessing a very anxious young man who looks frightened and is complaining of trouble breathing. His respiratory rate is 32 and deep. He states his fingers and hands are numb.

- What is the most likely cause?
- What blood levels would help you clarify what is going on?

Example Problem: Respiratory Infections (URIs, Influenza, and Pneumonia)

Respiratory infections interfere with gas exchange. They are among the most common causes of short-term disability in the United States. It is important to distinguish among respiratory infections because antiviral medications are effective for some conditions, but not others. Diagnosis can be difficult because many conditions start with cold-like symptoms (e.g., whooping cough, croup, allergies, measles, influenza, and pneumonia).

BOX 36-2 ■ Alterations in Gas Exchange

Hypoxemia—Low arterial blood oxygen levels

Etiology: Poor oxygen diffusion across the alveolar–capillary membrane into the blood (ineffective external respiration) due to lung or pulmonary circulation disorders. Hypoventilation predisposes to the development of hypoxemia and may lead to hypoxia.

Comments: Even if the blood is adequately oxygenated, hypoxia may still occur in the organs and tissues because of poor circulation.

Hypoxia—Inadequate oxygenation of organs and tissues

Etiology: Either hypoxemia or circulatory disorders

Comments: The effects of hypoxia depend on the organs affected. For example, hypoxic central nervous system tissue causes abnormal brain functioning (e.g., altered level of consciousness), whereas hypoxic renal tissue causes abnormal kidney functioning (e.g., poor urine output), and hypoxic limb tissue results in abnormal muscle functioning (e.g., muscle weakness and pain with exercise).

Hypercarbia (hypercapnia)—An excess of dissolved CO_2 in the blood

Etiology: Hypoventilation is caused by abnormalities affecting the lungs or chest cavity or by neuromuscular abnormalities that interfere with normal breathing. Hypercarbia can occur suddenly, as in acute airway obstruction or drug overdose, or chronically, as in chronic lung disease.

Comments: Very high blood levels of CO_2 have an anesthetic effect on the nervous system and can lead to somnolence progressing to coma and death, a syndrome known as carbon dioxide narcosis.

Hypocarbia (hypocapnia)—A low level of dissolved CO_2 in the blood

In most cases (except high altitude), blood O_2 levels remain normal.

Etiology: Hyperventilation

Comments: Severe hypocarbia stimulates the nervous system, leading to muscle twitching or spasm (especially in the hands and feet) and numbness and tingling in the face and lips.

URIs Most URIs, including the common cold, are caused by viruses. Symptoms of URIs include stuffy nose, sore throat, cough, sneezing, tearing, and a mild fever. Colds are more common in children, and tend to decline with age. They are rarely dangerous to healthy adults and children. There is no "cure" for the common cold.

Influenza Influenza (flu) is a highly infectious viral disease, usually more severe than the common cold, and may involve the lower airways. Most flu fatalities occur in children younger than age 2 years and in older adults, especially the frail elderly. In addition to cold symptoms, the patient may experience high fever, headache, myalgia (muscle pain or tenderness), weakness, exhaustion, nasal inflammation and discharge, sore throat, and cough. New strains of the virus continually emerge, so it is difficult to develop immunity to the disease. Influenza immunizations are manufactured for each season in an attempt to keep pace with the changing virus.

Lower Respiratory Tract Infections Pneumonia, acute bronchitis, respiratory syncytial virus (RSV), and tuberculosis are examples of lower respiratory tract infections. They occur more often and are more severe and more likely to be life threatening in children, older adults, and people with impaired immunity or lung function.

Pneumonia is an infection of the lungs caused by bacteria, fungi, or viruses. It occurs more often during winter months and often follows a recent URI or influenza. Pneumonia-causing organisms gain entry into the lungs from being released into the air with coughing, sneezing, or talking; from contaminated respiratory therapy equipment; transported from the blood to the lung; or from the nose and throat. The invading pathogen releases toxins that damage bronchial and alveolar–capillary membranes. A full-scale inflammatory response triggers edema in the small airways and deposits debris and exudate in the alveoli. Some toxins even cause lung tissue necrosis. The area of the lung affected becomes *consolidated* (solid rather than air filled).

Symptoms of pneumonia include cough, malaise, pleural pain from coughing, discolored sputum, fever, chills, dyspnea, and elevated WBC counts. Treatment includes antipyretics for fever, expectorants to enhance mobilization of secretions, humidity to moisten inhaled air, hydration to thin secretions, *pulmonary hygiene* (deep breathing, coughing, and chest percussion and vibration) to move secretions out of the airways, rest to conserve body energy stores, and, if needed, oxygen therapy. Curative therapy includes specific anti-infective agents to kill the causative organisms. Immunizations are available and are discussed in your textbook.

Pulmonary System Abnormalities

The following is a brief discussion of various pulmonary abnormalities that can lead to alterations in gas exchange.

Structural Abnormalities Structural abnormalities include anything that restricts or limits the free movement of the chest wall (e.g., fractured ribs, kyphosis), interruptions in the chest cavity that inhibit inflation of the lungs (e.g., pneumothorax), or a collection of fluid (blood, lymph, pus) in the pleural space that inhibits lung expansion.

Airway Inflammation and Obstruction Allergic reactions (e.g., asthma) or irritation from smoke or other irritants may cause airway inflammation. Obstruction may be mechanical, as with a foreign object or bolus of food, or due to spasm (e.g., laryngospasm). Swollen tonsils and a swollen epiglottis may also cause obstruction.

Alveolar–Capillary Membrane Disorders These disorders are characterized by a change in the consistency of the lung tissue, especially at the alveolar level. The alveoli become stiff and difficult to ventilate, and gas exchange is impaired. Pulmonary edema, acute respiratory distress syndrome (ARDS), and pulmonary fibrosis are examples.

Atelectasis Anything that reduces ventilation (e.g., tumor, obstructed airway) can cause **atelectasis**, or alveolar collapse.

Pulmonary Circulation Abnormalities

For gas exchange to occur in the alveoli, there must be adequate blood flow through the pulmonary circulation. The most common causes of impaired pulmonary circulation are pulmonary embolus and pulmonary hypertension. A **pulmonary embolus** is obstruction of pulmonary arterial circulation by a foreign substance (e.g., a blood clot, air, or fat).

Pulmonary hypertension is elevated pressure within the pulmonary arterial system. High pressure in the pulmonary circulation increases the workload of the heart. Over time, this causes right-sided heart failure, with a reduced amount of blood pumped into the pulmonary circulation. You will learn about the difference between right-sided and left-sided heart failure in a medical-surgical nursing course. However, if you need some information about it now,

 Go to Chapter 37, **Tables, Boxes, Figures: ESG Table 37-1,** on Davis*Plus.*

If you would like to see an animation demonstrating how blood is oxygenated in the heart and lungs,

 Go to **Cardiovascular/Pulmonary Animations: Blood Flow and Carbon Dioxide/Oxygen Transport,** on Davis*Plus.*

Central Nervous System Abnormalities

Any condition that injures or alters the function of the CNS can interfere with the regulation of breathing and, therefore, gas exchange. Trauma and stroke (cerebrovascular accident) are the most commonly seen CNS problems in adults. Spinal cord injuries interfere with nerve transmission between the brain and the area below the level of the injury and may, for example, limit diaphragm function. Immature breathing patterns, such as apnea or periodic breathing, are common in preterm and term infants.

Neuromuscular Abnormalities

Neuromuscular abnormalities can affect gas exchange by interfering with the regulation of breathing or by limiting movement of the muscles involved with breathing. Any condition that alters CNS function can interfere with the regulation of breathing. Trauma, stroke, and medications are the most common causes. Neuromuscular disorders that affect the nerves involved in breathing can also depress respiratory function (e.g., Guillain-Barré syndrome, amyotrophic lateral sclerosis, and myasthenia gravis).

KnowledgeCheck 36-6

- Identify four pathophysiological conditions that affect pulmonary function. How are they similar? How are they different?
- What types of injuries are most likely to cause oxygenation problems?

 ## ThinkLike a Nurse 36-6

You are the nursing supervisor on the night shift in a small community hospital. At the beginning of the shift, you have only one critical care bed available. During your shift, you receive calls for assistance on the following patients:

- Patient A has burns on her face, scalp, and chest and is coughing up sputum with black streaks.
- Patient B has pneumonia but has suddenly become confused.
- Patient C is short of breath and complaining that he can't breathe. His skin is cool and moist, and he is coughing up clear sputum with small bubbles in it.

Which patient would you admit to the critical care bed? Why?

Practical Knowledge
knowing how

In the remainder of the chapter, we discuss focused respiratory assessment and the nursing activities to maximize ventilation and gas exchange. In Chapter 20, the section Respiration provides more information about assessing respirations. Also,

 Go to Chapter 20, **Procedure 20-5: Assessing Respirations,** in Volume 2.

ASSESSMENT

Although this section focuses on respiratory assessments, recall that the pulmonary system is only a part of the concept of oxygenation. An evaluation of overall oxygenation includes a history and physical examination to assess lung, heart, and circulatory function. The order of data collection and the priorities of assessment vary with the patient's condition and the purpose of the assessment. For example, for someone in obvious respiratory distress, the immediate assessment focus is to ask simple questions about current symptoms while performing a quick examination to determine adequacy of breathing, circulation, and oxygenation. In contrast, assessment for risk of respiratory disease in a healthy person might include more extensive questions about occupation, smoking habits, and living environment; a medical history; and an extensive physical examination. For a respiratory assessment that is focused but thorough, you will need to identify risk factors, perform a physical examination, and be familiar with certain diagnostic tests.

Assessing for Risk Factors

A health history related to pulmonary function includes questions about the presence of risk factors that affect lung and airway function. Topics to assess include demographic data, health history, respiratory history, cardiovascular history, environmental history, and lifestyle. For a detailed list of interview questions for each of these topics,

 Go to Chapter 36, **Assessment Guidelines and Tools, Focused Assessment: Oxygenation,** in Volume 2.

Key Point: *All patients, not just those with oxygenation problems, should be asked whether they use tobacco and should have their tobacco-use status documented on a regular basis.*

Physical Examination

You will use all four examination techniques to assess respiratory function:

- *Inspect* to observe respiratory patterns, signs of respiratory distress, chest structures and movement, skin and mucous membrane color, presence or absence of edema, sputum characteristics, and overall general appearance. Refer to Chapter 22 to review the details of inspecting the skin and mucous membranes. Also

 Go to **Procedure 22-2: Assessing the Skin,** and **Procedure 22-12: Assessing the Chest and Lungs,** in Volume 2.

- *Palpate* pulses, skin temperature, heart pulsations through the chest wall, and areas of tenderness.
- *Percuss* over the lung fields to screen for areas of consolidation or excess air pockets in the lungs.
- *Auscultate* breath sounds, heart sounds, and vascular sounds. For a step-by-step discussion of how to assess the chest and lungs,

 Go to Chapter 22, **Procedure 22-12: Assessing the Chest and Lungs,** in Volume 2.

Assess breathing patterns, cough and associated symptoms, and respiratory effort, as follows. You may also need to monitor oxygenation and ventilation with pulse oximetry and capnography.

Poor peripheral circulation is characterized by weak or absent pulses; mottling (skin marbling); pale, ashen, or cyanotic skin and mucous membranes; and cool skin temperature. You can assess tissue oxygenation indirectly by determining whether organs are functioning normally. You will learn more about this in Chapter 37.

Assessing Breathing Patterns

Assess for normal and altered breathing patterns. They include the following: eupnea, bradypnea, tachypnea, apnea or periodic breathing, Kussmaul's breathing, Biot's breathing, and Cheyne-Stokes respirations. You can see a description of these patterns in Table 20-4. Most irregular breathing patterns result from brain injury or the effects of drugs on the brain.

- **Eupnea**—Normal breathing; rate about 12 to 20 breaths/min

- **Tachypnea**—Fast, shallow breathing; more than 24 breaths/min. Generally caused by hypoxemia or increased oxygen demand (e.g., exercise). Rapid, shallow respirations draw limited air into the alveoli and may result in hypoventilation.
- **Bradypnea**—Slow respirations; Fewer than 10 breaths/min. Bradypnea may cause poor gas exchange. Causes include sedative and opioid medications and neuromuscular dysfunction.
- **Kussmaul's respirations**—Regular but increased in rate and abnormally deep respirations. These may be a compensatory mechanism for metabolic disorders that lower blood pH, as well as a form of hyperventilation caused by fear, anxiety, or panic.
- **Biot's respirations**—Irregular respirations of variable depth (usually shallow), alternating with periods of apnea. This pattern is often associated with damage to the medullary respiratory center or high intracranial pressure due to brain injury.
- **Cheyne-Stokes respirations**—Gradual increase in depth of respirations, followed by a gradual decrease in depth, than a period of apnea. This pattern often results from damage to the medullary respiratory center or high intracranial pressure due to brain injury.
- **Apnea**—Absence of breathing. Respiratory arrest requires immediate cardiopulmonary resuscitation.

Recall that pain alters the rate and depth of respirations. Often patients in pain breathe shallowly and are at risk for atelectasis. Regularly assess all patients for pain. Once you have medicated the patient, reassess breath sounds, and encourage the patient to breathe deeply and cough.

Assessing Respiratory Effort/Dyspnea

A healthy person breathes effortlessly. A patient experiencing shortness of breath or dyspnea requires a thorough assessment. However, you must take care not to increase his respiratory effort. Use closed questions that the patient can answer with yes, no, or only a few words. Ask whether the shortness of breath began suddenly or gradually, how severe it is right now, and whether it is getting better or worse. At the same time, observe for or ask about the signs of increased respiratory effort discussed below. Note that these signs are most easily visible in infants and small children.

- **Nasal flaring**—The visible enlargement of the nostrils with inhalation. It helps reduce resistance to airflow in the nose and keep the nasal passages open to take in more air.
- **Retractions**—The visible "pulling in" of intercostal, supraclavicular, and subcostal tissue, caused by excessive negative pressures generated in the chest to try to increase the depth of inhalation.
- **Use of accessory muscles** during inspiration—The patient may use the intercostals, abdominal muscles, and muscles of the neck and shoulders when there is an increased demand for oxygen or problems with ventilation.
- **Grunting**—Noisy, difficult breathing. It is caused by forced expiration against a closed glottis, and by involuntary muscle contraction during expiration to help keep alveoli open and enhance gas exchange.
- **Body positioning** to facilitate respirations—The patient usually finds an upright posture the most comfortable. In the upright position, gravity pulls the abdominal organs down and allows the diaphragm more room to contract. Most patients with dyspnea cannot tolerate lying down. **Orthopnea** is the term used to describe difficulty breathing when lying down. Ask how the patient usually sleeps. Some patients may report sleeping in a recliner or chair.
- **Paroxysmal nocturnal dyspnea**—Sudden awakening due to shortness of breath that begins during sleep. The patient feels panic and extreme dyspnea and must sit upright to ease breathing.
- **Conversational dyspnea**—The inability to speak complete sentences without stopping to breathe. The more frequently the patient pauses when speaking, the more severe the dyspnea.
- **Stridor**—A high-pitched, harsh, crowing, inspiratory sound caused by partial obstruction of the larynx or trachea. You can hear it without a stethoscope. ✚ Partial airway obstruction can easily become complete airway obstruction. Therefore, the patient with stridor needs immediate care.
- **Wheezing**—A musical sound produced by air passing through partially obstructed small airways. It is often heard in patients with asthma and lung congestion.
- ✚ **Diminished or absent breath sounds**—In a patient experiencing dyspnea these are signs of worsening ventilation and oxygenation. Oxygen therapy and measures to restore adequate ventilation may be required.

Assessing Cough

Everyone coughs from time to time to remove small amounts of mucus and debris from the airways. Coughing is a normal protective response to known respiratory irritants (e.g., cigarette smoke, irritating fumes, dust particles) or when food or fluid accidentally gets into the airways. A cough becomes significant if it persists, is recurring, or is productive. A persistent or recurring cough may indicate ongoing or recurring airway irritation. Advise patients to obtain medical evaluation for a cough that lasts more than 3 weeks and cannot be explained.

Assess the Type of Cough Is it dry, productive, or hacking? When does the cough occur and how long has the patient been coughing? What makes it worse? What seems to help it? What has been used to treat the cough, and what were the effects?

Assess for Other Clinical Findings Associated With a Cough This helps determine its cause. A cough associated with nasal congestion, sneezing, or watery eyes or nose discharge is most likely due to allergies and may be successfully treated with OTC remedies. A cough occurring with fever, chest congestion, noisy breath sounds, and sputum production is more likely to be due to a URI, which may require antibiotics. A cough associated with dyspnea, chest tightness, and wheezing may be due to an airway obstruction disorder such as asthma, which requires corticosteroids and bronchodilating medications.

Assess the Sputum A cough is described as **productive** if it raises sputum (mucus and debris) up from the airways.

- **Sputum Appearance and Odor.** Sputum appearance and odor provide valuable *clues* about the cause and significance of a cough (see Box 36-3).
- **Sputum Amount.** The amount of sputum can vary from a teaspoon to pints. In general, sputum production increases with the severity of the underlying condition. However, limited sputum production does not always indicate that the problem is minor, because excess mucus and debris may be trapped in the airways and the patient is unable to cough it up and out of the body.
- **Sputum Timing.** Sputum production ranges from constant to once per day. Tobacco smokers often have a "morning cough," which helps clear their airways of mucus and debris accumulated overnight. In contrast, someone with a URI is more likely to produce sputum throughout the day.

BOX 36-3 ■ Significance of Sputum Appearance and Odor

Color/Appearance	Significance
White or clear	Usually present in viral infections (e.g., common cold, viral bronchitis), often requiring only supportive care
Yellow or green	A sign of infection
Black	Caused by coal dust, smoke, or soot inhalation
Rust colored	Associated with pneumococcal pneumonia, tuberculosis, and possibly the presence of blood
Hemoptysis	The coughing up of blood or bloody sputum. It may range from small streaks of blood to large amounts of frank blood.
Pink and frothy	Associated with pulmonary edema

Foul-smelling sputum usually indicates bacterial infection (e.g., pneumonia, lung abscess).

KnowledgeCheck 36-7

- What areas should you include in a nursing history for a patient with oxygenation concerns who is undergoing a comprehensive assessment?
- When is a cough significant? What aspects of a cough should be assessed?
- Identify at least five signs that you may observe in a patient experiencing dyspnea.
- A patient has a respiratory rate of 30 breaths/min that is rhythmic and moderate in depth. What term would you use to describe this breathing pattern?

 ThinkLike a Nurse 36-7

Review the patients presented in the Meet Your Patients scenario.

- Which patients are experiencing respiratory distress? Identify the signs of distress in these patients.
- Which patients require a comprehensive assessment, and which patients will need a rapid assessment and immediate treatment because of the severity of their symptoms?

Diagnostic Testing

Diagnostic testing helps clinicians identify the causes of impaired oxygenation and monitor patient responses to treatment. You will need to assist with and be familiar with the results of the tests of respiratory function. We discuss several of these tests in the next sections. For others,

 Go to Chapter 36, **Diagnostic Testing: Tests Related to Oxygenation,** in Volume 2.

Obtaining Sputum Samples

You may need to collect sputum samples. Sputum samples are examined microscopically and cultured in the lab to identify organisms and test for sensitivity to different anti-infective agents. For a summary of this procedure, see the Highlights of Procedures box. For the complete steps,

 Go to Chapter 36, **Procedure 36-1: Collecting a Sputum Specimen,** in Volume 2.

Skin Testing

To review a procedure for administering intradermal injections,

 Go to Chapter 26, **Procedure 26-11: Administering Intradermal Medications,** in Volume 2.

- **Tuberculin skin testing** is widely used to detect exposure and antibody formation to the tubercle bacillus. Annual screening is recommended for low-income populations, residents in congregate living conditions (e.g., dormitories, correctional facilities), immigrants from countries with a high prevalence of tuberculosis (TB), and healthcare workers. For the skin test to be effective, you must administer the antigen intradermally, not subcutaneously. Read the test site 48 to 72 hours after administration.

A positive skin test is defined as an area of induration (hardness) at the test site. The size of the induration that indicates a positive result depends on risk factors. Patients with positive TB skin tests must undergo further testing (chest x-ray study and sputum cultures) to determine whether they have merely been exposed to disease or whether they have active disease. For guidelines for interpreting test results,

 Go to Chapter 36, **Diagnostic Testing: Reading a Tuberculin Skin Result,** in Volume 2.

- **Allergy testing** uses skin testing to identify antigens that may cause hypersensitivity reactions in susceptible individuals. Testing is performed by scratching antigen samples onto the skin. The area is then observed for allergic skin reactions. Skin testing is performed in facilities with resuscitation equipment and personnel trained in its use, because life-threatening airway obstruction sometimes occurs in response to the allergens.

Pulse Oximetry

Pulse oximetry is a noninvasive estimate of arterial blood oxygen saturation (SaO_2). **SaO_2** reflects the percentage of hemoglobin molecules carrying oxygen. The normal value is 95% to 100%. Values below 94% are considered abnormal in healthy people and should be investigated to determine the cause. Well-oxygenated hemoglobin and deoxygenated hemoglobin absorb light differently. Using a light-emitting diode (LED), the oximeter is able to detect this difference and calculate the percentage of oxygenated hemoglobin.

Pulse oximetry is simple to perform, provides a rapid reading, and can be used intermittently or continuously (Fig. 36-5). Frequency of measurement depends on the

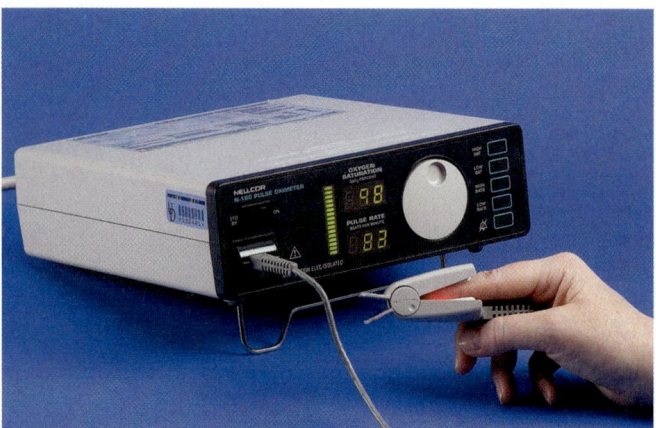

FIGURE 36-5 Pulse oximetry is a noninvasive estimate of arterial blood oxygen saturation (SaO_2). It uses a light-emitting diode (LED) probe to measure light absorption by hemoglobin in the circulating red blood cells.

clinical condition of the patient. Recent recommendations are that pulse oximetry can be used to screen newborns for critical congenital heart disease (American Academy of Pediatrics, 2011b).

Such factors as movement, acrylic fingernails, nail polish, or cold extremities can interfere with the accuracy of the readings. For the complete procedure,

 Go to Chapter 36, **Procedure 36-2: Monitoring Pulse Oximetry (Arterial Oxygen Saturation),** in Volume 2. Also, go to Chapter 36, **Clinical Insight 36-1: Tips for Obtaining Accurate Pulse Oximetry Readings,** in Volume 2.

Capnography

Capnography measures the carbon dioxide (CO_2) in inhaled and exhaled air. As a beam of infrared light passes through a sample of respiratory gases, more or less of it is absorbed depending on the amount of CO_2 that is present. The device displays the results digitally and prints out a graph showing CO_2 at various times in the breathing cycle. Capnography directly measures ventilation, and indirectly measures the partial pressure of CO_2 in the arterial blood. Normally the difference between arterial blood and expired CO_2 is very small.

Capnography is often used with pulse oximetry because (1) it provides information about ventilation because it shows accumulation or depletion of CO_2, whereas pulse oximetry reflects only oxygenation of the blood; and (2) capnography is a more reliable indicator of respiratory depression than is pulse oximetry. Examples of the situations in which capnography is used include the following: when a patient is receiving opioids, during general anesthesia, and for adjusting parameter settings in mechanically ventilated patients.

Although they do measure carbon dioxide, **CO_2 detectors** are different from capnography. They use chemically treated paper that changes color when exposed to CO_2. They do not give exact readings, but can measure only a range of values.

Spirometry

Spirometry is a measure of air that moves into and out of the lungs. To describe the events of pulmonary ventilation, the air in the lungs is divided into four volumes and four capacities. Normal lung volumes and capacities vary with body size, age, and exercise. Men, large people, and athletes have greater lung volume and capacity for ventilation. For a summary of this information,

 Go to Chapter 36, **Diagnostic Testing: Lung Volumes and Capacities,** in Volume 2.

 ThinkLike a **Nurse** 36-8

You hear a pulse oximeter alarm sound in a nearby patient room and find it reading 75%.

- What observations should you make?
- What actions should you take?

Arterial Blood Gases

Arterial blood gas (ABG) analysis measures the levels of oxygen and carbon dioxide in arterial blood. A blood sample is obtained from an artery (usually the brachial, radial, or femoral), either by arterial puncture or by withdrawal from an existing arterial line. Arteries are located deep under the skin and alongside nerves, making needle insertion painful. Nurses in critical care units routinely draw ABGs and monitor patients with invasive arterial monitoring; however, you may care for patients on medical-surgical units, or even outpatients, who will undergo periodic ABG evaluation. ABG analysis measures pH, partial pressure of oxygen (Po_2), partial pressure of carbon dioxide (Pco_2), saturation of oxygen (Sao_2), and bicarbonate (HCO_3) level. Here, we discuss only Po_2 and Pco_2. For a more thorough discussion of arterial blood gas values, see the discussion, Interpreting ABGs, and Table 38-6 in Chapter 38.

Measuring Arterial Blood Oxygen

Three values are important when assessing the degree to which the tissues are receiving oxygen:

- **Hemoglobin** is the iron-containing pigment of red blood cells that as *oxyhemoglobin* carries oxygen in the blood.
- **Po_2 (partial pressure of oxygen)** is the amount of oxygen available to combine with hemoglobin to make oxyhemoglobin.
- **Sao_2 (saturation of oxygen)** reflects oxygen that is actually bound to hemoglobin.

At sea level, the normal Po_2 range in arterial blood is 80 to 100 mm Hg. After tissues have extracted oxygen from arterial blood and the blood enters the veins to return to the heart, the venous blood Po_2 has fallen to around 40 mm Hg. The Sao_2, along with the Po_2 and hemoglobin level, indicates the degree to which the tissues are receiving oxygen. Small changes in Sao_2 are associated with large changes in Po_2. For blood gas values,

 Go to Chapter 38, **Diagnostic Testing: Assessing Fluid, Electrolyte, and Acid–Base Balance,** in Volume 2.

To fully interpret Po_2 and Sao_2 values, you need to know the percentage of oxygen in the air the patient is inhaling. This is known as the **fraction of inspired oxygen,** or **Fio_2**. At sea level, atmospheric air (commonly known as *room air*) is 21% oxygen ($Fio_2 = 21\%$). The norms quoted for Po_2 and Sao_2 are based on an Fio_2 of 21%. If a healthy patient receives 100% oxygen for a few minutes, the arterial Po_2 would rise to 500 to 600 mm Hg, and the Sao_2 would remain at 100%. The reason is that the Sao_2 measures the oxygen *bound to hemoglobin*—and of course the hemoglobin cannot be "filled" with oxygen to more than 100% capacity. When gas exchange is impaired as a result of disease or injury, Po_2 and Sao_2 levels fall. However, they can be kept at normal levels if supplemental oxygen is given.

Measuring Arterial Blood Carbon Dioxide

The **partial pressure of carbon dioxide (Pco_2)** is a measure of the CO_2 dissolved in the blood. Normal arterial Pco_2 is 35 to 45 mm Hg. Carbon dioxide readily diffuses across the alveolar–capillary membrane in the lungs even when there are obstacles such as alveolar fluid or thickened membranes. As a result, Pco_2 levels remain normal until a severe disorder interferes with all gas exchange. Once in the alveoli, the amount of carbon dioxide exhaled from the lungs is directly influenced by how well air is moving into and out of the lungs (ventilation).

- **Hypocarbia.** When a person hyperventilates, he exhales large amounts of CO_2, causing arterial Pco_2 values to fall. Hyperventilation brings more oxygen into the lungs, so unless it is triggered by hypoxemia, oxygen levels (Po_2) usually remain normal.
- **Hypercarbia.** Conversely, in hypoventilation less CO_2 moves into the alveoli for exhalation, leaving more CO_2 in the arterial blood. This causes Pco_2 values to rise. High Pco_2 levels (hypercarbia) suppress the respiratory drive, have an anesthetic effect on the nervous system, and can be toxic. Hypoventilation severe enough to cause hypercarbia is usually associated with hypoxemia because not enough oxygen is inhaled.

KnowledgeCheck 36-8

- What does a pulse oximetry reading tell you?
- What is the relationship between arterial Po_2 and Sao_2 levels?
- Identify normal Po_2, Sao_2, and Pco_2 levels.
- What effect does ventilation have on arterial Pco_2?
- How is Pco_2 related to oxygenation?

 ThinkLike a Nurse 36-9

You are caring for two patients, both of whom have a Po_2 of 95 mm Hg and Sao_2 of 99%. Do they have similar lung function? Explain your answer.

Peak Flow Monitoring

Peak expiratory flow rate (PEFR) measures the amount of air that can be exhaled with forcible effort. Patients with asthma use PEFR monitoring to detect subtle changes in their condition, often before symptoms occur. A peak flow meter is used to monitor these changes (Fig. 36-6). Peak flow is expressed in liters per minute. Patients with asthma are often asked to measure their peak flow daily and with the onset of any symptoms. Treatment protocols describe the use and frequency of medications based on individualized peak flow rates. The Home Care box Home Use of a Peak Flow Meter describes self-monitoring.

ANALYSIS/NURSING DIAGNOSIS

Alterations in pulmonary function may be nursing diagnoses, etiologies of other problems, or merely symptoms of other problems. In analyzing the assessment data, you must determine which. For example, suppose

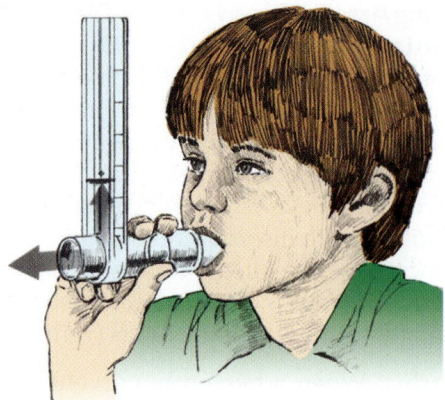

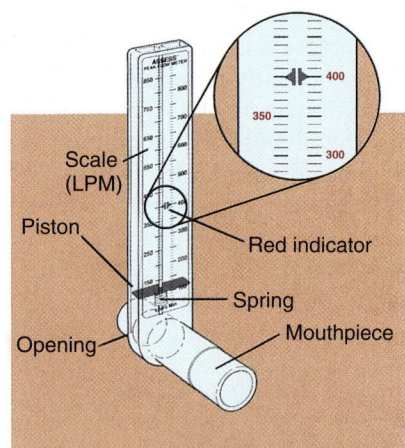

Scale (LPM)

Piston

Red indicator

Spring

Opening

Mouthpiece

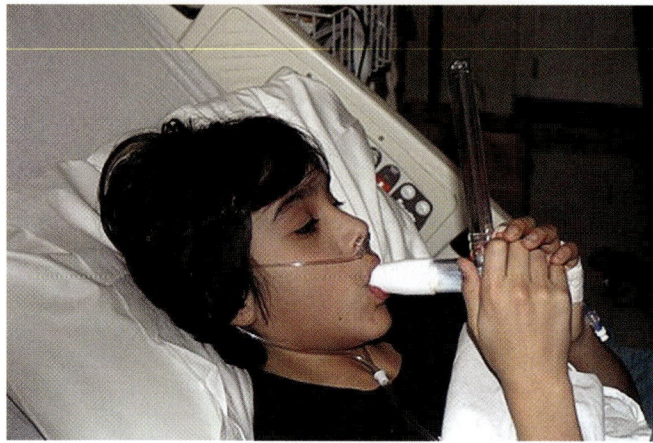

FIGURE 36-6 A patient with asthma using a peak flow meter to monitor peak expiratory flow rate (PEFR).

a patient is breathing shallowly and slowly. The pulmonary problem might be one of the following:

- **A nursing diagnosis:** *Ineffective Breathing Pattern (hypoventilation)* r/t pain secondary to rib fractures. In this case, you would provide pain relief; the desired outcome is that the patient will have effective (normal) ventilation. To sees a nursing care plan and care map for Ineffective Breathing Pattern,

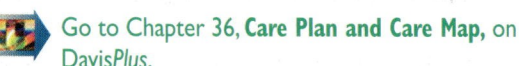

Go to Chapter 36, **Care Plan and Care Map,** on Davis*Plus.*

Home Care

Home Use of a Peak Flow Meter

People with asthma are often asked to monitor their peak flow readings at home and to compare their current readings with their baseline "personal best."

➤ Teach patients that to get an accurate reading, they need to take a deep breath and forcefully exhale.

➤ Teach patients to take a series of three readings and record the highest reading.

➤ Teach patients to maintain or adjust their medication according to their highest reading. They should follow the color-coded treatment protocols prescribed by their physician. These are individualized for each patient. Notice that these correspond to the color-coded markers on their peak flow meter.

*Green = **All clear: Baseline peak flow**—Peak flow is within 80% to 100% of personal best baseline.*

Treatment protocol calls for routine medication use.

*Yellow = **Caution: Peak flow is 50% to 80% of usual or "normal" rate.** Said another way, there is a 20% to 50% reduction in peak flow—This reading signals the onset of airway changes.*

Treatment protocols usually specify an increase in the dosage of maintenance medications, use of rescue therapies (e.g., fast-acting bronchodilators), or a call to the healthcare provider. These measures are designed to reverse acute exacerbations before they become severe.

*Red = **Medical alert: Peak flow is less than 50% of personal best baseline.** Severe reduction in peak flow.*

Treatment protocols usually specify immediate treatment with rescue medications and to seek emergency treatment if symptoms do not improve.

Source: Adapted from American Lung Association. (2013). *Six steps.* Retrieved from http://www.lungusa.org/lung-disease/asthma/living-with-asthma/take-control-of-your-asthma/AsthmaActionPlan-JUL2008-high-res.pdf

- **An etiology:** Risk for ineffective Cerebral Tissue Perfusion (Cerebral) *r/t Ineffective Breathing Pattern (hypoventilation).* In this case, you might address the etiology by administering oxygen; the desired outcome would be effective cerebral perfusion, evidenced by normal speech and alertness.

- **A symptom:** Decreased Intracranial Adaptive capacity r/t brain injury, *as manifested by Ineffective Breathing Pattern (hypoventilation), and baseline ICP ≥10 mm Hg.* In this situation, you would, of course, support ventilation (the symptom) until the problem subsides. However, the primary interventions would be directed toward the head trauma and increased intracranial pressure (ICP). Once these etiologies were corrected, the hypoventilation would disappear. The goal would be normal intracranial pressure, evidenced in part by a normal breathing pattern.

Problems of Ventilation and Gas Exchange Five NANDA International (NANDA-I) diagnoses directly describe problems with ventilation and gas exchange. Use these diagnoses when they are the central problem and you intend to use interventions to eliminate the cause of the problem.

- *Ineffective Airway Clearance* is the inability to maintain a clear airway.
- *Ineffective Breathing Pattern* is used to describe inadequate ventilation, such as hypoventilation, hyperventilation, tachypnea, or bradypnea.
- *Impaired Gas Exchange* is the appropriate diagnosis if the patient is ventilating adequately but diffusion of gases across the alveolar–capillary membrane is impaired.
- *Impaired Spontaneous Ventilation* describes a condition in which a patient, as a result of decreased energy reserves, is unable to maintain breathing adequate to support life.
- *Dysfunctional Ventilatory Weaning Response* represents a specific situation in which a patient who is being mechanically ventilated cannot adjust to lower levels of ventilator support, prolonging the ventilatory weaning process.
- *Risk for Aspiration* should be used when there is a risk for secretions, solids, or fluids entering into tracheobronchial passages (e.g., for patients who have had head or neck surgery or who have a reduced level of consciousness).

For further discussion of these diagnoses,

 Go to Chapter 36, **Standardized Language, Nursing Diagnoses Associated With Impaired Ventilation and Gas Exchange,** on Davis*Plus.*

PLANNING OUTCOMES/EVALUATION

NOC standardized outcomes appropriate for patients with pulmonary function problems include, for example, Mechanical Ventilation Weaning Response: Adult; Respiratory Status: Airway Patency; and Respiratory Status: Gas Exchange. For examples of other NOC outcomes and NIC interventions for selected oxygenation nursing diagnoses,

 Go to Chapter 36, **Standardized Language, Examples of NOC Outcomes and NIC Interventions Linked to Oxygenation Diagnoses,** on Davis*Plus.*

These provide a general care planning guide. Depending on individual patient needs, other NOC outcomes or NIC interventions may also be appropriate.

Individualized goals/outcome statements depend on the nursing diagnosis you identify. For diagnoses related to gas exchange, the following are examples of goals you might write:

Expectorates secretions effectively
No dyspnea or shortness of breath
Lungs clear; no adventitious sounds present

PLANNING INTERVENTIONS/IMPLEMENTATION

NIC standardized interventions related to oxygenation are found in the Respiratory Management category. They focus on maintaining a patent airway and promoting gas exchange, and include Airway Management, Airway Suction, Cough Enhancement, Oxygen Therapy, and Respiratory Monitoring.

Specific nursing interventions for patients with oxygenation problems include health promotion, prevention, and treatment activities. They are discussed in the sections that follow.

Administering Respiratory Medications

Respiratory medications promote ventilation and oxygenation by their effects on the respiratory system itself. Some need a prescription; others do not. Medications used to improve respiratory function include bronchodilators and anti-inflammatory agents such as corticosteroids, cough suppressants, expectorants, and decongestants.

See the accompanying Self-Care box Cough and Cold Medicines: Tips for Parents for assistance in administering such medications to children. Also refer to the accompanying CAM box for some common alternative cold remedies. For an extensive discussion of individual medications that either interfere with or improve respiratory function,

 Go to Chapter 36, **Supplemental Materials: Medications That Can Interfere With Oxygenation and Medications Used to Improve Oxygenation,** on Davis*Plus.*

Promoting Optimal Respiratory Function

Deep, regular breathing promotes ventilation and optimizes gas exchange. Other interventions to promote optimal function include preventing and treating URIs, influenza, and pneumonia (including immunizations); supporting smoking cessation; positioning; incentive spirometry; and preventing aspiration.

Example Problem: Upper Respiratory Infections (Prevention Interventions)

URIs may be viral or bacterial. Viral infections usually last about 10 to 21 days and are self-limiting. URIs may, however, lead to other respiratory diseases and seriously compromised oxygenation in children, older adults, and people who have other illnesses. Therefore, it is important to teach clients the importance of hand washing and other measures for preventing URIs. For teaching tips, see the Self-Care box Teaching Clients How to Prevent URIs, in Chapter 42.

Overuse of antibiotics to treat URIs has contributed to the current crisis of antimicrobial resistance. Teach clients that antibiotics should be used only as prescribed for diagnosed bacterial infections. This includes taking

Cough and Cold Medicines: Tips for Parents

➤ Do not give children medicines labeled for adults only.

➤ ✚ Do not give over-the-counter (OTC) cough and cold remedies to children younger than age 4 years. There is a risk of serious and even life-threatening side effects.

➤ Read labels! Some labels are marked "Do not use for children under age 4."

➤ The safety and effectiveness of OTC cough and cold remedies for children ages 2 through 11 years is still in question. It is not certain they are safe, and they may not be effective.

➤ Choose medications with safety caps. Close caps tightly and store out of sight and reach of children.

➤ Do not give more than one medicine with the same active ingredient. Check the "active ingredients" on the label. Your child could be harmed by getting too much of the ingredient.

➤ Carefully follow the directions on the label for how to use the medicine. Overuse or misuse can cause serious side effects (e.g., drowsiness, breathing problems, and seizures).

➤ Measure carefully. Do not use household spoons because they come in different sizes.

➤ Understand that OTC medicines do not cure the cold or cough. They only treat symptoms such as runny nose, congestion, fever, and aches. They do not shorten the length of time your child is sick.

Source: CDC (2009); U.S. Food and Drug Administration (2013).

Common Cold Remedies

➤ Cold care products containing *Pelargonium sidoides*, an extract of the South African geranium, may reduce the intensity of the common cold. However, more evidence is needed (Ross, 2012). In the United States, Zucol products are one example.

➤ ✚ Honey is more effective than dextromethorphan in children with nocturnal cough (Cohen, Rozen, Kristal, et al., 2012). However, avoid giving honey to children younger than the age of 1 year because it is a reservoir of *Clostridium botulinum* spores, and may cause botulism in infants.

➤ Vitamin C in daily doses of 200 mg or more has not been found to prevent colds, but it did reduce the length and severity of symptoms. Be aware that in amounts of 2,000 mg, it may cause diarrhea and gas (Hemilä & Chalker, 2013).

➤ A systematic review of research studies found there is no evidence that Echinacea preparations are effective for preventing and treating the common cold (Thomas, 2012).

➤ Although lab studies are preliminary, elderberry (*Sambucus nigra*), an herb, has been found to help combat viruses, specifically influenza. It is thought to strengthen the immune system and keep the flu virus from adhering to cells (Kinoshita, Hayashi, Katayama, et al., 2012).

---

the full course of prescribed antibiotics, even if symptoms are no longer present. Antibiotics are not without risks, and they are not effective for treating the common cold. Advise clients not to pressure clinicians for a prescription, nor to take any antibiotics left over from previous prescriptions or from others who might offer to share antibiotics.

Example Problem: Influenza (Prevention Interventions)

The most effective strategy for preventing influenza is annual vaccination. Vaccines are developed annually to closely match the major known strains of the virus that have evolved. Immunizations given to healthy young adults are 70% to 90% effective. Though less effective in preventing the disease in older adults, immunization decreases the severity of the disease, the development of secondary complications, and the incidence of death (American Academy of Pedriatics, 2011a; Fiore, Uyeki, Broder, et al., 2010).

Another prevention measure is to avoid exposure to the virus. That is, avoid being around people who are sick, if possible; and use recommended hand hygiene measures.

Infection rates are highest among children. Rates of serious illness and death are highest among older adults, children younger than age 2 years, and people with certain medical conditions. However, the CDC continues to recommend universal vaccination—that is, all people age 6 months and older receive annual influenza vaccination (CDC, 2013).

Example Problem: Pneumonia (Prevention Interventions)

Pneumonia is a leading cause of infectious death in the United States, with a mortality rate of approximately 50% in people older than age 65. Therefore, people who are most susceptible should be immunized against pneumonia. Historically this vaccine was thought to convey lifetime immunity, but recent data illustrate that this may not be so. As a result, the vaccine is recommended annually for high-risk groups, including the following (CDC, 2012b):

- Adults age 65 years or older
- Children younger than age 5 years
- Children age 6 through 18 years who have certain medical conditions
- People age 2 through 64 years who have chronic illnesses (e.g., those with heart disease, diabetes, pulmonary disease, alcoholism, HIV infection) or lowered resistance to infection
- Adults age 19 through 64 years who have asthma or are smokers

CDC recommended immunization schedules change periodically. To be certain you have the most current information, always check the CDC Web site at

 www.cdc.gov/vaccines/schedules/index.html

Healthcare-Associated Pneumonia Healthcare-associated pneumonia tends to be more complicated and to have a higher mortality rate than community-acquired pneumonia. Guidelines for preventing healthcare-associated pneumonia include following standard precautions for hand hygiene and gloving.

- ✚ Wear gloves when handling respiratory secretions or objects contaminated with respiratory secretions of all patients.
- Change gloves and decontaminate hands:
  - Between contacts with different patients
  - After handling respiratory secretions or contaminated objects and before contact with another patient, object, or environmental surface
  - Between contacts with a contaminated body site and the respiratory tract or respiratory device on the same patient (Allegranzi & Pittet, 2009)

Support Smoking Cessation

Smoking cessation is important in preventing and treating all respiratory problems, including the example problems (URIs, influenza, and pneumonia). Nurses can provide effective support to patients who want to quit smoking. When nurses offer smoking cessation advice, smokers are more likely to quit as compared with smokers who do not receive such advice from nurses (Rice & Stead, 2008; Rigotti, Clair, Munafò, et al., 2012). *All* patients, including school-age and adolescent children, should be asked whether they use tobacco. Furthermore, a systematic review of evidence indicates that their tobacco-use status should be documented regularly (e.g., by chart stickers or computer prompts) (Coffin, Klompas, Classen, et al. 2008). The U.S. Public Health Service guidelines suggest the "5A's" model for treating tobacco dependence (Box 36-4) (Fiore, Jaén, Baker, et al., 2008).

Motivational counseling includes discussion about the connection between tobacco use and current health status, the risks of continued tobacco use, the rewards of quitting, anticipated barriers to quitting, and strategies for addressing barriers. It may also be important to refer the person to a tobacco cessation program. Most smokers are not able to quit "cold turkey."

Combining medication and counseling is more effective than either used alone. Encourage patients to contact their primary care provider for nicotine replacement therapy (e.g., nicotine patch) or other medications (e.g., antidepressants, clonidine) to treat tobacco dependence. A recent study indicates that electronic cigarettes have been used as successfully as nicotine patches for smoking cessation (Bullen, Howe, Laugesen, et al., 2013). However, others (e.g., Grana, 2014) have found

BOX 36-4 ■ The 5A's for Treating Tobacco Dependence

Ask about tobacco use and document tobacco use status for every patient at every visit.

Advise to quit. Use a clear, strong, personalized approach to urge the patient to quit.

Assess willingness to make a quit attempt at this time.

Assist in a quit attempt. If the patient is willing, refer for counseling and medication. If the patient is not willing to quit at this time, provide interventions designed to increase future quit attempts.

Arrange follow-up. If the patient is willing to quit, make follow-up contacts beginning the first week after the quit date. If the patient is not willing to quit at this time, address tobacco dependence and willingness to quit at the next clinic (or other) visit.

Source: Adapted from Fiore, M., Jaén, C., Baker, T., et al. (2008). *Treating tobacco use and dependence: 2008 update.* Clinical Practice Guideline. Rockville, MD: U.S. Department of Health and Human Services. Public Health Service.

that e-cigarettes are not associated with higher rates of smoking cessation. For pregnant women, smokeless tobacco users, light smokers, and adolescents, medications may be contraindicated or may lack evidence of effectiveness (National Guideline Clearinghouse, 2013; Stead & Lancaster, 2012).

Box 36-1 highlights some of the benefits of smoking cessation. Share these and smoking cessation tips with patients (Self-Care: Smoking Cessation Tips).

Position for Maximum Ventilation

Position affects ventilation. An upright or elevated position pulls abdominal organs down, allowing maximum diaphragm excursion and lung expansion. Therefore, this intervention is applicable to almost all respiratory problems, including the example problems, URI, influenza, and pneumonia.

- If the patient is short of breath, provide an overbed table to lean forward on. Patients with impaired respiratory function adopt a tripod position to allow maximum expansion. They may need to rest their arms on an overbed table.
- When the patient is lying on her side, provide pillows to support the upper arm.
- Assist with frequent position changes to keep all areas of the lungs well ventilated, and ambulate as often as possible without creating fatigue.

Assist With Incentive Spirometry

Incentive spirometers are designed to encourage patients to take deep breaths by reaching a goal-directed volume of air. Incentive spirometry is usually reserved for patients at risk for developing atelectasis or pneumonia, for

Smoking Cessation Tips

➤ Identify several personal reasons to quit smoking, such as: "I'll live longer and be able to spend more time with my children and grandchildren," or "My father died of lung cancer. He really suffered. I have no desire to experience that."

➤ Plan a time to quit. Choose a time that will not require many additional demands on you.

➤ Talk with friends and coworkers who have successfully quit smoking.

➤ Tell several supportive people of your plan to quit. Ask them to help you be successful.

➤ Identify friends who do not smoke, and plan to spend time with them.

➤ Participate in a structured smoking cessation program, if possible.

➤ Tell your healthcare providers that you would like to quit smoking.

➤ Consider asking your healthcare provider about nicotine-replacement therapy, for instance, gum or patches.

➤ Before smoking, ask yourself, "What can I do instead of smoking this cigarette?"

➤ Have carrot sticks, celery, gum, or sunflower seeds available to chew instead of smoking a cigarette. These also help you cope with the increased hunger you may feel.

➤ Learn several relaxation techniques, such as meditation or visualization, to help you through the stress of quitting.

➤ Use positive affirmations daily. "I can successfully quit smoking. I am no longer a smoker."

➤ When you feel a craving to smoke, breathe deeply, find something to distract yourself, or call a supportive person.

➤ To help cope with irritability, use relaxation exercises or deep breathing; take a hot bath; or do something else you enjoy.

➤ Make a list of things you enjoy doing. Choose one of these items as a reward for not smoking.

➤ Save the money you would have spent on cigarettes. Treat yourself to an activity or event with the money you have saved.

example, patients who have had abdominal, chest, or pelvic surgery, patients on prolonged bedrest, or patients with a history of respiratory problems. Incentive spirometers offer various visual cues (such as elevation of a ball or piston) to show patients whether they are inhaling deeply enough. As a registered nurse (RN), you can delegate incentive spirometry coaching to licensed practical nurses (LPNs) and qualified nursing assistive personnel (NAPs). However, you are responsible for ensuring that incentive spirometry is carried out correctly and at required frequencies. You must also evaluate patient responses, airway clearance, and ventilation. See Figure 39-6 and Self-Care: Teaching Your Patient About Incentive Spirometry, in Chapter 39.

Take Aspiration Precautions

Aspiration is a risk for patients with a decreased level of consciousness, diminished gag or cough reflex, or difficulty with swallowing. Preventing aspiration requires you to have practical knowledge about positioning, enteral and oral feedings, and administering medications. For guidelines to use with at-risk patients,

 Go to Chapter 36, **Clinical Insight 36-2: Guidelines for Preventing Aspiration,** in Volume 2.

Many of the guidelines involve basic care and can be delegated to qualified LPNs and NAP. The RN is responsible for monitoring for aspiration. Record in the nursing notes any preventive measures taken.

KnowledgeCheck 36-9

Identify at least three nursing interventions to promote optimal respiratory function in a hospitalized patient with chronic lung disease.

ThinkLike a Nurse 36-10

■ Review the Meet Your Patients scenario. For which of these patients should you recommend annual flu or pneumonia immunizations? Why?

■ A 24-year-old nursing student has no previous hospitalizations or known chronic health problems, takes no medications, and has no current respiratory symptoms. On routine purified protein derivative, or PPD, testing (tuberculin skin testing), the student has an area of induration measuring 5 mm. How would you interpret these results?

Mobilizing Secretions

Coughing promotes deep inhalation and forceful expulsion of secretions. Interventions that help enhance coughing and mobilize secretions include deep breathing, coughing exercises, and hydration. Mobilizing secretions is useful for many respiratory conditions, including the example problems, UTI, influenza, and pneumonia.

Teach Deep Breathing and Coughing

Deep breathing promotes ventilation and gas exchange. Coughing after deep breathing mobilizes secretions, which keeps airways and alveoli open and provides greater surface area for gas exchange. This intervention is important, for example, in treating pneumonia and preventing stasis pneumonia postoperatively. For information about teaching patients to deep-breathe,

 Go to Chapter 36, **Procedure 36-1A: Collecting an Expectorated Sputum Specimen,** in Volume 2.

Alter this procedure for patients with chronic lung disease. Have the patient exhale through pursed lips and cough throughout expiration in several short bursts to avoid high expiratory pressures, which collapse diseased airways.

Maintain Hydration
The following activities are important to keep pulmonary secretions thin and mobile. (e.g., in infections such as influenza and pneumonia):

- *Maintain systemic hydration.* Encourage oral fluid intake as much as possible. Supplement oral intake by intravenous fluid administration if the patient cannot ingest adequate amounts of fluid. For guidelines to use in teaching patients to maintain hydration, refer to the Self-Care box Teaching Patients to Prevent Fluid and Electrolyte Imbalances in Chapter 38.
- *Humidify inhaled air.* You can accomplish this with humidification devices or nebulizers. A **humidifier** is a device that delivers small water droplets from a reservoir. Small humidifiers filled with sterile distilled water are attached to oxygen delivery systems to moisten the dry oxygen and keep secretions thin and mobile. A **nebulizer** is a device that turns liquids into an aerosol mist that can be inhaled directly into the lungs. Nebulizers are often used to deliver medications to the lungs, but they can also be used to deliver moisture to the airways and lungs. See Administering Respiratory Inhalations in Chapter 26, and Figures 26-11 and 26-12. Also,

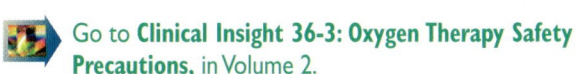 Go to **Clinical Insight 36-3: Oxygen Therapy Safety Precautions,** in Volume 2.

Perform Chest Physiotherapy
Chest physiotherapy moves secretions to the large, central airways for expectoration or suctioning (Fig. 36-7). It involves postural drainage, chest percussion, and chest vibration. In many institutions, respiratory therapists routinely perform chest physiotherapy. However, these procedures are briefly discussed below and in the Highlights of Procedures box. For detailed discussion,

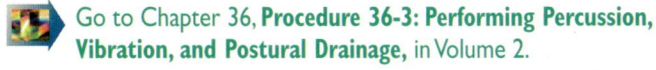 Go to Chapter 36, **Procedure 36-3: Performing Percussion, Vibration, and Postural Drainage,** in Volume 2.

- *Postural drainage* is the use of positioning to promote drainage from the lungs. Check chest x-ray results to see what segments of the lungs are affected. With this information, you can plan how to position your patient. Postural drainage uses gravity to drain the lungs, so you will position the affected area uppermost so that secretions will drain down toward the large, central airways. For example, if the patient has pneumonia of the right lower lobe, you would place her on her left side and elevate the foot of the bed to allow the right lower lobe to drain.

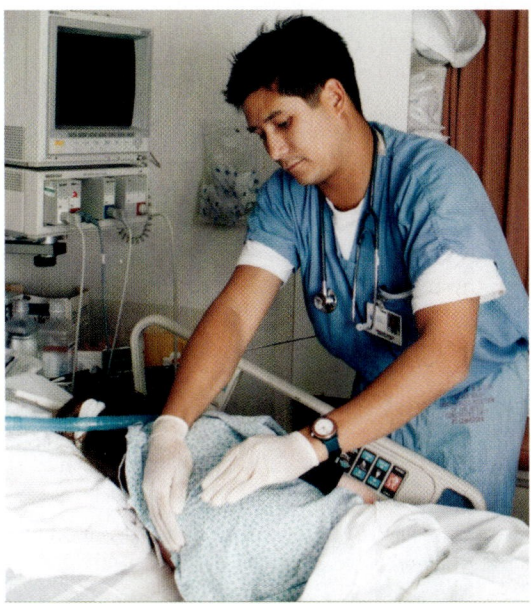

FIGURE 36-7 Patient receiving chest physiotherapy.

- *Chest percussion and chest vibration* are used in conjunction with postural drainage to loosen and mobilize secretions. **Chest percussion** is the rhythmic clapping of the chest wall using cupped hands. **Chest vibration** is the vibration of the chest wall with the palms of the hands. Vibration is a gentle procedure, so you can use it in frail patients who cannot tolerate percussion. You can use a vibrating machine, if one is available, instead of the palms of your hands. Have the patient assume the desired position for 10 to 15 minutes before percussing and vibrating.

 Think**Like a Nurse** 36-11
Your patient has pneumonia in the right lower lobe. She is mildly dyspneic with any activity. Plan how you would perform chest physiotherapy on this patient. What activities would you consider to make this procedure more tolerable for the patient?

Providing Oxygen Therapy
Oxygen therapy provides oxygen at concentrations greater than the level found in room air, which contains only about 21% oxygen. Because oxygen is a medication, it requires a medical prescription for dosage (concentration) and route. Many agencies have protocols with standing orders for oxygen administration in an emergency. (Note that oxygen therapy may be needed for the example problem, pneumonia.) Oxygen is supplied in several different ways.

- *Wall outlets* connected to a large central tank of oxygen are usually provided in healthcare facilities (Fig. 36-8).
- *Compressed O_2 in portable tanks* may also be available (Fig. 36-9).
- *Liquid oxygen units* are often used for home oxygen therapy (Fig. 36-10).

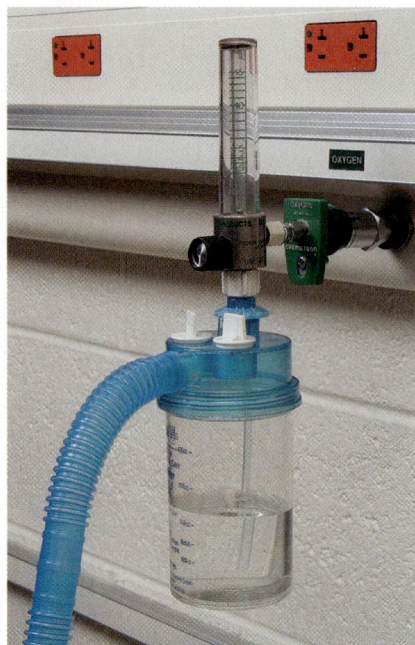

FIGURE 36-8 Healthcare facilities usually have oxygen available through wall outlets connected to a large central tank of oxygen.

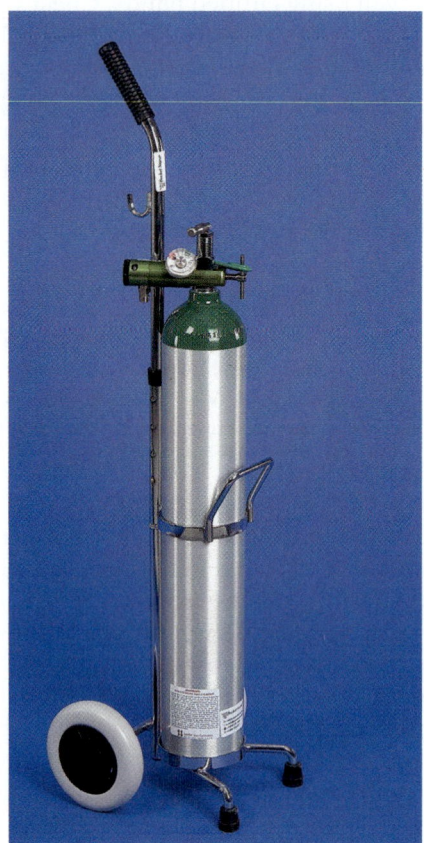

FIGURE 36-9 Portable oxygen tanks come in a variety of sizes.

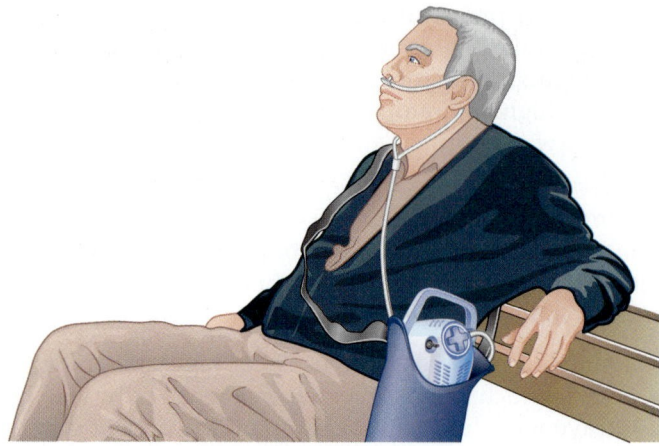

FIGURE 36-10 Liquid oxygen units are small and portable. They are ideal for home use.

■ An *oxygen concentrator* removes nitrogen from room air and concentrates O_2. It requires a battery pack or electrical outlet for power. Oxygen concentrators can deliver flow up to 4 liters per minute (L/min) to create an FIO_2 of approximately 36%. Concentrations are higher at lower flow rates (e.g., an FIO_2 of 95% at 1 L/min). These devices eliminate the need for buying oxygen cylinders, relieving clients' anxiety about running out of oxygen. However, they are expensive, noisy, and not portable; moreover, the client must still have backup oxygen in case of a power failure.

An oxygen flow meter must be connected to the oxygen source to control the flow rate of oxygen from its source to the patient. Flow meters are set in liters per minute.

Various devices (e.g., mask, cannula) are used to deliver oxygen to a patient. They differ in the amount of oxygen they can deliver and the degree to which they enclose the patient. Low-flow devices are the nasal cannula, simple face masks, and rebreather masks. High-flow devices include Venturi masks, aerosol face masks, face tents, and tracheostomy collars—all capable of reaching up to 100% oxygen concentration (Stich & Cassella, 2009).

The Highlights of Procedures box summarizes how to set up and apply oxygen therapy. For the complete procedure and to see the various types of masks,

 Go to Chapter 36, **Procedure 36-4: Administering Oxygen,** in Volume 2.

Oxygen administration is a nursing responsibility. NAP may assist in maintaining oxygen use (e.g., adjusting the face mask), but you are responsible for monitoring the patient's response to therapy.

Oxygen Hazards
The following risks are associated with oxygen therapy. For guidelines,

 Go to Chapter 36, **Clinical Insight 36-3: Oxygen Therapy Safety Precautions,** and **Procedure 36-4,** in Volume 2.

■ ✚ *Oxygen toxicity can develop* when O_2 concentrations of more than 50% are administered for longer than 48 to 72 hours. Prolonged use of high O_2 concentrations reduces surfactant production, which leads to alveolar collapse and reduced lung elasticity.

■ *Oxygen supports combustion,* although it does not burn. High concentrations of oxygen will turn a small spark or fire into a large fire. Fire prevention precautions must be used near oxygen delivery systems.

■ *Oxygen tanks contain oxygen under pressure.* If the tank ruptures or falls, compressed oxygen shoots forcefully from the tank, turning it into an unguided missile. Oxygen tanks have been known to hurtle through walls when ruptured.

Transtracheal Oxygen Delivery

A **tracheostomy** is a surgical opening into the trachea through the neck. It may be permanent or temporary. When a patient has a tracheostomy, inhaled air bypasses the upper airway, which normally warms and moistens air before it reaches the lower airway. Oxygen may be delivered through the tracheostomy via a collar or an adapter. A **transtracheal catheter** is a catheter placed into the tracheostomy to deliver O_2 directly into the trachea. Because oxygen cannot be humidified through this device, it is rarely used.

KnowledgeCheck 36-10

■ Why is oxygen humidified?
■ Which oxygen delivery method is appropriate for the following patients?
A patient prescribed to receive 2 L/min of oxygen
A patient who complains of being claustrophobic and requires low-flow humidified oxygen
A patient with chronic obstructive pulmonary disease (COPD) with an order for oxygen at an FIO$_2$ of 24%
A patient who wants to avoid intubation but requires an FIO$_2$ of 100%

Using Artificial Airways

Artificial airways provide an open airway for patients who have or who are at risk for airway obstruction. Airways may be placed into the pharynx or deeper, into the trachea.

Pharyngeal Airways

Pharyngeal airways provide an open air passage by holding the tongue away from the back of the pharynx. When artificial airways are properly placed, air can flow around and through them, and suction catheters can be passed through them. Pharyngeal airways may be placed through the mouth or the nose.

■ **Oropharyngeal airways** are C-shaped, hard plastic devices inserted through the mouth into the pharynx. To select the appropriate size, hold the airway next to the patient's face. The length of the airway should extend from the front of the teeth to the end

of the jawline (Fig. 36-11). If it is *too short,* it will not keep the tongue pulled forward; if it is *too long,* it may push the epiglottis against the laryngeal opening and completely obstruct the airway. To learn how to insert an oropharyngeal airway,

 Go to Chapter 36, **Procedure 36-12: Inserting an Oropharyngeal Airway,** in Volume 2.

■ **Nasopharyngeal airways** are flexible rubber tubes that are inserted through a nostril into the pharynx. Patients who are semiconscious can tolerate nasal airways because they do not stimulate the gag reflex. Nasopharyngeal airways are available in a variety of pediatric and adult sizes. Generally, the larger the internal diameter is, the longer the tube will be. To select the appropriate size, hold the airway next to the patient's face. The length of the airway should extend from the nares to the end of the jawline (Fig. 36-12). To learn about inserting a nasopharyngeal airway,

 Go to Chapter 36, **Procedure 36-13: Inserting a Nasopharyngeal Airway,** in Volume 2.

Endotracheal Airways

Patients who cannot breathe effectively because of airway obstruction or respiratory or cardiac failure need an airway inserted directly into the trachea. **Endotracheal**

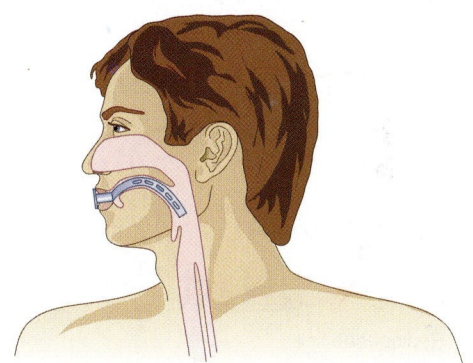

FIGURE 36-11 Oropharyngeal airway in place.

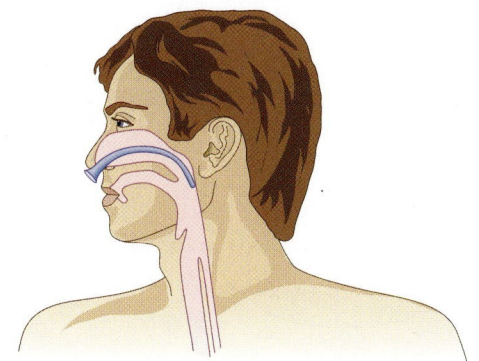

FIGURE 36-12 A nasopharyngeal airway in proper position.

airways are pliable tubes inserted into the trachea through the following routes:

Orotracheal tube—the mouth
Nasotracheal tube—the nose
Tracheostomy tube—an opening directly into the trachea

There are several types of tracheostomy tubes, made of various materials. They may be cuffed or uncuffed and may have a single or double lumen. A cuffed tube is used for patients who are being ventilated or who have difficulty swallowing. For self-care at home, a tube with an inner cannula is preferred because the inner tube can be removed and cleaned to avoid tube occlusion, primarily due to accumulation of secretions in the airway.

Because tracheostomy tubes bypass the upper airway, the patient inhales air directly into the lower airway without humidification, filtering, or warming. For this reason, devices that warm and humidify inhaled air are used with endotracheal airways. Figure 36-13A illustrates the parts of an endotracheal airway. Figure 36-13B shows the placement of an orotracheal tube. Nursing responsibilities related to endotracheal airways are to assist in their insertion, maintain stabilization, and provide routine suctioning and management.

Assisting With Endotracheal Airway Insertion

Insertion of endotracheal airways is within the scope of practice of certain specially trained nurses (e.g., nurse

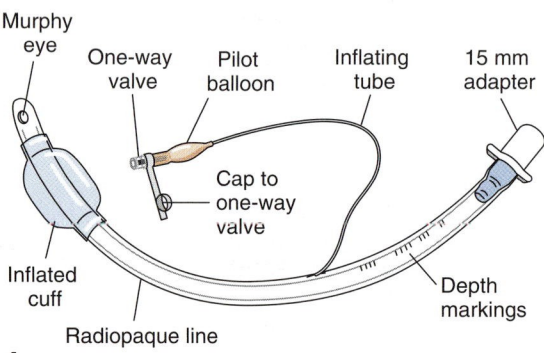

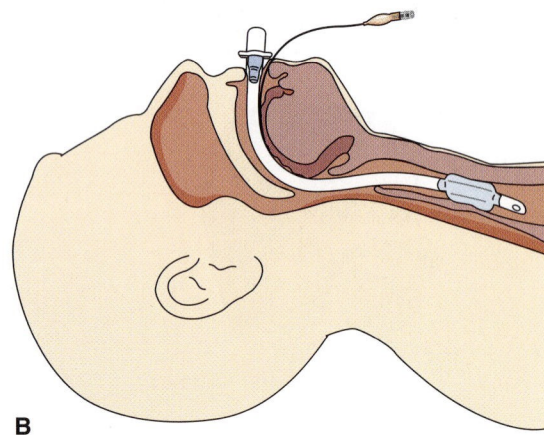

FIGURE 36-13 *A*, An endotracheal tube. *B*, Placement of an orotracheal tube.

anesthetist). As a general-practice nurse, you will assist with insertion by gathering equipment and preparing the patient. On most units, you will find intubation equipment in the resuscitation cart. Intubation must often be done quickly, in response to a temporary decline in the patient's respiratory function during a procedure. For more information about assisting with and managing endotracheal airways,

 Go to Chapter 36, **Clinical Insight 36-4: Caring for Patients With Endotracheal Airways,** in Volume 2.

Managing Endotracheal and Tracheostomy Tubes

Managing endotracheal and tracheostomy tubes generally requires the expertise of a respiratory therapist or an RN, but you can delegate this activity to specially trained and skilled LPNs, especially in critical care areas. Once the ostomy is well healed, the airway will not collapse if the tracheostomy tube is dislodged; so a NAP, or even the patient, can reinsert it if necessary. Many patients with permanent tracheostomies perform self-care at home.

Evidence is still mixed about whether to use sterile or clean gloves when performing endotracheal care. The following are the different levels of asepsis currently in use for tracheostomy care:

- **Sterile technique** is the use of a sterile suction catheter and other supplies with sterile gloves. For new tracheostomies, most facilities use sterile technique. However, some use sterile technique only for patients who have increased susceptibility to infection.
- **Modified sterile technique** is use of a sterile suction catheter and supplies, but with nonsterile procedure gloves. For healed tracheostomies, and in many institutions for all tracheostomies, the trend is toward a modified sterile technique.
- **Clean technique** is use of a clean catheter and clean hands or nonsterile gloves. The portion of the catheter that will be inserted in the tracheostomy tube is protected to avoid contact with unclean surfaces. Clean technique is the usual method in the home setting. Anyone who is not a family member and anyone concerned about acquiring an infection should wear nonsterile procedure gloves, even in the home setting.

You should follow the technique used in your healthcare facility or school. To learn a procedure and guidelines for tracheostomy care, respectively,

 Go to **Procedure 36-5: Performing Tracheostomy Care Using Sterile Technique** and **Clinical Insight 36-4: Caring for Patients With Endotracheal Airways,** in Volume 2.

KnowledgeCheck 36-11

- In what circumstances would you use an oropharyngeal airway? A nasopharyngeal airway?
- What facts should you record if a patient is intubated?
- Describe seven interventions associated with caring for a patient with an endotracheal tube.

Removing Barriers to Patient and Family Involvement in Care

Chapter Key Concepts: *Oxygenation, Ventilation*

Competency: *Patient-Centered Care (Knowledge, Skills, Attitudes); Teamwork (Knowledge)* *

Scenario: Mrs. Yablonski, a 66-year-old former smoker, has a permanent tracheostomy but can speak using an electromechanical device. The nurses want her to learn how to suction herself and change the tracheotomy dressing. For 3 days in a row, different nurses have tried to explain how to perform the care. Each time Mrs. Yablonski became tearful and frustrated. The nurse manager speaks with her to identify problems that may be occurring. Mrs. Yablonski cites several issues:

> "Sometimes it's me. I may just feel too overwhelmed or I may just not have any energy. But the nurses don't always ask me if I feel well enough to learn. None of them really know me, and they don't take enough time with me. And sometimes my nurse doesn't want me to help; she would rather just do it herself and get it over with.
>
> "There are too many nurses trying to teach me. They tell me different ways to do it or make me go over what I already know, so I get confused. I try to tell them what I already know, but they don't seem to listen. They want to do it their way. They should have this all written down somewhere.
>
> "I want my husband to learn how to do the trach care, but he can't be here during the day, and that's the only time anyone tries to show me how to do it. I asked the doctor about learning about it later on in his office but he didn't even want to talk about it. He said the nurses here would teach me."

Think about it: Including patients or their significant others as equal partners in care is the foundation of patient-centered care. Think about the following questions:

➤ What barriers to participating in her own care does Mrs. Yablonski identify?

➤ Are the barriers you identified applicable to other patient care scenarios?

➤ How is team communication affecting this situation?

➤ Does Mrs. Yablonski see herself as a valuable partner in her care?

➤ What might the effects be if Mrs. Yablonski felt more empowered?

➤ What are the potential negative outcomes if Mrs. Yablonski goes home before she masters her tracheostomy care?

➤ What can the nurse manager do to make Mrs. Yablonski's care more patient-centered?

*For specific Knowledge, Skills, and Attitudes,

Go to the QSEN Web site at http://qsen.org/ competencies/pre-licensure-ksas/

Source: Larsson, Sahlsten, Segesten, et al. (2011).

Suctioning Airways

Airways are suctioned to remove secretions and maintain patency. Signs that indicate the need for suctioning include agitation, gurgling sounds during respiration, restlessness, labored respirations, decreased oxygen saturation (SaO_2), increased heart and respiratory rates, and adventitious breath sounds on auscultation. Although suctioning helps remove secretions, it also removes air from the airways and causes the patient's O_2 levels to fall. Therefore, suctioning must be done quickly and is often accompanied by supplemental oxygen. Suctioning can also irritate mucous membranes if done too frequently.

Suction catheters may be open tipped or "whistle tipped" (Fig. 36-14A and B). Most suction catheters have a port on the side, over which you place your thumb to control the suction. A Yankauer tube (Fig. 36-14C) is a rigid device for suctioning the oral cavity.

Both respiratory therapists and nurses are responsible for suctioning and tracheostomy care. The respiratory therapist and the nurse should keep each other informed of changes in the patient's condition. Airway suctioning is usually performed by RNs and LPNs, but not by NAPs. NAPs may use a Yankauer tube to suction the oral cavity as part of maintaining hygiene and preventing aspiration of oral secretions.

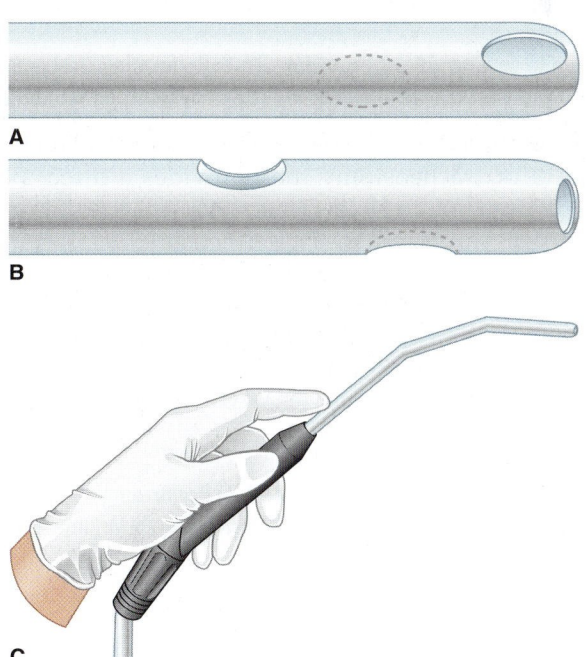

A

B

C

FIGURE 36-14 *A,* Whistle-tipped suction catheter. *B,* Open-tipped suction catheter. *C,* Yankauer (oral) suction tube.

Suctioning the Upper Airway

Pharyngeal suctioning is performed to prevent oral and nasal secretions from entering the lower airway when the patient is too weak to cough them up. Suctioning the pharynx triggers a cough, which helps loosen and mobilize secretions. The patient's condition determines whether you suction the pharynx through the mouth or nose. Most patients find oropharyngeal suctioning more comfortable than the nasal approach. However, if the patient is unable to cooperate and automatically bites down when anything is placed in his mouth, or if the jaw is wired, use a nasal approach. To learn how to suction the pharynx, see the summary in the Highlights of Procedures box. For the complete steps,

 Go to Chapter 36, **Procedure 36-9: Performing Upper Airway Suctioning,** in Volume 2.

Suctioning the Lower Airway

In tracheal suctioning, a catheter is passed beyond the pharynx into the trachea to remove secretions from the lower airways. The trachea may be suctioned through the mouth, nose, or an endotracheal airway. In the healthcare setting, deep tracheal suctioning is a sterile procedure.

Orotracheal or Nasotracheal (NT) Approach When suctioning through the nose or mouth, insert the catheter into the pharynx, and advance it into the trachea during inspiration. This prevents the catheter from entering the esophagus and causing the patient to gag or vomit. When the suction catheter enters the trachea, it will stimulate coughing. Except in an emergency, NT suctioning should be done through a nasopharyngeal airway. The Highlights of Procedures box provides a summary of this procedure. For the complete steps,

 Go to Chapter 36, **Procedure 36-8: Performing Orotracheal and Nasotracheal Suctioning (Open System),** in Volume 2.

Endotracheal or Tracheostomy Approach An endotracheal or tracheostomy tube provides a direct path into the trachea. To suction, insert the catheter through the artificial airway into the trachea. You do not need to insert the catheter as far into a tracheostomy tube, because you are bypassing the long upper airway. Before suctioning, make sure the airway is secured so it is not dislodged by coughing or suctioning. The Highlights of Procedures box summarizes this procedure. For the complete steps,

 Go to Chapter 36, **Procedure 36-6: Performing Tracheostomy Suctioning (Open System),** in Volume 2.

KnowledgeCheck 36-12

- Describe the difference between pharyngeal and tracheal suctioning.
- How can you ensure that the suction catheter enters the trachea and not the esophagus?

Caring for a Patient Requiring Mechanical Ventilation

A **mechanical ventilator** is a machine that assists a patient to breathe. The patient is intubated before he is connected to the ventilator. An endotracheal tube or a tracheostomy tube is connected by oxygen tubing to the ventilator. Before initiating ventilation, be certain that the healthcare team is aware of advance directives and consults with family members. Many patients do not wish to be mechanically ventilated if it might be a permanent intervention. Mechanical ventilation is indicated for acute or chronic respiratory failure, and may be a short- or long-term therapy.

Negative pressure ventilators consist of shells that fit externally around the chest. Negative pressure generated inside the shell pulls the chest outward and forces the patient to inhale air, similar to normal breathing. These ventilators are rarely used for acutely ill patients, but they are occasionally used for chronic conditions, for example, in patients with muscle weakness from neuromuscular disease.

Positive pressure ventilators (also called mechanical ventilation) are the most widely used type. They require the patient to have an artificial airway (Fig. 36-15). Positive pressure ventilation carries risks, including *barotrauma* (injury to the airways as a result of pressure changes) and drop in cardiac output as the positive pressure in the chest decreases venous return to the heart.

To care for a patient receiving mechanical ventilation you will need to be familiar with the types of ventilators in use. You need a thorough understanding of the ventilator you are using, its settings, and how to troubleshoot problems. In the event of a malfunction, if the repair is not readily obvious, manually ventilate the patient with an Ambu bag (resuscitation bag) connected to supplemental oxygen while a colleague troubleshoots the problem. The Highlights of Procedures box describes the care of a patient on a mechanical ventilator. For the

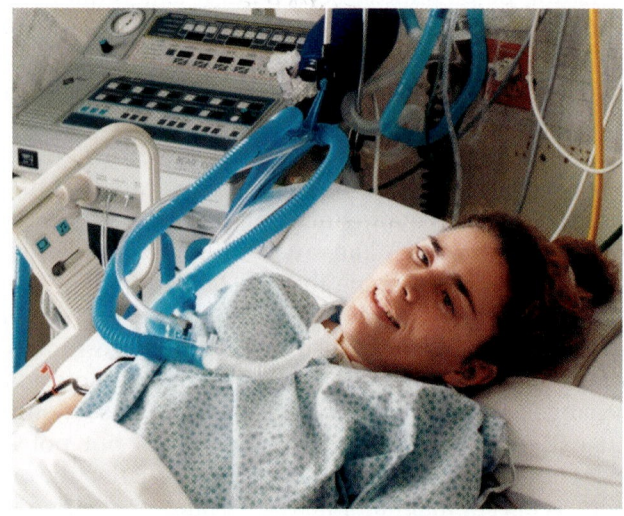

FIGURE 36-15 A patient being mechanically ventilated.

Toward Evidence-Based Practic

> Rello, J., Afonso, E., Lisboa, T., et al. (2012). A care bundle approach for prevention of ventilator-associated pneumonia. *Clinical Microbiology and Infection, 19*(4), 363–369.

This was a study of patients in three adult intensive care units who were intubated and mechanically ventilated. Nurses implemented ventilator-associated pneumonia (VAP) bundle (which includes elevating the head of the bed to 30° and other interventions). There was a significant reduction in VAP related to hand hygiene, intra-cuff pressure control, oral hygiene, and sedation. In addition there was a reduction of ICU length of stay (from 10 to 6 days) and duration of mechanical ventilation (from 8 to 4 days).

> Kelly, D. M. (2012). The organization of critical care nursing and outcomes of mechanically ventilated older adults. Scholarly Commons Repository. University of Pennsylvania. Paper AAI3542907. http://repository.upenn.edu/dissertations/AAI3542907

This was a multi-state analysis that examined the organization of critical care nursing and outcomes of 56,826 mechanically ventilated ICU patients cared for in 303 hospitals. Critical care nurse staffing, the practice environment, and hospital proportion of bachelor's prepared (BSN) nurses and specialty certified nurses were measured. Healthcare-associated infections were less likely to occur when staffing and resources in the critical care unit were higher, with greater proportion of BSN prepared nurses, and better practice environment.

> Mateoso, J., Gonzalez, N., Sadaba, M., et al. (2011). Nursing care in the prevention of ventilator-associated pneumonia. *Enferm Intensive, 22*(1), 22–30.

Researchers observed and described the care of 26 patients with more than 24 hours of invasive mechanical ventilation. They reported good nursing compliance with established protocols for oral hygiene, oropharyngeal suction, and turning of patients, and of patient tolerance of enteral nutrition. Incidence of VAP was low and well within internationally established ranges. They concluded, nevertheless, that incidence of VAP could be further reduced with better control of endotracheal tube cuff pressures and by elevating the head of the bed to between 30° and 45°.

1. Based on these study findings, list two interventions a staff nurse could do to help prevent VAP.

2. Which study might you use to convince a hospital administrator to hire more nurses?

 Go to Chapter 36, **Toward Evidence-Based Practice Suggested Responses,** on Davis*Plus.*

---

complete procedure, including ventilator terminology you will hear,

 Go to Chapter 36, **Procedure 36-10: Caring for Patients Requiring Mechanical Ventilation,** in Volume 2

Patients being mechanically ventilated, even for a short period, are at high risk for developing *ventilator-associated pneumonia (VAP)*. VAP is associated with high mortality rates. Procedure 36-10 includes guidelines for nursing interventions to help prevent VAP.

Caring for a Patient Requiring Chest Tubes

Normally there is negative pressure in the pleural space and only a thin layer of fluid between the membranes. Accumulation of fluid and blood in the pleural space (**hemothorax**) interferes with lung expansion, ventilation, and gas exchange. Air in the pleural space (**pneumothorax**) creates positive pressure, causing lung tissue to collapse. To see diagrams of different types of pneumothorax,

 Go to Chapter 36, **Tables, Boxes, Figures: ESG Figure 36-1, ESG Figure 36-2,** and **ESG Figure 36-3,** on DavisPlus.

The purpose of a chest-drainage system is to make room for the lungs to fully expand. This is done by removing air and fluid from the pleural space. A valve in the line or a water-sealed compartment prevents reentry of air and fluid. A chest-drainage system is composed of a chest tube inserted into the pleural space and a drainage collection system. The system usually is attached to some form of suction.

Flow of air and fluid must be in one direction: from the patient to the collection system. Think of the chest tube as an extension of the pleural space. To provide negative pressure within the chest tube, the open end of the tube is placed under water. With each exhalation, air is expelled through the chest tube into the water, but no air is drawn in during inhalation (Fig. 36-16). Once all air is expelled from the pleural space, negative pressure is reestablished and the lung can fully expand. When the lung tissue is re-expanded, the chest tube can be safely removed.

Types of Drainage Systems

Various chest drainage systems are available, including the older, reusable glass, three-bottle, water-seal system. However, you will most often use a disposable system. These are more compact and lightweight. Disposable systems may be water-seal or dry-seal, and may or may

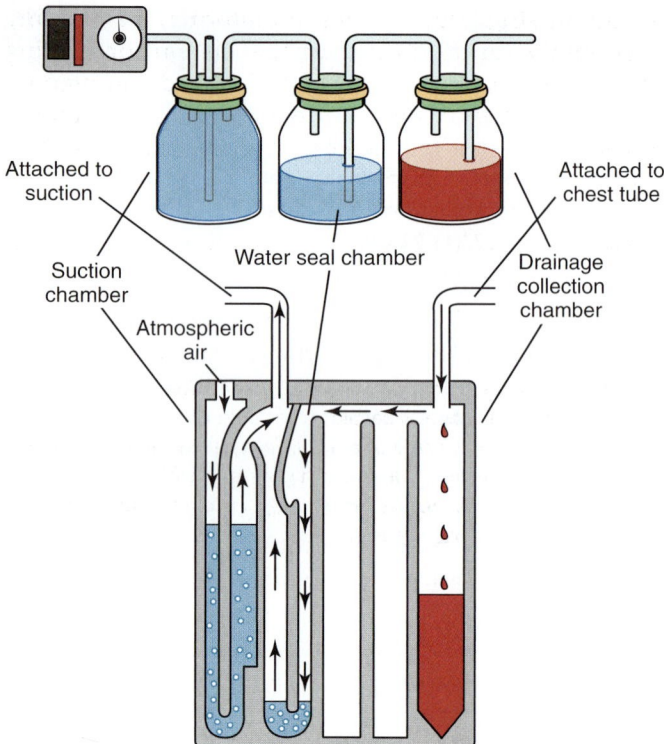

Attached to suction

Suction chamber

Atmospheric air

Water seal chamber

Attached to chest tube

Drainage collection chamber

FIGURE 36-16 A disposable chest drainage system.

not use suction. To learn how to set up disposable chest drainage systems

 Go to **Procedure 36-11: Setting Up Disposable Chest Drainage Systems**, in Volume 2.

Water-Seal Systems

Water-seal systems can consist of one, two, or three chambers (or bottles, in the traditional glass bottle system).

- **One-Chamber Device.** A one-chamber device is the simplest chest drainage system. The chest tube connects to one drainage chamber, which serves as both a collector and a water seal. This system can handle only small volumes of fluid or air. As fluid drains through the chest tube, it raises the fluid level in the chamber, making it harder for the patient to exhale. It is important that the device not be tipped over because the vent tube would no longer be below water and air would enter the pleural space.

- **Two-Chamber System.** A two-chamber system has one chamber that connects directly with the chest tube and serves as a collection bottle. The second chamber serves as the water seal; it maintains negative pressure as air flows through it. Because the chest drainage never enters the water-seal chamber, you can measure the amount of drainage more accurately. The two-chamber system can handle large amounts of fluid drainage, but its design can still contribute to labored breathing.

- **Three-Chamber System.** This system adds a third chamber, which connects to the water-seal chamber and

placed to suction (see Fig. 36-16). This creates controlled negative pressure within the system. The suction control chamber has three vent tubes: one connected to suction, one connected to the water seal chamber, and a long middle tube with one end open to air at the top. The amount of sterile water in the suction chamber determines the maximum suction possible within the system. Suction pressure is expressed in centimeters of water.

Adjusting the suction regulator does not increase the amount of suction. Instead, it simply draws more air in from the atmosphere and causes more bubbling within the bottle. This is a safety feature that prevents excessive negative pressure from being created in the system. For proper functioning, adjust the suction regulator to create gentle bubbling in the suction control bottle.

Dry-Seal Systems

Dry-seal systems are fairly new. They are a one-piece device with three chambers: fluid collection, dry seal, and dry suction control. They do not use water in the suction chamber, relying instead on a mechanical automatic control valve (ACV) and an air leak monitor. The valve allows air to pass out of the patient and prevents it from returning to the patient—even if the system is knocked over. Pressure is set by adjusting the rotary suction dial. The ACV keeps the pressure constant by adjusting to changes in air leaks and fluctuations in the suction source.

Portable Systems

Portable or mobile systems consist of a single, dry-seal chamber attached to the patient's chest tube (Fig. 36-17). It drains by gravity, but can be connected to wall suction. Portable systems improve ambulation and reduce the

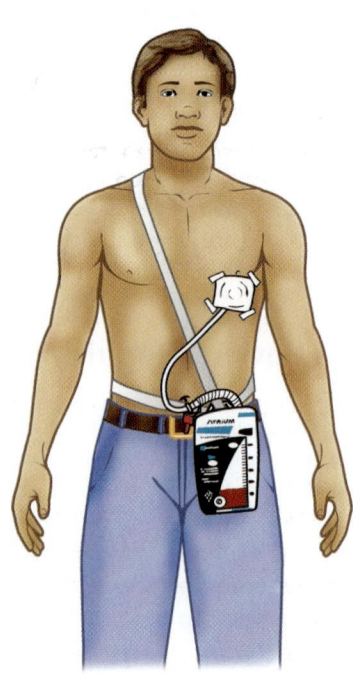

FIGURE 36-17 A one-chamber, dry-seal, portable chest drainage system.

risk of deep vein thrombosis and pulmonary embolism. They are thought to decrease the length of time a patient must stay in the hospital. The collection chamber holds a maximum of 500 mL, so portable systems are not practical for patients whose drainage is more than 500 mL daily.

For more information on how to set up disposable chest drainage system, see the Highlights of Procedures box, and

 Go to Chapter 36, **Procedure 36-11: Setting Disposable Chest Drainage Systems,** in Volume 2.

Preventing Complications of Chest Drainage

Drainage is usually greatest when the chest tube is initially inserted and decreases as the lung reexpands. Care of a patient with a chest drainage system involves four broad nursing interventions: monitoring, maintaining a properly functioning drainage system, promoting lung reexpansion, and recognizing and intervening promptly should complications develop. For guidelines to help you manage care for patients with chest tubes,

 Go to Chapter 36, **Clinical Insight 36-5: Managing Chest Tubes,** in Volume 2.

KnowledgeCheck 36-13

- What is the purpose of mechanical ventilation?
- Why is a chest tube inserted?
- What is the advantage of a three-chamber system (compared with a one-chamber or two-chamber system)?
- How does a portable chest drainage system compare to a water-seal drainage system?

Highlights of Procedures 36-1 Through 36-13

 For steps to follow in *all* procedures, refer to the Universal Steps for All Procedures found on the inside back cover of Volume 2. Go to the full procedures in Volume 2 to practice and learn the procedure steps. Use these procedure highlights later to help you review key points.

Procedure 36-1: Collecting a Sputum Specimen

Procedure 36-1A: Collecting an Expectorated Sputum Specimen

- Use a high- or semi-Fowler's position.
- Caution the patient not to touch the inside of the sterile container or lid.
- Instruct the patient to breathe deeply for three or four breaths, cough forcefully, then expectorate in the container.
- Label the specimen container with the patient's name, test name, and collection date and time.
- Place the specimen in a plastic bag with a biohazard label. Follow agency policy.
- Send the specimen to the laboratory immediately. If specimen transport is delayed, consult the lab; refrigeration may be required.

Procedure 36-1B: Collecting a Suctioned Sputum Specimen

- Position patient in a high- or semi-Fowler's position.
- Don protective eyewear.
- Attach the suction tubing to the male adapter of the inline sputum specimen container.
- Don sterile gloves.
- Attach the sterile suction catheter to the rubber tubing on the inline sputum specimen container.
- Lubricate the suction catheter with sterile saline solution.
- Insert the tip of the suction catheter through the nasopharynx, endotracheal tube, or tracheostomy tube. Advance into the trachea.

- When the patient begins coughing, apply suction for 5 to 10 seconds to collect the specimen.
- If an adequate specimen is not obtained, allow the patient to rest for 1 minute, and then repeat the procedure. Administer oxygen at this time, if indicated.
- When an adequate specimen is collected, discontinue suction, and gently remove the suction catheter.
- Label the specimen container.
- Place the specimen in a plastic bag with a biohazard label.
- Send the specimen to the laboratory immediately. If specimen transport is delayed, consult the lab; refrigeration may be required.

Procedure 36-2: Monitoring Pulse Oximetry (Arterial Oxygen Saturation)

- Choose a sensor that is appropriate for the patient's age, size, and weight and for the desired location.
- Attach the probe sensor to the site, with photodetector and light-emitting diodes facing each other.
- Connect the sensor probe to the oximeter, and turn it on.
- Read the SaO_2 measurement on the digital display when it reaches a constant value.
- If continuous monitoring is necessary, set and turn on the alarm limits for SaO_2 and pulse rate, according to the manufacturer's instructions, patient condition, and agency policy.
- When monitoring is no longer needed, remove the probe sensor, and turn off the oximeter.

Procedure 36-3: Performing Percussion, Vibration, and Postural Drainage

- Help the patient assume the appropriate position based on the lung field that requires drainage.

Continued

➤ Keep the patient in the desired position for 10 to 15 minutes.

➤ Using cupped hands, perform percussion over the affected lung area for 1 to 3 minutes while the patient is in the desired drainage position.

➤ Next, perform vibration.

➤ Assist the patient to sit up. Ask him to cough at the end of a deep inspiration to clear the airways of secretions.

➤ Repeat postural drainage, percussion, and vibration for each lung field that requires treatment. The entire treatment should not exceed 60 minutes.

➤ Provide mouth care.

Procedure 36-4: Administering Oxygen

➤ Attach the flow meter to the oxygen source.

➤ Assemble and apply the oxygen equipment according to the device prescribed (nasal cannula, face mask, or face tent).

➤ Turn on the oxygen using the flow meter, and adjust according to the prescribed flow rate.

➤ Double check that the oxygen equipment is set up correctly and functioning properly.

➤ Assess the patient's respiratory status before you leave the bedside.

Procedure 36-5: Performing Tracheostomy Care Using Sterile Technique

➤ Position the patient in a semi-Fowler's position.

➤ Don gown, eye protection, and sterile gloves.

➤ Suction the tracheostomy.

➤ Remove soiled dressing; remove gloves; wash hands.

➤ Set up sterile field and prepare the equipment, keeping supplies sterile.

➤ Don sterile gloves (procedure gloves for modified sterile technique).

➤ Remove the oxygen source, if the patient is receiving supplemental oxygen, and attach to outer cannula if possible. If not possible, clean and return the inner cannula before proceeding.

➤ Remove the inner cannula with your nondominant hand, and dispose of it (if it is a disposable cannula) or clean it (if it is a reusable cannula).

➤ Clean the stoma under the faceplate with the cotton-tip applicators.

➤ Clean the top surface of the faceplate and the skin around it with the gauze pads and cotton-tip applicators

➤ Dry the skin around the faceplate and stoma with dry sterile gauze.

➤ With the help of an assistant, remove soiled tracheostomy ties.

➤ Ask the patient to flex his neck, and apply new tracheostomy ties.

➤ Insert a precut, sterile tracheostomy dressing under the faceplate and new ties.

Procedure 36-6: Performing Tracheostomy Suctioning (Open System)

➤ Suction only when necessary.

➤ Use a suction catheter that is no more than half the internal diameter of the airway tube.

➤ Position the patient in a semi-Fowler's position.

➤ Adjust the suction regulator according to agency policy, using the lowest possible suction pressure.

Adults: 100 to 150 mm Hg

Children: 100 to 120 mm Hg

Infants: 50 to 95 mm Hg

➤ Don sterile gloves. (Dominant hand is sterile; nondominant is unsterile.)

➤ Using your dominant hand, attach the suction catheter to the connecting tubing.

➤ Hyperoxygenate the patient.

➤ Insert the catheter gently, without suction.

➤ Advance the suction catheter, gently aiming downward, no further than the carina tracheae (or a maximum of 6 inches).

Do not force the catheter.

Do not apply suction as you enter the airway.

➤ Apply continuous suction as you withdraw the catheter. Apply suction for no longer than 15 seconds.

➤ Avoid saline lavage during suctioning.

➤ Repeat suctioning as needed, allowing intervals of at least 30 seconds between suctioning. Hyperoxygenate the patient between each pass.

➤ Replace the oxygen source when finished.

➤ Provide mouth care and reposition the patient.

Procedure 36-7: Performing Tracheostomy or Endotracheal Suctioning (Inline Closed System)

➤ Position the patient in a semi-Fowler's position unless contraindicated.

➤ Adjust the suction regulator according to guidelines or agency policy.

➤ Hyperoxygenate the patient according to agency policy.

➤ Insert the suction catheter gently, with suction off.

➤ Advance the suction catheter gently, aiming downward, no farther than the carina trachea (premeasure). Do not force the catheter.

➤ Do not apply suction as you enter the airway.

➤ Apply continuous suction as you withdraw the catheter, but for no longer than 15 seconds.

➤ Avoid saline lavage during suctioning.

➤ Repeat suctioning as needed, allowing at least 30 seconds between each suctioning. Hyperoxygenate the patient between each pass.

➤ Withdraw suction catheter completely into the sleeve, until you see the indicator line.

➤ Use normal saline to clear secretions from the catheter.

➤ Lock the suction regulator port.

➤ Provide mouth care and reposition the patient.

Procedure 36-8: Performing Orotracheal and Nasotracheal Suctioning (Open System)

➤ Position the patient in a semi-Fowler's position.

➤ Adjust suction pressure according to guidelines or agency policy (typically 100 to 150 mm Hg for adults, 100 to 120 mm Hg for children, and 80 to 100 mm Hg for infants, and 60 to 80 mm Hg for neonates).

➤ Prepare the suction equipment. For the nasotracheal (NT) approach open the water-soluble lubricant.

➤ Don sterile glove(s), protective eye equipment, and gown.

➤ Holding the suction catheter in your dominant hand, attach it to the connection tubing.

➤ Approximate the depth to which the suction catheter should be inserted.

➤ Preoxygenate the patient, if indicated.

➤ Lubricate (for NT approach) and insert the catheter, and advance it to the pharynx as the patient inhales.

➤ Advance the catheter to the predetermined distance as the patient inhales.

➤ Apply suction (no longer than 15 seconds) while you withdraw the catheter, using a continuous rotating motion.

➤ Withdraw the catheter and clear it with sterile saline.

➤ Repeat lubrication and suctioning as needed, allowing intervals of at least 30 seconds between suctioning.

➤ Replace the oxygen source.

➤ Coil the suction catheter in your dominant hand. Pull the sterile glove off over the coiled catheter. Discard in a biohazard receptacle.

➤ Make sure new suction supplies are readily available for future suctioning.

➤ Provide mouth care.

Procedure 36-9: Performing Upper Airway Suctioning

➤ Position the patient in a semi-Fowler's position.

Oropharyngeal: Patient's face turned toward you

Nasopharyngeal: Neck hyperextended

➤ Adjust suction regulator according to agency policy (typically 100 to 120 mm Hg for adults, 95 to 110 mm Hg for children, and 50 to 95 mm Hg for infants).

➤ If using the nasal approach, open the water-soluble lubricant.

➤ Don procedure gloves.

➤ Using your dominant hand, attach the suction catheter to the connection tubing.

➤ Approximate the depth the suction catheter should be inserted.

➤ Remove the oxygen delivery device, if necessary.

➤ If the oxygen saturation is <94%, or if the patient is in distress, administer supplemental oxygen before, during, and after suctioning.

➤ Lubricate and insert the suction catheter.

➤ Gently advance the catheter the premeasured distance into the pharynx.

➤ Engage the suction and apply it while you withdraw the catheter, using a continuous rotating motion.

➤ Clear the catheter with sterile saline.

➤ Lubricate the catheter, and repeat suctioning as needed, allowing 20-second intervals between suctioning.

Procedure 36-10: Caring for Patients Requiring Mechanical Ventilation

➤ Prepare the resuscitation bag; keep it at the bedside.

➤ Wear protective eye covering and gown.

➤ Respiratory therapists are responsible for setting up mechanical ventilation in most agencies. If you must assume the responsibility, refer to the manufacturer's instructions and:

　➤ Verify ventilator settings with the medical prescription.

　➤ Make sure the ventilator alarm limits are set appropriately.

　➤ Don gloves.

　➤ Attach the ventilator tubing to the endotracheal tube or tracheostomy tube, and secure the ventilator tubing.

　➤ Attach capnography device, if available.

　➤ Prepare the inline suctioning equipment.

After the initial ventilator setup:

➤ Check arterial blood gases and assess respiratory status about 30 minutes after setup.

➤ Maintain the patient in a semirecumbent position (head of bed at 30° to 45°).

➤ Check the ventilator tubing frequently for condensation.

　Drain the condensate into a collection device, or briefly disconnect the patient from the ventilator and empty the tubing into a waste receptacle, according to agency policy.

　Never drain the condensate into the humidifier.

➤ Provide the patient with an alternative form of communication.

➤ Check ventilator and humidifier settings regularly.

➤ Check the inline thermometer.

➤ Give sedatives or anti-anxiety drugs as needed.

➤ Reposition the patient regularly (every 1 to 2 hours).

➤ Moisten the lips with a cool, damp cloth and water-based lubricant. Provide frequent antiseptic oral care.

➤ Ensure the call light is within reach; answer the call light and respond to ventilator alarms promptly.

➤ Monitor tracheostomy tube for proper cuff inflation.

➤ Monitor for gastric distention.

Procedure 36-11: Setting Up Disposable Chest Drainage Systems

➤ Position the patient according to the indicated insertion site.

➤ Set up the sterile field and supplies you will need for dressing the insertion site.

Continued

➤ Don mask, gown, and sterile gloves.

➤ As soon as the chest tube is inserted, attach it to the drainage system.

➤ Turn on the suction source (usually –80 mm Hg).

➤ Set the prescribed suction level on the chest drainage unit (CDU).

➤ Don a clean pair of sterile gloves.

➤ Using sterile technique, wrap petroleum gauze around the chest tube at the insertion site, and dress the site with two precut sterile drain dressings covered by a large drainage dressing.

➤ Apply an occlusive dressing over the insertion site (cover the dressing completely). Date, time, and initial the dressing.

➤ Using the spiral taping technique, wrap 1-inch silk tape around the connections. Wrap from top to bottom and bottom to top. (Or use locking connections, if available.)

➤ With an 8-inch-long piece of 2-inch tape, secure the top end of the drainage tube to the chest tube dressing.

➤ Make sure the tubing lies with no kinks and no dependent areas, in a straight line to the CDU.

➤ Prepare the patient for a portable chest x-ray exam.

➤ Keep emergency supplies at the bedside in the event of tube dislodgement or system failure.

➤ Maintenance: Prevent tubing kinks, ensure patency of the air vent, and keep the system below the level of the chest tube.

➤ Keep the head of the bed always elevated to at least 30°.

Procedure 36-12: Inserting an Oropharyngeal Airway

➤ You will need a variety of sizes of airway, procedure gloves, tongue blade, suction equipment, and possibly a handheld resuscitation bag and oxygen source.

➤ Measured on the outside of the cheek, the airway should extend from the front teeth to the end of the jaw line.

➤ Clear the mouth of debris and secretions. Suction if needed.

➤ Position patient in supine or semi-Fowler's position, neck hyperextended.

➤ Hold the tongue down with a tongue blade, as needed, and insert the airway in the upside-down position.

➤ Rotate the airway 180° and continue inserting until the front flange is flush with the lips.

➤ Keep the patient's head slightly tilted and chin elevated.

➤ Verify airway patency by auscultating breath sounds.

➤ Do not tape the airway in place.

➤ Keep suction available at the bedside.

➤ Suction the oropharynx as needed.

Procedure 36-13: Inserting a Nasopharyngeal Airway

➤ You will need a correctly sized nasopharyngeal airway, procedure gloves, tongue blade, water-soluble lubricant, suction equipment, and possibly a handheld resuscitation bag and oxygen source.

➤ Measured on the outside of the cheek, the airway should extend from the tip of the nose to the earlobe. It should be slightly smaller than the nares.

➤ Position patient in a supine or semi-Fowler's position, neck hyperextended.

➤ Lubricate the airway with water-soluble lubricant.

➤ Advance the airway through the naris until the outer flange rests on the nostril. Do not force.

➤ Visually inspect the top of the posterior pharynx; only the tip of the tube should be visible.

➤ Use your finger to check for air exchange at the naris.

➤ Auscultate the lungs bilaterally.

➤ Keep suction available at the bedside.

➤ Suction as needed.

ᴛo explore learning resources for this chapter,

Go to DavisPlus a DavisPl.us/Wilkinson3.

Chapter Resources for Chapter 36

  Response sheets for all learning activities

  Resources for Caregivers and Health Professionals

  Reading More About Oxygenation (suggested readings)

  Concept Map of chapter content

Interactive Case Studies

NCLEX-Style and Chapter Review Questions

Chapter Overview Podcasts

For references cited in this chapter,

  Go to Volume 2, **References Cited.**

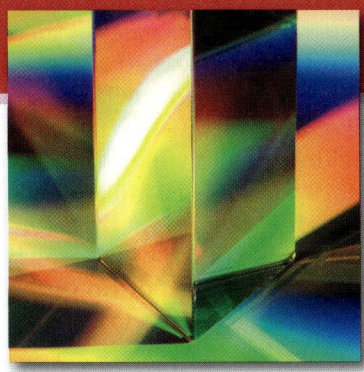

CHAPTER 37

Circulation

Learning Outcomes

After completing this chapter, you should be able to:

➤ Describe the structure and function of the cardiovascular system.
➤ Identify individual, environmental, and pathological factors that influence circulation and perfusion.
➤ Assess circulation and perfusion.
➤ Interpret diagnostic testing related to circulation and perfusion.
➤ Develop nursing diagnoses related to circulation and perfusion.

➤ Safely and correctly perform common nursing procedures related to circulation and perfusion.
➤ Evaluate adequacy of circulation and perfusion, and modify nursing activities appropriately based on outcomes.
➤ Provide measures to promote peripheral circulation.
➤ Recognize medications used to enhance cardiovascular function.

Key Concepts

Circulation
Perfusion

Related Concepts
See the Concept Map on Davis*Plus*.

Meet Your Patients

You are scheduled for a clinical placement in urgent care clinic. Your assignment is to (1) perform a focused assessment related to circulation, (2) perform common therapeutic interventions related to circulation, (3) identify desired outcomes and evaluate achievement of those outcomes, and (4) plan for follow-up and home care needs. One of your clients is Ms. Saunders, a 55-year-old accountant. She says she has been extremely tired, easily becomes short of breath, and is unable to complete her chores without frequent rest breaks. She is pale and moves slowly. Her vital signs are as follows: temperature, 98.4°F (36.7°C); pulse, 86 beats/min; respirations, 24 breaths/min and unlabored; BP, 136/78 mm Hg; and pulse oximetry, 98% on room air. She is now waiting for her lab results, which include a complete blood count (CBC).

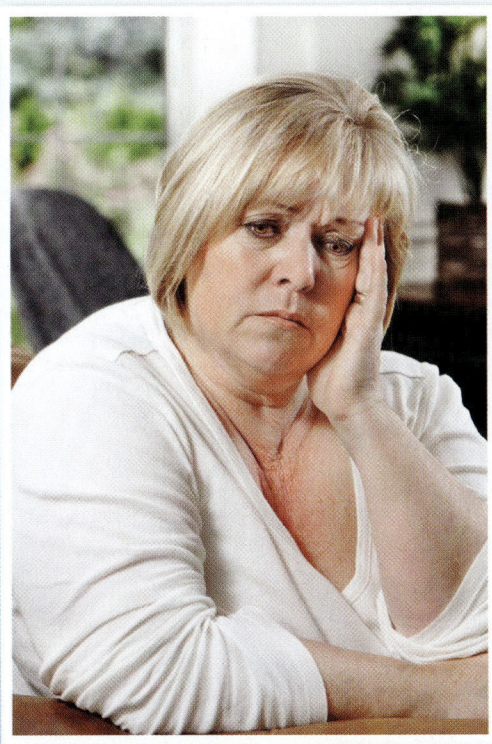

Theoretical Knowledge
knowing why

As you have you learned in Chapter 36, the pulmonary, cardiovascular, musculoskeletal, and neurological systems work together to achieve oxygenation. The lungs oxygenate the blood, and the heart circulates the blood throughout the body and back to the lungs. The circulatory system transports oxygenated blood throughout the body to meet the needs. Changes in one system create changes in the other. Theoretical knowledge in this chapter consists of the structures, functions, regulation, and factors affecting the cardiovascular system, as well as factors that affect cardiovascular function.

ABOUT THE KEY CONCEPTS

The concept of **circulation** refers to flow of blood throughout the heart and blood vessels. **Perfusion** describes blood flow to a capillary bed to provide nutrients and oxygen to tissues and organs. Although the distinction between these two concepts is subtle, they go hand in hand in explaining how a healthy circulatory system contributes to healthy functioning of every organ in the body.

WHAT ARE THE STRUCTURES OF THE CARDIOVASCULAR SYSTEM?

The structures of the cardiovascular system are the heart, the systemic and pulmonary blood vessels, and the coronary arteries.

The Heart

The heart is a four-chambered muscular organ encased in the **pericardium** (a sac of connective tissue) located inside the chest cavity. The two thin-walled **atria** receive blood into the heart, and the two thick-walled **ventricles** pump blood out of the heart. Valves between the heart chambers open widely to allow blood to flow easily and without turbulence from one chamber to another, and the valves close tightly to prevent backflow of blood. The **base**, or broadest side of the heart, which houses the atria, faces upward. The **apex**, or tip of the heart, which houses the ventricles, faces downward (Fig. 37-1).

A strong, efficient heartbeat keeps blood flowing through the vascular system. Deoxygenated blood from organs and tissues flows through the venous system into the right side of the heart and then into the pulmonary circulation. At the alveolar–capillary membrane, external gas exchange occurs. The newly oxygenated blood then flows from the lungs into the left side of the heart and out into the arterial circulation.

The Cardiac Cycle

The **cardiac cycle** is the sequence of mechanical events that occurs during a single heartbeat. Very simply, it is the simultaneous contraction of the two atria, followed a fraction of a second later by the simultaneous contraction of the ventricles—one cycle of diastole and systole. The electrical activity of the myocardium regulates the cardiac cycle (Fig. 37-2).

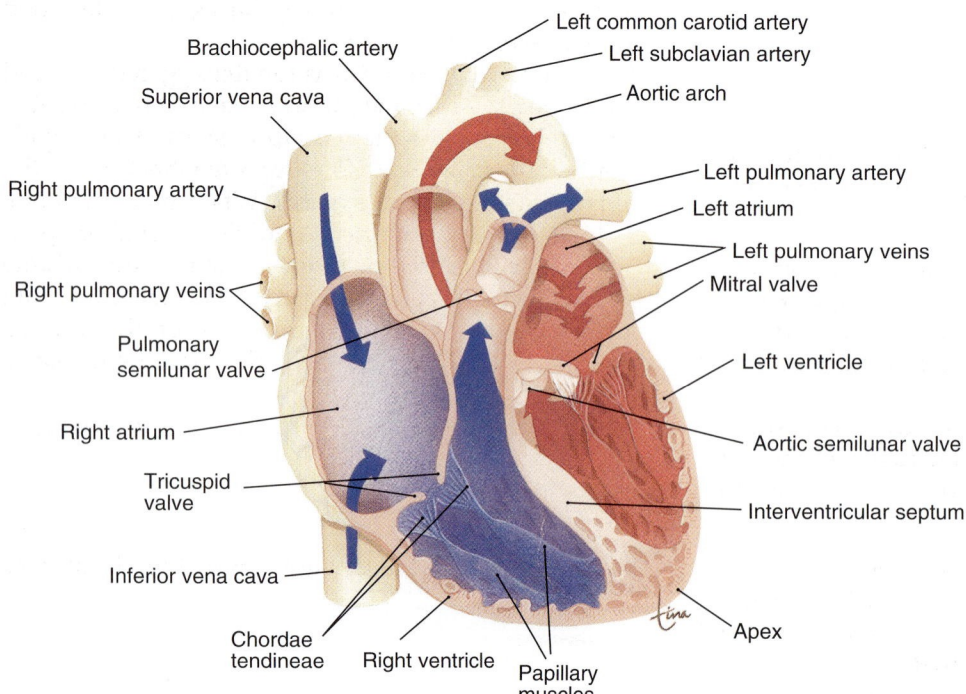

FIGURE 37-1 The atria receive blood into the heart; the ventricles pump blood out of the heart. Valves between the chambers allow blood to flow in one direction from one chamber to another without backflow.

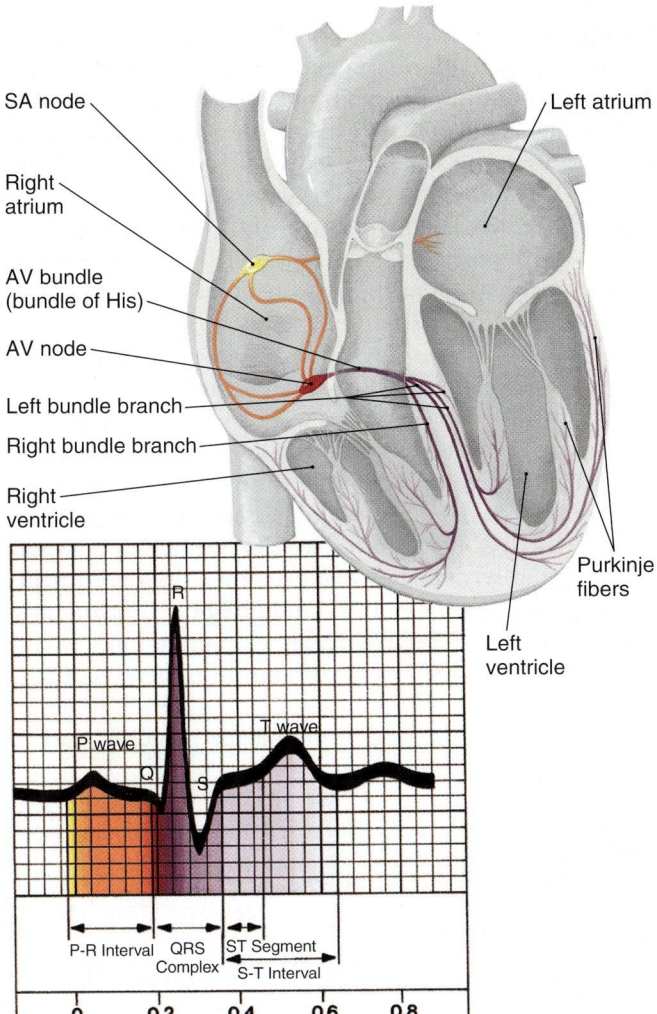

FIGURE 37-2 Conduction pathway of the heart. Anterior view of the interior of the heart. The electrocardiogram tracing is one of a normal heartbeat. See text for description.

Electrical Conduction

The heart contains specialized areas of nerve tissue that initiate electrical impulses without external nervous system stimulation

- The **sinoatrial (SA) node** acts as the pacemaker. Located in the right atrium, it initiates an impulse that triggers each heartbeat. The impulse travels rapidly down the atrial conduction system so that both atria contract as a unit.
- At the **atrioventricular (AV) node**, there is a slight delay. From the AV node, impulses pass into the left and right *bundles of His* and into the *Purkinje fibers* to the ventricles.

In this way, myocardial fibers are electrically stimulated almost simultaneously to create a unified cardiac muscle contraction strong enough to pump blood out of a heart chamber. This spontaneous rhythm of the heart is called **automaticity**. If there are defects in this electrical

system, impulses travel more slowly through the heart and some areas contract before others. This can lead to ineffective heart pumping and decreased cardiac output.

Normally, the SA node is in charge and initiates a rate of 60 to 100 beats/min, depending on the body's oxygen needs. If the SA node fails, the AV node can take over as the pacemaker, but it generally triggers a slower heart rate. If both the SA and AV nodes fail, the conduction fibers can initiate impulses. Ventricular conduction generates a very slow rate, usually less than 40 beats/min; however, this can be lifesaving if no other node or fiber is initiating an impulse.

Systemic and Pulmonary Blood Vessels

The vascular system is composed of three types of vessels: arteries, veins, and capillaries. All vessels are lined with a smooth endothelial layer that promotes nonturbulent blood flow and prevents platelets from sticking to the sides of the walls and beginning a clot.

- **Arteries** have thick, elastic walls that allow them to stretch during cardiac contraction (**systole**) and to recoil when the heart relaxes (**diastole**).
- **Arterioles** are smaller branches of arteries. They are primarily smooth muscle and thinner than arteries. Under the control of the sympathetic nervous system, the arterioles constrict or dilate to vary the amount of blood flowing into capillaries and help maintain blood pressure.
- **Capillaries** are microscopic vessels, created as arterioles branch into smaller and smaller vessels. Capillaries connect the arterial and venous systems and carry blood from arterioles to venules. Because they are only one cell thick, capillaries facilitate the exchange of gases, nutrients, and wastes between the tissue cells and the blood. Billions of capillaries provide blood flow to every cell in the body.
- The **venous system** returns the deoxygenated blood to the heart. **Veins** and **venules** have thin, muscular, but inelastic walls that collapse easily. These walls contract or relax in response to feedback from the sympathetic nervous system: When blood volume is low, the veins contract to provide a smaller space for smaller volume of blood; when blood volume is high, veins relax and enlarge to accommodate increased volume of blood. Think of the venous system as a holding tank for fluctuations in blood volume.

For illustrations of the systemic arteries and veins,

 Go to Chapter 37, **Tables, Boxes, Figures: ESG Figure 37-1** and **ESG Figure 37-2**, on Davis*Plus*.

To see an animated illustration of the circulatory system,

 Go to **Animations, Cardiovascular/Pulmonary Animations: Blood Flow**, on Davis*Plus*.

The Coronary Arteries

The heart has its own blood supply through the coronary arteries (Fig. 37-3). The coronary sinus (not shown), located just above the aortic valve, fills with blood during diastole. From the coronary sinus, blood flows into the two main coronary arteries, which branch into several sections to supply the heart muscle with blood. The coronary arteries are the only arteries in the body that fill during diastole. To see an animated illustration of the coronary circulation,

 Go to **Animations, Cardiovascular/Pulmonary Animations: Blood Flow Through the Heart,** on Davis*Plus*.

KnowledgeCheck 37-1

- Describe oxygenation and perfusion.
- Trace the path of normal electrical impulses in the heart.
- How do the walls of arteries, veins, and capillaries differ?
- What is the importance of diastole to perfusion of the heart?

ThinkLike a Nurse 37-1

Your patient has a condition that has caused the mitral valve to become stiff with only a narrow opening for blood flow. What type of problems related to oxygenation would you anticipate in this patient?

HOW ARE OXYGEN AND CARBON DIOXIDE TRANSPORTED?

The cardiovascular system circulates oxygenated blood to organs and tissues and returns deoxygenated blood to the heart. Maintaining this blood flow requires adequate

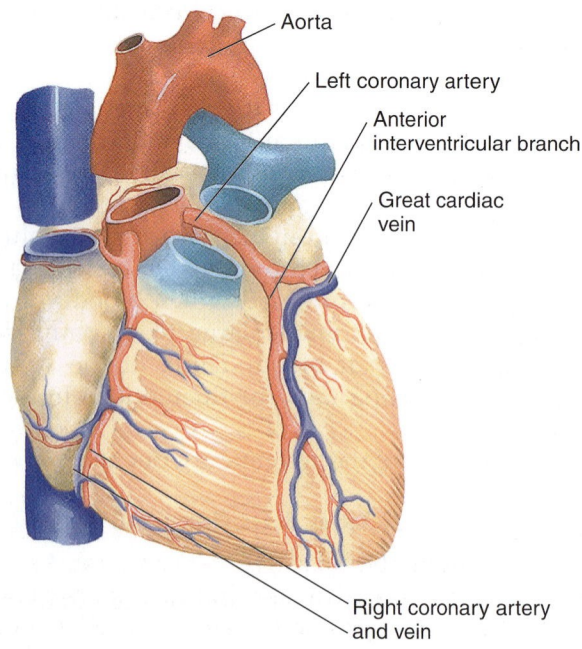

FIGURE 37-3 Coronary vessels in anterior view. The pulmonary artery has been cut to show the left coronary artery emerging from the ascending aorta.

circulation and effective regulation of cardiovascular function.

A full 97% of blood oxygen is bound to hemoglobin, the iron-containing protein in red blood cells; only 3% is in a dissolved state. At the tissue level, O_2 leaves the hemoglobin, becomes dissolved in the blood, and passes through the capillary membrane into the tissues. Only the dissolved form of O_2 can pass through capillary membranes. Hemoglobin thereby serves as a reservoir for oxygen until it is needed in the dissolved state.

Carbon dioxide is a waste product of normal aerobic tissue metabolism. Carbon dioxide can be carried in the blood in three ways: About 7% of CO_2 is dissolved in plasma, 23% attaches to hemoglobin, and 70% is converted into bicarbonate ions. However, CO_2 diffuses through cellular and alveolar–capillary membranes only in its dissolved state. The CO_2 bound to hemoglobin eventually detaches and becomes dissolved in the plasma for diffusion into the alveoli of the lungs. The bicarbonate ions in the plasma are converted back to CO_2, which becomes dissolved, diffuses into the alveoli, and is exhaled.

To see an animated explanation of CO_2 and O_2 transport,

 Go to **Animations, Cardiovascular/Pulmonary Animations: Carbon Dioxide/Oxygen Transport,** on Davis*Plus*.

HOW IS CARDIOVASCULAR FUNCTION REGULATED?

Cardiovascular function is regulated by the autonomic nervous system (ANS) and by control centers in the brainstem.

Autonomic Nervous System

The autonomic nervous system regulates cardiovascular function through its influence on cardiac rate and muscle contractility, as well as vascular tone.

Heart Through branches at the thoracic level of the spinal cord, *sympathetic fibers* stimulate the heart to beat faster and contract more strongly. *Parasympathetic fibers* innervate the heart through the vagus nerve. Parasympathetic stimulation results in a slowed heart rate, but it does not influence myocardial contractility.

Vascular System All blood vessels are innervated by *sympathetic fibers* that maintain them in a constant baseline state of partial contraction (**tone**). Vascular tone maintains blood pressure and blood flow even when a person is resting or asleep. Sympathetic stimulation above and beyond baseline tone varies in response to body needs. Increased sympathetic stimulation causes constriction of some vessels (e.g., skin, gastrointestinal tract, and kidneys) and dilation of other vessels (skeletal muscle). This shunts blood flow to the skeletal muscles for a fight-or-flight response. The *parasympathetic nervous system* has no significant control over blood vessels.

For more complete information, consult an anatomy and physiology text. For a brief overview of the nervous system,

 Go to Chapter 36, **Oxygenation, Supplemental Materials: The Nervous System,** on DavisPlus.

Brainstem Centers

The brainstem centers integrate feedback from baroreceptors and chemoreceptors in the body to regulate cardiac function and blood pressure. The *vasomotor center* controls sympathetic stimulation of the heart and vascular system. The *cardioinhibitory center* controls parasympathetic slowing of the heart rate.

Baroreceptors Baroreceptors located in the walls of the heart and blood vessels are sensitive to pressure changes. The aortic arch and carotid artery baroreceptors are particularly important in the regulation of heart rate and vascular tone. When baroreceptors sense even a small drop in pressure, they send messages to the brainstem centers to stimulate the sympathetic nervous system to increase heart rate and induce vasoconstriction. This mechanism allows us to change positions and maintain blood pressure.

Chemoreceptors Chemoreceptors located in the aortic arch and the carotid arteries are sensitive to changes in blood pH, oxygen levels, and carbon dioxide levels. Their main function is to regulate ventilation, but they also send information to the vasomotor center in response to lack of oxygen. The vasomotor center responds by activating sympathetic stimulation.

If you would like further review of nervous regulation of the heart,

 Go to Chapter 37, **Tables, Boxes, Figures: ESG Figure 37-3,** on DavisPlus.

KnowledgeCheck 37-2

- How are oxygen and carbon dioxide transported in the blood?
- How is the cardiovascular system regulated?
- Does poor peripheral perfusion increase the risk for hypoxemia (a low level of oxygen in the blood)?

 ## ThinkLike a Nurse 37-2

You are assigned the care of a 4-year-old girl with a history of asthma. She is receiving a nebulized treatment containing Proventil (albuterol) and Atrovent (ipratropium bromide). These medications stimulate the sympathetic nervous system.

- What cardiovascular side effects can you anticipate?
- How might these side effects affect oxygenation?
- What do you need to know about the patient's history to safely administer the drugs?

WHAT FACTORS INFLUENCE CARDIOVASCULAR FUNCTION?

Similar to respiratory function, cardiovascular function is influenced by developmental stage, environment, lifestyle, substance abuse, medications, and pathophysiological conditions.

Developmental Stage

Normal development influences heart and circulatory function. Developmental factors exert more of an influence on older adults than on young and middle adults.

Infants

Successful transition from life inside the uterus to the extrauterine environment depends on critical physiological changes that occur at birth. Prior to delivery, the fetus uses the placenta for gas and nutrient exchange. Fetal circulation bypasses the lungs. When the umbilical cord is clamped and the newborn takes the first breath, the resistance in the pulmonary vessels then markedly decreases. The lungs inflate, and blood circulates without shunting as it did during fetal life.

Preschool and School-Age Children

Preschool and school-age children have body systems mature enough to adapt to moderate stress and change, including the heart and circulatory systems. However, children as young as school age sometimes begin social habits, such as tobacco use, that can have long-term adverse effects on the cardiovascular system. A diet high in fats and sugars contributes to hyperlipidemia and the beginning of plaque lining the walls of blood vessels. Processed foods contain a great deal of salt and fat, which can contribute to high blood pressure and high cholesterol, even in children.

Adolescents

In adolescence, the heart and blood components develop adult characteristics. The average adolescent is developmentally at little risk for heart or circulatory disorders, although some athletes can be at risk for collapse and sudden cardiac dysrhythmia that is familial. New guidelines for health professionals performing sports assessments call for thorough investigation of the family history for fainting, collapse, or sudden death.

Some adolescents adopt behaviors and habits that can create risk throughout life. For instance, about half the adults who use tobacco were regular smokers by their 18th birthdays, and 20% of students in high schools report they have smoked cigarettes on one or more of the 30 days preceding the survey (American Lung Association, 2011; Centers for Disease Control and Prevention [CDC], 2012). Although obesity rates have fallen among preschoolers, the overall incidence of childhood obesity in the United States has risen to epidemic incidence. As a result, some adolescents exhibit signs of cardiovascular disease (e.g., high blood levels of lipids and cholesterol, a known factor in the development of high blood pressure, heart disease, and blockages in the arteries of the heart).

Young and Middle Adults

Lifestyle in young and middle adulthood can create cardiac risk factors. Some adults become "too busy" to prepare and eat nourishing foods, or more often simply prefer the taste of high-fat, high-sugar foods. A sedentary lifestyle, lack of aerobic exercise, and tobacco use also contribute to cardiovascular disorders in this group. Crack cocaine and methamphetamine abuse can lead to sudden cardiac failure. Family history of cardiovascular disease is yet another risk factor for this age group.

Older Adults

Cardiac efficiency gradually declines as the heart muscle loses contractile strength and heart valves become thicker and more rigid. The peripheral vessels become less elastic, which creates more resistance to ejection of blood from the heart. As a result of these changes, the heart becomes less able to respond to increased oxygen demands, and it needs longer recovery times after responding. For example, in response to exercise, an older adult's heart rate does not increase as much as a younger person's, but it does remain elevated longer. Thus, older adults have lower exercise tolerance, need more rest after exercise, and are more prone to orthostatic hypotension. Keep in mind, though, that endurance training and regular exercise slow the rate of these changes. In fact, an older person who is physically conditioned by regular exercise may have better heart and circulatory function than a younger adult who is not well conditioned.

Environment

Environmental factors, such as stress, allergic reactions, altitude, and temperature, affect cardiovascular function.

Stress

The stress response stimulates the release of catecholamines from the sympathetic nervous system. This results in increased heart rate and contractility, vasoconstriction, and increased tendency of blood to clot. Sustained stimulation of the sympathetic nervous system can lead to cardiovascular disease. In addition, a chronically suppressed immune and inflammatory response increases the risk for all infections. For additional information on the effects of stress, see Chapter 12.

Allergic Reactions and Air Quality

An **allergy** is a hypersensitivity, or overresponse, to an antigen. Inflammatory substances released during an allergic response (e.g., histamine, protease) cause the following cardiovascular events:

- Blood vessels dilate in areas affected (which increases blood flow to the areas).

- Eosinophils and neutrophils are attracted to the reaction site.
- Local tissues are damaged by protease.
- Capillaries become more permeable, resulting in fluid leak into tissues.
- Local (e.g., vascular) smooth muscle cells contract.

Altitude

Oxygen pressure falls proportionally with increased altitude (to review, refer to Chapter 36) making more oxygen available in the alveoli and at the tissue level. Over the long term, people who live at high altitudes undergo physiological changes that facilitate oxygenation. Among the cardiopulmonary changes are the following:

- Increased production of red blood cells (RBCs)
- Increased vascularity of body tissues
- Increased ability of tissue cells to use oxygen even when atmospheric oxygen pressure is low

Heat and Cold

Heat generally causes vasodilation, which increases cardiac output and oxygenation. However, heat also increases metabolism. As a result, people are naturally more sedentary in hot weather.

Cold slows cell metabolism, reducing O_2 demand. It also causes vasoconstriction, and slows the heart rate. Induced hypothermia is used in some medical and surgical procedures. As another example, victims of cold-water near-drowning have been revived after long periods of time, in part because of the reduced O_2 demands associated with hypothermia. Prolonged exposure to cold causes frostbite, loss of hypothalamic temperature regulation, and death.

Lifestyle

Lifestyle factors that affect cardiovascular function include pregnancy, nutrition, obesity, exercise, tobacco use, and substance abuse.

Pregnancy

During pregnancy, oxygen demand increases dramatically because of the needs of the fetus. Therefore, there is an approximate 15% increase in maternal metabolism during the last half of pregnancy. To compensate, the mother's blood volume increases by 30%. The woman requires additional iron to produce this blood as well as to meet fetal requirements. Failure to meet these iron demands can result in maternal anemia, reducing tissue oxygenation to the mother and fetus.

Nutrition

The body needs an appropriate balance of proteins, carbohydrates, fats, and other nutrients for proper immune function, resistance to disease and infection, normal cellular function and tissue repair, and maintenance of a healthy weight. A diet high in saturated fat predisposes to the development of atherosclerosis, coronary artery disease, and hypertension, all of which can compromise circulation and oxygenation. A low-fat, low-cholesterol, low-sodium diet is considered "heart healthy." Vitamins, minerals (especially iron), and protein are important to prevent anemia, which reduces blood-oxygen–carrying capacity. Green tea consumption has been associated with reduced mortality due to cardiovascular disease (Kokubo, Iso, Saito, et al., 2013).

Recent studies have demonstrated the relationship between the consumption of sugar-sweetened beverages and adverse changes in lipids, inflammatory factors, and increased waist circumference in both adults and children (deKoning, Malik, Kellog, et al., 2012; Kosova, Auinger, & Bremer, 2013). Consuming sugar-sweetened beverages such as cola has been associated with an increased risk for weight gain and type 2 diabetes, which are risk factors for coronary heart disease (CHD) (Sugiri, Hisatome, & Bahrudin, 2012).

Obesity

Obesity is a body mass index (BMI) above 30 (see Chapter 27). Obesity causes multiple health problems, many of which affect the heart and circulation. Obesity increases the risk of developing atherosclerosis and hypertension. Excess fat stores in and around the heart itself reduce its effectiveness as a pump. At the same time, the workload of the heart is increased by the need to perfuse the excess body tissues.

Exercise

Exercise improves blood circulation and delivery of oxygen to tissues and cells. It also increases metabolic demands. The body responds by increasing the heart rate and the rate and depth of breathing. Like skeletal muscles, the heart muscle is strengthened with regular aerobic exercise. As the heart becomes stronger, it becomes a more efficient pump. As a result, resting heart rate is slower because a higher heart rate is not required to maintain cardiac output. Lack of exercise has the opposite effect. A sedentary lifestyle reduces the efficiency of the heart and the capacity to increase ventilation in response to exercise.

Tobacco Use

Tobacco use is a major risk factor in several chronic cardiovascular conditions: stroke, peripheral arterial disease, aortic aneurysm, and heart disease. Smoking has been shown to cause atherosclerosis (fatty buildups in the arteries), hypertension, and decreased HDL (good) cholesterol—all of which lead to coronary heart disease and heart attack. The risk of coronary artery disease is four times higher in cigarette smokers than it is in non-smokers. Cigarette smoking doubles a person's risk for stroke. Older adults who smoke have a 73% higher chance of developing heart failure than non-smokers. Former smokers' risks are related to how long they have smoked. Even light smoking increases the risk of sudden cardiac death. Cigar and pipe smoking are also implicated, but not to the extent of cigarettes (American Heart Association, 2011a).

Substance Abuse

Substances that people abuse include over-the-counter (OTC) and prescription medications, commonly available commercial products, and illegal substances. Large amounts of alcohol depress respiratory, cardiac, and vasomotor centers of the brain. Chronic alcohol abuse causes fatty infiltration of the heart muscle, thrombi in the coronary arteries, heart enlargement, and dysrhythmias, all of which can ultimately lead to heart failure. Illicit drugs, including stimulants (e.g., methamphetamine, cocaine), hallucinogens (e.g., LSD [acid], mescaline [buttons]), and cannabinoids (e.g., marijuana), also have adverse effects on the cardiovascular system. For example, cocaine has been linked to myocardial dysfunction, dysrhythmias, endocarditis, and aortic dissection.

Medications

The U.S. Preventive Services Task Force (USPSTF) (Agency for Healthcare Research and Quality [AHRQ], 2009) recommends the use of aspirin for the primary prevention of cardiovascular disease (CVD). Aspirin fights pain and inflammation associated with heart disease by blocking the production of prostaglandin, a chemical that signals an injury and triggers pain. Prostaglandins also trigger clumping of platelets to form blood clots. Thus, when aspirin inhibits prostaglandins, it inhibits the formation of blood clots. Blood clots are harmful because they can clog the arteries supplying the heart muscle and brain, increasing the risk of heart attack and stroke. Aspirin has been shown to reduce the risk of heart attack and stroke and reduce the short-term risk of death among people suffering from heart attacks. Aspirin is recommended for men ages 45 to 79 years to reduce risk of myocardial infarction (MI) and for women ages 55 to 79 years to reduce risk of ischemic stroke.

Various other types of medication are used to improve cardiac output and tissue oxygenation. They act to slow the heart rate or reduce the force of myocardial contraction; ease the workload of the heart; dilate blood vessels and reduce blood pressure in the pulmonary circulation and systemically; rid the body of excess fluid accumulation; and block abnormal heart rhythms (American Heart Association, 2011b). See Table 37-1.

 Go to Chapter 37, **Supplemental Materials: Cardiovascular Medications,** on DavisPlus.

KnowledgeCheck 37-3

- What changes occur in the cardiovascular system with aging?
- How does smoking affect the cardiovascular system?

Table 37-1 ➤ Medications That Promote Circulation

CLASS	ACTION	EXAMPLES AND COMMENTS
Vasodilators	■ Enhance cardiac output, providing increased blood flow and oxygenation to organs and tissues. ■ Cause vessel dilation, which eases workload of the heart. ■ Control blood pressure. ■ Treat heart failure.	Angiotensin-converting enzyme (ACE) inhibitors Angiotensin II receptor blockers Nitrates
Beta-Adrenergic Blockers	■ Block norepinephrine and epinephrine (adrenaline) ■ Reduce the workload of the heart and oxygen consumption. ■ Control abnormal heart rhythms (dysrhythmias) by slowing conduction through the AV node. ■ Control blood pressure.	Beta$_1$-Selective: atenolol, metoprolol Nonselective: carvedilol, metoprolol, propranolol
Calcium-Channel Blockers	■ Block the flow of calcium into the cells of the heart and blood vessels. ■ Decrease blood pressure. ■ Reduce the strength of myocardial contraction; slow heart rate. ■ Dilate the arteries and arterioles.	Nifedipine
Positive Inotropic Agents	■ Improve the effectiveness of the heart's pumping action without creating excess cardiac workload and oxygen demand. ■ Reduce the heart muscle cells' ability to trigger their own contraction (automaticity). ■ Dilate blood vessels.	Cardiac glycosides: digoxin Phosphodiesterase (PSE) inhibitors: PDE3 inhibitors (congestive heart failure) PDE5 inhibitors (erectile dysfunction)
Diuretics	■ Remove sodium and water from the body through urine. ■ Reduce the volume of circulating blood. ■ Prevent accumulation of fluid in the pulmonary circulation and body tissues.	Thiazide diuretics: hydrochlorothiazide (HCTZ), metolazone Loop diuretics: furosemide Potassium-sparing diuretics: spironolactone Bumetanide Metolazone Triamterene

Pathophysiological Conditions

Alterations in circulation and perfusion at the tissue or cellular level may be life threatening, particularly when hypoxemia and acidosis occur. Refer to Chapter 36 to review the effect of poor oxygenation on body systems.

Cardiovascular Abnormalities

Alterations in gas exchange are caused by a number of disorders that affect the structure, function, and regulation of the cardiovascular system. Cardiovascular abnormalities interfere with the flow of oxygenated blood to organs and tissues, and continue to be the number one cause of death for adults in the United States (CDC, 2011). Major abnormalities are as follows:

- **Heart failure** occurs when the heart becomes an inefficient pump and is unable to meet the body's demands. Blood is oxygenated when it passes through the lungs, but it is not well circulated to the organs and tissues. Impaired circulation leads to systemic and pulmonary edema, which further impairs gas exchange.
- **Cardiomyopathy** is a heart muscle disorder that results in heart enlargement and impaired cardiac contractility.
- **Cardiac ischemia** occurs when oxygen requirements of the heart are unmet. Prolonged ischemia leads to

Toward Evidence-Based Practice

Mizuno, J., & Monteiro, H. L. (2012). An assessment of a sequence of yoga exercises to patients with arterial hypertension. *Journal of Bodywork and Movement Therapies,* *17*(1), 35–41.

This study describes the effects of a yoga sequence on patients with hypertension. Thirty-three volunteers participated in the study (control = 16 and yoga = 17) for 4 months. Blood pressure measurements and cardiac and respiratory rates were collected monthly. The yoga group showed a significant reduction of systolic blood pressure and heart and respiratory rates ($p < 0.05$). The authors concluded that yoga exercises should be implemented as a means of complementary non-pharmacological control of blood pressure in patients with hypertension.

Begum, M. N. (2013). To evaluate the effect of yoga on moderate degree hypertension and lipid profile. *National Journal of Integrated Research in Medicine, 4*(3), 109–114.

Sixty patients (30 females and 30 males) aged 40 years to 60 years with moderate degree hypertension were trained in asanas (postures), pranayama (breathing exercise), and relaxation techniques for 6 months. Blood pressure; serum total cholesterol; LDL, VLDL, HDL cholesterol; and total triglycerides were measured at the beginning and at the end of the study. The results demonstrated that yoga practice in patients with moderate degree hypertension leads to a decrease in blood pressure and lipid profile within the period of 6 months.

Deepa, T., Sethu, G., & Thirrunavukkarasu, N. (2012). Effect of yoga and meditation on mild to moderate essential hypertensives. *Journal of Clinical and Diagnostic Research,* *6*(1), 21–26.

This study evaluated the effect of yoga and meditation on mild to moderate essential hypertensive patients. Patients were divided in to two groups: (a) 15 patients treated with antihypertensive drugs along with yoga, (b) 15 patients with antihypertensive drugs alone. Yoga was practiced for 45 minutes daily in the morning and again in the evening. The study showed a significant fall of mean blood pressure after 3 months of yoga, suggesting that yoga can be used as adjunctive treatment with drug therapy for those with mild and moderate hypertension.

These three studies demonstrate that yoga may be a complementary therapy for use in patients with hypertension. Using what you know about yoga,

1. What may be some reasons for patients not participating in this type of exercise?

2. What strategies can you use to motivate patients to practice yoga?

 Go to Chapter 37, **Toward Evidence-Based Practice Suggested Responses,** on Davis*Plus.*

MI as parts of the heart *necrose* (die) from inadequate oxygen. **Angina pectoris** is transient chest pain due to myocardial ischemia. The tissue becomes injured but does not necrose.

- **Coronary artery disease**, a leading cause of cardiac ischemia, is a condition in which plaque builds up inside the coronary arteries. Plaque narrows the arteries, reducing blood flow to the heart muscle and making it more likely that clots will form and block the arteries. If you are interested in seeing animated explanations of plaque buildup and coronary artery disease, respectively,

 Go to **Animations: Atherosclerosis** and **Coronary Artery Disease,** on Davis*Plus.*

- **Dysrhythmias** (alterations in heart rate or rhythm) can lower cardiac output, decrease tissue oxygenation, and increase the risk of stroke
- **Heart valve abnormalities** create turbulent flow, leading to a decrease in cardiac output and compromised tissue oxygenation. Often there is an audible murmur. The valves most commonly affected are the mitral and aortic valves.

If you are interested in a more extensive discussion of cardiovascular abnormalities,

 Go to Chapter 37, **Supplemental Materials, Cardiovascular Abnormalities,** on Davis*Plus.*

Peripheral Vascular Abnormalities

Disorders of peripheral blood vessels impair blood flow to and from organs and tissues. Arterial abnormalities disrupt flow of oxygenated blood to tissues. When arterial blood flow is compromised, signs and symptoms include pallor, pain, weak or absent pulses, poor capillary refill, cool skin, and tissue dysfunction. Venous abnormalities disrupt blood return to the heart. Clinical signs of compromised venous blood flow include edema, brown skin discoloration, and tissue dysfunction (e.g., stasis ulcers). If you are interested in a more extensive discussion of peripheral vascular abnormalities,

 Go to Chapter 37, **Supplemental Materials, Peripheral Vascular Abnormalities,** on Davis*Plus.*

Oxygen Transport Abnormalities

Even if the heart is functioning well and arterial blood flow is intact, tissues can become hypoxic if the blood is unable to carry adequate amounts of oxygen. The most common causes are anemia and carbon monoxide poisoning. **Anemia** is an abnormally low level of red blood cells, hemoglobin, or both. **Carbon monoxide** is a colorless, odorless gas produced by the combustion of flammable materials and fuels. When inhaled, carbon monoxide binds tightly to hemoglobin at the oxygen receptor sites, making it impossible for hemoglobin to carry oxygen. If you are interested in a more extensive discussion of oxygen transport abnormalities,

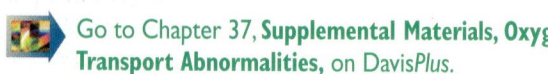 Go to Chapter 37, **Supplemental Materials, Oxygen Transport Abnormalities,** on DavisPlus.

PracticalKnowledge
knowing **how**

Nursing care for patients with cardiovascular problems is directed at assessing for and maximizing the effectiveness of the heart and circulatory system.

ASSESSMENT

Although this section focuses on cardiovascular assessments, evaluation of overall oxygenation status includes a history and examination that gathers information about lung, heart, and circulatory function. **Key Point:** *The patient's condition and the purpose of the assessment determine your priorities for assessment and the order in which you gather information.* For example, for someone with a cardiac emergency, the immediate assessment focus would be to ask simple questions about current symptoms while performing a quick examination to determine adequacy of breathing, circulation, and oxygenation. In contrast, the assessment for risk of coronary artery disease in a healthy individual might include more extensive questions about occupation and smoking habits, a medical history, and an extensive physical examination.

You will need information about the patient's past and present cardiovascular signs and symptoms, risk factors, medications, activity level, tolerance of activity, and lifestyle factors that affect cardiovascular functioning.

Assessing for Risk Factors

One aspect of improving cardiovascular health and quality of life is prevention, detection, and treatment of risk factors for heart attack and stroke (Healthy People 2020, 2010). A health history related to cardiovascular functioning includes questions about the presence of risk factors that affect the heart, and peripheral vascular function. Topics to assess include the following:

- Demographic data
- Health history
- Family history
- Respiratory history
- Cardiovascular history
- Environmental history
- Lifestyle

You should also assess the patient's anxiety level. Patients with cardiac or respiratory problems are almost certain to be anxious, and anxiety interferes with achieving good outcomes for these patients. Pay close attention to verbal cues because heart rate and blood pressure changes may not be useful in assessing acutely ill patients for anxiety (Van Beek, Mingels, Voshaar, et al., 2012). For a detailed list of interview questions for each of these topics,

 Go to Chapter 37, **Assessment Guidelines and Tools, Focused Assessment: Assessing Circulation,** in Volume 2.

Physical Examination

Start the physical exam by obtaining the patient's height and weight. BMI and waist circumference indicate obesity, which is a major risk factor for cardiovascular disease. Assessment of heart and peripheral vessels includes inspection, palpation, and auscultation (and occasionally percussion). Use inspection to observe for signs of distress (e.g., chest pain), skin and mucous membrane color, presence or absence of edema, and overall general appearance. Palpate pulses, skin temperature, edema, heart pulsations through the chest wall, and areas of tenderness. Auscultate heart sounds, vascular sounds, and blood pressure. Auscultate the lungs because adventitious sounds, such as rales, may signal decreased cardiac output. For a step-by-step discussion of how to assess the heart and vascular system,

 Go to Chapter 22, **Procedure 22-13: Assessing the Heart and Vascular System,** in Volume 2.

Assess Pain

If a patient has chest pain, evaluate it immediately because chest pain is the most common heart attack symptom. Ask the patient to describe the pain, its location, duration, frequency, and radiation. Chest pain may also be caused by musculoskeletal or respiratory conditions, for example, a fractured rib or pleuritis (inflammation in the pleural space). **Key Point:** *You can differentiate cardiac pain because it is usually in the center or on the left side of the chest and radiates to the left arm (most often in men). The pain typically lasts several minutes; it may go away and come back. Some women have milder chest pain, sometimes none at all. They are thought to be* *more likely than men are to experience other symptoms, such as jaw or back pain, nausea, fatigue, and shortness of breath. Cardiac pain typically does not change with inhalation or exhalation.* Ask the client to rate the pain on a scale of 0 to 10, with 0 representing no pain and 10 representing the worst possible pain. See Chapter 31 for pain assessment, as needed.

Patients experiencing chest pain are likely to be fearful—most people are aware that chest pain may signal a heart attack. You need to work quickly but calmly to instill confidence in the patient. If the person is experiencing a cardiac event, anxiety and stress can make it worse by increasing oxygen consumption, thereby extending hypoxic damage to the heart.

When assessing for a clot in the veins (deep vein thrombosis [DVT]), deep under the muscles of the leg, you will assess for pain, warmth, redness, and swelling of the leg. **Homan's sign** (pulling toes forward) and **Pratt's sign** (squeezing calf to trigger pain) have not been found to be reliable in diagnosing DVT. However, these signs may help confirm DVT when also considering the clinical signs of DVT, as well as the results of more accurate and specific diagnostic tests, such as ultrasound or venography (Naib & Salih, 2013).

Assess Fatigue

Fatigue is a subjective experience. The patient feels tired and lacks endurance. Fatigue is a common symptom of various oxygenation problems, including anemia and heart failure. Ask your patient to rate his fatigue on a 0 to 10 scale, as you do for pain.

Assess Dyspnea

Dyspnea (shortness of breath) is discussed in Chapter 36 in relation to respiratory conditions. Recall that dyspnea is a sign of hypoxia, which can be associated with cardiovascular diseases and anemia, as well as with respiratory problems. As with pain, dyspnea provokes anxiety.

Assess Peripheral Circulation

Even if the lungs and heart are functioning well, pathology in the arteries and veins can interfere with tissue perfusion. Palpate the peripheral pulses, assess skin color and temperature, and note the distribution of hair on the extremities. Weak pulses, cool feet, lack of hair, and shiny skin on lower legs and feet usually accompany peripheral vascular disease. Look for skin ulcers that often accompany severe venous or arterial disease. Check for edema of the feet and ankles; this is one symptom of heart failure.

KnowledgeCheck 37-4

Why would you auscultate the lungs as a part of your assessment of cardiac function?

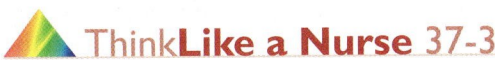

ThinkLike a Nurse 37-3

Why might it be more difficult to recognize a heart attack in a woman than in a man?

Diagnostic Testing

Diagnostic testing helps clinicians identify the causes of cardiovascular symptoms and monitor patient responses to treatment. We discuss several of these tests in the next sections. For others,

 Go to Chapter 37, **Diagnostic Testing: Tests Related to Circulation,** in Volume 2.

Tests of Blood Oxygenation

Pulse oximetry, capnography, and arterial blood gases were discussed in the Diagnostic Testing section of this chapter. You should understand, though, that results from all of those tests are pertinent to cardiac conditions. **Key Point:** *Remember: The heart and lungs work together to provide oxygenation; a problem in one creates a problem in the other.* For the complete procedure,

 Go to Chapter 36, **Procedure 36-2: Monitoring Pulse Oximetry (Arterial Oxygen Saturation),** in Volume 2.

To review (and use in clinical assignments) arterial blood gas values, see the section Interpreting ABGs, and Table 38-6 in Chapter 38.

Laboratory Testing

Cholesterol, lipid panel, C-reactive protein (CRP), and glucose testing are a valuable part of cardiovascular risk assessment. The National Heart, Lung, and Blood Institute (NHLBI) (2002, updated 2012) recommend testing total cholesterol, HDL and LDL, triglyceride levels every 5 years for adults over age 20. For adults with total cholesterol >200 mg/dL, a fasting measurement is recommended. The maximum LDL cholesterol would be 176 mg/dL. Glucose testing is indicated, particularly those at risk for metabolic syndrome, which includes heart disease. The CRP appears to be the most reliable marker for arterial inflammation currently available.

An Expert Panel appointed by the NHLBI (2011) is recommending aggressive cholesterol screening for all children, regardless of family history. The panel recommends that children undergo select lipid screening between the ages of 9 and 11 years age followed by another full lipid screening test between 18 and 21 years of age. The panel also recommends measuring fasting glucose levels to test for diabetes in children 10 years of age (or at the onset of puberty) who are overweight with other risk factors, including a family history, for type 2 diabetes mellitus.

Cardiac Monitoring

Cardiac monitoring is the continuous monitoring of the **electrocardiogram (ECG)**, a rendering of the electrical activity of the heart. Three to five electrodes placed on the skin of the chest display a waveform on a monitor screen or printout (Fig. 37-4). The ECG illustrates electrical activity, but not mechanical activity. In other words, the ECG reflects what the nerves are telling the heart muscle to do, but *not* what the heart muscle is actually doing in response.

The USPSTF (2012) recommends against screening with resting or exercise ECG for the prediction of CHD events in asymptomatic adults at low risk for CHD events. The current evidence is insufficient to balance the benefits and harms of screening for the prediction of CHD events.

The purposes of cardiac monitoring are to:

- Identify the patient's baseline rhythm and rate.
- Recognize significant changes in the baseline rhythm and rate.
- Recognize lethal dysrhythmias that require immediate intervention.

The ECG reading illustrates the complete cardiac cycle. Each part of the ECG complex has been given a letter to identify it: **P, Q, R, S,** and **T** (see Fig. 37-4).

- The **P wave** represents the firing of the SA node and conduction of the impulse through the atria. In the healthy heart, this leads to atrial contraction.
- The **QRS complex** represents *ventricular depolarization* and leads to ventricular contraction.
- The **T wave** represents the return of the ventricles to an electrical resting state so they can be stimulated again (*ventricular repolarization*). The atria also repolarize, but they do so during the time of ventricular depolarization; thus, they are obscured by the QRS complex and cannot be seen on the ECG complex.
- The **U wave** is not always seen on the ECG, but may be detected with electrolyte imbalance, such as hypokalemia or hypercalcemia. U waves sometimes occur in response to certain medication (e.g., digitalis, epinephrine). Inverted U wave may occur with ischemia to the cardiac muscle.

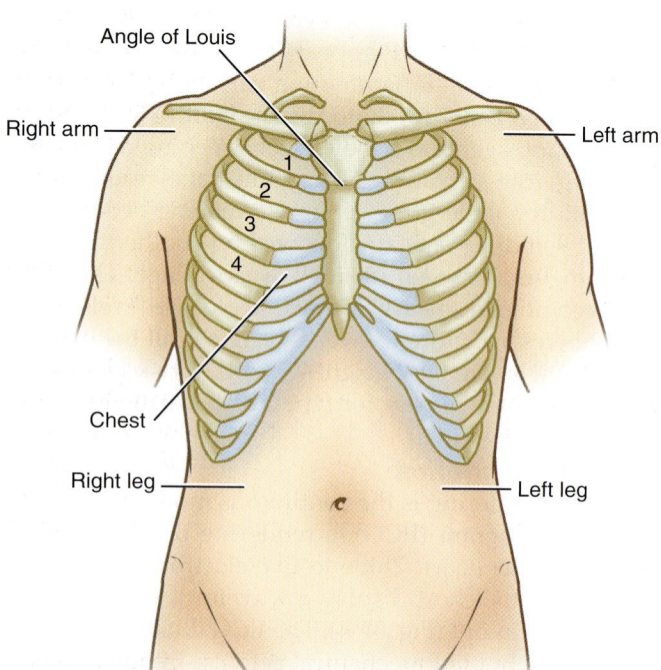

FIGURE 37-4 Electrodes placed for continuous cardiac monitoring.

Dysrhythmias are abnormal heart rhythms. Dysrhythmias can be broadly categorized according to rhythm as follows:

Tachydysrhythmias—Rates >100 beats/min
Bradydysrhythmias—Rates <60 beats/min
Ectopy—extra beats

Within each or those categories, dysrhythmias can be further classified by their site of origin:

Supraventricular—Above the ventricles
Junctional—Within the AV node
Ventricular—In the ventricles

Note that a tachy- or bradydysrhythmia depends on the patient's baseline heart rate. Some people have a low resting heart rate (fewer than 60 beats/min) without distress. Keep this in mind before assuming that the heart rate is abnormal.

All dysrhythmias have the potential to decrease cardiac output, resulting in hypotension and tissue hypoxia. Skill in identifying cardiac rhythms (both normal and abnormal) requires study and experience and is beyond the scope of this chapter. The Highlights of Procedure 37-1 box summarizes the activities involved in the care of a patient requiring a cardiac monitor. For the complete procedure,

Go to Chapter 37, **Procedure 37-1: Performing Cardiac Monitoring,** in Volume 2.

In contrast to cardiac monitoring, *electrocardiography* uses 12 "leads" (views of the heart). These are done by specially trained nurses or technicians. If you are interested in reading more about 12-lead ECGs,

Go to Chapter 37, **Supplemental Materials, 12-Lead Electrocardiography,** and **Tables, Boxes, Figures: ESG Figure 37-4** and **Figure 37-5,** on *DavisPlus*.

KnowledgeCheck 37-5

- What do the P wave, QRS complex, and T wave of an ECG complex represent?
- What kind of dysrhythmia would describe a heart rate of 140 beats per minute that originates in the ventricles?

■ ANALYSIS/NURSING DIAGNOSIS

Several nursing diagnoses address impaired circulation and tissue or organ hypoxia. They are briefly discussed below. For additional information,

Go to Chapter 37, **Standardized Language, Nursing Diagnoses Associated With Impaired Circulation,** on *DavisPlus*.

- *Decreased Cardiac Output* is the appropriate diagnosis when the heart is unable to pump adequate amounts of blood to meet the metabolic demands of the body. Definitive interventions for this problem are collaborative.

Highlights of Procedure 37-1

Procedure 37-1: Performing Cardiac Monitoring

➤ Identify electrode sites based on the monitoring system and the patient's anatomy.

➤ With an alcohol pad, clean the areas for electrode placement; allow to dry.

➤ Connect lead wires to electrodes.

➤ Apply the electrodes, pressing firmly.

➤ If the patient's chest is very hairy, shave the small areas for the electrodes.

➤ Check the ECG tracing on the monitor. If necessary, adjust the gain (sometimes called sensitivity) to increase the waveform size.

➤ Set the upper and lower heart rate alarm limits and turn them on.

➤ Obtain a rhythm strip by pressing the "record" button.

■ *Risk for Decreased Cardiac Tissue Perfusion* is appropriate for a patient who has no symptoms of decreased cardiac perfusion, but has risk factors such elevated C-reactive protein, cardiac surgery, taking birth control pills, hyperlipidemia, or substance abuse.

■ *Risk for Ineffective Cerebral, Gastrointestinal, or Renal Tissue Perfusion* is appropriate for a patient who is at risk for experiencing poor perfusion to those systems (e.g., a patient with a brain tumor, certain heart problems, embolism, substance abuse).

■ *Ineffective Peripheral Tissue Perfusion* is appropriate for a patient experiencing poor perfusion to the periphery that compromises health.

■ *Risk for Shock* should be used for patients who have inadequate blood flow to body tissues that may lead to life-threatening cellular dysfunction (e.g., patients with sepsis and hypovolemia).

Cardiovascular functioning can also be the etiology of other nursing diagnoses, such as the following examples:

■ Risk for Activity Intolerance related to decreased oxygen-carrying capacity of the blood secondary to anemia
■ Acute Pain secondary to myocardial ischemia
■ Anxiety related to shortness of breath
■ Death Anxiety related to diagnosis of myocardial infarction (heart attack)
■ Ineffective Coping related to hospitalization for oxygenation impairment

PLANNING OUTCOMES/EVALUATION

NOC standardized outcomes and evaluation criteria related to cardiovascular status are included in the Cardiopulmonary class of NOC Domain II: Physiologic Health. They include the following: Blood Loss Severity, Cardiac Pump Effectiveness, Circulation Status, Tissue Perfusion (Abdominal Organs, Cardiac, Peripheral, Pulmonary), and Vital Signs.

Individualized goals/outcome statements depend on the nursing diagnosis you identify. For diagnoses related to cardiac function or circulation, the following are examples of goals you might write:

■ No dyspnea or shortness of breath
■ Heart rate in expected range
■ Peripheral pulses strong and equal bilaterally
■ Brisk capillary refill
■ Normal skin color (no pallor or cyanosis)

For examples of NOC outcomes and NIC interventions for selected oxygenation nursing diagnoses,

 Go to Chapter 37 **Standardized Language, Examples of NOC Outcomes and NIC Interventions Linked to Circulation Diagnoses,** on Davis*Plus.*

PLANNING INTERVENTIONS/IMPLEMENTATION

NIC standardized interventions related to the cardiovascular system are found in NIC Domain 2: Physiological Interventions: Complex, in the subcategory of Tissue Perfusion Management. Tissue Perfusion Management focuses on optimizing circulation. These provide a general care planning guide. Depending on individual patient needs, other NOC outcomes or NIC interventions may also be appropriate.

Specific nursing interventions for patients with cardiovascular problems focus on relieving anxiety, promoting circulation, administering medications, and performing cardiopulmonary resuscitation (CPR).

Manage Anxiety

Almost everyone who experiences dyspnea or chest pain becomes anxious—some, extremely so. It is important to reduce anxiety because anxiety activates the sympathetic nervous system and triggers the stress response. Hormone changes occur, including the release of aldosterone, which promotes fluid retention and increases blood pressure. The heart rate and contraction force increase; peripheral and visceral vessels constrict; and the blood clots more readily. All of these make a cardiac or vascular condition more serious.

Prioritize your interventions. You will need to intervene first to prevent life-threatening situations. But try not to appear rushed, and speak calmly and quietly to the patient and to those around you. Do not leave the patient alone. Provide clear factual information and keep the patient and family informed about treatments being given. Many patients are reassured by the presence of a family member. If you need a review of detailed information about assessments and interventions for anxious patients, go to Chapter 13.

Promote Circulation

Adequate circulation ensures that oxygenated blood reaches tissues and organs and that venous blood returns to the heart. Two important nursing interventions are to promote venous return and prevent clot formation.

Promote Venous Return

Measures that promote venous return increase the flow of blood back to the vena cava and the right side of the heart.

- Elevate the patient's legs above the level of the heart. Gravity promotes venous return from the feet and legs.
- If a recliner is available, have the patient sit in one that elevates the legs rather than sitting upright in a chair with legs elevated on a stool. Flexion of the hips, legs, and knees constricts the veins and slows venous blood flow.
- Teach patients to avoid sitting with the legs crossed; this interferes with blood flow.
- Encourage and support early and frequent ambulation (e.g., after surgery). Contraction of the muscles in the legs moves blood upward against gravity.
- Encourage or provide range-of-motion (ROM) exercises, which increase venous blood flow through rhythmic massaging of the veins by the active muscles (see Chapter 32 to review ROM).
- Apply compression devices. **Antiembolism stockings (TED hose)** are elastic stockings that compress superficial leg veins and promote venous return. **Sequential compression devices (SCDs)**, also called *pneumatic compression devices*, are cuffs that surround the legs and alternately inflate and deflate to promote venous return to the heart. Antiembolism stockings and SCDs are frequently used in perioperative patients to promote venous return and prevent clot formation (Woo & Cowie, 2013). See Chapter 39 for further discussion and instructions on how to apply these stockings and appropriate follow-up care.

 Go to Chapter 39, **Procedure 39-2: Applying Antiembolism Stockings,** in Volume 2.

Promote Peripheral Arterial Circulation

Peripheral artery disease, usually found in the legs and feet, occurs when tissues do not receive enough blood flow to keep up with the demand for oxygen. It is caused by the buildup of fatty deposits and plaque within the arteries (atherosclerosis). When arteries that supply blood to the legs are narrowed, leg pain occurs, especially with walking. This is called **intermittent claudication**. As the blood flow becomes more restricted, pain occurs at rest, as well as numbness or a cold feeling to the leg or foot, especially on one side, weak pulse, change in color, hair loss or shiny skin on the legs, sores that won't heal, and erectile dysfunction in men. Teach the patient and family the following:

- Patients with poor peripheral circulation need to quit using tobacco because smoking restricts blood flow.
- When circulation is poor, healing is slower. It is especially important to take good care of feet and prevent injury to the feet. Even dry, cracked skin can result in a sore and become infected. Patients need to wear well-fitting shoes with smooth, dry socks.
- Regular exercise improves circulation and oxygen delivery to body tissue.
- Medication might be needed to control blood pressure, control pain, lower cholesterol, prevent clots, and control blood sugar if the patient has diabetes.
- Angioplasty using a mesh stent or graft bypass surgery might be necessary to create a new path for blood flow to go around the damaged area of the blood vessel.

When peripheral artery disease is treated properly, new, collateral blood vessels can form, allowing blood to circulate around the damaged area.

Prevent Clot Formation

A **thrombus** is a stationary clot adhering to the wall of a vessel. Clots can form after injury to vessels or in response to hypercoagulability. An **embolus** is a clot that travels in the bloodstream.

- Patients at high risk for thrombus formation may be prescribed anticoagulant mediations to help prevent abnormal clot formation. Anticoagulant medications include heparin and warfarin sodium (e.g., Coumadin). Newer anticoagulants (e.g., dabigatran, apixaban, and rivaroxaban) work by inhibiting thrombin or factor X in the clotting chain. They have the advantage of not requiring tests of blood levels. However, unlike heparin and warfarin, they have no specific antidote.

- Hospitalized patients are at particularly high risk for clot formation and may develop an asymptomatic DVT and die from pulmonary embolism (PE) even before the diagnosis is suspected. For this reason, The Joint Commission (TJC) (2013) identified thromboprophylaxis (anticoagulant therapy) against VTE as the "number one patient safety practice" for hospitalized patients. Of course, all the strategies to promote venous return also help prevent clot formation.

- Turn patients frequently; teach patients to change positions frequently. This prevents vessel injury from prolonged pressure in one position.
- Use scrupulous sterile technique when inserting or handling intravenous lines. This prevents infection that can damage the vessel lumens.
- Be sure intravenous medications are adequately diluted. This prevents chemical irritation of veins during IV medication therapy.
- Promote adequate hydration (i.e., monitor intake and output, assess hydration, manage fluid intake, teach patients to drink plenty of fluids). Unless contraindicated, adult fluid intake should be approximately 2,000 mL per day to keep urine output around 1,500 mL per day. Adequate hydration keeps respiratory secretions thin but also keeps the blood from becoming viscous ("thick"). Viscous blood clots more readily.
- Promote smoking cessation. Nicotine increases the risk for thrombus formation because of its constricting effects on vessel walls.

Administer Medications

Cardiovascular medications are used to prevent athero-sclerosis and to enhance cardiac output, thus providing increased blood flow and oxygenation to organs and tissues. They include vasodilators, beta-adrenergic blocking agents, diuretics, positive inotropes, and anti-cholesterol medications.

- *Vasodilators* cause vessel dilation, which eases the work of the heart. Drugs that dilate arterioles decrease the resistance against which the heart pumps (afterload). Drugs that dilate veins decrease venous return to the heart (preload). Vasodilating agents include angiotensin-converting enzyme (ACE) inhibitors, angiotensin II receptor blockers, and nitrates.

> ✚ Vasodilators can cause hypotension, especially when the person rises from a sitting or lying position. Patients should be warned of this effect. You will need to monitor the patient's blood pressure and observe for symptoms of hypotension.

- *Beta-adrenergic agents* block stimulation of beta receptors, which are located primarily in the heart, lungs, and blood vessels. Beta-1 selective agents are used to treat angina, acute myocardial infarction, and congestive heart failure (CHF). They decrease heart rate, slow conduction through the AV node, and decrease myocardial oxygen demand by reducing myocardial contractility.
- *Diuretics* increase removal of sodium and water from the body by increasing urine output. In patients with CHF, diuretics are used to reduce the volume of circulating blood and prevent accumulation of fluid in the pulmonary circulation.
- *Positive inotropes* increase cardiac contractility. They are used therapeutically to make the heart a more effective pump. The goal is to improve pumping effectiveness without creating excess heart work and oxygen demand. The two main classes of positive inotropes are cardiac glycosides and phosphodiesterase inhibitors.
- *Anticholesterol medications (statins)* are a class of drugs that protect against coronary artery disease by lowering the level of triglycerides and reduce the production of cholesterol by the liver. Statins block the liver enzyme that is responsible for making cholesterol. Statins are used for those who have an elevated LDL cholesterol level. For primary prevention recent guidelines recommend their use for all persons, even with a normal level, if they have diabetes or a high risk of cardiovascular disease (Ray, Kastelein, Boekholdt, et al., 2014; Stone, Robinson, Lichtenstein, et al., 2013.)

Performing Cardiopulmonary Resuscitation

All of the previously discussed interventions are designed to promote circulation and perfusion. However, the patient's condition can rapidly deteriorate.

You must be prepared to perform *cardiopulmonary resuscitation (CPR)* in the event your patient experiences a respiratory, cardiac, or cardiopulmonary arrest. **Cardiac arrest** is the cessation of heart function. Signs of cardiac arrest are pale, cool, grayish skin; absence of femoral or carotid pulses; apnea; and pupil dilation. In the event of cardiac arrest, you have only 4 to 6 minutes before the brain is damaged by lack of oxygen. **Respiratory (pulmonary) arrest** is cessation of breathing. It can be caused by a blocked airway or occur after a cardiac arrest; it may be sudden or preceded by increasingly labored breathing.

CPR procedures are regularly updated as new knowledge is gained. The American Heart Association provides training sessions for healthcare professionals to become certified in CPR. This is a prerequisite for employment and clinical practice. **Key Point: We recommend you obtain CPR training from certified professionals.** However, if you are already trained and just want to review the procedure,

 Go to Chapter 37, **ESG Procedure 37-1: Performing Basic Life Support for Healthcare Providers,** on DavisPlus.

Key points of the most recent guidelines *for trained professionals* include the following:

- Focus on effective, uninterrupted chest compressions.
- Push hard, push fast in the center of the chest.
- About 100 compressions per minute
- 30 compressions to 2 breaths—for all victims except newborns
- Give breaths over 1 second and make the chest rise visibly (Dumas, Rea, Fahrenbruch, et al., 2013; Sayre, Berg, Cave, et al., 2008).

In-Hospital Arrests

All agencies have procedures (called a "Code Blue" in many agencies) for announcing cardiac or respiratory arrest, and there is usually an emergency alert system in the patient rooms in acute care facilities. Activating the alert system (e.g., by pulling down a handle) summons a code team trained in CPR. However, you will probably need to begin CPR before they arrive. Begin CPR immediately after activating the alert, and use an automatic external defibrillator (AED) or manual defibrillator as soon as one is available. For a manual defibrillator, use a dose of 2 J/kg for the first shock and a dose of 4 J/kg for the second and subsequent shocks. Before beginning CPR, you are responsible for knowing whether your patient has an advance directive stating whether or not he would want CPR.

"Hands-Only" CPR

The American Heart Association (2011c) recommends different responses for laypersons, first responders, and CPR-trained professionals. The goal of these changes is to make it easier to learn, remember, and perform CPR. Referred to as "Hands-Only" CPR, the method is recommended for people who see an adult collapse suddenly in the community. It has only two steps:

1. Call 911, or send someone to make the call.
2. Push hard and fast in the center of the victim's chest.

See Self-Care: Teaching Your Client Hands-Only CPR for a more detailed description of CPR that you can teach to lay persons.

Rescuers should use Hands-Only CPR only for adults they observe to suddenly collapse. They should use CPR that combines breaths and compressions for:

Adults found already unconscious and not breathing normally
Victims of drowning or collapse due to breathing problems
All infants and children

KnowledgeCheck 37-6

- Identify three strategies that prevent clot formation.
- How do diuretics affect oxygenation?

To explore learning resources for this chapter,

 Go to Davis*Plus* at **DavisPl.us/Wilkinson3.**

Chapter Resources for Chapter 37:
  Response sheets for all learning activities
  Resources for Caregivers and Health Professionals
  Reading More About Circulation (suggested readings)
  Concept Map of chapter content
Interactive Case Studies
NCLEX-Style and Chapter Review Questions
Chapter Overview Podcasts
Sound files (e.g., for heart and blood pressure sounds)

For references cited in this chapter,

Go to Volume 2, **References Cited.**

Self-Care

Teaching Your Client Hands-Only CPR, for a Single Rescuer, Adult Victim

Witnessed Collapse

If you see an adult suddenly collapse in an "out-of-hospital" setting:

1. Call 911 (or send someone to do that).
2. Push hard and fast in the center of the chest (100 pumps per minute)
3. Continue until help arrives.

Unwitnessed Collapse

For an unwitnessed collapse of an adult victim:

1. Establish unresponsiveness (ask, "Are you okay?")
2. Call 911 (or send someone to do it).
3. Obtain an AED, if possible.
4. Start traditional CPR, if you know how, while waiting for the AED.

Traditional CPR

1. When the AED arrives, turn it on for rhythm analysis.
2. After turning on the AED, apply pads and await directions from AED.
3. Administer one shock and wait for the AED to tell you what to do next.
4. When the AED says to continue CPR, start alternating 30 compressions with 2 breaths. Continue until help arrives. Stop only to check the AED for rhythm.

Key point: *Remember: The most important action is to deliver uninterrupted, hard and fast chest compressions.*

Source: American Heart Association (2010); Morrison, L. J., Neumar, R. W., Zimmerman, J. L., et al. (2013).

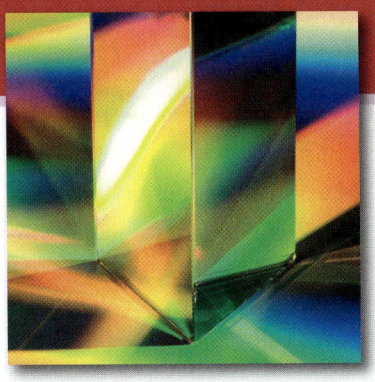

Fluids, Electrolytes, & Acid–Base Balance

Learning Outcomes

After completing this chapter, you should be able to:

➤ Identify the fluid compartments within the body.

➤ Describe the location and function of the major electrolytes of the body.

➤ Differentiate among active and passive transport, osmosis, diffusion, and filtration.

➤ Describe the body mechanisms for maintaining fluid and electrolyte balance.

➤ Summarize the major fluid and electrolyte balance disorders.

➤ Compare and contrast respiratory and metabolic acidosis and alkalosis.

➤ Describe compensatory mechanisms for acid–base imbalances.

➤ Provide nursing interventions for clients with fluid, electrolyte, and acid–base imbalances.

Key Concepts

Acid–base balance

Electrolyte balance

Fluid balance

Related Concepts

See the Concept Map on Davis*Plus*.

Example Problem

Fluids, electrolytes, and acid–base imbalance

Meet Your Patients

Your instructor has assigned you to care for Jackson LaGuardia, a 60-year-old man with end-stage renal disease. You arrive at the hospital to review his chart so you can provide care the following day. When you arrive on the unit, the charge nurse informs you that Mr. LaGuardia is still in the emergency department (ED) waiting to be admitted to the medical-surgical unit. You go to the ED to review his chart and gather data.

In the ED, you introduce yourself and explain your purpose. The charge nurse tells you that five members of the LaGuardia family have all come to the ED complaining of nausea, vomiting, and diarrhea related to severe gastroenteritis, a viral intestinal disorder. The family members include the following:

8-month-old Jason, grandson of Jackson
26-year-old Susanna, Jackson's daughter and Jason's mother

58-year-old Gemma, Jackson's wife
60-year-old Jackson
82-year-old Martha, Jackson's mother

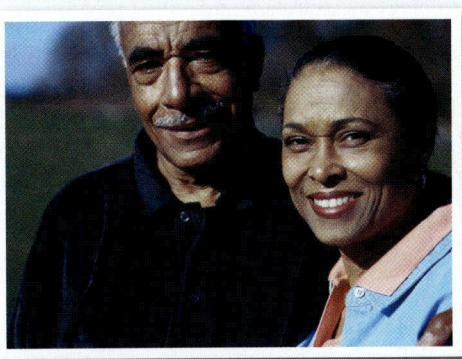

Jason, Jackson, and Martha are being admitted to the hospital. However, Susanna and Gemma have been asked to follow up tomorrow in the urgent care clinic. As you prepare for your clinical day, you think, "If they all have the same disorder, why are only three family members being admitted? What makes these patients different?" In this chapter, we follow the LaGuardias and answer these questions.

Theoretical Knowledge
knowing why

When we are healthy, the fluid and chemical state of our bodies is in balance. However, illness can disturb this balance and threaten our existence. In this chapter, we examine how fluid, electrolyte, and acid–base balances are maintained, as well as what happens when there are disturbances in each of these areas.

ABOUT THE KEY CONCEPTS

The concepts of **fluid balance** and **electrolyte balance** are intricately related. Usually, when one electrolyte changes, so does another; and often fluids shift with the electrolyte. Tipping the delicate balance among fluids and electrolytes leads to dysfunction and disease.

Likewise, the status of **acid–base balance** is a reflection of the overall body functioning. Disruption of the balance in pH (acidity and alkalinity) and other body chemicals has a profound effect on overall health. By the end of this chapter, you will become familiar with the various balances and imbalances among fluids, electrolytes, acids, and bases.

BODY FLUIDS AND SOLUTES

Body fluid is primarily water and is essential for proper functioning of the body organs. It contains gases (e.g., carbon dioxide and oxygen) and solid substances, called **solutes**, that dissolve in body fluids. Many solutes are **electrolytes**—substances (e.g., sodium, potassium) that develop an electrical charge when dissolved in water. Other solutes are nonelectrolytes. **Nonelectrolytes** (e.g., glucose, urea) do not conduct electricity. Body fluids perform several important functions:

- Maintain blood volume.
- Regulate body temperature.
- Transport material to and from cells.
- Serve as a medium for cellular metabolism.
- Assist with digestion of food.
- Serve as a medium for excreting waste.

Fluid makes up approximately 60% of an average adult's body weight. However, total body water content varies with the number of fat cells, age, and sex. Infants have very high body water content (70%–80%), and the percentage progressively decreases with age. Women have less body fluid than men because they have proportionately more body fat. An obese person has less fluid than a person of lean build. Table 38-1 presents the distribution of fluid based on age and gender.

What Are the Body Fluids Compartments?

Most body fluid is contained within two compartments. **Intracellular fluid (ICF)** is contained within the cells. It accounts for approximately 40% of body weight and is

Table 38-1 ▶ Total Body Fluid in Relation to Sex and Age	
AGE	**TOTAL BODY FLUID (% OF BODY WEIGHT)**
Full-term newborn	70%–80%
1 year old	64%
Young adult	Men: 60% Women: 50%–55%
Middle adult	Men: 55% Women: 45%–50%
Older adult	Men: 50% Women: 45%

essential for cell function and metabolism. **Extracellular fluid (ECF)** is outside the cells. It carries water, electrolytes, nutrients, and oxygen to the cells and removes the waste products of cellular metabolism. ECF accounts for 20% of body weight and exists in three main locations in the body:

- *Interstitial fluid* lies in the spaces between the body cells. Excess fluid within the interstitial space is called edema.
- *Intravascular fluid* is the plasma within the blood. Its main function is to transport blood cells.
- *Transcellular fluid* includes specialized fluids that are contained in body spaces (e.g., cerebrospinal, pleural, peritoneal, and synovial fluid); and digestive juices.

Figure 38-1 illustrates the distribution of body fluids. In times of illness, fluid may move into an area that makes it physiologically unavailable, such as the peritoneal space (a condition called *ascites*), the pericardial space (a condition called *pericardial effusion*), or the *vesicles* (blisters) produced by a burn wound. This type of fluid movement is known as **third spacing** because fluid is literally trapped in a third compartment—not within interstitial (cells) or the intravascular spaces (blood vessels).

What Electrolytes Are Present in Body Fluids?

In addition to water, body fluid is composed of oxygen, carbon dioxide, dissolved nutrients, metabolic waste products, and electrolytes. Electrolytes that carry a positive charge are called **cations**. Electrolytes that carry a negative charge are called **anions**. Electrolytes are measured in milliequivalents per liter (mEq/L) of water or milligrams per 100 mL (mg/100 mL or mg/dL). Note that 1 dL, or deciliter, equals 100 mL. *Milliequivalent* is a measure of chemical combining power, whereas *milligram* is a weight measure.

The composition of body fluids varies between compartments:

- **In the ICF**, the major cations are potassium and magnesium. The major anion is phosphate. Other electrolytes are present, but to a lesser degree.

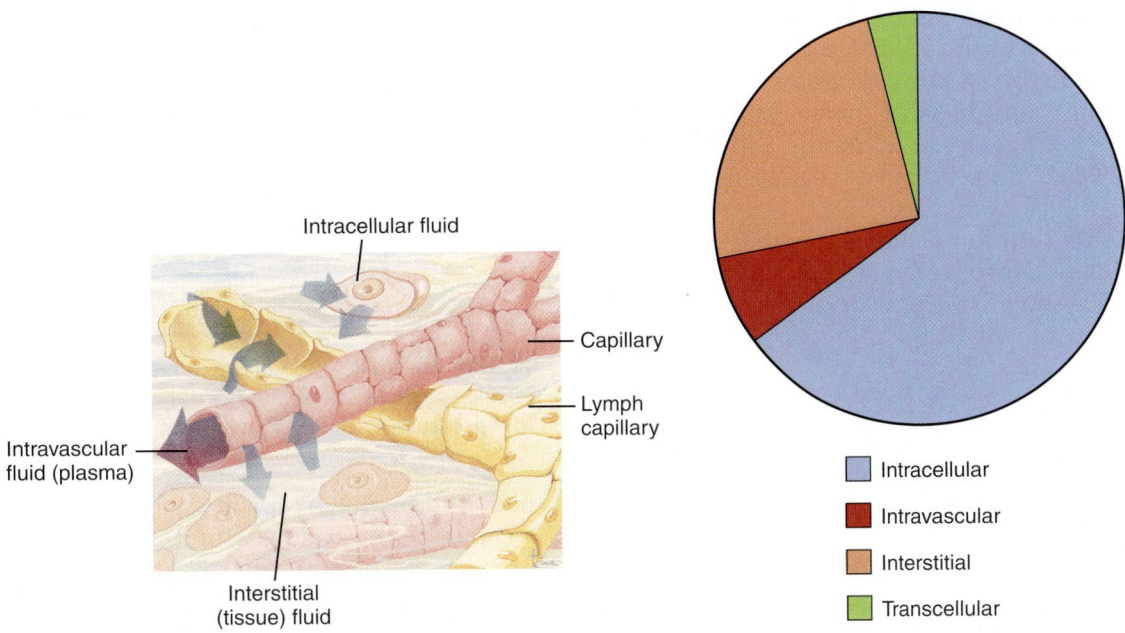

Intracellular fluid

Capillary

Lymph capillary

Intravascular fluid (plasma)

Interstitial (tissue) fluid

- Intracellular
- Intravascular
- Interstitial
- Transcellular

FIGURE 38-1 Normal distribution of body fluids. Transcellular fluid includes specialized fluids such as cerebrospinal and peritoneal fluid and digestive juices.

- **In the ECF,** the major electrolytes are sodium, chloride, and bicarbonate. Albumin is also present in the ECF, mostly in the intravascular fluid. Gastric and intestinal secretions (transcellular fluids) also contain electrolytes.

Severe electrolyte imbalances can occur if electrolytes move into a compartment they do not normally occupy or if they are lost in excess amounts from the body through perspiration, wounds, injury, or illness.

KnowledgeCheck 38-1

- Define *solute, electrolyte, intracellular fluid, extracellular fluid, cation,* and *anion.*
- Identify the major electrolytes in the ICF and ECF.

 ThinkLike a Nurse 38-1

- Based on the information presented in the Meet Your Patients scenario, rank the members of the LaGuardia family based on total body water content.
- Does this information help you understand which family members were admitted to the hospital?

How Do Fluids and Electrolytes Move in the Body?

The selectively permeable membranes of cells and capillaries separate ICF and ECF (see Fig. 38-1). Fluid and electrolytes move across these membranes by passive and active mechanisms. In **active transport,** movement of fluid and solutes requires energy. **Passive transport** requires no energy. The three passive transport systems are osmosis, diffusion, and filtration. To see an animated illustration of these three systems,

 Go to **Animations: Osmosis, Diffusion, Filtration, and Active Transport,** on Davis*Plus.*

Osmosis

Osmosis involves movement of water (or other pure solute) across a membrane from an area of a less concentrated solution to an area of more concentrated solution. Water moves across the membrane to dilute the higher concentration of solutes (Fig. 38-2). Recall that a solute is a substance dissolved in body fluid. Solutes may be crystalloids or colloids. **Crystalloids** are solutes that readily dissolve (e.g., electrolytes). **Colloids** are larger molecules that do not dissolve readily (e.g., proteins).

The concentration of solutes creating pressure in body fluid is called **osmolality.** **Osmols** refers to the number of particles of solute per kilogram of water and is expressed as milliosmoles per kilogram (mOsm/kg). Sodium is the greatest determinant of serum osmolality, and potassium is the greatest determinant of intracellular osmolality. Glucose and urea also contribute to osmolality in the ICF and ECF.

Another term for osmolality is **tonicity.**

- **An isotonic solution** is of the same osmolality as blood. An isotonic solution is often given by intravenous (IV)

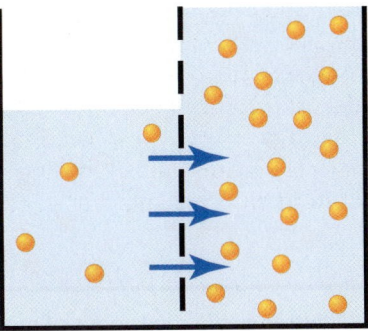

FIGURE 38-2 Osmosis is the movement of water across a membrane from a less concentrated solution to a more concentrated solution.

infusion if blood volume is low. Because the solution is the same concentration as blood, the fluid will remain in the vascular space, and no osmosis will occur.

- A **hypotonic solution** is of lower osmolality than blood. When a hypotonic solution is infused, water moves by osmosis from the vascular system into the cells.
- A **hypertonic solution** contains a higher concentration of solutes than does blood. When a hypertonic solution is given to a patient, water moves by osmosis from the cells into the ECF.

Diffusion

Diffusion is a passive process by which molecules of a solute move through a cell membrane from an area of higher concentration to an area of lower concentration. Movement occurs (Fig. 38-3) until the concentrations are equivalent on both sides of the membrane. For an example of diffusion, pour yourself a cup of coffee. Now add cream to the coffee. Initially, the cream is concentrated in the area where you have poured it. However, within a short time the cream is evenly dispersed throughout the coffee. If you stir the coffee, the cream disperses even more quickly. Fluids within the human body work on a similar principle; movement of the body speeds the diffusion of molecules.

The rate of diffusion varies according to the size of the molecules, the concentration of the solution, and the temperature of the solution. Small molecules move more rapidly than larger molecules. Large differences in concentration require a longer period of time to reach equilibration. Higher temperatures cause molecules to move faster, so that diffusion occurs more rapidly.

Filtration

Filtration is the movement of both water and smaller particles from an area of high pressure to one of low pressure (Fig. 38-4). **Hydrostatic pressure** is the force created by fluid within a closed system; it is responsible for normal circulation of blood. In other words, blood flows from the high-pressure arterial system to the lower pressure capillaries and veins. As fluid (plasma)

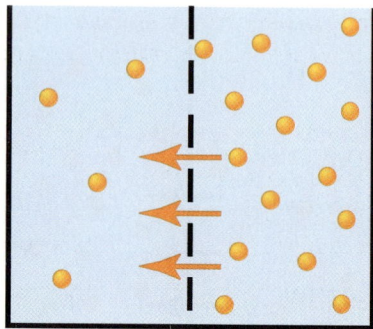

FIGURE 38-3 Diffusion is the movement of molecules of a solute through a cell membrane from an area of higher concentration to an area of lower concentration.

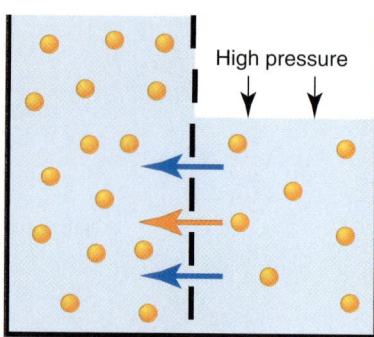

FIGURE 38-4 Filtration is the movement of water and smaller particles from an area of high pressure to an area of low pressure.

moves through the capillary membrane, only solutes of a certain size can flow with it. For example, the membrane pores of Bowman's capsule in the kidneys are very small, and only albumin, the smallest of the proteins, can be filtered through the membrane. By contrast, the membrane pores of liver cells are extremely large, so a variety of solutes can pass through and be metabolized.

Osmotic pressure is the power of a solution to draw water. A highly concentrated solution (with many molecules in solution) draws water and has a high osmotic pressure. The plasma proteins in the blood exert osmotic, or colloidal, pressure to help maintain fluid in the vascular space. However, when hydrostatic pressure exceeds osmotic pressure, fluid leaves the vessels. This difference, known as the **filtration pressure**, represents the net pressures that move fluid and solutes. The hydrostatic pressure is higher at the arteriole end of the capillary and lower at the venous end; thus, blood is forced out at the arteriole in and returned at the venule side.

Active Transport

Active transport occurs when molecules (e.g., electrolytes) move across cell membranes against a concentration gradient (from an area of low concentration to an area of high concentration). Active transport requires energy expenditure (Fig. 38-5). Adenosine triphosphate (ATP) is released from the cell to enable certain substances to acquire the energy needed to pass through the cell membrane. For example, sodium concentration is greater in ECF; therefore, sodium tends to enter by diffusion into the intracellular compartment. This tendency is offset by the sodium-potassium pump, which consists, in part, of transport proteins located on the cell membrane. In the presence of ATP, the sodium-potassium pump actively moves sodium from the cell into the ECF and potassium from the ECF into the cell. Active transport is vital for maintaining the unique composition of both the extracellular and intracellular compartments.

Table 38-2 summarizes the processes of fluid and electrolyte movement.

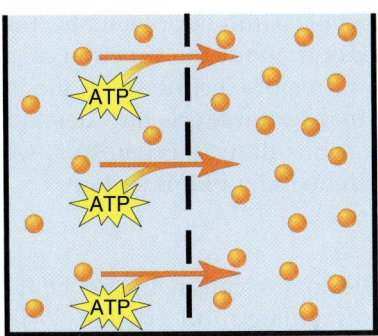

FIGURE 38-5 Active transport is the movement of electrolytes against a concentration gradient. For the movement to occur, active transport requires energy expenditure.

KnowledgeCheck 38-2

Identify the appropriate mechanism: osmosis, diffusion, filtration, or active transport:

- Molecules move across a membrane to equalize concentration.
- Fluid moves across a membrane to equalize concentration.
- Molecules move against a concentration gradient.
- Molecules move to equalize pressure.

How Does the Body Regulate Fluids?

A balance between fluid intake and output is essential to maintain homeostasis. Excesses or deficits of intake or output can lead to severe disorders.

Fluid Intake

You have undoubtedly been told to drink eight to ten glasses of water per day. Did you ever wonder where that recommendation came from or why that volume is important? Eight to ten 8-ounce glasses of water provide 1,920 to 2,400 mL of fluid. The Institute of Medicine (IOM) (2004), however, recommends a total fluid intake of 2,700 mL per day for women and 3,700 mL per day for men. The IOM states that we should obtain 80% of our intake from drinking fluids and the remaining 20% from food and cellular metabolism of foods. Prolonged exercise and heat exposure increase the requirements. The IOM did not set an upper limit on fluid intake.

 A daily intake of 1,500 to 2,000 mL of noncaffeinated fluids will maintain hydration in older adults (Miller, 2012).

Thirst is the major regulator of fluid intake. Changes in plasma osmolality signal the thirst center in the hypothalamus, which leads to the urge to drink. Situations that increase plasma osmolality (and promote thirst) include excessive fluid loss, excessive sodium intake, and decreased fluid intake. Situations that inhibit the thirst mechanism include a high intake of fluids, fluid retention, excessive IV infusion of hypotonic solutions, and low sodium intake.

Fluid Output

Fluid loss occurs throughout the day, creating a constant need to replenish fluid. In a healthy state, fluid losses are equivalent to fluid intake. **Sensible fluid loss** is measurable and perceived (e.g., urine, diarrhea, ostomy, and gastric drainage). **Insensible fluid loss** is loss that we do not perceive, is not easily measured, but accounts for about 900 mL per day. It occurs primarily by diffusion and evaporation through the skin, but also from the lungs. Insensible loss increases with open wounds, burns, or other breaks in the protective layer of the skin. The following are common sources of fluid loss:

- *Urine* (1,500 mL/day). Urine accounts for the greatest amount of fluid loss. Urine output varies according to intake and activity, but should remain at least 30 to 50 mL/hour. The volume of urine increases as intake increases, and it decreases to compensate for other fluid losses (e.g., vomiting and excessive perspiration).
- *Feces* (100 to 200 mL/day). Soft stools contain more water than hard stools. As stool frequency increases, water loss also increases.
- *Skin* (about 600 mL/day). **Sensible (perceived) fluid loss** through the skin occurs through perspiration, at 300 to 600 mL/day. Perspiration varies based on temperature, skeletal muscle activity, and metabolic activity. Fever, exercise, and some disease processes increase metabolic activity and heat production, leading to increased fluid loss.
- *Lungs* (about 300 mL/day). Insensible loss occurs through the lungs as water is exhaled with each breath. An increase in respiratory rate increases the amount of fluid lost.

Hormonal Regulation

The kidneys are the principal regulator of fluid and electrolyte balance. The following hormones are involved:

Table 38-2 ▶ Processes of Fluid and Electrolyte Movement			
PROCESS	**WHAT MOVES**	**FROM AREA OF**	**TO AREA OF**
Diffusion	Molecules (solute)	High concentration	Low concentration
Active transport	Molecules (solute)	Low concentration	High concentration
Osmosis	Water	Low concentration	High concentration
Filtration	Water and small particles	High pressure	Low pressure

Antidiuretic Hormone Pressure sensors in the vascular system stimulate or inhibit the release of **antidiuretic hormone (ADH)** from the pituitary gland. ADH causes the kidneys to retain fluid. If fluid volume within the vascular system is low, fluid pressures within the system decrease, and more ADH is released. If fluid volume (and therefore pressure) increases, less ADH is released, and the kidneys eliminate more fluid. ADH is also produced in response to a rise in serum osmolality, fever, pain, stress, and some opioids.

Renin–Angiotensin System When extracellular (i.e., intravascular) fluid volume is decreased, receptors in the glomeruli respond to the decreased perfusion of the kidneys by releasing renin. **Renin** is an enzyme responsible for the chain of reactions that converts angiotensinogen to angiotensin II. **Angiotensin II** acts on the nephrons to retain sodium and water and directs the adrenal cortex to release aldosterone.

Aldosterone When aldosterone is released, it stimulates the distal tubules of the kidneys to reabsorb sodium and excrete potassium. Sodium reabsorption results in passive reabsorption of water, thereby increasing plasma volume and improving kidney perfusion. When fluid excess is present, renin is not released, and this process stops.

Other Hormones Other hormones affect fluid and electrolyte balance by their effect on certain organs of the body:

- *Thyroid hormone* affects fluid volume by influencing cardiac output. An increase in thyroid hormone causes an increase in cardiac output, thereby increasing glomerular filtration rate and urine output. A decrease has the opposite effect.
- *Atrial natriuretic peptide (ANP), brain natriuretic peptide (BNP),* and *C-type natriuretic peptide (CNP)* are important in renal and cardiovascular regulation of fluid maintenance. **Natriuresis** (natriuretic) is the discharge of sodium through urine. BNP is actually released from both the brain and the right atrium. In clinical practice, BNP can be measured in the serum to help determine presence of heart failure with fluid excess and to distinguish heart failure from pulmonary edema. The test can be performed at the bedside.

ThinkLike a Nurse 38-2

Apply the information on fluid balance to the LaGuardia family (Meet Your Patients). What have you learned that helps you explain why some family members require hospitalization? What additional information do you need to be able to predict each person's fluid balance?

How Does the Body Regulate Electrolytes?

To maintain health, the body must balance electrolyte losses and intake. For example, potassium lost through diarrhea and vomiting must be replaced by dietary potassium or potassium supplements. Table 38-3 provides information about the function, regulation, and food sources of major electrolytes in the body. Maintenance of normal serum levels also depends on dietary intake and various other mechanisms, which are discussed in the remainder of this section.

Sodium (Na⁺)

Sodium is the major cation in the ECF. Its primary function is to regulate fluid volume. When sodium is reabsorbed in the kidney, water and potassium are also reabsorbed, thereby maintaining ECF volume. According to the *2010 Dietary Guidelines for Americans*, adults should limit the intake of salt to 2,300 mg/day. People (including children) with chronic diseases (e.g., hypertension, diabetes, chronic kidney disease), African Americans, and people older than age 51 are especially sensitive to the blood-pressuring raising effects of salt. They are advised to limit salt intake to 1,500 mg/day. This applies to nearly 50% of the U.S. population (U.S. Department of Agriculture [USDA], 2011).

Potassium (K⁺)

Potassium is the major cation of the ICF; it is a key electrolyte in cellular metabolism. Only 2% of body potassium is found in the extracellular fluid. The *2010 Dietary Guidelines for Americans* recommends that adults consume at least 4,700 mg/day. However, most people do not consume enough potassium. Most American women age 31 to 50 consume less than half this amount and intake is only moderately higher for men. Moderate potassium deficiency is associated with increases in blood pressure, salt sensitivity, risk of kidney stones, and risk of bone turnover (USDA, 2011). Because of its effect on blood pressure, low intake of dietary potassium is associated with increased risk of stroke.

The Dietary Reference Intakes (DRIs) do not specify an upper limit of potassium intake because there is no evidence of problems associated with higher potassium intake (IOM, 2004). In a healthy person, a high potassium intake does not result in a high serum potassium level (hyperkalemia) because the kidneys efficiently eliminate excess dietary potassium.

Calcium (Ca²⁺)

Calcium is responsible for bone health and neuromuscular and cardiac function. It is also an essential factor in blood clotting. About 99% of body calcium is located in the bones and teeth. The remaining 1% circulates in the blood and affects system functions. Because calcium is so vital for cardiac and muscle function, serum levels are tightly regulated. As serum levels drop, calcium leaches from the bones into the blood to compensate.

Prolonged insufficient dietary intake can cause bone loss that leads to osteoporosis. Half the women older than age 50, 90% of women older than age 75, and about 30% of men older than age 50 have osteoporosis. About half of all Caucasian women will suffer an osteoporosis-related fracture at some point in life, as will approximately 1 in 5 men. Because most Americans do not include the recommended amount of calcium in their diets, the chances of bone loss increase with age. Most calcium should be obtained from naturally calcium-rich foods, such as dairy products. Calcium-fortified foods and calcium supplements can be used as a secondary source.

Calcium requirements are highest during childhood, adolescence, pregnancy, and breastfeeding. People who are immobile are at increased risk for reduced bone density.

 Older adults are at risk for calcium deficiencies because of reduced absorption that occurs with aging and chronic medical conditions (National Osteoporosis Foundation, n.d.).

For recommended calcium intake by age group, see Table 38-4.

Magnesium (Mg²⁺)

Magnesium is a mineral used in more than 300 biochemical reactions in the body. Like calcium, only about 1% of magnesium is found in the blood. The remaining 99% is divided between the ICF and bone (in combination with calcium and phosphorus). Although magnesium deficiency is rare, you may find low levels in individuals who have a high alcohol intake. Some malabsorption disorders may also cause magnesium depletion (Crawford & Harris, 2011a).

Chloride (Cl⁻)

Chloride is the most abundant anion in the extracellular fluid. It is usually bound with other ions, especially sodium or potassium (e.g., as sodium chloride, or salt). A healthy adult between the ages of 19 and 50 should consume 2.3 grams of chloride each day along with 1.5 grams of sodium to replace daily losses and maintain serum blood levels (IOM, 2004).

Phosphorus (Phosphate [PO₄⁻])

Most phosphorus in the body is combined with oxygen, forming phosphate—mostly bound with calcium in teeth and bones as calcium phosphate. Phosphate is the most abundant intracellular anion. Phosphate and calcium exist in an inverse relationship; as one increases, the other one decreases. As a result, high blood phosphate levels decrease the movement of calcium from the bones. Phosphate in the ECF is known as **phosphorus**.

Bicarbonate (HCO₃⁻)

Bicarbonate is present in both ICF and ECF. The kidneys regulate extracellular bicarbonate to maintain acid–base balance. When serum levels rise, the kidneys excrete excess bicarbonate. If serum levels are low, the kidneys conserve bicarbonate. Bicarbonate is not consumed in the diet but is produced by the body to meet current needs.

KnowledgeCheck 38-3

- Identify the major functions of sodium, potassium, calcium, magnesium, chloride, phosphate, and bicarbonate.
- What are the major concerns associated with sodium and potassium intake?
- Identify at least five potassium-rich foods.
- Identify the ideal calcium intakes for each member of the LaGuardia family (Meet Your Patients).

 ## ThinkLike a Nurse 38-3

Based on the information you have learned about the major electrolytes of the body, which electrolytes are most likely to be out of balance in members of the LaGuardia family? Explain your answer.

How Is Acid–Base Balance Regulated?

Acids and bases are formed in the body as part of normal metabolic processes. An **acid** is any compound that contains hydrogen ions (H^+) that can be released. For this reason, acids are referred to as cation donors. A common strong acid is hydrochloric acid (HCl), which is present in gastric secretions. A **base** or **alkali** is a compound that combines with (accepts) hydrogen ions in solution. Therefore, bases are referred to as cation (a positively charged particle) acceptors. A strong base has a tendency to bind hydrogen ions, whereas a weak base binds only a small portion of the available hydrogen ions.

The amount of acid or base present in a solution is measured as **pH**. The pH is reported on a scale of 1 to 14: 1 to 6.9 is acidic, 7 is neutral, and 7.1 to 14 is basic, or alkaline. The stronger an acid, the lower the pH. In contrast, a strong base has a high pH. The pH is a *logarithmic* scale. For example, a pH of 4 is 10 times more acidic than a pH of 5. The body functions normally within a narrow range of pH values. Arterial blood and tissue fluid normally have a pH of 7.35 to 7.45; therefore, they are slightly alkaline. A serum pH below 7.30 or above 7.52 alters enzymatic activity and creates myocardial irritability. A serum pH below 6.9 or above 7.8 is usually fatal. Three complex mechanisms maintain acid–base balance: (1) buffers, (2) respiratory control of carbon dioxide, and (3) renal regulation of bicarbonate (HCO_3^-).

Buffers

Buffer systems prevent wide swings in pH. A buffer system consists of a weak acid and a weak base. Buffer molecules keep strong acids or bases from altering the pH either by absorbing or releasing free hydrogen ions.

Carbonic Acid–Sodium Bicarbonate System Carbonic acid (H_2CO_3) and sodium bicarbonate ($NaHCO_3$) buffer almost 90% of metabolic processes in the ECF. Blood and tissue fluid depend on this buffer system to maintain a relatively constant pH. During normal metabolism, blood and tissue fluids tend to become acidic; therefore, more sodium bicarbonate is required than carbonic acid. The usual ratio of $NaHCO_3$ to H_2CO_3 is 20:1.

Table 38-3 ➤ Major Electrolytes

ELECTROLYTE	FUNCTION	REGULATION	SOURCES
Sodium (Na⁺) Major cation in the ECF *Normal serum level is 135–145 mEq/L	Regulates fluid volume. Helps maintain blood volume. Interacts with calcium to maintain muscle contraction. Stimulates conduction of nerve impulses.	Moves by active transport across cell membranes. Regulated by aldosterone and ADH levels Reabsorbed and excreted through the kidneys Minimal loss through perspiration and feces Low sodium may be caused by excess water intake.	Table salt, soy sauce, cured pork, cheese, milk, processed foods, canned products, and foods preserved with salt
Potassium (K⁺) Major cation in the ICF Normal serum level is 3.5–5.0 mEq/L	Maintains ICF osmolality. Regulates conduction of cardiac rhythm. Transmits electrical impulses in multiple body systems. Assists with acid–base balance.	Regulated by aldosterone Excreted and conserved through the kidneys Lost through vomiting and diarrhea Loss triggered by many diuretics	Common food sources include bananas, oranges, apricots, figs, dates, carrots, potatoes, tomatoes, spinach, dairy products, and meats.
Calcium (Ca²⁺) Most abundant electrolyte in the body Normal serum level is 8.5–10.5 mg/dL	Promotes transmission of nerve impulses. Major component of bone and teeth Regulates muscle contractions. Maintains cardiac automaticity. Essential factor in the formation of blood clots Catalyst for many cellular activities	Combines with phosphorus to form the mineral salts of the teeth and bones. Calcium and phosphorus levels are inversely proportional Parathyroid hormone (PTH) stimulates release of calcium from bones and reabsorption from kidneys and intestines. Calcitonin (from the thyroid) blocks bone breakdown and lowers calcium levels. Absorption stimulated by vitamin D	See Table 38-4 for average daily requirements. Common food sources include milk, milk products, dark green, leafy vegetables, and salmon, as well as calcium-fortified foods such as breads and cereals.
Magnesium (Mg²⁺) Present in skeleton and ICF; second most abundant cation in ICF Normal serum level is 1.6–2.6 mEq/L	Involved in protein and carbohydrate metabolism Necessary for protein and DNA synthesis within the cell Maintains normal intracellular levels of potassium. Involved in electrical activity in nerve and muscle membranes, including the heart	Ingested in the diet and absorbed through the small intestine Excreted by kidneys Loss may be triggered by diuretics, poorly controlled diabetes mellitus, and excess alcohol intake.	Average daily requirement is 18–30 mEq. Found in most foods, but high levels are present in green vegetables, cereal grains, and nuts.

Table 38-3 ➤ Major Electrolytes—cont'd

ELECTROLYTE	FUNCTION	REGULATION	SOURCES
	May have a role in regulating blood pressure and may influence the release and activity of insulin (Crawford & Harris, 2011a; IOM, 2004).		
Chloride (Cl⁻) Major anion in the ECF Normal serum level is 95–105 mEq/L	Works with Na^+ to maintain osmotic pressure between fluid compartments. Essential for production of HCl for gastric secretions Functions as buffer in oxygen–carbon dioxide exchange in RBCs. Assists with acid–base balance.	Reabsorbed and excreted through the kidneys along with sodium Regulated by aldosterone and ADH levels Deficits lead to potassium deficits; potassium deficits lead to chloride deficits.	Found in foods high in sodium
Phosphate (PO₄⁻) Major anion in the ICF Normal serum level is 1.7–2.6 mEq/L	Serves as a catalyst for many intracellular activities Promotes muscle and nerve action Assists with acid–base balance Important for cell division and transmission of hereditary traits	Combines with calcium to form the mineral salts of the teeth and bones Calcium and phosphorus levels are inversely proportional Regulated by PTH; has inverse response to calcium Excreted and reabsorbed by the kidneys	Foods high in phosphorus are meat, fish, poultry, milk products, carbonated beverages, and legumes. Readily available in body as a result of metabolism
Bicarbonate (HCO₃⁻) Major buffer in the body In ECF and ICF Normal serum level is 22–26 mEq/L	Maintains acid–base balance by functioning as the primary buffer in the body	Lost through diarrhea, diuretics, renal insufficiency Excess possible if person ingests quantities of acid neutralizers	Present in acid neutralizers (e.g., sodium bicarbonate)

*Note that normal ranges may differ among references and in different laboratories.
ADH = antidiuretic hormone; ECF = extracellular fluid; ICF = intracellular fluid; PTH = parathyroid hormone; RBC = red blood cell.

As long as this ratio is maintained, the pH remains within its normal range. If bicarbonate is depleted while neutralizing a strong acid, the pH may drop below 7.35, resulting in a condition called **acidosis**. If a strong base is added to extracellular fluid and depletes carbonic acid, the pH may rise above 7.45, resulting in a condition called **alkalosis**.

Phosphate System The phosphate system helps regulate acid–base balance in intracellular fluids. The phosphate system works in the same way as the bicarbonate system but converts alkaline sodium phosphate (Na_2HPO_4) to acid sodium phosphate (NaH_2PO_4).

Protein System Plasma proteins and the globin portion of hemoglobin (in red blood cells) contain chemical groups that can either combine with or free up hydrogen ions. This system helps buffer intracellular fluid and plasma to maintain pH balance.

Respiratory Mechanisms

The lungs are the second line of defense to restore normal pH. They control the body's carbonic acid supply via carbon dioxide retention or removal to maintain the 20:1 ratio of base to acid. When the serum pH is too acidic (pH is low), the lungs remove carbon dioxide

Table 38-4 ➤ Recommended Daily Allowances (RDA) for Calcium and Vitamin D*

AGE	CALCIUM (MILLIGRAMS)	VITAMIN D* (INTERNATIONAL UNITS)
Birth to 6 months	200	400
6–12 months	260	400
1–3 years	700	600
4–8 years	1,000	600
9–13 years	1,300	600
14–18 years	1,300	600
19–30 years	1,000	600
31–50 years	1,000	600
51–70 years, males	1,000	600
51–70 years, females	1,200	600
Older than 70 years	1,200	800
Pregnant or Lactating Women		
18 years or younger pregnant or lactating	1,300	600
19–50 years	1,000	600

*Adequate intake of Vitamin D is necessary for absorption of calcium.
Source: Institute of Medicine of the National Academies. (2010, rev. 2011). Dietary reference intakes for calcium and vitamin D. Retrieved from http://www.iom.edu/~/media/Files/Report%20Files/2010/Dietary-Reference-Intakes-for-Calcium-and-Vitamin-D/Vitamin%20D%20and %20Calcium%202010%20Report%20Brief.pdf;
NIH Medline Plus. (2011). New recommended daily amounts of calcium and vitamin D. Retrieved from http://www.nlm.nih.gov/medlineplus/magazine/issues/winter11/articles/winter11pg12.html

through rapid, deep breathing. This reduces the amount of carbon dioxide available to make carbonic acid. If the serum pH is too alkaline (pH is high), the lungs try to conserve carbon dioxide through shallow respirations.

Renal Mechanisms

The last line of defense is the kidneys, which regulate the concentration of plasma bicarbonate. They can neutralize more acid or base than either the respiratory system or the chemical buffers. If the serum pH is too acidic, the kidneys conserve additional bicarbonate to neutralize the acid. If the serum pH is too alkaline, the kidneys excrete additional bicarbonate to lower the amount of base and thereby decrease the pH. The kidneys also buffer pH by forming acids and ammonium (a base).

Although the renal system is very effective at altering pH, it is slow. It may take up to 3 days to return the pH to normal limits. This process is known as *compensation*. The pH returns to normal, but the carbon dioxide or bicarbonate level is abnormal. Over time, or when the original problem is corrected, these levels also return to normal.

KnowledgeCheck 38-4

- Briefly describe the three mechanisms used to maintain pH.
- Rank in order the acid–base balance mechanisms from the most rapidly acting to the slowest acting.

Example Problem: Fluid, Electrolyte, and Acid–Base Imbalances

Illness or disease may lead to imbalances of fluid, electrolytes, or pH. These are discussed in the next sections. The Practical Knowledge section, later in this chapter, presents some interventions to correct these imbalances.

Fluid Imbalances

Fluid imbalances involve a deficit or excess in fluid volume or an alteration in distribution among the fluid compartments. Fluid deficit, regardless of the cause, is referred to as *hypovolemia*, whereas fluid excess, usually not blood, is referred to as *hypervolemia*.

Deficient Fluid Volume

Deficient fluid volume (hypovolemia) occurs when there is a proportional loss of fluid and electrolytes from the ECF. Loss of blood volume is called hypovolemia (*hypo* = low, *vol* = volume, *emia* pertains to blood). Hypovolemia may occur with surgery, trauma, or uterine rupture.

Dehydration

Dehydration describes a state of negative fluid balance in which there is a loss of water (*hydro* = water) from the intracellular, extracellular or intravascular spaces. Dehydration can be categorized by three causes:

- Insufficient intake of fluids (e.g., as may occur with depression, sedation, or alcohol abuse)
- Excessive fluid loss (e.g., bleeding, vomiting, diarrhea, nasogastric [NG] suction)
- Fluid shifts (e.g., intravascular fluid may leak into body tissues, burns).

When dehydration occurs from the loss of body fluids, electrolytes may also be lost. Fluid loss can also lead to an increase is serum osmolarity.

Early Symptoms of Dehydration The first symptom of volume loss is thirst. If the patient is able to recognize thirst and respond by drinking liquid, no further treatment may be required. If fluid is not available or the patient is unable to drink, or if blood loss continues faster than fluid is replaced (e.g., hemorrhage), fluid becomes deficient. Initially as fluid volume decreases, the heart rate increases and the blood vessels constrict. This increases the blood pressure, in order to continue to circulate the remaining fluid to meet the body's fluid demands.

Continuing Fluid Loss (Hypovolemic Shock)

If volume continues to be lost, the heart pumps faster but not as powerfully, resulting in a rapid, weak pulse, and orthostatic hypotension. This is known as **hypovolemic shock**. Orthostatic blood pressure is measured when the patient is lying, sitting, and standing. A drop in the systolic blood pressure (from lying or sitting to standing) greater or equal to 20 mm Hg is called **orthostatic hypotension**. Low fluid volume is just one of its causes.

As fluid loss continues, water is pulled from the interstitial spaces and the ICF into the vascular system, resulting in dry skin and mucous membranes, decreased skin and tongue turgor, decreased urine output, and flat neck veins. Patients complain of muscle weakness, fatigue, and feeling warm. Temperature increases because the body is less able to cool itself through perspiration. In an older adult, temperature will rise but may not be elevated above normal body temperature.

Assessing for and Preventing Deficient Fluid Volume

Weight is a sensitive measure of fluid loss. A sudden 5% loss of body weight is considered clinically significant. When loss approaches 8%, fluid loss is severe. A sudden loss of 15% of body weight due to fluid loss is usually fatal. The patient with fluid volume deficit usually has elevated blood urea nitrogen (BUN)–to-creatinine ratio and elevated hematocrit. Both values increase because there is less water in proportion to the solid substances being measured. Specific gravity of the urine increases as the kidneys attempt to conserve water, resulting in more concentrated urine.

You can help prevent fluid volume deficit by identifying patients who have the highest risk for developing this condition: older adults, infants, children, and any patients with conditions associated with fluid loss (e.g., diabetes insipidus, vomiting, diarrhea, fever). You will learn how to facilitate fluid intake and provide parenteral fluid replacement in the Planning Interventions/Implementation section, to follow.

Excess Fluid Volume

Excess fluid volume (hypervolemia) involves excessive retention of sodium and water in the ECF. Fluid volume excess can result from excessive salt intake, disease affecting kidney or liver function, or poor pumping action of the heart. The retained sodium increases osmotic pressure in the ECF. This pressure pulls fluid from the cells into the ECF.

Signs of Fluid Overload The vital sign changes in a patient with hypervolemia are the opposite of those seen in hypovolemia. The blood pressure is elevated, pulse is bounding, and respirations are increased and shallow. The neck veins may become distended. Along with increased intravascular volume, excess ECF may accumulate in the tissues, especially in dependent areas, as *edema*. The skin is pale and cool. Urine output becomes dilute, and volume increases. The patient rapidly gains weight. In severe fluid overload, the patient develops moist crackles in the lungs, dyspnea, and ascites (excess peritoneal fluid). Hemodilution causes BUN, hematocrit, and specific gravity of the urine to decrease.

Preventing Fluid Overload You can help prevent fluid overload by monitoring intake and output and carefully regulating intravenous infusions. The use of electronic infusion pumps controls the rate of infusion of intravenous fluid, thereby minimizing the risk of fluid overload (see Planning Interventions/Implementation).

KnowledgeCheck 38-5

- Define *deficient fluid volume* and *excess fluid volume*.
- Identify the signs and symptoms of deficient fluid volume and excess fluid volume.
- Describe dehydration and hypervolemia.

Electrolyte Imbalances

Any electrolyte may become imbalanced. Table 38-5 discusses the common causes; signs and symptoms; and treatment of sodium, potassium, calcium, magnesium,

Table 38-5 ➤ Electrolyte Imbalances

DISORDER	COMMON CAUSES	SIGNS AND SYMPTOMS	TREATMENT
Hyponatremia Na⁺ <135 mEq/L	Diuretics GI fluid loss Adrenal insufficiency Excessive intake of hypotonic solutions, such as water or D_5W IV fluids Syndrome of inappropriate ADH	Anorexia, nausea, and vomiting Weakness Lethargy Confusion Muscle cramps or twitching Seizures	Monitor I&O. Monitor sodium level. Increase oral sodium intake. Administer IV saline infusion and take seizure precautions, if severe.

Hypernatremia
Na⁺ >145 mEq/L
	Excessive sodium intake
	
	Water deprivation
	
	Increased water loss through profuse sweating, heat stroke, or diabetes insipidus
	
	Administration of hypertonic tube feeding
		Thirst
		
		Elevated temperature
		
		Dry mouth and sticky mucous membranes
		
		If severe:
		
		   Hallucinations
		
		   Irritability
		
		   Lethargy
		
		   Seizures
			Monitor I&O.
			
			Monitor sodium level.
			
			Monitor vital signs and level of consciousness.
			
			Restrict sodium in the diet.
			
			Beware of hidden sodium in foods and medications.
			
			Increase water intake.
			
			Administer IV solutions that do not contain sodium.

Hypokalemia K⁺ <3.5 mEq/L	Diuretics GI fluid loss through vomiting, gastric suction, or diarrhea Steroid administration Hyperaldosteronism Anorexia or bulimia	Fatigue Anorexia, nausea, and vomiting Muscle weakness Decreased GI motility Dysrhythmias Paresthesia Flat T wave on ECG Increased sensitivity to digitalis	Monitor I&O. Monitor potassium level. If the client is taking digoxin, monitor pulse and observe for toxicity. Encourage intake of foods rich in potassium. Administer potassium supplements ✚ (Note: IV potassium must be well diluted and administered into a central vein slowly.)
Hyperkalemia K⁺ >5.0 mEq/L	Renal failure Potassium-sparing diuretics Hypoaldosteronism High potassium intake coupled with renal insufficiency Acidosis Major trauma Hemolyzed serum sample produces pseudohyperkalemia	Muscle weakness Dysrhythmias Flaccid paralysis Intestinal colic Tall T waves on ECG	Monitor I&O. Monitor potassium level. Caution about potassium-rich food intake in patients with elevated creatinine levels.
Hypocalcemia Ca²⁺ <8.5 mq/dL	Hypoparathyroidism Malabsorption Pancreatitis	Diarrhea Numbness and tingling of extremities	Monitor I&O. Monitor serum calcium. Encourage increased

Table 38-5 ➤ Electrolyte Imbalances—cont'd

DISORDER	COMMON CAUSES	SIGNS AND SYMPTOMS	TREATMENT
	Alkalosis Vitamin D deficiency	Muscle cramps Tetany Convulsions Laryngeal spasms Cardiac irritability *Positive Trousseau's and Chvostek's signs	calcium intake. Administer calcium supplements. If severe, monitor patency of airway, institute seizure and safety precautions, and administer parenteral calcium.
Hypercalcemia Ca^{2+} >10.5 mq/dL	Hyperparathyroidism Malignant bone disease Prolonged immobilization Excess calcium supplementation Thiazide diuretics	Muscle weakness Constipation Anorexia, nausea, and vomiting Polyuria and polydipsia Kidney stones Bizarre behavior Bradycardia	Monitor I&O. Encourage fluid intake to prevent stone formation. Encourage fiber to prevent constipation. Eliminate calcium supplements and limit calcium-rich foods. Avoid calcium-based antacids. Renal dialysis may be required.
Hypomagnesemia Mg^{2+} <1.3 mEq/L	Chronic alcoholism Malabsorption Diabetic ketoacidosis Prolonged gastric suction	Neuromuscular irritability Disorientation Mood changes Dysrhythmias Increased sensitivity to digitalis	Monitor I&O. Encourage foods high in magnesium. Avoid alcohol intake. If the client is taking digoxin, monitor pulse and observe for toxicity.
Hypermagnesemia Mg^{2+} >2.1 mEq/L	Renal failure Adrenal insufficiency Excess replacement	Flushing and warmth of skin Hypotension Drowsiness, lethargy Hypoactive reflexes Depressed respirations Bradycardia	Monitor vital signs and airway. Monitor reflexes. Avoid magnesium-based antacids and laxatives. Restrict dietary intake of foods high in magnesium.
Hypophosphatemia PO_4^- <2.5 mg/dL	Refeeding after starvation Alcohol withdrawal Diabetic ketoacidosis Respiratory acidosis	Paresthesia Joint stiffness Seizures Cardiomyopathy Impaired tissue oxygenation	Monitor serum phosphorus level. Monitor calcium levels as phosphate is replaced. Start TPN slowly to avoid drops in phosphate.
Hyperphosphatemia PO_4^- >4.5 mg/dL	Renal failure Hyperthyroidism Chemotherapy Excess use of phosphate-based laxative	Short term: tetany symptoms—tingling of extremities and cramping Long term: Calcification in soft tissue	Monitor serum phosphorus level. Monitor for tetany. If severe, administer aluminum hydroxide with meals to bind phosphorus.

*See Clinical Insight 38-1: Assessing for Trousseau's and Chvostek's Signs
ADH = antidiuretic hormone; ECG = electrocardiogram; GI = gastrointestinal; I&O = intake and output; TPN = total parenteral nutrition
Source. Van Leeuwen, A., Poelhuis-Leth, D., & Bladh, M. (2011). *Davis's comprehensive handbook of laboratory and diagnostic tests with nursing implications* (4th ed.). Philadelphia: F. A. Davis.

and phosphate imbalances. Disorders affecting chloride ions occur along with sodium disorders. As sodium levels rise, chloride levels also rise. Decreases also occur simultaneously. Clinical signs and treatments are identical to sodium imbalances. Because of the role of bicarbonate as a buffer, bicarbonate levels rise and fall to maintain pH. You will find further discussion of abnormal bicarbonate levels in the section Acid–Base Imbalances, which follows.

We can apply the information in Table 38-5 to the LaGuardia family (Meet Your Patients). Jackson La-Guardia has end-stage renal disease (ESRD), or renal failure. As a result, he is at risk for imbalances in all of his electrolytes. Now he is experiencing nausea, vomiting, and diarrhea. This will further aggravate the imbalance of potassium and sodium. Because of his complex imbalances, he is a candidate for admission to the hospital. He will need careful rehydration and monitoring of his electrolytes. The remaining family members are likely to be experiencing sodium, potassium, and fluid deficits.

 ## ThinkLike a Nurse 38-4

Martha LaGuardia is taking the following medications: atenolol (Tenormin) 50 mg daily at bedtime, alendronate sodium (Fosamax) 10 mg daily, furosemide (Lasix) 20 mg every morning, and calcium carbonate 500 mg three times per day. She takes her medications regularly and sees her primary care provider monthly. Using your reference books, look up her prescribed medications. Given that Ms. LaGuardia is now experiencing nausea and vomiting, she may be at risk for developing problems and side effects related to her medications. Which medications may cause problems and what problems might they cause? Explain your rationale.

Acid–Base Imbalances

The two broad types of acid–base imbalance are acidosis and alkalosis. **Acidosis** occurs when the serum pH falls below 7.35. **Alkalosis** occurs when the serum pH increases above 7.45 (Fig. 38-6). Arterial blood gases (ABGs) are used to monitor acid–base balance. **ABG analysis** measures pH, partial pressure of oxygen (P_{O_2}),

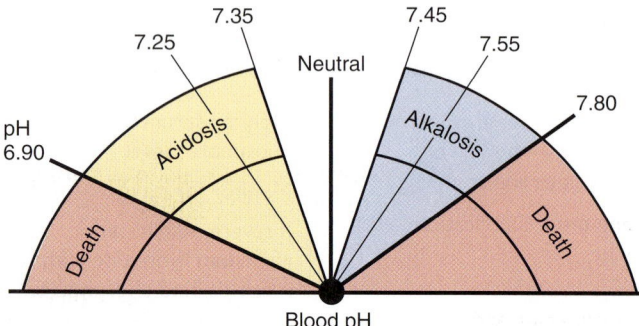

FIGURE 38-6 The pH scale ranges from 1 to 14. Normal blood pH is 7.35 to 7.45.

partial pressure of carbon dioxide (P_{CO_2}), saturation of oxygen (Sa_{O_2}), and bicarbonate (HCO_3^-) level. Acid–base balance is reflected by the pH, P_{CO_2}, and HCO_3 values.

A respiratory disturbance alters the carbonic acid portion of the buffering system, and the resulting imbalance is labeled **respiratory acidosis** or **respiratory alkalosis**. A metabolic disturbance alters the bicarbonate portion of the buffering system, so the resulting imbalance would be labeled as **metabolic acidosis** or **metabolic alkalosis**. Metabolic and respiratory problems can coexist, resulting in disturbances of both sides of the buffering system. Compensatory mechanisms may also produce both bicarbonate and carbon dioxide abnormalities.

Interpreting ABGs

To determine acid–base balance, you must examine the ABG results. The pH, P_{CO_2}, and HCO_3^- values are of primary importance (Table 38-6). The partial pressure of oxygen (P_{O_2}) and saturation of oxygen (Sa_{O_2}) are also part of the ABG result, but they do not affect acid–base balance. Instead, they affect tissue oxygenation. For further discussion on those two measures, see Chapter 36. Table 38-7 describes the causes, manifestations, ABG results, and treatments of acid–base imbalances. Use the following steps to interpret acid–base balance of blood.

> **Step 1: Examine the pH.** *Is it acidotic, alkalotic, or normal?*

- If the pH is low (<7.35), then the blood is *acidic*.
- If the pH is high (>7.45), then it is *alkalotic*.
- If the pH is between 7.35 and 7.45, then it is *normal*

Key Point: *Don't forget that the neutral pH is 7.4, which will be very important when we discuss compensation.*

> **Step 2: Check the amount of carbon dioxide in the blood (P_{CO_2}).** *Is there too little or too much?*

- If P_{CO_2} is <35 mm Hg, that means there is too little acid in the blood (respiratory alkalosis).
- If P_{CO_2} is >45 mm Hg, then there too much acid in the blood (respiratory acidosis).
- If P_{CO_2} is 35 to 45 mm Hg, then the cause for the abnormal pH is not respiratory.

> **Step 3: Think about the bicarbonate level (HCO_3).** *Is there too little or too much?*

- If HCO_3 is <22 mEq/L, that means there is too little base in the blood (metabolic acidosis).
- If HCO_3 is >26 mEq/L, then there too much base in the blood (metabolic alkalosis).
- If HCO_3 is 22 to 26 mEq/L, then the cause for the abnormal pH is not metabolic.

Table 38-6 ➤ Using ABGs To Assess Acid–Base Balance

EXPLANATION OF CHANGES	ABG COMPONENT	NORMAL RANGE	ACIDOSIS	ALKALOSIS
Indicates acidosis, alkalosis, or normal acid–base balance	pH	7.35–7.45 (7.4 is "neutral")	Low	High
Carbon dioxide ("acid"). Signals respiratory cause	P_{CO_2}	35–45 mm Hg	High	Low
Sodium bicarbonate ("base"). Signals metabolic cause	HCO_3^-	22–26 mEq/L	Low	High

Table 38-7 ➤ Acid–Base Imbalances

DISORDER	CLINICAL MANIFESTATIONS	INTERVENTIONS
Respiratory Acidosis May be caused by conditions or medications that impair gas exchange at the alveolar–capillary membrane, depressed respiratory rate and depth, or injury to the respiratory center in the brain.	*Acute:* Increased pulse and respiratory rate Headache, dizziness Confusion, decreased level of consciousness (LOC) Muscle twitching *Chronic:* Weakness Headache	Provide pulmonary hygiene. Institute measures to improve gas exchange, such as chest physiotherapy, bronchodilators, antibiotics possible. Provide supplemental oxygen. Maintain hydration.
Respiratory Alkalosis May be caused by hyperventilation resulting from anxiety, fever, sepsis, thyrotoxicosis, lesion in the respiratory center in the brain, or excessive ventilation with a mechanical ventilator.	Confusion, difficulty focusing Headache Tingling Palpitations Tremors	If caused by anxiety, encourage the patient to relax and breathe slowly. For other causes: Identify and treat the underlying disorder.
Metabolic Acidosis May be caused by retained acids in the blood resulting from renal impairment, poorly controlled diabetes mellitus, or starvation. Conditions that decrease bicarbonate, such as excessive GI loss, will also trigger metabolic acidosis. May be caused by excessive intake of acids, which may occur with aspirin poisoning, or by prolonged infusion of chloride-containing IV fluids.	Headache Confusion, drowsiness Weakness Peripheral vasodilatation Nausea and vomiting Kussmaul's breathing (rapid and deep) Frequently associated with hyperkalemia	Treatment is directed at correcting the underlying problem. Bicarbonate may be ordered.
Metabolic Alkalosis May be caused by excessive acid loss due to vomiting or gastric suction, use of potassium-wasting diuretics, hypokalemia, excess bicarbonate intake, or hyperaldosteronism.	Dizziness Tingling of extremities Hypertonic muscles Decreased respiratory rate and depth	Treatment is directed at correcting the underlying problem. Treatment often includes administration of NaCl-rich fluids.

UNCOMPENSATED ABG	pH	PaCO₂	HCO₃
Respiratory Acidosis	↓	↑	normal
Respiratory Alkalosis	↑	↓	normal
Metabolic Acidosis	↓	normal	↓
Metabolic Alkalosis	↑	normal	↑

> **Step 4: Is there compensation?** *If so, is it partially or fully?*

Now let's look at what happens when the acid–base imbalance continues for a period of time.

Key Point: *The body will naturally try to correct the unhealthy situation by using the lungs and kidneys to buffer the abnormality and return the pH into a normal range. If breathing is the reason for the abnormal pH, then the kidneys will pick up the slack and try to improve the situation. But if the problem is metabolic, then breathing (either faster and deeper or slower and more shallow) is the answer.*

- **No compensation.** If the pH is abnormal, no compensation has occurred. The following example shows low pH levels and high levels of carbon dioxide. This is respiratory acidosis with no compensation.

    pH = 7.30, PCO_2 = 50 mm Hg, HCO$_3^-$ = 24 mEq/L

- **Partial compensation.** Again, the pH will be abnormal unless it is fully compensated. If the *pH and one ABG component are abnormal*, with the second ABG value starting to change and the pH beginning to move toward normal, partial compensation is taking place. Compare the uncompensated blood gas (above) with the partially compensated blood gas below. Although below, the pH is increasing, it is still acidotic, while the PCO_2 remains high. Note that the HCO₃ is increasing to alkalosis to bring the pH closer to normal. This is partially compensated respiratory acidosis. In this same respiratory acidosis example the pH and PCO_2 are still abnormal in the ABG below. However, the HCO₃ has also become abnormal (high) and is pulling the pH toward normal. This example is *partially compensated respiratory acidosis.*

    pH = 7.32, PCO_2 = 50 mm Hg, HCO$_3^-$ = 28 mEq/L

PARTIAL COMPENSATION	pH	Paco₂	HCO₃
Respiratory Acidosis	↓	↑	↑
Respiratory Alkalosis	↑	↓	↓
Metabolic Acidosis	↓	↓	↓
Metabolic Alkalosis	↑	↑	↑

- **Full compensation.** Full compensation occurs when the *pH returns to normal range* and both other ABG components are abnormal. The initial causal component is still abnormal, and the second ABG component (that had the normal values) has changed enough to return the pH to normal. Note in the blood gas below, the pH is now in the normal range and the PCO_2 is still high. But the HCO₃ is now also high; it has moved enough to raise the pH into the normal range. The problem is now *fully compensated respiratory acidosis.*

    pH = 7.35, PCO_2 = 50 mm Hg, HCO$_3^-$ = 30 mEq/L

FULL COMPENSATION	pH	PaCO₂	HCO₃
Respiratory Acidosis	Normal, but <7.35	↑	↑
Respiratory Alkalosis	Normal, but >7.35	↓	↓
Metabolic Acidosis	Normal, but <7.35	↓	↓
Metabolic Alkalosis	Normal, but >7.35	↑	↑

KnowledgeCheck 38-6

Interpret the following ABG results:

pH = 7.53	PCO_2 = 26 mm Hg	HCO$_3^-$ = 22 mEq/L
pH = 7.40	PCO_2 = 39 mm Hg	HCO$_3^-$ = 25 mEq/L
pH = 7.30	PCO_2 = 70 mm Hg	HCO$_3^-$ = 30 mEq/L
pH = 7.48	PCO_2 = 46 mm Hg	HCO$_3^-$ = 30 mEq/L

PracticalKnowledge knowing **how**

In the remainder of this chapter, you will learn to apply theoretical knowledge of fluids, electrolytes, and acid–base balance to patient care.

ASSESSMENT

The purposes of a focused assessment of fluids, electrolytes, and acid–base status are to identify clients at risk for or already experiencing imbalances, to identify the nature of the disorder, and to evaluate responses to treatments.

Assessing for Example Problem: Fluids, Electrolytes, and Acid–Base Imbalances

Assessment for fluid, electrolyte, and acid–base imbalances includes collecting a focused nursing history, performing a physical assessment, and reviewing pertinent

PICOT

Early Treatment of Metabolic Acidosis

Situation: Several family members are being seen in the emergency department for suspected food poisoning. The grandfather, who has chronic kidney disease (CKD), is diagnosed with metabolic acidosis and admitted for treatment. The nurse wonders about the rationale for the treatments the patient receives.

PICOT Components:

P Population/client = Patients with CKD

I Intervention/indicator = Early metabolic acidosis treatment

C Comparator/control = Late or no treatment for metabolic acidosis

O Outcome = Reduced muscle wasting

T Time = The course of the disease

Searchable Question: Do _____(P) who receive/are exposed to _____(I), as compared to _____(C), demonstrate _____(O) during _____(T)?

Example of Evidence: The kidneys regulate fluid, electrolyte, and acid–base homeostasis. When these balances are altered, a client with CKD commonly develops chronic metabolic acidosis. This can lead to acceleration of the CKD, muscle wasting, development of bone disease, resistance to insulin, and increased mortality. Metabolic acidosis can be treated early in renal disease, with oral medications or the addition of bases to dialysate. This helps maintain a normal plasma bicarbonate level and prevent chronic CKD.

Practice Change: The nurse acquired new knowledge of the importance of early treatment of CKD and its potential for preventing muscle wasting and other CKD complications.

Source: Kraut, J., & Madias, N. (2011). Consequences and therapy of the metabolic acidosis of chronic kidney disease. *Pediatric Nephrology, 26*(1), 19–28.

laboratory tests. The purpose of the focused assessment is to identify clients at risk for or already experiencing imbalances, to identify the nature of the disorder, and to evaluate responses to treatments.

Focused Nursing History

A focused nursing history for fluids, electrolytes, and acid–base balance includes questions about demographic data, past medical history, current health concerns, food and fluid intake, fluid elimination, medications, and lifestyle. For questions to use in obtaining this focused nursing history,

 Go to Chapter 38, **Assessment Guidelines and Tools, Focused Assessment for Fluid, Electrolyte, and Acid–Base Balance, Nursing History,** in Volume 2.

Focused Physical Assessment

Correlate physical assessment data with the nursing history and laboratory studies. You will need to assess the following:

■ *Skin.* Assess for color, temperature, moisture content, continuity, turgor, and edema. To describe edema, see Chapter 22, Procedure 22-2, Assessing the Skin.
■ *Mucous membranes.* Inspect the tongue and buccal mucosa; assess the color, moisture, and continuity of the mucous membranes. Also assess tongue turgor in all age groups, since it is not affected by age.
■ *Cardiovascular system.* Pulse and blood pressure are affected by fluid and electrolyte status. Also assess for orthostatic hypotension, capillary refill, jugular venous distension, and peripheral edema.
■ *Respiratory system.* Assess respiratory rate, depth, and pattern, and breath sounds.
■ *Neurological system.* As described in Tables 38-5 and 38-7, neurological status (e.g., level of consciousness) provides cues to fluid, electrolyte, and acid–base imbalance.

In addition to the above assessments, you will track vital sign changes, monitor daily weights, and record intake and output. These are independent nursing assessments. They do not require a medical prescription. You may delegate these tasks to assistive personnel, but you remain responsible for evaluating the data. For complete guidelines for focused physical assessments and clinical observations,

 Go to Chapter 38, **Assessment Guidelines and Tools, Focused Assessment for Fluid, Electrolyte, and Acid–base Balance, Physical Assessments,** in Volume 2.

Vital Signs

All of the vital signs reflect information about fluid, electrolyte, and acid–base balance. These effects are briefly summarized below.

■ *Temperature.* An elevated body temperature increases the loss of body fluids. In hypernatremia, body temperature rises because the fluid available for sweating decreases. In uncomplicated fluid volume deficit, body temperature decreases.
■ *Pulse.* Tachycardia is an early sign of fluid volume deficit. Dysrhythmias can result from potassium, calcium, and magnesium imbalances. Fluid status directly affects the pulse volume: As fluid volume increases, the pulse volume also increases; similarly, a drop in fluid volume leads to a drop in pulse volume.
■ *Respiratory rate.* Alterations in respiratory rate may cause acid–base imbalances or be associated with compensation for a metabolic disorder.
■ *Blood pressure.* Blood pressure rises and falls with fluid volume. Postural hypotension occurs with dehydration. Blood pressure is also affected by electrolytes.

High sodium intake is a factor in hypertension, whereas high potassium and magnesium intake may lower blood pressure.

Daily Weights

Monitoring daily weight change is an accurate method of assessing fluid status. Weight changes over time are usually related to diet and exercise. In contrast, short-term changes usually indicate changes in fluid status. Each kilogram (2.2 lb) of weight is equivalent to 1 liter (1,000 mL) of fluid. Thus, in a client with diarrhea, a sudden drop in weight of 5 pounds is equivalent to a fluid loss of almost 2,300 mL.

Key Point: *For weight to accurately reflect fluid status, you must use the same balanced scale each time. Weigh the client at the same time each day, making sure that he is wearing the same amount of clothing.*

Clients undergoing hemodialysis (blood cleansing through an artificial kidney) are usually weighed before and after dialysis treatments. Many lose 3 to 4 kg (6.6 to 8.8 lb) over the course of several hours of dialysis. As a result, hypotension, tachycardia, and feelings of lightheadedness are common after a dialysis treatment.

Weight monitoring is especially valuable data when it is impractical or impossible to measure intake and output. For example, it is not easy to know for sure how much fluid a breastfed infant receives with each feeding nor how much fluid is lost in urine and stools. Incontinence, draining wounds, and limited resources may also make it difficult to monitor intake and output. Weight monitoring is a practical solution that may be initiated as a nursing order.

Fluid Intake and Output

Intake and output (I&O) are monitored to assess fluid status. I&O are usually tallied at the end of each shift, as well as for each 24-hour period. In intensive care units, I&O are measured at least hourly. To monitor I&O, measure all fluids the client consumes or excretes. You must correlate I&O with daily weights to accurately determine overall fluid status (Ladeserto, Chohan, Kasa, et al., 2009; Shepherd, 2011).

- **Output.** Fluid output includes urine, liquid stools, emesis, gastrointestinal fluids (e.g., from suction devices), and drainage (e.g., from wounds and pressure ulcers). Output also includes insensible losses through perspiration and respiration, but these are not usually measured. For more information about I&O, refer to the section Measuring Intake and Output in Chapter 28. For procedure steps,

 Go to Chapter 28, **Procedure 28-1: Measuring Urine,** in Volume 2.

- **Intake.** Measuring fluid intake includes a variety of sources (e.g., oral fluids, semiliquid foods, ice chips, parenteral fluids, enteral feedings, and irrigations

instilled and not withdrawn immediately). For more information about measuring intake,

 Go to Chapter 38, **Clinical Insight 38-2: Guidelines for Measuring Intake and Output (I&O),** in Volume 2.

Most healthcare facilities have standardized I&O forms for recording at the bedside and as a permanent part of the patient record (either paper or electronic). To see an electronic I&O record, see Figure 18-2 in Chapter 18. For an example of a paper I&O flow sheet,

 Go to Chapter 18, **Charting Forms: Intake and Output Sheet,** in Volume 2.

KnowledgeCheck 38-7

- Identify 10 physical assessment components that can be used to monitor fluid, electrolyte, and acid–base balance.
- What aspects should be evaluated in a nursing history focused on fluid, electrolyte, and acid–base balance?

ThinkLike a Nurse 38-5

What vital sign changes would you expect to find when assessing Jackson LaGuardia (Meet Your Patients)?

Laboratory Studies

Several laboratory tests are performed to evaluate fluid, electrolyte, and acid–base status.

Complete Blood Count Fluid status is reflected in a **complete blood count (CBC)**, which is a measure of red blood cells (RBCs), white blood cells (WBCs), and platelets. Included in the CBC is the hematocrit, a measure of the percentage of RBCs in whole blood. As fluid levels decrease, the percentage of blood made up by cells increases, and the hematocrit rises. Conversely, as fluid levels increase, the hematocrit falls.

Serum Electrolytes Venous blood samples are taken commonly to measure sodium, potassium, chloride, and bicarbonate levels. In many labs, a basic metabolic panel also includes calcium, BUN/creatinine ratio and glucose. BUN and creatinine are sensitive measures of fluid status and kidney function. Physical assessment can also reveal hypocalcemia; for information,

 Go to **Clinical Insight 38-1: Assessing for Trousseau's and Chvostek's Signs,** in Volume 2.

Serum Osmolality A measure of the solute concentration of the blood is **serum osmolality**. It is expressed as milliosmoles per kilogram (mOsm/kg). Sodium is the greatest determinant of serum osmolality. Glucose and urea also contribute to serum osmolality. Serum osmolality may be directly measured with venous blood or estimated by doubling the serum sodium level. A rise in serum osmolality indicates fluid volume deficit; a decrease indicates fluid volume excess. Changes in serum osmolality usually indicate alterations in sodium levels.

Urine Osmolality The solute concentration of urine is measured by **urine osmolality**. The body excretes nitrogenous wastes as well as electrolytes. As a result, urine osmolality is substantially higher than serum levels. Fluid volume deficit increases urine osmolality; fluid volume excess decreases urine osmolality. This test may call for a 24-hour urine specimen, or for discarding the first morning specimen and collecting a clean-catch specimen 2 hours later.

Urinalysis The routine screening test **urinalysis** includes a measure of urine pH and specific gravity. Urine pH normally ranges from 5.0 to 9.0, with an average of 6.0.

- *pH.* Urine becomes more acidic in respiratory or metabolic acidosis, starvation, or fluid volume deficit. Alkaline urine is associated with an alkaline state in the blood.
- *Specific gravity.* Specific gravity rises and falls in opposition to fluid status. A normal range is 1.001 to 1.029. A low specific gravity occurs when fluid is plentiful. When fluid levels decrease, urine becomes more concentrated, and specific gravity increases. For a procedure for testing specific gravity of urine,

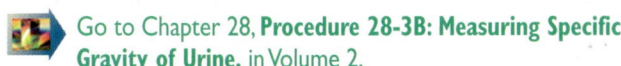
Go to Chapter 28, **Procedure 28-3B: Measuring Specific Gravity of Urine,** in Volume 2.

- ABGs. Interpretation of ABGs was discussed earlier in this chapter. For a list of these values, along with other lab studies discussed earlier,

Go to Chapter 38, **Diagnostic Testing: Assessing Fluid, Electrolyte, and Acid–Base Balance,** in Volume 2.

ANALYSIS/NURSING DIAGNOSIS

Nursing diagnoses directly related to fluid, electrolyte, and acid–base balance include: Deficient Fluid Volume, Excess Fluid Volume, Readiness for Enhanced Fluid Volume, Risk for Deficient Fluid Volume, Risk for Electrolyte Imbalance, Risk for Imbalanced Fluid Volume, and Risk for Vascular Trauma. For other defining characteristics and etiologies of these NANDA International (NANDA-I) diagnoses,

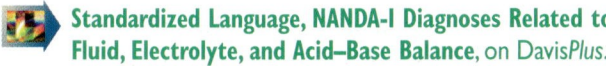
Standardized Language, NANDA-I Diagnoses Related to Fluid, Electrolyte, and Acid–Base Balance, on DavisPlus.

Diagnoses for Example Problem: Fluid, Electrolyte, and Acid–Base Imbalances

Impaired Gas Exchange is appropriate for a client with a disorder affecting gas exchange at the alveolar–capillary membrane in the lungs (see Chapter 36). This condition limits the effectiveness of the carbonic acid–bicarbonate buffer system and alters serum pH, predisposing the patient to acid–base imbalances.

Fluid, electrolyte, acid–base imbalances (e.g., dehydration, metabolic acidosis, respiratory alkalosis), and treatment imbalances may be etiologies of other nursing diagnoses. Below are a few examples:

- Activity Intolerance related to excess fluid and electrolyte loss through Diarrhea
- Impaired Oral Mucous Membrane related to Deficient Fluid Volume
- Decreased Cardiac Output related to Hypovolemia
- Risk for Vascular Trauma (from insertion of an IV catheter)

PLANNING OUTCOMES/EVALUATION

The overall goal for a client experiencing fluid, electrolytes, or acid–base imbalance is to restore balance.

Outcomes for Example Problem: Fluids, Electrolytes, and Acid–Base Imbalances

NOC standardized outcomes for describing fluid and electrolyte status include: Electrolyte & Acid/Base Balance, Fluid Balance, Fluid Overload Severity, and Hydration. For selected indicators for these outcomes,

Go to Chapter 38, **Standardized Language, Selected NOC Outcomes and NIC Interventions for Fluid and Electrolyte Problems,** on DavisPlus.

Individualized goals/outcome statements you might write for a client include the following examples:

- Maintains fluid balance, as evidenced by balanced 24-hour intake and output; good skin and tongue turgor; blood pressure and heart rate within normal limits; and no adventitious breath sounds.
- Electrolyte balance restored, as evidenced by alertness and cognitive orientation and no muscle cramping, seizures, or electrocardiogram changes.
- Drinks at least 2,500 mL in 24 hours.
- Urine specific gravity within normal limits.

PLANNING INTERVENTIONS/IMPLEMENTATION

The following sections describe nursing interventions and activities for preventing and treating fluid, electrolyte, and acid–base problems.

Interventions for Example Problem: Fluid, Electrolyte, and Acid–Base Imbalances

NIC standardized interventions related to fluid, electrolyte, and acid–base balance include Acid–Base Management, Electrolyte Management, and Fluid Management. For a listing of other interventions,

Go to Chapter 38, **Standardized Language, Selected NOC Outcomes and NIC Interventions for Fluid and Electrolyte Problems,** on Davis*Plus*.

Individualized interventions are aimed at correcting the underlying disorder that led to imbalance. Nursing care focuses on preventing imbalances, modifying oral intake, providing parenteral fluids, and transfusing blood products, all of which are discussed in the rest of this chapter.

Preventing Fluid and Electrolyte Imbalances

It is better to prevent imbalances than to treat them. Use the data obtained from your assessment to plan how to help your client avoid imbalances. Common strategies are listed in the accompanying Self-Care box Teaching Patients to Prevent Fluid and Electrolyte Imbalances.

Dietary Changes

To promote fluid and electrolyte balance, most people need to limit their sodium intake and increase their intake of dietary potassium and calcium. Some may need oral electrolytes supplements as well (see the Self-Care box Taking Oral Electrolyte Supplements). As previously discussed, most North Americans consume more sodium than they should and not enough potassium and calcium. Teach clients to eat foods rich in potassium and calcium every day and to avoid sodium-rich foods (e.g., processed foods) (see Chapter 27 to review foods, as needed). For example, instruct clients to read food labels, particularly when trying to limit sodium intake.

Self-Care

Teaching Patients to Prevent Fluid and Electrolyte Imbalances

➤ Teach the client about usual fluid needs and circumstances that increase fluid needs, such as high environmental temperature, fever, gastrointestinal (GI) fluid loss, or draining wounds. Base your teaching on the client's current intake and the changes required to meet fluid goals.

➤ Identify medications or conditions that place the client at risk for imbalances. For example, if the client is receiving a potassium-wasting diuretic, she will need to increase potassium intake, either by taking a supplement or by altering the diet.

Also teach clients to do the following:

➤ Drink at least eight to ten 8-ounce glasses of water per day unless your healthcare provider has told you to limit fluids.

➤ Healthy adults use thirst as a guide to fluid intake. However, adults older than age 50 may have diminished thirst sensation and cannot depend solely on thirst for fluid replacement.

➤ Colorless urine is also a guide to adequate hydration, whereas darker urine is associated with dehydration. You can also use a urine color chart to monitor hydration.

➤ Limit consumption of fluids high in salt, sugar, caffeine, or alcohol.

➤ Vigorous exercise may delay the thirst mechanism. Athletes should become accustomed to consuming fluids at regular intervals during training sessions and competition so that they do not experience dehydration.

➤ Drink water before, during, and after strenuous exercise.

➤ Avoid routine use of laxatives, antacids, weight-loss products, or enemas. These products may cause imbalances of fluids and electrolytes such as sodium and potassium.

➤ Weigh yourself daily if fluid balance is critical or if you are experiencing excessive loss or gain.

➤ Contact a health professional if there is a sudden change of weight, decreased urine output, swelling in dependent areas (e.g., hands and feet), shortness of breath, or dizziness.

➤ Contact a healthcare provider if you experience prolonged vomiting, diarrhea, or inability to tolerate liquids or food.

➤ Eat a well-balanced diet, including dairy products rich in calcium.

Self-Care

Taking Oral Electrolyte Supplements

➤ Encourage clients to take potassium supplements with juice to mask the taste.

➤ Teach clients to take supplements as prescribed to maintain electrolyte balance.

➤ Remind clients that supplements are medications and should be viewed as part of the treatment plan.

➤ If the client's medications are altered, review the continued need for supplements.

➤ Caution clients that salt substitutes contain potassium. If the client has been advised to use salt substitutes, evaluate the need for potassium supplements.

➤ Encourage clients who take calcium supplements to consume at least 2,500 mL of fluid per day to avoid constipation and reduce the risk of kidney stone formation.

CHAPTER 38 Fluids, Electrolytes, & Acid–Base Balance 1003

Oral Electrolyte Supplements

Many clients are unable to correct electrolyte disturbances with dietary changes alone. This is especially true for clients who have food intolerances, who rely on prepared meals, or who live in group settings. Such clients may need oral supplements to meet their dietary requirements. Potassium and calcium are among the most common supplements.

 Most adults, especially older adults, consume less dietary calcium per day than the 1,200 mg recommended amount. This further increases their risk for osteoporosis and fractures.

Calcium supplements come in many forms, including tablet, liquid, and chewable form. Potassium supplements are available in pill and liquid form. Many have an unpleasant taste. See the Self-Care box Taking Oral Electrolyte Supplements for suggested nursing activities to help improve your client's compliance.

KnowledgeCheck 38-8

- Identify laboratory tests that monitor fluid, electrolyte, and acid–base balance.
- Give at least five strategies to prevent fluid and electrolyte imbalance.

Modifying Oral Fluid Intake

Clients experiencing fluid imbalances may need to restrict or increase their daily oral intake to correct the underlying disorder.

Facilitating Fluid Intake

Clients with actual or potential fluid volume deficit may need to increase their fluid intake. Whenever possible, clients should take fluids by mouth. You may provide replacement through a nasogastric or feeding tube if the client is unable to meet his needs independently, but can tolerate fluids in the gastrointestinal tract. Parenteral fluid replacement is used only when enteral replacement cannot meet the client's fluid needs (for review, see Chapter 27).

To increase fluid intake successfully, you must first establish the desired amount of fluid intake for the client. The daily fluid goal reflects the client's current fluid balance and underlying condition. For example, if a client is dehydrated, an order might read: "Force fluids: 2,500 mL oral fluids per 24 hours." You can develop a plan to increase fluids from this order. Typically people drink more fluid during the day and early evening, when they are more likely to be active. A large volume of fluid late in the evening may interrupt sleep because it may prompt the need to urinate. Therefore, you should distribute fluids to reflect the time of day, for example:

0700 to 1500—1,300 mL
1500 to 2300—1,000 mL
2300 to 0700—200 mL

Strategies to increase fluid intake include the following:

- Assess the client's fluid preferences.
- Offer a variety of fluids throughout the day on a regular schedule. Vary hot and cold liquids, and offer a choice of juices and other drinks.
- Instruct nursing assistive personnel to make "fluids rounds" to offer and help with oral fluids.
- Each time you are at the bedside, remind the patient to drink.
- Break daily goals into hourly amounts. For example, in the preceding example, in the 8 hours between 0700 and 1500 have the patient drink 150 mL of fluid every hour. Give him a written schedule.
- Provide a glass or cup with milliliter markings on it so that the patient will know how much he is drinking.
- Always have fluid readily available to the patient. For example, keep a pitcher of water at the bedside.
- When possible, have the patient and family members participate in offering fluids and tracking fluid intake.
- Schedule diagnostic and surgical procedures to minimize the length of time the patient must be NPO.
- For ambulatory patients (e.g., residents in long-term care facilities) schedule "tea time" or "happy hour" to promote increased intake.

Facilitating Fluid Restriction

Patients may need to limit fluids for a variety of reasons (e.g., cardiovascular, liver, or renal impairment). To facilitate fluid restrictions effectively, teach patients and caregivers the reason for the restriction and the amount of fluid allowed. Typically, fluid volume is divided into amounts allotted per shift. However, fluid restrictions usually include *all* forms of intake, not only oral. For example, a prescription might read: "Limit total fluid intake to 1,500 mL per 24 hours." If the patient is receiving IV antibiotics four times per day, you must include that volume as a part of the total fluids. If 75 mL is infused with each administration, total IV fluids equal 300 mL. So, the oral intake must be limited to 1,200 mL per day. This amount may be distributed as 700 mL on the day shift, 400 mL on the evening shift, and 100 mL at night. Strategies to restrict fluid intake include the following:

- Do not offer liquids with meals. Reserve liquids for between meals.
- Limit intake of foods that increase thirst (e.g., dry, salty, or spicy foods).
- Offer ice chips to help quench thirst.
- Provide frequent oral hygiene.
- Keep liquids away from the bedside.
- Provide diversional activities for the patient.

Parenteral Replacement of Fluids and Electrolytes

When fluid loss is severe or the client cannot tolerate oral or tube feedings, fluid volume is replaced parenterally. The word *parenteral* refers to any route other than through the alimentary canal (passage from the mouth to the anus). **Intravenous (IV) therapy** is the administration of fluids, electrolytes, medications, or nutrients by the venous route. IV fluids are used to:

- Expand intravascular volume.
- Correct an underlying imbalance in fluids or electrolytes.
- Compensate for an ongoing problem that is affecting either fluid or electrolytes.

For instance, Martha LaGuardia (Meet Your Patients) is being treated in the emergency department (ED) for gastroenteritis. She is experiencing fluid loss from vomiting and diarrhea, complicated by her use of a diuretic. IV therapy will allow her to receive fluid to expand her intravascular volume and to maintain her hydration until the vomiting and diarrhea subside. It will also provide electrolyte replacement based on her laboratory results. Mrs. LaGuardia will continue to receive IV fluids until she can meet her fluid and electrolyte needs orally. All of the members of the LaGuardia family are experiencing fluid losses and would benefit from increasing their fluid intake. When fluid balance is fragile, or when the client cannot tolerate oral fluids, replacement may be supervised in an inpatient setting.

When initiating and maintaining intravenous infusions, always use careful aseptic technique. Remember that the IV catheter provides a portal of entry for pathogens directly into the bloodstream. You should know that Medicare will not reimburse a hospital for the expenses (e.g., antibiotics, extra hospital days) caused by catheter-related infections that occur during hospitalization. Excellent nursing technique can reduce IV catheter-associated infections.

Types of Intravenous Solutions

Solutions, including IV fluids, are classified according to how they compare to the osmolality of blood serum: IV fluids are classified as isotonic, hypotonic, and hypertonic solutions (Crawford & Harris, 2011b). To help you remember, here is a somewhat oversimplified summary. When infused:

- *Isotonic* fluids remain *in* the intravascular compartment.
- *Hypotonic* fluids pull body water *out* of the intravascular compartment.
- *Hypertonic* fluids pull body water *into* the intravascular compartment.

Isotonic Fluids Normal blood serum osmolality is 275 to 295 mOsm/kg. Isotonic solutions have similar tonicity (250 to 375 mOsm/L). Therefore, when infused, they remain inside the blood vessels. As a result, isotonic fluids are useful for clients with hypotension or hypovolemia. Commonly prescribed isotonic fluids are the following:

- 0.9% sodium chloride (0.9% NaCl), also called *normal saline (NS)*
- Lactated Ringer's (LR)

The solution, 5% dextrose in water (D_5W) may be classified as both isotonic and hypotonic. It is isotonic in the bag, but is not prescribed for isotonic use because after (rapid) metabolism, it is hypotonic in the body.

Clients who have congestive heart failure (CHF) must be closely monitored when they receive isotonic fluid replacement, because they may easily develop fluid overload.

Hypotonic Fluids The osmolality of a hypotonic solution is less than that of serum (less than 250 mOsm/L). Therefore, when infused, these solutions pull body water from the intravascular compartment into the interstitial fluid compartment. As the interstitial fluid is diluted, its osmolarity decreases, drawing water into the adjacent cells. Hypotonic fluid is used for hyperglycemic conditions, such as diabetic ketoacidosis, in which high serum glucose draws fluid out of the cells and into the vascular and interstitial compartments. Examples of hypotonic fluids include:

- 5% dextrose in water (D_5W). Recall that D_5W is isotonic in the bag, with an osmolality of 253 mOsm/L, but becomes hypotonic in the body.
- 0.45% NaCl (½ normal saline)
- 0.33% NaCl
- 0.2% NaCl

Administer hypotonic fluids carefully to prevent a sudden fluid shift from the intravascular space to the cells. Never give hypotonic solutions to patients at risk for increased intracranial pressure because they can cause or worsen cerebral edema.

Hypertonic Fluids The osmolality of hypertonic fluids is higher than that of serum. When administered, they pull fluids and electrolytes from the intracellular and interstitial compartments into the intravascular compartment. Hypertonic fluids can help stabilize blood pressure, increase urine output, and reduce edema. Volume expanders (e.g., dextran and serum albumin) are hypertonic, and used to increase blood volume following severe loss of blood or plasma, such as in major burns or hemorrhage. Following are examples of hypertonic fluids:

- D_5 0.9% NaCl (D_5 NS)
- D_5 0.45% NaCl (D_5 ½ NS)
- D_5 lactated Ringer's
- 3% NaCl and 5% NaCl—highly hypertonic; used only in critical situations.
- 10% dextrose in water ($D_{10}W$)
- $D_{20}W$—used as an osmotic diuretic to promote diuresis

For more information about these types of IV solutions,

Go to Chapter 38, **Supplemental Materials: Types of IV Fluids,** on Davis*Plus*.

Peripheral Vascular Access Devices

Intravenous therapy requires placement of a vascular access device (VAD). You will choose the type of device on the basis of the client's condition, type of fluid that will be infused, and the anticipated length of treatment.

Key Point: *IV catheters (and needles) are sized by their diameter, which is called the* **gauge**. *The smaller the diameter is, the larger the gauge will be (e.g., a 16-gauge catheter is larger than a 21-gauge catheter).*

Therefore, the smaller the gauge, the more rapidly fluid can be delivered. Various types of catheters are used to access peripheral veins, including the following:

Over-the-Needle Catheters These are also called **angiocaths**, short for angiocatheter (Fig. 38-7A). A polyurethane or Teflon catheter is threaded over a metal stylet (needle). You pierce the skin and vein with the needle, advance the catheter into the vein, and remove (or retract) the metal needle. In most cases, the plastic catheter is less than 7.5 cm (3 in.) in length. This type of access device is ideal for brief therapy. However, you cannot give highly irritating or hyperosmolar solutions through this type of catheter because it may cause severe damage to the vein. For an animated illustration of an over-the-needle IV catheter,

Go to **Animations: Insertion of an Over-the-Needle IV Catheter,** on Davis*Plus*.

Inside-the-Needle Catheters This type of catheter is similar to the over-the-needle catheter; however, the polyurethane or Teflon catheter lies inside the metal needle (Fig. 38-7B). After you advance the catheter into the vein, you withdraw the needle.

Butterfly Needle Also called a *scalp vein needle* or *wing-tipped catheter*, a **butterfly needle** is a short, beveled metal needle with flexible plastic flaps attached to the shaft (Fig. 38-8). You can pinch the flaps and hold them tightly together to facilitate insertion. After insertion, flatten them out and tape them against the skin to prevent dislodgement during the infusion process. These needles are commonly used for intermittent or short-term therapy for children and infants or for single-dose medications and drawing blood. Because the inflexible metal needle remains in the vein, a butterfly needle is more likely to **infiltrate** (damage the vein and allow fluid to leak into the interstitial spaces) than a flexible plastic catheter.

Midline Peripheral Catheter A **midline peripheral catheter** (midline VAD) is a peripherally inserted flexible IV catheter typically inserted into the antecubital fossa and then advanced into the larger vessels of the upper arm for greater hemodilution. It is 15 cm (6 in.) long, so it can be used for a longer period of time than a shorter, over-the-needle catheter—typically 1 to 4 weeks. A midline peripheral catheter should be changed only when there is a specific indicator (CDC, 2011a) (e.g., swelling, pain). A midline catheter is still considered a peripheral line, so you cannot administer highly osmolar and irritating solutions through it.

It is essential to distinguish a midline VAD from a peripherally placed central line (PICC). Because visual identification is not sufficient for identification, the type of VAD must be marked on the dressing label. If you are uncertain about the catheter type, consult the patient's health record.

In response to the Needlestick Safety and Prevention Act passed by Congress in 2000, the Occupational Safety and Health Administration (OSHA) requires the use of "needleless" systems (OSHA, 2011). Therefore, you will usually have available access devices with safety features to prevent accidental "sticks." But if you find you must use an older, nonsafety device, do not attempt to recap the needle after removing it from the vein.

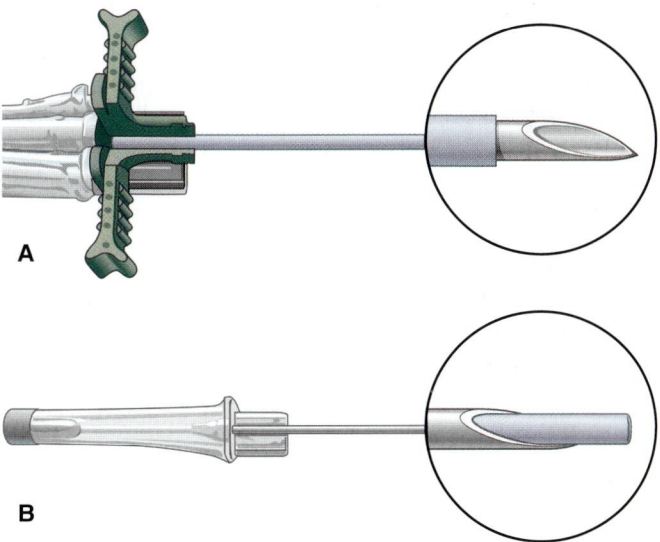

FIGURE 38-7 Typical IV access devices. *A,* An over-the-needle catheter. *B,* An inside-the-needle catheter.

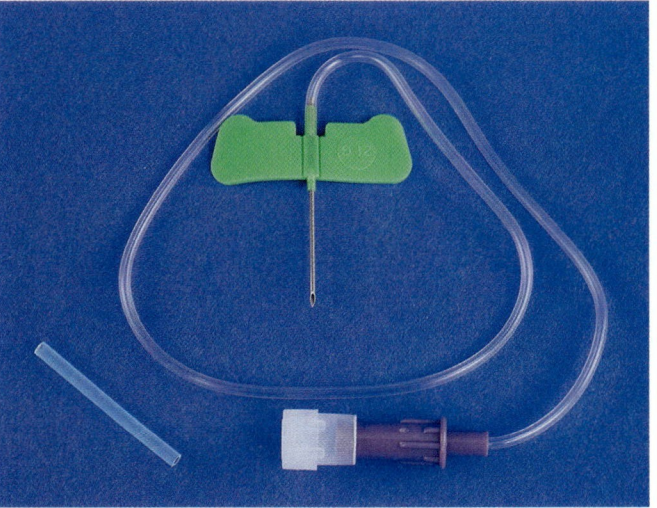

FIGURE 38-8 The butterfly, or scalp vein, needle is commonly used for intermittent or short-term therapy for children and infants.

Peripheral Intravenous Lock

A **peripheral intravenous lock** (also called a saline lock, a prn adapter, and sometimes a heparin lock) establishes a venous route as a precautionary measure for clients whose condition may change rapidly or who may require intermittent infusion therapy. A peripheral IV catheter or butterfly wing–tipped catheter is inserted into a vein, and cap the hub with a lock port (Fig. 38-9). Patency of the lock is maintained by injecting normal saline or a dilute heparin solution, depending on agency policy.

Central Venous Access Devices

A **central venous access device (CVAD)** is an intravenous line inserted into a major vein. Typically, the subclavian or internal jugular vein is used. Using surgical asepsis, a catheter is advanced from the insertion site into the superior vena cava. CVADs are used to administer large volumes of fluid or highly irritating medications, when peripheral sites are unavailable, for monitoring central venous pressure, and for frequent blood draws. You will likely care for patients with central lines, and you may need to assist with inserting them. To learn how to care for patients with central lines, see the Highlights of Procedures box for a summary, and

 Go to Chapter 38, **Clinical Insight 38-4: Caring for Patients With a Central Venous Access Device, Procedure 38-5B: Central Line Dressings,** and **Procedure 38-9: Assisting With Percutaneous Central Venous Catheter Placement,** in Volume 2.

Advantages of Central Lines A central line offers several advantages:

- A central vein can accommodate highly irritating and hyperosmolar solutions because the blood and solution mix rapidly at the infusion site.

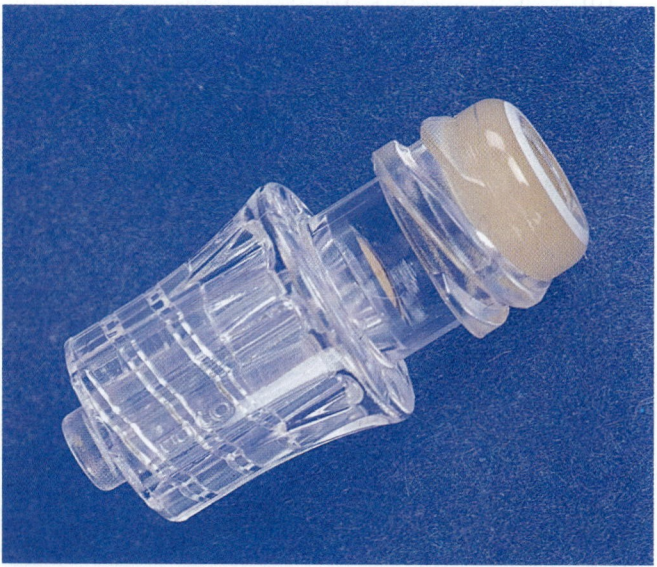

FIGURE 38-9 A peripheral intravenous lock establishes a venous route as a precautionary measure for clients whose condition may change rapidly or who may require intermittent infusion therapy.

- Central veins are accessible even if the patient is experiencing severe fluid depletion.
- Some types of central lines may also be used to monitor central venous pressure.
- Central lines can be left in longer than peripheral IVs, ranging from a week to long term, depending on the type of central line used.
- Nutrition can be given parenterally.
- Phlebitis, extravasation, and infiltration are less likely to occur with central lines.
- Central lines with extra ports allow you to withdraw blood from a port to use for laboratory tests.

Disadvantages of Central Lines Drawbacks to central lines include:

- Practitioners must have specialized training to insert the catheter.
- You must obtain patient consent.
- Placement must be confirmed by radiography.
- Placement is treated as a minor surgical procedure, requiring strict sterility.
- Dressing changes require strict sterile technique.
- When placed via the neck, especially though the subclavian vein, there is a risk of pneumothorax.
- There is a risk that the catheter will float into the right side of the heart, where it may cause ventricular dysrhythmias.
- There is a greater risk of air embolus and infection when compared to peripheral IVs.
- Associated costs are greater than with peripheral lines.
- The risk for sepsis is much higher than for peripheral sites. CVCs account for about 90% of catheter-related bloodstream infections.

Preventing Central Line–Associated Bloodstream Infections This is one of The Joint Commission's national patient safety goals for 2013, and is likely to be a continuing goal.

Key Point: *To help prevent CVC catheter-related infections, The Joint Commission recommends the following set of measures:*

- **Education and training**—regarding proper infection control measures to prevent intravascular catheter-related infections. Encourage patients to report any changes or new discomfort in their catheter site.
- **Hand hygiene**—Wearing gloves does not make handwashing unnecessary.
- **Maximal barrier precautions for insertion**—Includes sterile drape for patient, hat, mask, and sterile gown and gloves.
- **Chlorhexidine skin antisepsis**—Use 2% chlorhexidine gluconate in 70% isopropyl alcohol to prep the insertion site.
- **Optimal catheter site selection**—The subclavian vein has the lowest rate of infection. The femoral vein should be avoided if possible.
- **Type of catheter**—To reduce the risk of catheter-related infection, the catheter with the fewest number of ports or lumens needed to manage the patient is best.

- **Daily review of lines**—The CVC should be removed as soon as it is no longer necessary. Risk of infection is closely related to the length of time the CVC is in place (Institute for Healthcare Improvement [IHI], 2012; O'Grady, Alexander, Burns, et al., 2011)

Types of Central Venous Catheters

There are four types of CVADs: peripherally inserted central catheters, nontunneled CVCs, tunneled CVCs, and implanted ports.

Peripherally Inserted Central Catheters (PICC lines)

PICCs are long, soft, flexible catheters inserted at the antecubital fossa through the basilic or cephalic vein of the arm. The catheter is then advanced into the superior vena cava (Fig. 38-10). A physician or specially trained registered nurse performs the insertion. PICC lines are most commonly used for prolonged IV antibiotic therapy, parenteral nutrition, and chemotherapy. A PICC line is intended for intermediate to long-term use and does not need to be replaced unless the site appears infected or the catheter is no longer patent.

Nontunneled Central Venous Catheters

Nontunneled CVCs are inserted by a physician, specially trained nurse practitioner, or physician assistant through the skin into the jugular, subclavian, and, occasionally, femoral veins. They are sutured in place. Often these are referred to as single-, double-, triple-, or quadruple-lumen catheters, depending on the number of ports in the line (Fig. 38-11). These CVADs are intended for shorter use than a PICC line (less than 6 weeks); however, guidelines advise that nontunneled CVADs not be routinely replaced (CDC, 2011). They can be used to measure central venous pressure (CVP) to obtain information on blood volume. A low reading indicates hypovolemia and a high reading, hypervolemia.

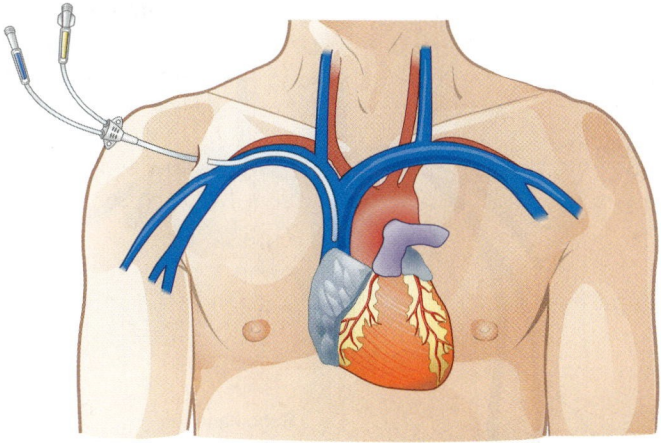

FIGURE 38-11 Nontunneled central venous catheters are inserted into the jugular, subclavian, and, occasionally, femoral veins.

Blood can also be drawn from a nontunneled CVAD for other diagnostic studies. However, if parenteral nutrition or blood is running in a port, you cannot use that same port for blood draws.

> *Example:* Imagine that you have a frail elderly patient who needs two different kinds of IV fluid, parenteral nutrition, and frequent blood draws for lab tests. This patient has fragile peripheral veins and is also at high risk for infection and other complications. With a multiple-lumen central catheter, the patient needs only one insertion site. You can run both fluids and the parenteral nutrition fluids, and still reserve one port for drawing blood. The patient has less risk for the catheter to become dislodged or infiltrate, or for phlebitis to develop.

Tunneled Central Venous Catheters

Tunneled CVCs are intended for long-term use. The catheter is inserted by a surgeon through a 7.5- to 15-cm (3- to 6-in.) subcutaneous tunnel in the chest wall and then into the jugular or subclavian vein (Fig. 38-12). The catheter can be sutured in place, with the sutures removed when fibrosis has developed around the catheter, or it can be secured with an IV securing device. Because CVCs are tunneled through the skin rather than through a vein, the risk of infection is less with their use than it is with PICCs or nontunneled central lines.

Implanted Ports

Implanted ports are devices made of a radiopaque silicone catheter and a plastic or stainless steel injection port with a self-sealing silicone-rubber septum. The catheter enters the internal jugular vein in the neck, and it may be tunneled or untunneled to a completely implanted subcutaneous reservoir (port) in the upper chest (Fig. 38-13). Implanted ports are placed by surgeons and only specially trained nurses are allowed to access an implanted port because of the risk of infiltration into the tissue if the needle placement is not correct. Implanted ports are intended for long-term use.

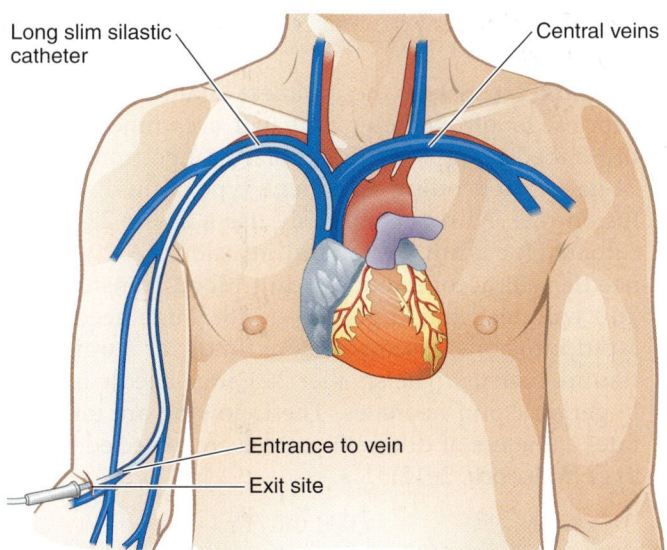

Long slim silastic catheter

Central veins

Entrance to vein

Exit site

FIGURE 38-10 A PICC line is a long, soft, flexible catheter inserted through a vein in the arm and threaded into a central vessel.

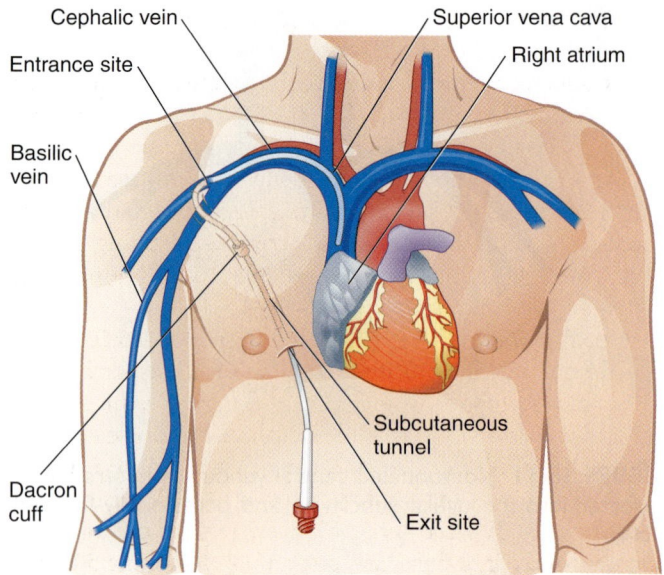

Cephalic vein
Superior vena cava
Right atrium
Entrance site
Basilic vein
Subcutaneous tunnel
Dacron cuff
Exit site

FIGURE 38-12 A tunneled central venous catheter is inserted through subcutaneous tissue in the chest wall into the jugular or subclavian vein.

 Avoid taking blood pressures or drawing blood in the extremity on the side of the chest where the implanted port has been placed.

The Highlights of Procedures box summarizes steps. For a procedure, for assisting with placement of a central venous catheter,

 Go to Chapter 38, **Procedure 38-9: Assisting With Percutaneous Central Venous Catheter Placement,** in Volume 2.

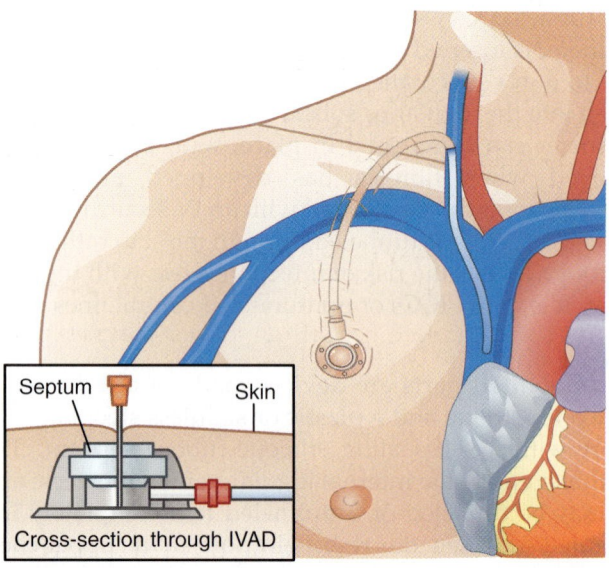

Septum   Skin

Cross-section through IVAD

FIGURE 38-13 An implanted venous access port (IVAD) is a CVAD that enters the internal jugular vein in the neck but is tunneled to a completely implanted subcutaneous reservoir (port) in the upper chest.

Intraosseous Devices

Designed for immediate access (within seconds) and short-term use (less than 24 hours), intraosseous (IO) access devices are used to administer fluids when a peripheral catheter cannot be inserted or when a central line insertion is not advisable, but especially in emergency situations. IOs are placed into the matrix of a bone. The venous sinusoids in the matrix can quickly absorb fluids to send to the central circulation. The most common access site is the proximal tibia in both children and adults. The sternum and the head of the humerus can also be used in adults. Osteomyelitis is a rare complication, occurring in fewer than 1% of cases. Contraindications for IO use include obesity, fracture, recent surgery, infection, or evidence of poor circulation at the proposed insertion site.

KnowledgeCheck 38-9

- What is the purpose of intravenous fluids?
- Describe the functions of the three types of IV solutions—isotonic, hypotonic, and hypertonic—and identify two commonly prescribed fluids in each category.
- Under what conditions would a central venous access device be preferable to a peripheral device?

ThinkLike a Nurse 38-6

What type of venous access device would you expect Martha LaGuardia (Meet Your Patients) to receive in the hospital? Why?

Starting an Intravenous Infusion

To start an IV infusion, you will need to gather equipment and supplies, set up the solution and administration set, select a venipuncture site, and perform venipuncture.

Obtain Equipment and Supplies

Venipuncture supplies and IV infusion equipment are sterile, prepackaged, and disposable. They vary based on manufacturers, so familiarize yourself with what is available in your facility. Set up the solution and administration set before performing the venipuncture.

- **IV Catheter.** Select the smallest diameter and the shortest length catheter that will accommodate the prescribed therapy. Catheter sizes range from 16- to 24-gauge, depending on patient, type of fluid, and infusion rate. Nurses commonly use a 20- or 22-gauge catheter for adult peripheral infusions. A 20-gauge needle will accommodate adult blood transfusions. You will need the larger 16- or 18-gauge needle for rapid infusions, viscous (thick) fluids, or surgical or trauma patients. The smaller 24-gauge needle is used in geriatric and neonates. The following are infusion rates catheters of different gauges are expected to deliver (Masoorli, 2012):

18 gauge	4,000 mL/hr
20 gauge	3,500 mL/hr
22 gauge	2,000 mL/hr
24 gauge	1,500 mL/hr

- *Administration Set (Infusion Kit).* The administration set connects the fluid container to the catheter inserted in the patient. The set consists of tubing with a plastic insertion spike, a drip chamber, a roller clamp to regulate the flow, an injection port, and a catheter adapter (hub) (Fig. 38-14). Both ends of the infusion set (the spike and the hub) are sterile and must remain sterile. You should remove the protective caps just before use and avoid touching the spike and hub when connecting the tubing to the solution container and the IV catheter in the patient's vein.

  The drip chamber is calibrated to allow a predictable amount of fluid to be delivered in each drop. The drop factor is indicated on the package. A roller clamp on the tubing controls the rate of flow.

  - A *macrodrip* delivers 10 to 20 drops per milliliter of solution, depending on the manufacturer; select a macrodrip for most adult infusions.

  - A *microdrip* delivers 60 drops per milliliter; use a microdrip for very slow infusion rates or for infants and children.

- *Extension Tubing and Filters.* The end of the IV tubing contains an adapter that attaches to the inserted sterile IV catheter. This should be a locking or screw-on connection, if one is available. You may use extension tubing to lengthen the primary tubing (e.g., for active patients) or to provide additional Y-injection ports for administration of multiple IV solutions or medications.

  Particulate matter may be generated when glass ampules are opened, or from additives or medications that have a tendency to clump. Occasionally, a filter will be used to remove particulate matter from the solution or to filter microorganisms. Some administration sets have built-in filters, or you may attach one to the end of the tubing. The finer the filter size is, the smaller the particles that are removed from the solution. Research on the use of IV filters to reduce the rate of phlebitis and bacteremia is inconclusive and at present, guidelines do not recommend using filters routinely for infection-control purposes (Niel-Neise, Stijnen, & van den Broek, 2010).

- *Injection Port.* Use the injection port to administer a secondary IV fluid or medication (see Chapter 26).

- *Solutions.* Inspect the solution container to be certain that it contains the desired fluid, the fluid is clear, the bag is intact, and the solution has not expired. Glass containers were the first containers for IV fluids, but today most IV fluids are packaged in plastic. Fluids for continuous infusions are packed in 1-liter or 500-mL bags. Smaller solution bags (50 mL, 100 mL, and 250 mL) are used for intermittent infusions, such as antibiotics or other medications. Plastic containers collapse as fluid infuses, so you can use a nonvented administration set. Glass bottles do not collapse and therefore require a vented administration set.

Select a Peripheral Intravenous Site

To select a venipuncture site, consider the following factors:

- *Age.* For adults, you will usually use veins in the hand or arm (Fig. 38-15); for infants, veins in the scalp or dorsum of the foot.

- *Type of solution.* For hypertonic solutions, viscous solutions, or irritating medications, use a large vein to cause the least amount of trauma.

- *Speed of infusion.* The faster the rate is, the larger the vein and the larger the IV catheter you will need. Use the largest vein available, keeping other selection criteria in mind.

- *Duration of infusion therapy.* To prevent bacterial colonization and phlebitis, some guidelines recommend changing short peripheral IV catheters every 72 to 96 hours (CDC, 2011a; while others recommend changing it as clinically indicated (Infusion Nurses Society [INS], 2011a).

- *Presence of disease or previous surgery.* For example, avoid areas with scarring or impaired circulation.

For more detailed guidelines for selecting an insertion site,

 Go to Chapter 38, **Clinical Insight 38-3: Guidelines for Selecting a Peripheral Venipuncture Site,** in Volume 2.

Perform Venipuncture

For a successful venipuncture, you need to be able to visualize or palpate the vein before attempting to insert the catheter. Use a vein viewer, if available, to aid in locating the vein. These instruments use infrared light and camera technology to project the patient's superficial

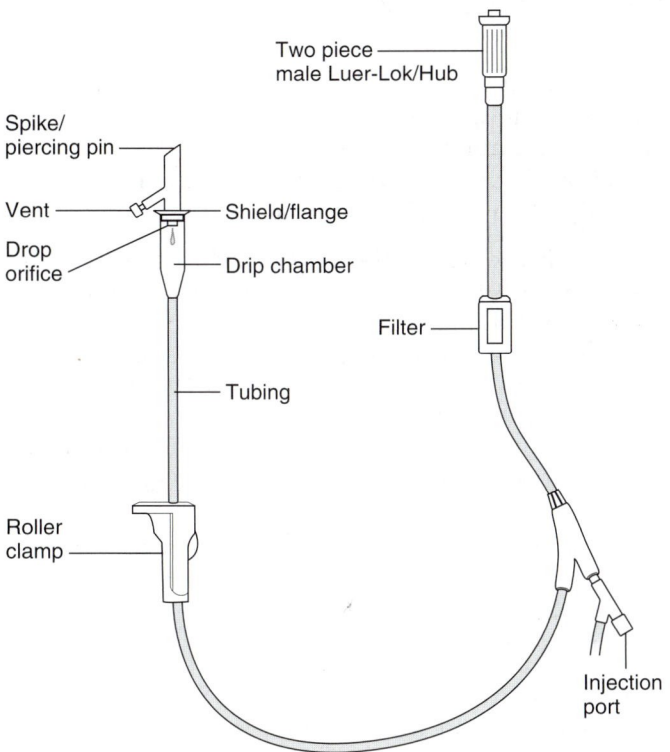

FIGURE 38-14 A basic administration set, or infusion kit.

Two piece male Luer-Lok/Hub

Spike/ piercing pin

Vent

Drop orifice

Shield/flange

Drip chamber

Filter

Tubing

Roller clamp

Injection port

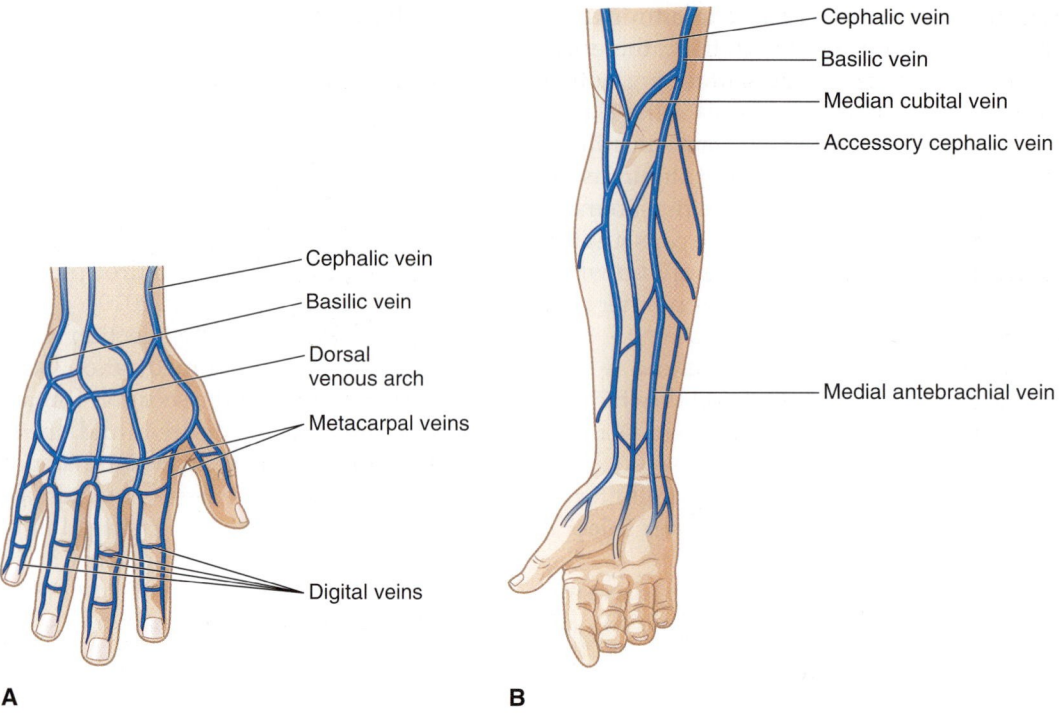

FIGURE 38-15 *A,* Superficial veins of the hand. *B,* Superficial veins of the forearm.

veins on to the skin surface. The Highlights of Procedures box summarizes the procedure for venipuncture. For other fine points of venipuncture (e.g., stabilizing the vein, angle of insertion, other techniques),

 Go to Chapter 38, **Procedure 38-1: Initiating a Peripheral Intravenous Infusion,** in Volume 2.

Key Point: *If you are not successful with the venipuncture, you can make a second attempt above the initial site or in the opposite extremity. But do not make more than two attempts to start an IV on a patient. Get help from a more experienced colleague.*

Regulating and Maintaining an Intravenous Infusion

Intravenous fluids can flow by gravity or be regulated by an electronic infusion-control device (pump). You are responsible for maintaining the correct rate of flow and for monitoring the client's response to the infusion. Many factors can influence the flow rate of an IV solution, especially when using gravity flow.

- *The height of the solution container.* The greater the distance between the height of the container and the patient's heart, the faster the flow will be. Check the flow rate each time the client or IV solution is repositioned to ensure that it is correct.
- *Client position.* Pressure on the IV site decreases flow. If an IV is infusing in the right arm and the patient is positioned on his right side, the pressure on the right arm will be greater than if the client were positioned supine or on the left.
- *Blood pressure.* As blood pressure rises, more force is required to infuse into the vein.

- *The internal diameter of the IV catheter.* The smaller the diameter (that is, the higher the gauge), the more you must open the roller clamp to achieve the flow rate desired.
- *Condition of the catheter and tubing.* If the catheter is dislodged from the vein, flow may stop entirely or continue at a slowed rate. A knot or kink at any point in the tubing will slow flow.

Gravity Flow

Most IV fluids are administered by a volume-control pump. However, you may still encounter instances when you will need to regulate the rate with the roller clamp on the tubing. You should check gravity infusion rates hourly and adjust the flow as needed. If the fluid is running too slowly, do not attempt to catch up by administering extra fluid rapidly. If the fluid is running too fast, slow the rate, and assess the client for signs of fluid volume excess.

If the client is ambulatory, attach the fluid container to a pole with wheels. Instruct the client to keep the solution container above the infusion site and to avoid pulling on the tubing or the infusion site. The Highlights of Procedures box summarizes how to regulate a gravity-flow IV. For the complete procedure,

 Go to Chapter 38, **Procedure 38-2: Regulating the IV Flow Rate,** Volume 2.

Volume-Control Set

A volume-control set (e.g., Buretrol, Soluset, Volutrol) is another method for regulating an IV infusion (see Fig. 26–35). You will drain a small amount of fluid from the larger IV solution container into the volume-control container. Typically, the volume placed in the volume-control container is equal to the prescribed hourly infusion rate. The rate is regulated in the same way as other administration sets (the drip factor is usually 60 gtts/mL [60 drops/mL]); however, the maximum amount of fluid that can enter a patient is limited to the volume in the volume-control set. You may use this type of equipment when the client is at risk for fluid volume excess and for infants and children, who require close supervision of fluid intake. However, more often, the policy will be to use an infusion pump for continuous infusions for such patients. An advantage of this system is that medications can be added to the volume-control set and diluted with IV fluid for intermittent administration.

Infusion Pump

If you are using an electronic volume-control device (pump), the machine will maintain the infusion rate after you program it. Most infusion pumps sound an alarm when the fluid bag is almost empty, when air is in the line, or when there is resistance to flow. Infusion-control devices save time and prevent accidental delivery of large amounts of fluid. They do not, however, excuse you from regularly monitoring the flow rate and assessing the needle insertion site.

✚ You should know that absence of an alarm does not mean there is no problem. For example, if the IV is infiltrated, the pump may keep infusing fluid into the tissues.

To learn more about how to regulate an IV using an infusion pump, see the Highlights of Procedures box and,

 Go to Chapter 38, **Procedure 38-3: Setting Up and Using Volume-Control Pumps,** in Volume 2.

KnowledgeCheck 38-10

- What factors should you consider when selecting an insertion site for a peripheral IV line?
- What are the preferred locations for peripheral IV lines?
- What equipment is needed when inserting an IV and starting an IV infusion?
- Identify three ways to regulate the flow rate of IV fluid.

Calculating Flow Rates

As you already know, intravenous administration sets are sized as microdrips or macrodrips. Microdrips deliver fluid at a rate of 60 drops/mL. Macrodrips deliver fluid at a rate of 10 to 20 drops/mL (depending on the manufacturer). To begin, you need to know the ordered infusion rate and the flow rate of the administration set in drops per minute. See Box 38-1 to learn how to calculate flow rates.

Managing Multiple Lines

When a patient has multiple IV solutions and multiple lines, you must label each line to identify what is infusing in it. Label the IV tubing close to the catheter so that it is easy to see which fluid is infusing in the line.

BOX 38-1 ■ Calculating IV Flow Rates

Microdrips = 60 drops/mL

Macrodrips = 10 to 20 drops/mL

You need to know drops per minute: the prescribed infusion rate and the flow rate of the administration set.

1. Multiply the hourly rate (number of mL to be infused in 60 minutes) by the drop factor (in drops per milliliter) to obtain the total drops per hour.

2. Then divide by 60 to get the drip rate in drops per minute. For example, an hourly rate of 100 mL multiplied by 15 drops per milliliter and divided by 60 equals the drip rate. Therefore, the drip rate equals 25 drops per minute.

Use this formula to calculate flow:

$$\frac{\text{Hourly rate in mL} \times \text{drop factor (drops/mL)}}{60 \text{ minutes}} = \text{drip rate}$$

Example: gtts/min

$$\frac{100 \text{ (mL per hour)} \times 15 \text{ (gtts/mL)}}{60 \text{ minutes}} = 25 \text{ gtts/min}$$

This is especially true when using double- and triple-lumen catheters. Multiple lines are often used because solutions are not compatible with each other (e.g., you can never infuse blood, parenteral nutrition, or lipids through a line with anything else; and you can never draw blood samples from these lines).

- *Record the name of each line in your nursing notes and the intake form.* For peripheral IVs, use RA for right arm, LA for left arm, and so on; and designate a number for each site because there may be more than one line or site in each arm (e.g., RA-1, RA-2, LA-1). If the lines are in separate arms, it may seem unnecessary to give each one a number; however, over the course of therapy, some lines may need to be discontinued and new ones started.

- *For multiport central lines, label each port, in addition to recording in nursing notes.* For example, with a triple-lumen central catheter, you might have named each lumen as proximal, mid, and distal, or CVAD-1, CVAD-2, CVAD-3. The finished labeling and nursing record may indicate "CVAD-1—TPN; CVAD-2—$D_5 1/2$ NS; CVAD-3—insulin."

- ✚ Always keep the lines untangled and know where your main IV fluid is (e.g., the D_5-½ NS), so that if a crisis occurs or intermittent infusions are needed, you can quickly identify the correct solution and tubing for use.

Complications of Intravenous Therapy

Complications at the IV site include infiltration, extravasation, infection, thrombus, and thrombophlebitis. Inserting an IV catheter breaks the body's first line of defense (the skin) and provides a portal of entry for microorganisms.

In addition, trauma roughens the vein wall and predisposes the person to platelet clumping and thrombus formation. Minimize this effect by swiftly piercing the skin and anchoring the catheter and tubing to reduce tissue trauma. Systemic complications occur less frequently than do local complications but may be life threatening. They include fluid volume excess, sepsis, and embolus. Table 38-8 describes potential complications of IV therapy. For more information on managing infiltration and extravasation,

 Go to **Clinical Insight 38-5: Managing Infiltration and Extravasation,** in Volume 2.

Changing Intravenous Solutions, Tubing, and Dressings

Follow practice guidelines and agency policies for changing IV solutions, tubing, and dressings. As with IV insertion, use meticulous aseptic technique.

Changing IV Solutions Hang a new container of fluid when the present container is nearly empty, but fluid still remains at the appropriate level in the drip chamber. The infusion rate dictates how often you need to change the IV solution. For example, a liter of IV fluid infusing at 125 mL/hr must be changed every 8 hours; a liter infusing at 50 mL/hr will hang for 20 hours. Evidence-based practice does not provide an exact length of time that an IV solution can hang before it has to be changed (CDC, 2011a); therefore, you should follow your agency's policy. For full instructions on the procedure for changing solutions, tubing, and dressings,

 Go to Chapter 38, **Procedure 38-4A: Changing the IV Solution, Procedure 38-4B: Changing the IV Administration Tubing and Solution,** and **Procedure 38-5: Changing IV Dressings,** in Volume 2.

Changing Administration Sets The INS (2011a) and the CDC (2011b) recommend that primary and secondary administration sets be changed no more frequently than 96 hours, but at least every 7 days; primary intermittent administration sets should be changed every 24 hours. This guideline applies to administration sets that are continuously used and the patient is not receiving blood, blood products, or fat emulsions. Administration sets used for parenteral nutrition are exposed to intravenous fat emulsions and should be changed every 24 hours and every 96 hours for non-lipid-containing parenteral nutrition solutions (INS, 2011).

Key Point: *As a rule, if you start an IV at a new site, use a new administration set. Reusing a set from a previous site increases the risk of contamination.*

Changing IV Dressings Change peripheral IV dressings routinely when the catheter is replaced, or as clinically indicated (e.g., when the dressing becomes

damp, soiled, or loose) (CDC, 2011). For central venous catheters (CVCs), The Infusion Nurses Society (INS, 2011a) recommends the following:

- For short-term CVCs, the dressing at the site must be changed every 2 days for gauze dressings and every 7 days for transparent dressing. In pediatric patients, if the risk of dislodging the catheter is high, the dressing can be left in place.
- For tunneled or implanted sites, unless soiled or loose, a transparent dressing is changed no more than once a week until the insertion site has healed.
- For long-term cuffed and tunneled CVS with well-healed sites, no recommendations are made. You should follow your agency's policy for dressing changes on these sites. In home care, the dressing may be left in place for 1 week. Change any dressing, regardless of site, when it becomes soiled, damp, or loosened.

Key Point. *It is best to dress both central and peripheral lines with transparent, semipermeable dressings.* These dressings allow direct visualization of the site between dressing changes, permit evaporation of moisture, and provide a secure anchor for the catheter. You may still sometimes see tape securing a catheter at the insertion site; however, the use of a catheter stabilization device is preferred over tape or sutures (INS, 2011a).

Converting to a Peripheral Intravenous Lock

The terms *peripheral lock, saline lock,* or *prn adapter* are used interchangeably. Recall that you may need a peripheral IV lock (PIV) for intermittent infusions or for venous access for emergencies. Also, when clients do not need the additional fluids provided by a constant infusion of solution, a peripheral infusion can be easily converted to a peripheral lock. To do this, you simply remove the tubing from the IV catheter and replace it with a sterile injection cap (see Fig. 38-9). Some IV locks also contain a short segment of tubing.

Each time you give a medication through the lock, you will need to disinfect and flush the lock before and after you administer the medication. The INS (2011a) recommends that 0.9% sodium chloride (USP) be used to flush the peripheral IV lock. A PIV should also be flushed and locked at least every 12 hours when not in use. The Highlights of Procedures box summarizes the procedure for converting to a PIV. For complete instructions,

 Go to Chapter 38, **Procedure 38-6: Converting a Primary Line to a Peripheral IV Lock,** in Volume 2.

Discontinuing an Intravenous Line

Discontinue the IV line and IV catheter when IV fluids and medications are no longer needed or if the integrity of the line is compromised. Inspect the catheter to ensure that it is intact when you remove it. The Highlights of Procedures box summarizes removal of an IV catheter. For the complete procedure,

Table 38-8 ➤ Complications of Intravenous Therapy

COMPLICATION	CAUSES	SIGNS AND SYMPTOMS	NURSING RESPONSE
Local Complications			
Hematoma—a localized mass of blood outside the blood vessel	Nicking the vein during an unsuccessful insertion, discontinuing an IV line without holding pressure over the site, or applying a tourniquet too tightly above a previously attempted venipuncture site	Ecchymosis, localized mass, discomfort	Be gentle with venipuncture technique. Apply pressure when discontinuing an IV.
*Infiltration—the seepage of nonvesicant solution or medication into surrounding tissues	IV catheter dislodges or the tip penetrates the vessel wall.	Slowed or stopped flow Swelling, tenderness, pallor, hardness and coolness at the site The patient may report a burning sensation in the area.	Stop the infusion immediately. Restart the IV infusion in a different vein, higher in the extremity or in another extremity. Elevate the affected arm on a pillow to promote absorption of excess fluid.
*Extravasation—seepage of a vesicant substance into the tissues. (A *vesicant* is a solution that causes the formation of blisters and subsequent tissue sloughing and necrosis.)	IV catheter dislodges, or the tip penetrates the vessel wall.	Slowed or stopped flow Pain, burning, and swelling at IV site, blanching and coolness of the surrounding skin Blistering is a late sign. If extravasation resulted from vasoconstricting medication may see necrosis (death) of dermis.	Treatment depends on the severity of the infiltration. Stop the IV infusion immediately. Administer an antidote, if one is available. (Antidotes alter the pH, alter DNA binding, neutralize the drug, or dilute the extravasated drug.) Apply cold compresses, and elevate the extremity.
Phlebitis—inflammation of the vein	May be due to mechanical irritation, infusion of solutions that are irritating to the vessel, or sepsis. Dextrose solutions, potassium chloride, antibiotics, and vitamin C are associated with a higher risk of phlebitis. Trauma to the vessel, compression of the line by client movement, or a low flow rate	Redness, pain, and warmth at the site, local swelling, palpable cord along the vein, sluggish infusion rate, and elevated temperature Slowed or stopped infusion, localized warmth at the site, inability to restart flow of IV	Discontinue the IV infusion and restart in a new location. Initially, apply cold compresses to the site if the site is warm and tender. Thereafter, use warm compresses. Assess for circulatory impairment. Consult the primary care provider if there is streaking or erythema along the vein or a palpable cord. *Prevention measures:* Use the smallest catheter practical (usually 22-gauge or 24-gauge thin-walled catheter). Use polyurethane catheters instead of Teflon.

Continued

Table 38-8 ➤ Complications of Intravenous Therapy—cont'd

COMPLICATION	CAUSES	SIGNS AND SYMPTOMS	NURSING RESPONSE
			Stabilize and secure the catheter to minimize movement in the vein.
			Rotate the site at least every 96 hours.
Thrombophlebitis—thrombosis and inflammation	Use of veins in the legs for infusion, use of a hypertonic or highly acidic solution; can be a result of untreated phlebitis	Sluggish flow rate, edema, tender and cord-like veins, warmth, and erythema at site	Discontinue the IV infusion, and restart in the opposite extremity, using all new equipment.
			Apply warm, moist compresses.
			Consult the primary care provider.
Local infection—mic-robial contamination of the cannula or IV site	Using poor technique when inserting the catheter, leaving the catheter in place for longer than 96 hours, or direct contamination	Redness, swelling, exudate, elevated temperature	Remove the IV line.
			Apply a sterile dressing over the site.
			Administer antibiotics, if necessary.
Nerve injury—a nerve is inadvertently injured during venipuncture (direct) or is compressed	Using veins on inner surface of the wrist and forearm; not anchoring the vein for puncture; using a large needle; advancing the needle across instead of with the vein; "probing" (excessive redirection of the needle at insertion); inserting too deeply and through the back wall of the vein; too many venipuncture attempts; infiltration, extravasation, tourniquet too tight or left on too long	*Direct injury*—sharp acute pain at the site or up and down the arm; pins and needles or electric shock sensation; pain, numbness, or tingling in fingers; pain that persists after the needle is removed. *Compression injury*—pain and tingling typically appear 24 to 96 hours after venipuncture.	Do not make more than 2 venipuncture attempts. *If patient complains of symptoms:* Stop the procedure and withdraw the catheter. Apply pressure to prevent hematoma. Report to supervisor and physician. Do not start a new IV in the affected arm. Treat infiltration if it occurs. **Fasciotomy** (incisions around the area to let blood or fluid seep out) is the usual treatment; or fluid may be expressed.
Systemic Complications			
Septicemia—the presence of microorganisms or their toxic products in the circulatory system	A break in aseptic technique, or contaminated IV solution	Fluctuating fever, chills, tachycardia, confusion, hypotension, altered mental status, elevated WBC count	Discontinue the IV infusion immediately. Consult the primary care provider. Treatment often involves antibiotics, fluids, and medications to support vital signs.

Table 38-8 ➤ Complications of Intravenous Therapy—cont'd

COMPLICATION	CAUSES	SIGNS AND SYMPTOMS	NURSING RESPONSE
Fluid overload	Infusing excessive amounts of IV fluids or administering fluid too rapidly.	Weight gain, edema, hypertension, shortness of breath, crackles, distended neck veins	Slow the IV flow rate. Place the client in high-Fowler's position. Monitor vital signs. Administer oxygen, if needed. If severe, diuretics may be ordered.
Air embolus—a rare complication involving the introduction of air into the vascular system	Loose connections, adding a new IV bag to a line that has run dry without clearing the line of air, air in tubing cassette of infusion pump	Palpitations, chest pain, light-headedness, dyspnea, cough, hypotension, tachycardia, sudden change in mental status	Call for help. Place client in Trendelenburg's position on the left side. Administer oxygen. Have emergency equipment available.
Catheter embolus—a piece of catheter breaks off and travels through the vascular system	Reinserting a catheter used in an unsuccessful insertion; removing and reinserting a stylet, causing shearing of the catheter; placing the catheter in a joint flexion	Sharp, sudden pain at IV site, jagged catheter end on removal, dyspnea, chest pain, tachycardia, hypotension	Apply a tourniquet above the site. Notify the physician and radiologist. Start a new IV line. Prepare the patient for radiographic examination.

*For more information about interventions for infiltration and extravasation,

 Go to Chapter 38, **Clinical Insight 38-5: Managing Infiltration and Extravasation,** in Volume 2.

Source: Phillips, L. D. (2010). *Manual of I.V. therapeutics* (5th ed.). Philadelphia: F.A. Davis.

 Go to Chapter 38, **Procedure 38-7: Discontinuing a Peripheral IV,** in Volume 2.

KnowledgeCheck 38-11

- The prescription reads, "5% dextrose in water/0.45% saline solution ($D_5\frac{1}{2}$ NS) with 20 mEq KCl; infuse 1 liter in 5 hours." Calculate the hourly rate and the drip rate using (1) a macrodrip administration set with 15 gtts/mL and (2) a microdrip set.
- Describe the difference between infiltration and extravasation as a complication of IV therapy.
- In general, how often are administration sets changed on peripheral IV lines? How often are administration sets changed when total parenteral nutrition (TPN) is being infused?

Replacement of Blood and Blood Products

Intravenous fluids can replace fluid volume, but they do not restore oxygen-carrying capacity or replace clotting factors. Blood products are infused when the patient has experienced significant blood loss, diminished oxygen-carrying capacity, or a deficiency in one of the blood components. The American Association of Blood Banks (AABB) estimates that 9.2 million volunteers donate blood each year; a total of 15.7 million units of whole blood and red blood cells was donated in 2011 (AABB, n.d.).

Each unit of donated blood is separated into multiple components, such as red blood cells, plasma, platelets, and clotting factors. Thus, one unit of donated blood may be used in the care of four clients. Unfortunately, fewer than 10% of eligible persons donate blood each year. To

For steps to follow in *all* procedures, refer to the Universal Steps for All Procedures found on the inside back cover of Volume 2. Go to the full procedures in Volume 2 to practice and learn the procedure steps. Use these procedural highlights later to help you review key points.

For all intravenous procedures, maintain scrupulous aseptic technique to prevent infection and possible sepsis.

Procedure 38-1: Initiating a Peripheral Intravenous Infusion

➤ Prepare the IV solution and administration set, including extension tubing and volume-control device if used. Prime the tubing.

➤ Label the IV solution container and place a time-tape on it with the infusion rate. Label the tubing with the date and time.

➤ Apply the tourniquet.

➤ Locate a vein. Then loosen the tourniquet. (As a rule, select the most distal vein in an upper extremity.)

➤ Don clean nonsterile gloves and open the catheter package. Keep the catheter sterile.

➤ Reapply the tourniquet and cleanse the site. Allow the antiseptic to dry on the skin.

➤ Inform the patient that you are about to insert the catheter.

➤ Stabilize the vein with your nondominant hand.

➤ Hold the catheter, bevel up, at a 30° to 45° angle and pierce the skin.

➤ Look for a flashback of blood. Lower the catheter so it is parallel to the skin, and advance into the vein.

➤ When the needle is at least halfway into the vein or when a steady backflow of blood occurs, gradually withdraw the needle while advancing the catheter fully into the vein.

➤ While holding the catheter in place with one hand, release the tourniquet with your other hand.

➤ Connect the IV administration set to the IV catheter.

➤ While stabilizing the catheter with your hand, adjust the flow rate according to the prescriber's order.

➤ Secure the connection; stabilize the catheter; and dress the IV insertion site.

➤ Label the dressing.

➤ Loop and tape the tubing to the skin.

➤ Place an arm board as needed.

Procedure 38-2: Regulating the IV Flow Rate

➤ Follow all "checks" and "rights" of medication administration, including:

Verify the prescription

Check the solution to make sure that you have the proper IV fluid with the prescribed additives.

Apply a time tape to the solution container. Mark the time the infusion was started.

Open the roller clamp so that the IV fluid begins to flow.

➤ Calculate the hourly rate and the drip rate; verify your calculations.

➤ Hold a watch beside the drip chamber; count the number of drops for 1 minute.

➤ Adjust the roller clamp, increasing or decreasing the flow until you achieve the prescribed drip rate.

➤ Monitor manually regulated infusion rates closely for the first 15 minutes after you begin the infusion; then monitor the rate hourly.

Procedure 38-3: Setting Up and Using Volume-Control Pumps

➤ Calculate and verify the infusion rate.

➤ Attach the volume-control pump to the IV pole, and plug it into the nearest electrical outlet.

➤ Close the clamp on the administration set and spike the port of the solution container. Attach a filter if one is needed.

➤ Label the tubing and solution container.

➤ Hang the solution container on the IV pole.

➤ Fill the drip chamber halfway.

➤ Place the electronic sensor on the drip chamber, if there is one. If not, consult the manufacturer's instructions.

➤ Prime the administration tubing, then close the clamp.

➤ Turn on the pump, and load the administration tubing into the pump.

➤ Program the pump with the hourly infusion rate, total hours, and the volume to be infused.

➤ Don clean nonsterile gloves and check the IV site for patency.

➤ Scrub the injection port; allow to dry.

➤ Connect the tubing adapter to the injection port.

➤ Unclamp the administration set tubing, and press the start button.

➤ Make sure that the alarms are turned on and audible.

➤ Check the pump regularly to make sure that the correct volume is infusing.

➤ At the end of your shift (or at the specified time), clear the pump of the volume infused and record the volume.

Procedure 38-4: Changing IV Solutions and Tubing

Procedure 38-4A: Changing the IV Solution

➤ Prepare and label your next container of IV solution at least 1 hour before the present infusion is scheduled to finish.

➤ Close the roller clamp on the infusing (empty) administration set.

➤ Wearing nonsterile gloves, remove the old IV solution container from the IV pole. Remove the spike from the bag, keeping the spike sterile.

➤ Spike the new IV solution container.

➤ Hang the new IV solution, and inspect the tubing for air.

➤ Adjust the drip rate.

➤ Place the time tape on the new IV solution container. Mark the times.

Procedure 38-4B: Changing the IV Administration Solution and Tubing

➤ Prepare and hang the new IV solution and tubing.

➤ Close the roller clamp on the old administration set.

➤ Wearing clean nonsterile gloves, stabilize the IV catheter while applying pressure over the vein just above the insertion site.

➤ Remove the protective cover from the distal end of the new administration set and connect the new tubing.

➤ Adjust the drip rate.

➤ Cleanse the IV site.

➤ Resecure the IV catheter and tubing connection; loop and tape the tubing.

➤ Label tubing and solution with date, initials, rate, and time tape.

Procedure 38-5: Changing IV Dressings

Procedure 38-5A: Peripheral IV Dressings

➤ Wearing clean procedure gloves, stabilize the catheter with your nondominant hand, and carefully remove the dressing.

➤ Inspect the insertion site.

➤ Don clean gloves. Cleanse the insertion site, following manufacturer's guidelines for product use

➤ Allow the antiseptic to dry on the skin.

➤ Perform hand hygiene and don nonsterile gloves.

➤ Apply a new sterile catheter stabilization device and dressing.

➤ Secure the connection between the catheter and the tubing.

➤ Loop and tape the tubing to the patient's skin.

➤ Label the dressing with the date and time of insertion, catheter size, the date the dressing was changed, and your initials.

Procedure 38-5B: Central Line Dressings

➤ Obtain sterile central line dressing kit (or equivalent supplies if there is no kit) and a mask for the patient, if one is needed.

➤ Place the patient in a semi-Fowler's position, if tolerated.

➤ Ask the patient to turn his head to the opposite side of the insertion site; if unable, place a mask on the patient.

➤ Don mask and clean nonsterile gloves.

➤ Carefully remove the old dressing and stabilization device.

➤ Inspect the site for signs of complications.

➤ Remove gloves and perform hand hygiene

➤ Set up a sterile field, open dressing change kit, and don sterile gloves.

➤ Arrange sterile supplies as needed.

➤ Scrub the insertion site with gentle friction for at least 30 seconds, using the antiseptic swabs contained in kit.

➤ Scrub the sutures (if any) and the catheter from insertion site to the hub or bifurcation with an antiseptic swab for at least 15 seconds.

➤ Allow the site to dry completely; do not fan.

➤ Apply the transparent dressing that comes in the kit.

➤ Apply the new catheter stabilization device, if one is used.

➤ Remove drape, if one was used.

➤ Loop the catheter gently and secure it with tape to the skin (do not tape it to the dressing).

➤ Label the dressing with the date changed, time, and your initials.

Procedure 38-5C: PICC Line Dressings

➤ Obtain sterile central line dressing kit (or equivalent supplies if there is no kit) and mask for the patient, if one is needed.

➤ Place the patient in a comfortable semi-Fowler's position.

➤ Explain the procedure to the patient

➤ Ask the patient to turn his head to the opposite side of the insertion site; if unable, place a mask on the patient, if consistent with agency policy.

➤ Inspect the site for signs and symptoms of infection.

➤ Don mask and nonsterile gloves

➤ Remove and discard your gloves along with the old dressing.

➤ Perform hand hygiene.

➤ Set up a sterile field, open dressing change kit, and don sterile gloves.

➤ Arrange sterile supplies, as needed.

➤ Use sterile tape, measure the external length of PICC to compare to base insertion length, if consistent with agency's policy.

➤ Scrub the catheter's insertion site and the surrounding skin that will be covered by the dressing for 30 seconds.

➤ Allow to air dry completely.

➤ Apply the stabilization device, if one is used.

➤ Apply the transparent dressing. Loop the catheter and injection camp so that it is pointing up.

➤ Label the dressing with the date, time, and your initials.

➤ Loop and anchor the catheter; secure with tape.

Procedure 38-6: Converting a Primary Line to a Peripheral IV Lock

➤ Maintain sterility of equipment throughout.

➤ Don clean nonsterile gloves.

➤ Remove the IV lock from the package, and flush the adapter, according to agency policy. Do not contaminate the lock.

Continued

➤ Remove the IV dressing and the tape that is securing the tubing.

➤ Close the roller clamp on the administration set.

➤ With your nondominant hand, apply pressure over the vein just above the insertion site; stabilize the catheter hub with your thumb and forefinger.

➤ Disengage the used tubing from the IV catheter.

➤ Quickly insert the lock adapter into the IV catheter and turn it to lock it in place.

➤ Scrub the adapter injection port and flush the lock again with the second syringe.

➤ Apply a sterile transparent semipermeable dressing; do not cover the catheter-tubing connection.

➤ Label the dressing with date and initials.

➤ Discard used supplies.

Procedure 38-7: Discontinuing a Peripheral IV

➤ Place a linen-saver pad under the extremity with the IV catheter.

➤ Don clean nonsterile gloves, and close the roller clamp on the administration set.

➤ Remove the dressing; scrub the catheter-skin junction with an antiseptic pad for 15 seconds.

➤ Place a sterile 2 in. × 2 in. gauze pad above the IV insertion site and gently remove the catheter.

➤ Apply firm pressure with the gauze pad; hold pressure for 1 to 3 minutes, or longer if bleeding persists.

➤ Replace the soiled 2 in. × 2 in. gauze pad with a new sterile one. Secure it with tape or use a transparent dressing.

Procedure 38-8: Administering a Blood Transfusion

Procedure 38-8A: Administering Blood and Blood Products

➤ Verify that informed consent has been obtained.

➤ Verify the physician's prescription, noting the indication, and rate of infusion.

➤ Administer any prescribed pretransfusion medications.

➤ Obtain a blood administration set and 250 mL of IV normal saline solution.

➤ Obtain infusion pump, if possible and blood warmer, if necessary.

➤ Obtain the blood product from the blood bank according to your institution's policy. Verify that the blood matches the prescription. Inspect it for abnormalities.

➤ With another qualified staff member (per agency policy) verify the patient and blood product identification (e.g., date of birth, hospital identification number, blood type). If all verifications are in agreement, both staff members should sign the blood bank form. Contact the blood bank immediately if there are discrepancies, and do not administer the blood product.

➤ Document on the blood bank form the date and time the transfusion is begun.

➤ Close all clamps on the blood administration set. Label the tubing.

➤ Hang the normal saline and prime the tubing.

➤ Gently invert the blood product container several times.

➤ Spike the blood product and hang the blood on the IV pole.

➤ Obtain a set of vital signs.

➤ Scrub the port with an alcohol swab or chlorhexidine/alcohol antiseptic product for at least 15 seconds before connecting to an existing line.

➤ Attach the administration set tubing to the IV catheter.

➤ Slowly open the roller clamp closest to the blood product. Infuse the first 50 mL slowly; if no reaction, set to the prescribed rate.

➤ Remain with the patient for the first 5 minutes. Measure vital signs in 5 minutes, 15 minutes, and 30 minutes; then hourly.

➤ Observe for and ask the patient to immediately report symptoms of transfusion reaction.

➤ When the blood has transfused, flush the line with the normal saline solution.

➤ Disconnect the tubing from the IV catheter, and dispose of the blood product container and tubing per agency policy.

➤ If a second unit of blood is to be transfused, the same administration set may be used.

➤ Administer any post-transfusion medications prescribed.

Procedure 38-8B: Managing a Transfusion Reaction

➤ If there are signs or symptoms of transfusion reaction, stop the transfusion immediately. Do not flush the tubing.

➤ Disconnect the administration set from the IV catheter.

➤ Call for help and prepare for emergency care.

➤ Obtain vital signs, and auscultate heart and breath sounds.

➤ Maintain patency of the IV catheter by hanging a new infusion of normal saline solution, using new tubing.

➤ Notify the primary care provider.

➤ Place the administration set and blood product container, with the blood bank form attached, inside a biohazard bag. Send the bag to the blood bank immediately.

➤ Obtain blood (in the extremity opposite the transfusion site) and urine specimens according to your institution's policy.

➤ Continue to monitor vital signs frequently.

➤ Administer medications, as prescribed.

Procedure 38-9: Assisting With Percutaneous Central Venous Catheter Placement

➤ Explain procedure to the patient and verify informed consent.

➤ Obtain vital signs.

➤ Gather supplies and perform meticulous hand hygiene.

➤ Position the table so it is easily accessible by the provider.

➤ Prepare sterile field and add supplies.

➤ Position the patient (Trendelenburg with a rolled towel between the shoulders).

➤ After the physician or advanced practice nurse performs hand hygiene, offer mask, gown, and sterile gloves (and possibly hat, depending on agency policy).

➤ Don mask and then sterile gloves.

➤ Prep an 8 in. × 10 in. area around the site, using applicators of 2% chlorhexidine gluconate in 70% alcohol, per agency guidelines.

➤ Place the large sterile drape to cover patient's head and chest.

➤ Have the patient turn his head opposite the direction of insertion.

➤ Observe while the physician inserts and sutures the catheter.

➤ Apply sterile transparent dressing, close any lumen clamps, and place tape across the lumens near the injection caps.

➤ Monitor for complications (especially respiratory distress).

➤ Obtain a chest x-ray.

---

be eligible to donate blood, a person must be in good health (no cold or flu, uncontrolled hypertension, anemia, or diabetes), at least 16 years of age (although some states permit younger people, with parental consent, to donate), have a hemoglobin of at least 12.5 gm/dL, and weigh at least 110 pounds. In addition, each potential donor is screened for travel to certain countries and for a variety of disorders, such as hepatitis, HIV, and Creutzfeldt-Jakob disease (the human form of mad cow disease).

Blood Groups

Human blood is classified into four main groups (A, B, AB, and O) based on the presence or absence of certain antigens and antibodies. You inherit the blood group you belong to from your parents.

If you belong to blood group A, you have A antigens on the surface of your red blood cells (RBCs), and B antibodies in your plasma. The opposite is true for persons with blood group B. Blood group AB has both antigens on the surface of the red blood cells and no antibodies at all in the plasma. In contrast, blood group O has neither A nor B antigens on the surface of the red blood cells but both A and B antibodies in the blood plasma (Table 38-9). Patients must receive only blood that is compatible with

their own blood group to prevent a hemolytic reaction (see Table 38-10).

An additional antigen, known as Rh factor, is also important with blood typing. If the antigen is present, you are referred to as Rh positive (Rh+). If it is absent, you are Rh negative (Rh-). Thus, you can belong to one of the following eight groups:

A Rh+   B Rh+   AB Rh+   O Rh+
A Rh-   B Rh-   AB Rh-   O Rh-

Blood Typing and Crossmatching

Once blood is donated, several tests are performed on the sample. First, the sample is tested for ABO group (blood type) and Rh type (positive or negative), as well as for any unexpected red blood cell antibodies that may cause problems in a recipient. Screening tests assess for evidence of donor infection with hepatitis B and C viruses, HIV, human T-lymphotropic viruses, West Nile virus, and syphilis. If all disease screens are negative, the blood is acceptable for transfusion and is placed in the pool of available products.

When a potential donor is identified, crossmatching is performed. **Crossmatching** identifies possible minor antigens that will affect the compatibility of the donor blood in the recipient. RBCs from the donor blood are

Table 38-9 ➤ Blood Transfusions				
BLOOD GROUP	**ANTIGENS**	**ANTIBODIES**	**CAN GIVE BLOOD TO**	**CAN RECEIVE BLOOD FROM**
AB	A and B	None	AB	AB, A, B, and O
A	A	B	A and AB	A and O
B	B	A	B and AB	B and O
O	None	A and B	AB, A, B, and O	O

mixed with plasma from the potential recipient. A reagent is added, and the sample is observed for clumping or agglutination. If no clumping is observed, the risk of transfusion reaction is low, and it is considered safe to transfuse the sample of blood. Table 38-9 summarizes blood group matching.

Key Point: *People with blood group O are considered universal donors, because of the absence of antigens, whereas people with blood group AB are considered universal recipients because of the absence of plasma antibodies.*

In regard to Rh factor, people who are Rh+ may receive blood with or without Rh factor. However, people who are Rh− may receive only Rh− blood.

When possible, **autologous** (self-donated) units of blood are given instead of blood from a donor. This negates the risk of a mismatch or exposure to undetected disease. The patient's blood is usually collected in the preoperative weeks for possible transfusion during elective surgery. Autologous donation is most often done with orthopedic, cardiac, and vascular surgery. The process of donating autologous blood stimulates the bone marrow to produce new blood cells. Given adequate time for recovery, the collected cells may be wholly or partially replaced prior to surgery.

Blood Products

Several blood products are available for transfusion:

- *Whole blood* contains RBCs, WBCs, and platelets suspended in plasma.
- *Red blood cells* are prepared from whole blood by removing the plasma. RBCs can raise the client's hematocrit and hemoglobin levels while minimizing an increase in volume. RBCs are available for transfusion as packed RBCs (PRBCs).
- *Plasma* is the liquid portion of the blood. It is 90% water and makes up about 55% of blood volume. Plasma may be transfused whole or may be separated into specific products, such as albumin, clotting factor concentrates, and immune globulins.
- *Platelets* help the clotting process by sticking to the lining of blood vessels. Units of platelets are prepared by using a centrifuge to separate the platelet-rich plasma from the donated unit of whole blood. The platelet-rich plasma is then centrifuged again to concentrate the platelets further. Platelets are used to treat clients who have a shortage of platelets or have abnormal platelet function.
- *White blood cells (WBCs),* specifically granulocytes, can be collected by centrifugation of whole blood. They are transfused within 24 hours after collection and are used for infections that are unresponsive to antibiotic therapy. The effectiveness of WBC transfusion is still being investigated.
- *Plasma derivatives* are concentrates of specific plasma proteins prepared from many units of plasma. Plasma derivatives include a variety of clotting factors, immune globulins, and albumin.

Initiating a Transfusion

 It is critical to identify the patient and the blood product when transfusing blood. Before beginning a transfusion, verify the written prescription for the blood product.

Obtain a set of vital signs 5 to 15 minutes before initiating the infusion. If the patient's temperature is elevated, inform the primary care provider before hanging the transfusion. Most patients experience a minor temperature elevation after a transfusion is given. A preexisting elevated temperature may exacerbate this response. Some patients will refuse a blood transfusion because of cultural, religious, or other beliefs. Be ready to discuss with them any available alternatives to whole blood administration.

Also inspect the IV site to be sure it is patent before hanging the blood product. Nurses commonly use a 20-gauge catheter to infuse blood and a larger size for rapid flow rates. There is evidence that a 22-gauge catheter can be used in adults without damage to the red blood cells (INS, 2011a). Certainly, for children and the frail elderly you will need a smaller, 22- or 24-gauge catheter. The Highlights of Procedures box summarizes the procedure for initiating and monitoring a blood transfusion. For the complete procedure,

Go to Chapter 38, **Procedure 38-8A: Administering Blood and Blood Products,** and **Procedure 38-8B: Managing a Transfusion Reaction,** in Volume 2.

Transfusion Reactions

Even though you use perfect technique, transfusion reactions can and do occur. Five types of reaction are possible: allergic, bacterial, febrile, or hemolytic reactions; and circulatory overload. Table 38-10 describes each of these reactions. To help prevent transfusion reactions, be extremely careful in identifying the patient and the blood, start the transfusion slowly, remain with the patient for the first 5 minutes of the transfusion, and assess again at 15 minutes (see Procedure 38-8, in Volume 2). Many physicians routinely prescribe acetaminophen (e.g., Tylenol) or diphenhydramine (e.g., Benadryl) before transfusions, with the goal of preventing febrile and minor allergic reactions. However, some question whether the risks of routine medication outweigh the benefits and suggest that more research is needed in this area (Geiger & Howard, 2007).

KnowledgeCheck 38-12

- Identify eight potential blood types.
- Describe the types of blood products that are available for transfusion.
- Identify and describe types of transfusion reactions.

Table 38-10 ➤ Transfusion Reactions

TYPE OF REACTION	SIGNS AND SYMPTOMS	NURSING RESPONSIBILITIES
Allergic—allergy to blood being transfused	Flushing, itching, wheezing, urticaria (hives); anaphylaxis, if severe	Stop the transfusion. Replace with a saline infusion. Notify the physician immediately. Administer prescribed antihistamine.
Bacterial—contamination of the blood	Fever, chills, vomiting, diarrhea, hypertension	Stop the transfusion. Replace with a saline infusion. Notify the physician. Administer antibiotics as ordered. Treat symptoms.
Febrile—temperature elevation due to sensitivity to WBCs, plasma proteins, or platelets	Fever, chills, warm, flushed skin, aches	Stop the transfusion. Replace with a saline infusion. Notify the physician. Treat symptoms.
Hemolytic reactions—destruction of RBCs as a result of infusing incompatible blood; occurs in 1 in 600,000 transfusions	Fever, chills, dyspnea, chest pain, tachycardia, hypotension; can be fatal	Stop the transfusion immediately. Replace with a saline infusion. Notify the physician immediately. Send the remaining blood, including tubing and filter; a sample of venous blood; and the first voided urine to the lab for analysis. Treat shock.
Circulatory overload—administering too great a volume or too rapidly	Persistent cough, crackles, hypertension, distended neck veins	Slow or stop the transfusion. Monitor vital signs. Place the client upright. Notify the physician.

Toward Evidence-Based Practice

Houck, D., & Whiteford, J. (2007). Transfusion with infusion pump for peripherally inserted central catheters and other vascular access devices. *Journal of Infusion Nursing, 30*(6), 341–344.

In a 500-bed community hospital, policy required that blood transfusions be infused by gravity flow using a peripheral IV (PIV). Nurses sought to show that using a peripherally inserted central catheter (PICC) line with an infusion pump was safe and efficient. A literature review showed no increased risk of hemolysis of red blood cells when given via pump as compared with gravity. A total of 169 units of blood products were infused via various types of PICCs and infusion ports, some using a pump and some using gravity flow. All PICC lines remained patent during transfusion and no problems with using a pump were identified. An overall reduction in cost was identified based on a 30-minute decrease in nursing time (starting and maintaining a PIV). Based on the study, the policy for blood administration via PICC lines was changed.

Galvey, J., Ibey, A., McConnell, G., et al. (2011). Infusion pumps for blood and blood products transfusions and administration. Retrieved from http://resna.org/conference/proceedings/2011/CMBEC34/galvey-69501.pdf

Based on evidence-based research and preferences by nurses, various regulatory and coordinating agencies investigated and developed standards for changing practice from blood transfusions using gravity sets to using infusion pumps. The change required reviewing manufacturers' research on infusing blood and blood products with various pumps, establishing preventive maintenance schedules, developing operating policies and procedures, and cost analysis. The average cost increase per infusion based on equipment and supplies was less than $20.

1. Based on these studies, how do you see that nurses can affect institution policy and procedure?

2. Are there any other concerns related to infusing blood via an infusion pump that you might have, and why?

3. What factors must be considered when implementing new changes in practice?

 Go to Chapter 38, **Toward Evidence-Based Practice Suggested Responses,** on Davis*Plus*.

Care**Planning** & **Mapping**Practice

For Care Planning and Care Mapping practice,

 Go to Student Resources, **Care Planning & Care Mapping Practice,** on Davis*Plus*.

DocumentationPractice

For a practice documentation exercise,

 Go to **Student Resources: Documentation Exercise,** on Davis*Plus*.

 Go to Davis*Plus* at **DavisPl.us/Wilkinson3.**

 To explore learning resources for this chapter,

 Go to Davis*Plus* a **DavisPl.us/Wilkinson3.**

Chapter Resources for Chapter 38:
   Response sheets for all learning activities
   Resources for Caregivers and Health Professionals
   Reading More About Fluids, Electrolytes, & Acid–Base Balance (suggested readings)
Interactive Case Studies
NCLEX-Style and Chapter Review Questions
Chapter Overview Podcasts

For references cited in this chapter,

 Go to Volume 2, **References Cited**.

Nursing Functions

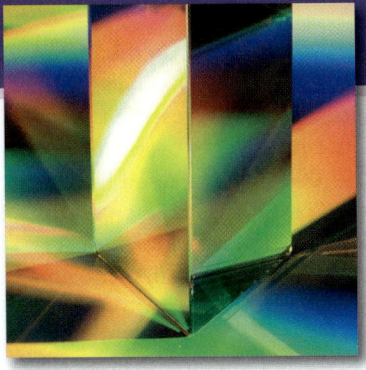

Perioperative Care

Learning Outcomes

After completing this chapter, you should be able to:

- ➤ Discuss the importance of perioperative safety.
- ➤ Name and differentiate the three phases of the perioperative period.
- ➤ Describe the ways in which surgeries can be classified.
- ➤ Discuss factors that affect the degree of risk of surgery.
- ➤ Describe nursing actions associated with the preoperative phase, including physical preparations for surgery, preoperative teaching, and surgical consent forms.
- ➤ Compare and contrast the roles of the circulating and scrub nurse.
- ➤ Compare and contrast general anesthesia, local anesthesia, regional anesthesia, and conscious sedation.

- ➤ Discuss common nursing interventions during the intraoperative phase, including skin preparation, positioning for surgery, and intraoperative safety measures.
- ➤ Describe nursing assessments appropriate for surgical clients on admission to the nursing unit.
- ➤ Provide nursing care to prevent postoperative complications, including application of elastic and sequential compression devices, use of incentive spirometry, and management of gastric suction.
- ➤ Use nursing diagnoses appropriately to describe a patient's unique needs during the preoperative, intraoperative, and postoperative periods.

Key Concepts

Perioperative nursing
Preoperative care
Intraoperative care
Postoperative care

Related Concepts

See the Concept Map on Davis*Plus*.

Meet Your Patient

Nishad Singh is a 68-year-old man who came to the emergency department (ED) with sudden onset of rectal bleeding. He tells the ED nurse, "I've been real tired and dragging for several months. This morning I felt a little worse than usual. When I went to the bathroom, there was a lot of blood. I've never had that before, and it scared me. I've had to go to the bathroom a couple times this morning, and it's all blood." The ED nurse collects the following data:

BP: 138/88 mm Hg
Pulse: 104 beats/min and regular
Respiratory rate: 20 breaths/min
Temperature: 36.7°C (98.0°F)
Oxygen saturation: 98%

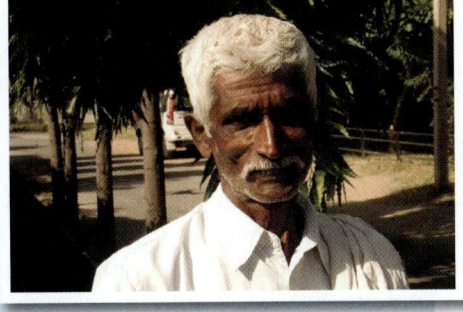

The ED nurse assesses that Mr. Singh is mildly anxious. His breath sounds are clear, but his abdomen is tender in the left lower quadrant (LLQ). The nurse draws blood to be sent to the lab. While they are waiting for the lab results, Mr. Singh tells the nurse, "My stomach is cramping down low, and I need to go to the bathroom." She provides him with a bedpan. He passes approximately 200 mL of bright red blood with a small amount of fecal material. He becomes sweaty and lightheaded after the BM. The nurse rechecks his vital signs and

(Continued)

Meet Your Patient (continued)

notes that his BP is now 120/76 mm Hg and that his pulse is up to 120 beats/min. The nurse shows the ED physician the bloody bowel movement and updates him on the change in vital signs. When the ED physician examines Mr. Singh, he tells Mr. Singh that he will need to be admitted to the hospital for further evaluation of the bleeding.

You are the nurse assigned to care for Mr. Singh on the medical-surgical unit. Mr. Singh has been sent from the ED directly to radiology for a computed tomography (CT)

scan of his abdomen. The scan reveals a tumor in the sigmoid colon. Since leaving the ED, Mr. Singh has had three more bloody bowel movements. His blood pressure is 100/72 mm Hg, and his pulse rate is now 134 beats/min. The physician prescribes a bolus of 1,000 mL of lactated Ringer's solution and a unit of packed red blood cells as soon as it is available. Mr. Singh is scheduled for colon resection surgery, which will occur as soon as the surgical team can be assembled and the room prepared.

ABOUT THE KEY CONCEPTS

The overarching concept for this chapter is **perioperative nursing**, which includes the key concepts of **preoperative**, **intraoperative**, and **postoperative care**. To help you understand and remember those concepts, we discuss in this chapter how to prepare a client for surgery and the activities that occur before, during, and after surgery, as we follow Mr. Singh (Meet Your Patient) through his perioperative experience. We will present definitions and examples of the key concepts as well as numerous sub-concepts that relate to each other in various ways. We begin with perioperative nursing.

PERIOPERATIVE NURSING

Perioperative nursing involves the care of clients before, during, and after surgery and some other invasive procedures. Historically, perioperative nursing practice was called "operating room nursing" and was limited to transferring patients into and out of operating rooms and handing instruments to surgeons during surgical procedures. Now nurses in all phases of the operative experience actively provide and manage care, teach, and study the care of perioperative patients.

The Association of periOperative Registered Nurses (AORN) is one of the most highly organized and influential specialty organizations within the nursing profession. AORN *Standards and Recommended Practices* (2009, updated 2011) keep perioperative nurses up to date on current practice. For additional information about AORN,

 Go to the **AORN Web site,** at http://www.aorn.org

Perioperative Safety

An important aspect of the perioperative nursing role is to help prevent complications of surgery. Hand hygiene is an important component of prevention (Box 39-1). Preventable perioperative errors cause 10% of surgery-related deaths, have an unfavorable financial impact on healthcare institutions, and result in physical and emotional harm to patients (Agency for Healthcare Research

and Quality [AHRQ], 2008). Various government and private organizations stress the importance of patient safety:

- *The Association of periOperative Registered Nurses (AORN, 2009, updated 2011).* Perioperative Safety is one of the four domains under which AORN organizes its perioperative patient outcomes (the others are Physiological Responses, Family and Individual

---

BOX 39-1 ■ Recommended Practices for Hand Hygiene

- Perform hand hygiene:

  Immediately before and after each patient contact

  After removing gloves. Wearing gloves does not substitute for hand hygiene.

  Anytime you may have come in contact with blood or potentially infectious substances

  Before and after eating

  After using the restroom

- Remove rings, watches, and bracelets before performing hand hygiene.
- Preferably, do not wear rings. They have been associated with a significant increase in skin microorganism count.
- Keep fingernails short and clean. They should not extend beyond the fingertips.
- Replace nail polish when it is chipped or at least every 4 days.
- Do not wear artificial nails. Fungal growth often occurs under them.
- Be certain there are no lesions or breaks in skin integrity on your hands.
- For handwashing and handrub procedures,

   Go to Chapter 23, **Procedure 23-1: Hand Hygiene,** in Volume 2.

Sources: Adapted from AORN (2009, updated 2011); Boyce & Pittet (2002); Siegel, Rhinehart, Jackson, et al. (2007).

Behavioral Responses, and Health System). Specific safety outcomes include prevention of injury and freedom from infection.

- *The Joint Commission (2012).* The Joint Commission National Patient Safety Goals for 2012 applicable to surgery include preventing infection, improving the accuracy of patient identification, using medication safely, and performing a time-out immediately before starting procedures to prevent mistakes in surgery (right surgery on right site on right patient).
- *The National Priorities Partnership (NPP) (2011).* The NPP National Quality Forum established a national priority that includes the aims of achieving better care, providing improved health for people and communities, and making quality care more affordable. One of its six national priorities and goals is making care safer by reducing harm caused in the delivery of care.
- *The Institute for Healthcare Improvement (IHI) (n.d., 2011).* This is an independent, not-for-profit organization that works to reduce morbidity and death in American healthcare, including perioperative care. One goal of its 100,000 Lives Campaign and its 5 Million Lives Campaign was to reduce surgical complications and specifically surgical infections. To see the entire list of IHI recommendations,

 Go to Chapter 23, **Tables, Boxes, Figures: ESG Box 23-1, The 100,000 Lives Campaign,** on Davis*Plus.*

"Never Events"

"Never events" are serious and costly errors resulting in severe consequences for the patient, and that are mostly preventable. Believing these events are reasonably preventable and should never happen in a hospital, Medicare will no longer reimburse institutions for care related to such complications (Centers for Medicare & Medicaid Services, 2006, updated 2008, 2011). Several of the never events (also called serious reportable events) are also targeted by the national organizations listed earlier. Among the never events important to perioperative care are

- Surgery on the wrong body part
- Surgery on the wrong patient
- Wrong surgery on a patient
- Deep vein thrombosis (DVT) or pulmonary embolism (PE) after total knee or hip replacement
- Foreign body left in a patient after surgery (e.g., sponge, clip for draping)
- Surgical site infections after certain elective procedures (e.g., bariatric surgery for obesity). AORN, The Joint Commission, NPP, and IHI extend that to include all infections. The Centers for Disease Control and Prevention (CDC) targeted certain antimicrobial-resistant bacterial infections.

You will see those themes recur in the theoretical and practical knowledge in the remainder of this chapter and in Volume 2.

PREOPERATIVE CARE

The **preoperative phase** begins with the client's decision to have surgery and ends when he enters the operating room.

Theoretical Knowledge
knowing **why**

Nursing care during the preoperative phase focuses on identifying existing health concerns, planning for intraoperative and postoperative needs, and providing preoperative teaching. Preoperative nursing care is delivered in a variety of settings. More than two-thirds of surgeries in the United States are performed in outpatient settings, such as endoscopy suites, physicians' offices, and ambulatory surgery centers (Cullen, Hall, & Golosinskiy, 2009). The length of the preoperative period and the extent of the patient teaching depend on the type of surgery to be done and the patient's overall health status.

How Are Surgeries Classified?

Knowing the type of surgery helps you identify the patient's perioperative needs and plan patient care. Surgeries can be classified by body system, purpose, level of urgency, and acuity. The classifications often overlap.

By Body System

The body system classification is useful for determining the postoperative risk of infection. For example, surgical incisions that enter the gastrointestinal, respiratory, or genitourinary tract have a higher risk for infection than does surgery of other body systems. However, if an organ ruptures or surgery is required to repair a penetrating injury, the risk of infection is very high regardless of the body system involved. Mr. Singh (Meet Your Patient) will have surgery of the gastrointestinal system.

By Purpose

See whether you can identify the purpose that describes Mr. Singh's (Meet Your Patient) surgery.

- **Ablative surgery** involves removal of a diseased body part. For example, a cholecystectomy removes a diseased gallbladder.
- **Diagnostic (exploratory) surgery** is done to confirm or rule out a diagnosis. Examples include a biopsy, a fine-needle aspiration, or invasive testing, such as a cardiac catheterization.
- **Palliative surgery** is performed to relieve discomfort or other disease symptoms without producing a cure. Examples include nerve root destruction for chronic pain.
- **Reconstructive surgery** is performed to restore function, for example, rotator cuff repair (repair of a torn ligament).

- **Cosmetic surgery** is done to improve appearance (e.g., a face-lift).
- **Transplant surgery** replaces a malfunctioning body part, tissue, or organ. Joint replacements and organ replacement procedures are included in this category.
- **Procurement surgery** is related to transplant surgery. An organ or tissue is harvested from someone pronounced brain dead for transplantation into another person.

By Degree of Urgency

Based on the following definitions, how would you describe the degree of urgency for Mr. Singh's surgery?

- **Emergency surgery** requires transport to the operating suite as soon as possible to preserve the patient's life or function. The surgical team is summoned and preparations are made rapidly. Internal hemorrhage, rupture of an organ, and trauma are common causes of emergency surgery.
- **Urgent surgery** is scheduled within 24 to 48 hours to alleviate symptoms, repair a body part, or restore function. Removal of a cancerous breast and internal fixation of a fracture are examples.
- **Elective surgery** is performed when surgery is the recommended course of action, but the condition is not time sensitive. The client may delay surgery to gather information, consider options, or organize care for the family. Examples include repair of a torn ligament, removal of rectal polyps, or a rhinoplasty (repair of the nose).

By Degree of Risk

There is an old adage that "the only minor surgery is someone else's surgery." This statement reflects the anxiety that often accompanies surgery. Nevertheless, surgery is defined as major or minor based on the degree of seriousness or risk associated with the procedure. The degree of risk varies with the condition of the client as well as with the type of surgery.

Major surgery is associated with a high degree of risk. For example, it may be associated with the potential for significant blood loss, involve vital organs, be a prolonged or complicated procedure, or have significant potential for postoperative complications. Some examples of major procedures are coronary artery bypass graft (CABG), organ transplantation, nephrectomy (removal of a kidney), and colon resection. **Minor surgery**, often performed on an outpatient basis, involves little risk and usually has few complications. Examples include arthroscopy, breast biopsy, and inguinal hernia repair.

What Factors Affect Surgical Risk?

The patient's age, general health, and personal habits can contribute to increased risk during any surgical procedure.

Age The very young and very old are at greatest risk during surgical procedures. *Infants* have limited ability to regulate temperature and have immature immune, cardiovascular, liver, and renal systems. They are also at greater risk for infection, excess fluid volume, and deficient fluid volume. Even minor blood loss may represent a substantial portion of the infant's blood. In addition, infants may have difficulty calming. They are unable to understand what is happening, so you cannot use verbal reassurance and explanations to comfort them.

Toddlers understand simple explanations but may be anxious about separation from parents or caregivers. Many have fear of the dark. *Preschoolers* fear damage to body parts. Fear of pain or of needles is common for children of any age. *Teens* might fear disfigurement resulting from scars. *Young adults* commonly are anxious about the cost associated with hospitalization or surgery.

Older adults are at increased risk because they have less physiological reserve and often have comorbid conditions (other illness not related to the surgery). Many of the physiological changes of aging predispose older adults to increased risk. Among these changes are decreased kidney function, diminished immune function, decreased bone and lean body mass, increased peripheral vascular resistance, decreased cardiac output, decreased cough reflex, and increased time required for wound healing.

Type of Wound Both preexisting wounds (e.g., from trauma) and the wounds (incisions) created by the surgical procedure can pose a risk for infection (Table 39-1). Risk to the patient increases along with the risk for or presence of infection. Which type of wound will Mr. Singh have immediately after surgery?

Preexisting Conditions The ideal surgical candidate is a healthy young adult who takes no medications. Unfortunately, many surgical clients have underlying acute or chronic disorders that increase surgical risk (Box 39-2). Also see the accompanying PICOT box.

Mental Status Patients with altered cognition, from either physical or mental illness, may be unable to comprehend preoperative instructions or give informed consent for surgical procedures. They may also require medications (e.g., antipsychotic agents) that interact with anesthetics and analgesics given in the perioperative period. Surgery and anesthesia may aggravate preexisting dementia, confusion, and disorientation.

Medications Both prescribed and over-the-counter medications may increase surgical risk (Box 39-3). For example, patients who self-prescribe vitamin E may be at increased risk for bleeding. Certain herbal and alternative medications can:

- Increase the risk for cardiac dysrhythmias secondary to potassium loss.
- Interfere with metabolism of anesthetics because of their effects on the liver.

Table 39-1 ➤ Wound Type and Potential for Infection

WOUND TYPE	WOUND CHARACTERISTICS	EXAMPLES OF SURGERY ASSOCIATED WITH THE WOUND
Clean Wounds	Uninfected; minimal inflammation; little risk of infection AND Surgery does not involve the gastrointestinal, respiratory, or genitourinary tract.	Face-lift, cataract surgery, joint replacement, breast biopsy, tonsillectomy
Clean-Contaminated Wounds	Not infected, but carry increased risk for infection	Surgical incisions that enter the gastrointestinal, respiratory, or genitourinary tracts
Contaminated Wounds	Not infected, but carry high risk for infection	Surgery to repair trauma to open wounds, such as compound fractures; surgery in which a major break in surgical asepsis occurred
Infected Wounds	Evidence of infection, such as purulent drainage, necrotic tissue, or bacterial counts above 100,000 organisms per gram of tissue	A postoperative surgical incision of any type that has evidence of infection

---

BOX 39-2 ■ Preexisting Conditions That Increase Surgical Risk

Chronic Conditions

Cardiovascular diseases (such as hypertension, congestive heart failure, and myocardial infarction) affect the ability of the heart to work as an efficient pump. If these disorders are well controlled (e.g., with blood pressure medications or cardiotonic medications), risk is limited.

Coagulation disorders delay clotting and increase blood loss, placing the patient at risk for hemorrhage and hypovolemic shock. In contrast, a hypercoagulation state increases the risk of stroke, embolism, or intravascular clotting.

Chronic respiratory disorders (such as emphysema, asthma, or bronchitis) decrease pulmonary function, increase the risk of respiratory infection, and may be exacerbated (made worse) by general anesthesia.

Renal disease affects the patient's ability to excrete many medications, including anesthetic agents. It also affects the ability to regulate fluid and electrolytes.

Diabetes mellitus delays wound healing and increases the risk of infection and cardiovascular disorders associated with diabetes.

Liver disease affects the body's ability to metabolize amino acids, carbohydrates, and fat; to manufacture prothrombin for clotting; and to detoxify medications. Therefore, the patient is at increased risk for poor wound healing, hemorrhage, and toxic reactions to anesthetics and medications.

Neurological disorders (such as paralysis or spinal cord injury) increase the risk for vasomotor instability and thus create the potential for wide swings in blood pressure. In addition, patients with seizure disorders are more likely to have a seizure in the perioperative period.

Nutritional disorders can affect surgical outcomes. Patients who are malnourished or obese are at risk for delayed wound healing, infection, and fatigue. Obese clients are also more prone to cardiovascular disorders and impaired pulmonary function.

Acute Conditions

Upper respiratory tract infections are associated with increased risk of postoperative pneumonia, especially if the patient receives a general anesthetic.

Acute infections tax the patient's energy and physiological reserves, increasing the risk for various postoperative complications.

- Increase the potential for excessive bleeding.
- Decrease cerebral blood flow.
- Cause hypertension.
- Increase the effects of opioids and sympathetic nervous system stimulants.

For a list of herbal products and associated surgical risks,

 Go to Chapter 39, **ESG Box 39-1,** on Davis*Plus.*

Personal Habits Substance abuse can increase surgical risk. Smoking affects pulmonary function; long-term alcohol use contributes to liver disease, predisposing the patient to bleeding. Alcohol and drugs interact with anesthetic agents and medications to create adverse effects. Also, habitual substance abusers may have a cross-tolerance to anesthetic and analgesic agents, causing them to need higher than normal doses.

Allergies Patients may be allergic to medications (e.g., antibiotics, such as penicillins or cephalosporins), analgesics (e.g., codeine), tape, latex, and solutions used in surgery. Reactions range from unpleasant to life-threatening.

BOX 39-3 ■ Medications That Increase Surgical Risk

Antibiotics	May potentiate the action of anesthetic agents.
Anticoagulants	Increase risk for bleeding.
Antidysrhythmics	May impair cardiac function during anesthesia.
Antihypertensives	Increase the risk for hypotension during surgery; may interact with anesthetic agents to cause bradycardia and impaired circulation.
Aspirin	Increases risk for bleeding.
Corticosteroids	Delay wound healing and increase risk for infection.
Diuretics	Alter fluid and electrolyte balance (especially potassium balance).
Opioids	Increase the risk of respiratory depression.
NSAIDs	Inhibit platelet aggregation, increasing the risk for bleeding.
Tranquilizers	Increase the risk of respiratory depression.

KnowledgeCheck 39-1

- Define *preoperative phase*.
- What are four ways surgery can be classified?
- What factors affect surgical risk?

 ### ThinkLike a Nurse 39-1

How would you evaluate Mr. Singh's (Meet Your Patient) surgical risk? What additional information do you need to answer this question?

PracticalKnowledge
knowing how

The nursing focus in the preoperative phase is to prepare the patient for surgery. You will use the nursing process to identify any unique nursing diagnoses a patient might have. However, many perioperative nursing interventions are routine preventive measures that you will use for *all* surgical patients.

Perioperative Nursing Data Set

The Perioperative Nursing Data Set (PNDS) is a standardized vocabulary specifically designed to describe the care of perioperative patients. It is the first nursing language developed by a specialty organization that has been recognized by the American Nurses Association (ANA). The latest update of PNDS reflects the nursing process including nursing assessment, diagnoses, identified nursing-sensitive outcomes, nursing interventions, and implementation and evaluation. The PDNS promotes better communication among nurses and other healthcare providers, increases visibility of

---

PICOT

Older Adults, Comorbidity, and Risk for Surgical Site Infection

Situation: The student is caring for an elderly patient who is four days postoperative after a colon resection. The abdominal incision is reddened, with purulent yellow drainage on the dressing. The patient has a history of chronic obstructive pulmonary disease (COPD), and obesity (BMI of 31).

PICOT Components

P	Population/patient	= Older adults
I	Intervention/indicator	= Chronic disease and comorbidity
C	Comparator/control	= No health problems
O	Outcome	= Increased risk of incision infection
T	Time	= After surgery

Searchable Question

Do _____ (P) who receive/are exposed to _____ (I), as compared to _____ (C), demonstrate _____ (O) during _____ (T)?

Example of Evidence: Surgical site infections (SSIs) account for roughly 11% of hospital-acquired infections in patients age 65 and older. Older people who experience SSIs tend to have a worse clinical outcome than do younger adults. Researchers evaluated cases of elderly patients with SSIs, and identified several independent predictors of surgical site infections. These include obesity, COPD, congestive heart failure, American Society of Anesthesiologists grade of ≥3, wound class >2, and socioeconomic factors.

Application to Practice: Patients with these risk factors can be identified preoperatively, and nursing care adjusted to decrease the potential for SSIs.

Source: Kaye, K., Sloane, R., Sexton, D., et al. (2006). Risk factors for surgical site infections in older people. *Journal of the American Geriatrics Society, 54*(3), 391–396. doi:http://dx.doi.org/10.1111

nursing interventions, improves patient care, and standardizes a way to evaluate nursing care outcomes (Peterson & Kleiner, 2011).

In this chapter, we continue to use the NANDA-I, NOC, and NIC standardized languages, to which you have already been introduced in previous chapters.

Perioperative Patient-Focused Model The PNDS is derived from the Perioperative Patient-Focused Model. The patient is at the center of the model and the focus of care. The perioperative nurse intervenes within the context of the healthcare system to assist the patient throughout the perioperative experience to achieve outcomes in the Health System domain and the Patient-Centered domains (which include Safety, Physiological Responses to Surgery, and Behavioral Responses to Surgery).

The Health System domain refers to the system in which perioperative care is given. It involves administrative and structural elements necessary for successful surgical outcomes—for example, equipment, supplies, staff, and policies (AORN, 2009, updated 2011).

ASSESSMENT

For patient safety, patient data must be correct and complete. To prevent omission of important information, many organizations have developed a preoperative checklist. Although the forms may vary at each institution, the areas for assessment are the same and are discussed in the sections that follow.

Focused Nursing History

It is essential to determine whether the client is physiologically, cognitively, and psychologically prepared for the intraoperative and postoperative phases of surgery. For an accurate nursing history, collect assessment data from the client, significant others, medical records, and other members of the healthcare team. Include the following topics in your preoperative assessment: health history, physical status, allergies, medications (including herbal products and over-the-counter medications), mental status, knowledge and understanding of the surgery and anesthesia, cultural and spiritual factors, access to social resources, coping strategies, and use of alcohol and drugs. It is also important to elicit patients' values and expressed needs (see the accompanying Quality and Safety Education for Nurses box).

To see an example of a preoperative assessment form developed by the AORN,

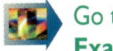 Go to Chapter 39, **Assessment Guidelines and Tools, Example of a Preoperative Checklist,** in Volume 2.

Additional assessments may be needed if the client is undergoing outpatient surgery or has a planned short stay after surgery (see the Home Care box Preoperative Assessment for the Surgical Client Who Will Be Discharged to Home).

Quality and Safety Education for Nurses

Quality and Safety for Perioperative Patients

Chapter Key Concepts: Perioperative Nursing, Preoperative Care, Intraoperative Care, Postoperative Care

Competency: Patient-Centered Care

Eliciting each patient's values, preferences, and expressed needs as part of the focused nursing history will assist you in meeting the QSEN (2012) competency of patient-centered care. You can then communicate patient values, preferences, and expressed needs to other members of the healthcare team to assure patient-centered care with sensitivity and respect for the diversity of individual patients.

Competency: Teamwork and Collaboration

To provide for effective participation within nursing and inter-professional teams, nurses must foster open communication, mutual respect, and shared decision making with the goal of quality patient care (Cronenwett, Sherwood, Pohl, et al., 2007).

Surgical briefings encourage team members to talk when there is no problem, so they are more likely to speak up when they have misgivings when problems occur (Hendrickson, Wadhera, & El Bardissi, 2008). Two-minute briefings led by the attending surgeon, using a standardized format, just before surgery have been found to improve communication and reduce delays and wrong-site surgery (Makary, Mukherjee, Sexton, et al., 2007).

To see a description of the knowledge, skills, and attitudes you need for achieving this competency,

 Go to the QSEN Web site, at www.qsen.org/ksas_ prelicensure.php

---

Home Care

Preoperative Assessment for the Surgical Client Who Will Be Discharged to Home

The type of surgery, the client's condition, and the support system determine whether it is safe to discharge a client to home after surgery. Your assessment for home care should focus on these questions:

➤ What kind of care will be needed?

➤ Is the client able to take care of himself? If not, who is available to assist with care?

➤ Does the caregiver have the necessary skills to provide care?

➤ If not, can these skills be taught before the client is discharged?

➤ What features in the home environment will facilitate the client's progress? What features will inhibit progress? For example, can the client get to the bathroom? Can the client negotiate the stairs in the house?

➤ How will the client be followed after discharge? That is, how soon should he visit his physician? Will he receive home nursing care?

Focused Physical Assessment

If you identify risk factors from the nursing history, focus on these aspects during your brief head-to-toe physical assessment. For example, if the patient states she had a cough last week, perform a focused assessment of the ear, nose, throat, and lungs to determine how the cough may affect the patient's risk. If the patient has lower airway congestion, as evidenced by rhonchi and productive cough, communicate these findings to the surgeon and the anesthesia team; if a general anesthetic is planned, it may be necessary to delay the surgery. For all patients, assess risk factors for thrombophlebitis, as venous thrombus is one of the never events that can lead to potentially life-threatening pulmonary emboli. For additional details on a brief (bedside) physical assessment, see Chapter 22.

 Recent guidelines state that optimal preoperative assessment of older adults include:

- cognitive ability
- capacity to understand the surgery
- nutritional status
- risk factors for postoperative delirium and pulmonary complications
- patient's treatment goals and expectations
- family and social support system
- depression
- cardiac status
- functional status
- history of falls
- detailed medication history, including polypharmacy
- baseline frailty score
- diagnostic tests specific to elderly patients (Chow, Ko, Rosenthal, et al., n.d.)

Diagnostic Testing

Preoperative screening tests are usually prescribed before surgical procedures. The type of testing depends on the patient's age, health history, and facility policies. For example, most institutions require a complete blood count and urinalysis before surgery, as well as an electrocardiogram for patients older than age 50. Routine chest radiology (x-ray) is not recommended for all patients prior to surgery. Chest x-ray incurs extra costs to the healthcare system and exposes patients to small risks from radiation exposure (National Guideline Clearinghouse [NGC], 2011). Patients with chronic health problems, including cardiopulmonary disease, may require additional testing.

 Age alone is not a risk factor for postoperative complications, but older adults with multiple comorbidities (other medical conditions), such as cardiovascular or pulmonary disease, may be at risk for postoperative complications. Further preoperative screening may be ordered for older adults to identify risk factors for perioperative and postoperative complications and to optimize patient condition prior to surgery.

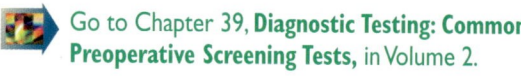
Go to Chapter 39, **Diagnostic Testing: Common Preoperative Screening Tests**, in Volume 2.

 KnowledgeCheck 39-2
- List the information you should gather in the preoperative nursing history.
- What type of physical assessment is performed as part of the preoperative assessment?
- What laboratory tests are most commonly prescribed before surgery?

ThinkLike a Nurse 39-2
- What factors will affect your preoperative assessment of Mr. Singh (Meet Your Patient)?
- Describe how you might perform the assessment as well as provide physical care. What modifications, if any, should you make in his assessment?

ANALYSIS/NURSING DIAGNOSIS

As you learned in Chapter 4, nursing diagnoses describe the individualized needs of patients. However, preoperative patients share a common set of needs, regardless of their individual differences and the type of surgery they are to have. Consider the following examples:

- All preoperative patients need preoperative teaching, so it's not necessary to write a nursing diagnosis of Deficient Knowledge for every patient. Agency protocols or critical pathways will almost certainly mandate teaching.
- Almost all surgical patients have at least mild anxiety, and many of your routine actions will help to relieve anxiety, so there is no need to always include a diagnosis of Anxiety.

Key Point: *Do not put any nursing diagnosis on the care plan unless you plan to address it with something other than the routine preoperative interventions.*

Individualized Nursing Diagnoses

Individualized nursing diagnoses for the preoperative patient evolve from your assessment. You should identify an actual nursing diagnosis only if the patient has the defining characteristics for it. Identify risk (potential) diagnoses only if the patient has an underlying condition that places him at higher risk than the average surgical patient. The following NANDA-I nursing diagnoses may be useful for certain preoperative patients:

- *Anxiety* may be mild, moderate, severe, or at panic level. In the preoperative client, anxiety may be related to the current change in health status or due to concerns about being unable to provide care for loved ones. Make this diagnosis only if the client has symptoms such as restlessness, trembling, increased pulse, and other defining characteristics.
- *Fear* is a common reaction to surgery. Fear may be related to the unknown outcome of the surgery, to learning the diagnosis after a diagnostic procedure, and to the prospect of pain during and after surgery. Fear

and Anxiety share several defining characteristics. Many of the routine preoperative interventions help to address Fear.

- **Ineffective airway clearance** may be used for patients who have a preexisting health problem, such as bronchitis or emphysema.
- **Disturbed Sleep Pattern** often results from anxiety about the upcoming surgery.
- **Ineffective Coping** may be appropriate for a patient with extreme anxiety and concerns about the outcomes of the surgery.
- **Latex Allergy Response** is appropriate for patients who have a known allergy to latex.
- **Risk for Latex Allergy Response** is appropriate for patients who have had multiple surgeries or urinary catheterizations; are in professions with daily exposure to latex; have a history of asthma; or are allergic to bananas, avocados, kiwi, chestnuts, or poinsettia plants. Do not use it routinely for all patients.
- **Deficient Knowledge.** As you know, you do not usually need a Deficient Knowledge diagnosis. If you believe the patient may not learn, or that the information is too complex to remember, then identify the problem likely to result from the Deficient Knowledge. For example:

Ineffective Management of Therapeutic Regimen related to Deficient Knowledge of postoperative medications and office visits

Risk for Infection related to Deficient Knowledge of wound care and asepsis

Special Risks for Older Adults

Older adults, especially those older than age 70 and the frail elderly, are likely to need some individualized nursing diagnoses. They present unique risks not only because they often have other illnesses, but also because of certain physiological changes of aging. For example, older adults metabolize anesthetic agents differently from younger adults (see Table 39-2)

ThinkLike a Nurse 39-3

Which, if any, of the preceding nursing diagnoses would be most appropriate for Mr. Singh (Meet Your Patient)? Do not use the potential complications in Table 39-2. Explain your reasoning.

Table 39-2 ▶ Special Risks for Older Adults

RISK FACTORS	POTENTIAL COMPLICATIONS (PC) AND NURSING DIAGNOSES
Most older adults have at least some degree of coronary artery disease.	■ PC: Hypotension ■ Risk for Falls secondary to orthostatic hypotension
Delirium is one of the most common surgical complications in older adults. Predisposing factors include being older than 75 years, preoperative hyperglycemia or hypoglycemia, psychological distress, preoperative cognitive impairment, inadequate nutrition, and functional impairment (Brooks, 2012)	■ PC: Delirium
Age-related respiratory changes, such as decreased chest wall compliance, forced vital capacity, and diaphragmatic strength	■ PC: Pneumonia ■ PC: Atelectasis
Age-related skin changes: Dry, fragile skin; decreased turgor and elasticity	■ Risk for Impaired Skin Integrity ■ Risk for Impaired Tissue Integrity
Age-related musculoskeletal changes: Decreased bone mass and muscle fiber mass	■ Risk for Impaired Mobility ■ Risk for Falls
Comorbidities of the central nervous system are more common in older adults. Some conditions may be aggravated by surgery and anesthesia.	■ PC: Dementia ■ Risk for Acute Confusion
Age-related decrease in gastrointestinal motility	■ PC: Ileus ■ Risk for Aspiration secondary to vomiting
Age-related decreases in genitourinary function: decreased bladder tone, elasticity, and tone; decreased renal function	■ PC: Side effects of medications ■ PC: Renal complications ■ PC: Urinary tract infection ■ Risk for Impaired Skin Integrity r/t urinary incontinence

PLANNING OUTCOMES/EVALUATION

The overall nursing goal in the preoperative phase is to prepare the patient adequately for surgery and to deliver him to the operating suite in the best condition possible. Outcomes that provide evidence of achieving this goal, and that are appropriate for nearly all preoperative patients, are that the patient:

- Is able to describe his surgical procedure in a basic manner.
- Provides informed consent.
- When asked, states what he can expect in the postoperative period.
- States he has very little anxiety.

Associated NOC outcomes for the preoperative nursing client depend, of course, on the nursing diagnoses you identify. For outcomes and goals using NOC terminology for the diagnoses Anxiety, Fear, Deficient Knowledge, and Disturbed Sleep Pattern, and for *individualized goals/ outcome statements* you might write for those diagnoses,

 Go to Chapter 39, **Standardized Language, Preoperative Patients—Selected Standardized Nursing Diagnoses, Outcomes, and Interventions,** in Volume 2.

PLANNING INTERVENTIONS/IMPLEMENTATION

For *NIC standardized interventions* designed to achieve the expected outcomes for the nursing diagnoses of Anxiety, Fear, Deficient Knowledge, and Disturbed Sleep Pattern,

 Go to Chapter 39, **Standardized Language, Preoperative Patients—Selected Standardized Nursing Diagnoses, Outcomes, and Interventions,** in Volume 2.

Many preoperative nursing activities are routine interventions to be used for *all* preoperative patients, regardless of their nursing diagnoses. NIC has a special Perioperative Care domain (category) for such interventions. The following are the preoperative NIC interventions in that domain:

- *Preoperative Coordination:* Facilitating preadmission diagnostic testing and preparation of the surgical patient. (Activity example: Notify the physician of abnormal diagnostic test results.)
- *Surgical Preparation:* Providing care to a patient immediately before surgery and verifying required procedures/tests and documentation in the clinical record. (Activity example: Complete the preoperative checklist.)
- *Teaching: Preoperative:* Assisting a patient to understand and mentally prepare for surgery and the postoperative recovery period. (Activity example: Correct unrealistic expectations of the surgery, as appropriate.)

The following sections explain in more detail how to carry out routine interventions such as obtaining informed consent for the surgery, providing preoperative teaching, communicating with the surgical team, preparing the client physically, and transferring to the operating suite. Be sure to include parents and caregivers in your plan of care.

Confirm That Surgical Consent Has Been Obtained

Before a surgical procedure is performed, professional standards and the law require the surgeon to obtain the patient's informed consent. The signed consent form verifies that the surgeon and patient have communicated adequately about the surgery (Dale, Rothrock, & McEwen, 2011). Once signed and witnessed, the consent form is part of the patient's record and accompanies him to the operating room.

Key Point: *The surgeon is responsible for (1) giving the patient the necessary information and (2) determining the patient's competence to make an informed decision about the surgery. You are responsible for verifying that the surgical consent form is signed and witnessed.*

Often you will obtain the signature and document on the preoperative checklist that you have done so. As a patient advocate, you should first verify with the patient that the physician has explained the procedure and answered all his questions: Ask the patient to state what he was told during the consent process. If the patient has questions or if you have any questions about the patient's competence, notify the surgeon, and delay sending the patient to surgery. Be sure to document these conversations, and document in the nursing notes that the surgeon was notified of any additional questions or concerns.

The surgical consent form includes the following information (The Joint Commission, 2010):

- The type of surgery being performed
- The name and qualifications of the person performing the surgery (e.g., Jason Esmar, MD) and the primary practitioner for the patient's care and treatment
- A statement that the risks and benefits of surgery, as well as reasonable alternatives, have been explained to the patient
- A statement of the relevant risks, benefits, and side effects of the alternatives
- The likelihood of achieving goals
- A statement that the patient has the right to refuse surgery or withdraw consent at any time
- When indicated, any limitations on the confidentiality of information about the patient

Informed consent requires that the patient understood the communication and was not coerced (pressured) to consent. The patient must be alert, rational, mentally competent, and not sedated when he signs; and the information must be given to him in a language and vocabulary that he can understand. Patients who are unconscious or have a mental disability; who have been judged insane; who cannot read, write, or hear; and those under the influence of sedative drugs or alcohol are generally not competent to give consent (Buppert, 2012). In most states a family member, conservator, or legal guardian may give consent for the procedure. If you would like more information on informed consent, see Chapters 44 and 45.

Informed consent helps protect patients from having a surgery they do not understand or want, and the signed document protects the healthcare agency and workers from later claims that the patient did not consent to have the procedure.

KnowledgeCheck 39-3

- Who is responsible for obtaining informed consent for the surgical procedure?
- What are the nursing responsibilities related to informed consent?

Provide Preoperative Teaching

Preoperative teaching prepares the patient for the surgical experience, allays fears, and decreases the risks of postoperative complications. See Chapter 19 as needed to review patient teaching.

What to Teach

The content of the teaching plan should focus on:

- What will happen before, during, and after surgery
- How the patient or caregiver can participate in the care
- Common feelings and concerns that patients have about surgery. This helps the patient feel supported and less anxious.
- What patients and families can do to prevent surgical site infection (The Joint Commission, 2012). Teach patients the content in the Self-Care box Teaching Patients How to Help Prevent Surgical Site Infections.

The type of surgery influences the content of your teaching. For example, if the patient is scheduled for an outpatient knee arthroscopy (visualization of the joint) under spinal anesthesia, the teaching plan needs to describe the procedure and the anticipated discharge of the patient within hours after surgery. This is different from the teaching for a patient who will have cardiac surgery and spend a number of days in the hospital. You will find specific teaching content in the teaching interventions for the Deficient Knowledge diagnosis, in the Standardized Language table in Volume 2. Also refer to Clinical Insight 39-1, in Volume 2.

 Go to Chapter 39, **Standardized Language, Preoperative Patients: Selected Standardized Nursing Diagnoses, Outcomes, and Interventions,** in Volume 2.

 Go to Chapter 39, **Clinical Insight 39-1: Preoperative Teaching,** in Volume 2.

Self-Care

Teaching Patients How to Help Prevent Surgical Site Infections

Before Surgery

➤ If you smoke, stop. Those who smoke are more likely to get infections.

➤ Discuss your health problems with your surgeon (e.g., diabetes, allergies). These can affect incision healing.

➤ Ask your surgeon whether you should have antibiotics before surgery.

➤ Don't shave near where you will have surgery. Not all procedures require hair removal, but if they do, it should be done with electric clippers. If someone starts to use a razor to shave you, speak up.

After Surgery

➤ Be sure family and friends wash their hands or use alcohol-based handrub before and after they visit you.

➤ When anyone examines you or checks your incision ask them if they have washed their hands (or used alcohol-based handrub).

➤ Wash your hands before and after caring for your own incision.

➤ Do not allow family and friends to touch your incision or the surgical dressing.

➤ Be sure you know how to care for your incision before you go home.

➤ If you have fever or redness, pain, or drainage at the surgery site, call your physician right away.

Source: Adapted from Centers for Disease Control and Prevention. (n.d., updated 2011). Having surgery? What you should know before you go. Retrieved from http://www.cdc.gov/features/SafeSurgery/

For the complete steps of deep breathing, coughing, moving in bed, and leg exercises,

 Go to Chapter 39, **Procedure 39-1: Teaching a Patient to Deep-Breathe, Cough, Move in Bed, and Perform Leg Exercises,** in Volume 2.

How to Teach

You can use written instructions, video presentations, phone contact, or face-to-face discussion to provide preoperative teaching. Teach in a language the patient understands and at a level that is easily understood. Use terms the patient understands clearly—that is, avoid medical jargon. See Chapter 19 if you need to review patient teaching techniques and information about health literacy.

Obtain an interpreter for translation if the patient speaks a language that you do not speak. When possible, avoid using family members as translators to protect the patient's privacy or avoid a bias in translation (see Chapter 15 if you need more information about language differences).

Include family members in the teaching as much as possible and as much as desired by the patient, especially if the patient is a child or dependent adult. So that the child better understands what will happen before, during, and after surgery, you might teach using dolls or age-appropriate toys. Play is an effective way for children to learn (e.g., have the child give medicine to her doll with an empty syringe or listen to its "heart" with your stethoscope). Simple language is a must! For example, you'd say to a young child, "Lie on your tummy, please."

Older adults may experience physical, psychological, and/or psychosocial issues that impair their ability to learn. Decreased hearing, vision, and sense of touch may interfere with their ability understand and remember information. To increase understanding, provide an environment conducive to learning, allow for more time for the patient to process information, and provide written material that clearly conveys the essentials.

When to Teach

For elective surgery, many patients have a scheduled preoperative assessment about a week before the surgery. The session may include preoperative testing, an appointment with the anesthesia staff, signing the consent form, and planned preoperative teaching.

Patients undergoing emergency surgery usually require extensive physical care preoperatively. You may need to give IV fluids, transfuse blood, treat for pain, and administer many medications, as in the case of Mr. Singh (Meet Your Patient). Because of the urgency of some surgeries, you may have limited time for preoperative teaching. However, you should always teach the patient as much as possible to prepare him for the surgical experience.

Prepare the Patient Physically for Surgery

Physical preparation of the patient for surgery involves several nursing concerns.

Maintaining Normothermia Recent evidence-based guidelines stress that maintaining a normal body temperature helps produce good surgical outcomes (Hooper, Chard, Clifford, et al., 2010; Joanna Briggs Institute, 2010). In addition to monitoring temperature, you can provide passive thermal care measures, such as providing blankets, socks, and head coverings; and keeping the room temperature at or above 75°F (24°C). If the patient is hypothermic you can use forced-air warming gowns or mattresses to pre-warm patients before surgery as well as in the intraoperative and postoperative periods.

Nutritional Status Anxiety and anesthesia reduce gastrointestinal motility. To decrease the risk of nausea and vomiting, patients usually fast, taking no food or liquids (NPO) for 8 hours before surgery. Stress to patients

and family the importance of fasting (for the prescribed length of time) to avoid the danger of aspiration. You should know, though, that years of evidence support shorter fasting times than you will see used in most institutions. The American Society of Anesthesiologists preoperative fasting guidelines for healthy patients recommends ingesting clear liquids up to 2 hours before surgery—and even a light meal up to 6 hours before surgery (Crenshaw, 2011; "Practice Guidelines for Preoperative Fasting," 2011).

Skin Preparation Depending on the surgery and facility, patients may be asked to shower or scrub the surgical site with soap or an antibacterial solution (e.g., 4% chlorhexadine gluconate, Betadine) the evening before surgery and the morning of the surgery. Studies demonstrate that this reduces bacterial colonization on the skin, but do not clearly prove that it reduces surgical infection (National Guideline Clearinghouse [NGC], 2008a; National Institute for Health and Clinical Excellence [NICE], 2008). Final skin preparation and hair removal, if done, should be completed before taking the patient into the surgical suite.

Bowel Preparation Enemas are now used primarily for surgical procedures of the colon, not for all surgeries. To empty the colon of feces, patients are asked to consume a low-residue diet for several days before surgery and are given a regimen of medications and/or enemas to clear the bowel. Stress the importance of adhering to the regimen to limit the risk of contaminating the operative site with feces.

Urinary Elimination Indwelling catheters are not routinely inserted for surgery. Catheterization may be prescribed if it is important to keep the bladder empty during surgery, if fluid status is being carefully monitored, or if surgery is expected to last for a prolonged period of time.

> ✚ If a catheter is not prescribed, have the patient void before receiving preoperative medications. The patient could fall if he gets out of bed to use the bathroom after being sedated or given opioids for pain.

Preoperative Medications The anesthesiologist may prescribe preoperative medications to relax the patient, reduce respiratory secretions, or reduce the risk of vomiting and aspiration (Table 39-3). If the surgery time is known, the medication is prescribed at a prearranged time (e.g., at 0615). If not, it may be prescribed to give "on call." You will give the on-call medication when the surgical suite staff notifies you it is time to do so.

Antibiotics are often administered prophylactically to help prevent postoperative infections in patients before:

- clean surgery involving the placement of a prosthesis or implant
- clean-contaminated surgery
- contaminated surgery

Table 39-3 ➤ Preoperative Medications

TYPE OF MEDICATION	USE	EXAMPLES
Antibiotics	Reduce the microbial burden of intraoperative contamination to a level that cannot overwhelm host defenses	Cephalosporins (e.g., cefazolin, cefoxitin), clindamycin, vancomycin
Anticholinergics (e.g., phenothiazines)	Reduce oral and pulmonary secretions, prevent laryngospasms, prevent bradycardia	Atropine (Atropisol), chlorpromazine (Thorazine), scopolamine (Hyoscine), glycopyrrolate (Robinul)
Anxiolytics (e.g., benzodiazepines)	Control anxiety, calming	Alprazolam (Xanax), clonazepam (Klonopin), diazepam (Valium), lorazepam (Ativan), midazolam (Versed)
Antihistamines	Provide sedation and antiemetic effects	Hydroxyzine (Vistaril), diphenhydramine (Benadryl)
Barbiturates	Provide sedation without significant cardiopulmonary depression	Secobarbital (Seconal), pentobarbital (Nembutal)
H_2 receptor antagonists	Reduce gastric acidity	Cimetidine (Tagamet), ranitidine (Zantac)
Hypnotics	Provide sedation and increase the duration of sleep	Temazepam (Restoril)
Neuroleptics	Provide sedative, antiemetic, and anticonvulsant effects	Droperidol (Inapsine), Innovar (fentanyl and droperidol)
Opioid analgesics	Provide pain relief and sedation; induce anesthesia	Fentanyl (Sublimaze), meperidine (Demerol), morphine (Duramorph)

You will usually administer the antibiotic intravenously timed so that a bactericidal concentration of the drug will be present in the serum and tissues by the time the incision is made (usually within the hour preceding incision, just as the patient is going to the surgical suite (NGC, 2008a; NICE, 2008). Antibiotics may, instead, be given at the start of anesthesia and repeated if the surgery is longer than the duration of the antibiotic.

Routine Medications Many routine medications are held (not administered) on the day of surgery. For example, an insulin-dependent diabetic patient may be instructed to hold her morning injection or administer half of the normal dose. The patient needs less insulin because her NPO status will keep her blood sugar lower than usual. The anesthesiologist will monitor the blood sugar in the operating room and give additional insulin if needed. Some patients may be instructed to stop routine medications several days before surgery. For example, a client receiving warfarin for anticoagulation may need to stop the medication 7 days before surgery.

Prostheses Before being transported to the operating suite, the patient must remove all artificial body parts, such as dentures, artificial limbs, or contact lenses. Wigs, eyeglasses, makeup, and jewelry must also be removed.

Antiembolism Stockings Also referred to as thromboembolic disorder hose (or "TED hose"), **antiembolism stockings** are elastic stockings that compress the veins of the legs and increase venous return to the heart (Fig. 39-1). They may be applied preoperatively to prevent venous pooling during surgery and decrease the risk of thrombus formation. Along with prophylactic medications (antithrombotics), antiembolism stockings aid in the prevention of DVT and PE (*Morbidity and Mortality Weekly Report*, June 8, 2012). However, hospitals are increasingly using sequential compression devices and anticoagulation therapy, instead of elastic stockings, to prevent DVT (Perry, Borchert, Burke, et al., 2012).

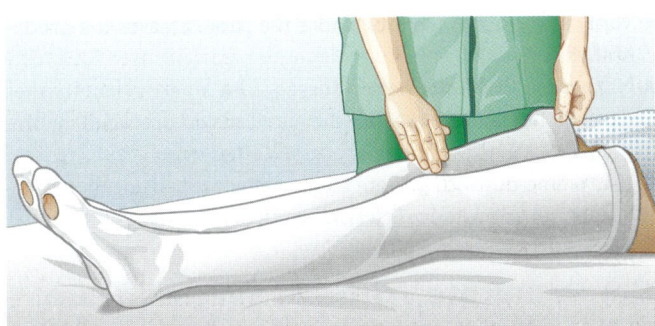

FIGURE 39-1 Antiembolism stockings compress the veins of the legs and increase venous return to the heart.

Older adults and those with risk factors for venous thromboembolism are most in need of antiembolism stockings (Bartley, 2006). Risk factors include the following conditions (AORN, 2009, updated 2011):

- Venous stasis (such as occurs with bedrest, lengthy surgery, varicose veins, and heart failure)
- Vascular wall injury, which initiates clotting (e.g., surgery, IV catheter, irritating IV drugs, prior DVT, smoking).
- Hypercoagulability (e.g., estrogen therapy, oral contraceptive use, cancer, dehydration, pregnancy)

 Older adults may be at higher risk for DVT because they have more than one of these risk factors. Safety measures to prevent DVT in older adults include range-of-motion (ROM) exercises and applying antiembolism stockings to prevent pooling of blood in the extremities (Bashaw & Scott, 2012)

Antiembolism stockings may extend from foot to knee, or foot to thigh, although the Institute for Clinical Systems Improvement (ICSI) suggests that thigh-high stockings be avoided because of their tendency to roll and restrict circulation (Perry, Borchert, Burke, et al., 2012). Some stockings have an opening at the toes that allows you to assess circulation in the feet.

Stockings must be sized and applied correctly to be effective. Stockings are contraindicated for some patients (e.g., those with peripheral arterial disease) (The Joanna Briggs Institute, 2008b; Winslow & Brosz, 2008).

The procedure for applying antiembolism stockings is summarized in the Highlights of Procedures box. For complete steps,

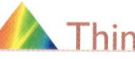 Go to Chapter 39, **Procedure 39-2: Applying Antiembolism Stockings,** in Volume 2.

Take Measures to Prevent Wrong Patient, Wrong Site, Wrong Surgery

The following safety measures will help prevent patient misidentification and wrong-site surgery (The Joint Commission, 2012; Reid, 2011):

- Use a preoperative checklist to confirm that appropriate documents are available and the appropriate activities have been performed.
- Verify the patient's identity before the patient leaves the preoperative area.
- Mark the surgical site before surgery. Use a permanent marker that will not be removed by the surgical skin prep, and involve the patient in the marking process.
- Take a time-out with all team members before starting the procedure (see Perioperative Safety, near the beginning of this chapter).

Communicate With the Surgical Team

The most common root cause of medical errors is communication failure (AHRQ, 2003). For this reason, good communication is essential for patient safety in perioperative care. The following are elements of successful communication among the surgical team. Team members:

- Receive a summary of the plan of care (e.g., a short briefing by the surgeon) and develop a shared understanding of the plan.
- Speak up and are assertive with concerns about the procedure or decisions.
- Ask questions to clarify confusion.
- Acknowledge that they have heard and understood.
- Ask for and provide feedback (e.g., read back) on critical information.
- Use standard terminology (e.g., checklists). In one large, long-term study, use of surgical checklists was found to reduce the number of deaths from surgery by more than 40% (Haynes, Weiser, Berry, et al., 2009).

Two-minute briefings just before surgery, led by the attending surgeon using a standardized format, have been found to improve communication and reduce delays and wrong-site surgery (Makary, Mukherjee, Sexton, et al., 2007). Surgical briefings encourage team members to talk when there is no problem, so they are more likely to speak up when they have misgivings or when problems occur (Hendrickson, Wadhera, & El Bardissi, 2008).

Also see the preceding Quality and Safety Education for Nurses box.

KnowledgeCheck 39-4

- Identify topics that should be discussed in preoperative teaching.
- Describe the typical physical preparation of a client undergoing surgery.

ThinkLike a Nurse 39-4

- What aspects of preoperative teaching should you stress when caring for Mr. Singh (Meet Your Patient)?
- A bowel preparation is typically part of preoperative preparation for a client having colon surgery. Do you think this will be part of Mr. Singh's physical preparation? Why or why not?

Transfer Patient to the Operative Suite

Once you have completed your preoperative care, the patient is ready for transport by stretcher to the operative area, usually to the surgical holding area (Fig. 39-2). The completed preoperative checklist and the patient's chart must accompany the patient. Lock up valuables according to agency policy, or have the patient's family keep them. Occasionally, especially if the patient has a significant sensory deficit, the patient can wear his hearing aid or glasses to the surgical suite. You will need to arrange this in advance with the surgical staff or anesthesia team.

Often children are permitted to bring a favorite toy with them to the operating room (OR) to provide comfort.

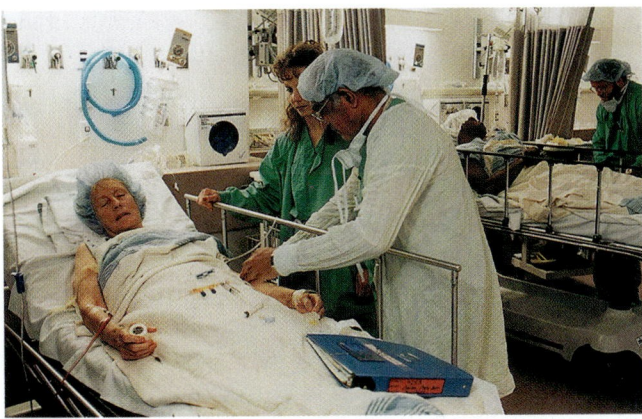

FIGURE 39-2 Surgical holding area.

Children may fear being separated from their parents, so arrange for parents to spend time with the child immediately before the surgery and as soon as possible after the surgery. Keep the parents informed, and let them know what to expect.

Prepare the Postoperative Room

If you transfer the patient to the surgical suite from a nursing unit in the hospital, you should prepare the room for the patient's return after surgery. Put clean linens on the bed and arrange the supplies and equipment you will need. For an illustration and complete instructions;

 Go to Chapter 39, **Clinical Insight 39-2: Preparing a Room for a Patient's Return From Surgery,** and Chapter 11, **Clinical Insight 11-1, Preparing the Room for a Newly Admitted Patient,** in Volume 2.

INTRAOPERATIVE CARE

The **intraoperative phase** begins when the patient enters the operating suite and ends when she is admitted to the postanesthesia care unit.

Theoretical Knowledge
knowing **why**

To provide intraoperative care, you will need theoretical knowledge of the roles of the various members of the intraoperative team and of the different types of anesthesia that are used.

Operative Personnel

The personnel who attend the client during the surgical procedure are called the *intraoperative team*. The team is divided into members who must use sterile technique and those who use clean technique (see Chapter 23 if you need to review medical and surgical asepsis). During the

intraoperative phase, a registered nurse can function as the scrub nurse, circulating nurse, or registered nurse first assistant. Each of these roles contributes to the safe care of surgical clients.

Sterile Team Members of the sterile intraoperative team include the surgeon, surgical assistant, and scrub person. Before beginning the surgery, they perform a surgical scrub of the hands and arms, dry with sterile towels, and don sterile gowns and gloves. To review these procedures, see Chapter 23.

The **scrub nurse** can be an RN, LVN/LPN, or a surgical technician. The scrub nurse sets up the sterile field, prepares the surgical instruments, assists with the sterile draping of the patient, anticipates and responds to the surgeon's needs, and maintains the integrity of the sterile field. The **registered nurse first assistant (RNFA)** is an RN with additional education and training in surgical technique and is also part of the sterile team. The RNFA serves as an assistant to the surgeon, a role that has historically been filled by physicians. The RNFA may be employed by the surgeon or the hospital.

Sterile team members are the only persons allowed to enter the sterile field. The sterile field encompasses the client and the area immediately surrounding the client. Creation of the operative field is explained in:

 Chapter 39, **Clinical Insight 39-3: Creating an Operative Field,** in Volume 2.

Clean Team Team members who abide by clean technique (medical asepsis) include the anesthesiologist or nurse anesthetist, the circulating RN, biomedical technicians, and radiology technicians. These personnel never enter the sterile field, but instead function around and beyond it.

An **anesthesiologist** or a **nurse anesthetist (CRNA)** induces amnesia, analgesia, and muscle relaxation or paralysis with anesthesia. His role is to continuously monitor and evaluate the patient's responses to the anesthetic agent and the surgical procedure. CRNAs administer more than half of all anesthetics in the United States.

The **circulating nurse** is a registered nurse who applies the nursing process to coordinate all activities in the operating room. She is a strong client advocate who continuously monitors the client and the sterile field. The circulating nurse maintains a safe, comfortable environment, communicates with appropriate personnel outside the operating room, manages care of the intraoperative client, and responds to emergencies. An important aspect of the circulating nurse's role is to attend to the patient during the induction of anesthesia.

KnowledgeCheck 39-5

- Identify the intraoperative nursing roles that are part of the sterile intraoperative team and those that are part of the clean intraoperative team.
- Which nursing roles are always held by a registered nurse?

Toward Evidence-Based Practice

White, J., Khan, W., & Smitham, P. (2011) Perioperative implications of surgery in elderly patients with hip fractures: An evidence-based review. *Journal of Perioperative Practice*, 21(6), 192–197.

Older adults are at higher risk for complications following surgery owing to many factors including comorbidities and a depressed physiological state. Older adults are also more likely to experience poor postoperative pain management, pressure ulcer development, venous thromboembolism, and postoperative confusion/dementia. The authors reviewed current research studies to develop an evidence-based approach to decrease complications in the postoperative period. To improve outcomes for older adults, the authors recommend that they are put in the best physiological state prior to having surgery, are cared for by a multidisciplinary team approach, and experience careful and frequent assessment to identify risks factors and changes in their condition. Evidence-based management of patient complications is essential to assure the best outcomes possible.

Egol, K. A., & Strauss, E. J. (2009). Perioperative considerations in geriatric patients with hip fracture: What is the evidence? *Journal of Orthopedic Trauma*, 23(6), 386–394.

Managing the care of geriatric patients with hip fractures is complex. Based on the findings from a review of current

research studies from the American Association of Orthopedic Surgeons' Task Force on Serving the Elderly Orthopedic Patient, the authors recommend a collaborative approach to care including the orthopedic surgeon, the geriatrician, the nursing staff, therapists, pharmacists, nutritionists, and pain management specialists. A collaborative approach has been shown to decrease the rate of perioperative complications, including deep vein thrombosis, uncontrolled pain, pressure ulcer development, malnutrition, and surgical site infection. The authors identified the goal of care of early mobilization as a way to minimize complications and help the patient attain the highest functional status possible.

1. As a nurse caring for older adults on your surgical unit, what could you include in your preoperative assessment that may help you to identify older adults at risk for postoperative complications?

2. Based on the information in the research articles and the Quality and Safety Education for Nurses (QSEN) project, identify ways you could address the QSEN competency of *Teamwork and Collaboration*.

 Go to Chapter 39, **Toward Evidence-Based Practice Suggested Responses**, on Davis*Plus*.

Types of Anesthesia

During surgery, anesthesia is used to obtain analgesia (control of pain), muscle relaxation or paralysis, and amnesia (memory loss). Anesthesia is classified as general, conscious sedation, or regional.

General Anesthesia

General anesthesia produces rapid unconsciousness and loss of sensation. The anesthesiologist or nurse anesthetist administers inhaled and intravenous medications that depress the patient's central nervous system (CNS) and relax the musculature. Muscle relaxants, paralyzing agents, narcotics, barbiturates, and inhaled gases are some of the agents used during general anesthesia.

Advantages of General Anesthesia

- The patient is unconscious, so she experiences no anxiety that might affect cardiac and respiratory functioning.
- The muscles are relaxed, so the patient remains completely motionless during the surgical procedure.
- Anesthesia can be adjusted to accommodate the length of the procedure and the patient's age and physical condition. For example, an older adult may require less anesthetic than anticipated; if so, the anesthetist can decrease the dosage without interrupting the procedure.

Also, if complications occur, the anesthesia can be continued for longer than originally planned.

Disadvantages of General Anesthesia

- The respiratory and circulatory muscles are depressed, so mechanical ventilation is needed while the patient is under the effects of the anesthetic agent(s). These effects predispose the patient to pneumonia and thrombophlebitis in the postoperative period.
- General anesthesia creates a risk for death, heart attack, stroke, and malignant hyperthermia. **Malignant hyperthermia** is a rare, often fatal, metabolic condition that can occur during the use of muscle relaxants and inhalation anesthesia. Metabolism increases in the skeletal muscles, and they become rigid. The temperature rises rapidly. Predisposition to this condition is inherited.
- Frequent minor complaints after general anesthesia include sore throat (from intubation), nausea and vomiting (from relaxation of gastrointestinal smooth muscle), headache, uncontrollable shivering, and confusion.

Conscious Sedation

Conscious sedation is an alternative form of anesthesia that provides intravenous sedation and analgesia without producing unconsciousness. During conscious sedation, the patient may feel sleepy but is aware of his surroundings, can be easily aroused by touch or speech, and can talk with the surgical team. Nevertheless, blood pressure, heart rate, respiratory rate, and oxygen saturation are monitored, and the patient usually receives oxygen via nasal cannula during the procedure. Because of the amnesic effect of many of the medications, the patient may not recall aspects of the procedure afterward. Advantages are that (1) pain and anxiety are adequately controlled without the risks of general anesthesia, and (2) recovery is rapid. Conscious sedation is used for procedures such as bronchoscopy and cosmetic surgery, but it is not practical for highly anxious patients.

Regional Anesthesia

Regional anesthesia prevents pain by interrupting nerve impulses to and from the area of the procedure. The patient remains alert but is numb in the involved area. Regional anesthesia may be administered by infiltration of the surgical site and surrounding tissue with local anesthetics, such as lidocaine (Xylocaine) or bupivacaine (Marcaine). These medications may also be injected into and around specific nerves to depress the sensory, motor, and/or sympathetic impulses of a limited area of the body.

Regional anesthesia is low in cost, is simple to administer, and requires a minimal recovery period. It is especially suitable for minor ambulatory procedures. However, many patients are apprehensive about being able to see and hear the procedure. Regional anesthesia may not be practical if the patient is highly anxious or if adequate pain control cannot be achieved. Techniques for achieving regional anesthesia include the following.

Peripheral Nerve Block

A **nerve block** is the injection of an anesthetic into and around a nerve or group of nerves (e.g., the facial nerve, the brachial plexus). A **Bier (intravenous) block** is a nerve block technique in which the anesthetist places a tourniquet on an arm or leg, and then injects a local anesthetic agent intravenously below the level of the tourniquet. The tourniquet is maintained at a pressure that limits venous return but continues to allow arterial circulation. The patient feels no pain in the extremity as long as the tourniquet is in place. Advantages of the Bier block are its rapid onset and recovery time. Also, the tourniquet decreases bleeding during the surgical procedure and prevents systemic absorption of the local anesthetic. However, when the procedure is finished, the tourniquet is deflated, and there is potential for systemic absorption of the anesthetic. To prevent tissue damage, the tourniquet must not be left in place for more than 2 hours.

Spinal Anesthesia

Spinal anesthesia is the injection of an anesthetic into the cerebrospinal fluid (CSF) in the subarachnoid space (Fig. 39-3A). This injection blocks sensation and movement below the level of the injection. Spinal anesthesia is often used for surgical procedures in the lower abdomen, pelvis, and lower extremities. This technique allows the patient to remain conscious during the procedure and usually does not depress respirations. Occasionally a higher level of spinal anesthesia is achieved than intended—that is, the medication may migrate upward in the spinal fluid. This can depress respirations and cardiac rate. Placing the patient in Fowler's position may prevent respiratory paralysis.

Side effects of spinal anesthesia include hypotension, nausea, vomiting, urinary retention, or a headache from leakage of CSF. A headache after spinal anesthesia must be closely monitored and may require additional treatment by the anesthesia staff.

The blood pressure may also decrease suddenly due to pervasive vasodilatation—the anesthesia blocks the sympathetic vasomotor nerves, which normally maintain muscle tone in peripheral blood vessels. Patients with these complications often require ventilation and support of blood pressure during surgery, so they must be carefully monitored during surgery and in the recovery period.

Epidural Anesthesia

Epidural anesthesia requires insertion of a thin catheter into the epidural space (Fig. 39-3B). Anesthetic agents are infused through the catheter to produce loss of sensation. Epidural anesthesia can be used as a surgical anesthetic and to provide postoperative analgesia. Advantages and disadvantages of epidural anesthesia are similar to those of spinal anesthesia. Epidural anesthesia is safer than spinal anesthesia because the anesthetic does not enter the subarachnoid space and the depth of anesthesia is not as great. However, drugs intended for epidural administration are of a higher concentration than those for spinal administration; so if the medication is inadvertently injected too deeply (into the subarachnoid space), hypotension and respiratory paralysis occur, and temporary mechanical ventilation is necessary.

Epidural anesthesia is ideal for obstetrics procedures (e.g., cesarean birth or pain control with vaginal birth) because the mother is awake to bond with the newborn, and her mobility is limited for only a short time.

Local Anesthesia

Local anesthesia produces loss of pain sensation at the desired site (e.g., a wound to be sutured, a skin growth to be removed). It is typically used for minor procedures. However, after finishing a major surgery, the surgeon may infiltrate the operative area with local anesthetics to provide postoperative pain relief. Local anesthetics may be applied topically or injected. A **topical anesthetic** is applied directly to the skin and mucous membranes. Lidocaine (Xylocaine) and benzocaine (Orajel, T-caine) are commonly used because they are rapidly absorbed and rapid-acting.

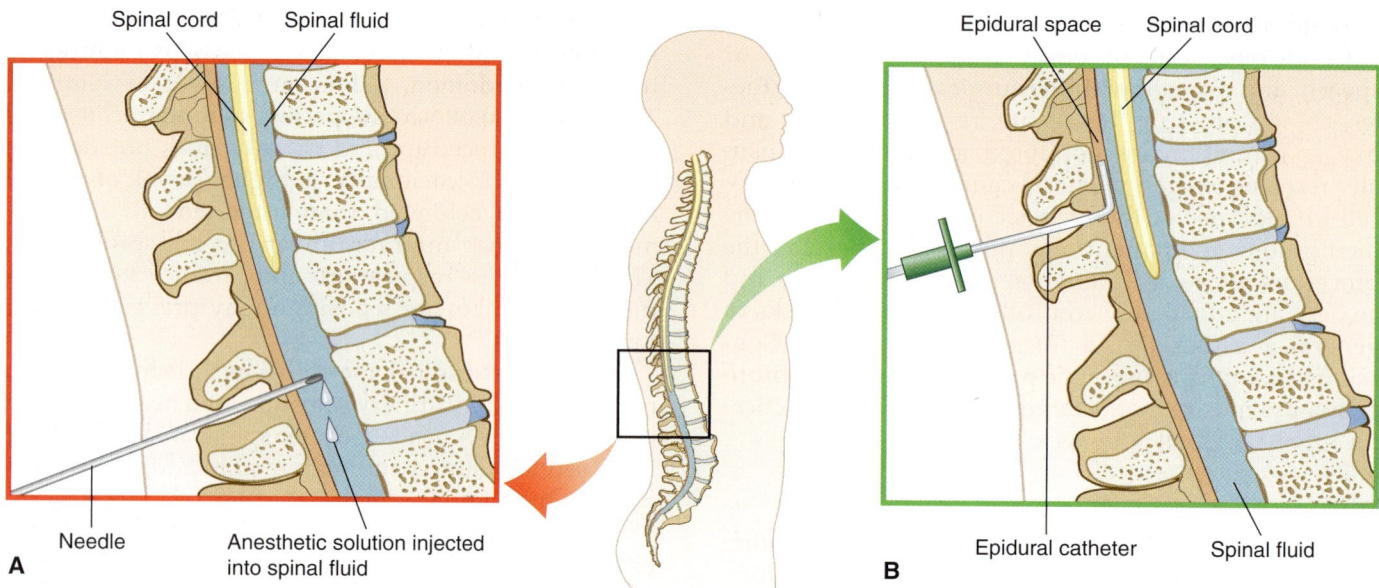

FIGURE 39-3 *A,* Spinal anesthesia is the injection of a local anesthetic into the subarachnoid space to block sensation and movement. *B,* Epidural anesthesia can also be used to provide continuous postoperative analgesia.

KnowledgeCheck 39-6

- What is the purpose of anesthesia?
- Under what type(s) of anesthesia does the client remain conscious?

 ThinkLike a Nurse 39-5

What form of anesthesia is Mr. Singh (Meet Your Patient) most likely to receive? Why?

PracticalKnowledge
knowing **how**

When a patient arrives in the surgical suite, the nurse verifies the information on the preoperative checklist and assesses the patient. The nursing focus is on safe and successful completion of the surgery.

ASSESSMENT

The circulating nurse greets the client in the preoperative holding area and performs a brief assessment. The nurse first verifies that the surgical consent has been signed and witnessed and that the preoperative checklist is complete. The nurse then assesses the client's anxiety level and physical condition. The next steps are to measure the vital signs; examine the surgical site; and inspect IV lines, drainage tubes, and catheters. Often the circulating nurse or the anesthetist starts an IV line in the holding area if one is not already present. A preoperative medication may be given in the holding area. Vital signs are monitored often, or even continuously, during the intraoperative period.

For common interview questions to use in the intraoperative period,

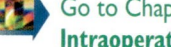 Go to Chapter 39, **Assessment Guidelines and Tools, Intraoperative Care Questionnaire,** in Volume 2.

In addition to the checklist completed in the preoperative period, the surgery team will also complete a checklist, with one staff member functioning as the checklist coordinator. The World Health Organization (WHO, 2009) checklist covers three phases of a surgical procedure:

- Before Induction of Anesthesia
- Before Skin Incision
- Before Patient Leaves the Operating Room

Commonly referred to as "sign in," "time out," and "sign out," the three phases of the surgical checklist are reviewed by the checklist coordinator, who verbally checks that each element was done. The goal of using a surgical checklist is to enhance communication, teamwork, and safety by addressing key activities that occur as part of the perioperative process.

To see the complete WHO checklist,

 Go to Chapter 39, **Assessment Guidelines and Tools, Example of a Surgical Safety Checklist,** in Volume 2.

ANALYSIS/NURSING DIAGNOSIS

As in the preoperative phase, most intraoperative nursing care consists of standard activities to be used for all patients. Most intraoperative patients, regardless of the surgery, have the following potential complications (collaborative problems) of surgery and anesthesia:

- Potential complications of surgery:
  Hypothermia
  Fluid and electrolyte imbalance
  Excessive bleeding or hemorrhage
  Musculoskeletal injury secondary to positioning
- Potential complications of anesthesia:
  Aspiration
  Vasomotor instability (and resultant hypotension and diminished peripheral perfusion)

Respiratory depression
Cardiovascular compromise

Except in unusual circumstances (e.g., a patient in poor nutritional status, a frail elderly patient), you may not need to identify nursing diagnoses for a patient because the standardized care addresses all the potential complications. However, for nurses who prefer to organize care according to nursing diagnoses, the following potential diagnoses apply to most patients having major surgery:

- *Risk for Imbalanced Body Temperature* related to exposure in cool environment and administration of cool IV fluids. This applies especially to very young, very old, and very thin patients.
- *Risk for Aspiration* related to depressed respirations and reflexes. For patients who have weak muscles for coughing or a poor gag reflex, this diagnosis is especially relevant.
- *Risk for Imbalanced Fluid Volume* related to NPO status and blood loss from surgery. Some patients are at higher than normal risk, for example, patients with renal or cardiac problems.
- *Risk for Perioperative Positioning Injury* related to patient factors such as edema, emaciation, obesity, and sensory perceptual disturbances secondary to anesthesia.

Use the following nursing diagnoses only if the patient has the necessary defining characteristics or risk factors. Do not use them for all patients.

- *Risk for Latex Allergy Response* related to multiple exposures (e.g., multiple surgeries, catheterizations) or history of related allergies
- *Latex Allergy Response* (needs no etiology)

PLANNING OUTCOMES/EVALUATION

The overarching goals in the intraoperative phase are that the patient will:

Be free from injury
Remain physiologically stable
Experience optimal surgical outcomes

For *associated NOC standardized outcomes* for intraoperative patients, along with examples of goals created with NOC indicators and scales,

 Go to Chapter 39, **Standardized Language, Intraoperative Patients: Selected Standardized Nursing Diagnoses, Outcomes, and Interventions,** in Volume 2.

Notice that the goals are appropriate for nearly all surgical patients.
Individualized goals/outcome statements are formulated from the patient's nursing diagnoses. The following are examples:

- Maintains body temperature within the normal range.
- Has clear lung sounds and patent airway.

- Has urine output of at least 30 mL/hr.
- Will have no skin, tissue, or neuromuscular injury as a result of positioning.
- Will not acquire healthcare-related infection.

PLANNING INTERVENTIONS/IMPLEMENTATION

Intraoperative care focuses on maintaining a safe environment and assisting the surgery team to provide appropriate care for the client. The nurse anesthetist manages the interventions for most of the patient's potential problems, for example, fluid volume status, airway protection, and vital signs monitoring.

NIC standardized interventions for the intraoperative period come from the domain of Perioperative Care. They include interventions for all intraoperative patients, regardless of their individual nursing diagnoses. One intervention, Anesthesia Administration, must be performed by an anesthesiologist or nurse anesthetist. The nurse assists in implementing a number of interventions:

- Anesthesia Administration
- Autotransfusion
- Infection Control: Intraoperative
- Positioning: Intraoperative
- Surgical Assistance
- Surgical Precautions
- Surgical Preparation
- Temperature Regulation: Intraoperative

For NIC *standardized interventions for specific intraoperative nursing diagnoses,*

 Go to Chapter 39, **Standardized Language, Introperative Patients: Selected Standardized Nursing Diagnoses, Outcomes, and Interventions,** in Volume 2.

Notice, however, that most of the interventions apply to all surgical patients and are subsumed by (or fall under) the preceding NIC Perioperative Care interventions. As in all patient care, you should be always mindful of using hand hygiene. Sterile asepsis is an important focus in the intraoperative period; you can review that in Chapter 23.

The following sections explain in more detail how to carry out "routine" interventions, such as providing skin preparation, positioning, and intraoperative safety measures. **Key Point:** *Note that "routine" in this context means that the activities are planned and performed for all patients. Nursing interventions are* **never** *routine in the general sense; they must always be performed with thought and skill.*

Skin Preparation

Surgical skin preparation reduces the risk of postoperative wound infection by reducing the microbial count at the operative site. Skin preparation may begin in the preoperative phase, when the client cleanses the skin with an antimicrobial solution the evening before and the morning of surgery. The intraoperative nurse provides additional skin preparation as follows:

Assess the Skin Assess skin for signs of infection, rash, or other forms of skin irritation. Document the condition of the skin on the intraoperative record.

Remove Hair From the Site Only If Necessary Historically, the surgical site was always shaved. Now, however, you will remove hair only if there is a large amount of it in the area of the surgery or if the surgeon specifies a preference for hair removal. Hair removal increases the risk of abrasions or nicks in the skin, which can provide a portal of entry for bacteria. If you do remove hair, you will likely do it in the preoperative holding area immediately before surgery to reduce the time for bacterial growth. Use clippers or depilatory cream to trim hair because they are less likely than a razor to cause skin irritation (The Joanna Briggs Institute, 2007).

Cleanse the Surgical Site In the operative suite, skin preparation precedes draping of the client. Using sterile technique, cleanse the surgical site and a generous part of surrounding area with the recommended anti-infective solution. Povidone-iodine (Betadine) is commonly used for the scrub; then the skin is painted with Betadine solution. ✚ If the client is allergic to iodine, use an alternative preparation solution.

Positioning

The position of the patient in the OR is determined by the surgical site, access to the patient's airway, the need to monitor vital signs, comfort, and safety. A position that is ideal for accessing the surgical site may not be used if any of the other factors are compromised. If the patient has preexisting injuries or discomfort, factor this information into the decision about how to position. For example, a patient with chronic cervical spine pain may be positioned using a neck roll.

The patient is usually positioned after anesthesia has begun. Use straps, wedges, pillows, and surgical table attachments to maintain the position during the surgery. To prevent shearing, lift—do not slide—the patient into position. In many cases, the surgical team assists with positioning.

The circulating nurse is responsible for preventing positioning injuries. Surgical patients often spend 3 to 4 hours, or even longer, in the same position. This places them at risk for pressure ulcer formation. Some anesthetic agents decrease tissue perfusion, further increasing the patient's risk for sustaining positioning injuries. Padding the bony prominences is one measure to protect the client during surgery. For nursing interventions to address the NANDA-I diagnosis Risk for Perioperative Positioning Injury,

 Go to Chapter 39, **Standardized Language, Intraoperative Patients: Selected Standardized Nursing Diagnoses, Outcomes, and Interventions,** in Volume 2.

Intraoperative Safety Measures

Just before starting any surgical or invasive procedure, you should conduct a final verification process to confirm the correct patient, procedure, and site (The Joint Commission, 2012). The circulating nurse is responsible for a variety of other measures that protect the patient in the intraoperative phase. These measures are briefly explained here.

Assist the Scrub Nurse to Prepare and Maintain the Sterile Field The circulating nurse gathers surgical supplies and equipment for use during surgery. She then works with the scrub nurse to transfer the supplies to the sterile field.

Provide Supplies and Materials During Surgery If additional supplies are needed during surgery, the circulating nurse obtains them and opens them on the sterile field. Supplies may include dressings, surgical equipment, medications, irrigating solutions, or sutures.

Monitor Intake and Output of the Client Together with the anesthetist, the circulating nurse monitors the fluid infused, urine output, drainage, and blood loss.

Handle Specimens The circulating nurse handles specimens and sends them to the lab or pathology for evaluation after the surgery is complete. The surgeon may sometimes obtain a tissue sample that must be analyzed during the operative procedure. The circulator receives the specimen, coordinates with the pathologist to review the sample, and reports the pathology findings to the surgeon.

Perform Sponge, Sharps, and Instrument Counts

✚ The circulating nurse and the scrub nurse count the material that is added to the sterile field. As the surgery comes to an end, a repeat count is performed to ensure that no instruments, sponges, or sharps are left inside the client. A retained sponge can lead to infection and additional surgeries. A major surgery, such as a heart surgery, can use several hundred sponges. Once soaked in blood, sponges can blend in with the body cavity and be difficult to see. Some agencies are now using sponges with barcodes, which the nurse scans before and after use. The system alerts the surgical team if they are left behind. In another system, chip-embedded sponges rely on radiofrequency identification technology to count sponges and locate any that are left behind.

Document Record the care provided and the client's response to care on the surgical record. Usually you will use a graphic or a checklist form, perhaps with some space for narrative notes about anything the form does not address.

KnowledgeCheck 39-7

- For what activities is the circulating nurse responsible in the surgical suite prior to the skin incision?
- Describe six intraoperative safety measures performed by the circulating nurse.

ThinkLike a Nurse 39-6

What special concerns, if any, do you have about Mr. Singh (Meet Your Patient) during the intraoperative phase of care?

POSTOPERATIVE CARE

The postoperative phase begins when the client enters the postanesthesia care unit and ends when he has healed from the surgical procedure. This phase consists of two parts: recovery from anesthesia and recovery from surgery.

TheoreticalKnowledge knowing **why**

When the surgical procedure is complete, members of the surgical team prepare the client for transfer to the postanesthesia care unit (PACU), also called the recovery room (Fig. 39-4).

Recovery From Anesthesia

The first postoperative phase is often known as the *postanesthesia phase* or the *immediate postoperative phase*. This phase begins when the client is transferred from the operating table to a bed (or gurney) for transport to the PACU. During this phase, the client is at high risk for respiratory and cardiovascular compromise. As a precaution, the anesthetist and the circulating nurse accompany the client and attend to her needs during transport to the PACU. They are also responsible for giving a comprehensive report to the PACU nurse.

The PACU, located near the OR, is typically an open unit that allows nurses to observe clients easily. PACU nurses have specialized education and experience in caring for postoperative clients. Commonly, nurses working in the PACU have experience in critical care. The PACU nurse receives a comprehensive report from the anesthesia provider and circulating nurse (see Box 39-4):

Recovery From Surgery

The second phase of postoperative care begins when the patient is discharged from the PACU and admitted to the surgical nursing unit. The patient is transported to the surgical unit only after he has recovered from anesthesia and his condition is stable. The goal of this phase is to facilitate healing and prevent postoperative complications.

PracticalKnowledge knowing **how**

In the next sections we discuss nursing care associated with both phases of postoperative care.

Nursing Care in the Postanesthesia Care Unit

The PACU nurse performs a quick, focused initial assessment of the surgical patient in the presence of the anesthesia provider and circulating nurse. After that, she assesses the patient every 5 to 15 minutes. AORN (2009, updated 2011) has identified the essential elements of assessment in the PACU.

For that information

 Go to Chapter 39, **Assessment Guidelines and Tools, Postanesthesia Assessment: Essential Elements,** in Volume 2.

BOX 39-4 ■ Information Contained in the Report From the Surgical Suite

- Procedure performed
- Type of anesthesia
- Medications administered in the surgical suite
- Duration of the procedure and anesthesia
- Postoperative vital signs
- Pulse oximetery values
- Allergies
- Lab values
- Estimated blood loss
- Fluid intake and output, including urine, stool, gastric losses
- Preoperative mobility status, skin integrity, and sensory perception abilities
- Surgical complications
- Presence of tubes, drains, catheters
- Existing IV lines
- Postoperative prescriptions

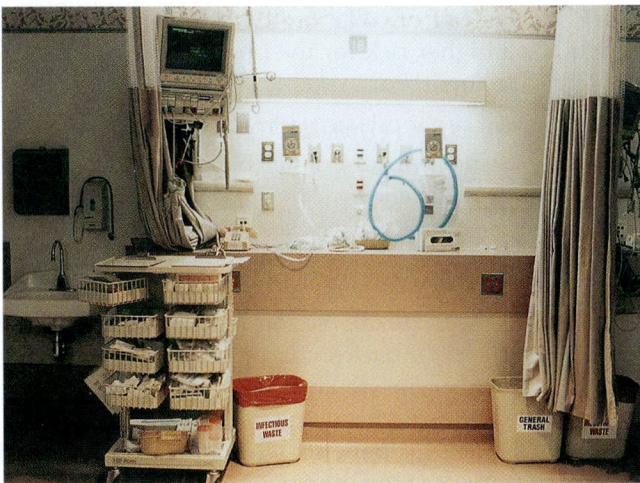

FIGURE 39-4 Postanesthesia care unit.

An unconscious client is usually positioned on his side to help maintain an open airway. This decreases the likelihood of aspirating mucus or saliva by allowing it to drain out instead of back into the throat. Elevating the superior arm on a pillow allows for good chest expansion so the patient can breathe deeply and expand the lungs fully.

NIC: Postanesthesia Care. The only postoperative intervention from NIC's Perioperative Care category is Postanesthesia Care. Postanesthesia Care encompasses the preceding assessments and adds measures such as providing for safety and administering oxygen. Many patients arrive in the PACU with an artificial airway or endotracheal tube in place. The client remains in the PACU until the PACU nurse determines that he has recovered from the effects of anesthesia (Box 39-5) and is able to maintain his own airway. She then removes the airway and transfers the patient to the surgical unit.

For *NIC interventions* for other postoperative nursing diagnoses:

Go to Chapter 39, **Standardized Language, Postoperative Patients: Selected Standardized Nursing Diagnoses, Outcomes, and Interventions,** in Volume 2.

BOX 39-5 ■ Evidence of Recovery From Anesthesia

Airway—The patient is able to maintain a patent airway independently and to deep-breathe, cough, and expectorate secretions.

Level of consciousness—The patient is conscious and easily reoriented. Often patients will drift off to sleep between arousals; however, they easily reorient and are generally aware of circumstances and surroundings.

Vital signs—Vital signs are stable and within an acceptable range. The blood pressure may be markedly different from that taken during the immediate preoperative measures, because BP is often elevated preoperatively. This can also be caused by anxiety, pain, and not administering routine BP medications because of NPO status. The patient may require medication to control pain or BP before he can be discharged from the PACU.

Mobility and sensation—The patient is able to move all extremities that he could move preoperatively. The patient regains movement and sensation once spinal or epidural anesthesia has worn off.

Fluid balance (I&O)—The patient is urinating at least 30 mL/hr and is in relative fluid balance. Consider blood loss, urine output, gastric drainage, and emesis when calculating fluid balance.

Dressings and drains—Dressings are dry and intact, or wound drainage is considered appropriate for the procedure. The patient should have no overt signs of excessive blood or fluid loss before he is transferred to the surgical unit.

Postoperative Nursing Care on the Surgical Unit

The assigned nurse admits the patient to the surgical unit. If the patient is transported by gurney, assist him to the bed. As soon as the patient has arrived, perform an assessment, and listen to a summary report from the PACU nurse (Box 39-4).

■ ASSESSMENT

The initial postoperative assessment is identical to the assessment performed by the PACU nurse. However, the patient has undergone a period of stabilization since surgery, so assessments can be less frequent than in the PACU, where the patient was assessed every 5 to 15 minutes. You may increase the frequency if the patient's condition changes. Of course agency protocols vary, but a common pattern is to assess the patient:

On arrival to the nursing unt
Every 15 minutes for the first hour
Every 30 minutes for the next 2 hours
Every hour for the next 4 hours
Then every 4 hours

KnowledgeCheck 39-8

- What are the two phases of the postoperative phase of care?
- How often is a patient typically assessed after surgery?
- What assessments are made?

■ ANALYSIS/NURSING DIAGNOSIS

If healing proceeds normally and no complications develop, most postoperative patients have a common set of collaborative problems (Table 39-4), regardless of the type of surgery they underwent. You will not need to write potential ("risk for") nursing diagnoses, except in special situations (e.g., patients with comorbid conditions, such as diabetes or asthma).

Potential Nursing Diagnoses Write potential nursing diagnoses (instead of collaborative problems) only if a patient has a higher risk for the problem than the average surgical patient. For example, you might use:

- *Risk for Ineffective Peripheral Tissue Perfusion* for patients who have a history of peripheral arterial disease or cardiac insufficiency.
- *Risk for Deficient Fluid Volume* for patients who have lost a large amount of blood in surgery or who are dehydrated on admission.
- *Risk for Ineffective Breathing Pattern* for patients with weak accessory muscles for breathing, with a decreased level of consciousness, or with a respiratory condition such as emphysema.
- *Risk for Infection* for patients who have compromised immune status or who may not be capable of managing their own wound care at home.

Actual Nursing Diagnoses Of course, you will use a nursing diagnosis whenever a problem becomes actual instead of merely potential. Nursing diagnoses will vary based on the surgical procedure and the client situation. There is no need for a *Deficient Knowledge* diagnosis because patient teaching is a routine intervention for all postoperative patients. Two common postoperative nursing diagnoses are:

- *Delayed Surgical Recovery*. This is appropriate when the patient requires more days to recover than the anticipated length of stay for the surgery.
- *Acute Pain*. There are independent nursing interventions to relieve pain (e.g., teaching the patient to splint the incision). However, they do not usually provide adequate relief in the early post-op period. You will nearly always need to administer analgesics, which require a medical prescription.

For other frequently used diagnoses,

 Go to Chapter 39, **Postoperative Patients: Selected Standardized Nursing Diagnoses, Outcomes, and Interventions,** in Volume 2.

■ PLANNING OUTCOMES/EVALUATION

A comprehensive plan of care for common postoperative nursing diagnoses includes NOC standardized outcomes as well as individualized goals. Because of shortened hospital stays, the postoperative period now extends well past the patient's discharge from the hospital. Often, especially for those who have had major or complex procedures, a home health nurse continues to follow the patient at home to facilitate a smoother transition through the postoperative process.

For postoperative *NOC standardized outcomes and individualized goals,*

 Go to Chapter 39, **Postoperative Patients: Selected Standardized Nursing Diagnoses, Outcomes, and Interventions,** in Volume 2.

■ PLANNING INTERVENTIONS/IMPLEMENTATION

Most postoperative interventions focus on prevention and early detection of potential complications (collaborative problems). Many such interventions are done as a part of the preoperative teaching. Others are described in Table 39-4. These are routines that are followed for all postoperative patients, regardless of type of surgery.

For *NIC interventions for postoperative nursing diagnoses,*

 Go to Chapter 39, **Postoperative Patients: Selected Standardized Nursing Diagnoses, Outcomes, and Interventions,** in Volume 2.

Specific nursing activities should be designed to relieve identified nursing diagnoses. In the next sections, we discuss pain management, routine postoperative teaching, and the use of sequential compression devices.

Pain Management

One systematic evidence synthesis has found that there is no strong evidence to support that any particular nursing intervention for relief of postoperative pain is better than any other. Interventions included medication administration, preoperative education, regular assessment and documentation of pain intensity, use of protocols and flowsheets, and nonpharmacological interventions (e.g., massage) in relieving postoperative pain (Crowe, Chang, Fraser, et al., 2008). Therefore, when interventions seem to be equally effective, you will need to weigh the potential benefits, possible adverse events, and patient preferences to decide which to use.

Postoperatively, a patient usually receives analgesics by more than one route. For example, in the immediate postoperative period, the patient may receive intravenous or epidural medications, progress to oral opioids in a day or two, and then move to nonopioid analgesics (e.g., acetaminophen).

 Providing sufficient pain control for older adults can be a challenge. Because of concerns about impaired cognition, medical comorbidities, drug interactions, and problems with appropriate dosing many older adults may be undermedicated and experience unnecessary pain (Egol & Strauss, 2009).

For a complete discussion of types of pain relief, refer to the section Routes of Administration for Opioid Analgesics in Chapter 31, and

 Go to Chapter 31, **Procedure 31-1: Setting Up and Managing Patient-Controlled Analgesia by Pump,** and **Clinical Insight 31-1: Nursing Care of the Patient with an Epidural Catheter,** in Volume 2.

Key Point: *Keep in mind that no one drug is likely to work with every person with pain.*

One recent development is a single-use pain relief pump that administers a continuous, regulated flow of local anesthetic through a thin catheter directly into the patient's surgical site. A dressing holds the tubing in

(text continues on page 1052)

CAM for Pain, Anxiety, and Tension

Massage Therapy for Postoperative Pain, Anxiety, and Tension

Cutshall, Wentworth, Engall, et al. (2010) collected data from 58 postoperative cardiovascular patients. Twenty-eight of the patients received 20 minutes of massage therapy in addition to the usual pain management during postoperative days 2 to 5. Statistically and clinically significant decreases in pain, anxiety, and tension were reported compared to the group of patient who did not receive massage therapy.

Table 39-4 ➤ Potential Postoperative Complications (Collaborative Problems)

POTENTIAL COMPLICATION	DESCRIPTION	CLINICAL SIGNS	INTERVENTIONS FOR PREVENTION AND EARLY DETECTION
Respiratory System			
Aspiration Pneumonia	Airway inflammation caused by inhaling gastric secretions (especially hydrochloric acid from the stomach) because of absent gag reflex secondary to anesthesia	Cough, fever, elevated WBC, decreased or absent breath sounds, decreased oxygen saturation (SaO_2), tachypnea, dyspnea, blood-tinged sputum	*Preoperative:* Institute NPO for at least 8 hours prior to surgery. *Postoperative:* Continue NPO until intestinal motility returns; carefully monitor sedated patient and place in side-lying position.
Atelectasis	Collapse of alveoli due to hypoventilation, airways blocked by mucous plugs, opioid analgesics, immobility	Decreased or absent breath sounds, noisy respirations, decreased O_2 saturation (SaO_2), chest asymmetry, sternal retractions, accessory muscle use, trachea deviated from midline, fever, tachypnea, dyspnea, tachycardia, diaphoresis, pleural pain, increased restlessness, anxiety	■ Monitor for clinical signs (Column 3) ■ Monitor rate, rhythm, depth, and effort of respirations. ■ Monitor ability to cough effectively. ■ Determine need for suctioning by listening for crackles and rhonchi over major airways. ■ Suction, as needed. Auscultate lung sounds after suctioning, and other respiratory treatments to determine effectiveness. ■ Encourage deep breathing, coughing, moving in bed, ambulation, use of incentive spirometry. ■ See interventions for NIC category Respiratory Monitoring.
Pneumonia	Inflammation of the alveoli due to infection with bacteria or viruses, toxins, or irritants. Caused by hypoventilation secondary to anesthesia and opioid analgesics, and by poor cough effort as a result of aging or weakness.	Productive cough with blood-tinged or purulent sputum, fever, elevated WBC, decreased or absent breath sounds, decreased SaO_2, chest pain, tachypnea, dyspnea	■ Monitor for clinical signs. ■ Encourage and assist with deep breathing, coughing, moving in bed, ambulation, use of incentive spirometry.
Pulmonary Embolus	A clot that occludes blood flow to a portion of the lungs; usually a result of clot formation in the lower extremities, which breaks loose and migrates to the lungs. May also be due to venous injuries, hypercoagulable state, use of high-dose estrogen, preexisting circulatory disorders.	Sudden onset of dyspnea, shortness of breath, chest pain, hypotension, tachycardia, decreased SaO_2, cyanosis	■ Prevent thrombophlebitis: Encourage and assist with leg exercises, early ambulation, antiembolism stockings, sequential compression devices, hydration. Go to Chapter 39, **Procedure 39-2: Applying Antiembolism Stockings**, and **Procedure 39-3: Applying Sequential Compression Devices,** in Volume 2. ■ If thrombophlebitis occurs, position and immobilize the limb; do not massage calves.

Table 39-4 ➤ Potential Postoperative Complications (Collaborative Problems)—cont'd

POTENTIAL COMPLICATION	DESCRIPTION	CLINICAL SIGNS	INTERVENTIONS FOR PREVENTION AND EARLY DETECTION
Cardiovascular System			
Thrombophlebitis	Blood clot and inflammation of a vein or artery, usually in the legs. Results from increased coagulability and venous stasis resulting from immobility during and after surgery.	*Superficial:* Vein is red, hard, and hot to touch. *Deep:* Limb is pale and edematous; aching, cramping in limb; Homans' sign (pain in calf when foot is dorsiflexed).	Refer to Pulmonary Embolism actions, above.
Embolus	■ Movement of a thrombus or foreign body from its original location. ■ Movement in the arterial system results in symptoms in the area affected (e.g., cerebrovascular accident, myocardial infarction, or loss of circulation to an area). ■ In the venous system, often results in pulmonary embolus (see Pulmonary Embolus, preceding).	See Pulmonary Embolus. For arterial emboli, symptoms depend on the location.	■ Monitor for clinical signs. ■ Prevent thrombophlebitis. If thrombophlebitis occurs, position and immobilize the limb. ■ Do not massage calves.
Hemorrhage	Bleeding may be internal or external. May be caused by slipped ligature, uncontrolled bleeder, or infection.	*If external:* Dressings saturated with bright red blood; increased output in drains or chest tubes *If internal:* Increased pain, increasing abdominal girth, ecchymosis or swelling around incision, tachycardia, hypotension	Frequently monitor vital signs, dressings, and wound drainage.
Hypovolemia	Decreased blood volume; may be due to blood loss during and after surgery, dehydration, or excess loss through vomiting, diarrhea, or drains	Hypotension, tachycardia, decreased urine output, fatigue, thirst, dehydration	■ Monitor vital signs and I&O. ■ Insert urinary catheter, if appropriate. ■ Monitor skin color, temperature, and moistness; central and peripheral cyanosis. ■ Identify possible causes of changes in vital signs. ■ Administer IV therapy as prescribed. ■ Promote oral intake when tolerated. ■ Prepare to administer blood or blood products, as prescribed.

Continued

Table 39-4 ▶ Potential Postoperative Complications (Collaborative Problems)—cont'd

POTENTIAL COMPLICATION	DESCRIPTION	CLINICAL SIGNS	INTERVENTIONS FOR PREVENTION AND EARLY DETECTION
Gastrointestinal System			
Nausea and Vomiting	Stomach upset or vomiting related to pain, anxiety, anesthesia, medications, or oral intake before peristalsis returns	Vomiting, retching, stated nausea	■ Have patient remain NPO until return of bowel sounds. ■ Advance diet slowly. ■ Treat pain.
Abdominal Distention (Tympanites)	Excess gas within the intestines; may be the result of a slow return of peristalsis or from handling of the intestines during surgery	Abdominal discomfort, bloating, hypoactive or absent bowel sounds	■ Encourage and assist to move in bed and ambulate. ■ Maintain NPO until return of bowel sounds; avoid drinking with a straw. ■ Provide fluids at room temperature.
Constipation	A decrease in the frequency of bowel movements, resulting in the passage of hard stool. Usually related to use of opioids, immobility, inadequate fluid intake, or low-fiber diet.	Abdominal discomfort, bloating, hypoactive or absent bowel sounds	Encourage and assist the patient to move in bed, ambulate, and increase fluid and fiber intake after bowel sounds return.
Ileus	Loss of the forward flow of intestinal contents because of decreased peristalsis secondary to anesthesia, handling of the intestines during surgery, electrolyte imbalances, infection, or ischemic bowel	Abdominal pain, distention, absent bowel sounds, vomiting	There are few independent preventive measures. Observe for symptoms; notify the surgeon.
Genitourinary System			
Renal Failure	Decreased or absent urine output owing to hypovolemia, shock, or toxic reaction to medications.	Urine output <30 mL/hr; rising BUN and creatinine levels	Carefully monitor I&O and lab values.
Urinary Retention	Accumulation of urine in the bladder. May result from poor muscle tone as a result of anesthesia and anticholinergic medications, handling of tissues during surgery, or inflammation in the pelvic region.	Bladder distention, suprapubic pain, diminished urine output or output less than fluid intake, inability to void or small frequent voidings, hypertension, restlessness	■ Monitor for clinical signs. ■ Provide privacy and adequate time to urinate. ■ Catheterize if needed.
Urinary Tract Infection	Infection in the urinary tract related to catheterization, stagnant urine in the bladder secondary to immobility or anticholinergic medications, or instrumentation of the urinary tract	Urinary frequency, suprapubic discomfort, burning on urination, cloudy urine	■ Monitor for clinical signs. ■ Monitor I&O. ■ Use aseptic technique with catheterization and perineal care. ■ Provide adequate IV and oral fluids.

Table 39-4 ➤ Potential Postoperative Complications (Collaborative Problems)—cont'd

POTENTIAL COMPLICATION	DESCRIPTION	CLINICAL SIGNS	INTERVENTIONS FOR PREVENTION AND EARLY DETECTION
Surgical Incision			
Dehiscence	Separation of one or more layers of the wound as a result of poor nutritional status, obesity, or other strain on suture line, inadequate closure of the muscles, or wound infection	A pop or tearing sensation, especially with sudden straining from coughing, vomiting, or changing positions in bed. Usually an immediate increase in serosanguinous drainage occurs.	▪ Provide adequate nutrition. ▪ Use binders to support the incision. ▪ Have client avoid strain. ▪ Monitor for infection.
Evisceration	Protrusion of organs or tissues through the separated incision. For causes, see Dehiscence.	Visible protrusion of organs through incision	Same as for Dehiscence
Wound Infection	Inflammation or drainage from a wound as a result of growth of microorganisms secondary to poor aseptic technique or pathogens already present in surgical area	Localized swelling, redness, heat, pain, fever (>100.4°F or 38°C), foul-smelling drainage, or a change in the color of the drainage.	▪ Effective skin prep in preoperative period ▪ Surgical scrub according to guidelines in the intraoperative period ▪ Monitor for systemic and localized signs and symptoms of infection. ▪ Inspect incision and drain areas for redness and extreme warmth. ▪ Inspect surgical dressings for drainage and odor. ▪ Monitor vital signs, especially temperature. ▪ Assess vulnerability to infection. ▪ Maintain aseptic nontouch technique with surgical dressing changes. ▪ Use and teach good hand hygiene. ▪ Use sterile saline for wound cleansing up to 48 hours post-op (NICE, 2008). ▪ See interventions for NIC category Infection Protection. ▪ Limit the number of visitors, as appropriate. ▪ Obtain cultures as needed. ▪ Encourage sufficient nutritional and fluid intake. ▪ Teach client about signs of infection.

place, and the pump can be carried in a small bag and used after the patient returns home. It reduces the need for opioids, thus reducing complications, such as nausea, vomiting, and respiratory depression. It is said to hasten ambulation and the return to normal activities. Depending on the type of pump, it is filled with 65 to 750 mL of medication and can remain in place for up to 5 days, depending on the amount of anesthetic included (Fig. 39-5).

Postoperative Teaching

Teaching is especially important postoperatively because most patients must perform quite a bit of self-care. Postoperative teaching should reinforce content taught preoperatively. In addition, you should teach the patient about the topics in the Self-Care box Postoperative Patient Teaching. To use time efficiently, try to do some teaching each time you are at the bedside for other care. Be sure the patient is comfortable but alert. Do not attempt teaching when the patient is in pain, needs to void, or is drowsy from opioid analgesics.

Incentive Spirometry

Incentive spirometry may be prescribed for patients who are at high risk for atelectasis and pneumonia (e.g., the patient has a history of lung problems or smoking or will experience a prolonged period of inactivity). Incentive spirometry facilitates deep breathing, increases lung volume, and promotes coughing to clear mucus from the respiratory tree. The equipment varies in appearance, but all devices include a gauge to monitor the patient's progress visibly (Fig. 39-6).

If incentive spirometry is prescribed postoperatively, explain its use to the patient (see the Self-Care box Teaching Your Patient About Incentive Spirometry). If

Self-Care

Postoperative Patient Teaching Topics

- ➤ Postoperative treatment regimen (e.g., dressing changes, exercises), including rationale for the treatments
- ➤ Self-management of the treatment regimen
- ➤ Expected results and effects of the surgery
- ➤ The prescribed diet, and how to select foods on the diet
- ➤ Prescribed activity
- ➤ Signs and symptoms of complications that require the patient to notify the surgeon or primary care provider
- ➤ Return office or clinic visits
- ➤ Lifestyle changes that may be needed
- ➤ Community resources available (e.g., Reach for Recovery)

See also the Complementary & Alternative Modalities box Massage Therapy on Pain, Anxiety, and Tension for an alternative approach to pain management.

you know in advance that the patient will be using an incentive spirometer postoperatively, include its use in your preoperative teaching.

Antiembolism Stockings and Sequential Compression Devices

More than half of all hospitalized patients are at risk for venous thromboembolism, and surgical patients seem to be at higher risk than medical patients (Cohen, Tapson, Bergman, et al., 2008). Preventive measures include anticoagulant medications (blood thinners),

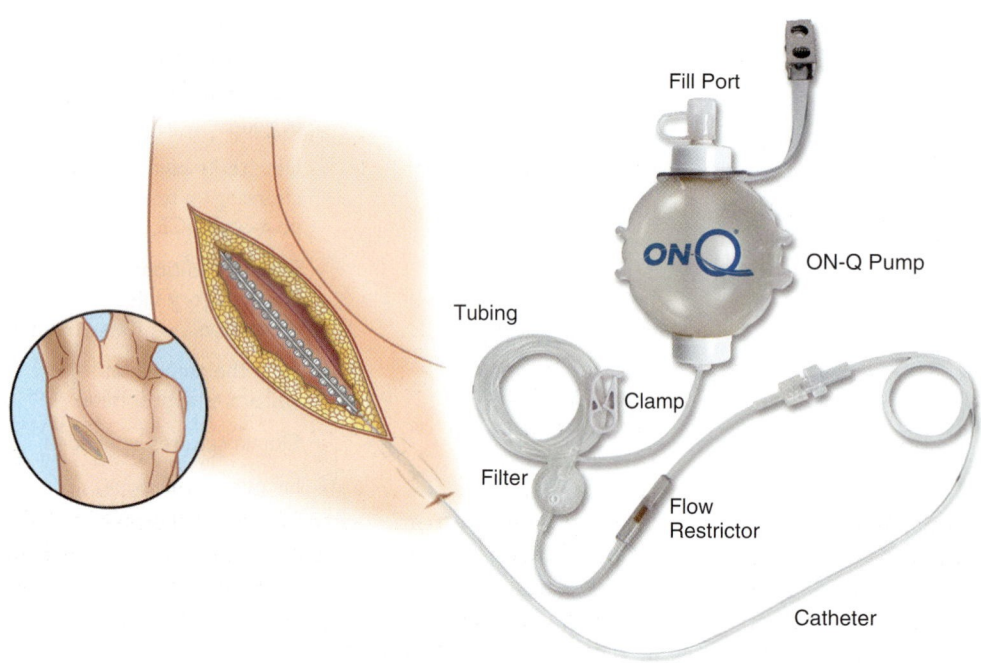

FIGURE 39-5 A single-use pain relief pump delivers a local anesthetic directly into the patient's surgical site.

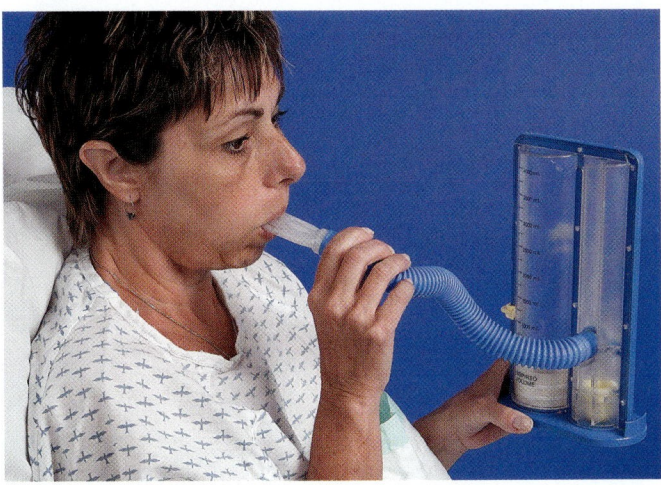

FIGURE 39-6 Incentive spirometry facilitates lung expansion and coughing to clear mucus from airways.

Teaching Your Patient About Incentive Spirometry

➤ Explain to the patient that the machine will enable him to monitor the depth of his breathing.

➤ Patients with abdominal or chest incisions may require pain medication to use the incentive spirometer.

➤ Assist the patient to an upright position in the bed or chair.

➤ Instruct the patient to do the following:

1. Breathe out normally.

2. Place the mouthpiece in the mouth and create a seal.

3. Breathe in slowly and as deeply as possible through the mouthpiece. Monitor the depth of inspiration by viewing the gauge. (Establish goals for the patient so that progress can be monitored.)

4. Hold your breath as long as possible, at least to a slow count of 3.

5. Remove the mouthpiece from your mouth, and exhale.

6. Rest for a few seconds

7. Repeat this process 10 times every hour while awake, if possible.

8. After each set of 10 deep breaths, cough to be sure lungs are clear. Support any incision when coughing by holding a pillow firmly against it.

postoperative exercises, and antiembolism stockings ("TED hose").

Antiembolism Stockings Antiembolism stockings were discussed previously as a preoperative care intervention in the Preoperative Care section Prepare the Patient Physically for Surgery. Encourage postoperative patients to ambulate as soon and as much as possible to promote peripheral circulation and prevent thrombophlebitis. **Key Point: Antiembolism stockings are not a substitute for activity. Early ambulation is essential to prevent postoperative complications.**

To learn how to apply antiembolism stockings,

 Go to Chapter 39, **Procedure 39-2: Applying Antiembolism Stockings,** in Volume 2.

Sequential Compression Devices (SCDs) In addition to antiembolism stockings, a sequential compression device (SCD) may be prescribed for patients at high risk for thrombophlebitis. The SCD is a plastic sleeve with chambers (Fig. 39-7). The sleeve is wrapped around the patient's legs and connected to an air pump that provides sequential pressure to the chambers of the plastic sleeve. Starting at the ankle, the first chamber is inflated. When the second chamber inflates, the first chamber deflates, and so on. SCDs apply brief pressure to each segment of the leg. This compresses the veins and promotes venous return to the heart. SCDs may extend from ankles to knees or up to the top of the thighs. To learn how to apply SCDs,

 Go to Chapter 39, **Procedure 39-3: Applying Sequential Compression Devices,** in Volume 2.

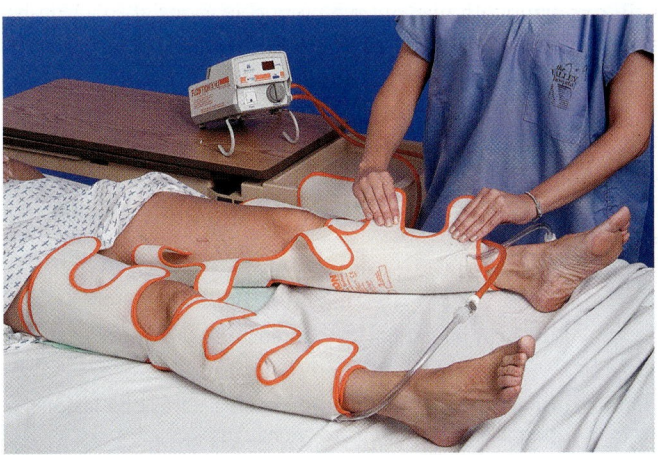

FIGURE 39-7 Sequential compression devices may be prescribed for clients at high risk for thrombophlebitis.

Gastrointestinal Suction

Patients having certain surgeries, such as a laparotomy to close a bowel perforation or surgery to relieve a bowel obstruction, are at high risk for abdominal distention. In addition to causing pain, distention can increase postoperative respiratory problems, place a strain on suture lines, and interfere with wound closure. Such patients will return from surgery with a nasogastric (NG) or nasointestinal tube in place for gastric or intestinal decompression. If prolonged intestinal decompression is anticipated, a gastrostomy may be performed instead of using a nasogastric tube.

Decompression tubes are typically connected to either intermittent or continuous suction to collect excess fluid and gas. Suction is continued until peristalsis resumes, bowel sounds are audible, and the patient is passing flatus. While suction is in place, the patient remains NPO. To review insertion and care of NG and nasoenteric tubes, see Chapter 27. To learn how to manage gastrointestinal suction, see the summary in the Highlights of Procedures box, and

 Go to Chapter 39, **Procedure 39-4: Managing Gastric Suction**, in Volume 2.

KnowledgeCheck 39-9

- Identify six potential postoperative complications.
- Why are sequential compression devices used?

CarePlanning & MappingPractice

For Care Planning/Care Mapping practice,

 Go to Student Resources, **Care Planning & Care Mapping Practice,** on Davis*Plus*.

Highlights of Procedures 39-1 through 39-4

 For steps to follow in *all* procedures, refer to the inside back cover of Volume 2. Go to the full procedures in Volume 2 to practice and learn the procedure steps. Use these procedure highlights later to help you review key points.

Procedure 39-1: Teaching a Patient to Deep-Breathe, Cough, Move in Bed, and Perform Leg Exercises

➤ Assess the patient's readiness to learn.

➤ Ensure that the patient is clear about the difference between coughing and merely clearing the throat.

➤ Demonstrate how to splint a potential chest or abdominal incision.

➤ Make sure the patient flexes her knees prior to turning on her side in bed.

➤ Support the patient who is unable to maintain a side-lying position with pillows.

➤ Teach the patient to alternately flex and extend the knees.

➤ Teach the patient to alternately dorsiflex and plantar flex the foot.

➤ Teach the patient to rotate her ankles in a complete circle.

Procedure 39-2: Applying Antiembolism Stockings

➤ Measure the patient's leg to ensure that you select stockings of the correct size.

➤ Inspect the legs and feet for edema, abrasions, lesions, open areas, and circulatory changes.

➤ Elevate the patient's legs for at least 15 minutes prior to applying stockings.

➤ Insert your hand and turn the stocking inside out to the level of the heel.

➤ Insert patient's foot into stocking. Gradually pull the remaining portion of the stocking up and over the leg.

   Keep knee-high stockings 2.5 to 5 cm (1 to 2 in.) below the joint.

   Do not apply thigh-high stockings if the thigh circumference is greater than 82 cm (32 in.).

➤ Make sure the stocking is free of wrinkles and is not rolled at the top or bunched.

Procedure 39-3: Applying Sequential Compression Devices

➤ Determine whether elastic stockings are to be used concurrently with the sequential device. If so, apply them (see Procedure 39–2).

➤ Place the regulating pump for the sequential compression in a location that will ensure patient safety.

➤ Place the patient in a supine position.

➤ If you are using SCD and PAS brand thigh-high compression sleeves, measure the thigh.

➤ Place the lower extremity on the open sleeve, ensuring that the compression chambers are located over the correct anatomical structure (e.g., knee opening is at the level of the joint).

➤ Leave one to two fingerbreadths between the sleeve and the extremity.

➤ Set the regulating pump to the correct pressure, as ordered.

➤ Instruct the patient to call for assistance in disconnecting the tubing from the sleeve.

Procedure 39-4: Managing Gastric Suction

Procedure 39-4A: Initial Equipment Setup

➤ Connect and secure the suction source, collection container, and drainage tubing.

➤ Don nonsterile gloves.

➤ Connect suction drainage tubing to nasogastric tubing.

➤ Secure the NG tube to the patient's nose and gown (if not already done).

➤ Turn on the suction.

Procedure 39-4B: Emptying the Suction Container

➤ Don nonsterile gloves.

➤ Turn off the suction; close the stopcock (or clamp the tubing).

➤ Empty the suction container and measure the contents.

➤ Empty and wash the graduated measuring container.

➤ Cleanse the suction container port and close the stopper; place the container back in the holder.

➤ Turn on the suction.

➤ Observe for proper functioning and tubing patency.

Procedure 39-4C: Irrigating the Nasogastric Tubing

➤ Prepare the irrigation set.

➤ Don nonsterile gloves.

➤ Place patient at a 30° to 45° degree elevation

➤ Check for NG tube placement.

➤ Fill the syringe with 10 to 30 mL of saline.

➤ Turn off the stopcock or clamp the NG tube.

➤ Disconnect the NG tube from drainage.

➤ Drain the suction tubing and turn off the suction source.

➤ Turn on the stopcock or unclamp the NG tube.

➤ Slowly instill and withdraw irrigant into the NG tube until fluid flows freely.

➤ Turn off the stopcock or reclamp the NG tube.

➤ Reconnect the NG tube.

➤ Turn on the stopcock or release the clamp.

Procedure 39-4D: Providing Comfort Measures

➤ Don nonsterile gloves.

➤ Provide mouth care.

➤ Remove nasal secretions.

➤ Apply water soluble lubricant to nostrils.

➤ Check that tape or tube fixation device is secure.

To explore learning resources for this chapter,

Go to Davis*Plus* at DavisPl.us/Wilkinson3.

Chapter Resources for Chapter 39:

    Response sheets for all learning exercises

    Resources for Caregivers and Health Professionals

    Reading More About Perioperative Care (suggested readings)

    Concept Map of chapter content

Interactive Case Studies

NCLEX-Style and Chapter Review Questions

Chapter Overview Podcasts

For references cited in this chapter,

Go to Volume 2, **References Cited**.

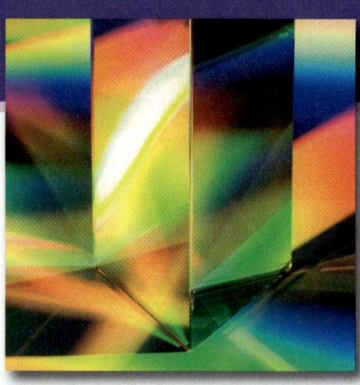

CHAPTER 40

Leading & Managing

Learning Outcomes

After completing this chapter, you should be able to:

- Distinguish leadership, followership, and management.
- Compare and contrast authoritarian, democratic, and laissez-faire leadership styles.
- Explain the differences between transactional and transformational theories.
- Discuss the qualities and behaviors that contribute to effective leadership and followership.
- Discuss the qualities and activities that contribute to effective management.
- Explain how a SWOT analysis or a SOAR analysis can help you prepare to become a leader and manager.
- Discuss the qualities of preceptors and mentors.
- Present strategies for effective followership.

- Describe the challenges presented to nurse managers by the economy and the nursing labor market.
- Define power and empowerment.
- Describe several ways in which nurses can be empowered.
- Explain why communication skills are important to nurse leaders and managers.
- Describe the change process.
- Identify methods of dealing with change.
- Describe the major concepts of conflict, conflict resolution, and informal negotiation.
- Describe the major concepts of safe and effective delegation.
- Establish short- and long-term personal and career goals.
- Develop effective time management strategies.

Key Concepts

Leadership
Management
Followership
Change

Related Concepts

See the Concept Map on Davis*Plus*.

Portions of this chapter were taken from D. K. Whitehead, S. A. Weiss, & R. M. Tappen (2010). *Essentials of nursing leadership and management* (5th ed.). Philadelphia: F. A. Davis. Used with permission.

Meet Your Peer

Mary is a student in a nursing program. She considers herself a "pretty good test-taker" and has a GPA of 3.4. She received her first test grade in the Nursing Fundamentals class, and it was a C. Mary is sure that she will never pass this course and that her dream of becoming a nurse will vanish. When discussing the test with her classmates, she realized there are several other disappointed students who have been used to making As and Bs on exams. The nursing exams seem different because they do not only ask students to recall memorized material but also apply what they have learned. Mary decides to get the group together and plan some strategies for study groups. She asks the instructor whether she will meet with them and go over their plan to make sure they are on the right track. Mary has exhibited some leadership qualities.

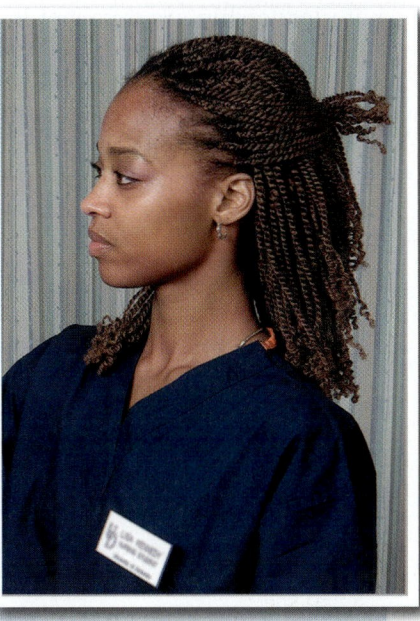

Theoretical Knowledge
knowing why

In this chapter, we discuss the challenges to nurses as they lead and manage others, and deal with change in organizations and the healthcare environment.

ABOUT THE KEY CONCEPTS

Have you ever heard the phrase, "Not every good leader can manage, and not every good manager can lead"? This chapter defines and differentiates between the key concepts of leadership and management. To lead and manage effectively, you will also need to grasp and apply the key concepts of **leadership**, **management**, **followership**, and **change**, as well as subconcepts such as power, empowerment, conflict resolution, delegation, and time management. As you study each of those concepts, try to grasp how they relate to leadership and management.

WHAT IS LEADERSHIP?

You may be thinking, "I just started in my nursing program. How can you expect me to be a leader now?" As a student, you do need time to learn how nurses function in a work environment. However, you can begin to assume some leadership skills as a new student. The essence of **leadership** is the ability to influence other people. Effective leaders enable people to move "in the same direction, toward the same destination, at the same speed, not because they have been forced to, but because they want to" (Lansdale, 2002, p. 63; Gonzalez, 2012). A leader in healthcare has three primary tasks:

- Set direction (i.e., help people develop vision, a mission, goals, and purpose).

- Build commitment (i.e., help people develop motivation, team spirit, and teamwork).
- Confront challenges that arise from innovation, change, and turbulence (Porter-O'Grady, 2011).

 Think **Like a Nurse** 40-1

1. Think of a goal your class might have. Obviously, each student wants to develop the skills necessary to provide excellent patient care and learn the theory content to pass the course and continue in the program. What other goals might you have, as a group? As a leader, how might you help the group members meet their goals?
2. Brainstorm with your peers to identify some shared goals of professional nurses.

Leadership Theories

How does a person become a leader? What type of leader is most effective? Although much research has been done to study these questions, no theory has yet emerged as the clear answer. The reason may be that different situations require different qualities and behaviors. In nursing, for example, some situations require quick thinking and fast action. Others require time to reflect on the best solution to a complicated problem. Let's look now at some of the best-known leadership theories, beginning with some of the older ones.

Trait Theories

Have you ever heard someone say, "Leaders are born, not made"? That implies some of us are natural leaders, but others of us are not. Much of the early leadership research was done in an attempt to identify the qualities, or **traits**, that distinguish a leader from a nonleader. The traits most often identified are intelligence and initiative. Other qualities that were found to be associated with leadership are excellent interpersonal skills, high self-esteem, creativity, willingness to take risks, and ability to tolerate the consequences of taking risks (Northouse, 2013; White & Lippitt, 1960). Leadership may come more easily to some than to others, but everyone can be a leader, at least in certain areas, if she develops the necessary knowledge and skills.

Behavioral Theories

The trait theories were concerned with what a leader *is*, whereas the behavior theories are concerned with what the leader *does*. One of the most influential of these behavioral theories is concerned with leadership style. Three styles have been identified (Northouse, 2012; White & Lippitt, 1960). Pavitt summed up the difference between these three leadership styles:

- A democratic leader tries to move the group *toward its goals*.
- An autocratic leader tries to move the group *toward the leader's goals*.
- A laissez-faire leader makes *little or no attempt* to move the group (Pavitt, 1999, p. 330; Zineldin & Hytter, 2012).

Authoritarian Leadership

This is also called *autocratic, directive, controlling*. The **authoritarian leader** gives orders, makes decisions for the group as a whole, and bears most of the responsibility for the outcomes. For example, when a decision needs to be made, an authoritarian leader would say, "I've given this a great deal of thought and decided this is the way we're going to solve our problem." Authoritarian leadership may be either punitive or kind and compassionate. This type of leadership can be an efficient way to run things when a group needs lots of direction in achieving high-quality and high-quantity outputs (Marquis & Huston, 2012). However when used long term, it tends to inhibit creativity and motivation.

Democratic Leadership

Democratic leadership is also called *participative leadership*. In contrast to the authoritarian leader, a democratic leader shares the planning, decision making, and responsibility for outcomes with members of the group. This type of leader tends to provide guidance rather than control. Although this is often a less efficient way to run things, it is more flexible and more likely to foster motivation and creativity. Group output tends to be of high quality.

Laissez-Faire Leadership

Also called *permissive or nondirective*, the **laissez-faire** ("let it alone") leader has a relatively inactive style and intervenes only when goals have not been met or a problem arises (Zineldin & Hytter, 2012). Laissez-faire leadership gives followers the majority of control in the decision-making process. Some mature individuals thrive under laissez-faire leadership because they need little guidance. However, in most instances, followers look to the leader for direction and may become confused and frustrated with no goal, guidance, or direction. The laissez-faire leader offers little feedback and support to the followers, postpones decision making, or never makes it at all, which leads to poor quality and inefficient work output.

KnowledgeCheck 40-1

- Identify the three common styles of leadership in the behavioral theories of leadership.
- Discuss the type of follower that would benefit from each style of leadership.

Task Versus Relationship Theories

Another important distinction in leadership style is that between a *task* focus and a *relationship* focus (Blake, Mouton, & Tapper, 1981; Havig, Skogstad, Kjekshus, et al., 2011). Some leaders emphasize the tasks (e.g., keeping the nursing station neat, getting charting done) and fail to realize that interpersonal relationships (e.g., attitude of physicians toward nursing staff, treating housekeeping staff with respect) have considerable impact on employee morale and productivity. Others focus on the interpersonal aspects and ignore the quality of job performance. The most effective leader is able to balance the two, attending to both the task and the relationship aspects of working together.

Emotional Intelligence Theory

Emotional intelligence (EI) theory focuses on the relationship aspects of leadership. In part, what sets leadership "stars" apart from ordinary leaders is that they consciously address the effect of people's feelings on the team. This is done by leaders who:

- Learn how to recognize, understand, and manage their own emotions; and how to stay clearheaded and suspend judgment until all the facts are in (Feather, 2009).
- Listen attentively, perceive and accurately interpret unspoken emotions, and acknowledge others' perspectives.
- Bring people together in an environment of respect and cooperation so they can direct their energies toward achieving team goals.

The emotionally intelligent leader's enthusiasm, caring, and support inspires the same feelings throughout the team (Feather, 2009; Sadri, 2012; Whitehead, Weiss, & Tappen, 2010).

Situational Theories

We know now that people and leadership situations are far more complex than the early theories recognized. Furthermore, situations may change rapidly, requiring even more complex theories to explain people's responses. Thus, less simplistic theories have evolved to replace the trait and behavioral theories.

Adaptability is the key to the situational approach (Flackman, Hansebo, & Kihlgren, 2009; Furtado, Batista, & Silva, 2011). Instead of assuming that one particular approach works in all situations, situational theories recognize the complexity of work situations and encourage the leader to consider a number of factors when deciding what action to take. Every situation is different. Situational theories emphasize that it is important to (1) understand all of the factors that affect a particular group of people in a particular environment, and (2) vary the type of leadership to meet the needs of the situation.

Transformational Theories

Although situational theories were an improvement over earlier theories in recognizing how complex the process of influencing others really is, they were still missing something. They did not address meaning, inspiration, and vision, which are the distinguishing features of transformational leadership theory. According to transformational theory, people need a sense of mission that goes beyond good interpersonal relationships or the reward for a job well done (Bass & Avolio, 1993; Salanova, Lorente, Chambel, et al., 2011). This is especially true in nursing. Caring for people, sick or well, is the goal of our profession. Most of us chose nursing for our vision: to do something for the good of humankind. One goal of nursing leadership is to guide us toward achieving that vision.

Transformational leadership involves the ability to inspire and motivate followers. The transformational leader creates a supportive climate, listens to followers, and acts as a coach and mentor. Transformational leaders communicate their vision in a way that is so meaningful and exciting that it reduces negativity and inspires commitment in the people with whom they work (Leach, 2005; Salanova, Lorente, Chambel, et al., 2011). Followers become motivated to go beyond their own self-interests for the good of the group or organization, often accomplishing more than what would normally be expected of them (Doody & Doody, 2012).

The American Nurses Credentialing Centers (ANCC) (2013) Magnet Recognition Program was developed to recognize healthcare organizations that provide the very best in nursing care. The ANCC expects leaders in Magnet organizations to demonstrate the transformational qualities listed in Table 40-1.

Transactional Theories

Whereas transformational leadership uses more of a "selling" style, transactional leadership uses more of a "telling" style. Transactional theory assumes that people are motivated by reward and punishment and that they work best within a clear chain of command. The leader creates structures to make clear what is required of subordinates and what the rewards are. The structure usually includes formal systems of discipline. These leaders monitor behaviors closely to point out errors and make

Table 40-1 ➤ Contrast of Traits in Transactional and Transformational Leadership	
TRANSACTIONAL LEADERSHIP	**TRANSFORMATIONAL LEADERSHIP**
Directive	Participative
Top down	Bottom up
Information	Conversation
Hierarchical communication	Matrix communication
Event oriented	Future oriented
Task focused	Overall experience focused
Directed	Facilitated
Rigid	Flexible
Here and now	Visions for the future
Traditional	Contemporary
Rules	Risk taking
Control	Creativity
Individual performance	Team and relationships
Responsibility	Accountability

Source: Used with permission of Patricia Davis, RN, DNP, MS, NEA-BC, CNL; Concord, CA.

corrective criticisms. They enforce rules to avoid mistakes (Jones & Rudd, 2007; Sabir, Sohail, & Khan, 2011). Transactional leadership is commonly used by managers, and in an organization, the "rewards" are salary and benefits (e.g., healthcare insurance). However, when the demand for a skill—or for workers of a particular type—is greater than the supply, the usual rewards may not be sufficient, and other types of leadership are more effective. Table 40-1 compares the traits of transactional and transformational leadership.

 Think**Like a Nurse** 40-2

Observe a nurse in one of the healthcare agencies at which you are doing a clinical rotation. What leadership qualities and behaviors do you see the nurse exhibiting? How do these behaviors help in planning nursing care?

WHAT IS MANAGEMENT?

Whereas leaders may or may not have official appointments to the position, managers are usually officially appointed. A **manager** is an employee of an organization who has the power, authority, and responsibility for enforcing decisions and for planning, organizing, coordinating, and directing the work of others. Every nurse should be a good leader and a good follower; however, not everyone can or should be a manager. You may notice the following discussion of management overlaps a great deal with the content on leadership you have just read. That is because managers must be leaders, and they have varying styles of leadership.

Key Point: *Not all leaders should be managers, but all managers should be leaders.*

You may be saying to yourself, "I don't want to be a manager. I just want to take care of patients." However, as a registered nurse, you will manage groups of patients, and you will be responsible for supervising nursing assistants, licensed practical nurses, and other ancillary staff. Even as a staff nurse, you will be a manager of care. You may be interested to know that the NCLEX-RN Testing Plan has an entire section devoted to management of care, which is not necessarily about managing the nurses or the nursing unit but rather organizing and delivering (i.e., managing) care to the patient. Questions address nursing activities, such as assessing clients to prioritize care, making appropriate referrals to the community, and acting as a client advocate.

Management Theories

Although there are many management theories, there are two major schools of thought in management: (1) scientific management and (2) the human relations approach to management. As you will see, the first emphasizes the task aspects of managing people, and the second emphasizes the relationship aspects.

Scientific Management

Almost 100 years ago, Frederick Taylor argued that most jobs could be done more efficiently if they were thoroughly analyzed (Lykins, 2011; Taylor, 1911/2011). Given a properly designed task and sufficient incentive to get the work done, workers would be more productive. For example, Taylor encouraged paying people "by the piece," that is, by the number of "widgets" made rather than by the number of hours worked. This encourages workers to get the most work done in the least amount of time. In healthcare, the equivalent of paying "by the piece" would be to pay for the number of clients bathed or monitored. In scientific management, the fastest way to do a job is usually thought to be the best way (Taylor, 1911/2011).

Which do you think would take the least amount of time and worker power: bringing patients to the radiology department or bringing a portable x-ray machine to the bedside? What about physical therapy: taking patients to the physical therapy department or having the therapist come to the patient's room? In healthcare, there has been much discussion about these kinds of questions. This type of thinking is the basis for the emphasis on eliminating excess staff and increasing the productivity of remaining employees.

Human Relations–Based Management

McGregor's (1960) Theory X and Theory Y are good examples of the difference between scientific management and human relations–oriented management (O'Leary, 2010).

Theory X managers believe that most people really do not want to work very hard and that the manager's job is to make sure that they do work hard. According to Theory X, a manager needs to use strict rules, constant supervision, and the threat of punishment (e.g., reprimands, withheld raises, and threats of job loss) to create industrious, conscientious workers. Theory X is similar to scientific management.

Theory Y managers believe that work itself can be motivating, that people want to do their jobs well, and that they will work hard if their managers provide a supportive atmosphere. Theory Y, a human relations–oriented theory, is the opposite viewpoint of Theory X. A Theory Y manager emphasizes guidance rather than control, development rather than close supervision, and reward rather than punishment.

A Theory Y nurse manager is concerned with keeping staff morale as high as possible, assuming that satisfied, motivated staff will do the best work. Employees' attitudes, opinions, hopes, and fears are important to this type of leader. Such a manager would make an effort to work out conflicts and promote mutual understanding among the staff to provide an atmosphere in which people can do their best work.

Servant Leadership

Despite its name, servant leadership applies more to supervisors and administrators than to nurses in staff positions. This type of management emphasizes interpersonal relationships, but goes one step further. The servant leadership manager believes people have value as people, not just as workers (O'Brien, 2011). The manager's attitude is employee first, and the manager is committed to improving the way each employee is treated at work. The servant-leader manager is there to remove barriers, make the work easier, and provide employees with whatever they need to provide the best patient care possible.

Qualities of an Effective Manager

Two-thirds of people who leave their jobs say the main reason was an ineffective or incompetent manager (Ripper, 2013). Given the high costs associated with orientation of new employees, nurse managers are challenged to retain staff nurses. A review of the nursing administration literature indicates that effective leadership styles of nurse managers and administrators enhance staff nurse retention (Duffield, Roche, Blay, et al., 2010). An effective nurse manager has the qualities of leadership, clinical expertise, and business sense. None of these alone is enough; it is the combination that prepares a person for the complex task of managing a group of healthcare providers. Let's look at each quality:

Leadership Leadership is the core of skills (e.g. people, leadership, influence) the nurse needs to function as an effective manager.

Clinical Expertise A nurse manager's role is to help others develop their skills and evaluate how well they have done; therefore, she needs a certain amount of clinical expertise. It is not necessary (or even possible) to know everything that every professional on the team knows, but it is important to be able to assess the effectiveness of the team's work in terms of client outcomes.

Business Sense Nurse managers need to be concerned with the "bottom line," that is, the cost of providing care, especially in comparison with the benefit received from that care. In other words, nurse managers need to be able to analyze how much time is spent to provide a given amount of client care, how effective that client care has been, how much will be paid to the institution for the care delivered, and who will pay for it (e.g., private insurance, government insurance, or the client). These are complex tasks that require knowledge of budgeting, staffing, and measuring patient outcomes, most of which are beyond the scope of this textbook.

Activities of an Effective Manager

Mintzberg (1989) divides the manager's activities into three categories: interpersonal, decisional, and informational. Whitehead, Weiss, and Tappen (2010) build on that work:

Interpersonal Activities

Interpersonal activities are important to both leaders and managers. In fact, one might say that interpersonal skills are important to everyone! From the beginning of your career in nursing school, you will have many opportunities to develop positive working relationships with members of other disciplines, departments, and units within the organization. Can you see how Mary (Meet Your Peer) would need interpersonal skills to accomplish her goals?

Interpersonal activities of managers include the following:

- *Networking.* Managers must clearly articulate nurses' roles in and value to the institution.
- *Conflict negotiation and resolution.* For example, conflict may arise on a unit over work schedules, especially on holidays.
- *Employee development.* This includes providing for continuing learning and upgrading employees' skills.
- *Rewards and punishments.* Examples include salary increases, time off, and praise.
- *Coaching.* The goal is to help the employee do a better job through learning. Some managers use a directive approach ("Let me show you how to do this"). Others use a nondirective approach ("How do you think we can improve our outcomes?").

Decisional Activities

From the very beginning of your career, you will be expected to develop critical-thinking, prioritizing, and decision-making skills in your clinical experiences. Even as a student, you will need to know what information to report to your instructor and when to provide it. Nurse managers' decisions include:

- *Employee evaluation* (e.g., conducting formal performance appraisals)
- *Resource allocation* (e.g., budgeting and how to use available funds wisely)
- *Personnel action* (e.g., hiring and terminating employees)
- *Planning for future changes* (e.g., in budgets or client populations)
- *Job analysis and redesign* (e.g., to make the units run as efficiently as possible)
- *Unit-based decisions* (e.g., staffing policies, space utilization)

What decisions did Mary (Meet Your Peer) make?

Informational Responsibilities

Side by side with decisional responsibilities are the informational responsibilities of a manager.

- *Spokesperson.* The manager relays information from administration to staff members, and speaks to administration on behalf of staff members.
- *Monitoring.* Managers monitor the activities of their units or departments (e.g., the number of clients seen, length of stay), as well as the staff (e.g., absenteeism) and the budget (e.g., money spent).
- *Public Relations.* Nurse managers share information with clients, staff members, and employers, for example, regarding new developments in healthcare and policy changes.

What kinds of information would Mary (Meet Your Peer) need to communicate to the students interested in forming a study group?

KnowledgeCheck 40-2

- How is transformational leadership different from the other theories of leadership?
- Define *manager*.
- In McGregor's management theory, which is more like scientific management: Theory X or Theory Y?

HOW CAN I PREPARE TO BECOME A LEADER AND MANAGER?

You may still be asking yourself, "What does all this leadership and management stuff have to do with me?" Besides learning the role of the registered nurse, you should begin right now to look at the skills employers think you need to be ready to work for them. Along with passing the NCLEX-RN examination to obtain nursing licensure, employers cite the skills listed in Box 40-1 as

BOX 40-1 ■ Desirable Job Candidate Skills

- Ability to assume responsibility
- Computer knowledge
- Critical-thinking and analytical skills
- Interpersonal skills
- Leadership abilities
- Motivation, initiative, and flexibility
- Oral and written communication skills
- Organizational skills
- Problem-solving and decision-making abilities
- Proficiency in field of study or technical competence
- Self-discipline
- Teamwork ability
- Willingness to work hard
- Ability to teach others
- Ability to adapt equipment to serve user needs
- Flexibility to adjust action in relation to others

desirable in job candidates (Ghannadian, 2013; Shingleton, 1994; Villarreal, 2002). Many of these skills have been identified in our discussion of leading and managing. It is not too early to begin to develop your abilities in these areas. These skills will assist you as you go through your nursing program, and will also make your adjustment to the RN role much easier.

One of the first steps in identifying what skills you already possess and which you need to develop is to do a brief SWOT analysis. A SWOT (strengths, weaknesses, opportunities, threats) analysis plan, borrowed from the corporate world, can guide you through an analysis of your own internal strengths and weaknesses and reveal external opportunities and threats that may help or hinder your leadership and management skills (Orr, 2013). Your SWOT analysis may include the factors listed as examples in Table 40-2, but certainly you will have others.

You might prefer to use the SOAR strategic planning model to help you prepare to become a leader and manager (Table 40-3). This model can be used to analyze any type of situation and create a plan to achieve personal and professional goals. With this model, you would use inquiry, imagination, innovation, and aspiration, and also focus on strengths, opportunities, aspirations, and results (Sprangel, 2011; Stavros, Cooperrider, & Kelly, 2007).

 ThinkLike a Nurse 40-3

Stop and think! Take some time to personalize the SWOT analysis in Table 40-2. What weaknesses do you need to minimize, or which strengths do you need to develop as you begin to develop your leadership and management skills?

How Can Mentors and Preceptors Help Me?

There are two aspects to consider as you get ready to become a leader and manager. The first, discussed earlier, consists of developing self. The second is really a combination of developing self and developing others: mentorship and preceptorship. A **mentor** is someone more experienced who provides career development assistance, such as coaching, sponsoring advancement, providing challenging assignments, protecting protégés from adversity, and promoting positive visibility. Mentors provide guidance to new students or recent graduates as they continue in the profession. They offer a constructive example as a role model to novices. Mentors can also fulfill psychosocial roles, such as personal support, friendship, acceptance, role modeling, and counseling.

Table 40-2 ➤ SWOT Analysis Plan—Examples

STRENGTHS	WEAKNESSES	OPPORTUNITIES	THREATS
Relevant work experience	Poor communication and people skills	Changes in healthcare	Changes in healthcare
Advanced education	Inflexibility	Availability of mentors and preceptors	Lack of time
Good communication and people skills	Lack of interest in self-learning	Variety of experiences in clinical rotations	Competition from other students and other nursing programs
Computer skills	Difficulty adapting to change	Many leadership and management books and self-learning programs available	

SWOT = strengths, weaknesses, opportunities, threats

Table 40-3 ➤ SOAR Strategic Planning

THE PROCESS: HOW TO SOAR	THE SOAR REPORT OR SUMMARY
To SOAR: Inquire, imagine, innovate, and inspire.	Use SOAR to report or tell your story.
Inquiry: Internal analysis of strengths and external analysis of opportunities	**Strengths.** My (or the group's) strengths are ... (Examples of strengths may be a supportive environment, individual strengths, a product that others need, and so on.)
Imagination: Co-create vision, values, and mission. Imagine desired outcomes. Imagine the best pathway to achieve the outcomes.	**Opportunities.** My values are ... (e.g., dedication, quality). As I imagine the future, my vision (for myself, for our group) is ... (e.g., to become a transformational manager on a nursing unit).
Innovation: Create initiatives, strategies, structures, and systems. Create plans for tactics.	**Aspirations.** Here is how I believe I (or we) can achieve the desired outcomes.
Inspiration: Inspire action-oriented activities that achieve results. Implement a plan for continuous improvement.	**Results.** To achieve your desired outcomes, you must be motivated (and possibly need to inspire others) to take the necessary actions.

SOAR = strengths, opportunities, aspirations, results

✚ You should always use sound judgment when following the advice of others. Do not blindly engage in behaviors or actions because others do them.

Many organizations have preceptors for new employees. A preceptor is someone with more experience who provides practical teaching and guidance for a student or new employee. As a student, you may be assigned an RN preceptor in your clinical rotations. You may work side by side with a preceptor to provide patient care as a student nurse and as a new graduate nurse (Fig. 40-1). In many instances, the preceptor will become your mentor. However, the mentor role is much more encompassing than the preceptor role. The mentor relationship is a voluntary one and is built on mutual respect and development of the mentee. Box 40-2 identifies responsibilities of the mentor and mentee in this relationship.

You should look for a mentor in the nursing program right now—someone to guide you as you grow into your professional role. A student who has already completed several semesters and appears to be a leader is a good choice. In some programs, you may be assigned a student preceptor while you are in the program. Although this student may or may not become your mentor, you will need to have leadership and management skills to work side by side effectively.

Will you assume the role of preceptor or mentor while you are still in school? We hope your response is yes. As you progress in the program, remember the feelings of uncertainty and anxiety that you may now have, and volunteer to mentor another new student. Through the mentoring process, you can continue to develop yourself as a leader. Mentoring and preceptoring are part of your professional responsibilities, as the American Nurses Association (ANA, 2010) Standard of Professional Performance 10 states:

Collegiality. The registered nurse interacts with and contributes to the professional development of peers and colleagues.

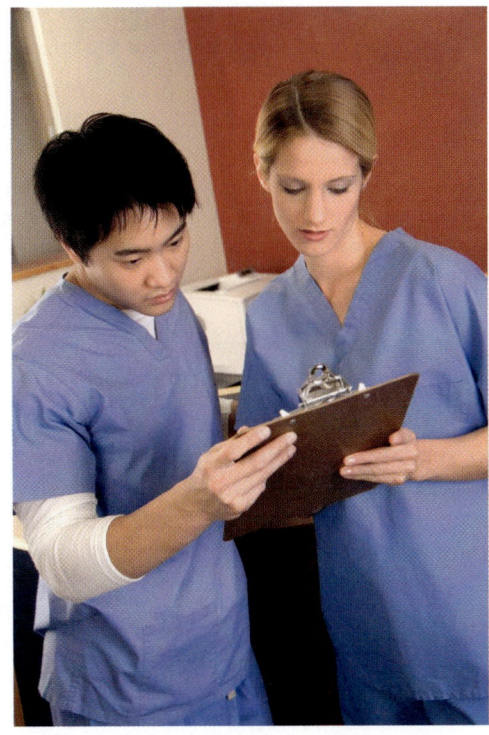

FIGURE 40-1 Nurse precepting a new graduate.

BOX 40-2 ■ Mentor and Mentee Responsibilities

Mentor Responsibilities

- Demonstrate excellent communication and listening skills.
- Be sensitive to the needs of nurses, patients, and the workplace.
- Encourage excellence in others.
- Share and provide counsel.
- Exhibit good decision-making skills.
- Demonstrate an understanding of power and politics.
- Demonstrate trustworthiness.

Mentee Responsibilities

- Demonstrate eagerness to learn.
- Participate actively in the relationship by keeping all appointments and commitments.
- Seek feedback, and use it to modify behaviors.
- Demonstrate flexibility and an ability to change.
- Be open in the relationship with the mentor.
- Demonstrate an ability to move toward independence.
- Evaluate choices and outcomes.

Source: Whitehead, D., Weiss, S., & Tappen, R. (2010). *Essentials of nursing leadership and management* (5th ed.). Philadelphia: F.A. Davis.

How Will Leadership Grow in My Nursing Career?

As you begin your nursing clinical experiences, your nursing instructor will supervise most of your decisions. As you continue to develop your knowledge and skills, you will begin working more as a member of the team. You will be expected to prioritize patient care, work with a variety of team members and families, and provide care for groups of clients. You may go to community agencies and network with community groups. To be successful in your continued role development as a nurse, you must work on perfecting the skills discussed in this chapter.

KnowledgeCheck 40-3

- Identify four skills that employers cite as desirable in job candidates.
- Identify three responsibilities of a mentor and three responsibilities of a mentee.

 ThinkLike a Nurse 40-4

Think about how you are working with your peers at this time. What mentor responsibilities are you exhibiting? Is there someone who is already mentoring you? If so, what qualities does this person exhibit?

WHAT IS FOLLOWERSHIP?

Leadership and followership are two separate concepts and two separate roles that are complementary, not competitive. Great leaders can create successful followers, and great followers create successful leaders. No one person can have the best strategy, the clearest vision, or identify the most effective approaches to solve problems. All participants need to be recognized as full partners in the organizational venture. If we define **followers** as individuals who take another person as a role model and who act in accordance with, imitate, support, and advocate the ideas and opinions of another (Grossman & Valiga, 2012), then we can define **followership** as the

willingness to work with others toward accomplishing the group mission. This term also refers to those who show a high degree of teamwork and build cohesion among the group (Ricketts, 2010).

An organization is a community of many leaders and many followers, frequently changing places depending on the particular activity that is occurring. Blindly following a leader without question or taking a passive role in one's work or professional organization will do little to advance the profession, promote individual growth, or achieve quality patient care. To participate fully and provide significant feedback, followers need to demonstrate a number of important qualities and behaviors (Grossman & Valiga, 2012; Kean, Haycock-Stuart, Baggaley, et al., 2011; Whitehead, Weiss, & Tappen, 2010):

- Suggest ways to improve client care.
- If you discover a problem, inform your team leader right away. Include a suggestion for solving the problem. If it is not accepted, your job is then to support—not undermine—the leader.
- Listen carefully and reflect on what the leader or manager says.
- Be truthful. Give honest feedback and constructive criticism, even if it means politely challenging the leader's ideas. Suggest alternative courses of action.
- If you feel you must have a "heated" discussion with the leader, do so privately. When you disagree, explain why.
- Freely invest your interest and energy in your work and in finding best solutions for the group.
- Function independently; be a self-starter; take on extra tasks without being asked.
- Be innovative, creative, and actively involved.
- Be responsible and hold up your end of the bargain; accept responsibility when it is offered.
- Be supportive of new ideas and directions suggested by others, but think critically about ideas that are proposed. Seek information so you can see the larger picture.
- Don't gossip.

- Think and act as a team; be cooperative and collaborative.
- Draw on and complement one another's and the leader's specialties, strengths, and areas of expertise.
- Work on behalf of the organization and the mutually agreed-on vision and goals.
- Continue to learn as much as you can about your specialty area; share what you learn with others.
- Know your own strengths and what your unique contributions to the effort can be.
- Know how to assume the role of the leader when necessary.
- Have a positive sense of self-worth and a "can do" attitude.
- Take care of yourself and your family. If you and they are unhappy, your job performance will suffer.

To find more suggestions for developing your skills as a follower,

 Go to Chapter 40, **Tables, Boxes, Figures: ESG Box 40-1, Developing Effective Follower Skills,** on *DavisPlus.*

WHAT ARE THE CHALLENGES TO BEING AN EFFECTIVE LEADER AND MANAGER?

Even after you have developed the skills necessary to become an effective leader or manager, challenges exist in the healthcare environment. These challenges include the economic climate of healthcare and the nursing labor market.

Economic Climate of Healthcare

For many years, decisions about care were based primarily on providing the best quality care, whatever the cost. More recently healthcare providers are pressured to seek methods of care delivery that achieve quality outcomes at lower costs. This economic perspective is rooted in three fundamental observations:

1. *Resources are scarce.* The scarcity of resources means that three decisions must be made:
   - How much do we spend on healthcare services, and what do those services consist of?
   - How will those healthcare services be produced?
   - How should, or can, we distribute healthcare? In other words, how are services apportioned within the population? For example, it is hard to believe that the healthcare needs of more than 47 million uninsured individuals in America are not being met because these people cannot afford to pay insurance premiums. How will this change with the Affordable Care Act?
2. *Resources have alternative uses.* Because resources are limited, a choice to spend resources in one area eliminates the allocation of those same resources for another use. If we wish to build more nursing homes, for example, we must be willing to accept fewer hospitals or less housing, education, or other uses of those same resources. In healthcare, an expanded program of immunization may mean limiting care for certain chronic illnesses or for certain age groups.
3. *Individuals want different things or have different preferences.* Some people choose alternative treatment modalities, such as acupuncture, herbal therapy, or massage therapy, rather than traditional healthcare. The assumption exists that preferences for products and services can be influenced—hence, the extensive marketing of healthcare services.

Nursing Labor Market

The number of registered nurses employed in the nurse workforce in the United States is at 2.6 million, and continues to grow. There are 62.2% registered nurses employed in hospitals (ANA, 2011). More than half of RNs work at least 40 hours a week in their principal position, and another 24% work 32 to 39 hours per week (U.S. Department of Health and Human Services [USDHSS], 2013).

The Bureau of Labor Statistics predicted there would be more than 1 million vacant positions for registered nurses by 2020 (Robert Wood Johnson Foundation, 2013). The need for nurses is expected to increase even more dramatically as the baby boomers reach their 60s, 70s, and beyond. From now until 2030, the population aged 65 and older will double. The questions are (1) whether there will be enough nurses available to fill those jobs, and (2) even if nurses are available, whether it will be economically feasible for organizations to hire as many as they need. The Affordable Care Act will present changes in the healthcare system in the United States. It is certain that the future supply and demand of nurses will be affected by this (Poghosyan, Lucero, Rauch, et al., 2012).

As in the past, cost control and demand for nursing services will most likely involve changing nurse staffing patterns, the model of care, or professional nursing practice (Douglas, 2009). All of these changes will affect you. Regardless, healthcare system changes will likely demand that the RN lead and manage personnel delivering patient care while maintaining fiscal responsibility. Healthcare is big business, even though it is heavily regulated by government and other agencies. You must juggle the needs of your patients with the needs of the organization. From time to time, think about how you might do that.

 Think**Like a Nurse** 40-5

Identify changes in your community that will affect you as you embark upon your nursing career. What will you do to prepare for these changes?

WHAT ARE POWER AND EMPOWERMENT?

The leadership and management techniques discussed so far will help you to achieve your goals. However, there are times when your attempts to influence others are overwhelmed by other forces or individuals. Where does this power come from? Who has it? Who does not?

Although people at the top of an organization have most of the *authority* in the organization, they do not have all of the *power*. In fact, the people at the bottom of the hierarchy also have some power. **Power** is the ability to influence other people despite resistance from them. In other words, one person or group can impose its will on another person or group (Haslam, Reicher, & Platow, 2011). Power may be actual or potential, intended or unintended. It may also be used for good or for evil, for serious purposes or for selfish ones.

Sources of Power

The sources of power vary from one situation to another. Some of these sources may be available to nurses (Kelly, 2012).

- **Authority:** The power granted to an individual or a group by virtue of position (within the organizational hierarchy, for example)
- **Reward:** The promise of money, goods, services, recognition, or other benefits to an individual or group to influence them to change.
- **Expert:** The power derived from knowledge and skills an individual is believed to possess. As Sir Francis Bacon said long ago, "Knowledge is power" (Bacon, 1597, quoted in Fitton, 1997, p. 150; Bacon, 2011).
- **Coercion:** The threat of pain or of harm, which may be physical, economic, or psychological

Let's look at various groups of people in a healthcare organization in terms of the types of power that may be available to them.

Managers are able to reward people with salary increases, promotions, and recognition. They can also use coercion—cause economic or psychological pain for the people who work for them, particularly through their authority to evaluate and fire people.

Patients at first appear to be relatively powerless in a healthcare organization. However, if patients refused to use the services of a particular organization, that organization would eventually cease to exist. Patients reward healthcare workers by praising them to their supervisors. They can also cause discomfort by complaining about them.

Registered nurses have expertise power, as well as authority to delegate appropriately to licensed practical nurses, nursing assistive personnel (NAPs), and other personnel by virtue of their position in the hierarchy and the state's nurse practice act. Nurses are essential to the operation of most healthcare organizations and could cause considerable disruption if they refused to work. These actions are another source of power (coercion) for nurses (Weydt, 2010).

Nurses have always had the power of information, or expertise. For example, Florence Nightingale showed very graphically in the 1800s that wherever her nurses were, far fewer patients died; and wherever they were not, far more died. Think of the power of that information. Immediately people were saying, "What would you like, Miss Nightingale? Would you like more money? Would you like a school of nursing? What else can we do for you?" (Fralic, 2000, p. 340). She had solid data, she knew how to collect, interpret and distribute the data in terms of things that people valued (Stanley & Sherratt, 2010).

Assistants and technicians may appear to have less power because of their position in an organization's "top-down" hierarchy. Imagine, though, how the work of the organization (e.g., hospital, nursing home) would grind to a halt if all the nursing assistants failed to appear one morning. Therefore, they have both expertise and coercive power.

KnowledgeCheck 40-4
What are the sources of power available to nurses?

Sources of Empowerment

How can nurses, either individually or collectively, maximize their power and increase their feelings of empowerment? To answer this question, you should first distinguish between the concepts of power and empowerment. Recall that power is the ability to influence other people despite resistance from them. **Empowerment** is a psychological state, a feeling of competence, control, and entitlement that a person experiences.

Key Point: *Given these definitions, it is possible to be powerful and yet not feel empowered. Power refers to action, and empowerment refers to feelings. Both are of interest to nursing leaders and managers.*

Feeling empowered includes the following:

- **Self-determination:** Feeling free to decide how to do your work
- **Meaning:** Caring about your work, enjoying it, and taking it seriously
- **Competence:** Confidence in your ability to do your work well
- **Impact:** Feeling that people listen to your ideas, that you can make a difference

Nurses, like most people, want to have some power and to feel empowered. You want to be heard, recognized, valued, and respected. You do not want to feel unimportant or insignificant to society or to the organization in which you work. The following contribute to your empowerment: (a) manageable, reasonable work assignments; (b) reward, recognition, and appreciation for a job well done; and (c) fair, consistent treatment of all staff.

Not all empowerment comes from others. You can become empowered by actively participating in professional nursing organizations, joining a collective bargaining unit, and seeking opportunities to be involved in decision making in your organization. Two other ways of empowering yourself are by enhancing and sharing expertise.

Enhancing Expertise

Nurses and other healthcare professionals are empowered to some degree by their own professional knowledge and competence. Following are some ways in which you can enhance your competence, thereby increasing your own sense of empowerment:

- Actively participate in interdisciplinary team conferences and patient-centered conferences on your unit.
- Attend continuing education activities to enhance your expertise. This might include local, regional, national, and international conferences sponsored by nursing organizations.
- Use evidence-based practice guidelines, current nursing journals, and books to make decisions regarding your nursing practice.
- Participate in nursing research projects related to your clinical area.
- Discuss with colleagues in nursing and other disciplines how to handle a difficult clinical situation.
- Observe the practice of experienced nurses.
- Continue education by earning additional degrees and certifications in nursing.

Although you have just begun your nursing career, it is not too early to begin thinking of ways to become empowered.

Sharing Expertise

The second part, becoming empowered through expertise, is to share with others the knowledge and experience you have. This means not only using your knowledge to improve your own practice, but also communicating what you have learned to other students and, later, to your colleagues in nursing. It also means letting your instructors and supervisors know that you have enhanced your professional competence. You can share your knowledge with your clients, empowering them as well. In the future, you may even reach the point at which you have learned more about a particular subject than most nurses have and want to write about it for publication.

PracticalKnowledge
knowinghow

As a leader or manager, you will need to get people to work together to make things happen. To do so, you will need to effectively communicate, delegate, deal with conflict and change, and manage your time appropriately. All of these can be thought of as skills or processes (practical knowledge).

COMMUNICATING

Leadership arises through relationships with other people, and leaders use communication to engage and support these relationships. Some view communication as a circular process that is affected by many factors. Thus, communication has both content and a relationship context. This means the activity is continuous, mutually interdependent, and influenced by the behaviors of each communicator. You need to use active listening to pick up all levels of meaning in a communication. Surface listening, or inattention, often causes a misinterpretation of the message. Your attitude also influences what you hear and how you interpret the message. Communication skills are taught extensively in Chapter 21, if you need to review them now.

To effectively manage client care, it is important to keep the lines of communication open on all levels. As a professional nurse, you will need to communicate client information to members of the nursing team, members of other disciplines, families, and individual clients. Trust and sincerity enhance communication among team members. Congruence (agreement) between your words and your deeds promotes trust. If team members feel that you are trustworthy and sincere, they will be more likely to ask questions and seek clarification when they are uncertain of something.

A leader is responsible for providing frequent evaluative feedback. Done poorly, evaluation can be stressful, even injurious. Done well, it promotes growth and employee satisfaction. Evaluative feedback is important because it:

- *Reinforces constructive behavior.* Positive feedback lets people know which behaviors are most productive and encourages them to continue the behaviors.
- *Discourages unproductive behavior.* Negative feedback prompts the person to correct inappropriate behavior.
- *Provides recognition.* Praise is an excellent motivator.

DELEGATING

An important aspect of leadership and management is learning how to delegate. You can apply the nursing process to delegating to safely provide client care.

- *Assess and diagnose.* Before deciding who should care for a particular client, you must assess each client's particular needs.
- *Plan goals and interventions.* Set client-specific goals, and identify the interventions required to achieve these goals. Mentally identify which staff member is best suited for the task or activities before delegating helps prevent problems later.
- *Implement.* Next, determine which personnel have the knowledge and skills to care for the client, and assign the tasks to the appropriate person.
- *Evaluate.* You must still oversee care and determine whether client care needs have been met. Be sure to

The Effect of Authority Gradients on Teamwork and Patient Safety

Chapter Key Concept: *Management, (Subconcept) Followership*

Competencies: *Teamwork and Collaboration (Knowledge, Skills, Attitudes); Patient-Centered Care (Skills)**

Teamwork and collaboration are influenced by the psychological distance a team member feels between him and others higher up in the team structure. This is called the *authority gradient*. The greater the authority gradient, the less likely a person is to feel part of a team, question those in authority, or communicate concerns. Minimizing the authority gradient has been shown to improve communication, which reduces errors.

The authority gradient between physicians and nurses is very steep and is reinforced by tradition, individual personalities, physicians' attitudes, and, at times, nurses' fears of being incorrect. What are the authority gradients between nurses and other members of the healthcare team, including nursing assistants and others over whom nurses have authority?

Education and Team Building. To flatten these gradients, facilities need to provide education and team-building activities to all staff, including physicians.

Team Briefings. Another strategy is to establish team briefings as an expected routine. Briefings promote clear, effective communication and include introductions all around, review of the patient's problems and the treatment plan, and specific requests by the physician (or other person with the most authority and accountability) for input. Briefings create a shared understanding and foster an environment in which team members can and do speak up about any concerns.

Individual Skills. Individually, you can develop your communication skills, adopt an attitude of collaboration, and learn more about how to become a capable team member. To begin this process, consider the following:

➤ What are your strengths or weaknesses as a team member? What Knowledge, Skills, and Attitudes can you acquire to become more effective?

➤ How can you gain the confidence to question a doctor's order or assert your perspective on a patient's treatment plan? Have you practiced assertive communication?

➤ Are you succinct when you communicate? What structured communication style can you adopt to keep your comments and requests clear?

➤ Do you consistently show respect for other team members and what they contribute to the patient's care?

➤ Can you communicate the patient's values, preferences, and expressed needs to the healthcare team?

Sources: Hamman, Beaudin-Seiler & Beaubien. (2010); The Joint Commission (2011); Magrane, Khan, Pigeon, et al. (2010); Manser, T. (2009).

*For specific Knowledge, Skills, and Attitudes,

 Go to the QSEN Web site, at http://qsen.org/ competencies/pre-licensure-ksas/

---

allow time for feedback during the day. This enables all personnel to see how they are doing and what they still need to do. If you must give negative feedback, do so privately.

You will find an extended discussion of delegation in Chapter 7. You might also find helpful the American Nurses Association and National Council of the State Boards of Nursing (NCSBN) (n.d.) joint statement on delegation and a decision tree to promote proper delegation. For the NCSBN (2009) checklist using the *Five Rights of Delegation,*

 Go to Chapter 7, **Implementation and Evaluation Tools, The Five Rights of Delegation-Checklist,** in Volume 2.

A manager must first determine the mix of personnel (RN, LVN/LPN, or NAP) required to deliver care on a unit before being able to delegate tasks to individuals. By looking at the needs of each client, you can make an educated decision about which staff members have the appropriate education and skill to deliver safe, quality care.

What If I Lack the Experience to Delegate?

The added responsibility of delegation often causes discomfort for new graduates. You may be used to providing total patient care for one or more clients, but lack the experience of organizing care for groups of clients with other team members. To overcome your discomfort, you need to observe how more experienced nurses delegate to others. Working with a preceptor will also give you experience in delegation.

Become familiar with nursing professional organization guidelines. The ANA has specified that RNs may not delegate the following tasks (Neumann, 2010):

- Initial nursing assessment; follow-up assessments if nursing judgment is indicated
- Nursing diagnosis
- Decisions and judgments about outcomes
- Formulation and approval of a patient plan of care
- Interventions that require professional nursing knowledge, decisions, or skills
- Decisions and judgments necessary for the evaluation of patient care

The ANA (2002, 2007) has issued a Position Statement on use of nursing assistive personnel (Plawecki & Amrhein, 2010). The list includes direct and indirect client care that may be delegated to NAPs (Fig. 40-2). Various other nursing personnel can also be used to meet patient care needs (Box 40-3).

What Are the Concerns About Delegating?

Today's healthcare environment requires nurses to delegate. Many nurses voice concerns about the personal

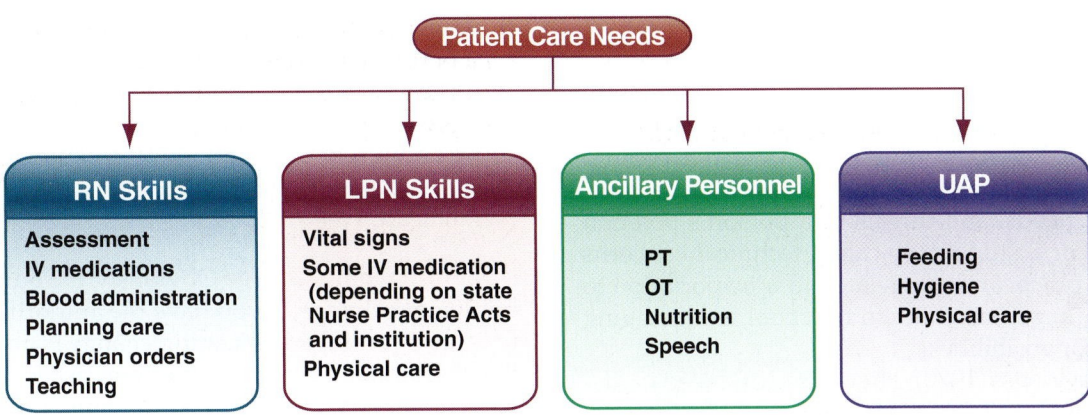

FIGURE 40-2 Patient care needs.

BOX 40-3 ■ Examples of Care That May Be Delegated to Nursing Assistive Personnel

Direct Client Care Activities

■ Assisting with activities of daily living: feeding, drinking, ambulation, grooming, toileting, dressing

■ Assisting with socializing

■ Taking vital signs

Indirect Client Care Activities

■ Providing a clean, safe environment

■ Providing transport for noncritical clients

■ Assisting with stocking nursing units

■ Providing messenger and delivery services

■ Making beds

■ Ordering supplies

risk to their licensure if they delegate inappropriately. The courts have usually ruled that nurses are not liable for the negligence of other workers, provided that the nurse delegated appropriately. Delegation is within the scope of nursing practice, according to the ANA. Refer to Chapter 45 for further discussion on the legal aspects of delegation.

Nurses have also expressed concern over the effects of delegation on the quality of client care. When you delegate, you control the delegation. You decide to whom and what you will delegate. Remember that there are levels of acceptable performance and that not every task needs to be done perfectly.

KnowledgeCheck 40-5

Explain the relationship of delegation and the nursing process.

MANAGING CHANGE

Change is a naturally occurring phenomenon, a part of everyone's life. Every day, we have new experiences, meet new people, and learn something new. We grow up, leave home, graduate from college, and begin a new career, and perhaps a new family as well. Some of these changes are milestones in our lives, ones we have prepared for and anticipated for some time. Others are entirely unexpected—sometimes welcome and sometimes not. Many are exciting, leading us to new opportunities and challenges. When change occurs too rapidly or with high demands, it can make us very uncomfortable.

The Comfort Zone

The basic stages of Lewin's change process are unfreezing, change, and refreezing (Doolin, Quinn, Bryant, et al., 2011; Lewin, 1951). Figure 40-3 shows the relationship among those stages and the concepts of comfort zone, discomfort zone, and a new comfort zone.

Let's assume that your daily routine was basically stable before you started nursing school. You took care of the family or worked during the day and took a class or two each term. You knew what to expect and how to deal with whatever problems arose in the course of a day. In other words, you were operating within your "comfort zone" (Farrell & Broude, 1987; Lapp, 2002; Ryder, 2013). A big change is likely to move you out of this comfort zone into disequilibrium, possibly into discomfort. Now you are most likely attending a full-time nursing program and juggling changes in finances, child-care arrangements, and planning options. This first stage in the change process is called *unfreezing*. You are moving out of your comfort zone.

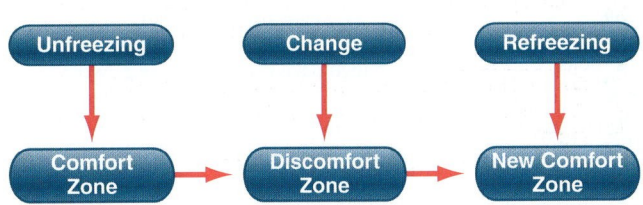

FIGURE 40-3 The change process. (Based on Doolin, C., Quinn, L., Bryant, L., et al., 2011; Farrell, K., & Broude, C., 1987; Lewin, K., 1951; Ryder, J., 2013.)

Resistance to Change

People resist change for a variety of reasons. For example, you may find that you can manage the change in class schedule, but that the child-care arrangements are more difficult. Resistance to change (and unfreezing) comes from three major sources: technical concerns, psychosocial needs, and threats to a person's position and power. For a student, so-called technical concerns may involve practical issues related to transportation to school or work, getting children to school, or managing household responsibilities.

Recall Maslow's (1970) Hierarchy of Needs, discussed in various chapters in this book. Maslow observed that the more basic needs (e.g., physiological and safety needs) must be at least partially met before a person is motivated to seek fulfillment of the higher-order needs. Change can make it more difficult for a person to meet any or all of these physiological and psychosocial needs (Cannon, 2013). Once status, power, and influence are gained within families and organizations, they are hard to give up. You may be the one in charge in the family and in the office, yet be a novice in the nursing program.

Recognizing Resistance

It is easy to recognize resistance to a change when it is expressed directly. When a person says to you, "That's not a very good idea," "I am going to quit if I can't get better grades," or "There's no way I'm going to do that," there is no doubt that you are meeting resistance. When resistance is less direct, however, you may not recognize it unless you know what to look for. Resistance may be active or passive.

- **Active resistance** can take the form of aggressive actions or outright refusals to comply (such as the statements in the previous paragraph), writing negative e-mails that attack and destroy the idea or the person who suggested it, quoting existing rules that make the change difficult or impossible to implement, or organizing resistance to the change (encouraging others to resist).
- **Passive approaches** involve avoidance: canceling appointments to discuss implementing the change; being "too busy" to make the change; agreeing to the change but doing nothing to effect it; and simply ignoring the entire process as much as possible.

 ThinkLike a Nurse 40-6

Recall one change that you have experienced that was put into effect by a command (or a new rule, policy, or law).

- What effects did this change have on your life (e.g., work, school, home)?
- How did the command make you feel?
- What would have made this change easier for you?

Lowering Resistance

Key Point: *A change that is welcomed by one group may be strongly resisted by another group. Resistance to change is affected by the leadership approach and the type of organizational structure.*

You can use various approaches to lower people's resistance to change. Strategies fall into four categories: commanding, disseminating information, refuting currently held beliefs, and providing psychological safety (Whitehead, Weiss, & Tappen, 2010).

Commanding Change Obviously, the quickest way to implement change, if you have the authority to do so, is to issue a command. Dictating change is not necessarily the best strategy, but it is sometimes necessary when the change must be made quickly. Commanding a change may not be effective if there are ways for people to resist, for example, when:

- Passive resistance can undermine the change
- High motivational levels are necessary to make the change successful
- People can refuse to obey the order without negative consequences

Sharing Information Much resistance is simply the result of misunderstandings about a proposed change. Sharing information is usually an effective way to reduce uncertainty and ease transition. Information about the change can be shared on a one-to-one basis, in group meetings, or through written materials distributed by print or electronic means. For you as a student, it is important that any changes in the program are communicated to you without delay. You should also communicate any changes in your plans to the appropriate people, such as other students, your nurse team leader, or your instructor. As a student nurse or staff member, you should treat client resistance to change in the same manner. The more information that you give the client, the more likely she will be to cooperate with the change.

Refuting Currently Held Beliefs You can sometimes increase a person's willingness to change by simply providing evidence that his actions or beliefs are inadequate, incorrect, or inefficient. For example, a patient may enter the hospital recalling horror stories from friends and family, but may then find that there was no basis for the stories. Consider the fact that your ideas about the nursing program have changed since you first began. What happened, or what information did you receive, that caused you to change your beliefs?

Providing Psychological Safety When a proposed change threatens basic human needs in some way, reducing that threat can lower resistance. This leaves people feeling more comfortable about the change. Although each situation poses different kinds of threats and requires different actions to reduce them, Box 40-4 identifies common strategies that help increase psychological safety and reduce resistance to change.

BOX 40-4 ■ Common Strategies to Increase Psychological Safety and Reduce Resistance to Change

- Point out similarities between old and new procedures.
- Suggest ways in which the change can provide new opportunities and challenges.
- Allow time for learning and practice of any new procedures, if possible, before a change is implemented.
- Recognize the competence and skill of the people involved.
- Involve as many people as possible in both the design and implementation of the change.
- Express approval of people's concern for providing the best care possible.
- Express the value of each individual's and group's contributions in general and to the proposed change.
- Provide a climate of trust and acceptance in which mistakes can be made without negative consequences for individuals.
- If possible, provide assurance that no one will lose his or her position because of the change.
- Provide opportunities for people to express their feelings and ask questions about the proposed change.

Implementing the Change

In planning for change, you will already have asked yourself these questions:

What is the purpose of this change? What are we trying to accomplish?

Is the change necessary?

Is the change technically correct?

Will the change work?

Is there a better way to do this?

After employing some unfreezing strategies, you are ready to make the change that has been so carefully planned. In addition to employing strategies to lower resistance, increase motivation, and help people work well together, you will want to consider the following characteristics of the change:

- **Magnitude of the Change.** Is this a major change that affects almost everything people do, or is it a minor one with little impact on what people do every day?
- **Complexity of the Change.** Is this a difficult change to make? Does it require much new knowledge or skills, or both? How long will it take for people to acquire the necessary knowledge and skills?
- **Pace of the Change.** How urgent is this change? Can it be done gradually, or must it be implemented all at once?
- **Stress Level of Those Involved.** What is the current stress level of the people involved in this change? Is this the only change that is taking place, or is it just one of many changes taking place? How stressful are these changes? How can I help people keep their stress levels within tolerable bounds?

As indicated earlier, some discomfort is likely to occur with almost any change, but it is important to keep it within tolerable limits. You need enough pressure to get people to pay attention to the change process, but not so much that they are overstressed by it. In other words, you want to raise the heat enough to get them moving, but not so high that they boil over (Battilana & Casciaro, 2013).

Integrating the Change

Integrating the change is the last step. After the change has been made, it is important to make sure that everyone has moved into a new comfort zone. Ask yourself:

- Is the change well integrated into everyday operations?
- Are people comfortable with it now?
- Is it well accepted and perceived as valuable? If not, why not? What can be done to increase acceptance?
- Is there any residual resistance that could still undermine full integration of the change? If there is, how can this resistance be overcome?

Change "sticks" when, instead of being the new way to do something, it has become "the way we always do things around here" (Kotter, 1999, p. 18; see also Dean, 2013).

Change is an inevitable part of living and working. Your leadership can influence how people respond to change, the amount of stress it causes, and the amount of resistance it provokes. Handled well, most changes can become opportunities for professional growth and development rather than just additional stressors for students, nurses, and their clients.

CONFLICT

Nursing education and healthcare settings bring together people of different ages, genders, income levels, statuses, ethnic groups, educational levels, lifestyles, and professions. They share the goal of maintaining people's health. Differences of opinion over how to best accomplish goals are a normal part of working with people of various skill levels and different segments of society. Each unique individual brings different experiences, beliefs, values, and habits to interactions with others. Various pressures and demands in the classroom, clinical setting, and workplace can also generate problems and conflicts. Any or all of these can interfere with your ability to work together.

Conflicts Occur at All Levels

Conflicts can occur at any level and involve any number of people, including your boss, subordinates, peers, patients, or families.

- On the *individual level*, they can occur between two people working together on a classroom or clinical project, between two people in different departments,

Toward Evidence-Based Practice

The Center for Health Design. (2009). Pebble Project data summary. Retrieved from http://www.healthdesign.org/pebble

Preliminary data from the Pebble Project include the following studies:

Weill Cornell Medical College, New York, New York. Conducted studies at six ambulatory sites to examine how wait times affect perceived quality and anxiety. Key findings include the following:

- The more attractive the environment is, the higher the perceived quality and the lower the anxiety will be.
- There was no significant relationship between *actual* wait times and perceived quality or anxiety.
- There was a significant relationship between *perceived* wait times and perceived quality and anxiety.

Paoli Hospital, Paoli, Pennsylvania. Results collected on a new patient pavilion found (Nash & Taylor, 2011):

- That patients feel the design features (e.g., private rooms, décor, increased room size, larger windows and natural light, and rooms with window views) positively affect their hospital experience. As a result patient satisfaction scores increased significantly.
- That staff feel the design features (e.g., materials, temperature, and noise) provide patient privacy and improve everyday work tasks except access to staff break rooms.
- That the rate of patient falls per 1,000 patient days was reduced by nearly 10% in the new pavilion, with an 86% reduction in the rate of falls with injury. Key features of the redesign included location of nurses work areas and visibility of the patient by the staff.
- That medication errors decreased by 19%. Design strategies included placing medications in a box outside each patient room with a closed door to minimize distractions during medication preparation.

Lake Health TriPoint Medical Center, Concord Township, Ohio. Results and data collected on new acute care hospital using state-of-the-art digital hospital design include the following (Gardiner, 2012):

- A 20% to 30% reduction in operating costs as a result of custom air-handling units and integrated controls solutions that delivered the desired temperature and humidity to both critical and non-critical spaces. The sustainable design also increased additional usable floor space.
- A long-term contingency emergency preparedness plan was developed that would minimize the amount of time the hospital would be out of service and would quickly restore productivity in operating rooms.

1. Imagine you are a nurse manager about to present at a budget meeting your ideas for why it would be cost effective to remodel the clinic lobby, including addition of skylights, plants, and a small fountain. List your rationale and state which of the healthcare agency studies supports each item. Be sure to tie your rationale to cost-effectiveness.

---

or even between a staff member and a client or family member.

- **On the *group level*,** conflict can occur between two or more teams, departments, or professional groups (e.g., nurses and social workers may conflict over who is responsible for discharge planning).
- **On the *organizational level*,** conflicts can occur between two or more hospitals, health agencies, or community organizations. *Gender-based* conflicts may involve equal pay for women and sexual harassment issues.

"Win–Win" Resolutions

Some people think about problems and conflicts in the same way as they think about a football game or tennis match: Someone has to win, and someone has to lose. There are some problems with this comparison to sports competition:

- In healthcare, our aim should be to work together more effectively, not to defeat the other party.

- The people who lose are likely to feel bad about losing. As a result, they may spend their time and energy preparing to win the next round, rather than on their work.
- A tie (neither side wins or loses) may be just a stalemate; no one has won or lost, but the problem is also still there and no gain is achieved.

So the answer to the question, "Win, lose, or draw?" is, "None of the above." Instead, a win-win result, in which both sides gain some benefit, is the best resolution (Haslam, Reicher, & Platow, 2011). People address conflict in various ways. Some avoid it, some make immediate decisions, others use an analysis approach.

When compared with their younger counterparts, older adults were more likely to choose the deferral option when presented with low and high conflict scenarios. Both groups were more likely to defer decisions in high conflict scenarios (Pethtel & Chen, 2013). You should accept that not everyone will address conflict.

Conflict Resolution

When differences and disagreements first arise, problem-solving may be sufficient. If the situation has already developed into a full-blown conflict, however, formal or informal negotiation of a settlement may be necessary. Using a problem-solving process, the goal is to find a solution that satisfies everyone involved.

Step 1 *Identify the problem or issue.* Ask people what they want (Hagemann & Stroope, 2012). Sometimes, if the issue is not a highly charged or highly political one, it is easy to identify the real issue or problem. At other times, however, some discussion and exploration of the issues are necessary before the real problem emerges. "It would be relaxing if what other people were really saying was always obvious, if all their essential thoughts were clearly labeled for us . . . and if all knowledgeable people agreed about answers to important questions" (Browne & Kelley, 2010, p. 6). Even though this is ideal, it may not happen. People are often vague about their real concern; sometimes they are genuinely uncertain about what the real problem is. Emotional involvement may further cloud the issue. All of this must be sorted out so that the problem is clearly identified and a solution can be sought.

Step 2 *Generate possible solutions.* Here creativity is especially important. As a leader, begin the process of trying to find new, creative solutions. It is natural for people to try to repeat something that worked well for them in the past, but solutions that were previously successful may not work in the future. Instead, encourage people to spend some time searching for innovative solutions. Think outside the box for new and better ways to handle things.

Step 3 *Evaluate suggested solutions.* An open-minded, objective evaluation of each suggestion is needed, but you may find that this is not always easy to accomplish. When a group engages in problem-solving, it is sometimes difficult to separate the suggestion from its source. For example, on a team, the status of the person who made the suggestion may influence whether the suggestion is judged to be useful. Judge the suggestion on its merits, not its source.

Step 4 *Choose the best solution.* Choose the solution that is most likely to work—one that will give you the best results with the fewest negative effects. A combination of suggestions is often the best solution.

Step 5 *Implement the solution chosen.* The true test of any solution is how well it actually works. Once a solution has been implemented, it is important to give it time to work. Impatience may lead you to abandon a good solution prematurely.

Step 6 *Evaluate—Is the problem resolved?* Not every problem is resolved successfully on the first attempt. If the problem has not been resolved, you need to resume the process with even greater attention to identifying the real problem and how it can be successfully resolved.

Informal Negotiation

If problem-solving does not resolve the conflict, you may have to move on to the next step—informal negotiation. The following steps may prove useful.

1. **Clarify the situation in your own mind.**
   What am I trying to achieve?
   What is the environment in which I am operating?
   What problems am I likely to encounter?
   What do both sides want?
2. **Set the stage.**
   This may involve confronting the two parties or groups with their behavior toward one another, making direct statements designed to open communication and challenge them to seek resolution of the situation.
3. **Conduct the negotiation.**
   Manage the emotions.
   Set the ground rules.
   Clarify the problem.
   Make your opening move.
4. **Continue with offers and counteroffers.**
5. **Agree on the resolution of the conflict.**

Conflict is inevitable within any large or diverse group of people who are trying to work together over an extended period of time. However, it does not have to be destructive, and it does not even have to be a negative experience if everyone handles it skillfully. In fact, conflict can stimulate people to learn more about each other and how to work together in more effective ways. Resolution of a conflict, when it is done well, can lead to improved relationships, more creative methods of problem-solving, and higher productivity.

TIME MANAGEMENT

Many of the personal management and workplace organizational skills focus on time management and scheduling. Although new nurses may have the required job skills, many lack personal management skills, specifically, time management. You might be able to handle conflict and change, delegate appropriately, and be a strong leader among your peers, your faculty, and staff. But if you can't organize and manage your time, you will never gain your full potential.

Many nurses "punch a time clock" that records the minute they enter and leave work, and management accepts very few excuses for being late. Timesheets and schedules are part of most healthcare workers' lives. We are expected to follow precisely set schedules and meet deadlines for virtually everything we do, from distributing medications to getting reports done on time. Many agencies analyze computer-generated data to determine the amount of time spent on various activities. Consider how you can use the following suggestions to improve your time management.

Setting Your Own Goals

It is difficult to decide how to spend your time, because there are so many things that need time. A good first step is to get an overview of the situation. Then ask yourself, "What are my goals?" Goals help clarify what you want and give you energy, direction, and focus. Once you know where you want to go, set priorities. This is not an easy task. In Lewis Carroll's (1865/2010) *Alice's Adventures in Wonderland*, the child heroine, Alice, becomes lost and asks for help from a fantasy creature, the Cheshire Cat. They have this conversation:

> "Would you tell me please, which way I ought to go from here?" asked Alice.
> "That depends a good deal on where you want to go to," said the Cat.
> "I don't care where," said Alice.
> "Then it doesn't matter which way you go," said the Cat.

How can you get somewhere if you do not know where you want to go? It is important to explore your personal and career goals. This can help you make decisions about the future. You can apply these ideas to daily activities as well as to career decisions. Spend some time thinking about what you want to accomplish over a particular time period.

To help organize your time, you need to set both short- and long-term goals. **Short-term goals** are goals that you wish to accomplish within the near future. Setting up your day in an organized fashion is a short-term goal, and so is scheduling a time to study. **Long-term goals** are goals you wish to complete over a long period of time. Advanced education and career goals are examples. A good question to ask yourself is, "What do I see myself doing 5 years from now?" Every choice you make requires a different allocation of time.

Organizing Your Work

Many healthcare professionals are linear, fast-tempo, achievement-oriented people. However, working at a rapid pace is not necessarily the same as accomplishing a great deal. You can use much energy in rushing around and stirring things up while actually achieving very little. Fast does not necessarily mean efficient or effective.

To "manage" time, you need to handle time with a measure of skill. Therefore, time management includes efficiently meeting client care needs during a nursing shift. Organizing your work can eliminate extra steps or serious delays in finishing. It can also reduce the amount of time you spend doing things that are neither productive nor satisfying. As you begin your nursing program, you may care for only one or two patients. However, as you develop time management skills, you will be able to handle a workload of care for seven or eight inpatients. The following are some suggestions:

Time Inventory To begin managing your time, you need to develop a clearer understanding of how you use your time. A personal time inventory helps you estimate how much time you spend in typical activities. Keeping the inventory for a week gives a fairly accurate estimate of how you spend your time. It also helps identify "time wasters." Set up a time log and enter your activities every half hour. Keep this record for about 3 days so you can see a pattern emerging. You may be interested to know that one study of 36 hospitals found that medical-surgical nurses spend their time in the following ways (Hendrich, Chow, Sklerczynski, et al., 2008; Robert Wood Johnson Foundation, 2009):

Documentation	27.5%
Care coordination	16.0%
Patient care activities	15.1%
Medication administration	13.4%
Assessments/vital signs	5.8%
Nonclinical	12.6%
Waste [of time]	6.8%
Unit-related functions	2.8%

Key Point: *Promoting the efficient use of nurses time is a top concern in unit redesigns.*

Energy Use Work on the most difficult tasks when you have the most energy. This decreases frustration later in the day, when you may be more tired and less efficient. Also consider your energy levels when beginning a big task. Start when levels are high and not at, say, 4 p.m., if that is when you find yourself winding down. For example, if you are a "morning person," plan your demanding work in the morning. If you get energy spurts later in the morning or early afternoon, plan to work on larger or heavier tasks at that time. Of course, this choice is not always within your control. Many nursing tasks are based on a schedule. If the wound care is due at 1 p.m., you must carry out the task then, even if you would prefer to eat lunch and rest. Analyze your work to determine which tasks are fixed and what you can manipulate to match your energy.

Lists and Schedules Make a "to do" list and prioritize the tasks in order of importance. Determine how much time each task will require, and when each must be completed. If you find yourself postponing an item for several days, decide whether to give it top priority the next day or drop it from the list altogether.

Daily Worksheet To help organize your day, provide yourself with reminders of various tasks and when they need to be done. Without some type of schedule, you are more likely to drift through a day or shift from one activity to another in a disorganized fashion. The risk in using schedules, however, is that the more they divide the day into discrete segments, the more they fragment the work and discourage a holistic approach. Use the schedule as an organizational tool, but focus on your clients. For a worksheet you can use,

Go to Chapter 7, **Tables, Boxes, Figures: ESG Figure 7-1, Worksheet for Organizing Nursing Care,** on *DavisPlus.*

Say "No" Take control to avoid time wasters. It is important to prevent endless activities and other people controlling you. Learn when to say no. Learn to say, "I would really like to help you; can it wait until I finish this?" Or, "I am sorry, I won't be able to help you with that."

Delegate See previous discussions about delegation.

Do Not Multitask Studies show that people who do many things at once do none of them well, even though they believe they do. Do not check your voicemail while documenting in the patient record, for example. Finish one task, then move on to the next one.

Streamline Your Work Many tasks cannot be eliminated or delegated, but they can be done more efficiently. Here are three wise sayings in time management:

- "Work smarter, not harder." This should appeal to nurses facing increasing demands on time (Box 40-5).
- "Never handle a piece of paper more than once." This philosophy can be used for patient care, as well as office work and schoolwork. Handle an issue now rather than putting it off until later.
- "A stitch in time saves nine." Preventive action saves time in the long run.

Plan the Night Before Take a few minutes before bedtime to lay out your clothing for the next day, set up the coffee pot, or whatever you need to do to avoid last-minute chaos in the morning.

Components of Time Management

Time can be your best friend or your worst enemy. It is important to identify how you feel about time and to assess your own time management skills. Nursing requires that you perform numerous activities within what often seems a very short period of time, so learn how to make the most of your day. Finally, remember that you should set aside 8 hours for sleep and a few more for personal or leisure time ("time off"). Use Table 40-4 to help you to review the necessary components of time management.

Table 40-4 ▶ Components of Time Management	
ACTION	**EXAMPLES**
Prioritize	List tasks in order of importance.
	Remember that some tasks must be done at specific times, whereas others can be done at any time.
	Emergencies take precedence.
	Identify events you control and events others control.
	Use critical-thinking skills to assign priorities.
Question	
▪ Effectiveness	▪ Did the task produce the desired outcome?
▪ Efficiency	▪ How can I accomplish the plan with the least expenditure of time? Is there a way to break this down into simpler tasks?
▪ Efficacy	▪ Do I have the skill and ability to obtain the desired effect?
Recheck	Mentally and physically recheck an unfinished or delegated task.
Practice Self-Reliance	Identify tasks that are within your control and those that are not.
	Use critical-thinking skills and adaptability to revise priorities
	"Go with the flow."
Treat	Treat yourself to a break when you can.
	Treat yourself to time off.
	Treat yourself to an educational experience: Commit yourself to excellence.
	Treat others with courtesy and respect.

BOX 40-5 ▪ Work Smarter, Not Harder

- Gather materials, such as bed linens, for all of your clients at one time. As you go to each room, leave the linen so that it will be there when you need it.
- While giving a bed bath or providing other personal care, perform some of the aspects of the physical assessment, such as taking vital signs, skin assessment, and parts of the neurological and musculoskeletal assessment.
- If a client does not "look right," do not ignore your instincts. The client is probably having a problem.
- Prevention is always a good idea. If you are not sure about a treatment or medication, ask before you proceed. It is usually less time consuming to prevent a problem than it is to resolve one.
- When you set aside time to do a specific task that has a high priority, stick to your schedule and complete it.
- Do not allow interruptions while you are completing any tasks (e.g., paperwork, medication administration). Focus on the task at hand.

KnowledgeCheck 40-6

- List the steps of conflict resolution.
- List several suggestions for organizing your work.
- State one "wise saying" to guide you in streamlining your work.

PUTTING IT ALL TOGETHER

You are just beginning your journey toward becoming a nurse. Undoubtedly you will want to function well within your organization and deliver high-quality patient care. Begin now to examine and work on your own strengths and weaknesses. As you work with your classmates, your instructors, and the clinical facilities, focus on developing the traits of a good leader. You will soon recognize that conflict and change are a normal part of life and your clinical practice, so learn to become proactive as issues arise. You will observe how "real" nurses delegate and manage their time. Take what is useful, and learn from their examples. There will be opportunities to be mentored; watch for those and make time to mentor others. Above all, remember that you may be the most important person in the life of your client during the time you are with him or her—a very big responsibility, but one you will meet with honor and courage.

To explore learning resources for this chapter,

    Go to DavisPlus at DavisPl.us/Wilkinson3.

Chapter Resources for Chapter 40:

Response Sheets for all learning activities

Resources for Caregivers and Health Professionals

Reading More About Leadership & Management (suggested readings)

Concept Map of chapter content

Interactive Case Studies

NCLEX-Style and Chapter Review Questions

Chapter Overview Podcasts

For references cited in this chapter,

    Go to Volume 2, **References Cited**.

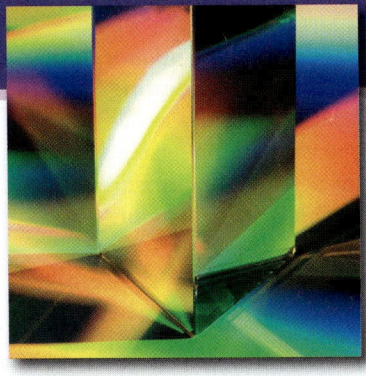

CHAPTER 41

Nursing Informatics

Learning Outcomes

After completing this chapter, you should be able to:

➤ Define informatics and its four components.

➤ Describe the importance of computers in evidence-based nursing practice.

➤ Explain the role of interoperability and standardized languages within the electronic health record system for exchanging health information.

➤ Discuss the benefits of the electronic health record.

➤ Discuss the impact of legislative efforts to encourage electronic health record adoption.

➤ Describe the importance of protecting personal health information.

➤ Explain the relationship between computers and standardized nursing languages.

➤ Identify at least two ways that automation decreases error in healthcare.

➤ Explain how computers can reduce some of the barriers to evidence-based practice.

➤ Identify at least four online sources of nursing research.

➤ Describe the process of literature database searching.

➤ Outline a process for evaluating evidence and determining a solution.

Key Concepts

Electronic communication

Informatics

Healthcare technology

Related Concepts

See the Concept Map on Davis*Plus*.

Meet Your Nurse Role Model

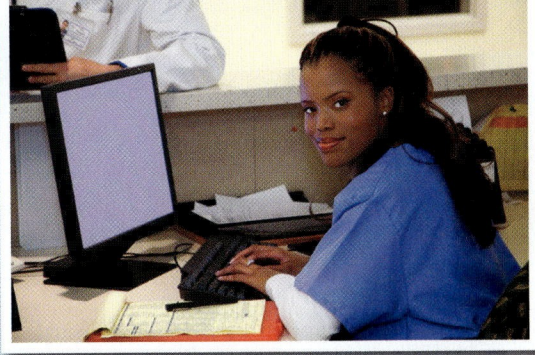

Six weeks ago, Ted Samuels, 67, a business executive, began experiencing headaches, occasional palpitations, blurred vision, and increased thirst. Mr. Samuels accesses the **patient web portal** of his **personal health record (PHR)** and sends an e-mail to his physician's scheduling service requesting an appointment. Within an hour, an appointment is confirmed with the family nurse practitioner (FNP) the next day.

The physician's office has just installed an **electronic health record system (EHR)** that is **integrated** with the hospital record for seamless communication among Mr. Samuel's caregivers. At his appointment, the FNP enters his insurance and personal contact information into the system, and explains that the system is **encrypted** (special security coding) to protect his privacy. In the exam room, the medical assistant weighs Mr. Samuels,

takes his vital signs, and enters the information in the EHR. Next, Karen Shock, FNP, arrives. As she takes Mr. Samuels's history and completes a physical examination, she updates the information in the computer. Noting his family history of diabetes, the increased thirst, and slight weight gain, she checks a random glucose via the office glucometer and finds a blood sugar level of 300 mg/dL. The **decision support algorithms** built into the software alert her that Mr. Samuels's blood pressure was also elevated at 170/98. The software suggests

(Continued)

Meet Your Nurse Role Model (continued)

possible medical diagnoses of hyperglycemia and hypertension. Following the evidence-based care guidelines in the computer, Ms. Shock uses **computerized provider order entry** (**CPOE**) to enter requests for a basic metabolic profile, lipid profile, electrocardiogram (ECG), blood urea nitrogen (BUN), creatinine, and Hgb A_{1c}. She asks that Mr. Samuels be fasting for the blood work, and prints patient education instructions. Ms. Shock instructs Mr. Samuels to check his blood pressure two to three times daily for 1 week and to enter the results in the online log in his PHR. She asks Mr. Samuels to grant viewing rights to the log for her and Dr. Gregg.

The next morning Mr. Samuels arrives at the hospital for his lab work and ECG. His registration information is automatically updated from the information provided with a previous health visit. The **online order requisitions** Ms. Shock entered yesterday provide the technicians with the information needed, the tests are completed, and Mr. Samuels is quickly on the way back to his office. At the end of the day, he receives an e-mail notification that his lab results are available for review. He logs into the PHR portal to view the results. He also finds a message from Ms. Shock confirming the preliminary diagnosis of type 2 diabetes. The office is scheduling diabetic instruction, and they have e-mailed a prescription to Mr. Samuels's pharmacy for metformin, an antidiabetes drug. An education leaflet explaining the medication and potential side effects is attached to the message. Mr. Samuels notices that metformin is now showing on his **medication list** in his PHR.

During the course of the week, Ms. Shock monitors Mr. Samuels's blood pressure log entries. A **trending graph** shows consistently high blood pressure readings. She orders Lisinopril, an antihypertensive, 5 mg daily, and requests that he continue to check his blood pressure frequently. A follow-up appointment is scheduled for 6 weeks.

A few weeks later, Mr. Samuels wakes up with severe chest pain and calls 911. En route to the emergency department (ED), the paramedic transmits an ECG tracing via satellite to the ED physician. Using telehealth technology, the physician interprets the ECG, determines that Mr. Samuels is having a myocardial infarction (MI), and notifies the cardiac catheterization team to be on standby. The ED physician sees that Mr. Samuels has recently completed tests at the hospital, and reviews his medication list, allergies, and medical history online. Within 30 minutes Mr. Samuels is sent to the cath lab for percutaneous transluminal coronary angioplasty.

Four hours later, Mr. Samuels is resting comfortably in the progressive care unit. Throughout the next 48 hours, the bedside nurse monitors Mr. Samuels's vital signs and cardiac rhythm. An **interface** allows the nurse to directly import vital signs data from the cardiac monitor directly into his electronic health record. Caregivers document electronically at the bedside, and the physician uses CPOE to manage Mr. Samuels's prescriptions. At discharge, the nurse gives Mr. Samuels a printed copy of his medication list, discharge instructions, and follow-up appointments are made with Dr. Gregg and the cardiologist.

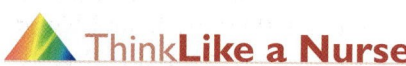 ThinkLike a Nurse 41-1

Reflect on this Meet Your Nurse Role Model scenario. Identify how information was managed and processed.

- What mechanisms for gathering and disseminating information were used?
- How did automation assist decision making?
- How was evidence used in decision making?
- What characteristics make it more likely for patients to use personal health records?

Theoretical Knowledge knowing why

Computers have become as much of a diagnostic tool as stethoscopes have been for the past century. The Meet Your Nurse Role Model scenario is an example of how healthcare professionals use these tools to make decisions in practice. This chapter gives you an overview of how this works.

ABOUT THE KEY CONCEPTS

You may already feel the push and pull on your time and knowledge. And why work harder, when you can work smarter using technology-based tools? In today's increasingly complex and ever-changing environment, healthcare professionals must be competent in the use of information technology to communicate effectively with the healthcare team, patients, and families; manage information; support clinical decision making; and reduce the risk of medical error.

Nursing informatics and **healthcare technology** (e.g., mechanical ventilators, implantable insulin pumps) support your passion for nursing and innovation, leading to improved patient outcomes and higher quality care. **Electronic communication** (e.g., electronic health records and telehealth) is also an important part of this equation.

WHAT IS NURSING INFORMATICS?

Whether you become a staff nurse, an administrator, a researcher, primary healthcare provider, or an educator, you will need current, accurate, and "best available" information to do your job well. The good news is that plenty of information is available. MEDLINE, a vast medical literature database supported through the National Institutes of Health (NIH), currently contains more than 18 million citations and is growing at the rate of more than 1.4 million new entries per year (NIH, 2013). If you read two new articles every day, by the end of the year you would be 918 years behind in keeping up with the literature. The bad news (if you want to call it that) is that we are drowning in information while still lacking in knowledge. Do you ever feel that way as a student?

It is not possible to keep all the necessary information in your head. No one can. We need critical thinking and tools to make it useful to us. No one can learn and retain all the information, so you must know how to find, process, and manage it to arrive at the best decisions for your practice. In essence, this is the definition of **informatics**: the managing and processing of information necessary to make decisions. **Nursing informatics** is informatics applied to nursing practice, education, and research. The first conceptual framework for informatics envisioned the elements ("stuff") of informatics as *data, information,* and *knowledge* (Graves & Corcoran, 1989). Full-spectrum nurses interact with all three of these elements in daily practice, so you need to understand how they interrelate.

Nursing informatics specialists (NIS) work with informatics technicians and others to provide clinical information and data analysis for effective patient care. In addition, they work with computers, data analysis systems, and nursing knowledge and experience to be sure the best possible care is provided. This role involves good understanding of basic nursing techniques and standards. Data collection, analysis of different types of data, information sharing, and research dissemination are functions of the NIS. The NIS also acts as a manager or team leader to bring together all aspects of treatment options and best practice research. In sum, the NIS uses nursing science, computer science, and information science to manage and communicate data, information, knowledge, and wisdom in nursing practice. The sections that follow describe these four elements of informatics.

Data

Data are "discrete entities that are described objectively without interpretation" (American Nurses Association [ANA], 2008). In other words, data are raw, unprocessed numbers, symbols, or words that have no meaning by themselves. For example, what does 101 mean? It could indicate the college course English 101; a piece of programming language; or someone's body temperature, pulse rate, weight, or age. Without a context, data are meaningless.

In nursing, we speak of data as the primary facts and observations acquired when providing services, such as the numerical value of a blood pressure measurement, or facts such as, "Father died of prostate cancer." Notice that even this information has no meaning until the nurse interprets it: The meaning of "Father died of prostate cancer" changes if the client is a healthy 24-year-old female sharing this information versus a 74-year-old male experiencing blood in his urine.

Information

Information consists of groupings of data processed into a meaningful, structured form (ANA, 2008). If you combine 300 with a unit of measure, you know that the number represents a blood sugar result. If other data—gender (male), age (67), and family history—are grouped together, information is formed. You now know that this man has most likely developed type 2 diabetes.

Data:	300 mg/dL glucose, male, 67, thirst
Grouped data:	Male gender, age 67, family history of diabetes
Information:	Man with probable new onset of diabetes

In the opening scenario, what information did the FNP receive that triggered an alert?

Knowledge

In the Meet Your Nurse Role Model scenario, what *information* did the FNP use to create knowledge of Mr. Samuels's condition? Take a minute to write your answer.

The answer to the question is that the FNP received information on the blood sugar (300 mg/dL) and blood pressure (170/98 mm Hg). Grouping this with other information (e.g., the history of headaches, blurred vision, palpitations, family history of diabetes), the FNP created *knowledge* of the potential for a diagnosis of type 2 diabetes and hypertension.

Knowledge is formed when data are grouped, creating meaningful information and relationships, which are then added to other structured information (ANA, 2008). The knowledge can either be previously known or new. In the preceding scenario of the 67-year-old man with the blood sugar of 300 mg/dL, we can add information about pathophysiology, pharmacokinetics (how medications work), patient history, and physical assessment, providing the knowledge to make an informed decision about the patient's current condition and further treatment.

Figure 41-1 depicts the transformation of data into knowledge. We have come to realize that the gathering

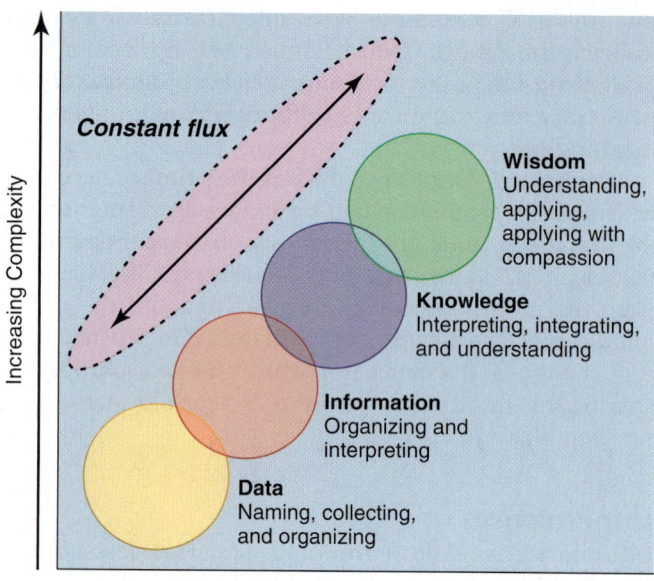

FIGURE 41-1 The relationship of data, information, knowledge, and wisdom. Each level increases in complexity. (Reprinted from Englebardt, S., & Nelson, R. *Health care informatics: An interdisciplinary approach.* Copyright 2002. With permission from Elsevier.)

of data and information to make decisions is never ending. Notice that the model shows overlapping circles and both forward and backward movement.

Wisdom

Nelson and Joos (1989) added *wisdom* to the Graves and Corcoran model. **Wisdom** is defined as the *appropriate use* of knowledge in managing or solving human problems. Wisdom develops as an outcome of your clinical experience, theoretical knowledge, critical thinking, and intuition—as you progress from novice to expert in the practice of full-spectrum nursing.

KnowledgeCheck 41-1

- What is the difference between knowledge and wisdom?
- Define the following: *data, information, knowledge.*
- Give an example of each: data, information, knowledge.

HOW DO NURSES USE INFORMATICS AT WORK?

Because computers are essential in healthcare, it is important that nurses develop a set of core computer competencies or skills (Hart, 2008; TIGER, 2009). These include a basic understanding of computer logic, data entry, data retrieval, information literacy, and troubleshooting basic hardware and software issues. In your work as a nurse, you will use computers not only to communicate, but also to provide and document patient care, seek information, examine evidence-based practice resources, and possibly conduct or participate in clinical research.

UNDERSTANDING COMPUTER BASICS

Computers are vital to the functioning in our daily lives. We rely on them for communication (e.g., e-mail, texting, blogs, social networking), access to information (e.g., personal and business contacts, education, general information), and business operations (e.g., scheduling, purchasing), to name but a few. By definition, a **computer** is an electronic device with four main functions: input, processing, output, and storage. Collectively, these operations are known as **information processing** (or *data processing*).

Key Point: *The power of a computer is based on the speed, accuracy, and reliability with which it operates, as well as the enormous amounts of data it can store and keep readily available for processing.*

Computers consist of hardware (machines and monitors), memory (data storage), processors (translators), and software (coded programs or applications that support specific functions). They can exist as a stand-alone device, or as part of a network of computers that share a common purpose. Power in computing is enhanced by the ability to connect to other computers. Devices can be either *wired* (connected with physical wires) or *wireless* (connected through electromagnetic waves). *Connectivity* is a term referring to the ways in which computers and other hardware communicate and share information.

Data are stored either internally (in the memory) or externally on some form of storage media (disc, flash drive, external hard drive, network drive, the Cloud). If you are a savvy computer user, you probably already know how a computer functions. See if you can answer questions about computer basics.

 Go to Chapter 41, **Supplemental Materials: Pretest Questions and Pretest Answer Key,** Davis*Plus*.

If you had difficulty answering the questions,

 Go to Chapter 41, **Supplemental Materials: How Does a Computer Work?** on Davis*Plus*.

Electronic Communication

Electronic communication, whether simple (e.g., text messaging), or complex (e.g., telehealth), can be a time-saver, but does reduce face-to-face interaction between people.

Electronic Mail and Text Messaging

In many facilities electronic mail (e-mail) is now a primary method for managers to communicate with staff. E-mail and text messaging allow for rapid, simultaneous distribution of information and messaging to individuals or a large number of recipients. Nurses and other healthcare providers can use e-mail to interact with patients; consult with colleagues; and communicate with insurance industry representatives, pharmacies, and hospitals. E-mail and text offer convenient, up-to-the-minute patient updates among nurses, other providers, and patients and their families; plus, it can be used to document communications between people or groups.

Key Point: *Protected information includes any individually identifiable health information; current, past, or potential physical or mental conditions; and any payment information. These transmissions occur only on secure or encrypted sites if personal patient information is involved, not in an e-mail.*

Be aware that privacy is not protected with electronic messaging. For example, it is entirely legal and not uncommon for employers to read incoming and outgoing employee messages when they are transmitted on company equipment. In addition, once a message has been sent, you have no control over who may read it or to whom it might be forwarded. You also don't know whether other people receive a blind copy of the message without your knowledge.

Key Point: *Most facilities have policies governing use of company e-mail for personal use. Always check facility policies before sharing e-mail addresses with persons outside of the organization.*

How was e-mail used to facilitate communication between the patient and providers in the Meet Your Nurse Role Model situation?

Web Conferencing and Webinars

Web conferencing is used to conduct or participate in live or synchronous meetings or presentations via the Internet. Attendees download a Internet-based application onto their local computers. These interactions are most often two-way communication. To access the meeting, an e-mail is distributed to the attendee(s) that contains a link to enter the conference at the arranged time. A **webinar,** or **webcast**, is a specific type of Web conference that is conducted in a one-way manner, from the speaker to the audience. These tools can be useful in helping staff obtain updated clinical information (e.g., continuing education, inservice) for patient care.

Electronic Mailing List

An electronic mailing list, often called a *listserv*, is essentially a large, undisclosed distribution list whose members share a specialty interest. The names and addresses of the people on the mailing list, called **subscribers**, are stored on a single server. A single address is then designated for the group to use. When a message is sent to that address, it is delivered to the mailing list server, which then distributes the message via e-mail to all subscribers.

Electronic mailing lists are a powerful communication tool. Communication is global and almost instantaneous. Ideas and protocols can be shared, questions asked and answered, and surveys taken. Everyone on the list has an opportunity to share in the discussion.

Key Point: *If you use an electronic mailing list, be aware that any message you send through the mailing list goes to everyone on the distribution list. So be careful when you hit the "Reply All" command!*

Numerous nursing mailing lists are available representing a wide variety of topics and health specialty areas. Use your favorite Internet search engine and search using the key words "nursing listservs." Look for a site that interests you. What kind of information do you see? Visit one of the sites. What kind of information do you see?

Social Networking

Social networking tools allow people to connect interactively with others who have similar interests. This can be done through **blogging** (posting open messages that can be read by anyone with permissions to access the site), sharing pictures, videos, or **texts**. Sites generally require you to register for the site, create a profile, and be granted access privileges by the Internet page administrator. Twitter, FaceBook, YouTube, CaringBridge, PatientsLikeMe, CureTogether, are examples of popular social networking sites. For instance, you can go to YouTube to view video demonstrations showing nursing skills. You will need to be cautious about whether the source of information is expert and reliable; for example, some of the YouTube skills videos have errors in the demonstrations. To find nursing videos, often it's easiest to search the specific topic, not simply "nursing videos."

As with many Internet-based tools, social networking sites are searchable by anyone with access. Many employers now regularly include searching these sites as part of their applicant verification process.

Key Point: *Never post anything on these sites that you would not want an employer to view. In addition, posting pictures or descriptions of patient information represents significant risk of violating federal privacy laws.*

Wikis are an increasingly popular way to exchange information. These are Internet pages that can either be public or limited to specific groups through user name and passwords. Many schools have created Wikis to support communication among student groups. Support group Wikis are becoming common for use by patients with chronic health conditions, such as diabetes and congestive heart failure.

✚ It is important to note that anyone with access can add information to these sites, creating the potential for you to find inaccurate information. It is useful to know whether support groups are being facilitated or at least monitored by a professional before recommending them to patients.

Interactive Gaming and Virtual Learning

As we are shifting from the Information Age to the Interaction Age, educators are adopting new, more engaging and collaborative methods for teaching and learning. One example is a Internet-based, three-dimensional virtual world called Second Life that digitally simulates the human experience. Residents, or participants in Second Life, also called **avatars**, can interact with one another in a social networking–type community that the residents refer to as the Grid. Educators use this game-like environment to simulate a nurse–patient experience and clinical care as well as to evaluate a variety of nursing skills.

Telehealth

Telehealth is the use of telecommunication to send healthcare information between patients and professionals at different locations (Fig. 41-2). It improves access to healthcare by providing long-distance clinical healthcare, patient and professional education, and health administration. For instance, the U.S. Department of Defense pioneered telehealth technology and now uses it to provide healthcare services to soldiers in combat and dependent families in outlying posts. The following are other examples of the use of telehealth.

- **Rural Healthcare.** In rural healthcare sites there may not be a specialist located in the area. Telecommunications equipment at the rural site and the specialist's

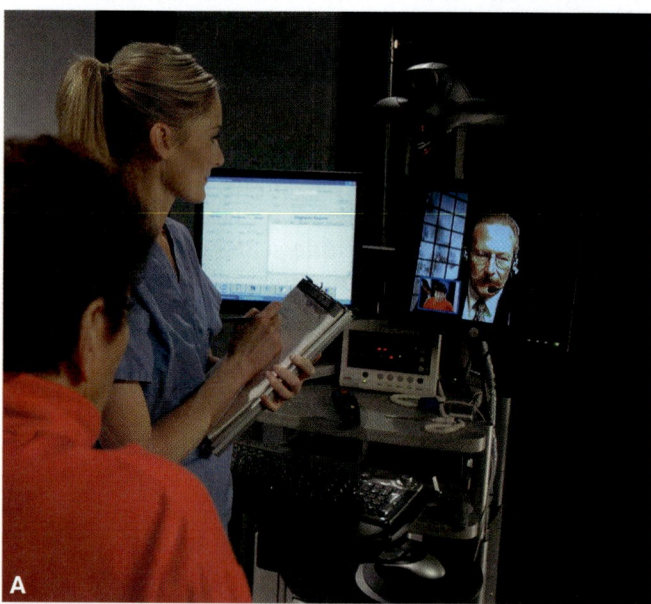

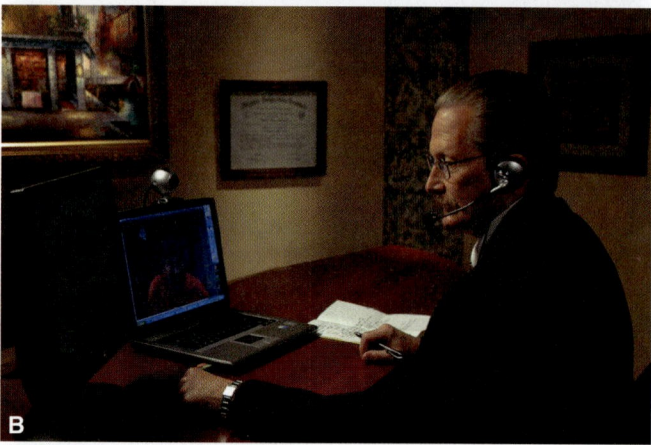

FIGURE 41-2 *A, B,* Telehealth improves access among healthcare providers at remote and central sites.

site allow the specialist and patient to see and talk to each other. The specialist can also view the health records, x-ray films, lab results, and so on. This reduces the cost of traveling to a distant site, and the stress on a patient who may not feel well enough to travel.

- **Home Health Monitoring.** A more common use of telehealth is the use of home health monitoring devices. These devices allow the healthcare professional to monitor vital signs and other indicators without physically entering a home or requiring a patient to make a clinic trip. Therefore, patients can be monitored more frequently, providing better follow-up care, and earlier discharge from the hospital. See the Home Care box Use of Informatics in Home Care.

- **Compensating for Shortage of Healthcare Providers.** In the hospital, critically ill patients can be remotely monitored by a hospital **intensivist** (physician employed by the hospital to provide healthcare to patients in intensive care) and critical care nurses from a central location. These systems enhance patient safety and provide an extra set of eyes for a busy nurse who cannot remain constantly at a patient's bedside.

- **Emergency Care Triage.** Some cities have incorporated telehealth nurse triage into their emergency 911 call system. Telenurses use a set of protocols to manage patient calls. These cities report a significant decrease in the need for ambulance services and emergency room visits (Enrado, 2009).

Despite barriers such as cost and issues surrounding licensing and reimbursement, telehealth applications will continue to expand in the future. For information about barriers that slow the growth of telehealth,

 Go to Chapter 41, **Supplemental Materials: Barriers to Telehealth,** Davis*Plus.*

Home Care

Use of Informatics in Home Care

A telephone application for documentation has been developed for home health aides. It reduces the amount of time the aide must spend in recording care, improves accuracy, and prevents lost documentation.

- ➤ **When arriving at a patient's home,** the aide uses the patient's phone to dial in to a central number and keys in her identification. The time of the call, telephone number from which it came, and identification of the worker are automatically recorded.

- ➤ **At the end of the visit,** the aide again calls from the patient's phone. Again, the location, time, and identification of the caller are recorded. Using the telephone keypad, the aide then keys in codes indicating the tasks accomplished. She never has to physically write a documentation record; it is accomplished using the telephone.

ThinkLike a Nurse 41-2

- As a patient, would you prefer a telehealth or a face-to-face consultation? Why?
- Now imagine that you are an accident victim brought to a rural clinic staffed only with paraprofessionals. Does your answer change? If so, why?

KnowledgeCheck 41-2

- What is personal health information, and why is it important to protect it?
- How is a listserv different from regular e-mail?

Computer-Based Tools for Providing and Managing Care

As a nurse, you will be called on to use a wide variety of computerized devices in the workplace such as digital thermometers, cardiorespiratory monitors, glucometers, smart IV pumps, barcode scanners, and electronic bedscales.

Tracking Patients and Equipment

Global positioning systems (GPS) allow real-time tracking, which can be used in select clinical situations in which wandering is a patient safety concern. The Alzheimer's Association promotes use of electronic tracking for some patients with dementia as a way to postpone the need for a more secure environment (McShane, 2013).

Some agencies are using Real Time Location Systems (RTLS) or Radio Frequency Identification Detectors (RFID) to assist in locating patient care equipment that may be dispersed throughout a building. These systems save nurses time, deter staff from storing equipment on a particular unit rather than a centrally accessible location, and decrease costs of lost equipment (Turisco & Rhoads, 2008). Other efficiency-enhancing devices include hands-free communication badges and wireless smart phones, which may be interfaced with alerts from bedside equipment.

Managing Workflow

Internet-based tools for staff scheduling, patient flow, access to evidence-based references, policy and procedures, and staff education are used for their efficiency and convenience. Many hospitals have developed internal resources, special intranet pages with references specific to nursing. Mobile digital devices, including tablet computers and personal digital assistants (PDAs), are efficient for bedside retrieval of patients' health information, prescribed medications and interventions, and test results in the electronic health record. They also are convenient for charting at the bedside or other locations (Prgomet, Georgiou, & Westbrook, 2009).

Reducing Error With Automation

As healthcare becomes more complex, the opportunities for error increase significantly. A hospital stay can be prolonged or injury and even death can result from a seemingly simple mistake such as administering incompatible medications, or erroneously transcribing a medication order. There are two types of errors:

- *Errors of commission*— when the wrong action occurs (e.g., giving an incorrect drug)
- *Errors of omission*—when the correct action does not occur (e.g., overlooking a serious medication allergy or failing to put up the bed rails for a confused patient)

Another way to look at errors is by asking whether the error was in planning or execution:

- *An error in planning* occurs when the original intended action or plan was not correct.
- An *error of execution* occurs when the correct action is taken but does not proceed as intended.

Toward Evidence-Based Practice

Duffy, M. (2012). Tablet technology for nurses. *American Journal of Nursing, 112*(9), 59–64.

This article explores the advantages and potential barriers for nurses' use of tablets in the clinical setting. Advantages include portability, the potential to teach patients at the patient bedside, and EHR documentation at the point of care. Barriers include cost, availability of wireless connectivity, and concerns about compromising HIPPA/patient confidentiality.

Mitchell, M. (2012). Nursing informatics. How mobile is your technology? *Nursing Management, 43*(9), 26–30.

This article examines the use of mobile technology (tablets and smart phones) by patients and healthcare providers. Patients use mobile technology, with a hospital-provided access code, to go to the portal for patient education and information about when medications are scheduled to be taken and what procedures are scheduled. Nurses use mobile technology to access healthcare references, including drug guides, and secure text-messaging capabilities between the nurse and the physician.

According to both Duffy and Mitchell,

1. What are the advantages of using tablets?

2. What barriers exist to the use of tablets in the healthcare setting?

3. How can the nurse assure that patient confidentiality is protected when using tablets and smart phones?

 Go to Chapter 41, **Toward Evidence-Based Practice Suggested Responses,** on Davis*Plus*.

Automation (e.g., EHR) provides a secure way to integrate all patient information, including allergy history, laboratory values, and other prescriptions. It improves communication among those who prescribe, dispense, and administer medication to patients. For example, new prescriptions are automatically checked for potential errors or problems. The system can detect dosing errors by flagging medication dilution or dosages that fall outside normal standards and alert providers of the possibility of a drug interaction, allergy, or incorrect dose. In addition, some drug names sound like other drugs, the EHR can notify prescribers and help avoid a serious drug error.

 Following are three examples of error-prevention technologies:

- **Computerized physician order entry (CPOE)** helps prevent errors in reading and transcribing orders.
- **Bar-coding medications at the unit-dose level** helps to prevent nurses from selecting an incorrect medication (Bell, 2009; Fowler, Sohler, & Zarillo, 2009).
- **Use of smart technologies (e.g., infusion devices) at the point of care** helps to ensure that the correct dose is delivered to the patient.

To read more about ways to decrease medication error,

 Go to Chapter 41, **Supplemental Materials: How Does Automation Decrease Medication Error?** on Davis*Plus*.

Aiding Patients in Self-Care

The convergence of personal health records with mobile communication devices (e.g., smart phones, mobile tablet personal computers) boosts patients' ability for self-care. Internet-based programs and applications (apps) for mobile devices provide patients with patient education (e.g., disease-specific information, or healthy habit tips, including nutritional information, meal planning, dietary tracking), patient-specific medication dose reminders (Fig. 41-3), and even medical bill-paying reminders, for instance.

The Pew Research Center (2013) found that roughly one-third of American adults have gone online to find healthcare-related information and figure out what medical condition they have. Patients who look for this information may be seeking information about conventional, alternative, or complementary therapies and treatments, or looking for shared experiences of others with similar conditions. Patients may not always share their findings from online searches with their healthcare providers, which can lead to confusion or adverse reactions to prescribed treatment.

You can help guide your patients in their searches by educating them about how to use online sources and choose reputable, trustworthy sites. You may also need to help them interpret information that they find. Many hospitals have patient education materials on their Internet sites that provide links to reputable sources

---

Quality and Safety Education for Nurses

Are Information Technologies Living Up to Their Promise?

Chapter Key Concept: Informatics

Competency: Informatics (Knowledge, Skills, Attitudes); Safety (Knowledge, Skills, Attitudes)

Billions of dollars have been allocated for the development of electronic information systems (which are made up of electronic health records, digitized images, decision-support systems, computerized provider order entry, communication systems, and more). The electronic health information system has been promised to enhance the quality and safety of healthcare and provide information for clinical research. But is it really possible to develop a reliable, error-proof system that everyone understands and uses correctly?

A recent article (Black, Car, Pagliari, et al., 2011) questions whether we should automatically assume the usefulness of an all-electronic information system. Using 53 high-quality studies, researchers evaluated the evidence to support the use of information technologies to improve the quality and safety of healthcare. They concluded that existing evidence was weak and inconsistent. Not only did very few of the promised benefits materialize, but also new sources of errors were created. They found one particularly troubling effect: the tendency for prescribing errors to occur, which resulted when prescribers overestimated the capabilities of clinical decision-support systems.

Think about it: The informatics competency stresses the need for nurses to understand the time, effort, and skill required for information technologies to become reliable, effective tools for patient care system. What do you see as the nurse's role in developing and evaluating the electronic health record?

Consider the following questions to help develop your knowledge and skills and shape your attitudes about informatics and safety:

➤ What thinking skills will be necessary for nurses and other providers to respond appropriately to decision supports and alerts?

➤ How will nurses in particular use an electronic health record?

➤ How might electronic health records be used to improve care?

➤ How might the electronic health record improve the safety of an individual patient's care?

➤ What information should be included in an electronic database to make it useful for clinical research?

Source: Black, A. D., Car, J., Pagliari, C., et al. (2011).

To learn about specific Knowledge, Skills, and Attitudes,

 Go to the QSEN Internet site at http://qsen.org/competencies/pre-licensure-ksas/

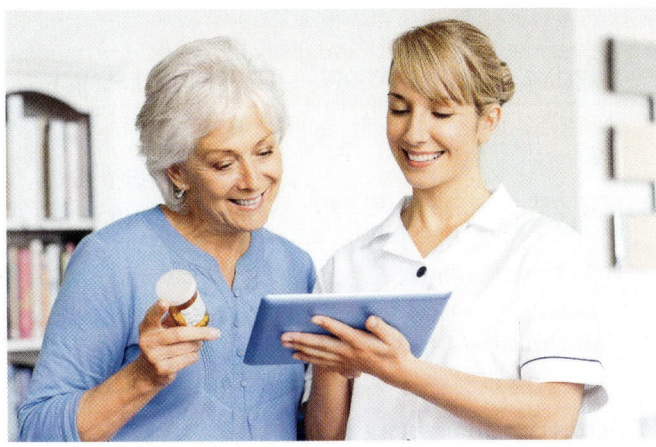

FIGURE 41-3 Nurse and senior client using a digital tablet for medication reminder and dose tracking.

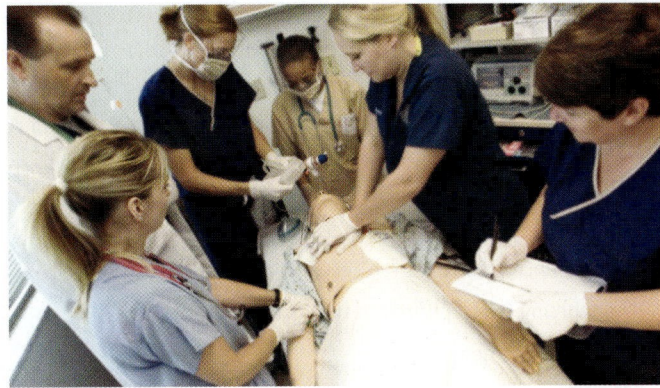

FIGURE 41-4 Human patient simulator offers practical experience before caring for patients or training special skills.

(Gee, Greenwood, Kim, et al., 2012). In addition, customizable digital products (e.g., ebooks, apps, games, Web worlds) provide patients with interactive ways to engage in their medical care. Gaming applications are available to motivate patients in taking medication doses and manage dietary intake, weight, activity, and other prescribed health habits.

Educating Nurses

The electronic learning environment continues to expand in nursing education. A few of the many ways that computers assist nursing students in learning include:

- *Communicating* with faculty, peers, and patients through text messaging, synchronous and asynchronous text-based discussions, Web logs (blogs), social media, and other social sources
- *Searching online databases and the Internet* for evidence-based support of clinical practice and other sources of health information
- *Performing and documenting course assignments, clinical tasks, and self-evaluation tasks* using learning management systems
- *Using clinical simulation mannequins* (Fig. 41-4) and other interactive gaming tools to emulate an authentic clinical environment prior to performing skills using live patients. You may have already been using clinical simulation mannequins in your nursing program. Would it surprise you to know that practicing nurses also use them in continuing education provided in their workplaces? What kind of computer programs and devices are available in your clinical setting?

ELECTRONIC HEALTH RECORDS

You have been introduced to several ways in which computer information systems are used in nursing care. In addition, this section discusses EHRs and the barriers to and benefits of their adoption. Table 41-1 summarizes the use of information systems in practice, education, administration, and research.

EHRs are a system for exchange of healthcare information. As a part of networked information systems software, EHRs allow clinicians to create, store, edit, and retrieve patient charts via the Internet or local intranet software. Patient demographics, progress notes, problems, medications, vital signs, past medical history, immunizations, laboratory data, and radiology reports are important components of the patient health record.

Figure 41-5 is an example of a computer screen using EHR software. Notice the electronic view uses combinations of tabs and icons to support logical navigation through the patient chart. These tabs are often named and arranged to match tabs in a traditional paper chart, including patients' clinical and personal data. A successful EHR project allows an organization to replace paper charts and care plans with electronic records.

Interoperability and Standardized Nursing Languages

In this section, we describe the role of informatics and standardized nursing languages in communicating health information in EHRs, nursing education, and evidence-based practice.

EHRs are a system for exchanging health information. **Interoperability** refers to the ability of many different kinds of computers and operating systems to talk with each other through standard languages or formats without losing the meaning of the information. For that to happen, consistent languages are needed—languages that all computers can understand. If information about heart rate is to be exchanged, consistent languages are needed. For example the EHR system in Hospital A might refer to "heart rate," while the EHR system in a physician's office might refer to "pulse rate." This could interfere with clear communication of meaning. Standardized nursing language facilitates communication among organizations and between nurses and the healthcare team.

Table 41-1 ► Use of Computer Information Systems in Nursing

NURSING PRACTICE	NURSING EDUCATION	NURSING ADMINISTRATION	NURSING RESEARCH
Literature access and retrieval (e.g., for evidence-based practice)	Literature access and retrieval	Quality assurance and utilization review	Literature review
Care planning	Computer-assisted instruction (CAI) programs	Employee records (e.g., to track licenses, immunizations)	Data collection
Client records (e.g., documenting, order entry, retrieving lab results)	Classroom technology	Staffing patterns, hiring	Data analysis (both qualitative and quantitative)
Telenursing (e.g., in home health)	Distance learning	Buildings and facilities management	Research dissemination
Case management	Testing and grading	Finance and budgets	Applying for grants
Documenting medications	Student records	Accreditation reviews (e.g., monitoring quality indicators for The Joint Commission)	
Transcribing orders	Development of electronic and learning communities using the World Wide Web		
Reordering medications			
Identifying drug interactions			
Warning practitioners about drug incompatibilities			

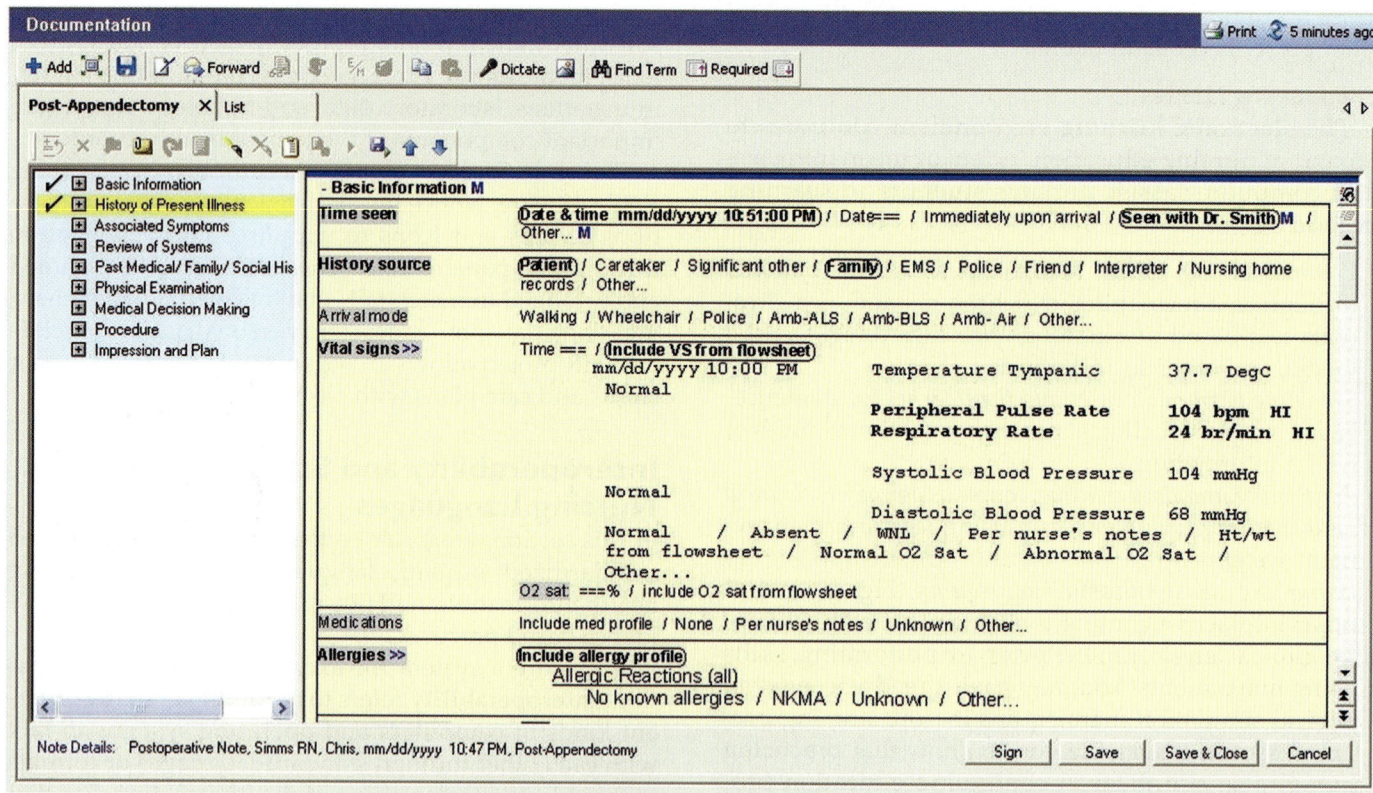

FIGURE 41-5 Computer screen from an electronic health record (Courtesy of Cerner Corporation, Kansas City, MO)

Standardized languages also support evidence-based practice. Suppose you wanted to find out how many patients on your hospital unit had a nursing diagnosis of Impaired Skin Integrity during the past year. If the hospital uses paper medical records, how could you find out? If patient records are computerized, would that make a difference?

You may have thought about pulling all patient charts within a select time period, and examined the nursing notes. Or perhaps you might search for the words *Impaired Skin Integrity* in the computerized records. That's a beginning—but this task would have been difficult because nurses use a variety of terms to describe the same data. For example, in some charts you would find the term *skin breakdown*; in others, *a reddened area*, *bedsore*, or a *stage III pressure ulcer*. Would you count all of these as Impaired Skin Integrity? What if the nurses used some terms you didn't think to search for?

Do you see how the lack of a standardized way to describe patient problems can hamper efforts to create and retrieve nursing data from automated documentation systems? Recall the goal for interoperability among EHR systems discussed above. **Standardized language—** using the same terms to describe a clinical condition in all EHRs—helps to achieve that goal. For more discussion about standardized language,

 Go to Chapter 41, **Standardized Language, American Nurses Association Recognized Languages for Nursing,** in Volume 2.

Electronic Health Record (EHR) Adoption

EHR usage among healthcare providers and hospitals has sharply increased since passage of the Health Information Technology for Economic and Clinical Health (HITECH) Act in 2009. The HITECH Act focuses on improving healthcare quality and efficiency. Approximately 80% of all eligible hospitals and more than half of physicians and other eligible healthcare professionals in the United States have received an incentive payment for adopting, implementing, upgrading, or meaningfully using an EHR (U.S. Department of Health and Human Services [USDHHS], 2013). The rationales for federal-funding support for a nationwide, interoperable system of health records are that EHRs are expected to provide higher-quality, patient-focused healthcare by improving care provider access to patients' health information; to improve population health by facilitating research and wider use of patient information; and to facilitate billing and record keeping.

Benefits of an Electronic Health Record

EHR systems improve the quality of care and reduce healthcare costs with technology-based tools for the exchange of health information exchange, computerized physician order entry (CPOE) systems, and clinical decision support (CDS) tools (Menachimi & Collum, 2011). These are discussed later in this section. Other benefits of EHRs include being able to easily access computerized records and to eliminate poor handwriting, which has historically been a potential source of error within the healthcare delivery system.

Improved Efficiency Improved access to patient health information can increase efficiency, productivity, and continuity of care. A paperless health record conveniently stores all patient information in one location rather than in bits and pieces in many different files and locations. Some EHR systems are designed for planning as well as for documenting care. Standardized care plans are typically incorporated in EHR systems. Other applications are designed to support efficient patient care workflow. Standardized coding for patient diagnoses and interventions allows for more accurate, convenient, and uniform billing.

Reduced Redundancy Allowing for the secure and potentially real-time sharing of patient information can reduce costly redundant tests. For example, diagnostic testing is often ordered because one provider (e.g., a family physician) does not have access to the clinical information stored at another provider's location (e.g., a cardiac specialist). Historically, providers relied on faxing or mailing each other pertinent information, which makes it difficult to access on site when and where it is needed.

Accessibility Have you ever needed to write your nursing notes before leaving the clinical setting, only to discover that the chart was in the x-ray department with the patient? Or that the physician was making rounds with it in her hands? In contrast to a paper record, any number of people in different locations can access a computerized record—and all at the same time. A physician can view lab results from the office at the same time a nurse views them in the hospital and a lab technician adds more data. Various types of hardware support access patient health information, from stationary bedside terminals, wireless laptops mounted on mobile carts, and handheld devices (Fig. 41-6).

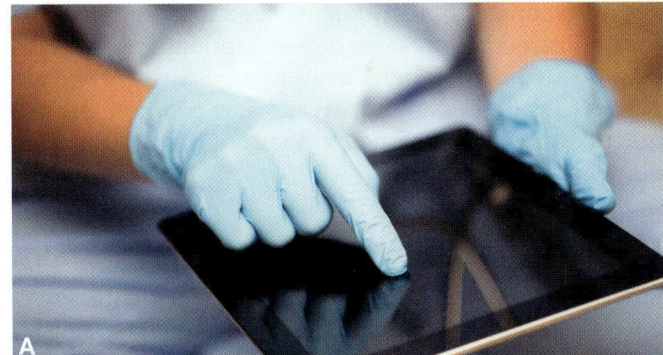
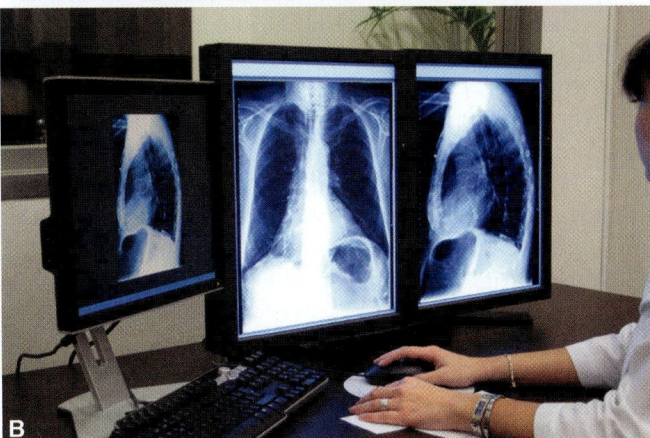

FIGURE 41-6 Point-of-access computing. A, Handheld device. B, Terminal unit for accessing patient data.

Clinical Support Tools (CST) EHRs equip providers with clinical support tools to conveniently access information to assist with clinical decision making. For example, a CST may offer current drug information; cross-reference a patient allergy to prescribed medication; and alerts prescribers and nurses to potential drug interactions and other patient risks.

Reduced Errors Computer physician order entry (CPOE) allows healthcare providers to enter orders via a computer instead of handwriting them, thus reducing errors resulting from illegible handwriting. It also makes the prescription process more efficient for nursing and pharmacy staffs by saving time in soliciting information missing from illegible or incomplete orders.

Privacy Access to sensitive patient information can be limited only to individuals with proper authorization, and each retrieval of data can be logged electronically—a vast improvement over the folders and charts that can pass through many hands without a record of who examines them.

Research and Public Health Benefits Computerized records place data in repositories (storage areas) so that the information can be sorted and analyzed to create the information and knowledge necessary to aid research to support decision making. For example, state health departments can access population-based medical information to track communicable diseases, possibly preventing epidemics. Health researchers and analysts can also use aggregate health information to judge which treatment is most effective for a disease. One possible outcome might be fewer prescriptions for unnecessary antibiotics (Hebert, Beaumont, Schwartz, et al., 2012). To protect patient privacy and promote ethical practice of research, review boards govern access to population data.

Barriers to EHR Adoption

There are numerous reasons why some providers and hospitals resist using an EHR. Some providers resist using an EHR because they fear of loss of autonomy. Some claim moving to an EHR will cause disruption in workflow or lead to errors, as some EHR products are hard to use and not well engineered for clinical workflow (Ford, Menachemi, Peterson, et al., 2009). Others object to EHRs because of the purchase and installation costs. The most prevalent reason, though, is computer illiteracy and discomfort with technology. User adoption and systems training are expensive, time consuming, and frustrating. This can be problematic in a demanding clinical environment.

Although the intent of computerization is to decrease cost by improving efficiency and communication, there may be unintended consequences of EHR implementation, such as diminished face-to-face communication among the healthcare team. Software upgrade and periodic new releases are inevitable, some of which may require more robust hardware than previous editions. New, expensive equipment to replace perfectly serviceable hardware, which has been rendered obsolete by the EHR, is a factor when considering the cost of an EHR.

The nurse informatics specialist, a nurse with additional education and experience in informatics, provides guidance for clinicians in identifying gaps between how the EHR system functions and how clinical processes work. Successful changes from paper to electronic systems are those that provide opportunities for nurses to have a voice in choosing systems and planning the change. Some people adopt change readily and some are more resistant. For more discussion about how people tend to respond to innovation,

 Go to **Chapter 41, Tables, Boxes, Figures: ESG Box 41-1, Adopters of Innovation,** on Davis*Plus*.

KnowledgeCheck 41-3

- What are some of the benefits of EHR implementation?
- List at least three ways in which computers can help reduce medication errors.

Ethical Use of Electronic Health Records

Medical records contain highly sensitive information. Patients confide in nurses and physicians, trusting that their information will remain private. Most facilities have disciplinary policies in place to manage security breaches and assign fines or prosecution when patient privacy is violated. Personal integrity and adherence to nursing and other codes of ethics are necessary to protect patient privacy within healthcare organizations.

With an automated record, many people can view the information at the same time, and they can be in many different locations. Nevertheless, in some ways the automated record is more secure than the paper record. Almost anyone in the clinical unit can view the paper record. There is no record to show who has seen the information. In contrast, several measures protect the confidentiality of the electronic health record.

Passwords

Passwords for all users are probably the most obvious protection. In most institutions, exposure to protected patient information is tied to the responsibilities of the job description. For example, as a rule, the business office does not see day-to-day clinical information; and nurses do not see any special arrangements a patient has made to pay a bill.

Although it is important to protect the privacy of healthcare records from outside observers, professionals who have password access but are not assigned to the patient to provide care make most breaches of confidentiality.

BOX 41-1 ■ Some Simple Rules for Password Management

- Never share passwords with others.
- The more complex the password is, the harder it is for hackers to break it. Use combinations of letters, numbers, and symbols for maximum protection.
- Don't use words or numbers that are easy to guess (e.g., pet names, birthdays).
- Change passwords frequently.
- Do not record passwords in easily accessible places.

Audit Trails

Organizations are required to have software that tracks each person who accesses information. This is called an **audit trail**. Anything a person adds to or changes in the record is recorded automatically on the audit trail and can be investigated.

HIPAA Regulations

Most health insurance plans and care providers must comply with the Department of Health and Human Services (HHS) Privacy Rule (also referred to as "the HIPAA regulations"). The Privacy Rule was mandated in response to the Health Insurance Portability and Accountability Act (HIPAA) of 1996. It was the first comprehensive federal protection for the privacy of individually identifiable health information. The two important requirements are that health plans and providers must:

- Obtain consent before disclosing health information used for treatment or payment options.
- Limit disclosure of information to the minimum necessary to accomplish intended purposes.

These rules were extended as part of the HITECH Act discussed earlier. New rules increase fines levied on organizations for each reported breach of personal health information, and give authority to individual states to monitor compliance with the rules. They apply to all forms of communication: electronic, written, and oral. For full information,

 Go to the **U.S. Department of Health and Human Services** Internet site at http://www.hhs.gov/ocr/hipaa/

If you would like further discussion of EHR privacy issues, review the section How Do I Maintain Confidentiality and Data Security? in Chapter 18.

KnowledgeCheck 41-4

- Discuss at least three measures to protect the confidentiality of patients' electronic health records.

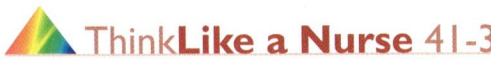 ThinkLike a Nurse 41-3

- How does automation contribute to or decrease errors in healthcare?

PracticalKnowledge knowing how

Professional standards require accountable practitioners to keep up to date with research and new knowledge. For example, criteria in the ANA Professional Standard 8 state the nurse should demonstrate a commitment to lifelong learning and seek experiences that reflect current practice to maintain skills and competence (ANA, 2010). You can accomplish this by knowing how to search literature databases efficiently and use Internet resources discriminatingly to complement your use of the EHR in providing quality patient care.

USING INFORMATICS TO SUPPORT EVIDENCE-BASED PRACTICE

The *traditional model of healthcare decision making* relies on each practitioner's personal experience and judgment. But healthcare is now so complex that problems routinely exceed the clinical decision-making capacity and reliability of individual practitioners. A better model of decision making is *evidence-based practice*. As you have learned in previous chapters, evidence-based practice involves (1) identifying a clinical question or need for change; (2) searching the literature for "best evidence," which can change quickly and continuously; (3) evaluating evidence; and (4) translating the results into practice (Majid, Foo, Luty, et al., 2011; Sackett, Rosenberg, Gray, et al., 1996).

Nurses require the most current, best-quality information for making decisions in their practice. It is not enough to find one journal article in support of an intervention, but rather to search broadly for high-quality, scientific evidence. Managing and processing information are essential for these tasks. Nurses need information on a wide variety of topics including clinical nursing issues, drug therapy, improving patient outcomes, innovative practice changes, and leadership skills. To find the current *best* evidence, you must be skilled in computer use and in searching relevant literature. These skills partially describe an information-literate person. Other qualities of an information-literate person are found in Box 41-2.

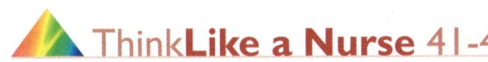 ThinkLike a Nurse 41-4

Analyze the Meet Your Nurse Role Model scenario. What example of evidence-based practice do you find in it?

Computers for Evidence-Based Practice

Most nurses are action oriented, preferring to learn by looking, listening, and talking. It may seem easier to seek information from colleagues, rely on past experience, draw on knowledge of pathophysiology, and read whatever references are closest at hand. However, in the clinical setting, the closest reference book may not

BOX 41-2 ■ Profile of an Information-Literate Person

An information-literate person *accesses* information:

- Recognizes the need for information
- Understands accurate and complete information is the basis for intelligent decision making
- Formulates questions based on information needs
- Identifies potential sources of information and selects those with credibility
- Accesses print and technology-based sources of information

An information-literate person *evaluates* information:

- Accepts authoritative, current reliable information
- Sorts information based on accuracy and relevance
- Distinguishes opinion from factual knowledge
- Rejects inaccurate and misleading information
- Rejects biased information
- Creates new information to replace inaccurate or missing information as needed

An information-literate person *manages* information:

- Develops successful search strategies
- Organizes information so the most important points are clear
- Breaks complex information into understandable chunks

- Sorts out language and technical points into meaningful terms
- Tracks sources of information responsibly and credits appropriately

An information-literate person *uses* information:

- Organizes information for practical application
- Integrates new information into an existing body of knowledge
- Applies information in critical thinking and problem-solving

Other characteristics:

- A resourceful and independent learner
- Competent reader
- Confident in his ability to solve problems
- Able to function independently and work well in groups
- Creative and able to adapt to change

Source: Adapted from: Association of College & Research Libraries. (2000). Information literacy competency standards for higher education. Retrieved from http://www.ala.org/acrl/standards/informationliteracycompetency; U.S. Department of Health and Human Services. (n.d.). *Quick guide to health literacy.* Retrieved from http://www.health.gov/communication/literacy/quickguide/quickguide.pdf

---

contain the most current information or the best possible evidence. Computers at the workplace help overcome this barrier to evidence-based practice by providing fast, easy access, 24 hours a day, to current practice information from around the world. For example, you could quickly use a computer to look up the latest tested interventions for a patient who is incontinent of urine.

How Do I Use Computers to Search the Literature?

Lack of literature-searching skills is another reason many nurses fail to take advantage of automated information available to enrich their practice. There are several steps to conducting an automated search of the literature:

- **Identify the information.** When you clearly define the information you want to gather and how it will be used, it is easier and more efficient to search, locate, evaluate, retrieve, organize, and manage the resources required to answer your question.
- **Formulate a precise definition of the problem.** This is usually in the form of a question, for example, "What are the leading causes of falls in older adults?" This question guides your search for information.
- **Conduct a search** of the most recent literature and most relevant studies. To learn about or review the PICOT method of defining and stating questions, go

to the section Formulate a Searchable Question and Box 8-4, in Chapter 8.

 ThinkLike a Nurse 41-5

Before reading the next section, see whether you can puzzle out the answers to the following two questions. Consult with your classmates and instructors, if necessary, after finishing the chapter.

- Why must a question be formed before initiating the search?
- The suggested question in the preceding section was "What are the leading causes of falls in older adults?" Why can't you use a general topic such as "falls" for your search topic?

Sources of Nursing Research Literature

You must evaluate the type of literature you need to answer the question. For instance, a research report provides better support for an intervention than does an opinion article. Although some information is classic and timeless, it is usually best to find the most current studies from reliable sources, such as government agencies, clinical organizations, or professional, refereed, peer-reviewed sources.

Textbooks   Textbooks are good for general information. However, they are not the most current source of information because of the time it takes to prepare them for publication.

Printed Journal Articles Printed journal articles are more current, but the information may still be 6 months to 2 years old by the time the article is published. Journals come in varying degrees of academic rigor. You must discriminate among scholarly, general interest, and popular periodical literature.

- *Scholarly Journals.* Scholarly journals contain tables and graphs, but are not as colorfully illustrated as general interest periodicals. A scholar, clinical expert, or scientific researcher in the field submits topical articles that adhere to professional standards, carefully footnoting and citing references. Articles submitted to scholarly journals are reviewed by a group of experts to determine whether they are suitable for publication. This process is known as a peer review. The main purpose of a scholarly journal is to report on original research to make the information available to others. Examples of scholarly journals include *Journal of Nursing Scholarship, Journal of Nursing Administration, Nursing Research,* and *International Journal of Nursing Terminologies and Classifications.*
- *General interest periodicals.* General interest periodicals are usually attractive. Articles tend to be heavily illustrated, commonly with photographs. News and general interest periodicals sometimes cite sources, but not always. Articles may be written by a member of the editorial staff, a scholar, or a freelance writer and are often peer reviewed. The language is geared to any educated audience. A specialty is not assumed. Some examples of general interest nursing periodicals include the *American Journal of Nursing, RN,* and *Nursing* [current year].
- *Popular periodicals.* Popular periodicals are usually slick and attractive in appearance. They include many graphics and photographs. These publications rarely, if ever, cite sources. Information in such journals is often second- or thirdhand, and the original source is sometimes obscure. Articles are usually short, lack depth, and are written in simple language and designed to meet a minimal education level. The main purpose is to promote a product or viewpoint. Examples include *Women's Health* and *Modern Healthcare.*

The World Wide Web The World Wide Web contains the most current information, from such sources as professional organizations (e.g., American Heart Association), government sources (e.g., Centers for Disease Control and Prevention), sites publishing clinical guidelines (e.g., Joanna Briggs Institute; National Guideline Clearinghouse), and various online nursing journals. New health information can be uploaded immediately on the Web for the entire world to see without the delay of print publishing.

Literature Databases

Literature databases are a powerful tool for finding information. Literature databases are catalogues of articles, usually sorted by discipline. Databases exist for engineering, education, law, medicine, nursing, and other disciplines. For example:

- MEDLINE is the largest medical database and lists internationally published articles from journals in all areas of biomedicine.
- The Cumulative Index for Nursing and Allied Health Literature (CINAHL) is a smaller database covering nursing, allied health, biomedical, and consumer health journal articles.

These databases often overlap—what is found in one database might also be found in another. Most of the articles in CINAHL are also listed in MEDLINE. If, however, you are looking for a nursing-focused article, it is more efficient to use CINAHL because the search is already narrowed to nursing and allied health.

Each entry in a database contains an article citation, subject headings describing the article, and a text summary of the article called an **abstract**. Other information about the article may also be included, such as the name of the author(s), the name of the institution at which the research was done, and the language in which the article was published (Box 41-3). Many full-text journal articles are available online, some free and some for a fee. Some are available in the school or hospital's library for nurses to access. Table 41-2 includes descriptions of some commonly used databases in healthcare. Do not limit your search to a single database. You will find valuable information in the databases of other disciplines (e.g., psychology, education, business, law).

How Do I Evaluate Evidence and Determine a Solution?

Evaluating the evidence is sometimes as simple as reading a descriptive research study and applying the results to your current situation. For example, when searching for information about falls in older adults, you may find research to indicate a number of safety measures that can be easily implemented to create a safer environment for your patients. At other times, evaluating evidence can be very complicated, requiring an understanding of statistics and research methodologies. Just because one study indicates that sugar causes cancer does not mean that the study was valid or reliable; therefore, you must not base conclusions on the results of only one study. Experience and further study about research will increase your ability to evaluate your findings in the literature.

Key Point: *Although an article you find on the Internet may be current, it is not necessarily complete, accurate, valid, or reliable.*

Many sites are created by individuals with questionable credentials or by companies attempting to sell their product or service. Such sites may not provide the best information to support your research; even

BOX 41-3 ■ Example of a Database Entry

Author(s):	Remsburg-Bell, E., Cook, V.	**Special Interests:**	Obstetric Care; Pediatric Care; Quality Assurance; Women's Health
Title:	Meaningful use: Staff led design for a new perinatal electronic health record	**ISSN:**	0884-2175
		MEDLINE Info:	NLM Unique Identifier: 8503123
Source:	Journal of Obstetric, Gynecologic & Neonatal Nursing (JOGNN), 42: Supplement: S59. 2013, June.	**Entry Date:**	20130628
		Revision Date:	20130628
Publication Type:	Journal article—abstract	**DOI:**	http://dx.doi.org.ezproxy.jccc.edu/ 10.1111/1552-6909.12137
ISSN:		**Accession Number:**	2012137648
Language:	English	**Database:**	CINAHL with Full Text
Major Subjects:	Perinatal Care		
	Computerized Patient Record		
Minor Subjects:	Posters; Quality Improvement		
Journal Subset:	Core Nursing; Nursing; Peer Reviewed; USA		

The search results may also contain an abstract of the article and in some instances the full-text article is available either for a fee or at no charge.

Table 41-2 ➤ Selected Databases for Health Literature

DATABASE	DESCRIPTION
CINAHL (Cumulative Index for Nursing and Allied Health Literature)	Covers nursing, allied health, biomedical, and consumer health journals; publications of the American Nursing Association; and the National League for Nursing. Coverage with abstracts is from January 1986 to the present. Coverage with indexing is from 1982 to the present. Updated monthly.
Cochrane Library	A regularly updated collection of evidence-based medicine databases, including systematic reviews, reviews of effectiveness, and a controlled-trials register. This is a source of reliable evidence about the effects of healthcare.
Health and Wellness Resource Center	Provides integrated access to medical, health, and wellness information from reference sources, magazine and journal articles, pamphlets, and some Internet resources. Quick Start links include a medical encyclopedia, dictionary, drug and herb finder, health organization directory, health assessment links, health news, and a few select medical Internet sites.
MEDLINE	Produced by the U.S. National Library of Medicine, MEDLINE is the world's largest medical library in all areas of biomedicine and healthcare.
PsycINFO 1887	Covers worldwide literature in psychology and related disciplines, such as psychiatry, sociology, anthropology, education, linguistics, and pharmacology. Journal articles, technical reports, and dissertations are included. Coverage is from 1887 to the present. Updated weekly.

---

worse, their information may be incomplete, inaccurate, biased, or unreliable. See Table 41-3 for suggestions on evaluating materials obtained from a Internet site. For ethical principles to guide health information Internet sites,

If you would like to review the process for evaluating the quality of research articles you find in your searches, or for a process to find the best evidence for a nursing intervention, refer to the section How Can I Base My Practice on the Best Evidence? in Chapter 8.

 Go to **Chapter 41, Tables, Boxes, Figures: ESG Box 41-2, Guiding Ethical Principles for Health Information Internet Sites,** on *DavisPlus.*

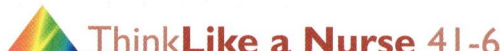 Think**Like a Nurse** 41-6

What factors can make the Internet an unreliable source of information? What factors can help you find reliable information?

Table 41-3 ➤ How to Evaluate a Health Information Web Site

Remember, anyone can publish anything on the Web. The information you obtain may have been created by an expert, but most World Wide Web sites are authored by nonexperts. They may contain fact or opinion. Do not believe everything you read on the Web! Use the following questions to guide your evaluation.

EVALUATE FOR	QUESTIONS TO ASK
Authority	■ *Who is the author?* What are his credentials and qualifications to speak on this topic? Are the sources of information stated? Don't confuse the author with the webmaster. ■ *Check the URL domain* (e.g., *www.nih.gov*). What institution published the document? The Web address provides clues to this: .com—a company. .mil—the U.S. military .edu—a school or university .net—a network of computers .gov—the U.S. government .org—a nonprofit organization ■ The domain symbols ~ or % or a name (e.g., jsmith), "users," or "members" indicate a personal web page. ■ *Who is the sponsor?* The name right after "www" will provide a clue (e.g., see "nih"), but the full name (e.g., National Institutes of Health) should be on the page. ■ *Can you contact the author* for clarification or more information?
Currency	■ *When was it produced?* For some topics, you need current information. ■ *When was it updated?* Note that the fact that the Web page was "updated" may not mean that the information was updated at the same time. It may simply mean that the physical file was changed in some way (e.g., a misspelled word corrected) ■ *Are the links up to date?* Check the links to see whether they work.
Purpose	■ *Why was the page put on the Web?* Remember that many sites are designed to promote a product or an idea. Other purposes may be to entertain, to give facts, to share humor, or to provide a forum for ideas and opinions. ■ *Look for words such as "about our company," "mission," "philosophy," "who am I,"* and so on. ■ *Who are the intended users* of the page? Students, experts, patients? ■ *Are there advertisements* on the page? This may be a clue.
Availability	■ *Can you view or download the information* without a special browser or special software? ■ *Are there fees* for viewing the full content?
Content quality (accuracy, objectivity, coverage)	■ *Are the sources documented* with footnotes or links? Are they scholarly links or information sources? ■ *Is the information provided by the site, or is it reproduced* from another source? ■ *Are there links to the original sources* (if they are online)? Or a reason for not providing a link? Do they work? ■ *Look for bias* (e.g., political or ideological), especially when you agree with it! Are there links to opposing views if it is an opinion page? ■ *Is the information reliable and error free?* Is there someone who verifies or checks the information? ■ *How in-depth* is the material? ■ *What does the page offer* that you can't find elsewhere? ■ *Look up the page* in a directory that evaluates the website contents. For example: ■ *www.ipl.org (the Librarians' Internet Index)* ■ *http://www.lib.umd.edu/guides/webcheck.html*
Usability	■ *Is it easy to read and navigate?* ■ *Are HELP screens available?* ■ *Is there a search engine on the site?* ■ *Is it frequently offline or slow to load?*

To explore learning resources for this chapter,

Go to DavisPlus at **DavisPl.us/Wilkinson3**

Chapter Resources for Chapter 41:
- Response sheets for all learning activities
- Resources for Caregivers and Health Professionals
- Reading More About Nursing Informatics (suggested readings)
- Concept Map of chapter content

Interactive Case Studies

NCLEX-Style and Chapter Review Questions

Chapter Overview Podcasts

For references cited in this chapter,

 Go to Volume 2, **References Cited**.

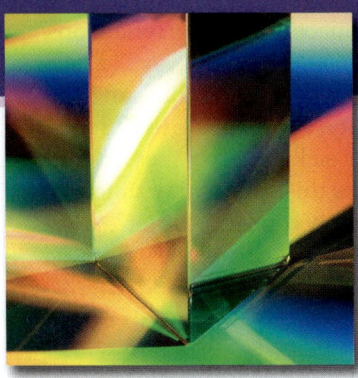

CHAPTER 42

Promoting Health

Learning Outcomes

After completing this chapter, you should be able to:

➤ Define *health*, *health promotion*, and *health protection*.

➤ Identify health prevention activities and categorize them as primary, secondary, or tertiary levels of prevention.

➤ Discuss the *Healthy People 2020* report in relation to leading causes of death and to health promotion strategies: nutrition, exercise, lifestyle, and environment.

➤ Apply Pender's Health Promotion Model to plan activities designed to change unhealthy behavior.

➤ Identify Prochaska and DiClemente's four stages of change.

➤ Identify specific health promotion strategies (including immunizations and screenings) across the life span.

➤ Discuss nurses' roles in health promotion, and list health promotion activities that a nurse may conduct in acute care facilities, in the workplace, in local communities, and in schools.

➤ Identify the areas of assessment in relation to developing a health promotion plan.

➤ Assess a client's cardiorespiratory function, muscle strength and endurance, joint flexibility, and nutrition (body mass index or body fat percentage).

➤ Construct a health promotion plan of care using the nursing process, NANDA-I taxonomy, Nursing Outcomes Classifications, and Nursing Interventions Classifications.

Key Concepts

Health promotion
Health protection
Illness prevention
Wellness

Related Concepts

See the Concept Map on Davis*Plus*.

Meet Your Peer

You have completed all your prerequisites and are now enrolled in your first nursing course. Aside from classroom work, you have a skills course and clinical rotation. You spend a lot of time reading, studying, preparing for clinical work, writing care plans, and completing follow-up assignments from your clinical rotation. You have other non-nursing course work and family responsibilities as well. Often, you stay up late and get up early, usually getting about 5 or 6 hours of sleep. By the end of the week, you're exhausted. You don't have time to cook so you pick up fast food several times a week. Even though it is not the healthiest choice, at least this way you can get something to eat. You have little time to exercise, and when you do have time, you feel too tired and uninterested. You use cigarettes to relax and help cope with stress. On the weekends, you let loose with friends, drinking beer and having a good time.

You spend most of your time learning about health and illness. Given your current lifestyle, do you consider yourself healthy? How did you make that decision? Your answer is based on your personal beliefs about health and what you have learned in your nursing course work. In this chapter, we explore health promotion. As you learn more about this topic, you may develop a plan to promote your own health as well as the health of clients.

Theoretical Knowledge
knowing why

To begin, we explore what others have written about the concepts. Various descriptions and definitions use the concepts health and wellness interchangeably, and we do the same in this chapter.

ABOUT THE KEY CONCEPTS

In Chapter 11, we considered the concepts of health, wellness, and illness. In this chapter, the emphasis is on strategies to support those concepts: **health promotion**, **health protection**, **illness prevention**, and **wellness**. As you study various concepts, such as health screening, role modeling, and health behaviors (to name a few examples), try to understand how they relate to the key concepts.

WHAT IS HEALTH PROMOTION?

To promote health, we must first identify what we mean by *health* and *wellness*. We will use the following definitions to synthesize a meaning.

World Health Organization The World Health Organization (WHO) defines health as "a state of complete physical, mental and social well-being and not merely the absence of disease or infirmity" (WHO, 1948). At the first conference for health promotion, WHO defined **health promotion** as the process of equipping people to have control over, and to improve, physical, emotional, and social health (WHO, 1986).

Jean Watson This nursing theorist proposed that health consists of three elements: (1) a high level of overall physical, mental, and social functioning; (2) a general adaptive-maintenance level of daily functioning; and (3) the absence of illness (or the presence of efforts that lead to its absence). She also refers to health as being a state of mind, the perception of the individual. A person may have a terminal illness and yet consider himself healthy (Watson, 1979).

Betty Neuman This nursing theorist describes health as an expression of living energy available to an individual. The energy is displayed as a continuum, with high energy (wellness) at one end and low energy (illness) at the opposite end. Individuals have varying levels of energy at various stages of life. When more energy is generated than expended, there is wellness. When more energy is expended than is generated, there is illness, possibly death (Neuman, 1995).

Myers, Sweeney, and Witmer In 2000 these theorists defined wellness as "a way of life oriented toward optimal health and well-being in which body, mind, and spirit are integrated by the individual to live more fully within the human and natural community" (p. 252). This definition includes lifestyles and habits as components

of health and permits people who have been diagnosed with disease to be considered healthy.

Synthesis Applying aspects of these reflections on health, **health promotion** means finding ways to help individuals develop a state of physical, spiritual, and mental well-being. Health promotion activities are useful to all individuals, whether well or sick, because they encourage optimal function. How does this compare with the WHO definition of health promotion you read earlier?

Health Promotion Versus Health Protection

For the most part, the activities that promote health also protect health. Nevertheless, the ideas behind health promotion and health protection differ subtly but significantly. Pender, Murdaugh, and Parsons (2010) explain that motivation is what distinguishes the two activities.

- Health promotion is motivated by the desire to increase well-being.
- Health protection is motivated by a desire to avoid illness.

For instance the 40-year-old who begins an exercise program to improve strength and endurance is motivated by the benefits of health promotion. If he starts exercising because his father died of a heart attack at age 50, he may be motivated by the need to protect his health.

Levels of Prevention

Leavell and Clark (1965) identified three levels of activities for health protection (illness prevention): primary, secondary, and tertiary. Interventions are classified according to their purpose in different stages of the disease process. This timing directs the types of interventions needed.

- **Primary prevention** activities are designed to prevent or slow the onset of disease. Examples include eating healthy foods, exercising, wearing sunscreen, obeying seat belt laws, and keeping up with immunizations.
- **Secondary prevention** involves screening activities and education for detecting illnesses in the early stages. Examples are breast self-examination, testicular exams, regular physical examinations, blood pressure and diabetes screenings, and tuberculosis skin tests.
- **Tertiary prevention** focuses on stopping the disease from progressing and returning the individual to the pre-illness phase. Rehabilitation is the main intervention during this level.

Patients and health providers move among these levels of prevention. For example, a patient hospitalized for a total hip replacement would receive tertiary prevention—care focused on helping her recover from surgery, preventing complications of surgery, and, later on, helping her regain her strength and learn to walk again. Secondary prevention strategies may have been used previously, for example, to screen for osteoporosis that leads to bone fragility and fractures. When she goes home, if she decides to limit her salt intake and eat a balanced diet that is low in fat and refined sugar, these activities would be primary prevention strategies.

Health Behaviors

For the population overall, life expectancy (at birth) reached a record high of 78.7 years, up from 75.4 years in 1990. The gap between men and women has narrowed from 7.0 years in 1990 to 4.8 years in 2010 (Centers for Disease Control and Prevention [CDC], 2013). Health status is affected by health behavior, such as weight management, increasing the amount of physical activity, safer sex, moderate alcohol use, and avoidance of tobacco and drugs.

Teen Pregnancy

Pregnant teenagers are less likely to receive early prenatal care. They are more likely to drop out of school and to live in poverty than are older pregnant women. The birth rate for teenagers aged 15 to 19 years dropped 8% from 2010 to 2011, to 31.3%, a historic low for the United States. Rates fell for all races including in those of Hispanic origin (CDC, 2013).

Abuse of Alcohol and Illicit Drugs

The risk of disease, injuries, and intentional death (suicide and homicide) increases with substance abuse.

- An estimated 30% of the U.S. population is affected by alcohol misuse; most of the 30% engage in risky use. More than 85,000 deaths per year are attributable to alcohol misuse, which is the estimated third leading cause of preventable deaths in the United States. The U.S. Preventive Service Task Force (USPSTF) (2013) recommends that clinicians screen adults aged 18 years or older for alcohol misuse and provide persons engaged in risky or hazardous drinking with brief behavioral counseling interventions to reduce alcohol misuse.
- In 2011, 8.1% of students reported having tried marijuana before the age of 13 years, and 20.7% reported nonmedical use of prescription drugs. (*Morbidity and Mortality Weekly Report*, 2012).

✚ Substance abuse in adolescents is associated with a greater frequency of suicide attempts, more lethal (successful) attempts, an increased seriousness of intent, and greater suicidal ideation.

Tobacco Use

Cigarette smoking increases the risk of lung cancer, tuberculosis, heart disease, emphysema, and other diseases.

- The percentage of middle and high school students who reported smoking cigarettes in the past month was 7.1% and 23.2%, respectively (CDC, 2012).
- "Ever use" of electronic cigarettes among students in grades 6 to 12 increased from 3.3% to 6.8% during 2011–2012. Those who said they are "currently using" them increased from 1.1% to 2.1% (*Morbidity & Mortality Weekly Report*, 2013).

- Overall the percentage of high school students and adults who reported smoking cigarettes remained stable at 20% to 23%, after declining from 36% in the previous decade.
- Men were more likely to be current cigarette smokers than were women (24% compared with 18%) (CDC, 2010).
- The highest percentage of tobacco users are in the South (CDC, 2009a).
- Smoking as few as three cigarettes a day can increase the risk for cardiovascular disease by more than 60% (Pope, Burnett, Krewski, et al., 2009). The risk of active tuberculosis is nearly doubled with tobacco use (Linn, Ezzati, Chang, et al., 2009).

Obesity

The risk of heart disease, diabetes, and stroke increases with obesity.

- In 2009–2010, more than 16% of U.S. children and adolescents were obese. The prevalence of obesity was higher among adolescents than among preschool-aged children and higher among boys (18.6%) than girls (15%) (CDC, 2012).
- More than 35% of U.S. men and women were obese in 2009–2010. There was no significant difference in prevalence between men and women at any age. Overall, adults aged 60 years and over were more likely to be obese than younger adults (CDC, 2012).
- With the U.S. obesity trend, only 7.5% of Americans now have five low-risk factors for cardiovascular disease—no tobacco use, normal blood pressure, normal weight, low blood cholesterol, no diabetes, and age younger than 75 years (Ford, van Dam, & Fonarow, 2009).

Sedentary Lifestyle

Exercise reduces the risk of disease and enhances mental and physical health. American adults have made no substantial progress toward achieving recommended levels of physical activity or strength training. Between 1995 and 2006, the percentage of adults 18 years of age and older engaged in regular leisure-time physical activity or strength-training activities remained level.

KnowledgeCheck 42-1

- How does health promotion differ from health protection?
- Which level of prevention is represented by the following activities?
  Mumps, measles, rubella (MMR) vaccination
  Tuberculosis (TB) skin test
  Physical therapy after repair of a hip fracture

Health Promotion Models

A model illustrates a system or framework to help explain what you see in clinical practice. The most common frameworks used for designing health promotion programs are described next.

Pender's Health Promotion Model

Pender's Health Promotion Model (HPM) (Fig. 42-1) identifies three groups of variables that affect health promotion: (1) individual characteristics and experiences, (2) behavior-specific cognitions and affect, and (3) behavioral outcome. The HPM is based on seven assumptions that reflect both nursing and behavioral science perspectives (Pender, Murdaugh, & Parsons, 2010). Two general assumptions are about the interpersonal environment:

1. Health professionals constitute a part of the interpersonal environment, which exerts influence on persons throughout their life span.
2. Self-initiated reconfiguration of person–environment interactive patterns is essential to behavior change.

The other five assumptions are characteristics of people, who the theorists assume:

1. Seek to create conditions of living through which they can express their unique human health potential.
2. Have the capacity for reflective self-awareness, including assessment of their own competencies.
3. Value growth in directions viewed as positive and attempt to achieve a personally acceptable balance between change and stability.

4. Seek to actively regulate their own behavior.
5. In all their biopsychosocial complexity interact with the environment, progressively transforming the environment and being transformed over time.

Pender's model has been used extensively in several disciplines in research and professional practice focused on health promotion. As a nurse, you should find Pender's focus applicable to your work.

▲ Think**Like a Nurse 42-1**

- How might peers influence health behaviors? At what age might peers have more influence?
- Apply Pender's model to a person trying to lose weight. What might be some perceived barriers (see Fig. 42-1)?

Wheel of Wellness

Several authors have likened the different facets of health to the spokes of a wheel (Hettler, 1984; Myers, Sweeney, & Witmer, 2000; Witmer & Sweeney, 1992). If one of the spokes is weak, the whole wheel is weak. The "spokes" of the health wheel represent the dimensions of health: emotional, intellectual, physical, spiritual, social/family, and occupational (Fig. 42-2). The level of

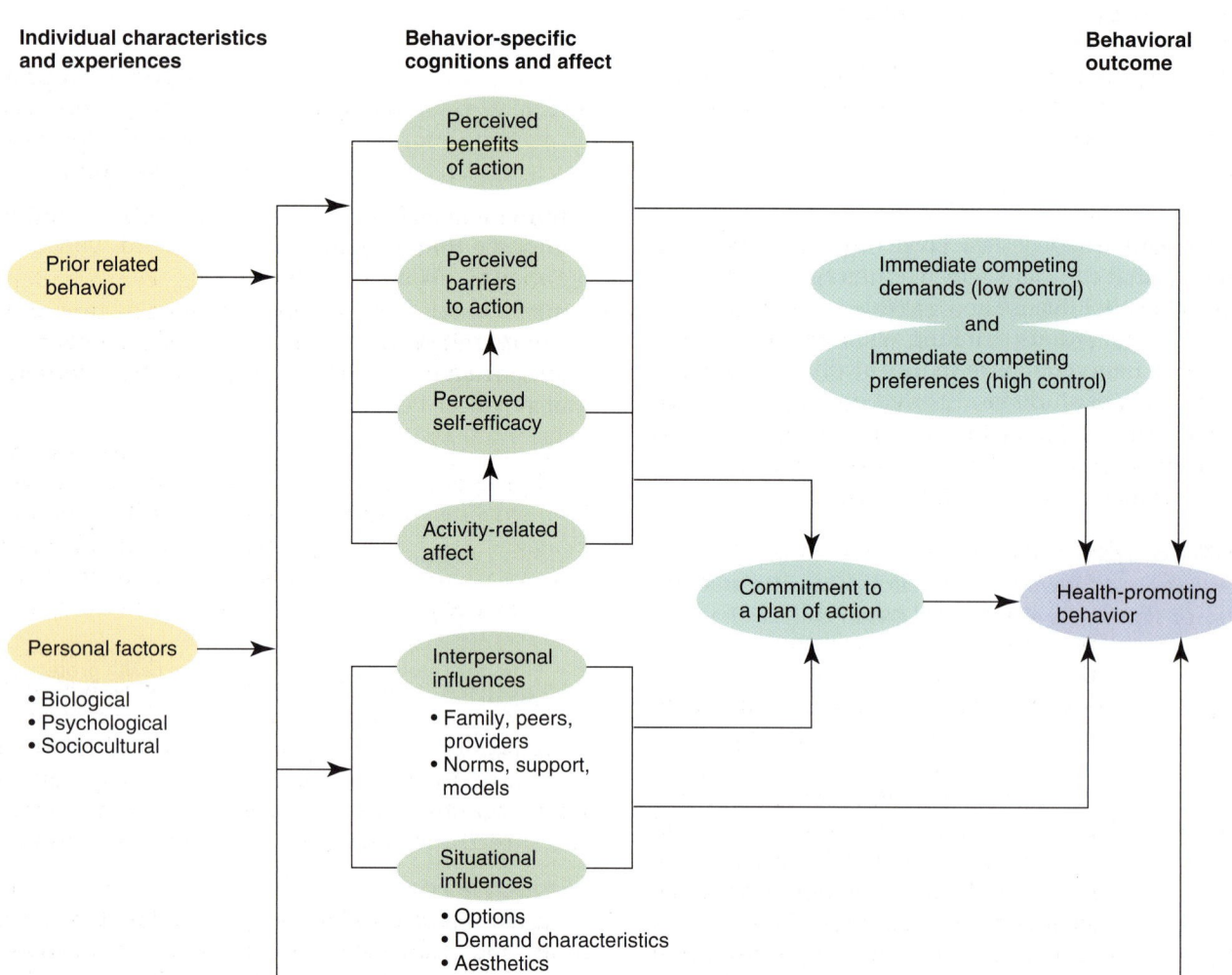

FIGURE 42-1 Pender's Health Promotion Model.

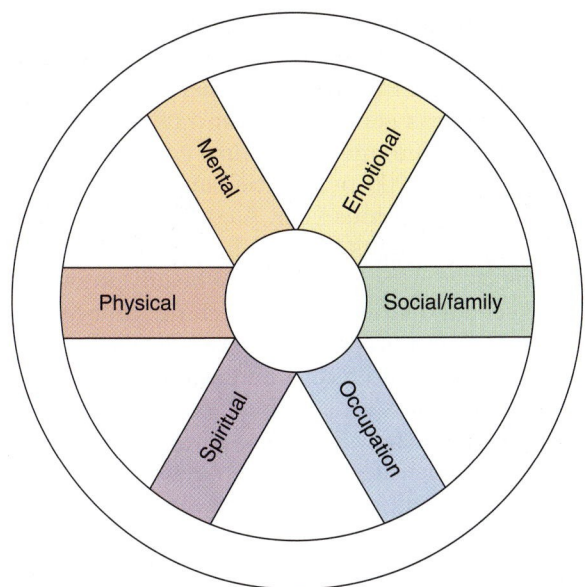

FIGURE 42-2 Wheel of Wellness.

wellness progresses from the center to the outer part of the wheel. The center represents the least amount of wellness, and the outer part represents optimal wellness. If one area of a person's life is not functioning at optimal level, life will not be as fulfilling as it could be. As a nurse, you should assess each dimension for strengths and weaknesses.

Transtheoretical Model of Change

The transtheoretical model of change (Prochaska & DiClemente, 1982) may serve as a means to alter unhealthy behaviors. Health promotion and protection involve either changing the individual's response to the illness-producing stimuli or changing the environment so that the person will be less likely to encounter illness-producing stimuli. Either idea involves change. In this model, change occurs in five stages (six, if you do not include termination in the maintenance stage):

Stage 1	**Precontemplation** is the stage in which there is no intention to change behavior in the foreseeable future, because patients are unaware or underaware of their problems.
Stage 2	**Contemplation** is the stage in which patients are seriously thinking about overcoming a problem but have not yet made a commitment to take action.
Stage 3	**Preparation** is the stage in which individuals are intending to take action in the next month and are reporting some small behavioral changes ("baby steps").
Stage 4	**The action stage** is the implementation of the plan and requires considerable commitment of time and energy.

Stage 5	**The maintenance stage** allows the changed behavior to be reinforced.
Stage 6	**The termination stage** completes the maintenance. A person who enters the termination stage has changed the behavior and is not in danger of relapse.

Ideally, the stages would progress in this order. Realistically, a person may progress and regress in any of the stages. The change process in persons with some unhealthy habits (e.g., cigarette smoking, substance abuse, and excessive eating) may best be described as a revolving door. An individual may exit at any point as the door goes around. If the exit occurs during or at the end of the maintenance period, the behavioral change is successful. If the exit occurs before the end of the maintenance period, relapse will occur, and the individual will return to the previous lifestyle.

Health Promotion Programs

Health promotion programs help a person advance toward optimal health. In the sections that follow we discuss several types. For further discussion of individual activities that promote health,

 Go to Chapter 42, **Supplemental Materials: Individual Health Promotion Activities,** on DavisPlus.

Disseminating Information To recognize a problem and understand the options for change, people need information. Information may be disseminated at three levels, as illustrated in the following examples:

- Individual level—Teaching a client how to modify his personal dietary intake
- Group level—Classes offered at the local hospital, prenatal education programs, and worksite programs
- Community level—A billboard that presents the dangers of smoking, health blogs on the Internet, and health fairs

Changing Lifestyle and Behavior These are group-level programs. They focus on activities such as weight loss, smoking cessation, exercise, nutrition, and stress management. These programs usually provide information and offer support. Many times, they include a maintenance program to help solidify the change.

Protecting the Environment The term *environment* refers to air, water, and soil as well as social and political surroundings. Environmental control programs promote health by working to create a healthy environment. Programs focus on air and water quality, toxic waste, healthy homes and communities, infrastructure and surveillance, and global environmental health.

Assessing Wellness and Appraising Health Risk These programs focus on identifying behaviors that promote health and create the risk for disease. A wellness assessment tends to focus on the healthy behaviors. It supports positive change to improve health. A health risk appraisal identifies risky behaviors that promote disease. These programs are readily available on the Internet, in magazines, and at fitness centers.

KnowledgeCheck 42-2

- What are the six dimensions of health represented by the spokes on the wellness wheel?
- Identify the stages of change identified by Prochaska and DiClemente.
- Describe the four main types of health promotion programs.

 ThinkLike a Nurse 42-2

J.T. drinks a vodka and tonic while eating lunch with his coworkers. He keeps a bottle of vodka in his office desk for use during the day. Later, he stops at a local bar for a drink on the way home. At home, he drinks a six-pack of beer while watching the game. What information do you need to determine which of Prochaska and DiClemente's stages of change he is experiencing? How would you get this information?

Settings for Health Promotion Programs

The most common sites for health promotion programs are health facilities, worksites, and schools. Healthcare settings, such as clinics, physician offices, or hospitals, are natural settings for health promotion. Remember, each interaction between patient and healthcare provider is an opportunity for health promotion. Unfortunately, most interactions focus on the disease process and compliance with treatments. You will need to make a conscious effort to help clients focus on behaviors that prevent illness and promote health.

Nurses work in health clinics within large companies or may be contracted to provide specific health promotion programs, such as smoking cessation, stress management, weight reduction, and fitness training. Employers have found that health programs decrease work-related injuries and sick leave. For instance, one study demonstrated that employees classified as high risk (according to body fat, blood pressure, anxiety, and other measures) who received cardiac rehabilitation and exercise training from an expert team were converted to low-risk status by the end of a 6-month program. Furthermore, medical claims costs had declined by more than $1,000 per participant, compared with those from the previous year. A control group showed no such improvements (Berry, Mirabito, & Baun, 2010).

Another setting for community health promotion is the local school district. Health teaching can begin at an early age, and nurses and teachers can regularly reinforce healthy behaviors and redirect unhealthy behaviors. The school setting allows for continued exposure to information. Interventions may be directed at general health promotion issues, such as physical activity, or they may focus on specific health risks, such as tobacco and alcohol use. Ideally, parents and families are included in the learning. School nurses work closely with teachers and parents to provide health promotion services in the schools.

Health Promotion Throughout the Life Span

Health promotion is a lifelong process that begins at conception. Table 42-1 describes the focus of health promotion programs at each developmental stage, as well as the types of screenings recommended for each age group.

PracticalKnowledge
knowing **how**

Pender, Murdaugh, and Parsons (2010) summarized the health promotion process as a series of nine steps that involve the client and the nurse. Notice that many steps of this process are similar to the nursing process:

1. Review and summarize data from assessment.
2. Reinforce the client's strengths and abilities.

Table 42-1 ➤ Health Promotion Throughout the Life Span			
HEALTH PROMOTION FOCUS	**HEALTH SCREENINGS**	**HEALTH PROMOTION FOCUS**	**HEALTH SCREENINGS**
Conception to Birth		Infancy	
Education about pregnancy	Alpha-fetoprotein level	Nutrition (breast versus bottle)	Hearing evaluation
Abstinence from alcohol, cigarettes, and illicit drugs	Screening for gestational diabetes	Introduction of solid foods	Screening for birth defects
Nutrition, including folic acid and iron requirements	Prenatal care	Placing the infant on her back for sleep without a pillow to reduce the risk of sudden infant death syndrome (SIDS)	Blood work to rule out certain metabolic conditions
Exercise to maintain strength and muscle tone and to control weight gain	Abuse Additional screenings that may be offered:		Monthly examinations until at least 6 months of age
	■ Ultrasound	Sensory stimulation	After age 6 months, visits every 2 or 3 months
Parenting education	■ Amniocentesis	Safety	
	■ Chorionic villus sampling	Motor vehicle safety	Growth and development
		Oral health	Abuse

Table 42-1 ➤ Health Promotion Throughout the Life Span—cont'd

HEALTH PROMOTION FOCUS	HEALTH SCREENINGS	HEALTH PROMOTION FOCUS	HEALTH SCREENINGS
Toddler and Preschool		**Middle Adult**	
Adequate supervision	Annual examinations	Physical activity	Comprehensive exam at least every 3 years to age 40, yearly after age 40
Safety, including storage of poisons	Growth and development	Safety	
Toilet training	Cognitive skills	Obesity	BP screening
Motor vehicle safety	Abuse	Sexuality	Lipid panel
Nutrition	Kindergarten readiness	Lifestyle	Blood glucose
Immunizations		Update of immunizations	Stress
Oral health		Oral health	Mammograms yearly and clinical breast exam for women over age 40
Sleep and rest		Substance use and abuse	
School Age			Digital rectal exam for prostate evaluation in men
Nutrition	Annual examinations		PSA for men yearly over age 50 (as decided with provider)
Physical activity	Growth and development		
Safety	Cognitive skills		Annual eye exam
Sexuality	Abuse		Sigmoidoscopy or colonoscopy
Stranger danger			Stool for occult blood with comprehensive exam
Oral health			
Adolescence			Bone density
Peer pressure	Growth and development		Abuse
Motor vehicle safety		**Older Adult**	
Safety	Sexually transmitted infection (STI) screening	Physical activity	Functional skills (ADLs and IADLs)
Self-esteem		Nutrition	
Physical activity	Breast self-exam	Safety	Hearing
Suicide and depression	Testicular self-exam	Obesity	Falls risk
Firearm safety	Mental health	Sexuality	Stress
Violence	Stress	Lifestyle	Annual eye exam
Sexuality	Alcohol and drug use	Update of immunizations	BP screening
Substance use and abuse	Abuse	Oral health	Lipid panel
Limiting sun exposure		Changes associated with aging	Blood glucose
Update of immunizations			Mammograms and clinical breast exam (as decided by provider and patient)
Oral health			
Young Adult			Digital rectal exam for prostate evaluation in men
Physical activity	Comprehensive exam at least every 3 years		PSA for men (as decided with provider)
Motor vehicle safety	Lifestyle		
Safety	Pap smear		Stool for occult blood
Violence	STI screening		Bone density
Sexuality	Breast self-exam monthly		Follow-up sigmoidoscopy or colonoscopy
Substance use and abuse	Testicular self-exam monthly		
Limiting sun exposure	Mental health		Mental health
Update immunizations	Stress		Abuse
Oral health	Alcohol and drug use		
	Abuse		

3. Identify health goals and related behavioral change options.
4. Identify behavioral or health outcomes that will indicate that the plan has been successful from the client's perspective.
5. Develop a behavior change plan based on the client's preferences, on the stages of change, and on "state-of-the-science" knowledge about effective interventions.
6. Reiterate benefits of change, and identify incentives for change from the client's perspective.
7. Address environmental and interpersonal facilitators and barriers to behavior change.
8. Determine a time frame for implementation.
9. Commit to behavior-change goals, and structure the support needed to accomplish them.

ASSESSMENT

A health promotion assessment involves obtaining a health history, physical examination, fitness assessment, lifestyle and risk appraisal, life stress review, analysis of health beliefs, nutritional assessment, and screening activities.

History and Physical Examination

Assessment should begin with a thorough health history, review of body systems, and a physical examination. Ask the client about family history of various health disorders and cause of death of family members. Keep in mind the accuracy of reporting is higher for relatives without, rather than those affected by, a given disease (Qureshi, Wilson, Santaguida, et al., 2009). Gather the history directly from the client. As always, provide privacy and comfort while conducting the history and exam.

The level of detail of the physical examination depends on the health history. At a minimum, the exam should include vital signs, weight, body mass index (BMI) or waist circumference, auscultation and palpation of the chest and abdomen, inspection of the skin, and palpation of peripheral pulses. The exam may be accompanied by laboratory studies. Recommended lab work depends on the history and exam findings. For most adult clients, a screening lab consists of a complete blood count, comprehensive metabolic panel (also known as a chem 20 panel), lipid panel, thyroid function panel, and urinalysis (American College of Sports Medicine [ACSM], 2013). In clients with known cardiac or pulmonary disease, additional disease-specific studies may be performed (e.g., electrocardiogram [ECG], carotid ultrasound, or pulmonary function tests).

Physical Fitness Assessment

Regular physical activity each week, sustained for months and years, can produce long-term health benefits. Regular physical activity is linked with a lower risk for heart disease, stroke, type 2 diabetes, hypertension, high cholesterol, metabolic syndrome, certain types of cancer, and depression. Regular physical activity also prevents weight gain; improves cardiorespiratory and muscular fitness; prevents falls by increasing muscle tone, strength, and balance; and promotes better memory and cognition in older adults (ACSM, 2013). A physical fitness assessment includes the following:

- *Cardiorespiratory fitness* is reflected in the ability to perform large-muscle, moderate- to high-intensity exercise for prolonged periods of time (ACSM, 2013). There are many different modes of testing, such as field tests (walking or running), treadmills, stationary bicycles, and step testing. Results depend on age and gender.
- *Muscular fitness* refers to both muscle strength and endurance. Muscle strength is a measure of the amount of weight a muscle (or group of muscles) can move at one time. Muscle endurance refers to the ability of a muscle to perform repeated movements.
- *Flexibility* is the ability to move a joint through its range of motion. The most common assessment is to evaluate low back and hip (trunk) flexion.

For information and guidelines for assessing physical fitness,

 Go to Chapter 42, **Assessment Guidelines and Tools, Focused Assessment—Cardiorespiratory Fitness, Muscular Fitness Assessment, and Flexibility Assessment** in Volume 2.

Lifestyle and Risk Appraisal

Lifestyle refers to the manner in which a person conducts his life: physically, emotionally, spiritually, and mentally. Personal habits, recreation, and occupation are part of one's lifestyle. In the context of health and wellness, lifestyle includes all of the activities that promote optimal living, such as taking responsibility for one's health, physical activity, nutrition, interpersonal relations, spiritual growth, and stress management. You can gather this information by interview or by using a variety of questionnaires. A **health risk appraisal (HRA)** is a questionnaire that evaluates risk for disease based on current demographic data, lifestyle, and health behaviors. There are many HRA tools available; many are online. For one example of an HRA,

 Go to Chapter 42, **Assessment Guidelines and Tools, Focused Assessment: Lifestyle and Risk Assessment,** in Volume 2.

 Think**Like a Nurse** 42-3

- Evaluate your own compliance with recommended health screenings for your age group. What activities should you incorporate into your own health promotion plan?
- Answer the questions in the Lifestyle and Risk Assessment in Volume 2. How did you score? What additional activities should be added to your health promotion plan?

Life Stress Review

In 1976, Hans Selye proposed that stress triggers physiological responses that may, over time, induce illness. Likewise, Richard Rahe (1974) identified some stress-inducing life change events and researched their possible effects on health. He attached numeric values for each change based on the degree of disruption or stress produced by the event. Rahe discovered that a high score on a life-change event scale is associated with a greater likelihood of a negative health change. To see and use a life-change event scale,

 Go to Chapter 12, **Assessment Guidelines and Tools, The Holmes-Rahe Social Readjustment Scale,** in Volume 2.

Other researchers have focused on daily stresses and their effects on actual health or on one's perception of health. Daily stresses involve travel to and from work, taking children to activities, daily chores, waiting in lines at shops, raising teenagers, and traffic jams. Researchers have found these stresses may gradually erode one's coping mechanisms, producing an inability to cope with daily events and an increased likelihood of illness.

Hardiness Research has also demonstrated that in the face of life events, some people develop hardiness rather than vulnerability (Maddi, Koshaba, Fazel, et al., 2009). Kobasa (1979) identified hardiness as a quality in which an individual experiences high levels of stress yet does not fall ill. There are three general characteristics of the hardy person:

- **Control**—belief in the ability to control the experience
- **Commitment**—feeling deeply involved in the activity producing stress
- **Challenge**—the ability to view the change as a challenge to grow

These traits are associated with a strong resistance to negative feelings that occur under adverse circumstances (Escolas, Pitts, Safer, et al., 2013). If you need additional information on hardiness, review Chapter 11.

 ThinkLike a Nurse 42-4

- Undoubtedly you are experiencing stress as a student in a nursing program. How would you rate your level of hardiness?
- What statements would demonstrate a hardy personality in each area (commitment, control, challenge)?

Health Beliefs

A health promotion assessment would not be complete without investigating an individual's health beliefs. Health beliefs are embedded in one's culture and personal experiences. Culture consists of characteristics, beliefs, and behaviors of an individual or group (Chapter 15)—all the experiences, biases, beliefs, and rituals. Culture influences beliefs and practices affecting wellness and disease prevention. For example, some people may use certain foods (e.g., garlic to prevent heart disease, orange juice to prevent a cold) or herbs to protect or restore health. Why do you think it is important for you to respect cultural and religious views regarding health while working with clients to adopt personal health goals?

It will be helpful to know whether health outcomes are a result of actions the person takes, actions of powerful others, or chance. The Multidimensional Health Locus of Control scale (MHLC), developed by Wallston, Wallston, and DeVellis (1978), helps you obtain this information. The MHLC measures the person's perception of the extent of control from each source. The person rates her level of agreement with statements such as "I am in control of my health," "No matter what I do, if I am going to get sick, I will get sick," and "Regarding my health, I can only do what my doctor tells me to do." Identifying a patient's locus of control is of practical importance for several reasons:

- People who feel powerless about preventing illness are least likely to engage in health promotion activities.
- People who respond to direction from respected authorities often prefer a health promotion program that is supervised by a healthcare provider.
- Clients who feel in charge of their own health are the easiest to motivate toward positive change.

For a copy of the MHLC you can print out and use with your patients,

 Go to Chapter 42, **Resources for Caregivers and Health Professionals, Vanderbilt University Web Site,** on DavisPlus.

Nutritional Assessment

A nutritional assessment is a key component of an overall wellness assessment. Unhealthy eating habits occur across all ages, ethnicities, and socioeconomic classes. The assessment involves an evaluation of typical eating patterns correlated with physical examination findings and BMI. Body composition is important in identifying health risks. The usual methods for determining body fat composition clinically are by measuring height, weight, circumferences, and skinfolds (see Chapter 27 to review these).

The pattern of body fat distribution is an important predictor of health risks. People with fat stored around the trunk and abdominal area have a higher incidence of metabolic syndrome, hypertension, hyperlipidemia, heart disease, type 2 diabetes, and premature death than those who have the fat stored in the extremities (Ashwell, Gunn, & Gibson, 2012). Traditionally, the waist-to-height ratio has been used as a method for determining fat patterns in the body. More recently, the focus has shifted to waist circumference alone.

Health Screening Activities

Health screening activities are secondary prevention activities designed to diagnose specific diseases at an early stage so that treatment can begin before there is an opportunity for the disease to spread or become debilitating. Many of these screening activities are part of your usual care. For example, each time you check a client's blood pressure, you are performing a screen for hypertension. Table 42-1 identifies the typical health screening activities with each developmental stage. For further information about selected health screening activities.

 Go to **Assessment Guidelines and Tools: Selected Health Screening Activities,** in Volume 2.

Screening for Breast Cancer   Currently, there is some controversy about whether we should encourage breast self-examination (BSE) (American Academy of Family Physicians [AAFP], 2012; Tria, 2013). In studies around the world, BSE was found not to reduce mortality resulting from breast cancer, and may even cause false security and delayed diagnosis when lumps that are present are not detected. Because of the ongoing uncertainty raised by such studies and the fact some women do self-detect lumps that signal cancer, the American Cancer Society continues to advise women that BSE is an optional screening tool but plays only a small role in finding breast cancer (American Cancer Society, 2012). However, BSE can be a useful screening strategy when used in combination with regular physical exams and mammography. So until evidence is conclusive, it seems reasonable to continue to encourage and teach BSE.

Screening for Prostate Cancer   The issue of whether to perform mass prostate-specific antigen (PSA) and digital rectal exam screening for prostate cancer is also unsettled. The U.S. Preventive Services Task Force (USPSTF) (2012) recommends against PSA-based screening for prostate cancer but understands that some patients may request testing. PSA screening should be done only if it includes shared decision making that enables an informed choice by patients.

For points to include when teaching breast and testicular self-examination,

 Go to **Assessment Guidelines and Tools: Breast Self-Exam and Testicular Self-Exam,** in Chapter 9.

KnowledgeCheck 42-3

- Identify at least three common sites for health promotion activities.
- What assessments are parts of a health promotion assessment?
- What role does stress play in health promotion?

 ThinkLike a Nurse 42-5

Your 55-year-old aunt tells you she hasn't had a physical examination in 20 years. She is a registered nurse. "I don't need one because I feel fine and I can take care of myself." How would you respond?

ANALYSIS/NURSING DIAGNOSIS

"Health promotion diagnoses describe clinical judgment about a person's, family's, group's, or community's motivation and desire to increase well-being and actualize human health potential" (NANDA International, 2012, p. 96). Health promotion diagnoses can be used in any health status and do not require a current level of wellness. NANDA-I health promotion labels are specific behaviors preceded by the phrase *Readiness for Enhanced*, and will be one-part statements with no etiology (e.g., Readiness for Enhanced Parenting, and Readiness for Enhanced Nutrition). For specific NANDA-I labels you can use to describe health promotion diagnoses,

 Go to Chapter 42, **Standardized Language, Examples of NANDA-I Health Promotion Diagnoses,** in Volume 2.

PLANNING OUTCOMES/EVALUATION

NOC standardized outcomes related to health promotion vary depending on the focus area. For example, if the nursing diagnosis is Readiness for Enhanced Nutrition, a NOC outcome might be Nutritional Status. For examples of other NOC health promotion outcomes,

 Go to Chapter 42, **Standardized Language, Examples of NOC Standardized Health Promotion Outcomes,** on DavisPlus.

Individualized goals and outcomes might include losing 20 pounds or exercising for 30 minutes five times per week. The nurse's role in health promotion primarily is to motivate clients and facilitate change. Clients are independently responsible for most of their health promotion activities. You may need to help them identify goals, but it is essential that the goals be the clients', not yours.

Healthy People 2020 Goals. You may need aggregate wellness goals for groups as well as individualized goals. The following are four broad goals for the U.S. population set by the *Healthy People 2020* initiative (U.S. Department of Health and Human Services [USDHHS], 2009, p. 2):

- Attain high-quality, longer lives free of preventable disease, disability, injury, and premature death.
- Achieve health equity, eliminate disparities, and improve the health of all groups.
- Create social and physical environments that promote good health for all.
- Promote quality of life, healthy development, and healthy behaviors all life stages.

Interventions to achieve these goals are targeted at the 37 focus areas shown in Box 42-1.

Public health agencies at the local, state, and federal levels use these focus areas as a blueprint to design programs aimed at improving the health status of the community (USDHHS, 2009). To view those objectives,

 Go to the ***Healthy People 2020* Web site,** at http://www.healthypeople.gov/Search/objectives.htm

BOX 42-1 ■ Focus Areas of *Healthy People 2020*

1. Access to health services
2. Adolescent health
3. Arthritis, osteoporosis, and chronic back conditions
4. Blood disorders and blood safety
5. Cancer
6. Chronic kidney disease
7. Diabetes
8. Disability and secondary conditions
9. Early and middle childhood
10. Educational and community-based programs
11. Environmental health
12. Family planning
13. Food safety
14. Genomics
15. Global health
16. Health communication and health IT
17. Healthcare-associated infections
18. Hearing and other sensory or communication disorders
19. Heart disease and stroke
20. HIV
21. Immunization and infectious diseases
22. Injury and violence prevention
23. Maternal, infant, and child health
24. Medical product safety
25. Mental health and mental disorders
26. Nutrition and overweight
27. Occupational safety and health
28. Older adults
29. Oral health
30. Physical activity and fitness
31. Public health infrastructure
32. Respiratory diseases
33. Sexually transmitted infections
34. Social determinants of health
35. Substance abuse
36. Tobacco use
37. Vision

Source: U.S. Department of Health and Human Services, Office of Disease Prevention & Health Promotion and Human Services. (2009, October 30, revised). *Healthy People 2020* topics and objectives. Retrieved from http://www.healthypeople.gov/hp2020/Objectives/TopicAreas.aspx

---

Whether standardized or individualized, expected outcomes for wellness diagnoses describe behaviors or responses that demonstrate health maintenance or achievement of an even higher level of health. For example:

> During the next year, Mr. Needham will continue to eat a balanced diet, with more emphasis on including whole grains and fiber.

By using the highest number (5) on the rating scale, you can use the NOC to write wellness outcomes. For example:

> *Nursing diagnosis:* Readiness for Enhanced Nutrition
> *Expected outcome:* Nutritional Status: (5) Not compromised

PLANNING INTERVENTIONS/IMPLEMENTATION

Community and public health nurses focus on the problems contributing to disease, such as poor housing conditions, poor sanitation, poor nutrition, poverty, and substance abuse. The wellness focus in acute care is to educate patients about health and disease.

Once the client identifies his goals, help him to identify the steps that he must take to reach the goals. Change occurs in stages. To create positive change, the client will need to understand the benefits of change, overcome the barriers to change, and make a commitment to follow through on the plan.

For *NIC standardized interventions* and activities for health promotion,

 Go to Chapter 42, **Standardized Language, Selected NIC Health Promotion Interventions,** in Volume 2.

NIC does not have a special domain, or grouping, for wellness interventions. Instead, they are found throughout all areas of the taxonomy, particularly in the Behavioral, Safety, Family, Health System, and Community domains. Specific NIC nursing activities for health promotion include those in the following four subsections. The remainder of the chapter provides some strategies to promote their use (see the accompanying PICOT box).

Nutrition To guide people in making nutritional choices that promote health and prevent disease, the U.S. Department of Agriculture (USDA) and the USDHHS revised the *Dietary Guidelines for Americans* (you will find these in Chapter 27) to include My Plate, a symbol of a plate that is divided into four sections—fruits, vegetables, grains, and protein. It replaces the familiar pyramid image, which was first introduced in 1992 and revised in 2005 but had become too complicated for people to understand easily. Instead, My Plate is a quick, simple reminder to people to be more mindful of the foods they eat. The symbol is part of a healthy eating initiative that conveys seven key messages: Enjoy food but eat less; avoid oversized portions; make half of the plate fruits and vegetables; drink water instead of sugary drinks; switch to fat-free or low-fat (1%) milk; compare sodium in foods; and make at least half your grains whole grains. From a practical point of

Health Promotion

Situation: The student has noticed that many of his classmates have gained significant amounts of weight as the program has advance. In addition, it seems as though there is always someone who is sick in class. Students are complaining about the cost of co-payments and over-the-counter medications. The student wonders whether there are practical ways to improve this situation at his school.

PICOT Components

P	Population/client	= Young adult students
I	Intervention/indicator	= Health promotion information
C	Comparator/control	= None
O	Outcome	= Decreased risk of health problems
T	Time	= None

Searchable Question

Do _____ (P) who receive/are exposed to _____ (I) demonstrate _____ (O) as compared to _____ (C) during _____ (T)?

Example of Evidence: The World Health Organization defined health promotion as the process that enables people to improve their own health by improving control over the determinants of health. Health promotion is an important nursing activity. Healthcare spending in the United States exceeded $2 trillion in 2006. America's worsening health habits, particularly obesity, are contributing to this massive growth in spending. Cost-effective health promotion measures include educating people about preventable health problems such as obesity, diabetes, hypertension, and other chronic diseases. Nursing educators will be at the forefront in evaluating nursing programs and teaching future nurses according to the needs of global health.

Practice Changes: The student talks to his professor about organizing a wellness group to share health promotion ideas.

Source: Jadelhack, R. (2012). Health promotion in nursing and cost-effectiveness, *Journal of Cultural Diversity, 19*(2), 65–68.

---

view, the plate image will help people make better food choices.

Exercise Encourage the development of physical fitness lifestyle habits in people of all ages and abilities. Most health benefits occur with at least 150 minutes (2 hours and 30 minutes) a week of moderate-intensity physical activity, such as brisk walking. Additional benefits occur with more physical activity (USDHHS, 2008). Children and teens should engage in at least 1 hour of age-appropriate, physical activity daily. Activity should be vigorous in intensity and varied in type, not only to prevent boredom but also to promote muscle and bone strengthening as well as flexibility (Fig. 42-3). For more information,

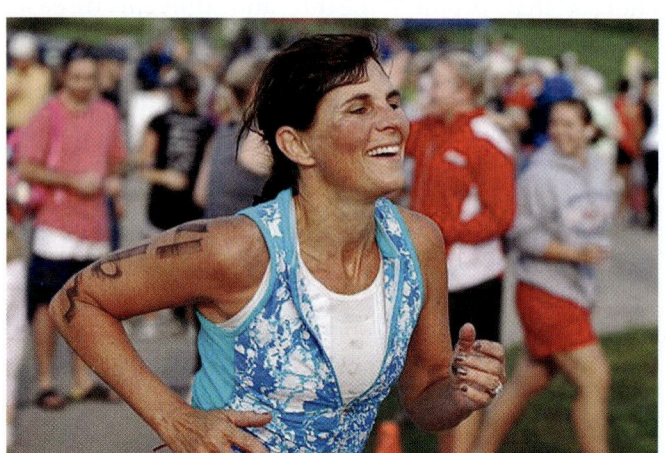

FIGURE 42-3 Vigorous-intensity exercise promotes muscle and bone strength and improves cardiovascular health.

 Go to the **President's Challenge Web site,** at http://www.presidentschallenge.org

Lifestyle Changes For healthy living, adults and teens choose a lifestyle without drugs, including tobacco, and little alcohol. Getting enough sleep, and managing stress are also important.

Sleep In general, adults need 6 to 9 hours of sleep a night. Children need more sleep (see Chapter 34). Inadequate sleep is linked to weight gain and obesity.

For an expanded discussion of these areas for health promotion,

 Go to Chapter 42, **Supplemental Materials: Individual Health Promotion Activities,** on Davis*Plus.*

Role Modeling

A role model teaches by example, demonstrating the behaviors and/or attitudes to be learned. Models provide inspiration and strategies for health promotion behavior. Clients select their own role models, often without making a conscious decision to do so. For example, a morbidly obese female joins a weight loss group led by a woman who has lost nearly 100 pounds. She admires the leader for her determination and success and selects her as a role model.

It may sometimes be helpful for you to facilitate the client's choice. When suggesting a model, consider the client's age, culture, values, and preferred activities. The model should be someone with whom the client identifies. Ideally, the role model should be someone accessible to the client during the early stages of change.

This allows for interacting and for exchanging information. Nurses also serve as role models. As a result, we should provide an example of healthy behaviors. It is difficult to advocate for healthy behavior if you do not follow the behavior you recommend to clients. Imagine the trust a client loses when he finds out that the nurse who tells him not to smoke cigarettes has a two-pack per day habit. To what extent do you role model healthy behaviors?

Providing Counseling

Counseling is an interpersonal communication process that helps a client to identify problems and make changes. In the context of health promotion, counseling promotes personal growth and helps clients change their lifestyle. Counseling may be formal one-to-one or small-group discussion, or it may be informal discussion with the client at a healthcare encounter. Each meeting with a client is a potential counseling session. In addition to face-to-face contact, counseling may be offered via telephone or even by e-mail.

Individual Counseling

Face-to-face interaction may be helpful when clients are attempting major lifestyle change. In an individual session, you can customize and map out the steps required to meet the client's goals. This may include writing a contract detailing the client's expected behaviors. Print the contract, and have the client sign it to reinforce his commitment. Suggest the client post the plan in a location he sees often so that it serves as a frequent reminder.

During counseling sessions, remember to reinforce health-promoting behaviors that have already been established. For example, the client who uses tobacco may eat a balanced diet; reinforce the healthy habit to boost self-esteem. Stress to the client that although the behavior to be changed may be unhealthy, you believe the client can succeed in making the change.

Telephone Counseling

Telephone counseling may be used as a primary counseling approach or as follow-up. Many clients with hectic schedules find it easier to arrange telephone counseling than to schedule a face-to-face interaction. The disadvantage is that telephone counseling does not allow you to observe nonverbal communication.

When using telephone counseling, you will set goals and map out the strategy for change just as you would in face-to-face counseling. Let the client know how

Toward Evidence-Based Practice

Cooley, M. E., Finn, K. T., Wang, Q., et al. (2013). Health behaviors, readiness to change, and interest in health promotion programs among smokers with lung cancer and their family members: A pilot study. *Cancer Nursing, 36*(2), 145–154

Data were collected once from 37 lung cancer patient–family member dyads. Lung cancer patients and their family members had high rates of continued smoking, low intake of fruits and vegetables, and high rates of physical inactivity. Patients and family members indicated readiness to change behaviors within the next 6 months and interest in participating in a behavioral risk reduction program.

Hoffman, A. J., Brintnall, R. A., Brown, J. K., et al. (2013). Too sick not to exercise: Using a 6-week, home-based exercise intervention for cancer-related fatigue self-management for postsurgical non-small cell lung cancer patients. *Cancer Nursing, 36*(3), 175–188.

Seven participants with early-stage lung cancer performed light-intensity walking and balance exercises using the Nintendo Wii Fit Plus. Exercise started the first week after hospitalization for surgical removal of the tumor and continued for 6 weeks. The intervention positively impacted cancer-related fatigue severity; fatigue self-management; walking, and balance; fatigue self-management behaviors; and functional performance (number of steps taken per day). Researchers concluded that a home-based, light-intensity

exercise intervention for patients after surgery for lung cancer is feasible, safe, well tolerated, and highly acceptable, showing positive changes in cancer-related fatigue self-management.

Cooley, M. E., Emmons, K. M., Haddad, R., et al. (2011). Patient-reported receipt of and interest in smoking cessation interventions after a diagnosis of cancer. *Cancer, 117*(13), 2961–2969.

Data were collected from questionnaires and medical records from 160 smokers or recent quitters with lung or head and neck cancer. Eighty-six percent of smokers and 75% of recent quitters reported that healthcare providers gave advice to quit smoking. Fifty-one percent of smokers and 20% of recent quitters expressed an interest in a smoking-cessation program. An individualized smoking-cessation program was the preferred type of program. Among smokers, younger patients with early stage disease and those with partners who were smokers were more interested in programs.

1. Based on these studies, why is it important to assess a patient's interest in smoking-cessation programs?

2. Why do you think a patient's diagnosis of lung cancer might influence his willingness to participate in healthy activities?

3. In light of the research, what might you do to facilitate health promotion in your patient with a lung cancer diagnosis?

and when you can be reached if questions arise. If you are using the telephone for follow-up counseling, it is best to schedule a time to speak. Having an appointment helps keep the client accountable to the expected behavior and to reinforce the information.

Providing Health Education

Health education may focus on self-care strategies, caregiver concerns, or how to be an effective healthcare consumer. Self-care programs typically cover nutrition, exercise, stress management, or disease prevention. Programs may consist of lectures, printed material, billboards, or posters. For example, the accompanying Self-Care box Teaching Clients How to Prevent Upper Respiratory Infections might be reproduced and posted in the lounge, rest rooms, or locker areas of a worksite during cold and flu season to decrease absenteeism. Caregiver education programs may teach caregivers how to perform nursing tasks or prevent injuries, or they may provide a list of community resources for respite care. Nurses can teach clients how to be effective healthcare consumers, how to interact with healthcare providers, and how to maneuver through the healthcare system. For a review of teaching and learning, see Chapter 19.

Providing and Facilitating Support for Lifestyle Change

Changing one's lifestyle is difficult. Most clients need support to make the change. You can provide support during your interactions and counseling sessions. You can also help the client to identify available support and resources within the community as well as from family, friends, coworkers, and others.

Group support exists for a variety of lifestyle changes. For example, Weight Watchers is a group support program for clients who want to lose weight; Alcoholics Anonymous is a group support program for clients who want to become and stay sober; various cancer support groups help clients deal with the common issues and fears associated with dealing with a potentially life-threatening disease. Group support provides clients with a chance to meet people experiencing the same difficulties and perhaps to find a role model. As a nurse, you should be familiar with various programs available in your community and refer clients to them.

KnowledgeCheck 42-4

Identify four strategies to help a client engage in positive lifestyle change.

Documentation Practice

To practice charting health promotion interventions and patient responses,

 Go to Chapter 42, **Documentation Exercises,** on Davis*Plus.*

CarePlanning & CareMapping Practice

To practice care mapping for Effective Therapeutic Regimen Management,

 Go to Chapter 42, **Care Planning and Care Mapping Practice,** on Davis*Plus.*

Self-Care

Teaching Clients How to Prevent Upper Respiratory Infections

➤ **Maintain a healthy lifestyle.** That means get adequate sleep, ensure good nutrition, and engage in physical exercise. A balanced diet and physical fitness can boost your immune system to fight infection if it occurs.

➤ **Wash your hands often, and teach children to do so.** This helps prevent spread of infection. When using public restrooms, wash your hands. Then turn off the faucet with a paper towel. Also use a paper towel to open the door as you leave the room.

➤ **Avoid touching your eyes, nose, and mouth,** because doing so spreads any virus your hands have contacted (e.g., on doorknobs).

➤ **Avoid crowds when there is a cold or influenza epidemic.**

➤ **Throw away tissues as soon as you use them.**

➤ **When someone in the family has a cold,** keep bathrooms and the kitchen very clean and do not drink from the same glass or use the same utensils.

➤ **When someone at home or at work has a cold,** wipe telephone receivers with soap and water or an antibacterial solution.

➤ **If a child has a cold,** wash his toys and commonly used items well.

➤ **When choosing childcare,** look for a clean environment; ask what rules the facility or individual has about keeping the children clean (e.g., washing hands before snack time).

➤ **Don't smoke.** Cigarette smoke can irritate the respiratory tract, making you more susceptible to colds and illness.

➤ **Control stress.** People experiencing emotional stress tend to have weakened immunity to fight infection.

➤ **Consider taking echinacea,** although conclusive evidence of its effectiveness does not exist at this time. Consult your primary healthcare provider.

To explore learning resources for this chapter,

Go to DavisPlus at DavisPl.us/Wilkinson3.

Chapter Resources for Chapter 42:

> **Response sheets for all learning activities**
>
> **Resources for Caregivers and Health Professionals**
>
> **Reading More About Promoting Health (suggested readings)**
>
> **Concept Map of chapter content**

Interactive Case Studies

NCLEX-Style and Chapter Review Questions

Chapter Overview Podcasts

For references cited in this chapter,

Go to Volume 2, **References Cited**.

The Context for Nurses' Work

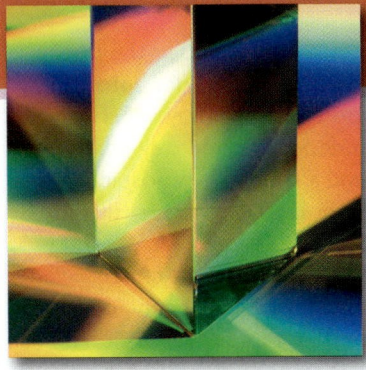

CHAPTER 43

Community & Home Health Nursing

Learning Outcomes

After completing this chapter, you should be able to:

➤ Define the meaning of community.

➤ Identify at least four factors by which you can recognize a healthy community.

➤ Discuss factors that create vulnerability for a population.

➤ Compare and contrast community-based care, community health nursing, public health nursing, and community-oriented nursing.

➤ Distinguish primary, secondary, and tertiary interventions in regard to a community health scenario.

➤ Discuss at least three strategies that nurses use to gather community data.

➤ Describe the roles of nurses in the community setting.

➤ Use standardized nursing language taxonomies (NANDA-I, NOC, NIC, Omaha, and CCC) to describe care planning in community and home care.

➤ Identify the primary goal of home care.

➤ Describe ways in which home healthcare differs from hospital nursing.

➤ Categorize the various agencies that deliver home healthcare according to purpose, client served, and funding source.

➤ Describe how the nurse's emphasis differs in hospice nursing as compared to home health nursing.

➤ List at least four criteria clients must meet for home care to be reimbursed by Medicare.

➤ Outline the steps required to prepare for a home visit, including considerations for the nurse's safety.

➤ Discuss ways in which the assessment process is unique in home care.

➤ Explain the role of the nurse in helping clients and families manage medications and treatments in the home setting.

➤ Describe how infection control measures differ in the home and in the hospital.

➤ State two important safety concerns in home care that arise out of The Joint Commission 2014 home care safety goals.

➤ Describe the nurse's role in treating caregiver strain.

Key Concepts

Community nursing
Home healthcare
Population

Related Concepts

See the Concept Map on DavisPlus.

Meet Your Patients

Your Neighbor, Tanya

You are nearing completion of your fundamentals course. One night while you are preparing for your next clinical, the telephone rings. It is your neighbor, Tanya. Her 5-year-old son, Jacob, came home from kindergarten with a letter from the school nurse stating that a classmate was ill with H1N1 influenza and that all the students in the class had been exposed to the disease.

Tanya is concerned about the risks to Jacob and the rest of the family. Tanya is 8 months pregnant, and the

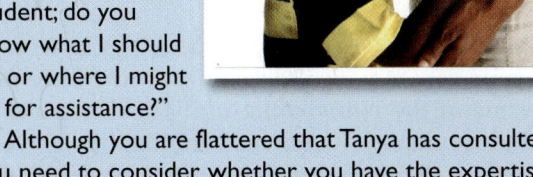

family has no health insurance. She says, "You are a nursing student; do you know what I should do or where I might go for assistance?"

Although you are flattered that Tanya has consulted you, you need to consider whether you have the expertise to answer her questions. This situation requires knowledge

(Continued)

Meet Your Patients (continued)

from many aspects of nursing (e.g., immunizations, pregnancy, microbiology, pathophysiology). Though you may not have all of the information you need to answer her questions, you should be able to help your neighbor resolve her concerns. You will need to consider the following questions:

- What is going on in the situation that may influence the outcome?
- Who should be involved to improve the outcome?
- What theoretical knowledge do I need to answer my neighbor's questions? Where would I find this information?
- What additional data do I need to collect from my neighbor?
- What suggestions and/or referrals should I offer to my neighbor?

Your Patients, the Escobars

Flora Escobar is 78 years old. She lives at home with her husband, Roland, age 78. Both enjoyed good health until Roland was hospitalized for a cerebrovascular accident (CVA, or stroke) 3 weeks ago. He then spent 2 weeks in a skilled nursing facility (SNF). He returned home yesterday and will be followed by the local home health agency for physical therapy and nursing care.

At your initial visit, Mrs. Escobar greets you at the door. She is a petite woman who looks exhausted. Her apron pockets are stuffed with pill bottles. The hallway is partially blocked with a bedside commode, walker, and tray table. Mr. Escobar, wearing pajamas and a robe, is in a hospital bed in the living room. He is a tall, stocky man who is sitting up in bed but is slumped and leaning to the left.

After introducing yourself, you ask an open-ended question to build rapport: "How have things been going since you came home yesterday?" Mrs. Escobar sighs, and says, "I'm worried that I'm doing things wrong. I have a hard time helping him move. He is so much bigger than me, and I don't want to hurt him. He is frustrated with me, but he has difficulty talking and can't tell me what he needs." Tears fill Mrs. Escobar's eyes. Her husband turns away to avoid eye contact with you. To refocus their attention, you suggest that you go over some information and then begin to look at what additional services might be helpful.

Imagine how stressed Mrs. Escobar must feel. How do you think you could best help this family? In this chapter, as you read the section on home health nursing, you should find it easier to answer those questions.

Theoretical Knowledge
knowing why

In the past couple of decades, the population has aged and hospital stays have become shorter in an effort to reduce costs. As a result, community-based healthcare, including home nursing care, has grown rapidly. Community and public health nurses regularly deal with such concerns as health screening and preventing disease. Home-care nurses provide care to clients with complex, chronic, or terminal illness in the home. They promote self-care and independence with activities of daily living, regardless of the level of functioning. In this chapter, we discuss communities and community and home nursing care. We also explore the roles, interventions, and career opportunities for nurses who work in communities.

ABOUT THE KEY CONCEPTS

Perhaps your career path will lead you to caring for clients in one of the many community healthcare settings, including clients' own homes. In this chapter, you will learn about the concepts of **community health** and **home health** and how different **populations** have unique healthcare needs. You will learn how these concepts are related to each other and to subconcepts, such

as public health nursing, vulnerable populations, and home visits.

UNDERSTANDING THE CONCEPT OF COMMUNITY

The word **community** comes from the Latin term *communis*, meaning the "gift or fellowship of common relations and feelings." Historically, it meant a body of like-minded people or the inhabitants of a town. Then and now, the term suggests a general sense of selflessness, sharing, relationship, and doing good that comes from working together. Most members of a community share a common language, certain rituals, and special customs.

In contrast to community, we tend to think of a **population** as a certain geographic region. But the term *population* has other meanings, as well.

- It can mean the group of people of a particular race or class in a specified place (e.g., "There are 1,500 Latino people living in Edwards County").
- It can also mean *any* group of people subject to statistical or other study (e.g., all the homeless people in Edwards County, or all the pregnant adolescents living in Edwards County).

The U.S. Bureau of the Census conducts a survey and count of the American people (the population of the

United States) every 10 years. The most recent census is the one conducted in the year 2010. For results,

Go to the **U.S. Census Bureau Web site,** at www.census.gov/2010census/

When the census is completed, the U.S. Census Bureau groups the data into sections of 1,500 to 8,000 people, known as **census tracts**. The area of individual census tracts varies according to the density of the population. In urban centers, a census tract covers a small area. Rural census tracts are large. Census tracts are useful to public officials, market analysts, and anyone—including community nurses who study the characteristics and concerns of smaller sections of people.

Maps and census tracts show the *geopolitical* boundaries of a community. But as we noted earlier, a community can also be a group of people with a common purpose. They may live in different geographical areas, but they have a "sense of belonging" to their group (community). For a comparison of geopolitical boundaries and census tracts,

Go to Chapter 43, **Tables, Boxes, Figures: ESG Figure 43-1,** Geopolitical Boundaries and Census Tract Data on Davis*Plus*.

An **aggregate** is a group of individuals with at least one shared characteristic, either personal or environmental. For example, a community health nurse may work with a class of high school girls to reduce the incidence of adolescent pregnancy. The shared characteristics of this aggregate are that they are female, of childbearing age, and attend a particular school. As another example, the nursing students in your school are an aggregate. What characteristics and goals do you share?

KnowledgeCheck 43-1

- Give several examples of a community.
- How is a population different from a community?

ThinkLike a Nurse 43-1

- Why might the boundaries of a census tract change every 10 years?
- How could you figure out what census tract you live or go to school in?

What Are the Components of a Community?

To understand a particular community and its needs, you will need information about its three components: the concepts of structure, status, and process.

- **Structure** refers to the general characteristics of a community. These include demographic data, such as gender, age, ethnicity, and educational and income levels, as well as data about healthcare services, such as the number of primary care providers or emergency care facilities in the area.

- **Status** describes the biological, emotional, and social outcome components of a community. *Biological* data include morbidity (illness) and mortality (death) rates, life expectancy ratios, and risk factor profiles for the respective age groups within a community. *Emotional* data include general indications of mental health and consumer satisfaction survey results about various aspects of the community as compared to other locales. *Social* data include crime rates, citizenship involvement in community-wide activities, and general functioning levels of the community members.

- **Process** describes the overall effectiveness level of the community. For example, do the members of the community perceive that they are part of a group with common purpose, values, or interests? What is the extent of interaction among community members? Does the community have an established forum for conflict resolution?

What Makes a Community Healthy?

As with individuals, the meaning and perception of health varies among aggregates. For nurses, it is important to understand what a particular community defines (and values) as health rather than relying on personal definitions.

When determining what makes a community healthy from a traditional biomedical perspective, the national consensus paper *Healthy People 2020* provides useful guidelines. That document is based on the understanding that many of the health problems of Americans were preventable. *Healthy People 2020* identifies leading indicators for measuring the health of our nation (U.S. Department of Health and Human Services [USDHHS], 2008). Some examples affecting community health include:

- Physical activity
- Overweight and obesity
- Tobacco use
- Substance abuse
- Sexual behavior
- Mental health
- Injury and violence
- Environmental quality
- Immunizations
- Access to healthcare

For the complete list of indicators, see Box 42-1, Focus Areas of *Healthy People 2020*.

The four overarching goals of the *Healthy People 2020* initiative are to (1) attain high-quality, longer lives free of preventable disease, disability, injury, and premature death; (2) achieve health equity, eliminate health disparities, and improve the health of all groups; (3) create social and physical environments that promote good health for all; and (4) promote quality of life, healthy development, and healthy behaviors across all life stages. These aggregate goals are to be achieved through promoting healthy behaviors, increasing access to quality healthcare, and strengthening community health resources. For more information,

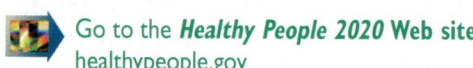 Go to the *Healthy People 2020* **Web site**, *at* http://www. healthypeople.gov

KnowledgeCheck 43-2

- What makes up the "structure" of a community?
- What is community "status"?
- What is community "process"?
- Use the guidelines from *Healthy People 2020* to compile a list of several characteristics that make a community healthy.

What Makes a Population Vulnerable?

The concept of **vulnerable population** is defined as an aggregate that is at increased risk of adverse health outcomes. Members of vulnerable populations have a higher probability of developing illness than do members of the general population. Because of their increased risk for developing health problems, vulnerable populations are a major focus of community health efforts. Vulnerability involves multiple factors:

Limited Economic Resources Income is a major predictor of health risk. People with higher incomes typically have greater access to health services and greater selection of providers, treatment options, and location of health services. In contrast, the more limited a person's income is, the more limited her healthcare options will be. Many persons with low income forgo preventive care and seek healthcare only when they are quite ill.

Limited Social Resources Friends and family are valuable resources to help a person deal with day-to-day stress and demands of an illness. They can provide feedback, listen to concerns, and offer emotional and physical assistance. Unfortunately, not everyone has social resources. Older adults who live alone and people with mental illness are examples of groups at increased risk because of social isolation.

Age The very young and the very old are less able to adapt to physiological stress and are at increased risk of disease. They are more prone to infections and may not be able to protect themselves against environmental hazards, such as cold or heat. These age groups are also more often living in poverty.

Chronic Disease and Obesity People who have chronic diseases are at greater risk of health problems. For example, people with obesity are at increased risk of heart disease, diabetes, impaired mobility, joint pain, and other complications. People with diabetes are at risk of blindness, impaired wound healing, kidney failure, poor peripheral circulation, heart disease, and other complications.

History of Abuse or Trauma People who have experienced abuse or traumatic events often feel they have limited control over their health and circumstances. They may feel powerless or hopeless, and be unable to take actions that promote health or lead to early treatment of illness. Abuse and trauma also tax a person's reserves, placing them at risk of mental health problems.

Other Factors Other vulnerable populations include people who are poor or homeless, migrant workers, people with disabilities, premature infants, women with a high-risk pregnancy and pregnant adolescents, people with communicable disease, people who abuse substances, members of certain ethnic/racial groups, and the untreated mentally ill.

UNDERSTANDING THE CONCEPT OF COMMUNITY-BASED NURSING

A community can be either a *site* for healthcare delivery or a *recipient* of healthcare services. In fact, the first hospitals in the United States were established only in the late 1860s to protect society from contagious disease. Several decades passed before hospitals and other freestanding clinics became the predominant settings for providing healthcare. However, as the technological advances of the past 30 years have escalated the costs of delivering health services, efforts to lower costs have resulted in a move back to more community-based care, including complementary and alternative care.

Community-based care refers to healthcare or rehabilitative services performed in clinics, offices, mobile care units, and other facilities in the community—rather than in acute care settings, such as hospitals (although acute care settings also exist within the community). For example, many surgeries and diagnostic procedures are now performed in privately owned surgical centers, health clinics, and physicians' offices rather than in hospitals. People also receive mental, physical, cardiac, and pulmonary rehabilitation services in outpatient settings. Extended care facilities, or nursing homes, commonly provide rehabilitative care for patients after acute traumatic injuries as well as continuous skilled care for older adults and people with chronic illness. The following sections describe three approaches to community-based nursing care: community health nursing, public health nursing, and community-oriented nursing.

Community Health Nursing

Although many people use the terms *community health nursing* and *public health nursing* interchangeably, the two are not identical. **Community health nursing** focuses on how the health of individuals, families, and groups affects the community as a whole. Community health nurses strive to promote, protect, preserve, and maintain the health of the population through the delivery of personal health services to individuals, families, and groups. For example, a community health nurse may work in a prenatal clinic providing free services for low-income women. The nurse provides a direct service

Complementary & Alternative Modalities (CAM)

Using CAM for Preventing Illness

Barrett, B., Muller, H. M, Ward, A, et al. (2012). Meditation or exercise for preventing acute respiratory infection: A randomized controlled trial. *Annals of Family Medicine,* *10*(4), 337–463.

In a study designed to evaluate the potential preventive effects of meditation or exercise, 154 adults 50 years and older were recruited from the community and randomized into one of three groups: (1) those who received 8 weeks of training in mindful meditation, (2) a matched group involved in 8 weeks of training in moderate-intensity and sustained exercise, and (3) an observational group.

Researchers found fewer episodes and reduced severity of acute respiratory infection (ARI) in the meditation and exercise groups.

within the federal government. Some examples of successful public health programs are human papillomavirus (HPV) immunizations for adolescents, smoking cessation for healthcare workers, motor vehicle and infant car-seat safety, and obesity prevention programs for children. For additional information on the USPHS,

 Go to Chapter 43, **Supplemental Materials: United States Public Health Service,** on Davis*Plus.*

Community-Oriented Nursing

Community-oriented nursing combines components of community and public health. It focuses on health promotion, illness prevention, early detection, and treatment provided within the community setting. The practice is evidence-based and collaborative with other community health disciplines. The approach is a comprehensive look at the individual, family, group, and community at large. For example, a nurse with a community-oriented approach might work in an adolescent prenatal program. The nurse provides individual care at the local clinic 2 days per week. While at the clinic, she gathers data from adolescent clients about the schools they attend; their knowledge of birth control, pregnancy, and childbirth; and the issues these girls face with pregnancy. On the remaining 3 days, she meets with school officials to identify pregnant teens who need prenatal care; teaches a class about sexuality in the local high school; works with teachers to identify strategies to keep pregnant teens in school; provides parenting education to adolescents who have children; and advocates changing a bus route so that teens can easily get to the local clinic. Each aspect of care allows the nurse to gather more data about the needs of the individuals and the community as a whole. Figure 43-1 provides a schematic of the relationship of the various community-based nursing approaches identified in this section.

to each pregnant woman, yet she is doing so to improve the general health of the entire community. By encouraging the mother to eat balanced meals, exercise, and avoid harmful substances, the nurse improves the health of both mother and baby—who are members of the community—and therefore improves the overall health of the community.

Public Health Nursing

Public health nursing focuses on the community as a whole and the eventual effect of the community's health status on the health of individuals, families, and groups. The goal of public health is to prevent individual disease and disability, in addition to promoting and protecting the overall health of the community. Today's public health nurses functioning in a health promotion role must process important skills, such as community assessment, cultural competence, program planning, communication, financial planning and management, leadership and systems thinking, and policy development, for example (Quad Council of Public Health Nursing Organizations, 2011).

For example, a public health nurse may be employed by a county health department to provide surveillance services to monitor for tuberculosis (TB). The nurse helps to protect the entire community by screening for TB at the local school, by testing high-risk individuals for TB, and by identifying and tracking clients with active disease to ensure that they complete the prescribed 6- to 9-month medication regimen.

Because public health focuses on large-scale programs for the entire community, government-based agencies often provide these services. The U.S. Public Health Service (USPHS) is an example of a public health agency

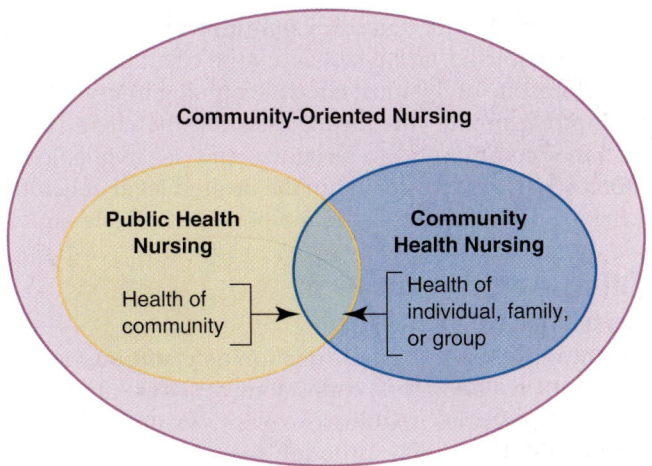

FIGURE 43-1 Schematic relationship of community nursing approaches.

KnowledgeCheck 43-3

- What is the distinction between an aggregate population and a vulnerable population?
- Identify practice differences between a community-based nurse and an acute care nurse.
- How is public health nursing different from community health nursing? How is it the same?
- How is community-oriented nursing related to community health nursing and public health nursing?

ThinkLike a Nurse 43-2

Review the scenario of Tanya and Jacob (Meet Your Patients). Which form of community-based nursing would be most appropriate to address their concerns?

Who Were Some Pioneers of Community Nursing?

The following are some of the most notable people who have contributed to the development of community-based nursing care.

- *Florence Nightingale*—Established the importance of promoting health by manipulating the environment (e.g., light, warmth, sanitation, cleanliness) and nursing the whole person.
- *Lillian Wald*—Known as the first community health nurse; founded the first visiting nurses association in New York.
- *Clara Barton*—Founder of the American Red Cross.
- *Margaret Sanger*—Founded the International Planned Parenthood Federation. Pioneered the use of family planning and birth control education.

If you would like to learn more about the achievements of these community health pioneers,

 Go to Chapter 43, **Supplemental Materials: Pioneers of Community-Based Nursing,** on Davis*Plus.*

WORKING WITHIN COMMUNITIES

Community nurses' roles vary depending on the community and its identified needs. Community nursing care is by nature holistic, and it serves a large client population. Therefore, one of the most effective nursing interventions is **empowerment**. This means assisting the client (individual or community) to recognize and use available resources to achieve or maintain the desired level of health, achieve autonomy, and maintain positive self-esteem.

What Are the Roles of Community Nurses?

Community health nurses function as client advocates, educators, collaborators, counselors, and case managers. All of these roles require excellent written and oral communication skills. Although the widespread use of electronic health records, e-mail, text messaging, and other forms of electronic communication have made it possible to communicate efficiently with large numbers

of people, computer or Internet access might be a problem in some areas. In addition, there are still some people with limited or no computer skills.

Client Advocate The effective community health nurse consistently supports the identified or expressed concerns of the client and/or community. Advocating for a community often requires political involvement at the local, state, or national level. The challenge is in knowing whom to approach for political support and how to gain their support. As a community health nurse you can effect change by getting involved in your local student nurses association, professional nursing organizations, school board, and citizen committees, or by attending council meetings.

Educator Because community nursing focuses on wellness and disease prevention, much of what the nurse does involves client education—of individuals, aggregates at risk of disease, politicians, or a community. It is difficult to evaluate the effect of the health education because people may not act on the knowledge for months or years after the teaching moment. When planning teaching, you must be aware of the stage of development, educational level, and learning style of the community group you intend to educate. The best learning programs are short; provide relevant, practical information; and can be easily incorporated into the learner's daily routine. For more information about teaching clients, see Chapter 19.

Collaborator A primary role of a community health nurse is to serve as a collaborator Consider the following example: A community health nurse is concerned about poor compliance with recommended immunization schedules for 2-year-olds in a particular community. After surveying some of the parents, the nurse discovers that the clinic's operating hours are limited and the automated call routing system is frustrating for people trying to set an appointment; and the clinic does not offer online scheduling. The nurse also discovers that some offices do not send reminders to clients, nor follow up to reschedule missed appointments. The nurse schedules a meeting of clinic staff, practice managers, and patients to resolve these issues. At the meeting, some larger issues are revealed, such as the insufficient number of Medicaid providers to serve the community, and the failure of state Medicaid agencies to reimburse the providers adequately and in a timely manner. Partnerships and coalitions can effectively address common concerns among different communities, as well as those within a single community.

Counselor Once you have established rapport with a group, members may consult you about a variety of health- and non–health-related concerns. Be careful to offer counsel only in areas within your scope of practice and make recommendations that are practical yet meet the needs of the community. Often, you may need only to serve as a witness to the group's concerns. Letting clients discuss or work through issues empowers them and fosters self-reliance.

Case Manager Community nurses commonly make referrals to or collaborate with various health and social agencies. Be aware when referring clients to these resources that agency policies and financing change frequently. Also, because community agencies often operate on grants and time-limited funding, a program that is available at one time may be dissolved at another. As a community health nurse, you will need to remain informed about the community services in your area. For example, a local group has established a healthcare program at a minimal charge for low-income families. Providers and nurses volunteer their time to provide the care. Pharmaceutical representatives donate the medical supplies and routine medications. Local specialists (e.g., surgeons) provide services to those with complex or specialized needs. However, in such a clinic the appointment times fill up quickly, and often clients have to wait more than a month or two for an appointment. Before enrolling families in the program, you would need to be aware of these limitations and share this information with clients.

KnowledgeCheck 43-4

Give an example of a nursing activity involved in each of the following community health roles: educator, advocate, case manager, counselor, and collaborator.

How Are Community Nursing Interventions Classified?

There are three basic levels of care in which nursing interventions can be classified: primary, secondary, and tertiary. Most community-oriented nursing practices are aimed at the primary (prevention) level.

Primary Interventions

The goal of **primary (first-level) interventions** is to promote health and prevent disease. Educating susceptible individuals with no known disease process is a routine, primary intervention that community health nurses practice. For example, a nurse may educate ninth-grade students about the risk of hepatitis B and HPV, the benefits of vaccination, and strategies to reduce the likelihood of exposure to contaminated body fluids. Other examples include collaborating with local agencies to provide clean and secure temporary housing for migrant farm workers, or lobbying elected representatives for a ban on smoking in restaurants and other public places.

Secondary Interventions

Secondary (second-level) interventions aim to reduce the impact of the disease process by early detection and treatment. For example, a community health nurse may screen a sexually active adolescent girl for hepatitis B and/or HPV. She has known risk factors for sexually transmitted infection (STI) but no apparent disease symptoms. The nurse will also teach the client how to protect herself from STIs, hepatitis B, and HIV in the future. Other examples of secondary interventions include providing outreach screening programs offering mammography, scoliosis screening, lipid testing, or prostate-specific antigen (PSA) testing for prostate cancer (Fig. 43-2).

Quality and Safety Education for Nurses

Promoting Patient-Centered Care in Community Health

Chapter Key Concept: *Community Nursing*
Competency: *Patient-Centered Care (Knowledge, Skills, Attitudes)**

Scenario: Nurses at a public clinic note an increased number of Hispanic clients seeking services. To best serve this growing community, one of the nurses researches healthcare issues affecting urban Hispanic populations. Latino men are more likely to be diagnosed with late-stage prostate cancer and to die from the disease than non-Latino men. Clinic staff plan to develop a flyer about prostate cancer screening, directed at Hispanic men aged 50 and older. The nurse asks a coworker, Mr. Sanchez, what cultural norms might influence health behaviors. He says that many Latino men view seeking healthcare as a sign of weakness. He explains "machismo" and "caballerismo," concepts of manliness in the Latino culture that value courage, honor, and dignity. This means that for many Latino men, a digital rectal exam would be emasculating, embarrassing, and an affront to dignity.

The nurse searches the literature for more information and learns that many Hispanic men feel healthcare providers do not understand their culture and do not take time to develop a relationship with them. After synthesizing the literature, the nurses decided to adopt the following strategies:

➤ They will create educational materials, which will be available in Spanish.

➤ Educational materials will specifically address culture-based fears that the exam is a threat to manliness.

➤ To reach the men (who tend to avoid healthcare), nurses will educate the women in the family. They believe the women will then encourage their men to get screened.

➤ The nurses will use community leaders, public service announcements, and churches to spread information.

Think about it:

➤ In what ways did the nurses make the planned educational materials patient-centered?

➤ How could the nurses evaluate the patient-centeredness of the educational materials? What information would they need? Where might they obtain the information?

➤ Patient-centered care often correlates to improvements in care. How can the clinic staff evaluate improvements in the healthcare of Latino men in their community after the educational campaign?

What goals are reasonable for this educational effort?

What assessments would be used to determine effectiveness?

Source: Agency for Healthcare Research and Quality (2010); Center for Research Strategies (2002); Rivera-Ramos & Buki (2011).

*For specific Knowledge, Skills, and Attitudes,

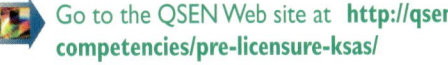 Go to the QSEN Web site at **http://qsen.org/ competencies/pre-licensure-ksas/**

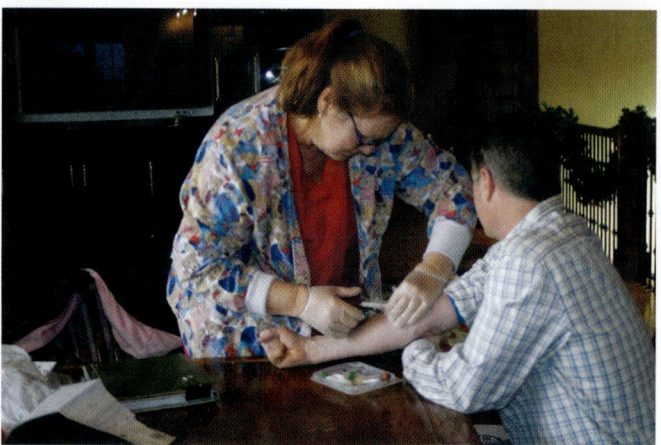

FIGURE 43-2 Secondary interventions. Early detection of heart disease with lipid screening.

Tertiary Interventions

The goal of **tertiary (third-level) intervention** is to halt disease progression and/or restore client functioning to the pre-disease state. The disease process is clinically apparent and client debilitation, including death, is likely without intervention. Tertiary-level interventions require the nurse to collaborate with members of other healthcare providers to provide treatment. For example, a student may report to a school nurse that she has been involved in unprotected sexual activities. The school nurse may refer the student to the public health clinic for a pelvic exam and lab testing to detect STI, and hepatitis B, HPV, and HIV screening. The student has an abnormal Pap smear, showing cells suggestive of HPV exposure. The clinic nurse, in collaboration with the provider, administers medical treatment. There is no cure for HPV, so the teen also needs to learn how to prevent the spread of the disease to others, get immunized with the HPV vaccine, and obtain regular Pap and pelvic exams to detect cervical cancer and other STIs.

 ThinkLike a Nurse 43-3

What level of intervention is required to address the concerns of Tanya and Jacob (Meet Your Patients)? Discuss your response.

KnowledgeCheck 43-5

For each of the nursing actions listed, identify the level of the nursing intervention as primary, secondary, or tertiary.

- Taking a client's blood pressure at a health fair
- Administering insulin to an elderly person at an extended care facility
- Teaching second-grade students to wash their hands correctly

Toward Evidence-Based Practice

Jones-Cooper, S. N., & Walton-Moss, B. (2012). Using reminder/recall systems to improve influenza immunization rates in children with asthma. *Journal of Pediatric Health Care,* 27(5), 327–333. doi:org/10.1016/j.pedhc.2011.11.005

This literature review examined the effectiveness of reminder systems in improving immunization rates in children with asthma. Healthcare providers provided verbal and mailed reminders, electronically generated alerts, and year-round scheduling of flu vaccination appointments. Although the reminder methods improved vaccination, the gain was only modest using these traditional strategies. More effective alert systems are needed.

Abbas, A. H. (2011, November 23). Children vaccination reminder via SMS alert. *International Conference on Research and Innovation in Information Systems,* 1–5. doi:10.1109/ICRIIS.2011.612575

This study presents a reminder system for parents of children due for vaccination using short message service (SMS). The existing practice for notifying the vaccination schedule was via written appointment. Results show the benefit of having reminders sent via SMS in improving vaccination compliance and reducing missed appointments.

Pereira, J. A., Quach, S., Heidebrecht, C. L., et al. (2012). Barriers to the use of reminder/recall interventions for immunizations: A systematic review. *BMC Medical Informatics and Decision-Making, 12,* 145. doi:10.1186/1472-6947-12-145

Researchers conducted a systematic review of 10 evidence-based articles examining healthcare providers' perceptions of the barriers in implementing electronic reminder systems to improve vaccination. The most reported barriers were limited staffing (time and willingness to implement vaccination reminders) and the expense of electronic software. The accuracy of patient immunization records was questionable given the lack of data sharing among numerous immunization providers.

1. In spite of reminders, what would you anticipate to be patient-related obstacles to optimal vaccine coverage?

2. What would you anticipate to be some other factors in the medical clinic or office practice that could contribute to a less-effective immunization program?

3. What are some ideas you have to improve the effectiveness of an immunization program in the setting in which you might work?

What Career Opportunities Are Available for Community-Based Nurses?

The following are only a few of the many career opportunities for those who want to practice community-based nursing.

School Nursing

Nursing practice in the school setting began when educators realized that children with health problems had more difficulty learning. School nurses provide direct care for children with chronic health conditions such as asthma, attention deficit disorder, and diabetes. They also help children who need routine procedures, such as catheterization, during the school day. School nurses perform vision and hearing screenings. They also administer prescribed medication and ensure that age-appropriate immunizations are documented. Some school nurses offer health education on topics such as nutrition, physical activity, and sexual and reproductive health. The nurse may also serve as a role model for students who lack parental support or who are struggling with peer pressure. For the most part, a school nurse is autonomous and must be capable of prioritizing and making decisions (American Nurses Association [ANA] and the National Association of School Nurses [NASN], 2011).

Occupational Health

Occupational health nurses work primarily in industrial or corporate settings. They provide health promotion programs for employees and their families in an effort to reduce absentee hours, increase productivity, and reduce illness and complications. Occupational health nurses also complete required medical documentation for disability claims or occupational hazardous events. They conduct new-hire and annual screenings, provide care to injured or ill workers, obtain random drug testing, and file worker's compensation claims. To reduce costs, some industries contract a staffing agency to provide trained occupational health nurses. Nursing autonomy and responsibility vary with the employer and the negotiated contract.

Parish Nursing

Parish nursing is a specialized area of nursing practice that focuses on the promotion of health within the context of the values and beliefs, and practices of a faith community. Integrating faith with health, parish nurses act as educators of holistic health (e.g., parenting issues, use of medications, choosing healthcare providers). In the role as personal health counselor, parish nurses increase awareness of the interrelationship between lifestyle, personal habits, attitudes, and faith (Fig. 43-3). Parish nurses develop support groups, provide information through seminars and printed or electronic materials, train volunteers, and

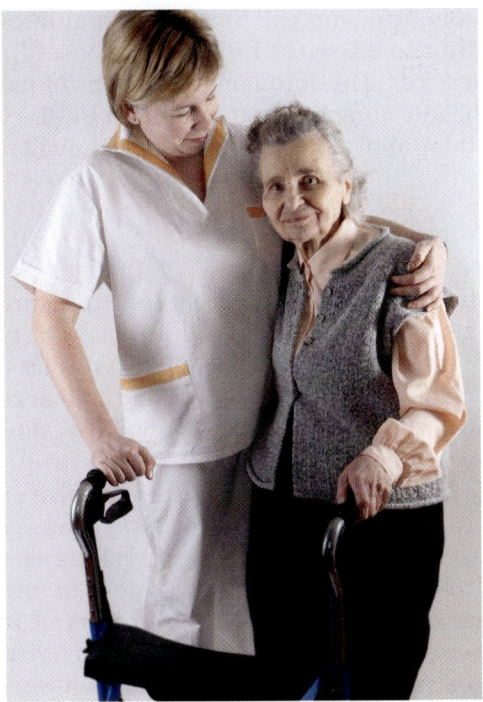

FIGURE 43-3 Parish nursing. Caring for an elderly woman in her home.

act as a liaison to community services as needed (Health Ministry Association/American Nurses Association, 1998). The level of autonomy and responsibility of parish nurses varies, depending on the faith community setting.

Nursing in Correctional Facilities

Corrections nurses deliver healthcare within the criminal justice system, for example, in juvenile detention, substance abuse treatment facilities, and prisons. The nurse provides primary care services to people of all ages in an unbiased and nonjudgmental manner (ANA, 2013a). Nurses have a high level of autonomy in most correctional or substance rehabilitation facilities. Correctional facilities employ providers who conduct routine examinations and acute and chronic healthcare on a scheduled or as-needed basis. The nurse also commonly performs occupational health duties for facility staff. For personal safety, nurses must meet certain physical requirements and complete special weapons training before working in most correctional facilities.

Public Health Clinics

Many community nurses practice within local and state departments of health, including public health clinics. Services offered by health departments can range from basic to comprehensive, based on the needs of the community and funding. Large cities tend to have many nurses who may specialize in an area, such as immunizations, prenatal health, school health, or epidemiological survey. Smaller communities may have only one nurse (or full-time equivalent) providing all services. The autonomy and scope of practice of public health nurses are often limited by the philosophy of the political administration and availability of funding.

Disaster Services Nursing

A disaster is any event or catastrophe inflicting widespread loss of life, health, and destruction of property. Features characterizing a disaster typically involve unpredictability, urgency, threat, speed, and uncertainty. They may develop as sudden-onset or slow-onset. *Human-generated disasters* might be the result of acts such as a terrorist attack, war, or use of nuclear energy to cause harm or fear. *Technological disasters* cause damage or disruption on a large scale (e.g., computer systems failure, mass power outage, explosion, or hazardous substance exposure). Examples of *natural or ecological disasters* include hurricanes, earthquakes, tsunamis, and floods, or even environmental degradation, such as deforestation. *Biological disaster* may involve exposure to pathogenic microorganism, toxin, or other bioactive substance, for instance an outbreak of endemic disease or plant contagion.

Community-oriented nursing emphasizes community assessment and education to reduce the number of casualties when disasters occur and to achieve the best possible level of health for the people and community involved in a disaster.

Disasters affect the health status of a community in the following ways:

- Lead to premature death, illness, or injury.
- Disrupt healthcare services offered within the community.
- Cause environmental issues, such as outbreaks of communicable disease or food/water-borne illness.
- Cause shortages of safe food and drinking water.
- Burden other healthcare systems when displaced populations shift to a host community for basic needs (Veenema, 2013).

In large-scale disasters, nurses practicing in special circumstances and disaster conditions are typically needed to:

- Rapidly assess the overall situation and that of individual victims.
- Triage care and initiate life-saving measures first.
- Adapt nursing skills to the disaster situation, considering available equipment, supplies, and personnel.
- Evaluate the safety of the environment and remove health hazards.
- Provide leadership in coordinating care, assigning priorities for care, and transporting victims.
- Prevent further injury or illness.

- Provide compassionate support to victims and their families.

Good Samaritan laws protect nurses when volunteering—in any state—as long as actions are reasonable.

For additional information on disaster preparedness and preparation for terrorist attacks,

 Go to Student Resources, Chapter 43, **Supplemental Materials: Disaster Preparedness,** on Davis*Plus*.

International Nursing

Nurses working internationally commonly provide relief services after a natural or man-made disaster. They may also offer health or human aid services through a medical clinic, faith-based mission, orphanage, or other international relief program. International nursing requires a high level of autonomy, flexibility, and ingenuity, depending on community needs and available resources. Common problems affecting the health of international communities are poor sanitation, contaminated food and water, waste management, limited or dangerous transportation, communicable disease, parasitic infections, cultural practices, and limited education. Nurses working globally commonly treat people with malnutrition, dehydration, mosquito and other insect-related illnesses, parasitic infestation, hepatitis and HIV, to name a few (Fig. 43-4). Because of poor access to healthcare and limited or no resources to pay for medication, many people do not receive adequate healthcare.

BOX 43-1 ■ What You Should Do During a Disaster Event

- Remain calm and be patient.
- Follow the advice of local emergency officials.
- Listen to your radio or television for news and instructions.
- If the disaster occurs near you, check for injuries. Give first aid, and get help for seriously injured people.
- If the disaster occurs near your home while you are there, check for damage using a flashlight. Do not light matches or candles or turn on electrical switches. Check for fires, fire hazards, and other household hazards. Sniff for gas leaks, starting at the water heater. If you smell gas or suspect a leak, turn off the main gas valve, open windows, and get everyone outside quickly.
- Shut off any other damaged utilities.
- Confine or secure your pets.
- Call your family contact—do not use the telephone again unless it is a life-threatening emergency.
- Check on your neighbors, especially those who are older or disabled.

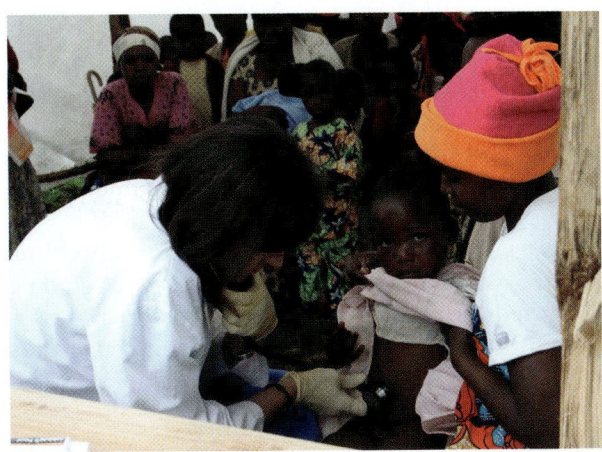

FIGURE 43-4 International nursing. Health and nutrition program for women and children at an African health clinic.

 Think**Like a Nurse** 43-4

Increase your self-knowledge: Assume you are going to be a community-based nurse. Of the many career opportunities available, which work do you think you would rather do? Explain why.

PracticalKnowledge
knowing **how**

The American Nurses Association, in the *Standards for Community Health Nursing* (1986), describes the goal of community health nursing as the promotion and preservation of the health of the community population as a whole, defined groups, families, and individuals. Community nursing care should be delivered in a practical, culturally sensitive manner (Kulbok, Thatcher, Park, et al., 2012).

For more information about community health nursing standards,

 Go to Chapter 43, Student Resources, **Supplemental Materials, American Nurses Association Standards of Community Health Nursing Practice,** on Davis*Plus*.

▰ ASSESSMENT

The nursing process follows the same steps you have studied in the previous chapters but uses different forms and different language when your client is a community. Community assessment is usually ongoing and requires the nurse to collaborate with and compile information from a variety of sources. The assessment approach is based on the type of community, the purpose of the assessment, and personal preference. Most beginning students elect to assess a geopolitical community because the data are more readily available than data from aggregate groups. Therefore, we focus on the geopolitical community assessment procedure.

Windshield Survey Community assessment usually begins with a windshield survey. A **windshield survey** is performed by observing the community through your automobile window, while walking, or otherwise being physically present in the area. It is similar to general observation of the individual client in that it provides an overview and allows you to see the community in its natural state. As you observe, make note of the condition of buildings and public facilities, residences, religious facilities, streets and sewers, modes of transportation, lighting, outward signs of crime or violence, pollution, waste disposal, and other signs of the well-being of the community. Protective services, such as police and fire services, should be included. You may need to repeat the survey over a period of time at different times of the day, month, or year to get an accurate picture of the community. For more reliable survey results, observers should be trained.

- Begin by describing the neighborhood and the people you see in the community.
- Strive to remain objective in your observations; avoid using personal opinions and biases
- Route your course prior to conducting the visit.
- Record your findings as soon as possible after your survey.
- Document the observation with photographs and videography when possible.

Databases and Public Records You can also obtain data from publicly available resources, such as birth records, marriage licenses, local news publications, and community Internet sites. Internet search engines can help you obtain demographic information, morbidity and mortality data, vital statistics, educational levels, criminal activity, political leadership issues, and/or information about community resources.

Client Perceptions You will also gather information about how individuals in the community perceive the community and its state of health. Through community gatherings and informal conversations, you can assess a cross section of the population. This is not only an important part of your assessment, but also an excellent way to establish rapport, convey your concerns, and develop a working relationship with key community members.

▰ ANALYSIS/NURSING DIAGNOSIS

After a thorough assessment, you will analyze the complete set of data and compile a list of community strengths and limitations. Work with the community to develop a list of their priorities, considering needs identified by the client, and based on availability of funding and political feasibility.

The NANDA-International Taxonomy

In community practice, you need nursing diagnoses that describe the health status of individuals, families, groups, and entire communities. Recall from Chapter 4 that the NANDA-I taxonomy of nursing diagnoses can be used in any nursing setting or specialty. You would simply add the term *community* to other NANDA-I labels when creating a community-based diagnosis: for example, Decisional Conflict (Community) related to safety needs of the homeless population. In addition, the NANDA-I taxonomy includes four diagnoses that specifically describe the health status of a community:

- Deficient Community Health
- Ineffective Community Coping
- Readiness for Enhanced Community Coping
- Ineffective Management of Community Therapeutic Regimen

The Omaha Problem Classification System

The Omaha system was developed specifically for use in community settings (Martin & Norris, 1996). In addition to nursing diagnoses, it contains standardized terminology for outcomes and interventions. For a thorough overview,

 Go to the **Omaha System Web site,** at http://www.omahasystem.org/

For an expanded discussion of the Omaha problem classification scheme and for examples of diagnosis (problem) labels, and problem modifiers, and examples of creating a diagnostic statement,

 Go to **Standardized Language, Omaha Problem Classification Scheme,** in Volume 2.

PLANNING OUTCOMES/EVALUATION

In the community you will need to write goals and outcomes for aggregates. The *Healthy People 2020* goals are aggregate goals. The NOC and Omaha taxonomies provide standardized terms for stating community goals. For guidelines in using these two taxonomies,

 Go to Chapter 43, **Standardized Language, Using the NOC and Omaha Systems to Write Aggregate Goals,** in Volume 2.

PLANNING INTERVENTIONS/IMPLEMENTATION

As a community health nurse, you will need interventions to promote and preserve the health of individuals, aggregates, and communities. Both NIC and the Omaha system provide standardized vocabularies for aggregate interventions.

The NIC taxonomy includes 18 interventions specifically designed for community health. The Omaha taxonomy provides four intervention categories that can be used in community-oriented nursing practice. For guidelines,

 Go to Chapter 43, **Standardized Language, Using the NIC and Omaha Interventions Labels,** in Volume 2.

APPLYING THE NURSING PROCESS IN COMMUNITY-BASED CARE

Community assessment and care planning may at first seem different from what you have been doing for individual patients. But it does follow the same problem-solving process, as illustrated following:

Scenario: As a nurse employed by a local immunization clinic, you have been hired into a new position created by federal and state grant monies to investigate why immunization levels are low among 2-year-olds in Census Tract 15. You would begin with an assessment.

1. **Gather data about the community.**
   - *Define the community.* For instance, determine the physical boundaries of Census Tract 15, a geopolitical community.
   - *Learn the community.* Start interacting with the community to build rapport. Begin the ongoing assessment by conducting windshield surveys, searching for information through reputable databases, and talking with community members.
   - *Focus the data collection.* Focus on the information that will help you determine possible causes of low immunization rates. In this case, the priority problem has already been defined by the financing agency.

 Think**Like a Nurse 43-5**

What data would you want to look at? What are possible reasons for low immunization rates?

2. **Analyze the Data.** Next, examine the characteristics of the families failing to provide immediate immunization for children, including:
   - Family demographics
   - Age of children
   - Number of immunizations needed and the cost
   - Beliefs about negative effects of vaccines
   - Availability of transportation
   - Public sites providing vaccinations
   - Overall continuity of general healthcare for children

   Assume that after working with the community for 6 months, you have spoken at parenting classes about the need to vaccinate children. Several community members have told you they thought their child had already received all necessary immunizations or that their healthcare provider had said to wait until they have better insurance. You will need to arrange a meeting with the local providers to discuss low immunization status. They explain that many vaccinations are too expensive to provide based on the reimbursement they receive from government funding sources.

3. **Plan care.** Your next move is to do some planning. Using the Omaha system you could generate a care plan to address some of the issues raised by community members and physicians.

4. **Evaluate results and follow up.** Community assessment is never complete because the community is constantly changing. However, you need to define the identified needs and desired outcomes during a given period of time, based on best data available at the time of collection. In this case, you would share with local healthcare providers, the health department, and local health policy committee your approach to addressing the factors suspected of contributing to poor immunization compliance. An important part of your role as a community health nurse is to continue to monitor and evaluate the data and provide updates to the appropriate groups.

Now that you have some understanding of community healthcare, the rest of the chapter focuses on a specific type of community nursing: delivering healthcare in the patient's home.

TheoreticalKnowledge
knowing **why**

UNDERSTANDING THE CONCEPT OF HOME HEALTHCARE

Recall that community-based healthcare refers to services performed outside of acute care settings. Home healthcare is one such service. **Home healthcare** is the delivery of health-related services in the client's home. Home healthcare is appropriate when a client needs ongoing care that exceeds the abilities of friends and family, as in the following situations:

- To supplement the skills a family member is providing
- To serve as a backup for safety or additional assessment

- For older adults who need ongoing care but want to avoid moving to a skilled nursing facility
- For people of any age who require home-care service when they are recovering from illness or surgery or when they are terminally ill
- For ongoing care of chronically ill adults and children to avoid hospitalization

Goals of Home Healthcare

Nurses provide home care to clients with complex, chronic, or terminal illness. The primary goals in home healthcare are that (1) the client's self-care ability and Independence will improve and (2) caregivers gain the ability to assist the client with ongoing health needs.

This approach may be very different from what you have experienced in other clinical settings. For example, as the nurse in the Meet Your Patients scenario, you would help the couple manage Mr. Escobar's care independently at home. Initially you might show Mrs. Escobar how to administer medications and explain their function, and demonstrate strategies for moving and turning Mr. Escobar. However, your goal would be for her to progress to handling these tasks independently.

Distinctive Features of Home Healthcare

Home health nursing differs from hospital nursing in several ways. The hospital environment is controlled. Surfaces are regularly disinfected; supplies are stocked; and foods, medications, and other therapies are readily available. Computers are conveniently located with information easily accessible about the patient. In addition, the hospital-based nurse can consult almost immediately with a team of healthcare providers (i.e., other nurses, the primary care provider, various therapists, social workers, a pastoral care provider, and even a business office staff to ensure that reimbursement will be forthcoming).

In contrast, when you are in a patient's home, surprisingly little is within your control. The home may be spotless or filthy, food plentiful or scarce, and supplies readily available or unreliable. The television or music may be loud; a dog may bark continually; or several young children may be playing nearby and repeatedly interrupting your interactions with the client or caregiver. You will find nursing care in the home environment to be different from inpatient settings in the following ways:

- You are a guest in the client's home. The client and family determine whether they are willing to let you enter the home to deliver care.
- You are responsible for making the assessments and determining whether to advise the primary care provider of client changes.
- You must bring all necessary supplies or arrange to have them delivered ahead of time.
- You must be able to distinguish between skilled services, which are eligible for reimbursement from Medicare, and homemaker services. **Skilled services** are services that must be performed or supervised by a licensed healthcare professional (Box 43-2). **Homemaker services** (e.g., cleaning, meal preparation) are reimbursed to clients only if the principal reason for home care is a skilled service. These services are provided by home health aides.
- You must be more self-sufficient and function more independently. Often there are no other team members immediately available for support, assistance, or consultation.
- You must be aware of and comfortable with the family observing you as you provide care.
- You will need to adapt to varying family relationships and some home environments that are difficult or even dysfunctional.
- You will need to encourage the family to help in providing care and in taking over care when you leave the home. Be aware that overburdened caregivers may need your help as much as does the client.

BOX 43-2 ■ Skilled Nursing Services

Medicare defines *skilled nursing care* as services and care that can be done safely and correctly only by a licensed registered or practical nurse. The services must be reasonable and necessary for the treatment of the illness or injury.

- Patient assessment
- Ongoing monitoring of patient status
- Management and coordination of the patient's plan of care
- Evaluation of response to medications or treatment
- Medication instruction
- Teaching patients or caregivers to provide care or therapies
- Disease-related teaching (e.g., diabetes education)
- Complex tasks, such as injections, insertion of urinary catheters, infusion therapy, wound care, tube feedings, or ventilator management

- You must preplan your visit by figuring out the directions to sites in advance and arranging appointments efficiently.

- ✚ Your personal safety may be more of a concern when making home visits. You must always be aware of the environment around you and alert to possible dangers.

- As things do not always go as planned in a less controlled home environment, you will need to be flexible and learn to modify your plan.

One advantage of home healthcare is that it allows you to expand your understanding of the concept of *client*. The home is a window into the client's life, through which you can see his personal environment: how he lives, eats, and negotiates his world (Fig. 43-5). The photos, mementos, personal belongings, and other things the client values and cherishes make cultural beliefs and practices more visible. These things provide clues to his lifestyle, strengths, resources, and motivation.

Home health nursing also differs from community healthcare. Community health nurses provide care for individuals, families, and groups with an emphasis on population-based care. In contrast, home health nursing focuses on the individual and his support system.

KnowledgeCheck 43-6

Identify at least four skilled services that may be provided in the home.

WHO PROVIDES HOME HEALTHCARE?

Home healthcare is provided by a variety of healthcare professionals employed by or working in cooperation with home healthcare agencies.

Home Health Agencies

Home health agencies coordinate the services of various professionals and paraprofessionals. They may be categorized by purpose, by type of client served, or by funding source.

Purpose In this category, **direct care agencies** are the most common. They focus on direct client interaction by providing skilled care, associated therapies and health services, home health aides, chore workers, and delivery of **respite care** (relief for family caregivers). **Indirect service agencies** also play a vital role in home healthcare. Examples of indirect home services include pharmaceutical and infusion companies and suppliers of durable medical equipment. **Durable medical equipment (DME)** is reusable equipment (e.g., walkers, wheelchairs, apnea monitors). Medicare pays for some, but not all, such devices. It is expensive, so before ordering it, be sure the DME is covered or the client is able to pay for it.

Type of Client Served An important specialty home service agency is hospice care. This may be a separate agency or a division of a home health agency. Still other agencies specialize in caring for patients with complex diseases, such as AIDS, or ventilator-dependent clients, or patients of a certain age group (services for older adults or chronically ill children).

Funding Source Agencies may take on many forms based on funding source, profit or nonprofit status, and relationship with other healthcare organizations.

- **Public agencies** are official or governmental agencies organized at the city, county, state, or national level. They are usually funded by taxes, along with reimbursement from insurance companies. The local health department is a good example of a public agency. Health departments focus chiefly on community needs, although they often also offer some home health services, especially when tracking clients in some of their disease management programs.
- **Voluntary agencies** are prominent in the delivery of home healthcare. These agencies are normally governed by a board of directors and funded by donations,

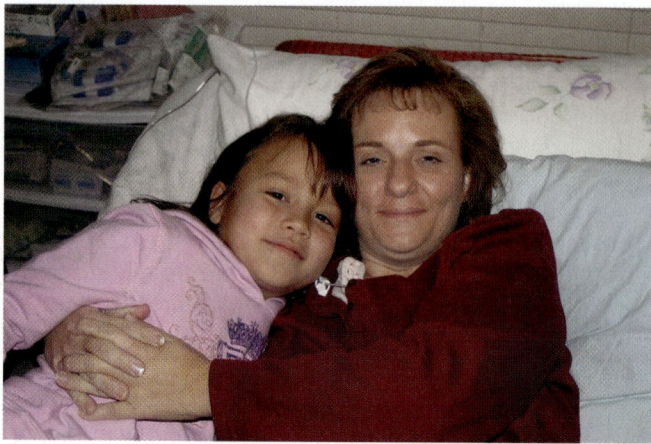

FIGURE 43-5 The home is a window into the client's life.

endowments, and third-party (insurance) reimbursement. Many **hospice organizations** (groups that provide care for people who are frail, terminally ill, dying, or not expected to improve) are voluntary organizations.

■ **Proprietary organizations** are corporate or privately owned businesses that aim to make a profit. These agencies receive payment from insurance companies but also accept private-pay clients. Proprietary organizations may provide traditional home health services as well as private-duty care and other services that assist individuals to remain independent.

■ **Hospital-based agencies** are an extension of the services provided by a hospital. Clients who no longer meet the criteria for continued hospitalization may be transferred to home care for continued services. A benefit of this type of home health agency is in the ease of transition between hospital and home.

The Home Health Team

In home healthcare, the registered nurse serves as the coordinator of health services, but other members of the healthcare team may also provide care. The team varies according to the needs of the client but is usually multidisciplinary. It may include physicians; nurse practitioners; registered nurses; licensed practical (vocational) nurses; home health aides; physical, speech, occupational, or respiratory therapists; nutritionists; social workers; pharmacists; podiatrists; dentists; chaplains; and family members.

Home Health Nurses

To succeed in home healthcare, you must have the ability to work independently and collaboratively, be flexible and resourceful, and adapt to different home environments and family interactions. The ANA asserts that because of the level of independence, knowledge, and expertise required to meet the demands of home care, baccalaureate nurses are better prepared for that role. However, it also says that the necessary knowledge and skills can be developed through formal orientation programs, structured preceptor programs, and guided clinical experiences (ANA, 2008, p. 8).

Home health nurses provide a broad range of services to clients of all ages. Your principal roles as a home health nurse (also called visiting nurse) are discussed in this section. Each role requires you to function as a skillful communicator. Communication is crucial in home care because of the need to establish good rapport with the client and family and to communicate frequently with other members of the healthcare team.

Direct Care Provider As a direct care provider, you may administer medications, dress wounds, or perform other skilled, complex tasks.

Client and Family Educator Recall that the goal of home healthcare is to promote self-care. Instead of focusing on performing the procedures, you will be helping the client or family take over the care. You can easily see the need to communicate skillfully in this role. You must be able to clearly explain the care required, the rationale for it, and how to safely perform the care. This requires patience, skill, and repetition.

Client Advocate In home care, the client and family are directly in charge of the plan of care. As client advocate, you support the client's right to make healthcare decisions yet protect the client from harm if he is unable to make decisions. In the event family members disagree, remember that as the client's advocate, you must try to see that his choices are respected and his rights upheld. You must also advocate for services the client needs. This may mean trying to secure additional home health support to avoid hospitalization, or it may mean advocating for another level of service, such as referral to hospice or placement in the hospital, based on your assessment of the client and discussion with the client and family.

Care Coordinator Home health nurses must manage and coordinate care among an array of healthcare providers. Therefore, as the case manager, you will need to gather data at an initial visit and develop a plan of care that addresses the client's needs. Your plan may require you to make additional visits as well as specify and perhaps arrange delivery of therapies and services by other professionals in the home.

KnowledgeCheck 43-7

What roles does the nurse assume in home care? List and describe them.

Hospice Nurses

As you learned in Chapter 17, **hospice nursing** focuses on care of patients who are dying or whose condition is not expected to improve. Hospice services are provided in the home, in the hospital, in nursing homes, and in homes specifically designed as hospices. The goal of hospice care is to promote comfort and quality of life. For these reasons, most hospice services are provided in the client's home. Because the client is not expected to recover, the focus of home hospice care is quite different from traditional home care. More than promoting self-care and independence, hospice care focuses on providing comfort and managing symptoms (Table 43-1).

The roles of hospice nurse and home health nurse differ mainly in their emphasis. As a direct care provider, the hospice nurse assesses the client's condition and monitors responses to interventions aimed at relieving distress. As an educator, the hospice nurse teaches the client and family how to adjust medications and care to control pain and other symptoms. The roles of communicator and client advocate assume prime importance as the client's condition deteriorates. The nurse shares these roles with the family and other home caregivers. Generally, there is less coordination of multiple services

Table 43-1 ➤ Home Healthcare and Home Hospice Care

	HOME HEALTHCARE	HOME HOSPICE CARE
Purpose	Promote self-care and independence.	Promote comfort and quality of life.
Focus of Nursing Interventions	Teach the family or other caregivers to assist the client with ongoing health needs and activities of daily living.	Provide comfort and manage symptoms.

in home hospice care. Instead, there may be greater emphasis on pain management. If you need more information on hospice care, see Chapter 17.

WHO PAYS FOR HOME HEALTHCARE?

Medicare, Medicaid, other government funded or mandated coverage, private insurance, and individual payments (private pay) help pay for home-care services. Medicare and Medicaid are the largest payors for home healthcare. Keep in mind the federal healthcare act passed in 2010 will likely change reimbursement in a variety of ways over the coming years (111th Congress, 1st session, 2010).

Medicare is a federally funded healthcare system designed to provide health coverage for persons who are older than 65 years and younger people who are disabled or diagnosed with end-stage renal disease or amyotrophic lateral sclerosis.

Medicare Reimbursement

Reimbursement by Medicare for home care depends on the following, strictly applied criteria:

- *The client must need skilled care.* See Box 43-2. Other services may also be provided, but the primary purpose for establishing care must be based on a skilled care need. This means that Medicare will not pay for personal care such as bathing and dressing when this is the only care the client needs.
- *The client must be homebound.* This means (1) the client must have a condition that restricts the ability to leave the home; and (2) leaving the home requires special assistance, transportation, supportive devices, or an escort.
- *The client must require nursing care that is part-time and intermittent.* This means Medicare will pay for a limited number of hours per day or days per week that the client can get skilled nursing care or home health aide services.
- *The plan of care must be authorized by the physician and recertified every 62 days.* For the client to continue to receive care, there must be evidence of continued need that remains acute.
- *The care must be medically necessary and reasonable.* The plan of care must address the client's health concerns and have clearly delineated outcomes. The expectations of the patient must be reasonable.

- *Medicare will pay only for interventions identified on the treatment plan.* The payer may periodically request patient health records to verify that the care was given.
- *The home health agency must be approved by Medicare.* An agency must show that it meets the Medicare definitions and requirements to become Medicare certified.

Medicaid is a program sponsored jointly by the federal government and the states to provide services to people whose income is below a mandated level. In many states, the criteria for reimbursement are the same as those required by Medicare. However, each state at present determines what services will be part of its medical assistance plan.

Private Insurance and Self-Payment

Private insurance companies may also offer home health services. The type and extent of covered services are specified in each separate insurance group and plan.

Many people require assistance in the home but do not meet criteria for reimbursement from Medicare, Medicaid, or their private insurer. Others simply do not have health insurance. (This was true when this book was published, but it is likely to change during the next few years as the new federal healthcare regulations are gradually put into effect.) Frequently, older clients require home health assistance but may not need skilled services. For example, they may need assistance with grocery shopping, meal planning and preparation, or transportation. The client or family may contact an agency to provide assistance for these services. Services are billed directly to the client.

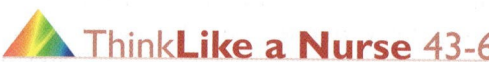 **ThinkLike a Nurse 43-6**

Review the scenario focused on Mr. Escobar (Meet Your Patients). What members of the home health team may be required to provide care? Why?

HOW ARE CLIENTS REFERRED TO HOME HEALTHCARE?

Referrals to home healthcare come from a variety of sources. However, for home care to begin, there must be a medical prescription and a physician-approved treatment plan.

Hospital-based agencies have a built-in referral base. If the primary provider or nursing staff determine that the client would benefit from home health services, they refer the patient to the agency for evaluation while he is still hospitalized. Many agencies have *intake coordinators* who work in the hospital and review clients for suitability of services, gathering information from the chart, the client, the family, and the hospital team. Home services are arranged before discharge from an inpatient facility. Ideally, a discharge planner gathers information, secures the prescription from the provider, and makes arrangements. In some smaller hospitals, this task falls to the staff nurse providing predischarge care.

Referrals may also come from doctors, nurses, primary care offices and clinics, mental health workers, and other healthcare providers in the community, as well as directly from families and clients. Most home health agencies evaluate clients to determine whether they are eligible for services that are reimbursable by insurance. They may also offer services that the client may pay for independently.

WHAT IS THE FUTURE OF HOME HEALTHCARE?

Healthcare analysts have predicted several changes in home care during the next few decades:

- **Increased need for home healthcare.** During the next several decades, the demand for home care is expected to rise. Considering the growing number of older adults in the United States, it is more cost effective to provide healthcare in the home than in an inpatient setting.
- **Increased use of the home for hospice care.** Public acceptance of the home as a place of comfort and care, as well as concerns about the cost of inpatient care, has increased the number of persons who choose this compassionate option for end-of-life and palliative care.
- **Increased technology.** Technological advances, such as online resources or telemedicine consultation, make it safer and more affordable to deliver complex care in the home and allow home health nurses to deliver information and provide support (Bradford, Armfield, Young, et al., 2013). Computerized monitoring and documentation allow home health agencies to better coordinate care, receive needed supplies, and manage costs.
- **Continued research.** Research is needed in the area of strategies to improve the effectiveness of care, identify predictors of need for rehospitalization, and integrate home care into overall community-based services.

Practical Knowledge
knowing *how*

As a home healthcare nurse, your days will vary. Normally your caseload will be contained within a limited geographic boundary, so that you can schedule your visits efficiently, spending less time driving to visits, and have more time for delivering care. If you want to envision what it would be like to be a home health nurse, you need only to look at the list of services Medicare recognizes as skilled, in Box 43-2.

HOW DO I MAKE A HOME VISIT?

The home visit has three phases: preparation before the visit, nursing care during the visit, and evaluation after the visit.

Before the Visit

First review the client's chart and referral form to determine why you are making the visit. You may also need to review material about the client's health problem, medications, or treatment plan. Then you can begin to plan for the visit. What supplies will you need? What teaching materials will you need? What are the goals of the visit? Does the agency require additional client information, such as insurance data, to provide care? The agency will probably have a set of forms (e.g., HIPAA privacy forms, billing information) for you to complete during the first visit. Be sure you have those with you.

Before the visit you will need to find the address, get directions to the home, and determine whether there are safety concerns. Contact the client to notify him of the planned date and time of the visit and to determine whether his health status has changed since the referral was made. This will allow you to bring additional equipment or personnel along if needed.

Prepare Supplies

Home health nurses usually carry a nursing bag (Fig. 43-6). The nursing bag is often customized to the needs of the

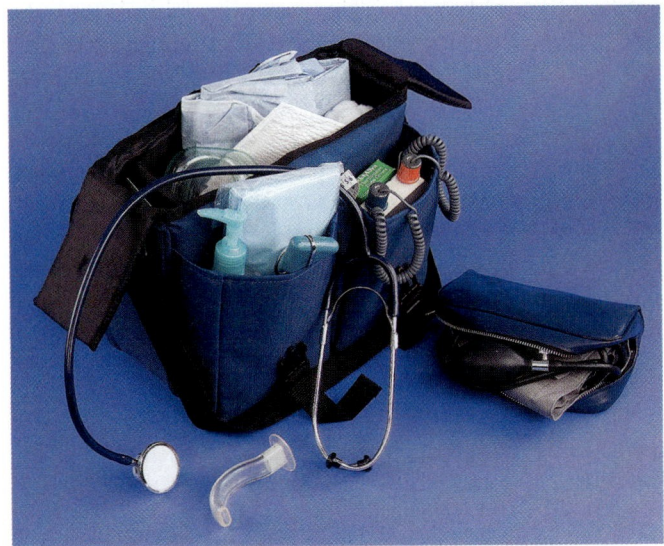

FIGURE 43-6 The home health nursing bag contains some standard items but is usually customized according to the requirements of the clients in the nurse's caseload.

clients in the nurse's caseload, and normally contains the following:

- Handwashing supplies (e.g., soap or antibacterial handrub, paper towels)
- Stethoscope
- Sphygmomanometers (with cuffs in a variety of sizes)
- Thermometers (oral and rectal)
- Small equipment (scissors, forceps, penlight, staple remover)
- Tape measure (with plastic coating that can be cleaned, or several disposable ones)
- Plastic apron
- Gloves, sterile and clean
- An assortment of gauze dressings, tape, and cotton balls
- Occupational Safety and Health Administration (OSHA) supplies: mask, protective eyewear, disinfectant spray, disposable gowns to protect clothing
- A variety of syringes and safety needles (this varies widely among agencies)
- Venipuncture supplies
- Airway and resuscitation mask
- Miscellaneous supplies (e.g., specimen cups, sealable bag to transport specimen, agency forms, business cards)

You may need other supplies, such as medications, a scale, and a transfer belt, depending on the requirements of the clients in your caseload. If the client needs frequent dressing changes or supplies for treatments (e.g., tube feedings), it is best to have the supplies delivered directly to the client's house to reduce the number of materials you must carry. Note that in some states nurses are not permitted to carry medications because of safety concerns. You will need to check on the rules that apply to your state.

Provide for Your Safety

 As you drive to the home, begin to make your assessment. Locate the stores, hospital, and community resources. What is the overall character of the neighborhood? Does this appear to be a safe neighborhood? What are the conditions of the approach to the home?

Safety for yourself and the client is an essential consideration in home healthcare. Bring your impressions about neighborhood safety and home safety with you into the home. You should evaluate whether the environment contributes to the client's health problems. In addition, you must also assess the implications for your own safety. You should provide your agency with your patient care schedule for the day. For suggestions about the safe delivery of home healthcare,

Go to **Clinical Insight 43-1: Safety Considerations in Home Care,** in Volume 2.

KnowledgeCheck 43-8

What are the major tasks that must be completed before making a home visit?

At the Visit

When you arrive at the home, you must remember this is the client's domain. Knock or ring the doorbell, and wait to be invited in. Introduce yourself to the client and family. Be respectful of their home, as well as their beliefs, values, practices, and cultural preferences.

The first few minutes of the initial visit set the tone for the relationship among client, family, nurse, and agency. This is your opportunity to develop rapport and trust. Introducing yourself, waiting for permission to enter, and treating the client and family members with respect are ways to help to establish rapport (Fig. 43-7).

You should also offer your card to identify yourself, and provide contact information for the home health agency. Generally, agencies have information packets that include the client's bill of rights, client responsibilities, billing information, information on the frequency and duration of services, how to reach the agency, and the date and time of the next visit.

As you do all this, you also gather data. Who answered your questions? What is the relationship between the caregiver and the client? How do they interact? What other people live there? What is the condition of the home? If this is an initial visit, you may need to verify or complete client data on the referral form. In the hospital, admissions personnel usually gather admitting data and obtain consent for treatment. In home care you need to collect and document this information.

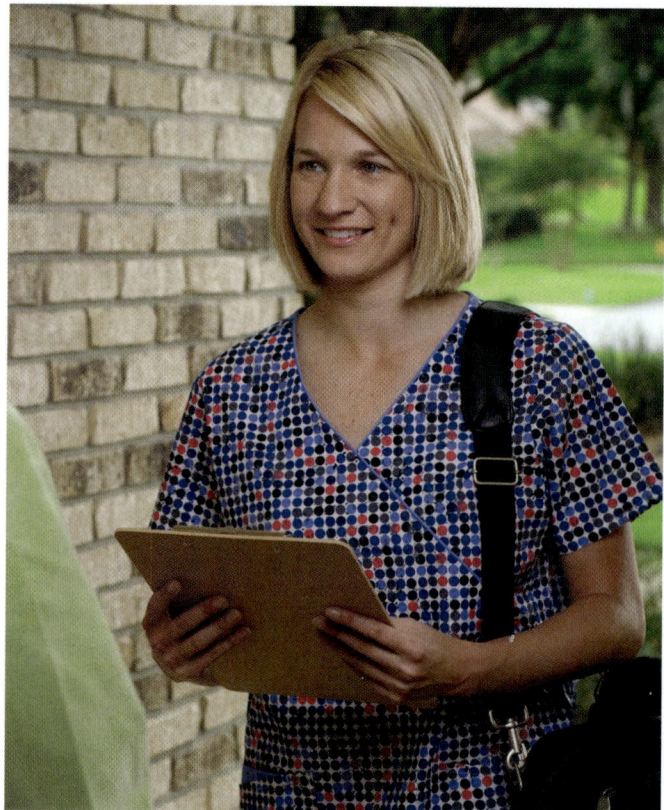

FIGURE 43-7 The first few minutes of the initial visit set the tone for the relationship among client, family, nurse, and agency.

At a home visit, you might do a variety of things, such as performing physical care; drawing blood sample for lab work; checking weight; administering medication, IV fluid, or tube feedings; providing wound or ostomy care; or whatever is needed.

ThinkLike a Nurse 43-7

Review the case of Mr. Escobar (Meet Your Patients). What information did you gain from the first few minutes of the visit?

- Both Mr. and Mrs. Escobar are in need of nursing interventions. However, this is your agency's first home visit to them, and you have other clients you must visit today, so you will need to prioritize. What must the home health nurse do during the initial visit to a client?
- In addition to completing your assessment and talking about a plan of care with the Escobars, what do you think is the single most important thing you can do for them today? Explain your thinking.
- When Mrs. Escobar meets you at the door and brings you into the living room, you notice a large German shepherd dog lying beside Mr. Escobar's bed. Mrs. Escobar says, "Stay, King"; and then to you, "Roland likes having him nearby." What should you do?

After the Visit

After you leave the home, there is still a lot of work for you to do. Often you will need to complete the documentation for the visit. In Chapter 18, you learned about documentation techniques, various forms of charting, and legal aspects of documentation. In home care all of these rules apply; however, some aspects of home-care documentation are unique.

Home health agencies use Medicare's Outcome and Assessment Information Set (OASIS) to record initial assessment data. To continue to provide needed services to the client, you must include in your documentation: (1) evidence of homebound status, and (2) evidence of continued need for skilled care.

Other post-visit activities include ordering supplies needed for the next visit, making referrals to additional services (e.g., occupational therapy), coordinating care among the various services, and scheduling the next visit.

NURSING PROCESS IN HOME CARE

The nursing process moves through the same phases in all patient care settings. The difference in home care is that you must use forms structured to satisfy Medicare and other insurance requirements. Nevertheless, you need to assess the client, the family, the home, and the community to identify nursing diagnoses and other health problems. You will work from a plan of care prescribed by a medical provider, but individualize it with suitable nursing diagnoses and interventions. Periodically, you must evaluate the client's continued homebound status and ongoing need for medical treatment and skilled nursing care.

ASSESSMENT

On the initial visit, you need to perform an assessment to establish a baseline and determine the type of care required. This assessment includes a health history, review of all medications—prescribed, over-the-counter, and alternative—pertinent family and social history, mental status, functional ability, availability of family and informal support and caregivers, nutritional status, and assessment of the home environment. Typically a full assessment requires multiple visits.

Medicare requires home health agencies to collect specific information for all Medicare clients they serve. The OASIS data must be collected at the start of care, with each recertification (every 60 days), and at the termination of care. Medicare uses these data to determine the effectiveness of care and to monitor client outcomes. In addition to the required OASIS information, many agencies use other assessment tools created specifically for their needs. For an example of the OASIS form,

 Go to Student Resources, Chapter 18, **Tables, Boxes, Figures: ESG Figure 18-3, Outcome and Assessment Information Set (OASIS),** on DavisPlus.

It is also important to assess the needs of the caregivers—the family members, friends, and support system in the home. To be successful in home care, you must work *with* the caregivers. Take time at each visit to speak with them, making sure to include them in your assessment, plan of care, and teaching. Assessment of the caregivers often allows you to determine what services are needed in the home. Caregivers may have health problems of their own that affect their ability to provide care for another. This is common among older couples.

ANALYSIS/NURSING DIAGNOSIS

As in any setting, the nursing diagnoses are based on the client's responses to illness and care. As a home healthcare nurse, you will work with clients with numerous medical and nursing diagnoses. Two frequently used nursing diagnoses, Caregiver Role Strain and Deficient Knowledge, are discussed below. Safety and Risk for Infection, also key concerns in the home, are thoroughly discussed in Chapters 24 and 23, respectively. Infection control measures in the home are also presented in a following section, Infection Control in the Home.

Caregiver Role Strain Providing care to a loved one at home can be a challenge, especially when finances don't allow a family to hire home health aides. Around-the-clock caregiving duties can lead to physical exhaustion, social isolation, resentment, sadness, or depression. In addition, family members themselves may become seriously ill and no longer be able to function as caregiver. These role changes may be difficult for both the ill person and the caregiver. For example, imagine that your mother suddenly became very ill and you became her primary caregiver. This would be a reversal of the roles you both are used to, and it would be emotionally taxing, especially if you are already exhausted and isolated from your friends and other support. In addition, a primary caregiver may worry that caring for the client interferes with other responsibilities (e.g., as a parent, spouse, friend, student, worker).

Given these factors, it is not surprising that the two nursing diagnoses most commonly applicable to loved ones providing care at home are Caregiver Role Strain and Risk for Caregiver Role Strain. These diagnoses identify those for whom the burden of delivering care has become—or is at risk of becoming—overwhelming. Common signs of caregiver role strain include difficulty adjusting to role changes, fatigue, isolation, depression, and difficulty in performing routine care for the client.

Deficient Knowledge Client and family teaching is especially important in home care because most of the caregiving is performed by the client and significant others. You will spend much of your time teaching them the skills necessary for self-care (e.g., how to administer insulin, how to manage the oxygen equipment). Recall that to be eligible for home nursing care, clients must require skilled nursing care. Client education is a service for which Medicare and other insurers will reimburse. You must be certain to include a Deficient Knowledge diagnosis on the care plan to ensure the client's continued eligibility and reimbursement for the service.

Key Point: *In other chapters we caution against indiscriminate use of the Deficient Knowledge diagnosis. However, an exception must be made for home care because of Medicare regulations.*

KnowledgeCheck 43-9

- Why are the first few minutes of the initial visit so important?
- Identify five things that should be assessed at an initial home visit.

 ## ThinkLike a Nurse 43-8

- Based on the information in the scenario, what nursing diagnoses might Mr. Escobar (Meet Your Patients) have? There may not be enough data to make definite diagnoses, but what probable diagnoses are there for which you would want to gather confirming data? Do not include potential diagnoses, such as Risk for Imbalanced Nutrition.
- Mr. Escobar has a potential problem, Risk for Falls. What are two interventions you would probably be able to do today to reduce his falls risk?
- What, if any, evidence of caregiver strain does Mrs. Escobar exhibit?

Standardized Terminology for Home Health Nursing Diagnoses

Recall from the nursing process chapters that various disciplines, including nursing, have developed classifications of standardized terminology (also called taxonomies, vocabularies, and standardized languages) for describing their work and for planning and documenting care. You are familiar with the NANDA-I

taxonomy of nursing diagnoses; however, home-care nurses more commonly use the Clinical Care Classification (CCC) because it is closely related to the OASIS reporting forms required by Medicare. If you need to review the concept of standardized nursing language, see Chapters 4, 5, and 6.

The CCC also contains 176 diagnostic concepts—60 major categories and/or 116 subcategories—that describe nursing diagnoses and patient problems (Saba, 2012). Approximately 50 labels are also NANDA-I diagnostic categories that are especially applicable to home healthcare. Common CCC nursing diagnoses used in the home include:

Activities of Daily Living (ADLs) Alteration
Caregiver Role Strain
Family Processes Alteration
Home Maintenance Alteration
Knowledge Deficit
Physical Mobility Impairment
Self-Care Deficit

The CCC system consists of 21 care components to classify diagnoses and interventions. An accompanying coding structure and framework parallel the steps of the nursing process and link the CCC diagnoses to interventions and outcomes. To see the CCC Care Components and an example of a CCC nursing diagnosis with interventions, respectively,

 Go to **Standardized Language**, **Clinical Care Classification System for Home Healthcare,** and **An Example of a CCC Nursing Diagnosis and Interventions**, in Volume 2.

For complete information on the CCC and complete lists of diagnoses, outcomes, and interventions,

 Go to the **Clinical Care Classification Web site,** at http://www.sabacare.com

PLANNING OUTCOMES/EVALUATION

Each Nursing Diagnosis requires an Expected Outcome, which is the anticipated goal of the nursing actions planned to care for the patient's condition (Saba, 2012). To formulate a goal/outcome in the CCC system, attach one of the three CCC "modifiers" (*improve, stabilize, deteriorate*) to the diagnosis. The outcome describes the *desired* client health status. To evaluate client progress, you again use one of the three modifiers to describe the client's *actual* health status. The following is an example:

CCC nursing diagnosis:	Knowledge Deficit
Goal/expected outcome:	Knowledge Deficit, Improve
Actual status on evaluation:	Knowledge Deficit, Stabilized

Medicare requires that the client's status be evaluated and coded as improved, stabilized, or deteriorated, the same as the CCC system. In your nursing notes, you would include additional narrative to support your evaluation.

The Nursing Outcomes Classification (NOC) can also be used in home health nursing (Moorhead, Johnson, Maas, et al., 2013). A few of the outcomes that pertain to home and families are Caregiver Home Care Readiness, Caregiver Performance: Direct Care, Caregiver Stressors, Family Coping, and Family Functioning.

To prepare the client and family for self-care, inform them of the needs you have identified, and involve them in setting goals and planning care. They may be able to identify strategies to solve problems or to help you identify needs that are not readily apparent.

PLANNING INTERVENTIONS/IMPLEMENTATION

Medicare requires that the physician-prescribed plan of care include the following, as applicable:

- Parameters for notifying the primary provider of changes in vital signs and other clinical findings
- Diabetic foot care, including education
- Falls prevention interventions
- Depression interventions
- Interventions to monitor and treat pain
- Interventions to prevent pressure ulcers
- Pressure ulcer treatments

Once the plan of care has been agreed on, you will document it and forward it to the client's physician for certification. At the first visit, you will determine the specific skilled care required and make referrals to other required services such as physical, occupational, or speech therapy, social services, nutritional support, or home health aide services.

Standardized Nursing Interventions

The CCC system is commonly used in planning and recording home care, but the NIC taxonomy is also an option.

CCC Nursing Interventions The CCC contains 201 nursing interventions organized according to the care components. For an example,

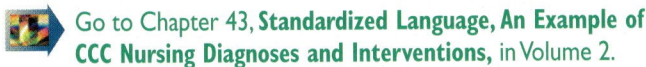

Go to Chapter 43, **Standardized Language, An Example of CCC Nursing Diagnoses and Interventions,** in Volume 2.

An intervention consists of a label (e.g., Activity Care) and a definition (e.g., Actions performed to carry out physiological or psychological daily activities). In addition to the label, you must specify the type of intervention action from among four qualifiers:

Assess/Monitor/Evaluate/Observe
Care/Perform/Provide/Assist
Teach/Educate/Instruct/Supervise
Manage/Refer/Contact/Notify

The CCC nursing interventions include only skilled services because this type of service is the only type of care reimbursed by Medicare and most insurers in home health. In the Meet Your Patients scenario, Mrs. Escobar is clearly experiencing Caregiver Strain. This is a nursing

diagnosis under the Care Component of Coping. Several interventions are possible:

> **Coping Support:** Actions to sustain a person dealing with responsibilities, problems, or difficulties
> Assess for Caregiver Strain.
> Provide (perform) emotional support.
> Refer to community services: caregiver support groups, Meals on Wheels, and respite care services.

NIC Interventions for Home Health The Nursing Interventions Classification (NIC) may also be used in home health nursing (Bulechek, Butcher, & Dochterman, 2012). A few of the interventions that pertain to home and families are Caregiver Support, Family Integrity Promotion, Home Maintenance Assistance, and Respite Care.

Assisting With Medication Management

One of The Joint Commission 2014 safety goals for home care is to use medications safely. This includes preventing errors with look-alike and sound-alike medications, educating patients about anticoagulant therapy, and keeping a current list and reconciling medications when a client transfers from one agency to another. Nurses in the home setting must be careful to avoid error when recording and communicating information about patients' medications. The Joint Commission also advises nurses to diligently compare those medications the patient is already taking with new ones to be given in the home. Make sure your patients know about medications they take at home and that they should bring a complete and updated list every time they visit a healthcare provider.

Some patients, particularly older adults, have visual and motor deficits that limit their ability to read labels and manipulate bottle caps, syringes, and so on. Other reasons for noncompliance include lack of outward symptoms, inability to tolerate side effects, pain, forgetfulness, low motivation, and impaired mental capacity. Always investigate the patient's reasons for nonadherence so that you can take appropriate actions.

You may need to teach clients and caregivers skills, such as measuring dosages, giving injections, and managing intravenous therapy. Or they may need tips on how to help clients with difficulty swallowing take oral medications. For example, for some clients, pills may be crushed and mixed in a small amount of applesauce or pudding.

Involve family members in the care of the older adult as needed, including giving medication. Older adults and caregivers may have difficulty remembering when to take their pills, which ones to take, and even whether they have already taken them. Suggest they use a medication organizer with a compartment for each day of the week. You may need to prepare a week's worth of oral medications for them during your visits. To help them remember which drug is used for each of their illnesses or symptoms, write the medical condition, names of medication, and doses, and how and when to take the medication on a large card. Then use clear tape to attach a sample of each drug next to its name on the card.

Because improperly disposed medication may end up in the water supply, it is important to inform clients about how to safely dispose of medications in the home. Teach them to return unwanted or expired prescription and over-the-counter drugs to a drug take-back program. Some counties offer household hazardous waste collection sites where drugs are accepted. Expired or unused prescription and over-the-counter drugs should never be flushed down the toilet or poured into a drain unless the label or accompanying patient information specifies that it is safe to do so (Environmental Protection Agency, 2011).

For more information about ways to properly discard medication,

 Go to Chapter 24, **Home Care: Preventing Poisoning in the Home**

Controlling Infection in the Home

 The Joint Commission (2014) safety goals for home care include reducing the risk of healthcare-associated infections. In the hospital, you have ready access to supplies that facilitate infection control. The home presents unique challenges.

Hand hygiene is one of the most important home interventions to prevent the transmission of infection. You will need to follow Standard Precautions but recognize how to modify infection control techniques for the home environment. For suggestions to help you maintain infection control during a home visit,

 Go to **Clinical Insight 43-2, Infection Control in the Home,** in Volume 2.

Homes and conditions vary widely. Do not assume that a client lives in clean surroundings or that running water and electricity are readily available. Some people with limited financial resources, especially in urban environments, live in single-room occupancy hotels (SROs). Residents of SROs live in a small room with shared bath and shower areas. To provide optimal care, you need to bring infection control supplies and personal protective equipment to the visit or order them to be delivered to the home.

Barrier Precautions

 The reason you implement barrier precautions in the home setting differs from use in hospital practice. As a rule, you will use gowns, gloves, and masks in home care to protect yourself, rather than the patient. You will need to use standard precautions, but will usually need a mask only when caring for clients who have pulmonary tuberculosis, airborne pathogens, or multidrug-resistant infections. Such organisms may be transmitted to other home-care patients through inanimate objects or hands, so use appropriate barrier precautions (Lescure, Locher, Eveillard, et al., 2009). See Chapter 23 if you need to review infection control.

Clean and Sterile Technique

Infection control in home care is different in many ways from that in acute care. In acute care, the patient is exposed to invasive interventions and environmental risks, including other patients and contaminated inanimate objects. Generally, patients have developed some resistance to the microorganisms in their own homes and are less likely to acquire infections there than in the hospital environment. You may find differences in how you handle home infusion therapy, urinary tract care, respiratory care, wound care, and enteral therapy. It is safe, in many instances, to replace sterile with clean technique, as in some of the following examples:

- **Intravenous therapy.** Sterile practices should be the same at home as in the hospital because the associated risk of sepsis is so high.
- **Insulin injections.** Many people (e.g., those who have diabetes) must give themselves repeated injections, perhaps several each day. Supplies for home use are expensive. Insurance may or may not cover the cost, or the person may not have insurance. Therefore, manufacturers recommend that disposable syringes and needles be used only once and discarded in a puncture-proof container, and it is safest to do that. Nevertheless, some people find it practical to reuse needles and syringes. For guidelines for teaching patients about this,

 Go to **Clinical Insight 26-1, Reusing Needles and Syringes: Home Care,** in Volume 2.

- **Urinary catheters.** Clients and family typically use clean, rather than sterile, gloves to perform catheterization. In the home, clients frequently interrupt the drainage system to empty a leg bag, or to change or disinfect the drainage bag. They may also disinfect and reuse urinary catheters.
- **Respiratory care.** As an example, tracheostomy care in the home is nearly always performed using clean, not sterile, technique.
- **Wound care.** Procedures for wound care should be based on the potential for contamination and infection. Usually clean technique is adequate. For example, a surgical site that is primarily closed and has no drains should be low risk for home-care-acquired infection. However, if the incision has drains or is open, the risk for infection increases, and your wound-care procedures must address the risk. Also, you do not need to arbitrarily "always" discard irrigation fluids at set intervals (e.g., every 24 hours). Order for them, or guide caregivers to buy, small containers (e.g., no more than 500 mL) that can be used up in two or three visits. Teach them how to avoid contaminating the fluids (e.g., how to handle the cap, always recap the bottle, and store the bottle away from children and pets).
- **Enteral therapy.** Emphasize the need to refrigerate the feedings after opening and store solutions until expiration. Teach caregivers to keep the kitchen appliances (e.g., blenders) and tools used in preparation meticulously clean. Sterilization of blender parts, measuring cups, and spoons is probably not necessary, but they should be washed in a hot water dishwasher after use.

KnowledgeCheck 43-10

Identify three infection control supplies that you should bring in your nursing bag on a home health visit.

Promoting Home Safety

The following two The Joint Commission 2014 home-care safety goals are important to keep in mind.

- *Reduce the risk of client harm resulting from falls.* Assess the client and the home for risk factors (e.g., dimly lit stairs, clutter on the floors) and teach caregivers falls reduction measures. Educate the patient concerning the potential for their medications to make them feel weak, dizzy, or sleepy. You will find extensive discussion of falls prevention in Chapter 24 if you need more information about that.

- *Identify risks associated with oxygen therapy* (e.g., *fire*). Be certain the home has working smoke detectors, fire extinguishers, and a fire safety plan. Assess the client and family's ability to understand and comply with fire prevention activities, and report any concerns to the physician.

If you need a checklist to use in assessing for safety hazards in the home,

Go to Chapter 24, **Tables, Boxes, and Figures: ESG Figure 24-2, Home Safety Checklist,** on Davis*Plus.*

Supporting Caregivers

Even when the client is receiving in-home care from an agency, it is not usually around-the-clock care. If the client cannot perform self-care, most of the duties fall to family members. One study found that even with short-term formal services, family caregivers provided three-fourths of the care of homebound patients. Half of the caregivers said they were not adequately prepared when it was time for their home health services to be discontinued. And at all stages, they expressed significant isolation, anxiety, and depression (Levine, Albert, Hokenstad, et al., 2006).

Unrelieved caregiving duties are physically and emotionally taxing. Caregivers may become depressed, physically exhausted, isolated from friends, and neglectful of their own health. If the primary caregiver becomes unable to function, the client must be institutionalized. Clearly, it is important to provide caregiver support.

There is some evidence to indicate that caregiver support and training workshops can relieve depression, reduce the perceived burden of caregiving, and better prepare the caregivers for their role. However, the most improvement in adaptation to the caregiver role was shown by those with more independent lives and social support (Huynh-Hohnbaum, Villa, Aranda, et al., 2008). See Box 43-3 for suggestions to help caregivers.

BOX 43-3 ■ Ways to Help Caregivers

Provide a listening ear. Encourage caregivers to talk about what they do and how they feel, and listen actively to their concerns. Find time to focus on the caregiver's needs, rather than on those of the care recipient.

Give positive feedback and validate their importance to the client's health.

Help the caregiver identify people who may be able to help, for example, family members living outside the home, neighbors, church members, community support groups.

Talk with family and friends, if the caregiver wishes. Teach them how to support the caregiver, for example, by telephoning regularly, visiting, sending cards, or staying with the client a few hours (or days) so the caregiver can rest or take a vacation. Encourage them to listen to the caregiver without giving advice, and to help her feel appreciated (e.g., "I really appreciate all you do for Dad.")

Arrange for a home health aide, if possible. This relieves the caregiver of housekeeping and grocery shopping.

Remind family members and significant others to take care of themselves. Explain that their health is important to both them and the patient. Even the most devoted and self-sacrificing person may understand when you explain, "You must take care of yourself so that you are able to take care of your loved one."

- Stress the need for the person to eat nutritious meals. Arrange for meals to be delivered to the home, if needed.

- Encourage the caregiver to rest as much as possible, perhaps while the home health aide is there; or ask family

members and acquaintances to take turns staying an hour or two with the patient while the caregiver rests or "gets away." Help contact those offering respite care and make a schedule, if needed.

- Stress the need for the caregivers to take some time for themselves, even if it is just an hour alone, or coffee with a neighbor.

- Encourage caregivers to take a vacation, if they can afford it, even if the getaway is close to home or for a short time. Reassure them that competent help can be obtained and that it is okay to delegate caregiving to others for a while.

- Some agencies have a weekend respite program for caregivers. The client is admitted to a skilled care unit for 2 or 3 days so the caregiver can have a break.

Encourage the caregiver to maintain spiritual connections, for example, to take time to go to church; or ask the spiritual adviser to visit the home.

Communicate medical updates about the client—lab results, new treatment plans, and so on.

Help the family understand the goals of care and solve problems when needed.

Teach the family what to expect with regard to medications, treatments, and signs of approaching death. If family members know what is normal, they will be less likely to panic or fear the inevitable.

Follow up with other healthcare team members promptly if the family has questions that are outside your scope of practice.

To explore learning resources for this chapter,

Go to DavisPlus at DavisPl.us/Wilkinson3.

Chapter Resources for Chapter 43:

    Response sheets for all learning activities

    Resources for Caregivers and Health Professionals

    Reading More About Community & Home Nursing (suggested readings)

    Concept Map of chapter content

Interactive Case Studies

NCLEX-Style and Chapter Review Questions

Chapter Overview Podcasts

For references cited,

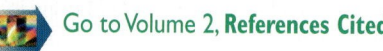

Go to Volume 2, **References Cited**.

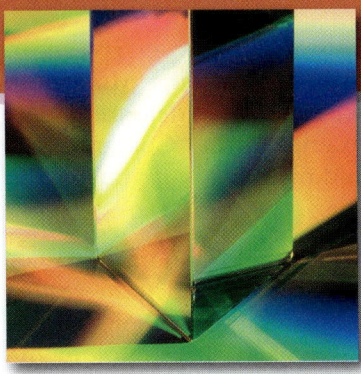

CHAPTER 44

Ethics & Values

Learning Outcomes

After completing this chapter, you should be able to:

➤ Define *morals*, *ethics*, *bioethics*, and *nursing ethics*.

➤ Discuss what is meant by *ethical agency*.

➤ Identify at least four factors that contribute to the frequency of nurses' moral problems.

➤ Differentiate personal values and morality from professional values.

➤ Explain how developmental stages, values, moral frameworks, professional guidelines, and moral principles affect moral decisions.

➤ Describe five major ethical principles that are used in reasoning about healthcare.

➤ Compare and contrast four ethical frameworks: consequentialism (e.g., utilitarianism), deontology, an ethics of care, and feminist ethics.

➤ Identify the ethical issues and principles involved in a given ethical situation.

➤ Describe a systematic approach for resolving ethical dilemmas.

➤ Discuss the concept of an integrity-producing compromise.

➤ Describe the nurse's obligations in ethical decisions.

➤ Discuss the role of the nurse as client advocate in the delivery of ethical nursing care.

➤ Apply the steps identified in the MORAL model to make ethical decisions in patient care.

Key Concepts

Morals
Nursing ethics
Values

Related Concepts

See the Concept Map on Davis*Plus*.

Example Problems

Moral distress
Whistleblowing

Meet Your Patients

Angie and Edward Frese are a couple with two teenage children. They are a close and loving family with a large network of family and friends. Alan, 15 years old, has just been severely injured in a high school soccer game. At the hospital, Angie and Edward are told that Alan has multiple bone fractures and active internal bleeding.

The surgeon informs the distressed parents that Alan will need a blood transfusion to survive. Although genuinely devastated, the parents adamantly refuse to consent to a lifesaving blood transfusion, stating they are Jehovah's Witnesses and that receiving blood is against their religious beliefs. The surgeon asks you, Alan's nurse, to get the parents to change their minds right away. You talk with the couple, but they continue to refuse a blood transfusion. You immediately contact your charge nurse. Try to answer the following critical-thinking questions about Alan and his parents. You may not have the experience or theoretical knowledge to answer them all—you will acquire that in this and the following chapter—but do your best based on the background you have.

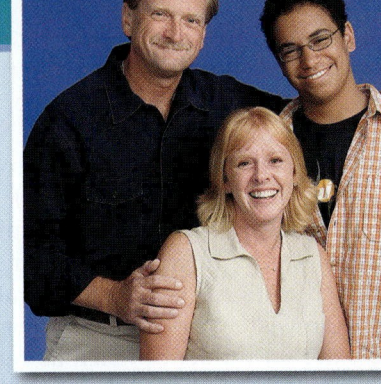

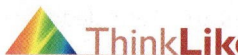

ThinkLike a Nurse 44-1

- Do Alan's parents have the right to refuse a blood transfusion based on their religious beliefs?
- Do you think the fact that Alan is a minor (age less than 18 years) may make a difference in this situation?
- What actions do you think the charge nurse should take?
- Can an ethical conflict such as this be resolved to everyone's satisfaction?

Theoretical Knowledge
knowing why

The theoretical knowledge you will need to begin professional practice includes an understanding of the nature of morals and ethics (and especially nursing ethics) and basic information about factors that affect moral decisions (i.e., values, moral frameworks, professional guidelines, and ethical principles).

ABOUT THE KEY CONCEPTS

Nursing ethics, morals, and **values** are key concepts in this chapter because everything in the chapter is related to those concepts in some way—as you will discover. The subconcepts of *advocacy* and *compromise*, for example, are intimately integrated in the implementation of nursing ethics in clinical practice. Remember to use the key concepts to help you organize chapter content in your mind. As you read, try to understand how each subconcept you encounter relates to nursing ethics, morals, and values.

ETHICS AND MORALS

To understand ethics, we must first understand the broader meaning of ethics. Although the terms *ethics* and *morals* have similar meanings, in modern theory **morals** refers to private, personal, or group standards that consider in a broad, general manner what is good or bad, right or wrong (e.g., "In general, it is wrong to steal"). Ethics answers the question "What should I do in a given situation?" (e.g., "Is it wrong to steal if you have to do it to feed your children?").

Morals are learned from external influences and communicated through various systems (e.g., religious, political, educational, societal). **Moral behavior** is that which is consistent with customs or traditions based on the external influence (such as religious beliefs). A person whose behavior is inconsistent with traditional notions of right and wrong is labeled as immoral. Consider the conversation between two nurses discussing a teenager who assaulted and robbed a wheelchair-bound 92-year-old woman.

> Nurse A: "I cannot believe someone would be so heartless as to attack an innocent, helpless elderly woman."

> Nurse B: "I agree—that person is immoral. Absolutely no morals."

You may agree with this, because you have been taught to respect and protect older adults. Morals are linked to a person's character and often determine how we treat others. Another example is the "Golden Rule," which states that you should treat others as you wish to be treated.

> Can you think of another example of moral behavior that you may have learned as a child?
> Can you identify any morals that are evident in the scenario about Alan at the beginning of the chapter?
> How do his parents' morals influence Alan's care?

Ethics, in contrast, is the study of a system of moral principles and standards, or the process of using them to decide your conduct and actions. Ethics helps us to decide what is right or wrong and what actions should be taken in certain circumstances. While a nurse's moral code would find the act of driving under the influence thoughtless and reprehensible, his ethics as a nurse would require him to provide care to the driver for the injuries received in the motor vehicle accident. In the case of Alan and his family (Meet Your Patients), the ethical decision making is quite different from the moral perspective of Alan's parents. The parents believe a blood transfusion is morally wrong; this fits with their religious beliefs. The surgeon and the nurse, however, believe withholding blood from Alan would be unethical.

Ethics and Law How are laws related to ethics and morals? In some situations, there is a fine line between law and ethics. Think about the following:

- *Law:* It is illegal to drive faster than the speed limit.
  Situation: A child is bleeding profusely and may have cut an artery. The driver drives very fast and even drives through a red light.
  Question: Was that illegal? Was it immoral?
- *Law:* In the United States, it is legal in certain situations to have an abortion.
  Fact: Although everyone would have to agree that the act is legal, people are about evenly divided about whether they believe it is moral.

The adage "Courts are ill equipped to deal with ethical issues" reflects the difficulty of trying to decide a case on a continuum of right and wrong (ethics) versus applying strict legal principles (law). Although ethics is rooted in the religious, political, customs, and other values of a society, you should be able to see now that ethics is not the same as law, religion, institutional practices, or customs. An action that is legal or customary may not be morally right or ethically justifiable. The same holds true of religion. You cannot assume that an accepted practice of a certain religion is an ethical practice in every situation.

What Is Nursing Ethics?

Bioethics refers to the application of ethical principles to healthcare. Bioethics is concerned with every area of healthcare, including direct care of patients, allocation of resources, utilization of staff, and medical and nursing research. **Nursing ethics** is a subset of bioethics. It refers to ethical questions that arise out of nursing practice. The first things to come to your mind may be the dramatic questions such as, "Should we turn off the ventilator and allow this patient to die? Should this baby have surgery even though his quality of life will probably never be good?" "Is abortion moral?" In reality, you may have some input, but the patient, physician, and family will make the final decision in such situations. As a nurse, you are responsible for deciding the nature and extent of your own participation in each situation, and you must support patients who are making ethical decisions or perhaps coping with the results of decisions made by others. Consider the following true story paraphrased from Curtin and Flaherty (1982, pp. 3–4):

A woman took her 6-year-old son to the emergency department (ED) to have a scalp laceration sutured. She tried to calm him by telling him that the doctors would "numb" him and no one would hurt him "on purpose." On arrival, they were placed in a cubicle next to another little boy who was awaiting treatment for a similar laceration. His father was also trying to reassure his son.

In the cubicle of the father and son, a nurse roughly cleansed the cut with no explanation or words of comfort. The physician came and sewed the laceration without a word and without waiting for the local anesthetic to take effect. The boy screamed in pain and terror the whole time. The woman was horrified, and her son was scared. But when the same nurse approached the woman and her son, she was kind and gentle. The same physician carefully injected a local anesthetic and waited for it to take effect before suturing.

Can you think of reasons for the stark differences in the treatment? Was it because the man and boy appeared to be of lower socioeconomic status? Was it the presence of a father rather than a mother? Was it because the father and son were from a minority group and the woman and son were not? It may have been all of these reasons or none of them. Regardless of why it happened, what makes this case important? After all, both boys received medical treatment; both incisions will heal; no one's life or health was threatened; no life-and-death decisions were made. But notice that the first child's humanity and dignity were violated, and the actions were not fair.

Key Point: *This case is a perfect example of nursing ethics: questions that have to do with the nurse's actions, not the actions of others. The nurse did not need a medical prescription or permission from hospital administration to act ethically.*

In the Meet Your Patients scenario, you, as the nurse, are not responsible for deciding the broad questions: "Is blood transfusion right or wrong?" "Do the parents have a right to refuse blood transfusion?" *Your* decision is "What should *I* do? Should I try to persuade the parents to change their minds, as the surgeon directs, or not?" That is the *nursing ethics* question. And in that scenario, you will need to deal with the effects of the final decision on Alan. He may be frightened; he may be angry; he may die. The nurse is there for patients' most human and vulnerable moments.

Why Should Nurses Study Ethics?

Nurses should study ethics for a variety of reasons. This section will help you understand those reasons.

- *You will encounter ethical problems frequently in your work.* A consciously made, informed decision must surely be better than one made without awareness of the ethical issues involved. The most difficult questions you will face as a nurse will not be "How do I do this?" but "Should I do this?"
- *Ethics is central to nursing.* Commitment to caring for other human beings supports the claim that nursing is a moral art (Butts & Rich, 2012). Caring for the sick, promoting health, and practicing with care and compassion are central values in nursing.
- *Multidisciplinary input is important.* No one profession is responsible for an ethical decision. As situations become more complex, multidisciplinary input becomes increasingly important. For example, surgeons are responsible for knowing what surgery to perform and obtaining consent, but the nurse has a part in being sure the patient is adequately informed so that true consent is obtained.
- *Ethical knowledge is necessary for professional competence.* Being a professional includes being accountable to others in the profession for the ethical conduct of your work. Using professional expertise for social good is one hallmark of a profession. Therefore, to conduct our work well and have it stand the test of public scrutiny, we need to be clear about the ethics of our work.
- *Ethical reasoning is necessary for nursing credibility among other disciplines.* For your opinion to be valued by others, you must be able to clearly express your moral position in a logical way. To be a truly accountable practitioner, you must be able to (1) understand your own values as they relate to basic morality and (2) use ethical reasoning to articulate your moral position.
- *Ethical proficiency is essential for providing holistic care.* Nurses deal with the whole person—that includes providing support for spiritual and moral concerns.
- *Nurses have a responsibility to be advocates for patients.* **Advocacy** is the communication and defense of the rights and interests of another. Since the 1960s, schools have socialized nurses to include patient advocacy in their role conceptions. Currently, the American Nurses Association (ANA) Code of Ethics for Nurses

(2001), provision 3, states: "The nurse promotes, advocates for and strives to protect the health, safety and rights of the patient."

Advocacy includes protecting patients' legal or moral rights (e.g., taking appropriate action when the actions of a healthcare team member jeopardize the patient's rights or best interests). However, you can advocate for patients in everyday practice, for example, by contacting a primary provider to request a new prescription when a pain medication is not effective. To advocate for patients in ethical situations, you must be able to identify the ethical issues, know your resources, and communicate the patient's wishes.

- *Studying ethics will help you to make better decisions.* The study of ethics prepares you to analyze moral problems from multiple perspectives rather than relying entirely on your personal values, intuition, and emotions. Practice in analyzing ethical dilemmas will help you to become an informed decision maker, capable of understanding the perspectives of all the people in each situation—to understand, for example, why the Freses (Meet Your Patients) are refusing a blood transfusion.

Most nursing problems have more than one acceptable answer. This is especially true of ethical problems. Each situation is unique in its details—for example, the people are different in how they evaluate what is and is not beneficial for themselves. By thinking it through critically from several different perspectives, you will be assured that you have done all that you can to provide your client with the highest quality of ethical care.

KnowledgeCheck 44-1

- Define *morals*, and give an example that is not in the text.
- Define *ethics*, and give an example that is not in the text.
- How is bioethics different from ethics?
- Why do nurses need to study ethics?

What Is Ethical Agency?

Moral agency or **ethical agency** for nurses is the ability to base their practice on professional standards of ethical conduct and to participate in ethical decision making. Simply stated, it means that nurses have choices and are responsible for their actions. An ethical agent must be able to:

- Perceive the difference between right and wrong.
- Understand abstract moral principles.
- Reason and apply moral principles to make decisions, weigh alternatives, and plan sound ways to achieve goals.
- Decide and choose freely.
- Act according to choice (this assumes both the power and the capability to act).

For a more expanded discussion of ethical agency,

 Go to Chapter 44, **Supplemental Materials: Elements of Ethical Agency,** on Davis*Plus.*

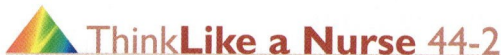 Think**Like a Nurse 44-2**

Consider the five components of ethical agency. To what extent do you believe nurses possess those abilities? Explain your thinking.

Example Problem: Moral Distress

In practice, nurses may find themselves in situations in which they feel morally responsible and have identified an ethically acceptable course of action, but are unable to implement their moral decisions. A seminal study by Wilkinson (1987/1988) identified this as **moral distress**. Situational pressures (constraints) influence nurses' moral decisions as well as their ability to carry out their decisions. These constraints can be internal (e.g., relationships with physicians, power of nurse administrators, support from other nurses, perception or impact on the patient and family members, or threat of lawsuits) or external (e.g., being socialized to follow orders or policies, doubting their own knowledge, lack of courage, concern of other's opinions, or hope for miracles). Whether these constraints are real or merely perceived, nurses in various studies have named these factors as obstacles to carrying out their moral decisions (Burston & Tuckett, 2012; Jameton, 1984; Varcoe, Pauly, Storch, et al., 2012; Villers & DeVon, 2012; Wiegand & Funk, 2012).

The fact is that even if you make a logical, carefully considered moral decision, you may not be able to do what you believe to be right. This problem is not unique to nurses, and recent studies describe moral distress among other healthcare professionals (e.g., Allen, Judkins-Cohn, deValasco, et al., 2013; Milton, Peacock, Storch, et al., 2010). No one is 100% "free" to choose and act. Actions always have consequences: for you and for others. Nevertheless, if you are confident you have made a good decision and can express it logically and clearly to others, you can at least enter into a conversation with nurse administrators, physicians, and families about what ought to be done.

You should clearly identify the source of your moral distress and initiate actions based on reasoned choices and not emotions. In addition to discussing your concerns with those who can address the issues or provide solutions, you should develop a network of supportive colleagues. Because many sources of moral distress are not limited to nursing, you should involve members from other disciplines to can speak on work environmental issues (Epstein & Delgado, 2010). These approaches should give you a sense of comfort knowing that you have done all you could do, even if it is not all you wished to do.

If you would like an optional, expanded discussion of moral distress,

 Go to Chapter 44, **Supplemental Materials: Moral Distress,** on Davis*Plus.*

Example Problem: Whistleblowing

Nurses experience **moral outrage** when they perceive that others are behaving immorally (Wilkinson, 1987/1988).

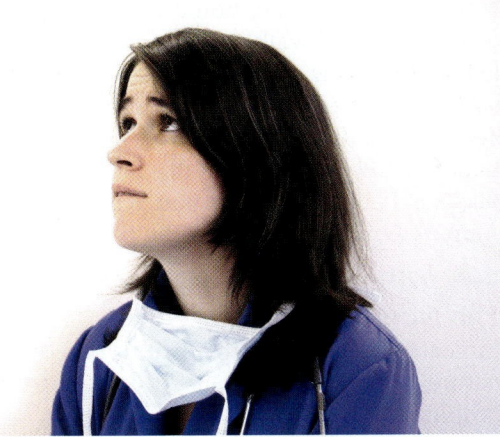

FIGURE 44-1 Ethical problems can create moral distress.

Moral outrage is similar to moral distress, except that in cases of moral outrage, nurses do not participate in the act. Therefore, they do not believe that they are responsible for doing wrong, but that they are powerless to prevent it (Burkhardt & Nathaniel, 2014; O'Mara, Jackson, Batson, et al., 2011). A nurse may respond to moral outrage by "blowing the whistle."

A **whistleblower** is person who reveals information about the practices of others that he reasonably believes is corruption; mismanagement; fraud; abuse; illegal; or harmful to the health, safety, and welfare of the general public. The "others" in question may be an individual or an entire organization. When the wrongdoing involves an organization, the whistleblower must hold the situation up to public scrutiny, for example, by going to the news media or pursuing legal recourse.

At some point in your nursing career, you may become aware that a team member is doing something illegal, unethical, or incompetent. It is difficult to know what to do. You will need to consider the nature of the action, the likelihood of immediate harm, and the accuracy and completeness of your data. If it involves an immediate threat to the health, safety, and well-being of others, you should report it immediately. In other situations, you should follow **THINK**:

Talk with an attorney or other legal representative.

Have concrete and credible evidence of the violation or wrongdoing.

Institute a survival plan, if your job is put in jeopardy or you are fired.

Note the nature and consequences of the problem—its type, severity, and potential impact. Weigh the risks against the benefits.

Know your reporting options and support systems. The systems involve that can correct the problems.

Impaired Nursing Practice Whistleblowing is difficult in the case of an impaired colleague. **Impaired nursing practice** occurs when the nurse's ability to perform the essential functions of nursing is diminished by chemical dependence on drugs or alcohol or by mental illness. Impairment is a threat to patients, and the impaired nurse may have difficulty being accountable to herself or in assessing her self-competence. The Code of Ethics for Nurses guides that as a compassionate colleague, you must ensure that an impaired nurse receives assistance in regaining optimal function by reporting the behaviors to the appropriate entity within the employment setting (ANA, 2001)

Toward Evidence-Based Practice

Attree, M. (2007). Factors influencing nurses' decisions to raise concerns about care quality. *Journal of Nursing Management, 15*(4), 392–402.

Professional ethics require nurses to raise concerns about standards of practice; however, underreporting is the norm. This qualitative study analyzed data from interviews with 142 nurses and found that nurses perceived reporting concerns to be a high-risk, low-benefit action. They lacked confidence in reporting systems. Nurses named fear of repercussions, retribution, labeling, and blame as reasons for not raising concerns, as well as the belief that nothing would be done about the concerns.

Peters, K., Luck, L., Hutchinson, M., et al. (2011). The emotional sequelae of whistleblowing: Findings from a qualitative study. *Journal of Clinical Nursing, 20* (19/20), 2907–2014.

Fourteen nurses who were either whistleblowers or the subject of a whistleblowing episode identify persistent, severe emotional distress after the incident due to a lack of social support and an unwelcoming work environment. Three major themes emerged from their interviews: (1) feelings of overwhelming distress, sadness, and depression; (2) physical symptoms associated with anxiety, insomnia, and hypervigilance; and (3) constant thoughts about the situation, resulting in nightmares and constant stress. While moral distress may cause nurses to become whistleblowers, the act itself can create long lasting emotional distress.

1. What type of moral situation (for the nurse) is best illustrated by the Peters study: moral distress or whistleblowing? Explain your reasoning.

2. How does the Peters study impact your thoughts of becoming a whistleblower?

KnowledgeCheck 44-2

- Define *ethical agency*.
- What five abilities must be present for ethical agency to exist?
- List at least three constraints that can keep nurses from carrying out their moral decisions.

What Are Some Sources of Ethical Problems for Nurses?

Several factors contribute to the frequency of nurses' ethical problems, including societal factors, the nature of nursing work, and the nature of the nursing profession itself.

Societal Factors

This section discusses how some ethical problems for nurses are created by the ever-changing nature of our dynamic, multicultural society.

Increased Consumer Awareness Historically, the healthcare system operated in a paternalistic manner. Sick people sought and followed the advice of a physician without question. Now, the Internet has increased consumer awareness and availability of information online, and consumers are more actively involved in healthcare decisions. Providers are now expected to share knowledge with patients, defend treatment choices different from those found on the Internet, and obtain truly informed consent for treatments.

Technological Advances New technology brings new ethical issues. For example, in vitro fertilization and embryo transfer methods raise questions about the disposal of embryos that are not implanted into a uterus: Who owns them? If implanted, child support issues may arise. Other ethical questions surround the topics of late-term abortions when amniocentesis reveals fetal defects, genetic engineering, human embryonic stem cell research, costs versus quality of life for ventilator-dependent patients, and security of electronic healthcare records (EHRs).

Multicultural Population We live in a multicultural, multifaith society. You cannot assume that your values and beliefs are similar to those of your patient, other providers, and your colleagues. You will need to respect a variety of belief systems, and serve as a patient advocate even when the patient's value system is strikingly different from your own. There are nursing theories that can help you recognize various cultural values, for example, Leininger's (2002) theory of Cultural Care Diversity and Universality (for a review, see Chapters 8 and 15).

Cost Containment The emphasis on reducing healthcare costs creates many morally questionable situations. For example, patients are being sent home from the hospital while they still require considerable nursing care. On being discharged, they may discover that insurance payments are limited for services outside the hospital, including specialists, home care, and medical supplies (e.g., bandages, walkers). Cost containment efforts have led healthcare agencies to increase the number of patients each nurse is assigned. You will undoubtedly find yourself in situations in which fewer nurses are available than patient acuity requires. You will have to make personal decisions about how far you will stretch your own resources to maintain patient safety.

The Nature of Nursing Work

Ethical problems exist in all kinds of work. However, the nature of nursing work itself can create unique ethical problems.

Nurses' Moral Problems

Nurses' moral problems are immediate, serious, and frequent. In the classroom, you have the luxury to leave questions unsettled. In the real world, you must always decide: Either you take action or you do not. For a nurse, deciding *not* to act is, in effect, an act. For example, suppose the family wishes a patient to have aggressive resuscitation efforts (code). However, you know the patient does not wish to be "coded." When the patient's heart stops, whether or not you know the "right" thing to do, you must decide immediately to carry out or not carry out the code. If you wait too long to ponder the ethical issues, the patient may die before you decide. If you do not decide, the effect is the same as though you had decided it was wrong to code.

Nurses' Unique Position in Healthcare Organizations

Nurses have multiple obligations and relationships, and sometimes conflicting loyalties. They are employees (with a relationship with the agency) as well as professionals (with a special relationship with patients). In addition, they have peer relationships and a unique relationship with providers. Although nurses are usually not employed by a physician, they are expected to follow physician prescriptions for patient care. In addition, in most organizations, providers are higher on the power and status hierarchy than are nurses. Ethical questions arise when nurses experience conflicts among their loyalties to patients, families, physicians, employers, and other nurses. Consider the following example: A patient wants to know his test results; but the provider is reluctant to tell him. What are the conflicting loyalties? Should the nurse give the patient the information or not? There are two options:

Tell. By providing the test results, the nurse would honor the principle of personal autonomy and her obligation to the patient. But this might harm the patient's relationship with the provider, which is important to the patient's well-being. Furthermore, if the nurse tells the patient his test results, it may create problems between the provider and the employer (e.g., the hospital). In addition, this action may in some instances violate hospital policies, and, therefore, harm the nurse's relationship with the hospital. It will certainly affect her relationship with the provider.

Don't tell. The nurse could preserve the patient–provider relationship by withholding the test results from the patient. This choice does not honor her relationship with the patient. Also, if the nurse does not tell the patient his test results, the patient may find out anyway and be angry with the hospital, the physician, and the nurse.

According to professional ethics, your first allegiance is to the patient. However, the patient's needs often conflict with institutional policies, family desires, or even laws of the state. There may also be conflicts in your relationships with the patient and his family. You can see an example of this in the Meet Your Patients scenario, wherein the nurse finds it impossible to honor the parents' autonomy and at the same time advocate for Alan. You may also encounter this type of conflict when a patient does not want any heroic measures and wishes only to die peacefully, but the family has not yet been able to accept the imminent death and are insisting on full resuscitation.

The Nature of the Nursing Profession

Some ethical problems arise because of value conflicts and a lack of clarity within the nursing profession. We have unresolved questions about the nature, scope, and goals of our practice, as well as our professional values (values are discussed later in the chapter). In most of the following examples, we value both of the opposites. We would not wish to give up either one. But specific situations require us to choose between them, and that is one source of our discomfort.

- ***Caring versus time spent with patients.*** Nursing values caring, humanistic care, and nurse–patient relationships—but nurses now spend less time with the patient than ever before. One reason is understaffing and heavier patient loads, but there are other factors: the use of technology; the need for careful documentation; and the emphasis on leading, managing, and delegating instead of hands-on care.
- ***Autonomy versus escaping hard choices.*** On one hand, we believe nurses should have an equal status with other healthcare professionals—on the other hand, many nurses want to escape hard choices by "letting the provider decide."
- ***Higher pay versus cost-effectiveness.*** Most nurses believe we deserve higher pay—yet, we claim nurses are cost effective because we work less expensively than do physicians and other providers.
- ***Professionalism versus caring.*** On one hand, we claim the nurse is a professional, citing critical thinking, knowledge, and management skills—on the other hand, we emphasize caring, with the nurse at the bedside offering comfort and doing hands-on tasks.

WHAT FACTORS AFFECT MORAL DECISIONS?

By now, you should have an idea of the nature of morals and ethics and of the need to study nursing ethics. We turn our focus now to some basic theoretical knowledge about factors that are involved in making moral decisions: developmental stages, values, moral frameworks, ethical principles, and professional guidelines. As you learn about each of these concepts, consider how it affects moral decision making.

Developmental Stage

A person's stage of moral development affects the way he reasons about moral issues. We learn and internalize our morals throughout the life span, beginning in childhood. Kohlberg's (1968, 1981) research led him to conclude that children go through a sequence of moral reasoning ability, proceeding through several stages. In stage I, they base moral reasoning on avoiding punishment and personal interest; in stage II, principles focus on pleasing others and following rules. In stage III, the final level in adulthood, people base moral principles on universal and impartial principles of justice (see Moral Development Theory: Kohlberg in Chapter 9). If you would like to have an expanded version of that theory and examples of Kohlberg's stages,

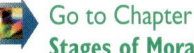 Go to Chapter 44, **Tables, Boxes, Figures: ESG Table 44-1, Stages of Moral Development,** on Davis*Plus.*

The stages overlap. Kohlberg found that more than half of a person's thinking always reflects the stage he is in, with the remainder at the stage he is leaving or the stage into which he is moving. Although some people never achieve Kohlberg's highest levels, progression through the stages is always forward—except in extreme trauma, it is never backward—and people do not skip stages.

Gilligan (1993) challenged Kohlberg's perspective of moral development, citing it as male biased. Gilligan found through her research that girls develop morally by paying attention to community and to relationships, whereas boys tend to process dilemmas through more abstract ideals or principles. If you need a review of Gilligan's three stages—caring for oneself, caring for others, and caring for self and others—refer to Chapter 9.

Values, Attitudes, and Beliefs

Your values influence what you think and do. This is important to know because values are entangled in all ethical situations. If asked, could you say what your values are? Could you explain how they affect your decisions about right and wrong in a given situation? If so, that's a great beginning. If not, you will learn more as you move through this section.

What Are Values? A **value** is a belief about the worth of something; it serves as a principle or a standard that influences decision making. Values are ideals, beliefs, customs, modes of conduct, qualities, or goals that are highly prized or preferred by individuals, groups, or society. You can value an idea, a person, a way of doing things, or even an object (e.g., money). People express their values through behaviors, feelings, knowledge, and decisions. For example, the nurse who values compassion will interact with patients in a sensitive, caring manner.

Your **value set** is your "list" of values. It gives direction for your life and forms a basis for behavior. Your **value system** is your value set ranked from the most important value to the least important. Your value system begins to emerge shortly after birth and continues throughout your life, as various sources (parents, teachers, religious figures, peers, and so on) influence your values. The total number of values a person has is rather small. The number of significant ones is even smaller. It is easy enough to identify values—for example, love, freedom, courage, and responsibility—but how many of them have a consistent and predictable impact on your actions? Those are the significant values.

Values are highly individualized. They can vary and change with new experiences. As you progress through your study of nursing, you will incorporate the professional values associated with the practice of a registered nurse (e.g., caring, compassion, human dignity). You will experience role conflict when your values are different from practice expectations.

KnowledgeCheck 44-3

- What are values?
- What are three characteristics of values?

 ## ThinkLike a Nurse 44-3

- Think about what you value personally in your own life. What are the five ideals, principles, or things that are most important to you?
- Now refer to Chapter 15, where you were asked to list five ideals, principles, or things that were most important to you. What did you list then? Is your list any different now that you have gained some clinical experience and theoretical knowledge?

What Are Attitudes? **Attitudes** are mental dispositions or feelings toward a person, object, or idea. They have three components: cognitive (thinking), affective (feeling), and behavioral (doing). These make up our way of responding to situations or things. For example, you might have a positive *attitude* about cleanliness—that is, you may think it is a good thing (e.g., "The floor is clean. That's nice.") But if you *value* cleanliness, you would be willing to scrub the floor. You would also wash your hands at appropriate times, bathe regularly, and teach others about hygiene.

What Are Beliefs? A **belief** is something that one accepts as true (e.g., "I believe that germs cause disease and that by washing my hands I remove germs"). Beliefs are sometimes based on faith and sometimes on facts. A belief may or may not be true.

 Our beliefs can be altered by acquiring knowledge and experiences. Research shows that nursing students' attitudes toward and beliefs about older adults changed when they spent quality time with older adults and were given the appropriate geriatric assessment tools. The students' misperceptions were replaced with an understanding of the unique needs, abilities, and desires of geriatric clients (Potter, Clarke, Hackett, et al., 2013).

Beliefs may or may not involve values. Consider the following statements of belief.

"I believe the Earth is round." (Does not involve a value)

"Working hard to achieve goals is important to me; therefore, I believe that I must work during the summer to save money for college." (Involves a value)

From those examples, can you see how values, beliefs, and behaviors are related?

How Are Values and Ethics Related? Values and morals are learned in conscious and unconscious ways and become a part of your makeup. When we evaluate right and wrong, or good and bad, we are using moral judgment. Therefore, our individual preferences (values) of right or wrong become our moral values. Whether or not you are aware of it, your values shape the manner in which you make ethical decisions in your nursing practice (Burkhardt & Nathaniel, 2014; Butts & Rich, 2012).

So, although ethics are based on a structured set of principles and theories, and ethical decisions are publicly stated in terms of possible alternative behaviors, such decisions are always influenced unconsciously by our own personal and moral values.

Key Point: *It is important to clarify the influence of your values each time you enter into a situation in which you are called on to be objective in your decision making.*

 ## ThinkLike a Nurse 44-4

- Think about Alan and his family (Meet Your Patients). What do you think were the values of Alan's parents that influenced their behavior at the hospital? First, identify their behaviors specifically. Then speculate about the values underlying each behavior.
- How do you think values can influence health?

KnowledgeCheck 44-4

- Define *belief*; give a new example.
- Define *attitude*; give a new example

Professional Versus Personal Values

Your **personal value system** is a set of values that you have reflected on and chosen that will help you to lead a good life (Purtilo, 2010). You have internalized some *societal values* and have come to perceive them as your own (e.g., good manners, such as saying "Please" and "Thank you"). In addition, you probably have some *personal values* (e.g., friendship, fairness, creativity) that are important to you but may or may not be important to society at large.

As you move forward in your profession, you will integrate what you learn and experience and form **professional values** (e.g., caring, autonomy, veracity, competence, justice). Many of these will simply expand your personal values. The American Association of Colleges of Nursing (AACN) has identified six professional values. These are included in Table 44-1, along with other professional values. Personal and professional values are not always congruent, though. Consider the following situation:

> Alexandra Jensen is a 17-year-old pregnant girl who comes in to your ambulatory surgical center for a voluntary termination of an early pregnancy. You are assigned to admit her to your unit and get her ready for this procedure. Imagine that your personal value in this situation is that you do not believe in abortion but that your professional value is guided by the ANA standards of professional practice, which state that the nurse "delivers care in a manner that preserves and protects patient autonomy, dignity, rights, values and beliefs" (ANA, 2010, p. 137). It is difficult to hold a personal value in high regard while under pressure to assume a conflicting professional value. How might you feel in the situation just described?

Do you think that your personal and professional values need to be compatible in order for you to be a competent nurse? Do you think that you should have the absolute right to refuse to participate in a situation (such as the one above) that may violate your personal values?

ThinkLike a Nurse 44-5

- Name some other examples of societal values.
- What groups and social experiences have helped to form your values?
- Examine your personal values to see whether they match the AACN's professional values (see Table 44-1).
  Which of those values, if any, do you not share? Explain your thinking.
  Name a few of your personal values that are not found on this list of professional values.

KnowledgeCheck 44-5

- What is the difference between personal and professional values?
- What is an example of professional values?
- What are some other types of values?

How Are Values Transmitted?

As you have learned, we acquire values from social interaction. So how does that work? How are values transmitted? Table 44-2 outlines the methods of value transmission. Research reports the reciprocal transmission of values between parents and adolescents and that the presence of a receptive and supportive parent makes value transmission more likely (Pinquart & Silbereisen, 2004). Another study found only a marginally positive relationship between maternal and adolescent values. However, when adolescents' basic needs (i.e., for autonomy, competence, and relatedness) were satisfied within the home, their values were more aligned with maternal values (Lekes, Joussemet, Koestner, et al., 2011).

What Is Value Neutrality?

You have probably been taught that nurses need to be nonjudgmental in working with their clients. As a nurse, you have a duty to provide the best care to clients. You should not assume that your personal values are right, and you should not judge the client's values as right or wrong on the basis of whether they agree with your value system. Think back to the discussion regarding Alexandra, who was seeking to terminate her pregnancy. A nurse who does not believe in abortion could still provide competent nursing care to Alexandra even though his personal values regarding abortion are different from Alexandra's. **Value neutrality** means that we attempt to understand our own values regarding an issue and to know when to put them aside, if necessary, to become nonjudgmental when providing care to clients. However, you should know that some healthcare professionals believe value neutrality is not possible to achieve. Further, they say it is not even desirable because it obligates healthcare providers to suppress or modify their own deepest moral and religious beliefs (Balch, 2006; Clark, 2006).

KnowledgeCheck 44-6

- What are some ways that values can be transmitted?
- What is value neutrality?

Ethical Frameworks

Ethics uses specific rules, theories, principles, and perspectives to inquire into the justification of an individual's actions in a particular situation. **Ethical** (or **moral**) **frameworks** are systems of thought (theories) that are the basis for the differing perspectives people have in ethical situations. Many such philosophical frameworks are rooted in ancient works, for example, of the Greek philosophers Plato and Aristotle. See Chapter 8 if you need to review the purposes and uses of theories.

There is no single "best" theory that will provide the one "true" answer to an ethical problem, as the value of theories is that each one provides a different perspective. Using more than one framework to analyze a situation enables you to perform a more comprehensive analysis of the problem.

Key Point: *No matter how well you know the theories, they will not provide the "right" answers for what to do in a specific patient situation. They merely offer a lens through which you can examine an ethical problem.*

Table 44-1 ➤ American Association of Colleges of Nursing (AACN) and Other Professional Nursing Values and Behaviors

VALUES	SAMPLE PROFESSIONAL BEHAVIORS
Altruism	
Concern for the welfare and well-being of others. Altruism is reflected by the nurse's concern for the welfare of patients, other nurses, and other healthcare providers. Includes patient advocacy.	■ Demonstrates understanding of cultures, beliefs, and perspectives of others. ■ Advocates for patients, particularly the most vulnerable. ■ Takes risks on behalf of patients and colleagues. ■ Mentors other professionals.
Autonomy	
The right to self-determination—to choose and act on that choice. Every competent person has the right to decide his own course of action.	■ Plans care in partnership with patients. ■ Honors the right of patients and families to make decisions about healthcare. ■ Provides information so that patients can make informed choices. ■ Informs patients about details of their care (e.g., test results).
Human Dignity	
Respect for the inherent worth and uniqueness of individuals and populations.	■ Provides culturally competent and sensitive care. ■ Protects the patient's privacy. ■ Preserves the confidentiality of patients and healthcare providers. ■ Designs care with sensitivity to individual patient needs. ■ Values and respects colleagues and patients.
Integrity	
Acting in accordance with an appropriate code of ethics and accepted standards of practice. Includes honesty.	■ Provides honest information to patients and the public. ■ Documents care accurately and honestly. ■ Seeks to remedy errors made by self or others. ■ Demonstrates accountability for own actions.
Social Justice	
Upholding moral, legal, and humanistic principles. Treating others fairly regardless of race, age, citizenship, economic status, disability, or sexual orientation. This value is reflected in professional practice when the nurse works to ensure equal treatment under the law and equal access to quality healthcare.	■ Supports fairness and nondiscrimination in the delivery of care. ■ Promotes universal access to healthcare. ■ Encourages legislation and policy consistent with the advancement of nursing care and healthcare. ■ Works to ensure equal treatment under the law.

Additional professional values frequently cited for nursing

■ Caring

■ Diversity

■ Equality (having the same rights, privileges, or status)

■ Aesthetics (qualities of objects or people that are pleasing)

■ Freedom (capacity to choose)

■ Truth (faithfulness to fact or reality)

■ Service (commitment to work useful to others)

Table 44-1 ➤ American Association of Colleges of Nursing (AACN) and Other Professional Nursing Values and Behaviors—cont'd

VALUES	SAMPLE PROFESSIONAL BEHAVIORS
■ Education (basic and lifelong continuing education for nurses)	
■ Holism	
■ Competence, excellence (skill, knowledge, performance of nursing work)	
■ Loyalty (feeling of duty or attachment to other nurses)	

Sources: American Association of Colleges of Nursing (AACN). (2008). The essentials of baccalaureate education for professional nursing practice. Washington, DC: Author. Retrieved from http://www.aacn.nche.edu/Education/pdf/BaccEssentials08.pdf; Jameton, A. (1984). *Nursing practice: The ethical issues.* Englewood Cliffs, NJ: Prentice Hall; National League for Nursing. (2007). Core values. Retrieved from http://www.nln.org/aboutnln/corevalues.htm; Paquin, S. (2011). Social justice advocacy in nursing: What is it? How do we get there? *Creative Nursing, 17*(2), 63–67; Park, M. (2009). The legal basis of nursing ethics education. *Journal of Nursing Law, 13*(4), 106–113.

Table 44-2 ➤ Modes of Value Transmission

MODE	DESCRIPTION
Modeling	Children learn values from a variety of role models (parents, peers, rock stars, significant others) by observation. This modeling may lead to socially acceptable or unacceptable behaviors.
Moralizing	"This way is the only way." Children are taught a complete set of values in an authoritarian approach. If the child does not conform, the parent may inflict guilt and fear on him. This approach by parents, teachers, church leaders, and other authorities may make it difficult for young people to make independent choices because they have no experience selecting values that are good for them.
Laissez-faire	"Doing your own thing." Children are allowed to explore differing sets of values on their own with little guidance or discipline. This may lead to conflict and confusion on the part of the child.
Reward and punishment	The child's behavior is controlled by offering rewards for certain valued behaviors and punishing the child who fails to comply. Rewards can strengthen behavior, whereas physical punishment may teach that violence is an acceptable behavior.
Responsible choice	A balance of freedom and restriction allows children to select the values, explore new behaviors, and experience the consequences. This can lead to personal satisfaction and parental support.

What Is Consequentialism?

In **consequentialist** theories, the rightness or wrongness of an action depends on the consequences of the act rather than on the act itself. **Utilitarianism**, the most familiar consequentialist theory, asserts that the value of an action is determined by its usefulness. The *principle of utility* states that an act must result in the greatest good (positive benefit) for the greatest number of people. Any act can then become the ethical choice if it delivers "good" results. In healthcare, the principle of "first, do no harm," is consequentialist in nature. Because of this principle, we are always concerned about weighing the risks and benefits of our care (e.g., a medication may kill cancer cells, but side effects may harm the patient's quality of life).

Using utilitarianism to resolve an ethical problem requires you to engage in a risk-benefit analysis. You evaluate every alternative action for its potential outcomes, both positive (pros) and negative (cons)—similar to a technique you may already use when making other decisions. You would then select the action that results in the most benefits for the greatest number of people involved in the situation. The following is an example of utilitarian reasoning: The practice of triage is used in a disaster when emergency workers sort patients to determine who will be treated first or who will receive limited resources (e.g., oxygen or intravenous therapy). If a victim has little potential for survival, he may not be treated at all, or his treatment may be postponed to allow the healthcare team to treat those victims with the greatest potential to survive. (i.e., "the greatest number")

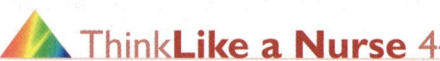

ThinkLike a Nurse 44-6

- Describe a time in your life when you used consequentialism to resolve a difficult situation.
- What types of clinical dilemmas might be best resolved using this theory?

What Is Deontology?

Deontology is based on rules and principles and uses the language of rights and duties. Unlike the utilitarian theory, deontology considers an action to be right or wrong regardless of its consequences. Such decisions are based on moral rules and unchanging principles. There is a variety of deontological theories, but you will commonly find they make use of the following, or similar, principles: ·

The Categorical Imperative This principle, established by the philosopher Immanuel Kant (1724–1804), states that one should act only if the action is based on a principle that is universal—or in other words, if you believe that everyone should act in the same way in a similar situation.

Treat People as Ends and Never as Means This means that the person is more important than the goal you may be trying to accomplish. Can you imagine the ethical concerns created if research subjects were exposed to some amount of risk (e.g., a new surgical procedure) to find a drug or treatment that will benefit many other people?

Moral Rules and Principles When using a deontological model, you would critically examine a situation to determine which actions are right or wrong according to moral rules and principles (e.g., justice, autonomy, doing good, and doing no harm). These principles are regarded as unchanging and absolute, and they come from the same universal values that underlie all major religions.

Rights and Duties Deontological frameworks also emphasize rights (e.g., the right to freedom, the right of self-determination) and duties (obligations). For example, you must help someone in need because you have a duty to help others, not because helping will produce good consequences. In fact, you have a duty to help even if your helping may produce some bad consequences.

Additional Considerations The following are two issues that may arise when using a deontology framework:

- **Conflict of Universal Principles.** Sometimes you must choose between conflicting universal principles. It is not always clear which principle to honor. Allowing Alan's parents (Meet Your Patients) to refuse to provide him with blood honors the principle of autonomy, but their

decision may interfere with a right: Alan's right to life. Can you see that it might be difficult to decide which is the appropriate principle to honor?
- **Evaluating Motives.** In deontology, it is important to consider motives. It is one thing for Alan's parents to refuse a blood transfusion because they are honoring a religious principle; it would be quite another thing if they refused the transfusion because they stood to inherit a large trust fund left to Alan by his grandfather. Motives may place more weight on one of the conflicting universal principles over the other and make a decision clearer. Unfortunately, it is sometimes hard to recognize your own motives, much less to be sure about the motives of others.

Key Point: *As a nurse, you will almost never be able to decide only on the basis of principles and rules; you will always need to consider the consequences of your actions.*

KnowledgeCheck 44-7

- Describe utilitarianism.
- Define *deontology*.

What Is Feminist Ethics?

Feminist ethics is based on the belief that traditional ethical models provide a mostly masculine perspective and that they devalue the moral experience of women (Butts & Rich, 2012). Traditional deontological models focus on abstract principles such as fairness, justice, and rights, which are more typical of male reasoning. In contrast, virtues such as love, relationships, caring, nurturing, and sympathy are more relevant to women but are rarely seen in traditional theories (Butts & Rich, 2012). Feminists assert that focusing on deontological principles distracts one from dealing with larger social issues. Feminist ethical reasoning uses relationships and stories rather than universal principles. Feminists argue that it is impossible to avoid being influenced by one's relationships. They see that influence as positive and believe it should not be lessened by an attempt to be objective—and in any case, that objectivity is impossible anyway.

Feminist theories do use principles and consequences, but they also ask you to look at social issues in the ethical situation to ensure that social facts are considered (Tong & Williams, 2009). The point is to address issues of gender inequality within each situation. This means that part of your reasoning would be to think, "How is this decision affecting the woman?" Consider an example of deciding whether to allocate federally funded healthcare resources to younger people or to older adults. Feminist reasoning on this question might say that, all other considerations being equal:

- In the United States older women outnumber older men.
- Older women tend to be poorer and are more likely to be alone than are men.

- Therefore, if healthcare for older adults were to be rationed, it would negatively affect women more than men.
- Thus, more healthcare resources should be allocated to older adults, especially women.

What Is Ethics of Care?

An **ethics-of-care** nursing philosophy directs attention to the specific situations of individual patients, viewed within the context of their life narrative. You would ask: "What is the story of this person's life? What is going on right now in his life? And what does that have to do with the morality of the action I'm considering?" Care theories (which grew out of feminist ethics) integrate the notion that caring is a natural human quality with the commitment and responsibility that you assume by entering into a helping profession (Lachman, 2012). An ethics of care emphasizes the role of feelings, but also includes some of the principles that are part of traditional ethics, such as *autonomy* (self-determination) or *beneficence* (doing good), responsibility, and commitment.

Using an ethics of care, nurses have a responsibility to care as a part of their professional behavior, consistent with the ANA Code of Ethics. Some aspects of care include the ability and duty to appreciate, understand, and even share the patient's pain or condition. Using a caring framework, your ethical analysis would focus on relationships and client stories. The following guidance is derived from an ethics-of-care philosophy (Edwards, 2009, 2011; Lachman, 2012; Vanlaere & Gastman, 2011):

- View caring as the central force in nursing.
- Promote dignity and respect for patients as people.
- Attend to a person's real needs and maintain the competence to fully address those needs.
- Cultivate a habit of care.
- Redefine fundamental moral principles to include virtues such as kindness, attentiveness, empathy, compassion, and reliability.

Using the caring perspective and patient stories tends to focus discussion at the level at which the relationships are located, rather than on an intellectual plane. Critics of the ethics of care suggest that the term *caring* can be misconstrued to become too sentimental and, therefore, ineffective. Further, unless the sentiment of care is associated with a universal principle, such as justice, favoritism or separateness can occur (Vanlaere & Gastman, 2011).

Ethics-of-care models provide a refreshingly new perspective into moral situations. As you gain more clinical experience, revisit these philosophies and reflect on how they apply to your nursing practice.

KnowledgeCheck 44-8

- How does feminist ethics affect ethical decision making?
- What do ethics-of-care philosophies emphasize?

Ethical Concepts and Principles

Remember from Chapter 8 that theories are made up of concepts and principles. The same is true for ethical theories. Although theories differ, they share some of the same principles. Therefore, ethical concepts and principles are useful in patient care discussions because they provide a common language for healthcare professionals to identify the issues. Even if people disagree about which action is right in a situation, they can agree on which principles apply. Agreement "in principle" can provide common ground for a compromise or other resolution of the problem. We will discuss the ethical principles of autonomy, nonmaleficence, beneficence, fidelity, veracity, and justice.

Autonomy

Autonomy refers to a person's right to choose and ability to act on that choice. It is based on respect for human dignity. You demonstrate respect for autonomy when you treat patients with consideration, believe their stories about the course and symptoms of their illnesses, and protect those who are unable to decide for themselves. You honor autonomy when you respect the patient's or surrogate decision maker's right to decide, without judgment, even when you believe those choices are not in the patient's best interest.

In the Meet Your Patients scenario, if you believed autonomy to be the most important principle in the situation, you would respect Alan's parents' decision to refuse blood products for their son. If respect for autonomy was not your dominant ethical principle, you would probably try to persuade them to change their minds.

Informed Consent. The principle of autonomy underlies informed consent—the right of competent patients to decide for themselves whether to agree to a proposed treatment.

Key Point: *Remember this general nursing principle: "Every competent adult has the right to accept or refuse treatment and should be provided all the information needed to make an informed decision."*

To ensure truly informed consent, patients need to know the diagnosis and related information, the recommended treatment, alternative treatment options, the risks and benefits associated with each, and the providers involved in the treatment regimen. The nurse's role is to verify that the patient understands and to obtain her signature.

Key Point: *The nurse should notify the provider if the patient does not understand the treatment, before obtaining her signature.*

Advance directives help to ensure that treatment given to an incompetent person is in accordance with his previous wishes. They were created to allow adults while they are competent to make decisions about their healthcare that will guide their care when they are incompetent. You can help support autonomy by informing patients about advance directives: the living will and durable powers of attorney for healthcare.

Privacy and Confidentiality The principles of **privacy** and **confidentiality** are also partly derived from the principle of autonomy. An autonomous person has control over the collection of, use of, and access to her personal information. Many patients share sensitive information with nurses that they would not share with others, and it is important to maintain the patient's trust. This means that you should not discuss patients in the elevator, halls, lunchroom, or anywhere it can be overheard, even if the discussion is relevant to the patient's care. You should communicate to those involved in the patient's care only the information needed to provide healthcare. Share other information only with the patient's consent.

You should also be careful not to post pictures of yourself with patients or post patient information on social media sites. Even inadvertently capturing patients in photographs has led to harsh disciplinary actions against the nurse.

Key Point: *A person who knowingly violates the privacy and confidentiality requirements of the Health Insurance Portability and Accountability Act (HIPAA) can face imprisonment of 1 to 10 years and a monetary fine of $50,000 to $250,000, depending on motive.*

If you would like more information about privacy and confidentiality, see Chapters 18 and 45; also

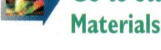 Go to Student Resources, Chapter 44, **Supplemental Materials: Confidentiality and Privacy,** on *DavisPlus.*

Nonmaleficence

The principle of **nonmaleficence** is the twofold duty to do no harm and to prevent harm. Nonmaleficence refers to both actual harm and risk of harm, as well as to intentional and unintentional harm. Both the physicians' Hippocratic Oath and the nurses' Nightingale Pledge state that care providers have a duty to cause no harm to patients. When you are careful to prevent medication errors, or a patient fall by providing a walker, or using an ambulation belt for mobility, you honor the nonmaleficence principle. In nursing it is rare to find intentional harm, but unintentional harm does occur as a result of incompetence or failure to adhere to each component of the nursing process (Beauchamp & Childress, 2012).

Nonmaleficence requires that you think critically and identify the potential risks and benefits in the treatment plan. When using nonmaleficence to guide treatment regimens, ask the question, "Does this treatment cause more harm or more good to the patient?"

- **Risk of harm is not always clear.** Suppose you are about to get a patient out of bed for the first time after surgery. The benefit clearly is that this will prevent postoperative complications such as pneumonia and thrombophlebitis; but the risks, in terms of excessive pain or unintentional damage to the operative site, may be less clear.
- **Weighing risks and benefits is a value-laden exercise.** Who is to say what amount of pain is excessive—you or

the patient? To honor the principle of nonmaleficence in this situation, you would need to be sure to premedicate the patient and carefully assess his status during ambulation.

Respect for Dignity The value of respect for human dignity derives in part from the duty to do no harm. **Respect for dignity** refers to the nurse's respect for the intrinsic worth of each person, without respect to age, race, religion, medical condition, or any other factors. Respect for dignity recognizes that patients are vulnerable, and that nurses should not abuse their relationships for personal gain or exploit or enter into romantic, sexual, or other relationships with their patients. The nurse should at all times maintain professional boundaries. To read more about professional boundaries,

 Student Resources, Chapter 44, **Supplemental Materials: Professional Boundaries,** on *DavisPlus.*

 ThinkLike a Nurse 44-7

Think about the Meet Your Patients scenario in terms of nonmaleficence. The parents refuse to allow a blood transfusion. You, the nurse, have tried to persuade them to change their minds. You do not need to decide what you ought to do; just analyze the situation in terms of the risks.

- What is it that creates the risk for harm to Alan?
- What is the risk for harm to Alan's parents because of the nurse's actions?

Beneficence

Beneficence is the duty to do or promote good. You can think of this principle as being on a continuum with nonmaleficence. At one end of the continuum is beneficence, the duty to bring about positive good; at the other end is the duty to do no harm. The following examples illustrate the duties in priority order:

- Do no harm. (Don't push the man into the river.)
- Prevent harm when you can. (If the man is getting dangerously close to the river's edge, warn him that he is about to fall into the river.)

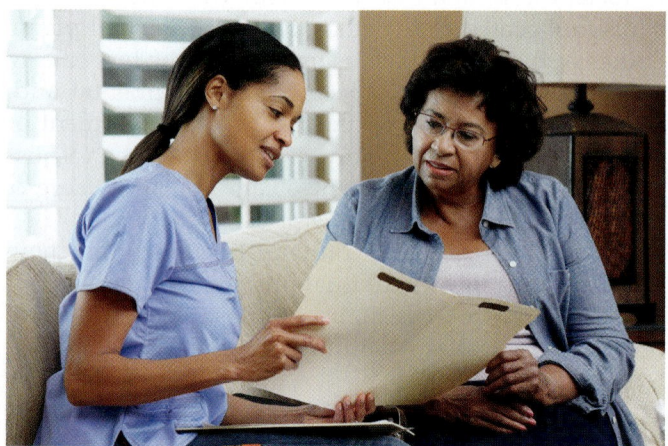

FIGURE 44-2 Nurse involves the patient in her plan of care.

- Remove harm when it is being inflicted. (If you see a struggle and someone is trying to push the man into the river, interfere and try to stop it if you can do so without undue harm to yourself.)
- Bring about positive good. (If the man has fallen in the river, jump in and try to save him, or toss him a lifeline and call 911 if you can't swim.)

When weighing the risks and benefits of an action, you are actually balancing nonmaleficence with beneficence. Keep in mind that patients, family members, and other professionals may identify benefits and harms differently. A benefit to one may represent a burden to another. For example, in Meet Your Patients, you may see a blood transfusion as a benefit to Alan, but to the parents it may represent harm. Doing good very much depends on the context and the rights of the person for whom the action is being taken.

Paternalism   Although beneficence seems like such a positive goal, it can have negative consequences. One such outcome is **paternalism** (treating others like children). This would occur, for example, if you think you know what is best for a competent client and then coerce the client to act as you wish rather than to act as she wishes. Saying to a patient, for example, "Trust us; we know what is best for you to do in this situation," may seem to be beneficent because you are trying to support the patient. But it is actually paternalistic behavior that lacks respect for the patient's autonomy (and therefore represents "harm").

Fidelity

Fidelity (faithfulness) is the duty to keep promises. It is a basic part of every patient care situation. Sometimes the promises are of major significance, such as promising not to share certain information with other members of the healthcare team. At other times it may be only a promise to come back to check the effectiveness of a pain medication or to bring a requested item back to the client's room.

In practice, you will often find that competing tasks prevent you from being able to deliver something exactly as you have promised. Instead of "I'll be right back with your medication," you might be a bit more vague and say, "I'll get back with your medication as quickly as I can" or "I must go help another patient for a few minutes, but I'll get here with your medication as quickly as I can."

Key Point: *The duty to keep a promise is the same regardless of its level of importance. Make promises in a thoughtful, careful manner to maximize the likelihood that you can keep them.*

Veracity

Veracity is the duty to tell the truth. This seems straightforward, but there are times when veracity presents a challenge. For example, should you tell the truth when you know that it might cause harm to the client? Would it be appropriate to tell a lie to relieve extreme patient anxiety? Most nurses would agree that it isn't hard to tell the truth, but at times it may be very hard to determine how *much* of the truth to tell. For example, healthcare professionals may feel uncomfortable giving families "bad news." So instead of saying, "Your father has a fatal illness and is unlikely to live for more than a month," they may say, "Your father is very ill, but we will do everything we possibly can for him." In this, as in most situations, the risk of losing patient trust outweighs any benefit of withholding the truth.

Although you always presume the value of telling the truth, there may be times when you are justified to withhold information. In the United States, we tend to place a high value on autonomy. However, in some cultures, families go to great lengths to protect a dying patient from the harsh truth of his prognosis, and the patient himself may not wish to know. In such a situation, you need to be culturally sensitive so that you may act on the family's values, not on the dominant cultural values. Always consider the context.

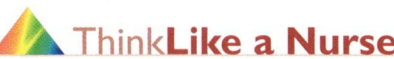

ThinkLike a Nurse 44-8

Review the Meet Your Patients scenario. Alan will not survive without a blood transfusion, yet the parents refuse to allow one. He asks the nurse, "Am I going to die?" You do not need to decide which response is best; just write an example that illustrates each of the following. What might the nurse say if she wishes to:

- Tell Alan the truth?
- Withhold or partially disclose the truth?
- Answer with an untruth?

Justice

Justice is the obligation to be fair. It implies equal treatment of all patients. Questions of justice will become a part of your everyday experience in patient care, from deciding how to allocate your time among patients to larger decisions, such as how to allocate limited healthcare resources.

Distributive Justice

Distributive justice requires fair distribution of both benefits and burdens (Butts & Rich, 2012). It is especially relevant to healthcare, as in the following issues.

- *Allocating resources.* Distributive justice questions come up when more than one person or group competes for the same resources. For example, consider organ transplantation. Human organs are scarce resources. How do we decide which patient should receive an available organ? Is an 18-year-old more deserving of a kidney than a 75-year-old? Is a person with liver disease due to alcoholism less deserving of a liver than someone with liver disease not caused by alcoholism? The decision of who should live and who may die is never an easy decision. In the United States, a national committee sets criteria for how organs will be distributed so the standard of justice is considered.

■ *Fair access to care.* Access to care is a specific kind of healthcare resource. The principle of distributive justice holds that we should provide equal access to healthcare for all. As the baby boomer generation ages and these nurses retire, there will be fewer nurses to care for more aging patients at a time when national healthcare dollars are stretched very thin. How will the nation decide where to spend the limited dollars? How will nurse managers decide how to provide adequate care when they do not have enough nurses on their staff? The ability to develop sound criteria on which to base the allocation of resources is the challenge of distributive justice.

Compensatory Justice

Compensatory justice focuses on making amends for wrongs that have been done to individuals or groups. Malpractice lawsuits consider this type of justice when they decide how much money to award a victim who has been harmed. Groups of citizens may also be harmed. For instance, if a company's unintentional pollution of water was proved to cause cancer in members of the community, a monetary settlement might be made.

Procedural Justice

Procedural justice is important in processes that require ranking or ordering (Landwehr, 2013). For example, institutional policies are written to ensure that the same procedures apply to all clients or employees in the same way (e.g., visiting hours, working on holidays, sick leave). Can you think of an example of procedural justice that you have experienced during your nursing education?

 ThinkLike a Nurse 44-9

Look again at the emergency department situation described in What Is Nursing Ethics? at the beginning of this chapter. In this scenario, two little boys were treated for lacerations. Which principle of justice was violated: distributive, compensatory, or procedural? Explain your thinking.

KnowledgeCheck 44-9

List the definition of each of the six ethical principles.

Professional Guidelines

You should consult professional guidelines when making ethical decisions. Healthcare professionals have an obligation to society to be competent in their field; to allow only qualified persons entry into the profession; to discipline members of the profession who do not practice at an acceptable level; to do no harm; and to use high moral and ethical standards to resolve dilemmas (Husted & Husted, 2008; Landwehr, 2013). You can find ethical standards for nurses in codes of ethics, standards of practice, statements of patients' rights, and in various laws.

Nursing Codes of Ethics

Professional codes of ethics are formal statements of a group's expectations and standards for professional behavior generally accepted by members of the profession. Codes of ethics set forth ideal behaviors, but they are only as effective as the behaviors of the nurses who live up to the codes. The purposes of a nursing code of ethics are to:

■ Inform the public about the profession's minimum standards.
■ Demonstrate nursing's commitment to the public it serves.
■ Outline major ethical considerations of nursing.
■ Provide general guidelines for professional behavior.
■ Guide the profession's self-regulating functions.
■ Remind us of the special responsibility we assume in caring for the sick.

Nursing codes are not legally binding. However, they often exceed legal obligations. In most states, the state board of nursing uses the nursing code of ethics as the standard against which to evaluate a nurse's ethical behavior. The board has the legal authority to censure or reprimand the nurse who does not practice within the boundaries of ethical practice. The following nursing organizations have had long-standing codes to guide nurses' ethical decision making. The codes differ in specific details, but are based on similar principles.

International Council of Nurses The International Council of Nurses (ICN) first adopted its Code of Ethics for Nurses in 1953 as "a guide for action based on social values and needs" (ICN, revised 2012). The ICN Code has since served as the standard for nurses worldwide. The ICN Code stresses respect for human rights, including cultural rights, the right to life and choice, the right to dignity, and the right to be treated with respect. The code is designed to guide nurses in everyday choices, and supports their refusal to participate in activities that conflict with caring and healing. If you wish to see the revised code,

 Go to Student Resources, Chapter 44, **Tables, Boxes, Figures: ESG Box 44-1, ICN Code of Ethics,** on Davis*Plus*.

The American Nurses Association The ANA revised its Code of Ethics for Nurses in 2001 (Box 44-1). The ANA used input from a wide range of nurses and groups to ensure that the revised code would be relevant in many practice settings and reflect current ethical situations. The code has nine provisions, followed by interpretive statements to explain what is meant by each provision. If you would like more information about the ANA Code,

 Go to the **ANA Web site,** at http://www.nursingworld.org/MainMenuCategories/EthicsStandards/CodeofEthicsforNurses

BOX 44-1 ■ American Nurses Association Code of Ethics for Nurses

1. The nurse, in all professional relationships, practices with compassion and respect for the inherent dignity, worth, and uniqueness of every individual, unrestricted by considerations of social or economic status, personal attributes, or the nature of health problems.

2. The nurse's primary commitment is to the patient, whether an individual, family, group, or community.

3. The nurse promotes, advocates for, and strives to protect the health, safety, and rights of the patient.

4. The nurse is responsible and accountable for individual nursing practice and determines the appropriate delegation of tasks consistent with the nurse's obligation to provide optimum patient care.

5. The nurse owes the same duties to self as to others, including the responsibility to preserve integrity and safety, to maintain competence, and to continue personal and professional growth.

6. The nurse participates in establishing, maintaining, and improving healthcare environments and conditions of employment conducive to the provision of quality healthcare and consistent with the values of the profession through individual and collective action.

7. The nurse participates in the advancement of the profession through contributions to practice, education, administration, and knowledge development.

8. The nurse collaborates with other health professionals and the public in promoting community, national, and international efforts to meet health needs.

9. The profession of nursing, as represented by associations and their members, is responsible for articulating nursing values for maintaining the integrity of the profession and its practice, and for shaping social policy.

Source: Reprinted with permission from American Nurses Association, *Code of ethics for nurses with interpretive statements,* ©2001, Nursebooks.org, American Nurses Association, Washington, DC. Used with permission.

BOX 44-2 ■ American Nurses Association Standards of Professional Performance Standard 7. Ethics

Definition: The registered nurse integrates ethical provisions in all areas of practice.

Measurement Criteria

The registered nurse:

- Uses the Code of Ethics for Nurses With Interpretive Statements (ANA, 2001) to guide practice.
- Delivers care in a manner that preserves and protects patient autonomy, dignity, and rights.
- Respects the centrality of the patient/family as core members of any healthcare team.
- Upholds and advocates for patient confidentiality within legal and regulatory parameters.
- Serves as a patient advocate assisting patients in developing skills for self-advocacy and informed decision making.
- Maintains a therapeutic and professional patient–nurse relationship with appropriate professional role boundaries.
- Demonstrates a commitment to practicing self-care, managing stress, and connecting with self and others.
- Contributes to resolving ethical issues of patients, colleagues, community groups, systems, and other stakeholders.
- Takes appropriate action regarding instances of illegal, unethical, or inappropriate behavior that can endanger or jeopardize the best interests of the patient or situation.
- Cooperates in an interprofessional team to make ethical decisions regarding the application of technologies and the acquisition and sharing of data.
- Demonstrates professional comportment (openness, honesty, integrity, and authenticity) (Massachusetts Department of Higher Education, 2010).
- Speaks up when appropriate to question healthcare practice when necessary for safety and quality improvement.

Source: Excerpted from American Nurses Association. (2010). *Nursing: Scope and standards of practice* (2nd ed.). Silver Spring, MD: Author.

ANA Standards of Care

In addition to its Code of Ethics, the ANA sets standards for all aspects of clinical practice. In *Nursing: Scope and Standards of Practice* (2010), standard 7 focuses on ethical practice. This standard (see Box 44-2) directs nurses to practice within the parameters described in the Code of Ethics for Nurses. Standard 7 speaks to the nurse's responsibilities to patients and directs nurses to manage ethical dilemmas and to report practices that are illegal, incompetent, or impaired.

The Patient Care Partnership

When patients are admitted to hospitals or to extended care facilities, they are entitled to specific rights in terms of their treatment: the right to make their own decisions, to be active partners in the treatment process, and to be treated with dignity and respect. Because rights are rooted in values, and because values are derived from culture, patient rights are different throughout the world. In the United States, the American Hospital Association (AHA) published *Patient Care Partnership* (2003). Instead of using "rights" language, this document is written in terms of patient expectations and responsibilities. The *Patient Care Partnership* encourages healthcare providers to be more aware of the need to treat patients in an ethical manner and to protect their rights (Box 44-3).

BOX 44-3 ■ American Hospital Association: The Patient Care Partnership

Patients, when hospitalized, should expect the following:

- High-quality care, including the right to know the identity of caregivers
- A clean, safe environment, including safety, freedom from abuse and neglect, and discussion of any changes in care
- Respect for healthcare goals, values, and spiritual beliefs
- To be involved in making decisions about their care and treatment. This includes receiving information about:

  Health condition and treatments

  The benefits and risks of treatments, and whether a treatment is experimental or part of a research study

  What the patient and family will need to do regarding treatment follow-up after leaving the hospital

- Information about the right to make decisions and to refuse care, including advance directives and counselors or chaplains available to help with decision making
- Protection of their privacy and confidentiality
- Help reviewing the bill and filing insurance claims
- Preparation and information when leaving the hospital, including:

  Identification of sources for follow-up care and whether the hospital has a financial interest in any of the referrals

  Coordination of hospital activities with caregivers outside the hospital

  Information and training about the self-care the person will need at home

Source: Excerpted and adapted from American Hospital Association. (2003). *The patient care partnership: Understanding expectations, rights and responsibilities.* Chicago: Author.

To see the complete brochure,

 Go to **The American Hospital Association Web site, The Patient Care Partnership,** at http://www.aha.org/aha/issues/Communicating-With-Patients/pt-care-partnership.html

The Joint Commission Accreditation Standards

The Joint Commission standards contain sections on organizational ethics and individual rights. The section on organizational ethics requires ethical behavior in care, treatment, services, and business practices. The patient's values, preferences, need for information, and other factors that promote autonomy must be considered in her plan of care. It includes a statement about the need to provide for meeting patient needs in the event care must be denied in the institution. In meeting the patient's needs, you must also consider the organization's legal responsibility.

KnowledgeCheck 44-10
- How would the nurse use a professional guideline or code of ethics to assist in the ethical decision-making process?
- What are some examples of such resources?

ETHICAL ISSUES IN HEALTHCARE

As a nurse, you are likely to encounter several ethical issues that occur in healthcare. For example, ethical questions arise in the following situations:

Abortion

Acquired immune deficiency syndrome (AIDS)

Advance directives

Allocation of healthcare goods and services

Compelling unwanted treatment

Confidentiality and privacy (e.g., reporting gunshot wounds and child abuse)

Do Not Attempt Resuscitation (DNAR) orders

Euthanasia, assisted suicide, aid in dying, extraordinary (heroic) measures to prolong life

Informed consent

Organ transplantation

Reproductive technology (e.g., in vitro fertilization, surrogate mothering, sex preselection)

Withdrawing or withholding life-sustaining treatments (e.g., ventilators, artificial nutrition, and hydration)

Extended discussion of those specific issues is best addressed in an ethics text or an ethics course. However, if you wish to learn some basic information about these situations and the ethical conflicts surrounding them,

 Go to Student Resources, Chapter 44, **Supplemental Materials: Ethical Issues in Healthcare,** on Davis*Plus.*

PracticalKnowledge knowing **how**

To fulfill your professional obligations for ethical practice, you will need practical knowledge of the processes of values clarification, ethical decision making, patient advocacy, and integrity-producing compromise.

■ ASSESSMENT/ANALYSIS/DIAGNOSIS

A holistic, comprehensive patient assessment will help you establish the context in which ethical decisions are made. For patients struggling with moral (ethical) issues, the following diagnoses may apply:

- *Decisional Conflict*—Use this label when the patient is uncertain about which course of action to take. The patient may verbalize distress and uncertainty, may delay decision making, may show physical signs of distress (e.g., increased heart rate), and may question moral rules and values and personal beliefs.
- *Moral Distress*—Use this label when the patient has made a moral decision but is unable to carry out the

chosen action. Cues include expressions of powerlessness, guilt, frustration, anxiety, self-doubt, and fear.

NANDA-I also lists other diagnoses in the Value/Belief/Action Congruence class, including Spiritual Distress and Risk for Spiritual Distress.

VALUES CLARIFICATION

Values clarification refers to the process of becoming conscious of and naming one's values (Burkhardt & Nathaniel, 2014). If you are clear about your values, you will be more able to make good decisions and to avoid imposing your values on others. Because each person has his own unique values set, it is important that you appreciate how others' values influence their decisions. Clarifying values should be a positive process of growth that results in more awareness, empathy, and insight (Peate, Watts, & Wakefield, 2013; Roberts, 2012). A values clarification process does not tell you what your values ought to be; it merely helps you discover what they are. Values change over time, so you may need to repeat the process more than once in your lifetime.

How Can I Clarify My Values?

As a nurse, you will need to examine your values regarding life, death, wellness, and illness. A good place to start is to ask yourself questions about situations that you think you may be uncomfortable with, such as caring for a substance abuser seeking drugs in the emergency department, an unwed adolescent mother pregnant for the second time in 11 months, or parents such as the Freses (Meet Your Patients), who refuse treatment for a child because of religious beliefs. Ask yourself questions such as:

- Could I take care of this person?
- Does this bother me?
- What would I do if confronted with such a situation?
- Could I provide the same quality care as for my other patients?

If you would like to use some exercises that can help you begin to clarify your values related to healthcare,

 Go to Student Resources, Chapter 44, **Tables, Boxes, Figures: ESG Box 44-2, Rank-Ordering Values** and **ESG Box 44-3, Values Preference Exercise,** on Davis*Plus.*

Remember that there are no right or wrong answers to values clarification exercises. They are designed to assist you to identify your values and examine their relevance in your personal and professional life.

How Can I Help Clients to Clarify Their Values?

Some clients may exhibit behaviors that indicate that their values are not clear. Consider this example:

Jon White is the chief executive officer of a large healthcare facility. Jon has had two myocardial infarctions (heart attacks) in the past 5 years. He also has hypercholesterolemia (high cholesterol) and hypertension (high blood pressure). Jon's physician has prescribed a heart medicine, low-dose aspirin, and medications to control his hypertension and cholesterol. Jon has repeatedly been taught about his diet, medications, and activity. He insists he is compliant. Jon's wife tells you that he has stopped exercising and is eating whatever he wants, including saturated fats. Jon tells her it is okay to eat what he wants because he is taking a "cholesterol-buster" pill.

The following patient behaviors may indicate that a patient needs values clarification:

- Ignoring the advice of a health professional
- Patient's words not consistent with his actions
- Numerous admissions for the same problem
- Uncertainty or confusion about which action to take

Which of those behaviors did Jon exhibit? To help Jon clarify his values, you might ask him to list the three things that are most important to him in life. Or you might help him work through the steps in Table 44-3 (choosing, prizing, and acting).

KnowledgeCheck 44-11

- What is values clarification?
- What are the steps in values clarification?

ETHICAL DECISION MAKING

Decision models used in bioethics do not offer easy decisions, but they do provide a guiding structure to help you arrive at the best answer in specific situations. Decision models can help you decide on a course of action even if they do not tell you absolutely that the action is right or wrong.

How Can I Recognize Ethical Issues? We have said it is important to be aware of the ethical issues in patient care situations, but how will you recognize them? The key is that there is usually a conflict:

- About the right action to take
- Among the duties and obligations of healthcare professionals (or they are unclear)
- Between the needs and interests of an individual and a group of clients
- Between what the family wants and what the client wants or needs
- Between the family and health professionals
- Among ethical principles or values (e.g., autonomy versus nonmaleficence, as in the Meet Your Patients scenario)

Problem or Dilemma?

In the best of all possible worlds, you could easily apply ethical principles and decide what to do. However, often in moral situations one ethical principle is in conflict with another equally important principle. It

Table 44-3 ➤ Values Clarification

STEP AND DESCRIPTION	QUESTIONS TO ASK YOUR PATIENT
Choosing (cognitive)	
Beliefs are chosen:	Do (did) you have any choice about what you do?
Freely (allows you to cherish your choice)	Do you have any control over what happens?
From alternatives	What have you decided to do?
After considering all consequences (ensures that the alternative is right for you)	Can you list some alternative actions?
	What are your options?
	What could you do instead of ...?
	What do you think will happen if you do that?
	What will you gain by doing that?
	What is the disadvantage of doing that?
Prizing (affective)	
Beliefs and behaviors that are chosen are prized:	How do you feel about your decision?
With pride (feeling good about your choice)	People sometimes feel good after making such a decision. Others feel pressured. How is it for you?
With public affirmation	How do you intend to tell your family (friends) about this decision?
	What will you say to your wife (friends, family)?
	When will you announce your decision to ...?
Acting (behavioral)	
Beliefs are acted on:	Try to determine whether the client will act on the decision:
By incorporating the choice into one's own behavior	▪ How do you think your wife (significant other) will react when you do that?
With consistency and repetition	▪ When will you actually carry out this decision?
	▪ Try to predict consistent behavior by asking:
	• How many times in the past have you ...?
	• What kind of schedule have you worked out? How often and when will you ...?

Source: Adapted from Raths, L. E., Harmin M., & Simon, S. B. (1978). *Values and teaching: Working with values in the classroom.* Columbus, OH: Merrill.

is also possible for a philosophical framework to produce more than one acceptable option. An **ethical dilemma** is a situation in which a choice must be made between two equally undesirable actions. There is no clearly right or wrong option. Such situations are emotionally painful for everyone in the situation, as you can see from the Meet Your Patients scenario at the beginning of this chapter. If you support Alan's parents' right to refuse a blood transfusion, you honor the principle of autonomy, but at the expense of the principle of nonmaleficence, which says we should prevent harm to Alan.

Fortunately, not all moral problems are dilemmas nor are they complex and difficult. In fact, you will confront a true dilemma only occasionally. Some questions are easily answered (e.g., "Should I take the patient's morphine to relieve my back pain?"). It is probably more accurate, then, to talk about "moral questions," "moral problems," or "moral situations" and not use the term *dilemma* loosely. Only problems that pose a question between competing and equally valuable interests are true dilemmas. You may never or only occasionally confront a true emotional dilemma.

Ethical behavior and decision making do not deal only with dilemmas. They really involve choosing to be ethical in the everyday aspects of your practice: for example, treating colleagues and patients with respect, not passing by a room when you see a patient crying, or helping out a new graduate who is frustrated and anxious. The scenario (in What Is Nursing Ethics?) about the two little boys in the emergency department is more representative of everyday ethics than is the Meet Your Patients scenario.

How Do I Work Through an Ethical Problem?

Once you have identified an ethical problem, a decision model can help you logically decide the best action to take. Still, in the case of a true ethical dilemma, you will probably not be comfortable with any course of action, no matter how logically you think it through.

Ethical decision-making models will help you carefully consider several perspectives, guide your reasoning, and explain the reasons for your final action. Each approach may produce a different solution. One of the easiest to remember and use is the MORAL model. This model has been credited to two different authors: Thiroux (1977) and Crisham (in Scott, 1985). The letters MORAL will remind you of the steps in this model, which is described in the following section. To use the model in clinical settings,

 Go to **Clinical Insight 44-1: Using the MORAL Model for Ethical Decision Making,** in Volume 2.

First, Use Problem-Solving

As a first step in ethical decision making, use the nursing process approach to describe the problem and alternative approaches:

- *Assessment—What are the relevant facts?* Alan needs a blood transfusion to survive. Both you and the surgeon have tried to persuade the parents to consent, but they still refuse. The parents' religion prohibits blood transfusions. Alan is 15 years old (a minor), so you cannot administer a transfusion without his parents' consent.
- *Analysis/Diagnosis—Identify the problem; state the conflict.* There is a values conflict: The healthcare professionals value preserving physical life; the parents place more value on preserving the soul. There is an ethical dilemma, as well: If no transfusion is given, you violate the principle of nonmaleficence (harm to Alan); if you somehow coerce the parents to consent, you have violated the principle of autonomy (respect for their values and their freedom to choose). So the decision to be made is whether to (a) follow the parents' wishes, (b) find a legal way to transfuse without their consent, or (c) find some compromise that will work.

Next, Use the MORAL Model

Now use the MORAL model to come up with alternative solutions for the Frese family.

M—Massage the Dilemma

1. *First identify and define the issues in the dilemma, and consider the values and options of all the major*

players: Mr. and Mrs. Frese, Alan, the surgeon, possibly a member of the clergy, and you (the nurse). You have already identified the values in the problem-solving approach: physical life versus spiritual life. You and the surgeon also value the principles of autonomy and nonmaleficence.

2. *Then identify the information gaps.* In massaging the situation, you should ask yourself:
   - Do I fully understand the situation that is causing the need for blood?
   - How much time is available to make this decision— do the parents have to decide within a few minutes, or do they have enough time to discuss this with their congregational elders?
   - Does the physician know that the family members are Jehovah's Witnesses?
   - Does the surgeon have any treatment that could be used to stabilize Alan while the parents discuss the situation?
   - Do Alan's parents fully understand the nature of Alan's physical emergency?
   - In the Freses' religious view, what is the consequence of receiving blood?
   - Do they understand what might happen if blood is not administered (i.e., do they understand the consequence of their action or inaction)?
   - Is this what Alan would want? Has Alan discussed in the past how he feels about blood transfusions? Have they ever had family discussions when other young Jehovah's Witnesses have been faced with such a decision? Where did Alan stand in those discussions?
   - How is this situation like other situations they have experienced in their lives?
   - Have they thought about their opposing duties: the duty to uphold their religious values and the duty to protect their son from harm?
   - Has everyone's voice been heard?
   - Have the parents contacted their congregational elders and discussed the situation?
   - What emotions are coming into play in this situation?
   - How is this decision affecting the parents as individuals? Are they in agreement on the issue, or is there dissension? If there is dissension, are both sides being supported fairly?
   - Is there some common ground between what the surgeon wants and what the parents feel they need to do to uphold their religious convictions?

O—Outline the Options

At this step in the MORAL model, you (or the charge nurse or a member of the ethics committee) should outline all of the options to all parties, including those that are less realistic and conflicting. You might ask a member of the ethics committee or the hospital chaplain to help the family and the doctor understand the opposing viewpoints.

The surgeon needs to outline the state of emergency that exists for Alan and to explain what the limited medical options are: to transfuse blood or, if no blood is given, what other treatments are available (e.g., volume enhancers). The surgeon will need to say how soon the decision must be made based on Alan's condition. He should clearly describe the consequences of each action. Carefully, and with as little emotion as possible, explain the consequences of each action to the parents. The physician should state whether one administration of blood will likely fix the situation or whether continued administration may be required.

The family (or the congregational elders) should explain for the doctor and nurse the basis for their refusal to consent and what they believe the consequence would be if blood were given.

R—Resolve the Dilemma

Now carefully review the issues and options. Apply basic ethical principles. If you can, also look at the situation using alternate ethical frameworks.

- **Autonomy.** By their refusing to give consent, the Freses are exercising their autonomy. How far will we go to honor their autonomy?
- **Beneficence and Nonmaleficence.** How are we defining "good" (beneficence) and "harm" (nonmaleficence) in this situation? The physician defines "good" as Alan receiving the needed blood. He defines "harm" as the outcome for Alan without the blood, even if he uses a less effective alternative. Alan's parents would define "good" as following their religious mandates and making sure their son will remain pure in the eyes of God. They might explain that a Jehovah's Witness who willingly accepts a blood transfusion might forfeit his or her eternal life. The Freses might believe the taking of blood to be more harmful than death, because they believe that would affect Alan's eternal life, not just his physical life.
- **Fidelity.** The surgeon is being loyal (exhibiting fidelity) to the principles of medicine and evidence-based practice, which mandate the administration of the blood. To the parents, their loyalty to their religious principles to ensure that Alan has eternal life may be more important than the loss of the physical life itself.
- **Veracity.** The principle of veracity holds that the surgeon should not exaggerate the need for the blood, and he should be honest with the parents in terms of the consequences of the alternative actions. Another question of veracity involves the parents: Are they being honest with each other regarding their feelings?

Your role as a nurse is to be an advocate for the patient and the family. Talk with the family and their religious representative, if available, about what they are thinking about their opposing duties: the duty to uphold their religious values and the duty to protect their son from physical harm. Explain to the surgeon the reasoned position of Alan's parents, if you can do so.

Key Point: *Ensure that everyone's viewpoint has been respected and considered. This may be as important as the final decision that is reached. In this and other difficult situations, always look for the opportunity for a good compromise (to be discussed later in this chapter).*

A—Act by Applying the Chosen Option

This step is the first one that actually requires action. The hospital is bound to follow the parents' decision because Alan is a minor. However, if there is time, many agencies might refer this situation to the hospital ethics committee. The hospital might also ask a legal court authority to resolve the situation. If an emergency requires an immediate decision, the only *legal* action is to follow the parents' decision, whether or not you consider it the best moral action.

Whatever happens, Alan's parents will need emotional support. If they decide to refuse the blood transfusion, you must remain nonjudgmental in supporting them, even if you do not agree with their decision. If they, or the courts, decide that the blood will be given, they may need even more support. They may feel overwhelming guilt, and they may fear that Alan will be forever burdened with guilt at the realization that they violated church doctrine with the medical care. If their extended family is not present, you could volunteer to call in extended family, friends, and church members if they wish. They will need a quiet, private place to await the outcome of the treatment.

L—Look Back and Evaluate

This phase calls for evaluation of the entire process, not just the consequence of the decided action.

- How well did the process work? Were processes in place for the dilemma to be discussed respectfully without undue delay in treatment?
- Were all parties' expectations realistic?
- How are all of the affected parties feeling now (doctor, parents, family, Alan, you)? Regardless of the outcome of the decision, do all involved feel they had a voice and their views were respected?
- How well did you do in the situation? Did you act as an effective advocate for the rights of Alan and his parents? Did the power and authority of the physician or hospital in the situation unduly influence you?
- Were policies and procedures in place to guide you in the process of working out this situation?
- Has anything changed since the dilemma came to light? Has a greater good been achieved for future situations? Have future situations been made easier as a result of the things learned in this situation? Has any aspect of this ethical decision now become a universal policy at the institution?
- Are further actions required in terms of this or like situations?

For guidelines to help you avoid common errors when making ethical decisions,

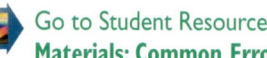 Go to Student Resources, Chapter 44, **Supplemental Materials: Common Errors in Decision Making,** on DavisPlus.

Look for a Good Compromise

Even if you believe you know the right thing to do, others may not agree with you, or there may be constraints that prevent you from doing it. For example, in the case of Alan, even if you decided the right thing to do is give him a blood transfusion, (1) his parents do not agree with you, and (2) the law says you cannot do so without his parents' consent. This will happen often—much more often than a true dilemma, in which you cannot *decide* the right thing to do. No matter how well we work together, there will always be ethical problems and disagreements. Many cases are full of complexity and uncertainty, and sometimes the price of acting on your beliefs is extremely high. For example, what might have happened if the surgeon had infused blood without the Freses' consent? What might have happened if you had refused to talk to the parents as the surgeon asked you?

Many times, it will be possible to reach a "good" compromise. A **good compromise** is one that preserves the integrity of all parties. This means that:

- **The discussions are carried out in a spirit of mutual respect**—that all viewpoints are respected and considered.
- **The compromise solution itself is ethically sound**; that is, you should be able to provide a principles-based rationale for the compromise, as well as for each of the opposing positions. In the case of Alan and his parents, there probably is no compromise position between "give blood" and "don't give blood." Perhaps the parents would agree to one, but no more than one, transfusion; but that is hard to justify ethically. If one transfusion is acceptable (to honor nonmaleficence), why not two or three? If two transfusions are against their religious beliefs, why would one be acceptable? Nevertheless, in many cases compromise is possible.

So how do you compromise without losing moral integrity? First, realize there is more at stake than the issue itself ("Is a blood transfusion right or wrong?"). There are some things that are inherently good in compromising.

- **First, it is never good to settle things by force** (as you would if you got a court order to transfuse Alan without his parents' consent). You have probably heard the old saying "Might doesn't make right." A compromise can preserve the rights of the less powerful party in a disagreement.
- **Keeping peace on a nursing unit is good for both the nurses and patients.** When there is upheaval and moral suffering, care quality throughout the unit can suffer. A compromise can bring peace.
- **There is intrinsic good in taking part in a process in which we try to see things from others' points of view.** It may make us more open minded, more creative, and less judgmental.
- **Keep in mind that most issues do contain room for reasonable differences of opinion.** In the Meet Your Patients scenario, can you see that both sides are people of good will who have ethical reasons to justify their opinion? Also, there is often room for doubt, on your own part, about the morally best action to take.
- **A compromise may achieve mutual respect.** It is a significant thing to reach a settlement in which each party feels assured of the other's respect for its seriousness and sincerity.

Given all those ideas, a person of good will might want to reexamine and back away from a very strong opinion. Remember, sometimes your position isn't all that strong, and the other position isn't all that weak (as in the case of Alan). There is also always the chance that you may have made an error in your reasoning or have not completely understood some facts of the case. Ethical disputes can be settled only if you are willing to engage in discussion and admit that the other people might have a point! There may be cases in which you cannot compromise (perhaps Alan's case is one), but don't listen to people who say, "You can never reach agreement on ethical issues. They are too complex." It is possible to achieve integrity-producing compromises, and in nursing it is often necessary.

What Are My Obligations in Ethical Situations?

As you can see, in making ethical decisions, nurses rarely act alone. Usually you will be one of several healthcare professionals and family members who will jointly arrive at the best decision. Your role when an ethical decision is needed includes the following:

- *Be aware of and sensitive to issues* so you can identify them when they arise. Educate yourself—attend workshops, read, and talk to other nurses.
- *Assume responsibility for your own moral actions.* Even if you do not have the "last word" about what happens to a patient or about what others do, you are always responsible for your own actions in every situation.
- *Function as a team member* when ethical problems arise. Realize you should have input—no one profession has full moral expertise—and realize that your input can be valuable.
- *Support the patient and family members* while they are making the decision and afterward. Listen. Ask questions. Provide unbiased information. Be helpful without being too directive or judgmental.
- *Support patients who are not being allowed to decide.* For example, in the Meet Your Patients scenario, you would want to be sure Alan's wishes were considered, if possible. However, if the parents insist on deciding for him, against his wishes, he may need a great deal of emotional support.
- *Use and participate in institutional ethics committees* if you are given the opportunity.
- *Most important, advocate for your client.* You may need to balance your client's autonomy with the

wishes of family members or the responsibilities of other healthcare professionals to the patient. As an advocate, you may find yourself in conflict with other team members or family members. Frequently you and the others involved will have different ethical perspectives.

■ *Continually strive to improve your ethical decision making.*

Use and Participate in Institutional Ethics Committees

There is no easy way to decide which principle should outrank another principle, or which person's values are best in a given situation. For this reason, many healthcare institutions have ethics committees. These interdisciplinary committees typically include nurses, doctors, clergy, ethicists, and lay representatives. Ethics committees develop guidelines and policies, provide education and counseling, and, in the case of ethical dilemmas, review the case and provide a forum for the expression of the diverse perspectives of those involved. Ethics committees usually follow one of three models when discussing a dilemma: the autonomy model, the patient benefit model, and the social justice model.

Autonomy Model The **autonomy model** is useful when the patient is competent to decide. This model emphasizes patient autonomy and choice as the highest value. For example, if this committee knew Alan's (Meet Your Patients) wishes, they might be inclined to try to persuade his parents to do as Alan wants.

Patient Benefit Model The **patient benefit model** assists in decision making for the incompetent patient by using substituted judgment (i.e., what the patient would want for himself if he were capable of making these issues known). If Alan is unconscious and cannot say what he wants, this committee would probably ask Alan's parents, family, and friends, "What do you think Alan would want? Have you ever heard him talk about a situation such as this?"

Social Justice Model The **social justice model** focuses more on broad social issues involving the entire institution, rather than on a single patient issue (Yoder-Wise, 2010). Such a committee might consider whether, in general, an institution ought ever to seek a legal order to act against the wishes of the parents. Or they might discuss whether supporting parents' religious beliefs in this instance might have implications for supporting other types of religious beliefs in future cases.

KnowledgeCheck 44-12

- Define *ethical dilemma.*
- How can you recognize an ethical problem?
- What is an integrity-producing compromise?
- What are the functions of an ethics committee?
- What does the mnemonic MORAL stand for?

Be a Patient Advocate

The role of advocates is to safeguard clients against abuse and violation of their rights. When you think of the rights and values described, for example, in the *Patient Care Partnership* and in nursing codes of ethics, you can see how important this role is. Be aware that advocacy in everyday clinical practice is less about the patient's legal rights and ethical theory, and more about such seemingly "routine" measures as obtaining a new prescription when an analgesic is ineffective, even if it does mean telephoning the prescriber for the third time on your shift. The advocacy role requires you to be respectful, considerate, courageous, persistent, and concerned with justice.

Why do you think advocacy is so important? Why can't patients do these things for themselves? The following are some of the reasons.

You Have Special Knowledge That the Patient Does Not Have Diseases, treatments, and the healthcare system are so complex that when clients become ill, they may not have the energy to deal with the complexity, even if they do have the necessary knowledge. You may need to help them to "jump through the necessary hoops" to get what they need. When patients' rights are denied or when patients do not have the ability to exert their rights, nurses have a responsibility to step in. "Without the advocacy and protection of rights there really are no rights" (Bandman & Bandman, 2002, p. 23).

One Aspect of Your Professional Role Is to Defend Patients' Autonomous Decisions Recall that the ANA Code of Ethics requires you to be a patient advocate (see Boxes 44-1, 44-2, and 44-3). As a nurse, you will be called on to defend your patients' autonomous decisions, even if you do not agree with them and even if they conflict with the opinions of others involved in the patient's care. You may find yourself the sole supporter of a patient's right to choose for himself the direction of his care.

Nurses Have a Special Relationship With Patients You may find that you are able to obtain information about a patient that is not available to professionals of other disciplines. In general, nurses interact with patients over longer time intervals and are involved in very personal activities, especially in inpatient settings. They often become the most trusted caregivers. Details about family life, coping styles, personal preferences, fears, and insecurities are all more likely to be discussed during the time involved in nursing interventions than in the brief minutes of interaction when a physician makes rounds. In addition, patients may perceive less social distance between themselves and the nurse and, therefore, feel freer to confide in them. The nurses' point of view can be a valuable asset to resolving an ethical problem satisfactorily. Of course, many providers have long-standing relationships with their patients; however, this does not negate the importance of the nurse's input, which may provide a different perspective.

Your Role as an Advocate Is to Inform, Support, and Communicate You should inform clients of their rights and provide the information they need to make informed decisions, if they are capable of doing so. Then you must remain objective and support them in the decisions they make, even if (perhaps especially if), you do not agree with the patient's decision. If others are not respecting client choices, you will need to intervene. This may simply be a matter of conveying information and clarifying the client's wishes to family or healthcare professionals (e.g., "I know how hard it is for you to let him go, but your dad says he has made peace and is ready to die. His treatments make him feel even more ill, and he simply does not want to fight anymore."). Advocacy may require you to arrange for the client to consult with a religious leader or an attorney for advice and support, or may require you to consult an institutional ethics committee.

Inform Patients About Advance Directives Data reveal that 28% of home healthcare patients, 65% of nursing home residents, and 88% of discharged hospice patients had at least one advance directive on file (Jones, Moss, & Harris-Kojetin, 2011), so there is work to be done with certain populations. An important advocacy intervention is to ask patients whether they have an advance directive and to inform them about advance directives if they do not. Even people who have an advance directive do not always, or even often, understand the statements they have checked in the boxes on the form. Take the time to go over the form with them if they are able to do so. See Chapters 17 and 45 if you need further discussion of advance directives.

For guidelines that will help you to function effectively as an advocate,

 Go to Chapter 44, **Clinical Insight 44-2: Guidelines for Advocacy**, in Volume 2.

Improve Your Ethical Decision Making

By now, you should understand that you cannot avoid making moral decisions in nursing. A recent study pointed out the need to promote nurses' development from the conventional (rules-bound) to the post-conventional (reasoning) stage of moral development. The study found that when nurses were faced with ethical dilemmas they tended to use conventions (e.g., rules, procedures) as criteria for decision making rather than patients' personal needs and well-being (Dierckx de Casterlé, Izumi, Godfrey, et al., 2008). As a full-spectrum nurse, you should use the following suggestions so you will be prepared when ethical issues arise.

- **Use Theoretical Knowledge.** Review nursing and other literature for discussion of cases and experiences of other nurses. This will give you a broader view of the problems you may confront and the strategies for managing them. Become familiar with the various codes of ethics, the *Patient Care Partnership*, and ethical frameworks and principles.

- **Use Self-Knowledge.** Examine your personal value system. Explore the influences of your religion, cultural beliefs, and personal experiences. This will help you to recognize your comfort zone with specific ethical issues.

- **Use Practical Knowledge.** While still a student, you should ask to attend either ethical rounds or an ethics committee meeting. As a graduate nurse, you could volunteer to be a member of your institution's ethics committee or plan to attend nursing ethics rounds to familiarize yourself with the types of ethical problems that occur at your institution.

- **Consult Reliable Sources.** Attend ethics education programs and talk about issues with other healthcare providers. Attorneys, ethicists, and members of the clergy can provide helpful perspectives.

- **Share.** Regularly engage in discussions with the staff on your unit to determine differences in value systems and to collaborate proactively to work out methods that can be used to resolve ethical dilemmas effectively. When you are faced with a difficult moral decision, consult with peers, coworkers, and teachers. Seek guidance and support.

- **Evaluate.** After the situation is resolved, evaluate your decision and the effects of your actions. You should be able to learn from even the worst decision. And when everything goes well, you can file your strategies away to use in future similar situations.

KnowledgeCheck 44-13

- What are three reasons patients may need a nurse advocate?
- Briefly describe the nurse's role as a patient advocate.

 To explore learning resources for this chapter,

 Go to Davis*Plus* at **DavisPl.us/Wilkinson3.**

Chapter Resources for Chapter 44:
  Response sheets for all learning activities
  Resources for Caregivers and Health Professionals
  Reading More About Ethics & Values (suggested readings)
  Concept Map of chapter content
Interactive Case Studies
NCLEX-Style and Chapter Review Questions
Chapter Overview Podcasts

For references cited in this chapter,

 Go to Volume 2, **References Cited.**

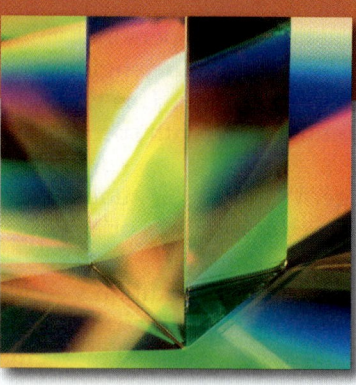

CHAPTER 45

Legal Accountability

Learning Outcomes

After completing this chapter, you should be able to:

- Identify four basic sources of law.
- Discuss direct implications of the Nurses' Bill of Rights to practice.
- Relate the impact of the Health Insurance Portability and Accountability Act (HIPAA) to patient rights and protections.
- Discuss the effects of the Patient Self-Determination Act on healthcare practices.
- Describe accommodations that conform to the Americans With Disability Act (ADA).
- Apply state mandatory reporting laws to patient care situations.
- Apply the concepts of Good Samaritan laws to nurses' actions.
- Identify seven rights of nurses within the healthcare workplace.

- Discuss how nurse practice acts provide the foundation for nursing practice.
- Explain disciplinary actions for unacceptable nursing decisions or actions.
- Discuss basic principles of criminal law that affect nursing practice.
- Compare and contrast intentional and unintentional torts.
- Discuss common causes of malpractice litigation.
- Describe the phases of the litigation process in a nursing malpractice case.
- Identify strategies to minimize liability in nursing practice.

Key Concepts

Law
Liability
Malpractice

Related Concepts

See the Concept Map on Davis*Plus*.

Disclaimer: The material contained in this chapter is intended to convey information on topics of interest to nursing students. Although prepared by a nurse attorney, this chapter should not be used as a substitute for legal counseling. No one should act on the information contained in this chapter without professional guidance. These materials should not be considered legal advice or a legal opinion.

Meet Your Nurse Role Model

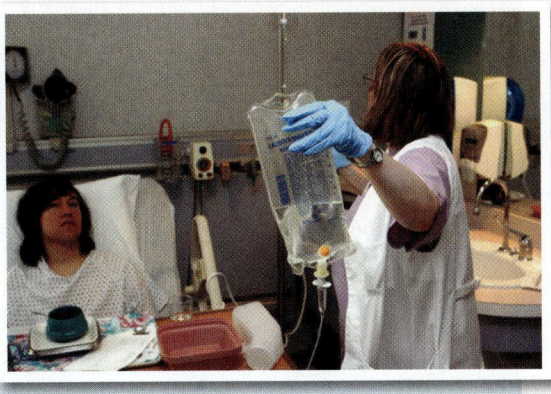

A nurse with 3 years of experience on a medical-surgical unit arrives at work and discovers that two of her colleagues called in sick, including the charge nurse. The nursing supervisor informs her that she will need to assume the charge nurse role, in addition to assuming care for three patients. Feeling frustrated, the nurse ponders whether she should just quit and find another job, but, nevertheless, decides to accept the assignment. Two hours into the shift, one of her patients begins to experience complications, requiring blood glucose checks every 2 hours and frequent monitoring. In addition, one of the nurses becomes ill and is replaced by a float nurse from the labor and delivery unit. The nurse contacts the nursing supervisor and requests additional assistance, but is told no other nurse is available and that the supervisor is involved with an emergency situation on another unit. The nurse begins to analyze this situation from a legal perspective to determine the best course of action.

- Should the nurse have accepted the assignment? If yes, what factors should the nurse have considered before accepting the assignment?
- If the nurse should not have accepted the assignment, could she have been charged with abandonment?
- How should the nurse handle this situation?

Theoretical Knowledge
knowing why

In clinical practice, nurses are often confronted with situations that present legal issues. You must have an understanding of the legal guidelines governing nursing practice to protect yourself, your patients, your colleagues, and your employers. The theoretical knowledge in this chapter, combined with the critical thinking model in Chapter 2, will help you to answer questions related to the Meet Your Nurse Role Model scenario.

ABOUT THE KEY CONCEPTS

The concept of **law** can be described as a binding practice, rule, or code of conduct that guides appropriate actions and defensible decisions of an individual or a group. Laws protect society by establishing acceptable patterns of behaviors and are enforceable by a controlling authority. Nurses are legally responsible for their own actions and this responsibility cannot be delegated—this is the basis for liability in nursing practice. **Liability** means that the person is financially or legally responsible for something. **Malpractice** is one source of legal liability. It means that a professional person has failed to act in a reasonable and prudent manner. If someone is harmed, the professional may be held liable.

WHAT ARE THE SOURCES AND TYPES OF LAW?

The U.S. Constitution establishes three branches of government: executive, legislative, and judicial. Each branch has specified powers that are designed to equalize power among the three and to provide a system of checks and balances. Laws are derived primarily from four sources: (1) the Constitution, (2) statutes, (3) administrative bodies, and (4) the courts (Table 45-1).

Constitutional Law A **constitution** is a system of fundamental laws and principles that prescribes the nature, functions, and limits of a government. The U.S. Constitution is the superior law of the land and applies to all states throughout the United States. Thus, all state and federal laws must be consistent with the U.S. Constitution. The U.S. Constitution limits the powers of the federal government and gives each state the power to govern itself and to pass laws to promote the health, welfare, order, and security of its citizens (police power). Each state has a similar structure that likewise establishes the governing system for the state, its cities, and municipalities. Any law that conflicts with the U.S. Constitution is considered invalid or void. If you would like to see the seven articles of the Constitution,

 Go to Chapter 45, **Tables, Boxes, Figures: ESG Box 45-1, Articles of the United States Constitution.**

Statutory Law A **statute** is a law passed by Congress or by a state legislative body. Congress passes laws for the benefit of society as a whole, whereas states use their police power to pass laws to ensure the general health, safety, and welfare of their citizens. Nurse practice acts (NPAs) are examples of statutory law. NPAs, passed by the legislative body of each state, are regulations that govern the profession of nursing.

Administrative Law Formally defined, **administrative law** refers to the laws that govern the activities of administrative agencies. Administrative agencies are created at

Table 45-1. Branches of Government and Sources of Law

Branches of government		
	EXAMPLES	**DESCRIPTION**
Executive	U.S. president, attorney general, secretary of state, state governors	Authority to execute and enforce laws.
Legislative	Congress (House of Representatives + Senate)	Make or formulate laws.
Judicial	U.S. Supreme Court; state and local courts	Interpret statutory law and decide cases and controversies.
Type/sources of law		
	EXAMPLE	**QUESTION POSED**
Constitutional Law	Freedom of speech	Can an employer prevent internationally educated nurses from speaking in their native language in the work environment?
Statutory Law	Definition of nursing	What is the nurse's scope of practice (duties and responsibilities)?
Administrative Law	Delegation and supervision	Is the registered nurse legally responsible for tasks or assignments delegated to other nurses?
Common Law	Affirmative duty	Does a registered nurse have a responsibility to exercise an independent judgment to prevent harm to patients?

the federal level by Congress and at the state level by its legislative bodies. As applied to nursing, within each state's nurse practice act, the legislative body created a board of nursing to enforce the NPA. The board creates rules and regulations that define and expand on the provisions in the NPA necessary to ensure compliance with its statutory mission—to regulate the practice of nursing.

Common (Judicial) Law   A compilation of laws made by judges or courts is known as **common law**. Also referred to as *case law*, common law is based on common customs and traditions. It comes from legal principles and guidelines that judges use to determine the outcome of legal cases.

WHAT LAWS AND REGULATIONS GUIDE NURSING PRACTICE?

As a professional nurse, you will need to understand the various laws and regulations that guide nursing practice. Laws and regulations at the federal and state levels have a direct impact on the nurse's actions and decisions.

Federal Law

Several federal statutes have direct implications for professional nursing practice. Many NPAs require nurses to have knowledge of such laws. This section presents some federal laws.

Bill of Rights

The first 10 amendments to the U.S. Constitution are known as the *Bill of Rights*. It clearly identifies, and in many ways limits, the role of government in individuals' lives. Many of these rights have direct implications for healthcare, including the rights of nurses and of patients. For example, protecting patients' privacy rights is a fundamental role of the professional nurse that is derived from the Fourth Amendment to the U.S. Constitution. If you would like to review all the amendments in the Bill of Rights,

 Go to Chapter 45, **Tables, Boxes, Figures: ESG Box 45-2, The Bill of Rights, Amendments 1–10 of the Constitution,** on *DavisPlus*.

 Think**Like a Nurse** 45-1

- Develop a scenario illustrating how a nurse might protect a patient's right to privacy.
- What is one thing a nurse can do to respect a patient's property rights?

Health Insurance Portability and Accountability Act (HIPAA)

The Health Insurance Portability and Accountability Act (HIPAA) was passed by Congress in 1996 to:

- Protect health insurance benefits for workers who lose or change their jobs

- Protect coverage to persons with preexisting medical conditions
- Establish standards to protect the privacy of personal health information

Under HIPAA rules, healthcare agencies and their employees must take steps to ensure the confidentiality of the patient information and medical records. Nurses and other healthcare providers must protect the patient's right to privacy by not sharing patient information with unauthorized individuals. In addition, HIPAA allows patients to see, make corrections to, and obtain copies of their medical records. The cases in the following box highlight the importance of understanding and complying with the safeguards created under HIPAA.

Case: Violation of a Patient's Privacy

- A nursing assistant spent 8 days in jail after being convicted of invasion of personal property for posting graphic photos of elderly and disabled patients on Facebook.
- Several emergency room nurses were fired after painting the face of an unconscious obese patient with charcoal, making unprofessional comments, and taking pictures of him with their cell phones.
- A man who received the registration face sheets of patients admitted to the hospital from the manager of the hospital's trauma unit and provided them to personal injury attorneys was sentenced to 33 months in federal prison for violation of HIPAA.

Emergency Medical Treatment and Active Labor Act (EMTALA)

The Emergency Medical Treatment and Active Labor Act (EMTALA) requires healthcare facilities to provide emergency medical treatment to patients who seek healthcare in the emergency department (ED), regardless of their ability to pay, legal status, or citizenship status. The obligation is for the medical facility to provide medical screening to determine whether an emergency exists and to stabilize the patient before transferring him or her to another healthcare facility.

Case: EMTALA

A patient presented to the ED with complaints of chest pain. Per protocol, the triage nurse obtained information on the onset and severity of the pain and medications taken by the patient. She then completed a focused history and assessment, obtained a pulse oximeter reading, and ordered an electrocardiogram (ECG) and lab work. She reported the results to the ED physician, who consulted a cardiologist. The patient initiated a lawsuit alleging he suffered heart damage because of a delay in treatment. Ruling in favor of the hospital and nurse, the court noted that the care received via protocol was the same as that of any patient with similar complaints (*Byrne v. Chester Co. Hospital*, 2013).

 **Think**Like a Nurse** 45-2**

A 54-year-old uninsured and unemployed woman arrives at the ED of a small private hospital complaining of chest pain and nausea. The triage nurse calls the on-call physician, who instructs the nurse to send the patient to the county hospital several blocks away. The nurse assesses the patient and contacts her supervisor, who tells her to contact the medical chief of staff to inform him that the patient is in need of emergency treatment.

- Discuss whether the nurse's action was appropriate or inappropriate.

Patient Self-Determination Act

The Patient Self-Determination Act (PSDA) of 1991 recognizes the patient's right to make decisions regarding his own healthcare, based on the information provided to him by the healthcare provider, regarding the medical or surgical treatment options available, the benefits, risks, and alternatives. Box 45-1 describes agency and healthcare workers' responsibilities under the PSDA.

There are two types of legal written advance directives: the living will and the durable power of attorney for healthcare.

A **durable power of attorney for healthcare (DPOA)** identifies a person who will make healthcare decisions in the event the patient is unable to do so. The person given the right to make decisions is called the *surrogate decision maker*. The surrogate has the right to make the medical decisions for as long as the person is not able to do so for himself (is incompetent).

Case: Durable Power of Attorney

Mr. Green was in a coma as a result of head trauma experienced in a motor vehicle accident. In his DPOA, he had designated his brother, Joey, as his surrogate. Although Mr. Green is married with two adult children, Joey is the person legally recognized to make decisions regarding Mr. Green's healthcare. Two weeks later, Mr. Green came out of the coma and regained the ability to make decisions. At that point, Mr. Green no longer required Joey as a surrogate.

BOX 45-1 ■ The Patient Self-Determination Act

The Patient Self-Determination Act requires healthcare facilities to:

- Provide written information to each patient regarding the right to make decisions, including the right to accept or to refuse medical treatment and the right to make advance directives.
- Document in the patient's medical record the presence or absence of advance directives.
- Provide education to the staff, healthcare providers, and community on advance directives.
- Follow state law as it relates to advance directives.
- Treat everyone the same regardless of the presence or absence of advance directives. (Facilities may not discriminate.)

A **living will** is prepared by an alert and oriented (competent) individual that gives directions to others about the person's wishes regarding life-prolonging treatments if the person becomes unable to make those decisions. As a legal document, the requirements may vary from state to state. However, language common in the living will gives the person the opportunity to specify treatment in numerous areas (Box 45-2).

The American Nurses Association (ANA, 2010a) highlighted the nurse's role in advance care planning and counseling in a 2010 position statement. As a nurse, you have the following responsibilities:

- Listen to patients to identify their concerns, expectations, and hopes regarding end-of-life care.
- Review patients' documented preferences upon admission to healthcare facilities.
- Recognize that advance care planning is a continual process and not a one-time execution of documents.
- Encourage patient and family participation in healthcare decisions about advance directives and end-of-life decisions.

You might want to ask the following questions about advance directives as a part of your nursing admission assessment:

What is your understanding of an advance directive, including the living will and durable power of attorney for healthcare?

Do you have an advance care directive?

If you have an advance care directive, do you have a copy with you?

Do you wish to initiate an advance care directive?

Who will make your healthcare decisions if you are unable to do so? Have you discussed your end-of-life choices with this person, significant others, and your provider?

BOX 45-2 ■ Sample Living Will Language

If I am in a terminal condition, irreversible coma, or in a persistent vegetative state, my wishes are as follows:

I ☐ **do** ☐ **do not** want to be in or taken to a hospital.

I ☐ **do** ☐ **do not** want pain medications to keep me comfortable.

I ☐ **do** ☐ **do not** want cardiac resuscitation, including drugs and electrical shock.

I ☐ **do** ☐ **do not** want mechanical respiration/artificial respiration.

I ☐ **do** ☐ **do not** want tube feeding or any other artificial or invasive form of nutrition (food).

I ☐ **do** ☐ **do not** want hydration (water), via tube or intravenous.

I ☐ **do** ☐ **do not** want blood or blood products.

I ☐ **do** ☐ **do not** want any form of surgery or invasive diagnostic tests.

I ☐ **do** ☐ **do not** want kidney dialysis.

I ☐ **do** ☐ **do not** want antibiotics.

Case: Durable Power of Attorney

Mrs. Terry Schiavo collapsed in her Florida home in 1990 after a suspected potassium imbalance secondary to bulimia, and was without oxygen for about 5 minutes. She suffered severe brain damage. Terry Schiavo did not have a living will. According to Florida law, her husband became her legal guardian, and thus the decision maker regarding her medical treatments. In November 1992, Mr. Schiavo won a medical malpractice lawsuit for $1 million from her physician on the theory that he failed to diagnose Mrs. Schiavo's bulimia. In 2000, Mr. Schiavo petitioned the court to have her feeding tube removed. Her parents opposed the action. During the next 5 years, extensive legal battles ensued. Finally, the court ruled in favor of removing the feeding tube. Mrs. Schiavo died on March 31, 2005. It was lack of a living will that (1) allowed this situation to go on for so long and (2) made it impossible to know for sure what Terry Schiavo would have wanted. It's all guesswork without a documented living will (Shepard, 2009).

Americans With Disabilities Act

The Americans With Disabilities Act (ADA) of 1990 provides protection against discrimination of individuals with disabilities. A person has a *disability* if he has a physical or mental impairment that substantially limits one or more major life activities, has a record of such impairment, or is regarded as having an impairment (ADA Amendments Act of 2008). In general, the ADA says that employers must provide reasonable accommodations within the work setting to allow employees with disabilities to perform their jobs.

Case: ADA Accommodations

- A nurse with a substance abuse addiction was caught using illegal drugs. She was allowed to return to work after rehabilitation. Her employer had a policy that provided employees with a last-chance agreement. When the nurse returned to work, she was reassigned to a job that did not require her to dispense medication. She was given periodic drug tests.
- A nurse with fibromyalgia syndrome was provided accommodations to help her overcome extreme fatigue and pain at work. She switched from evening to day shift to better regulate her sleep pattern, eliminated working two consecutive 12-hour shifts, and changed from full-time to part-time employment status.
- A nurse with insulin-dependent diabetes had difficulty maintaining glucose control. Her employer provided consistent times for breaks and lunch and privacy to check blood sugars and administer insulin as needed (Job Accommodation Network, n.d.).

To read about strategies to accommodate disabilities and follow the Job Accommodation Network link,

 Go to Chapter 45, **Resources for Caregivers & Health Professionals,** on Davis*Plus.*

KnowledgeCheck 45-1

- Which federal law requires healthcare agencies to provide patients with information about advance directives?
- Which federal law ensures that patients can receive emergency treatment regardless of their ability to pay?
- What protections are provided to patients by the Department of Health and Human Services "privacy rule" of HIPAA?

State Laws

In addition to federal law, many states have laws that directly impact nurses' actions and behaviors. These include mandatory reporting laws, Good Samaritan laws, nurse practice acts, and medical malpractice statutes.

Mandatory Reporting Laws

The law in various states requires healthcare workers to report communicable diseases. You also have a duty to report physical, sexual, or emotional abuse or neglect of vulnerable individuals (e.g., children, older adults, the mentally ill), whether you suspect it or have actual evidence of it. The intent is to protect people who cannot protect themselves and to protect society against the spread of communicable diseases. Mandatory reporting laws also protect you when reporting abuse. In most instances, the identity of the reporter is kept confidential. If you fail to report certain communicable diseases or child abuse, you can be charged with a criminal misdemeanor or be subject to disciplinary action by the board of nursing.

The duty to report takes priority over the patient's right to privacy. Therefore, if you report abuse or neglect, you cannot be charged with violating a patient's right to privacy (e.g., under HIPAA). Since the mandatory reporting laws vary from state to state, you should be familiar with the law in your state.

Case: Mandatory Reporting

A high school principal and superintendent were arrested and charged with failure to report child abuse for allegedly failing to notify the Department for Children and Families of a student allegation of inappropriate touching by a teacher. State law mandates that allegations of child abuse be reported within 24 hours after allegations are brought (Wellington, 2013).

Good Samaritan Laws

Good Samaritan laws are designed to protect from liability those who provide emergency care to someone who is in need of medical services. To successfully use the Good Samaritan defense, the following elements must be present:

- Care was provided in an emergency situation.
- Person(s) providing the care did not cause the emergency or injury.
- Care was provided in a reasonably competent manner.
- Care provided must be voluntary (not paid or eligible for payment).
- Person receiving care did not object to receiving care.

Additional guidelines nurses should follow to ensure their protection by Good Samaritan laws include the following:

- Call 911, or have someone else call, as soon as you can.
- Do not leave the person unless you transfer care to an equally competent professional.
- Place the person under the care of emergency personnel, physicians, or advanced practice nurses as soon as possible and follow their instructions.
- Do not accept money or any other form of compensation for the services provided.

Good Samaritan laws vary from state to state. You should be familiar with the law in your state. A typical case involving Good Samaritan laws is as follows:

Case: Good Samaritan

A registered nurse is leaving the hospital after working a 12-hour shift, when she witnesses a single-person motor vehicle accident. She calls 911, stops, and approaches the accident scene, where she smells gasoline. Fearing that the car will explode, she pulls the accident victim from the car, places him flat on the ground, and assesses his injuries. She puts pressure on his bleeding femoral artery and stays with him until the ambulance arrives. The victim has spinal cord injuries and sues the nurse for removing him from the car. The nurse is protected from liability by the Good Samaritan law.

Nurses working in healthcare environments may not be protected by Good Samaritan laws if they already have a responsibility to provide care to those in need.

Case: Good Samaritan

The court denied the Good Samaritan defense for two physicians who were sued for malpractice. The physicians were salaried employees of a college of medicine that contracted with a community health clinic to provide backup emergency services for medically complex cases. The college of medicine received a fixed amount of money from the clinic for such services. The two physicians were called to assist with a complicated delivery that resulted in the death of an infant from injuries received during birth. One physician billed the clinic for her services and the

(Continued)

court ruled that, based on the relationship, the physician rendered emergency services for a fee. The other physician deviated from policy and did not submit a bill. However, the court ruled that a provider who is eligible for payment is not protected from liability under the Good Samaritan doctrine simply because he does not bill for his services (Rodas v. Seidlin, 2011).

Nurse Practice Acts

Nurse practice acts (NPAs) are statutory laws passed by each state's legislative body that define the practice of nursing. Nurse practice acts are designed to:

- Regulate nursing practice to protect the health, safety, and welfare of the general public.
- Define the scope of nursing practice.
- Approve programs providing prelicensure nursing education to students.

The components of NPAs are discussed in more detail later in the chapter.

Medical Malpractice Statutes

Medical malpractice refers to a lawsuit brought against a healthcare provider for damages (e.g., money) when there has been death of, injury to, or other loss to the person being treated. Laws governing medical malpractice vary from state to state, primarily regarding the time frame for bringing a lawsuit (statute of limitations) and the amount of monetary compensation allowed. To protect themselves from personal losses, many healthcare providers purchase malpractice insurance, which provides them with an attorney to defend against the claim and pay the damages (money) awarded to the claimant by a judge or jury. Malpractice is discussed in more detail later in this chapter.

Other Guidelines for Practice

In addition to federal and state laws, other practice guidelines may define what constitutes reasonable and prudent nursing care.

Institutional Policies and Procedures

Institutional policies and procedures usually are more specific and detailed than standards set by professional organizations. They describe care that is reasonable, appropriate, and expected in the context of that facility. You must be familiar with these policies and procedures because they can be used as evidence of a violation of a standard of care if you failed to follow them. Healthcare facilities should not have policies and procedures that conflict with the nurse practice act, professional standards of practice, the ANA Code of Ethics for Nurses, and other documents that guide nursing practice. If you encounter conflicts, or if a policy is not working well,

you should bring the matter to your supervisor's attention and/or contact the board of nursing in your state for an advisory opinion.

American Nurses Association Code of Ethics

The ANA Code of Ethics (2001) describes the standards of professional responsibility for nurses and provides insight into ethical and acceptable behavior. It describes nurses' obligations for safe, compassionate, nondiscriminatory, and quality care while defining commitments to self, the patient, the employer, and the profession.

The Code of Ethics is not a law, and therefore you would not be charged with criminal offenses for violating the code's provisions. In many situations, there is a fine line between what is legal and what is ethical. When confronted with a situation, to avoid legal jeopardy you should ask yourself, "Is there a law that relates to this situation?" If the answer is yes, you should understand the guidance provided by the law. If you cannot follow the law in good conscience, talk with your supervisor or seek legal advice. If there is no law, or if it seems immoral or unethical to you, ask, "What guidance is provided under the Code of Ethics?" Your action should be consistent with the code, if at all possible. The ANA code guarantees the patient the right to dignity, privacy, and safety. And that the nurse will:

- Be accountable and competent
- Use informed judgment
- Maintain employment conditions conducive to quality patient care
- Protect the client from misinformation and misrepresentation
- Collaborate with other healthcare professions to meet the patient's healthcare needs

A nurse who violates a provision of the Code of Ethics may have to defend her action to the state board of nursing. Also, in a malpractice suit, courts may look to these codes to judge whether the nurse's action was at the level expected by the profession. However, you must understand that the code will not likely protect you if you break a law or fail to follow agency policies, even if you believe the law to be immoral. If you need more information on nursing codes of ethics, see Chapter 44.

Patient Care Partnership

The Patient Care Partnership (PCP) replaced the American Hospital Association's Patient Bill of Rights. The PCP brochure is available in eight languages that explain in detail to patients that during hospitalization, they should expect:

- High-quality care
- A clean and safe environment
- Involvement in care
- Protection of privacy
- Help when leaving the hospital
- Help with billing claims

Like the ANA Code of Ethics, these rights are not necessarily legally binding, but they can provide evidence by which to judge whether the patient's care and environment met reasonable and appropriate standards. For more information on the Patient Care Partnership, see Box 44-3.

American Nurses Association Nurses' Bill of Rights

The Nurses' Bill of Rights is a policy statement adopted by the ANA to identify the seven conditions that nurses should expect from their workplace that are necessary for sound professional practice. It provides a framework for employers to understand what nurses need for a safe work environment and to support nurses as they address such issues as unsafe staffing, workplace violence, and mandatory overtime (ANA, n.d.a). The Nurses' Bill of Rights highlights that nurses have the right to:

- Practice in a manner that fulfills their obligations to society and to those who receive nursing care
- Practice in environments that allow them to act in accordance with professional standards and legally authorized scopes of practice
- A work environment that supports and facilitates ethical practice as defined by the Code of Ethics for Nurses
- Freely and openly advocate for themselves and their patients, without fear of retribution
- Fair compensation for their work, consistent with their knowledge, experience, and professional responsibilities
- A work environment that is safe for themselves and for their patients
- Negotiate the conditions of their employment, either as individuals or collectively, in all practice settings

American Nurses Association Standards of Practice

The ANA (2010b) Standards of Practice have three components:

1. *Professional standards of care* that incorporate the nursing process in the diagnostic, intervention, and evaluation aspect of patient care
2. *Professional performance standards* that identify the various role functions of the nurse in direct patient care, quality of practice, ethics, education, communication, research, leadership, collaboration, resource management, collegiality, and environmental health
3. *Practice guidelines* for the various specialty areas that are developed by professional organizations (e.g., American Association of Critical Care Nurses).

If you need to review the ANA Standards of Clinical Nursing Practice, refer to Chapter 1, Table 1-3. Standards establish the minimum level of competency for nurses. Nurses are expected to follow the standards that apply to their specialty areas. For a list of the Scope and Standards of Practice for the various clinical areas published by ANA,

 Go to Chapter 45, **Resources for Caregivers and Health Professionals,** on Davis*Plus*.

 ## ThinkLike a Nurse 45-3

Recall the Meet Your Nurse Role Model scenario. Would the nurse have done the right thing if she had decided not to accept the assignment and leave the facility immediately?

- What standards, guidelines, and laws would apply to determine whether the nurse's behavior was in accordance with standards of practice?
- Which statements in the ANA Nurses' Bill of Rights might the nurse use to justify her actions?

Nurse Practice Acts

As you have learned, nurse practice acts (NPAs) contain a provision that creates and empowers a state board of nursing to regulate the practice of nursing in that state. All 50 states, the District of Columbia, and the four U.S. territories have established boards of nursing. Although NPAs can vary from state to state, they all have common components, because states used ANA guidelines in developing their regulations. A state's nurse practice act usually includes the following:

- The authority of the board of nursing, its composition, and powers
- A definition of *nursing* and the boundaries of nursing practice
- Standards for the approval of nursing education programs
- The requirements for licensure of nurses
- Grounds for disciplinary action against a nurse's license

If you would like to see specific standards of care found in a typical nurse practice act,

 Go to Chapter 45, **Tables, Boxes, Figures: ESG Box 45-4, Minimum Acceptable Standards of Care Required by a Typical State Nurse Practice Act,** on Davis*Plus*.

Case: Nurse Practice Act

Mejonus X Institute is advertising an associate degree nursing program that can be completed in 12 months at a cost of $45,000. You are interested in the program, but are not sure whether the program is legitimate. Your initial investigation of the program should start with the state board of nursing, which approves nursing education programs. A list of approved nursing programs can usually be found on the state board of nursing Web site in many states.

Requirements for Licensure

Perhaps the most important function of state boards of nursing is establishing and enforcing the requirements for licensure. Unlicensed health providers pose a danger to the health, safety, and welfare of the general public because they have not met the specified standards to ensure a minimum level of competency to enter the nursing profession. In most states, the applicant for licensure must:

- Graduate from an approved or accredited nursing program
- Meet the established character criteria
- Undergo a criminal background check and fingerprinting
- Pass the NCLEX-RN or -PN exam
- Pay an application fee
- Some states, such as Texas, may require applicants to pass a jurisprudence examination before receiving a permanent license.

Case: Applicant for Licensure With a Criminal Conviction

An RN applicant for licensure was convicted 3 years earlier of a misdemeanor theft. He was sentenced to 12 months in jail, with 11 months of the sentence suspended; 2 years of probation; 180 hours of community service, and $1,200 in fines. The board of nursing approved his application for licensure by examination and reprimanded him for the criminal conviction.

Special Cases of Licensure

To protect the public, licensing is meant to ensure that practicing nurses have met the minimum competencies set by the state.

Mutual Recognition Model (MRM)/Nurse Licensure Compact Certain states, through a multistate agreement, allow nurses whose primary state of residency is in a compact state to practice in other compact states without obtaining a new license. You must obtain licensure "by endorsement" if you change your state of residency to another compact state or if your state of residency is not a member of the compact. To be *licensed by endorsement*, you do not have to retake the NCLEX examination, but must apply to the new state and fulfill any of that state's application requirements such as fingerprinting, background check, transcripts, and fees.

Case: Multi-State Compact

Roberto is a clinical nurse residing in Overland Park, Kansas (his primary state of residency), and originally licensed in Kansas after passing the NCLEX-RN exam. He is now employed at the Children's Hospital on the other side of the state line in Missouri. Roberto is required to maintain active licensure in the state where he is employed. He received an RN licensure by endorsement in the state of Missouri by meeting the requirements of the Missouri State Board of Nursing, but did not have to retake the NCLEX-RN.

Government/Military Personnel Another special case of licensure involves nurses employed by the military, Veterans Administration, Public Health Service, or other entities of the federal government. These nurses may practice in other states without obtaining a new license as long as they are practicing within the scope of their employment.

Case: Special Case of Licensure

Jane is a clinical nurse in the U.S. Air Force Reserve. She is licensed in the state of Texas, but is assigned to a military hospital in Nevada for her 2-week annual military tour. Jane will not need to obtain a license in the state of Nevada to practice at the military hospital.

Scope of Practice

The scope of nursing practice is found in the definition of nursing at the various levels. Nurses must be familiar with the definition of *nursing* at their level to plan and implement care that is consistent with their scope of practice. A nurse who practices outside the scope of practice can be charged with violation of the nurse practice act.

Nurse practice acts vary slightly state by state. However, in most states, the licensed practical nurse (LPN) scope of practice is limited in assessment privileges and interpretation of clinical data. Typically, LPN/LVNs do not have authority to alter nursing care plans. You must know the requirements of your state because they determine the legal limits of your practice. The following landmark case should make clear that no one, including an employer or physician, can increase a nurse's legal scope of practice.

Case: Scope of Practice

A physician delegated to an LPN the task of administering a polio booster to a 2-year-old boy. The nurse put the boy over her knee and proceeded to give the injection. The boy moved and the needle broke off in his buttocks, where it remained for 9 months despite attempts to surgically remove it. Since the Washington State Nurse Practice Act at that time did not allow LPNs to give injections, the nurse was in violation of the Nurse Practice Act by performing a task that was outside of her legal limits (Barber v. Reinking, 1966).

For the ANA (n.d.b) model of professional practice regulation,

 Go to Chapter 45, **Resources for Caregivers and Health Professionals,** on DavisPlus.

Disciplinary Actions

The state board of nursing can take disciplinary actions against your license for violation of the NPA.

A disciplinary action usually involves some or all of the following:

- The process begins with a complaint from an individual, employer, or professional organization that the nurse has engaged in unprofessional conduct.
- The complaint is then assigned to an investigator to determine its legitimacy or validity.
  If the investigator decides the complaint is invalid or does not constitute a violation of the NPA, it will be dismissed.
  If the complaint may violate the NPA, the investigator gathers additional information by contacting the nurse, interviewing witnesses, and reviewing documents and records.
- The case may be heard by the board of nursing members, who will decide whether the nurse violated the NPA and the appropriate punishment. To fulfill the due process requirements of the Fourteenth Amendment, the board of nursing must provide you with:
  Notice of the charges against you
  Evidence that supports the charges
  A hearing in which you have the opportunity to cross-examine the witnesses and to present your own evidence and witnesses
- If you are not satisfied with the board's actions and punishment, you can appeal your case to the appropriate state court.
- At every stage during the disciplinary process, you have the right to have an attorney present. Questions that you should ask of a potential attorney include the following: (1) How many of your cases were in the area of administrative law and procedures? (2) How many times have you represented clients in front of professional boards, such as the board of nursing?

For examples of nursing actions that constitute unprofessional conduct,

 Go to **Tables, Boxes, Figures: ESG Box 45-3, Actions, Behaviors, or Omissions That Constitute Unprofessional Conduct,** on Davis*Plus.*

 Think**Like a Nurse** 45-4

A registered nurse was assigned to care for a 76-year-old patient who had a stroke (brain attack). On entering the room, the nurse found the patient surrounded by 10 family members. The nurse requested the family members leave the room so she could conduct her initial assessment and perform any related treatments. They did so. The nurse provided care in a professional, unhurried, and gentle manner. As she was leaving, the patient said, "Thank you. You are a wonderful nurse." Later, the nursing supervisor told her the patient told his family members that the nurse had spoken harshly to him and had yanked his arms. The family stated they would file a complaint with the hospital administrator and the board of nursing.

- Are there grounds for disciplinary actions? What should the nurse do?

Knowledge**Check** 45-2
How does each of the following protect patients?
- The Patient Care Partnership (PCP)
- Nursing codes of ethics
- Mandatory reporting laws

Credentialing

Many healthcare disciplines, including nursing, use a voluntary form of self-regulation called **credentialing**. In the legal sense, credentialing includes accreditation and certification. Having credentials implies that the person or agency has met higher standards than the minimum (e.g., licensure).

Accreditation Most nursing boards establish educational requirements for nursing programs and continuing education courses within a given state. The board usually requires that for a nursing program to be approved, it must meet the requirements for accreditation established by the Accreditation Commission for Education in Nursing or the Commission on Collegiate Nursing Education and by the state NPA. This helps ensure students receive education that meets the minimum standard for quality and that patients are cared for by safe practitioners.

Accreditation also applies to institutions other than educational facilities; for example, hospitals seek accreditation by The Joint Commission. This is intended to ensure a minimum standard quality of care is provided.

Certification Another form of credentialing is **certification**. Through certification and licensing, the board identifies nurses who are qualified for advanced practice (e.g., clinical nurse specialists, midwives, and nurse practitioners) or for certification in a subspecialty, such as emergency nursing or pediatric nursing. In some states, the board establishes the criteria for certification, including (1) educational preparation, (2) clinical experience, and (3) certification by other professional organizations. In other states, the nurse may obtain an advanced practice license only if she is first certified by a national organization, such as the American Nurses Credentialing Corporation or a specialty organization. Not all states require certification for advanced practice nurses.

WHAT IS CRIMINAL LAW?

Criminal law deals with wrongs or offenses against society. It may result in prosecution (legal action) by the state or federal government for engaging in behavior that constitutes a crime. A **crime** is a violation of a law as defined by a legislative body. The legislature also specifies the punishments for the crime. State-level criminal laws vary from state to state.

There are two "levels" of crimes: misdemeanors and felonies. The primary difference is the possible punishment.

- **Felonies** involve crimes punishable by more than 1 year in jail (e.g., murder, assisted suicide, rape/sexual assault, stealing drugs and equipment, felony abuse). A person convicted of a felony loses the right to vote, hold public office, serve on a jury, and possess firearms. The person may also lose any professional license.

- A **misdemeanor**, compared with a felony, is a minor charge. Misdemeanors involve less than a year in jail. They include crimes such as assault, battery, and petty theft. You may also lose your nursing license if you are convicted of a misdemeanor that involves crimes against persons or that can cause harm to others.

An emerging issue in the nursing profession is whether nurses who accidentally cause harm to patients should be charged with criminal offenses (e.g., a nurse accidentally administers the wrong drug to a patient and the patient dies). In the past, these cases have been dealt with under civil law and by the board of nursing. Now state prosecutors are beginning to bring felony and misdemeanor charges against these nurses.

Case: Criminal Law

Several patients complained that their pain medication was not working. A review of the health records of the patients assigned to the nurse revealed that all but one of her patients who received pain medication had similar complaints. When confronted, the nurse admitted to stealing the patients' pain medication and giving them saline. She also admitted to using other nurses' passwords to steal narcotics. The nurse was terminated and reported to the board of nursing. She refused to enter an impaired nurse's program. Her license was revoked after a hearing. She also faced criminal charges for theft of controlled substances.

Case: Criminal Law

Joan, RN, was arrested for stealing computer equipment and wound supplies from the hospital that were valued at $55,000. She was charged with grand larceny, a felony. Two weeks before her trial, she entered into a plea deal that reduced the charge to a misdemeanor with probation for 6 months.

For an expanded discussion of criminal law,

 Go to Chapter 45, **Supplemental Materials: Criminal Law,** on Davis*Plus.*

WHAT IS CIVIL LAW?

In contrast to criminal law, in which the state or federal government brings charges against a person, civil law involves a dispute between individuals or entities. A settlement in civil law often results in the guilty party paying monetary damages. The two types of civil law are contract law and tort law.

- **Contract law** involves a written or oral agreement between two parties in which one party accepts an offer made by the other party to perform (or not perform)

certain acts in exchange for something of value. A breach of contract occurs if either party does not comply with the terms of the agreement. An example would be an employment contract.

- **Tort law**, in comparison, deals with wrongs done to one person by another person that do not involve contracts. A tort is a civil wrong and there are three types of tort: quasi-intentional torts, intentional torts, and unintentional torts.

What Are Quasi-Intentional Torts?

Quasi-intentional torts involve actions that injure a person's reputation. The overall concept for these torts is defamation of character. All four of the following essential elements of **defamation of character** must be present. The communication (written or oral) about the person:

- Was false
- Was made to another person or persons
- Caused the defamed person to experience shame and ridicule and had a negative impact on the person's reputation
- Was made as a statement of fact rather than as an opinion

Libel is the written or published form of defamation of character. **Slander** is the spoken or verbal form of defamation of character. A person is not guilty of defamation of character if the statement made about the other person is true or if the person has the protection of a "privilege," such as reporting possible child abuse.

Case: Quasi-Intentional Torts

The nursing supervisor calls you into a conference room and states, "I know that you have been stealing (diverting) narcotics from the unit and injecting yourself with it while at work. It shows, because your work is sloppy and you are falsifying your documentation. You are a poor excuse for a nurse." Before you can defend yourself, the supervisor turns and leaves. The statements are not true. Nurses in the conference room try to console you. The supervisor has committed slander.

What Are Intentional Torts?

An **intentional tort** is an action taken by one person with the intent to harm another person. The harm does not have to be violent, hostile, or cause a significant amount of pain or distress to the other person. The person must have merely intended to cause harm or known the action would bring about the harm. Intentional torts may also be prosecuted under criminal law. For example, a nurse who is sued for malpractice in civil court may also be charged with a homicide if a patient died because of the nurse's actions. Intentional torts most commonly encountered in nursing are assault, battery, false imprisonment, and invasion of privacy.

Assault

An assault occurs when a nurse intentionally places a patient in immediate fear of personal violence or offensive contact. An assault must include words expressing an intention to cause harm and some type of action. For example, a nurse has committed an assault if she says to the patient "I will slap you" and raises her hand as if to slap the patient. The combination of the words and action causes the patient to believe the threat will be carried out.

Battery

A **battery** is committed when (1) an offensive or harmful physical contact is made to the patient without his consent, or (2) there is unauthorized touching of a person's body by another person. To avoid charges of battery, always obtain informed consent before providing certain treatments. On admission to healthcare facilities, patients sign a general consent form, which usually covers routine aspects of nursing care, such as vital signs and patient assessments. However, when performing any invasive procedure, such as inserting a catheter or intravenous line, you should always explain the procedure to the patient and obtain his consent before beginning.

Case: Battery—Withdrawal of Consent During the Procedure

A patient having blood drawn experienced severe pain and requested the technician to stop while he was attempting to fill a second vial of blood. The technician continued and filled the second vial. Ruling in favor of the technician, the court noted that the patient did not allege that stopping the treatment was feasible and without harm. No battery is committed if, at the patient's request, the procedure cannot be stopped without creating harm (*Pallacovitch v. Waterbury Hosp.*, 2012).

Assault and Battery

An **assault and battery** occurs when there is the intent to cause a person fear combined with an offensive or harmful contact.

Case: Assault and Battery

A patient admitted for an elective surgical procedure complained that the automatic blood pressure cuff was causing her extreme pain and demanded it be removed. The nurse did not immediately remove the cuff as requested by the patient. The nurse was guilty of a battery, but not assault, because there was no evidence the nurse intended to create or cause fear or pain (*Coulter v. Thomas*, 2000).

False Imprisonment

False imprisonment is the restraining of a person without proper legal authorization. It includes any type of unjustified restriction on a person's freedom of movement—for example, when nurses restrain patients without their permission or when patients are involuntarily committed to mental health units. False imprisonment can involve the use of physical restraints (e.g., vest or wrist restraints) or chemical restraints (e.g., sedatives or opioids). You may restrain patients who pose an immediate threat to themselves or others. However, you must immediately obtain the proper authorization to continue the restraint.

Against Medical Advice If a competent patient wishes to leave the healthcare facility, you should contact the nursing supervisor and the primary care provider. The patient must be informed of the risks associated with leaving, and given the choice to stay and receive treatment or to sign out against medical advice (AMA). You need to be aware of the hospital policy and procedures on AMA discharges.

Invasion of Privacy

Invasion of privacy violates a person's right to be left alone. The law recognizes that a person's personal life should not be opened up for public scrutiny and the person has the right to freedom from unwanted interference in her private affairs. A person has the right to:

- Have her private information protected
- Not be falsely portrayed or intentionally misrepresented in character, beliefs, or actions
- Be free from unwanted intrusion (spying, eavesdropping).

Examples of violating right to privacy include discussing patients in public places (e.g., elevators, cafeterias), photographing patients without their permission, providing information to news media without consent, searching a patient's personal belongings without permission, and releasing medical information without the patient's consent.

Fraud

Fraud is the false representation of significant facts by words or by conduct. It can occur, through making false statements, falsifying documentation, or concealing information that should have been disclosed. It is intentionally misleading or deceiving another person to act (or not act) for the personal gain of the one committing the fraud.

Case: Fraud

A home health nurse was terminated from her salaried position after she refused to falsify Medicare documentation. She was instructed to bill patients for more visits than actually occurred, alter care records to prolong a patient's eligibility for home services, and admit a non-homebound patient to homebound therapy (*Admore v. Nurse Connection, Inc.*, 2009). An award of damages and attorney fees in her favor was upheld by the court of appeals (*Nurse Connection, Inc. v. Admore*, 2010).

What Are Unintentional Torts?

The most common type of unintentional tort involving healthcare professionals is negligence or malpractice. **Negligence** is the failure to use ordinary or reasonable care or the failure to act in a reasonable and prudent (careful) manner. *Malpractice* has a similar definition, but applies only to professionals, such as nurses and physicians. It is defined as the failure of a professional person to act in a reasonable and prudent manner. A malpractice lawsuit may occur when such actions cause injury or death to the patient. The person bringing the lawsuit is the **plaintiff** and the person who must defend against the lawsuit is the **defendant**.

Malpractice/Negligence Liability

To win and recover damages (money) in a malpractice lawsuit, the plaintiff must prove four elements (duty, breach of duty, causation, and damages). The elements must be proved by a "preponderance of the evidence," in other words, with enough evidence to tip the scale in his or her favor.

Duty The nurse–patient relationship creates this legal obligation. A duty forms when the patient is assigned to the nurse or seeks treatment from the nurse, or when the nurse observes another person doing something that could harm the patient.

Breach of Duty A breach of duty occurs when the nurse fails to meet standards of care. Attorneys look to several sources of information to identify the standards of care and to determine what a reasonable and prudent (careful) nurse would have done in the situation. These sources include the NPA, job descriptions, hospital policies and procedures, textbooks, professional standards and guidelines developed by professional organizations, and the nursing code of ethics.

The attorney will usually hire an **expert witness** who is a nurse with advanced education or experience. The purpose of an expert witness is to educate the judge and jury on the local practice of nursing and how the nurse's actions or omissions failed to meet acceptable practice for nurses.

Causation The breach of duty or deviation from acceptable standards of care by the nurse must be the direct and proximate cause of the injury suffered by the patient. Causation is usually established based on the testimony of experts, such as physicians, advanced practice nurses, or other healthcare professionals, who can clearly show the connection between the nurse's action or omission and the resulting injury to the patient.

Case: Causation

A nurse forgot to change the patient's dressing at the scheduled time, but changed it 3 hours later. The hospital policy reads that nurses must administer medications or perform prescribed treatments within 30 minutes before or 30 minutes after the scheduled time. The patient did not experience any harm or infection.

In this case, there were both existence of and a breach of duty, but the breach of duty did not cause any harm or injury to the patient. Therefore, if a malpractice action had been brought, the plaintiff would not have received an award. Nurses are encouraged to report medication and treatment errors as promptly as possible so that actions can be taken to prevent and/or minimize injury to the patient.

Damages In civil cases, the remedy for the harm the patient suffered is money. The judge or jury will award the plaintiff money to compensate him for pain and suffering, lost wages, additional medical bills, and other losses. In some cases, the plaintiff may be awarded punitive damages (additional money) for grossly negligent or wrongful behavior by the healthcare provider.

Case: Damages

The plaintiff began to bleed excessively after a non-emergency cesarean section delivery. The nursing staff notified the provider of the bleeding, decreased blood pressure and oxygen level, and increased heart rate. The patient had surgery to repair a uterine laceration and returned to the recovery room, where additional blood products and fundal massage were prescribed. The obstetrician indicated that nurses did not notify him that the patient's pulse rate was high and the blood pressure and blood oxygen content remained low. He admitted that he had not read the monitor. The nurses did not notify the physician because they assumed he reviewed and interpreted the monitor readings each time he visited the patient. Two hours after being admitted to the recovery room, the patient arrested, was resuscitated, but suffered severe brain damage. She died 6 months later when mechanical ventilation was removed.

Analysis of the Case:
Duty: Based on the nurse–patient relationship
Breach of Duty: Failure to communicate to the provider; failure to intervene to counteract the patient's deteriorating condition
Causation: Appropriate medical care was not provided based on the patient's signs and symptoms
Damages: In the above case, a settlement was reached with a present value of about $1.35 million.
(Nurses Service Organization, 2013a)

KnowledgeCheck 45-3

- Distinguish negligence from malpractice.
- Distinguish civil law from criminal law.
- Under which type of law (constitutional, statutory, administrative, or common law) does each of the following fall?
  A defendant claiming the right not to incriminate himself under the Fifth Amendment
  A nurse having her license revoked by the state board of nursing
  The wording of a state nurse practice act
- Define *plaintiff* and *defendant* in the context of civil law.

Toward Evidence-Based Practice

Falls: Care plan not updated, Jury finds negligence (2010). Legal Eagle Eye Newsletter for the Nursing Profession. Retrieved from www.nursinglaw.com/fallcareplan4.pdf

A 51-year-old male with a below-the-knee amputation, kidney failure, and liver disease was placed in a nursing facility. He had short-term memory deficit and problems with balance. He was able to ambulate with a prosthesis and cane, but spent most of his time in a wheelchair. After falling on five previous occasions, he fell and broke his hip and died 9 months after the hip repair surgery. The expert witness, testifying about the breaches of duty, indicated that each fall required more than documentation of the fall in the resident's medical record. Likewise, given his short-term memory deficits, reminding him to ring his call bell was not an effective safety measure; he required new safety equipment (e.g., wheelchair tipping guards, bed brakes).

O'Dea v. Cardinal Cook Care Center, 2010 WL 3232844 (Sup. Ct. New York Co., New York, June 20, 2010).

1. Nurses knew the patient suffered from short-term memory deficits. What do you think was the basis for the court decision that the patient's injury was due to negligence of the nurse?

Nurses Service Organization. (2011). August 2011 Legal Case Study. Retrieved from http://www.nso.com/case-studies/article/293.jsp

A 74-year-old female was admitted to the hospital for repair of a T4 fracture from a fall that occurred in her kitchen. She had a rheumatoid arthritis with hand and feet deformities and osteoporosis. After an uncomplicated surgery, the patient was transferred to the orthopedic unit. The next morning, after completing a physical and fall risk assessment, the nurse assisted the patient to the bedside commode. She instructed the patient to call her when finished to be assisted back to bed and left the room. The commode collapsed and came apart, causing the patient to fall and fracture her tibia, which required additional surgery. She was discharged to a skilled nursing facility for 7 weeks and required the assistance of a walker or wheelchair. The patient sued, alleging that the nurse breached the standard of care by not staying with her or providing her with a bedpan. A verdict was returned in favor of the nurse.

2. What factors led to a defense verdict in this case?

Nurses Service Organization. (2013c). Woman falls while home health nurse is weighing her—fractured leg— surgery, rehab and need for continuing care— $791,573 verdict. January 2013 Legal Case Study. Retrieved from http://www.nso.com/case-studies/casestudy-article/315.jsp

A 74-year-old patient was receiving home healthcare services after a total knee replacement. The nurse instructed the patient to stand on a scale in the bathroom to obtain her weight. The patient fell and broke the fibula and tibia in one leg. Her injuries required additional surgery, hospitalizations, and continuing 24-hour home care. She sued the nurse, alleging a breach of duty by not providing her with proper support given her unstable balance and weighing her in a confined space. The jury rejected the nurse's defense that proper support was given and weighing her in the bathroom was reasonable.

3. In this case, what was the basis for the jury's decision that the patient's injury was the result of the nurse's negligence of the nurse?

 ThinkLike a Nurse 45-5

- Give one nursing example of each: negligence, malpractice, damages.
- Can you think of one nonfraudulent example of a nurse's being untruthful with a patient? Do you think that the circumstances described in your example make the untruthfulness justifiable?
- Can you think of an example of a nurse's committing assault, other than the one given in the text?

Vicarious Liability

You are legally accountable for your actions or inactions. This is a common legal principle that should guide your behavior. It means that you can be sued for behavior or omissions that deviate from acceptable standards. In certain circumstances, though, the law will assign liability to a person or entity that did not directly cause the injury but with whom you have a special kind of relationship. This type of liability is known as **vicarious** or **substituted liability**. The various types of vicarious liability existing under common law are discussed below.

Captain of the Ship This principle applies to situations in which a physician (e.g., surgeon or obstetrician) is held liable for the negligence of another healthcare provider. *Captain of the ship* usually applies to surgical suite situations. Many states no longer recognize it as protection for the nurse because the nurse is still liable for her own actions.

Borrowed Servant Doctrine This doctrine relieves the primary employer of liability for the actions or omission of its employee when the employee was borrowed by another person. In theory, the borrower becomes liable for the actions of the employee. This would apply, for example, to agency nurses.

Respondeat Superior The Latin term **respondeat superior** means "let the master answer." The employer must answer for the negligent acts or omissions of its employees, who are functioning within the scope of their employment. For example, a nurse working within the scope of her practice as a labor and delivery nurse makes a medication error; the hospital can be sued for the nurse's error.

KnowledgeCheck 45-4

- Define these terms: *assault, battery, fraud, slander, libel, negligence, malpractice.*
- State the four elements of malpractice.

LITIGATION IN CIVIL CLAIMS

Litigation is the formal process wherein the legal issues, rights, and duties between the parties are heard and decided (adjudicated). The litigation process follows several stages: (1) pleading and pretrial motions, (2) discovery, (3) alternative dispute resolution, (4) trial, and (5) appeal.

Pleading and Pretrial Motions

The litigation process starts when the plaintiff files a complaint. A **complaint** is a legal document outlining how the plaintiff has been harmed by another person. Once the case is filed with the court, the complaint is served on (delivered to) the defendant. The complaint identifies the plaintiff, the specific allegations and time frame, the standards allegedly breached (e.g., behavior[s] or omissions), the persons (defendants) involved, and the harm suffered.

If you are served with a complaint, you must immediately notify your employer. In addition, if you have malpractice insurance, you must also notify your insurance company. You will need an attorney to defend you. Your attorney has a specified time within which to file an answer (response) to the complaint. The answer addresses each of the allegations (unproven accusations). As a defendant, you should not contact the plaintiff or the plaintiff's attorney or discuss the case with coworkers or friends. The facility's risk manager and your attorney will advise you. Cooperate fully and be honest in all your answers.

Discovery Phase

The discovery process allows for both parties to gather facts and evidence about the case that can be used at trial. Discovery is designed to make sure there are no "surprises" during the trial. Attorneys may obtain discovery through written questions (*interrogatories*), requests for documents and other evidence, and by *depositions* (attorneys orally question parties to the lawsuit under oath, as though they were testifying in court). You may be deposed (questioned) as either a

fact witness, a party to the lawsuit (defendant), or an expert witness. A *fact witness* is someone who was present when the incident occurred, whereas the defendant will testify about the care provided and the actions taken.

Deposition may occur several years after the incident, so you may not remember specific information. You should prepare for the deposition by reviewing the medical records and any other evidence that may exist regarding the lawsuit. During the deposition, listen to your attorney, do not volunteer information, take your time before answering each question, and provide only objective information. Always tell the truth, but base your answers on facts; do not speculate. If your attorney objects to any question, immediately stop and do not provide an answer unless directed by your attorney.

Alternative Dispute Resolution

Lawyers and involved parties usually try to resolve disputes before going to trial. The three most common methods of alternative dispute resolution are as follows:

- **Negotiation** takes place informally between the lawyers for the plaintiff and the defendant in an attempt to settle the case prior to trial.
- **Mediation** is the attempt to resolve the dispute using a neutral third party. The primary role of the mediator is to help the parties focus on the issues and to facilitate communication to identify what is needed to reach a resolution.
- **Arbitration** involves a third party making a decision after hearing the evidence and information from both parties.

Trial Process

If the dispute cannot be resolved and is not dismissed by the court during pretrial motions, the case goes to trial. Malpractice cases are usually heard by a jury. After hearing all the evidence and reviewing submitted documents, the judge or jury makes a decision, which is either dismissal or the award of damages.

Appeal

After the judge or jury has made a decision, either party has the opportunity to present post-trial motions, move for a new trial, or appeal the verdict and/or damages to a court of appeals. The court of appeals will review the transcript and documents from the trial and determine whether errors (e.g., improper evidence allowed, proper evidence denied, improper jury instructions) were made during that trial that resulted in an unfair verdict. The court of appeals can uphold the verdict or dismiss the verdict, in part or in whole, and remand (send back) the case to the trial court with special instructions.

KnowledgeCheck 45-5

- Identify the phases of the trial process.
- How is arbitration different from mediation?

PracticalKnowledge
knowing **how**

To decrease your chances of being involved in a malpractice suit, you should know the most common causes of malpractice claims and some practical preventive actions you can take. Keep in mind that causes are often difficult to categorize because they overlap; an error usually results from interlocking causes.

WHAT ARE THE MOST COMMON MALPRACTICE CLAIMS?

Nurses must use the nursing process to provide safe and efficient care to patients. The most common causes of nursing malpractice claims (Box 45-3) can be categorized according to where they fall in the nursing process: failure to assess and diagnose, failure to plan, failure to implement, and failure to evaluate (O'Keefe, 2001; Reising, 2012).

Failure to Assess and Diagnose

As the first step in the nursing process, the failure to conduct an adequate assessment can lead to numerous breaches of duty. Failure to analyze the data and make correct nursing diagnoses can lead to incorrect actions, no action, or improper delegation.

Case: Failure to Assess and Diagnose

In an actual case, a 67-year-old patient who had a total knee replacement had an epidural catheter inserted for pain management. After successful treatment of an episode of hypotension in the postanesthesia care unit, he was transferred to the medical-surgical unit. The registered nurses assessed the patient and delegated direct care to an LPN, although this was denied by the LPN. Three hours later, the patient experienced nausea and vomiting. The patient was found cyanotic and unresponsive 10 minutes later and subsequently died from anoxic encephalopathy. Many facts were disputed among the numerous codefendants and documentation was poor (Nurses Service Organization, 2012).

Safe and competent assessment and diagnosis practices require the nurse to:

- Perform an admission assessment. This duty cannot be delegated to a nursing assistant.
- Analyze the assessment data to clearly identify problems.
- Apply theoretical knowledge to ensure a correct diagnosis. The presenting signs and symptoms should be consistent with the disease process or medical problem. Remember that the nursing diagnosis consists of Patient Response r/t Etiology. When the assessment reveals adverse symptoms, the nurse must report the symptoms to the appropriate provider and carry out the standard nursing care and prescribed interventions.
- Conduct frequent focused assessments until the end of your shift or until the problem is resolved.

BOX 45-3 ■ Common Causes of Malpractice Litigation

Failure to respond, such as not intervening to care for the patient's specific symptoms or expressed request for care.

Failure to educate, such as not answering questions, not teaching self-care measures, or not explaining procedures or equipment adequately on the patient's discharge.

Failure to follow standards of care and institutional policies and procedures. This most commonly occurs in the form of medication errors and failure to follow a provider's orders. It also frequently occurs from failure to use equipment responsibly. Among other reasons, a nurse may fail to follow standards of care when the unit is understaffed or the nurse is inexperienced.

Failure to communicate often comes up when a nurse fails to seek medical authorization for a treatment or fails to notify a physician in a timely manner when a patient's condition warrants action.

Failure to document the following in the patient's record: assessment data (e.g., drug allergies), patient injuries, medication administration details, patient progress and response to treatment, physicians' orders, and telephone conversations with physicians.

Failure to act as an advocate. Nurses must frequently intervene to prevent harm to the patient by other healthcare providers and by relatives and significant others. The following are examples of advocacy errors:

- *Medical and discharge orders.* As an example of failure to advocate, suppose two physicians order the same drug for a patient, but under different brand names. The nurse does not recognize that two drugs are the same, so the patient receives twice the normal amount and has a toxic reaction. Other errors occur when the nurse does not question incomplete or illegible orders or does not question discharge orders when she believes the patient is not well enough to be discharged.

- *Impaired nurses.* You have a duty under most state nursing practice acts to report impaired nursing practice (e.g., as a result of alcoholism or mental illness) to the appropriate licensing agency. Failure to do so is a failure to advocate for patients.

- *Family and significant others.* Advocacy includes reporting neglect and intentional injuries to children, the elderly, and the disabled. Failure to do so may constitute negligence and/or violation of state statutes.

Failure to Plan

The ANA standards specifically requires nurses to formulate a plan of care. The plan of care may be written or unwritten depending on state regulations. Many agencies require nurses to complete nursing care plans or patient care tools as a means of measuring patient outcomes and progress. The plan of care should be consistent with standards of treatments acceptable for the given diagnosis or problem. Safe and competent practices in this category require the nurse to:

- Know the correct approach to treat patient actual or potential problems.
- Have the theoretical knowledge base to successfully plan nursing care for patients.
- Develop a plan of care that is individualized to the patient.

Failure to Implement a Plan of Care

Implementation is the nursing process step in which the nurse performs the care or nursing interventions. Failure to implement encompasses a variety of actions, shown in Box 45-3, Common Causes of Malpractice Litigation.

Failure to Evaluate

Evaluation is the last step in the nursing process. It requires you to make a decision or judgment about the success of your interventions in addressing the client's problems. The duty to evaluate requires an ongoing cycle of the following:

- *Observing for changes* after interventions and treatments. You must know the expected outcomes and side effects of medications and treatments, so you can accurately interpret and document anticipated and adverse responses.
- *Recognizing significance of the change.* For example, if Mr. Adkins's blood pressure (BP) is usually 140/88, a change to 150/90 after exercise would not be significant for him. But for Mrs. Jonas, whose BP is usually 100/64, a change to 150/90 would be cause for concern.
- *Documenting or reporting symptoms* to the appropriate person. If a change is significant, you have a legal duty to report the change to the appropriate provider and to document this change in the appropriate medical record.
- *Following up on patient responses* to nursing interventions requires you to know the expected outcomes and side effects of medications and treatments.

KnowledgeCheck 45-6

- State the four requirements of the nurse's duty to assess.
- State four ways in which the nurse may fail to implement a plan of care.
- Give one example of the duty to advocate for a patient.
- List the four components of the nurse's legal duty to evaluate.

Quality and Safety Education for Nurses

Fall Prevention and the Nurse's Legal Responsibilities

Chapter Key Concepts: Law, Liability, Malpractice, Negligence

Competency: Safety (Knowledge, Skills, Attitudes)*

Background: The beginning nursing student needs to acquire knowledge about the legal implications in nursing and develop the skills "necessary to make critical legal and personal accountability decisions about quality of care and patient safety" (March, Cassandra, Adams, et al., 2011, p. 68). Patient falls are considered a hospital-acquired condition, a priority issue for hospitals, and a threat to patient safety (Spoelstra, Given, & Given, 2012). A fall risk assessment and strategies to reduce falls are required to meet The Joint Commission standard.

Scenario: The student nurse is caring for a patient and leaves the bedside to prepare for medication administration. The student fails to return the bed to low position before leaving. The patient attempts to get out of bed, falls, and sustains a hip fracture.

Think About It: In the scenario, what are the legal responsibilities of the student, the faculty member, and the staff nurse?

➤ Using the American Nurses Association's *Scope and Standards of Clinical Nursing Practice*, identify which standard of care has been violated.

➤ Does the scenario constitute negligence/malpractice on the part of the student?

➤ Make a simple Concept Map showing how the following are related:

The key concept, Malpractice

The QSEN competency, Safety

Fall prevention

Discuss answers to the Think About It questions with your peers—if you have difficulty with any of the questions, consult your instructor.

 Go to the QSEN Web site, at **http://qsen.org/ competencies/pre-licensure-ksas/**

*As reference for your QSEN log box, the QSEN KSA that is most pertinent is:

Demonstrate effective use of strategies to reduce risk of harm to self or others.

HOW CAN YOU MINIMIZE YOUR MALPRACTICE RISKS?

The best way to minimize your risk of malpractice is to practice in a safe and competent manner. You must have the appropriate body of theoretical knowledge for clinical practice, which you are already beginning to acquire. You should also be familiar with your state's nurse practice act, professional standards of practice, and institutional policies and procedures. These provide the legal framework for your practice and help you to evaluate the quality of the care you deliver. Ignorance of the law and of practice standards is no excuse for failing to comply with the law, and it is no defense in a malpractice suit.

You may significantly reduce your risk exposures when you follow these three guidelines:

- Perform timely patient assessments and document your findings for every patient interaction.
- Communicate all changes in your patient's status to the primary healthcare provider and document those changes.
- Use the proper chain of command to ensure appropriate and timely care when the primary healthcare provider is not available (Banford & Budake, 2012).

You will find discussion of other helpful suggestions in the remainder of this chapter. For more tips,

 Go to Chapter 45, **Clinical Insight 45-2: Tips for Avoiding Malpractice,** in Volume 2.

If you would like to see the typical standards of care found in a nurse practice act,

 Go to Chapter 45, **Tables, Boxes, Figures: ESG Box 45-4, Minimum Acceptable Standards of Care Required by a Typical State Nurse Practice Act,** on DavisPlus.

Use the Nursing Process and Follow Professional Standards of Care

The nursing process provides you with a systematic approach to patient care and is the legally acceptable model of decision making in nursing practice. Your documentation should reveal that you have assessed, diagnosed, planned, implemented, and evaluated care based on current and acceptable standards.

Avoid Medication and Treatment Errors

Medication errors are among the most common healthcare errors. To administer medications accurately, you must know the rationale for administering the drug, safe dosage ranges, side effects of the medications, and relevant information to teach the patient about the medication. To prevent medication errors, you should:

- Follow the "rights of medication administration" (see Chapter 26).
- Investigate any patient concerns before giving the medication (e.g., the patient might say, "Is this a new medication? I have not taken this one before.").

- Question prescriptions that are incomplete or that seem inappropriate.
- Make sure the equipment used to administer drugs is working properly.
- Use the correct technique to provide patient treatment (e.g., maintain a sterile field during wound care to prevent an infection).

For tips to help you use equipment properly and safely,

 Go to Chapter 45, **Clinical Insight 45-1: Using Equipment Safely,** in Volume 2.

Report and Document

For every suggestion for minimizing malpractice risk, add the reminder "Document what happened." Remember the old adage "If it isn't documented, it wasn't done." If you are ever required to appear in court, the patient record may be the only proof you have of the care you gave. It is unlawful to make false entries or destroy entries in medical records, but do carefully record in detail all care you provide.

Cases: Documentation Can Make a Difference

In an actual case, the plaintiff alleged that the nurse had violated numerous standards of practice including the failure to properly assess the patient, failure to properly monitor vital signs and intake/output, and failure to recognize and respond to signs and symptoms of sepsis. A settlement was reached for $706,250. Weaknesses in documentation revealed that the patient's blood pressure was not documented until day 14 of home care, and evidence of infection—wound appearance and size, amount and appearance of drainage—was not consistently documented by the nurses caring for the patient (Nurses Service Organization, n.d.)

In another actual case, the nurse was accused of failure to properly assess and monitor an impaired, restrained patient and failure to provide proper care in a safe environment. The patient suffered severe burns over 25 percent of his body when the bed linen ignited as he attempted to burn off the restraints with a lighter. A verdict was rendered in favor of the nurse. Strengths in documentation showed that the nurse performed patient monitoring and assessments every 15 minutes as prescribed, missing one time to care for a critical patient. The assessment findings at each check were fully documented in the patient's medical records (Nurses Service Organization, 2013b)

Charting

Key Point: *A basic principle of charting is that a third person should be able to read your documentation and form a mental picture of your patient and the care provided during your shift.* Record all interactions with clients, as well as patients' refusal of or noncompliance with treatment. Document telephone conversations with primary care providers, including time, content of the conversation and the action you took. Document the facts; do not editorialize (e.g., do not write, "I could not check on the patient as often as ordered because we were understaffed"). Refer to Chapter 18 for a review of your documentation responsibilities, and use the letters F-A-C-T-U-A-L as a reminder when charting.

F—Your information must be **factual** and objective. Don't chart your opinions.

A—You must be **accurate**: For example, record the vital signs accurately.

C—Your information must be **complete**: Don't omit any important information.

T—You must be **timely**: Chart care as soon as possible after doing it; don't wait until the end of your shift and then try to remember everything that happened.

U—You must be **diligent**. Always document **unusual occurrences**.

A—You must document your **assessment data** and the plan of care.

L—Remember that the patient's chart is a **legal record** and is subpoenaed in a malpractice case.

 Go to Chapter 45, **Clinical Insight 45-3: Guidelines for Documenting Care,** in Volume 2.

Incident Reports

If a standard of care is breached or an unusual incident occurs (e.g., a visitor or patient falls or is injured), you should complete an **incident report** (also called *variance report* or *occurrence report*). These reports are used, in part, for quality improvement in the agency and should not be used to discipline staff members or be placed in employees' files. The goal is to prevent the incident from occurring again. In many states, the incident report is not made available as a part of discovery in litigation. It becomes discoverable (available to the plaintiff) if it is mentioned in the medical records. You can prevent an otherwise confidential report from becoming evidence by not writing "Incident report completed" in the patient record.

When reporting an incident, be sure to clearly identify the patient, date, time, and location. Briefly describe the incident in factual terms. Use the exact words of the patient or persons involved and put the information in quotes. Do not speculate, draw conclusions, or place blame. Identify any witnesses to the event or equipment involved. For example:

1900	Demerol 50 mg given intramuscularly. Physician order: Demerol 15 mg.
1930	Patient's respirations: 8 breaths/min; BP 100/60; skin pale.
2000	Called Dr. Smith. Prescription for naloxone (Narcan) 1 mg IV STAT
2005	Narcan given as prescribed. Resp 12 breaths/min, BP 118/70

You should be prepared to discuss the 30-minute delay between the patient's findings and contacting the physician. The standard of care would require that the physician be notified immediately. Chapter 18 presents additional information on occurrence (incident) reports.

Obtain Informed Consent

Informed consent is the permission for any and all types of care given by the patient with full knowledge of the risks, benefits, costs, and alternatives. For hospital admission and for invasive or specialized treatments or diagnostic procedures, the consent must be written and signed by the patient or the person legally responsible for the patient. The law provides for implied or assumed consent in emergency situations; therefore, written consent is not necessary in an emergency if experts would agree that there was an immediate threat to life or health.

Elements of Consent

To be legally valid, the informed consent should fulfill the following requirements:

- **Completeness.** Healthcare consumers need adequate information to make educated decisions regarding their treatment. Be sure they get information on the nature of the procedure, risks, benefits, post-procedure care and considerations, and treatment alternatives.
- **Clarity and Comprehension.** Language should be appropriate to the patient's educational level, so the patient (or his surrogate decision maker) can understand the explanation. Always ask the patient to describe in his own words the procedure to which he is consenting. If the patient asks, "What will the doctor do during surgery?" the nurse is aware that the patient does not understand the nature of the surgery. She could contact the surgeon.
- **Voluntariness.** The patient must be free to accept or reject the treatment. He must not be pressured or coerced to give consent. There must be no actual or implied threat by anyone to force the patient into having the surgery (e.g., "Mom, if you don't let them do this, I'm never coming back to see you."). Otherwise, the consent is not valid.
- **Competence.** The person must have the ability to understand the information and make a choice about the particular situation (e.g., the ability to decide what clothing to wear does not necessarily mean that the person is competent to decide whether to have surgery). If the person is confused and disoriented, you should contact the case manager or your supervisor for guidance. State law identifies the order of individuals who can make decisions for individuals who are judged incompetent. It is usually the spouse, then parents, then sisters and brothers, and so on. If the person does not have relatives, the court will appoint a legal guardian to make healthcare decisions.

Generally speaking, a competent adult has the legal right to consent to or refuse any treatment. However, this right does not always extend to situations in which an adult is making the decision for a minor. A court sometimes will authorize treatment of a child against his parents' wishes. In some states, a minor who is married or living independently is considered emancipated and can make his/her own healthcare decisions.

The Nurse's Role

As a nurse, your legal role regarding written consent is to collaborate with the primary provider, usually a physician or advanced practice nurse. You may witness a patient's signature on a consent form, but you are not legally responsible for explaining the treatments and options or for evaluating whether the provider has adequately explained them. You must, however, determine that the elements of a valid informed consent are in place, communicate the patient's needs for more information to the care provider, and provide feedback if the patient wishes to change her consent.

Be sure you have the patient's informal, verbal consent for nursing interventions that you perform (e.g., urinary catheterization). Coming to the agency for healthcare implies that the patient consents to usual treatment, such as injections and vital signs. However, you should explain all procedures to the patient before their implementation. If the patient objects, identify the reasons for the refusal, correct any misinformation, and explain the benefits of the treatment. If the patient still objects or refuses, do not proceed. Contact the primary care provider.

In addition to state statutes, case law, and agency policy, The Joint Commission standards provide valuable guidance regarding informed participation in decision making. See Chapter 44 for discussion of informed consent from an ethical perspective.

Maintain Patient Safety

 Falls are by far the most common incident reported in hospitals and long-term care facilities. On admission to the facility, all patients should be assessed for risks of falls and "fall precautions" instituted when needed. Simply raising the siderails on the bed is not enough to prevent falls. You may still be found negligent if the patient falls because he called for help and no one came to assist him out of bed, or if the call device was not placed within the patient's reach and he was unable to call for assistance. Several useful tools have been developed for assessing falls, including the Morse Fall Scale. See Chapter 24 for information about meeting patients' safety needs, including falls and use of restraints. For a falls risk tool,

 Go to Chapter 24, **Tables, Boxes, Figures: ESG Figure 24-1, Falls Risk Assessment Using the Morse Scale,** on DavisPlus.

Maintain Confidentiality and Privacy

Always maintain patient confidentiality unless directed by law to do otherwise (e.g., when a patient is threatening to harm someone). Family members and significant others do not have an automatic right to information about the patient. For example, parents do not have an automatic right to see the medical records of their adult child or minor child who is married or emancipated. Of course,

you need to discuss clients' medical conditions with other health team members, but this does not include chatting about the client's personal life or talking about the patient in the lunchroom. **Key Point: *You should discuss the patient's health status with those who have a need to know (those involved in the patient's care).***

Another aspect of privacy is to maintain the confidentiality of patient records (e.g., do not leave a patient's health record in locations that are accessible to visitors or nonauthorized staff). Do not give information about patients over the phone unless the agency has a system that enables you to know that you are speaking to a person authorized by the patient. Refer to Chapter 41 if you require advice about maintaining confidentiality of electronic records. Also,

Go to Chapter 18, **Clinical Insight 18-3: Guidelines for Documenting in the Electronic Health Record,** in Volume 2.

Provide Education and Counseling

Part of your role as a nurse is to provide information to patients and caregivers about their illness, medications, and other treatments. This helps to fulfill informed consent requirements and to involve patients in their own healthcare. Use teaching-learning principles to make sure the patient understands, retains the knowledge, and can demonstrate any skills. Ask the patient to repeat instructions to you or to provide a return demonstration of a skill, such as self-injection of insulin. To reinforce understanding, always review written information with the patient. Refer to Chapter 19 for more information on teaching patients.

Delegate According to Guidelines

As a nurse, you are expected to properly delegate to ensure patients receive timely and quality care. This involves implementing the five rights of delegation: delegating the right task to the right person, under the right circumstances, using the right directions and communication, and practicing the right supervision and evaluation. To do this safely, you (the delegator) must know the education background, knowledge, experience, and physical and emotional capability of those to whom you delegate (delegatee). You must also know the scope of practice of the delegatee as determined by the state board of nursing. In addition, you must consider the condition and requirements of the patient. The registered nurse should not delegate to LPNs or nursing assistive personnel patients whose care is complex, unpredictable, require nursing judgment, or involve a high level of interaction.

When delegating, be sure the delegatee understands the assignment. The Case feature "Failure to Assess and Diagnose" identifies numerous breakdowns in the delegation process. The duty to delegate has a corresponding duty to supervise the care and evaluate the outcome. For example, if you assign an LPN to provide direct care for a new postoperative patient, you should obtain hourly updates on the patient's status. If you need to review specific guidelines for delegating, see

Chapter 7. For the ANA and other relevant Web sites on delegation,

 Go to Chapter 45, **Resources for Caregivers and Health Professionals,** on DavisPlus.

Accept Assignments for Which You Are Qualified

As a nurse, when you accept an assignment, you must consider whether the assignment is within your level of education, experience, and physical and emotional capability. The refusal to accept an assignment does not mean that you have abandoned the patient. Your duty to the patient begins once you accept the assignment. **Key Point:** *You are legally responsible for the assignment that you accept. If your assignment becomes overwhelming and unmanageable, immediately contact the charge nurse or nursing supervisor for assistance.*

Nursing supervisors have a duty to ensure adequate staffing and patient coverage. This means that you must report to the nurse in charge when leaving the patient care unit. Failure to do this may result in charges of patient abandonment. A nurse should never leave the patient care unit without making certain there is another nurse available to provide care to the patient. This does not mean that you must work overtime (e.g., a double shift), as long as you follow established policies and procedures, which will include giving notice and explaining your reasoning (e.g., that you are too fatigued to provide safe care).

If you work a double shift or if a unit is understaffed, you are still liable for any malpractice that you commit. Unfortunately, being "busy" and overwhelmed is not a defense for error. In addition, you have the duty to tell supervisors that staffing is inadequate; be sure to do it in writing. You should know and follow agency policy on how to address short-staff issues.

Participate in Continuing Education

As a nurse, you have a duty to participate in ongoing education in your area of practice and to keep up with new laws, equipment, treatments, and procedures. Be sure to obtain documentation of your attendance. In some states, continuing education is mandatory for license renewal. In states where it is not mandatory, other standards of care still require that you obtain the education and training necessary to implement current nursing procedures and practices. In malpractice cases, the nurse's competency in providing nursing care is frequently an issue. Continuing education is available "for credit" through colleges and universities, other healthcare agencies, conferences, in some nursing journals (e.g., *The American Journal of Nursing*), and online.

Observe Professional Boundaries

Nurses must be careful to maintain professional boundaries, not only with the patient but also with other healthcare providers. Do not accept gifts from patients or encourage attempts to have close personal relationships outside the healthcare setting. Violations of professional boundaries may be physical, sexual, emotional, or financial in nature. Cues to possible overstepped boundaries are listed in Box 45-4.

If you would like more specific information on professional boundaries,

 Go to the **National Council on State Boards of Nursing Web site,** at https://www.ncsbn.org/Professional Boundariesbrochure.pdf

Sexual Harassment Be aware of and report the behaviors of staff members who commit sexual harassment. **Sexual harassment** involves the use of power over people lower in the power structure of the organization. It is defined as "unwelcome sexual advances, requests for sexual favors, and other verbal or physical conduct of a sexual nature" if submission (1) is a condition of employment, (2) interferes with job performance, (3) is the basis for employment decisions, or (4) creates a hostile and intimidating work environment (Equal Employment Opportunity Commission, n.d.).

If you witness or experience sexual harassment, your first step is to consult the agency's sexual harassment policy. Every agency receiving federal funding must have such a policy in place. It will tell you how to file a grievance, what forms you need to use, to whom the incident is reported, and what the procedure is for hearing and resolution.

BOX 45-4 ■ Potential Boundary Violations Between Nurse and Client

Excessive Self-Disclosure—Discussing personal problems or intimate details with the client

Flirtation—Communication that is sexual in nature or reveals personal attraction between client and nurse

Secretive Behavior—When the nurse is defensive or guarded about the interaction between client and nurse

"Super Nurse" Attitude—The nurse who acts as though she is the only one who understands and can meet the client's needs

Excessive Attention to Client—When the nurse spends much more time with a particular client than is required by his needs; personal gifts, off-duty visits, or trading assignments are signs of boundary violation.

Unclear Communication—When only part of the story is told with client care. The client might repeatedly seek out the nurse, even when not assigned to his care.

Source: Used with permission from the National Council of State Boards of Nursing. (n.d.). Professional boundaries: A nurse's guide to the importance of appropriate professional boundaries. Retrieved from https://www.ncsbn.org/ProfessionalBoundariesbrochure.pdf

Observe Mandatory Reporting Regulations

As noted earlier in the chapter, most states have laws requiring the nurse to report communicable diseases, known or suspected abuse of patients, and impaired or unsafe professional practice. When you observe violations of the state's licensing regulations, you have a professional and legal responsibility to report them to the appropriate authority. The "authority" varies among states; it may be your immediate supervisor, the board of nursing, or a peer assistance program, often sponsored by the state nurses association. See the section Mandatory Reporting Laws, earlier in the chapter, and the following discussion of reportable situations.

Impaired Nurses

Nurses who come to work under the influence of alcohol or mind-altering substances pose a danger to the health, safety, and welfare of the patients. You have a legal obligation to protect patients from impaired nurses. Always pay attention to the possibility of a coworker using or stealing narcotics. Impaired nurses account for a major percentage of disciplinary actions against nurses. The board of nursing in many states has programs that provide monitoring and support to nurses with substance addictions who seek help as an alternative to disciplinary actions against their license. See Box 45-5 for signs of chemical dependence in the workplace. To determine the magnitude of the problem in your state, go to the state board of nursing's Web site and click on *disciplinary actions*.

BOX 45-5 ■ Signs of Possible Chemical Dependence in the Workplace

Absenteeism

- Frequent unscheduled absences with improbable excuses
- Frequent late arrivals or early departures
- Absences after payday or days off
- Higher than average absences for cold, flu, and minor illnesses

Absent "On the Job"

- Long shift breaks
- Brief, unexplained absences from the nursing unit
- "Locked door syndrome" (excessively long use of restroom)
- Frequent visits to Occupational Health Services for illness on the job

Difficulty Concentrating

- Errors, particularly involving medication or with taking and transcribing verbal orders
- Omitted, illogical, incomplete, or illegible charting
- Taking more time to carry out assignments than is expected given the nurse's skill and experience
- Deterioration of handwriting during the shift
- Overlooking the signs of patient's deteriorating condition

Inconsistent Work Patterns

- Alternating periods of high and low efficiency
- Minimal or substandard work compared with that of peers
- Frequent requests for help with patient assignments
- Altered judgment in patient care decisions

Physical or Emotional Problems

- Nervousness, excessive sweating, tremors of the hands
- Physical or emotional condition changes during shift
- Deteriorating personal appearance, grooming, and hygiene
- Weight gain or loss

Decreasing Efficiency

- Omitting treatments; making bad decisions; showing poor judgment related to patient care
- Requests to be changed to a less supervised shift

Poor Relationships on the Job

- Mood swings, from isolation to angry outbursts
- Uncooperativeness
- Avoidance of contact with supervisors
- Patient complaints of irritability, roughness, or verbal abuse
- Lethargy and hyperactivity
- Emotional hypersensitivity
- Isolation from others

Medication-Centered Problems

- Excessive use of prn psychoactive medications or narcotics recorded for patients
- Increased waste or breakage of controlled substances
- Missing drugs, unaccounted-for doses
- Omission of dates or times from narcotic sign-out sheets
- Patient complaints about lack of pain relief

Personal Life Interferes With Job

- Frequent or excessively long phone calls
- Visitors or unexplained errands during work shift
- Legal problems
- Increased number of accidents

Source: Georgia Nurses Association. (n.d.). Nurse Advocate Program. The impaired nurse: Checklist for detecting potential chemical dependence in an employee. Retrieved from http://www.georgianurses.org/impaired_nurse.htm#pabi; Thomas, C., & Siela, D. (2011). The impaired nurse: Would you know what to do if you suspected substance abuse? *American Nurse Today*, 6(8). Retrieved from http://www.americannursetoday.com/article.aspx?id=8114&fid=8078

Unauthorized Practice

Your employer will require you to submit verification of current licensure in the state where you are working. If your license expires and you continue to practice nursing, you can be charged with unauthorized practice of nursing. You must report the unauthorized practice of nursing, which means reporting persons practicing nursing without a proper license. In addition, you must know the scope of practice for yourself, LPNs/LVNs, and nursing assistive personnel to ensure practice within professional boundaries. For example, unlicensed personnel cannot perform the initial patient assessment on a newly admitted patient.

Abuse and Communicable Diseases

State laws also require you to report known or suspected child, elder, and spousal abuse and communicable disease. Since state laws may vary, you need to be familiar with them to know what and to whom to report in your area. If you are working for a healthcare agency when you suspect abuse, always report it to your supervisor. If you need to review signs of abuse,

 Go to Chapter 9, **Procedure 9-1: Assessing for Abuse,** in Volume 2.

Other Safeguards for Nurses

In addition to the Good Samaritan laws and the ANA Nurses' Bill of Rights (previously discussed), safe harbor laws and professional liability insurance offer some legal protection for nurses.

Safe Harbor Laws

Safe harbor laws, found in the nurse practice act or other state laws, provide for exceptions to certain laws. They protect you from being suspended, terminated, disciplined, or discriminated against for refusing to do (or not do) something you believe would be harmful to a patient. Under these laws, you also have a right to ask for peer review of either the situation or directives that you believe would violate the nursing practice act. You must follow the guidelines required under the safe harbor provisions.

Case: Prepping a Patient for a Surgical Procedure

The nurse cannot find documentation in the patient's medical record for informed consent. Knowing her legal role in informed consent, she refuses to assist with treatment when a patient has not given informed consent. Safe harbor laws protect her from dismissal for denying the surgeon's request for her to obtain informed consent.

Professional Liability Insurance

If you are sued for malpractice, the insurance company pays for the attorney's fees and for any judgment or settlement, up to the policy limits. You should carefully review your insurance policy because most insurance policies have **exclusions** (items not covered by the policy). If the patient's claim arises out of excluded activities, the insurance company will not pay for the costs of litigation and damages. The following are examples of exclusions:

- Sexual abuse of a patient, assault and battery, and other intentional torts
- Injury caused while the nurse is under the influence of drugs or alcohol
- Criminal activity
- Transmission of acquired immunodeficiency syndrome from the nurse to a patient
- Actions that can lead to an award of punitive damages (damages awarded to punish the defendant for egregious acts or omissions)

Types of Coverage

There are two types of malpractice coverage. **Occurrence-type insurance** is most often recommended for nurses, because this policy covers malpractice claims for any injury or damage that occurred during the time the policy was in force, regardless of when the claim was reported and the lawsuit occurred. In contrast, **claims-made insurance** covers only those claims in which the negligent action or omission occurred and the claim was filed or reported during the policy period. To maintain coverage under a claims-made policy after it has lapsed or been canceled, some insurers will offer "tail" insurance. You should consult an attorney to decide which type of policy is best for you.

As a rule, if you work for a hospital or other institution, you will be covered by the institution's insurance. However, it covers you only while you are working within the scope of your employment. For example, you would not be covered during the one day a week that you volunteer at a free clinic. Some legal experts recommend that you purchase individual liability insurance in addition to the coverage provided by your employer. Again, consult an attorney before making a decision.

ThinkLike a Nurse 45-6

Susan, RN, was employed by Landold Nursing Service and assigned to Alvalup Hospital from June 1, 2012, to May 30, 2013. Susan carried her own professional liability claims-made policy during this time. She decided to attend real estate school and not renew her policy. On August 10, 2013, a medical malpractice claim was filed against Susan. Based on this scenario, would Susan have coverage under her policy? What kind of policy should she have obtained to have coverage for the claim made against her?

Student Responsibilities

As a student, you are held to the same standards of care as are licensed nurses. You must be familiar not only with your state's standards of practice, but also with the policies and procedures in the agency in which you have your clinical experiences. Your instructor is responsible for making assignments that are within your competence and for providing clinical supervision. However, this does not release you from your own legal responsibilities. To help protect yourself and your patients:

- Prepare carefully for each clinical experience.
- Never attempt a procedure or make a judgment about which you feel unsure. If you lack the theoretical or practical knowledge for an assignment, notify your clinical instructor immediately.
- Notify your instructor or a staff nurse if your patient's condition changes significantly.
- Unless otherwise arranged, take instructions only from your clinical instructor.

Your nursing school may require you to carry personal professional liability insurance. The school's policy will cover you only for the nursing care you give in your educational experiences. If you are employed as a nursing assistant, for example, the school's policy will not provide coverage for you at work. Furthermore, you are legally permitted to perform only the procedures contained in your job description. For example, even though you administer injections in your student role, you are not licensed to do so in your role as a nursing assistant.

SUMMARY

Ethical and legal issues are a major source of conflict for nursing practice. This chapter discusses only the legal aspects of the major issues. See Chapter 44 for ethical considerations. It is important to be clear in your mind that what is *legal* and what is *ethical* are not always the same thing. On the one hand, an act may be legal (e.g., abortion), even if you consider it unethical. On the other hand, you may believe an action (e.g., assisted suicide) is ethically necessary, but the law may forbid it. You should be aware of the legal consequences that your ethical decisions may bring about. For a more detailed discussion of some major legal issues in nursing (e.g., stem cell research, cloning, reproductive issues, life-sustaining medical treatment),

 Go to Chapter 45, **Supplemental Materials: What Are the Major Legal Issues in Nursing Practice?,** on DavisPlus.

 To explore learning resources for this chapter,

 Go to DavisPlus at **DavisPl.us/Wilkinson3.**

Chapter Resources for Chapter 45:
  Response sheets for all learning activities
  Resources for Caregivers and Health Professionals
  Reading More About Legal Issues (suggested readings)
  Concept Map of chapter content
Interactive Case Studies
NCLEX-Style and Chapter Review Questions
Chapter Overview Podcasts

For references cited in this chapter,

 Go to Volume 2, **References Cited.**

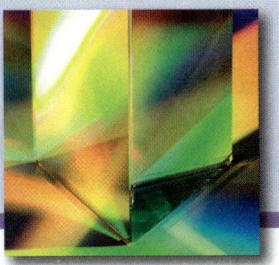

Credits

Note: Unless cited below, text credits appear within the text.

CHAPTER 1

Meet Your Patient 1-1: The National Library of Medicine
Meet Your Patient 1-2: Everyday Faces, BananaStock
Figure 1-2: © Stephen Mahar, www.photos.com
Figure 1-3: © Cynthia Farmer, www.photos.com
Figure 1-4: © iStock/Getty Images
Figure 1-5: © DNY59/iStock/Getty Images

CHAPTER 2

Meet Your Patient: © Corbis Images

CHAPTER 3

Meet Your Patient: © Everyday Faces, PhotoDisc
Figure 3-2: Wilkinson, J. M., *Nursing process and critical thinking* (5th ed.), © 2012. Electronically reproduced by permission of Pearson Education, Inc., Upper Saddle River, New Jersey.
Figure 3-3: © Getty Images
Figure 3-4: Courtesy of Smith Northview Hospital, Valdosta, GA.
Figure 3-5: Courtesy of Shore Memorial Hospital, Somers Point, NJ.

CHAPTER 4

Meet Your Patient: Photo © BananaStock
Figure 4-6: Adapted from Maslow, A. (1971). *The farther reaches of human nature.* New York: Viking Press; and Maslow A., & Lowery, R. (Eds.). (1998). *Toward a psychology of being* (3rd ed.). New York: Wiley & Sons.

CHAPTER 5

Meet Your Patient: © Ryan McVay/Photodisc/Punchstock
Figure 5-3: Courtesy of Shawnee Mission Health System, Shawnee Mission, KS.
Figure 5:4: Adapted from Genesis Medical Center, Davenport, IA. Used with permission.
Figure 5-5: Hospital of the University of Pennsylvania, Philadelphia, PA. Used with permission.

CHAPTER 6

Meet Your Patient: © Ryan McVay/Photodisc/Punchstock
Figure 6-2: Courtesy of J. A. Fain. (2008). *Reading, understanding and applying nursing research: A text and workbook* (3rd ed.). Philadelphia: F. A. Davis.
Figure 6-4: Copyright © Ergo Partners, L.C. All rights reserved. Used with permission.

CHAPTER 7

Meet Your Patient: © Thinkstock/Getty Images
Figure 7-2: Courtesy of Ergo Partners, L.C., Boulder, CO. Used with permission.

CHAPTER 8

Figure 8-2: Courtesy Dr. Jean Watson.
Figure 8-5: Adapted from Maslow, A. (1971). *The farther reaches of human nature.* New York: Viking Press; and Maslow, A., & Lowery, R. (Eds.). (1998). *Toward a psychology of being* (3rd ed.). New York: Wiley & Sons.

CHAPTER 9

Meet Your Patients: Photodisc Blue/Getty Images
Figures 9-1 and 9-2: From Dillon, P. M. (2007). *Nursing health assessment: A critical thinking case studies approach* (2nd ed.). Philadelphia: F. A. Davis.
Figure 9-3: From Polan, E., & Taylor, D. (2007). *Journey across the lifespan* (3rd ed.). Philadelphia: F. A. Davis.
Figures 9-4A through D: From Dillon, P. M. (2007). *Nursing health assessment: A critical thinking case studies approach* (2nd ed.). Philadelphia: F.A. Davis.
Figure 9-5: © Getty Images
Figure 9-6: © Robert Dant/iStock/Getty Images
Figure 9-7: © punchstock.com
Figure 9-8: © Photodisc Red/Getty Images, Scott T. Baxter
Figure 9-9: © Everyday Faces, Photodisc
Figure 9-10: © Photodisc Green/Getty Images, Anderson Ross.

CHAPTER 10

Figure 10-1: Source: Vincent, G., & Victoria, A. (2010). *The next four decades, the older population in the United States: 2010 to 2050, current population reports* (pp. 25–1138).

Washington, DC: U.S. Census Bureau. Retrieved December 9, 2012, from http://census.gov/prod/2010pubs/p25-1138.pdf

Figure 10-2: © Photodisc, Getty Images

Figure 10-3: Courtesy of V. Rempusheski, PhD.

Figure 10-4: Source: U.S. Department of Health & Human Services, Centers for Disease Control and Prevention

CHAPTER 11

Meet Your Patient: © Silvia Jansen/iStock/Getty Images

Figure 11-2: Adapted from Dunn, H. L. (1959). High level wellness for man and society. *American Journal of Public Health, 49*(6), 786–788.

Figures 11-3A and B: Adapted from Neuman, B. (1995). The Neuman systems model. In B. Neuman, *The Neuman systems model* (3rd ed., pp. 3–61) East Norwalk, CT: Appleton and Lange.

Figure 11-4: © Kali9/iStock/Getty Images

CHAPTER 12

Meet Your Patients: © Family Health, BananaStock

CHAPTER 14

Figure 14-3: © Punchstock, Photodisc

Figure 14-4: © PhotoDisc, Senior Lifestyles

Figure 14-6: From Dillon, P. M. (2007). *Nursing health assessment: A critical thinking case studies approach* (2nd ed.). Philadelphia: F. A. Davis Company.

CHAPTER 16

Meet Your Patient: © Photodisc, Senior Lifestyles

Figure 16-1: © Photodisc/Getty

Figure 16-4: Adapted from Millsppaugh, C. D. (2005). "Assessment and response to spiritual pain: Part II." *Journal of Palliative Medicine, 8*(6), 1110–1117.

Figure 16-5: Used with permission of Jonas Ngirinshuti

CHAPTER 17

Figure 17-1: © iStock/Getty Images

Figure 17-2: From U.S. Department of Health and Human Services. Retrieved from http://www.organdonor.gov

CHAPTER 18

Meet Your Patient: © Photodisc/Getty

Figures 18-2, 18-3, 18-5, 18-7, and 18-8: Courtesy of Cerner Corporation.

CHAPTER 19

Meet Your Patient: Photo © Bananastock

Figure 19-3: Courtesy of Laerdal Medical Corp., Wappingers Falls, NY.

Figure 19-4: Courtesy of Merck & Co., Inc. #994795(1)-05-COZ.

CHAPTER 20

Meet Your Patient: Photo © BananaStock

CHAPTER 22

Figures 22-1, 22-3 through 22-8, 22-10A through C, 22-12A through D, 22-16, 22-20, and Figures a through c and f through 1 in Table 22-1: From Dillon, P. M. (2007). *Nursing health assessment: A critical case studies thinking approach* (2nd ed.). Philadelphia: F. A. Davis.

Figure 22-17: From Scanlon, V. C., & Sanders, T. (2011). *Essentials of anatomy & physiology* (6th ed.). Philadelphia: F. A. Davis.

CHAPTER 23

Meet Your Patient: © Maliketh/iStock/Getty Images

Box 23-1: Photos © photos.com Figures 23-2 and 23-3: From Scanlon, V. C., & Sanders, T. (2003). *Essentials of anatomy & physiology* (4th ed.). Philadelphia: F. A. Davis.

Figure 23-4: © Wavebreak/iStock/Getty Images

CHAPTER 24

Meet Your Patient: © Jay Fries/Digital Vision/Getty Images

Figure 24-03: © webking/iStock/Getty Images

Safety Assessment Scale: Source: Dr. Louise Poulin de Courval © CL Cote-des-Nieges. Used with permission.

CHAPTER 25

Figures 25-2A and B: Courtesy of Invacare Corporation, Elyria, Ohio.

Figures 25-3 and 25-4: From Dillon, P. M. (2007). *Nursing health assessment: A critical thinking case studies approach* (2nd ed.). Philadelphia: F. A. Davis.

CHAPTER 26

Figure 26-17: Courtesy of Hospira, Lake Forest, IL.

Figure 26-29: Used by permission of the National Extravasation Information Service (UK). www.extravasation.org.uk

Figure 26-30: Courtesy of Medi-Dose® Inc., EPS® Inc.

Figure 26-34: Courtesy of Dr. Donna Clarren and Dr. Brian Oxhorn, Roseman College of Nursing.

CHAPTER 27

Figure 27-1: U.S. Department of Agriculture. (2005).

Figure 27-2: U.S. Department of Agriculture. (2005).

Figure 27-3: Text by Reed Mangels, PhD, RD. Design by Lindsey Siferd. The Vegetarian Resource Group, P.O. Box 1463, Baltimore, MD 21203; www.vrg.org

Figures 27-4 and 27-6A and B: Courtesy of Covidien, Mansfield, MA.

CHAPTER 28

Meet Your Patient: © BananaStock

Figures 28-1 through 28-3: From Scanlon, V. C., & Sanders, T. (2011). *Essentials of anatomy and physiology* (6th ed.). Philadelphia: F. A. Davis.

Figure 28-5: Courtesy of Atago, USA, Inc.

Figure 28-10: From Williams, L., & Hopper, P. (2011). *Understanding medical surgical nursing* (4th ed.). Philadelphia: F. A. Davis.

CHAPTER 29

Meet Your Patient: © thelinke/iStock/Getty Images

Figures 29-1 through 29-4: From Scanlon, V., & Sanders, T. (2011). *Essentials of anatomy and physiology* (6th ed.). Philadelphia: F. A. Davis Company. Used with permission.

Figures 29-8 through 29-10: Courtesy of Hollister Incorporated, Libertyville, IL.

CHAPTER 30

Meet Your Patient: © Aguru/iStock/Getty Images

Figures 30-1 and 30-2: From Scanlon, V., & Sanders, T. (2011). *Essentials of anatomy and physiology* (6th ed.). Philadelphia: F. A. Davis Company. Used with permission.

CHAPTER 31

Meet Your Patient: © Photos.com/Jupiter Images

Figures 31-1, 31-2, and 31-5: From Scanlon, V., & Sanders, T. (2011). *Essentials of anatomy and physiology* (6th ed.). Philadelphia: F. A. Davis Company. Used with permission.

Figure 31-4: Developed by the World Health Organization (WHO). *Cancer pain relief and palliative care: Report of a WHO expert committee* (WHO Tech. Rep. Series No. 804). Geneva, Switzerland: Author. Used with permission.

CHAPTER 32

Meet Your Patient: © Christopher Futcher/iStock/Getty Images

Figures 32-1 and 32-2: From Scanlon, V., & Sanders, T. (2011). *Essentials of anatomy and physiology* (6th ed.). Philadelphia: F. A. Davis Company.

Figures 32-9, 32-10, and 32-12 through 32-14: Courtesy of EZ Way, Inc., Clarinda, IA.

CHAPTER 33

Meet Your Patients: © iStock/Getty Images, © SteveLuker/iStock/Getty Images, and © iStock/Getty Images

Figures 33-1 through 33-4: From Scanlon, V. C., & Saunders, T. (2007). *Essentials of anatomy & physiology* (5th ed.). Philadelphia: F. A. Davis Company.

Figure 33-5: © iStock/Getty Images

Figure 33-8: © iofoto/iStock/Getty Images

CHAPTER 34

Meet Your Patient: Meet Your Patient: © Diane Diederich/iStock/Getty Images

Figure 34-5: From Hall, J. E. (2011). *Guyton and Hall textbook of medical physiology* (12th ed.). New York: Saunders.

CHAPTER 35

Meet Your Patient: © PhotoDisc, Everyday Faces

Figure 35-1: Adapted from Scanlon, V. C., & Saunders, T. (2011). *Essentials of anatomy & physiology* (6th ed.). Philadelphia: F. A. Davis Company.

Figure 35-10: Adapted from AHRQ Clinical Practice Guidelines.

Table 35-3: Photos © Gordian Medical, Inc. dba American Medical Technologies.

CHAPTER 36

Meet Your Patient: Photo Copyright BananaStock.

Figures 36-1 through 36-4: Adapted from Scanlon, V. C., & Sanders, T. (2003). *Essentials of anatomy and physiology*. Philadelphia: F. A. Davis Company.

Figures 36-6, 36-7, 36-13, and 36-15: From Williams, L., & Hopper, P. (2007). *Understanding medical surgical nursing* (2nd ed.). Philadelphia: F. A. Davis Company.

CHAPTER 37

Meet Your Patient: © iStock/Getty Images

Figures 37-1 through 37-4: From Scanlon, V. C., & Sanders, T. (2003). *Essentials of anatomy and physiology*. Philadelphia: F. A. Davis Company.

CHAPTER 38

Meet Your Patient: © Getty Images, Photodisc

Figure 38-1: Adapted from Scanlon, V. C., & Sanders, T. (2011). *Essentials of anatomy and physiology* (6th ed.). Philadelphia: F. A. Davis Company.

CHAPTER 39

Meet Your Patient: © Vikram Raghuvanshi/iStock/Getty Images

Figures 39-2 and 39-4: From Williams, L., & Hopper, P. (2011). *Understanding medical surgical nursing* (4th ed.). Philadelphia: F. A. Davis Company.

Figure 39-5: Courtesy of I-Flow Corporation, Lake Forest, CA.

CHAPTER 40

Figure 40-1: © iStock/Getty Images

Figures 40-2 and 40-3: From Whitehead, D., Weiss, S., & Tappen, R. (2007). *Essentials of nursing leadership and management* (4th ed.). Philadelphia: F. A. Davis.

CHAPTER 41

Meet Your Nursing Role Model: © istockphoto.com, Image ID: 2086476

Figure 41-1: Adapted from Englebardt, S., & Nelson, R. *Health care informatics: An interdisciplinary approach*. Copyright 2002. With permission from Elsevier.

Figures 41-2: Courtesy Doctors Telehealth Network, Newport Beach, CA.

Figure 41-3: © iStock/Getty Images

Figure 41-4: Courtesy Laerdal Medical Corp., Wappingers Falls, NY.

Figure 41-5: Courtesy Cerner Corporation.

Figure 41-6A and 41-6B: © Adivin/iStock/Getty Images

CHAPTER 42

Meet Your Patient: © Thomas_EyeDesign/iStock/Getty Images

CHAPTER 43

Meet Your Patient: © Photo Euphoria/iStock/Getty Images

Figure 43-3: © Alexander Raths/iStock/Getty Images

Figure 43-7: © iStock/Getty Images

CHAPTER 44

Figures 44-1 and 44-2: © iStock/Getty Images

CHAPTER 45

Meet Your Patient: © ntmw/iStock/Getty Images

CHAPTER 46

Meet Your Patient: © monkeybusinessimages/iStock/Getty Images

Figures 46-5 and 46-6: Courtesy of National Center for Complementary and Alternative Medicine.

INDEX

Note: Page number followed by *f* refer to figures; page numbers followed by *t* refer to tables; page numbers followed by *b* refer to boxes; page numbers followed by *p* refer to procedures.

A

A-delta fibers, (V1) 793–794, (V1) 793*f*

Abbreviations
  for documentation, (V1) 378, (V2) 169–170
  drug name, error-prone, (V2) 480*t*
  error-prone, (V2) 478–479*t*
  medication-related, (V2) 477–478*t*

ABCDEE pain assessment, (V1) 799*b*

Abdellah, Faye G., nursing theory of, (V1) 146*t*

Abdomen
  assessment of, (V1) 504–505, (V1) 504*f*, (V1) 505*f*, (V1) 514*p*, (V2) 271–277*p*
  auscultation of, (V1) 505
  inspection of, (V1) 504–505, (V1) 505*f*
  movement of, in respiration, (V1) 445
  palpation of, (V1) 505
  percussion of, (V1) 505
  postoperative distention of, (V1) 1050*t*

Abdominal binder, (V1) 929, (V1) 930–931*p*, (V2) 697–699*p*

Abducens nerve (VI), testing, (V2) 288*p*

ABG analysis, (V1) 996, (V1) 997*t*, (V1) 998

Ablative surgery, (V1) 1027

ABO blood groups, (V1) 1019, (V1) 1019*t*

Abrasion, (V1) 581, (V1) 902*t*

Abscess, (V1) 902*t*. *See also* Infection(s)

Absorption, medication, (V1) 609–614. *See also* Medication(s), absorption of

Abstinence, (V1) 862, (V2) 654

Abstract, (V1) 1091

Abstract thinking, assessing, (V2) 286–287*p*

Abuse
  of adolescents, (V1) 191
  of alcohol, (V1) 1097
  assessing for, (V2) 63–66
    documentation of, (V2) 66–67
    evaluation in, (V2) 66
    focused health history in, (V2) 63–64
    focused physical assessment in, (V2) 64–65
    follow-up in, (V2) 65
    home care in, (V2) 66
    patient teaching in, (V2) 66
    for psychological abuse, (V2) 64
  of child, (V1) 183–184
    assessing for, (V2) 65–66
  history of, population vulnerability and, (V1) 1116
  identification of, (V2) 62
  of infant, (V1) 177
    assessing for, (V1) 178*b*
    detection and prevention of, (V1) 178*b*
  of older adult, (V1) 211
    assessing for, (V1) 214, (V2) 66
  of opioids, (V1) 806
  reporting regulations on, (V1) 1184
  sexual, (V1) 864–865
  substance. *See* Substance abuse

Abusive head trauma (AHT), to infant, (V1) 177

Acceptance
  in communication, (V1) 233
  as stage of dying, (V1) 353*b*

Accessory muscles, during inspiration, (V1) 946

Accessory nerve (XI), testing, (V2) 290*p*

Accidents, motor vehicle
  prevention of, (V1) 564–565
  risk factors for, (V1) 551

Accommodation
  in cognitive development, (V1) 167
  in culturally competent care, (V1) 323
  pupil, (V1) 494
    testing of, (V2) 243*p*

Accountability
  for decisions and actions, (V1) 107
  legal, (V1) 1162–1185, (V2) 905–911

Accreditation, (V1) 1171

Accreditation Commission on Education in Nursing (ACEN), (V1) 22

Accrediting bodies, for nursing education, (V1) 22

Acculturation, (V1) 305–306

Acetaminophen, (V1) 805

Achilles reflex, testing, (V2) 294*p*

Achondroplasia, (V1) 827

Acid, (V1) 989

Acid-base balance
  assessment of, (V1) 998–1001, (V2) 815–817
  critical thinking about, (V2) 818–819
  disorders of, (V1) 996, (V1) 997*t*
    nursing diagnosis for, (V1) 1001
    nursing interventions for, (V1) 1001–1015
    nursing outcomes for, (V1) 1001
  full-spectrum nursing and, (V2) 817–818
  knowledge map for, (V2) 821
  regulation of, (V1) 989, (V1) 991–992

Acidosis, (V1) 991, (V1) 996
  metabolic, (V1) 996, (V1) 997*t*, (V1) 999
  respiratory, (V1) 996, (V1) 997*t*

Acne, (V1) 581

Acoustic nerve (VIII) testing, (V2) 289*p*

Acrochordons, (V1) 491, (V2) 228

Acromegaly, head size and, (V1) 493

Actigraph, (V1) 891

Acting, in values clarification, (V1) 1156*t*

Active listening
  for enhancing therapeutic communication, (V1) 473–474, (V1) 474*f*
  for spirituality diagnoses, (V1) 340

Active range of motion (AROM), (V1) 820. *See also* Range of motion (ROM)
  for mobility, (V1) 843–844

Active transport, (V1) 985, (V1) 986, (V1) 987*f*, (V1) 987*t*

Activities of Daily Living (ADLs)
  for ambulation conditioning, (V1) 844, (V2) 638
  in older adult assessment, (V1) 213

Activity
  in infection prevention, (V1) 532–533

level of
  bowel elimination and, (V1) 749
  energy expended by, (V1) 681*t*
  urinary function and, (V1) 719

Activity intolerance, (V1) 834
  exercise and, (V1) 834
  postoperative, (V2) 851
  sexuality and, (V1) 867

Activity theory, of psychosocial development of older adults, (V1) 207, (V1) 209, (V1) 209*f*

Actual nursing diagnosis, (V1) 66*t*
  goals for, (V1) 98, (V1) 99*t*
  intervention type related to, (V1) 110*t*

Acupressure, for pain, (V1) 802

Acupuncture
  for pain, (V1) 802
  in stress management, (V1) 259

Acute pain, (V1) 792, (V1) 797*b*
  postoperative, (V2) 851–852

Acute renal failure (ARF), definition of, (V1) 725*b*

Acute wound, (V1) 902

Adaptation(s)
  in cognitive development, (V1) 167
  definition of, (V1) 240
  hardiness and, (V1) 244
  health status and, (V1) 244
  in leadership, (V1) 1059
  as outcome of stress, (V1) 243
  perception of stressor and, (V1) 244
  personal factors influencing, (V1) 243–244
  stress and, (V1) 239–261, (V2) 92–101. *See also* Stress, adaptation to
  support system and, (V1) 244

Adapted physical activity (APA) programs, (V1) 206

Adaptive coping, (V1) 243

Addiction, (V1) 806. *See also* Substance abuse

Adhesive tape/strips, (V1) 905, (V1) 924, (V1) 929*p*

Adipose tissue, (V1) 898*f*, (V1) 899

Adjuvant analgesics, (V1) 805–806

Administrative law, (V1) 1163–1164

Admission, to nursing unit, (V1) 237*p*, (V2) 77–79*p*

Admission assessment, (V1) 47

Admission data form, (V1) 382–383, (V2) 171

Adolescent(s), (V1) 188–194
  abuse, neglect and violence involving, (V1) 191
  alcohol use by, (V1) 189–190
  anorexia nervosa in, (V1) 190
  assessment of, (V1) 191–193
  bulimia in, (V1) 190
  cardiovascular system in, (V1) 971–972
  cigarette smoking by, (V1) 971
  communication by, (V1) 465
  condom use by, (V1) 191
  depression in, (V1) 190
  development of
    cognitive, (V1) 168*t*, (V1) 189
    physical, (V1) 188–189, (V1) 188*b*